VOLUME 2

OPERATIVE HAND SURGERY

THIRD EDITION

VOLUME 2

OPERATIVE HAND SURGERY

THIRD EDITION

Edited by

David P. Green, M.D.

Clinical Professor
Department of Orthopaedics
University of Texas Health Science Center
at San Antonio
San Antonio, Texas

Assistant Editor
for Microvascular Surgery

Robert N. Hotchkiss, M.D.

Assistant Professor
Department of Orthopaedic Surgery
Cornell University Medical College
New York, New York

Churchill Livingstone
New York, Edinburgh, London, Melbourne, Tokyo

Library of Congress Cataloging-in-Publication Data
Operative hand surgery / edited by David P. Green. — 3rd ed.
p. cm.
Includes bibliographical references and index.
ISBN 0-443-08803-9
1. Hand—Surgery. I. Green, David P.
[DNLM: 1. Hand—surgery. WE 830 O61]
RD559.O63 1993
617.5 ' 75059—dc20
DNLM/DLC
for Library of Congress 92-48739
CIP

Distributed in the United Kingdom by Churchill Livingstone, Robert Stevenson House, 1–3 Baxter's Place, Leith Walk, Edinburgh EH1 3AF, and by associated companies, branches, and representatives throughout the world.

Accurate indications, adverse reactions, and dosage schedules for drugs are provided in this book, but it is possible that they may change. The reader is urged to review the package information data of the manufacturers of the medications mentioned.

The Publishers have made every effort to trace the copyright holders for borrowed material. If they have inadvertently overlooked any, they will be pleased to make the necessary arrangements at the first opportunity.

Acquisitions Editors: *Toni M. Tracy, Leslie Burgess*
Copy Editor: *Paul Bernstein*
Production Designer: *Jody L. Ouellette*
Production Supervisor: *Sharon Tuder*
Cover Design: *Paul Moran*

Printed in the United States of America

First published in 1993 7 6 5 4 3 2 1

Dedicated to my father,

J. Leighton Green, M.D.
(1899 –1986)

A physician and surgeon worthy of emulation

And to my mother,

Virginia Peeler Green
(1905–)

An equally exemplary role model

Contributors

Peter C. Amadio, M.D.
Associate Professor, Department of Orthopedic Surgery, Mayo Medical School; Consultant, Department of Orthopedic Surgery and Surgery of the Hand, Mayo Clinic, Rochester, Minnesota

Alexander C. Angelides, M.D.
Attending Hand Surgeon, Palmetto General Hospital, Hialeah, Florida

Loui G. Bayne, M.D.
Clinical Professor, Department of Orthopaedics, Emory University School of Medicine; Director, Hand Clinic, Scottish Rite Children's Hospital, Atlanta, Georgia

Robert D. Beckenbaugh. M.D.
Professor, Department of Orthopedics, Mayo Medical School; Consultant, Department of Orthopedic Surgery and Surgery of the Hand, Mayo Clinic, Rochester, Minnesota

William H. Bowers, M.D., M.S.
Associate Professor, Departments of Orthopedic and Plastic Surgery, Virginia Commonwealth University Medical College of Virginia School of Medicine; Chief, Children's Hospital Hand Service; Private Practice, Hand Surgery Specialists Ltd., Richmond, Virginia

Richard M. Braun, M.D.
Associate Clinical Professor, Department of Orthopaedic Surgery, University of California, San Diego, School of Medicine, La Jolla, California; Instructor, Department of Orthopaedic Surgery, University of Southern California School of Medicine, Los Angeles, California; Consultant in Upper Limb Rehabilitation, Rancho Los Amigos Hospital, Downey, California; Director of Upper Extremity Rehabilitation, Donald N. Sharp Memorial Community Hospital Rehabilitation Center, San Diego, California

Jürg Brennwald, M.D.
Assistant Professor, Surgery Department, University of Basel, Basel, Switzerland; Academic Staff, AO-Research Institute; Consultant for Hand and Microsurgery, Davos Hospital, Davos, Switzerland

Roberta Brockman, M.D.
Assistant Professor, Department of Orthopaedic Surgery, Cornell University Medical College; Assistant Attending Orthopedic Surgeon, Hospital for Special Surgery, New York, New York

Paul W. Brown, M.D.
Clinical Professor, Departments of Orthopedics and Rehabilitation and Plastic and Reconstructive Surgery, Yale University School of Medicine, New Haven, Connecticut; Consultant in Hand Surgery, Veteran's Administration Hospital, West Haven, Connecticut; Chief, Hand Surgery, Department of Surgery, St. Vincent's Medical Center, Bridgeport, Connecticut; Colonel, Medical Corps, United States Army, Retired

Richard E. Brown, M.D.
Assistant Professor and Chief, Section of Hand Surgery, Division of Plastic and Reconstructive Surgery, Department of Surgery, Southern Illinois University School of Medicine, Springfield, Illinois

Earl Z. Browne, Jr., M.D.
Head, Section of Research, Division of Plastic and Reconstructive Surgery, The Cleveland Clinic Foundation, Cleveland, Ohio

Thomas M. Brushart, M.D.
Assistant Professor, Departments of Orthopaedics and Neurology, The Johns Hopkins University School of Medicine; Attending Surgeon, Raymond M. Curtis Hand Center, The Union Memorial Hospital, Baltimore, Maryland

Ueli Büchler, M.D., Ph.D.
Chief, Division of Hand Surgery, University of Bern Hospital, Bern, Switzerland

*William E. Burkhalter, M.D.**
Professor Emeritus and Former Chief, Division of Hand Surgery, Department of Orthopaedics and Rehabilitation, University of Miami School of Medicine, Miami, Florida

Richard I. Burton, M.D.
Professor and Chairman, Department of Orthopaedics, University of Rochester School of Medicine; Co-Director, Hand Service, University of Rochester Medical Center, Rochester, New York

Stephen J. Chabon, P.A.C.
Instructor, Department of Orthopaedic Surgery, Bowman Gray School of Medicine of Wake Forest University, Winston-Salem, North Carolina

Harkeerat S. Dhillon, M.D., M.Sc.Orth.
Clinical Associate, Department of Orthopaedics, University of Connecticut School of Medicine, Farmington, Connecticut; Hand Fellow, Connecticut Combined Hand Surgery Service, Hartford, Connecticut

Harold M. Dick, M.D.
Frank E. Stinchfield Professor and Chairman, Department of Orthopedic Surgery, Columbia University College of Physicians and Surgeons; Director, Department of Orthopedic Surgery, Columbia-Presbyterian Medical Center, New York, New York

George Peter Dingeldein, M.D.
Private Practice, Plastic and Reconstructive Surgery, Texarkana, Texas

James H. Dobyns, M.D.
Professor Emeritus, Department of Orthopedics, Mayo Medical School, Rochester, Minnesota; Clinical Professor, Department of Orthopedics, University of Texas Health Science Center at San Antonio, San Antonio, Texas; Consultant Emeritus, Mayo Clinic, Rochester, Minnesota; Consultant, The Audie Murphy Veterans Administration Hospital, San Antonio, Texas; Consultant, The Hand Center, San Antonio, Texas

James R. Doyle, M.D.
Professor and Chairman, Division of Orthopedic Surgery, Department of Surgery, University of Hawaii John A. Burns School of Medicine, Honolulu, Hawaii

Gregory J. Dray, M.D.
Attending Hand Surgeon, Carolina Hand Surgery Associates, Asheville, North Carolina

Richard G. Eaton, M.D.
Professor, Department of Surgery, Columbia University College of Physicians and Surgeons; Director, Hand Surgery Center, The Roosevelt Hospital, St. Luke's-Roosevelt Hospital Center, New York, New York

William W. Eversmann, Jr., M.D.
Hand Surgeon, Iowa Medical Clinic, Cedar Rapids, Iowa

Paul Feldon, M.D.
Associate Clinical Professor, Department of Orthopedic Surgery, Tufts University School of Medicine; Chief, Hand Surgery Service, St. Elizabeth's Hospital, Boston, Massachusetts

Donald C. Ferlic, M.D.
Associate Clinical Professor, Department of Orthopedics, University of Colorado School of Medicine, Denver, Colorado

Michael O. Fidler, M.D.
Clinical Assistant Professor, Department of Orthopedic Surgery, West Virginia University School of Medicine; Surgeon, Department of Orthopedics, Charleston Area Medical Center, Charleston, West Virginia

Earl J. Fleegler, M.D.
Head, Section of Hand Surgery, Division of Plastic and Reconstructive Surgery, The Cleveland Clinic Foundation, Cleveland, Ohio

Guy Foucher, M.D.
Head, Emergency Hand Unit, S.O.S. Main, Strasbourg, France

Avrum I. Froimson, M.D.
Clinical Professor, Department of Orthopedics, Case Western Reserve University School of Medicine; Director, Department of Orthopedic Surgery, Mount Sinai Medical Center, Cleveland, Ohio

*Deceased.

Harris Gellman, M.D.
Associate Clinical Professor, Department of Orthopedic Surgery, University of Southern California School of Medicine, Los Angeles, California

Leonard Gordon, M.D.
Lecturer, Department of Anatomy, University of California, San Francisco, School of Medicine; Attending Surgeon and Director, Hand and Microsurgery Research Laboratory, California Pacific Medical Center, San Francisco, California

David P. Green, M.D.
Clinical Professor, Department of Orthopaedics, University of Texas Health Science Center at San Antonio; President, The Hand Center of San Antonio, San Antonio, Texas

Hill Hastings II, M.D.
Clinical Associate Professor, Department of Orthopaedic Surgery, Indiana University School of Medicine; Department of Hand Surgery, St. Vincent Hospital and Health Care Center; The Indiana Hand Center, Indianapolis, Indiana

Vincent R. Hentz, M.D.
Professor, Department of Surgery, Stanford University School of Medicine; Chief, Division of Hand Surgery, Stanford University Hospital, Palo Alto, California

James H. Herndon, M.D.
Professor and Chairman, Department of Orthopedic Surgery, University of Pittsburgh School of Medicine; Chief, Department of Orthopaedics and Rehabilitation, Presbyterian and Montefiore University Hospital, Pittsburgh, Pennsylvania

Rosemary Hickey, M.D.
Associate Professor, Department of Anesthesiology, University of Texas Health Science Center at San Antonio, San Antonio, Texas

M. Mark Hoffer, M.D.
Professor and Chief, Division of Orthopedics, Department of Surgery, University of California, Irvine, California College of Medicine, Irvine, California; Chief, Department of Children's Orthopaedics, Rancho Los Amigos Medical Center, Downey, California

Robert N. Hotchkiss, M.D.
Assistant Professor, Department of Orthopaedic Surgery, Cornell University Medical College; Chief, Hand Surgery, Hospital for Special Surgery, New York, New York

James H. House, M.D.
Professor and Director of Hand Surgery, Department of Orthopaedic Surgery, University of Minnesota Medical School—Minneapolis; Chief, Hand Surgery Service, University of Minnesota Hospital and Clinic, Minneapolis, Minnesota

James M. Hunter, M.D.
Distinguished Professor, Division of Hand Surgery, Department of Orthopedic Surgery, Jefferson Medical College of Thomas Jefferson University, Philadelphia, Pennsylvania

William B. Kleinman, M.D.
Clinical Professor, Department of Orthopaedic Surgery, Indiana University School of Medicine; Director, Congenital Upper Limb Deformity Clinic, The James Whitcomb Riley Hospital for Children, Indiana University Medical Center; Senior Attending Hand Surgeon, The Indiana Hand Center, Indianapolis, Indiana

L. Andrew Koman, M.D.
Professor, Department of Orthopaedic Surgery, Bowman Gray School of Medicine of Wake Forest University, Winston-Salem, North Carolina

L. Lee Lankford, M.D.
Clinical Professor, Department of Orthopedic Surgery, University of Texas Southwestern Medical Center at Dallas Southwestern School of Medicine; Teaching Staff, Department of Orthopedics, Baylor College of Medicine; Founding Director, Parkland Memorial Hospital Hand Service, Dallas, Texas

Joseph P. Leddy, M.D.
Clinical Professor and Chief, Section of Hand Surgery, Division of Orthopaedic Surgery, Department of Surgery, University of Medicine and Dentistry of New Jersey Robert Wood Johnson Medical School, New Brunswick, New Jersey

Robert D. Leffert, M.D.
Professor, Department of Orthopaedic Surgery, Harvard Medical School; Chief, Surgical Upper Extremity Rehabilitation Unit, Massachusetts General Hospital, Boston, Massachusetts

Ronald L. Linscheid, M.D.
Professor, Department of Orthopedics, Mayo Medical School; Consultant, Department of Orthopedic Surgery and Surgery of the Hand, Mayo Clinic, Rochester, Minnesota

Graham D. Lister, M.B., Ch.B
Professor, Department of Surgery, University of Utah School of Medicine; Chief, Division of Plastic and Reconstructive Surgery, University of Utah Medical Center, Salt Lake City, Utah

Dean S. Louis, M.D.
Professor, Department of Surgery, University of Michigan School of Medicine; Chief, Hand Surgery, Section of Orthopedics, University of Michigan Hospitals, Ann Arbor, Michigan

Ralph T. Manktelow, M.D.
Professor and Chairman, Division of Plastic Surgery, Department of Surgery, University of Toronto Faculty of Medicine; Head, Division of Plastic Surgery, Toronto General Hospital, Toronto, Ontario, Canada

Charles L. McDowell, M.D.
Clinical Professor, Division of Orthopedic Surgery, Virginia Commonwealth University Medical College of Virginia School of Medicine; Chief, Upper Extremity Surgery, Spinal Cord Injury Unit, McGuire Veterans Administration Medical Center, Richmond, Virginia

Robert M. McFarlane, M.D., M.Sc.
Professor and Chief, Division of Plastic Surgery, Department of Surgery, University of Western Ontario; Surgeon, Hand and Upper Limb Centre, St. Joseph's Health Centre, London, Ontario, Canada

Lewis H. Millender, M.D.
Clinical Professor, Department of Orthopedic Surgery, Tufts University School of Medicine; Assistant Chief, Hand Surgery Service, New England Baptist Hospital, Boston, Massachusetts

Owen J. Moy, M.D.
Assistant Professor, Department of Orthopaedic Surgery, State University of New York at Buffalo School of Medicine and Biomedical Sciences; Attending Physician, Department of Orthopaedic Surgery, Millard Fillmore Hospital, Buffalo, New York

Edward A. Nalebuff, M.D.
Clinical Professor, Department of Orthopedic Surgery, Tufts University School of Medicine; Chief, Hand Surgery Service, New England Baptist Hospital, Boston, Massachusetts

Robert J. Neviaser, M.D.
Professor and Chairman, Department of Orthopaedic Surgery, George Washington School of Medicine and Health Sciences; Director, Hand and Upper Extremity Division, George Washington University Medical Center, Washington, D.C.

William L. Newmeyer, M.D.
Associate Clinical Professor, Department of Surgery, University of California, San Francisco, School of Medicine, San Francisco, California

George E. Omer, Jr., M.D., M.S.
Professor and Chairman Emeritus, Department of Orthopedics and Rehabilitation, University of New Mexico School of Medicine; Consultant in Hand Surgery, The Carrie Tingley Hospital, Albuquerque, New Mexico

Andrew K. Palmer, M.D.
Professor, Department of Orthopedic Surgery, State University of New York Health Science Center at Syracuse College of Medicine; Director of Hand Surgery, State University of New York Health Science Center at Syracuse, Syracuse, New York

Clayton A. Peimer, M.D.
Associate Professor, Department of Orthopaedic Surgery, Clinical Assistant Professor, Departments of Anatomical Sciences and Rehabilitation Medicine, State University of New York at Buffalo School of Medicine and Biomedical Sciences; Chief of Hand Surgery, Millard Fillmore Hospital, Buffalo, New York

Gary G. Poehling, M.D.
Professor and Chairman, Department of Orthopaedic Surgery, Bowman Gray School of Medicine of Wake Forest University, Winston-Salem, North Carolina

Somayaji Ramamurthy, M.D.
Professor, Department of Anesthesiology, University of Texas Health Science Center at San Antonio; Chief, Anesthesia Pain Management Clinic, San Antonio, Texas

Spencer A. Rowland, M.D., M.S.
Clinical Professor, Department of Orthopaedics, University of Texas Health Science Center at San Antonio, San Antonio, Texas

Roger E. Salisbury, M.D.
Professor and Chief, Division of Plastic and Reconstructive Surgery, Department of Surgery, New York Medical College; Director, Burn Center, Westchester Country Medical Center, Valhalla, New York

William E. Sanders, M.D.
Clinical Associate Professor, Department of Orthopaedics, University of Texas Medical School at San Antonio, San Antonio, Texas

Lawrence H. Schneider, M.D.
Clinical Professor, Department of Orthopedic Surgery, Jefferson Medical College of Thomas Jefferson University; Director, Division of Hand Surgery, Department of Orthopaedic Surgery, Thomas Jefferson University Hospital, Philadelphia, Pennsylvania

David B. Siegel, M.D.
Assistant Professor, Department of Orthopaedic Surgery, Bowman Gray School of Medicine at Wake Forest University, Winston-Salem, North Carolina

*Richard J. Smith, M.D.**
Clinical Professor, Department of Orthopedic Surgery, Harvard Medical School; Chief, Section of Hand Surgery, Department of Orthopedics, Massachusetts General Hospital, Boston, Massachusetts

Peter J. Stern, M.D.
Professor and Chairman, Department of Orthopedic Surgery, University of Cincinnati College of Medicine; Attending Physician, University of Cincinnati Hospital, Cincinnati, Ohio

James W. Strickland, M.D.
Clinical Professor, Department of Orthopaedic Surgery, Indiana University School of Medicine; Chairman, Department of Hand Surgery, St. Vincent Hospital and Health Care Center; Senior Attending Hand Surgeon, The Indiana Hand Center, Indianapolis, Indiana

Julio Taleisnik, M.D.
Clinical Professor, Division of Orthopedics, Department of Surgery, University of California, Irvine, School of Medicine, Irvine, California

Kenya Tsuge, M.D.
Emeritus Professor, Department of Orthopaedic Surgery, Hiroshima University School of Medicine; Director, Hiroshima Prefectural Rehabilitation Center, Higashi-Hiroshima, Japan

James R. Urbaniak, M.D.
Professor and Chief, Division of Orthopaedic Surgery, Department of Surgery, Duke University School of Medicine, Durham, North Carolina

H. Kirk Watson, M.D.
Associate Clinical Professor, Department of Orthopaedics, University of Connecticut School of Medicine, Farmington, Connecticut; Associate Professor, Departments of Orthopedics and Surgery, University of Massachusetts Medical School, Worcester, Massachusetts; Assistant Clinical Professor, Division of Plastic and Reconstructive Surgery, Department of Surgery, Yale University School of Medicine, New Haven, Connecticut; Chief, Connecticut Combined Hand Service, Hartford, Connecticut; Chief, Hand Service, Newington Children's Hospital, Newington, Connecticut; Senior Staff, Department of Orthopaedics, Hartford Hospital, Hartford, Connecticut

Andrew J. Weiland, M.D.
Professor, Department of Orthopaedic Surgery, Cornell University Medical College; Surgeon-in-Chief, Hospital for Special Surgery, New York, New York

E.F. Shaw Wilgis, M.D.
Associate Professor, Division of Orthopedic and Plastic Surgery, Department of Surgery, The Johns Hopkins University School of Medicine; Chief, Division of Hand Surgery, Director, Raymond M. Curtis Hand Center, The Union Memorial Hospital, Baltimore, Maryland

Virchel E. Wood, M.D.
Professor, Department of Orthopedic Surgery, Loma Linda University School of Medicine; Chief, Hand Surgery Service, Loma Linda University Medical Center, Loma Linda, California

Elvin G. Zook, M.D.
Professor and Chairman, Division of Plastic and Reconstructive Surgery, Department of Surgery, Southern Illinois University School of Medicine, Springfield, Illinois

Preface to the Third Edition

The reader does not need to be reminded how very difficult it is to "keep up." There are too many journals to read, too many meetings to attend, and too many good ideas cropping up all over the world. From its inception, the goal of this book has been to provide the reader with a comprehensive reference work to be used as a starting point for study. Not all the answers will be found in these pages, because some of the problems we face as hand surgeons have not yet been solved. However, a major effort has been made to compile and summarize what *is* known, and to provide all the references (at least in the English language literature) for the reader to pursue if more in-depth study is desired.

As in the Second Edition, I have updated the book to include current advances in hand and upper extremity surgery. In choosing new subjects, I have intentionally limited new material to areas in which sufficient progress has been made to provide the reader with appropriate guidance, but have left out those brand new subjects for which the pathway is still a bit murky. Accordingly, a superb new chapter, Arthoscopy of the Wrist and Elbow, has been added, but I felt that not enough has been done on the upper extremity with Ilizarov techniques to include that subject—it will have to wait until the Fourth Edition.

I am not a microvascular surgeon, and therefore I enlisted the help of my good friend Bob Hotchkiss to serve as Assistant Editor for the Microvascular Surgery section. Bob loves the craft of writing, and he accepted this task with his typical enthusiasm, keen insight, and thorough preparation. He consolidated some of the chapters in previous editions, added several new authors, and by trying to anticipate what the reader will want to know, asked each contributor to include his own answers to many practical and clinically pertinent questions.

Readers from all over the world continue to give me comments in a variety of forms ranging from praise to criticism; I relish the former, but the latter serves a more useful purpose in helping to improve the quality of this text. The perfect book cannot be written, but with sustained feedback from friends and readers, we can continue to make this one better.

David P. Green, M.D.

Preface to the First Edition

Considering the recent flood of new books that has inundated the medical world, one might justifiably ask, "Why yet *another* book on hand surgery?" It is true that there are already a number of books on hand surgery, many of them quite good. In my opinion, however, a comprehensive book dedicated primarily to operative techniques in hand surgery, combined with an extensive bibliography, is not available. The goal of this book has thus been to compile this type of single comprehensive reference work for the reader.

It is hoped that this book will prove useful to all serious students of hand surgery, ranging from residents to expreienced practitioners. The breadth of hand surgery has expanded so widely during the past 35 years that few hand surgeons can hope to remain expert in all phases of what was once a relatively narrow surgical subspecialty. It is for this reason that this book was produced in a multi-author format. Prior to writing his chapter, each author had already established his credentials and expertise in the area about which he was selected to write.

The major emphasis in this book is on operative technique, but possessing the technical skill to perform an operation is obviously not an indication to do that operation. Surgical judgment cannot be learned entirely from a book, but an effort has been made here to put each operative procedure into proper perspective. There are often many different ways to manage a given clinical situation, and selecting the most appropriate method for a specific problem in an individual patient frequently poses a perplexing dilemma for the surgeon. For this reason, each author has been encouraged to describe a variety of well-accepted procedures, indicating which of these he prefers, and why.

The general format and organization of the book will be more apparent to the reader if he or she takes a few moments to scan the Contents page. In addition, the running heads at the top of each page contain the title, author, and number of each chapter to aid the reader in locating a specific topic.

Finally, we must all keep in mind that concepts, operations, and even our knowledge of anatomy change, and no written word should be considered inviolate. I am frequently reminded of an admonition that one of my former teachers, Harrison McLaughlin, inscribed in his classic book on trauma: "To the New York Orthopaedic residents: Don't believe everything you read."

David P. Green, M.D.

Acknowledgments

Writing a chapter for a book falls into the category of thankless tasks. To do the job well requires a minimum of six months' hard labor and so many hours robbed from family and pursuits of pleasure that one doesn't like to add them up. I continue to be amazed at the dedication to this task shown by our contributors, and remain genuinely appreciative of their unstinting investments of time and energy. When you read something in this book, I hope you will take a moment to look at the running head at the top of the page and be grateful to the author who fulfilled an enormous commitment in writing that particular chapter.

Every editor needs a research assistant who is more compulsive and nitpicky than he is. By some stroke of luck, such a person came to work with me, and Lorie Sanders has done a truly remarkable job in tending to the thousands of tiny details that critically affect the ultimate quality of a book such as this. In a short period of time, she has become a first-rate sleuth in tracking down incorrect references, and she has raised to a higher level than ever the standards for accuracy that we have tried to maintain.

One of the major reasons that this book has been successful is the talent of medical illustrator Elizabeth Roselius, who in this addition has added many new drawings that continue to add immeasurably to the understanding of the text. Readers should know that the Second Edition of *Operative Hand Surgery* was given an award as the best clinical text at the 1988 meeting of the Association of Medical Illustrators. Such recognition by her peers unmistakably distinguishes Elizabeth as one of the very best in her field.

Churchill Livingstone has continued to provide me with outstanding support. Toni Tracy, the President of Churchill, is a consummate professional who runs a truly first-class organization.

David P. Green, M.D.

Contents

Contractures

Dystrophy

Fasciotomy

Fractures and Dislocations

Infections

Microvascular Surgery

Index

VOLUME 2

Nails

Nerve Injury and Repair

Nerve Reconstruction

Open Injuries

Rheumatoid Arthritis

Skin

Tendons

Extensor Tendons

30

Vascularized Bone Grafts

Andrew J. Weiland
Robert N. Hotchkiss

Advances over the past decade in the field of microsurgery have made it possible to provide continuing circulation to bone grafts used in the reconstruction of extremities with massive segmental bone loss following trauma or secondary to tumor resection. To appreciate the significance of transferring segmental autogenous bone grafts on vascular pedicles in reconstructive surgery, the surgeon should have a knowledge of the methods traditionally used and their historical development.

BACKGROUND

The introduction of bone grafting in the late nineteenth century by Barth led to its use in the treatment of nonunions,[1,16,27,35,47] arthrodesis of joints, the filling of bone cavities secondary to infection or of bone loss secondary to trauma or tumor resection.[5,25,31,37,65,67,68,72,77,95,102,116] The various techniques employed have evolved into the following: (1) massive autogenous corticocancellous bone obtained from the ilium, tibia, or fibula,[1,16] (2) transfer of whole bone segments,[27,56] (3) allograft bone transplants,[1,36,66,87–89] and (4) free vascularized bone grafts.[106,109–112,123–125]

Autogenous Bone Grafts

In 1895, Barth[8] characterized the replacement of dead bone by new, living bone as *creeping substitution (schleinchender Ersatz).* He described the process where old bone is removed and new bone is deposited in its place at the site of contact. The term *creeping substitution* was introduced into the English language literature by Phemister in 1914.[89]

Autogenous transplants are better tolerated and heal more rapidly than any other bone grafts.[2,41,48,49,57,71,72,91] The mechanisms involved in bone formation by autogenous grafts are still unresolved, but two concepts have evolved. One theory is that new bone formation results from the functional activity of osteogenic cells that survive in the graft (osteogenesis).[42] Supporting this notion, Lane et al[61a] have induced bone formation using collagen impregnated with bone marrow alone. However, in most cancellous grafts, only a small percentage of osteocytes and osteoblasts survive transplantation, leading to speculation about another mechanism of bone induction, referred to as the *metaplasia theory.*[9,57,58,64,65,96,97,98] This theory proposes that bone transformation occurs under the influence of osteogenesis-inducing substances that diffuse from the transplant site into the host's connective tissue.[37] Both mechanisms proposed probably play a role in bone formation; that is, a combination of the right cell in the right environment.

Surviving cells in autogenous grafts are entirely dependent on nourishment from the surrounding soft tissue bed after transfer. The superiority of autogenous cancellous bone grafts is directly related to their open structure, which facilitates diffusion of nutrient substances necessary for osteocyte and osteoblastic survival. The open, porous structure also permits the ingrowth of vessels from the host bed carrying undifferentiated mesenchymal cells that differentiate into osteogenic cells.[46] Conversely, dense cortical bone acts as a barrier to diffusion, inhibiting cell survival. Since the majority of cells in autogenous grafts do not survive transplantation, they must be replaced by new bone. The ultimate incorporation of autogenous grafts requires adequate circulation in the recipient bed, where new bone formation can occur in the presence of cells with an osteogenic capacity.

Allograft Bone Transplants

Although it has been shown repeatedly that allografts and xenografts are not as effective in providing an environment conducive for osteogenesis as fresh autogenous bone, there is limited autogenous donor graft available. In addition, the iliac crest cannot be used to replace large osteochondral defects after resections for tumor.[48] The reconstruction of large bone defects with allograft transplantations have been reported by Ottolenghi,[86] D'Aubigne, Meary, and Thomine,[36] Mankin and colleagues,[72] Lexer,[66-69] Parrish,[87,88] and Volkov.[116] Complications associated with these procedures include nonunion between the graft and the recipient bone, resorption, collapse of articular segments, and fracture of the graft. Prolonged immobilization for 8 to 24 months is required for partial incorporation of the graft and healing.

To reduce the immunogenicity of allografts, several investigators have demonstrated a reduction in antigentic properties in freeze-dried and fresh frozen allografts.[26,34,48,51,52] This process does reduce antigenicity but also kills the osteoprogenitor cells in the graft. Allografts are inferior to autografts during the early stages of repair due to the cellular response of the host tissue, as well as the impairment of vascularization of the graft.[41]

Vascularized Bone Grafts

The ideal bone graft is an autogenous graft that remains alive, resists resorption and maintains its physical characteristics—adapting structure as needed to the mechanical demands of the limb. In order to achieve this ideal, unimpaired microcirculation of bone is necessary for continued life and function of all bone cells and is only achieved by preservation or immediate reconstitution of the primary blood supply to the bone graft. The concept of a vascularized, "living" bone graft is not new. As early as 1905, Huntington[56] recognized the advantages of using a bone graft with its nutrient blood supply intact—a vascularized bone graft in the reconstruction of large tibial defects.

Blood Supply of Cortical Bone

The circulation and blood supply of bone must be understood in order to prepare a vascularized bone graft, whether on a pedicle or using microvascular transfer. Well-defined nutrient arteries penetrate the cortex through the nutrient foramen and nutrient canal.[63-92] After entering the diaphysis, the nutrient artery divides into ascending and descending branches to become the medullary arteries. These vessels have radially oriented branches that supply the diaphyseal cortex by further branching in a longitudinal direction.[113,114] Epiphyseal and metaphyseal arteries are found at the ends of long bones and supply their respective areas. Finally, the bones are surrounded by a periosteal vascular bed, emerging from the vessels that supply the neighboring muscles.[3] From the studies of Trueta and Caladias[114] Rhinelander,[94] and Johnson,[61] it is evident that the blood flow through cortical bone depends predominantly on an intact medullary blood supply, while the periosteal arteries play a minor role in direct cortical nutrition. Under normal circumstances, arterial blood flow passes centrifugally from the medullary system into the cortical arterioles and into the periosteal system.[19] Venous drainage most likely occurs in a centripetal direction, although this point is somewhat controversial. In pathologic or ischemic situations, blood flow may be reversed; a centripetal periosteal supply then assumes the role of a collateral circulatory system.[17-19]

The Advent of Microsurgery

> The idea of replacing diseased organs by sound ones, of putting back an amputated limb, or even of grafting a new limb on a patient having undergone an amputation is doubtless very old. The performance of such operations, however, was completely prevented by the lack of a method for uniting vessels, and thus, reestablishing a normal circulation through the transplanted structure. The feasibility of these grafts depended on the development of the technique.
>
> *Alexis Carrel*[28]

This statement, taken from Alexis Carrel's classic paper of 1908, heralded the birth of vascular surgery. Following World War II, the first vascular stapling machine was developed in Russia by Androsov.[6] Various mechanical devices were thereafter designed and tested.[40,56,78] Jacobson and Suarez[60] pioneered microvascular surgery by demonstrating the value of the operating microscope in 1960. Salmon and Assimacopoulos,[98] Buncke and co-workers,[21-23] Holt and Lewis,[54] and Cobbett[32] were responsible for the improvement in instrumentation and early experimental work in free vascularized tissue transfer. The first clinically successful transfer of an island flap by microvascular anastomoses was reported by Daniel and Taylor in 1973.[35] In the ensuing years, the scope of free tissue transfer has expanded rapidly to include free muscle transfers.[73,104,105]

Free Vascularized Bone Grafts

In 1975,[106,109] Taylor reported the first clinically successful free bone graft with microvascular anastomoses in which a fibular segment was transferred from the contralateral leg to reconstruct a large tibial defect. Since this historic report, many centers have reported on their clinical results with this procedure.[43,55,83,107,117,118,122,126] Similarly, vascularized rib grafts were used for treatment of a nonunion of a mandible following radical resection of a tumor.[100] Free osteocutaneous flaps consisting of the rib and overlying soft tissue have been transferred by Buncke[21] and O'Brien[82]; Taylor and Watson[112] have reported on the one-stage repair of a compound leg defect with an osteocutaneous flap from the groin. Weiland, Daniel and Riley, and other authors have extended the application of free vascularized bone grafts to the treatment of malignant or aggressive bone tumors,[76,77,123,124,126] and the technique has been used in the treatment of congenital pseudarthrosis of the tibia.[30,45,121] The advantages of transferring segmental autogenous bone grafts on vascular pedicles for the treatment of upper extremity lesions have also been reported.[4,53,90,103,125]

In selected patients, free vascularized bone grafts offer significant advantages over conventional methods of treatment, since a massive segment of bone, along with its accompanying nutrient vessels, can be detached from its donor site and transferred to a distant recipient site with preservation of the nutrient blood supply by microvascular anastomoses to recipient vessels. With the nutrient blood supply preserved, osteocytes and osteoblasts in the graft can survive, and healing of the graft to the recipient bone will be facilitated without the usual replacement of the graft by creeping substitution. This concept has been validated by many authors who have reported experimental studies concerning the various factors affecting the survival of vascularized bone grafts.[7,11-14,38,70,101,119,127] Thus, with vascularized bone grafts the surgeon can achieve more rapid stabilization of bone fragments separated by a large defect without sacrificing viability. This is especially significant when the defect is situated in a highly traumatized or irradiated area with significant scarring and relative avascularity of the surrounding tissue, impeding incorporation of a conventional autogenous graft.

INDICATIONS FOR USE OF VASCULARIZED BONE GRAFTS

Several factors should be considered before choosing a vascularized graft over conventional grafting techniques. A surgical team that is thoroughly familiar with microsurgical techniques must be available, since these procedures are often long and tedious, lasting 5 to 6 hours. In patients with a history of severe trauma, irradiation, or infection, the likelihood of significant damage to recipient vessels in the extremity must be carefully weighed, since the possibility of failure due to poor arterial inflow and venous outflow is greater in these cases.

General Considerations

Health, Age, and Long-Term Goals

As with any reconstructive procedures, the benefits of limb reconstruction must be weighed against the risks of a long surgical procedure, prolonged limb protection, and the possibility of complications. In the upper limb, if a viable functional hand exists, every effort should be made to create a stable, painless limb. For the lower limb, the decision can be more vexing, and the amputation may be simpler and in the best interest of the patient.

There is no age limit—young or old—for microsurgery, including vascularized bone grafts. Children tend to have a much greater capacity to revascularize segments of bone graft if a normal bed is present. Unfortunately, many of the conditions that create bone defects in the young—tumors and severe trauma—may be associated with a poor blood supply in the recipient bed. In the elderly, life expectancy, limb function, and realistic demands must all be considered.

Alternatives

Before considering a vascularized bone graft, all alternative methods of reconstruction should be considered. Should a conventional graft be used? Is there a salvage procedure that will result in similar function, such as a one bone forearm? If other structures have been irrevocably damaged, such as tendons and nerves, should amputation be considered? Each situation demands careful consideration and discussion with the patient and family.

Bone Transport (Ilizarov)

When Ilizarov first explained and demonstrated his technique using distraction osteogenesis, he created a viable alternative to grafting of segmental bone defects.[58] His method of bone transport, slowly translating a small segment of bone the length of the defect leaving a contrail of healing regenerating bone, required no microsurgical expertise. In this country, his method has proven quite useful in the treatment of tibial defects and to a lesser extent in the femur. Some surgeons supplement the transport procedure with cancellous bone grafting at the docking site once transport is complete (Herzenberg J: personal communication). The technical difficulties of bone transport are substantial and numerous. In the humerus and forearm, great care must be taken to keep the wires or pins in the transport segment free of nerve and tendon. The tibia is optimal because of the large subcutaneous soft tissue envelope. The time of consolidation in bone transport can be quite prolonged, often requiring several months of frame use. Great patience is required.

As an alternative to bone transport, Grishin et al[44] reported the use of the Ilizarov frame in conjunction with free vascularized bone reconstruction in 71 patients using the frame for skeletal fixation. Instead of using internal fixation, casts, and splints after vascularized grafting, Grishin recommended establishing appropriate skeletal length and alignment, spanning the defect with a vascularized bone graft, then using the fixator for stability. The technique for this alternative is discussed below (see page 1191).

Defect Size and Location

The size of the defect must be considered with the function of the limb in mind. In the lower extremity, limb length equality is important for gait, and shortening greater than 2 cm is often not acceptable. In the humerus, shortening is better tolerated and an actual defect of 6 cm may be converted to 3 or 4 cm and conventional grafting used. In the forearm, defects of the radius or ulna must be made up to equalize the other bone or converted to a single bone forearm. A nonvascularized iliac crest segment has been successfully grafted in defects up to 6 cm.

For large segmental bone defects in the hand and wrist we have *not* found it necessary to employ vascularized bone grafts.

Nonvascularized iliac grafts covered by healthy soft tissue are revascularized and heal with stability in 6 to 12 weeks. For specialized circumstances, such as scaphoid nonunion, several pedicle bone grafts have been described to enhance healing, but these have not been used on a regular basis (see Chapter 22).

Recipient Soft Tissue Bed

Creeping substitution is a centripetal, circumferential process. If the bed of tissue surrounding the bone defect is scarred and poorly vascularized, the reason for vascularized bone grafting becomes more compelling. In irradiated beds or those subjected to cryosurgery following tumor extirpation, vascularized bone grafts should strongly be considered.

In cases of long-standing osteomyelitis or trauma (Fig. 30-1), the soft tissue may be scarred and relatively avascular. In most cases, the scarred soft tissue bed can be completely excised, a free muscle flap used to revitalize the recipient bed, and conventional bone grafting sued to heal the bone defect and span the gap. If the defect in these circumstances is 6 cm or greater, a vascularized bone graft should strongly be considered.

Contraindications

There are few absolute contraindications to vascularized bone grafting. Most decisions not to proceed with vascularized grafting are based on an unsuitable limb for reconstruction. The presence of active infection is an absolute contraindication for grafting. Other reasons not to proceed are (1) unsuitable vascular pedicle at recipient site, (2) unsuitable donor graft, and (3) severe systemic illness (chronic renal disease, chronic heart disease).

DONOR SITES—CHOOSING THE RIGHT SOURCE

The ideal donor source for a vascularized bone would contain a long, reliable pedicle with the exact shape and size of the bony defect in order to provide immediate skeletal stability. Most defects in the upper extremity are long and tubular, as with diaphyseal defects in the radius.

There have been many donor sites for vascularized bone grafts reported; each has its advantages and disadvantages. Most often mentioned (in order to descending utility) are the fibula, iliac crest, first metatarsal, and rib. The rib is the least useful because of its size and bone quality. Most often it has been employed in mandibular reconstruction. For the first metatarsal, the donor site morbidity is considerable and should only be considered in extreme circumstances.

Since most defects requiring vascularized bone grafts in the upper extremity are diaphyseal, the fibula is usually optimal. Occasionally the iliac crest is necessary because trauma to the lower extremities has damaged the fibula or a composite flap with skin and bone is needed. Then the iliac crest with skin, based on the deep circumflex iliac artery can be used. The curvature of the iliac crest usually limits its applicability to bone defects of 10 cm or less. Table 30-1 summarizes donor sites. For defects that require a block of bone, the iliac crest is preferable to the fibula.

OPERATIVE TECHNIQUE

Preoperative Planning

If the anatomy of the fibular bone graft is unfamiliar, it can be quite helpful to dissect the graft in the anatomy laboratory before clinical application. The surgeon should be comfortable with the vascular anatomy of the upper and lower extremities. In addition, the surgical team must be thoroughly acquainted with the various techniques of microvascular surgery and must be able to perform microvascular anastomoses with facility (see Chapter 26).

Angiography

Preoperative arteriograms of both donor and recipient sites should be obtained to identify possible vascular abnormalities resulting from congenital malformations or from trauma in the recipient extremity. Clinical experience has taught us that significant problems with arterial inflow may exist in patients with traumatic defects even when preoperative arteriograms appear normal. This finding reflects the fact that the zone of injury to the extremity often extends a significant distance from the obvious bone defect and results in vascular damage that jeopardizes successful microvascular anastomoses.

Arteriograms of the donor site for the fibula are mandatory. The vascular anomalies associated with trifucation of the anterior tibial, posterior tibial, and peroneal arteries are common. For instance, the patient may lack an anterior tibial artery. It is also helpful to know the level of the take-off of the peroneal artery. At times this can be quite low, which places the pedicle in the middle of the graft. This location may require adjustment in the recipient vascular site or the use of vein grafts.

Patient Preparation

The night before surgery, the patient is given 325 mg of aspirin. The patient should also be well hydrated. Most of the time, IV fluids are given at 80 to 100 cc/hr several hours before surgery.

The Operating Room, Equipment, and Staff

In situations where a microvascular surgical team is available to perform free tissue transfer, significant time is saved by using a two-team approach in which one team works on the recipient site and the other on the donor site.

The operating room should have adequate space to accommodate two surgical teams and the operating microscope. The room and patient should be kept warm to avoid vasoconstriction. If possible, we prefer to use regional anesthesia in the limb

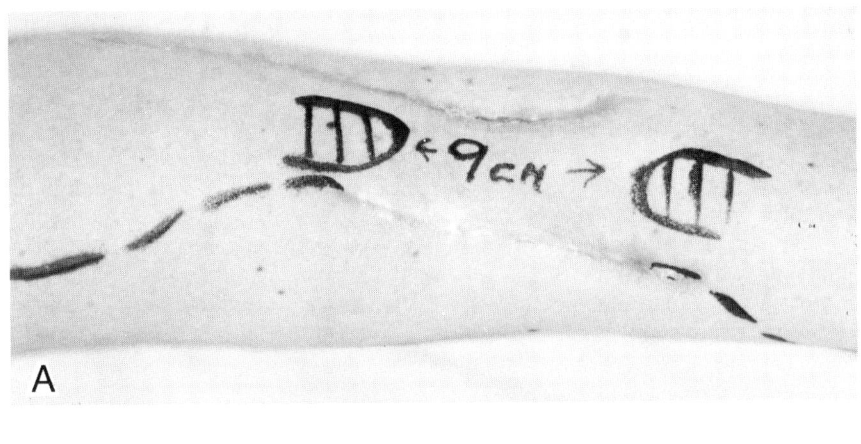

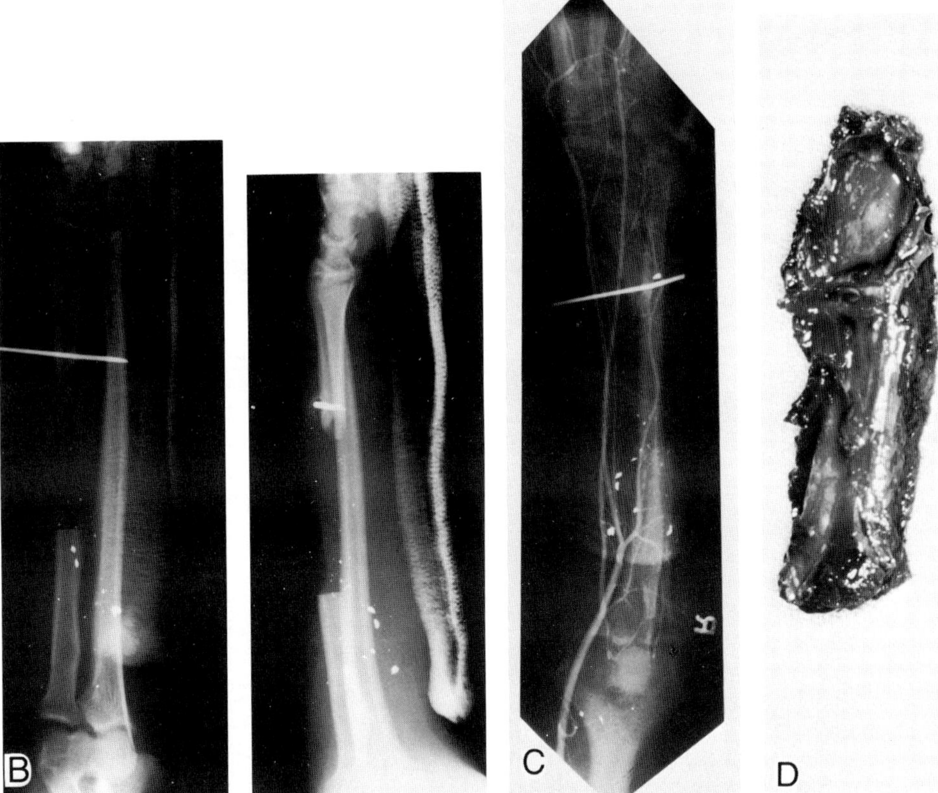

Fig. 30-1. **(A)** The preoperative clinical appearance of the left forearm in a 17-year-old male with a segmental 9-cm bony defect in the radius secondary to a shotgun wound (Case 2). **(B)** Preoperative radiographs of the left forearm. **(C)** Preoperative arteriogram demonstrating normal vascular anatomy supplying the forearm. **(D)** A 9-cm fibular graft with the surrounding 0.7-cm to 1.0-cm muscle cuff and peroneal vessels preserved. *(Figure continues.)*

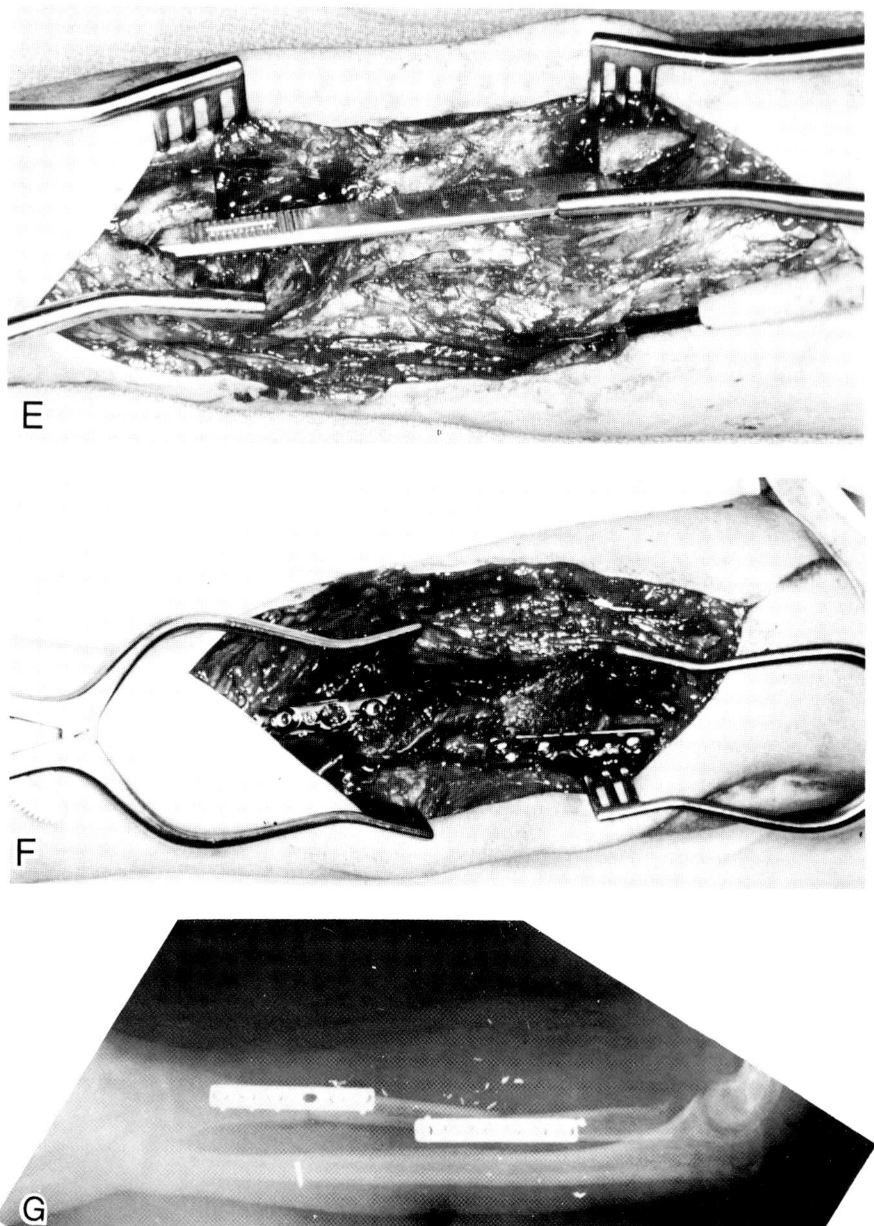

Fig. 30-1 *(Continued).* **(E)** The radial defect as seen at the time of operation. **(F)** The 9-cm fibular graft has been attached to the proximal and distal radius with two one-third tubular plates. **(G)** A radiograph taken immediately after operation, showing the fibular graft in place. *(Figure continues.)*

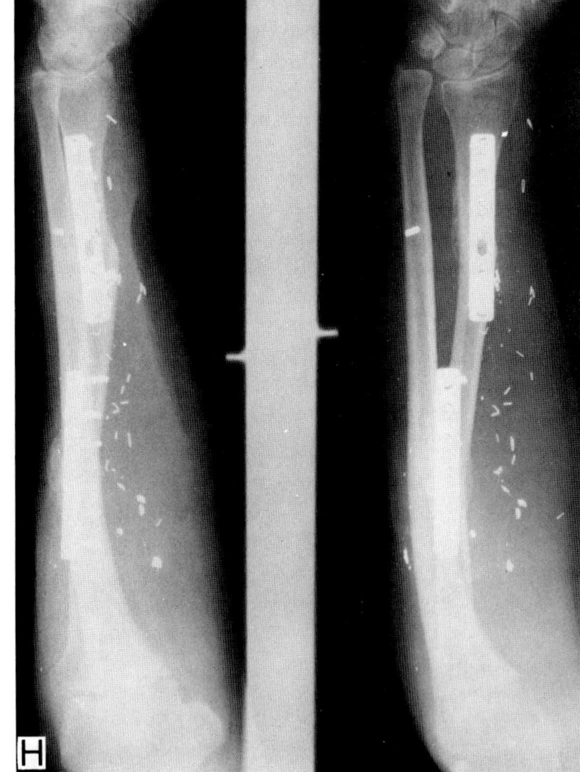

Fig. 30-1 *(Continued).* **(H)** Radiographs at 3 months show solid union of the fibular graft proximally and distally. (From Weiland and Daniel,[122] with permission.)

Table 30-1. Free Bone Transfers

Characteristics	Fibula	Rib	Iliac Crest
Bone			
Length (maximum)	22–26 cm	30 cm	10 cm
Shape	Straight	Curved	Slightly curved
Structure	Cortical, straight	Membranous, malleable	Corticocancellous, fixed
Vessels			
Artery	Peroneal (1.5–2.5 mm)	Posterior intercostal (1.5–2.0 mm)	Superficial circumflex iliac (0.8–3.0 mm)
Vein	Two venae comitantes (2.0–3.0 mm)	One intercostal (1.2–2.5 mm)	Superficial inferior epigastric (1.5–3.0 mm)
Vascular stalk	Short (1.0–3.0 cm)	Long (3.0–5.0 cm)	Moderate (1.0–5.0 cm)
Dissection	Superficial, simple, tedious	Deep, difficult, quick	Superficial, meticulous
Options			
Articular surface	Yes	Yes	No
Epiphysis	Yes	No	No
Adjacent muscle	Yes	Yes	No (nonfunctional)
Overlying skin	No	Yes	Yes
Nerve	No	Yes	Yes
Complications	Minimal	Thoracotomy Venous inadequacy and thrombosis	Abdominal wall hernia
Applications	Long bone defects (extremities)	Mandibular reconstruction; composite bone-skin replacement	Composite bone and skin (extremities); mandibular reconstruction

of the graft because of the sympatholytic effect on the local circulation. If the graft is to the lower extremity, an indwelling epidural catheter can maintain analgesia and vasodilation for 2 to 3 days after operation.

For dissection of the graft and isolation of the recipient pedicle, small hemoclips are especially useful, reducing time and danger to the microvasculature from electrocautery.

It is helpful to plan the method of fixation and to consider a back-up technique if necessary. Rounding up the necessary equipment during surgery can be stressful for the entire staff. It is therefore necessary to select the plate you plan to use and have a longer and shorter version available. External fixation systems may also need to be gathered.

Cancellous bone graft from the iliac crest needs to be harvested on nearly every patient to enhance healing at the proximal and distal junctions. The graft can be harvested at any time and stored on the back table. We usually harvest the cancellous graft after the vascularized graft is taken.

Free Fibula Graft (Fig. 30-2)

Introduction

The operation usually begins under tourniquet control at the recipient site where the vessels are identified and isolated. If a tumor is involved, the tumor is excised en bloc, incorporating any biopsy site, and the size of the defect is determined. Where a nonunion or infection exists, the bone ends are debrided and prepared proximally and distally in order to receive the fibular graft. It is imperative that the bone be resected back to normal tissue.

After the recipient vessels are identified, the defect measured, and the technical feasibility of the free fibular transfer determined, the free fibular graft is harvested from the donor leg.

We have not established the upper limits of the length of the fibular graft that may be harvested from the donor extremity. However, the distal ankle mortise with the anterior and posterior talofibular and calcanealfibular ligaments must be preserved and not harvested with the graft. Grafts as long as 24 cm have survived completely. This is not surprising when one considers that the periosteal and medullary blood supply to the bone is preserved. The technique for dissection of the fibula described below is a modification of that employed by Gilbert.[42]

Anatomy

The nutrient artery of the fibula (Fig. 30-2A) arises as a branch of the peroneal artery, which in turn originates from the posterior tibial trunk. The peroneal artery gives off several periosteal branches before giving origin to the nutrient artery that supplies the medullary nutrient blood flow to the fibula. Penetration through the fibular cortex usually occurs at the middiaphyseal level with a variation of 2.5 cm proximally or distally. The length of the nutrient artery external to the fibula ranges from 2 to 5 cm; the diameter is commonly 2.5 mm but may range from 1 to 3 mm.[114] The peroneal artery continues distally along the medial and posterior aspect of the fibular diaphysis (Fig. 30-2B) and provides direct musculoperiosteal branches. Preservation of the medullary and periosteal supply to the straight cortical bone is, therefore, possible by isolation of the peroneal artery at its origin from the posterior tibial peroneal trunk. The venous drainage closely parallels the arterial supply and occurs through the venae comitantes of the peroneal artery and medullary sinusoidal system.

Patient Position

Dissection of the fibula is performed under epidural (preferably) or general anesthesia with the patient supine and the donor extremity flexed approximately 135 degrees at the knee and 60 degrees at the hip. The surgeon and first assistant stand on the lateral side of the leg with the second assistant positioned medially, supporting the extremity in the flexed position. A tourniquet is used during the course of the dissection, which is performed under 2.5× to 4.0× loupe magnification.

Dissection of the Graft

For descriptive purposes, the procedure can be divided into eight steps. Figure 30-2B illustrates the plane of dissection.

Step I. A longitudinal skin incision is made along the lateral aspect of the fibula extending from the neck as far distally as needed.[50] The incision is carried through the skin and subcutaneous tissue to the superficial fascia overlying the interval between the peroneus longus and soleus muscles. The fascia is then split longitudinally for the length of the graft required.

Step II. The interval between the peroneus longus and soleus muscles is identified and the deep fascia incised over the entire length of the incision along this interval. Using a blunt elevator, this interval between the peroneus longus and soleus muscles is developed. The peroneus longus and soleus muscles are then reflected from the fibular diaphysis anteriorly and posteriorly respectively, using an extraperiosteal dissection technique.

Step III. The lateral border of the fibula is now exposed. There are three perforating vessels to the skin lying immediately posterior in the fascia overlying the soleus muscle. If the skin is to be harvested with the fibula, then these branches must be preserved. When the bone alone is to be transferred, these vessels should be ligated.

Step IV. Beginning proximally, the peroneus longus and brevis muscles are elevated from the anterior border of the fibula, using a blunt elevator until the anterior crural septum is reached while staying extraperiosteal. Some preserved muscle tissue is harvested with the fibular graft, but the 1-cm cuff of muscle surrounding the fibula as previously

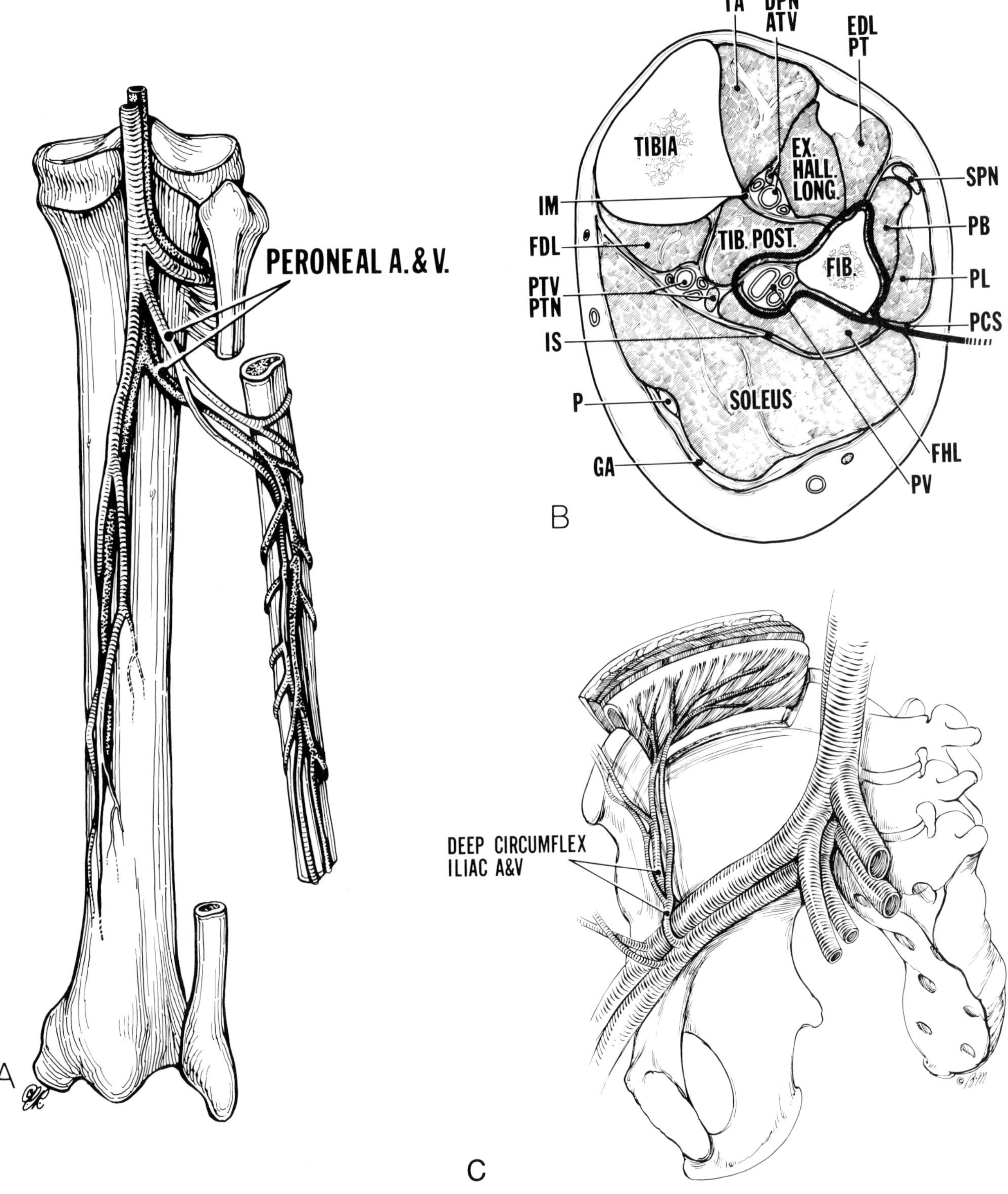

Fig. 30-2. **(A)** The free vascularized fibular graft isolated on the peroneal vessels. **(B)** Cross section of the leg illustrating the plane of dissection for harvesting a fibular graft *(solid black line)*. (*TA*, tibialis anterior; *DPN*, deep peroneal nerve; *ATV*, anterior tibial vessels; *EDL*, extensor digitorum longus; *PT*, peroneus tertius; *SPN*, superficial peroneal nerve; *PB*, peroneus brevis; *PL*, peroneus longus; *PCS*, posterior crural septum; *FHL*, flexor hallucis longus; *PV*, peroneal vessels; *GA*, gastrocnemius aponeurosis; *P*, plantaris; *IS*, intermuscular septum; *PTV*, posterior tibial vessels; *PTN*, posterior tibial nerve; *FDL*, flexor digitorum longus; *IM*, interosseous membrane.) **(C)** The osteocutaneous groin flap based on the deep circumflex iliac artery and vein.

described is no longer used.[121] In the event that the vascularized graft fails, the cuff of muscle will become necrotic and possibly serve as a nidus for infection. In addition, it will delay replacement of the graft by creeping substitution. The anterior crural septum is divided along the length of the graft, and the extensor group of muscles (extensor digitorum longus, peroneus tertius, and extensor hallucis longus) are dissected off of the interosseous membrane. Throughout the course of this portion of the dissection, the anterior tibial artery and nerve should be identified and protected by blunt retractors.

Step V. The posterior crural membrane is divided the entire length of the graft. Using careful extraperiosteal dissection techniques, the soleus and flexor hallucis muscles are reflected off the posterior border of the fibula, taking care to preserve the nerve to the flexor hallucis muscle. The dissection continues until the peroneal vessels are encountered. The vessels must be left attached to the posterior surface of the intermuscular septum to prevent separation from the fibular graft. Dissection is continued anteriorly and posteriorly for the length of the graft required. During the posterior dissection, any branches arising from the peroneal artery that will not be taken with the graft must be coagulated. Two of three large branches arising from the peroneal artery will supply a significant portion of the soleus muscle and must be preserved if a composite soleus and fibular graft is desired. Additional branches to the skin can also be preserved if the surgeon desires to monitor circulation to the graft. However, orientation of the skin flap can be difficult, especially when the bone defect is not located in a subcutaneous area. In the distal one-third of the fibula, the peroneal artery lies directly on the posterior surface of the bone; care should be taken to avoid damage to the artery during the osteotomy.

Step VI. The length of graft needed is measured and marked with methylene blue. The distal 6 cm of the fibula should be preserved to maintain integrity of the lateral aspect of the ankle joint. In children less than 10 years of age, a transfixation screw between the distal fibular segment and tibia is employed, and a formal synostosis of the tibia and fibula is performed distally to preserve the integrity of the ankle mortice and prevent possible proximal migration of the distal fibula, which could lead to valgus instability.

A hole is then made in the intermuscular septum, sufficiently large to allow a 1.5-cm malleable retractor to be placed around the bone, protecting the vessels that lie posterior to the retractor. At this point, an oscillating saw is used to cut the distal margin of the graft. A similar procedure is carried out at the proximal end of the graft, again taking great care to preserve the peroneal vascular bundle. The peroneal vessels at the distal end of the graft are then ligated with hemoclips.

Step VII. A small bone hook is placed in the medullary canal of the distal portion of the fibular graft. As the graft is retracted posteriorly and laterally, division of the interosseous membrane is performed along the entire length of the graft. The graft is then carefully retracted anteriorly, and the tibialis posterior muscle is dissected off the posterior aspect of the graft in the middle third where it has remained attached to the fibula. *Care should be taken at this step to identify and protect the nerve to the flexor hallucis muscle.* On completion of this step, the fibular graft is isolated on its vascular pedicle.

Step VIII. The peroneal artery is traced proximally to its junction with the posterior tibial artery. A vessel loop is placed around the peroneal artery and vein. The fibula is placed back into the bed until the recipient site is prepared. The tourniquet is deflated, permitting circulation to the graft. This portion of the dissection should take about 1½ hours to complete. On completion of the dissection in the recipient bed, the tourniquet is reinflated and the fibula is harvested and placed in the defect.

Skeletal Fixation

The transferred bone must be rigidly fixed in the recipient site before microvascular anastomoses are begun. Adequate bony fixation and alignment of the fibular graft is crucial to healing and graft incorporation.

The junction of the graft and recipient should be fashioned to maximize bone contact and stability. It is helpful to take time and craft the bone appropriately. The cross-sectional size of the fibular graft when compared to the recipient junctions usually determines the configuration of fixation at the proximal and distal junctions. For instance, when the humerus is grafted, the fibula can be inserted into the medullary canal of the humerus after enlarging the recipient bone with a small motorized burr. A small amount of the edge of the triangle can be burred from the fibular graft, but as little trimming of the graft as possible should be performed. When the graft more closely matches the diameter of the recipient site, as in the midshaft radius, a step cut can be made in the fibula and the radius to create overlap and the possibility of lag screw fixation. This provides better rotational stability. The fibular graft should be long enough to restore tension in the muscle tendon envelope by spanning the gap with adequate length (Fig. 30-3). The tension in the soft tissue envelope loads the graft, enhancing stability. This should be done whether internal or external fixation is employed.

Method of Fixation

The decision to use internal or external fixation depends on the patient, location of the defect, and the quality of bone. If the defect is middiaphyseal and the bone on either end of the graft is healthy, internal fixation with a plate spanning the

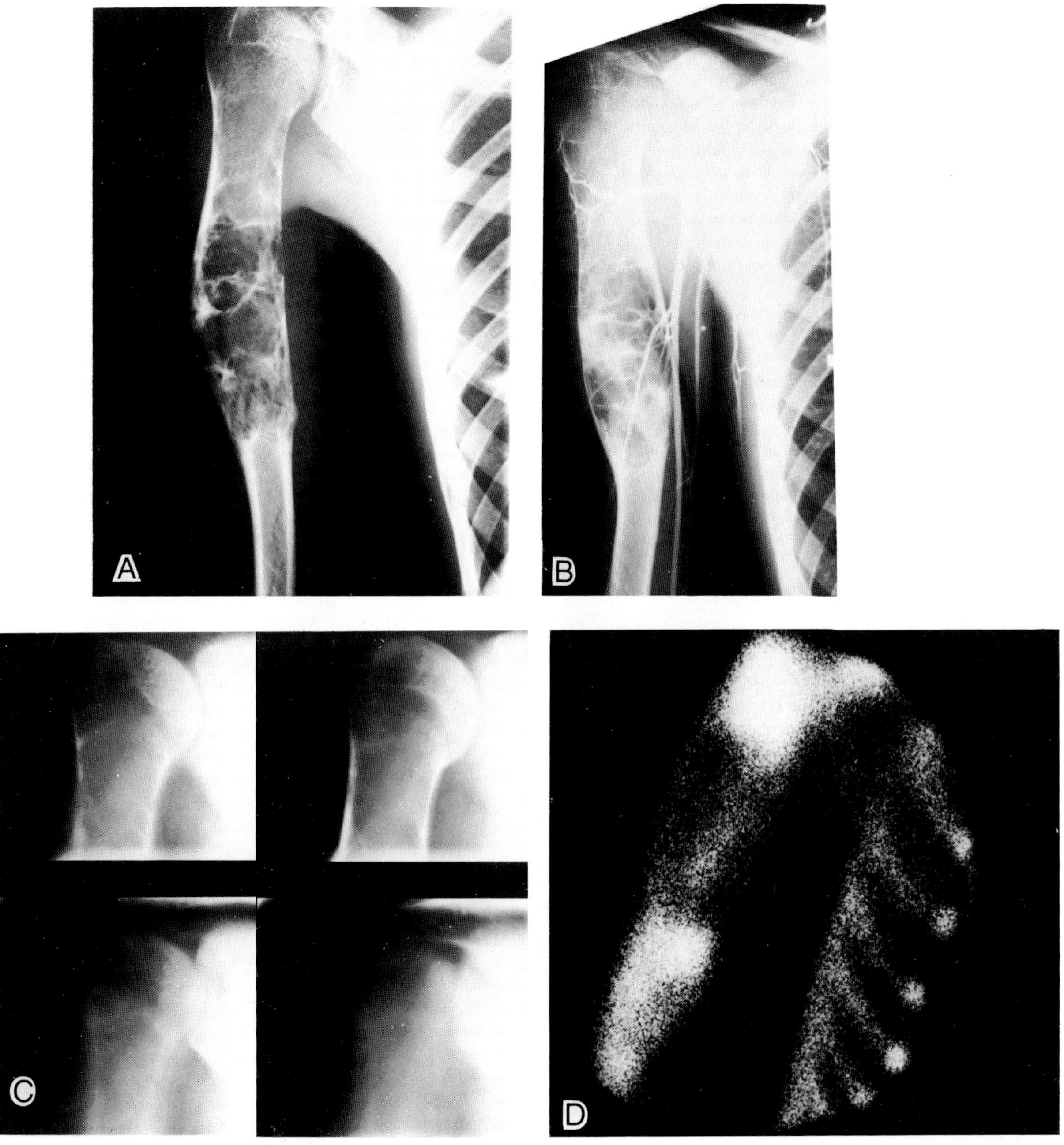

Fig. 30-3. **(A)** A unicameral bone cyst in the right humerus of a 17-year-old male (Case 1). **(B)** A preoperative arteriogram of the right upper extremity demonstrated the circumflex humeral artery proximally and the profunda brachii artery distally. **(C)** Tomograms revealed that only 1 cm of normal bone was present in the proximal humerus. **(D)** A bone scan demonstrated that sufficient bone stock was present proximally to allow fixation of the humerus with the Wagner apparatus. *(Figure continues.)*

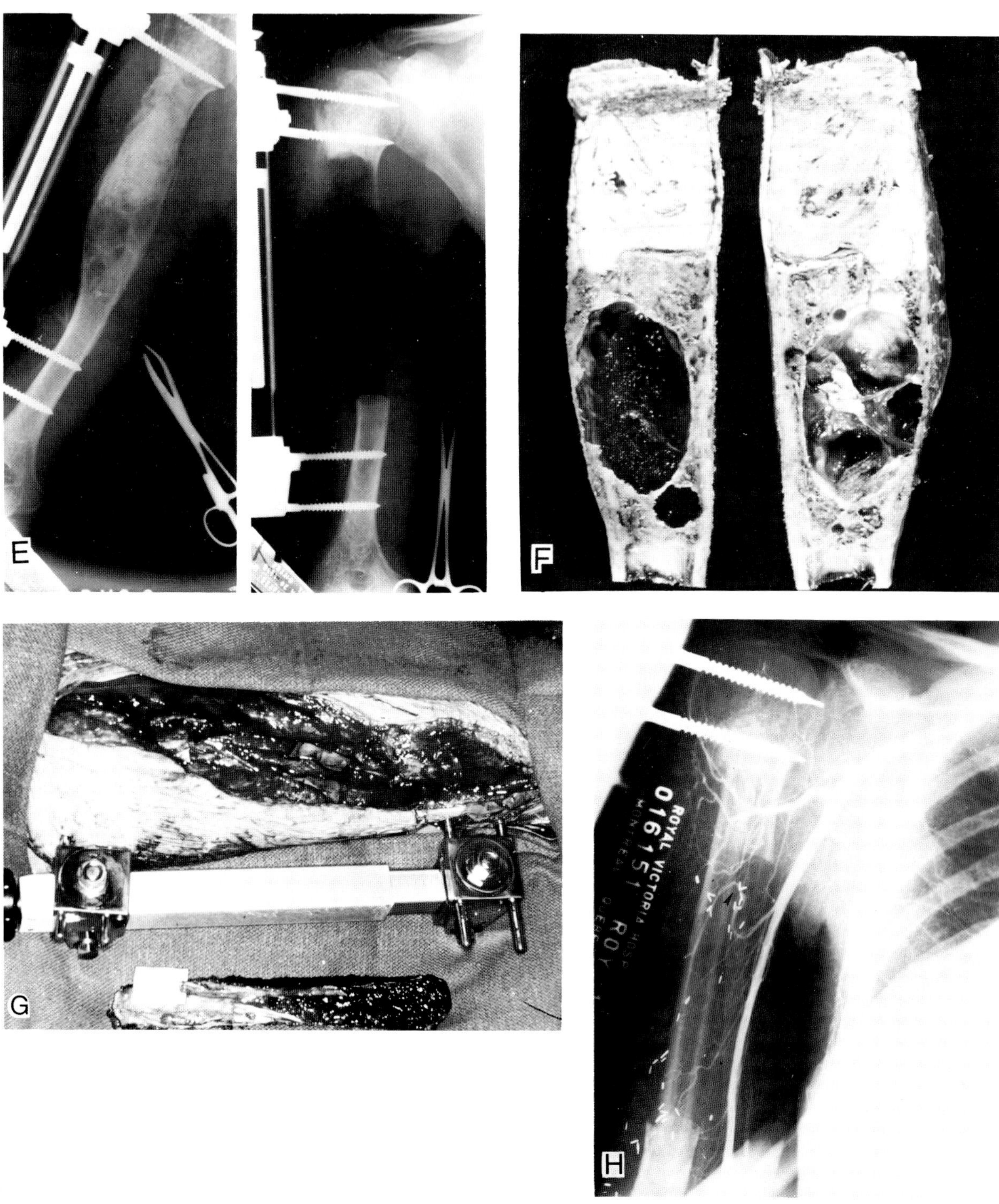

Fig. 30-3 *(Continued).* (E) Radiographs showing the Wagner apparatus in place prior to and after resection of the unicameral cyst. **(F)** The resected specimen, with the methylmethacrylate-packed portion of the tumor seen at the top of the picture and the remaining cyst seen distally. **(G)** Intraoperative photograph of the fibular graft just prior to insertion into the humeral defect. **(H)** An arteriogram at 6 weeks revealed a patent arterial anastomosis between the peroneal artery and the profunda brachii artery *(arrow)*; microclips are seen surrounding the graft. *(Figure continues.)*

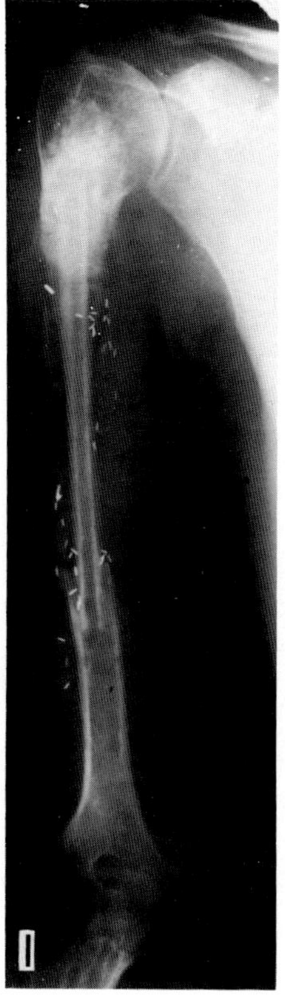
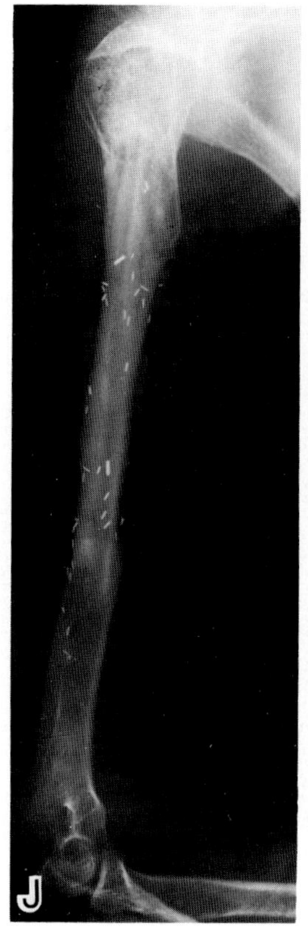
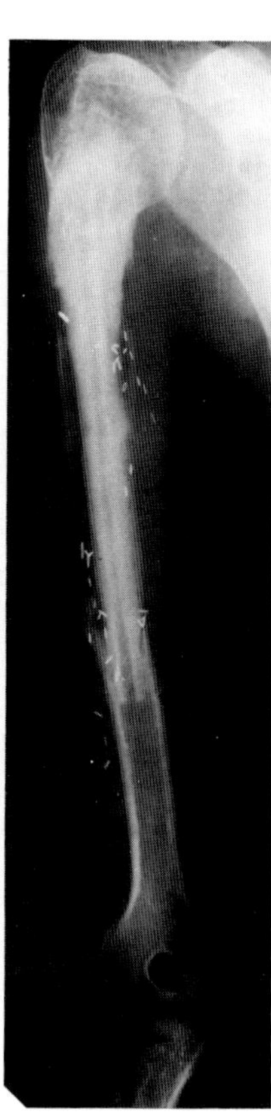

Fig. 30-3 *(Continued).* Radiographs at **(I)** 6 months and **(J)** 12 months, showing progressive hypertrophy of the free vascularized fibular graft. (From Weiland and Daniel,[122] with permission.)

defect is optimal. Two plates can also be used (Fig. 30-4). If the graft is placed into metaphyseal bone that has become soft and will not hold screws, external fixation may be the best option. It is often helpful to plan for both, in case you need to change plans during surgery.

Intramedullary fixation disrupts the medullary blood supply to the graft and should not be used.

Internal Fixation. Internal fixation of the fibular graft is more easily used when the bone defect is mid-diaphyseal. Both DC plates or recon plates (AO/ASIF) can be used to span the defect. Only one or two screws should be used in the graft, *avoiding the nutrient artery and pedicle at all costs.* The plate should also not lie on top of the nutrient artery. Screws through the distal and proximal junction can be placed to incorporate the recipient bone, fibular graft and plate. If the proximal or distal metaphysis is included, T-plates can be used. Liberal concellous bone graft should be applied at both the proximal and distal bone graft sites.

It is important to use a plate of adequate length with at least four (preferably six) cortices proximally and distally. Two plates securing the graft at either end can be used, but care must be taken to protect the vascular pedicle.

External Fixation. The use of external fixation has changed since the introduction of the Ilizarov ring external fixator. In those cases where inadequate bone quality or location precluded secure internal fixation, we have used the Ilizarov ring external fixator with success. In 1990, Grishin et al[44] published a series of vascularized fibular grafts in 71 cases using the Ilizarov ring fixator. Grishin used the frame to establish length and correct alignment, then placed the fibular graft. He also described lengthening, once the graft was in place. We have no experience with lengthening over a vascularized graft. Jupiter[62] has reported the use in the humerus using the frame similarly to Grishin in the humerus.

Although there are several different designs of external fixators, the Ilizarov frame offers multiplanar control and a variety of options of configuration. Both half-pins and transosseous wires can be used in the same frame, in a variety of locations as needed. Once the graft is in place, wires can be used to secure the graft to the recipient bone. Wires can be passed from the ring to the recipient bone and through the intussucepted fibular graft. The greatest difficulty lies in planning the frame so that access for the microsurgical anastomoses is not blocked by the frame. This can usually be managed by creating a half-shell frame that is fully assembled with additional wires and pins after the fibula is keyed into position and the microsurgery completed. This frame is especially useful in the humerus and the distal tibia. The other axial external fixation systems can also be used with success. We have also used the AO external fixation device and the Hoffman device because of their ease of application.

Vascularized Iliac Crest Graft—With or Without Skin Flap

If a large block of bone is needed or the fibular graft is unavailable, the iliac crest can be harvested with the deep circumflex iliac artery. In patients presenting with bone massive skin

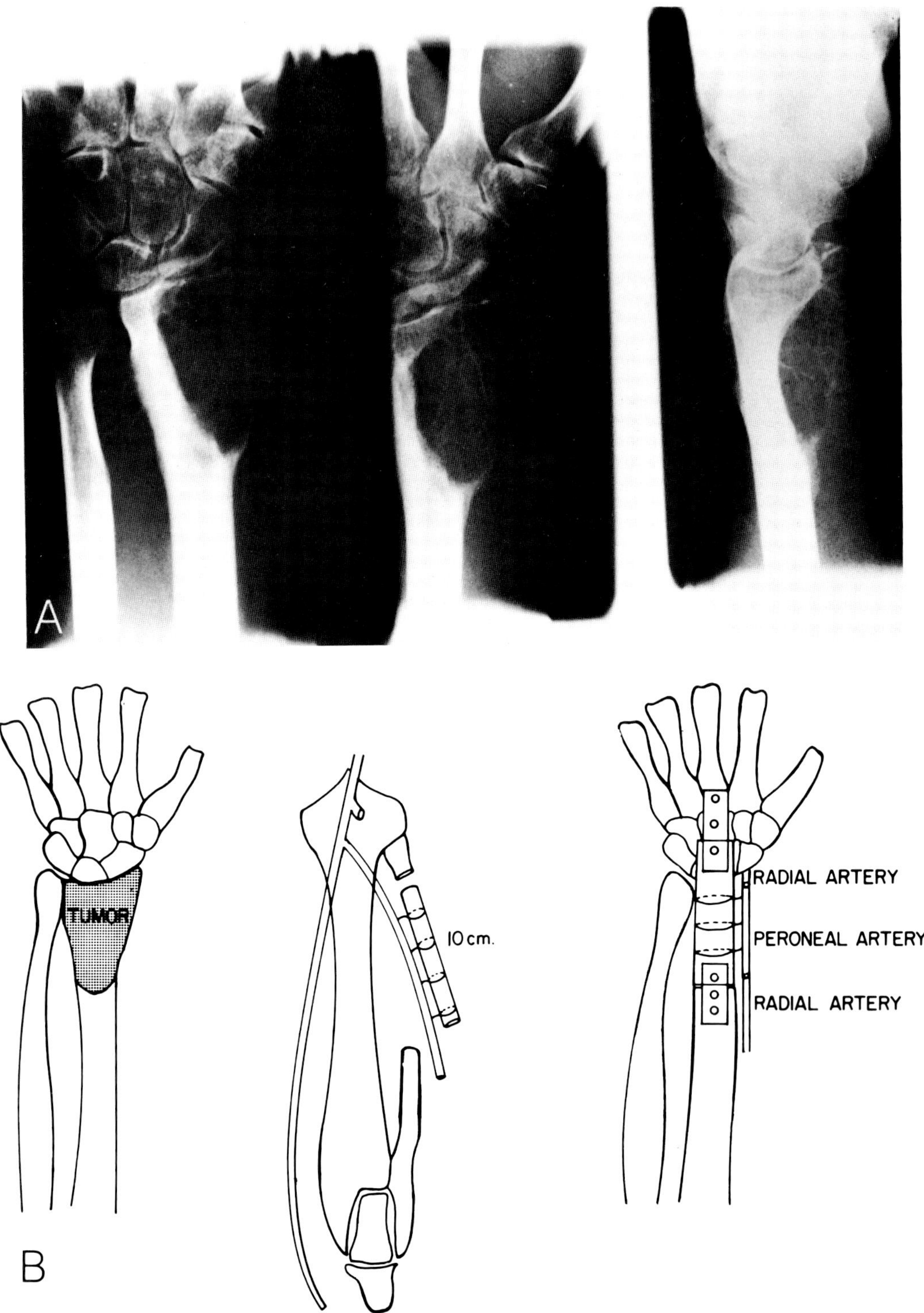

Fig. 30-4. **(A)** Radiographs of the left distal radius revealing a lesion compatible with giant cell tumor (Case 3). **(B)** Diagram of the free vascularized bone graft transfer. The tumor *(left)*. Isolation of the fibula on its vascular pedicle *(center)*. The free vascularized graft in place with anastomosis of the peroneal artery as an interposition graft between the radial artery proximally and distally *(right)*. *(Figure continues.)*

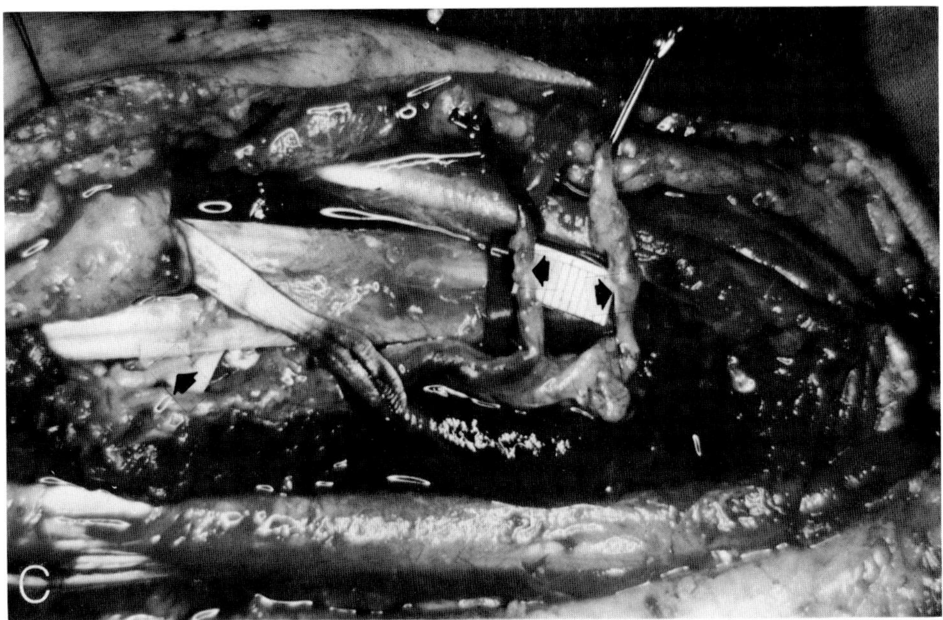

Fig. 30-4 *(Continued).* **(C)** Microvascular anastomosis of the peroneal artery to the radial artery *(left arrow)* and the two venae comitantes *(right arrows).* **(D)** Arteriogram showing patent anatomoses of the peroneal artery and radial artery 6 weeks after operation *(arrows).* **(E)** Bone biopsy of the vascularized graft at 6 months showing viable cortical bone. *(Figure continues.)*

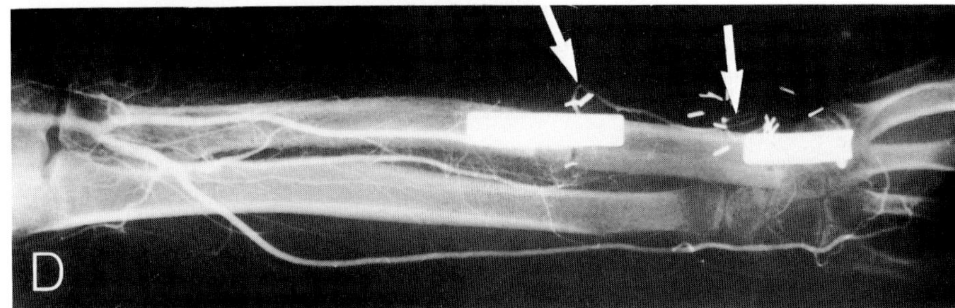

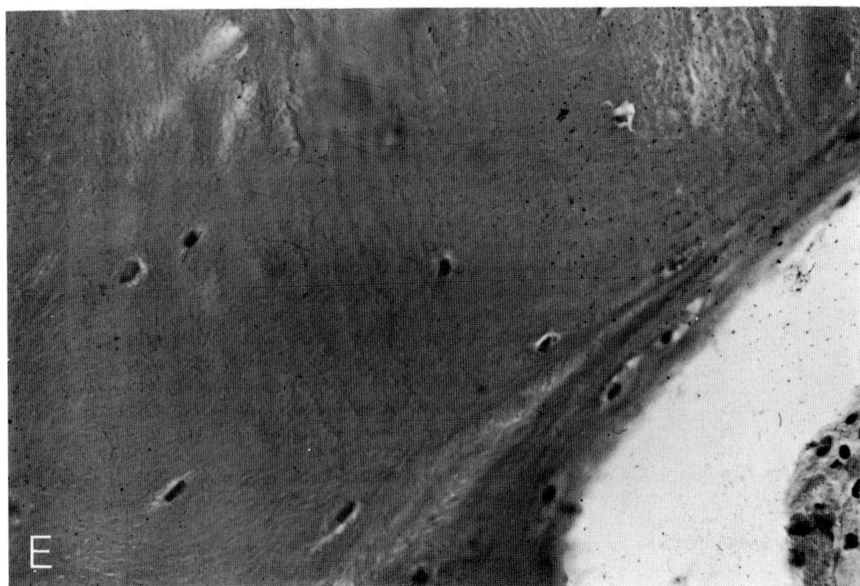

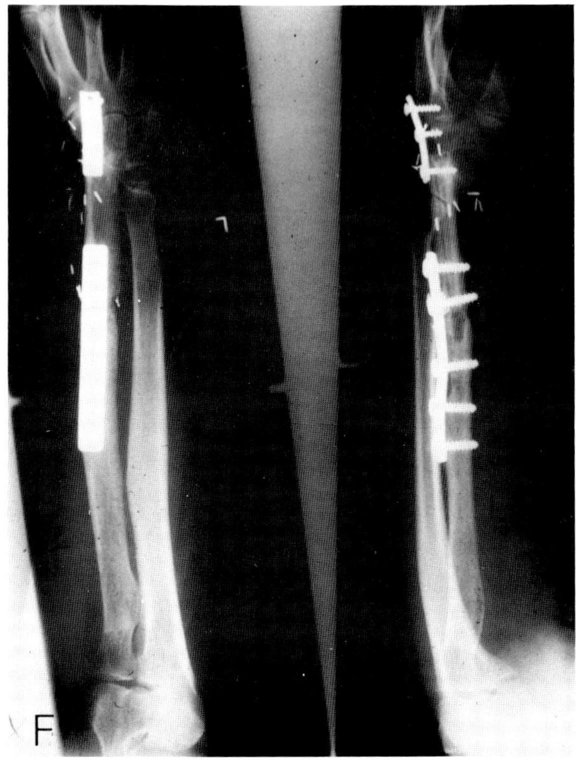

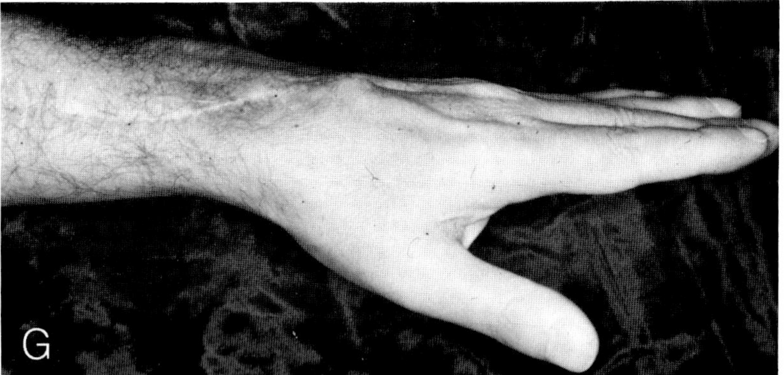

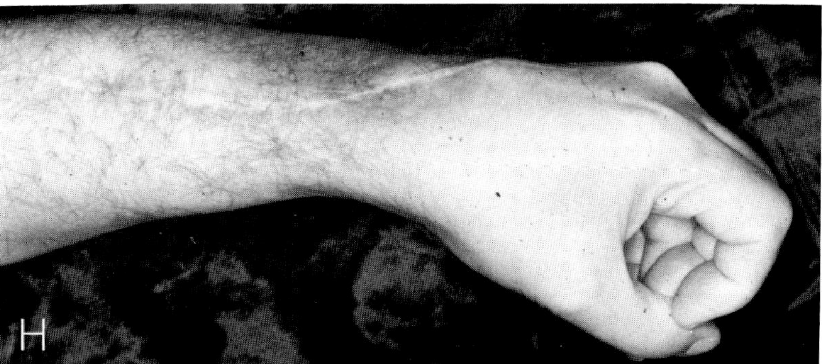

Fig. 30-4 *(Continued).* **(F)** Radiograph at 2 years, showing complete bony healing. **(G&H)** Clinical appearance of the left hand and forearm showing flexion and extension of the wrist and fingers. (Figs. **A–F** from Weiland et al,[125] with permission.)

and bone loss in an extremity, we have used also used the free osteocutaneous groin flap, again, based on the deep circumflex iliac system as described by Taylor[110-112] (Fig. 30-2C).

Patient Position

The patient is positioned supine with a small bump of towels under the ilium. The table should be able to be flexed after taking the flap to facilitate closure.

Dissection of the Graft

An incision is made from the femoral artery to a point about 10 cm posterior to the anterior iliac spine. If skin is to be harvested with the flap, the pattern should be made at this time. The superficial circumflex artery can be identified near the inguinal ligament as a branch off the femoral artery. After identifying the superficial circumflex iliac artery and vein and the inferior epigastric vein, dissection proceeds superior to the inguinal ligament, where the deep circumflex iliac artery and vein are identified arising from the external iliac artery and vein, respectively. Sharp and blunt dissection is used to expose the preperitoneal fascia after incisions are made in the external oblique, internal oblique, and transversus abdominis muscles, thereby allowing the posterior aspect of the inner table of the iliac crest with its iliacus muscle to be seen. The vessel runs approximately two finger breadths below the iliac crest on its internal margin. In men, the spermatic cord and vascular structures are carefully preserved, as well as the genitofemoral branch of the femoral nerve. The size of the flap is then outlined based on the deep circumflex iliac artery. Attention is turned to the lateral margin of the iliac crest where an oscillating saw is used to cut through the crest, preserving a depth of 2.5 cm in the graft. The cut is then continued medially with the osteocutaneous flap finally isolated on its vascular pedicle, consisting of the deep circumflex iliac artery and vein. The attachment of the overlying skin and subcutaneous tissue to the iliac crest must be carefully preserved to avoid accidental shearing of the small nutrient vessels supplying the skin.

Due to the curvature of the ilium, grafts larger than 10 cm usually cannot be obtained. A portion of the origin of the tensor fascia lata and gluteus medius can be preserved on the out table of the iliac crest, but this is not necessary; however, a similar sleeve of iliacus must be retained on the inner table in order to preserve the nutrient blood supply to the bone. The donor site is closed primarily with the hip flexed approximately 30 degrees.[110]

Skeletal Fixation

Since spanning lengths more than 8 cm is rare, most iliac crest grafts can be shaped and slotted to key into the bony defect and secured with internal fixation. For further discussion, see the section above on Skeletal Fixation for the fibula.

Microvascular Anastomoses

Once the graft is rigidly in place, the operating microscope is positioned, and microvascular anastomoses of one artery and one vein are performed (Fig. 30-4), the latter often representing a confluence of both venae comitantes. The size of the venae comitantes of the fibular graft can exceed 3 mm; it is helpful to find as large a vein as possible on the recipient side. Success of the anastomoses is evidenced by bright, red bleeding from the preserved muscle sleeve and good venous return. Unlike muscle or skin flaps, the venous return is often slow to develop in a vascularized bone graft due to the drainage from the medullary canal.

Postoperative Care and Monitoring

Postoperative management does not differ significantly from conventional bone grafting techniques. Anticoagulation is not routinely used, except for aspirin, 325 mg every other day. Heparin is not used.

Because the fibular graft is subcutaneous and not available for direct monitoring, immediate postoperative assessment of circulation to the graft is difficult. Although bone scans during the first 24 to 72 hours do afford reasonable assurance that circulation is intact, revision of anastomoses at this stage is not feasible if circulation is not adequate. More effective methods for monitoring patency of anastomoses, such as thermocouples and laser Doppler flowmeters, may provide more accurate evaluation of graft circulation. A small island of skin can be taken with the fibular graft based on the perforating vessels from the peroneal artery serving as a visual perfusion monitor. We do not routinely use this.

For the lower extremity, bed rest and elevation of the affected limb are prescribed for 2 weeks, and dressing changes are performed as necessary. For upper extremity cases, internal fixation with plate and screws is most often employed. Patients are allowed to ambulate on the donor extremity 3 to 5 days following surgery, and physical and occupational therapy is instituted to mobilize the upper extremity at that time. The average period of hospitalization has been 10 days.

Incorporation of the graft at the proximal and distal juncture sites is usually achieved within 3 to 4 months. In lower extremity cases partial weight bearing is then allowed, progressing to full weight bearing as the graft undergoes progressive hypertrophy. For upper extremity cases, unrestricted active range of motion of the extremity is permitted as soon as bone union is achieved (3 to 4 months).

Complications and Problems

Nonunion

Nonunion of the graft to the recipient site occurs in about 10 percent of cases. This problem should be discussed with the patient. When the graft shows no incorporation within 4 to 5 months, or shows signs of loss of fixation, cancellous bone

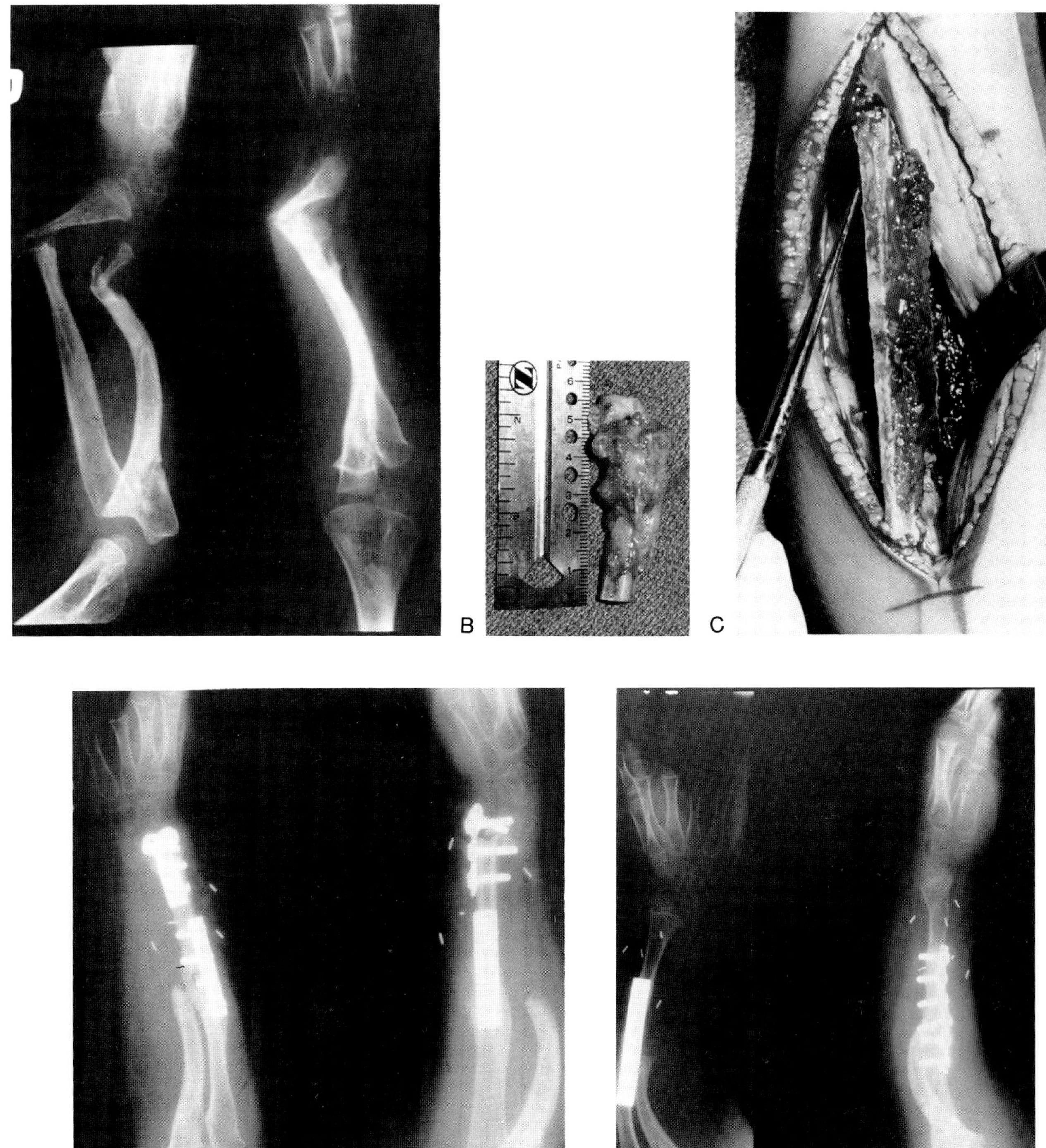

Fig. 30-5. (**A**) A 4-year-old with congenital pseudarthrosis of the radius and ulna. (**B**) Excised specimen of radius containing the pseudarthrosis. (**C**) Fibular graft in place before plating. (**D**) Radiograph 1 year after plating with proximal nonunion. (**E**) Replating and bone grafting 1 year following using longer plate. Note that the distal growth plate of radius was preserved.

grafting with internal fixation should be performed. In most cases, the graft will unite after reoperation. Infection of the graft should be treated as any infection—drainage and debridement should be used as needed.

Special Situations

Congenital Pseudarthrosis

The successful treatment of congenital pseudarthrosis (Fig. 30-5) depends on the excision of all involved bone and soft tissue. If the resection is complete, recurrence is rare.[30,45,99,121,122,123,124]

As recommended by Grishin,[44] we are now using the Ilizarov fixation frame for fixation of the tibia. The frame allows preoperative correction and lengthening as needed. Because of the inherent stability of the frame, supplemental fixation is seldom required. Application of the frame is not simple and does add to the complexity of the procedure.

SUMMARY

In dealing with upper extremity segmental bone defects, the surgeon should be familiar with conventional techniques available to achieve skeletal continuity. Shortening of the humerus up to 5 cm and forearm up to 4 cm can result in acceptable function. For forearm bone defects, the option of creating a one bone forearm should always be kept in mind despite the limitation of loss of forearm rotation.

REFERENCES

1. Albee FH: Transplantation of a portion of the tibia into the spine for Pott's disease. Clin Orthop 87:5–8, 1972
2. Allgower M, Blocker TG Jr, Engley BWD: Some immunological aspects of auto- and homografts in rabbits tested in vivo and in vitro techniques. Plast Reconstr Surg 9:1–21, 1952
3. Alm A, Stromberg B: Vascular anatomy of the patellar and cruciate ligaments: A microangiographic and histologic investigation in the dog. Acta Chir Scand suppl 445, 1974
4. American Replantation Mission to China: Replantation surgery in China. Plast Reconstr Surg 52:176, 1973
5. Anderssonn GBJ, Gaechter A, Galante JO, Rostoker W: Segmental replacement of long bones in baboons using a fiber titanium implant. J Bone Joint Surg 60A:31–40, 1978
6. Androsov PI: New methods of surgical treatment of blood vessel lesions. Arch Surg 73:902, 1956
7. Arata MA, Wood MB, Cooney WP III: Revascularized segmental diaphyseal bone transfers in the canine. An analysis of viability. J Reconstr Microsurg 1:11–19, 1984
8. Barth H: Histologische Untersuchungen uber Knochentransplantation. Beitr Path Anat Allg Path 17:65–142, 1895
9. Baschkerzew NJ, Petrow NN: Beitrage zur freien Knochenuberpflanzung. Dtsch Chir 113:490–531, 1912
10. Baudet J: The composite fibula and soleus free transfer. Int J Microsurg 4:10–14, 1982
11. Berggren A, Weiland AJ, Dorfman HD: Free vascularized bone grafts: Factors affecting their survival and ability to heal to recipient bone defects. Plast Reconstr Surg 69:19–29, 1982
12. Berggren A, Weiland AJ, Ostrup LT: Bone scintigraphy in evaluating the viability of composite bone grafts revascularized by microvascular anastomoses, conventional autogenous bone grafts and free nonrevascularized periosteal grafts. J Bone Joint Surg 64A:799–809, 1982
13. Berggren A, Weiland AJ, Ostrup LT, Dorfman HD: The effects of storage media and perfusion on osteoblast and osteocyte survival in free composite bone grafts. J Microsurg 2:273–282, 1981
14. Berggren A, Weiland AJ, Ostrup LT, Dorfman HD: Microvascular free bone transfer with revascularization of the medullary and periosteal circulation of the periosteal circulation alone. J Bone Joint Surg 64A:73–87, 1982
15. Bonfiglio M: Repair of bone transplant fractures. J Bone Joint Surg 40A:446–456, 1958
16. Boyd HB: The treatment of difficult and unusual non-unions. J Bone Joint Surg 25:535–552, 1943
17. Brookes M: The vascular architecture of tubular bone in the rat. Anat Rec 132:25–48, 1958
18. Brookes M: The vascularization of long bones in the human foetus. J Anat 92:261–267, 1958
19. Brookes M: The Blood Supply of Bone. Butterworths, London, 1971
20. Brown K, Marie P, Lyszakowski T, Daniel R, Cruess R: Epiphyseal growth after free fibular transfer with and without microvascular anastomosis. Experimental study in the dog. J Bone Joint Surg 65B:493–501, 1983
21. Buncke HJ, Furnas DW, Gordon L, Achauer BM: Free osteocutaneous flap from a rib to the tibia. Plast Reconstr Surg 59:799–805, 1977
22. Buncke HJ, Schulz WP: Experimental digital amputation and reimplantation. Plast Reconstr Surg 36:62, 1965
23. Buncke HJ, Schulz WP: Total ear re-implantation in the rabbit utilizing microminiature vascular anastomosis. Br J Plast Surg 19:15, 1966
24. Burrows HJ, Wilson JN, Scales JT: Excision of tumors of humerus and femur, with restoration by internal prosthesis. J Bone Joint Surg 57B:148–159, 1975
25. Burwell RG: Studies in the transplantation of bone VII. The fresh composite homograft-autograft of cancellous bone: An analysis of factors leading to osteogenesis in marrow transplants and in marrow containing bone grafts. J Bone Joint Surg 46B:110–140, 1961
26. Burwell RG: Biological mechanisms in foreign bone transplantation. In Modern Trends in Orthopaedics. Vol. 4. Butterworths, Washington, D.C., 1964
27. Campbell WC: Transference of the fibula as an adjunct free bone graft in tibial deficiency. J Orthop Surg 7:625–631, 1919
28. Carrel A: Results of the transplantation of blood vessels, organs and limbs. JAMA 51:1662–1667, 1908
29. Chalmers J: Transplantation immunity in bone homografting. J Bone Joint Surg 41B:160–179, 1959
30. Chen CW, Yu ZJ, Wang Y: A new method of treatment of congenital tibial pseudarthrosis using free vascularized fibular grafts. A preliminary report. Ann Acad Med Singapore 8:465–473, 1979
31. Clark K: A case of replacement of the upper end of the humerus by a fibular graft: Reviewed after 29 years. J Bone Surg 41B:365–368, 1959
32. Cobbett JR: Microvascular surgery. Surg Clin North Am 47:521–542, 1967
33. Crenshaw AH: Campbell's Operative Orthopaedics. 5th Ed. CV Mosby, St. Louis, 1971
34. Curtis PH Jr, Powell AE, Herndon CH: Immunological factors in

homogenous bone transplantation III. The inability of homogenous rabbit bone to induce circulating antibodies in rabbits. J Bone Joint Surg 41A:1482-1488, 1959
35. Daniel RK, Taylor GI: Distant transfer of an island flap by microvascular anastomoses. Plast Reconstr Surg 52:111-117, 1973
36. D'Aubigne RM, Meary R, Thomine JM: La resection dans le traitment des tumeurs des os. Rev Chir Orthop 52:305-324, 1966
37. DeBruyn PH, Kabisch WT: Bone formation by fresh and frozen autogenous and homogenous transplants of bone, bone marrow and periosteum. Am J Anat 96:375-417, 1955
38. Dee P, Lambruschi PG, Hiebert JM: The use of Tc-99m MDP bone scanning in the study of vascularized bone implants. Concise communication. J Nucl Med 22:522-525, 1981
39. Donski PK, O'Brien BMcC: Free microvascular epiphyseal transplantation: An experimental study in dogs. Br J Plast Surg 33:169-178, 1980
40. Eadie DGA, DeTakats G: The early fate of autogenous grafts in the canine femoral vein. J Cardiovasc Surg 7:148, 1966
41. Enneking WF, Burchardt H, Puhl JJ, Piotrowski G: Physical and biological aspects of repair in dog cortical bone transplants. J Bone Joint Surg 57A:237-251, 1975
42. Gilbert A: Vascularized transfer of the fibular shaft. Int J Microsurg 1(2):100-102, Apr 1979
43. Gilbert A: Free vascularized bone grafts. Int Surg 66:27-31, 1981
44. Grishin IG, Golubev VG, Goncharenko IV, Evgrafov AV, Kafarov FM: Transfer of free vascularized bone and skin-bone autografts: experience in application of external fixation apparatus. J Reconstr Microsurg 6(1):1-11, 1990
45. Hagan KF, Buncke JH: Treatment of congenital pseudarthrosis of the tibia with free vascularized bone graft. Clin Orthop 166:34-44, 1982
46. Ham A, Gordon S: The origin of bone that forms in association with cancellous chips transplanted into muscle. Br J Plast Surg 5:154-160, 1952
47. Harmon PH: A simplified surgical approach to the posterior tibia for bone grafting and fibular transference. J Bone Joint Surg 27:496-498, 1945
48. Heiple KG, Chase SW, Herndon CH: A comparative study of the healing process following different types of bone transplantation. J Bone Joint Surg 45A:1593-1616, 1963
49. Helsop BF, Zeiss IM, Nesbet NW: Studies on transference of bone. I. A comparison of autologous and homologous bone implants with reference to osteocyte survival, osteogenesis and host reaction. Br J Exp Pathol 41:269-287, 1960
50. Henry AK: Extensile Exposure. 2nd Ed. pp. 241-276. E & S Livingstone, London 1966
51. Herndon CH, Chase SW: Experimental studies in the transplantation of whole joints. J Bone Joint Surg 34A:564-578, 1952
52. Herndon CH, Chase SW: The fate of massive autogenous and homogenous bone grafts including articular surfaces. Surg Gynecol Obstet 98:273-290, 1954
53. Hirayama T, Suematsu N, Inoue K, Baitoh C, Takemitsu Y: Free vascularized bone grafts in reconstruction of the upper extremity. J Hand Surg 10B:169-175, 1985
54. Holt GP, Lewis FT: A new technique for end to end anastomosis for small arteries. Surg Forum 11:242, 1960
55. Hu CT, Chang CW, Su KL, Shen CC, Shen S: Free vascularized bone graft using microvascular technique. Ann Acad Med Singapore 8:459-464, 1979
56. Huntington TW: Case of bone transference. Ann Surg 41:249-256, 1905
57. Hutchinson J: The fate of experimental bone autografts and homografts. Br J Surg 39:552-561, 1952
58. Ilizarov GA: Transosseous Osteosynthesis. Springer-Verlag, Berlin, 1992
59. Jackson RW, MacNab I: Fractures of the shaft of the tibia: A clinical and experimental study. Am J Surg 97:543-557, 1959
60. Jacobson JH, Suarez EL: Microsurgery in anastomoses of small vessels. Surg Forum 11:243, 1960
61. Johnson RW Jr: A physiological study of the blood supply of the diaphysis. J Bone Joint Surg 9:153-184, 1927
61a. Lane JM, Sandhu HS: Current approaches to experimental bone grafts. Orthop Clin North Am 18:213, 1987
62. Jupiter JB, Kour AK: Reconstruction of the humerus by soft tissue distraction and vascularized fibula transfer. J Hand Surg 16A (5), 1991
63. Kelly PJ: Anatomy, physiology and pathology of the blood supply of bones. J Bone Joint Surg 50A:766-783, 1968
64. Lacroix P: Recent investigations on the growth of bone. Nature 156:576, 1945
65. Levander G: A study of bone regeneration. Surg Gynecol Obstet 67:705-714, 1938
66. Lexer E: Die Entstehung entzundlicher Knochenherde und ihre Beziehung zu den Arterien Versweigungen der Knochen. Arch Klin Chir 81:1, 1903
67. Lexer E: Substitution of whole or half joints from freshly amputated extremities by free plastic operation. Surg Gynecol Obstet 6:601-607, 1908
68. Lexer E: Blutige Vereiningung von Knochenbruchen. Dtsch Z Chir 133:1970, 1915
69. Lexer E, Kuliga, Turk: Untersuchungen uber Knochenarterien. Hirschwold, Berlin 1904
70. Lukash FN, Zingaro EA, Salig J: The survival of free nonvascularized bone grafts in irradiated areas by wrapping in muscle flaps. Plast Reconstr Surg 74:783-788, 1984
71. Maatz R, Lentz W, Graf R: Spongiosa test of bone grafts for transplantation. J Bone Joint Surg 36A:721-731, 1954
72. Mankin JH, Fogelson FS, Thrasher AZ, Jaffer F: Massive resection and allograft transplantation in the treatment of malignant bone tumors. N Engl J Med 194:1247-1255, 1976
73. Manktelow RT, McKee NH: Free muscle transplantation to provide active finger flexion. J Hand Surg 3(5):416-426, 1978
74. Marchand: Zur Kenntniss des Knochen-Transplantation. Verh Dtsch Ges Pathol 2:368-375, 1900
75. Mathes SJ, Buchannan R, Weeks PM: Microvascular joint transplantation with epiphyseal growth. J Hand Surg 5:586-589, 1980
76. Metaizeau JP, Olive D, Bey P, Bordigoni P, Plenat F, Prevot J: Resection of tumor followed by vascularized bone autograft in patients with possible recurrence of malignant bone tumors after conservative treatment. J Pediatr Surg 19:116-120, 1984
77. Miller RC, Phalen GS: The repair of defects of the radius with fibular bone grafts. J Bone Joint Surg 29:629-636, 1947
78. Nakayama K, Tamiya T, Yamamoto K, Alimoto S: A simple new apparatus for small vessel anastomoses (free autograft of the sigmoid included). Surgery 52:918-931, 1962
79. Nettelblad H, Randolph MA, Weiland AJ: Free microvascular epiphyseal plate transplantation. An experimental study in dogs. J Bone Joint Surg 66A:1421-1430, 1984
80. Nettelblad H, Randolph MA, Weiland AJ: Physiologic isolation of the canine proximal fibular epiphysis on a vascular pedicle. Microsurgery 5:98-101, 1984
81. Nettelblad H, Randolph MA, Weiland AJ: Heteroptic microvascular growth plate transplantation of the proximal fibula: An experimental canine model. Plastic Reconstr Surg 77:814-820, 1986
82. O'Brien BM: Microvascular free bone and joint transfer. pp. 267-289. In Microvascular Reconstructive Surgery. Churchill Livingstone, Edinburgh, 1977
83. Osterman AL, Bora FW: Free vascularized bone grafting for

large-gap nonunion of long bones. Orthop Clin North Am 15:131-142, 1984

84. Ostrup LT: The free, living bone graft—An experimental study. Kinkoping University Medical Dissertations, Linkoping, Sweden, 1975
85. Ostrup LT, Fredrickson JM: Distant transfer of a free, living bone graft by microvascular anastomoses: An experimental study. Plast Reconstr Surg 54:274-285, 1974
86. Ottolenghi CE: Massive osteo and osteo-articular bone grafts: Technique results in 62 cases. Clin Orthop 87:156-164, Technique results in 62 cases. Clin Orthop 87:156-164, 1972
87. Parrish FF: Treatment of bone tumors by total excision and replacement with massive autologous and homologous grafts. J Bone Joint Surg 48A:968-990, 1966
88. Parrish FF: Allograft replacement of all or part of the end of a long bone following excision of a tumor: Report of twenty-one cases. J Bone Joint Surg 55A:1-22, 1973
89. Phemister DB: The fate of transplanted bone and regenerative power of various constituents. Surg Gynecol Obstet 19:303-333, 1914
90. Pho RWH: Malignant giant-cell tumors of the distal end of the radius treated by a free vascularized fibular transplant. J Bone Joint Surg 63A:877-884, 1981
91. Ray RD, Degge J, Gloyd P, Mooney G: Bone regeneration. An experimental study of bone grafting materials. J Bone Joint Surg 34A:638-647, 1952
92. Reichel SM: Vascular system of the long bones of the rat. Surgery 22:146-157, 1947
93. Restrepo J, Katz A, Gilbert A: Arterial vascularization to the proximal epiphysis and the diaphysis of the fibula. Int J Microsurg 2:49-54, 1980
94. Rhinelander RW: Effects of medullary nailing on the normal blood supply of diaphyseal cortex. pp. 161-187. AAOS Instructional Course Lectures. Vol. 22. CV Mosby, St Louis, 1973
95. Riordan DC: Congenital absence of the radius. J Bone Joint Surg 37A:1129-1140, 1955
96. Rohlich K: Bildung neuer Knochensubstanz in Abgetoteten Knochentransplantation. Mikrosk Anat Forsch 50:132-145, 1941
97. Rohlich K: Uber die transplantation Periost-und markloses Knochenstucke. Mikrost Anat Forsch 51:636-653, 1942
98. Salmon PA, Assimacopoulos CA: A pneumatic needle holder suitable for microsurgical procedures. Surgery 55:446, 1964
99. Sellers DS, Sowa DT, Moore JR, Weiland AJ: Congenital pseudarthrosis of the forearm. J Hand Surg 13A(1):89-92, 1988
100. Serafin D, Villarreal-Rois A, Georgiade NG: A rib containing free flap to reconstruct mandibular defects. Br J Plast Surg 30:263-266, 1977
101. Shima I, Yamauchi S, Matsumoto T, Kunishita M, Sinoda K, Yoshimizu N, Nomura S, Yoshimura M: A new method for monitoring circulation of grafted bone by use of electrochemically generated hydrogen. Clin Orthop 198:244-249, 1985
102. Starr DE: Congenital absence of the radius. A method of surgical correction. J Bone Joint Surg 27:572-577, 1945
103. Swartz WM: Immediate reconstruction of the wrist and dorsum of the hand with a free osteocutaneous groin flap. J Hand Surg 9A:18-21, 1984
104. Tamai S, Komatsu S, Sakamoto H, Sano S, Sasauchi N, Hori Y, Tatsumi Y, Okuda H: Free muscle transplants in dogs with microsurgical neurovascular anastomoses. Plast Reconstr Surg 46:219-225, 1970
105. Tamai S, Sasauchi N, Hori Y, Tatsumi Y, Okuda H: Microvascular surgery in orthopaedics and traumatology. J Bone Joint Surg 54B:637-647, 1972
106. Taylor GI: Microvascular free bone transfer. A clinical technique. Orthop Clin North Am 8:425-447, 1977
107. Taylor GI: The current status of free vascularized bone grafts. Clin Plast Surg 10:185-209, 1983
108. Taylor GI, Daniel RK: The free flap: Composite tissue transfer by vascular anastomosis. Aust NZJ Surg 43:1-3, 1973
109. Taylor GI, Miller GDH, Ham FJ: The free vascularized bone graft. A clinical extension of microvascular techniques. Plast Reconstr Surg 55:533-544, 1975
110. Taylor GI, Townsend P, Corlett R: Superiority of the deep circumflex iliac vessels as the supply for free groin flaps: Clinical work. Plast Reconstr Surg 64:745-759, 1979
111. Taylor GI, Townsend P, Corlett R: Superiority of the deep circumflex iliac vessels as the supply for free groin flaps: Experimental work. Plast Reconstr Surg 64:595-605, 1979
112. Taylor GI, Watson N: One-stage repair of compound leg defects with free revascularized flaps of groin, skin and iliac bone. Plast Reconstr Surg 61:494-506, 1978
113. Trias A, Fery A: Cortical circulation of long bones. J Bone Joint Surg 61A:1052-1059, 1979
114. Trueta J, Caladias AX: A study of the blood supply of the long bones. Surg Gynecol Obstet 118:485-498, 1964
115. Urist M, McLean FC: Osteogenetic potency and new-bone formation by induction in transplants to the anterior chamber of the eye. J Bone Joint Surg 34A:443-470, 1952
116. Volkov M: Allotransplantation of joints. J Bone Joint Surg 52B:49-53, 1970
117. Weiland AJ: Current concepts review: Vascularized free bone transplants. J Bone Joint Surg 63A:166-169, 1981
118. Weiland AJ: Vascularized bone transfers. pp. 446-460. AAOS Instructional Course Lectures. Vol. 33. CV Mosby, St Louis, 1984
119. Weiland AJ, Berggren A, Jones L: The acute effects of blocking medullary blood supply on regional cortical blood flow in canine ribs as measured by the hydrogen washout technique. Clin Orthop 165:265-272, 1982
120. Weiland AJ, Daniel RK: Microvascular anatomoses for bone grafts in the treatment of massive defects in bone. J Bone Joint Surg 61A:98-104, 1979
121. Weiland AJ, Daniel RK: Congenital pseudarthrosis of the tibia: Treatment with vascularized autogenous fibular grafts. A preliminary report. Johns Hopkins Med J 147:89-95, 1980
122. Weiland AJ, Daniel RK: Clinical technique of segmental autogenous bone grafting in vascular pedicles. pp. 646-679. In Mears DC (ed): External Skeletal Fixation. Williams & Wilkins, Baltimore, 1983
123. Weiland AJ, Daniel RK, Riley LH Jr: Application of the free vascularized bone graft in the treatment of malignant or aggressive bone tumors. Johns Hopkins Med J 140:85-96, 1977
124. Weiland AJ, Kleinert HE, Kutz JE, Daniel RK: Free vascularized bone grafts in surgery of the upper extremity. J Hand Surg 4:129-144, 1979
125. Weiland AJ, Kleinert HE, Kutz JE, Daniel RK: Vascularized bone grafts in the upper extremity. pp. 605-625. In Serafin D, Buncke JH Jr (eds): Microsurgical Composite Tissue Transplantation. CV Mosby, St. Louis 1979
126. Weiland AJ, Moore JR, Daniel RK: Vascularized bone autografts. Experience with 41 cases. Clin Orthop 174:87-95, 1983
127. Weiland AJ, Phillips TW, Randolph MA: Bone Grafts: A radiologic, histologic and biomechanical model comparing autografts, allografts, and free vascularized bone grafts. Plast Reconstr Surg 74:368-379, 1984
128. Weiland AJ, Weiss APC, Moore JR, Tolo VT: Vascularized fibular grafts in the treatment of congenital pseudarthrosis of the tibia. J Bone Joint Surg 72A(5):654-662, 1990

31

Vascularized Joint Transfers

Guy Foucher

INTRODUCTION

Finger joints play a critical role in the function of the hand. Their function, however, can be absent, disturbed, or destroyed because of congenital malformation, trauma, or disease. Three main levels can be involved: the proximal interphalangeal joint (PIPJ), the metacarpophalangeal joint (MPJ), or the trapeziometacarpal joint (TMJ). In a recent study[67] the useful range of motion for 11 daily activities was 61 degrees for the MPJ, 60 degrees for the PIPJ and 39 degrees for the DIPJ. Many methods of joint reconstruction have been developed, but all of these fall short of the ideal requirements, which are a painless, stable, strong, durable joint with full range of motion and, in children, potential for growth.

The alternatives for treatment of damaged joints include amputation, fusion, prothesis, spacers, nonvascularized joint transfer (NVJT), and vascularized joint transfer (VJT) (free or island).

Finger amputation is rarely indicated for joint damage except in the case of complex associated lesions involving a single finger. Fusion can afford relief of pain with stability, durability, and, usually, good strength, but at the cost of mobility. Arthrodesis must still be thought of as a good operation, at least in adults and in certain joints, such as the thumb MPJ or carpometacarpal joint (CMC), but in other locations fusion may disturb the overall function of the hand, especially with multiple PIPJ or MPJ involvement. Despite constant improvement, prosthetic implants or spacers still present significant problems of stability, durability, and mobility, and they remain contraindicated in young patients.

HISTORY OF OSTEOCHONDRAL JOINT TRANSPLANTATION

Surgeons have long sought to provide a biologic joint replacement using specialized tissues with a similar anatomic configuration. These attempts fall into three major categories: perichondrial joint grafts, allografts, and autografts (vascularized or nonvascularized half- or whole-joint transfers).

There are several basic problems that are common to all biologic reconstructions. Successful transplantation of functioning organs depends upon rapid reestablishment of the circulatory perfusion of their tissues if the transplants are to survive and to function. Curiously, when bone and cartilage are transplanted, difficulties begin when the process of revascularization is established.[55] Ischemic loss of synovium is responsible for poor production of synovial fluid, which is the sole means of nutrition of the articular cartilage.[72] Moreover, the circulation of synovial fluid depends on movement of the joint, and prolonged immobilization causes trophic changes in the articular cartilage.[28,83] The role of denervation in degenerative change in transplanted joints, although poorly documented,[23,76] is probably relatively unimportant.[4]

Nonvascularized joint autografts and allografts have been extensively studied, but sound clinical series providing long-term results concerning ranges of motion, degenerative changes, and/or percentage of growth in young patients are scarce.

In our experience[35] and throughout the literature[71] results of periochondrial autografts have been quite unpredictable. This operation is applicable only to very limited problems in which damage is confined to the articular cartilage, in the presence of normal bone structure.

Allografts

Allografts have been the least successful method experimentally. However, most research with allografts has been concentrated on large weight-bearing joints, such as the knee. In 1908, Lexer[80] reported successful cases of homografts of half and whole joints taken from freshly amputated extremities. In 1925[81] he reviewed the long-term results (knee, shoulder, hip) and concluded that function could remain satisfactory for many years despite obvious degenerative changes in these joints. Subsequent series[6–8,63,88,97,114,127] demonstrated a high rate of failure. Whereas bone is strongly antigenic compared to cartilage, homografts of the latter, although antigenic as well, have been shown to survive longer than any tissue except the cornea. It has been demonstrated[112] that in a grafted bone at least 5 mm thick,[8,15,81,96,112] the joint space is relatively well maintained until collapse of subchondral bone occurs. In one study,[63] it was shown that most of the cells (bone and cartilage) in the joints died. Revascularization and active osteogenesis were slow. The transplants functioned for 6 to 8 months; then degenerative changes progressed to complete disintegration of the joint.

Autografts (Nonvascularized)

Nonvascularized replantations or autografts of half and whole joints have also been studied extensively, experimentally as well as clinically. Tietze,[120] in 1902, is thought to have been the first to use a proximal phalanx taken from the big toe, while Goebell[50] reported the substitution of a finger joint by a toe joint in 1913. Since then, many small series with short follow-up have been published. Experimental, radiologic, and histologic studies have demonstrated degenerative changes of cartilage, with survival of only scattered deep layers and progressive replacement with fibrotic tissue.[23,25,63,75,78] Small clinical series have been published concerning whole joint replacement using a toe,[10,11,23,26,53,56,81,87,100] or transposition of a normal joint from an otherwise irreparably damaged digit as a free whole-joint transfer.[23,24,85,98] Technically, several points have been stressed. The smaller the graft, the sooner revascularization takes place. On the other hand, bone periosteum and joint capsule have to be kept intact. Several authors have demonstrated that limited but satisfactory joint motion usually occurs after half and whole-joint transfer independently of articular cartilage survival.[23,25,63,77,81]

Growth Potential in Nonvascularized Transfers

The growth of such transfers in young patients remains controversial. In experiments several authors have demonstrated some growth,[26,62,66,106] while others have not.[61,62] Clinically, isolated successful cases have been published.[44,45,56,116,126,130] Two short but encouraging series[51,131] stressed that the reasons for success or failure of growth were not apparent. Age (the optimum was 6 months) and technique (conservation of periosteum) seem to be important contributing factors.

Vascularized Joint Transfer

Taking into account that most problems in NVJT arise from delay in bone revascularization, it seemed logical in 1966 that preservation or reestablishment of nutrient vessels could be the solution. The technical feasibility of whole, vascularized free-joint transfer was demonstrated experimentally in a dog's knee model; in 1968, long-term survival was demonstrated. These findings were soon confirmed by other investigators. Vascularized grafts are histologically indistinguishable from normal joints with viable subchondral bone. Functionally, only slight to moderate hyperplasia of the synovium with some restricted motion was demonstrated. Survival of the epiphyseal plate with growth has been demonstrated experimentally and clinically. Vascularized transfers based only on metaphyseal blood supply provde some (but not normal) growth. It seems advisable to use epiphyseal vessels to obtain normal growth. It is necessary to keep in mind that overgrowth may be seen after fractures or in association with inflammatory conditions, and that decreased growth may result in cases of chronic disease or prolonged immobilization.

Clinically, the first island, vascularized joint transfer was performed by Buncke[4] in 1967; we presented the first free, compound toe-joint transfer in 1976. Since then, few cases have been published.[33,35,36,38,40,76,124,125]

VASCULARIZED JOINT TRANSFER

The hand remains the ideal source to provide a similar joint. Three techniques can be used: hetero-digital transfer from a "bank" finger (an otherwise sacrificed finger due to complex lesions), either an island or free transfer (from a nonreplantable digit), or a homo-digital DIPJ to PIPJ island transfer.

The vascularization of the PIPJ and DIPJ is provided mainly through the palmar system. The palmar collateral arteries give retrotendinous metaphyseal and epiphyseal branches anastomosed with each other; small twigs arise going to bone, volar plate and ligaments. The dorsal skin is also vascularized through the palmar system and can be harvested along with the extensor mechanism as a compound tissue transfer.

The technique is the same whatever joint is transferred (either the MPJ, PIPJ, or DIPJ), and whatever the recipient level is (PIPJ or MPJ), but becomes more demanding when the donor finger is not sacrificed.

Transfers Between Fingers (Hetero-digital Transfers)

Hetero-digital Island Transfer

This technique can be used acutely or secondarily as a reconstructive procedure. First, the recipient site is prepared with skin debridement, extensor and intrinsic tendon preparation, and bone cut. The volar plate is thinned, taking care not to violate the flexor sheath. On the donor finger, a dorsal skin flap is outlined avoiding a circular scar; two or three dorsal veins are dissected proximally and retracted to harvest enough extensor tendon to allow an overlapping suture. Then one digital artery is dissected free, keeping as much fat as possible; the accompanying nerve can be used as a vascularized nerve if needed. This nerve, however, is not necessary for joint preservation, and no Charcot disease has been published to the best of our knowledge. Distally, the artery is cut at the level of the future bone section. Then a double osteotomy isolates the joint while keeping the volar plate intact and preserving the vascular bundle. The length of the intercalated segment has to be shorter than the actual recipient defect to avoid a natural tendency toward a flexion deformity due to increased flexor tendon tension.

The compound transfer remains attached solely by its veins and artery and can be transferred to the recipient site, usually through a dorsal subcutaneous route, in order to decrease dorsal scarring. Bone stabilization can be done in many ways, but we favor bone penetration in case of discrepancy combined with interosseous wiring or K-wire. When the fragment is a very small one (for example when the DIPJ is used as a donor), a single longitudinal K-wire has been most frequently used to stabilize the transferred joint in extension. Then the flexor sheath is reattached to the donor volar plate to decrease the mechanical advantage and the extensor tendon is secured by overlapping.

At the PIPJ level, the extensor is divided into two slips, one being secured to the central slip and the other one to a lateral band. Finally, the donor finger is treated according to its potential function either by arthrodesis, shortening, or ray amputation.

Mobilization begins usually at 4 to 6 weeks with dynamic extension splinting to avoid attenuation of the extensor suture. Splinting in flexion is postponed until 8 weeks.

Free Hetero-digital Island Transfer

This technique is basically the same as that described above, except that a microsurgical step is necessary. A DIPJ to PIPJ acute transfer from a nonreplantable finger is demonstrated in Figure 31-1. Usually arterial anastomosis is performed in situ with a collateral digital artery. The proximal veins of the skin flap are sutured to the distal veins of the recipient finger. This technique can provide a quite acceptable range of motion (Fig.

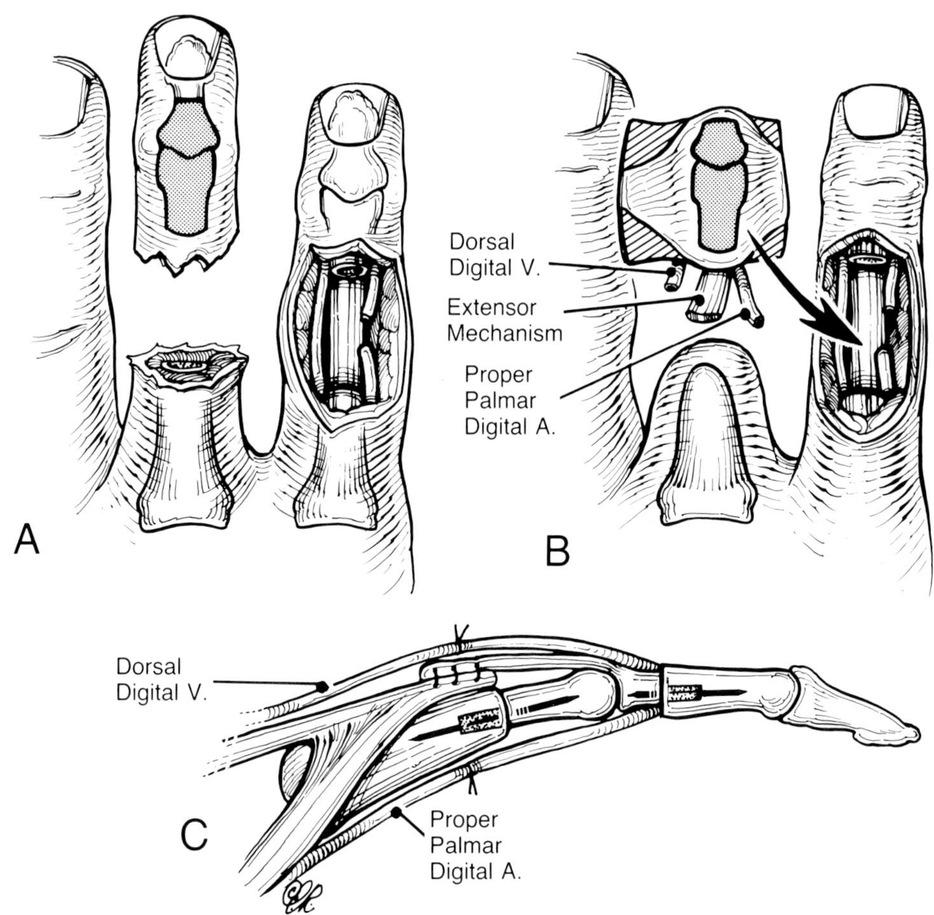

Fig. 31-1. **(A)** A destroyed PIP joint of the index finger with an intact flexor tendon. The third finger is not suitable for replantation, but the DIP joint is intact. **(B)** The third-finger DIP joint is harvested as a compound transfer for index finger PIP joint reconstruction. **(C)** The proper digital artery of the long finger is sutured to the recipient artery of the index finger.

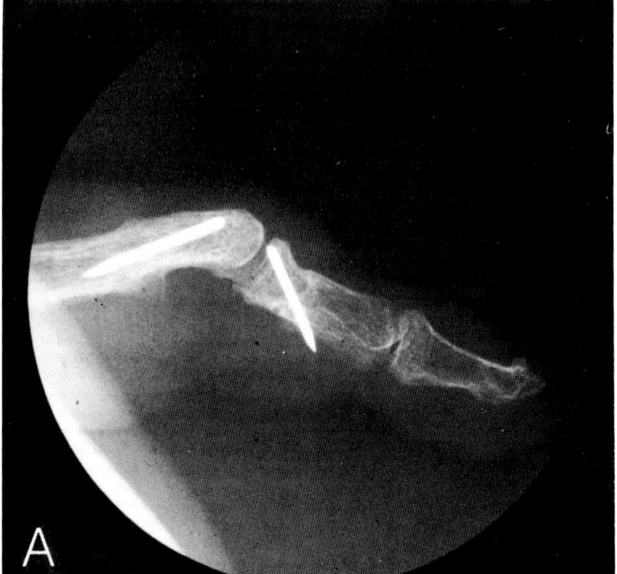

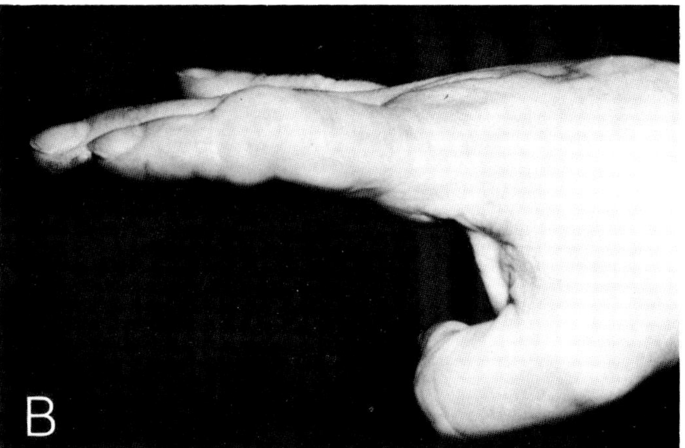

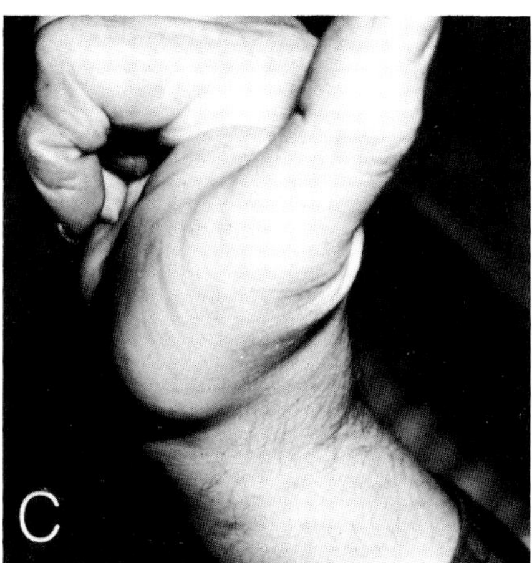

Fig. 31-2. **(A)** Radiograph of a transferred DIP joint at the PIP level. Final range of motion, showing **(B)** extension and **(C)** flexion.

31-2), challenging successfully the acute transfer of a toe VJT as proposed by Tsai.[124]

Transfers in the Same Finger (Homo-digital Transfers)

DIP to PIP

The principle of this transfer is derived from the fact that the DIPJ represents only 15 percent of the arc of finger joint mobility compared to 80 percent for the PIPJ. The finger is simplified to become a two-joint system, but the mobility provided more proximally avoids the finger catching in the way.

The technique differs only slightly from the hetero-digital island transfer, due to conservation of the finger, and a precise technique is mandatory. A functioning flexor tendon and two patent digital arteries are necessary prerequisites. Four incisions are drawn (Fig. 31-3), one longitudinally from the DIPJ down to the web to allow dissection of the sacrificed artery and to prepare some proximal space to accommodate the folded vessel. Three transverse incisions are used, two to isolate a dorsal skin flap at the DIPJ level and one at the PIPJ level to fit the transfer. The dorsal hinged flap of the middle phalanx is gently lifted, saving two or more dorsal veins for the transfer and allowing the cutting of the extensor tendon close to the PIPJ. Then the DIPJ is harvested by two transverse osteotomies 6 to 8 mm apart, avoiding the nail matrix distally and the insertion of the volar plate proximally. Then the collateral artery is severed at the distal bone cut level and the compound island transferred at PIPJ level as previously described.

Distally, an arthrodesis is performed along with reinsertion of the flexor profundus to maintain strength (this is particularly relevant for the fifth finger). Finally, the vessels are folded and buried in the web before skin closure.

Free Vascularized Toe Joint Transfer

Two types of joints are available: the PIPJ and the metatarsophalangeal joint (MTPJ) of the second and/or third toe.

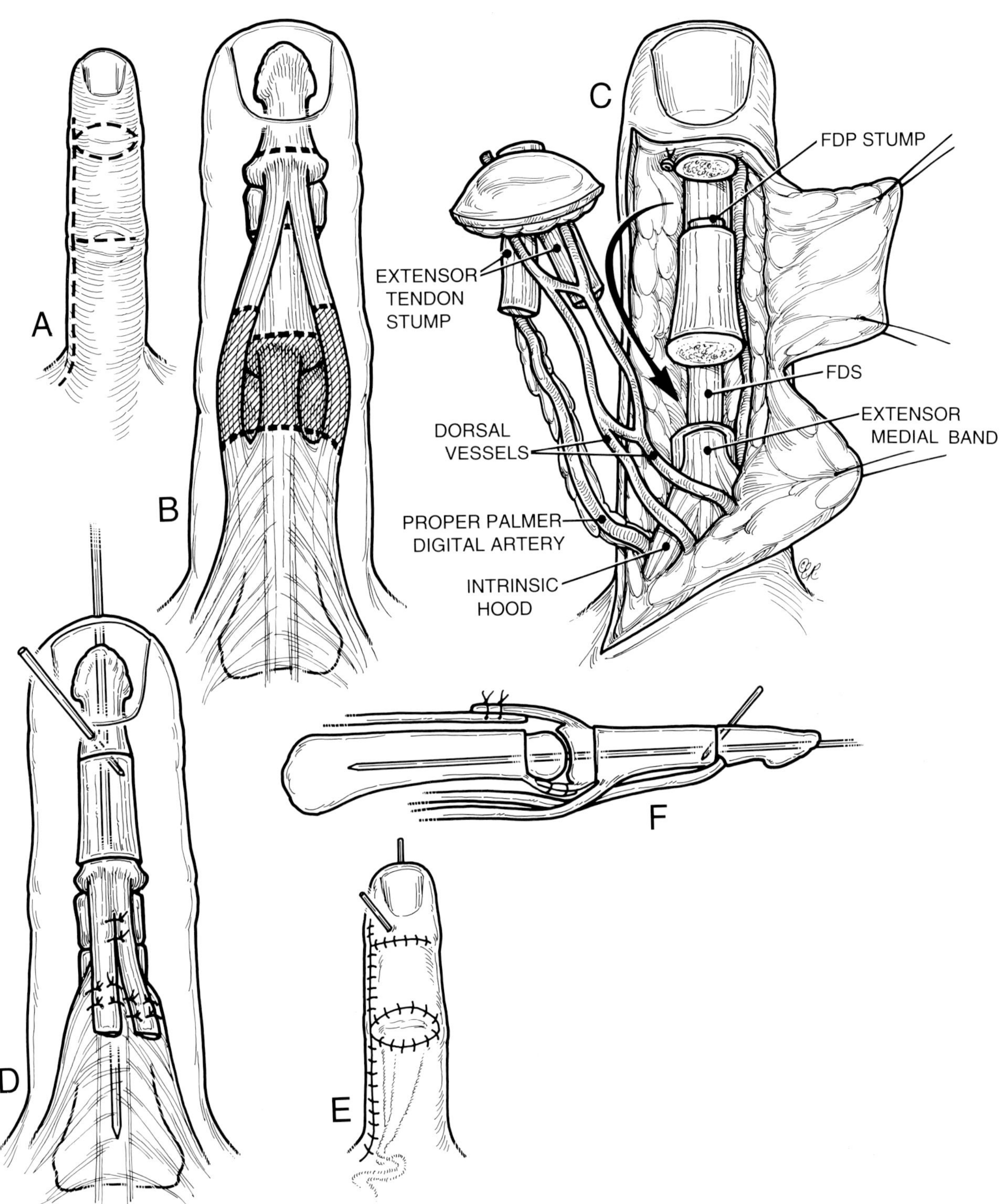

Fig. 31-3. **(A–F)** Technique of homodigital island transfer of the DIP joint to PIP level.

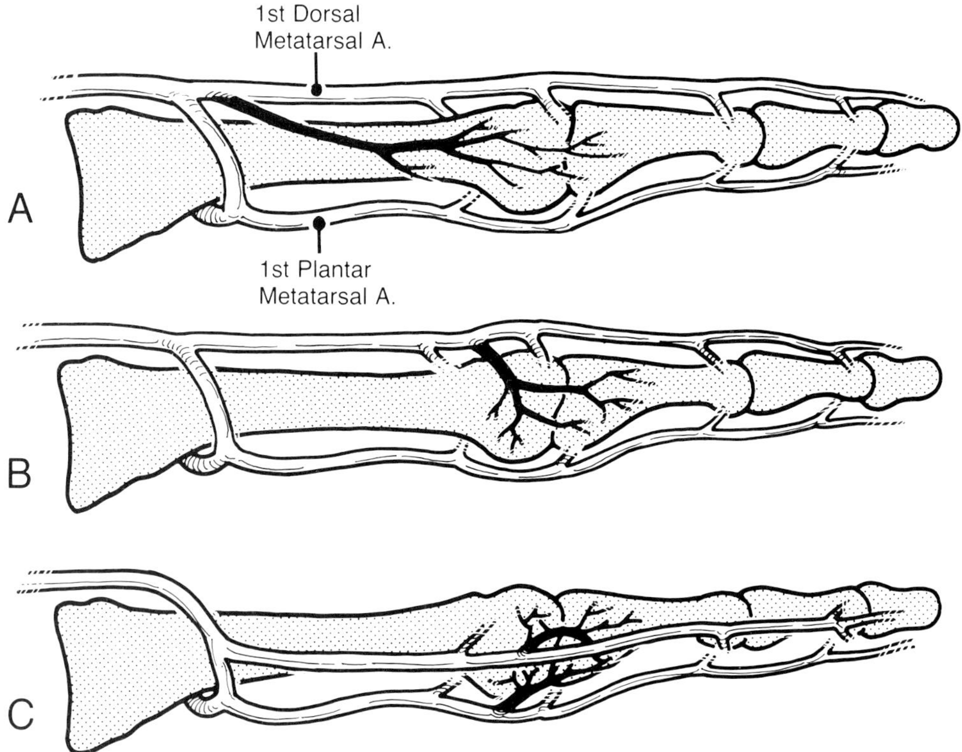

Fig. 31-4. PIP and MTP joint vascularization patterns according to Kuo et al.[79]

General Anatomy

Although its anatomy is similar, the toe PIPJ is rather small compared to the PIPJ of the finger. Mobility in flexion is good, but frequently there is a slight claw deformity that may be reduced by passive flexion of the MTPJ. In the child, only one growth plate is present, located at the base of the middle phalanx.

The MTPJ is larger and quite similar to the MPJ, possessing good lateral stability but a limited range of flexion compared to the range of hyperextension. Two growth plates are present, one on each side of the joint.

The extensor and flexor mechanisms are similar to those of the hand. The innervation of the MTPJ arises from the terminal branch of the peroneal profundus nerve running along the dorsalis pedis artery, and from the cutaneous dorsal medical branch of the superficial peroneal nerve.[76]

The vascularization pattern of the second toe has been known for a long time,[48,58,79,86] but only a few studies have been devoted to the vascular pattern of the joints.[76,137] A Chinese study[76] demonstrated that the blood supply of the MTPJ was mainly dependent on the articular branch of the first metatarsal artery. This constant artery presents three different patterns (Fig. 31-4): (1) most commonly (60 percent of cases), the artery branches off the first dorsal metatarsal artery at the distal third of the metatarsal bone; (2) in 18 percent of cases, the articular

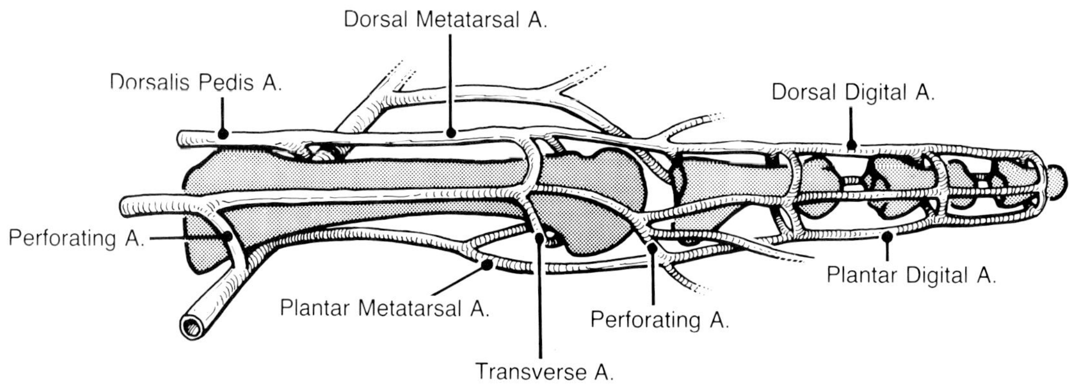

Fig. 31-5. PIP and MTP joint vascularization according to Yoshizu et al.[138]

vessel arises from the origin of the first dorsal metatarsal artery; or (3) in the case of a first dorsal metatarsal artery passing beneath the interosseous muscle, the articular vessel branches off close to the joint. The authors found additional branches emerging from the first plantar metatarsal artery, but they were inconstant and always communicated with the dorsal system. A Japanese study[137] and personal unpublished data stressed that vascularization of the PIPJ and MTPJ of the second toe is provided by both the dorsal and plantar vessels, which do communicate (Fig. 31-5). Furthermore, our study [31,43] underlined the role of a fundamental vessel that has been overlooked in the literature: the second plantar metatarsal artery (Fig. 31-6), which is a constant, reliable vessel passing in close contact to the volar plate of the MTPJ.

Specific Transfers

Several transfer techniques have been described: (1) toe PIPJ transfer for finger MPJ and PIPJ reconstruction; (2) MTPJ transfer for MPJ or TMJ reconstruction; (3) double transfer of PIPJ[125] for MPJ reconstruction; and (4) "twisted toe flap" technique to add a joint in a "wraparound" thumb reconstruction.[38,42,43]

Toe PIP to Finger PIP

There are only a few papers available on this topic.[38,125] The technique as described by Tsai is as follows:

Preoperatively, routine radiographs and selective angiography are performed on the foot and the hand.

Under general anesthesia, the donor and recipient sites are prepared simultaneously by two surgical teams. Through a longitudinal dorsal approach, the dorsalis pedis and first dorsal metatarsal arteries are dissected, along with the dorsal veins.[39] A small skin island over the tibial and dorsal aspect of the PIPJ of the second toe is preserved as a visible monitor of the underlying circulation (Fig. 31-7). The tibial side digital artery is divided distally at the level of the DIPJ, preserving the articular and metaphyseal branches. The fibular side artery is preserved by ligating its articular and metaphyseal branches. The extensor mechanism is then cut proximally and distally, and the joint is isolated by distal disarticulation through the DIPJ and by proximal osteotomy through the first phalanx. The hand is prepared, the involved PIPJ is excised, and a suitable artery is prepared.

The joint is transferred and stabilized with an intraosseous wire and longitudinal K-wire. The extensor mechanism is then reconstructed and the arterial suture is done usually by end-to-

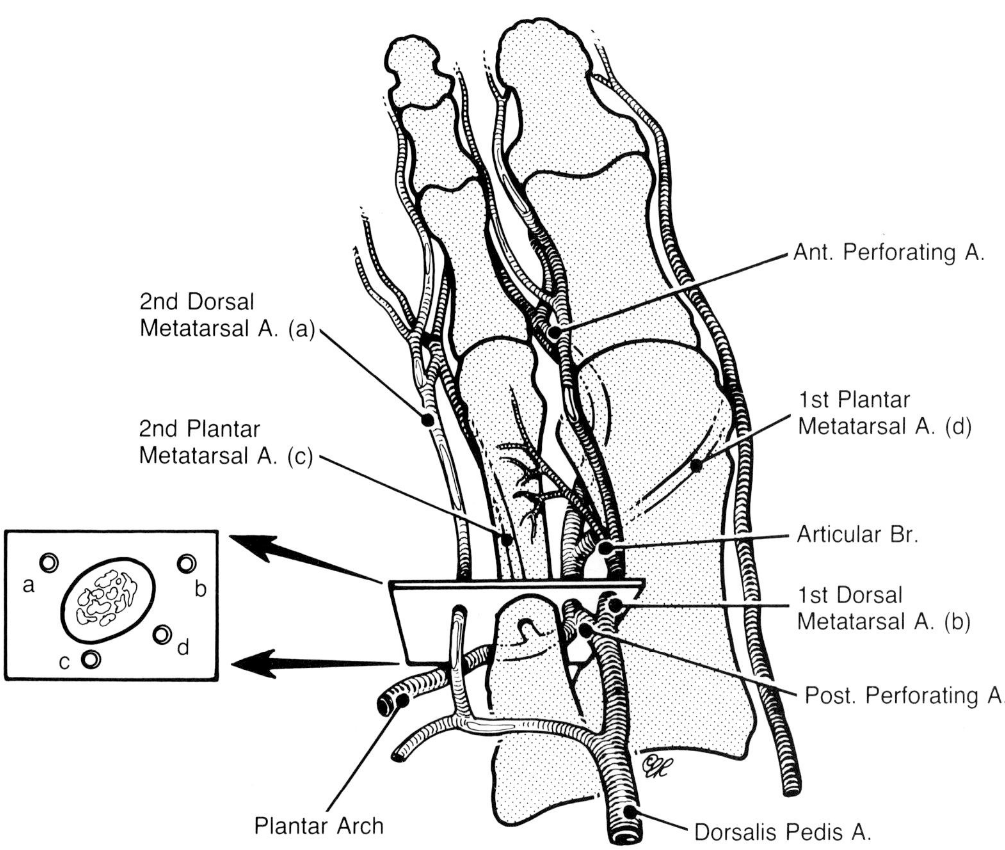

Fig. 31-6. The vascular pattern of the second web space in the foot, which has been overlooked in the literature. The second plantar and/or dorsal artery can frequently be used.

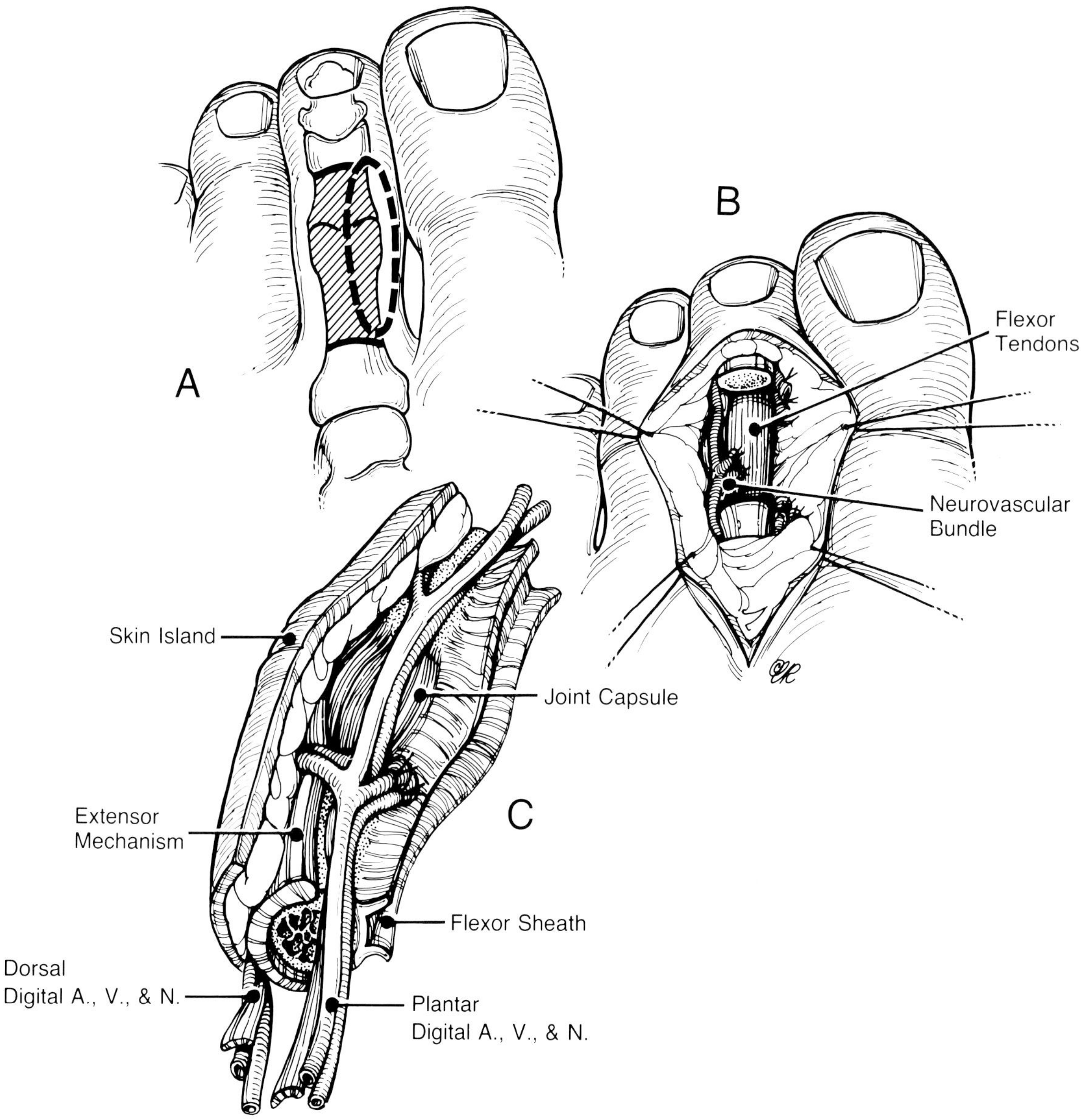

Fig. 31-7. Technique of second toe PIP joint transfer according to Tsai et al,[126] using a small skin island as a visible monitor of viability.

side anastomosis. At least two veins, including the saphenous vein, are sutured.

The foot defect may be managed as a resection arthroplasty or, preferably, by bone graft using the removed joint of the finger. Nothing was mentioned by the researchers[122] concerning postoperative management.

The technique described by Yoshizu[138] is similar, except that the second toe PIPJ graft is taken with the medial plantar digital artery, which is anastomosed to a common volar digital artery.

Toe MP to Hand MP

Under epidural and brachial plexus block anesthesia[76] this operation is comprised of four steps:

1. The joint is exposed at the recipient site through a curved skin incision. The ulnar side of the extensor hood is incised, retracted and the joint resected. The radial artery and the cephalic vein are approached through a separate incision. A small branch of the superficial radial nerve is dissected at the wrist level to be sutured to the nerve of the transplanted joint.
2. The donor site is prepared by dissection of the great saphenous vein and first dorsal metatarsal artery. The terminal branch of the deep peroneal nerve is also dissected.
3. The graft is turned 180 degrees around its longitudinal axis; that is, dorsal to volar. Bone fixation is done with a K-wire, and the vessels are anasto-

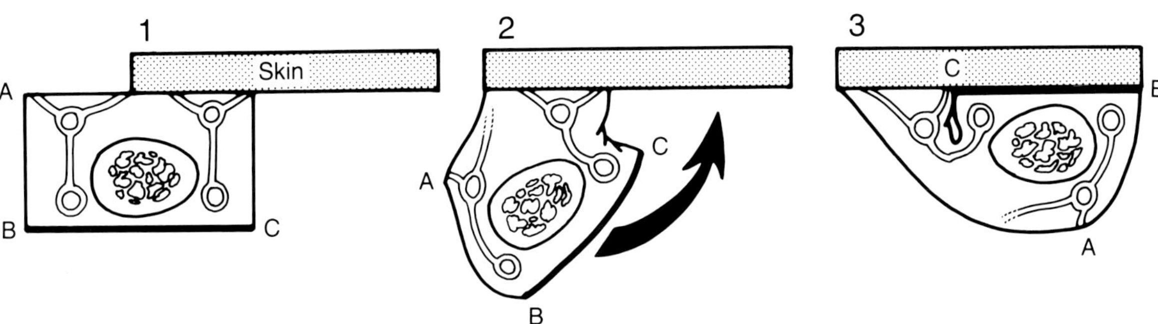

Fig. 31-8. A skin flap can be harvested with the MTP joint after turning the joint upside down (Smith and Jones[118]).

mosed: the dorsalis pedis to the radial artery, the great saphenous vein to the cephalic vein, and the deep peroneal nerve to the superfical branch of radial nerve. Last, the extensor mechanism is sutured and the skin closed.

4. At the donor site, the defect in the toe is filled by either the finger joint or by a cancellous bone graft.

Postoperative treatment includes prophylactic antiobiotics and low molecular Dextran for several days. The K-wires are removed at 4 weeks and functional exercises are then encouraged. The cast on the foot is removed at 4 weeks and walking is allowed.

One of the major shortcomings in this type of MTPJ transfer has been the difficulty with which a skin flap could be incorporated due to the rotation of the transfer. In an effort to solve this problem, Smith and Jones[117] described a technique using an eccentrically placed dorsalis pedis flap (Fig. 31-8). The non-dominant lateral digital artery is freed from its attachment to the skin flap. With this maneuver, the flap remains dorsal after rotation of the joint.

AUTHOR'S PREFERRED METHOD

Indications

The potential advantages of vascularized joint transfers are several.

A useful range of motion in an acceptable arc can be obtained with good lateral stability providing strong opposition to the thumb in pinch.

Despite a rather short follow-up period (13 years for our first case),[37] clinical durability has been found to corroborate experimental data with persistence of cartilage space.

Nevertheless, the two main advantages of this technique are the possibility of growth in young patients and the unique possibility of a compound transfer, providing not only joint but also bone stock, extensor mechanism, and skin, and allowing one-stage reconstruction as well.

However, several disadvantages must be emphasized as well, mainly as far as VJT from the toes is concerned: (1) the procedure is long, lasting 3½ hours on average; (2) it must be performed under general anesthesia with hospitalization required (average 5.3 days), and (3) the danger of failure, as in other microsurgical procedures, exists.

Finger Joint Reconstruction

PIP Joint

In our opinion, at the PIPJ level, toe VJT falls short of its goal due to restricted range of motion. We think that it is not a definite answer in adults, but remains useful, mainly in multiple PIP joint involvement, in young growing patients, and in large and complex losses (skin, bone, extensor tendon) with a normal flexor tendon.

MP Joint

At the MPJ level indications are similar, but in the case of double reconstruction, it seems better to reconstruct skin cover first. As for the PIPJ, the second and third rays are reconstructed most frequently. These radial fingers are more exigent for lateral stability than for amplitude, contrary to ulnar digits. The alternate transfer of a finger joint remains appealing when possible. In multiple digital injuries we carefully assess the possibility of an island or free vascularized finger joint transfer from a nonsalvagable segment. In a series of 16 cases[36] the average total active motion (TAM) was 45 degrees for MPJ reconstruction and 42 degrees for PIPJ. Otherwise the island transfer of a DIP at the PIPJ level[40] is now a preferred method when possible due to a mean TAM of 57 degrees (with a mean extension lack of 18 degrees). However our series (8 cases) and our follow-up (mean 15 months) are much too short to draw definite conclusions.

Thumb Reconstruction

The MTJ transfer provides an acceptable solution to some cases of congenital thumb ray hypoplasia (second degree in Blauth's classification.[1] As we have already stressed, it improves the cosmetic aspect, allows growth and provides satisfactory stability and mobility (usually after muscle or tendon transfer). In thumb reconstruction, the "twisted two toes" technique is indicated in some amputations located close to the

MPJ. It has several advantages over the classic "wrap-around"[91] and total second toe transfer in that it provides (1) a vascularized skeleton (avoiding resorption) with two phalanges (matching the normal thumb), (2) one joint (plus a proximal hemi-joint when necessary) with extensor and flexor mechanism; (3) firm support for the nail, and (4) a growth plate in children.

Specific Transfers

PIP Joint Reconstruction

For PIP joint reconstruction, we continue to use the technique that we described originally[37,38] using the second toe and which was modified later by Tsai. Specific details must be emphasized.

We do not use any preoperative angiography. The operation is performed under general anesthesia by one team only. The one-team approach avoids most of the pitfalls concerning matching of length and size of arteries, veins, nerves and tendons.

The first step is the toe dissection. A cutaneous flap is drawn distally to the DIPJ, and proximally a long tail is taken from the dorsum of the foot. A dorsal approach only is sufficient.[31,34,42,43] After dissection of the venous arch and the great saphenous vein, the dorsalis pedis artery is dissected just beneath the extensor hallucis longus tendon. The field of dissection then moves to the first web, looking for the dorsal metatarsal artery, superficial to the intermetatarsal ligament. If the diameter of this artery is not sufficient, we proceed with extensor tendon section and proximal osteotomy of the second metatarsal, which is then lifted with a bone hook. This osteot-

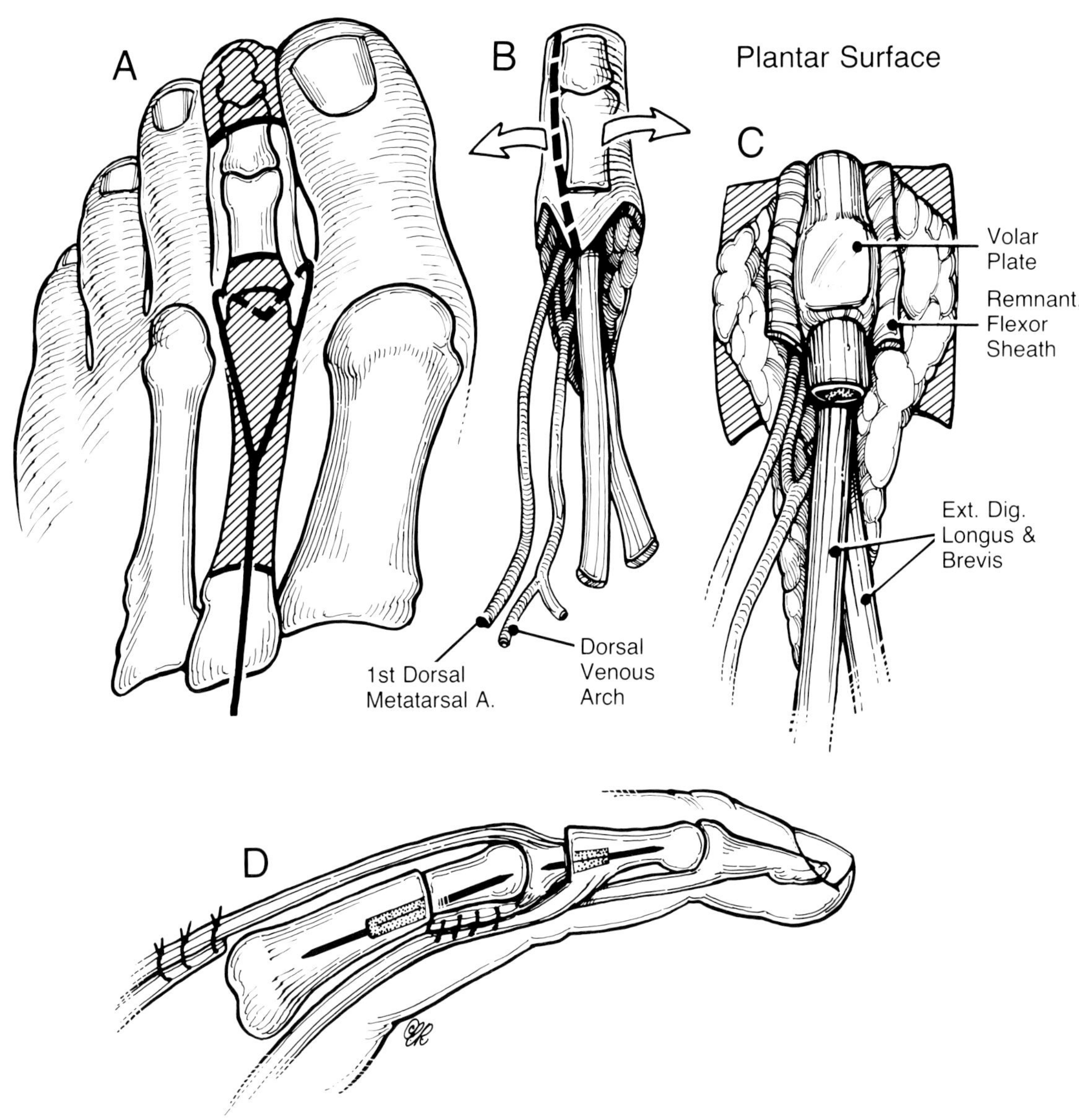

Fig. 31-9. Author's technique for PIP toe joint compound transfer. **(A)** A large flap is harvested. **(B)** The plantar skin is split on the midplantar aspect. **(C)** Two lateral flaps are reflected and the flexor mechanism removed, with preservation of part of the sheath for later repair. **(D)** Intramedullary bone penetration and suture of the recipient's flexor sheath to the rims of the donor site pulleys. *(Figure continues.)*

omy has two advantages: (1) it provides a wide approach to the plantar arterial system of the first and second space, and (2) it facilitates closure of the donor site.

When none of the arteries possess a suitable diameter, two (or even three) are taken in continuity with the dorsalis pedis artery. Then the toe is divided distally through the DIPJ. The skin is split on the medial line of the plantar aspect and two lateral flaps are reflected until reaching the vascular bundle (Fig. 31-9). The flexor sheath is then opened longitudinally and medially to remove the flexor mechanism, with care being taken to avoid injuring the retrotendinous vessels and the vascularization of the plantar plate. The first phalanx is osteotomized according to the length needed. A bone peg can be harvested from the discarded from the discarded metatarsal for bone stabilization either at the donor or recipient sites. When the compound transfer is pedicled only on its artery (or arteries) and vein, the tourniquet is released. Local topic vasodilator (lidocaine 2 percent) is applied to the artery, and the foot is wrapped with hot wet drapes.

Preparation of the hand is made through a classic longitudinal dorsal incision, but extensive excision of scarred tissue is possible because of the large skin flap of the compound transfer. The flexor sheath is cleared out and the remaining volar plate is made thinner. The bone ends and the extensor mechanism are prepared. A separate approach (ideally horizontal) is performed in the first intermetacarpal space, with dissection of the radial artery and one superficial vein. The skin is undermined between the two incisions, providing a sufficient channel for the vascular bundle. The length of missing bone and vessels needed is measured and the dissection of the foot is completed. The phalanges of the toe are usually trimmed in a step fashion to allow intramedullary penetration at the recipient site. Then the vein and the artery are divided. When length permits, the dorsalis pedis artery and the proxi-

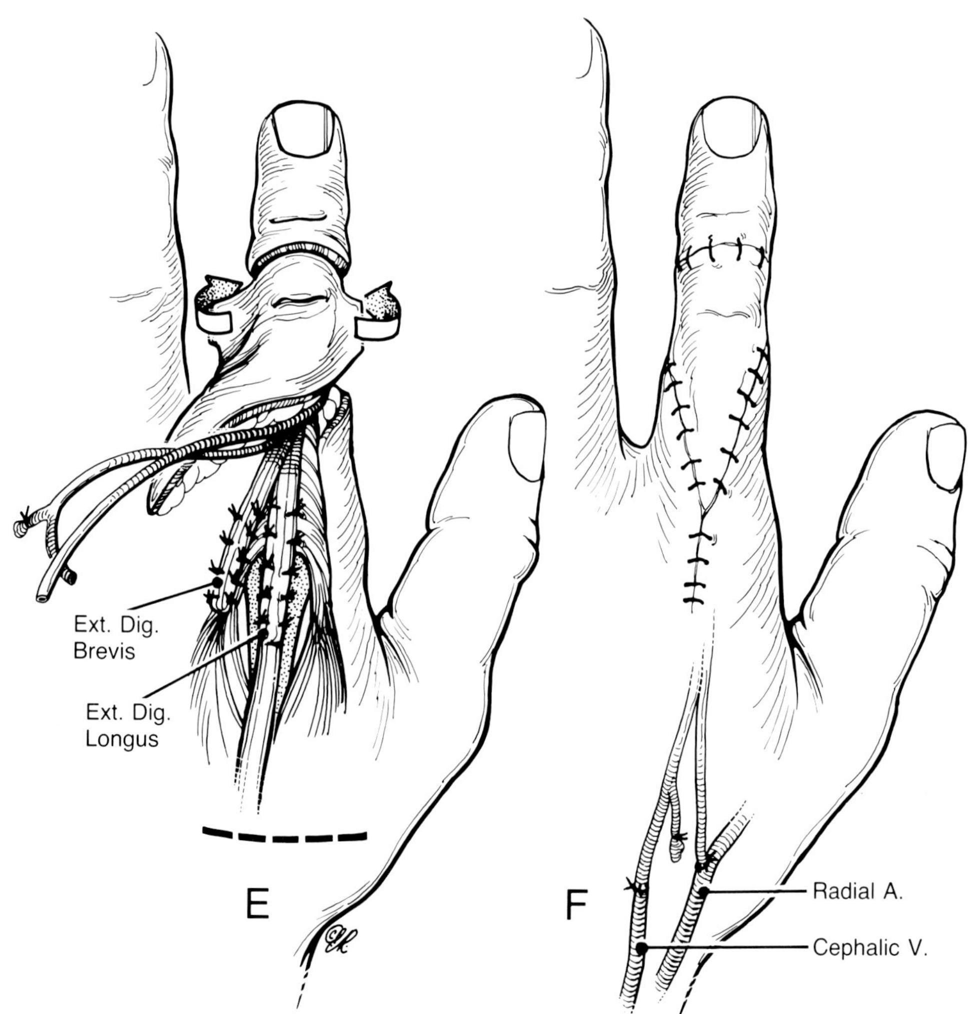

Fig. 31-9 *(Continued).* **(E)** Extensor tendon suture. The extensor brevis is sutured to the intrinsic mechanism, and the longus is sutured to the extrinsic extensor tendon. **(F)** Vessel anastomoses. End-to-side suture with the radial artery and end-to-end suture with the cephalic vein.

mal plantar arch are harvested so that the latter can be intercalated as a T-shaped graft (Fig. 31-10).

The compound joint is then transferred to the recipient finger and the bone secured. We have used different types of osteosynthesis (intramedullary screw, K-wire, bone peg, and wiring); there has been no specific correlation with the final range of motion depending on the type of fixation, and we have not noted any difference in postoperative motion when comparing methods or techniques of internal fixation. Most frequently, we have used a buried intramedullary pin and an oblique K-wire. Care has to be taken not to make the intercalated segment too long (it is preferable that it be too short).

The remnant of flexor sheath of the toe is sutured to the rim of the recipient sheath to prevent bowstringing of the flexor tendon. The extensor mechanism is sutured with overlapping, with the joint in full extension. The extensor hallucis longus is secured to the medial tendon on the dorsum of the first phalanx and the extensor brevis to the intrinsic tendon. The bundle is then passed through the subcutaneous tunnel, avoiding any twisting, and the skin flap is carefully trimmed, inserted, and sutured. The vessels are then sutured end-to-side or end-to-end (T-shaped) for the artery and end-to-end for the sole vein (Fig. 31-9F). The tourniquet is then removed and the donor site is closed after hemostasis. Intermetatarsal ligament reconstruction is performed and the skin closed with drainage tubes.

Our policy of second ray amputation is based on problems encountered following donor site grafting (nonunion and delayed walking). On the other hand, a study by a foot surgeon based on 20 cases of second toe amputation[92] has demonstrated that when the metatarsal was left in place, there was a consistent tendency to hallux valgus deformity. This decreased after ray amputation except when the angle between the first and second metatarsals was greater than 20 degrees. In such cases, reconstruction of the second toe has to be considered.

The last steps are assessment of viability of the flap at the recipient site after release of tourniquet and application of the dressing.

Moderate elevation is prescribed postoperatively, and visualization of the skin allows direct monitoring of the transfer. Low molecular Dextran is infused for 5 days with 1 g of aspirin daily. No antibiotics are given. The patient can be discharged from the hospital on the fifth day. A clinical trail of early mobilization with a dynamic dorsal splint did not correlate with the final range of motion; therefore, we routinely prescribe 3 weeks immobilization followed by active motion with dynamic extension splinting. Nightly passive flexion splinting is delayed until the fifth week. The pins are usually removed at 4 weeks. An illustrative case is shown in Figure 31-11.

Other Transfers

Three other techniques are worthy of mention:

1. Double transfer for MPJ or PIPJ reconstruction
2. TM joint reconstruction by MTPJ transfer
3. "Twisted two toes" for thumb reconstruction

Double Transfer of MT and PIP (Toe) Joint to Adjacent MP Joints

The MPJ can be reconstructed by using either the PIPJ or MTPJ of the toe. When two adjacent MPJs have to be reconstructed, it is possible to harvest both vascularized joints from

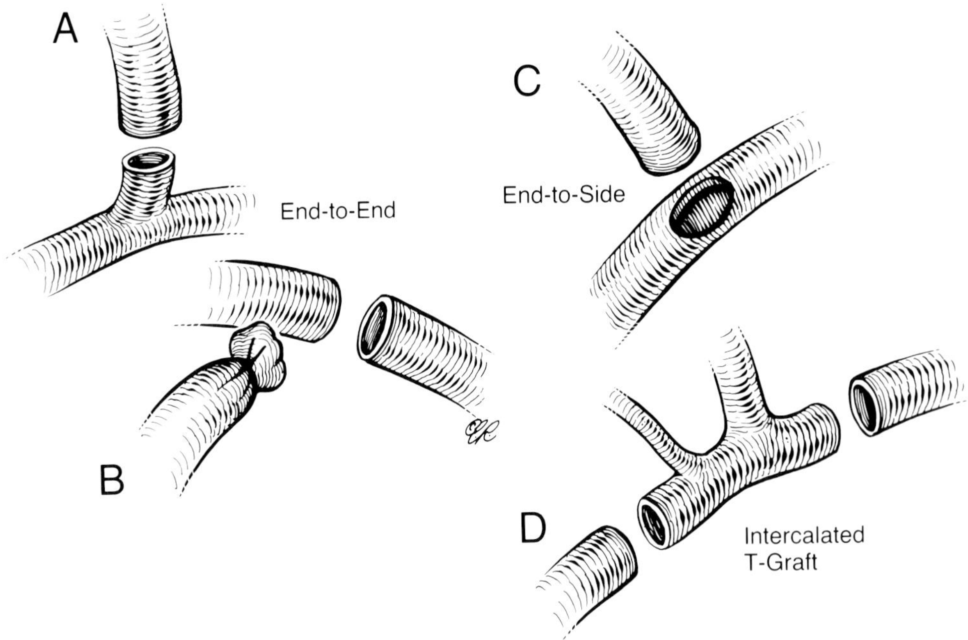

Fig. 31-10. Four types of arterial suture can be performed. **(A)** End-to-end suture with the princeps pollicis artery. **(B)** End-to-end suture with the radial artery. **(C)** End-to-side suture with the radial artery. **(D)** The dorsalis pedis artery in continuity with the plantar arch is intercalated as a T-shaped graft (in this case, two feeding arteries have been harvested from the foot).

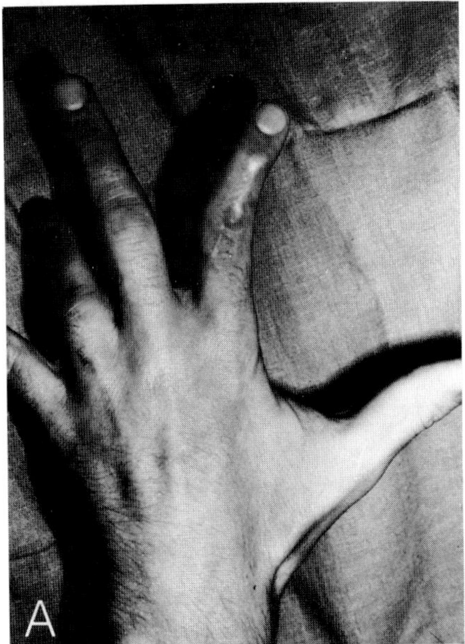

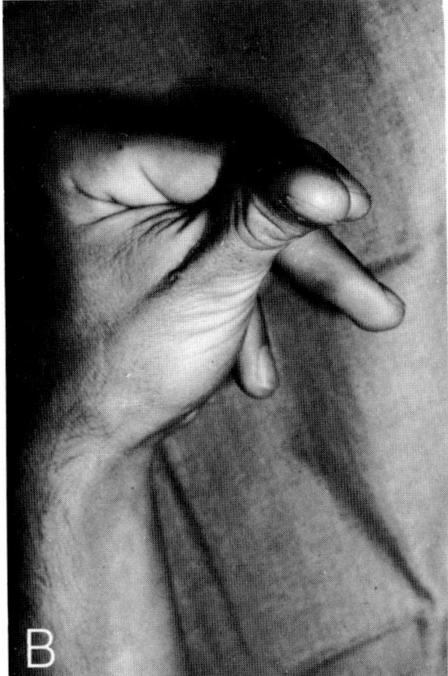

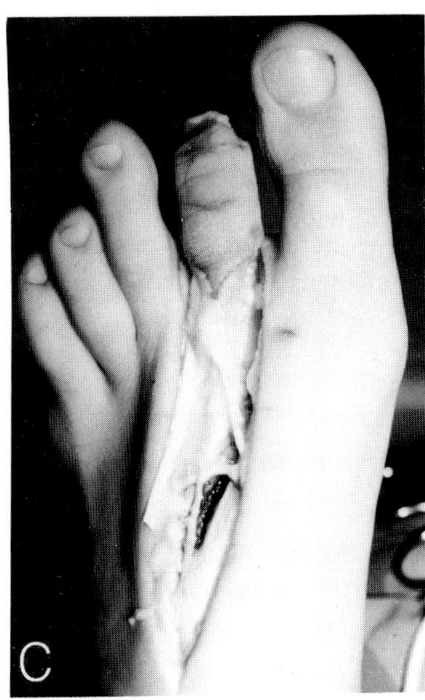

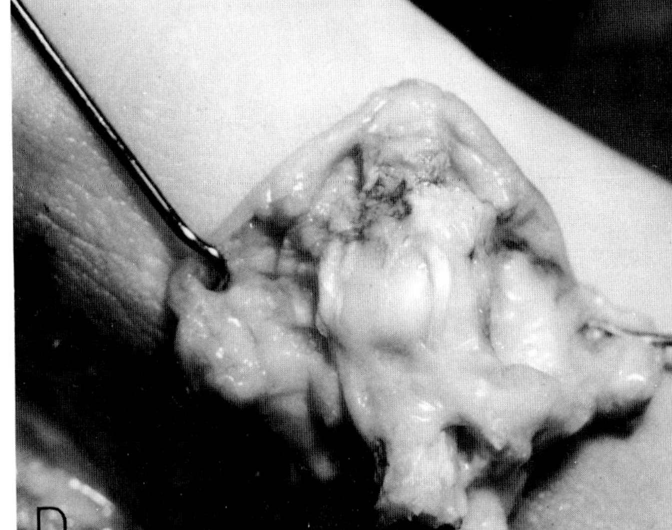

Fig. 31-11. An example of compound PIP joint transfer using the author's technique. **(A&B)** Multifinger involvement with a destroyed PIP joint of the second and fourth digits. **(C)** Preparation of a compound transfer of the PIP joint of the second toe. The first dorsal artery is visible proximally. **(D)** Plantar aspect of the transfer with intact volar plate. *(Figure continues.)*

the second toe (Fig. 31-12). The MTPJ is raised on the second plantar metatarsal artery and rotated 180 degrees on its axis. The PIPJ is raised on the first dorsal (or plantar) artery. This technique calls for a good extensor mechanism and good skin coverage.

Tranfer of Adjacent PIP (Toe) Joints to PIP Joint of Hand

For reconstruction of an adjacent PIPJ, Tsai[125] has used the PIP joints of the second and third toes with partial syndactylization. To avoid this major cosmetic drawback, we prefer to harvest each joint on a separate pedicle (Fig. 31-13): a first plantar or dorsal metatarsal artery for the PIPJ of the second toe and the second plantar metatarsal artery for the third toe. In such cases, we amputate the second ray and use part of the second metatarsal for reconstruction of the third toe.

MT Joint of (Second Toe) to CMC Joint of Thumb

Reconstruction of the CMC in certain cases of congenital thumb ray hypoplasia can be provided by an MTPJ transfer that provides bone stock, mobility, stability, and growth plates. The technique is not much different from that described above, except that it is implanted on the carpus in hyperextension as described by Buck-Gramcko[3] in his pollicization technique. A skin flap can be transferred at the same time to improve the thenar eminence, thus facilitating an abductor digiti minimi opponensplasty.

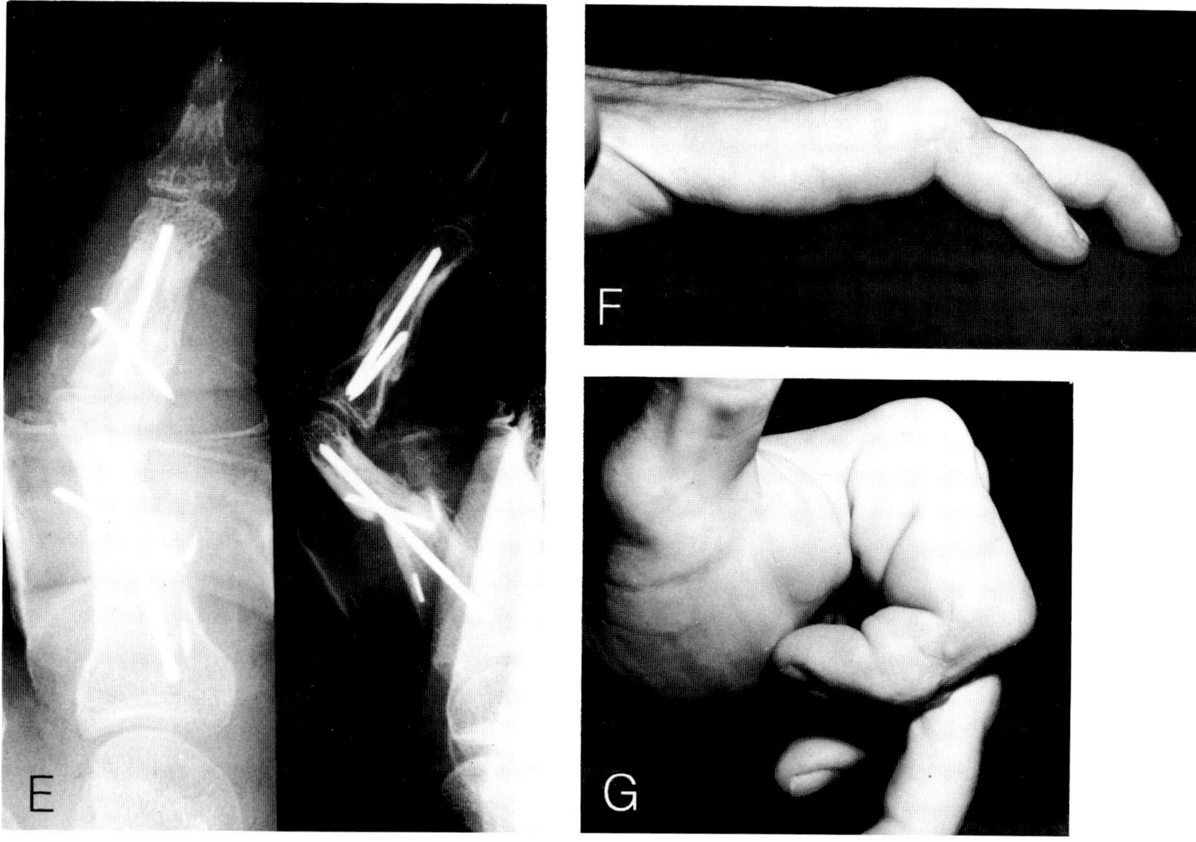

Fig. 31-11 *(Continued).* **(E)** A radiograph of the transferred joint in the PIP joint of the index finger. **(F&G)** Final range of motion 3 years after operation.

"Twisted Two Toes" Transfer

Finally, a VJT can be incorporated into a wraparound technique for thumb reconstruction in a "twisted two toes" (TTT) technique.[38,43] The skin and nail complex are taken from the ipsilateral big toe based on the first dorsal (or plantar) metatarsal artery. A piece of vascularized bone is incorporated into the flap to avoid bone resorption and to provide nail support. The PIP joint is lifted en bloc with the first and second phalanx on the second plantar (or, rarely, dorsal) metatarsal artery, the superficialis flexor, and the extensor mechanisms being harvested at the same time. Both arteries are taken in continuity with the dorsalis pedis artery, which is used for a T-shaped intercalated graft. The joint is buried into the big toe flap and the second phalanx is attached to the bone of the big toe by a K-wire (Fig. 31-14). In this way, a two phalanx "custom-made" thumb is constructed and then may be transferred to the thumb stump in the standard manner. Either a graft or an ulnar-based flap, tailored from the stump, is used to cover the ulnar side of the filleted big toe skin. At the donor site, the proximal part of the second metatarsal bone is removed, the intermetatarsal ligament repaired, and the filleted second toe skin wrapped around the skeleton of the big toe with a Z-plasty.

Postoperative Complications

Thrombosis of the vessels is a classic complication of microvascular procedures that can be managed by careful monitoring of the skin flap incorporated into the transfer. In case of skin necrosis, mainly in very young patients, the transfer can be saved by moving a remote flap on to the "non" vascularized joint. Infection, although not mentioned in the literature, should be managed with standard techniques.

Delayed bone healing does not seem to be a problem at the hand level, but has been mentioned frequently in the foot.[58,125,137] Stiffness of the VJT remains a major problem. We tried to improve joint mobility preoperatively in the foot by splinting at night, but without success. Even when early mobilization was employed, limitation of both active and passive extension as mentioned in total second toe transfers was found consistently after the toe VJT.[35,37,38,41,43,58,125,137] There are several possible reasons for this: (1) preexisting claw deformity of the donor toe, (2) deficient or insufficient tension on the extensor mechanism, (3) an overly long intercalated bony segment, and (4) bowstringing of flexor tendons, increasing the lever arm as seen in digits with damaged pulleys.

As noted previously, only some of these factors can be

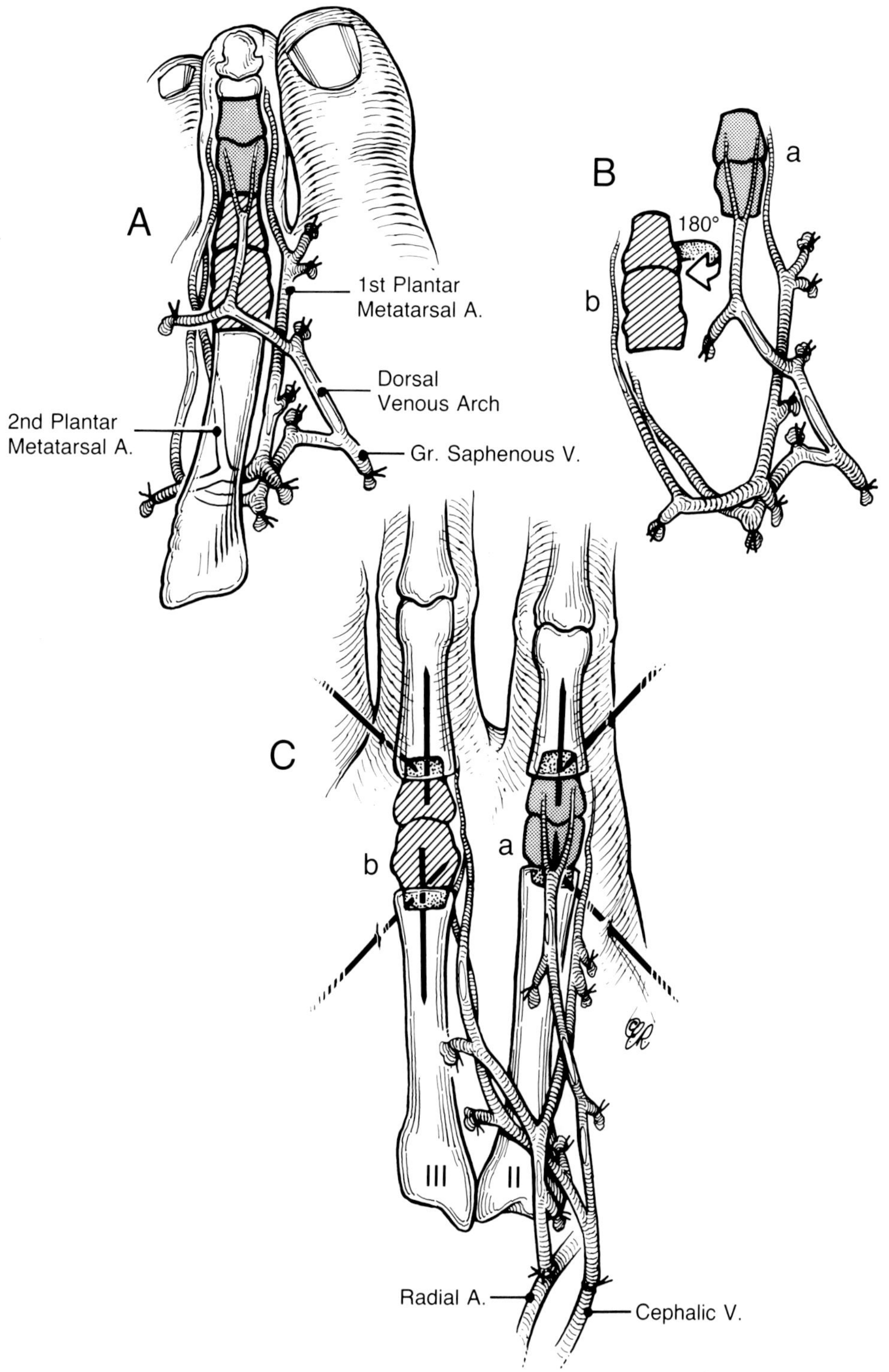

Fig. 31-12. The MTP joint and PIP joint of the second toe are lifted on separate bundles, allowing double MP joint reconstruction.

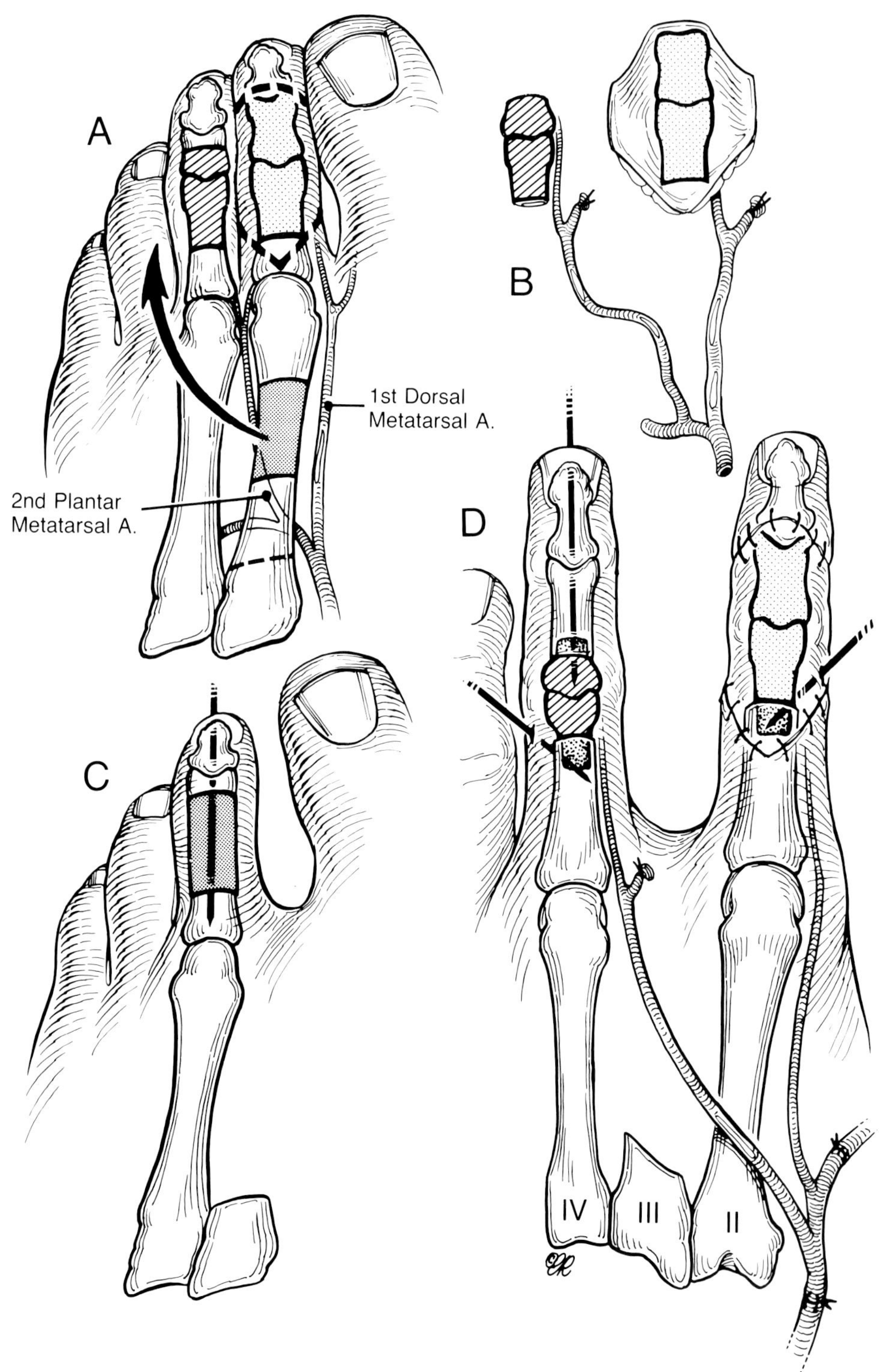

Fig. 31-13. The PIP joints of the second and third toes are harvested on separate bundles, which allows double PIP joint reconstruction.

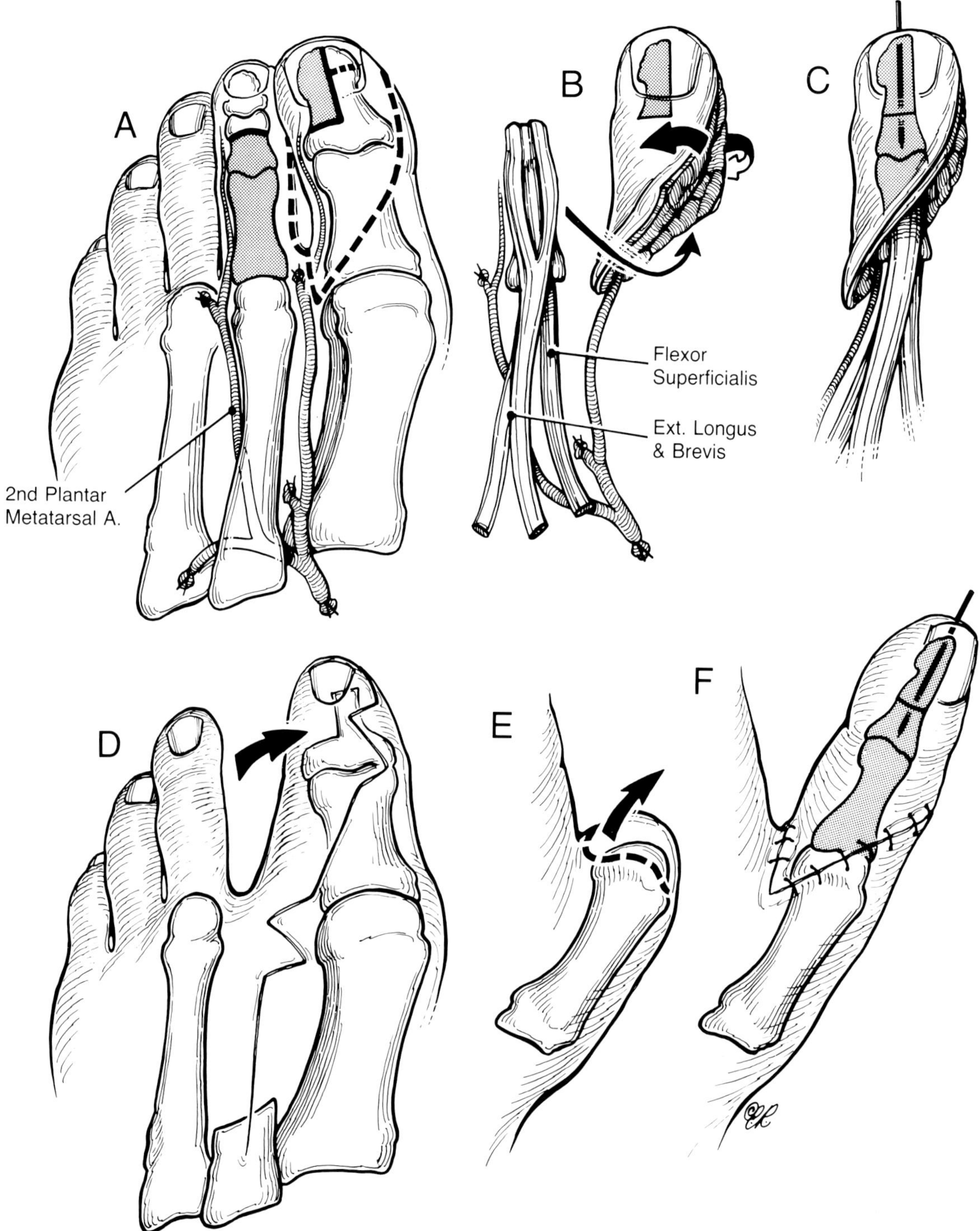

Fig. 31-14. "Twisted two toes" technique. **(A&B)** A sheath of skin, the nail complex, and a piece of loose bone are taken from the great toe; the PIP joint with extensor and flexor tendons is harvested from the second toe. **(C)** The bones of the first and second toes are joined by a K-wire and the skin wrapped around. **(D)** The filleted flap of the second toe covers the great toe defect. **(E&F)** A lateral flap is elevated from the thumb stump to cover the lateral aspect of the transfer.

avoided by surgical technique. Tsai has studied the mobility of 50 normal second toe PIPJ [123] and found that lack of extension correlates with age ranging from 0 degrees to 20 degrees with a TAM of 27 degrees to 69 degrees.

In our published series of 25 patients,[32] complications were as follows: two failures (7.1 percent), one successful reexploration for arterial thrombosis, one pin tract infection, and one discrete area of skin slough resulting in secondary scarring. With a mean follow-up of 54 months (14 months to 13 years) our MPJ reconstructions have a mean TAM of 35 degrees (20 degrees to 50 degrees) with a mean extension lag of 45 degrees; PIPJ, a TAM of 23 degrees (ranging from 0 degrees to 60 degrees with an average of 55 degrees lack of extension). The only good news concerns the absence of radiologic deterioration and the persistance of cartilage growth plates in children. The other "large" series published by Tsai[123] of 29 patients with an average follow-up of 1.9 years gives a complication rate of 48.4 percent; no motion was recorded in 28 percent and in successful cases the TAM was 46 degrees.

SUMMARY

Vascularized joint transfer may be indicated for PIPJ, MPJ, and TMJ reconstruction mainly in complex situations even if all the proposed techniques fall short of necessary range of motion for daily activities. Here again the aphorism of Bunnell is worth keeping in mind: "When there is nothing, a little is a lot," especially when this "little" is painless and stable in space and time. This technique provides the unique advantage of a compound transfer of skin, bone, joint, tendons, and growth plate. Until vascularized homografts become clinically available, this is a worthwhile technique in limited complex situations.

REFERENCES

1. Blauth W, Schneider-Sickert F: Congenital deformities of the Hand. An Atlas of Their Surgical Treatment, pp. 136–153. Springer-Verlag, Berlin, Heidelberg, New York, 1980
2. Boyes JH: Bunnell's Surgery of the Hand. 4th Ed. pp. 318–320. JB Lippincott, Philadelphia, 1964
3. Buck-Gramcko D: Pollicization of the index finger. Method and results in aplasia and hypoplasia of the thumb. J Bone Joint Surg 53A:1605–1617, 1971
4. Buncke HJ, Daniller AI, Schulz WP, Chase RA: The fate of autogenous whole joints transplanted by microvascular anastomoses. Plast Reconstr Surg 39:333–341, 1967
5. Bunnell S: Surgical repair of joints. pp. 300–304. In Surgery of the Hand. JB Lippincott, Philadelphia, 1948
6. Burwell RG: Skeletal allografts for synovial joint reconstruction (editorial). J Bone Joint Surg 52B:10–13, 1970
7. Campbell CJ: Homotransplantation of a half or whole joint. Clin Orthop 87:146–155, 1972
8. Campbell CJ, Ishida H, Takahoashi H, Kelly F: The transplantation of articular cartilage. An experimental study in dogs. J Bone Joint Surg 45A:1579–1592, 1963
9. Carroll RE, Green DP: Reconstruction of hypoplastic digits using toe phalanges (Abstract). J Bone Joint Surg 57A:727, 1975
10. Colson P: Osteo articular transplants in the hand. Vol. II. pp. 678–684. Ed. Tubiana Masson, Paris, 1984
11. Colson P, Hovot R: Chirurgie réparatrice du pouce. Greffe articulaire. Lyon Chir 42:721–724, 1947
12. Comtet JJ, Bertrand HG, Moyen B: Free autogenous composite joint graft use in multiple finger injuries. Int J Microsurg 2:121–124, 1980
13. Cuthbert JB: The late treatment of dorsal injuries of the hand associated with loss of skin. Br J Surg 33:66–71, 1945
14. Daniel G, Entin MA, Kahn DS: Autogenous transplantation in the dog of a metacarpophalangeal joint with preserved neurovascular bundle. Can J Surg 14:253–259, 1971
15. DePalma AF, Sawyer B, Hoffmann JD: Fate of osteochondral grafts. Clin Orthop 22:217–220, 1962
16. DePalma AF, Tsaltas TT, Mauler GG: Viability of osteochondral grafts as determined by uptake of S^{35}. J Bone Joint Surg 45A:1565–1578, 1963
17. Dingman RO, Grabb WC: Reconstruction of both mandibular condyles with metatarsal bone grafts. Plast Reconstr Surg 34:441–451, 1964. Dingman RO: Follow-up. Clinic Plast Reconstr Surg 47:594, 1971
18. Donski PK, Carwell GR, Sharzer LA: Growth in revascularized bone grafts in young puppies. Plast Reconstr Surg 64:239–243, 1979
19. Donski PK, O'Brien MMc C: Free microvascular epiphyseal transplantation. An experimental study in dogs. Br J Plast Surg 33:169–178, 1980
20. Ducuing J: Contribution expérimentale à l'étude des greffes articulaires totales. Masson Edit, Paris, 1912
21. Eades JW, Peacock EE: Autogenous transplantation of an interphalangeal joint and proximal phalangeal epiphysis. Case report and ten year follow-up. J Bone Joint Surg 48A:775–778, 1966
22. Edwards EA: Anatomy of the small arteries of the foot and toes. Acta Anat 41:81–96, 1960
23. Entin MA, Alger JR, Baird RM: Experimental and clinical transplantation of autogenous whole joints. J Bone Joint Surg 44A:1518–1536, 1962
24. Entin MA, Daniel G, Kahn D: Transplantation of autogenous half-joints. Arch Surg 96:359–368, 1968
25. Erdelyi R: Experimental autotransplantation of small joints. Plast Reconstr Surg 31:129–139, 1963
26. Erdelyi R: Reconstruction of ankylosed finger joints by means of transplantation of joints from the foot. Plast Reconstr Surg 31:140–150, 1963
27. Ferlic DC, Clayton ML, Holloway M: Complications of silicone implant surgery in the metacarpophalangeal joint. J Bone Joint Surg 57A:991–994, 1975
28. Field PL, Hueston JT: Articular cartilage loss in long-standing immobilisation of interphalangeal joints. Br J Plast Surg 1970, 23:186–191, 1970
29. Flatt AE: Studies in finger joint replacement. A review of the present position. Arch Surg 107:437–443, 1973
30. Foucher G: Vascularized joint transfer. pp. 1271–1293. In Green DP (ed): Operative Hand Surgery. 2nd Ed. Churchill Livingstone, New York, 1988
31. Foucher G, Braun FM, Merle M, Michon J: Le transert du deuxième orteil dans la chirurgie reconstructive des doigts longs. Rev Chir Orthop 67:235–240, 1981
32. Foucher G, Citron N, Merle M, Dury M: Free compound transfer of the distal interphalangeal joint. A case report. J Reconstr Microsurg 3:297–300, 1987
33. Foucher G, Citron E, Sammut D: Compound vascularized island joint transfer in hand surgery. A report of 16 cases. French J Orthop Surg 5:32–39, 1991
34. Foucher G, Denuit P, Braun FM, Merle M, Michon J: Le trans-

fert total ou partiel du deuxième orteil dans la reconstruction digitale. A propos de 32 cas. Acta Orthop Belg 47:854-866, 1981
35. Foucher G, Hoang P, Citron N, Merle M, Dury M: Joint reconstruction following trauma: Comparison of microsurgical transfer and conventional methods: A report of 61 cases. J Hand Surg 11B:388-393, 1986
36. Foucher G, Lenoble E, Sammut D: Transfer of a composite island homodigital distal interphalangeal joint to replace the proximal interphalangeal joint. Ann Hand Surg 9:369-375, 1990
37. Foucher G, Merle M: Transfert articulaire au niveau d'un doigt en microchirurgie. G.A.M., lettre d'information du GAM, 1976, n° 7
38. Foucher G, Merle M, Maneaud M, Michon J: Microsurgical free partial toe transfer in hand reconstruction, a report of 12 cases. Plast Reconstr Surg 65:616-626, 1980
39. Foucher G, Norris RW: The dorsal approach in harvesting the second toe. J Reconstr Microsurg 4:185-187, 1988
40. Foucher G, Sammut D, Citron N: Free vascularized toe-joint transfer in hand reconstruction: A series of 25 patients. J Reconstr Microsurg 6:201-207, 1990
41. Foucher G, Schuind F, Hoang P: Free vascularized joint transfers. Presented at the 1st meeting, American Society for Reconstructive Microsurgery, Las Vegas, 1985
42. Foucher G, Van Genechten F, Merle M, Denuit P, Braun FM, Debry R, Sur H: Le transfert à partir d'orteil dans la chirurgie reconstructrive de la main. A propos de soixante et onze cas. Ann Chir Main 3:124-138, 1984
43. Foucher G, Van Genechten F, Morrison WA: Composite tissue transfer to the hand from the foot. pp. 65-82. In Jackson IT, Sommerlad BC (eds): Recent Advances in Plastic Surgery. Churchill Livingstone, New York, 1985
44. Freeman BS: Reconstruction of thumb by toe transfer. Plast Reconstr Surg 17:393-398, 1956
45. Freeman BS: Growth studies of transplanted epiphysis. Plast Reconstr Surg 23:584-588, 1959
46. Freeman BS: Results of epiphyseal transplants by flap and by free graft. A brief survey. Plast Reconstr Surg 36:227-230, 1965 (Follow-up Clinic, 48:72, 1971)
47. Furnas DW: Growth and development in replanted forelimbs. Plast Reconstr Surg 46:445-453, 1970
48. Gibson T, Davis WB, Curran RC: The long-term survival of cartilage homografts in man. Br J Plast Surg 11:177-187, 1958
49. Gilbert A: Composite tissue transfers from the foot: Anatomic basis and surgical technique. pp. 230-242. In Daniller AL, Strauch B (eds): Symposium on Microsurgery. CV Mosby, St. Louis, 1976
50. Gill AB: Transplantation of entire bones with their joint surfaces. Ann Surg 61:658-660, 1915
51. Goebbel R: Ersatz von Fingergelenken durch Zehengelenke. München Med. Wehnschi 60:1598-1601, 1913
52. Goldberg NH, Watson HK: Composite toe (phalanx and epiphysis) transfers in the reconstruction of the aphalangic hand. J Hand Surg 7:454-459, 1982
53. Goldberg VM, Heiple KG: Experimental hemi-joint and whole-joint transplantation. A preliminary report. Clin Orthop 174:43-53, 1983
54. Goldberg VM, Porter BB, Lance EM: Transplantation of the canine knee joint on a vascular pedicle. J Bone Joint Surg 62:414-424, 1980
55. Graham WC: Transplantation of joints to replace diseased or damaged articulations in the hands. Am J Surg 88:136-141, 1954
56. Graham WC, Riordan DC: Reconstruction of a metacarpophalangeal joint with a metatarsal transplant. J Bone Joint Surg 30A:848-853, 1948
57. Gregory CF: The current status of bone and joint transplants. Clin Orthop 87:165-166, 1972
58. Gross AE, McKee NH, Pritzker KPH, Langer F: Reconstruction of skeletal defects at the knee. A comprehensive osteochondral transplant program. Clin Orthop 174:96-106, 1983
59. Gu YD, Wu MM, Zheng YL, Yang DY, Li HR: Vascular variations and their treatment in toe transplantation. J Reconstr Microsurg 1:227-232, 1985
60. Haas SL: Experimental transplantation of the epiphysis with observations on the longitudinal growth of bone. JAMA 65:1965, 1915
61. Haas SL: The transplantation of the articular end of bone including the epiphyseal cartilage line. Surg Gynecol Obstet 23:301-332, 1916
62. Haas SL: Further observation on the transplantation of the epiphyseal cartilage plate. Surg Gynecol Obstet 52:958-963, 1931
63. Harris WR, Martin R, Tile M: Transplantation of epiphyseal plates. An experimental study. J Bone Joint Surg 47A:897-914, 1965
64. Herndon CH, Chase SW: Experimental studies in the transplantation of whole joints. J Bone Joint Surg 34A:564-578, 1952
65. Hoffman S, Siffert RS, Simon BE: Experimental and clinical experience in epiphyseal transplantation. Plast Reconstr Surg 50:58-65, 1972
66. Huang SL, Hou MZ, Yan CL: Reconstruction of the thumb by a free pedal neurovascular flap and composite phalanx-joint-tendon homograft: A preliminary report. J Reconstr Microsurg 1:299-303, 1985
67. Hume MC, Gellman H, McKellop H, Brumfield RH Jr: Functional range of motion of the joints of the hand. J Hand Surg 15A:240-243, 1990
68. Hurwitz PJ: Experimental transplantation of small joints by microvascular anastomoses. Plast Reconstr Surg 64:221-231, 1979
69. Imamaliev AS: Transplantation of hemjoint in experiment. First report. Ortop Traum Protez 21:43-46, 1960
70. Imamaliev AS: Hemi-articular transplantation in experimental and clinical conditions.Ortop Traum Protez 23:9-15, 1962
71. Impallomeni G: Sul trapianto delle articolazioni. Arch Orthop 28:342-368, 1911
72. Johansson SH, Engkvist O: Small joint reconstruction by perichondreal arthroplasty. Clin Plast Surg 8:107-114, 1981
73. Judet H: Essai sur la greffe des tissus articulaires. CR Acad Sci Paris 146:193-196, 600-603, 1908
74. Judet H, Padovani JP: Transplantation d'articulation complète avec rétablissement circulatoire immédiat par anastomoses artérielle et veineuse. Mem Acad Chir 94:520-526, 1968
75. Judet H, Padovani JP: Transplantation d'articulation complète avec rétablissement circulatoire immédiat par anastomoses artérielle et veineuse chez le chien. Rev Chir Orthop 59:125-128, 1973
76. Kettelkamp DB: Experimental autologous joint transplantation. Clin Orthop 87:138-145, 1972
77. Kettelkamp DB, Alexander HH, Dolan J: A comparison of experimental arthroplasty and metacarpal head replacement. J Bone Joint Surg 50A:1564-1576, 1968
78. Kettelkamp DB, Ramsey P: Experimental and clinical autogenous distal metacarpal reconstruction. Clin Orthop 74:129-137, 1971
79. Kuo ET, Ji ZL, Zhao YC, Zhang ML: Reconstruction of metacarpophalangeal joint by free vascularised autogenous metatarsophalangeal joint transplant. J Reconstr Microsurg 1:65-74, 1984
80. Leung PC, Kok LC: Transplantation of the second toe. A preliminary report of sixteen cases. J Bone Joint Surg 62A:990-996, 1980

81. Lexer E: Substitution of whole or half-joints from freshly amputated extremities by free plastic operation. Surg Gynecol Obstet 6:601, 1908
82. Lexer E: Joint transplantations and arthroplasty. Surg Gynecol Obstet 40:782-809, 1925
83. Lloyd GJ, McTavish DR, Soriano S, Wiley AM, Young MH: Fate of articular cartilage in joint transplantation. Can J Surg 16:306-320, 1973
84. Lopez A: Articular grafts. Med Exper 47:501-507, 1962
85. Lugnegard H: Autologous transplantation of a finger phalanx with articular surface. Report of a case. Acta Chir Scand 126:185-190, 1963
86. Mathes SJ, Buchannan R, Weeks PM: Microvascular joint transplantation with epiphyseal growth. J Hand Surg 5:586-589, 1980
87. May H: The regeneration of joint transplants and intracapsular fragments. Ann Surg 116:297-303, 1942
88. May JW, Chait LA, Cohen BE, O'Brien BMcC: Free neurovascular flap from the first web of the foot in hand reconstruction. J Hand Surg 2:387-393, 1977
89. McKeever F: In discussion. Herndon and Chase. J Bone Joint Surg 34A:578-582, 1952
90. Menon J: Reconstruction of the metacarpophalangeal joint with autogenous metatarsal. J Hand Surg 8:443-446, 1983
91. Monney V, Ferguson AB: The influence of immobilisation and motion on the formation of fibro-cartilage after joint resection in the rabbit. J Bone Joint Surg 48A:6-10, 1966
92. Morrison WA, O'Brien BMcC, McLeod AM: Thumb reconstruction with a free neurovascular wrap-around flap from the big toe. J Hand Surg 5:575-583, 1980
93. Moyen B: Paper at the 8th International Meeting of Microsurgery. Panel on toe transfer. May 1982, (unpublished).
94. Nettelblad H, Randolph MA, Weiland AJ: Free microvascular epiphyseal-plate transplantation. An experimental study in dogs. J Bone Joint Surg 66A:1421-1430, 1984
95. O'Brien BMcC: Microvascular free small joint transfer. pp. 284-289. In Microvascular Reconstructive Surgery, Churchill Livingstone, New York, 1977
96. O'Brien BMcC, Gould JS, Morrison WA, Russel RC, MacLeod AM, Pribaz JJ: Free vascularized small joint transfer to the hand. J Hand Surg 9A:634-641, 1984
97. Pap K, Kronpecher S: Arthroplasty of the knee. Experimental and clinical experiences. J Bone Joint Surg 43A:523-530, 1961
98. Parrish FF: Treatment of bone tumours by total excision and replacement with massive autogenous and homologous grafts. J Bone Joint Surg 48A:968-972, 1966
99. Peacock EE: Reconstructive surgery of hands with injured metacarpophalangeal Joints. J Bone Joint Surg 38A:291-302, 1956
100. Planas J: Free transplantation of the finger joints. Rev Espan Cir Plast 1:21-26, 1968
101. Porter BB, Lance EL: Limb and joint transplantation. A review of research and clinical experience. Clin Orthop 104:249-274, 1974
102. Pritzker KPH, Gross AE, Langer F, Luk SC, Houpt JB: Articular cartilage transplantation. Hum Pathol 8:635-651, 1977
103. Rank BK: Long term results of epiphyseal transplants in congenital deformities of the hand. Plast Reconstr Surg 61:321-329, 1978
104. Reeves B: Studies of vascularized homotransplants of the knee joint. J Bone Joint Surg 1968, 50B:226-227
105. Reeves B: Orthotopic transplantation of vascularised whole knee-joints in dogs. Lancet 1:500-502, 1969
106. Rinaldi E: Metacarpal loss treated by metatarsal substitution. Ital J Orthop Trauma 2:335-340, 1976
107. Ring PA: Transplantation of epiphyseal cartilage; an experimental study. J Bone Joint Surg 37B:642-647, 1955
108. Roffe JL, Latil F, Chamant M, Huguet JF, Bureau H: Intérêt chirurgical de l'etude radio-anatomique de la vascularisation artérielle de l'avant-pied. Ann Chir Main 1:84-87, 1982
109. Rutishauser E, Taillard W: L'ischémie articulaire en pathologie humaine et expérimentale. La notion de pannus vasculaire. Rev Chir Orthop 52:197-223, 1966
110. Sarrafian SK, Topouzian LK: Anatomy and physiology of the extensor apparatus of the toes. J Bone Joint Surg 51A:669-679, 1969
111. Schreiber A, Walker N, Nishikawa M: Autologe Gelenkenstransplantationen mit mikrochirurgischer Gefassplastik. Helv Chir Acta 43:151-155, 1976
112. Schreiber A, Walker N, Nishikawa M, Yargarsil MG: Transplantation d'articulation avec la technique de microchirurgie vasculaire. Acta Orthop Belg 45:403-411, 1979
113. Seki T, Yoshizu T, Shibata M, Tanaka H, Tajima T: Long term follow-up of free vascularized toe joint to the hand in children (abstract). J Reconstr Microsurg 4:457, 1988
114. Seligman GM, George E, Yablon I, Nutik G, Cruess RL: Transplantation of whole knee joints in the dog. Clin Orthop 87:332-334, 1972
115. Singer DI, O'Brien BMcC: McLeod AM, Morrison WA, Angel MF: Long-term follow-up of free vascularized joint transfers to the hand in children. J Hand Surg 13A:776-783, 1988
116. Slome D, Reeves B: Experimental homotransplantation of the knee-joint. Lancet 2:205, 1966
117. Smith PJ, Jones BM: Free vascularised transfer of a metatarsophalangeal joint to the hand. A technical modification. J Hand Surg 10B:109-112, 1985
118. Snowdy HA, Omer GE, Sherman FC: Longitudinal growth of a free toe phalanx transplant to a finger. J Hand Surg 5:71-73, 1980
119. Straub GF: Anatomical survival, growth and physiological function of an epiphyseal bone transplant. Surg Gynecol Obstet 48:687-690, 1929
120. Swanson AB: Arthroplasty in traumatic arthritis of the joints of the hand. Orthop Clin North Am 1:285-298, 1970
121. Tietze A: Ersatz des Resezierten Unteren Radiusendes durch eine Grosszehenphalange. Chir Kongre Verhandl 1:77-81, 1902
122. Tomita Y, Tsai T-M, Steyers C, Ogden L, Jupiter JB, Kutz JE: The role of the epiphyseal and metaphyseal circulations on longitudinal growth in the dog: An experimental study. J Hand Surg 11A: 375-382
123. Tsai T-M, Hanna D: Free vascularized joint transfers. pp. 397-402. In Brunelli G (ed): Textbook of Microsurgery. Masson, Milano, 1988
124. Tsai T-M, Jupiter JB, Kutz JE, Kleinert HE: Vascularized autogenous whole joint transfer in the hand. A clinical study. J Hand Surg 7:335-342, 1982
125. Tsai T-M, Ogden L, Jaeger SH, Okubo K: Experimental vascularized total joint autografts: A primate study. J Hand Surg 7:140-146, 1982
126. Tsai T-M, Singer R, Elliott E, Klein H: Immediate free vascularized joint transfer from second toe to index finger proximal interphalangeal joint. A case report. J Hand Surg 10B:85-89, 1985
127. Vercauteren ME, Van Vynckt C: A free total toe phalanx transplant to a finger. A case report. J Hand Surg 8:336-339, 1983
128. Volkov M: Allotransplantation of joints. J Bone Joint Surg 52B:49-53, 1970
129. Watanabe M, Katsumi M, Yoshizu T, Tajima T: Experimental study of autogenous toe-joint transplantation. Anatomic study of vascular pattern of toe joints as a base of vascularised autogenous joint transplantation. Orthop Surg 29:1317-1320, 1978

130. Watanabe M, Katsumi M, Yoshizu T, Tajima T: Experimental study and clinical application of free toe-joint transplantation with vascular pedicle. Orthop Surg 31:1411-1416, 1980
131. Whitesides ES: Normal growth in a transplanted epiphysis. Case report with 13 year follow-up. J Bone Joint Surg 59A:546-547, 1977
132. Wilson JN: Epiphyseal transplantation. A clinical study. J Bone Joint Surg 48A:245-256, 1966
133. Wilson JN, Smith CF: Transplantation of whole autogenous joints in the hand. J Bone Joint Surg 48A:1651-1654, 1966
134. Worsing RA, Engber WD, Lange TA: Reactive synovitis from particulate silastic. J Bone Joint Surg 64A:581-585, 1982
135. Wray RC, Mathes SM, Young VL, Weeks PM: Free vascularized whole joint transplants with ununited epiphyses. Plast Reconstr Surg 67:519-525, 1981
136. Wray RC, Young VL: Drug treatment and flap survival. Plast Reconstr Surg 73:939-942, 1984
137. Yablon IG, Brandt KD, Delellis R, Covall D: Destruction of joint homografts. An experimental study. Arthritis Rheum 20:1526-1537, 1977
138. Yoshizu T, Watanabe M, Tajima T: Etude expérimentale et applications cliniques des transferts libres d'articulation d'orteil avec anastomoses vasculaires. pp. 539-551. In Chirurgie de la Main, Tome II. Ed. Tubiana, Masson, Paris, 1984
139. Zaleske DJ: Revascularized joint transplants. pp. 377-385. In Friedlender, Mankin, Sell (eds): Osteochondreal Allografts. Little Brown, Boston, 1983
140. Zaleske DJ, Ehrlich MG, Piliero C, May JW, Mankin HJ: Growth plate behavior in whole joint replantation in the rabbit. J Bone Joint Surg 64A:249-258, 1982
141. Zrubecky: Freie Verpflanzung von zehengelenken in der Hand. Hand Chirurgie 2:67-71, 1970

32

Microneural Reconstruction of the Brachial Plexus

Vincent R. Hentz

Advances in the reconstruction of complex nerve lesions have paralleled somewhat the advances in small vessel or microsurgery, benefiting from the same technical achievements in optics, sutures, and microsurgical instruments that have made microsurgery possible. While it is somewhat erroneous to associate the use of nerve grafts with the development of the operating microscope (Bunnell[10] reported on his experience in nerve grafts for reconstructing digital nerve injuries in 1926), clearly the major forward thrust in microneurosurgical reconstruction for nerve lesions of the hand and upper limb has come about because of the surgeon's ability to better visualize anatomic detail. Fine instruments have allowed the dissection of the delicate structures of a multifascicular nerve without causing or extending injury. Magnification has allowed the distinguishing between injured and healthy nerve more readily. Indeed the entire concept of interfascicular nerve repair and interfascicular nerve grafting owes its existence to the development of microsurgical techniques and technology.

The significant early advances in the reconstruction of nerve lesions are attributed to Hanno Millesi[45] of Vienna, Austria, who, in 1972, published in the English literature his results using interfascicular nerve graft techniques in a series of complex injuries of the median and ulnar nerve. Although the first mention of a clinical attempt at grafting a large defect in a peripheral nerve predates this article by more than 100 years,[27] Millesi's results[45,46] set the standard for years to come, and many consider him the father of microneurosurgical reconstruction of complex injuries of the upper limb.

Associated with the development of microneurosurgical techniques have been advances in the clinician's ability to diagnose the extent of peripheral nerve lesions, especially those that would benefit from early surgical intervention. Modern electrodiagnostic methods,[9,39,69,70] diagnostic imaging techniques,[12] and intraoperative histochemical analyses[11,18,25,26,55] have measurably improved surgical decision-making. These improvements, together with the associated advances in surgical techniques, in many instances have altered previously pessimistic attitudes about a number of complex nerve lesions.

INJURIES SUITABLE FOR MICRONEURAL RECONSTRUCTION

While microneurosurgical techniques are appropriate for the repair of almost any nerve lesion (i.e., atraumatic handling of tissues that magnification permits, fine sutures, and others), the application of these techniques in several complex peripheral nerve lesions has resulted in significant changes in the philosophy of management of such challenging problems as injuries to the brachial plexus in both infants and adults, and the management of very long peripheral nerve defects following trauma or associated with tumor ablation and limb salvage procedures. The remainder of this chapter will be devoted to a discussion of the management of several representative problems.

RECONSTRUCTION OF TRACTION INJURIES

Pathology of The Lesion

Traction injuries of the brachial plexus may be associated with varying amounts of energy imparted to the plexus.[38] Low energy injuries, such as a fall onto the shoulder, typically cause more or less reversible injuries such as neuropraxia[59] (Sunderland[62] level I) or various degrees of axonotmesis (Sunderland levels II–IV.) High energy injuries—for example, being thrown from a speeding motorcycle—are associated with more significant injuries, including rupture of plexal segments at any level (Sunderland level V), or avulsions of nerve roots from the spinal cord (Fig. 32-1). While some spontaneous recovery may occur in these circumstances, it is for these patients that microneurosurgical reconstruction may play a role.

The typical candidate for microneural reconstruction is the young man who falls from his motorcycle.[4] Although his helmet saves his life, it cannot prevent his shoulder from being driven downward and posteriorly and his neck from being driven in the opposite direction as he strikes the ground, guardrail, or fencepost. The force of the blow is imparted first to those structures having the most direct or straightest course from spine to arm, in this case, the C8 and T1 roots and their continuation as the interior trunk. The lowest energy and tension is imparted to the C5 and C6 roots because of the comparitively longer course and greater distance between points of fixation in the neck and arm.[61] The C7 root and associated middle trunk is intermediate in its course. Anatomic studies have also determined that the supporting tissues anchoring the upper roots to the vertebral foramina are significantly stronger about the C5 and C6 roots than more distally.[35] This anatomic arrangement predicts that the lower structures of the brachial plexus would suffer more significant injuries than more proximally located roots, trunks, and cords, and this is what has been observed clinically. The T1 and C8 roots are more likely to be avulsed from the spinal cord,[31] while the C6 and C5 roots are more likely to stretch or rupture in-continuity after exiting the spinal foramina (Table 32-1). The principle factor determining the extent of injury is the energy of the blow and, to a lesser degree, the direction and the relationship of arm to body.

Table 32-1. Operative Findings for Each Root

Root	Ruptured	Avulsed	Other
C5	59	14	40
C6	44	35	35
C7	39	53	20
C8	11	67	31
T1	11	61	37

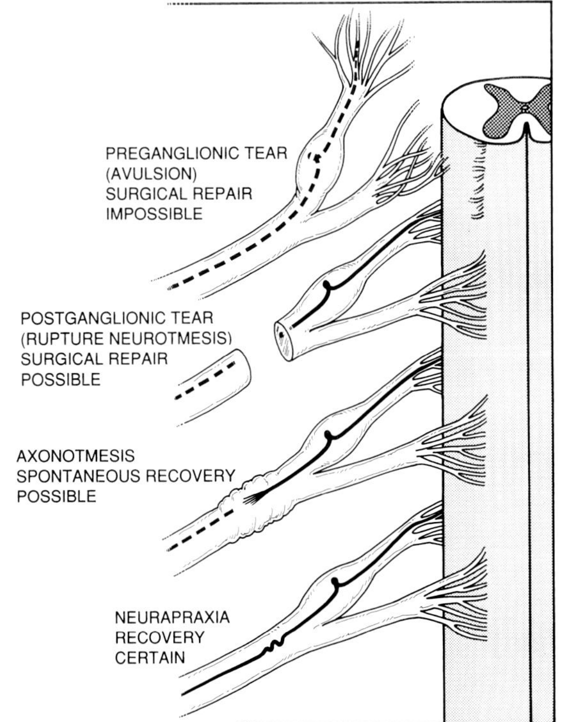

Fig. 32-1. In the same patient, a severe traction to the brachial plexus may cause nerve injuries of varying severity, including avulsion of the nerve root from the spinal cord (nonrepairable), extraforaminal rupture of the root or trunk (surgically repairable), or an intraneural rupture of fascicles (some spontaneous recovery possible.)

In the same patient, essentially every Sunderland level of injury, plus root avulsion can occur (Fig. 32-1). For example, the T1 and C8 roots may be avulsed, the C7 root or middle trunk ruptured (Sunderland V), with the upper trunk remaining intact but with varying degrees of internal damage, including some axon populations that are merely confused, and other fascicles having suffered various levels of axonotmesis injury (Sunderland II–IV.) No spontaneous recovery will occur in the C7, C8, or T1 derived muscles and sensory end organs, while varying degrees of spontaneous recovery *may* occur in those structures receiving innervation from axons of the upper trunk, again over widely varying periods of time, depending on whether or not the axon must regenerate to the motor endplate or the sensory end organ (a few weeks to a few years.)

The same energy may also fracture the transverse processes of the cervical vertebrae (though this is more likely an avulsion of the origins of scaleneus muscles), the clavicle, and the scapula. All are associated with a high-energy injury and concomitantly, significant injury to the brachial plexus.

Evaluation of the Patient

History

The typical candidate for microneural reconstruction presents with a total or near total unilateral palsy of the brachial plexus. For this patient, the goal of the examination is to determine, as accurately as possible, the extent of the nerve injury, and from this, determine whether or not he is a candidate for either early surgical reconstruction of the brachial plexus or a period of further observation. As mentioned in the preceding section, a good history of the mechanism of injury is helpful in determining the severity of injury. If associated with serious injury, a thorough search for more life-threatening injuries should be conducted before concentrating on the obvious. Germane are questions regarding loss of consciousness, and the presence of paresthesias or weakness in other extremities. Loss of consciousness may suggest the presence of an associated head injury. Occasionally, injury to the brain or to the cervical spinal cord may mimic a brachial plexus injury. In this situation there may be other long tract signs, such as weakness in other extremities. These signs must be evaluated both immediately after injury and at a later time, such as the initial outpatient consultation.

Special Physical Signs

One important indicator of severity of injury is the presence of a Horner's sign (Fig. 32-2) on the affected side. This may be present immediately, but occasionally is not readily apparent for 3 to 4 days following injury. A Horner's sign indicates severe injury to the C8 and T1 roots, and has been strongly correlated with avulsion of one or both of these roots.[31] Severe pain in an anesthetic extremity is also a sign of poor prognosis, indicating some degree of deafferentiation of the limb, and strongly correlates with root avulsion. Additional special presentations include a shift of the head on the shoulder away from the injured side. The patient may present with an abnormal posture of the head and neck characterized by a shift of the head and neck toward the unaffected side, almost like the position of the Balinese dancer, and caused by an imbalance in the unopposed pull of the contralateral paraspinous muscles. This is evidence of denervation of the paraspinous muscles on the side of the lesion, also strongly associated with severe nerve injury such as root avulsion.

Stability of the glenohumeral joint should also be assessed. Shoulder dislocation occurs frequently with trauma associated with brachial plexus injuries, and an inferior or posterior dislocation may add to the severity of the nerve injury by avulsing the axillary nerve from the deltoid muscle or rupturing it in its posterior course around the humerus.

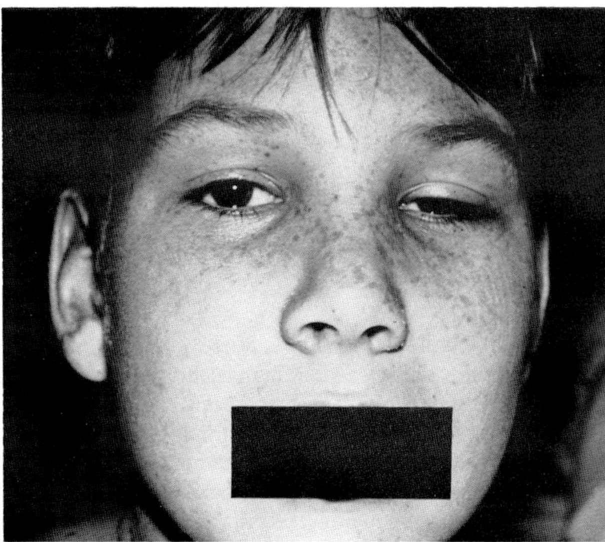

Fig. 32-2. The presence of a Horner's sign, (lagopthalmus, meiosis, and anhydrosis) is felt to indicate probable avulsion of the C8, T1 roots.

Motor and Sensory Examination

The metameric organization of innervation of the muscles of the upper extremity is well known, and there exist many charts or maps of sensory or motor innervation to assist in predicting the location of nerve lesions. It is not usually necessary to test all individual muscles; rather, it is more helpful to assess functional groups of muscles, such as the external or internal rotators of the shoulder, flexers of the elbow, and others. Two important indicators of the level of injury, especially for the patient with near total palsy, are the presence or absence of activity of the rhomboids, and serratus anterior muscles. Likewise, we are usually unconcerned with definitive tests for sensation, such as two-point discrimination, depending more on rapidly accomplished tests such as sharp-dull discrimination.

Several systems useful in recording the result of the examination of the injured brachial plexus have been published[49] (Fig. 32-3). It must be kept in mind that these charts represent the idealized or average situation, and that individual variations in plexus anatomy exist. For example, significant innervation may come from the C4 root, termed a prefixed plexus, or from the T2 root, termed a postfixed plexus.

Radiography

It is necessary to x-ray the cervical spine and frequently the chest, clavicle, and scapula. The chest x-ray should include an inspiration and expiration AP view to determine the activity of the diaphragm. A paralyzed diaphragm is an indicator of severe injury to the upper roots of the plexus. The presence of fractures of the transverse processes, as mentioned above, is also strong evidence of a high energy injury.

Imaging Studies for Plexus Injuries: Computed Tomography, Magnetic Resonance Imaging, Myelography

Modern imaging techniques have improved the clinician's ability to predict what the microneurosurgeon will find at exploration. Traditional myelography using metrizimide[38] contrast has been largely supplanted by computed tomography (CT) or magnetic resonance imaging (MRI) examinations, performed with and without contrast agents (Fig. 32-4). Both CT and MRI are useful. MRI reformatting provides a better picture of the soft tissues, particularly the T2-weighted images that highlight the fat content of the cervical spinal cord and nerve roots, but also the T1-image highlighting the water content associated with a pseudomeningocoele. The value of MRI is still very technique-dependent, and a technically excellent study is more difficult to obtain than a technically competent CT scan, especially one with intradural contrast. We continue to obtain MRI evaluations in order to learn more about the proper indications for these techniques. I suggest consulting

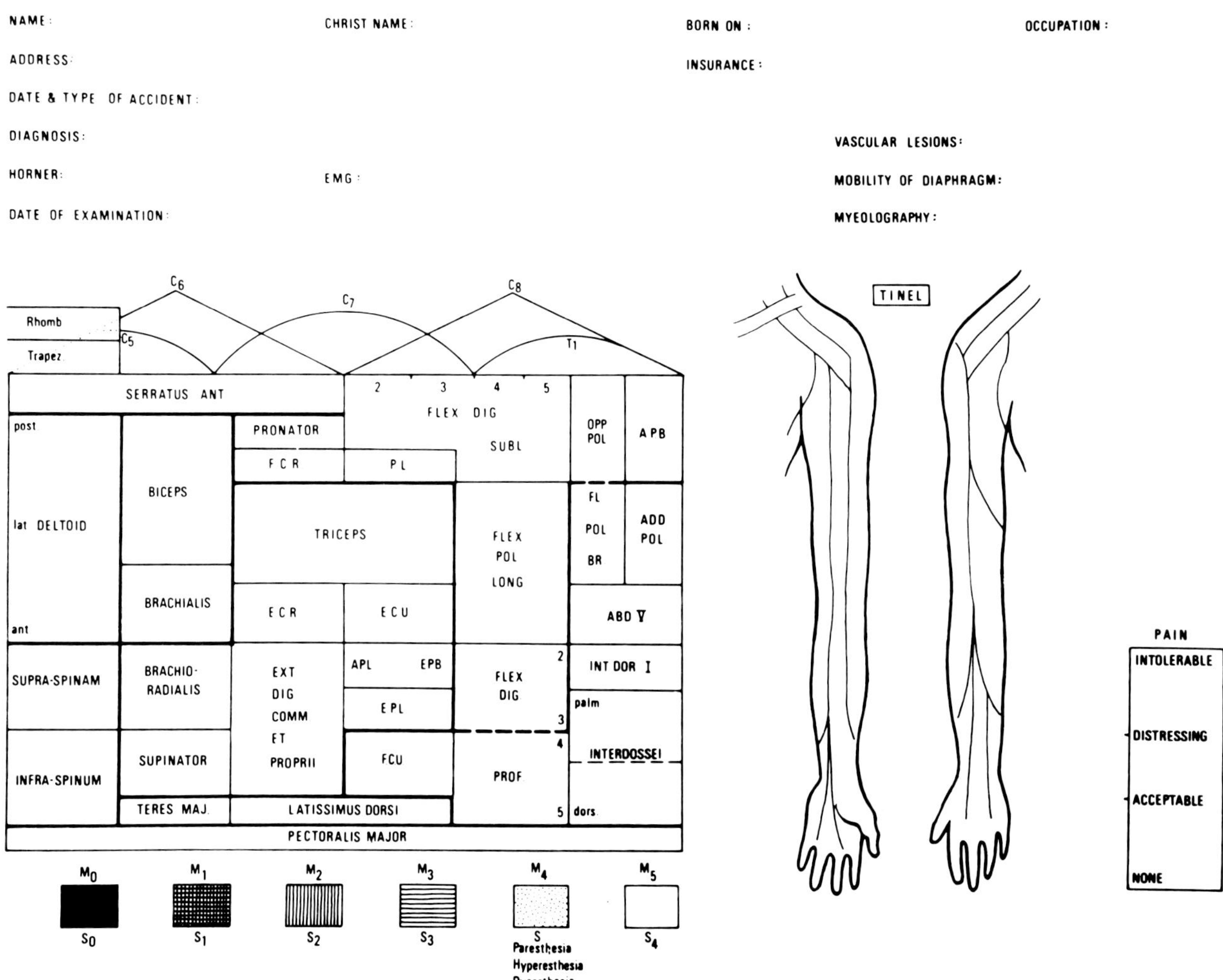

Fig. 32-3. It is critical to document accurately the motor and sensory findings prior to surgery and the progression of change following injury and/or surgery. Most surgeons use some variation of this format introduced by Merle d'Aubinge to record the data.

with your neuroradiologist regarding which technique they feel is more appropriate and more reliable in their hands.

The presence of a pseudomeningocoele has been strongly correlated with avulsion of the corresponding root (Fig. 32-5). When these tests are performed within a few days of injury, especially with contrast, there may be a higher incidence of false-positive interpretations because the contrast agent may leak through small tears in the dura, not necessarily associated with avulsion of the root.

Other evidence of significant injury include empty-appearing root sleeves, or a shift of the cord in one direction or another away from the midline. Almost all this information is obtained from the coronal views of the cervical spine. It is frequently difficult to obtain sufficient concentration of the contrast agent to clearly visualize the C4 and occasionally the C5 root area,[5] however. Some centers have been able to generate beautiful fronted plane orthographic representations of the entire brachial plexus that might allow a very detailed analysis of the extent of injury. With improvements in coil design and software, these reformats may become more available.

Sensory and Motor Evoked Potentials

These tests should be carried out after several days to weeks following injury, to allow Wallerian degeneration to proceed. Several different tests may be helpful in determining the severity of the injury. Standard electromyography (EMG) is not as helpful for severe injuries as sensory evoked potentials, corticosensory evoked potentials, and spinograms.[37] For example, if the sensory evoked potential examination demonstrates that the ulnar nerve is capable of conducting a compound action potential in the presence of electrically unexcitable muscles and ulnar anesthesia, this is strong evidence that a pregangli-

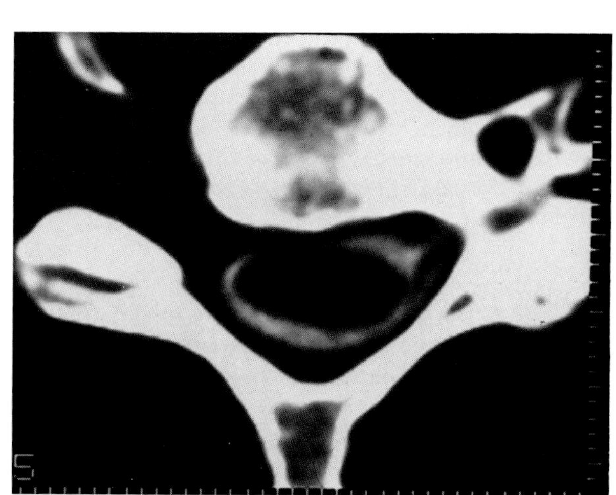

A

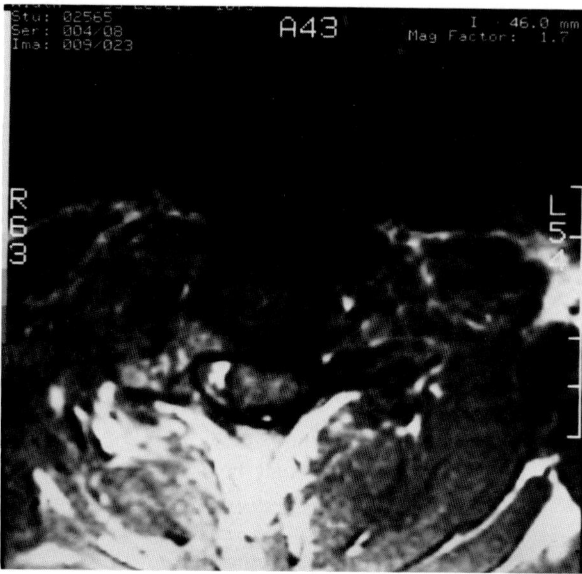

B

Fig. 32-4. **(A)** Computed tomography of the cervical spine with contrast demonstrates avulsion of a part of the transverse process and absence of a root shadow at the C6 level. This appearance suggests that the C6 root has been avulsed. **(B)** The MRI image with contrast demonstrates a pool of contrast where the root should be, indicating the presence of a small pseudomeningocoele and probable avulsion of the root.

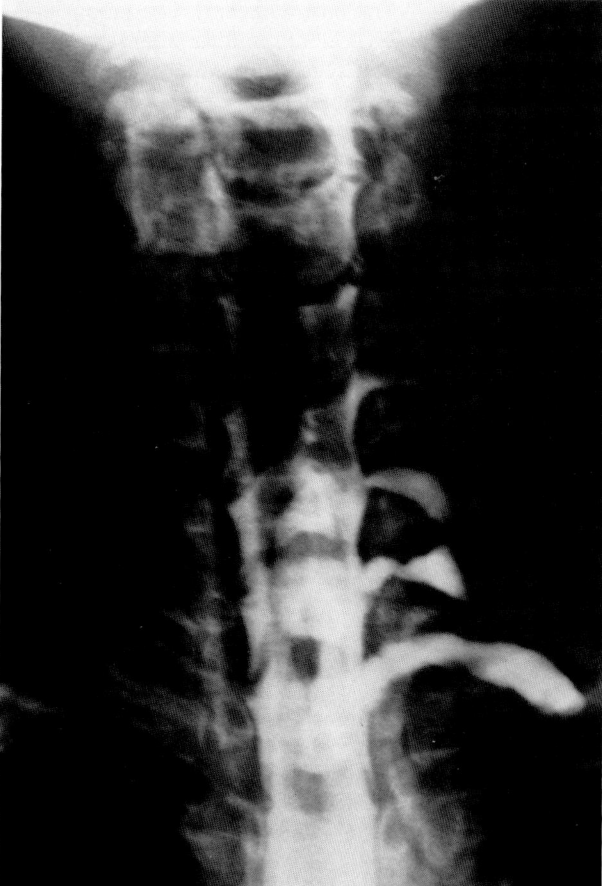

Fig. 32-5. Standard cervical myelogram demonstrating multiple large pseudomeningocoeles at several levels. Note the normal root shadows on the contralateral side.

onic injury, usually signifying root avulsion, exists. In this case, some of the sensory axons remain capable of conducting (they haven't undergone Wallerian degeneration because they are still connected to their dorsal root ganglion cells) but they are disconnected from the spinal cord and thus the brain. Similarly, stimulating over Erb's point in the supraclavicular fossa and recording signals from the cortex using scalp electrodes is evidence that some roots may still be in continuity with the spinal cord.

The spinogram can determine information about the level of innervation of the paraspinous muscles. Since these are innervated by the posterior primary rami of the plexus, paralysis of these muscles indicates a very proximal injury, but does not tell the examiner whether the injury is associated with avulsion, rupture, or axonotmesis.

No one test can be the conclusive basis for surgical decision-making. All the information must be assimilated and, most importantly, be viewed within the context of the presumed energy of the trauma.

Indications for Surgery

A sufficient number of reviews of the results of exploration of traction injuries of the brachial plexus have now been published to allow us to make some assessment as to the indications for and value of plexus reconstruction.[1,2,42,43,49,51,56,60] Most of these series attest to the inverse relationship between time from injury to operation to outcome. In cautious and skilled hands, exploration seldom results in extension of the injury. Even when total palsy exists, less than 20 percent of patients demonstrate avulsions of all five roots (Table 32-2) of the plexus,[31] meaning that for the great majority the surgeon will find something to repair, graft, and/or neurotize with a non-plexus nerve source. If neurotization is considered, then virtually 100 percent of patients might theoretically benefit from microneural reconstruction. These factors imply that when there is a strong suspicion of significant damage to the plexus, in the form of root avulsions and nerve ruptures, surgical exploration is warranted.

Controversial Indications

Occasionally a patient presents with a partial C8 and complete T1 lesion, with some finger flexers working, but with essentially an intrinsic palsy and anesthesia in the C8 and/or T1 distribution. This represents somewhat of a dilemma in decision-making because it seems almost impossible to recover intrinsic muscle function in the adult and, when injured, the C8 and T1 nerve roots are so often avulsed from the spinal cord that it is unlikely that anything repairable or even worth repairing will be found at surgery. Beyond the age of 15, I have preferred to reserve plexus surgery with the partial C8 and T1 lesion for the patient experiencing extraordinary and disabling pain. I and others[53] have found that an occasional patient has less pain following exploration, even if minimal reconstruction can be performed. For the others, I offer more standard muscle-tendon transfers.

Table 32-2. Frequently Occurring Patterns of Injury in Total Palsy (107 cases)

C5 ruptured; C6–T1 avulsed	9
C5, 6 ruptured; C7–T1 avulsed	13
C5–7 ruptured; C8, T1 avulsed	13
All roots avulsed	8
All roots ruptured	6
All roots intact (distal injury)	14

Contraindications

A key question is, "Are there contraindications to exploration of the brachial plexus?" Is the age of the patient an absolute contraindication? Aside from such issues as general health, there are few contraindications in terms of risk to still functioning nerve elements, at least in experienced hands. Surgeons involved in plexus injuries uniformly express agreement that, in the adult, loss of function secondary to nerve exploration is unusual, and in experienced hands, it is a minimal risk. The surgery, while sometimes lengthy, is not particularly stressful, at least to the patient. Clearly the value of exploration must be weighed against the potential gain, and this is a multifactorial analysis that must take into account such variables as the time since injury and the distance between injured nerve and functional end organ, among others. There is no hard rule regarding the value and timing of exploration, only the guidelines presented above, guidelines very similar to those governing our management of any peripheral nerve injury.

Timing of Surgery

Immediate Surgery

The timing of exploration is controversial. Immediate surgery is indicated for essentially any patient with a plexus injury of almost any degree of severity secondary to a penetrating injury, such as a stab wound, or following an iatrogenic injury, such as known or suspected injury to the plexus at the time of first rib resection for the treatment of thoracic outlet syndrome. Occasionally, the reconstructive surgeon is afforded the opportunity to make an early assessment of the degree of damage, for example, when vascular reconstruction of a ruptured subclavian or axillary artery is to be performed by the vascular surgeons at the time of injury. In this instance the vascular surgeon's incisions may be extended as described below, the supraclavicular fossa explored, the degree of damage mapped, various structures tagged by metal markers such as vascular clips, and preliminary plans for secondary reconstruction begun. It is critical that the reconstructive surgeon be involved in this emergency procedure, both to take advantage of the opportunity afforded to assess nerve damage, and also to guide the vascular surgeon in the dissection of the distal vessel in its intimate association with the components of the plexus, and in his placement of any vein grafts that might be necessary in vascular reconstruction. Few surgical procedures are more tedious than reopening a wound several weeks or months later and dissecting a relatively thin-walled vein graft that has been placed in the most direct and convenient (for the vascular surgeon) spot, (i.e., always superficial to the plexus). With your help and guidance, the vascular surgeon can pass the vein graft deep to the injured elements of the plexus, keeping this structure out of the reconstructive surgeon's eventual path to the plexus, and thus out of harm's way.

There are many arguments against immediate reconstruction of the plexus in traction injuries. Most surgeons[2,43,51] feel that some period of time must pass to permit the surgeon to be able to delineate injured from noninjured nerve. If events convince me that exploration is indicated after the typical motorcycle accident, I prefer to wait about 6 to 8 weeks following injury, both to allow time for diagnostic tests and to permit the patient some period of time in which to "live" with the injury. This includes the presence of features associated with a high energy injury in the context of a total plexus palsy. If the initial assessment proves incorrect, (i.e., the patient begins to recover function in previously paralyzed muscles), then a further period of observation is indicated. On the other hand, if more distal muscles begin to recover in the absence of any recovery in more proximal muscles, this also is a strong indication for early exploration. The value of sequential EMG studies is not clear to me because these almost always overestimate the potential for functional recovery. A sequential clinical exam is far more valuable.

Because the functional results of reconstruction of severe plexus injuries are, on average, so disappointing when compared to the function of the normal limb, having lived with a flail limb for some time may create a better acceptance of the ultimate functional limitations of microneural reconstruction.

Early Surgery

Early surgery is indicated for patients who present with total or near total palsy, or an injury associated with high energy levels. It is also indicated for gunshot wounds to the plexus. For those injuries associated with lower levels of energy and those associated with partial upper level palsy, I prefer to follow the course of recovery for 3 to 6 months, leaning toward operation if recovery seems to plateau as determined by several successive evaluations carried out at monthly intervals. These patients are more likely to have suffered in-continuity stretch lesions that are associated with a reasonable probability of useful spontaneous regeneration. The key to decision-making is a careful exam and a careful recording of the results by the same observer. The presence or absence of an advancing Tinel's sign can be a useful guide. The absence of a Tinel's sign in the supraclavicular fossa in the face of a nearly complete C5–6 level palsy is a poor prognostic sign for spontaneous recovery and warrants an early exploration, with the likelihood that C5 and C6 nerve roots may be avulsed. In this case, neurotization will be necessary. An alternative is to turn immediately to such secondary salvage procedures as shoulder fusion and perhaps muscle tendon transfers for elbow flexion, if these are possible.

Operative Technique

Patient Preparation and Informed Consent

The patient and family must be made aware of the relative low order of performance expected following surgery. They also must be made aware of the long period of waiting for reinnervation of muscles, when essentially nothing happens that the patient can appreciate. Prior to surgery, the patient should have been taught the exercises necessary to maintain a normal range of motion of the paralyzed joints, rather than depending on another person such as the therapist to perform these exercises for him. The therapist can teach and advise and record progress, but the patient must accept responsibility for performing the exercises.

Only if the patient has had a previous subclavian artery reconstruction, will I obtain a unit of autologous blood prior to surgery. Even so, the need for intraoperative or postoperative transfusion is rare. Otherwise, no special preoperative preparations are necessary.

Positioning of the Patient and Microscope

If possible, the electrodes for intraoperative corticosensory evoked potentials are placed prior to the patient's arrival in the operating room. This permits the neurologist or technician to test the equipment, electrodes, and electrode placement. Once the scalp electrode positions are confirmed, we occasionally remove the adhesive-backed electrodes and replace them with a spiral barbed electrode that is less likely to be displaced during movement of the patient's head. These are placed after induction of anesthesia.

The nature of the case, particularly the indeterminate length of the procedure and the need to perform intraoperative stimulation and recordings, are discussed with the anesthesiologist well ahead of time. This allows the anesthesiologist to alter techniques and agents. There are few more disconcerting moments than to find that the patient has been given a relatively long-acting paralytic agent as you are about to begin nerve stimulation. The anesthesiologist is instructed in the need to reposition the patient's head at intervals to avoid the possibility of causing scalp ischemia and hair loss.

The patient is placed supine on the operating table with the head supported on a circular roll or head rest. A small roll is placed behind the scapula. The head is turned somewhat away from the side of the lesion and the neck is extended. It is important not to maximally turn the head, as this distorts the anatomy and tenses muscles, making retraction difficult. The ipsilateral shoulder is retracted downward to lower the clavicle in preparation for the supraclavicular dissection. The affected limb is draped free and supported on one armboard that is maintained parallel to the operating table. Extending the armboard at right angles to the operating table creates an impediment about the field. A formal hand table is an even bigger nuisance. The endotracheal tube is brought directly over the patient's nose and central forehead; its profile is kept as low as possible so that the assistant opposite the surgeon does not have to work over this.

A well-padded tourniquet is placed on both thighs in preparation for harvesting sural nerve grafts and both legs are draped free to the tourniquet. Other surgeons[21,47] have recommended that if the likelihood of using sural nerve grafts is high, that the operation begin by initially placing the patient prone, harvesting both sural nerves, closing these wounds, applying dressings and then turning the patient to the supine position as described above. This may be reasonable if the surgeon lacks a sufficient number of assistants. We usually have a second team harvesting the sural nerve grafts after the need has been established, and while the initial surgeons prepare the recipient sites.

I use a combination of vertical and horizontal incisions over the course of the sural nerve; harvesting both the sural nerve and its peroneal derived branch[71] is relatively rapid. The distal portion of the nerve can be harvested by flexing and maximally internally rotating the hip. The upper portion is dissected as one assistant holds the leg elevated by resting it on his shoulder, assisting with skin retraction while the other assistant harvests the nerve. This part of the operation is carried out under tourniquet control. The skin wounds are rapidly closed with skin staples, and the legs are wrapped in elastic bandages and slightly elevated prior to releasing the tourniquet. It is the responsibility of all the surgeons and other OR personnel to make certain that the leg tourniquets are deflated after harvesting the nerve grafts.

We employ an operating microscope with a longer than usual arm and position it at the head of the table on the side opposite the lesion. The microscope stand serves as an anchor for one side of the surgical drapes, and the microscope's head can be easily swung into position at the appropriate times. We frequently move the microscope head in and out of the field to assist in decision-making. A few minutes spent at the beginning of the case in properly positioning the microscope for both surgeon and assistant comfort pays huge dividends later in the case. The microscope head frequently must be angled in one direction or another for good visualization; this can usually be predetermined.

Incisions and Surgical Dissection

A relatively standard incision is employed by most surgeons and is pictured in Figure 32-6. I routinely infiltrate the proposed line of the incision with an 1 : 200,000 solution of epinephrine prior to the skin preparation and scratch a few cross hatch marks at key points to assist in properly closing the incision. The skin is so lax in the neck and axilla that accurate closure can be difficult without these roadmaps. Crosshatching the line of incision with a marking pen is usually fruitless. The marks have long since disappeared at closing time.

The superior limb of the incision parallels the posterior border of the stemocleidmastoid muscle but angles away from the inferior border as depicted. The incision then parallels the clavicle, crossing the clavicle at the level of the coracoid process. A slightly zigzagged limb more or less parallels the deltopectoral groove to the anterior axillary fold, where it parallels the axillary fossa to the midpoint of the medial upper arm. At this point it turns distally, paralleling the brachial artery. The entire incision drawn though the dissection is occasionally limited to only the supraclavicular area.

The initial incision splits the platysma muscle, avoiding the external jugular vein. The platysma is elevated to expose the fibers of the sternocleidomastoid (SCM) muscle. The muscle is rolled somewhat medially exposing the superficial layer of the deep cervical fascia. Several landmarks are helpful in centering the dissection over the appropriate area. The rami of the cervical plexus are visualized as they exit the fascia along the posterior border of the SCM. The largest of these usually arises from the fourth or occasionally the fifth cervical root. As the superficial layer of the deep cervical fascia is opened, the cervical fat pad and the omohyoid muscle is encountered (Fig. 32-6). The muscle is divided between ties; the fat pad can be pushed both medially and inferiorly and will usually separate unless the area was affected by a hematoma during the injury. It is an error to try to pull this fatty tissue superiorly because this fat is in association with the mediastinal fat pad and is virtually unending. Only a few small vessels are encountered to this point. With separation of the fat pad the transverse cervical artery and veni comitanti appear. These need to be ligated and divided and the deep layer of the deep cervical fascia opened to expose the anterior and middle scalene muscles (Fig. 32-7). An angled laminectomy-type self-retaining retractor is placed to maintain the exposure.

Normally, one would come upon the superior trunk and suprascapular nerve. In severe traction injuries one finds instead a sheet of whitish scar tissue and fibrotic surfaces of the scaleni. A helpful landmark (Fig. 32-7) in identifying the locations of root stumps in cases of rupture is, for the C5 root, the phrenic nerve (Fig. 32-8). This is found on the surface of the anterior scalene muscle, running parallel to its fibers. A nerve stimulator is helpful in identifying this small nerve. It receives contributions from the C5 root and, by following the nerve superiorly, one may encounter the C5 root or superior trunk. Another approach is to follow medially the large cervical rami which leads to the C4 or occasionally the C5 root level. If the root has ruptures near the foramen, the search can be tedious, with fascicles of injured muscle easily mistaken for nerve. Typically, the C5 root is smaller than the C6 root, which can be found slightly inferiorly and posteriorly to the C5 root. The C5 root may be serpentine in its course, and the C6 and C5 root relationship distorted. Only experience can teach shortcuts to this difficult dissection.

The C7 root is frequently intimately associated with the transverse scapular artery, which may run over the C7 root or middle trunk. The C8 root arises again just inferiorly and posteriorly to the C7 root, and is very slightly above or even with the clavicle. The T1 root is intimately associated with the subclavian artery and appears just posterior to it. If a vascular anastomosis has been done at this level, I typically forego any intensive search for the T1 root, because of the danger of entering the vein graft and the great likelihood that T1 is avulsed. To visualize these lower roots, it is necessary to mobilize the clavicle. It is seldom necessary to osteotomize the clavicle in the adult. Rather, a finger can be inserted under the clavicle to free the tissues, the dissection continued inferior to the clavicle to mobilize the origin of the lateral border of the pectoralis major off the clavicle, and the small subclavius muscle divided and its ends tagged. The finger then penetrates the clavipectoral fascia, and by gently enlarging this tunnel under the clavicle and di-

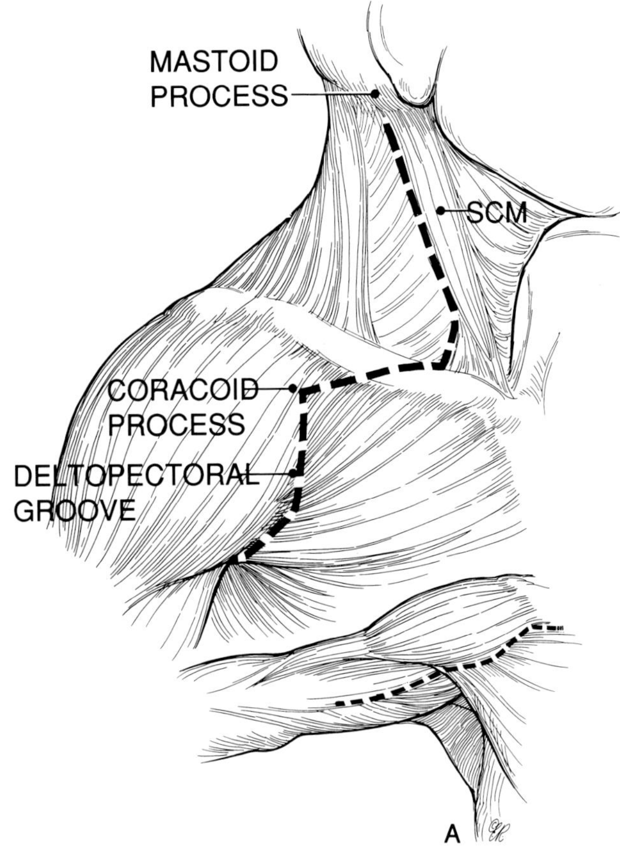

Fig. 32-6. (A) The entire incision is usually made in an adult traction injury. This is necessary to expose adequately the elements of the brachial plexus from vertebral foramen to branch level (B).

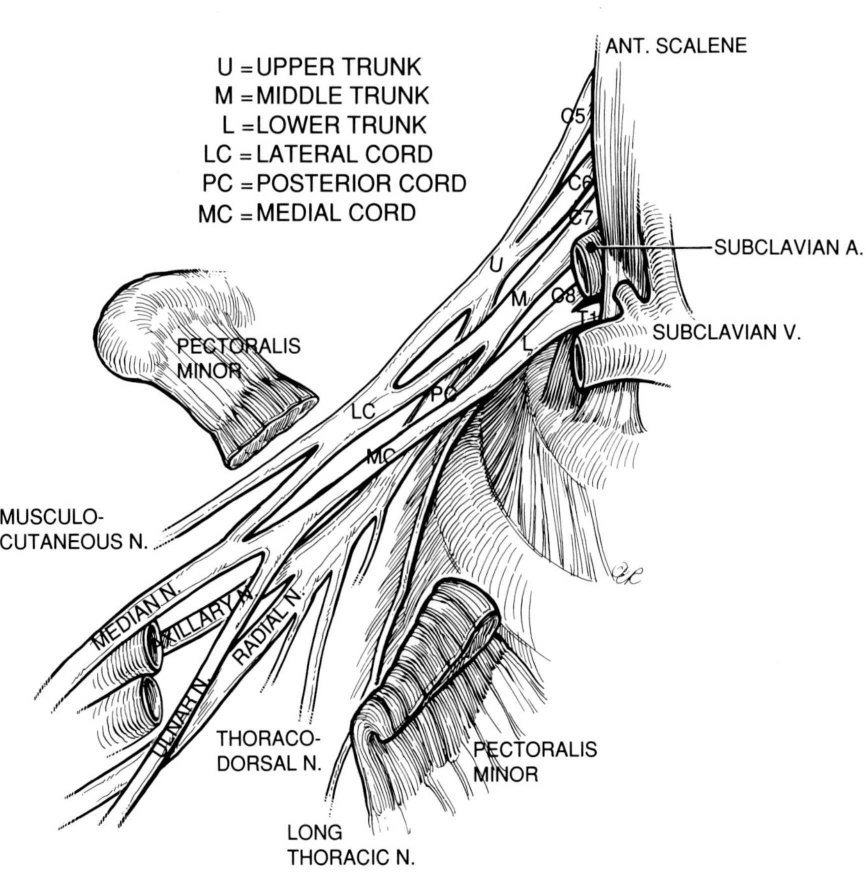

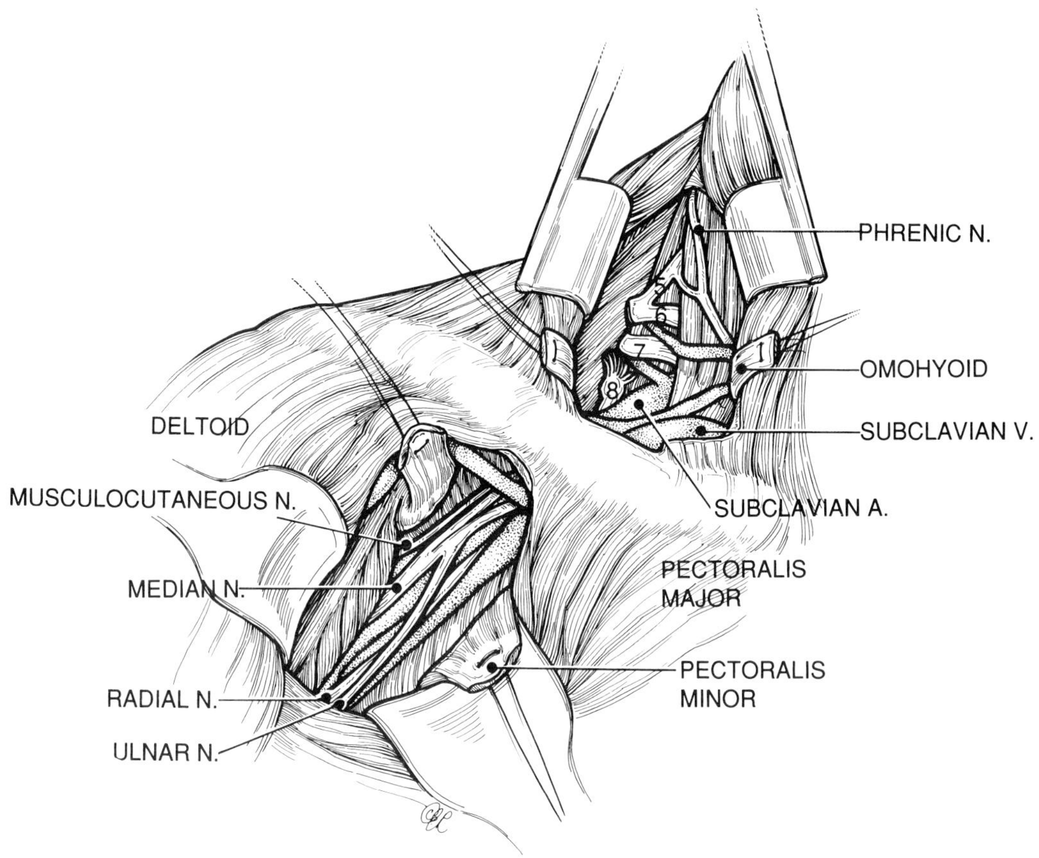

Fig. 32-7. Several key anatomic landmarks to the dissection include the omohyoid muscle and the pectoralis minor muscle, which are divided between ligatures for later reapproximation. The C8 root is located just above and posterior to the subclavian artery while the T1 root is almost directly posterior to the artery. With dissection of the deltopectoral groove, the lateral cord is the most superficial of the structures. The findings of a representative dissection are illustrated. Here, there is a rupture of the superior trunk, and the C7 root. In addition, the C8 root has been avulsed as evidenced by the appearance of rootlets attached to the swollen dorsal root ganglion.

rectly superiorly to the course of the plexus, a moistened 4 × 4 gauze for several turns of umbilical tape can slipped under the clavicle to be used as a retractor. By pulling downward or upwards, the structures deep to the clavicle are better visualized.

A variety of presentations may be seen. If the upper roots are avulsed, the rootlets and swollen dorsal root ganglion may be found twisted, and lying either behind the clavicle or slightly above it in the region of the C8 root (Fig. 32-9). If the upper roots or superior trunk and/or the middle trunk has ruptured, the distal ends typically lie behind the clavicle. The avulsed (often) or ruptured (infrequently) C8 and T1 structures are usually found much closer to their respective foramina than is the case with C5 or C6.

Essentially any combination of injuries may occur, including avulsion, rupture, and a neuroma-in-continuity. The supraclavicular dissection usually allows this assessment. However, it is critical to complete the remainder of the dissection if the findings above favor some type of reconstruction by nerve grafting. There exist a sufficient number of lesions occurring at two levels to encourage this compulsion. For example, rupture of the superior trunk in combination with avulsion of the axillary nerve from the deltoid, or rupture of the musculocutaneous nerve at the level of the shoulder; is not uncommon. Therefore, the deltopectoral groove (Fig. 32-7) is exposed, maintaining the cephalic vein superiorly; the deltoid and pectoralis major separated, exposing the clavipectoral fascia at this level; and the fascia divided, along with some of the dense insertion of the pectoralis major muscle. This space is widened until the origin of the pectoralis minor muscle at the coracoid process is visualized. The separation between pectoralis minor and the coracobrachialis muscle is developed, and a finger slipped behind the pectoralis minor insertion. Two sutures are placed a small distance apart and the tendon of the muscle divided between the two markers. The first structures encountered deep to this are the lateral cord and the subclavian-axillary artery. The remainder of the plexus can be dissected as far distally as is necessary. Additional helpful landmarks include the subscapular trunk off the axillary artery, useful in locating the posterior cord and the posterior branches from the posterior cord, such as the thoracodorsal nerve; and the cir-

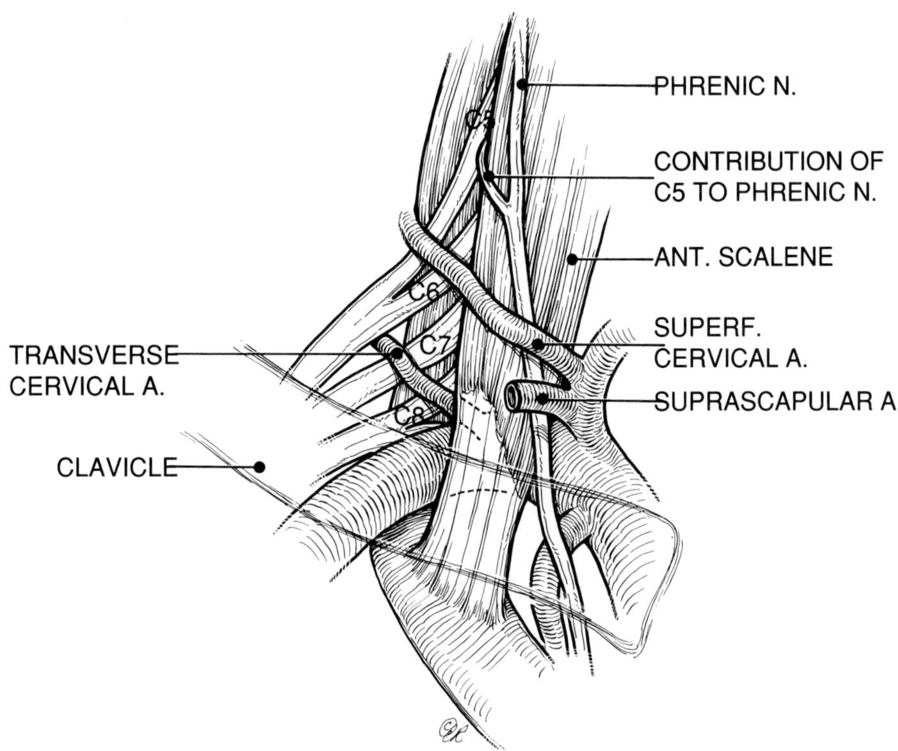

Fig. 32-8. Additional landmarks helpful in identifying the various roots include the phrenic nerve contributions from the C5 root and the transverse cervical (scapular) artery, which frequently cross over the C7 root.

cumflex humeral artery, useful in locating the axillary nerve. By using different colored silicon vessel loops, the various components can be identified. I have found it useful to bring a sterilized drawing of the normal plexus (Fig. 32-6) and to make a sketch of the operative findings on this. We use the same map in planning the priorities in reconstruction; this map is also useful in describing what reconstruction was performed. It is a mistake to depend on memory in dictating the operative note.

Intraoperative Evoked Potentials

At this time we perform intraoperative corticosensory evoked potentials on all structures appearing in-continuity with the spinal cord. For example, what appears to be a ruptured root is placed on electrodes and either 64, 128, or 256 stimulations performed and averaged (Fig. 32-10). We have come to depend heavily on this examination in determining when, for example, an intraforaminal avulsion (uncommon) versus rupture has occurred, or to tell us whether we have found only an empty root sleeve, i.e., only connective tissue with no axons therein (more common.) We also will perform evoked potential studies on neuroma-in-continuity both orthodromically and antidromically. These studies are not as predictable if surgery is carried out soon after injury; however, by 2 to 3 months post injury, we feel these studies are reliable in assisting in decision-making. As suggested by Kline (personal communication, 1989), when stimulating and recording across a neuroma-in-continuity, we no longer feel it necessary to average a large number of stimulations. If we cannot see a response above the noise level we resect the neuroma and *adjacent* damaged nerve, using the microscope to assist in determining when debridement is adequate, and place nerve grafts in the resultant defect. If we can see a clear signal above the background noise, we will perform a neurolysis under magnification. In Kline's experience (personal communication), having to average the recordings to bring a small response out of the background noise implies that too few axons have begun to regenerate or are still in-continuity to allow ultimate recovery of useful function. Table 32-1 describes the operative findings in 114 patients who presented with total plexus palsy and Table 32-2 describes several common patterns of injury in this cohort.

Intraoperative Decisions and Priorities of Repair

The influence of several adjuncts, such as intraoperative evoked potential studies, have been mentioned. I have followed the recommendations of Narakas and others in developing a sequence of reconstruction based on functional priorities (Table 32-3). What type of microneural reconstruction is performed depends on the intraoperative assessment of the damage and this predetermined list of priorities.

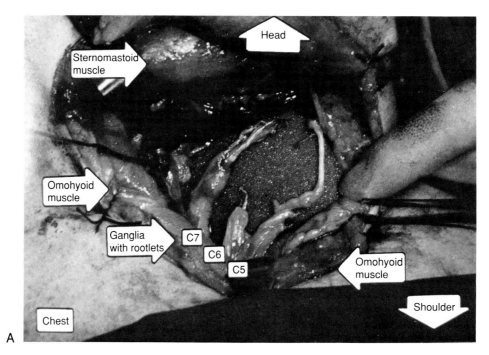

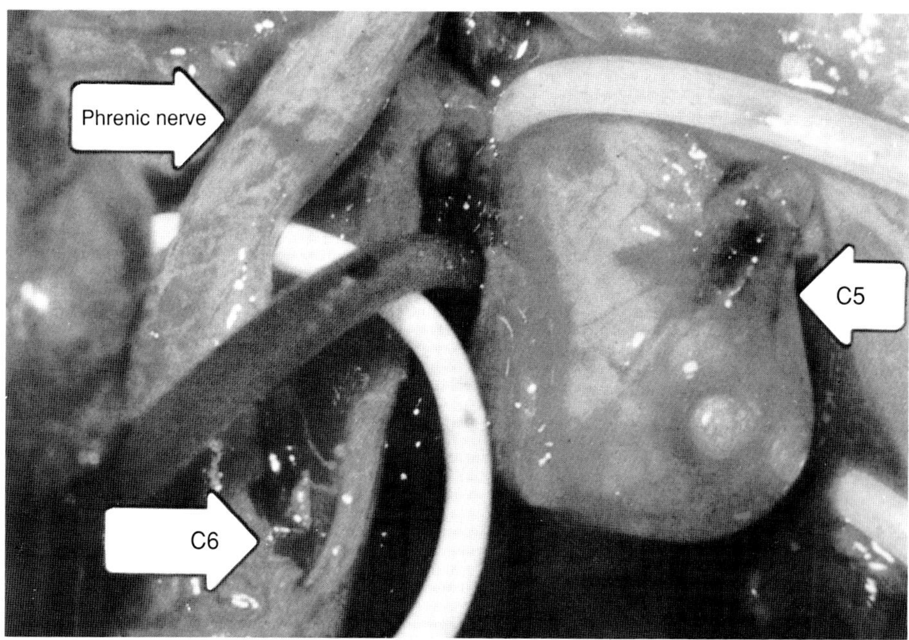

Fig. 32-9. The photographs from two clinical cases demonstrate the appearance of avulsed nerve roots (**A**) and the appearance of a ruptured C5 root (**B**). (Courtesy of Mr. Rolfe Birch, Royal National Orthopedic Hospital, London.)

When the patient presents with essentially total brachial plexus palsy, the priorities of repair include:

1. Elbow flexion—by biceps/brachialis muscle reinnervation
2. Shoulder stabilization, abduction and external rotation—by suprascapular nerve reinnervation
3. Brachiothoracic pinch (adduction of the arm against the chest)—by reinnervation of the pectoralis major muscle
4. Sensation below the elbow in the C6–7 area—by reinnervation of the lateral cord
5. Wrist extension and finger flexion—by reinnervation of the lateral and posterior cord

If the injury is limited to the upper roots (C5, C6) the priorities

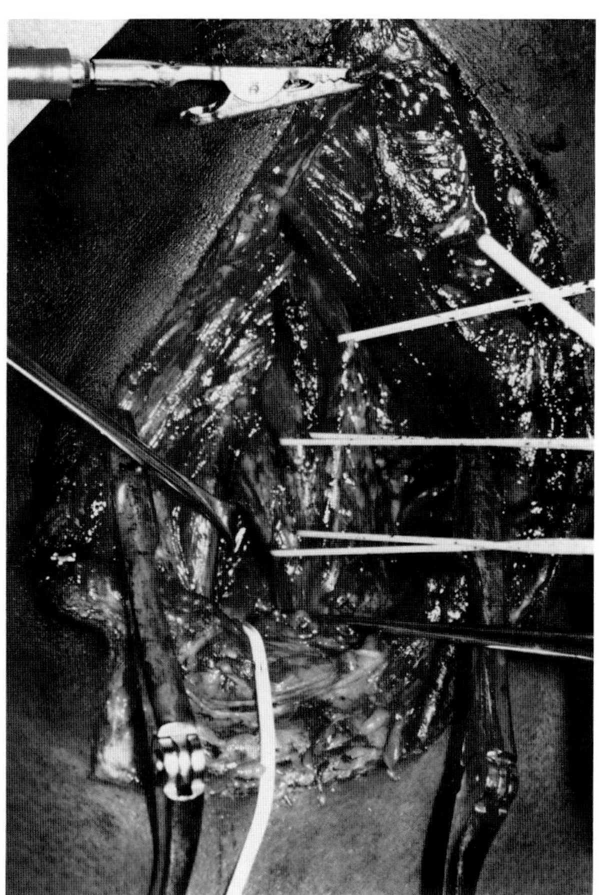

Fig. 32-10. At exploration, we found the C5, 6 and 7 roots (marked by Silastic tapes) scarred and stretched **(A)** but in-continuity. However, evoked potential studies **(B&C)** demonstrated no cortical activity with stimulation of these roots, while stimulation of the C8 root gave rise to a response of large amplitude, indicating a probable intraforaminal avulsion of C5, 6, and 7. In this case only neurotiation of several important nerves using extraplexal donor nerves was possible.

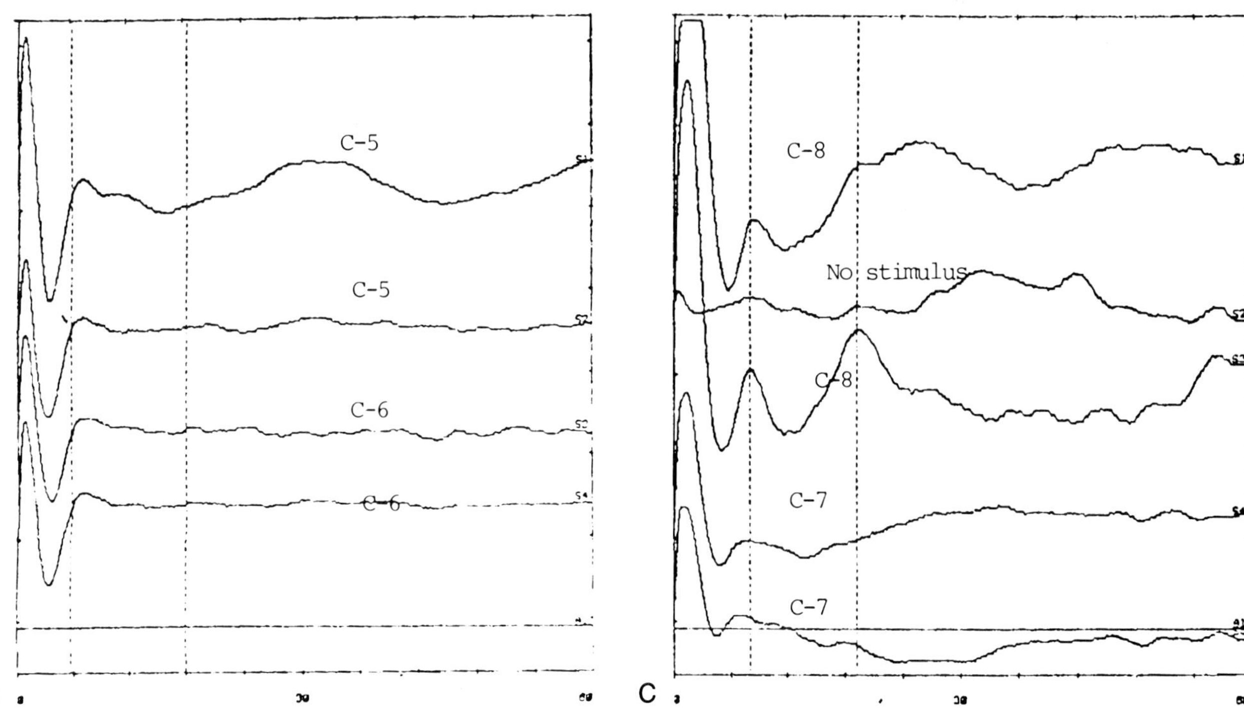

Table 32-3. Treatment Algorithm in Obstetrical Palsy

Ruptured/Avulsed Roots	Recipient Site	Functional Goal
C5, C6/0	Superior trunk	Shoulder control Elbow control Wrist control
C5–C7/0	Superior trunk Middle trunk	Above Finger extension
C5–7/C8, T1	Posterior cord Lateral cord Medial cord	Shoulder control Elbow control Finger flex+?intrinsics
C5, 6/C7, 8, T1	Lateral cord Medial cord ?Suprascapular nerve	Elbow control Finger flex+?intrinsics Should control
C5/C6–8, T1	Musculocutaneous nerve Suprascapular nerve IC (2–5) to lateral cord	Elbow control Shoulder control Sensation
0/C8, T1	Graft from C6 to medial cord	Finger flex+?intrinsics
0/C5, 6	Graft from medial pec nerve to musculocutaneous nerve	Elbow control

are numbers 1 and 2 above, plus possibly some effort at achieving recovery of wrist extension. The decisions regarding the rare patient with an injury limited to the lower elements of the plexus have already been discussed. These priorities have been chosen for three reasons; the first is their functional significance, the second relates to the likelihood of obtaining the chosen function by nerve reconstruction (more proximal muscles will be reinnervated more successfully than very distal muscles), and the third relates to the degree of difficulty in achieving the individual functions listed above by secondary surgery. For example, in the adult there is no reliable muscle tendon transfer to restore shoulder abduction.

Surgical Techniques for Plexo-Plexal Nerve Reconstruction

The microscope is again placed over the neck and the structures, having been already identified and tested electrically, are debrided back to healthy-appearing nerve. If the consistency and color of the structure are not changing as additional millimeters of nerve are sharply sliced away, we stop the debridement. If the cut end continually looks better and better we continue to debride, even back to the level of the bony foremen, where we stop. The former seconario is the more typical finding. Next, we assess the number of strands of sural nerve graft necessary to completely cover the proximal components to be grafted. This is determined by the number of structures, usually roots or trunks, still in-continuity with the spinal cord and their health. A robust C5 or C6 root may require six strands of sural nerve graft to completely cover the prepared face of the root, while a poor root may be covered by only 1 to 2 strands of graft. We try to take advantage of the knowledge gained by others[40,42] in internally mapping the plexus (Fig. 32-11). At the root level, we try to delineate the posterior and anterior division bound areas and try to guide these axons to appropriate target nerves. Next, the distal targets are dissected. These usually include the suprascapular nerve, which is frequently difficult to find, the lateral cord, and the posterior cord. As mentioned above, there are far more targets for nerve grafts than proximal resources. The target may be the lateral cord when several good roots are present, and thus room for many nerve grafts exists, or the target may be the musculocutaneous nerve dissected from the lateral cord as far proximal as possible, if few proximal resources exist. Every case must be individualized. The presence of the clavicle dictates somewhat the surgical strategy. The clavicle frequently must be retracted superiorly and the shoulder elevated to visualize the sites of some of the distal nerve junctures, and vice versa for some of the proximal sites.

Choice of Nerve Grafts—Conventional and Vascularized

Conventional Nerve Grafts

We use both standard fascicular grafts and, for certain cases, vascularized nerve grafts. The technique for harvesting both components of the sural nerve has been mentioned. Other

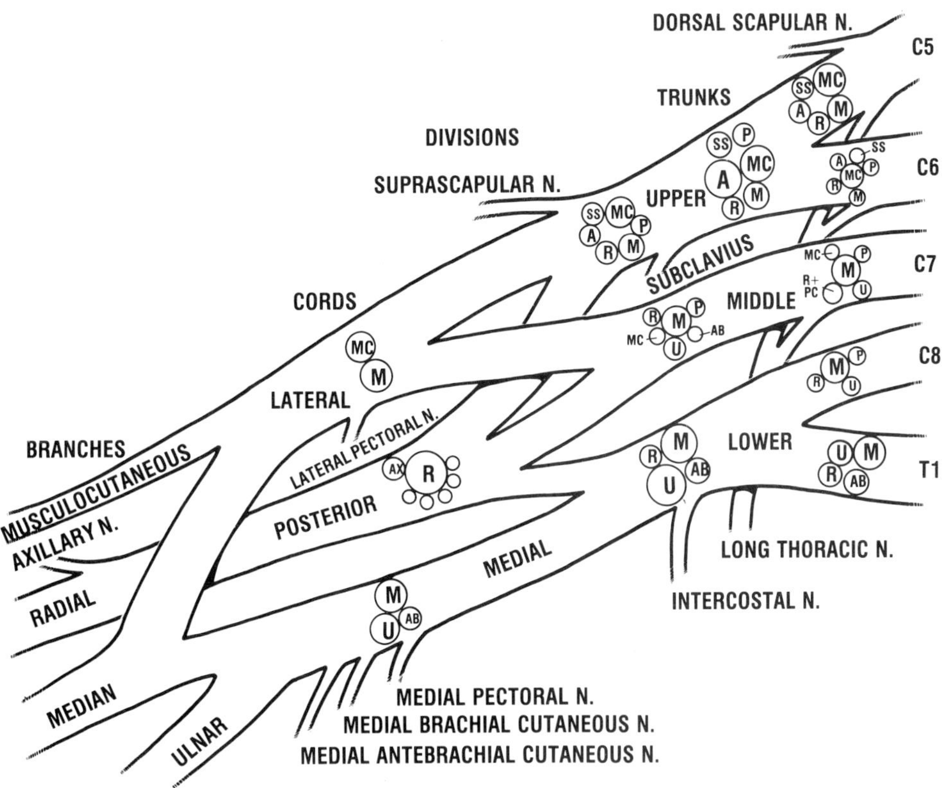

Fig. 32-11. The intraneural fascicular distribution within the brachial plexus. *M*, median nerve; *MC*, musculocutaneous nerve; *R*, radial nerve; *U*, ulnar nerve; *AB*, medial brachial and antebrachial cutaneous nerves, *PC*, posterior cord; *SS*, suprascapular nerve. A, anterior division; Ax, axillary 1; P, posterior. (Adapted from Narakas,[49] with permission.)

donor sites for standard grafts include both medial brachial and medial antebrachial cutaneous nerves. These can be dissected well into the medial cord to obtain some additional length, and far distally in the upper arm. We have also used the dorsal sensory branch of the radial nerve and the lateral antebrachial cutaneous nerve. Leffert[38] mentions using larger nerves that are not to be reinnervated, such as the ulnar nerve, as a source of autograft. He recommends dissecting the nerve to open it so that revascularization is hastened.

Vascularized Nerve Grafts

Since the mid-1980s there has been considerable interest in the possibility of enhancing nerve regeneration following nerve grafting by the use of nerve grafts that are themselves transferred as a "free flap," based on their mesoneurial blood supply. A number of anatomic and experimental studies in animals and some clinical studies in humans have been performed.[5-7,13,19,27,34,54,65,67] Termed vascularized nerve grafts, their role in plexus reconstruction remains controversial. Some advocates believe that the rate of axonal regeneration is enhanced but that the ultimate functional outcome is not altered (Birch, personal communication, 1986; Merle, personal communication, 1985). I believe that the principle reason to consider a vascularize nerve graft in plexus reconstruction is to maximize the amount of nerve graft material for reconstruction. Additional reasons given to support its use include situations where a long nerve graft is necessary, (e.g., to overcome a gap greater than 6 cm).[31] Perhaps its more traditional use in a less than adequately vascularized bed is met in the unusual case of severe trauma to the region, such as after a shotgun injury to the neck, or as part of reconstruction in an irradiation injury, but in most instances of traction injury, the bed for the nerve grafts is very adequate to support rapid revascularization of nonvascularized grafts.

The best indication for a vascularized graft in plexus reconstruction is a case involving proven avulsion of C8 and T1 in association with large root stumps of the remaining plexus. In this case, there is no possibility of spontaneous recovery of the ulnar nerve innervated structures or areas, and it makes little sense to waste precious proximal axons to recover some sensibility in the ulnar side of the hand (intrinsic muscle recovery is essentially never seen in the adult when C8 and T1 have been badly injured.) In this instance, the best source of a vascularized nerve graft is the ulnar nerve itself, based in the upper arm on one of several branches of the brachial artery, usually the superior ulnar collateral artery (Fig. 32-12). Based on this vessel, we have demonstrated bleeding from the ulnar nerve as far distal as the elbow (a 10- to 12-cm segment of nerve). The ulnar nerve in the forearm can also be dissected as a vascularized nerve graft, based on its accompanying ulnar artery and veni comitantes. The dorsal sensory branch of the radial nerve has been described as a source of a vascularized nerve graft, as has the sural, the anterior tibial, the superficial peroneal, and the saphenous nerve.[6] However, I strongly prefer to use the ulnar nerve in the circumstances described above, using the sural

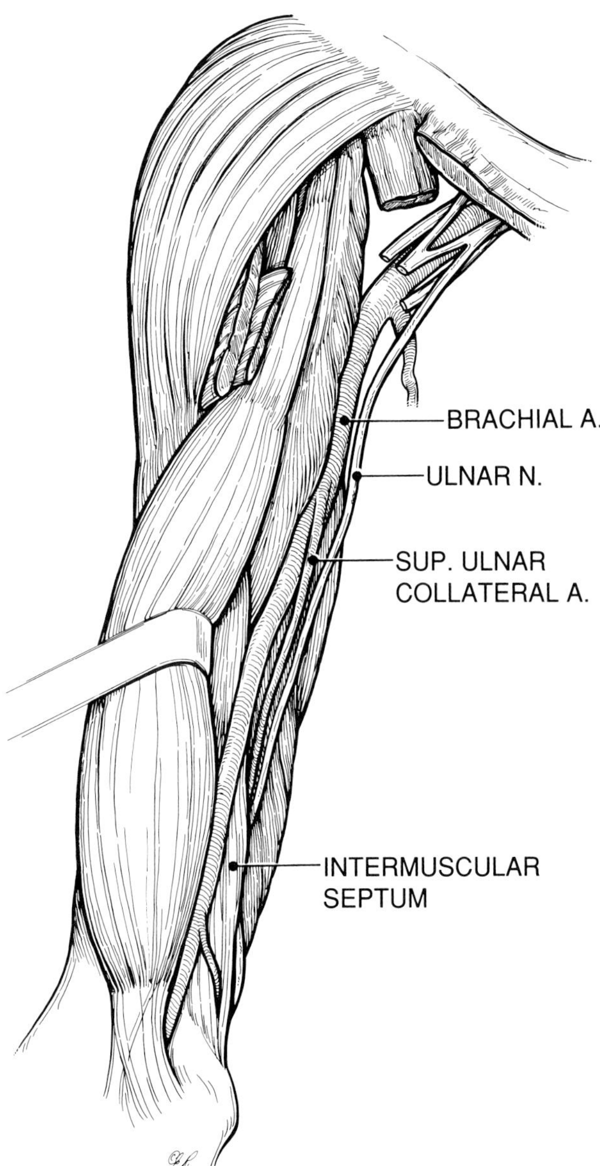

Fig. 32-12. The anatomic relationship between the ulnar artery and the superior ulnar collateral artery in the upper arm is demonstrated. The ulnar nerve may be harvested as a vascularized nerve graft from the paralyzed limb in cases of C8, T1 avulsion.

nerve as a nonvascularized graft for the bulk of the reconstruction. I will use the vascularized graft for the longest segment to be grafted, depending on the anatomy. There are typically only a few large fascicles in the proximal ulnar nerve, and their orientation can be assessed so that the anterior/posterior relationship at the root level can be honored.

The ideal recipient vessel for anastomosis is the transverse scapular artery. The large accompanying vein may be too large as a recipient vein, especially if veni comitantes are used as the donor veins. However, there is no shortage of appropriately sized veins encountered in the neck dissection. The proximal end of the vascularized nerve graft is sutured first to the proximal nerve source, the vessel arrangement checked, and if the donor and recipient vessels are well arranged, the distal end of the vascularized graft is passed under the clavicle, and the fascicles distributed as predetermined. The microvascular part of the repair is done last.

Grafting Methods

Most surgeons use the fascicular nerve graft suturing techniques attributed to Millesi[45] and described in detail in Chapter 35. In Europe, where tissue adhesives have been commercially available for some time, surgeons[48] have demonstrated simplified techniques for approximating bundles of nerve grafts to the donor and recipient site (Fig. 32-13). Whether functional recovery is enhanced has not been proven, but the results seem at least equal to suture repair methods, and with some experience, the nonsuture technique is performed faster and with much less frustration. Because the tissue adhesives are made from pooled plasma, they have not been found acceptable in the United States. However, many blood banks have the capability of manufacturing adequate amounts of fibrinogen from a unit of the patient's preoperatively donated blood. Wood (personal communication, 1989), from the Mayo Clinic, has reported his favorable experience with this method.

If sutures are to be used, I prefer to measure and precut the sural nerve segments. I dye both ends of the grafts destined for the posterior cord with methylene blue to assist in orientation of the infraclavicular part of the junctures, then begin the supraclavicular neurorraphies with the most distally situated root, trunk, etc., working my way superiorly. The posterior grafts are placed before anterior ones. I find it helpful to thread the distal ends of the grafts that are bound for similar subclavicular sites into a large bore catheter.

When all the proximal junctures are completed, the first catheter is passed deep to the clavicle toward the destination for the grafts contained within. This has helped to keep the multiple strands of graft separated into functional destinations. After the grafts have been passed under the clavicle, the superior junctures are checked a final time to be certain that no inadvertent disruption has occurred in passing the grafts under the clavicle. The microscope is moved over the subclavicular repair site and these nerve junctures are performed. It is beneficial to make a sketch of both the operative findings and the origin, destination, length, and number of nerve grafts (Fig. 32-14).

Once plexo-plexal nerve grafting, or extraplexal neurotization (see below) has been completed, the surgical wounds are closed as follows: the subclavius and omohyoid muscles are repaired, as these act as a buffer between nerve grafts and the clavicle; the supraclavicular fat pad is replaced, further protecting the nerve grafts; and a suction drain is placed somewhat away from the course of the grafts so that they are not dislodged when the drain is removed. The platysma is reapproximated and the skin closed.

Subclavicularly, the pectoralis minor is repaired, as is the clavipectoral fascia, and the skin incisions here closed.

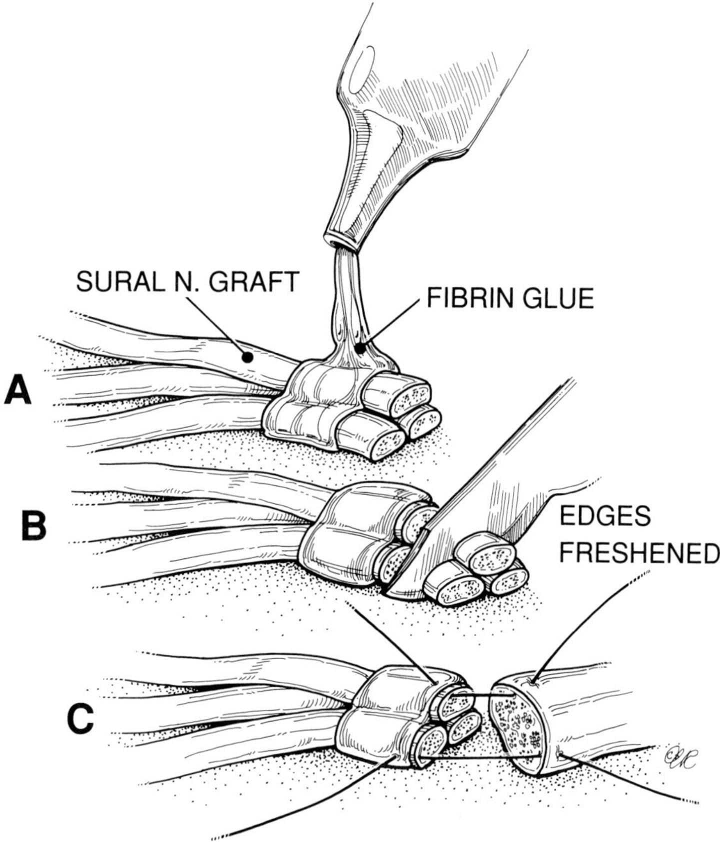

Fig. 32-13. Tissue adhesives can simplify the approximation of multiple strands of graft nerve proximally to a single large root stump or distally to a trunk or cord. The graft strands are first glued together (**A**), the graft ends are freshened (**B**), and the mass is then approximated to the correct recipient site with a few microsutures passed through the glue and epineurium (**C**). Additional glue can be used to reinforce this juncture.

Surgical Techniques for Neurotization

In the most severe injuries, those with all or most nerve roots avulsed, there are insufficient numbers of proximal axon resources from the remaining parts of the plexus still in-continuity with the spinal cord. In these cases, it has been necessary to turn to extraplexal sources of especially motor and also sensory axons. Many different nerves have been advocated by knowledgable surgeons.[2,8,12,15,45,53,69] However, the most common sources of extraplexal motor axons have been the spinal accessory nerve (SAN) and the intercostal nerves (ICN) from C3-6 (Fig. 32-15). Other authors report using motor branches of the cervical rami or even cross-chest grafts from branches of the contralateral plexus, such as a branch from the lateral pectoral nerve.[20] I have had greater success using the SAN, but several Japanese authors[47] have reported good results using IC neurotization. I believe the most appropriate targets for neurotization are the suprascapular nerve (shoulder abduction and external rotation), the musculocutaneous nerve (elbow flexion) or the lateral pectoral nerve (thoracohumeral pinch.) therefore, if insufficient root stumps are found, for example, or if all five roots are avulsed, I favor SAN grafted to the suprascapular nerve, (this can usually be done without a nerve graft) 2 to 3 ICNs to the musculocutaneous nerve, and one or two intercostals to the lateral pectoral nerve in hopes of achieving some adduction and thus thoracic-humeral pinch. In addition, I will neurotize the median nerve portion of the lateral cord with nerve grafts from the cervical plexus. If a small root stump of C5 remains, its axons are led to the musculocutaneous nerve, the SAN axons to the suprascapular nerve, and intercostals to the posterior cord. If good C5 and C6 stumps are found, I prefer not to perform neurotization in addition to nerve grafts.

The SAN is located just as it leaves the SCM muscle in the plane between the SCM and the anterior border of trapezium. A nerve stimulator is absolutely necessary. It is followed distally until it is joined by accessory branches coming from C2 to C3. These must be spared, or else total denervation of the trapezium will occur. By careful dissection under magnification those fascicles coming from the SAN can be separated. Usually there is sufficient length to allow its divided end to just reach the dissected portion of the suprascapular nerve. The suprascapular nerve has a great deal of connective tissue

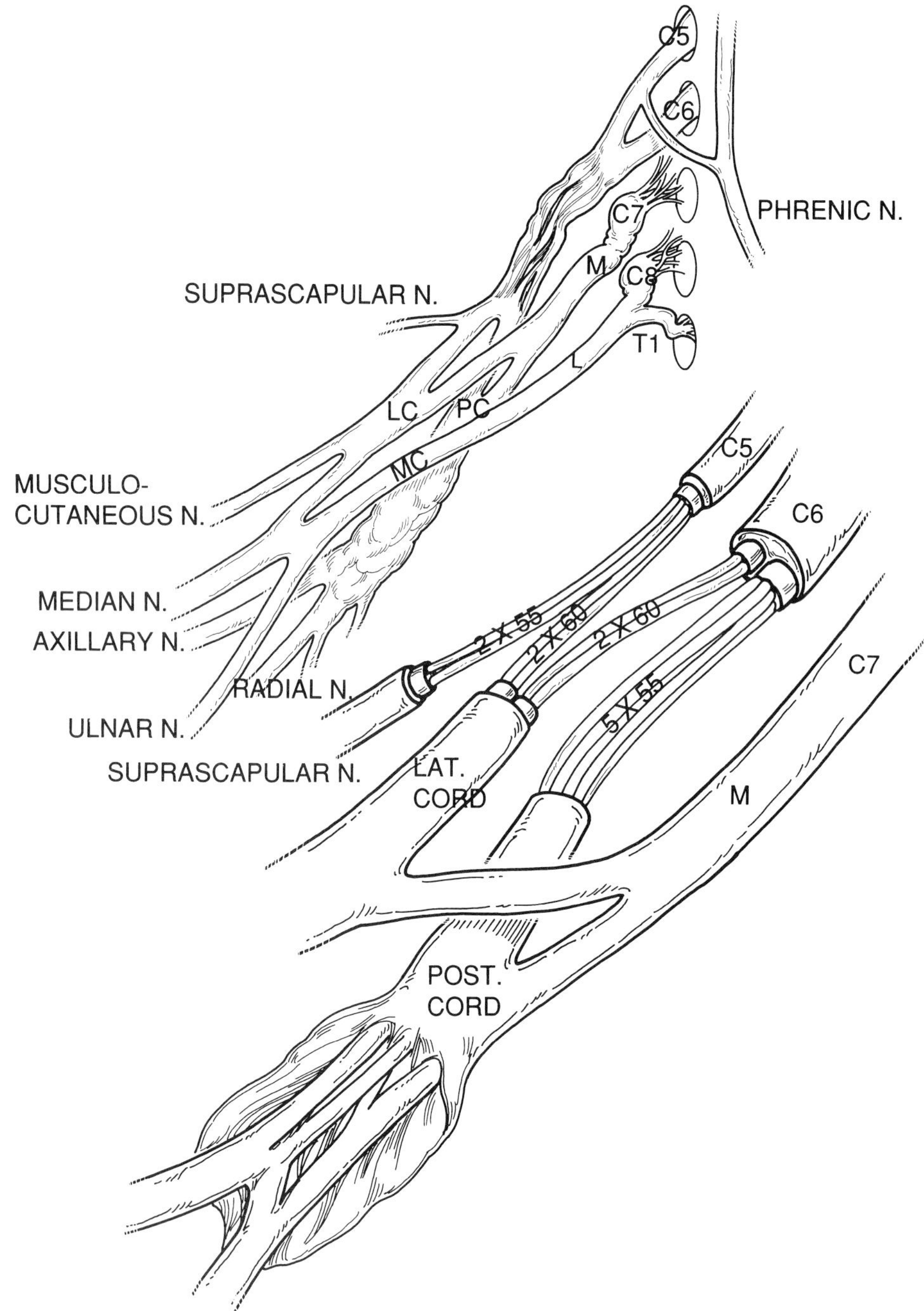

Fig. 32-14. It is useful to sketch the operative findings and the repair method, detailing the distribution of nerve grafts, including length and number and the source and destination of neurotization procedures.

surrounding the fascicles; this tissue should be dissected away prior to suturing. Here tissue glues seem less helpful.

The intercostal nerves are exposed through an oblique incision beginning just inferior to the point where the initial incision tums into the axillary fold. In line with the posterior axillary fold or mid-axilla, the serratus muscle is separated over the rib, the inferior muscle fibers sharply cut away from the rib, and a blunt elevator used to strip the intercostal muscle fibers inferiorly. A nerve hook is more or less blindly inserted and the hook tumed superiorly and scraped against the inferior surface of the rib. This will usually "hook" the neurovascular pedicle, allowing the nerve to be separated from the artery. The nerve is

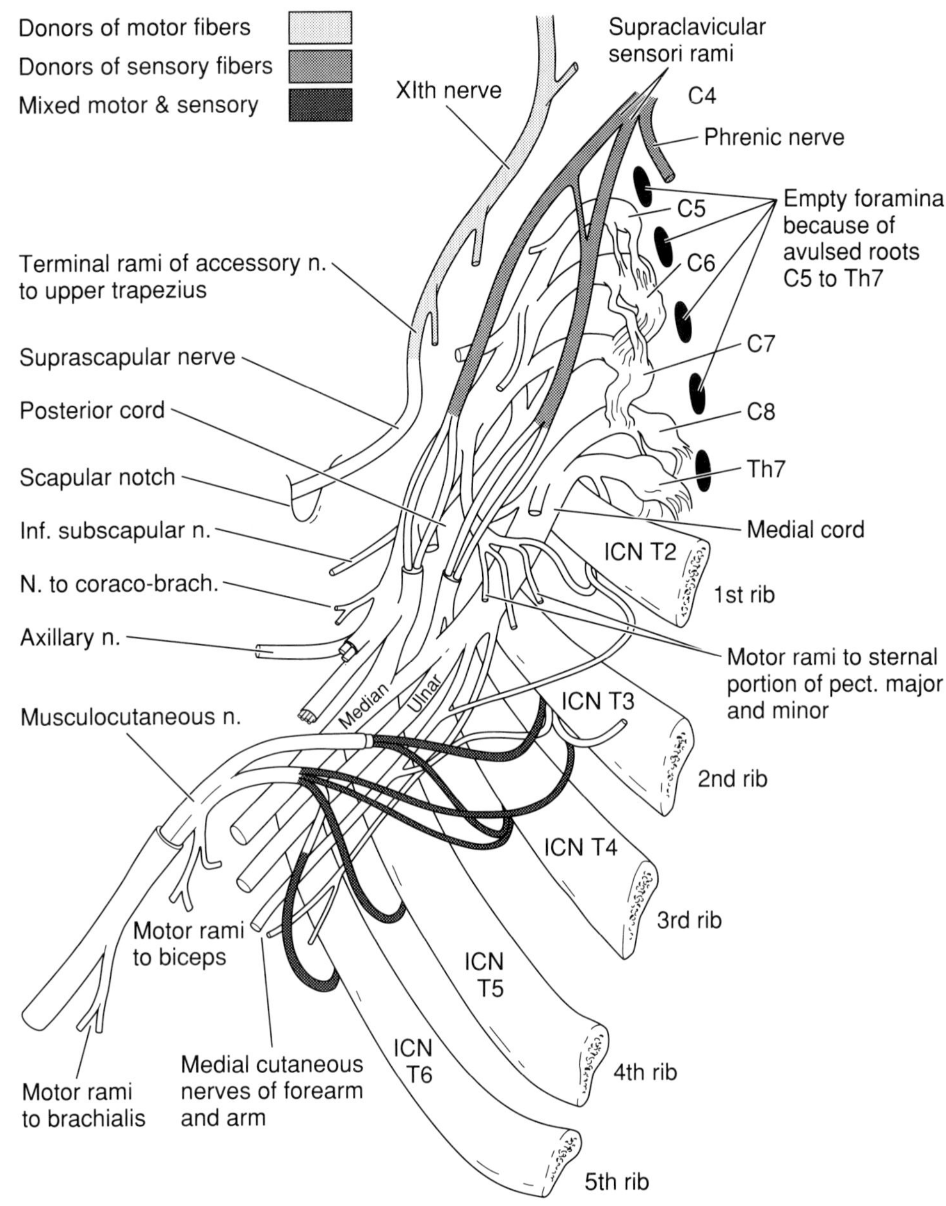

Fig. 32-15. The donor nerves and their destinations in a case of avulsion of all five roots is illustrated. (From Narakas and Hentz,[53] with permission.)

stimulated to determine that it contains motor axons. The nerve can be dissected toward the anterior axillary line. Much more medial to this point, the nerve becomes primarily sensory.[17] Some authors routinely dissect enough nerve to avoid the need for an interpositional nerve graft[8] but I have not always been successful in this. If neurotization is to be performed, it is crucial to dissect the musculocutaneous nerve as far proximal as possible, rather than risk "diluting" the motor axon resources by grafting to the lateral cord.

Neurotization in the Neglected Plexus Injury

Several authors have reported their results in combining microneural reconstruction with free vascularized functional muscle transfers for neglected cases of total brachial plexus palsy. In these cases, the time since injury is so long as to preclude successful neurotization or reinnervation of previously denervated muscles. In the adult, this is certainly true for injuries treated after 2 years and for all practical purposes, probably for those seen after significantly less time (1 year) has elapsed as well. Several strategies have evolved, with the Japanese authors presenting the largest experience. One strategy for the patient with total root avulsion is to preform a preliminary nerve graft between an available motor nerve, such as the SAN or IC nerves. The distal end of the graft is led to the vicinity of the shoulder or proximal arm. After allowing some period of time for axon regeneration to occur (e.g., 12 months), and with the presence of a Tinel's sign at the area of the distal end of the long nerve graft indicating axon regeneration to this point, the second operation is performed. This involves the transfer of a healthy muscle, either the opposite latissimus dorsi, the gracilis or another muscle, to the shoulder and arm by microvascular free transfer. The most common muscle used to date is the gracilis. The coracoid process is used to anchor the proximal tendon of the muscle, and the distal tendon is woven into the tendon of the biceps under proper tension as described by Manktelow in Chapter 29. Typically, the circumflex humeral or profunda brachial artery serves as the recipient artery. The motor nerve of the transferred muscle is joined to the previously placed nerve graft. Other strategies employ any available remaining nerve root as the source of proximal axons, but the use of an injured root carries the distinct possibility that regeneration will be poor and nonspecific, (i.e., perhaps provide more sensory than motor axons). Some surgeons recommend performing a preliminary operation, at which time the distal end of the previously placed nerve graft is biopsied and axon staining performed to document the presence of sufficient numbers of axons. Perhaps acetylcholinesterase stains for the presence of motor axons would be a better test.

Postoperative Care

At the completion of the operation, a cervical collar is fitted about the neck to restrict neck motion. The shoulder and elbow are immobilized, the shoulder in adduction and the elbow in 90 degrees flexion. Sandbags are placed on either side of the patient's head to further restrict excessive motion until the patient is fully awake and are used at night for several additional days. The neck and shoulder immobilizers are worn for 2 weeks; range of motion exercises are then renewed without restrictions. After initial healing, the progress of nerve regeneration is assessed about every 3 months. At least 2 and perhaps 3 years are necessary before the results of nerve reconstruction can be assessed.

Results of Nerve Reconstruction by Graft and Neurotization

In his 1963 address to the Royal College of Surgeons, Seddon[40] stated that repair of traction injuries of the brachial plexus was sufficiently disappointing as to essentially preclude it. More modern thought regarding the potential of reconstruction began with more favorable reports by Samii and Kahn[56] Millesi,[42] and Narakas.[51] These authors and others[3,32] reported their results following neural reconstruction of traction injuries to the brachial plexus. However, no systematic scheme of analysis was employed and it is difficult to compare one series with another. Table 32-4 summarizes the results of several published series for repair by both plexoplexal grafts, plus or minus, where necessary, by neurotization. Table 32-5 summa-

Table 32-4. Results of Reconstruction with Total Supraclavicular Palsy

Author	No. or Patients	Developed Useful Function[a]
Millesi[43]	20	10/20 (50%)[b]
Sedel[60]	26[c]	22/26

[a] Grade III = 11, grade IV = 12, grade V = 3
[b] Shoulder 5/8, Elbow flexion 9/18, Wrist/finger 2/18
[c] Additional 6 patients operated but nothing repaired

Results of Reconstruction with Partial Palsy

Author	No. of Patients	Developed Useful Function
Millesi[44]	11 (Supraclavicular lesion) 12 (Infraclavicular lesion)	9/11 10/12
Sedel[60] Narakas[49]	23	20/23

Table 32-5. Results of Neurotization For Elbow Flexion

Nerve	Author	No. of Patients Followed	Results	
			Good	Nil
SAN	Allieu[2]	15	3	12
	Narakas[54]	3	2	1
	Merle[54]	7	3	4
ICN	Millesi[45]	22	11	11
	Narakas[53]	24	9	15
	Nagano[53]	117	80	37

Abbreviations: SAN, spinal accessory nerve; ICN, intercostal nerve.

rizes the results as compiled by Narakas and Hentz[53] for neurotization using either the SAN or IC neurotization.

Analysis of these series by several authors[31,38,53] leads to several conclusions. Repair does improve the prognosis. Infraclavicular injuries have a better prognosis than supraclavicular. Supraclavicular injuries associated with at least two repairable roots have a better prognosis, partial injuries more so than complete ones. The results of neurotization have been more mixed. Figure 32-16 demonstrates the functional outcome in a patient with an upper root injury secondary to a shotgun wound, while Figure 32-17 demonstrates the functional result in a case of total root avulsion.

MICRONEURAL RECONSTRUCTION FOR OBSTETRIC PALSY

The approach to the infant who has suffered a traction injury of the brachial plexus differs somewhat from the approach to the adult. This section will be devoted only to a discussion of the differences because the mechanism of injury is absolutely similar, involving excessive direct traction on the brachial plexus associated typically with a difficult delivery[18] or perhaps with compression of the plexus by the first rib.[16] In most cases a similar set of circumstances prevail, including a high birth weight, usually greater than 4000 grams (frequently associated with maternal diabetes or short, heavy mothers), a difficult presentation (shoulder dystocia) cephalo-pelvic dysproportion, or forceps delivery.[22] Since the first reported attempts at repair by Kennedy[33] in 1903, the role of surgical reconstruction has been far more controversial than for the adult cases, and remains so to this day. The principle reason behind the controversy regarding the role of microneural reconstruction lies in the lack of a uniform system of evaluation. Most studies[24,28] lack reliable data on the initial clinical picture and there is no consensus on what constitutes a good result. For most studies, a good result translates into a well-functioning hand regardless of the condition of the shoulder, which frequently lacks normal external rotation and abduction. However, the hand is frequently spared because a majority of lesions involve C5 and C6 (plus or minus the C7) roots.[20,21] Most of these cases retain or regain good hand function. The recent interest in operating on infants has been stimulated primarily by the favorable reports of Gilbert[19,20,22] and others,[41,66] and by a better appreciation of the natural history of the spontaneous evolution following injury provided by several longitudinal studies.[63]

Current Recommendations For Obstetric Palsy

The tenets of the present regimen have been derived in large part from observations of a number of Gilbert's cases, and have been strongly influenced by a study of 44 children suffering birth palsies who were followed for more than 10 years at the St. Vincent DePaul Hospital in Paris,[63] and a more recent study of 25 children followed at the Scottish Rite Hospital in Dallas, Texas, and the Children's Hospital at Stanford.[29,30] These children were examined shortly after birth, then serially. None had surgical intervention. The results of the St. Vincent DePaul study are presented in the thesis of Tassin.[63] From this study, three groups emerged, labelled "complete recovery," "near complete recovery," and "others." An analysis of these groups demonstrated that there are several important clues to the eventual level of recovery:

1. Complete recovery seems possible only if the biceps and deltoid have reached the M1 stage by the second month.
2. The results, though still good, are nevertheless incomplete if initial contracting of these two muscles requires 3 to 3.5 months.
3. If the biceps is not at stage M3 by 5 months, the results will be highly unsatisfactory.

Preoperative Evaluation

The posture of the newborn is frequently diagnostic, with either a flail limb indicting complete palsy, or an internally rotated, adducted limb with the forearm pronated and the wrist flexed, indicating an upper root problem (Fig. 32-18). A precise muscle or sensory exam at this age is difficult, and requires patience on the part of the examiner. With a few simple tools, the examiner tries to stimulate movement of various muscles while palpating the muscle between two fingers. Like Gilbert, I have modified the usual muscle classification when examining infants so that:

M0 = no contraction

M1 = contraction without movement

M2 = slight or greater movement with the weight of the arm supported against the effects of gravity

M3 = complete movement against gravity

The sensory exam is even less precise. I test the reaction to pinching the skin only. Other signs to be observed include evidence of trophic changes, such as differences in hair growth or color, and the presence of a Horner's sign. Radiography is

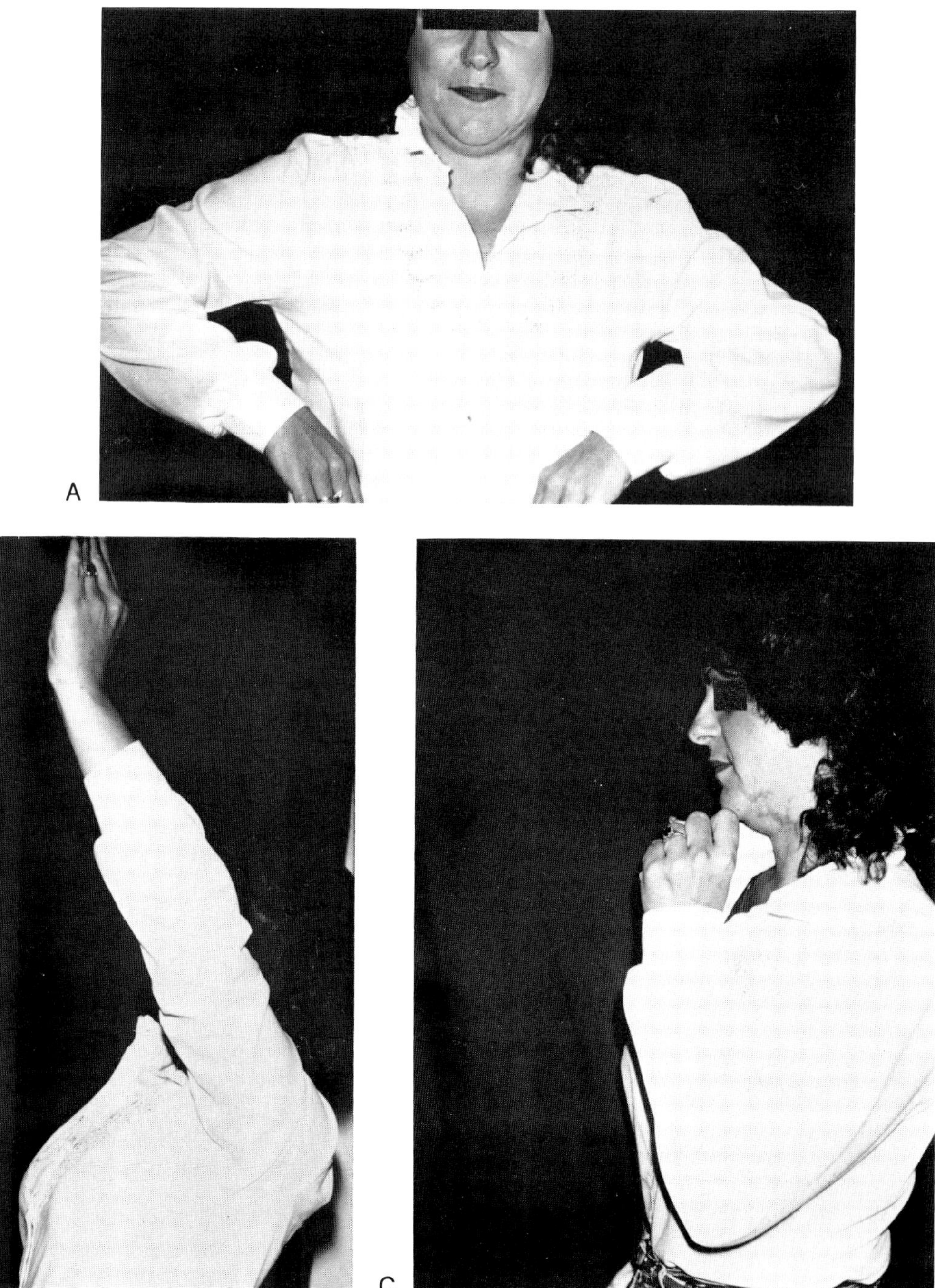

Fig. 32-16. **(A–C)** This 33-year-old woman suffered a shotgun injury to her left brachial plexus that resulted in a C5, 6 and 7 palsy. At exploration, the C5 root was ruptured, the C6 root avulsed, and the C7 root, and middle trunk was fibrotic but in-continuity. Nerve grafts were placed between C5 and the residual superior trunk and C7 was neurolysed. One year following surgery she had recovered good shoulder rotation and abduction, essentially normal elbow function, and good wrist flexion.

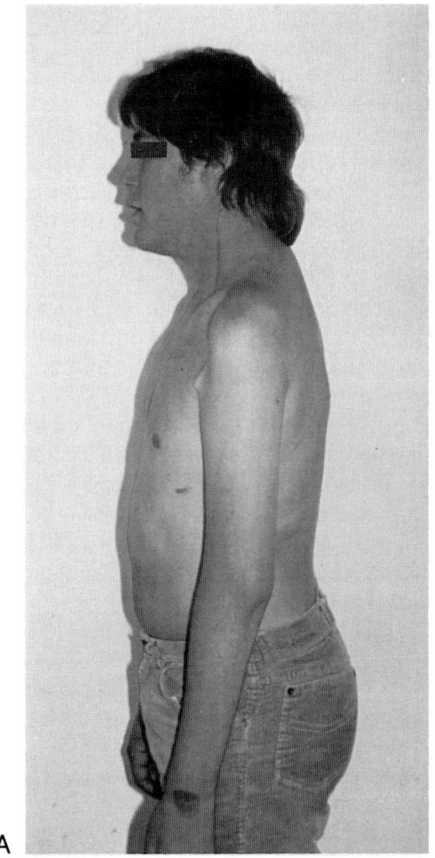

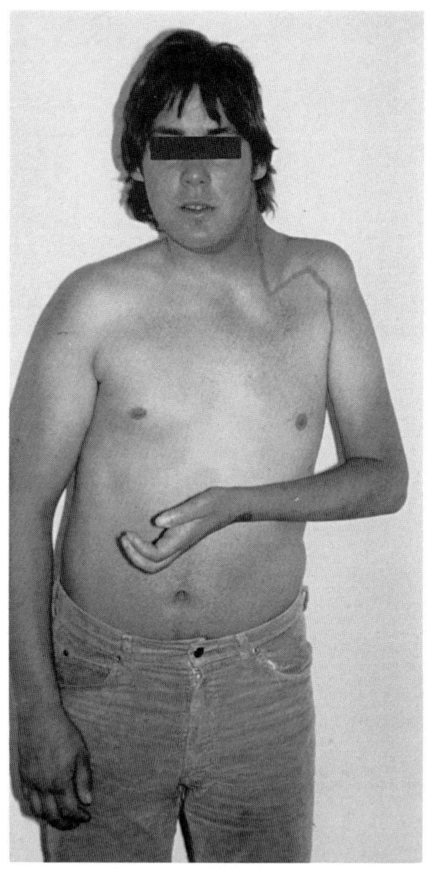

Fig. 32-17. (A&B) This patient suffered complete brachial plexus root avulsion. Reconstruction consisted of neurotization alone. The spinal accessory nerve was led to the musculocutaneous by way of a short interpositional nerve graft and intercostal nerves were used to neurotize his pectoralis major muscle. Two years following surgery he could flex his elbow (Grade IV strength), and could hold objects against his chest using his pectoralis muscle for thoracohumeral pinch.

helpful in differentiating the only other condition mimicking an upper root lesion (i.e., epiphyseal separation of the humeral head,[57]), although this examination is only conclusive after 2 to 3 weeks of age in association with the appearance of calcification of the humeral head. Ultrasound in the newborn may provide the same information at an earlier date. EMGs are not obtained until later.

The infant is reexamined at 1 month of age. Recovery may already be evident and will probably ultimately be complete. For the remaining babies, several presentations are evident:

1. If the palsy is still total and is associated with a Horner's sign, the outlook for spontaneous recovery is poor and a date for surgery, generally at around 2 months of age, is agreed on with the parents.
2. If the hand is recovering but no biceps or shoulder recovery is evident, there is still a chance for spontaneous recovery. A third evaluation prior to 3 months of age will be necessary to determine indications for surgery.

At 3 months of age, the child is retested. If any biceps function is evident, surgery is not recommended. For those without biceps function, an EMG is scheduled, although the results of EMG have been difficult to correlate with final outcome. However, total absence of electrical evidence of reinnervation at this time indicates avulsion of the corresponding roots. A final evaluation is cervical myelography. In skilled hands, there is minimal morbidity, and the absence of a pseudomeningocoele essentially confirms the presence of an extraforaminal lesion. In contrast, in a study of 108 patients undergoing myelography,[22] there were 14 false-positive studies (i.e., a pseudomeningocoele in the presence of an intact root).

The decision to operate is based on all the above studies, though the clinical exam is most important. For example, we propose surgery if the biceps is clinically inactive at 3.5 months, even if the EMG shows signs of electrical activity. There is no consensus on the timing of surgery, however. Terzis,[66] reporting on 17 infants, found videotaping of the exam helpful, and the EMG more predictable. She chooses to await evidence of plateauing of clinical improvement. Conversely, Meyer and Rudisill,[41] reporting on 20 babies, followed the guidelines of Gilbert.

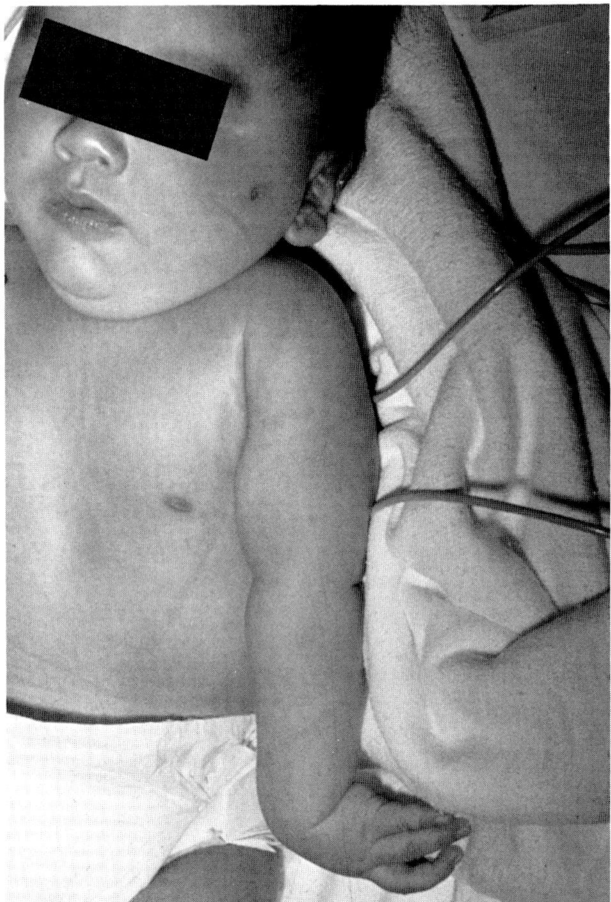

Fig. 32-18. A typical presentation of an infant with an upper plexus birth palsy. The arm is held by the side, the elbow extended, the forearm held in pronation, and the wrist in flexion. Depending upon the remaining function of the C7 root, the fingers may be extended or flexed.

Preoperative Preparation

Perhaps the most important aspect of preoperative preparation is a very thorough and usually repeated discussion with the family regarding the outcome and the time involved for recovery. In the United States, almost every one of these cases is associated with litigation over the question of causation and factors associated with birth trauma. Prior to surgery, the child is seen by the occupational therapist, who constructs, from a thermoplastic material, a molded half "clam-shell" that encompasses the infant's head, shoulder, and chest.

Surgical Approach

The surgical approach differs from that used for the adult. No curare or other long-acting muscle relaxants are used. Scalp needle electrodes are inserted, and tourniquets applied to both thighs. A dilute solution of vasoconstrictor is injected along the proposed incision. With this regimen, no infant has required transfusion. The upper part of the incision alone will usually suffice for C5,6, and 7 palsies. Otherwise, the dissection is the same as that described for the adult. The operative findings (Table 32-6) differ from the adult in that a neuroma-in-continuity is far more frequently encountered in the infant, typically at the level of the superior trunk (Fig. 32-19A). If C7 is affected, it is usually adherent to this neuroma. The clavicle can be lifted up off the plexus, allowing exposure of the divisions and the proximal cords. The suprascapular nerve can frequently be found exiting the neuroma. When all roots have been identified, they are sequentially stimulated and the evoked potentials measured. Gilbert and Razaboni[22] reports that he has yet to find a root both injured extraforaminally, and also avulsed from the cord. Even C8 and T1 can be visualized from the supraclavicular approach. In cases of total palsy, if these roots are normal by electrical studies, then an infraclavicular injury must be suspected and the infraclavicular portion of the incision made. If grafting from a supraclavicular to infraclavicular location is to be done, the clavicle is sectioned obliquely. When fibrous scar extends into the subclavicular region, the surgeon can expect to find one or two avulsed roots curled within the scar.

Surgical Decision-making

With the presence of a neuroma, it is tempting to perform only a neurolysis. However, Gilbert, Hentz, and Tassin[20] reported disappointing results with only neurolysis. In most instances, a purposeful decision to resect the neuroma and perform interpositional nerve grafts is made (Fig. 32-19B). Gilbert and Razaboni[21] reported that in 20 consecutive cases, essentially no healthy-appearing nerve fibers were found in the distal neuroma on serial histology, and Meyer and Rudisill[41] confirmed these findings in his cases.

Occasionally, we find a slack-appearing root, but on stimulation, a small evoked potential is obtained. This may mean that only some posterior rootlets remain intact. However, when the surgical examination and electrical studies disagree, we prefer to leave the root alone and await further spontaneous recovery. Meyer and Rudisill[41] believe that rapid staining techniques may supplant evoked potential studies. Where the exam and electrical studies correspond, we proceed with reconstruction either by plexoplexal grafts or by neurotization. Usually, the decisions are simple. For example, the freshly prepared C5 and C6 root stumps are joined by suture or tissue adhesives to freshly prepared superior trunk or their corresponding divisions, or others (Fig. 32-19B). In those cases with

Table 32-6. Surgical Results in Subtotal Obstetric Palsy

Rupture C5, 6[a]	2 years p.o.	50% Level IV or V
	5 years p.o.	70% Level IV or V
Rupture C5, 6, 7[b]	2 years p.o.	35% Level IV or V
	5 years p.o.	45% Level IV or V

[a] In contrast, in the Tassin control group, all achieved Grade III function; no patient obtained Grade IV or V shoulder function.

[b] In contrast, in the conservatively treated patients, the shoulder achieved Grade II in 30% and Grade III in 70%.

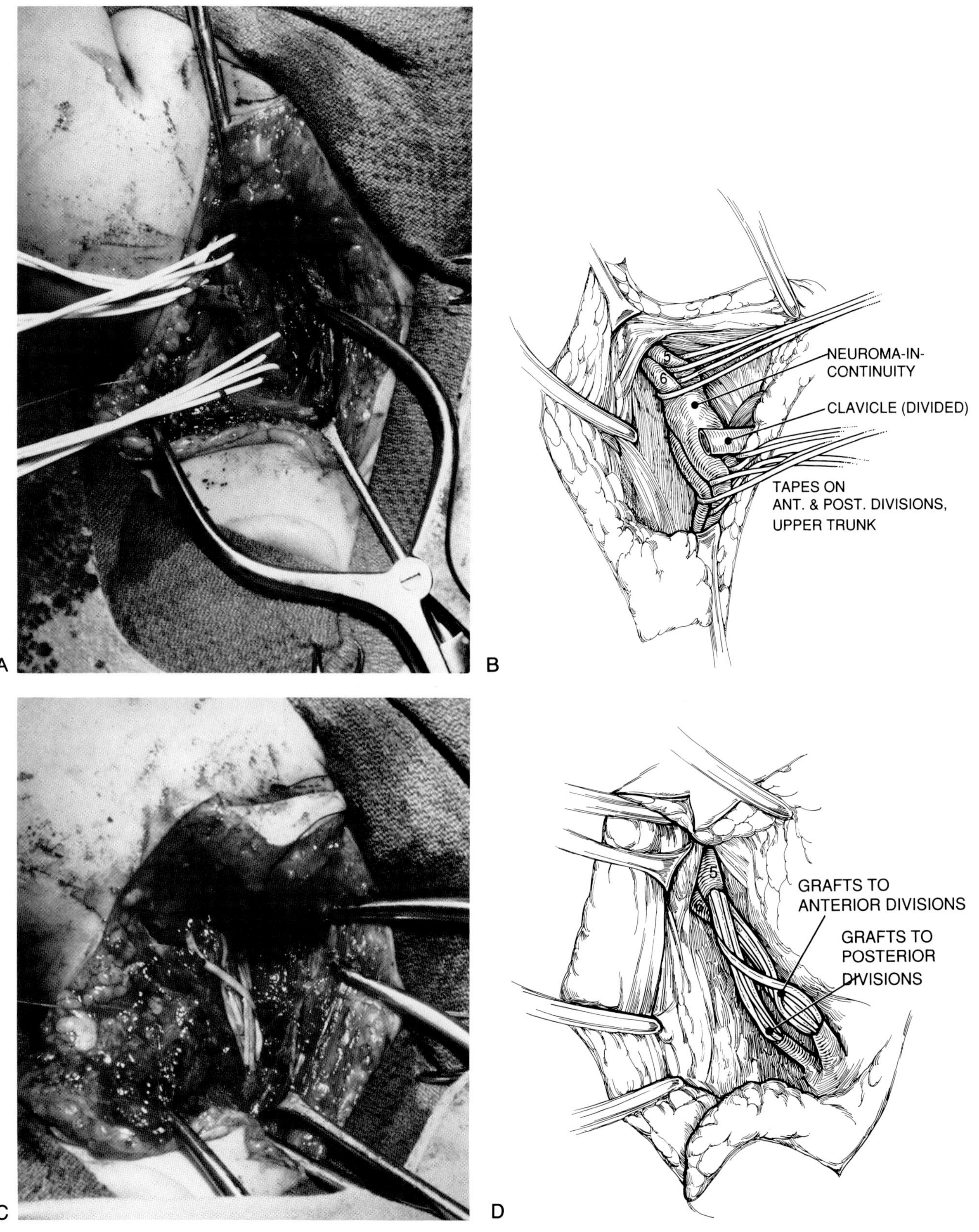

Fig. 32-19. **(A&B)** Dissection of the plexus in an infant suffering from apparent C5, 6, and 7 palsy. The C5 and 6 roots enter a large firm neuroma just as the exit the foramina. The clavicle has been sectioned to allow access to the distal superior trunk and their anterior and posterior divisions. **(C&D)** The neuroma has been excised and nerve grafts placed between residual roots and anterior and posterior divisions. Grafts placed on the posterior face of the residual roots are led to the posterior division, and those on the anterior face, to the anterior division.

total palsy, at least one root has always been found avulsed, though never all five roots (unlike the adult situation). The most commonly avulsed roots have been C8 and T1, occasionally in conjunction with C7 and even C6. In such cases, reconstruction depends on the number and location of remaining proximal neural resources. The plan and priorities of reconstruction differ from the adult in that we frequently make an attempt to reinnervate the inferior trunk or medial cord, because intrinsic muscle recovery has been seen in the infant plexus cases.

In summary, for subtotal lesions, lesions of C5, 6, and 7 are nearly always extraforaminal ruptures—frequently in-continuity lesions—which may be repaired. The lesions are all above the clavicle and may be repaired through limited incisions. For complete palsy, C8 and T1 are almost always avulsed, and there is always at least one root available for reconstruction. To us, this justifies systematic surgical intervention. No isolated lower root injuries without injury to the upper roots were found.

Postoperative Care

Postoperative care is essentially that for the adult, except that the infant is placed into his clam-shell splint for approximately 3 weeks (Fig. 32-20). Exercises aimed at maintaining

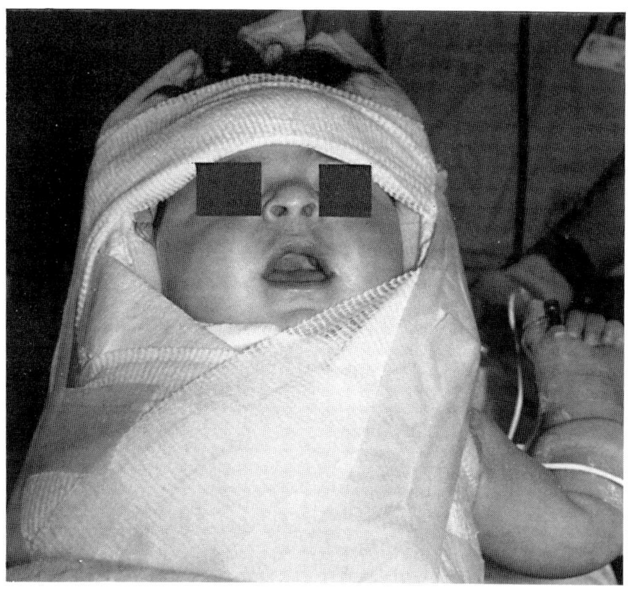

Fig. 32-20. Postoperatively, the infant is placed in a prefabricated "clam-shell" orthosis that limits motion of the head and neck, shoulder, and arm.

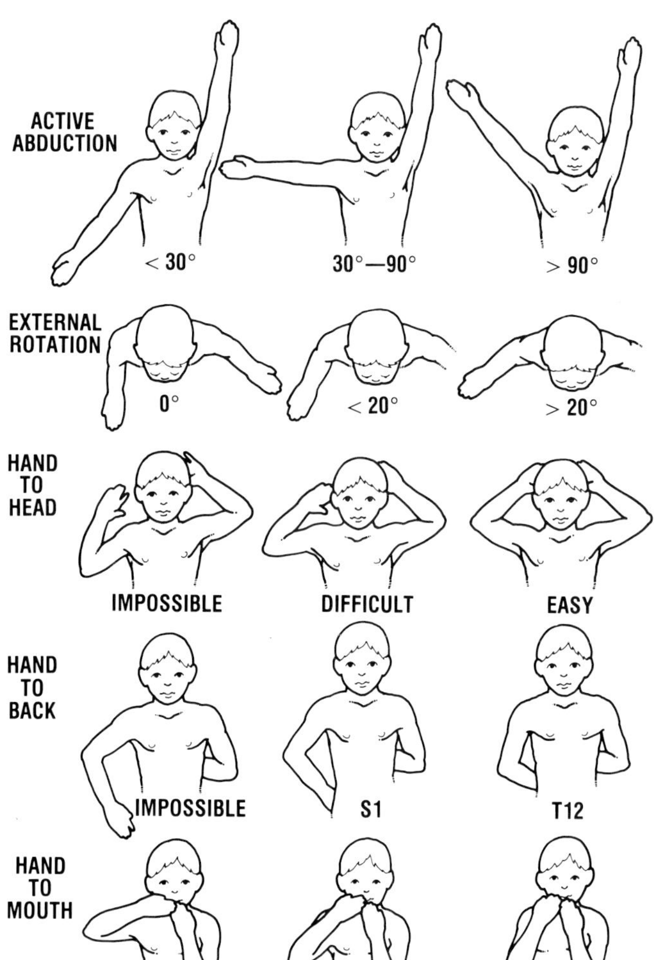

Fig. 32-21. Mallet's system for grading shoulder function in the child. (From Gilbert et al,[20] with permission.)

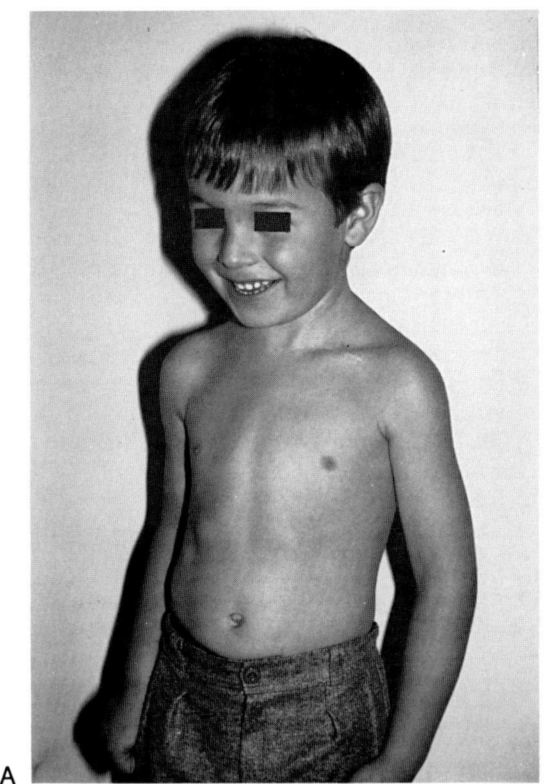
A

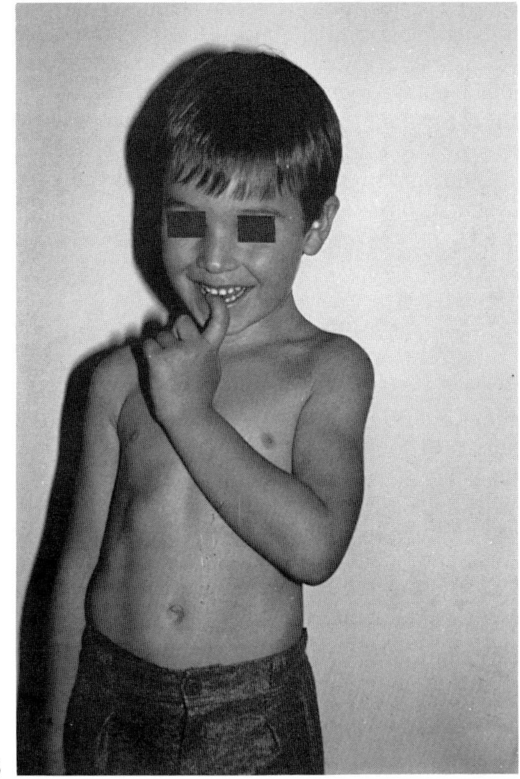
B

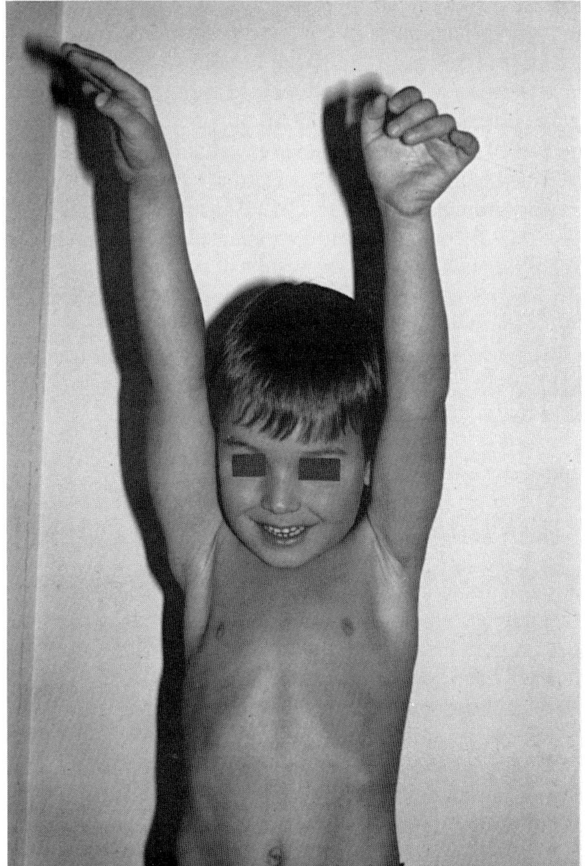
C

Fig. 32-22. **(A–C)** This child was initially seen with evidence of lesions of C5 and 6. At surgery, the fifth and sixth roots were found ruptured and were grafted. His level of recovery is illustrated at age 7. Hand function is normal.

good shoulder external rotation and abduction, elbow extension, and forearm rotation are initiated at 3 weeks. Clinical evaluation occurs every 3 months. The date of appearance of biceps reinnervation is a good prognostic sign. If this occurs by the fifth to sixth month postoperatively, the patient will go on to good recovery. Concern for the appearance of shoulder stiffness is of paramount importance. Surgical intervention is required if vigorous physical therapy fails.

Results of Surgery

The results of surgery must be categorized according to the severity of the initial presentation and surgical findings. Table 32-6 outlines Gilbert's results following reconstruction in subtotal palsy in the largest series published to date. Since the principal problems seen with spontaneous evolution have been shoulder problems, Gilbert[21-23] (personal communication, 1984) has adopted Mallet's[39] classification (Fig. 32-21) of shoulder function as the basis of his system of evaluation. These results indicate that two-thirds of Gilbert's operated group achieved a better functional result than had they been allowed to evolve spontaneously. Meyer and Rudisill[41] reported on five infants with C5 and 6 ruptured and C7 damaged. Four had a Grade IV biceps and deltoid, with Mallet level IV shoulder function, by 3 years postoperatively. Terzis, Liberson and Levine[66] reported six cases who had achieved Grade III shoulder and biceps strength by 3 years. Terzis[64] recently reported that reconstruction of the infant plexus results in improved growth of the affected limb, but not, however, to normal. Too few cases of total palsy are available for review. However, in contrast to the adult situation, where neurotization of muscles of the hand has almost been abandoned, in the infant, it is possible in more than 50 percent of cases to recover some intrinsic muscle activity, and in 90 percent to obtain some active digital flexion. When compared to the group allowed to spontaneously evolve, the results of surgery are fundamentally improved. These hands are functional and are used. In our experience, no patient in the operative group lost function. In Terzis' experience, it appeared that no child was downgraded by surgery. Figure 32-22 demonstrates a postoperative result from Gilbert's series.

Later Management

Frequent and systematic follow-up is necessary to identify the development of pathologic contractures, for reconstruction towards optimal functional is greatly simplified if joints remain supple. Those patients who have developed contractures, or subluxation of the glenohumeral joint or the radial head, represent difficult problems. Leffert[38] reviewed the history and indications for most of the commonly performed secondary reconstructive operations. The important contributions of L'Episcopo,[36] Hoffer, Wickenden, and Roper,[32] Zancolli,[72] and others should be noted. A description of all procedures useful in the child is beyond the scope of this chapter.

Summary

For the infant with obstetric palsy, the following points have emerged:

1. The typical palsy is a traumatic traction injury caused by forced lowering of the shoulder during delivery.
2. While the lesion may affect all roots, the upper roots are usually ruptures, while lower roots are frequently avulsed.
3. Spontaneous recovery is possible, but its quality depends greatly on how early recovery begins.
4. Microneural reconstruction is always possible, usually by grafting or by neurotization.
5. The results of surgery are better than the results of spontaneous evolution.
6. Palliative treatment of the sequellae of birth palsies is difficult, and the results obtained are rarely totally satisfactory.

For these reasons, the initial surgical intervention should be on the plexus itself in those cases meeting the criteria described above. It is important to make this decision as quickly as possible, before neuroplasticity is diminished and joint contracts have occurred.

REFERENCES

1. Allieu Y: Exploration et traitement direct des lesions nerveuses dans les paralysies traumatiques par elongation du plexus brachial chez l'adulte. Rev Chir Orthop 63:107–122, 1977
2. Allieu Y, Privat JM, Bonnel F: Paralysis in root avulsion of the brachial plexus. Neurotization by the spinal accessory nerve. Clin Plast Surg 11:133–136, 1984
3. Alnot JY, Jolly A, Frot B: Traitement direct des lésions nerveuses dans les paralysies traumatiques du plexus brachial chez l'adulte. Int Orthop 5:151–168, 1981
4. Bonney G: Prognosis in traction lesions of the brachial plexus. J Bone Joint Surg 41B:4–35, 1959
5. Bonney G, Birch R, Jamieson AM, Eames RA: Experience with vascularized nerve grafts. pp. 403–414. In Terzis JK (ed): Microreconstruction of Nerve Injuries. WB Saunders, Philadelphia, 1987
6. Breidenbach WC, Terzis JK: Vascularized nerve grafts: An experimental and clinical review. Ann Plast Surg 18:137–146, 1987
7. Breidenbach WC, Terzis JK: The blood supply of vascularized nerve grafts. J Reconstr Microsurg 3:43–55, 1986
8. Brunelli G: Neurotization of avulsed roots of the brachial plexus by means of anterior nerves of the cervical plexus. Int J Microsurg 2:55, 1980
9. Bufalini C, Pescatori G: Posterior cervical electromyography in the diagnosis and prognosis of brachial plexus injuries. J Bone Joint Surg 51B:627–631, 1969
10. Bunnell S: Surgery of the nerves of the hand. Surg Gynecol Obstet 44:145–152, 1927
11. Carson KA, Terzis JK: Carbonic anhydrase histochemistry: A potential diagnostic method for peripheral nerve repair. Clin Plast Surg 12:227–232, 1985
12. Celli L, Balli A, de Luise G, Rovesta C: La neurotizzazione degli ultimi nervi intercostali, mediante trapianto nervoso peduncu-

lato, nelle avulsioni radicolari del plesso brachiale. Chir Organi Mov 64:461, 1978

13. Doi K, Kuwata N, Kawakami F, Tamaru K, Kawai S: The free vascularized sural nerve graft. Microsurgery 5:175-184, 1984
14. Dolenc V: Intercostal neurotization of the peripheral nerves in avulsions plexus injuries. Clin Plast Surg 11:143-147, 1984
15. Duchenne G: De L'electrisation localisee et de son application a la pathologie et a la therapeutique. Bailliere, Paris, 1872
16. Erb W: Veber eine eigen thumliche localisation von lahmungen in plexus brachialis. Verh Dtsch 2:130, 1874
17. Freilinger G, Holle J, Sulzgruber SC: Distribution of motor and sensory fibers in the intercostal nerves. Plast Reconstr Surg 62:240-244, 1978
18. Ganel A, Engel J, Rimon S: Intraoperative identification of peripheral nerve fascicle. Use of a new rapid biochemical assay technique. Orthop Rev 15:669-672, 1986
19. Gilbert A: Vascularized sural nerve grafts. pp. 117-126. In Terzis JK (ed): Microreconstruction of Nerve Injuries. WB Saunders, Philadelphia, 1987
20. Gilbert A, Hentz VR, Tassin JL: Brachial plexus reconstruction in obstetric palsy: operative indications and postoperative results. pp. 348-364. In Urbaniak JR (ed): Microsurgery for Major Limb Reconstruction. CV Mosby, St. Louis, 1987
21. Gilbert A, Razaboni R: Etiology and pathology of obstetrical brachial plexus palsy—a review of 100 operated cases. 39th Annual Meeting of the American Society for Surgery of the Hand, San Antonio, October 1984
22. Gilbert A, Razaboni R: Ten years of surgical treatment of brachial plexus injuries—a review of 185 cases. 42nd Annual Meeting of the American Society for Surgery of the Hand, San Antonio, September 1987
23. Gilbert A, Tassin J: Reparation chirurgicale du plexus brachial dan la paralysie obstetricale. Chirurgie 110:70, 1984
24. Greenwald AG, Schute PC, Shiveley JL: Brachial plexus birth palsy: A 10-year report on the incidence and prognosis. J Pediatr Orthop 4:689-692, 1984
25. Gruber H, Freilinger G, Holle J, Mandl H: Identification of motor and sensory funiculi in cut nerves and their selective reunion. Br J Plast Surg 29:70-73, 1976
26. Gruber H, Zenker W: Acetylcholinesterase: Histochemical differentiation between motor and sensory nerve fibers. Brain Res 51:207-214, 1973
27. Gu Y-D, Wu M-M, Zheng Y-L, Li H-R, Xu Y-N: Arterialized venous free sural nerve grafting. Ann Plast Surg 15:332-339, 1985
28. Hardy AE: Birth injuries of the brachial plexus: Incidence and prognosis. J Bone Joint Surg 63B:98-101, 1981
29. Hentz VR: Operative repair of the brachial plexus in infants and children. pp. 1369-1383. In Gelbermen RH (ed): Operative Nerve Repair and Reconstruction. JB Lippincott, Philadelphia, 1991
30. Hentz VR Meyer RD: Brachial plexus microsurgery in children. Microsurgery 12:175-185, 1991
31. Hentz VR, Narakas A: The results of microneurosurgical reconstruction in complete brachial plexus palsy. Assessing outcome and predicting results. Orthop Clin North Am 19:107-114, 1988
32. Hoffer MM, Wickenden R, Roper B: Brachial plexus birth palsies. Results of tendon transfers to the rotator cuff. J Bone Joint Surg 60A:691-695, 1978
33. Kennedy R: Suture of the brachial plexus in birth paralysis of the upper extremity. Br Med, 1:298, 1903
34. Kline DG, Judice DJ: Operative management of selected brachial plexus lesions. J Neurosurg 58:631-649, 1983
35. Koshima I, Harii K: Experimental study of vascularized nerve grafts. Multifactorial analyses of axonal regeneration of nerves transplanted into an acute burn wound. J Hand Surg 10A:64-72, 1985
36. L'Episcopo JB: Tendon transplantation in obstetrical paralysis. Am J Surg 25:122-125, 1934
37. Landi A, Copland SA, Wynn-Parry CB, Jones SJ: The role of somatosensory evoked potentials and nerve conduction studies in the surgical management of brachial plexus injuries. J Bone Joint Surg 62B:492-496, 1980
38. Leffert RD: Brachial Plexus Injuries. Churchill Livingstone, New York, 1985
39. Mallet J: Paralysie obstetricale du plexus brachial symposium: Traitement des séquelles: Primauté du traitement de l'épaule—méthode d'expression des resultats. Rev Chir Orthop 58(suppl 1):166-168, 1972
40. Mansat M: Anatomie topographique chirurgical du plexus brachial. Rev Chir Orthop 63:20-26, 1977
41. Meyer R, Rudisill L: Early treatment of obstetrical palsy. 44th Annual Meeting of the American Society for Surgery of the Hand, Seattle, September 1989
42. Millesi H: Indications et résultats des interventions directes. Rev Chir Orthop 63:82-87, 1977
43. Millesi H: Surgical management of brachial plexus injuries. J Hand Surg 2:367-379, 1977
44. Millesi H: Neurotisation ladierter nerven unter heranzeihung gesunder nervenstamme. Handchirurgie. Nigst Ed. Georg Thieme, Stuttgart, 1983
45. Millesi H, Meissl G, Berger A: The interfascicular nerve-grafting of the median and ulnar nerves. J Bone Joint Surg 54A:727-750, 1972
46. Millesi H, Meissl G, Berger A: further experience with interfascicular grafting of the median, ulnar, and radial nerves. J Bone Joint Surg 58A:209-218, 1976
47. Minami M, Ishii S: Satisfactory elbow flexion in complete (preganglionic) brachial plexus injuries: Produced by suture of third and fourth intercostal nerves to musculocutaneous nerve. J Hand Surg 12A:1114-1118, 1987
48. Moy OJ, Peimer CA Koniuch MP, Howard C, Zielezny M, Katikaneni PR: Fibrin seal adhesive versus noabsorbable microsuture in peripheral nerve repair. J Hand Surg 13A:273-278, 1988
49. Narakas A: Brachial plexus surgery. Orthop Clin North Am 12:303-323, 1981
50. Narakas A: Indications et résultats du traitement chirugical direct dans les lésions par élongation du plexus brachial. Rev Chir Orthop 63:88-106, 1977
51. Narakas A: Les lésions dans les élongations du plexus brachial. Différentes possibilities et associations lésionnelles. Rev Chir Orthop 63:44-54, 1977
52. Narakas AO: Thoughts on neurotization or nerve transfers in irreparable nerve lesions. Clin Plast Surg 11:153-159, 1984
53. Narakas AO, Hentz VR: Neurotization in brachial plexus injuries. Indication and results. Clin Orthop 237:43-56, 1988
54. Restrepo Y, Merle M, Michon J, Folliguet B, Barrat E: Free vascularized nerve grafts: An experimental study in the rabbit. Microsurgery 6:78-84, 1985
55. Riley DA, Lang DH: Carbonic anhydrase activity of human peripheral nerves: A possible histochemical aid to nerve repair. J Hand Surg 9A:112-120, 1984
56. Samii M, Kahl R: Clinische resultate der autologen nerven transplantation. Melssunger Med Mittel 46:197, 1972
57. Scaglietti O: The obstetrical shoulder trauma. Surg Gynecol Obstet 66:868-877, 1938
58. Seddon HJ: The use of autogenous grafts for the repair of large gaps in peripheral nerves. Br J Surg 35:151-167, 1947
59. Seddon H: Surgical Disorders of the Peripheral nerves. 2nd Ed. Churchill Livingstone, Edinburgh, 1975
60. Sedel L: Results of surgical repair in brachial plexus injuries. J Bone Joint Surg 64B:54-66, 1982

61. Stevens JH: Brachial plexus paralysis. pp. 332–381. In Codman EA (ed): The Shoulder. G. Miller, New York, 1934
62. Sunderland S: Nerves and Nerve Injuries. 2nd Ed. Churchill Livingstone, Edinburgh, 1978
63. Tassin J: Paralysies obstetricales du plexus brachial: Evolution spontanee, resultats des interventions reparatrices process. Thesis, Universite Paris VII, 1983
64. Terzis JK: Microreconstruction of 50 cases of obstetrical brachial plexus paralysis. Presented at the ASSH 45th Annual meeting, Toronto, September 1990
65. Terzis JK, Breidenbach W: The anatomy of free vascularized nerve grafts. pp. 101–116. In Terzis JK (ed): Microreconstruction of Nerve Injuries. WB Saunders, Philadelphia, 1987
66. Terzis JK, Liberson WT, Levine R: Obstetric brachial plexus palsy. Hand Clin 2(4):773–786, 1986
67. Townsend PLG, Taylor GI: Vascularised nerve grafts using composite arterialised neuro-venous systems. Br J Plast Surg 37:1–17, 1984
68. Tsuyama N, Hara T: Intercostal nerve transfer in the treatment of brachial plexus injury of the root avulsion type. Excerpta Medica. 291:351, 1972
69. Van Beek AL, Massac E Jr., Smith DO: The use of the signal averaging computer for evaluation of peripheral nerve problems. Clin Plast Surg 13:407–418, 1986
70. Van Beek AL: Electrodiagnostic evaluation of peripheral nerve injuries. Hand Clin 2(4):747–760, 1986
71. Wilgis EFS: Nerve repair and grafting. In Green DP (ed): Operative Hand Surgery. 2nd Ed. Churchill Livingstone, New York, 1988
72. Zancolli EA: Classification and management of the shoulder in birth palsy. Orthop Clin North Am 12:433–457, 1981

33

Toe-To-Thumb Transplantation

Leonard Gordon

INTRODUCTION

Replantation of an amputated thumb has become a reliable operation that is feasible even after a crush or avulsion injury. Replantation can restore much of the thumb's original function and appearance and should be done if at all possible. In cases where replantation is not possible, the principle of restoring "like with like" calls for reconstruction using the next closest tissue. With this principle in mind, Nicoladoni attempted to transfer the great toe to the thumb in 1898.[84,85] He performed a two-stage procedure in which the great toe was used as a composite transfer that was held attached to the hand for 3 weeks, after which the pedicle was divided to complete the transfer. Understandably, this procedure did not gain wide acceptance because there were obvious difficulties with discomfort and positioning and the functional result was poor.

In 1966, Jacobsen described the anastomosis of 1-mm vessels, giving birth to the modern era of microsurgery. This and other animal research in the 1960s[4] culminated in the first human great toe-to-thumb transplant by Cobbett in 1968.[15] In 1973, the American Replantation Mission to China[1] reported that Yang had performed the first successful clinical transfer of a second toe to the thumb in 1966. Many reports of successful toe-to-thumb transplantation followed during the 1970s.[5,7,8,13,76,77,87–89,92,101,102,119]

Since it was first performed, complete or partial toe transfer has proved effective in reconstructing the absent or deficient thumb, and it has become established as the best thumb reconstruction in many circumstances.

An absent thumb represents a tremendous functional loss because the thumb is essential for grasping large objects, fine manipulation, and opposing the fingers.[12,100] In a hand that has been mutilated by damage to the fingers, an opposable and sensate thumb is even more important.[78] The goal of thumb reconstruction is to restore pinch and grasp by creating a thumb of ideal length and appearance with a maximum of strength, stability, movement, and sensation. In one operation, toe transplantation can restore all of these features, because the toe has strong skeletal support, a nail, glabrous skin that can be reinnervated, and mobile joints. It also has the potential for growth, which is important in children. The great toe is, however, approximately 20 percent larger than the thumb in all dimensions[115] (Fig. 33-1); methods have been developed to correct this discrepancy (see page 1275).

INDICATIONS

Etiology of the Defect

Traumatic Defects

The most common indication for toe-to-thumb transplantation is *traumatic loss of the thumb.* It is important to know the facts surrounding the injury, such as the presence of infection at the time of the original injury and whether there was damage to the vessels and nerves proximal to the site of amputation. Following burns, one must be aware that superficial veins may be destroyed, and a vena comitans will likely be needed as the recipient vein.

Tumors

Following *thumb amputation to resect an aggressive tumor,* toe transplantation can be used to restore thumb function. In these patients, the primary concern is appropriate treatment of

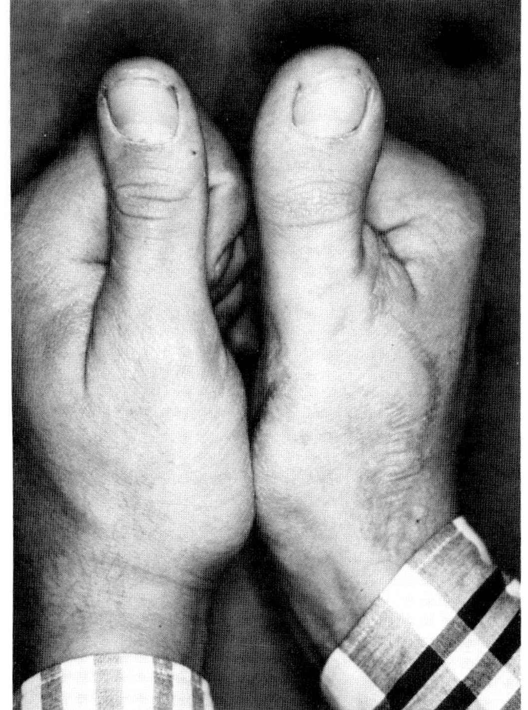

A

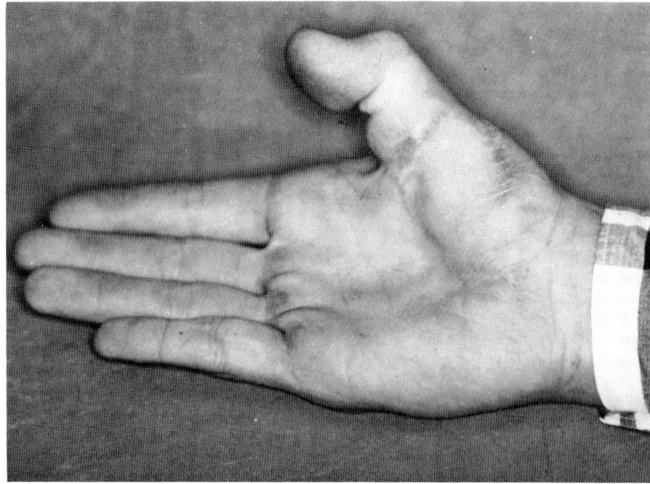

B

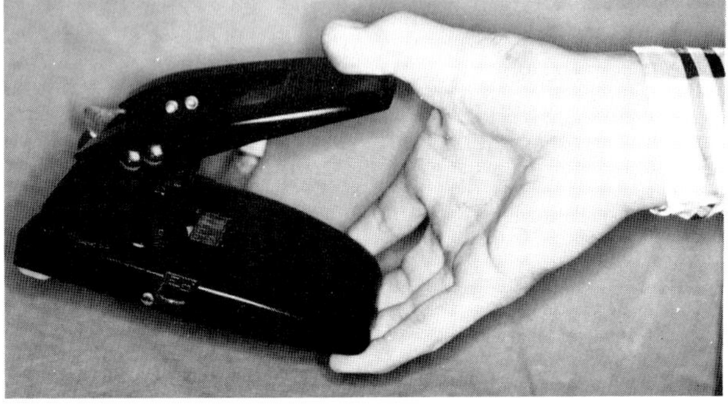

C

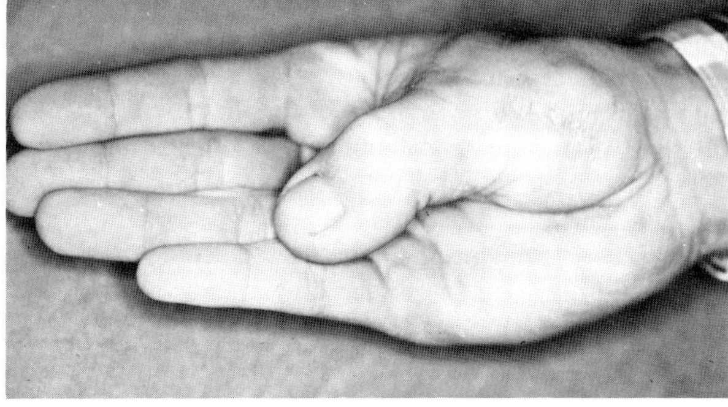

D

Fig. 33-1. The results of great toe transplantation. **(A)** The new thumb is slightly broader than the normal thumb but this difference in size is only noticeable when the two are seen side by side. If the ipsilateral toe is used, the new thumb is angled slightly toward the ulnar side. **(B)** Good motion at the interphalangeal joint is important, especially if there is no motion at the metacarpophalangeal joint. Fifteen to 30 degrees of motion can usually be achieved. **(C)** Good large object grasp is restored. **(D)** If intrinsic thumb muscles are present, the new thumb will have excellent opposition and dexterity. (From Gordon,[38] with permission.)

the tumor, which, in the majority of cases, should be completed with temporary cover prior to embarking on toe transplantation. Depending on the type and location of the tumor, toe transplantation can occasionally be performed at the time of amputation.[52]

Congenital Defects

Most *congenital defects* in which the thumb is absent are best reconstructed by pollicization of the index finger (see Chapter 57), especially if three or more digits are present.[21,34,78] Patients who do not have an adequate digit for pollicization may be candidates for second-toe transplantation. Considerations for such transfers depend on the etiology of the defect, the functional deficit, whether or not the deficit is bilateral, and age.[21] The procedure can be done in children who have longitudinal defects such as hypoplasia, isolated aplasia with or without radial club hand, or transverse defects such as symbrachydactyly, constriction ring syndrome, and true transverse arrest.[33,34] In patients who have longitudinal defects, all of the structures may be abnormal with multitendinous short fleshy muscles; the vessels may be absent or aplastic.

The vessels in symbrachydactyly and true transverse arrest are unpredictable.[34] In contrast, patients who have amniotic band syndrome have larger vessels out to the point of amputation, making toe transfer possible.[34] For this reason, it is important to dissect the hand before embarking on the toe dissection to ensure that adequate recipient structures are present, especially in patients who have longitudinal deformities. Arteriography can establish the presence of vessels but is unreliable in establishing their size.[33,34] Some surgeons advocate preoperative arteriography,[72,105] while others feel that this should not be done routinely.[40,57,66,81]

The advantage of toe transplantation over other techniques of thumb reconstruction is the inclusion of a viable growth plate, which enables an 85 percent rate of growth compared with the opposite thumb.[33,34] Ischemia time and age at operation do not affect growth.[33] The wraparound technique does not include a growth plate and therefore should not be considered in children.

Toe transplantation can be done in children over the age of 1 year. Children under 18 months have not yet established patterns of hand use and tend to incorporate the reconstructed thumb better than older children. This developmental timing is very important to remember in patients who have unilateral defects.[21,66] In hands that have no fingers, the goal of reconstruction is to provide sensation with two-finger pinch. The great or second toe from one foot can be transferred for use as the thumb to pinch against one or two minor toes from the opposite side. Some hands require transfer of only a single toe because one or more fingers are already present to oppose the transplant. There are alternative methods of reconstruction, such as web space deepening or metacarpal lengthening, which can create a post for pinch with the toe transplant.

The success of toe transfer for congenital defects depends on two factors. One is the presence of a mobile carpometacarpal joint in the recipient hand. This joint ensures good motion. If it is absent, its reconstruction can be attempted at the time of toe transplantation, but motion in the reconstructed thumb will be relatively limited. The other factor influencing the success of toe transfer is whether or not the defect is bilateral. As stated above, the goal of reconstruction in children who have no fingers is to provide sensate two-finger pinch. If the defect is bilateral, there is a compelling reason to do such complex reconstruction, and toe transfer is often indicated. In unilateral cases, one must realize that the reconstructed hand will be used in an assistive role. In patients who require a foot amputation because of concomitant congenital lower extremity problems, toe-to-thumb transplantation may make good use of structures that would otherwise be discarded, and the indications can be liberalized because there is no additional donor site deficit.[79] The second toe is generally preferred for thumb reconstruction in children[21,38,66] because the appearance of the donor site is nearly normal and the likelihood of subsequent growth and gait problems is minimal.

Considerations in the Hand

General Factors

Three questions must be answered before embarking on a toe transplant: Is a toe transplant the best method of reconstruction? (see Table 33-1), When should the procedure be done?, and Which toe transplant procedure is indicated? (see Table 33-2).

Many other methods of thumb reconstruction are described in great detail in Chapter 57, and the reader should be aware of the ramifications of alternative methods in a given situation. The myriad procedures available are evidence that no single procedure is appropriate for all cases of thumb amputation; each technique has advantages and drawbacks.[3,4,10,11,16,22,23,68,69,80,100] Toe transplantation has the obvious disadvantages of toe loss and the need for a long and complex operation. Nevertheless, the transplanted toe mimics the structure and function of a normal thumb more closely than does a thumb reconstructed by any other procedure (Table 33-1).

The *timing* of thumb reconstruction is important. Replacing the lost thumb soon after the injury has the obvious appeal of quickly restoring function, and some surgeons have advocated doing so.[96] However, there are several reasons to resist this temptation. The functional capability of a hand with a shortened or absent thumb is not immediately apparent, and the patient may find the new length of the thumb more or less functional, depending on his or her vocational and avocational requirements. Also, the patient may not fully understand the potential deficit in the foot. Therefore, in most cases, one should wait until the patient's condition has stabilized, the emotional frenzy of the injury has subsided, and the wounds have healed before discussing the option of toe transplantation, the donor site deficit, and possible alternatives. An exception to this general rule is when part of the thumb has been acutely injured and partial toe transplantation will avoid further thumb loss. An example of such a circumstance is when the soft tissues have been avulsed, leaving an exposed distal and middle phalanx that would be amenable to a wraparound flap (see Fig. 33-13). Similarly, if the soft tissues of the palmar region have been lost, an emergency partial toe flap may be the best option (see Fig. 33-13).

In cases where more than one toe transplant procedure is anticipated, the timing of reconstruction is often a dilemma. Double toe transplantation, which can be used to treat traumatic or congenital adactyly (Fig. 33-2), is usually best done in

Table 33-1. Evaluation of Toe Transplantation for Thumb Reconstruction

Advantages
Single operation
Good mobility and strength (depends on level of amputation)
Good sensation
Similar to the thumb in appearance
Glabrous skin; nail support
Growth potential
Disadvantages
Loss of a toe
Requires microvascular expertise
Lengthy operation

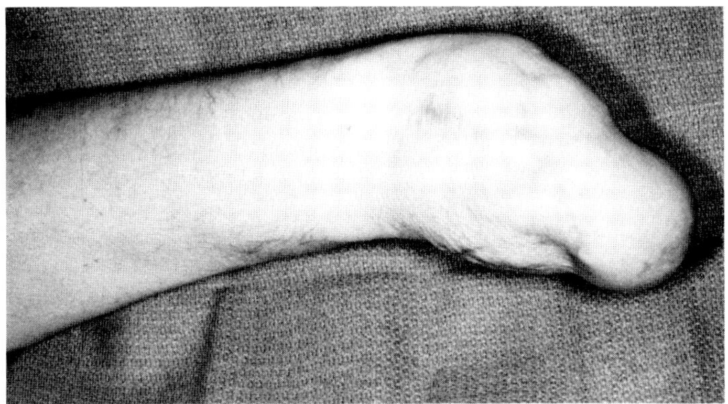

A

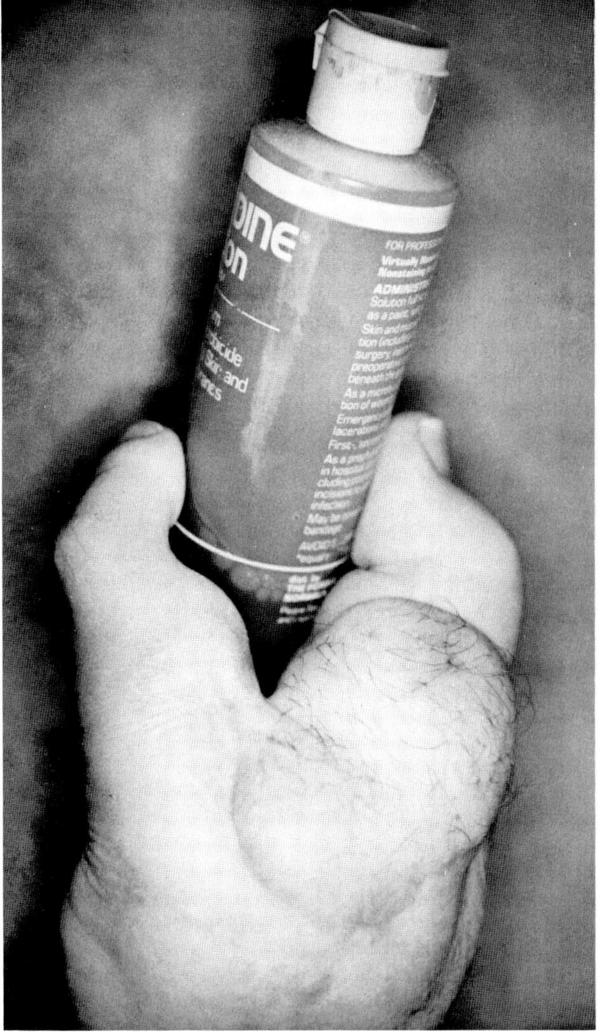

B

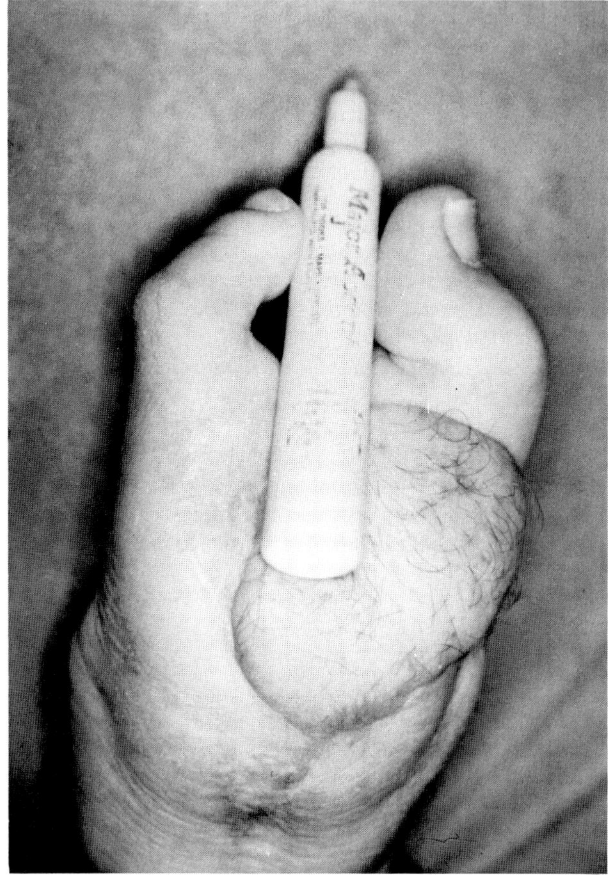

C

Fig. 33-2. **(A–C)** In post-traumatic adactyly, the hand can be reconstructed using a great toe from one foot and a second toe from the other. This approach limits the donor site deficit in each foot and restores limited pinch and grasp. The hand is used in an assistive role. (From Gordon,[38] with permission.)

two separate operations, but both transfers can be done simultaneously if a large enough operating team is available.[40] The great toe from one foot is used to replace the thumb, and a second toe from the opposite foot is placed in an opposable position.[40,63,93,114,116,123]

There are four toe transplant options for thumb reconstruction (Table 33-2): (1) whole great toe transfer (Fig. 33-1); (2) second-toe transfer (see Fig. 33-14); (3) the wraparound procedure, wherein a bone graft (usually from the iliac crest) is "wrapped" with the soft tissues from the great toe, including the nail and pulp (Fig. 33-13); and (4) partial toe transplantation, wherein parts of the toe such as the pulp, nail, or joint are used to remedy specific deficits (see Figs. 33-15, 33-16).

The method of thumb reconstruction must be individualized, with consideration given to the patient's general outlook and motivation, age, handedness, and functional requirements at work and home. A detailed analysis of the injured hand should then be done that includes a determination of the *status of the remaining digits.* Toe transplantation can be performed in individuals who are at least 1 year of *age;* there is no upper age limit with regard to either the technical feasibility of this operation or the ultimate function of the reconstructed thumb. It is important to remember that the wraparound procedure has no growth potential, and, for that reason, is not advisable for children. Nerve return in older individuals is less satisfactory than that in younger patients (Chapter 35).

Toe-to-thumb transplantation is indicated for both *dominant and nondominant hands.* In the vast majority of cases, thumb reconstruction is performed in patients who have a normal opposite extremity. In patients who have a bilateral deficit, the restoration of sensation, pinch, and grasp on at least one side is obviously of even greater importance. The *functional needs* of the patient must be carefully considered. Many patients require strength and dexterity, and appearance may be especially important for someone who is constantly in the public eye. Of course, some factors are subjective or may relate to culture. For example, loss of the great toe in some Asian patients may be unacceptable because it will preclude their wearing open style thongs. For this reason, the medical literature from these cultures often favors second-toe transfer.[119] A frank discussion with the patient is vital.

Level of Thumb Amputation (Fig. 33-3)

At or distal to the interphalangeal joint. If the amputation is distal to the interphalangeal joint, the thumb usually has adequate function and no reconstruction is necessary. If a longer thumb is desired for better function or appearance, metacarpal lengthening with first web space deepening may be considered, but neither of these methods provide a nail, glabrous skin, or additional motion. The great toe is often too bulbous if placed this far distal on a narrow proximal phalanx, and the second toe is too narrow. The *wraparound* (see Fig. 33-13) or *trimmed toe procedure* should be considered because either can restore length, sensibility, and near-normal appearance. The level at which amputation leaves enough length and dexterity for adequate function depends on the patient's motivation and functional requirements, and, for that reason, must be individualized. In a comparison of amputations and replantations, Goldner et al found that function after replantation distal to the proximal third of the proximal phalanx did not "demonstrate uniform superiority" over amputation closure.[37]

Through the proximal phalanx, with an intact metacarpo-

Table 33-2. Toe-to-Thumb Transplantation for Thumb Reconstruction: Comparison of Various Methods

Procedure	Function: Mobility	Function: Sensation	Strength	Appearance
Whole great toe	Optimal	++++ (broad contact area)	++++	++ (Best with a great toe of moderate size)
Second toe	Adequate	++++ (narrow contact area)	++	+ (Best with a large second toe)
Trimmed great toe	Optimal	++++	++++	++++
Wraparound	None	++++	+++	++++

Procedure	Amputation Level	Donor Site	Complications/ Disadvantages	Complexity of the Procedure
Whole great toe	Distal metacarpal; proximal phalanx	Function +++ Appearance +	None	Easy
Second toe	Proximal part of metacarpal w/ absent thenar muscles; pediatric patients	Function ++++ Appearance ++++	Mallet deformity of the distal joint	Easy
Trimmed great toe	Distal metacarpal; proximal phalanx	Function +++ Appearance +	None	One additional step
Wraparound	Distal to functioning MP joint	Variable ++	Bone resorption; No growth; No motion	More difficult; requires iliac crest graft in hand and skin graft on foot

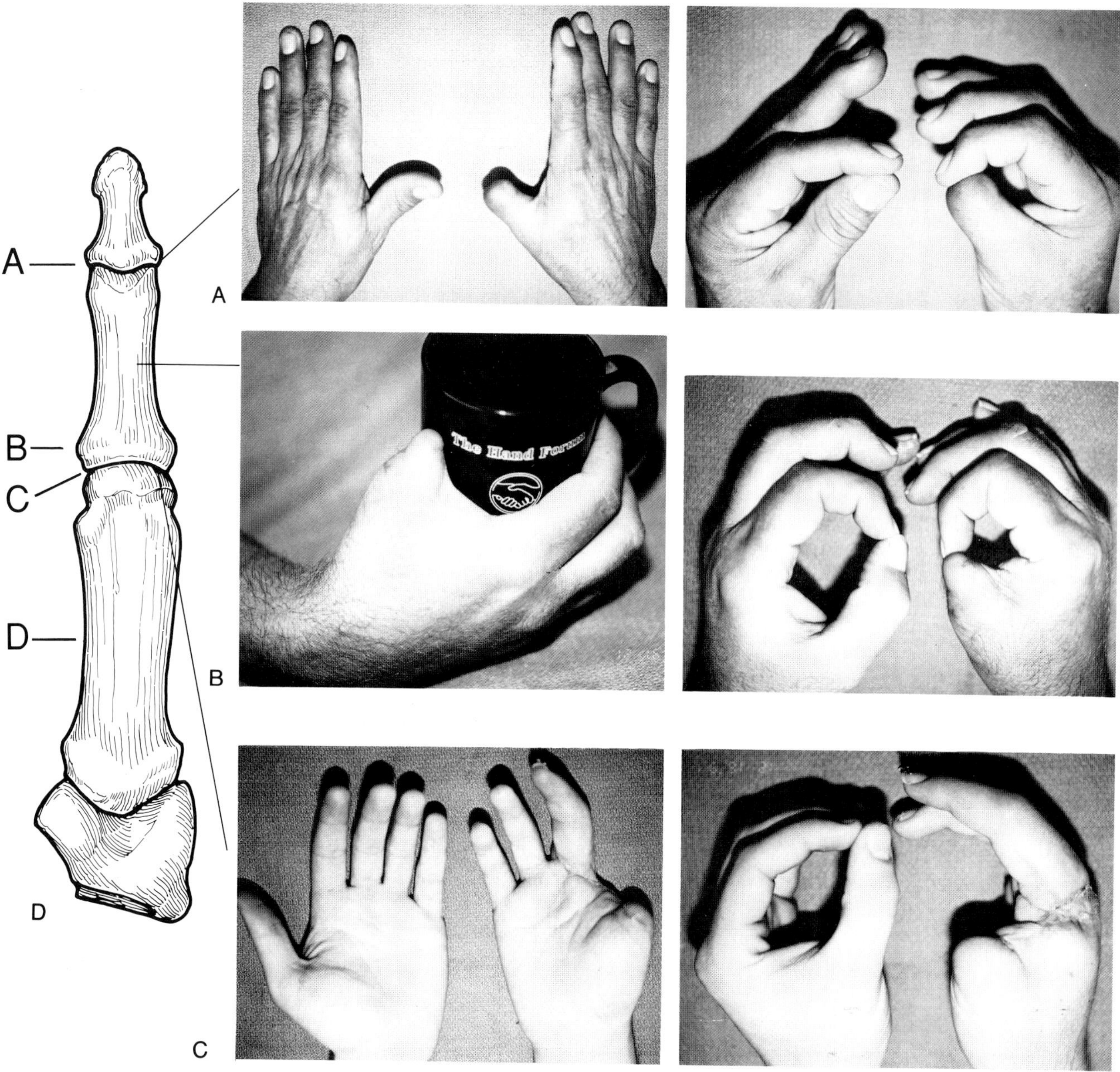

Fig. 33-3. The options for toe-to-thumb transplantation depend on the level of amputation (see page 1257). **(A)** Amputation at the interphalangeal joint level. The thumb may or may not require reconstruction. The wraparound procedure is done if reconstruction is necessary. **(B)** Amputation at the level of the proximal phalanx, with a functional metacarpophalangeal joint. Reconstruction will restore the ability to grasp large objects and improve pinch. Either whole great toe transfer, second-toe transfer, or the wraparound procedure may be used. **(C)** Amputation at the metacarpophalangeal level. No thumb function remains. Either whole great toe transfer or second-toe transfer may be used. **(D)** Amputation proximal to the midmetacarpal level. Second-toe transfer is needed.

phalangeal joint. Because motion is possible at the trapeziometacarpal joint as well as at the metacarpophalangeal joint, restoring motion at the interphalangeal joint is desirable but not essential. The *wraparound procedure* (see Fig. 33-13) provides a narrower thumb and better appearance than does a great toe transplant. However, no motion is possible at the interphalangeal joint because this transplant uses an iliac crest graft as the osseous support. The wraparound procedure should not be used in children because the transplant has no growth potential. Absorption of the iliac crest graft occasionally occurs, but this complication can be minimized if a small amount of the distal phalanx of the great toe is included with the transplant. The *trimmed toe* transplant also provides a narrower thumb than does the whole great toe but without the aforementioned disadvantages. The *second toe* (see Fig. 33-14) is narrower than the thumb and provides the least satisfactory appearance of all the options. Mobility at the interphalangeal joints is limited, and a flexion (mallet) deformity may result from incompetence of the extensors and intrinsics, compromising appearance and function. To avoid this complication, temporary pinning of the interphalangeal joint in extension for 2 to 3 weeks is advisable.

The *great toe* (Figs. 33-1 and 33-4) offers the best motion and strength of all the options. Its pulp is broader and it provides stronger pinch and grasp than does the second toe. The great toe must be taken distal to the metatarsophalangeal joint to avoid creating a thumb that is too long. Part of the proximal phalanx of the great toe must be removed to shorten the transplant, or else the toe phalanx can be hollowed out to create a mortise and tenon joint (see page 1270).

Any one of these options provides good opposition because of the level of the amputation. I prefer to use the great toe

A

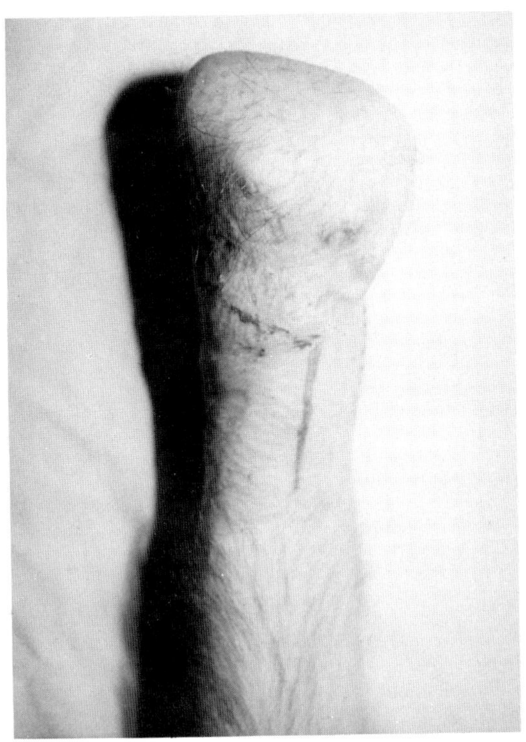

B

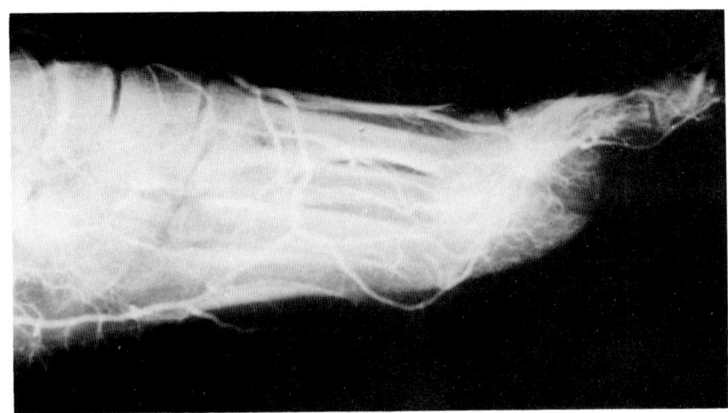

C

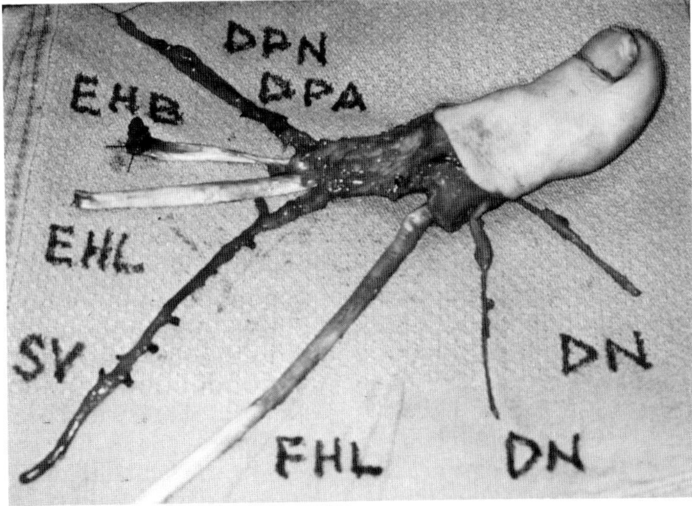

Fig. 33-4. Great toe transfer is performed in a case of traumatic adactyly to provide fine pinch and large object grasp with an orthosis. **(A)** Preoperative appearance of the hand. **(B)** A preoperative oblique arteriogram confirms the presence of a large first dorsal metatarsal artery. **(C)** The toe is now ready for transplantation. The dorsalis pedis artery *(DPA)*, deep peroneal nerve *(DPN)*, extensor hallucis brevis *(EHB)*, extensor hallucis longus *(EHL)*, saphenous vein *(SV)*, flexor hallucis longus *(FHL)*, and digital nerves *(DN)* have been dissected to appropriate lengths, which were determined by the available structures in the hand. *(Figure continues.)*

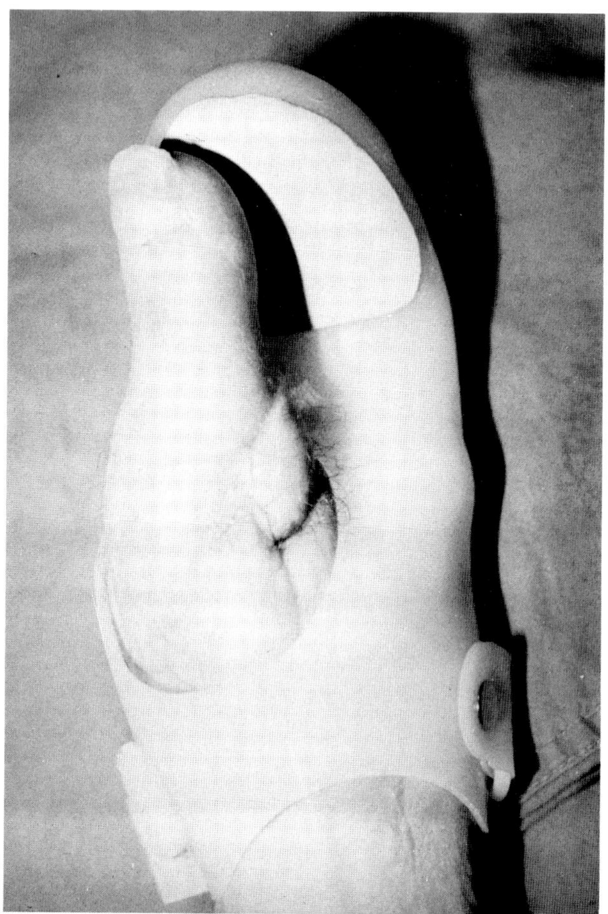

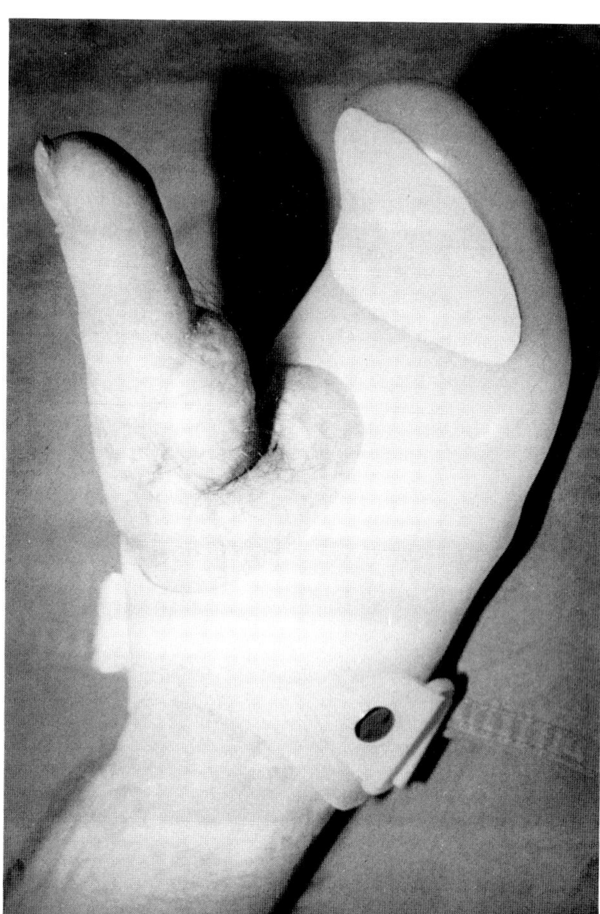

Fig. 33-4 *(Continued).* **(D&E)** Because the basal joint of the thumb was intact, the new thumb had good mobility. (Courtesy of Richard J. Smith, M.D., deceased.) (From Gordon,[38] with permission.)

transplant and reserve the wraparound flap or the trimmed-toe technique for patients who have a large bulbous great toe and feel that appearance is of paramount importance.

The distal half of the metacarpal to the metacarpophalangeal joint. Because the metacarpophalangeal joint is absent, it is important to restore some motion in the transplanted toe. This requirement is essential if there is any question of damage or limited motion at the trapeziometacarpal joint. Because the *wraparound procedure* provides no motion, the only motion in the reconstructed thumb will be at the carpometacarpal joint. If the amputation is fairly close to the metacarpophalangeal joint, the best option is the *great toe transplant* (Fig. 33-1). The great toe must not be removed proximal to the metatarsophalangeal joint (see page 1279) or else there will be subsequent problems with balance and push-off when walking. An angled osteotomy retains the metatarsal head and sesamoid bones and provides motion at the new metacarpophalangeal joint (see Fig. 33-7). For amputations at the metacarpophalangeal joint, the great toe can be removed at the metatarsophalangeal joint and a "composite" joint constructed using the articular surface of the hand metacarpal head and the toe proximal phalanx. The joint capsule is repaired using tissue from the metatarsophalangeal joint capsule.[118] If this repair is done, the new thumb will be slightly longer than is optimal. If the great toe is too short to be taken at the metatarsophalangeal joint, the *second toe* (see Fig. 33-14) should be used, because it can be taken with whatever length of second metatarsal is needed to provide appropriate thumb length. If possible, either the thenar muscle insertion should be reconstructed or an opposition transfer should be done to provide opposition. A better result will also be achieved if adduction of the thumb can be restored by repairing the adductor pollicis.

Proximal to the midportion of the metacarpal. Thumb reconstruction following amputations at this level are difficult and should be done with the *second toe.* If the second metatarsal is used to provide adequate thumb length, there may be difficulty with soft tissue cover in the region and the transplant may lack active opposition and abduction. The distance between the web space and the ends of the toes is shorter than the distance between the first web space and the end of the thumb in the hand. Because of this difference, placement of the second toe and its metatarsal in the thumb position will result in inadequate skin cover over the metatarsal and the surrounding interosseous muscle. Some of the muscle can be covered with a

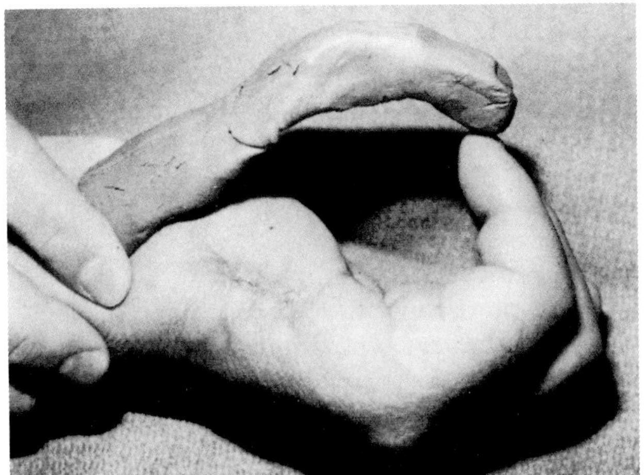

A

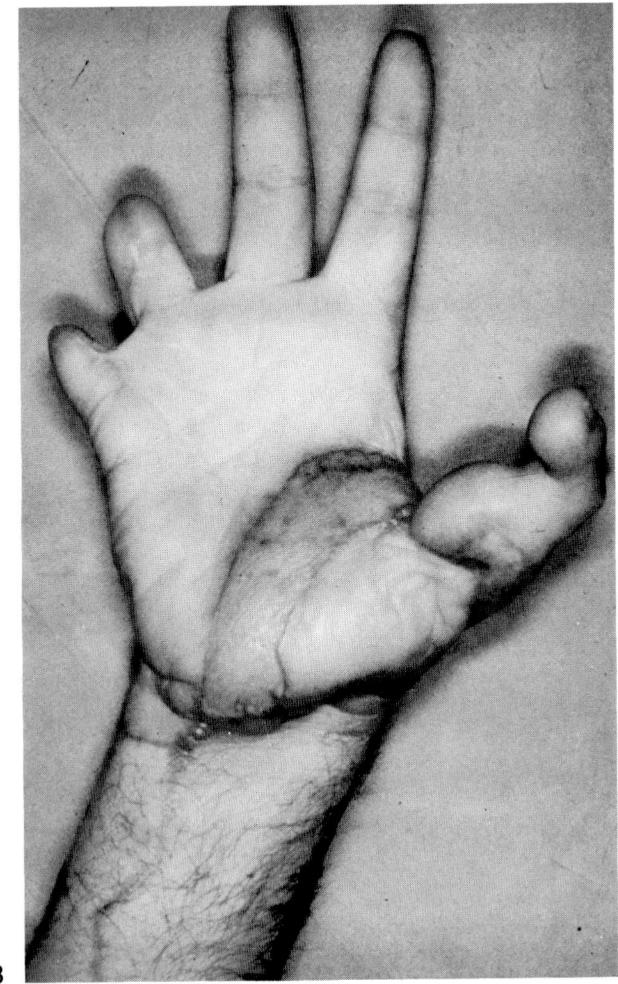

B

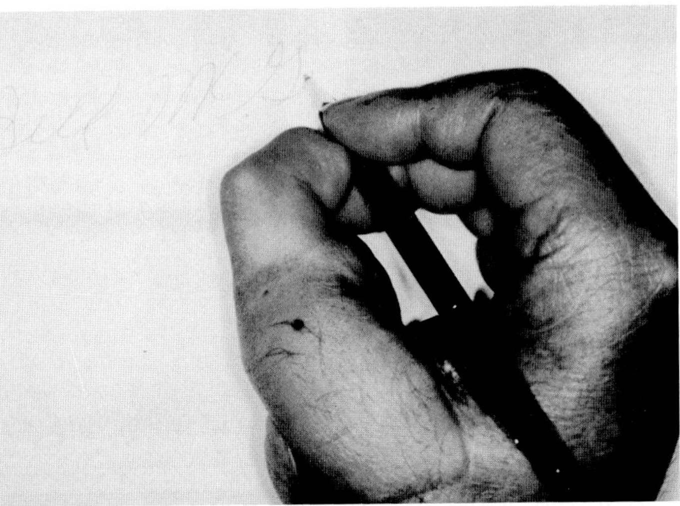

C

Fig. 33-5. When the entire first metacarpal is missing and fingers are not available for pollicization, thumb reconstruction is difficult. **(A)** A clay model is used to plan the second-toe transfer. **(B)** After second-toe transfer, a serratus anterior muscle flap was used to widen the first web space, and an opposition transfer was done to provide thumb abduction and opposition. Good grasp of large objects was restored. **(C)** Good pinch and dexterity were achieved. (From Gordon,[38] with permission.)

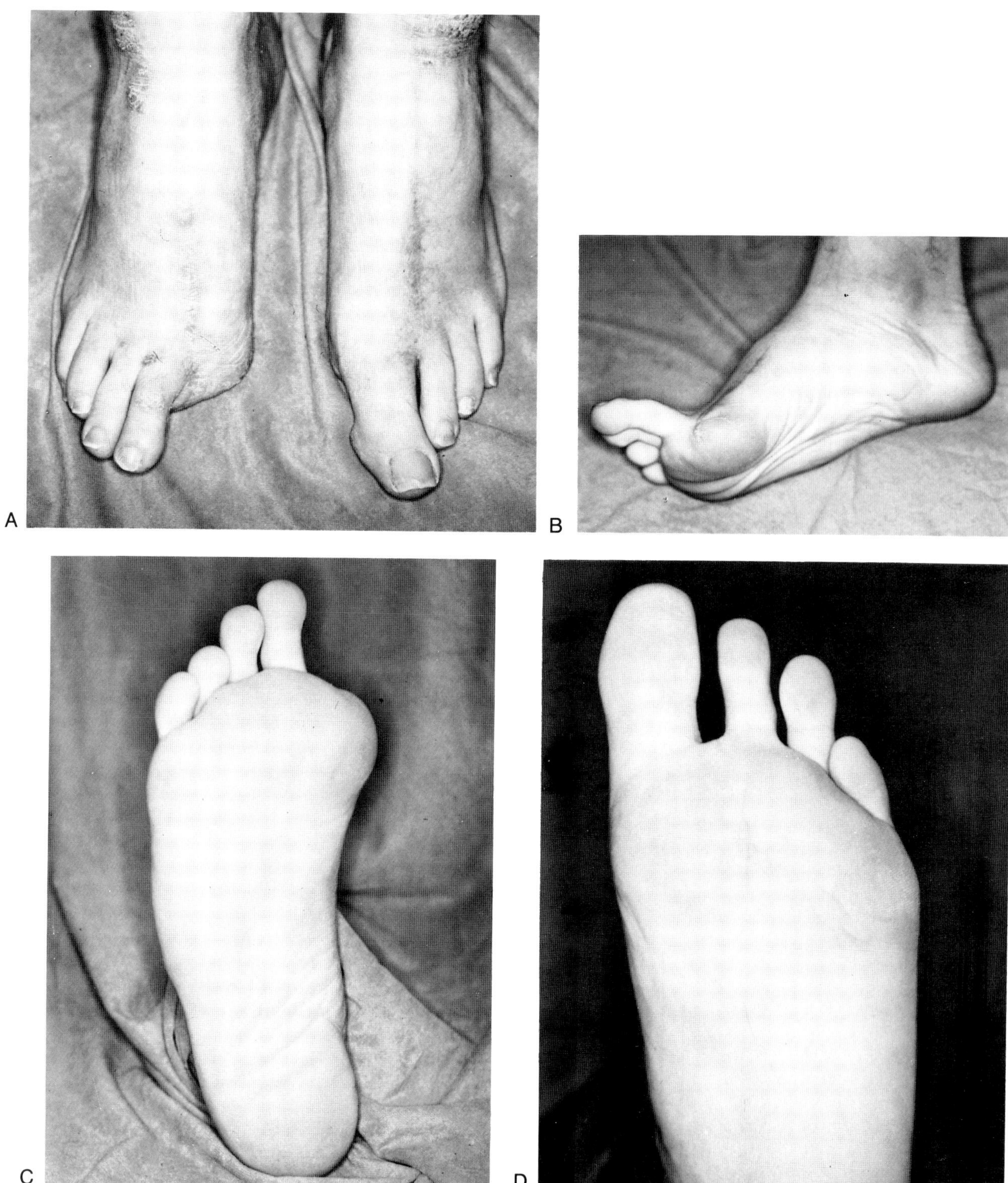

Fig. 33-6. Appearance of the donor site following toe-to-thumb transplantation. **(A)** The feet are shown from the dorsal aspect following great toe and second toe transplantation. **(B&C)** The foot is seen from the plantar surface following great toe transplantation. Retaining the sesamoid bone and maintaining the length of the first metatarsal are important for weight bearing; this is evidenced by the callus formation under the metatarsal head, which continues to be used for weight bearing and balance. **(D)** The foot is seen from the plantar surface following second-toe transplantation. *(Figure continues.)*

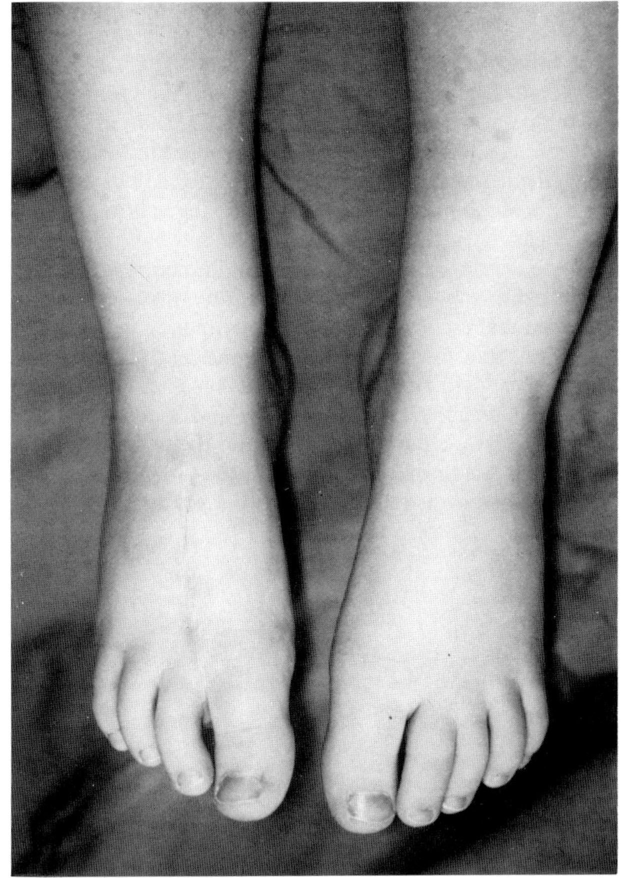

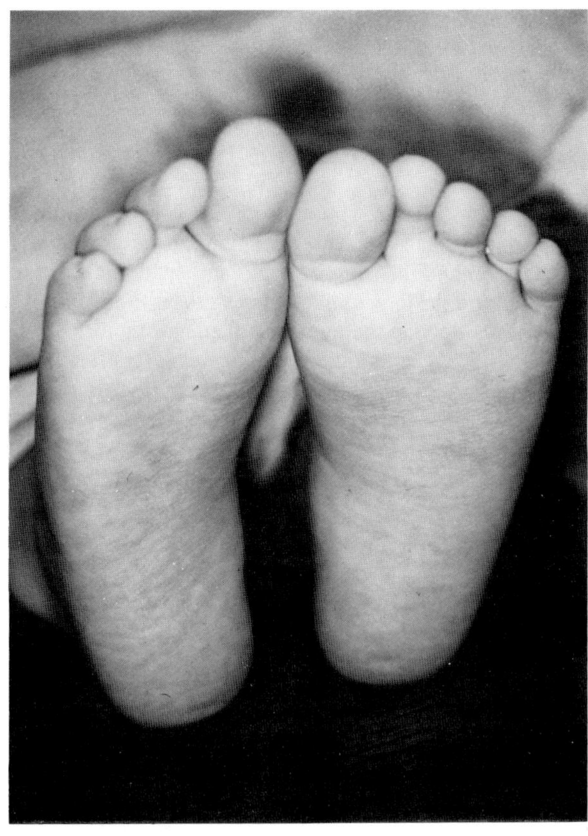

E F

Fig. 33-6 *(Continued).* **(E&F)** The donor foot is compared with the opposite side following second-toe transplantation in a 22-month-old child. (From Gordon,[38] with permission.)

split-thickness skin graft, but careful preoperative planning is essential and a preliminary skin or muscle flap will often be needed to provide adequate skin cover. An opposition transfer (see page 1279) can be done either at the time of the transplantation or as a secondary procedure. Cover and active opposition can be provided with a functional muscle microvascular flap.[41]

Proximal to the metacarpal (Fig. 33-5). Thumb reconstruction is a difficult challenge when none of the metacarpal remains.[41,104] After most such amputations, *pollicization of the index finger* is the best choice, especially if the index finger is slightly damaged or shortened as a result of the injury. If multiple digits have been injured, this option may not be possible and a toe transplant is then needed. The *second toe,* including the metatarsal, is used in these cases. The base of the metatarsal is placed on the trapezium and pinned temporarily. This junction forms a pseudojoint over time. Toe transplants of this type have also been placed on the distal radius in unusual cases of adactyly.[30,111,122]

Patients who have suffered bilateral traumatic amputations at the wrist or distal forearm level have undergone reconstruction[30,46,71,111,122] using a variety of innovative methods, such as toe transfer to a radial stump combined with osteoplastic lengthening of the ulna. The goal of such surgery is to provide rudimentary pinch. Only a few such cases are reported in the literature because these procedures are very rarely indicated. Pinch can be restored to the hand without digits by using a complex microvascular procedure in which many toes are transferred from the foot.[111,122,123] However, the deficit in the foot after such a procedure is substantial. The details of these complex procedures are beyond the scope of this chapter and the reader is referred to the original literature.

Partial thumb loss. When part of the thumb has been lost, the missing portion can be replaced with a partial toe transplant, or vascularized "spare part." The largest of the partial toe transplants is the *wraparound flap* (see Fig. 33-13). There is actually a myriad of bone, joint, and soft tissue defects that can be remedied in this way.[24,25,26,48,53,73,90,91,103] For example, a segment of the *metatarsophalangeal joint* can replace the metacarpophalangeal joint,[26,47,48,54,73,90,103] using the overlying skin to widen the first web space (Fig. 33-16). Parts of the toe, including *soft tissue and nail,* can be transferred.[24,25,53] When the pulp of the thumb has been lost and scar tissue or a split-thickness skin graft does not provide adequate cover or sensation, a segment of the *pulp of the toe*[24,25] can be transplanted to provide a better surface (Fig. 33-15). A toe pulp flap that includes the digital nerve will restore sensation if there is a scarred or damaged thumb pulp or if nerve damage precludes nerve repair and makes nerve grafting difficult. The pulp flap can be taken with a long segment of the digital nerve. Of course, flaps from the dorsum of the index finger and hand must also be considered for such reconstruction (see Chapter 12).

Considerations in the Foot (Fig. 33-6)

When contemplating the appropriateness of a toe transplant or trying to decide which toe transplant procedure to use, both the surgeon and the patient should anticipate the effect of the operation on the foot. When the *great toe* is used, amputation is generally done at the metatarsophalangeal joint. The problems that occur with amputation at this level are minor and infrequent. Analysis of gait and foot function following this procedure have shown that the most striking but expected change is a shift in weight bearing toward the lateral side of the foot.[64,94] It is important to retain the sesamoid bones and the head of the first metatarsal to better preserve balance and push-off[29] (Fig. 33-7).

Removal of the *second toe* causes less of a cosmetic defect than does removal of the great toe[29] (Fig. 33-6). After second toe removal, a ray amputation should be performed that leaves only the base of the metatarsal. The first and third metatarsals can then be approximated, after which the intermetatarsal ligament is reconstructed. The foot is somewhat narrower with only four toes, but its appearance and function are excellent.

Initially, the *wraparound procedure* was presented as a method that retains some length and function in the great toe. After this transplant is harvested, a considerable amount of the bone is exposed and the toe requires reconstruction. This reconstruction requires skin grafting, and some surgeons perform a cross-toe flap from the second toe to provide cover.[81] Although length may be preserved, the function and appearance of the reconstructed toe may not justify the effort. Usu-

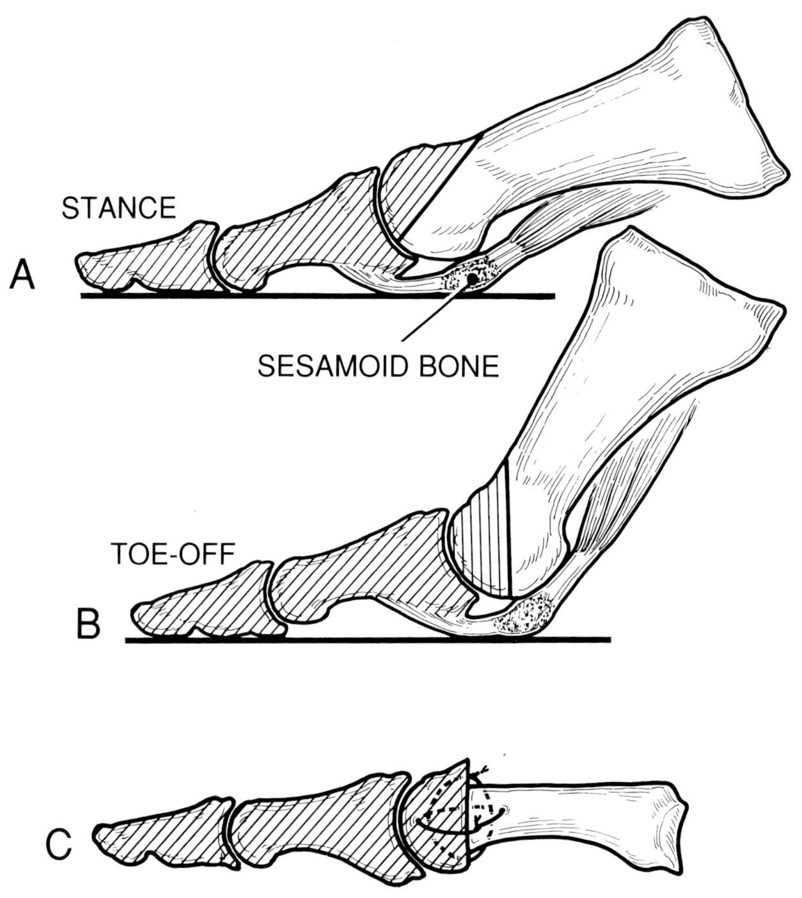

Fig. 33-7. The first metatarsal head and sesamoid bones should not be removed when the great toe is transplanted. A portion of the dorsal surface of the first metatarsal may be removed without affecting the weight-bearing surface. The plantar surface of the first metatarsal head and the sesamoid bones are important during the **(A)** stance and **(B)** toe-off phases of the gait cycle. **(C)** If this angled osteotomy is fixed to the first metacarpal with the metatarsophalangeal joint in an extended position, the joint will only be able to flex. Thus, the joint is converted from one that hyperextends into one that flexes. (Modified from Gordon,[38] with permission.)

ally, the donor site is only marginally better than if the toe were to be amputated at the metatarsophalangeal joint, and one should not choose to do the wraparound procedure because of donor site considerations alone.

There are two reasons for using the *ipsilateral great toe* to reconstruct the thumb. First, the vascular pedicle that lies in the first intermetatarsal space will be positioned on the appropriate side of the transplanted toe for suture to the radial artery on the dorsal aspect of the first web space of the hand. Second, the great toe generally has a 10- to 15-degree angle toward the lateral side at the metatarsophalangeal and interphalangeal joints. Following transplantation, this angle will provide better pinch and opposition with the fingers.

ANATOMY (Figs. 33-8, 33-9)

Regardless of which part of the foot is used, a thorough knowledge of the anatomy, including variations and anomalies, is essential before embarking on any of these procedures. The great toe is stouter than the thumb by approximately 20 percent, and the second toe is considerably narrower. The great

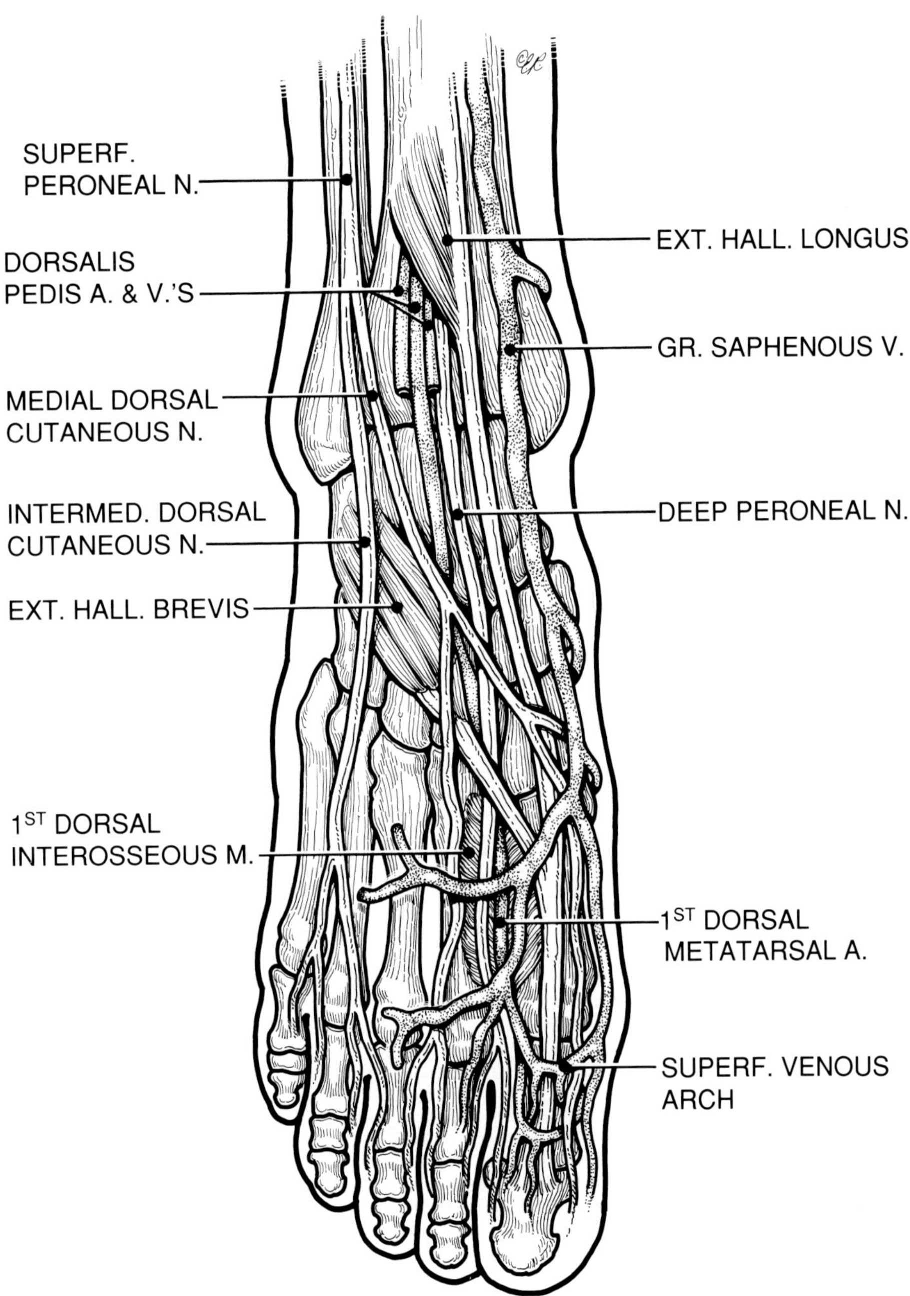

Fig. 33-8. Anatomy of the dorsum of the foot. (Modified from Gordon,[38] with permission.)

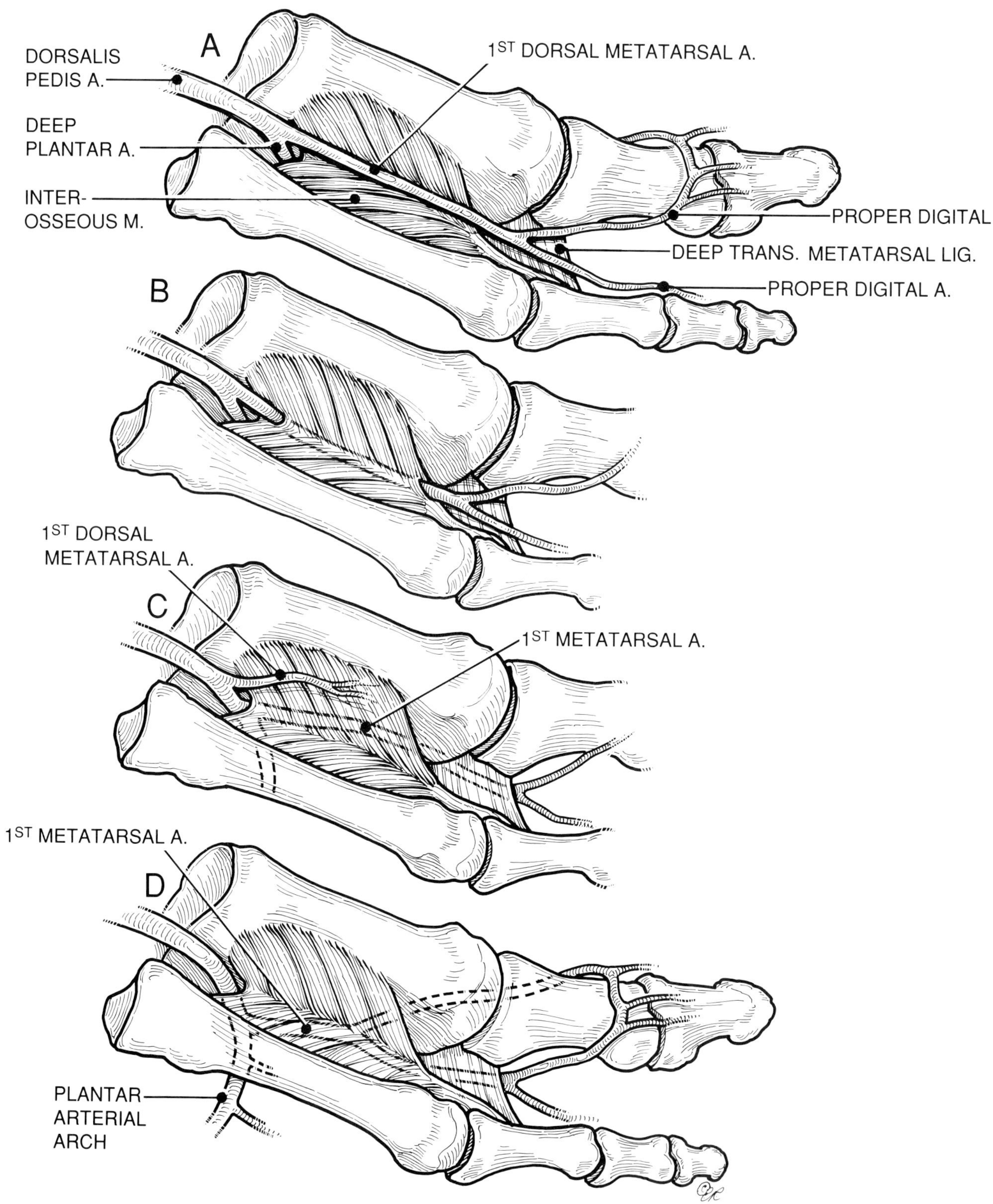

Fig. 33-9. Anatomic variations of the first dorsal metatarsal artery *(FDMA)*. **(A)** The dorsalis pedis artery divides into the deep plantar artery and the FDMA. The FDMA continues superficial to the interosseous muscle and deep transverse metatarsal ligament and divides into the proper digital arteries supplying the adjacent sides of the first web space. **(B)** The FDMA can travel in or deep to the interosseous muscle, but it remains superficial to the deep transverse metatarsal ligament. **(C)** The FDMA is a small and inadequate supply for the toes. The metatarsal artery originates from either the dorsalis pedis artery or the deep plantar artery and runs deep to the interosseous muscle and deep transverse metatarsal ligament. This artery tends to curve under the first metatarsal bone. **(D)** The first metatarsal artery emanates from the plantar arterial arch and runs deep to the interosseous muscle and deep transverse metatarsal ligament. The FDMA is small or absent.

toenail is often broader than the thumbnail but it is also shorter, although there is considerable variation in these relative dimensions. The great and second toes are hyperextended at the metatarsophalangeal joint, slightly flexed at the proximal interphalangeal joint, and extended at the distal interphalangeal joint (Fig. 33-7). The longitudinal arch of the foot ends at the metatarsal heads, which bear weight during gait. The longitudinal arch in the hand terminates at the end of the fingers. The web spaces in the foot are located more distally than they are in the hand.

The *superficial transverse metatarsal ligament* connects the digital slips of the plantar aponeurosis. The plantar ligament is analogous to the palmar plate of the fingers. In the great toe, it is largely replaced by the sesamoid bones, with a strong interconnecting ligament between. The plantar ligaments are connected by the *deep transverse metatarsal ligaments.* The articular capsule of the metatarsophalangeal joint is loose. Dorsally, it is reinforced by fibers from the extensor tendon and is attached closer to the articular border than it is on the plantar side. A collateral ligament lies on each side of the joint.

The foot has two arterial arches: the *dorsal arterial arch* arising from the dorsalis pedis artery, and the *plantar arterial arch* arising from the medial and lateral branches of the posterior tibial artery. The dorsal arch can be easily dissected through the dorsum of the foot, and it is almost always used in toe transplantation. The *anterior tibial artery* lies between the extensor hallucis longus and the extensor digitorum longus tendons. At the ankle, this vessel becomes the dorsalis pedis artery, passing over the dorsum of the foot to the first intermetatarsal space. Just proximal to this space, the artery is crossed by the extensor hallucis brevis tendon. Dividing this tendon and dissecting beneath it will provide easy access to the vessels.

At the base of the first intermetatarsal space, the *dorsalis pedis artery* divides into the deep plantar artery (also called the perforating branch) and the first dorsal metatarsal artery, which proceeds distally in the first intermetatarsal space (Fig. 33-9A). Distally, the *first dorsal metatarsal artery* divides into two branches that supply the adjacent sides of the great and second toes. The neurovascular bundles of the toes lie just plantar to their midaxial line. The lateral neurovascular bundle of the great toe is generally larger than the medial and reliably supplies good circulation.

The origin and course of the first dorsal metatarsal artery is the key to the vascular anatomy relevant to dissecting the great toe, second toe, and partial toe flaps. This anatomy is variable (Fig. 33-9).[32,42,44,62] In about two-thirds of patients, the first dorsal metatarsal artery emanates from the dorsalis pedis artery and travels in a relatively dorsal plane (Figs. 33-9A and B). This course can be dorsal to the interosseous muscle (Fig. 33-9A), within the muscle, or deep to it (Fig. 33-9B), but the artery courses dorsal to the deep transverse metatarsal ligament (Figs. 33-9A and B). Other configurations are seen in about one-third of patients. The first dorsal metatarsal artery may arise from the dorsalis pedis or deep plantar artery, but the principal vessel to the toes runs deep to the deep transverse metatarsal ligament (Fig. 33-9C). Occasionally, the vessels to the great and second toes may arise from the plantar arterial arch[44,51,57] (Fig. 33-9D). There is actually no consensus on the incidence of a dominant dorsal or plantar first metatarsal artery.[32,42,44,51,62,75,77,102] The first metatarsal artery reportedly travels dorsal to the deep transverse metatarsal ligament in 50[9,110] to 80 percent of feet.

Two levels of *veins* can be used for toe transplantation. Usually, the superficial veins on the dorsum of the foot form a network that will provide excellent drainage from the toe or dorsal foot flap. This superficial venous arch drains into the saphenous venous system on the medial side of the ankle. The other option is the vena comitans of the dorsalis pedis artery. Although the vena comitans can be used for drainage of a toe transplant, the superficial system is generally easier to dissect and larger, and a long pedicle can be obtained without difficulty.

Distal to the ankle, the *deep peroneal nerve* divides into medial and lateral branches. The medial branch passes distally just lateral to the dorsalis pedis artery, although it sometimes travels on the medial side. This nerve divides into two dorsal digital nerves that supply the adjacent sides of the first web space. The *superficial peroneal nerve* pierces the deep fascia proximal to the ankle joint, between the peroneus longus and the extensor digitorum longus. It divides into the medial and intermediate dorsal cutaneous nerves, which cross the ankle to supply the dorsum of the foot. Nerve supply to the plantar surface of the medial $3\frac{1}{2}$ toes arises from the medial plantar nerve. This nerve gives off a *proper digital nerve* to the medial side of the great toe, and *common digital nerves,* which pass between the divisions of the plantar aponeurosis. These common digital nerves then divide into proper digital nerves that pass plantar to the digital arteries along the sides of each toe.

PREOPERATIVE PREPARATION

Toe-to-thumb transplantation is a difficult procedure, even for an experienced surgeon. To ensure a smooth operation, meticulous planning is imperative and presumes a thorough knowledge of the pertinent anatomy and surgical procedure. Planning must address the following considerations.

General Appearance and Skin Flaps (Fig. 33-10)

The anticipated appearance of the toe transplant should be carefully planned and presented to the patient before the procedure. The shape and size of the toe transplant can be fashioned from clay and placed on the hand in the appropriate position. This model is also extremely helpful in determining the size and shape of the skin flaps needed to fit the defect in the hand. The location of the dorsalis pedis and first dorsal metatarsal arteries can be planned at this time to ensure easy positioning of the donor and recipient vessels for the microvascular anastomoses.

In planning the skin flaps, adjustments are made for soft tissue problems that may be present. For example, if the first web space is contracted, tissue from the ulnar side of the thumb stump can be mobilized, allowing skin to recede into the first web space and release the contracture. The toe transplant must, then, have more skin on the lateral side to provide ade-

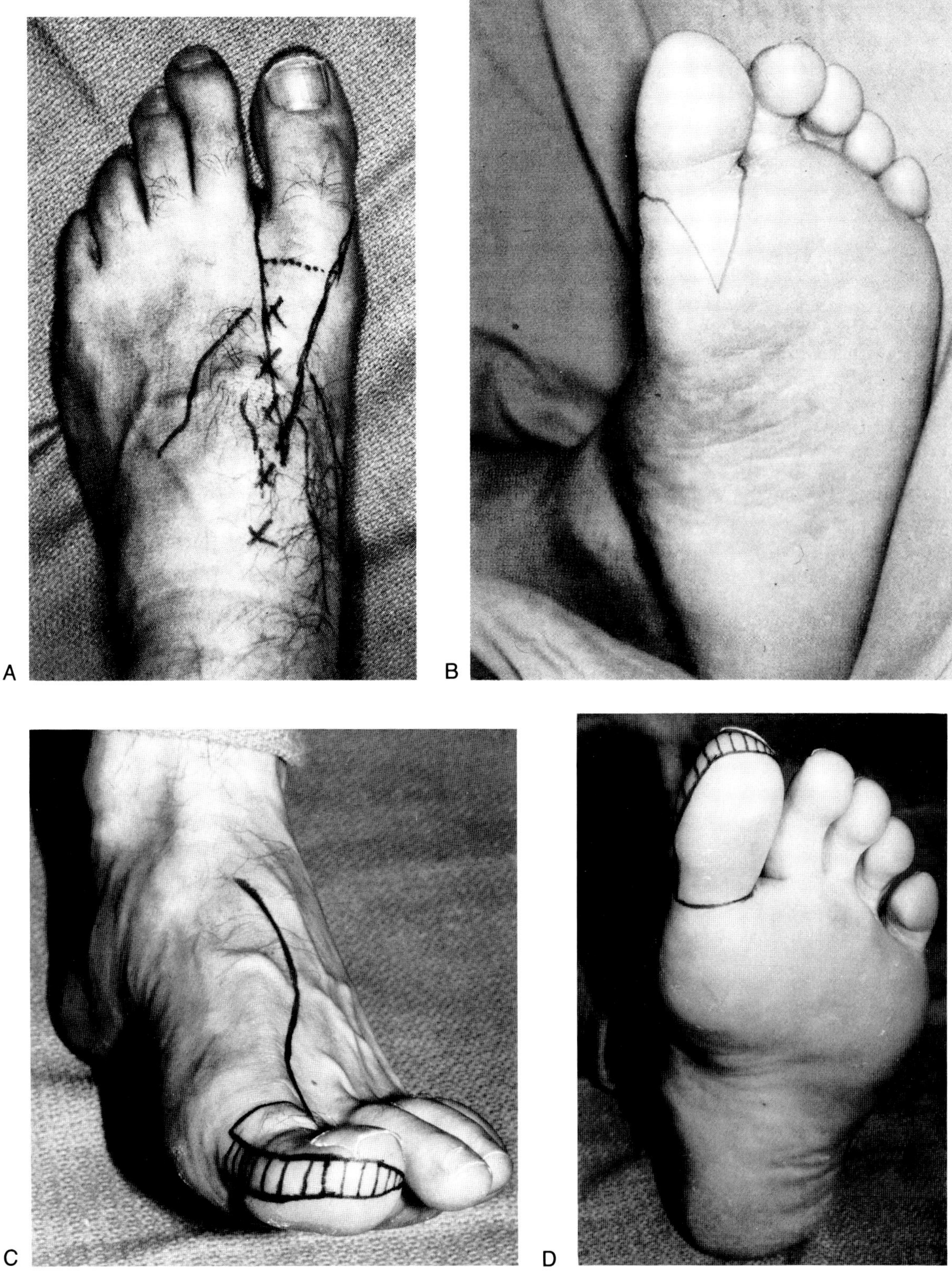

Fig. 33-10. Incisions for toe transplantation. Arterial pulse is located with a Doppler and marked, as are the veins emanating from the transplant and the proposed site of the osteotomy. **(A&B)** Great toe. **(C&D)** Wraparound flap. The shaded area is retained on the foot. *(Figure continues.)*

quate cover. This means that the ipsilateral toe with this skin is better suited to cover the first web space than is the contralateral toe.

The *ipsilateral great toe* is usually used because (1) it can be taken with some skin from the first web space to provide better cover for the first web space in the hand; (2) it will be angled about 10 degrees toward the index finger at the interphalangeal joint, affording better pinch but possibly compromising large object grasp to a slight degree (Fig. 33-1); and (3) as explained earlier, the arteries will be in the correct position for suture to the radial artery in the dorsum of the hand.

Arterial System

Because the vascular anatomy of the foot is variable, a lateral or oblique projection *arteriogram* (see Fig. 33-4) is useful in establishing the course and size of the vessels to the great toe.[42,44,50,62,105] Either a general anesthetic (in children) or an intraarterial vasodilator such as tolazoline (12.5 mg/70 kg body weight) is used to eliminate arterial spasm.[42] It is also important to investigate the vessels in the hand because some may be damaged or anomalous. In the thumb, the ulnar digital artery is larger than the radial and is the dominant digital artery. It is important to establish whether the hand has a dominant supply by the radial artery or independent radial and ulnar arterial supplies (see Chapter 62). A *Doppler* may be used to outline the course of the vessels in the hand and foot. However, if the results of the Doppler and physical examination are inconclusive, arteriography should be performed. Arteriograms of the foot and hand can be done simultaneously through a transfemoral approach.

Venous System

Before the procedure, a tourniquet is placed on the upper thigh and upper arm and elevated to a pressure between systolic and diastolic. As the subcutaneous veins dilate on the dorsum of the hand and foot, the largest and most conveniently positioned vessels are chosen and outlined with a marking pen. Except in patients with burns, these veins are generally of large caliber and make excellent donor and recipient vessels.

Osteosynthesis

The method of osteosynthesis should allow as much motion as possible in the adjacent joints, especially when the amputation is just distal to the metacarpophalangeal joint. Therefore,

E 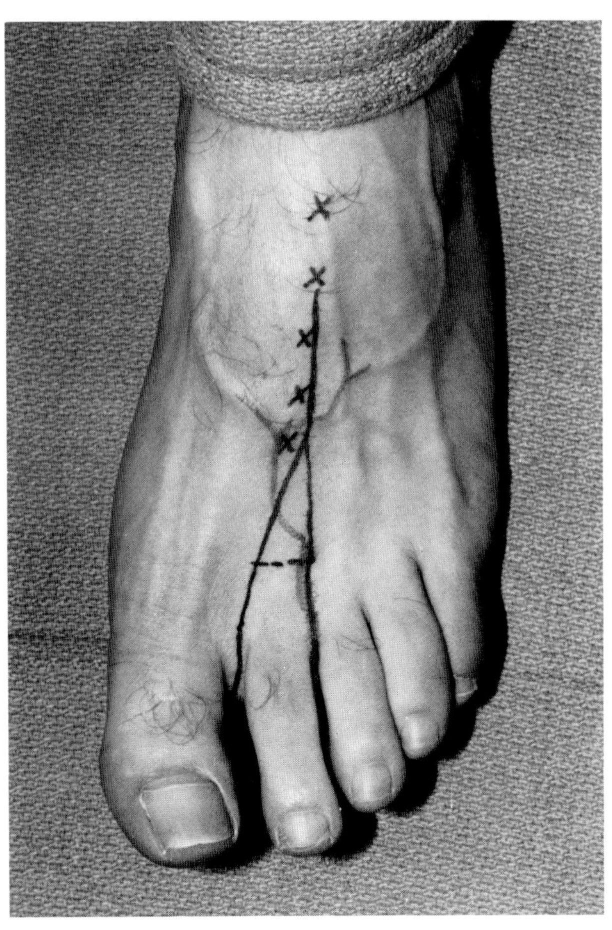

F 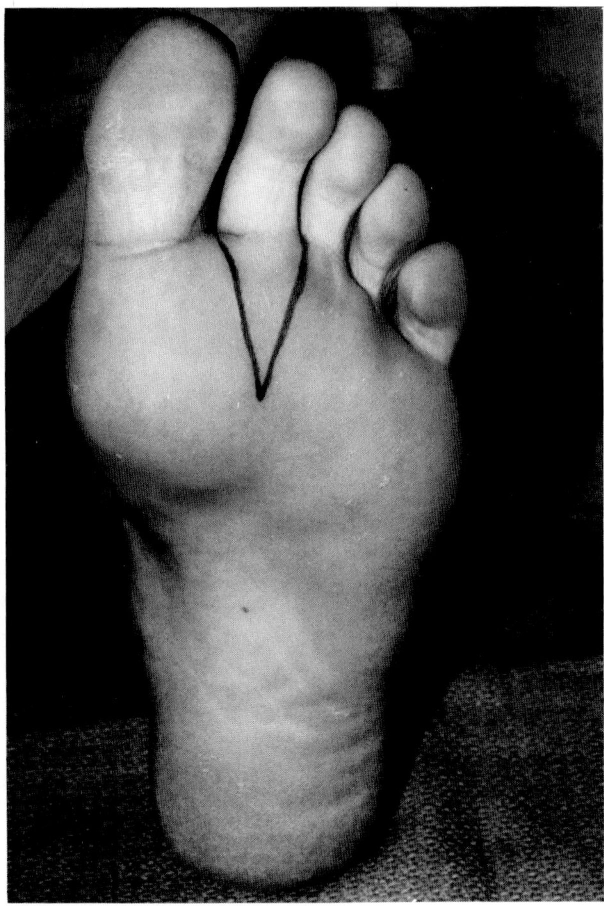

Fig. 33-10 *(Continued).* **(E&F)** Second toe.

the technique used should leave this joint unencumbered. Interosseous wiring is the best means of achieving this goal. A step-cut osteotomy with overlapping bone ends is sometimes effective. Another overlapping technique involves hollowing out the toe bone and fashioning a peg on the thumb to create a mortise and tenon joint. This connection has good bone contact and is secured with a single oblique K-wire to control rotation. An overlapping method will affect the ultimate length of the toe transplant, and this should be taken into account when planning the length of the reconstructed thumb. Length is a key factor in appearance and function. Ideally, the reconstructed thumb should be slightly shorter than its counterpart on the normal hand.

SURGICAL TECHNIQUE

Whole Great Toe Transfer (Figs. 33-1, 33-11, 33-12)

A model of the toe and skin flaps is fashioned from clay, and the positions of the arteries and veins are marked on it. This model is then transferred to the hand to ensure that the skin flaps will cover the vascular pedicle appropriately and that the length and position of the toe are perfect. The vascular pedicle is marked on the hand in the location where the anastomosis is planned.

The patient is positioned supine with tourniquets placed on the upper arm and thigh. The veins are mapped out as described above on page 1269 (Fig. 33-10). The dorsalis pedis artery, the first dorsal metatarsal artery, and the digital vessels are located with a Doppler and their position is marked on the skin (Fig. 33-10). An Esmarch bandage is used to partially exsanguinate the leg; some blood is left in the veins to make the dissection easier.

Toe-to-hand transplantation should be performed with the patient under general anesthesia in a warm operating room. The anesthesiologist should make a concerted effort to keep the patient warm before the operation as well as throughout the procedure to prevent peripheral vascular spasm. It is best for two teams to work simultaneously to reduce the operating time. Four- to six-power loupes are used for the dissection. Both the hand and foot are dissected under tourniquet control. Because toe transplantation is complex and requires multiple surgical teams, the tourniquets must be monitored diligently and the leg tourniquet released as soon as the dissection has been completed. In patients who have congenital hand problems, the hand should be dissected first to determine whether recipient structures of appropriate size are present.

Hand Dissection

To a great extent, the *incision* for exposing the thumb bone, tendons, and neurovascular structures depends on the nature of the injury or deformity. Most often, a sagittal incision is made middorsal to midvolar over the distal end of the thumb stump. This incision raises radial and ulnar flaps, readily exposing the bone and allowing the ulnar flap to settle into the first web space. Dorsally, the dissection is carried back to the radial artery on the dorsal aspect of the first web space, and the artery is easily located by palpation or Doppler. On the palmar side, the incision is made around the thenar crease, and, if

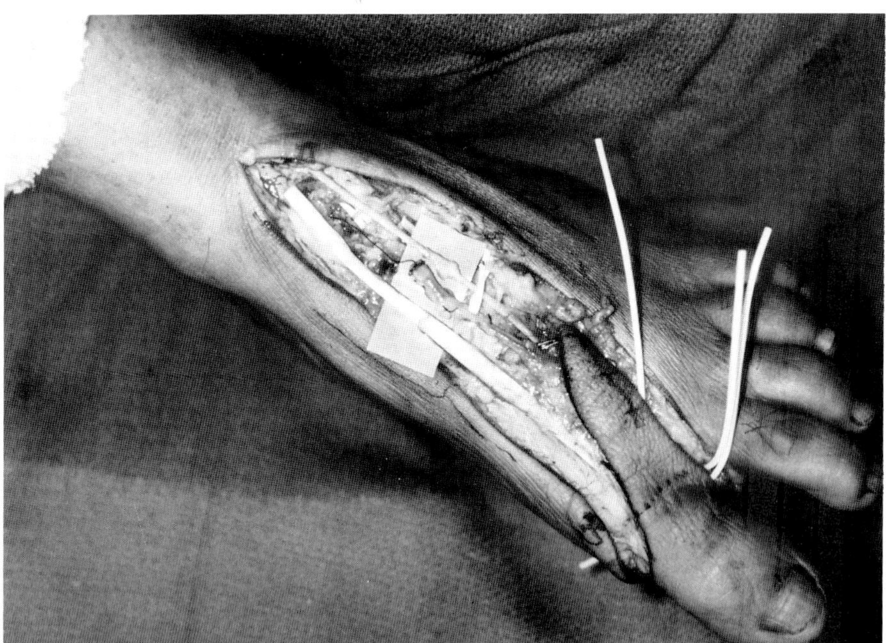

Fig. 33-11. Dorsal dissection of the foot is similar in great toe, second-toe, and partial toe transplantation and in the wraparound procedure. Superficial dorsal veins, the dorsalis pedis and first dorsal metatarsal arteries, the deep peroneal nerve, and the extensor tendons are dissected. (From Gordon,[38] with permission.)

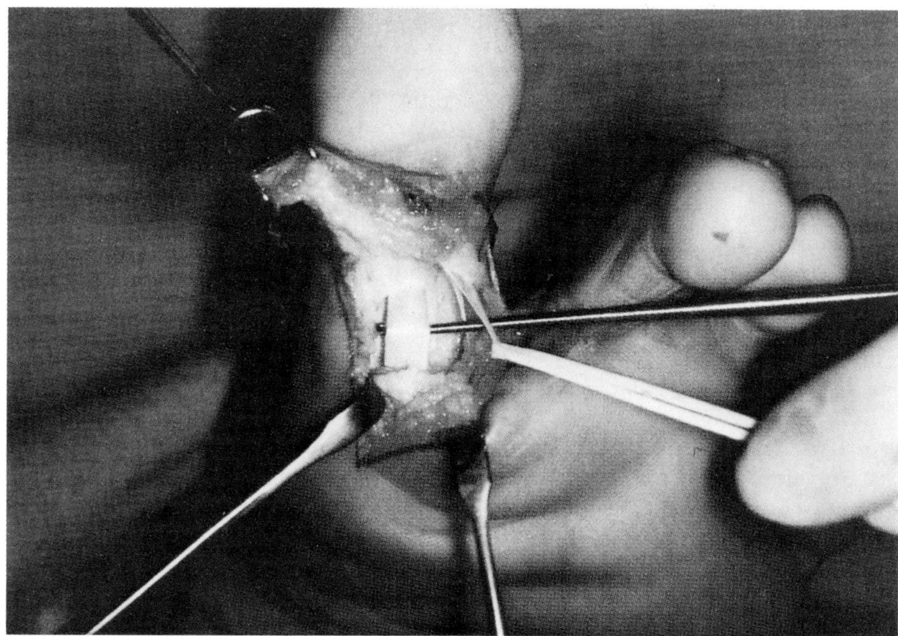

Fig. 33-12. The flexor tendon and digital nerves are dissected through the plantar incision. (From Gordon,[38] with permission.)

necessary, into the region of the carpal tunnel to expose the flexor pollicis longus tendon and the digital nerves. The incisions are carefully planned to receive the dorsal and plantar flaps being dissected in the foot. The *bone* is prepared to accept the transplant according to the planned method of osteosynthesis.

The flexor pollicis longus *tendon* is dissected close to the site of amputation, or, if necessary, in the palm or through a separate incision at the wrist. Similarly, the extensor pollicis longus and extensor pollicis brevis are dissected either on the dorsal aspect of the first metacarpal or more proximally. If these tendons are not available, tendon transfers may be necessary. For example, the extensor indicis proprius may be transferred to the thumb for use as the extensor, or the brachioradialis may be used as the thumb flexor. The digital *nerves* are dissected as close as possible to the thumb amputation. If the nerves have been damaged or avulsed from the median nerve, more proximal dissection is required. Sometimes, it may even be necessary to transfer the dorsal branch of the radial nerve, a nerve from another digit, or a nerve from another amputation stump to use as a recipient nerve.

A long *vein* is extremely easy to dissect in the foot and allows anastomosis to a large patulous recipient vein in the proximal part of the hand or even the wrist or forearm. The recipient artery—usually the radial artery on the dorsal aspect of the first web space—is then dissected. The *ulnar digital artery* is the dominant digital artery supplying the toe and can be used as a recipient vessel, but it is considerably smaller than the radial artery and may lie near or within the zone of injury. When this artery is used, positioning of the hand for the anastomosis is difficult. This digital vessel is more prone to spasm than is the larger radial artery. Thus, it is preferable but not essential to use the radial artery on the dorsal aspect of the first web space. Each of the dissected structures should be tagged for easy retrieval after the tourniquet has been released.

As each structure in the hand is dissected, the required length of each complementary structure in the toe becomes known and should be relayed to the team dissecting the foot. Making a list of structures and their required length is helpful. This coordination ensures that all structures will match perfectly.

Foot Dissection (Figs. 33-11, 33-12)

The skin incision follows the course of the dorsalis pedis artery and the first dorsal metatarsal artery with dorsal and plantar flaps (Fig. 33-10). On the dorsal surface, the triangular flap is fashioned to cover the arteries beneath. A shorter triangular flap is used on the plantar surface proximal to the flexion crease (Fig. 33-10). The lateral flap can include a part of the first web space of the foot and the skin on the medial aspect of the second toe if cover is needed in the first web space of the hand. It is generally better to plan to use less skin from the foot to enable primary closure of the donor site. If necessary, a skin graft can be used in the hand.

I usually do the dorsal dissection first (Fig. 33-11). Subcutaneous dorsal veins are dissected on the dorsal aspect of the foot. These veins must emanate from the region to be transplanted. The dorsal tendons and arteries should be dissected next. The extensor hallucis longus tendon is dissected to the appropriate length. The extensor hallucis brevis tendon is identified and divided. Located beneath it are the deep peroneal nerve and the origin of the first dorsal metatarsal artery from the dorsalis pedis artery and its venae comitantes. The vessels and deep peroneal nerve are dissected distally, with care taken to maintain the connections between these vessels and the dorsal skin flap.

The key to harvesting a great toe transplant lies in dissecting the first dorsal metatarsal artery from its origin, i.e., the dorsalis pedis or deep plantar artery, 6 to 7 cm to the point where it divides into the proper digital vessels to the toe. As described above (Fig. 33-9), the first dorsal metatarsal artery may take one of several courses. If it lies superficial, the dissection is straightforward. If it lies deep, the dissection is more challenging. Sometimes, the vessel will require dissection into the first dorsal interosseous muscle or deep to it. If the vessel is deep, small, and difficult to dissect, one can begin to dissect distally on the dorsal surface of the first web space. Here, the digital artery to the great and second toes can be identified, and the vessels can then be followed in a proximal direction. If the vessels travel plantarward, an additional plantar incision may be required.

If the first dorsal metatarsal artery is absent, the common digital vessel must be dissected deep to the transverse metatarsal ligament, which means that this ligament must be divided. The artery is then dissected from distal to proximal, which may be easier to do through a plantar incision. The dissection is carried back to a point where the artery is of adequate size for anastomosis.[51] Sometimes, it is easiest to dissect this artery 3 to 4 cm and extend it with a vein graft rather than proceed with the difficult dissection deep in the plantar region of the foot. As one proceeds with the dissection of the arteries in this region, it is important to ligate even the smallest branches to prevent later spasm of the vessels.

The digital nerves (Fig. 33-12), which lie just plantar to the vessels, are located within the plantar incision. These nerves are often close and adherent to the capsule of the metatarsophalangeal joint. As the lateral nerve is dissected back to the plantar surface of the first web space, care is required to dissect it from the nerve that supplies the medial aspect of the second toe. This dissection is done by gently retracting the proper digital nerves from the adjacent sides of the first web space away from each other as they emanate from the common digital nerve. The common digital nerve is carefully separated to produce a nerve pedicle that is long enough for easy suture in the hand. The deep peroneal nerve supplies the first web space and should be included with the transplant for later suture to terminal branches of the radial nerve.

The flexor tendon can be dissected through the plantar incision for 4 to 5 cm. If a longer tendon is needed, a medial midfoot incision is necessary and dissection is carried across the foot to identify the flexor hallucis longus and divide it more proximally. If tendon length to the ankle is required, a medial ankle incision is used to dissect the tendon at this level, and it can then be stripped from the other toe flexors using a vein stripper.

When all of these structures have been dissected, either the bone or the capsule of the metatarsophalangeal joint is divided in a manner complementary to the hand dissection. At this point, the artery and veins are the only structures not yet divided, and the tourniquet is released to allow circulation to return to the toe. This release is important to confirm that the dissected vessels will adequately supply the toe and skin flaps, and it also ends the period of ischemia, giving the toe a "drink" before transfer to the hand, which will require further ischemia.

Often, the dissected toe will not pink up as rapidly as the other toes in the foot. If this happens, the following steps should be taken: (1) the surgeon should ensure that the operating room is warm, and the anesthesiologist must confirm that the patient's body temperature and mode of anesthesia will maximize peripheral vasodilation; (2) warm soaks should be placed on the toe, and vasodilating agents such as bupivacaine should be placed on the vessel; (3) all unsatisfied branches of the artery, however small, should be ligated. The toe will generally pink up within 10 to 15 minutes, and it should be given another 15 to 20 minutes of circulation prior to transplantation.

Toe-To-Thumb Attachment

If the procedure has been well planned, attachment of the thumb should be straightforward and rapid. As mentioned above, any one of several methods of osteosynthesis can be used. I prefer coronal and sagittal interosseous wiring because this method leaves adjacent joints free and does not hamper tendon function. K-wires can also be used alone or in combination with a single interosseous wire.

At the level of the proximal phalanx, several methods of fixation can be used. A transverse osteotomy or step-cut osteotomy can be fixed with either interosseous wires or K-wires. Alternatively, the proximal phalanx of the thumb can be fashioned into a peg to fit into the proximal phalanx of the great toe after the latter has been hollowed out with a curette. This mortise and tenon joint is then fixed with a single K-wire or cross K-wires to control rotation.

At the level of the metacarpophalangeal joint, the proximal phalanx of the great toe can be placed onto the distal articular surface of the first metacarpal.[118] If this attachment is chosen, one should retain as much of the capsule and soft tissue from the first metacarpal and first metatarsophalangeal joints as is necessary to suture the capsule. Following this "composite" joint reconstruction, the toe will be slightly longer than the thumb on the opposite hand.

At the level of the distal metacarpal, a transverse osteotomy or step-cut osteotomy can be used, producing a toe that has motion at the carpometacarpal and interphalangeal joints but none at the metacarpophalangeal joint. Alternatively, at this distal metacarpal level, the metatarsophalangeal joint can be transferred. This is a hyperextension joint, whereas the metacarpophalangeal joint requires flexion. For this reason, the distal metatarsal is osteotomized at a 45-degree angle, starting proximal and dorsal and ending just distal to the sesamoid bone on the plantar aspect of the distal metatarsal. When this joint is transferred to the hand, the small segment of the distal metatarsal is internally fixed to the distal part of the metacarpal, with the joint in hyperextension. This position now represents neutral (Fig. 33-7),[75] and the joint can flex from this position. Thus, it has been converted from a hyperextension joint into one that will flex. Interosseous wiring is the best type of fixation for this transfer because it does not prevent motion at the new metacarpophalangeal joint.

The tendons are sutured using the strongest repair method possible. If adequate tendon is available, a Pulvertaft weave stitch (Chapter 51) can be used for the flexor tendon, and a similar technique or an overlapping repair can be used on the extensor side. Typically, the extensor hallucis longus is repaired to the extensor pollicis longus, and the extensor hallucis brevis is repaired to the extensor pollicis brevis. The flexor hallucis longus is sutured to the flexor pollicis longus. Occasionally, these tendons will not be available in the hand and various tendon transfers such as the flexor digitorum superficialis or brachioradialis will be needed to substitute (see page 1271).

Tendon repairs are usually done in the palm, but they are sometimes done at the wrist level. If thenar muscles and the adductor pollicis muscle are present, they should be sutured to the extensor mechanism proximal to the metacarpophalangeal joint. In the absence of thenar muscles, the abductor pollicis brevis can be left long for suture of an opposition transfer,[75] which is usually performed at a subsequent operation. Because the flexor is stronger than the extensor tendon, care should be taken not to suture the flexor too tight or a mallet deformity will develop. When the tendon repairs have been completed, the thumb should be "balanced" with the interphalangeal joint in an extended position.

On the dorsal surface, the dorsalis pedis artery is anastomosed either end-to-end or end-to-side to the radial artery. If an end-to-end anastomosis is done, the ulnar artery must be confirmed to provide adequate circulation to all of the fingers. One or two veins on the dorsal surface are anastomosed. The deep peroneal nerve is sutured to a branch of the radial nerve, if one is present. The digital nerves are sutured in the palm. Finally, the skin flaps are closed. Small skin grafts are often necessary for this purpose. Grafts are tolerated well in the hand and generally heal without problems, even if placed over the vascular structures.

Donor Site Closure

Closure of the donor site in the foot must be done meticulously. As mentioned earlier, it is important to maintain the head of the first metatarsal for push-off and stability during gait (see Fig. 33-7). The sesamoid bones are sutured into their previous position (through drill holes in the metatarsal head if necessary), and the deep transverse metatarsal ligament is repaired. If necessary, the position of the first and second metatarsals can be temporarily maintained with K-wires.

If the skin closure is too tight, the condyles and part of the dorsal bone should be trimmed so that the skin can be closed primarily. A drain is placed prior to closure to prevent hematoma formation, and a bulky soft dressing with a splint is used. Following closure, the limb should be well elevated while the toe is being attached to the hand.

Wraparound Procedure[18,20,70,81,86,109] (Fig. 33-13)

The size of the great toe varies considerably from patient to patient, but it is larger than the thumb in every aspect; the pulp is broader, the nail is wider, and its circumference is approximately 20 percent greater. For this reason, some surgeons have advocated modifications of the great toe transplant procedure to create a narrower reconstructed thumb for improved appearance. The wraparound and trimmed great toe procedures are two such modifications.

In the wraparound procedure, a soft tissue flap and nail from the great toe are transferred, and the osseous support is supplied by an iliac crest bone graft rather than by the phalanges of the great toe. These differences allow the soft tissues to be narrowed down to the size of a normal thumb, but there is no potential for growth or movement because no epiphysis or joint is transferred. This procedure should therefore not be used in children or when there is no motion remaining at the metacarpophalangeal joint of the injured thumb. Instead, it should be reserved for amputations distal to the metacarpophalangeal joint. The iliac crest bone graft has the potential to resorb. Transferring the distal phalanx of the great toe with the wraparound flap and placing it distal to the iliac graft decreases the likelihood of resorption. As the plantar skin is separated from the underlying bone, the septae between the phalanges of the great toe and the skin are destroyed, which occasionally causes scarring and immobility of the skin of the thumb pulp.

The skin incision is determined by measuring the circumference of the opposite (normal) thumb at the base of the nail. This measurement is transferred to the dorsal plantar and lateral sides of the great toe to be transplanted, leaving a medial bridge of skin on the foot. This bridge represents the difference between the circumferences of the great toe and thumb (See Fig. 33-10). The toe flap is a degloving of the great toe that includes the nail, but this medial strip of skin remains on the foot for closure.

Dissection of the vessels, nerves, and tendons is identical to that for whole great toe transfer, and, because the ulnar vessels of the thumb are dominant, the ipsilateral toe is used. Use of the ipsilateral toe allows the first dorsal metatarsal artery to be brought to the ulnar side of the thumb for anastomosis to the radial artery on the dorsal aspect of the hand between the first two metacarpals. As the wraparound flap is dissected, the skin flap and nail are dissected from the underlying bone of the great toe. When dissecting the dorsal flap under the nail, care should be taken to avoid disrupting the germinal matrix. The paratenon of the extensor tendon should be carefully retained on the foot. As with whole great toe transfer, the transplant will contain a dorsal venous system, both neurovascular bundles, both digital nerves, the lateral digital artery (which continues proximally as the first dorsal metatarsal artery), the dorsalis pedis vessel, and the deep peroneal nerve. The middle and proximal phalanges are not included in the tissue to be transplanted; most surgeons now include the distal phalanx to decrease the likelihood of iliac crest bone graft resorption.

The defect in the transplanted flap that corresponds to the medial aspect of the great toe is closed, creating a structure with dimensions similar to those of the contralateral thumb. At this stage, the nail can be narrowed, and the medial eponychial fold is brought over the medial aspect of the nail to reconstruct this fold. The bone of the distal phalanx is trimmed down to the desired size by removing the condylar flares.

A corticocancellous bone graft is harvested and wired to either the proximal phalanx or the metacarpal. The flap is then "wrapped around" the iliac crest graft, and K-wires are used to

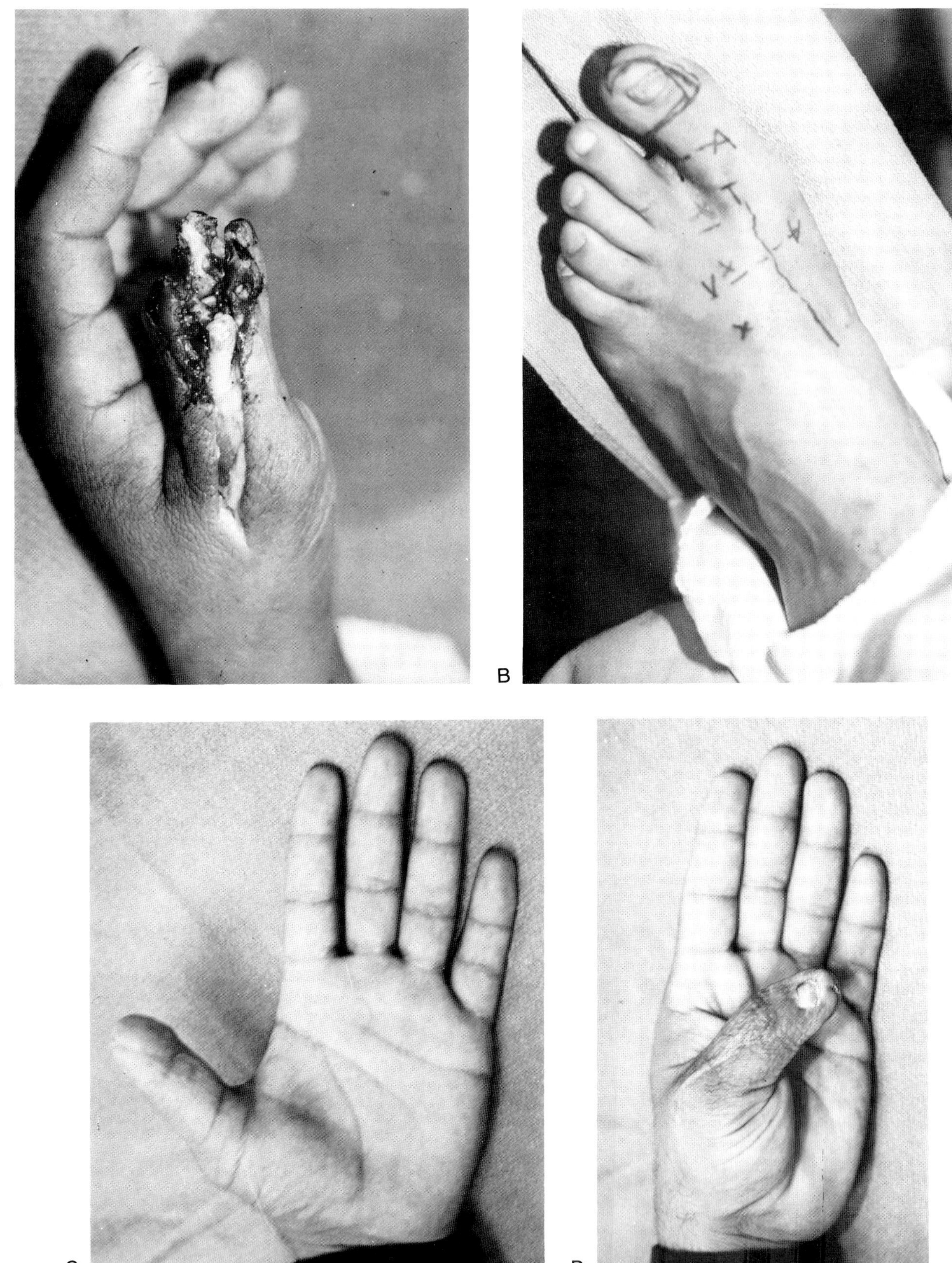

Fig. 33-13. This patient avulsed the soft tissues from the distal bone of the thumb. A wraparound flap was planned to salvage length and restore function. **(A)** Because the bone was exposed, the procedure was done just 2 days after the injury. **(B)** A small wraparound flap is marked on the foot. The first dorsal metatarsal artery, veins, and tendons are outlined. **(C&D)** The new thumb is similar in size to the opposite thumb. Good motion at the metacarpophalangeal joint was maintained.

fix the latter to the distal phalanx. All of the tendons, nerves, and vessels are repaired as in whole great toe transfer, and the skin incisions are closed.

Donor Site Closure

The medial bridge of skin retained on the foot is advanced over the bone of the great toe. This bridge provides adequate cover only if all of the phalanges are removed. As originally described, only the distal half of the distal phalanx is removed in this procedure, and a cross-toe flap from the plantar surface of the second toe is used to cover the dorsal defect. The remainder, including the plantar surface of the second toe, is covered with split-thickness skin graft.[81] Most surgeons prefer to compromise by shortening the donor great toe substantially so that the remaining medial flap and a split-thickness skin graft provide adequate cover. Some length is retained in the great toe and no cross-toe flap is needed.

Trimmed Toe Technique[106,107,115]

The disadvantage of the whole great toe transfer is its size, and the drawback of the wraparound procedure is that it provides no motion. The trimmed toe technique combines the assets of each in that it produces a smaller structure that is capable of motion. Although the great toe is trimmed to the dimensions of the opposite thumb, the joints are preserved. Motion is still not as good as that provided by whole great toe transfer. Bone resorption is not a problem because no iliac crest graft is used. Like the wraparound procedure, the trimmed toe transfer is primarily used for thumb loss distal to the metacarpophalangeal joint and when the great toe is too large. It should not be used in children because the growth plates will be damaged.

The normal thumb on the contralateral side is measured as it is in the wraparound technique, and this measurement is transferred to the great toe[106] to outline a similar skin incision. The medial toe flap (i.e., that which is to be retained on the donor foot) is elevated just superficial to the periosteum, with care taken not to injure the medial plantar neurovascular bundle.

The medial collateral ligament is raised at its distal insertion distal to the interphalangeal joint, including some periosteum. A proximally based "flap" is thus created, and the dissection is carried proximally to the level of the proximal part of the proximal phalanx. The proximal and distal phalanges of the great toe are longitudinally reduced along the radial border by removing a 4- to 6-mm-wide strip of bone plus the medial joint prominence. The elevated collateral ligament along with the periosteum distally is then replaced. As in the wraparound procedure, the skin is brought around the narrowed osseous structure, and the nail is trimmed on its medial aspect. The medial eponychial fold is retained and used to reconstruct this fold once the toe nail has been narrowed.

Second-Toe Transplantation (Figs. 33-10, 33-14)

The advantage of using the second toe for thumb reconstruction is that the second metatarsal and metatarsophalangeal joint can be included in the transplant.[58] These features make second-toe transplantation the best reconstructive option for amputations at the level of the proximal metacarpal.[41,104] Appearance and function of the donor site in the foot are better than they are following either great toe transplanta-

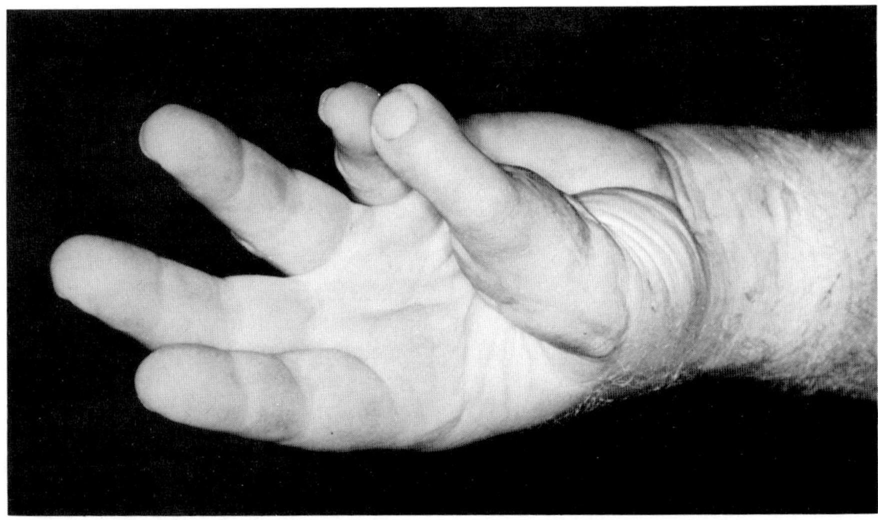

Fig. 33-14. This patient chose to have a second-toe rather than a great toe transplant because the appearance of the donor site is better. The transplant is narrower than the normal thumb and is flexed at the interphalangeal joint. Despite the narrower pulp and lesser strength, the patient regained good function and was satisfied with the result. (From Gordon,[38] with permission.)

tion or the wraparound flap, but the reconstructed thumb is more narrow than a normal thumb and is not as strong as a thumb reconstructed by any other technique described in this chapter (see Table 33-2). If a patient cannot accept losing a great toe because of personal or cultural preferences, the second toe may also be used to reconstruct the thumb at a more distal level.

When the thumb is reconstructed proximal to the midportion of the metacarpal, a length of the second metatarsal must be included for adequate thumb length. Skin cover is usually a problem because the skin flap taken with the transplant is not adequate to cover the metatarsal and surrounding interosseous muscle. Therefore, a preliminary flap is often needed for soft tissue cover. Although a dorsalis pedis flap can be included, I do not recommend that this be done because it can lead to prolonged healing problems in the foot. In addition, when reconstruction is at the level of the proximal metacarpal, thenar muscles are not available and either reattachment of the thenar muscles or an opposition transfer is necessary.

The technique is basically similar to that of whole great toe transfer. A clay model is helpful in planning dorsal and plantar flaps and the position of the first dorsal metatarsal artery. If the second metatarsal is to be taken, a long dorsal skin flap should be included to cover the vascular pedicle, and a split-thickness skin graft will usually be needed on the hand in addition. The flap should be planned so that primary closure following ray amputation of the second toe can be achieved (Fig. 33-10).

Dissection of the veins, dorsalis pedis artery, and first dorsal metatarsal artery is identical to that in great toe transplantation. The artery should be dissected on its medial side without disturbing any of the branches emanating laterally toward the second toe and skin flap. As the first web space is reached, care should be taken not to injure the digital branches traveling to the second toe. The branch supplying the great toe is ligated and divided.

If the metatarsal is included, a sizeable cuff of interosseous muscle should be taken with it because a split-thickness skin graft is often possible on this muscle. The tendons should be dissected and divided, and care should be taken to preserve as many of the pulleys of the flexor tendon as possible. The toe is transplanted to the hand, using the same repairs as those in whole great toe transfer. The distal interphalangeal joint should be pinned in a position of extension for 2 to 3 weeks to avoid a mallet deformity of the distal phalanx.

Donor Site Closure

Following second toe transplantation, a ray amputation will provide excellent appearance and function in the donor foot. The metatarsal is resected, leaving only the base, and a ray amputation is performed. The intermetatarsal ligament should be preserved and repaired at this time, approximating the third metatarsal to the first metatarsal. K-wires may be helpful in holding the first and third metatarsals in position; this can also be accomplished by placing a strong suture around both bones. Care must be taken to properly space the great toe and not bring it too close to the second toe. The toes should also be rotated properly. A drain is placed in the foot wound.

Partial Toe Transplantation (Figs. 33-15, 33-16)

Once the anatomy of the region is clearly understood, parts of the great toe or second toe can be dissected to replace parts of a damaged thumb. Such transplants can include (1) the second metatarsophalangeal joint or interphalangeal joint with or without an overlying skin paddle[26,47,48,54,73,90,103] (Fig. 33-16); (2) the skin of the first web space, including part of the great or second toe[91]; (3) the pulp skin of the great or second toe to provide sensibility[24,49] (Fig. 33-15); and/or (4) the nail and dorsal skin with or without underlying bone or soft tissue flaps.[24,53] Harvesting these "spare parts" may often require the toe to be sacrificed. Therefore, a decision must be made before operating about whether the trade-off in thumb reconstruction is worthwhile.

Dissection of the first dorsal metatarsal artery, dorsalis pedis artery, digital nerves, skin flaps, and joint is identical to that in great toe transfer. To maintain optimal vascularity, care must be taken not to disturb branches from the arteries and veins to the part to be transplanted. The particular transplant to be used among the myriad that are feasible depends on the anatomic and functional deficit in the hand, and the surgeon can tailor the transplant to precisely conform to the recipient site (Figs. 33-15, 33-16).

POSTOPERATIVE CARE

In the immediate postoperative period, the transplant should receive the same kind of care and monitoring as amputated parts that have been replanted (see Chapter 27). The patient's room should be warm and the patient should be kept maximally vasodilated, well hydrated, and comfortable. Both the hand and foot should be well elevated.

Each surgeon should have an anticoagulation protocol for managing patients who have undergone replantation or toe transplantation. I begin an infusion of low molecular weight dextran (30 cc/hour/70 kg body weight) in the operating room when the toe is transferred to the hand; this is maintained for 5 days postoperatively. Occasionally, if there has been a problem with the vascular anastomosis or if there appears to be a higher risk of thrombosis, I use heparin. One day before the dextran or heparin is stopped, aspirin (325 mg daily) is given and continued for one month for its antiplatelet effect.

The toe transplant should be monitored on an hourly basis, using either skin temperature monitoring, laser Doppler flowometry, or fluorimetry—depending on the availability of equipment and expertise (see Chapter 26). Thrombosis of the arterial or venous anastomosis occurs in 10 to 15 percent of patients,[38,55,56] but if this complication is recognized within a few hours, reanastomosis should be able to salvage the transfer a majority of the time. Clinical vigilance is therefore vital.

The dressing is changed at 5 to 7 days, at which time gentle hand therapy can be initiated. The hand therapist provides a protective splint and begins restoring joint motion and tendon gliding. The amount of passive and active motion that can be

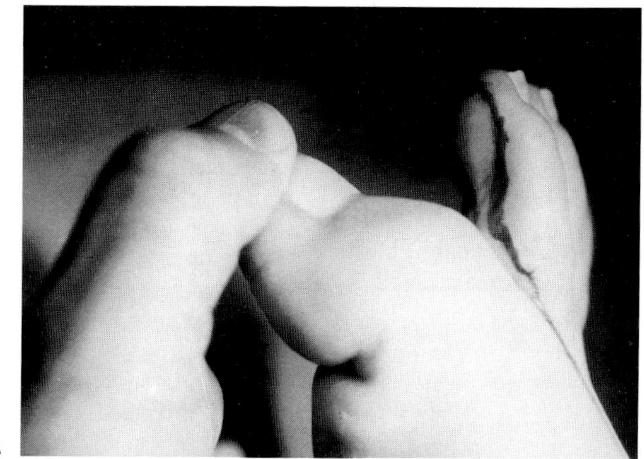

A

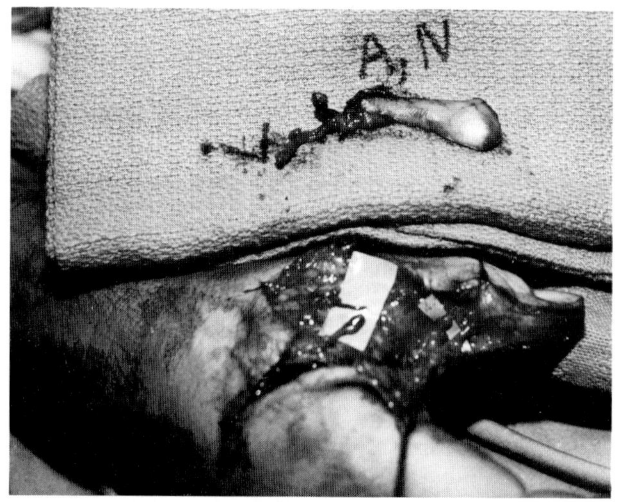

B

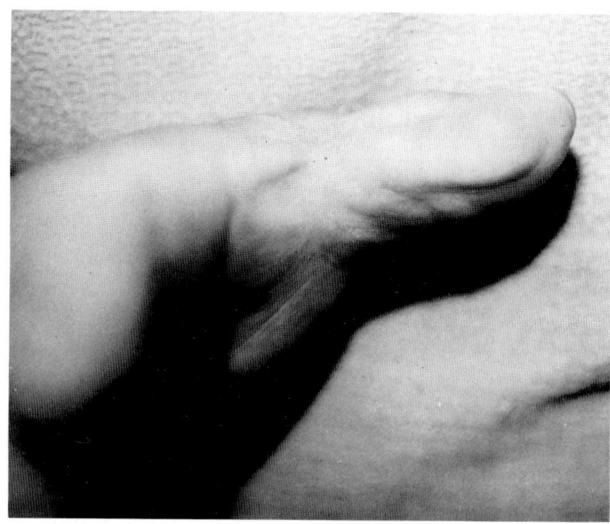

C

Fig. 33-15. Partial toe transplant. **(A)** A second-toe pulp transfer is outlined. The donor site in the toe is closed primarily and sustains minimal or no morbidity. **(B)** This flap includes the digital nerve and vessels. **(C)** The flap was used to resurface the pad of the thumb. Nerve repair to the thumb digital nerve restored 6-mm two-point discrimination.

done at this stage depends on the strength of the tendon repairs. After approximately 3 weeks, therapy can generally follow a tendon repair protocol. Sensation in the new thumb returns in about 4 to 6 months. At this time, the patient will start to feel as though the transplant is actually a thumb and begin to incorporate it into daily activities.

The donor foot requires careful treatment during the postoperative period. Initially, it should be continuously elevated for 2 weeks to permit healing and prevent swelling. The patient should avoid bearing weight for another 2 weeks, after which graduated ambulation is begun. Some patients may be able to start walking sooner, but the frequency of breakdown and other difficulties disallow an earlier schedule as a matter of routine.

SECONDARY SURGERY

Most patients require late secondary surgery of some type after toe-to-thumb transplantation.[65] Flexor tenolysis is the most common procedure, but bone grafting, osteotomy, nerve grafting, web deepening, or other minor procedures are frequently needed. Motion may be improved by tendon transfers. Either an opposition transfer or an adductorplasty may be necessary.

RESULTS

Survival

Survival of the toe transplant should be achieved in more than 95 percent of patients.[65,94] Similar survival rates should be achieved in children who have been treated for trauma-related or congenital defects.[33,34] In the 10 to 15 percent of cases where vascular problems arise, appropriate monitoring and clinical vigilance are needed to promptly return the patient to the operating room to redo the anastomosis.[43] Typically, vein grafts are required when this occurs. In general, the new thumb heals

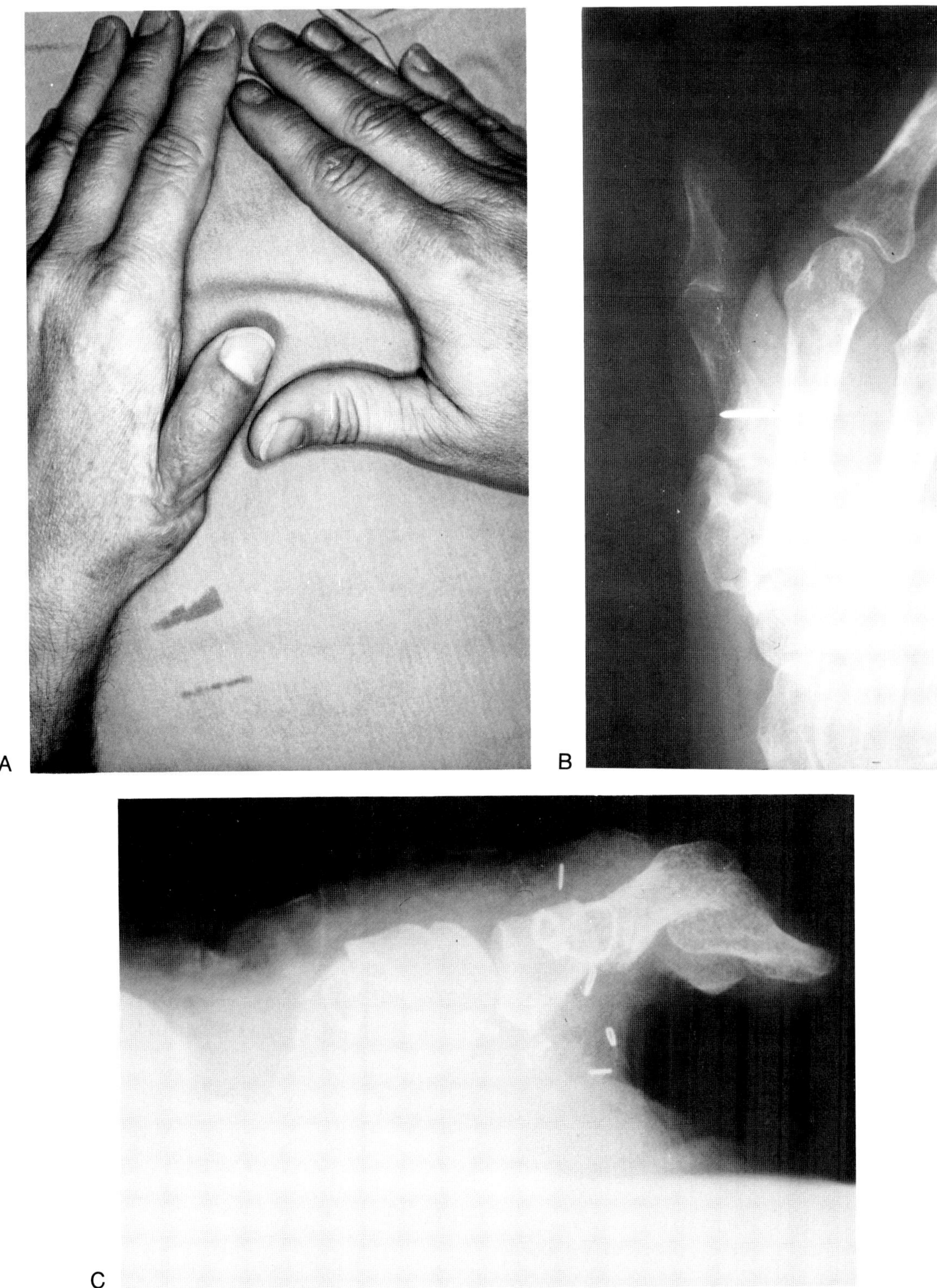

Fig. 33-16. Partial toe transplant. **(A)** A rifle injury destroyed the metacarpophalangeal joint of this thumb, producing a short thumb with an adduction contracture and no motion. The thumb needed lengthening, a metacarpophalangeal joint, extensor tendons for motion, and a skin flap to release the first web contracture. A custom-made partial second-toe transplant was planned to contain the metatarsophalangeal joint, the extensor tendon, and a skin flap. **(B)** X-rays show the bone deficit. **(C)** Postoperative x-rays show the joint wired into place. *(Figure continues.)*

rapidly, at a rate approaching that for isolated fracture, tendon, nerve, or skin flap repair.

Sensibility

Initially, the reconstructed thumb "feels like a toe" to the patient. This state is experienced before sensibility returns, and it lasts for about 4 to 6 months. After this period, most patients report that they have begun to use the new thumb and that it feels like part of the hand. Sensibility is largely restored in about 9 months but does not reach its maximum for about 2 years.[65]

Return of sensibility is related to the patient's age and is similar to that in isolated digital nerve repair.[17,94] Approximately half of patients develop two-point discrimination under 10 mm[29,39,49,59,65,94,112] that is often superior to that in the normal great toe on the contralateral side.[94]

Range of Motion

Following toe transplantation in which the carpometacarpal joint remains intact, both radial and palmar abduction are usually within 10 degrees of normal.[94] Flexion of the thumb to the base of the small finger is close to normal in most patients[9] (Fig. 33-1). When osseous stabilization is performed distal to the metacarpophalangeal joint, range of motion averages 25 degrees (range, 0 to 61 degrees)[39,94] and interphalangeal joint motion averages 29 degrees.

Pinch and Grip Strength[65,94]

In my view, the great toe transplant provides the strongest reconstructed thumb of all the methods described. The degree of strength largely depends on the extent of associated injury in the hand[94] and the presence or absence of thenar muscles.[29] In cases of isolated thumb loss, however, strength is largely restored after reconstruction; grip strength is 80 to 100 percent of the opposite side and key pinch 65 to 169 percent of the opposite side.[94] Lister found power grip and pinch to be 28.5 and 26.6 percent of the opposite, normal hand, respectively; however, pinch strength provided by the second toe was less than half that following great toe transfer.[65,67]

Subjective Evaluation

Patients are usually quite satisfied with their new thumb, and social acceptance following toe transplantation is high. The wraparound procedure produces the best cosmetic result because the reconstructed thumb has the dimensions most similar to those of the thumb on the opposite side. Appearance following whole great toe transplantation is acceptable.

Analysis of the Donor Site

Several investigators have carefully analyzed the donor foot, which, of course, is the greatest disadvantage of toe transplantation compared with other methods of thumb reconstruction. Following great toe transfer, there is a descent of the first metatarsal head that can be demonstrated radiographically but there is no change in either the ankle subtalar or midtarsal joint. Gait is usually close to normal, and functional problems in the foot are rare.[29,64,94] In general, weightbearing shifts toward the lateral side of the foot, centering between the second and third metatarsal heads and along the lateral border of the foot and heel.[94] Approximately one-half of the patients report some weakness in push-off and cutting, but there is no apparent problem with running long distances on level ground. An occasional patient will complain of difficulty with climbing or balancing on a narrow beam. Frykman et al[29] found that 11 of 12 patients were able to walk and run normally, but 6 were unable to wear thongs, heavy boots, or their regular shoes.

D 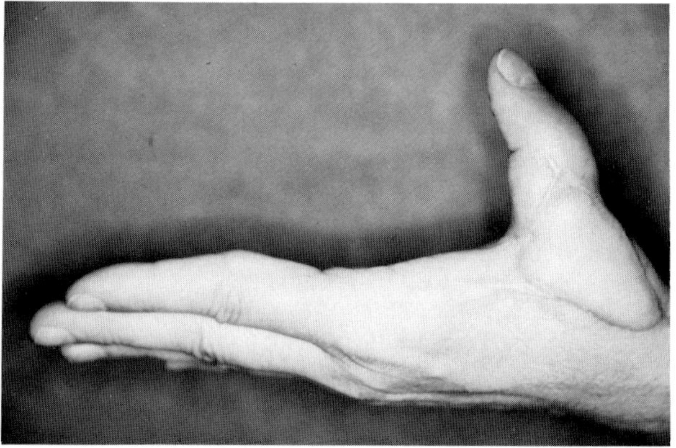

E 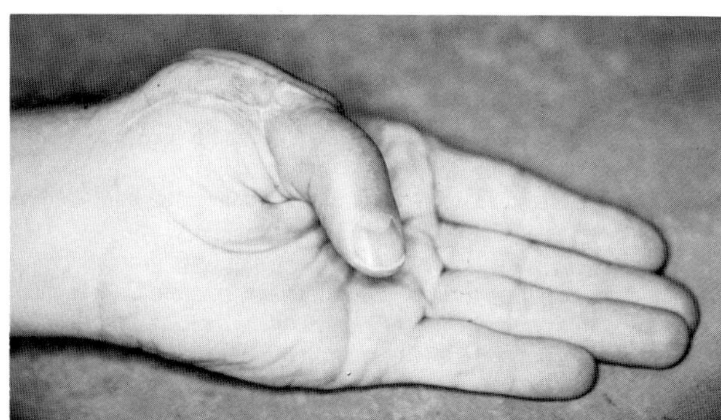

Fig. 33-16 *(Continued).* **(D&E)** Good abduction, length, and flexion are restored. (From Gordon,[38] with permission.)

REFERENCES

1. American Replantation Mission to China: Replantation surgery in China. Plast Reconstr Surg 52:476–489, 1973
2. Brown PW: Adduction-flexion contracture of the thumb. Correction with dorsal rotation flap and release of contracture. Clin Orthop 88:161–168, 1972
3. Buck-Gramcko D: Pollicization of the index finger; method and results in aplasia and hypoplasia of the thumb. J Bone Joint Surg 53A:1605–1617, 1971
4. Buckley PD, Smith P III, Dell PC: Thumb amputation: A review of reconstructive alternatives. Microsurgery 8:140–145, 1987
5. Buncke HJ: Toe digital transfer. Clin Plast Surg 3:49–57, 1976
6. Buncke HJ Jr, Buncke CM, Schulz WP: Immediate Nicoladoni procedure in the rhesus monkey, or hallux-to-hand transplantation, utilising microminiature vascular anastomoses. Br J Plast Surg 19:332–337, 1966
7. Buncke HJ Jr, McLean DH, Geroge PT, Creech BJ, Chater NL, Commons GW: Thumb replacement: Great toe transplantation by microvascular anastomosis. Br J Plast Surg 26:194–201, 1973
8. Buncke HJ, Rose EH: Free toe-to-fingertip neurovascular flaps. Plast Reconst Surg 63:607–612, 1979
9. Buncke HJ, Valauri FA, Buncke GM: Toe to hand. pp. 305–318. In Brunelli G: Textbook of Microsurgery. Masson, Milano, 1988
10. Bunnell S: Physiological reconstruction of a thumb after total loss. Surg Gynecol Obstet 52:245, 1931
11. Campbell-Reid DA: Reconstruction of the thumb. J Bone Joint Surg 42B:444–465, 1960
12. Campbell-Reid DA: The importance of the thumb in the human hand. pp. 1–6. In Campbell-Reid DA: Surgery of the Thumb. Butterworths, 1986
13. Chait LA, Fleming J, Becker H: Hallux-to-thumb transfer by microvascular anastomoses. S Afr Med J 52:249–432, 1977
14. Chase RA: An alternate to pollicization in subtotal thumb reconstruction. Plast Reconstr Surg 44:421, 1969
15. Cobbett JR: Free digital transfer: Report of a case of transfer of a great toe to replace an amputated thumb. J Bone Joint Surg 51B:677–679, 1969
16. Coleman DA, Urbaniak JR: Osteocutaneous flaps for thumb and digit reconstruction in unique situations. Hand Clin 1:717–728, 1985
17. Dellon AL: Sensory recovery in replanted digits and transplanted toes: A review. J Reconstr Microsurg 2:123–129, 1986
18. Doi K: Long term results of the wrap-around free flap for reconstruction of amputated thumbs. (Japanese) Jpn J Plast Reconstr Surg 27:23, 1984
19. Doi K, Hattori S, Kawai S, Nakamura S, Kotani H, Matsuoka A, Sunago K: New procedure on making a thumb—One-stage reconstruction with free neurovascular flap and iliac bone graft. J Hand Surg 6:346–350, 1981
20. Doi K, Kuwata N, Kawai S: Reconstruction of the thumb with a free wraparound flap from the big toe and an iliac-bone graft. J Bone Joint Surg 67A:439–445, 1985
21. Eaton CJ, Lister GD: Toe transfer for congenital hand defects. Microsurgery 12:186–195, 1991
22. Finseth F, May JW Jr, Smith RJ: Composite groin flap with iliac-bone flap for primary thumb reconstruction. Case report. J Bone Joint Surg 58A:130–132, 1976
23. Flynn JE, Burden CN: Reconstruction of the thumb. Arch Surg 85:56, 1962
24. Foucher G, Braun FM, Smith DJ Jr: Custom-made free vascularized compound toe transfer for traumatic dorsal loss of the thumb. Plast Reconstr Surg 87:310–314, 1991
25. Foucher G, Merle M, Maneaud M, Michon J: Microsurgical free partial toe transfer in hand reconstruction: A report of 12 cases. Plast Reconstr Surg 65:616–627, 1980
26. Foucher G, Sammut D, Citron N: Free vascularized toe-joint transfer in hand reconstruction: A series of 25 patients. J Reconstr Microsurg 6:201–207, 1990
27. Foucher G, Van Genechten F, Merle M, Denuit P, Braun FM, Debry R, Sur H: Toe-to-thumb transfers in reconstructive surgery of the hand. Experience with seventy-one cases. Ann Chir Main 3:124–138, 1984
28. Freeman BS: Reconstruction of thumb by toe transfer. Plast Reconstr Surg 17:393–398, 1956
29. Frykman GK, O'Brien BMcC, Morrison WA, MacLeod AM, Ciurleo A: Functional evaluation of the hand and foot after one-stage toe-to-hand transfer. J Hand Surg 11A:9–17, 1986
30. Furnas DW, Achauer BM: Microsurgical transfer of the great toe to the radius to provide prehension after partial avulsion of the hand. J Hand Surg 8:453–460, 1983
31. Ganske JG: Toe-to-hand transfer as an option for thumb reconstruction. Iowa Med J 77:596–599, 1987
32. Gilbert A: Composite tissue transfers from the foot: Anatomic basis and surgical technique. pp. 230–242. In Daniller AI, Strauch B (eds): Symposium on Microsurgery. CV Mosby, St Louis, 1976
33. Gilbert A: Toe transfers for congenital hand defects. J Hand Surg 7:118–124, 1982
34. Gilbert A: Congenital absence of the thumb and digits. J Hand Surg 14B:6–17, 1989
35. Gillies H, Reid DAC: Autograft of the amputated digit. Br J Plast Surg 7:338, 1955
36. Goldberg NH, Watson HK: Composite toe (phalanx and epiphysis) transfers in the reconstruction of the aphalangic hand. J Hand Surg 7:454–459, 1982
37. Goldner RD, Howson MP, Nunley JA, Fitch RD, Belding NR, Urbaniak JR: One hundred eleven thumb amputations: Replantation versus revision. Microsurgery 11:243–250, 1990
38. Gordon L: Microsurgical Reconstruction of the Extremities–Indications, Technique, and Postoperative Care. Springer-Verlag, New York, 1988
39. Gordon L, Buncke HJ, Alpert BS, Poppen NK, Norris TR: Great toe-to-thumb transfer: Indications and results in forty-one cases. pp. 239–242. In Buncke HJ, Furnas DW (eds): Symposium on Clinical Frontiers in Reconstructive Microsurgery. CV Mosby, St. Louis, 1984
40. Gordon L, Leitner DW, Buncke HJ, Alpert BS: Hand reconstruction for multiple amputations by double microsurgical toe transplantation. J Hand Surg 10A:218–225, 1985
41. Gordon L, Rosen J, Alpert BS, Buncke HJ: Free microvascular transfer of second toe ray and serratus anterior muscle for management of thumb loss at the carpometacarpal joint level. J Hand Surg 9A:642–644, 1984
42. Greenberg BM, May JW Jr: Great toe-to-hand transfer: Role of the preoperative lateral arteriogram of foot. J Hand Surg 13A:411–414, 1988
43. Gu Y, Wu M, Li H: Circulatory crisis in free toe-to-hand transfer and its management: 1. Clinical experience. J Reconstr Microsurg 5:111–114, 1989
44. Gu Y-D, Wu M-M, Zheng Y-L, Yang D-Y, Li H-R: Vascular variations and their treatment in toe transplantation. J Reconstr Microsurg 1:227–232, 1985
45. Hastings H II: Dual innervated index to thumb cross finger or island flap reconstruction. Microsurgery 8:168–172, 1987
46. Holle J, Freilinger G, Mandl H, Frey M: Grip reconstruction by double-toe transplantation in cases of a fingerless hand and a handless arm. Plast Reconstr Surg 69:962–968, 1982

47. Huang S-L, Hou M-Z, Yan C-L: Reconstruction of the thumb by a free pedal neurovascular flap and composite phalanx-joint-tendon homograft: A preliminary report. J Reconstr Microsurg 1:299-303, 1985
48. Ishida O, Tsai T-M: Free vascularized whole joint transfer in children. Microsurgery 12:196-206, 1991
49. Kato H, Ogino T, Minami A, Usui M: Restoration of sensibility in fingers repaired with free sensory flaps from the toe. J Hand Surg 14A:49-54, 1989
50. Koman LA, Pospisil RF, Nunley JA, Urbaniak JR: Value of contrast arteriography in composite tissue transfer. Clin Orthop 172:195-206, 1983
51. Koman LA, Weiland AJ, Moore JR: Toe-to-hand transfer based on the medial plantar artery. J Hand Surg 10A:561-566, 1985
52. Koshima I, Moriguchi T, Soeda S: One-stage reconstruction for amputated thumbs with melanoma. J Reconstr Microsurg 7:113-117, 1991
53. Koshima I, Soeda S, Takase T, Yamasaki M: Free vascularized nail grafts. J Hand Surg 13A:29-32, 1988
54. Kuo E-T, Ji Z-L, Zhao Y-C, Zhang M-L: Reconstruction of metacarpophalangeal joint by free vascularized autogenous metatarsophalangeal joint transplant. J Reconstr Microsurg 1:65-74, 1984
55. Leung PC: The "throbbing sign"—an indication of early venous congestion in replantation surgery. J Hand Surg 4:409-411, 1979
56. Leung PC: Problems in toe-to-hand transfers. Ann Acad Med Singapore 12(suppl 2):377-381, 1983
57. Leung PC: Thumb reconstruction using second-toe transfer. Hand 15:15-21, 1983
58. Leung PC: Thumb reconstruction using second-toe transfer. Hand Clin 1(2):285-295, 1985
59. Leung PC: Sensory recovery in transplanted toes. Microsurgery 10:242-244, 1989
60. Leung PC, Kok LC: Transplantation of the second toe to the hand. A preliminary report of sixteen cases. J Bone Joint Surg 62A:990-996, 1980
61. Leung PC, Ma F-Y: Digital reconstruction using the toe flap—Report of 10 cases. J Hand Surg 7:366-370, 1982
62. Leung PC, Wong WL: The vessels of the first metatarsal web space. An operative and radiographic study. J Bone Joint Surg 65A:235-238, 1983
63. Lichtman DM, Ahbel DE, Murphy RB, Buncke HJ Jr: Microvascular double toe transfer for opposable digits—Case report and rationale for treatment. J Hand Surg 7:279-283, 1982
64. Lipton HA, May JW Jr, Simon SR: Preoperative and postoperative gait analyses of patients undergoing great toe-to-thumb transfer. J Hand Surg 12A:66-69, 1987
65. Lister G: The choice of procedure following thumb amputation. Clin Orthop 195:45-51, 1985
66. Lister G: Microsurgical transfer of the second toe for congenital deficiency of the thumb. Plast Reconstr Surg 82:658-665, 1988
67. Lister GD, Kalisman M, Tsai T-M: Reconstruction of the hand with free microneurovascular toe-to-hand transfer: Experience with 54 toe transfers. Plast Reconstr Surg 71:372-384, 1983
68. Littler JW: The neurovascular pedicle method of digital transposition for reconstruction of the thumb. Plast Reconstr Surg 12:303-319, 1953
69. Littler JW: On making a thumb: One hundred years of surgical effort. J Hand Surg 1:35-51, 1976
70. Lowdon IMR, Nunley JA, Goldner RD, Urbaniak JR: The wraparound procedure for thumb and finger reconstruction. Microsurgery 8:154-157, 1987
71. Maillard G-F, Meredith P: Bilateral pinch reconstruction: Versatility of the Masquelet-Zancolli flap and the Wilkki operation. Plast Reconstr Surg 87:165-169, 1991
72. Mantero R, Rossello MI, Grandis C: Digital subtraction angiography in preoperative examination of congenital hand malformations. J Hand Surg 14A:351-352, 1989
73. Mathes SJ, Buchannan R, Weeks PM: Microvascular joint transplantation with epiphyseal growth. J Hand Surg 5:586-589, 1980
74. May JW Jr: Aesthetic and functional thumb reconstruction: Great toe to hand transfer. Clin Plast Surg 8:357-362, 1981
75. May JW Jr, Bartlett SP: Great toe-to-hand free tissue transfer for thumb reconstruction. Hand Clin 1:271-284, 1985
76. May JW Jr, Chait LA, Cohen BE, O'Brien BMcC: Free neurovascular flap from the first web of the foot in hand reconstruction. J Hand Surg 2:387-393, 1977
77. May JW Jr, Daniel RK: Great toe to hand free tissue transfer. Clin Orthop 133:140-153, 1978
78. May JW Jr, Smith RJ, Peimer CA: Toe-to-hand free tissue transfer for thumb construction with multiple digit aplasia. Plast Reconstr Surg 67:205-213, 1981
79. Meals RA, Lesavoy MA: Hallux-to-thumb transplant during ankle disarticulation for multiple limb anomalies. JAMA 249:72, 1983
80. Michon J, Merle M, Bouchon Y, Foucher G: Functional comparison between pollicization and toe-to-hand transfer for thumb reconstruction. J Reconstr Microsurg 1:103-112, 1984
81. Morrison WA, O'Brien BMcC, MacLeod AM: Thumb reconstruction with a free neurovascular wrap-around flap from the big toe. J Hand Surg 5:575-583, 1980
82. Morrison WA, O'Brien BMcC, MacLeod AM: Experience with thumb reconstruction. J Hand Surg 9B:223-233, 1984
83. Morrison WA, O'Brien BMcC, MacLeod AM: Ring finger transfer in reconstruction of transmetacarpal amputations. J Hand Surg 9A:4-11, 1984
84. Nicoladoni C: Daumenplastik: Wien Klin Wochnschr 10:663-665, 1897
85. Nicoladoni C: Daumenplastik fund organischer ersatz der fingerspitze. (Anticheiro-plastik und daktyloplastik). Arch Chir 61:606, 1900
86. Nunley JA, Goldner RD, Urbaniak JR: Thumb reconstruction by the wrap-around method. Clin Orthop 195:97-103, 1985
87. O'Brien B, MacLeod AM, Sykes PJ, Browning FSC, Threlfall GN: Microvascular second toe transfer for digital reconstruction. J Hand Surg 3:123-133, 1978
88. O'Brien BMcC, MacLeod AM, Sykes PJ, Donahoe S: Hallux-to-hand transfer. Hand 7:128-133, 1975
89. O'Brien BMcC: Microvascular Reconstructive Surgery. Churchill Livingstone, Edinburgh, 1977
90. O'Brien BMcC, Gould JS, Morrison WA, Russell RC, MacLeod AM, Pribaz JJ: Free vascularized small joint transfer to the hand. J Hand Surg 9A:634-641, 1984
91. Ohmori K, Harii K: Free dorsalis pedis sensory flap to the hand, with microneurovascular anastomoses. Plast Reconstr Surg 58:546-554, 1976
92. Ohtsuka H, Torigai K, Shioya N: Two toe-to-finger transplants in one hand. Plast Reconstr Surg 60:561-565, 1977
93. Pisarek W: Transfer of the third, fourth and fifth toes for one-stage reconstruction of the thumb and two fingers. Br J Plast Surg 43:244-246, 1990
94. Poppen NK, Norris TR, Buncke HJ Jr: Evaluation of sensibility and function with microsurgical free tissue transfer of the great toe to the hand for thumb reconstruction. J Hand Surg 8:516-531, 1983
95. Robbins F, Reece T: Hand rehabilitation after great toe trans-

fer for thumb reconstruction. Arch Phys Med Rehabil 66:109, 1985

96. Rose EH, Hendel P: Primary toe-to-thumb transfer in the acutely avulsed thumb. Plast Reconstr Surg 67:214–217, 1981
97. Stern PJ: Free neurovascular cutaneous toe pulp transfer for thumb reconstruction. Microsurgery 8:158–161, 1987
98. Stice RC, Wood MB: Neurovascular island skin flaps in the hand: Functional and sensibility evaluations. Microsurgery 8:162–167, 1987
99. Stirrat CR, Seaber AV, Urbaniak JR, Bright DS: Temperature monitoring in digital replantation. J Hand Surg 3:342–347, 1978
100. Strickland JW: Restoration of thumb function following partial or total amputation. pp. 379–406. In Hunter JM, Schneider LH, Mackin EJ, Bell JA (eds): Rehabilitation of the Hand. CV Mosby, St Louis, 1978
101. Tamai S, Hori Y, Tatsumi Y, Okuda H: Hallux-to-thumb transfer with microsurgical technique: A case report in a 45-year-old woman. J Hand Surg 2:152–155, 1977
102. Ti-Sheng C, Wei W, Jin-Bao W: Free transfer of the second toe combined with dorsalis pedis flap using microvascular technique for reconstruction of the thumb and other fingers. Ann Acad Singapore 8:404–412, 1979
103. Tsai T-M, Jupiter JB, Kutz JE, Kleinert HE: Vascularized autogenous whole joint transfer in the hand—A clinical study. J Hand Surg 7:335–342, 1982
104. Tsai T-M, McCabe S, Beatty ME: Second toe transfer for thumb reconstruction in multiple digit amputations including thumb and basal joint. Microsurgery 8:146–153, 1987
105. Ueba Y: Arteriography in the treatment for congenital anomalies of the hand. J Jpn Surg Hand 1:269–272, 1984
106. Upton J, Mutimer K: A modification of the great-toe transfer for thumb reconstruction. Plast Reconstr Surg 82:535–538, 1988
107. Upton J, Mutimer KL: A modified great toe transfer for thumb reconstruction: a more aesthetically pleasing reconstruction. pp. 319–322. In Brunelli G (ed): Textbook of Microsurgery. Masson, Milano, 1988
108. Urbaniak JR: Elective microsurgery for orthopaedic reconstruction. Part II. Thumb reconstruction by microsurgery. AAOS Instructional Course Lectures 33:425–446, 1984
109. Urbaniak JR: Wrap-around procedure for thumb reconstruction. Hand Clin 1:259–269, 1985
110. Urbaniak JR: Other microvascular reconstruction of the thumb. pp. 1311–1330. In Green DP (ed): Operative Hand Surgery. 2nd Ed., Churchill Livingstone, New York, 1988
111. Vilkki SK: Toe to antebrachial stump transplantation. Functional results after new grip reconstruction. pp. 329–333. In Brunelli G: Textbook of Microsurgery. Masson, Milano, 1988
112. Vitkus K, Vitkus M, Krivulin A: Long-term measurement of innervation density in second toe-to-thumb transfers receiving immediate postoperative sensory reeducation. Microsurgery 10:245–247, 1989
113. Wang W: Keys to successful second toe-to-hand transfer: A review of 30 cases. J Hand Surg 8:902–906, 1983
114. Wei F-C, Chen H-C, Chuang C-C, Noordhoff MS: Reconstruction of a hand, amputated at the metacarpophalangeal level, by means of combined second and third toes from each foot: A case report. J Hand Surg 11A:340–344, 1986
115. Wei F-C, Chen H-C, Chuang C-C, Noordhoff MS: Reconstruction of the thumb with a trimmed-toe transfer technique. Plast Reconstr Surg 82:506–515, 1988
116. Wei F-C, Chen H-C, Chuang C-C, Noordhoff MS: Simultaneous multiple toe transfers in hand reconstruction. Plast Reconstr Surg 81:366–377, 1988
117. Wei F-C, Colony LH: Microsurgical reconstruction of opposable digits in mutilating hand injuries. Clin Plast Surg 16:491–504, 1989
118. Wilson CS, Buncke HJ, Alpert BS, Gordon L: Composite metacarpophalangeal joint reconstruction in great toe-to-hand free tissue transfers. J Hand Surg 9A:645–649, 1984
119. Yang D, Yudong G: Thumb reconstruction utilizing second toe transplantation by microvascular anastomosis. Report of 78 cases. Chinese Med J 92:295–301, 1979
120. Yoshimura M: Toe-to-hand transfer. Plast Reconstr Surg 66:74–83, 1980
121. Zhong-jia Y, Ho H-G: Bilateral hand reconstruction: Report of three cases. J Reconstr Microsurg 1:253–261, 1985
122. Zhong-jia Y, Ho H-G, Chen TC-H: Microsurgical reconstruction of the amputated hand. J Reconstr Microsurg 1:161–165, 1984
123. Zhong-jia Y: Reconstruction of a digitless hand. J Hand Surg 12A:722–726, 1987

34

The Perionychium

Elvin G. Zook
Richard E. Brown

Fingernails are used for scratching, in defense and, more obviously, by humans to pick up small objects. However, the nail also protects the fingertip, contributes to tactile sensation,[41,45,66,80] and plays an important role in regulation of the peripheral circulation.[66] An abnormal nail is both a cosmetic and a functional problem, in that it catches on objects, particularly cloth, causing finger pain and damage to the object. Although nail injuries are among the most common of those of the hand,[47] until recently they have received little attention in the standard textbooks on hand surgery.[15,30,58]

ANATOMY

The perionychium consists of the paronychium and the nail bed[54] and has been described by many authors.[10,45,53,55,66,70,71,83,89,93,95] The nail anatomy is shown in diagrammatic form in Figure 34-1. The proximal nail fits into a depression called the *nail fold.* The skin over the dorsum of the nail fold is the *nail wall.* The thin membrane extending from the nail wall onto the dorsum of the nail is the *eponychium.* The *lunula* is the curved, white opacity in the nail found just distal to the eponychium and is roughly at the junction of the intermediate (germinal) and ventral (sterile) matrixes.

The nail fold is divided into the dorsal roof and the ventral floor by the nail. The *nail bed (matrix)* is all the soft tissue immediately beneath the nail that participates in nail generation and migration. The mass of keratin between the distal nail and the nail bed is the *hyponychium.* This is very resistant to infection, as shown by the fact that bacterial contamination in the area is heavy, yet infections are uncommon.

The embryology of the nail bed has been described by several authors.[45,54,55]

The nail is made up of material from three areas of the nail bed.[42] Lewis[54] attributed production of the vast majority of the nail volume to the ventral floor *(germinal matrix)* of the nail fold. He also suggested that the tissue produced by the dorsal roof and the ventral nail bed *(sterile matrix)* are nail (Fig. 34-2). This is in spite of the fact that the contributions to the nail are produced in two different ways. Zaias[89] stated that only the portion produced by the ventral floor (germinal matrix) is true nail (Fig. 34-3). There is little doubt that some material is added to the undersurface of the nail by the "sterile matrix" as it progresses distally, since the distal nail is thicker than the proximal portion[10] and a subungual hematoma that starts proximally beneath the nail becomes incorporated into the nail as it grows distally.[59] This argument, however, is primarily theoretical and has little effect on the practical care of the nail bed.

The arterial blood supply to the nail bed comes from two terminal branches of the volar digital artery (Fig. 34-4). They communicate in the nail bed to form blood sinuses that are surrounded by muscle fibers and help to regulate the blood pressure and blood supply to the extremities.[66]

The venous drainage of the perionychium coalesces in the proximal portion of the nail bed and the skin proximal to the nail fold, and the veins then course in a random fashion over the dorsum of the finger.[60,100] Lymphatic vessels are more numerous in the nail bed,[81] particularly in the area of the hyponychium, than in any other dermal area.[91]

The nerve supply to the perionychium comes from the dorsal branch of the volar digital nerve. Varying patterns of branching[88,100] have been reported.

Physiology

Complete longitudinal nail growth takes between 70 and 160 days,[45,66] at a rate of approximately 0.1 mm a day,[5] 25 mm a week,[39] or 1.5 inches a year.[22] Baden[3] described a 21-day

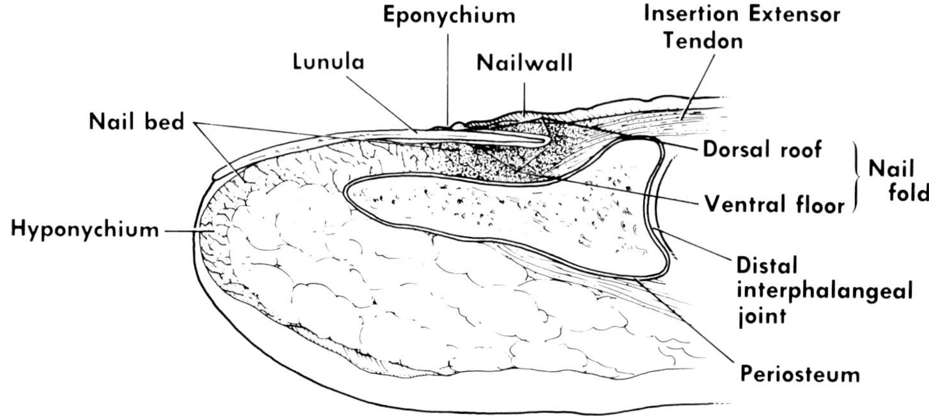

Fig. 34-1. The anatomy of the nail bed is shown in sagittal section.

delay in distal growth of the nail after injury, during which time it thickens proximal to the injury site. Nail generation continues to be greater than normal for the next 50 days and then is less for 30 subsequent days. This accounts for the bulge in the surface of a regrowing nail. Nail growth, therefore, is not physiologically normal for 100 days following injury. Nail growth is slower in children younger than 3 years and then is progressively faster until approximately age 30. After 30 it gradually slows as the individual ages. Fingernails grow more rapidly than do toenails by a ratio of 4 : 1, and grow progressively faster on the longer fingers.[66]

The nail progresses distally because of the confinement of the nail fold. As the matrix cells enlarge they are flattened by the pressure of newly forming cells beneath them. As this pressure is exerted, restriction of the nail fold results in a distal vector. Kligman[51] has shown that a germinal matrix graft placed on the forearm will grow upward in a vertical cylinder.

The material produced by the roof of the nail fold is responsible for the shiny surface of the nail. If the dorsal roof is removed, the nail surface will be dull in appearance[100] (Fig. 34-5). Hashimoto[36] has shown in monkeys that a smooth nail bed is essential for regrowth of a normal nail. Scar does not produce any type of nail, so if the nail bed is not accurately approximated, primary healing with minimal scar cannot result and deformity may occur.

If the scar is on the dorsal roof, a dull streak may appear; if it is in the intermediate nail (germinal matrix), a split or absent nail may occur; and if it is in the ventral nail (sterile matrix), a split or nonadherence of the nail beyond the scar may occur.

TREATMENT OF ACUTE INJURIES

Twenty years ago Ashbell et al[4] classified nail bed injuries, but made no mention of subungual hematomas, although blood beneath the nail comes from disruption of the nail bed blood vessels. We will use a simplified classification of simple lacerations, stellate lacerations, severe crush, and avulsion.[98]

Late reconstruction of the nail bed is unpredictable and frequently little, if any improvement, is obtained. It is therefore preferable to treat the injury early and properly to prevent deformity. "There's never time to do it right, but there is always time to do it over" (Meskimen's Law of Bureaucracies)[57] is an adage that should *not* be applied to the treatment of nail bed injuries.

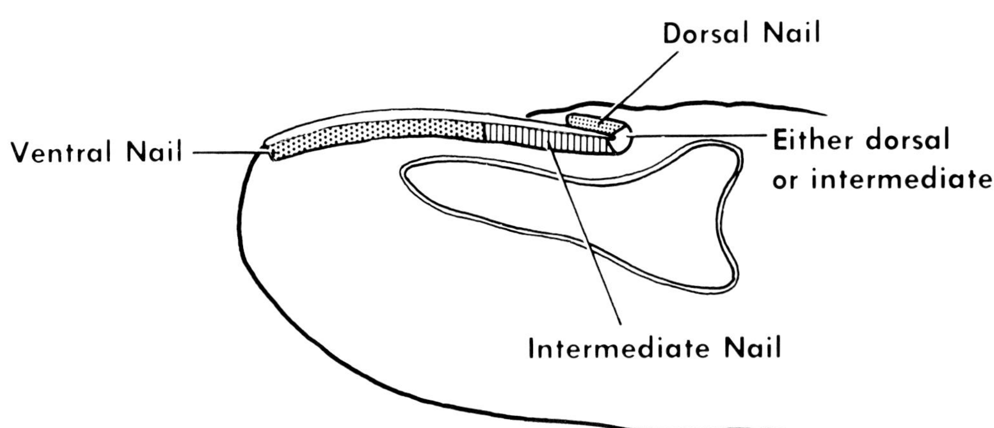

Fig. 34-2. The three areas that contribute to nail production are shown.

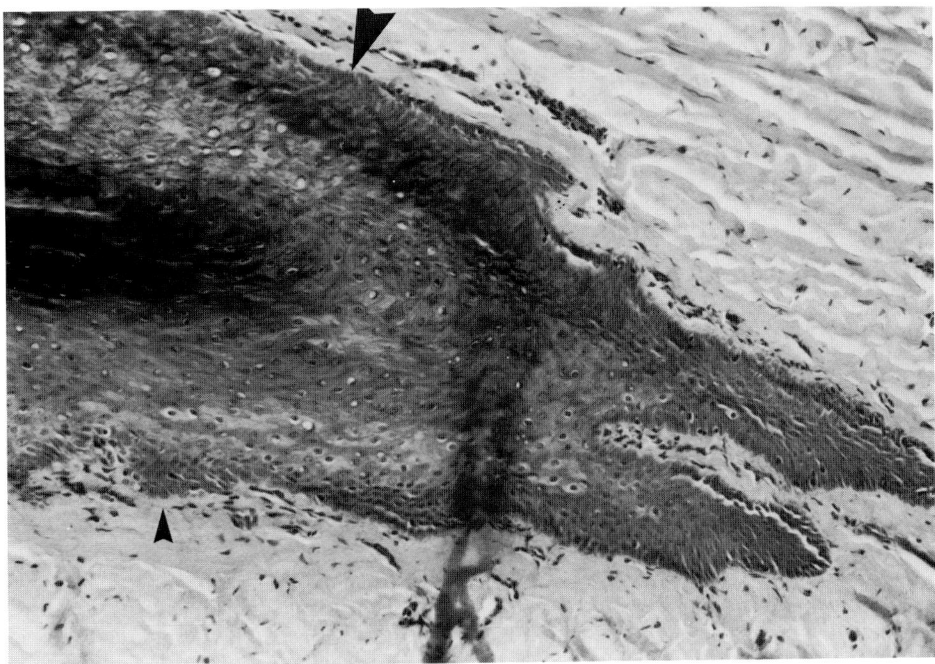

Fig. 34-3. The small arrow denotes intermediate nail production by the ventral floor and the large arrow shows the nail production of the dorsal roof, which contributes the shine of the nail.

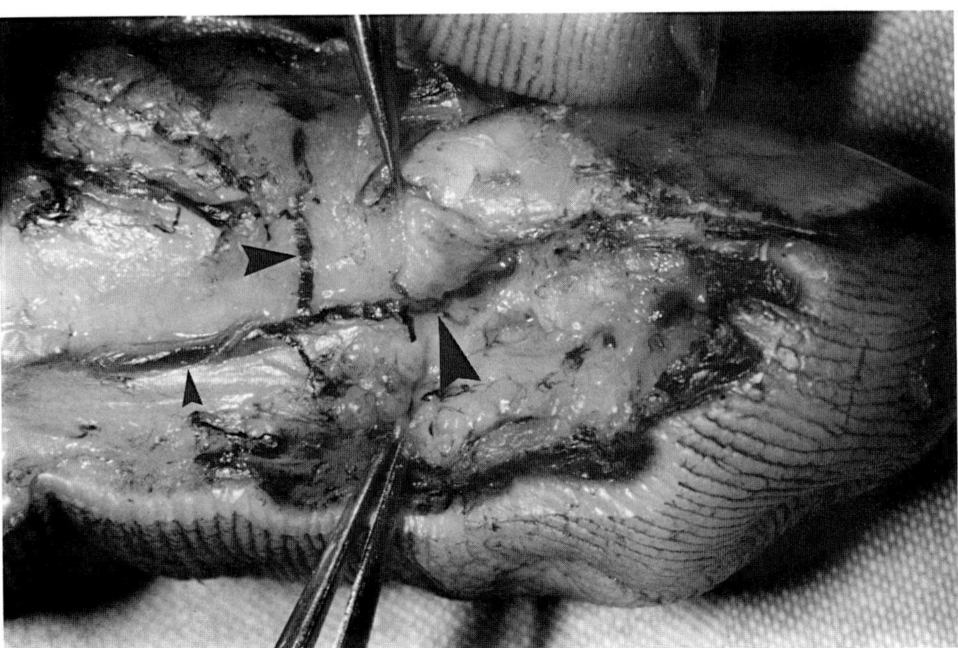

Fig. 34-4. The small arrow shows the common volar digital artery, the intermediate arrow the dorsal branch to the nail fold, and the large arrow the artery that progresses along the paronychium giving branches to the nail bed. The terminal branch to the pad of the finger is not shown. (From Zook et al,[100] with permission.)

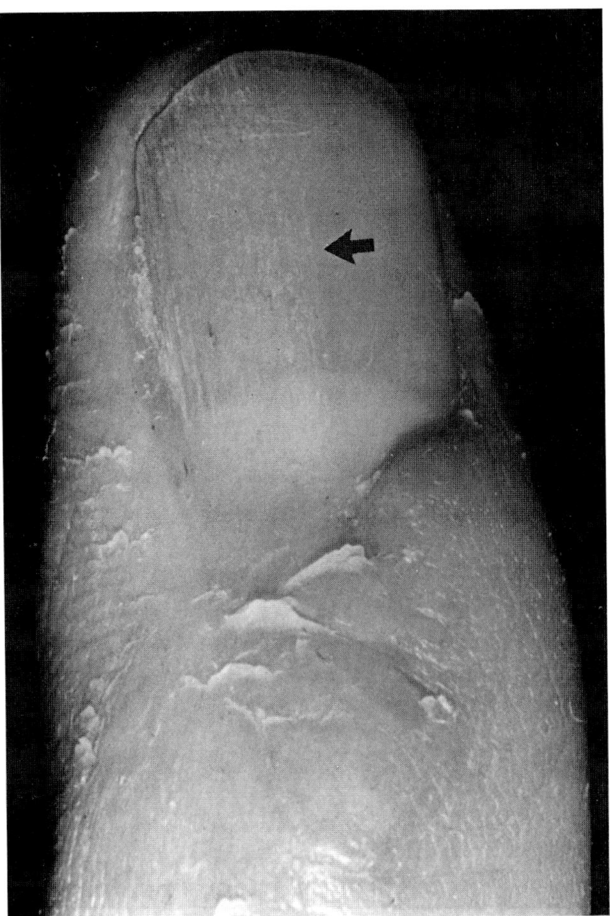

Fig. 34-5. A nail that has sustained avulsion of the nailproducing tissue of the dorsal roof from one side of the nail fold has lost its normal shine. (From Zook,[90] with permission.)

Epidemiology of the Injury

Nail deformities can occur secondary to anything that causes injury or deformation of the nail bed. This may include infection, self-mutilation, tumor, or trauma. Doors are the most common source of injury, followed by smashing between two objects, saws, and lawn mowers. The age groups most commonly injured are older children and young adults. The digits of the left and right hand are injured with equal frequency. The long finger, being the longest and most exposed, is the most frequently injured, with the ring, index, small, and thumb following in that order. Injuries to the nail bed alone are six times less common than injuries that involve the paronychium and tip. The most common type of injury is the simple laceration, followed by stellate laceration, crush, and avulsion in decreasing frequency. The middle and distal third of the nail bed are the most frequent site of injury, and 50 percent of injuries involve fracture of the distal phalanx and/or tuft.[33,96,98]

Injuries of the nail bed most commonly result from localized trauma to the nail that causes compression of the nail bed between the bent or broken nail and the bone (Fig. 34-6A). This causes a straight or stellate, tearing laceration of the nail bed. When the nail is compressed between a larger object and the bone, an exploding type of injury results in stellate lacerations or multiple fragments of nail bed (severe crush and/or avulsion; Fig. 34-6B). It is rare to have a truly sharp laceration of the nail bed. More commonly when a sharp object strikes the nail hard enough to perforate it, it goes through and amputates the tip.[98]

Subungual Hematoma

The nail bed is a highly vascular structure. A compression laceration of the nail bed secondary to a blow causes bleeding. If the nail is not broken or the edge dislodged, the pressure of the hematoma beneath the nail will frequently cause severe throbbing pain, and evacuation of the hematoma is indicated. If more than 25 to 50 percent of the visible portion of the nail is undermined by hematoma, it is best to remove the nail, inspect the nail bed, and repair the injury.[86,90,91,92] It is essential to surgically scrub the finger prior to perforation of the nail to prevent contamination of the subungual area and the subsequent risk of infection and potential osteomyelitis. We prefer a Betadine soap scrub for 5 minutes followed by Betadine solution application.

Use of a drill, needle,[61] or paper clip heated in an alcohol lamp or Bunsen burner until red hot, has been advocated (Fig.

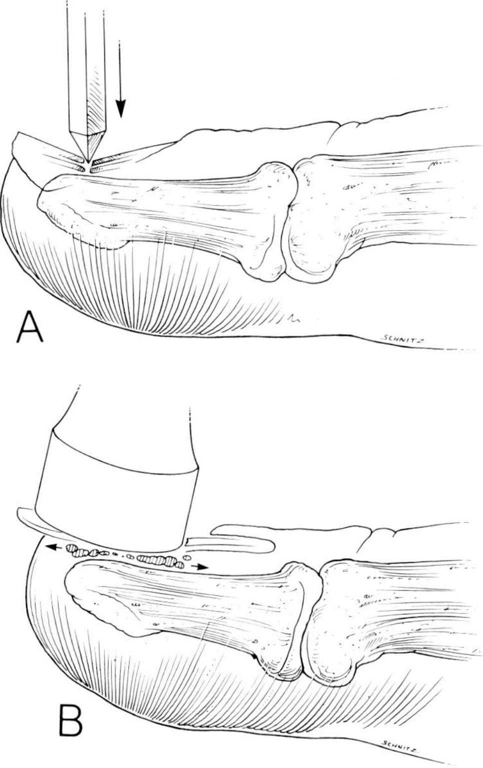

Fig. 34-6. (A) A relatively sharp object compressing the nail between the nail and bone causes a splitting laceration. (B) A wider area of compression of the nail bed between the nail and the bone causes an exploding-type injury that results in multiple fragments.

34-7A) for making a hole in the nail. We prefer the battery-powered microcautery unit available in most emergency rooms (Fig. 34-7B). The heated tip passes through the nail, is cooled by the hematoma, and does not injure the nail bed. The hole burned in the nail must be large enough to allow prolonged drainage. Some methods create a small hole that decompresses the hematoma immediately, but the hematoma re-forms when clot seals the hole.

Simple Lacerations

A simple laceration is the most common injury. Warning signs of significant injury to the nail bed other than the obvious are subungual hematoma involving over 25 percent of the visible nail and/or avulsion of the nail from the nail fold or paronychium (see Fig. 34-13A). A surgical prep and finger tourniquet are necessary to allow an adequate view of the nail bed. The nail is removed by gently opening and closing iris scissors inserted beneath the free edge of the nail and working them proximally. A small periosteal elevator may also be worked proximally from the hyponychium to free the nail. We find the Kutz periosteal elevator to be better than the Freer, since the former is smaller and does less damage to the nail bed. After the nail is removed it is cleaned by scraping the residual soft tissue from its undersurface and soaked in Betadine solution while the nail bed is being repaired.

The nail bed is explored with loupe magnification and the injury is evaluated to estimate the degree of crush and irregularity of the edges (Fig. 34-8A). Irregularities are trimmed, if it can be done without sacrificing so much tissue that tension on the repair occurs. If this is in doubt, it is usually advisable not to trim the edges. One millimeter of undermining of the nail bed from the periosteum will allow slight eversion of the wound edges and accurate wound approximation. Both 5-0 chromic catgut[87] and 6-0 plain catgut[4] have been advocated for suture. We prefer 7-0 chromic on a micropoint spatula, double-arm, GS-9, ophthalmic needle (Ethicon). The curve of this needle allows easier passage through the nail bed that is adherent to the periosteum, and the double needle provides a spare in case one is bent or broken. After the nail bed is accurately approximated (Fig. 34-8B), a round hole is drilled or burned through the nail at a point not over the repair site, to allow drainage of serum or hematoma from the subungual area after the nail is

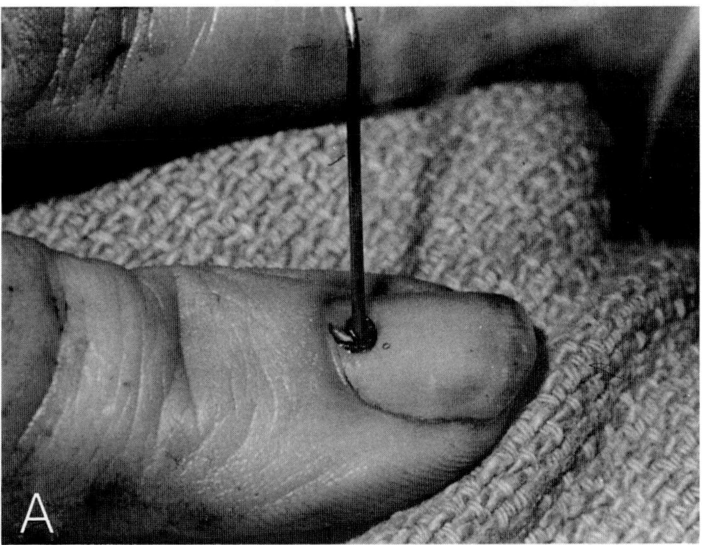

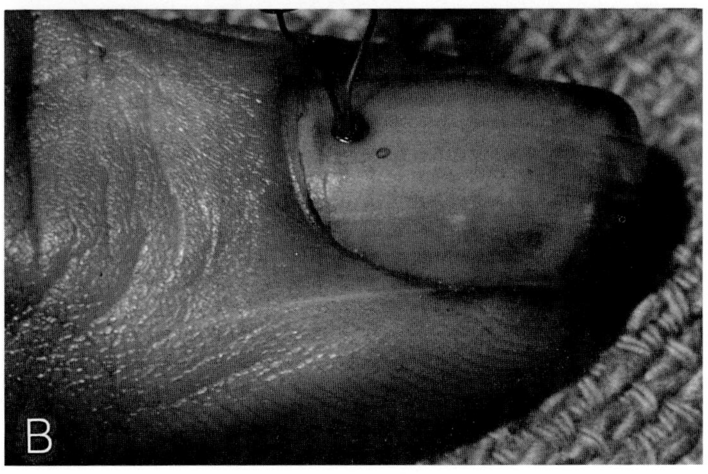

Fig. 34-7. **(A)** A time-honored method of burning a hole through the nail is with a heated paper clip. **(B)** The authors' preferred method of burning a hole through the nail is with an ophthalmic battery-powered cautery.

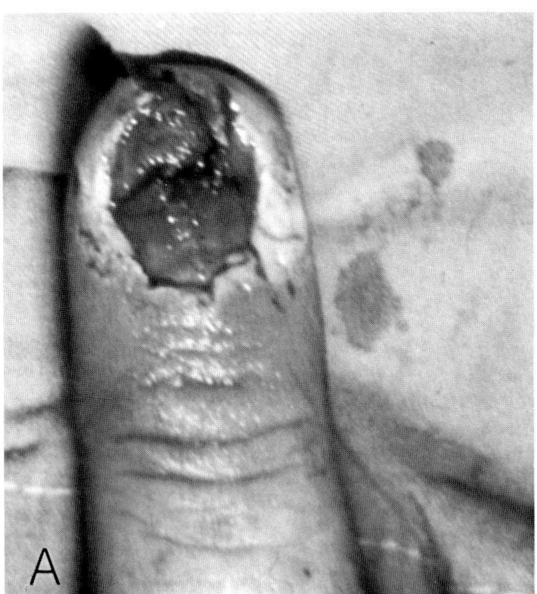

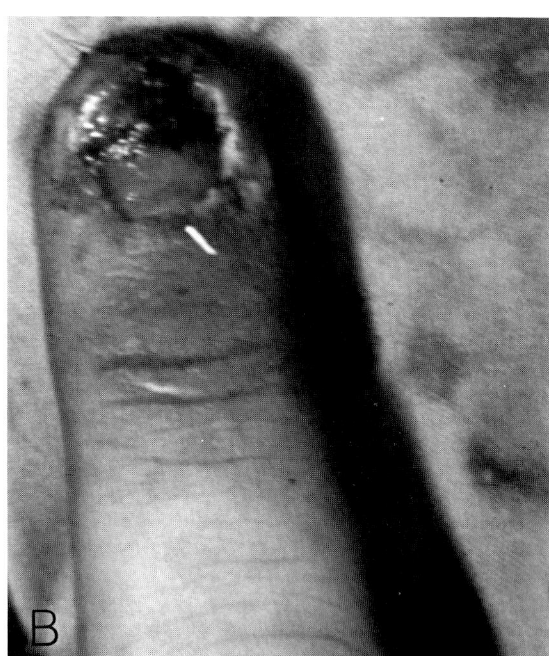

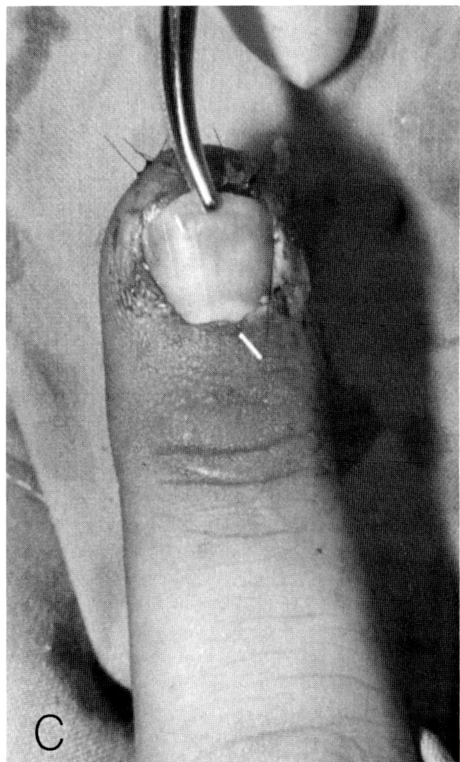

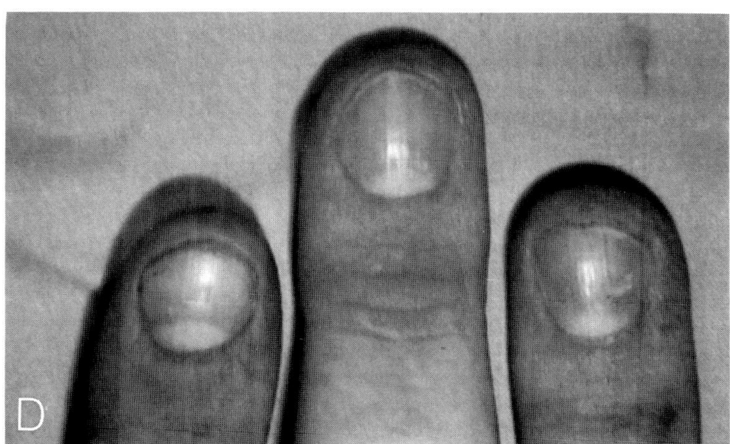

Fig. 34-8. **(A)** An injury in the simple laceration category. This laceration, although straight, is a crushing type of injury. **(B)** The nail bed has been sutured with 7-0 chromic sutures under magnification. **(C)** The nail, after it has been cleaned and soaked in Betadine, is replaced into the nail fold. A hole will be drilled in the nail to allow drainage, although it is easier to do this before the nail is reinserted into the nail fold. **(D)** The nail 1 year postinjury. (From Zook,[92] with permission.)

reinserted into the nail fold. Schiller in 1957[72] described replacing the fingernail into the nail fold to keep the fold open and better mold the edges of the repair (Fig. 34-8C). We hold the nail in place with a 5–0 monofilament nylon suture placed through the fingertip and the distal free border of the nail. The fingertip is then dressed with nonadherent gauze, a small dressing, and a splint that immobilizes the DIP joint and protects the tip. The dressing is changed in 5 to 7 days and the nail checked for subungual seroma or hematoma. If present, the hole is reopened or the nail raised at the paronychium to permit drainage. The suture is removed from the tip at 2 to 3 weeks. The nail will frequently adhere to the nail bed for 1 to 3 months until pushed off by the new nail. Replacement of the nail creates a much less tender fingertip while a new nail is growing (Fig. 34-8D).

If the nail is unavailable or too badly damaged for a portion of it to be replaced, a nail-shaped sheet of 0.020-inch reinforced silicone may be used as a substitute. A 6–0 nylon suture is brought from the nail wall through the proximal portion of the nail fold, placed through the edge of the silicone sheet at each corner, and returned through the nail fold onto the dorsum of the finger (Fig. 34-9). The silicone sheet molds the edges of the repair and keeps the nail fold open. If a suture is not used proximally to hold the silicone sheet in the nail fold, the softness of the sheet may allow it to slip out; however, the use of more firm prosthetic materials[63] does not allow the accurate conformational smoothing of the nail bed desired, and is more expensive.

A single thickness of nail-shaped Adaptic or other nonadherent gauze may be placed in the nail fold if the nail is not available. It will adhere adequately to stay in place and will loosen after healing has occurred. We start t.i.d. soapy water soaks 7 days after injury to clean the wound.

If the nail is avulsed with a distal base, sutures should be placed through the proximal portion of the fold into the free margin of the nail bed and brought back out through the dorsal roof of the nail fold, drawing the nail back into the nail fold (Fig. 34-10A and B). Accurate nailbed approximation in the nail fold may require an incision in the eponychium. The incision should be made perpendicular to the lateral curved portion of the eponychial fold and may be necessary on both sides (Fig. 34-11).

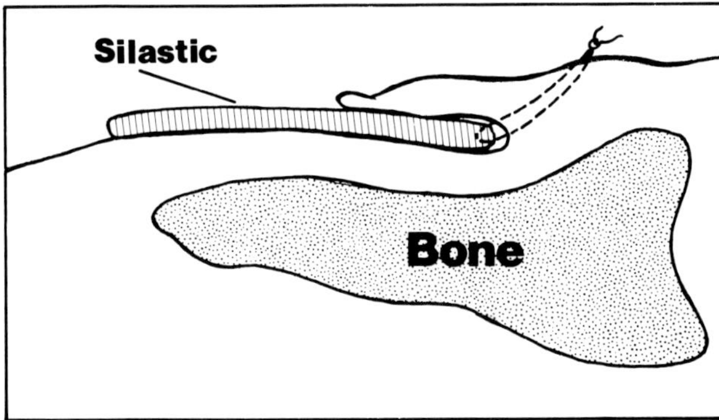

Fig. 34-9. A horizontal mattress suture through the nail wall is used to hold a silicone sheet into the nail fold.

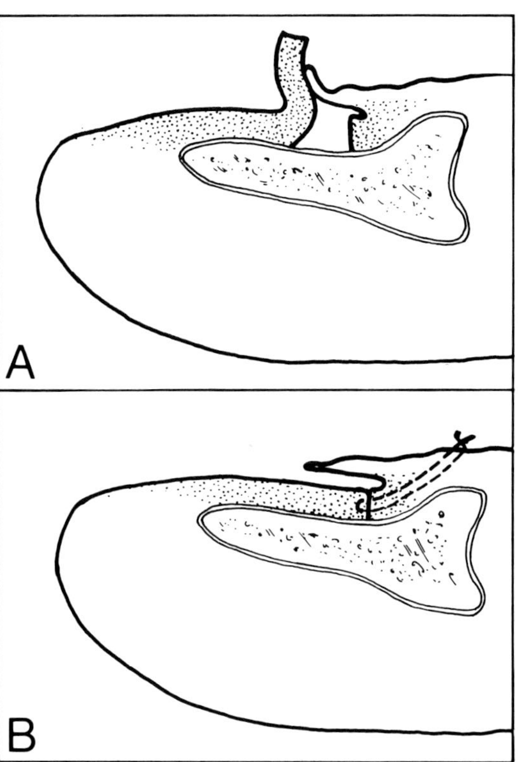

Fig. 34-10. **(A)** The nail bed has been torn in the proximal nail fold and stripped from the nail fold. **(B)** A horizontal mattress suture through the nail wall is used to replace the nail bed. The nail is then returned to the nail fold to mold the wound edges.

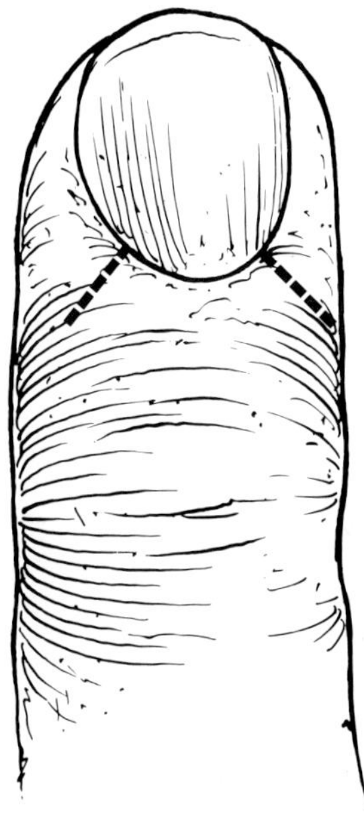

Fig. 34-11. When incisions are made in the eponychium, they should be made at 90-degree angles from the eponychium to prevent deformity.

If the laceration involves the dorsal roof and the ventral floor, it is important that both be similarly repaired. The fine chromic catgut sutures approximating the nail bed should have the knots placed in the nail fold, not buried in the soft tissue of the nail wall or matrix. The nail wall (skin) is then approximated with 6-0 nonabsorbable sutures. It is especially important with this type of injury to place the nail, silicone sheet, or gauze in the nail fold to prevent adhesions (Fig. 34-12A and B).

Stellate Lacerations

The etiology of stellate lacerations is similar to simple lacerations, but is caused by a more widely distributed force that involves more of the nail surface. Accurate approximation of the stellate points is necessary (Fig. 34-13C). Meticulous repair plus the use of the nail, silicone sheet, or nonadherent gauze as described previously will in most cases give a surprisingly good result (Fig. 34-13). The use of porcine xenografts[26] has been published showing good results. We have had no experience with this method.

Severe Crushing Injuries

Severe crushing injuries carry a poorer prognosis[98] than do the previously described injuries. In the severe crushing injury it is important that all fragments of the nail bed be returned to the nail bed and repaired as accurately as possible (Fig. 34-14A-C). Any fragments attached by tissue strands should be accurately replaced. Any segments of nail bed attached to the detached nail should be removed with a small periosteal elevator and used as free grafts to complete the nail bed. Nail, silicone sheet, or Adaptic is used to mold the edges and maintain the nail fold open until healing results.

Lacerations Associated with Fractures of the Distal Phalanx

Approximately 50 percent of nail bed injuries have an accompanying fracture of the distal phalanx.[98] If the fracture is nondisplaced, the nail bed should be repaired and the nail replaced as a splint. The replaced nail, due to its close proximity to the periosteum, makes an excellent splint to maintain fracture reduction. Displaced fractures are accurately reduced and fixed with fine longitudinal or crossed K-wires if unstable.

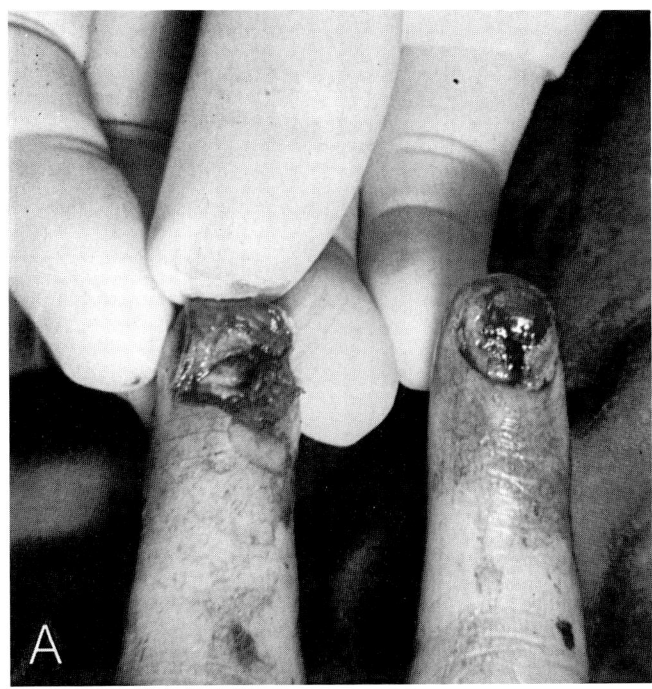

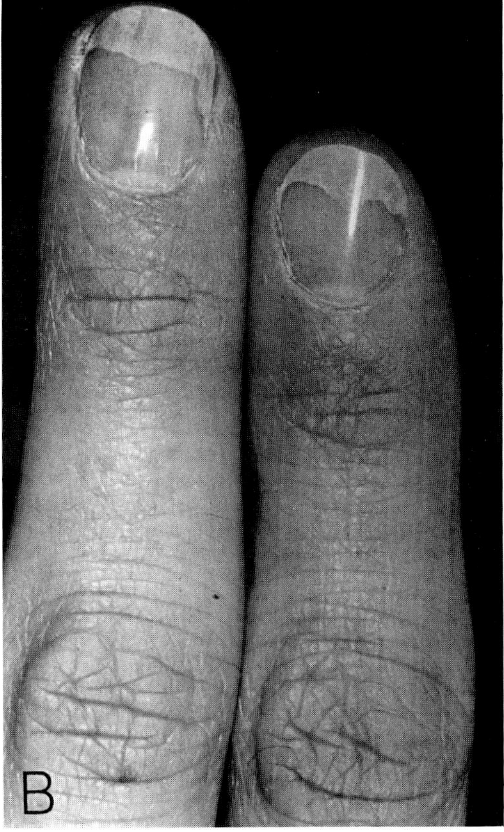

Fig. 34-12. **(A)** This through-and-through laceration of the nail fold was repaired as described in the text. **(B)** The nail 1 year postinjury. (From Zook,[92] with permission.)

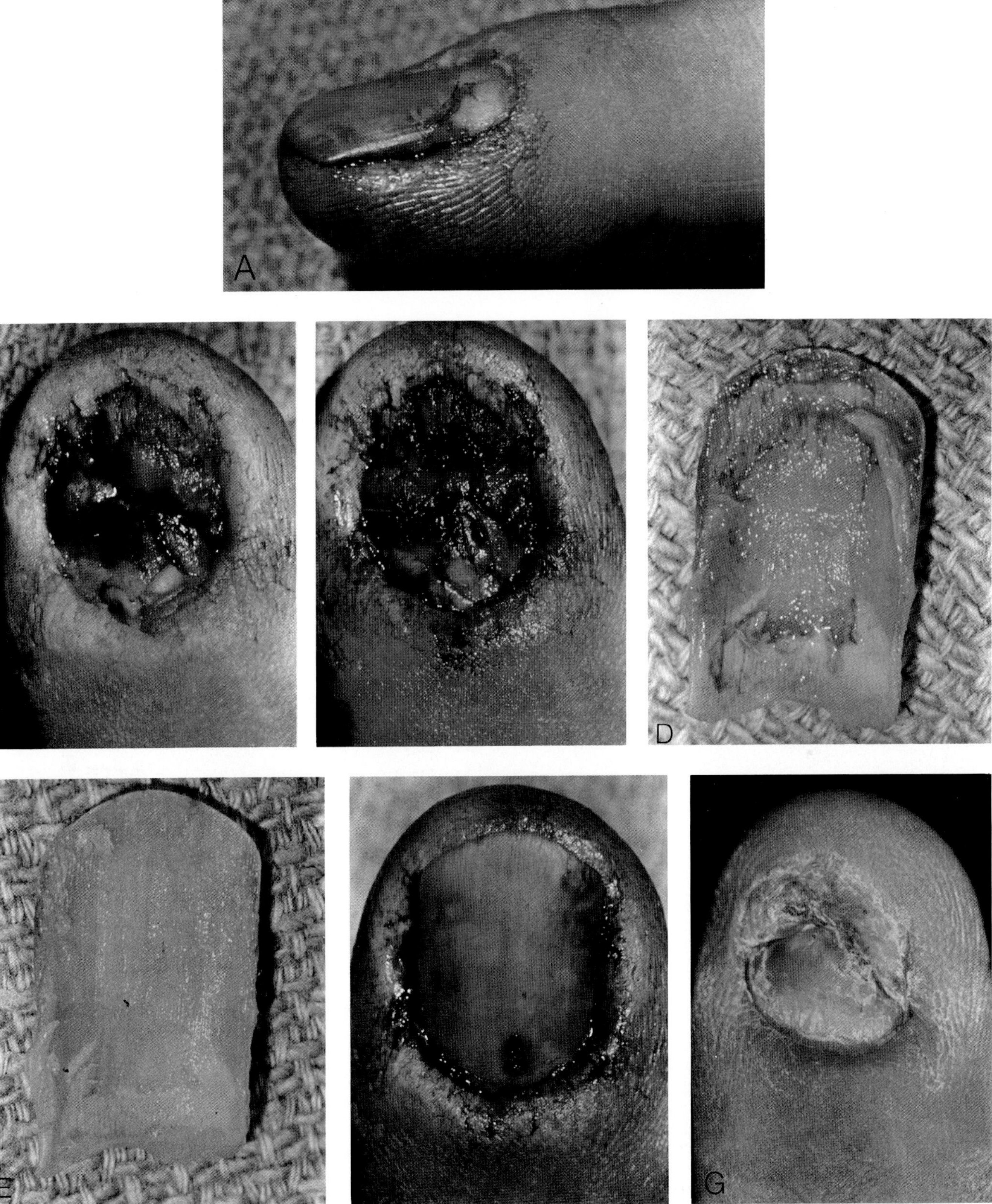

Fig. 34-13. **(A)** Avulsion of the proximal nail from the nail fold. **(B)** A stellate laceration of the nail bed is visible only after the nail has been removed. **(C)** The lacerations are approximated as accurately as possible with fine (7–0) chromic sutures and using magnification. **(D)** The undersurface of the nail after it has been removed from the nail bed, showing the residual soft tissue that is usually present. **(E)** The undersurface of the nail after it has been cleaned and soaked. **(F)** A hole large enough to allow drainage has been burned through the nail, and the nail has been inserted back into the nail fold. **(G)** The nail 2 months after the injury. *(Figure continues.)*

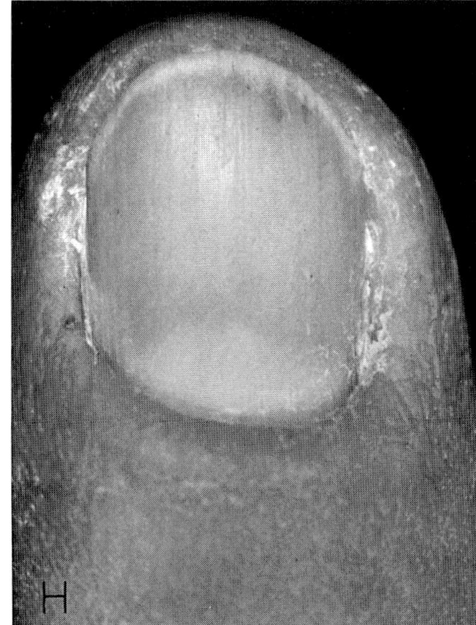

Fig. 34-13 *(Continued).* **(H)** The nail 1 year postinjury. (From Zook,[90] with permission.)

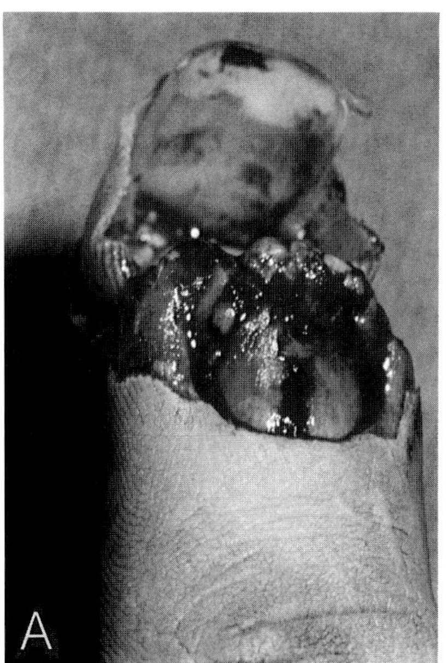

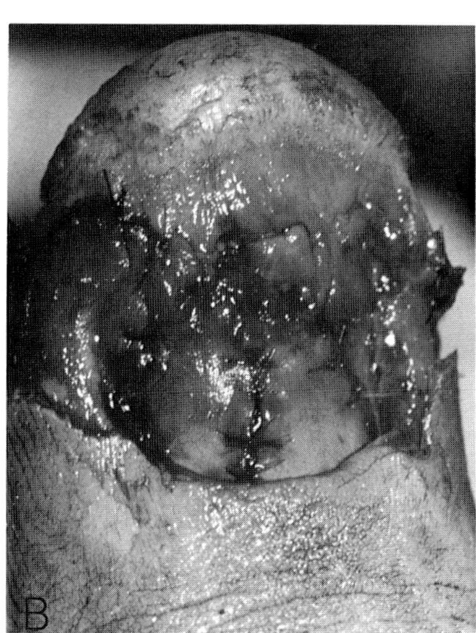

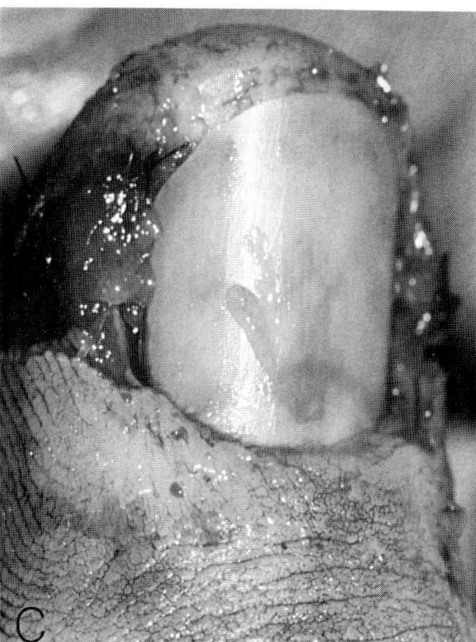

Fig. 34-14. **(A)** A severe crushing injury of the nail bed with avulsion of the nail and laceration of the tip. **(B)** The nail bed is approximated and sutured as accurately as possible. **(C)** The nail is replaced to maintain reduction of the fracture and to mold the edges of the nail bed.

If the patient is seen late with a displaced fracture that has not been reduced prior to a recent nail bed repair, the wound should be opened unless contraindicated by the presence of infection. The fracture should be accurately reduced, pinned if necessary to maintain reduction, and the nail bed re-repaired. If the dorsal cortex of the distal phalanx is left uneven it will cause a nail bed deformity.

Avulsion of the Nail Bed

Nail bed avulsion frequently leaves the fragment of nail bed attached to the undersurface of the avulsed nail. An attempt should be made to find the nail if it does not accompany the patient. Schiller[72] suggested that the nail to which the nail bed is attached is the optimum shape and tension to aid inosculation of the nail bed. It is therefore advisable to replace the nail as accurately as possible onto the avulsion site. One to two millimeters of nail may be freed and trimmed from the nail bed in the area to be sutured if the fragment is large (Fig. 34-15). This allows easier and more accurate placement of sutures.

Further injury to the nail bed might ensue if attempts are made to remove a fragment of nail bed from a small piece of nail. Therefore the nail should be replaced accurately without attempting to separate the nail and nail bed (Fig. 34-16).

Free Nail Bed Graft

All retrievable fragments of nail bed should be replaced as free grafts. A graft 1 cm in diameter will usually live by inosculation and ingrowth of circulation from the periphery, even on the bare cortex of the distal phalanx. Iselin[40] recommended storing the avulsed fragment in mild antiseptic solution for 2 to 4 days prior to replacement to determine viability of the bed. Swanker in 1947 advocated allowing small areas of nail bed

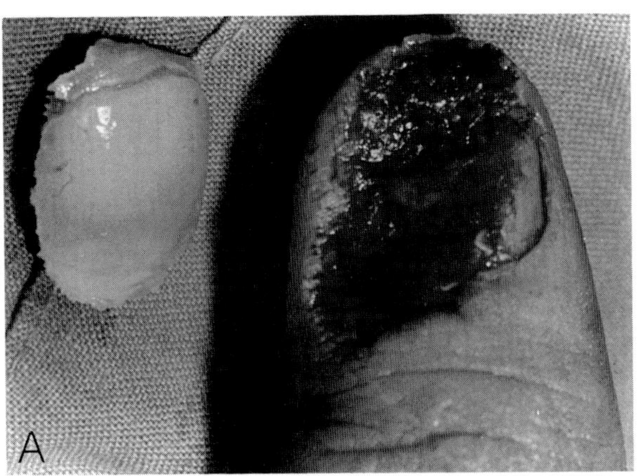

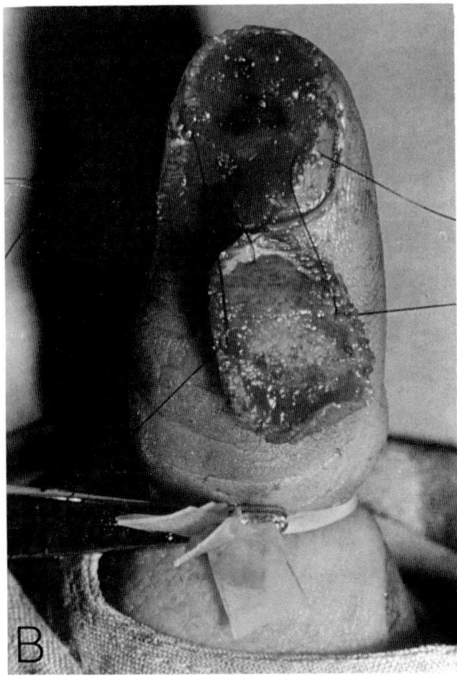

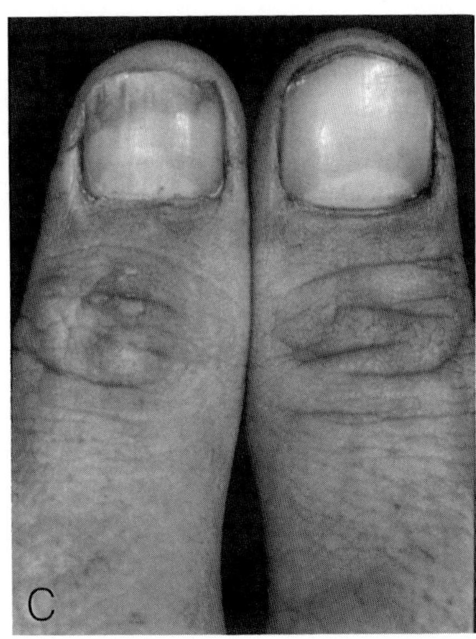

Fig. 34-15. **(A)** An avulsion of approximately 80 percent of the nail and nail bed. The nail bed is still attached to the nail. **(B)** The nail is dissected from the outer 2 mm of the nail bed to allow accurate suture placement, and the nail bed is replaced. **(C)** The repaired nail 1 year later with satisfactory growth, but with some lack of complete adherence distally, compared with the normal side. (From Zook,[92] with permission.)

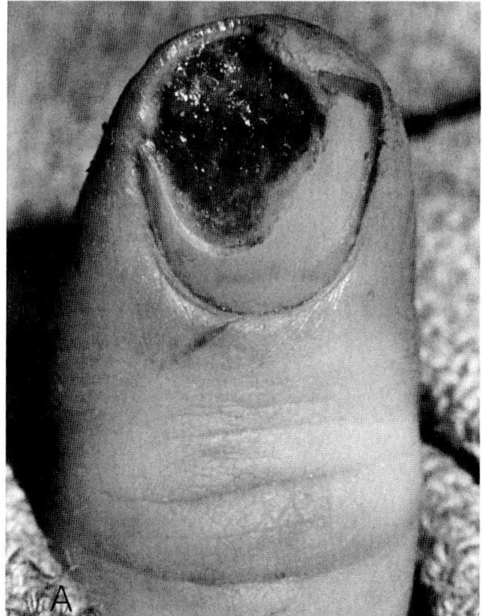

Fig. 34-16. (A) Avulsion of a small portion of the nail and nail bed. (B) The undersurface of the nail fragment with the attached nail bed is shown. (C) Only that portion of the nail that is overhanging the nail bed is removed. No attempt is made to dissect nail bed from the nail on small pieces. *(Figure continues.)*

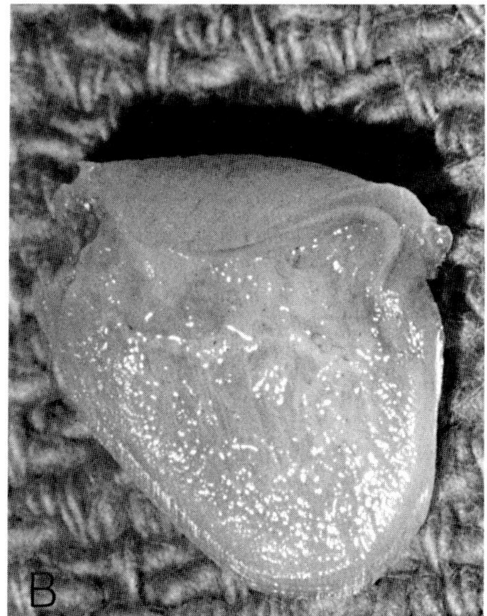

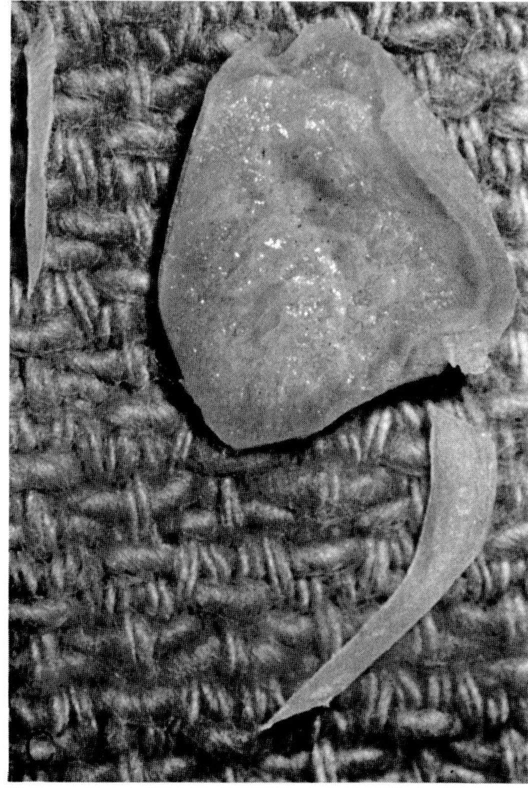

avulsion to heal by secondary intention while covered by tantalum sheet. Both increase the amount of scarring, and we believe that it decreases the chances of adherence of the nail. He also advocated the use of full-thickness nail bed grafts from an adjacent amputated finger or a 0.020-inch split-thickness nail bed graft from another finger to replace large avulsed segments.[84] Horner and Cohen,[39] Flatt,[27,28] and Hanrahan[35] advocate split-thickness skin grafts, while Ashbell et al[4] and Clayburgh et al[23] advocate using reverse dermal grafts.

If an adjacent finger has been amputated or is so severely crushed that it is to be amputated, removal of a full-thickness nail bed graft or split-thickness nail bed graft is a good choice for coverage of avulsions. Saita et al[69] have shown excellent results using free full-thickness nail bed grafts from toes in the acute nail bed avulsion injury. These have the disadvantage of causing deformity of a toenail and contradict Iselin's[40] suggestion of delay.

Shepard[76,77] demonstrated excellent results using split-thickness sterile matrix grafts from the adjacent nail bed of the injured finger or from a toe nail bed. It has been our experience

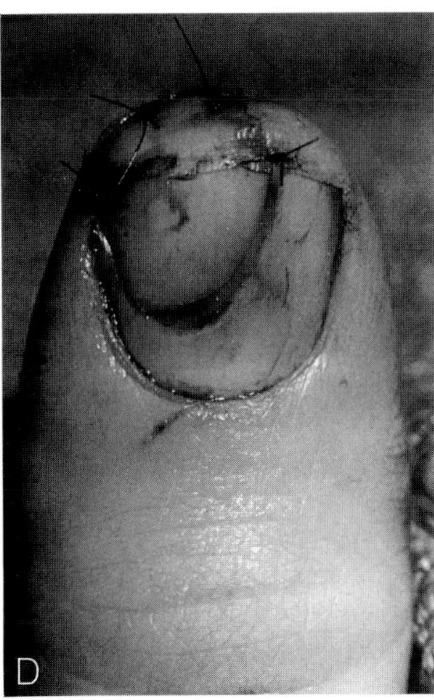

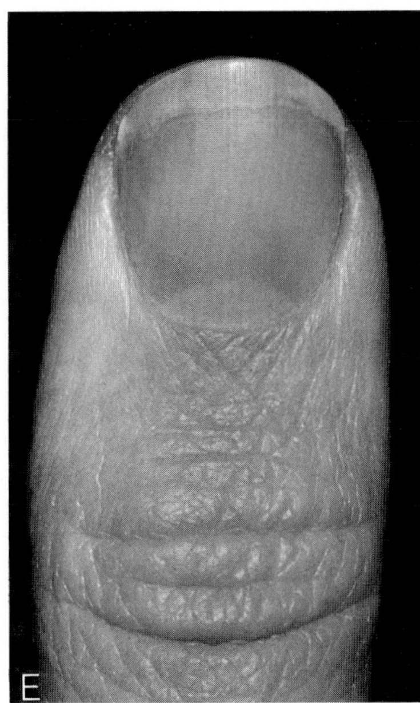

Fig. 34-16 *(Continued).* **(D)** The nail with attached nail bed is then accurately approximated and held in place with a few fine chromic sutures. **(E)** The nail 12 months postinjury.

that if there is inadequate undamaged area on the injured nail bed from which a split-thickness nail bed graft can be harvested, one must go to the large toe to acquire a large enough graft (Fig. 34-17A and B).

The toenail is removed from the great toe with a periosteal elevator under toe block anesthesia. A split-thickness nail bed graft (we suggest approximately 0.010 inches thick, but no one knows the best thickness) of the toenail bed is removed with a surgical blade. It is better for the graft to be too thin than too thick. A surgical blade can be used with a back-and-forth sawing technique to tangentially remove a small fragment of nail bed (Fig. 34-17C and D). The curve of the nail bed makes it impossible to obtain a large fragment with this technique. If a larger sterile matrix graft is needed, it is necessary to use the tip of the blade while picking up the edge of the graft being removed with fine forceps. The graft is sutured into the defect with fine chromic catgut sutures (Fig. 34-17E and F), and if the nail is available, it is replaced. The toenail is replaced into the nail fold after perforation and sutured distally as previously described.

A fragment of the tip is often avulsed with the nail bed in children. In such cases, we accurately approximate the edges of the nail bed and tip skin as a composite graft. Debridement should be minimal as the maximum possible inosculation effect is essential. The younger the child, the better the changes for "take" of a composite graft.

Delayed Treatment of Acute Injuries

Occasionally an injury of the nail bed will be seen hours or days following the injury. It may have received no care, inadequate care, or good care. The first decision must be whether the initial care was adequate, and if it was not, whether more should be done.

If there is any question the nail bed should be explored and accurately approximated. This can usually be done up to 7 days postinjury. Although the chance of infection may be greater, a nail deformity will occur if nothing is done and the risk is worth taking.[97]

LATE RECONSTRUCTION OF THE NAIL BED

Reconstructive procedures of the nail bed are commonly not as successful as the surgeon or the patient would desire. These less than satisfactory results have discouraged attempts at reconstruction and hindered progress of knowledge. Every reconstructive problem of the nail bed is different and must be approached individually. Unfortunately, no one has reported a large series and knowledge is limited. A thorough knowledge of the anatomy and physiology of the nail bed of the fingers and toes is essential to devise a treatment plan and carry it out.

Reconstruction can be divided into problems involving the sterile and germinal matrix. They may also be divided into deformity categories such as nonadherence, split nails, absence of nail, and so on.

Ridges

Nail ridges are caused by scar beneath the nail bed or an irregularly healed fracture. Since nail growth follows the shape of the nail bed, a nail ridge occurs. If an underlying ridge is transverse, the deformity can range from a transverse nail

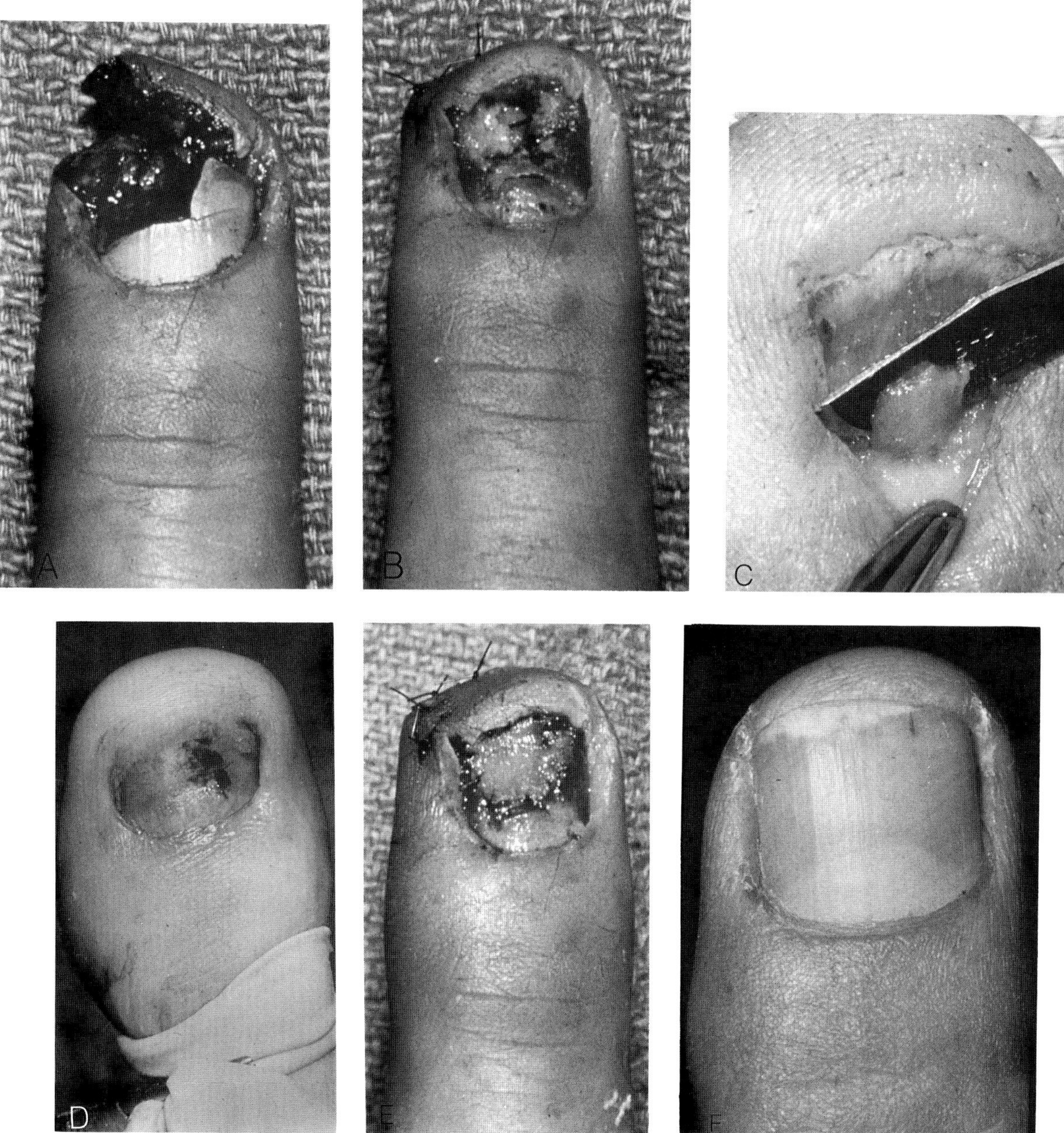

Fig. 34-17. **(A)** A nail bed and fingertip injury with avulsion of approximately 25 percent of the nail bed. **(B)** The tip skin and nail bed surrounding the avulsion have been repaired. The white area at the distal left portion of the nail bed is bare cortical bone of the distal tuft. **(C)** The technique of harvesting a small, split-thickness nail bed graft. **(D)** The large toe after the nail has been removed and a split-thickness graft has been removed from the sterile matrix. The germinal matrix should not be included in a split-thickness graft. **(E)** The split graft of sterile matrix is sutured in place on the nail bed. **(F)** The fingernail 1 year later.

groove to distal nonadherence. If the ridge is longitudinal, a longitudinal nail ridge will result. Correction of the ridged nail requires surgical excision of the scar and/or smoothing the irregularity of the bone to create a flat nail bed.[4,85]

Minor transverse ridges of the nail are frequently seen following hypoxic illnesses or use of the arm tourniquet for upper extremity surgical procedures. These resolve as new nail grows out to replace the deformed area.

Split Nail

A split nail may be caused by a ridge or longitudinal scar in the germinal and/or sterile matrix. Since scar does not produce nail cells, there is a blank area between the regions of normal nail production and a subsequent split. Carter in 1928[19] and 1930[20] and Seckel in 1986[73] reported successful treatment of distal split nails. Seckel's technique, a piece of 0.20-inch silicone sheet between the nail and nail bed, seems to be the most reasonable approach to us.

If the scar involves the sterile matrix, it can be treated by resection of the scar and closure of the adjacent edges of matrix. However, in our experience, if the scar is wide enough to cause a split nail, it is frequently too wide to approximate the defect without significant tension and recurrence of the split. In such cases, we recommend resection of the scar of the nail bed and replacement with a split-thickness nail bed graft from an adjacent portion of the same nail or from a toenail.

If the split is due to scar in the germinal matrix with lack of nail production, the scar must be eliminated and replaced. The eponychium should be elevated with incisions at right angles from the corners (see Fig. 34-11). The nail is removed, and under magnification the scar identified and resected. Johnson[43] has advocated incisions in the lateral paronychial folds with advancement of the germinal matrix toward the center of the nail, but we have had little success with this technique. Our preference is to use a germinal matrix graft from a toe (usually the second) similar in size and shape to the resected scar as a free composite graft (Fig. 34-18). This requires elimination of an entire toenail bed, but this is more acceptable to most individuals, particularly women, than having significant deformity of the large toenail.[5,7,21] Split-thickness grafts of germinal ma-

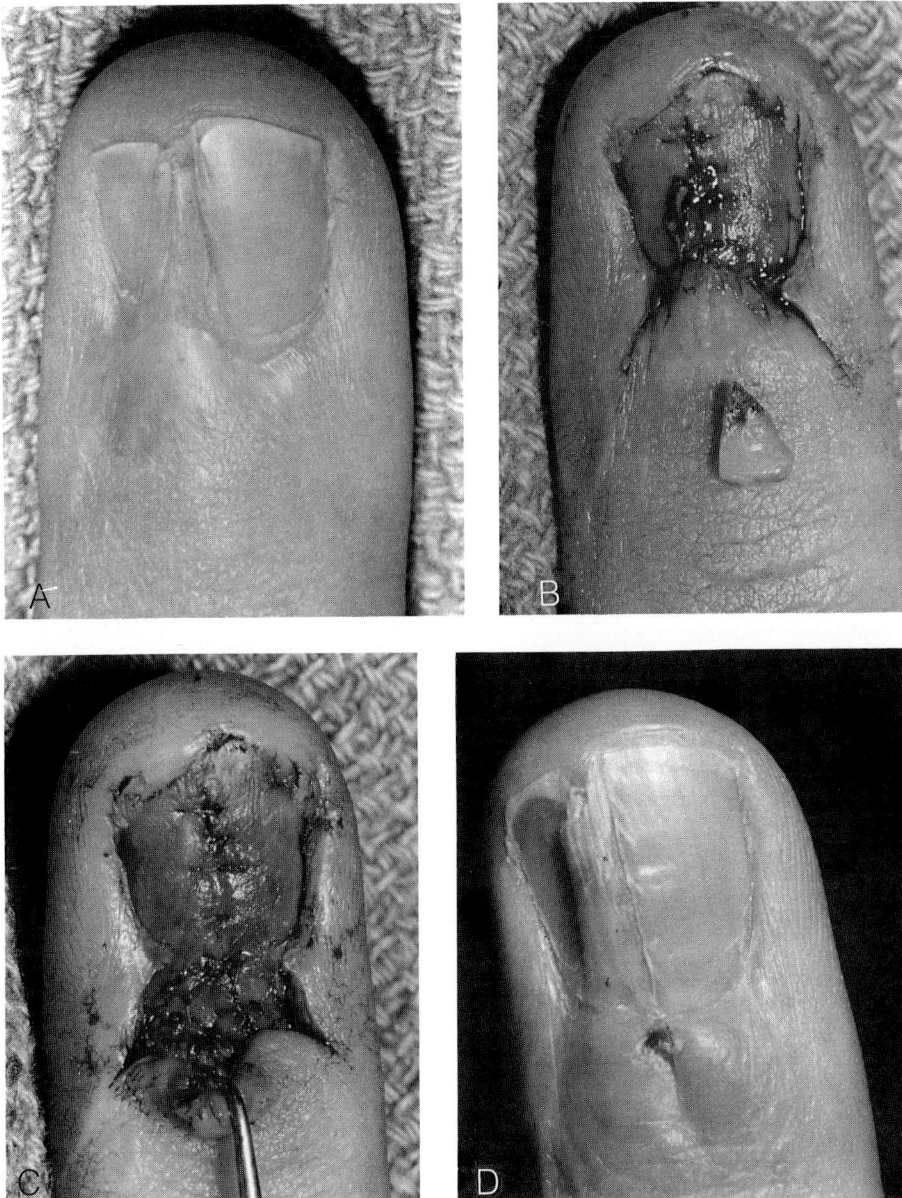

Fig. 34-18. **(A)** A split nail with a pterygium due to scar of the germinal matrix. **(B)** The scar of the germinal matrix has been removed and a fragment of germinal matrix from the second toe cut to shape to fit the defect. **(C)** The germinal matrix graft sutured in place. **(D)** Six months later, nail can be seen growing from the germinal matrix graft.

trix will *not* produce nail. If nail production is necessary, full-thickness germinal matrix grafts are essential.[67,77]

Nonadherence

When the scars of the sterile matrix are transverse or diagonal and wide, the non-nail producing scar may cause the nail to loosen and not re-adhere distal to the scar. Resection of the scar is essential. Our preference for replacement is a split-thickness sterile matrix graft from either an adjacent area of the nail bed or from a toenail bed (Fig. 34-19). If the majority of the sterile matrix is lost, a split- or full-thickness nail bed graft may be applied after the scar is excised.[99] A satisfactory result can be obtained with this technique (Fig. 34-20).

Absence

Absence of a nail may be congenital or may result from avulsion, severe crush, infection, or burn, among other things, and is a disconcerting deformity to the patient and/or the family.

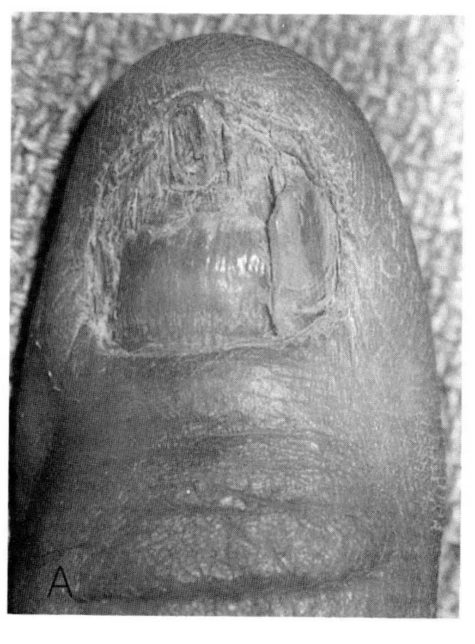

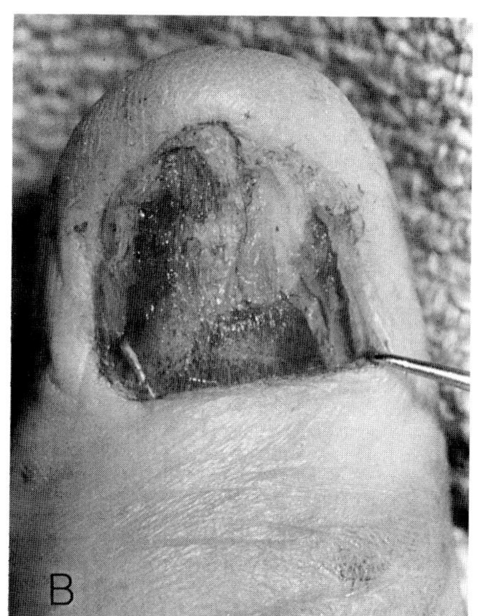

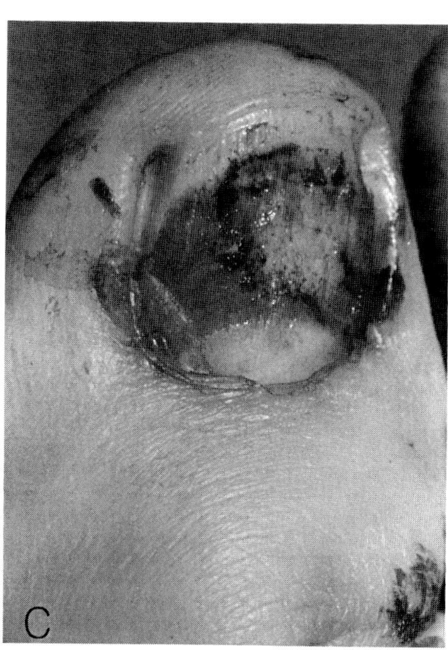

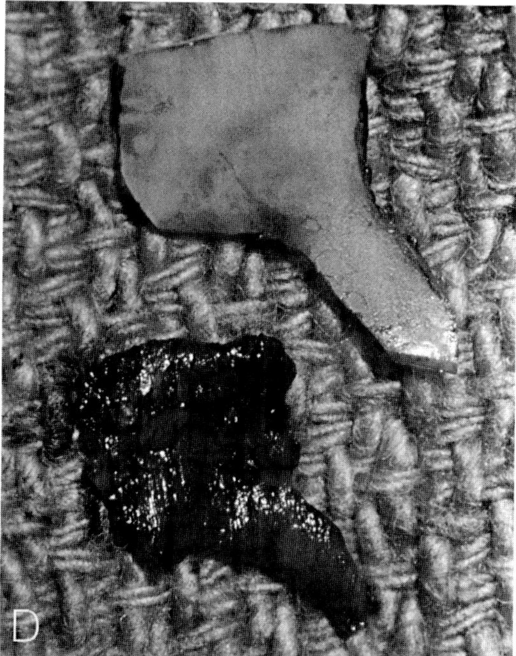

Fig. 34-19. **(A)** Preoperative view of a thumbnail following injury by a car door. The nail grows out and beomes nonadherent every 2 to 3 months. **(B)** The nail remnant has been removed and scar can be seen in the nail bed on the right side. **(C)** The scar of the nail bed is marked for excision. **(D)** An exact template in the configuration of the scar is used to shape a split-thickness nail bed graft from sterile matrix of the toe. *(Figure continues.)*

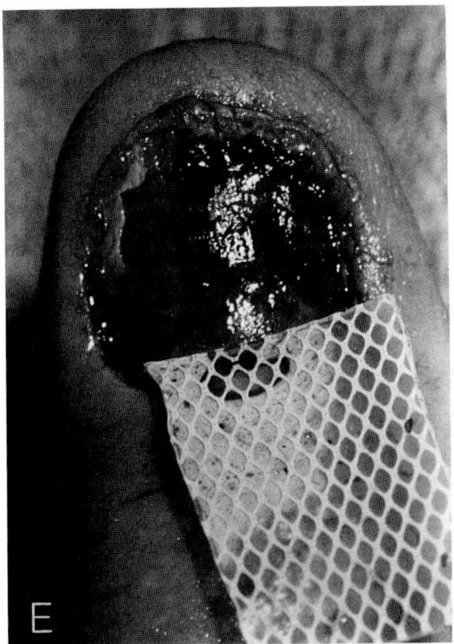

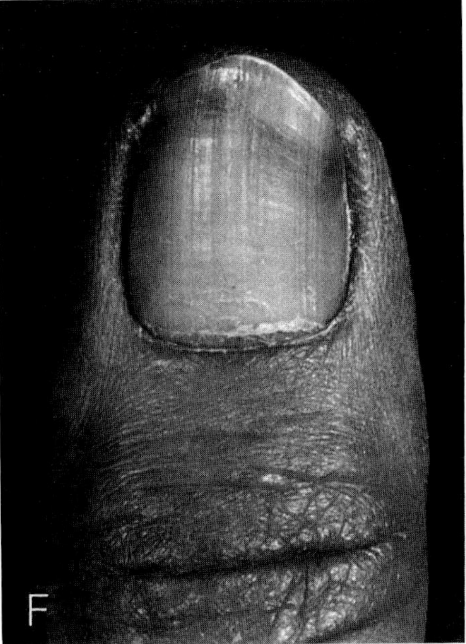

Fig. 34-19 *(Continued).* **(E)** The split-thickness nail bed graft has been sutured in place and a silicone sheet placed over it and into the nail fold. **(F)** The nail 11 months postoperative showing complete adherence of the nail.

We find that the simplest treatment is to resect an area of skin in the shape of a slightly-larger-than-normal nail. A full- or split-thickness skin graft is applied, and after healing, it mimics to some degree the appearance of a nail. The graft may also be done along with reconstruction of a pouch, into which an artificial nail can be placed.[8,17] However, in our experience this type of reconstructed nail fold is only satisfactory initially. As time passes, it becomes obliterated and will not hold the edge of the prosthetic nail. A free vascularized toenail bed graft is another potential alternative.[79]

Composite Nail Bed Grafts

Good results with composite toenail grafts have been reported.[13,65,75] The reported cases are few, and composite nail bed grafts are unpredictable in adults, but in our experience

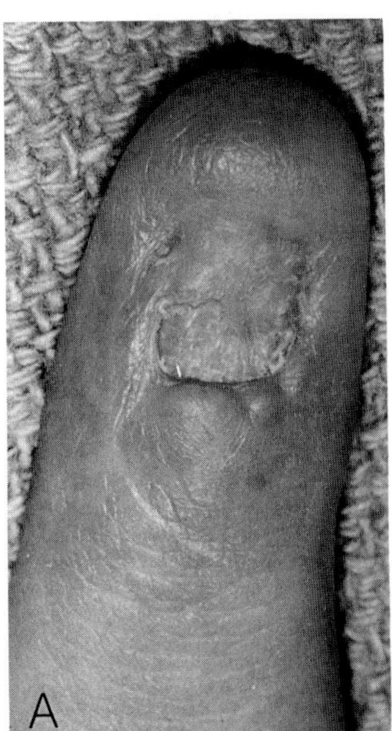

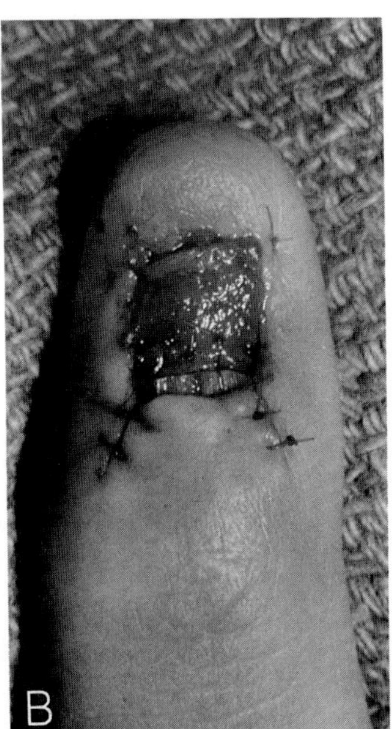

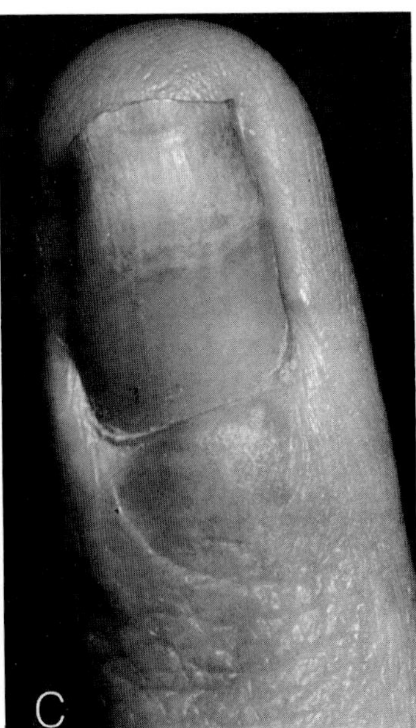

Fig. 34-20. **(A)** A finger with normal germinal matrix but absent sterile matrix for adherence of the nail. The patient had had repeated infections beneath the nail. **(B)** The scarred nail bed has been removed and a full-thickness sterile matrix graft from the second toe used to replace it. **(C)** One year later, the nail adheres to the full-thickness toenail graft but does not adhere to the distal scar. (From Zook,[90] with permission.)

give fairly good results in children. The younger the child, the better the results. We do not know the age at which the success rate falls significantly. However, the chances of free composite toenail grafts in adults having a satisfactory result are less. The patient must therefore be warned and willing to accept a toenail deformity for a potentially suboptimal result. In our earlier experience,[94] the results in adults were not as good. However, more recent results have shown sufficient success to warrant their use in the informed patient.

In selecting a donor site for composite grafts, we prefer to use the second toe, since it is usually approximately the width of the fingernail. A toenail is, however, not as long as the fingernail, and a split-thickness sterile matrix graft from another toe needs to be placed distal to the germinal matrix graft to lengthen the attachment area (Fig. 34-21). The large toenail or a portion of it is necessary for thumbnail reconstruction with composite grafts.

Free Microvascular Grafts

Free microvascular transfer of the dorsal tip of the toe, including the nail bed, is the most reliable treatment to produce a growing nail in adults (Fig. 34-22). However, this requires very skilled microvascular care, has some risk of failure, and leaves significant scars on the foot, toe, and finger.[52,59,79]

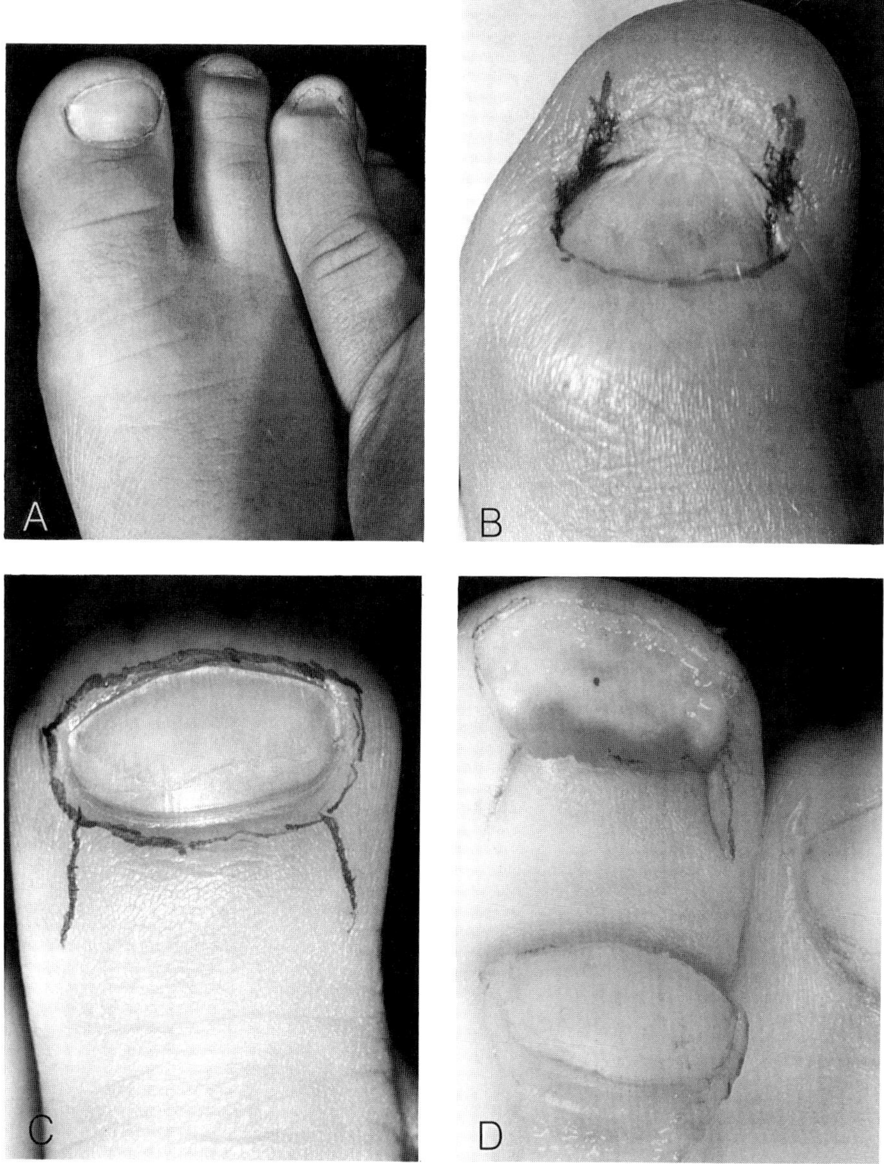

Fig. 34-21. **(A)** A 7-year-old child with post-traumatic absence of the index nail, showing the comparison in width of the fingernail and the second toe nail. **(B)** The nail bed is seen close-up at the time of the surgery. **(C)** The second toe is marked for removal of the composite nail and nail bed graft. **(D)** The composite graft excised. *(Figure continues.)*

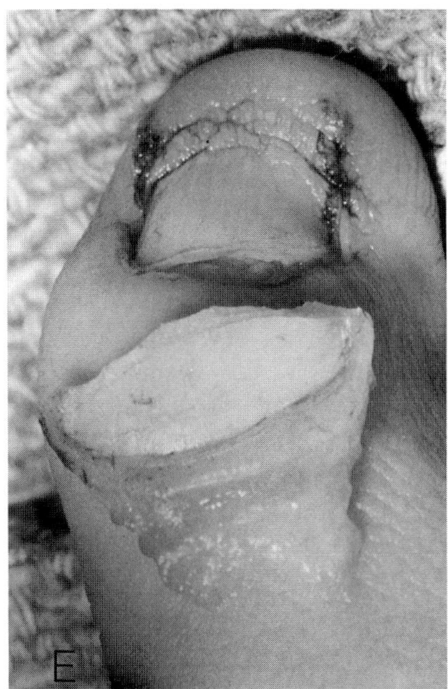

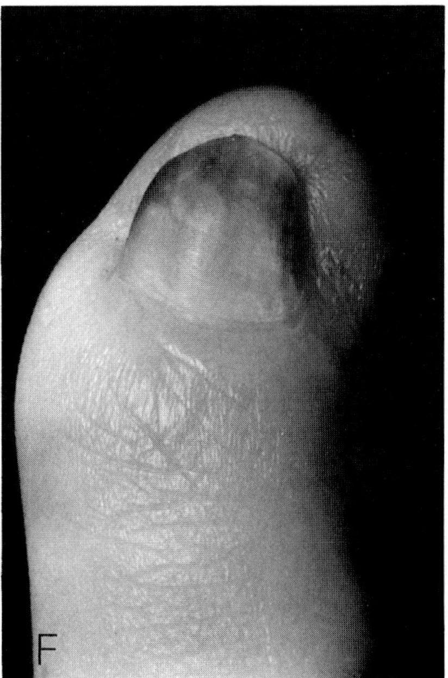

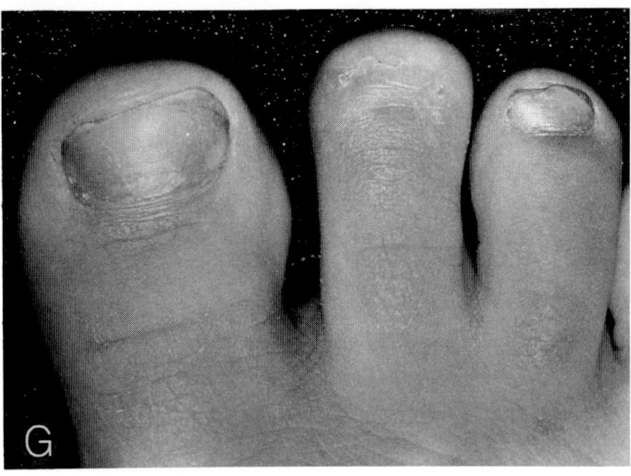

Fig. 34-21 *(Continued).* **(E)** The composite graft placed on the dorsum of the finger after the nail fold has been created. Note that the toenail does not have as much length as the normal fingernail. The sterile matrix was advanced distally to create a recipient site for the graft. **(F)** The nail 1 year postoperative. **(G)** Postoperative view of the second toe. A split-thickness skin graft was applied to the periosteum.

Pterygium and Eponychium Deformities

A pterygium of either the eponychium or hyponychium may occur secondary to trauma or ischemia. Pterygia of the hyponychial area may follow denervation injuries or ischemic injuries of the upper extremity. The pad of the finger becomes atrophic, and the hyponychial attachment to the nail becomes painful and tender. This is treated by removing the distal 5 mm of nail from the nail bed and hyponychial area. A strip of nail bed and hyponychium 3 to 4 mm wide is resected and replaced by a split-thickness skin graft. This causes nonadherence in the hyponychial area and usually provides relief of pain.

A persistent pterygium of the eponychium is treated by freeing the dorsal roof of the nail fold from the nail and inserting a small piece of silicone sheet with a horizontal mattress suture as shown in Figure 34-9. The undersurface of the nail fold epithelializes, releasing the adherence. If this is unsuccessful, a more complex approach is to separate the dorsal roof from the nail and place a thin split-thickness skin graft on the undersurface of the eponychium to prevent the adherence. Shepard[78] showed good results by using split-thickness sterile matrix grafts to cover the raw surface on the dorsal roof of the nail fold after release.

A notched eponychium may be reconstructed by a composite toe eponychial graft, the helical rim of the ear,[68] or rotation flaps. Eponychial deformities following burns of the finger are difficult to correct. The deformity varies from pulling on the eponychium to total destruction of the nail bed.[82] Reconstruction of the eponychium is still not good as desired, but newer techniques are progressively improving the results.[1,3,8,37,46,62,82]

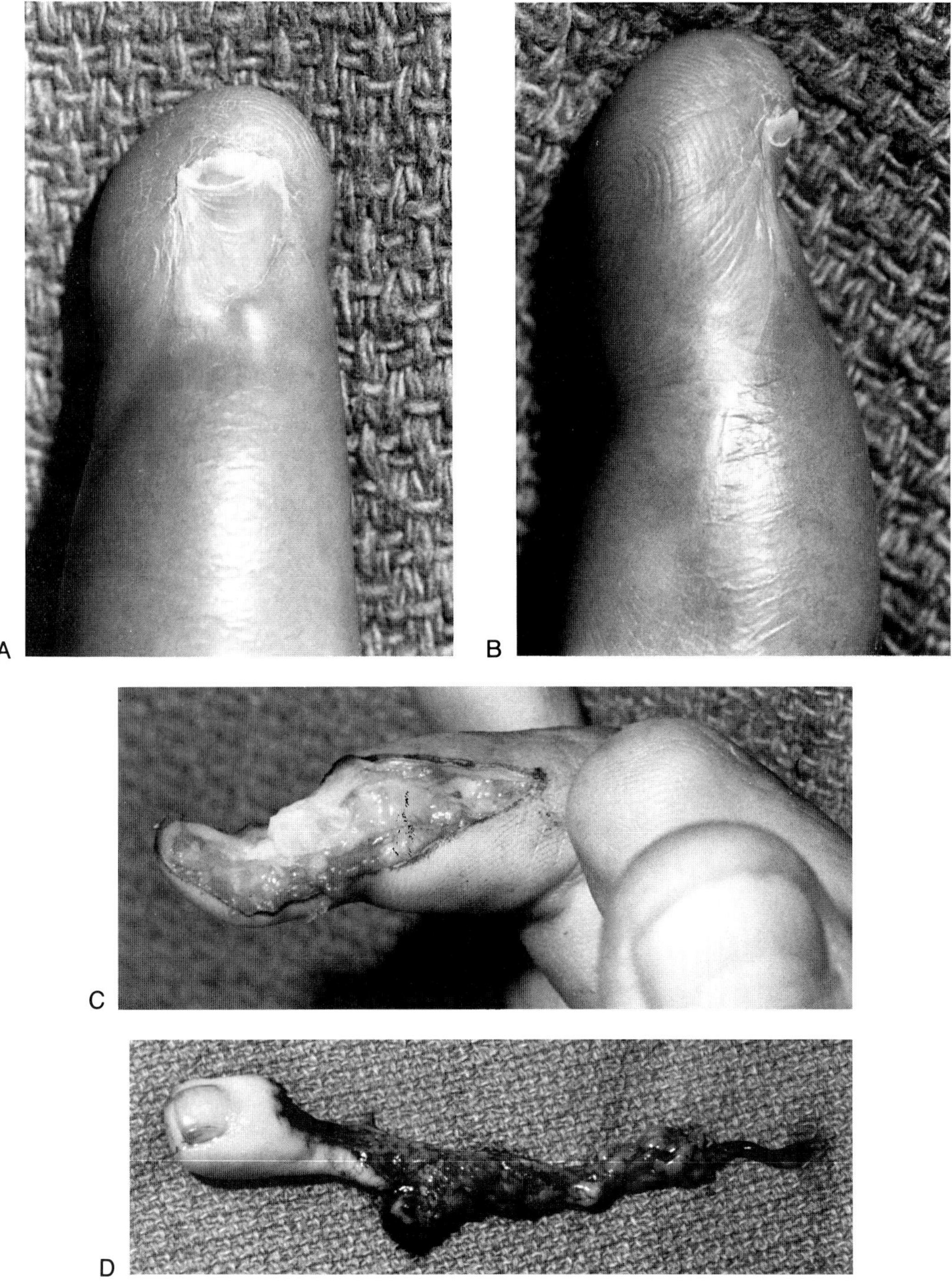

Fig. 34-22. **(A&B)** Minimal nail growth and soft tissue loss following an oblique amputation of the ring finger tip. **(C)** The defect following excision of the scarred nail bed and tip. **(D)** Partial second toe free flap. *(Figure continues.)*

Cornified Nail Bed

When the germinal matrix is removed to eliminate growth, the patient frequently has continued problems with keratinized material growing from the sterile matrix. To relieve this, the sterile matrix is excised and a split-thickness skin graft applied.

Nail Spikes and Cysts

Nail cysts most commonly occur following amputation of a fingertip and failure to remove all of the germinal matrix from the nail fold (Fig. 34-23A). Complete resection of the nail cyst and its wall is curative.

Nail spikes are also the result of incomplete removal of ger-

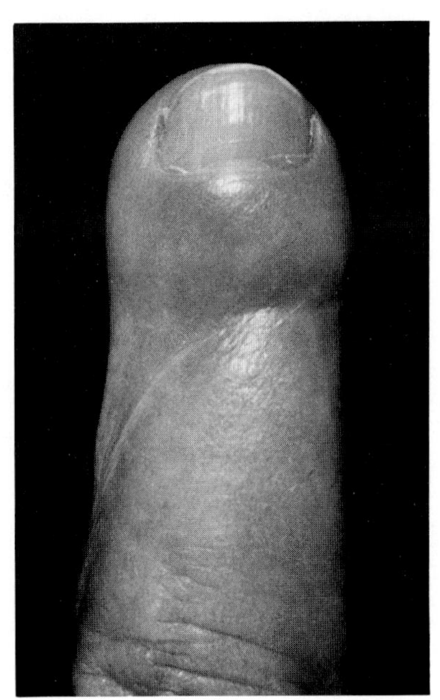

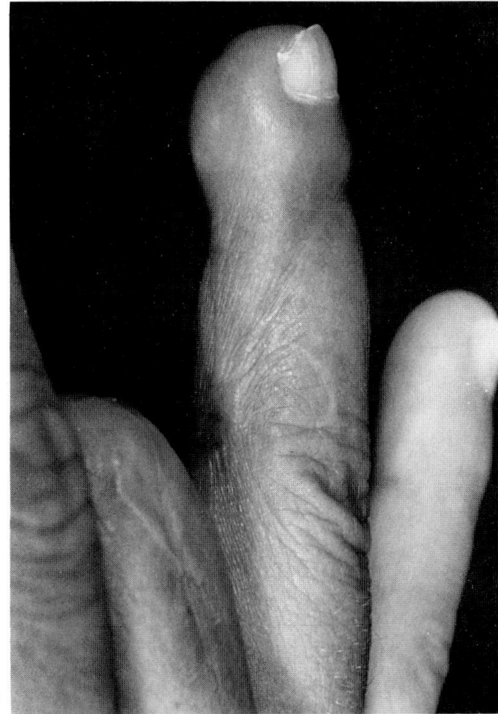

Fig. 34-22 *(Continued).* **(E&F)** Postoperative appearance of the ring finger.

minal matrix and are similar to nail cysts, except that they grow distally (Fig. 34-23B). They are a frequent occurrence following removal of the side of a nail and nail bed for ingrown toenail. The treatment is complete removal of the spike and the germinal matrix creating it.

Hooked Nail

The growing nail follows the nail matrix. The hooked nail is most commonly caused by either tight closure of a fingertip amputation (Fig. 34-24A) and/or loss of bony support for the nail bed (Fig. 34-24B). The nail bed should not be pulled over the distal phalanx to close a fingertip amputation, as this will almost surely cause a hooked nail. When the bone is absent, it must either be replaced or the nail bed trimmed back to the end of the bone so that the nail bed does not curve over the end and cause hooking.

When a hooked nail is present, a decision must be made whether to shorten the bone or attempt to add support to the nail bed. If the distal nail bed has been pulled over the end of the finger, a V-Y advancement flap, cross-finger flap, or full-thickness skin graft can be used to replace the soft tissue of the tip, allowing replacement of the nail bed onto the dorsum of the bone. This usually improves the hook, although complete correction is uncommon.

Correction of the hooked nail with maintenance of nail length requires replacement of the distal phalanx or tuft with a bone graft. This may require additional tip soft tissue prior to or at the time of the bone graft. Initially, bone grafts support the nail bed satisfactorily, but as with most bone grafts that do not have bone apposition on both ends, in time they tend to resorb and lose the correction. A free vascularized transfer of second toe tip, distal phalanx and nail may be the best although complex solution.

When the nail and/or tip are deformed the patient may choose a prosthesis rather than a reconstruction which in many instances may give a very satisfactory solution to the problem.[11]

INFECTION

Fungal Infections

Perionychial infections of the subungual area are the most common infections in the hand. These are most frequently chronic fungal infections, although superimposed bacterial infections may occur[88] and are usually treated medically by dermatologists.[6,7,88] The medical treatment may require surgical removal of the nail to reach the subungual infection. After removal of an isolated nail, we have the patient apply 4 percent Mycolog with Vioform ointment twice a day to the nail bed until the nail has completely regrown. Griseofulvin or other systemic antifungal agents may also be used, if indicated.

Bacterial Infections

Bacterial infections of the nail most commonly involve the paronychium. The dermal and epidermal layers of the paronychium are arranged in an overlapping fashion, much like the

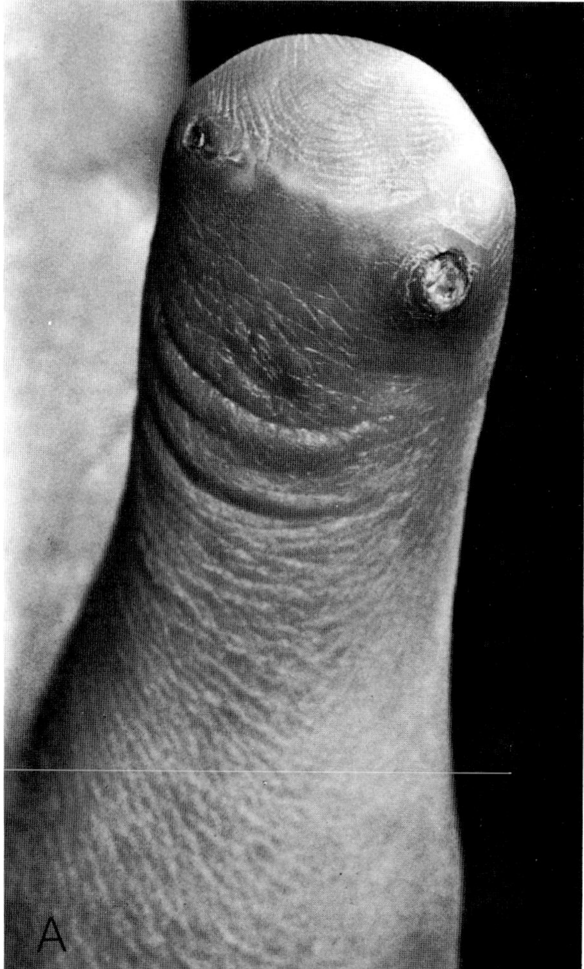

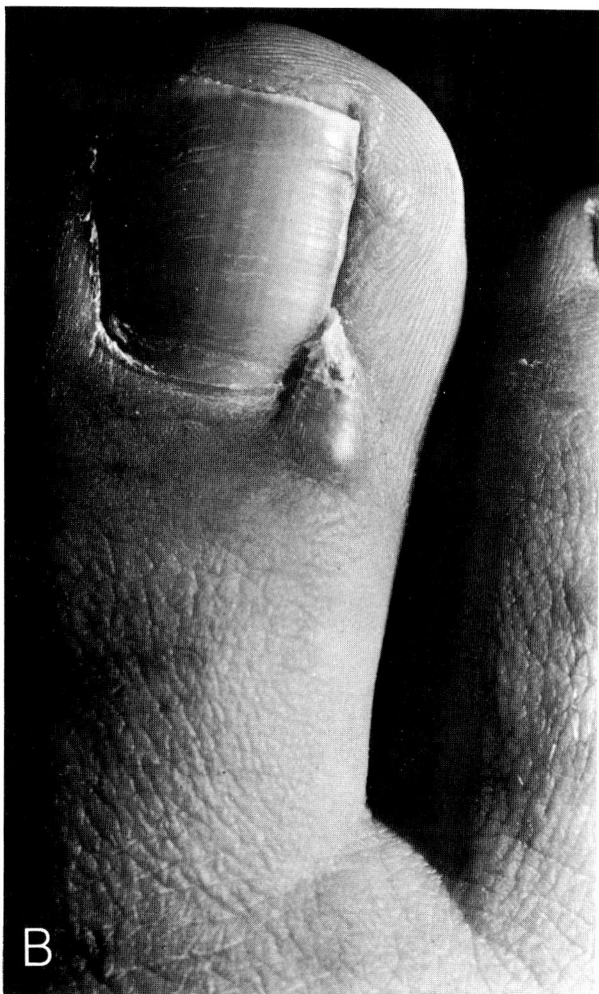

Fig. 34-23. **(A)** Nail cysts following amputation of the fingertip without complete removal of the nail bed. **(B)** A nail spike resulting from incomplete removal of nail bed after resection of an ingrown toenail.

shingles of a house. When one of these layers is pulled up, an open wound (hangnail) is created. *Staphylococcus aureus* most frequently cause the infection.[56] If the infection involves the paronychium but is above the nail, it can be drained by lifting the paronychium away from the nail, followed by soaks to encourage adequate drainage.

If the infection and purulence have progressed beneath the edge of the nail (Fig. 34-25A), a portion of the nail must be removed to permit adequate drainage. The nail is dissected from the underlying nail bed and the overlying proximal eponychium with fine scissors or a periosteal elevator (Fig. 34-25B). The nail is then split longitudinally and the undermined portion removed to allow drainage. (Fig. 34-25C–E). Adequate open drainage is maintained with soapy water soaks three to four times a day. Antibiotics are indicated if there is tissue cellulitis.

If the abscess dissects beneath the dorsal roof of the nail fold or beneath the nail in the nail fold, the proximal portion of the nail must be removed. The distal portion of the nail may be left in place to decrease discomfort.

In our opinion, in neither of these instances should incisions be made in the eponychium to drain the infection. The incision will frequently not heal primarily in the face of infection, and a notch or square corner in the eponychium may result. We have never seen a paronychia or a runaround that could not be adequately drained without incision in the eponychium.

Chronic Paronychia

Chronic paronychia usually occur between the nail and the dorsal roof of the nail fold. They are chronic in nature and are tender, erythematous, and swollen (Fig. 34-26A). The infection is most commonly caused by mixed gram negative organisms with an occasional fungus. The treatment is an arc-sharped excision of the nail wall that is allowed to heal secondarily[12,48,49] (Fig. 34-26B and C). We have found this treatment to be generally successful (Fig. 34-26D).

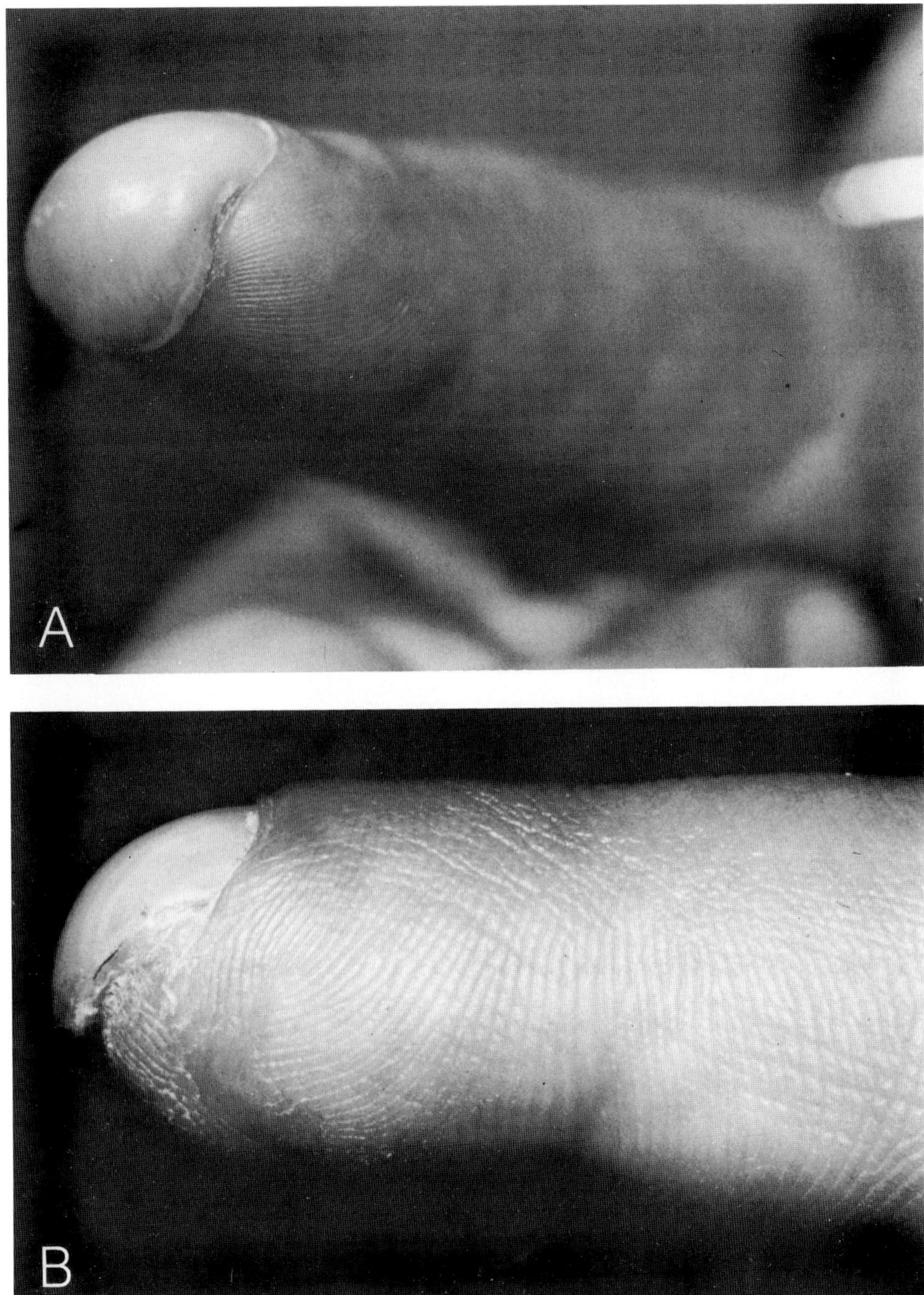

Fig. 34-24. **(A)** A hooked nail deformity due partially to some loss of bony support, but primarily to the nail bed being pulled over the tip to close the amputation. **(B)** Loss of bony support to hold the nail bed flat.

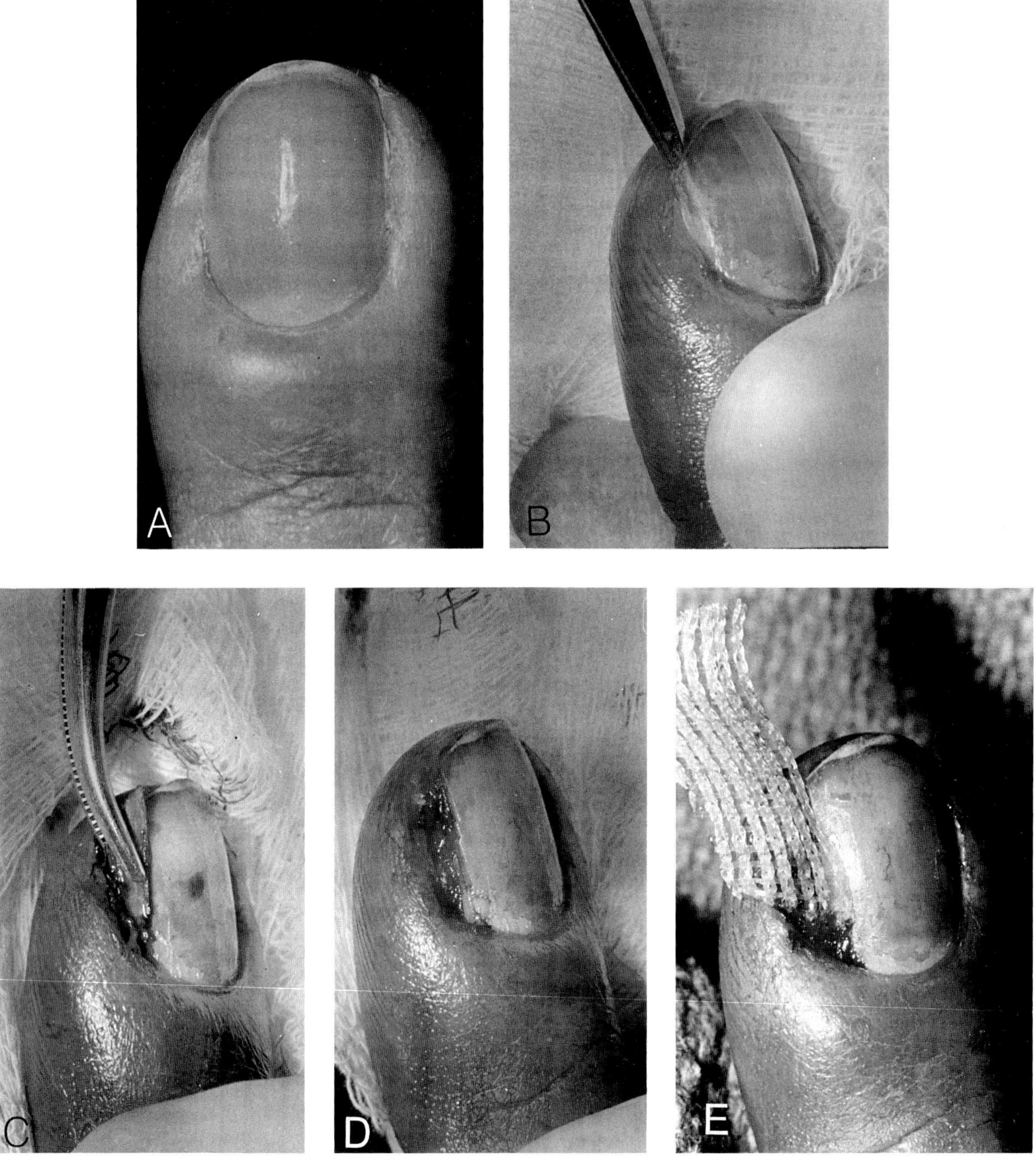

Fig. 34-25. **(A)** A paronychia is seen on the left side of this nail, with pus extending beneath the nail. **(B)** A fine pair of iris scissors is used to elevate the side of the nail from the nail bed and the eponychium from the dorsum of the nail. **(C)** The loosened fragment of nail is then split longitudinally and removed from the nail fold. **(D)** Adequate drainage of the paronychia after partial removal of the nail. **(E)** A small wick of gauze is used to promote drainage.

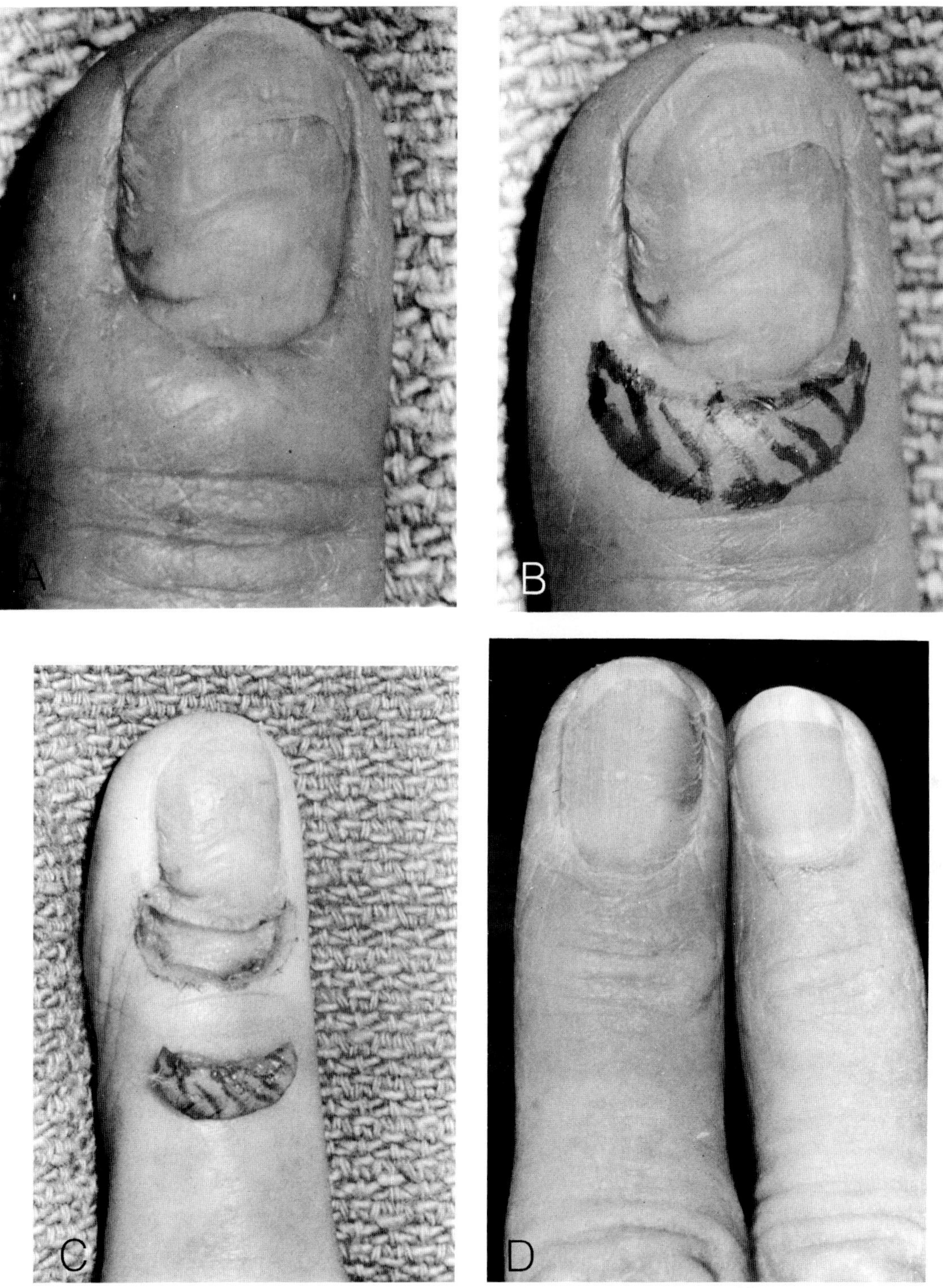

Fig. 34-26. **(A)** A chronic paronychia that has been present for 2 years. **(B)** The area on the dorsal roof is marked for excision. **(C)** The dorsal roof of the nail fold has been removed down to the nail. **(D)** The appearance 1 year postinjury with no further infection.

Pyogenic Granuloma

Pyogenic granulomas manifest themselves as a rapidly growing lesion with a round red elevated area similar to granulation tissue growing through the nail (Fig. 34-27). They are usually the result of perforations of the nail by trauma or iatrogenic causes. The treatment is repeated silver nitrate cauterization or hyfurcation, but some nail deformity usually results. The differential diagnosis is squamous cell carcinoma or amelanotic melanoma.

BENIGN TUMORS

Subungual Nevi

Nevi of the nail bed are not uncommon. The nail produced by the nail bed involved by a pigmented nevus will be pigmented. Roughening of the nail surface usually does not occur, but elevation and ridging of the nail may (Fig. 34-28). A nevus is frequently present at birth or is noticed shortly thereafter and as years pass they may become lighter or darker in color. Samman[70] in 1938 remarked that if a dark streak was present at birth or shortly thereafter, removal of the nail and biopsy of the nail bed might leave a nail deformity. He therefore recommended a watch and wait policy for at least the thumb and index finger. Fleegler and Zeinowicz[29] now believe that the danger of malignant degeneration at puberty is significant, and recommend nail bed biopsy prior to that time. If atypical cells are present, they recommend removal of the involved portion of the nail bed.

Bands of pigmentation may develop after trauma, particularly in black people with darkly pigmented skin. Areas of adult onset subungual pigment formation must be followed closely. If there is any question, a biopsy should be carried out. The most common differential diagnosis is subungual hematoma, even if no injury is known. In this case, we make a cut into the surface of the nail at the proximal and distal borders of the pigmented area (Fig. 34-29). If the pigmentation is a hematoma, it will progress toward the free edge of the nail with the scratches. If the pigment is a foreign body, nevus, or melanoma in the nail bed, the scratches will progress distally away from the area of pigmentation enough in 3 weeks to make a determination.

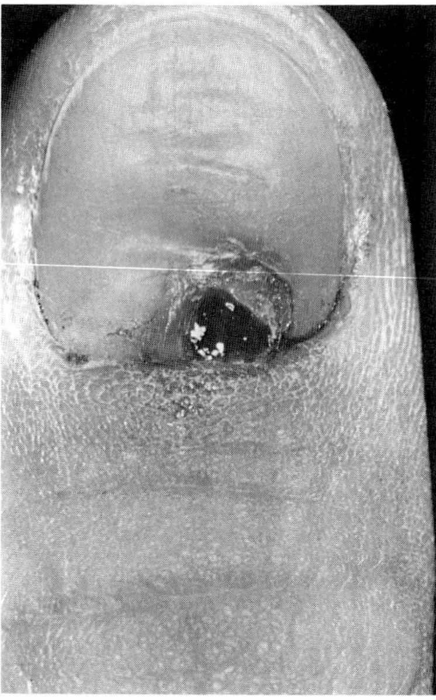

Fig. 34-27. A pyogenic granuloma growing through the nail following perforation of the nail with cuticle sissors.

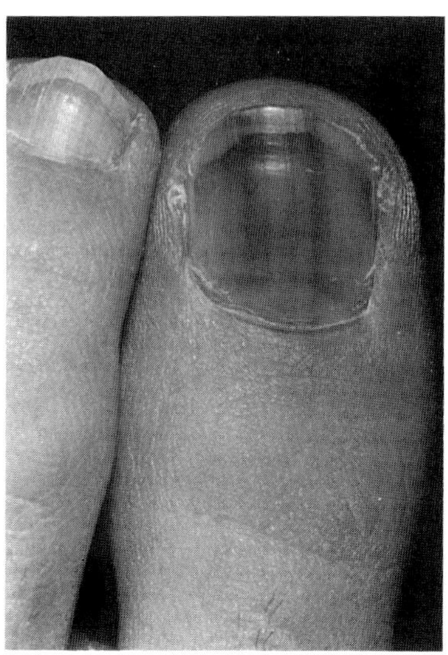

Fig. 34-28. A pigmented nevus of the large toenail present since birth that was biopsied at puberty and showed atypical melanocytes. The entire nail bed was excised.

Viral Warts (Verruca Vulgaris)

Viral warts, although not a common occurrence in the perionychium, are a significant cosmetic problem. Treatment with subsequent nail deformity and disfigurement is frequent. Halpern and Lane[34] recommended treatment with monochloroacetic acid and 40 percent salicylic acid plaster as well as the use of 3 percent formalin. Removal of the nail may be necessary to allow treatment of the underlying warts. We have had some success with cauterizing perionychial warts with the CO_2 laser. One should err on the side of treating too superficially rather than too deeply, and therefore multiple applications of the laser may be necessary. For some unexplained reason, spontaneous remission of warts after application of the CO_2 laser to other warts may occur. Unfortunately, many patients seen by the hand surgeon have been treated unsuccessfully by other methods, creating sufficient scar tissue to prevent return of normal nail growth after eradication of the wart.

Ganglions (Mucous Cysts)

Ganglions are the most common tumors that deform the nail bed. They have been called clear cysts, mucous cysts, and other names.[60,89]

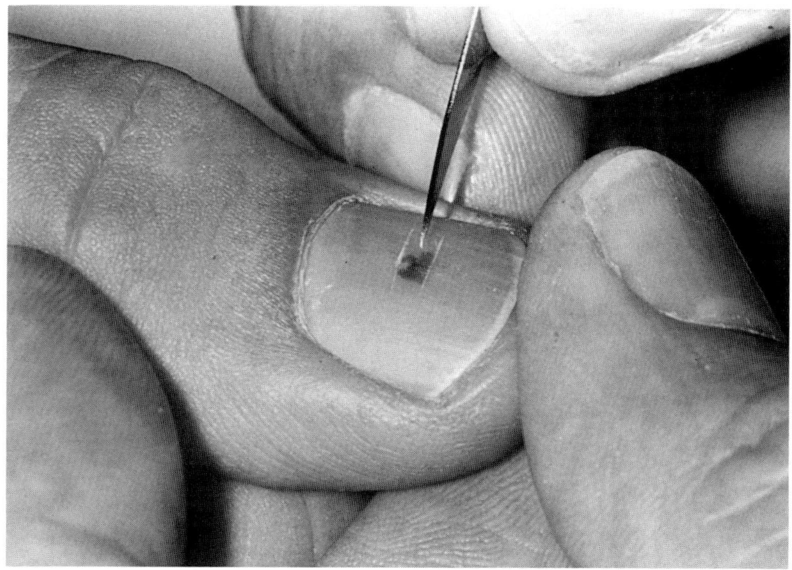

Fig. 34-29. Marking the nail over a pigmented area to measure changes in relation with growth (see text).

Kleinert[50] reported a communication between these cysts and the DIP joint in the area of an arthritic spur.

When the cystic expansion of the ganglion is between the floor of the nail fold and the periosteum, the upward pressure on the nail bed causes a ridge in the nail, a curve of the entire nail, or a ragged nail (Fig. 34-30). If the cyst is in the dorsal roof of the nail fold the pressure is downward on the nail, and a groove, thinning, or roughening may occur (Fig. 34-31).

If there is a severe nail deformity, we believe that the best treatment is removal of the nail followed by resection of the ganglion through an incision over the DIP joint. Even if the skin over the ganglion is very thin, the ganglion can usually be resected without perforation of the skin. If the skin is perforated, it is draped over the defect and will rapidly heal. After the cyst is removed, we place a piece of 0.020-inch silicone sheet into the nail fold to flatten the nail bed back into its normal position if the nail was removed. The joint osteophytes should be removed to prevent recurrence.[16] At the present time, we are debriding the osteophytes and evacuating the cyst without attempting to remove the cyst wall. Early results indicate less residual nail deformity.

Ganglions occasionally rupture and drain through the nail fold or the overlying skin. If infection occurs, permanent nail deformity and limitation of joint motion may result. If the

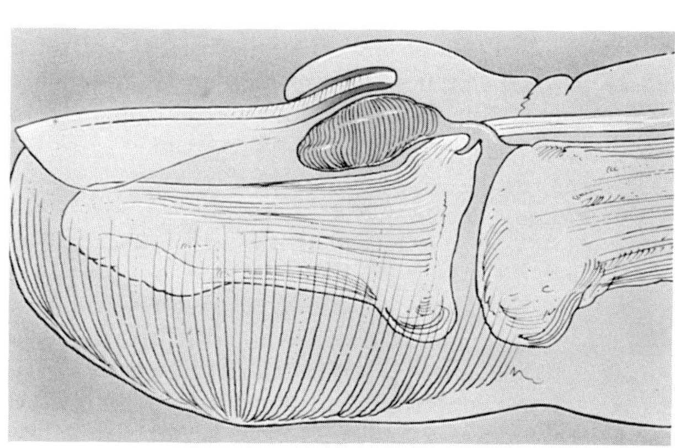

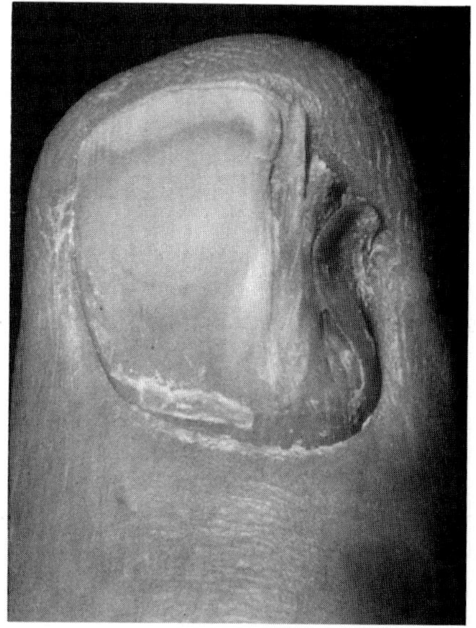

Fig. 34-30. **(A)** Dissection of a ganglion between the periosteum of the distal phalanx and the nail bed. **(B)** The typical (but somewhat extreme) longitudinal groove deformity that results when the ganglion is located as shown in A.

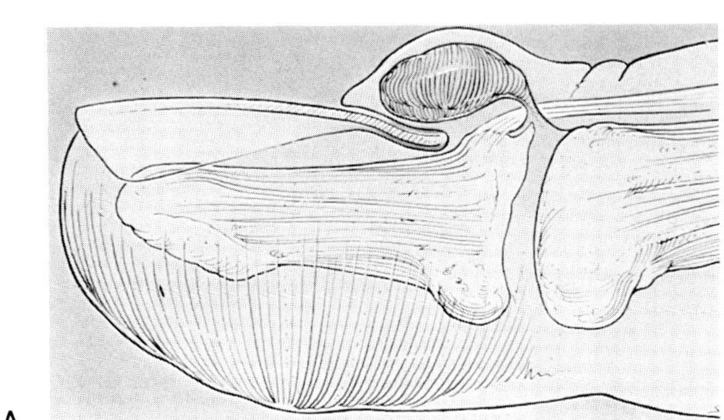

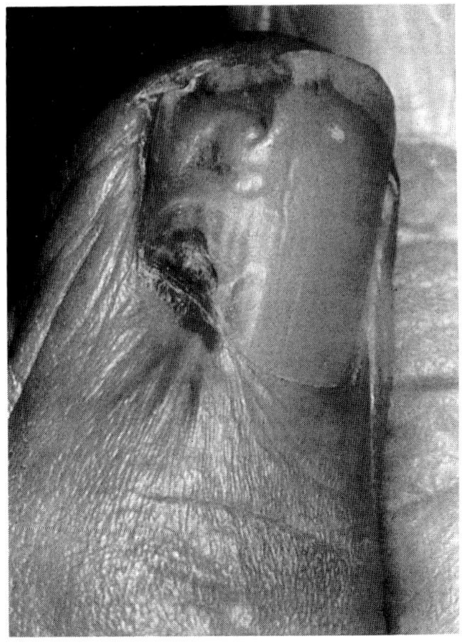

A B

Fig. 34-31. **(A)** Dissection of a ganglion into the dorsal roof of the nail fold compresses the nail bed volarly. **(B)** An irregular breakup of the nail (or a longitudinal groove) is the deformity frequently caused by the ganglion (shown in A).

ganglion ruptures, the appropriate treatment is antibiotics until the skin is closed, followed by surgical removal before the ganglion reruptures. A ganglion should not be surgically resected while it is actively draining, since this may lead to subsequent joint infection and greater deformity.

Subungual Glomus Tumor

The glomus tumor first described in 1924 by Barre and Masson,[9] while greatly publicized, is rare. It is formed from the vasculo-musculo-neuro "glomus" elements of the nail bed that affect regulation of the blood flow.[21] Proliferation of this angiomatous tissue may cause pressure on the nerve plexuses and exquisite pain. The nail may be tender to pressure, and temperature changes (particularly cold) may cause pain. There may be a bluish discoloration beneath the nail in the area of the glomus. The entire nail bed should be carefully examined for multiple tumors after the nail is removed.

Treatment consists of removal of the nail, identification of the glomus tumor or tumors, and surgical excision. If the glomus is small in the sterile matrix, the defect can be closed primarily (Fig. 34-32). A split-thickness nail bed graft from another portion of the same nail or a toenail will be required for larger defects. A full-thickness sterile matrix graft from a toe can be used, but causes significant toenail deformity.

Resection will usually cause deformity if the glomus is in the germinal matrix. The defect may be closed primarily by using relaxing incisions in the lateral paronychial fold or by a free germinal matrix graft from a toe. In the nonscarred nail bed, relaxing incisions are much more successful than in post-traumatic deformities, such as the split nail discussed on page 1294.

Giant Cell Tumors (Nodular Synovitis)

Enlargement of this benign synovial tumor that arises distal to the DIP joint may cause pressure on the nail-forming elements, with resultant nail plate deformities. The treatment is complete resection of the tumor and removal of the nail plate if necessary for complete resection of the tumor.

MALIGNANT TUMORS

Basal Cell Carcinoma

Basal cell carcinoma is rare in the hand and even more so in the finger.[2,38] Complete resection of the tumor with frozen section examination of the margins to ensure complete removal is necessary, even if a nail deformity is the result. Split-thickness skin graft coverage is usually necessary. Basal cell carcinomas most frequently occur after radiation exposure or other chronic problems of the nail bed, and some deformity of the nail is frequently present prior to resection. If the bone of the distal phalanx is involved, amputation at the DIP joint level is necessary.

Squamous Cell Carcinoma

Squamous cell carcinomas, although infrequent, are the most common malignant tumor of the perionychium[44] and are common secondary to radiation exposure[2,18,74] (Fig. 34-33).

Squamous cell carcinomas are frequently misdiagnosed as paronychia, and the average length of time between appearance and treatment was 4 years in Carroll's series.[18] Squamous cell carcinomas are more common in males, and the thumb is

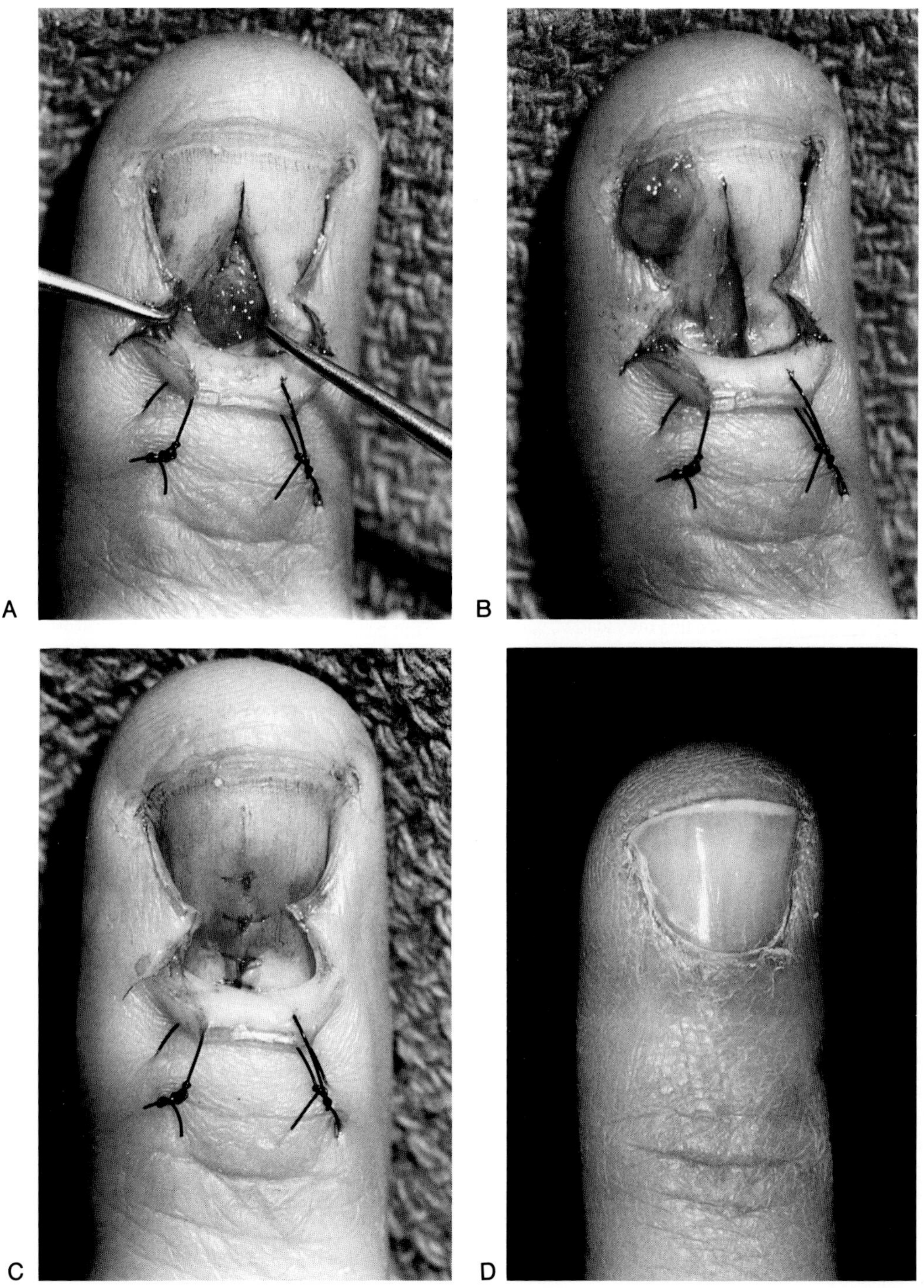

Fig. 34-32. **(A)** A glomus tumor exposed at the junction of the germinal and sterile matrices. The approach is through a longitudinal incision in the nailbed after removal of the nail. **(B)** Following excision of the tumor. **(C)** The nail bed is meticulously repaired. **(D)** Normal nail growth 6 months later.

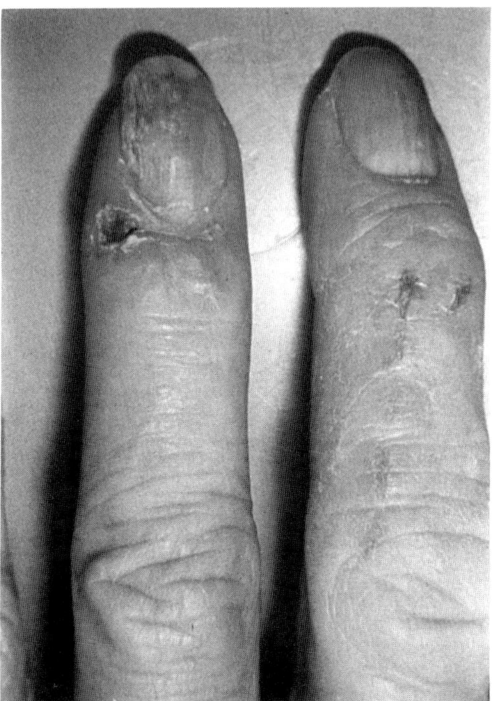

Fig. 34-33. A veterinarian with many years of radiation exposure to his fingers presented with a squamous cell carcinoma of the perionychium.

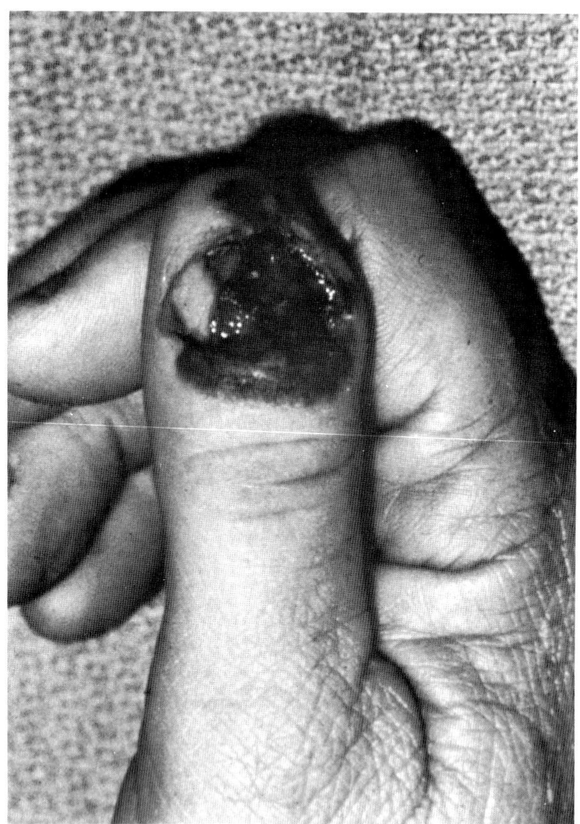

Fig. 34-34. A malignant melanoma of the nail bed.

the most frequently involved digit.[18] Dentists' hands are commonly involved due to repeated radiation exposure.[74]

A perionychial squamous cell carcinoma with no bone involvement necessitates resection of the entire lesion with adequate margins, frequently requiring a skin graft. If the carcinoma has a long existence, is large, or bony changes are present, amputation of the distal phalanx or even more proximally if necessary is indicated. Node dissection is indicated only if nodes do not disappear after amputation, since most nodal enlargements appear to be inflammatory.[25,74]

Subungual Melanoma

Melanomas of the hands and feet have a poorer prognosis than those elsewhere on the body.[24] They are almost always pigmented with or without nail deformity (Fig. 34-34). Melanoma of the nail bed is frequently mimicked by other paronychial conditions, and the diagnosis may be delayed.[32] Pack and Oropeza[64] reported on subungual melanoma in 72 patients. Forty of these were of the fingernail and 32 were of the toenails. Almost two-thirds occurred in the thumb or large toe. Almost all of the patients had fair complexions, red or sandy hair, and blue or hazel eyes. Of the cases involving subungual melanomas, 18.5 percent occurred in blacks. Pigmented areas had been present beneath the nail for many years in 29 percent of their patients. Nodal involvement was found in 36 percent of the patients.

The recommended treatment for stage I (local disease only) subungual melanoma is metacarpal or metatarsal ray amputation after the diagnosis is made.[32,64] Opinions vary on the advisability of node dissection and timing of regional node dissection.[14,31] Pack and Oropeza[64] reported that patients with nonpalpable nodes but with microscopic evidence of tumor in resected nodes were found to have a cure rate twice that of individuals in whom node dissection was not done. They recommended amputation of the digit and node dissection when nodes are palpable. (See Chapter 59 for further discussion of melanomas.)

REFERENCES

1. Achauer BM, Welk RA: One-stage reconstruction of the postburn nailfold contracture. Plast Reconstr Surg 85:937–940, 1990
2. Alport LI, Zak FG, Werthamer S: Subungual basal cell epithelioma. Arch Dermatol 106:595, 1972
3. Alsbjörn BF, Metz P, Ebbehøj J: Nailfold retraction due to burn wound contracture. A surgical procedure. Burns 11:166–167, 1985
4. Ashbell TS, Kleinert HK, Putcha S, Kutz JE: The deformed fingernail, a frequent result of failure to repair nail bed injuries. J Trauma 7:177–190, 1967
5. Baden HP: Regeneration of the nail. Arch Dermatol 91:619–620, 1965
6. Baran R: Onychia and paronychia of mycotic, microbial and parasite origin. Chapter 6. In Pierre M (ed): The Nail. Churchill Livingstone, New York, 1981

7. Baran R, Zais N: The Nail In Health and Disease. SP Medical and Scientific Book, New York, 1980
8. Barford B: Reconstruction of the nail fold. Hand 4:85-87, 1972
9. Barre JA, Masson PV: Anatomy-clinical study of certain painful subungual tumors (Tumors of the neuromyo-arterial glomus of the extremities). Bull Soc Frac de Dermat et Symph 31:148, 1924
10. Barron JN: The structure and function of the skin of the hand. Hand 2:93-96, 1970
11. Beasley RW, deBeze GM: Prosthetic substitution for fingernails. Hand Clin 6:105-111, 1990
12. Bednar MS, Lane LB: Eponychial marsupialization and nail removal for surgical treatment of chronic paronychia. J Hand Surg 16A:314-317, 1991
13. Berson MI: Reconstruction of index finger with nail transplantation. Surg 27:594-599, 1950
14. Booher RJ, Pack GT: Malignant melanoma of the feet and hands. Surg 42:1084-1121, 1957
15. Boyes JH: Bunnell's Surgery of the Hand. 5th Ed. JB Lippincott, Philadelphia, 1970
16. Brown RE, Zook EG, Russell RC, Kucan JO, Smoot EC: Fingernail deformities secondary to ganglions of the distal interphalangeal joint (mucous cysts). Plast Reconstr Surg 87:718-725, 1991
17. Buncke HJ, Gonzalez RI: Fingernail reconstruction. Plast Reconstr Surg 30:452-461, 1962
18. Carroll RE: Squamous cell carcinoma of the nail bed. J Hand Surg 1:92-97, 1976
19. Carter WW: Treatment for split fingernails. JAMA 90:1619-1620, 1928
20. Carter WW: Treatment of split fingernails. Med J Rec 131:599-600, 1930
21. Clark WE, Buxton LHD: Studies in nail growth. Br J Dermatol 52:21, 1938
22. Clark WE, LeGros-Buston LHD: Studies in nail growth. Br J Dermatol 50:221-235, 1938
23. Clayburgh RH, Wood MB, Cooney WP: Nail bed repair and reconstruction by reverse dermal grafts. J Hand Surg 8:594-599, 1983
24. Day CL, Lew RA, Mihn MC et al: A multi-variate analysis of prognotic factors for melanoma patients with lesions more than 3.65 millimeters in thickness. Ann Surg 195:44, 1982
25. Ellis VH: Squamous cell carcinoma of the nail bed. J Bone Joint Surg 30B:656-658, 1948
26. Ersek RA, Gadaria U, Denton DR: Nail bed avulsions treated with porcine xenografts. J Hand Surg 10A:152-153, 1985
27. Flatt AE: Minor hand injuries. J Bone Joint Surg 37B:117-125, 1955
28. Flatt AE: Nail-bed injuries. Br J Plast Surg 8:34-37, 1956
29. Fleegler EJ, Zeinowicz RJ: Tumors of the perionychium. Hand Clin 6:113-136, 1990
30. Flynn IE: Hand Surgery. Williams & Wilkins, Baltimore, 1966
31. Fortner JG, Booher RJ, Pack GT: Results of groin dissection for malignant melanoma in 220 patients. Surg 55:485-494, 1964
32. Goldsmith HS: Melanoma: An overview. CA Cancer J for Clinicians 29:194-215, 1979
33. Guy RJ: The etiologies and mechanisms of nail bed injuries. Hand Clin 6:9-21, 1990
34. Halpern LK, Lane CW: Treatment of periungual warts. Mo Med 50:765, 1953
35. Hanrahan EM: The split-thickness skin graft as a covering following removal of a fingernail. Surg 20:398-400, 1946
36. Hashimoto H: Experimental study of histogenesis of the nail and its surrounding tissue. Niigate Med J 82:254, 1971
37. Hayes CW: One-stage nail fold reconstruction. Hand 6:74-75, 1974
38. Hoffman S: Basal cell carcinoma of the nail bed. Arch Dermatol 108:828, 1973
39. Horner RL, Cohen BI: Injuries to the fingernail. Rocky Mt Med J 63:60-62, 1966
40. Iselin M: Avulsion injuries of the nail. Chapter 15. In Pierre M (ed): The Nail. Churchill Livingstone, Edinburgh, 1981
41. Iselin M, Iselin F: Treatise on Surgery of the Hand. Medicales Flammarion, Paris, 1967
42. Jarrett A, Spearman RIC: The histochemistry of the human nail. Arch Derm 94:652-657, 1966
43. Johnson RK: Nailplasty. Plast Reconstr Surg 47:275-276, 1971
44. John HG: Primary skin cancer of the fingers stimulating chronic infection. Lancet 1:662, 1956
45. Jones FW: The Principles of Anatomy as Seen in the Hand. 2nd Ed. Bailliere, Tindall, and Cox, London, 1941
46. Kasai K, Ogawa Y: Nailplasty using a distally based ulnar finger dorsum flap. Aesthetic Plast Surg 13:125-128, 1989
47. Kelsey JL, Pastides H, Kreiger N, Harris C, Chernow RA: Upper Extremity Disorders: A Survey of Their Frequency and Cost in the United States. CV Mosby, St. Louis, 1980
48. Keyser JJ, Eaton RG: Surgical care of chronic paronychia by eponychial marsupialization. Plast Reconstr Surg 58:66-70, 1976
49. Keyser JJ, Littler JW, Eaton RG: Surgical treatment of infections and lesions of the perionychium. Hand Clin 6:137-157, 1990
50. Kleinert HE, Kutz JE, Fishman JH, McGraw LH: Etiology and treatment of the so-called mucous cyst of the finger. J Bone Joint Surg 54A:1455-1458, 1972
51. Kligman AM: Why do nails grow out instead of up? Arch Dermatol 84:313-315, 1961
52. Koshima I, Soeda S, Takase T, Yamasaki M: Free vascularized nail grafts. J Hand Surg 13A:29-32, 1988
53. Lewin K: The normal finger nail. Br J Dermatol 77:421-430, 1965
54. Lewis BL: Microscopic studies of fetal and mature nail and surrounding soft tissue. AMA Arch Dermatol 70:732-747, 1954
55. McCash CR: Free nail grafting. Br J Plast Surg 8:19-33, 1956
56. McGinley KJ, Larson EL, Leyden JJ: Composition and density of microflora in the subungual space of the hand. J Clin Microbiol 26:950-953, 1988
57. Meskinen JK: p. 117. In Dickson P (ed): The Official Rules. Delacorte Press, New York 1978
58. Milford L: The Hand. CV Mosby, St. Louis, 1971
59. Morrison WA: Microvascular nail transfer. Hand Clin 6:69-76, 1990
60. Moss SH, Schwartz KS, von Drasek-Ascher G, Ogden LL, Wheeler CS, Lister GD: Digital venous anatomy. J Hand Surg 10A:473-482, 1985
61. Newmeyer WL, Kilgore ES: Common injuries of the fingernail and nail bed. Am Fam Physician 16:93-95, 1977
62. Ngim RCK, Soin K: Postburn nailfold retraction: A reconstructive technique. J Hand Surg 11B:385-387, 1986
63. Ogunro EO: External fixation of injured nail bed with the INRO surgical nail splint. J Hand Surg 14A:236-241, 1989
64. Pack GT, Oropeza R: Subungual melanoma. Surg Gynecol Obstet 124:571-582, 1967
65. Papavassiliou NP: Transplantation of the nail: A case report. Br J Plast Surg 22:274-280, 1969
66. Pardo-Castello V: Disease of the Nail. 3rd Ed. Charles C Thomas, Springfield, IL, 1960
67. Pessa JE, Tsai T-M, Li Y, Kleinert HE: The repair of nail deformities with the nonvascularized nail bed graft: Indications and results. J Hand Surg 15A:466-470, 1990
68. Rose EH: Nailplasty utilizing a free composite graft from the helical rim of the ear. Plast Reconstr Surg 66:23-29, 1980

69. Saita H, Suzuki Y, Fujino K, Tajima T: Free nail bed graft for treatment of nail bed injuries of the hand. J Hand Surg 8:171-178, 1983
70. Samman PD: The Nails and Disease. 3rd Ed. Year Book Medical Publishers, Chicago, 1938
71. Sammon PD: The Nails in Disease. 2nd Ed. Charles C Thomas, Springfield, IL, 1972
72. Schiller C: Nail replacement in fingertip injuries. Plast Reconstr Surg 19:521-530, 1957
73. Seckel BR: Self advancing silicone rubber splint for repair of split nail deformity. J Hand Surg 11A:143-144, 1986
74. Shapiro L, Baraf CS: Subungual epidermoid carcinoma and keratocanthoma. Cancer 25:141, 1970
75. Sheehan JE: Replacement of thumb nail. JAMA 92:1253-1255, 1929
76. Shepard GH: Treatment of nail bed avulsions with split thickness nail bed grafts. J Hand Surg 8:49-54, 1983
77. Shepard GH: Management of acute nail bed avulsions. Hand Clin 6:39-56, 1990
78. Shepard GH: Nail grafts for reconstruction. Hand Clin 6:79-102, 1990
79. Shibata M, Seki T, Yoshizu T, Saito H, Tajima T: Microsurgical toenail transfer to the hand. Plast Reconstr Surg 88:102-109, 1991
80. Shoemaker JV: Some notes on the nails. JAMA 15:427-428, 1890
81. Smith DO, Oura C, Kimura C, Toshimori K: The distal venous anatomy of the finger. J Hand Surg 16A:303-307, 1991
82. Spauwen PHM, Brown IF, Sauër EW, Klasen HJ: Management of fingernail deformities after thermal injury. Scand J Plast Reconstr Surg 21:253-255, 1987
83. Stone OJ, Mullins JF: The distal course of nail matrix hemorrhage. Arch Dermatol 88:186-187, 1963
84. Swanker WA: Reconstructive surgery of the injured nail. Am J Surg 74:341-345, 1947
85. Tajima T: Treatment of open crushing type of industrial injuries of the hand and forearm: Degloving, open circumferential, heat press and nail bed injuries. J Trauma 14:995-1011, 1974
86. VanBeek AL, Kassan MA, Adson MH, Dale V: Management of acute fingernail injuries. Hand Clin 6:23-35, 1990
87. Weckesser EC: Treatment of Hand Injuries: Presentation and Restoration of Function. Year Book Medical Publishers, Chicago, 1974
88. Wilgis EFS, Maxwell GP: Distal digital nerve graft: Clinical and anatomical studies. J Hand Surg 4:439-443, 1979
89. Zaias N: The Nail in Health and Disease. Spectrum Publications, Jamaica, NY, 1980
90. Zook EG: The perionychium: Anatomy, physiology, and care of injuries. Clin Plast Surg 8:21-31, 1981
91. Zook EG: Injuries of the fingernail. In Green DP (ed): Operative Hand Surgery. New York, Churchill Livingstone, 1982
92. Zook EG: Fingernail injuries. In Strickland JW, Steichen JB (ed): Difficult Problems in Hand Surgery. CV Mosby, St. Louis, 1982
93. Zook EG: Nail bed injuries. Hand Clin 1:701-716, 1985
94. Zook EG: Complications of the perionychium. Hand Clin 2:407-427, 1986
95. Zook EG: Anatomy and physiology of the perionychium. Hand Clin 6:1-7, 1990
96. Zook EG: Discussion of "The etiologies and mechanisms of nail bed injury." Hand Clin 6:21, 1990
97. Zook EG: Discussion of "Management of acute fingernail injuries." Hand Clin 6:37-38, 1990
98. Zook EG, Guy RJ, Russell RC: A study of nail bed injuries: Causes, treatment and prognosis. J Hand Surg 9A:247-252, 1984
99. Zook EG, Russell RC: Reconstruction of a functional and esthetic nail. Hand Clin 6:59-68, 1990
100. Zook EG, Van Beek AL, Russell RC, Beatty ME: Anatomy and physiology of the perionychium: A review of the literature and anatomic study. J Hand Surg 5:528-536, 1980

35

Nerve Repair and Grafting

E. F. Shaw Wilgis
Thomas M. Brushart

HISTORICAL REVIEW

Treatment of severed peripheral nerve by direct repair has gained acceptance only in the past two centuries. Galen (130–201 A.D.) believed peripheral nerve to be incapable of regeneration,[37] and this view dictated therapy into the Middle Ages. However, nerve suture was clearly practiced by the time of Guy de Chaulic (1300–1370), who observed in young patients that ". . . cut nerves and tendons have been so well restored by suture and other remedies that afterward one could not believe that they had been cut."[21] In spite of these early observations, nerve suture again fell into disrepute, and by the late eighteenth century it was commonly believed that nerves did not regenerate.[94]

Scientific confirmation of peripheral nerve regeneration was first sought by Cruikshank, who evaluated the effects of vagotomy in the dog.[25] Simultaneous bilateral vagotomy was uniformly fatal, but survival could be prolonged by delaying the second vagotomy for 3 weeks, presumably allowing for healing of the first nerve. Hindsight reveals this "success" to have resulted from a variable response to vagotomy rather than true nerve regeneration; it remained for Haighton[46] to demonstrate that a delay of 6 weeks between vagotomies, an adequate time for true regeneration, resulted in indefinite survival. Both sets of observations were published in the *Transactions* of the Royal Society in 1795. Regeneration was confirmed by Muller's simultaneous observations of functional return and (aided by Schwann) the presence of axons in the distal stump after section of the rabbit sciatic nerve.[94]

The nineteenth century was a time of bitter debate over the source of axons in the distal nerve stump.[146] The Monogenists believed these axons to be prolongations of those in the proximal stump, and thus part of the same parent neuron. This view was championed by Waller. Experimenting on the glossopharyngeal nerve of frogs, he observed dissolution of myelin in the entire nerve distal to a transection, not just that portion adjacent to the injury.[102] Further study of selective root lesions in kittens led him to firmly state that portions of the nerve still connected to the cell body remain viable, while those separated from the cell degenerate. The Polygenist hypothesis, in contrast, held that fibers of the distal stump survived and were reconnected to those of the proximal stump. This view was fueled by observations of rapid return of function after nerve section, such as Paget's description of a boy in whom most median nerve function returned 1 month after transection.[105] The controversy was finally laid to rest by Ramon y Cajal's direct observations of regenerating axons, made with a new technique of silver staining.[106]

The first organized clinical observation of nerve injuries was directed by Mitchell during the Civil War. This work, including Mitchell's description of causalgia, was summarized in *Injuries of Nerves and Their Consequences,* a book that laid the foundation for modern studies of peripheral nerve injury.[90] Subsequent military conflicts provided additional material for study. Treatment of World War I nerve injuries led Tinel to describe the "tingling" sign that bears his name; he clearly differentiated tingling, a sign of regenerating axons, from pain, a sign of nerve irritation.[141] Tinel was also active during World War II, and was imprisoned for 2 years because of his aid to the French Resistance. The tradition established by Mitchell and Tinel was continued in World War II by Sir Herbert Seddon in Britain and Barnes Woodhall in the United States. Seddon studied and reported on lesions of the peripheral nervous system from brachial plexus to digital nerve.[115] Both Seddon and Woodhall performed and studied bridge grafts, cable grafts, and primary and secondary repair. Their work defined the standards for modern nerve repair and grafting procedures, and firmly established the principle of secondary suture.[117,154]

Further pioneering contributions were made in the years following World War II. Sir Sidney Sunderland of Australia provided detailed accounts of the internal architecture of the major peripheral nerves (summarized in ref. 131), work that led to modern concepts of grouped fascicular repair and reconstruction. Eric Moberg, working in Goteborg, Sweden, emphasized the importance of sensibility for hand function. He coined the term "tactile gnosis" to describe "the complex sensibility that gives the grip sight," and recommended two-point discrimination as the most valid test of this function.[91,92]

We are currently involved in the next phase of peripheral nerve study, the definition of the events of repair and regeneration at the molecular level. A thorough understanding of these events will suggest pharmacologic and genetic manipulations to alter the basic processes of degeneration and regeneration, and thus ultimately lead to fundamental improvements in treatment of peripheral nerve injuries.

ANATOMY AND TERMINOLOGY

Detailed knowledge of the surgical anatomy of peripheral nerve and its response to injury is a prerequisite for rational planning of nerve repair or reconstruction. This knowledge aids recognition of the individual factors acting in a given patient, understanding of the likely interaction of these factors, and use of this understanding to formulate a plan of treatment.

Epineurium

Epineurium is a loose, collagenous connective tissue. The internal epineurium permeates the nerve, surrounding individual fascicles. The external epineurium is a condensation of this tissue that ensheaths the fascicles as a group (Fig. 35-1). It is often encased within loose areolar tissue,[126] and adheres to nutrient vessels as they enter the nerve. Internal epineurium cushions the fascicles from external pressure and allows movement of one relative to another; external epineurium contains the fascicles while allowing the nerve both longitudinal and lateral movement within its bed. Both layers absorb longitudinal stress before the undulating fasciculi are straightened enough to accept tension.[133]

The percentage of nerve cross-sectional area occupied by epineurium varies along each nerve, from nerve to nerve, and from individual to individual.[129] This variability is often extreme, with from 25 percent to 75 percent of the nerve being composed of epineurium.[134] The higher percentages are often found in the areas of joints, where extra padding is needed. Epineurial fibroblasts respond vigorously to injury; the external epineurium may reach a thickness of 2 to 3 mm in chronically inflamed nerves, and much of the scar formed after nerve transection results from brisk proliferation of these cells.[59]

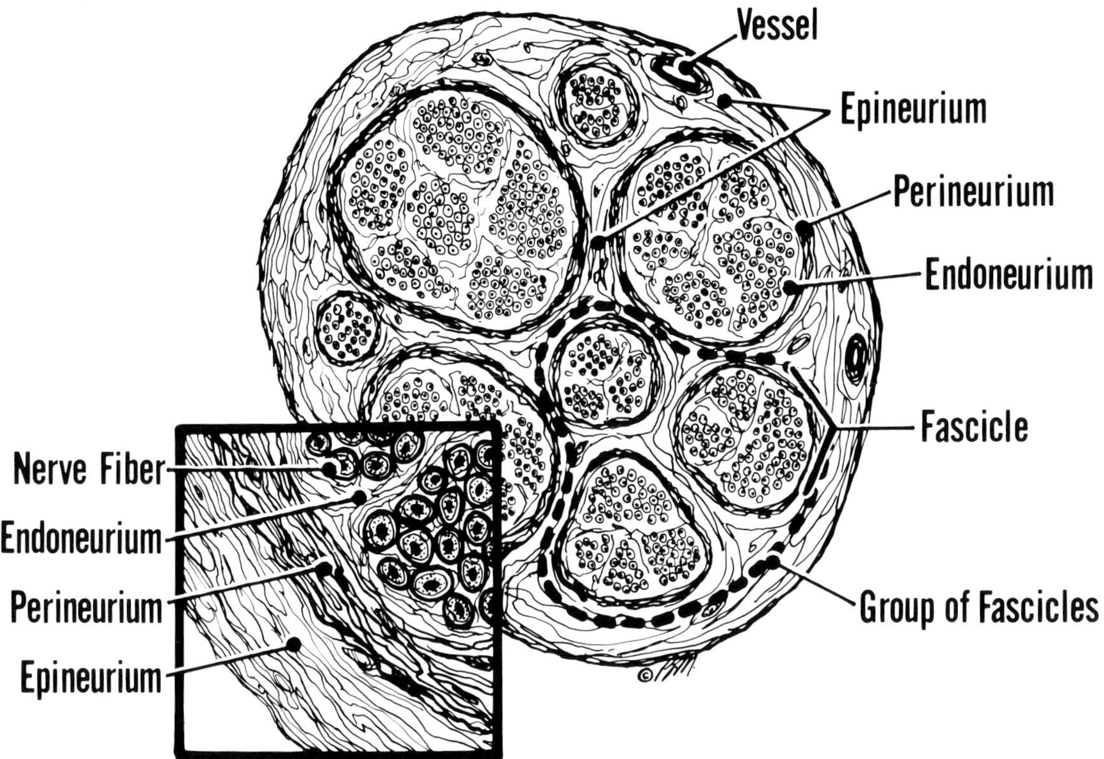

Fig. 35-1. Cross-sectional anatomy of a peripheral nerve.

Perineurium

The perineurium is the tissue layer surrounding individual fascicles (Fig. 35-1). It is composed of up to 10 concentric lamellae of flattened cells with prominent basement membranes that are "dovetailed" together and linked with tight junctions.[139] Longitudinally and obliquely oriented collagen fibers occupy the space between lamellae.[140] The perineurium functions as an extension of the blood-brain barrier, controlling the intraneural ionic environment by limiting diffusion, blocking the spread of infection to the endoneurium,[120] and maintaining a slightly positive intrafascicular pressure.[95] Removal of the perineurium results in cessation of neural function; removal of the epineurium, in contrast, has few immediate consequences. Mechanically, the perineurium strongly resists longitudinal traction; the elastic properties of a nerve undergoing elongation are retained as long as the perineurium remains intact.[127]

Endoneurium

The endoneurium is the collagenous tissue that serves as the "packing" among axons within the perineurium. There is no elastin, and endoneurial fibroblasts are infrequent. Endoneurium also participates in formation of the "Schwann Cell Tube" (or "endoneurial tube"), the cylindrical structure that contains the myelinated axon and its associated Schwann cells. Larger myelinated axons are invested by two layers of collagen, the outer longitudinally oriented and the inner arranged randomly and associated with carbohydrate-rich reticulin.[139] Small myelinated axons possess only the outer, longitudinal layer. The Schwann cell basement membrane forms the inner lining of this tubular structure. Endoneurial collagen resists longitudinal stress, while the Schwann cell participates in a complex homeostatic relationship with the axon.

Vascular Supply

Peripheral nerve is richly vascularized.[72] Segmental nutrient vessels join a plexus of predominately longitudinal vessels in the epineurium. These in turn supply a second plexus that lies among the lamellae of the perineurium. Perineurial vessels may travel for long distances before entering the endoneurium at a characteristically oblique angle, placing them at risk for occlusion if endoneurial pressure is raised.[75] The endoneurial vascular network consists of capillaries, arterioles, and venules. This network appears to be continuous throughout the length of the fascicle, and the direction of flow in any portion can be rapidly changed in response to injury. There are no lymphatics within the endoneurium. By virtue of the interconnecting longitudinal vascular plexi, a peripheral nerve may survive extensive mobilization from its bed.[74] The effect of nerve mobilization on the regeneration of transected axons has yet to be clearly defined. Extensive mobilization of the monkey tibial nerve did not impair subsequent regeneration after nerve transection and repair,[64] while mobilization of the monkey median nerve for 5 cm proximal and distal to a midforearm laceration adversely affected the outcome of repair.[123]

Fascicles

A fascicle (termed *funiculus* by Sunderland) is the smallest unit of nerve structure that can be manipulated surgically. It contains a group of axons, packed within endoneurium and enclosed within a sheath of perineurium (see Fig. 35-1). The number of fascicular subunits within a given nerve varies throughout its course; great variations are also seen among individuals. In his series of dissections, Sunderland found as few as 3 and as many as 36 fascicles in the median nerve.[130] Fascicles are not separate "cables" that run in parallel throughout the length of the nerve; instead, they undergo numerous interconnections that result in the formation of an intraneural plexus. This plexus formation is variable in its extent. It is most prominent in nerves to the proximal portion of the extremity, such as the musculocutaneous, where it may result in a complex web of interfascicular connections.[130] However, few interconnections are present in the distal portions of the median and ulnar nerves. The fascicles of the thenar motor branch may remain separate within the median nerve for up to 5.6 cm.[55]

The degree to which functionally related axons (defined by termination within a single nerve branch) are grouped together in proximal portions of the nerve has been controversial throughout this century.[18] On the basis of dissections, Sunderland has stated that there is no localization of functionally related axons in the proximal limb. "As the nerve proceeds distally, the fascicular plexuses effect a sorting out of the different branch fiber systems (axons ending in a particular nerve branch) until, finally, the fibers for a particular branch are collected into their own fasciculus, or group of fasciculi, which then leaves the nerve as a definitive branch."[133] This pessimistic view of intraneural organization at proximal levels has undergone recent modifications. In further dissections, Jabaley et al[55] found that terminal fascicles often maintain their integrity for greater distances than those found by Sunderland. Jabaley et al deemphasized the role of the intraneural plexus in axon sorting, stating that "fiber and funicular behavior, at least in the more distal portions of nerves, is rather purposeful . . . it is the random wandering of epineurium which is responsible for much of the change observed."

An entirely new perspective has been added by the development of neurophysiologic and histochemical techniques, which allow one to trace axons directly rather than infer their behavior from fascicular architecture. When stimulating median nerve axons in awake humans, Schady and his coworkers[112] found that 42 percent of fascicles studied in the upper arm projected only to skin, and within these, 67 percent of sensations elicited were confined to a single digital interspace. With refinements in technique, Hallin has gone one step further to demonstrate somatotopic arrangement of axons within individual fascicles.[48] These findings have been confirmed by studies in which histochemical techniques were used to trace digital nerve axons throughout the median nerves of rhesus monkeys.[18] The long-accepted picture of intraneural chaos, which reflects the limitations of dissection technique, is thus replaced by a view of partial localization of distal function at proximal levels.

Fascicular Groups

Recent awareness of functional localization within proximal segments of human nerve has had little impact on clinical practice; we do not yet possess the techniques to precisely identify and align related axon groups. However, a more immediately useful concept has been that of fascicular groups. In many areas of peripheral nerve, fascicles are not evenly spaced within the epineurium, but clustered into groups of three to six (see Fig. 35-1). These groups are bound together by partial condensations of the inner epineurium. Fascicular groups can be isolated over much greater distances than can individual fascicles; whereas interfascicular connections are common within a fascicular group, they are much less frequent between fascicular groups.[55,145,150] When injury has resulted in loss of neural substance, correct matching of fascicles in the proximal and distal stump is usually impossible. However, fascicular *groups* may still be identified and matched after losses of several centimeters. For this reason, knowledge of fascicular group anatomy is a cornerstone of modern peripheral nerve repair and grafting.

Longitudinal Excursion of Nerves

Peripheral nerve rarely crosses a joint at its axis of motion; the length of the peripheral nerve bed will therefore change with limb movement. The resulting longitudinal excursion of upper extremity peripheral nerves has been studied electrophysiologically and anatomically. McLellan and Swash[80] recorded median nerve action potentials before and during active and passive motion of the arm. Active and passive excursions were equal. Extension of the wrist and digits produced 7.4 mm of excursion, with an additional 4.3 mm resulting from elbow flexion. Displacement of the median nerve during wrist and digital flexion was 2 to 4 times greater at the wrist than in the upper arm. Wilgis and Murphy[149] dissected the peripheral nerves of 15 fresh adult cadaver arms to study their excursion anatomically. The brachial plexus had an average excursion of 15 mm in the frontal plane during abduction of the arm. The median and ulnar nerves moved an average of 7.3 and 9.8 mm, respectively, through a full range of elbow motion. Full wrist flexion/extension produced the greatest excursion, 15.5 mm in the median nerve and 14.8 mm in the ulnar nerve, as measured at the proximal edge of the carpal tunnel. The excursion was much lower in the palm and digits.

Normal nerve excursion in response to joint motion is made possible by the nerve's inherent elasticity and its ability to glide smoothly through its bed, redistributing focal stresses to the entire nerve. Awareness of the requirement for nerve excursion is important in the planning of neural reconstruction. A neuroma-in-continuity is often scarred to its adjacent bed; longitudinal stresses can no longer be distributed throughout the nerve, but are focused on the area of injury, increasing the resultant symptoms. Restoration of neural gliding to diffuse these forces is thus an important part of treating the neuroma-in-continuity. Similarly, management of the nerve gap must take into account postoperative demands for excursion. This is especially important in secondary repair.[86] One must overcome (1) the original gap due to substance loss, (2) the gap created by secondary neuroma excision, and (3) the elastic retraction and subsequent fibrotic fixation of the nerve. It may be possible to close the gap by flexing adjacent joints and suturing the nerve under tension. However, these maneuvers will exhaust the nerve's excursion. Joint mobilization will cause stretch injury to the nerve, hampering or altogether preventing axon regeneration.[49] Successful prevention of this problem requires the addition of neural length, either by nerve grafting or maneuvers such as anterior transposition of the ulnar nerve at the elbow.

DEGENERATION AND REGENERATION

Wallerian Degeneration

The molecular and cellular events of Wallerian degeneration have recently been extensively reviewed.[3,35,73] The process of Wallerian degeneration serves to clear the distal stump of axoplasm and myelin, preparing the way for subsequent axon regeneration. It is initiated by ingrowth of macrophages, which trigger Schwann cell proliferation. This proliferation peaks 3 days after nerve transection and continues for 2 weeks. The proliferating Schwann cells, aided by macrophages, clear the Schwann cell tubes of debris, forming Bands of Bunger, longitudinal columns of Schwann cells that remain within the Schwann cell basement membrane. As the axoplasm and myelin are cleared away, the contents of the Schwann cell tube decrease in volume, and the diameter of the tube shrinks. Deposition of new endoneurial collagen around the shrunken tube reduces its ability to expand when a regenerating axon reoccupies the lumen.[140]

Degeneration: Sensory End Organs

Sensory end organs may survive years of denervation. However, end organ survival is only the first step in restoration of function. In the primate, Pacinian corpuscles are reinnervated less often than Meissner's corpuscles.[153] This has been attributed to mechanical obstruction of the Pacinian endoneurial tube by myelin debris and fibrosis.[68] Reinervation of Meissner's corpuscles is also imperfect. Biopsy of human fingertips after repair and regeneration of the innervating nerve found reinnervation of Meissner's corpuscles in only 16 of 23 digits; furthermore, the presence or absence of reinnervation did not correlate with either clinical testing or subjective impressions of sensibility.[54] These findings presage the current debate concerning the ability of regenerated sensory axons to transduce sensory information from the bare axon tip, without end organ contact. Clinical studies have not clearly defined a period of denervation after which useful sensation cannot be restored. In a long-term follow-up of World War II injuries, there was no correlation between delay in nerve repair and ultimate sensory recovery.[103] However, protective sensibility with little two-point discrimination is often the most realistic goal after denervation periods of greater than 1 year.

Degeneration: Muscle

The time course of denervation changes within muscle and their consequences for recovery of function have been studied in both experimental animals and humans. Sunderland and Ray[136] found that denervated opossum muscle lost 50 percent to 60 percent of its weight by 60 days, a time at which the average fiber cross-sectional area was reduced by 70 percent. Fibroblastic proliferation peaked at 89 days and resulted in deposition of collagen, first in the perimysium and later in the endomysium. The result was separation of each atrophied fiber from its neighbors by a thickened endomysium, and separation of adjoining fiber groups (fasciculi) by a thickened perimysium. In human biopsy studies, significant fibrosis was also found as early as 3 months,[1] progressing in proportion to the total period of denervation. Most muscle fibers had undergone moderate or severe atrophy by 3 months, while moderate to severe fibrosis was usually present after 11 months. Overall, there was a wide range of variation amongst individuals. Bowden and Gutmann[12] performed 140 muscle biopsies on the patients of Sir Herbert Seddon. During the first 3 postdenervation years they found progressive atrophy and fibrosis, the degree of which was often affected by sepsis, muscle stretching, muscle nutrition, or patient age. Beyond 3 years they found progressive fragmentation and disintegration of muscle fibers, leading to their replacement by fibrous tissue.

Gutmann also studied the effects of various periods of denervation on ultimate muscle function.[44] In the rabbit model, he found that deficits of muscle function after up to 8 months of denervation reflected deficient maturation of nerve fibers or motor endplates; after 8 months muscle fiber atrophy became the limiting factor. Subsequent analysis of clinical cases demonstrated "complete or very good restoration of function" after muscle denervation of up to 12 months.[128] In summary, ideal reinnervation can be expected after 1 to 3 months of denervation, functional reinnervation can be expected for up to 1 year, and no reinnervation can be expected after 3 years.

Recent experiments have assessed the retardation of muscle atrophy after denervation by both pharmacologic and electrical means. Influx of calcium ions may trigger muscle atrophy through activation of the enzyme calcium-activated neutral protease. Treatment of primates after nerve repair with an inhibitor of this enzyme, leupeptin, improves functional reinnervation of muscle.[4] Multiple factors are involved, and the effect on nerve appears to predominate over that on muscle itself. Electrical stimulation of denervated muscle has been controversial since Gutmann and Gutmann[45] showed that it could retard atrophy of denervated rabbit muscle. However, stimulation with implanted electrodes is sufficiently promising to warrant continued study.[98,100]

Neuronal Response to Axotomy

The most dramatic neuronal response to axotomy is death of the parent neuron, decreasing the pool of neurons available for regeneration. The severity of neuronal death is highest in young animals and after proximal lesions. Neuronal loss after axotomy has been quantified in rats. Most injured motoneurons die after neonatal sciatic nerve transection, while a similar lesion in adults produces little or no detectable loss.[113] In young adults, proximal sciatic transection resulted in a 27 percent reduction in the number of sensory neurons in the affected dorsal root ganglia, while only a 7 percent loss was found after distal lesions.[157] Neonatal sciatic crush in midthigh caused a 60 percent decrease in sensory neurons.[9] Surviving neurons undergo "chromatolysis," or dispersal of Nissl substance (polyribosomes) within the cell body, a change that results from breakdown of the rough endoplasmic reticulum.[41,81] The cell body and nucleolus enlarge, the nucleus becomes eccentric, and the dendritic tree shrinks. The metabolism of the cell shifts from production of cytoskeletal components and neurotransmitters to the production of proteins needed for regeneration. Synthesis of neurofilament, a structural protein, is decreased;[50] synthesis of tubulin, actin, and growth-associated proteins (GAPS) are enhanced (reviewed in ref. 35). A prominent example is GAP-43, an axonally transported phosphoprotein concentrated in the growth cones of developing and regenerating axons.[121] Its concentration increases 100-fold after axotomy, returning to normal after cessation of regeneration.

Axon Regeneration

Transected axons form sprouts that enter the distal nerve stump and regenerate through it to contact and reinnervate peripheral end organs. After the minimal trauma of sharp transection, sprouts are generated at the most distal remaining node of Ranvier.[93] However, after the more diffuse trauma of a blast or stretch injury, the sprouts may originate several centimeters proximal to the severed nerve end. The sprouts from a single axon extend distally as the "regenerating unit."[93] Usually two to five sprouts persist as axon collaterals in the distal stump during the intermediate stages of regeneration.[56] The collateral sprouts that establish end organ contact survive, while most of those that do not are pruned away.[2] The collateral sprouts from a single "regenerating unit" may enter separate, and often unrelated, Schwann cell tubes in the distal nerve stump, leading them to different end organs. Collaterals of a single motor axon may reinnervate separate muscles,[34,70] and collaterals of a single sensory axon may supply separate cutaneous receptive fields.[51] Motor axon collaterals may also enter old sensory Schwann cell tubes; their selective pruning from this "inappropriate" environment has been recently described as the basis for sensor/motor specificity (see below).[14]

Transected axons begin to sprout within hours of injury. Initial sprouts are usually resorbed; permanent sprouts, with internal cytoskeletons, are formed within 27 hours.[82] The distal progress of these sprouts is retarded at the site of transection ("scar delay"). This delay may be as short as 48 hours in rats,[36] but may be several weeks in chimpanzees and humans.[62] Some regenerating axons fail to cross the repair site and form a local neuroma, while others cross but enter only interfascicular epineurium; both groups are excluded from functional reinnervation of the periphery. Most axons that contact distal Schwann cell tubes propagate within them, coursing between the inner surface of the tube and the longitudinal column of Schwann cells, Band of Bunger, which remains within the tube after Wallerian degeneration.[97] Regenerating axons have a definite preference for the inner surface of the Schwann cell basal lamina when experimentally given equal access to both sides.[52] The rate of axon propagation within the distal stump is again species dependent. Rodent axons may regenerate at 2 to 3.5 mm/day,[7,26] while the maximum human rate is 1 to 2 mm/day,[19,119] with progressive slowing as the axon nears the periphery.

The specificity with which regenerating axons are directed to appropriate end organs has profound functional consequences (reviewed in ref. 17). Axons may regenerate in normal numbers, but little or no useful function will result when they reach inappropriate targets. For example, motor axons that regenerate into cutaneous nerves cannot reinnervate muscle, and will block appropriate axons from the pathways they occupy. The specificity of axon regeneration may be viewed in an hierarchical framework, proceeding from gross through progressively finer discriminations (reviewed in refs. 14,17). Tissue specificity, the preferential growth of axons towards nervous versus other forms of tissue, has been known since the time of Ramon y Cajal. Growth of regenerating axons en mass toward a neural target probably reflects the action of neurotropism, or directed regeneration up a concentration gradient of a substance diffusing from the neural "target." Neurotropism may also influence specificity at the nerve trunk level. Selective reinnervation of appropriate distal nerve trunks has been demonstrated in a "Y" tube model, but not after routine nerve repair. Sensory/motor specificity, in contrast, directly influences the outcome of peripheral nerve suture.[14,16] Motor axons regenerating in mixed nerve will preferentially reinnervate a distal motor branch, even if the nerve stumps are intentionally misaligned or separated by a gap. Sensory/motor specificity is probably generated through neurotrophic (nutritive) support of motor axon collaterals that reinnervate old motor Schwann cell tubes in the distal nerve stump. This support is not provided to collaterals of the same axons that have entered old sensory Schwann cell tubes, and they are selectively pruned back, leaving only the correct projection to the motor nerve. Within both sensory and motor systems, there is a potential for topographic and end organ specificity. Topographic specificity describes reinnervation of the correct muscle within the motor system or the correct patch of skin within the sensory system; end organ specificity involves reinnervation of the correct type of sensory end organ within the sensory system, and the correct fiber type (fast versus slow, motor end plate versus muscle spindle) in the motor system. In nerve repair, the degree of topographic specificity is proportional to the mechanical accuracy with which related axon groups are aligned in proximal and distal nerve stumps.[15,17] Regenerating axons do not appear to have an inherent mechanism for selectively returning to topographically appropriate areas. End organ specificity does not appear to be under even mechanical control. Frequent reinnervation of appropriate end organs is found after repair of nerves which innervate only a few receptor types, but essentially random behavior is found after repair of larger mixed nerves (reviewed in ref. 17). Interestingly, some forms of inherent topographic and end organ specificity are found in neonatal animals; this developmental "holdover" may partially explain the superior results of nerve repair in juveniles.

In summary, it is crucial to recognize that the various forms of potential specificity may be controlled by entirely different factors, or not controlled at all. The forces that generate sensory/motor specificity in spite of an interstump gap are powerless when it comes to topographic specificity; axons cannot "find their way" to the appropriate topographic area. Accurate alignment of axons in proximal and distal stumps thus remains a primary goal of the peripheral nerve surgeon.

NERVE REPAIR

Primary Versus Secondary Repair

Primary repair includes immediate repair, within hours of injury, and "delayed primary" repair, within the first 5 to 7 days. Any repair performed more than 1 week after injury is termed "secondary." Secondary repair was initially developed in response to the limitations of wartime surgery (see Historical Review). Wounds were often contaminated, and nerve repair was not a priority for patient or limb survival. However, a delay of 2 to 3 weeks was later advocated in the treatment of clean, sharp civilian injuries.[33] This delay was timed to coincide with the peak of neuronal metabolic activity. In theory, a "primed" neuron would regenerate more readily. Subsequent research has confirmed the theoretical advantages of this approach (reviewed in ref. 81); a higher speed of axonal regeneration is attained by axons that have been injured previously (the "conditioning effect"). Conditioning is thought to increase the synthesis of growth associated proteins and the speed with which they are transported to the axonal growth cone. However, in spite of these theoretical advantages, delay has not been found to alter the final outcome of nerve repair. The results of primary suture of sharp lacerations are superior to the results of delayed repair in rats,[142] rabbits,[8] and monkeys.[40] Clinically, primary repair of ulnar and median nerve injuries has produced results clearly superior to those of delayed suture.[6,83]

Primary nerve repair has emerged as the treatment of choice when conditions permit. However, several criteria must be met before primary suture is chosen. These include

1. Sharp nerve transection. Any element of crush must be clearly localized, and small enough to permit coaptation of the nerve ends after it is resected. If significant crush or avulsion components are present, it is better to return later when their extent can be clearly defined and all damaged nerve excised.
2. Minimal contamination of the wound. Historically, the greatest improvement in the results of nerve repair has resulted from control of surgical infection.
3. A bed of viable, well-perfused muscle, fat, or tenosynovium. Crushed or devitalized tissue becomes progressively fibrotic, both constricting the nerve and tethering it to the underlying bed (see Nerve

Excursion). Regeneration may be impeded, and traction on the neuroma may produce painful dysesthesias. These symptoms may be more of a problem than the lack of nerve function itself. In this situation, the bed must be improved by bringing in distant tissue, or alternatively, the nerve must be moved into an uninjured area.
4. Absence of associated injuries that preclude concomitant restoration of circulation, skeletal stability, or soft tissue cover.
5. Surgical magnification and operating room staff familiar with microsurgical techniques.[83,152]
6. A patient in suitable metabolic and emotional condition to undergo surgery. An intoxicated patient who can be neither adequately studied nor reliably anesthetized is not a candidate for primary neurorrhaphy. Similarly, the emotional condition of a patient who has just attempted suicide often precludes major surgery.

If these conditions cannot be met, it is better to elect a delayed repair. Secondary neurorrhaphy under favorable conditions will give better results than primary neurorrhaphy under unfavorable ones. It is not sufficient to "throw in a few stitches and see how it does" (one should, however, tack the nerve ends together to prevent elastic retraction and facilitate a planned secondary operation). Several months must pass before a tentative repair can be evaluated properly, months during which the parent neuron is expending its regenerative potential and end organs are undergoing progressive atrophy. In peripheral nerve surgery, the first repair must be the best repair possible.[32]

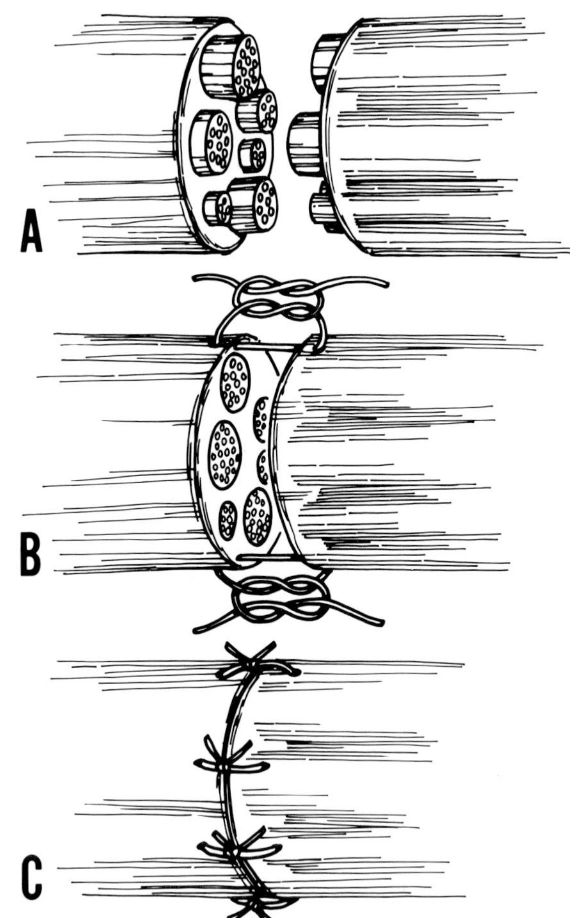

Fig. 35-2. Primary or secondary epineurial repair.

Techniques of Repair

As previously discussed, the anatomy of peripheral nerve varies tremendously, both along the course of any given nerve and from one nerve to another. The degree of functional localization, the mix of sensory and motor fibers, the number and size of fascicles, and the percentage of epineurial tissue are all factors that influence the choice of repair technique. No one technique is best for all situations; the surgeon must be comfortable with different techniques of varying complexity before undertaking the repair of any peripheral nerve.

Epineurial Suture

Preparation for any nerve suture begins with adequate anesthesia; the surgeon should not be "racing the clock," and must feel confident that the arm will not be suddenly withdrawn, destroying the repair. Use of magnification improves the outcome of nerve suture.[152] While some surgeons use high-powered loupes, most prefer the convenience and flexibility of the operating microscope. Surgery itself begins with isolation of proximal and distal nerve stumps on background material in a bloodless field (Fig. 35-2). Each stump is gently elevated by the assistant and inspected about its circumference, looking for fascicular or vascular landmarks and trimming away any fat that may obscure the epineurial margin. Epineurial suture is governed by the principles of hydraulics. Epineurial sleeves are joined in such a way as to oppose their contents, multiple independent "fluid" fascicles, under minimal, uniform pressure. Any focal increase in pressure will result in lateral bulging of fascicles and poor axonal alignment. The stump surfaces must be trimmed perpendicular to the long axis of the nerve so that pressure will be evenly distributed when the surfaces are joined. All damaged tissue should be removed. It is difficult to cleanly transect a large nerve, as evidenced by the multiple surgical devices available for this purpose. The nerve must be gently immobilized with a circumferential Penrose drain or slotted metal tube and cut transversely with a sharp blade. Serrated scissors are effective when trimming individual fascicles, but cannot be used to cut multiple fascicles within epineurium. Once the transection has been performed, all traction on the nerve stumps should be toward the repair; distracting forces will increase mushrooming of fascicles from the epineurium, making their alignment much more difficult. Epineurial vessels are coagulated with bipolar microforceps, and the nerve stumps are aligned using fascicular groupings and vascular landmarks. Every effort must be made to align related axon groups in proximal and distal stumps. A single suture is used to join the epineurial edges farthest from the surgeon. A second suture is then placed 180 degrees from the first one. The placement of this second suture is crucial to the completion of the repair. If the nerve is properly bisected into anterior and posterior halves, and the faces are cut perpendicular, the compression forces will be uniform and the nerve will assume a rounded appearance. The sutures should be just tight enough to produce contact between proximal and distal stumps, but not so tight as to produce buckling of the fascicles or lateral bulging of tissue. If the sutures do not bisect the nerve, the fascicles will bulge out the side where the sutures are farthest apart. This is usually the back, and considerable effort must be expended to rebalance the forces with multiple sutures before a good result can be obtained. It is often easier to replace the second suture. 8–0 suture is used for the first two stitches in a major peripheral nerve, and the tails are left long to facilitate rotation of the nerve. If the nerve stumps cannot be brought together with 8–0 suture, the tension is excessive and either further mobilization or grafting should be considered. 10–0 suture is used for additional sutures in large nerves, and all sutures in smaller nerves. The third and fourth sutures bisect the distance between the initial 180-degree sutures; additional sutures are placed sparingly to improve alignment where necessary and prevent protrusion of fascicles from the suture line. It is not necessary to perform a watertight closure of the epineurium, as only the amount of traction needed to oppose the fascicles is necessary.

Group Fascicular Suture

Group fascicular suture demands higher magnification and more delicate instruments than are required for epineurial suture. It is also more difficult to perform under tension, since traction forces are transmitted directly to fascicles rather than to the thick external epineurium. The proximal and distal stump surfaces are inspected to ascertain the outlines of fascicular groups, a process aided by slight rotation of the external epineurium. Fascicles of a single group are tightly joined and will move together, while fascicular groups will slide on their neighbors. The assistant then gently elevates the nerve stump by grasping the external epineurium, permitting the surgeon to place lateral traction on a fascicular group and sever the internal epineurium that binds it to its neighbors. This process is most easily performed with delicate curved microscissors that are kept extremely sharp and used only for intraneural dissection. A fascicular group should be isolated over just the distance required to reflect it from the main nerve trunk, usually 3 to 4 mm. Matching fascicular groups are dissected from proximal and distal stumps. It is often possible to begin the repair with suture of the posterior epineurium to alleviate tension on the more delicate group fascicular junctures. Beginning on the back of the nerve furthest from the surgeon, the fascicular groups are then trimmed perpendicular to their long axes and joined by sutures placed through the internal epineurium where possible and through the perineurium of the fascicle when this is the only structure available. Since the fascicular group is irregular in outline, considerable judgment must be exercised to place the minimum number of sutures in positions that will produce uniform apposition pressure across the face of the fascicular group.

Individual Fascicular Suture

When individual fascicular suture is chosen (Fig. 35-3), dissection is initiated as described above, but is continued to include the internal epineurium separating individual fascicles. Care must be taken to avoid cutting interfascicular connections. The process of repair is initiated by trimming and joining the fascicular stumps on the back of the nerve farthest from the surgeon. It may be possible to use a single suture for each fascicle if tension can be relaxed by partial repair of the epineurium. If not, two 10–0 sutures placed 180 degrees apart are required for each fascicle. Individual fascicular suture may be combined with epineurial repair in some situations (Fig. 35-4).

Fascicular Matching Techniques

Several techniques have been described for matching fascicles in proximal and distal nerve stumps. However, they provide only incomplete information, and must be supplemented by intraneural dissection of the distal stump or an educated guess based on intraneural maps. Their greatest value lies in separation of predominately sensory and motor fascicles.

Fascicular stimulation in the awake patient was described by Hakstian[47] and has been applied in several small clinical

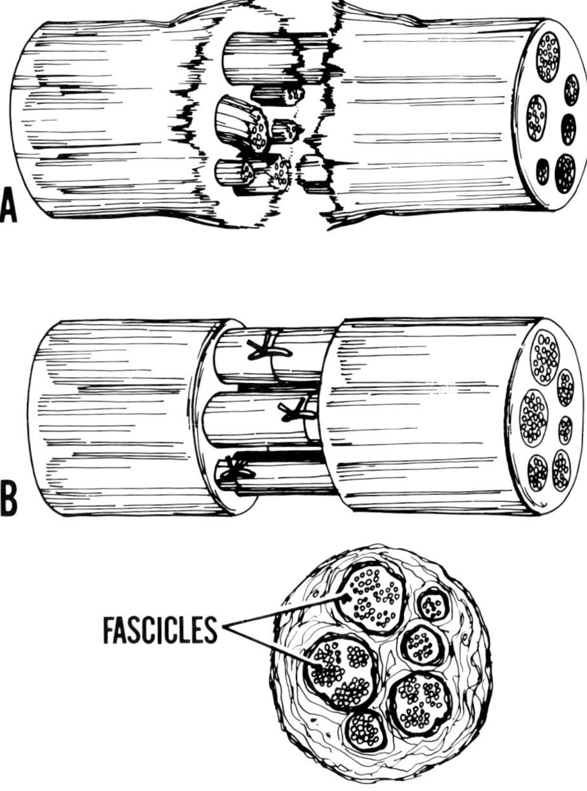

Fig. 35-3. Primary fascicular, or funicular, repair.

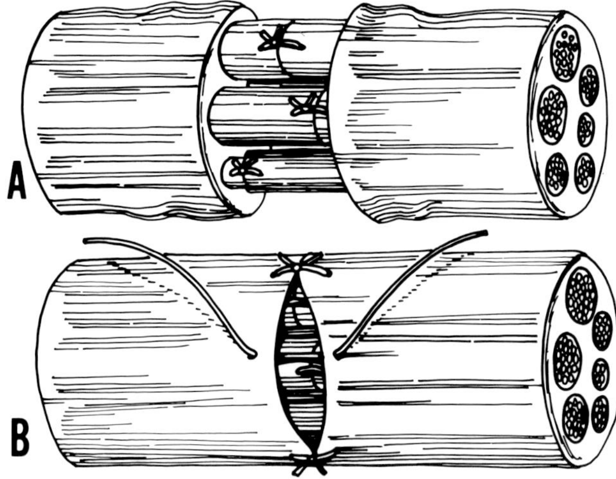

Fig. 35-4. Mixed fascicular and epineurial repair.

series.[53,96,144] The technique should only be attempted on patients who fully understand and feel comfortable with their pivotal role as described preoperatively by the surgeon. Initial wound debridement and fascicular dissection are performed under 0.5 percent plain lidocaine Bier block, and wound edges are infiltrated with 0.25 percent bupivacaine 10 minutes before tourniquet deflation. The tourniquet is then released for 15 minutes to completely reverse nerve ischemia. Stimulation is performed with the patient sedated but awake. A stimulus of 0.2 mA to 0.5 mA is delivered to each proximal fascicle with a standard nerve stimulator, and the patient is questioned as to the sensation elicited. Beginning with the lowest intensity and working up, an intensity is chosen that produces a reproducible, well-localized response. Sensory fascicles are then mapped as to their distal termination, based on the portion of the hand to which the patient localizes the stimulus. Proximal motor fascicle stimulation will produce no response at lower intensities, and poorly localized pain at higher levels. Stimulation of the distal stump will produce a motor contraction in the first 1 to 3 days postinjury, and nothing thereafter. Electrical stimulation is thus most useful in treating acute lacerations, but may be helpful at later times if distal motor branches can be identified anatomically. At the completion of mapping, a general anesthetic is administered and the nerve fascicles or fascicular groups are selectively reunited based on the proximal and distal maps.

This technique positively identifies only proximal sensory fascicles and distal motor fascicles. It is easy to infer the general character of motor fascicles in the proximal stump through their lack of response, but their specific destination remains unknown. In the distal stump, specific motor termination is known, but sensory fascicles must be dissected out for positive identification. The technique is thus most readily applicable just proximal to areas of nerve branching, and for primary or early delayed primary repair when distal motor axons have not degenerated.

Individual motor and sensory fibers can be identified in proximal stumps, and in distal stumps for up to 9 days after axotomy,[111] through histochemical identification of the enzymes acetylcholinesterase (AChE)[43] and carbonic anhydrase (CA).[108] AChE is present in the axoplasm of myelinated motor axons and many small unmyelinated axons, but not myelinated sensory axons. CA activity is found in myelin, and in the axoplasm of myelinated sensory axons. Nerve tissue must be sacrificed from both proximal and distal stumps for histochemical processing, running the risk of significantly altering the fascicular patterns, and a minimum of 1 to 2 hours are required for the most rapid techniques.[69,159] However, patient cooperation is not necessary. Histochemical techniques for labeling motor and sensory fascicles were initially described separately,[43,108] but their combined use may increase the accuracy of fascicular identification.[111] These techniques identify fascicles on cross section as predominately sensory or motor, but give no clue as to their topographic destination. There is no point in dissecting out distal motor fascicles to determine their precise destination, since this information is not available for the proximal stump. However, in late cases it is necessary to dissect the distal stump to make a sensory/motor determination on anatomic grounds.

Histochemical techniques of fascicular matching are in routine use in some centers, but no comparative clinical series have established their efficacy to date. We routinely use AChE stain during late reconstructive procedures, when nerve tissue must be trimmed from the proximal stump, but avoid removal of nerve tissue for assay in the acute setting.

Authors' Preferred Method

Rationale

Guidance of regenerating axons to appropriate end organs is the primary goal of nerve repair. This is best accomplished by surgical alignment of functionally and topographically related axons of the proximal stump with their old Schwann cell tubes in the distal stump. Tropic and trophic interactions may occur during axon regeneration, but mechanical alignment is the primary determinant of regeneration specificity.[17] Restoration of specific connections between peripheral end organs and the central nervous system (CNS) is crucial for the return of function. The complex disorganization of nerve impulses reaching the CNS after miswiring thousands of these connections is not like the switching of discrete functions with tendon transfer, and cannot be adequately overcome by CNS reorganization.[17] To maximize appropriate reinnervation, one should selectively reunite portions of the proximal and distal stump that serve discrete functions, *but only if they can be positively identified and matched.* Precise reunion of unrelated fascicles will lead regenerating axons to functionally inappropriate destinations, and exclude appropriate axons from the pathways they occupy. The recommendations of Sunderland,[132] based on dissection studies, limit selective reunion to anatomically clear branch fiber systems. Modern histochemical and electrophysiologic techniques allow us to localize these systems at more proximal levels, broadening the indications for selective reunion techniques. However, as we have just seen, current methods of fascicular matching often provide only generic information. Situations will thus frequently arise in which many or all injured fascicles remain incompletely characterized. In most instances, "selective reunion" currently refers to sensory versus motor, and not to finer anatomic discriminations. It should also be emphasized that this approach to nerve repair, though backed by experimental evidence, common sense, and small clinical series[38,47,144] has not yet been subjected to adequate clinical trial.

Primary Suture

Having established our conceptual approach to nerve repair, we will now apply it to specific areas of the ulnar and median nerves. The proper digital nerve represents a discrete function and contains relatively few fascicles; epineurial suture provides alignment that cannot be surpassed by fascicular techniques.[158] The common digital nerves are readily divisible into proper digital subunits, and group fascicular technique should be applied to each of these. Every effort should be made to precisely align fascicles within the ulnar and median motor branches, since motor function is well-localized at this distal level. Group fascicular technique will often adequately align individual fascicles, but one should not hesitate to repair them separately when visual matching is possible.

Repair of the ulnar and median nerves in the wrist and distal forearm presents a unique challenge to the microsurgeon. These injuries are frequent, and they lie within an area where discrete sensory or motor functions are often localized to individual fascicles or fascicular groups, an area in which technique can be expected to make a difference. Median nerve transection in the proximal palm often presents a dilemma, as one is faced with a single nerve trunk proximally but several branches distally. Each distal branch should be matched with the appropriate fascicular group in the proximal stump. If matching cannot be achieved visually, this is an ideal situation for awake stimulation; little or no dissection is required distally to establish the destination of the branches, and they can be precisely matched with topographically appropriate fascicular groups in the proximal stump. The appeal of stimulation technique for alignment of sensory fascicles decreases as one moves proximally out of the carpal tunnel. Dissection of terminal fascicular groups becomes progressively more invasive and risks injury to the nerve. In the distal third of the forearm, individual or group fascicular technique is used on the thenar motor branch. Visual matching is often possible, tracing the branch distally from the thenar eminence along its superficial course on the volaradial aspect of the nerve. When visual tracing is impossible, awake stimulation may be considered. Histochemical techniques are less appropriate in the acute situation, as they involve sacrifice of nerve tissue and exacerbate the problems of fascicular matching. Once the thenar motor fibers have been reunited, the remainder of the median nerve is repaired. Three fascicular groups are usually present at this level, one on the radial aspect containing thenar motor and sensory fibers to the thumb and first web space, and two on the ulnar aspect containing sensory fibers to the second and third web space common digital nerves.[24] Group fascicular technique is thus usually possible.

The ulnar nerve in the wrist and distal forearm is an even more fruitful area for fascicular matching than the median nerve. The dorsal sensory branch should be excluded and repaired with epineurial technique to prevent its fibers from entering the adjacent motor fascicles.[23] It can be separated from the main nerve trunk throughout the forearm if necessary. Motor fibers should then be precisely matched and reunited, using electrical stimulation if visual matching will not suffice. Because of the relatively high segregation of the motor branch and its large size and complex make-up, electrical stimulation may be useful for up to 9 cm proximal to the radial styloid.[23] The remaining sensory fascicles are then repaired as a group.

In the proximal forearm and elbow areas, the most prominent fiber localization results from formation of motor branches to the forearm musculature. These branches can often be localized for several centimeters proximal to their departure from the nerve, and every effort should be made to do so. Group fascicular technique is used on identifiable branches, and epineurial suture for the remainder of the nerve. The one prominent exception to this is the ulnar nerve at the elbow. There are often only three or four fascicles posterior to the epicondyle, and these may be individually matched and sutured. Epineurial suture is most useful proximal to the incorporation of motor branches into the main body of the nerve.

Partial nerve injuries often result from knife or glass lacerations. They are particularly amenable to group or even individual fascicular technique, since orientation is maintained by the intact portion of the nerve and there are fewer injured fascicles to match.

Secondary Repair

The delay of secondary repair imposes conditions that are not encountered with primary suture. The tissue that must be resected to expose healthy axoplasm now includes a neuroma, often involving tissue not initially damaged. Severed nerve ends have also undergone elastic retraction, and are usually fixed in the retracted position by fibrous proliferation. By the time the nerve ends are prepared for suture, they are often separated by several centimeters. Because of the tension required to close this defect, fascicular or group fascicular suture are rarely possible. Epineurial suture, advocated by Seddon[115,117] for secondary repair, remains the standard technique in this setting.

When undertaking secondary repair, one must separate the tasks of preparation and reconstruction. It is imperative to trim the proximal stump back to healthy axoplasm; the success of this maneuver can be assessed with vital dyes or frozen sections. Once stumps are prepared, then worry about how to bridge the gap. It is far better to graft between two healthy stumps than to join two fibrous scars under excessive tension.

Nerve gaps may be overcome by mobilization of the nerve, transposition of the nerve into a new bed, flexing adjacent joints, or shortening the extremity. The extreme limits of mobilization were reported by Zachary,[160] who demonstrated that the median nerve can be mobilized 7 to 9 cm, the ulnar nerve a similar distance routinely and as much as 13 cm when the nerve is transposed. However, Nicholson and Seddon[99] found that extensive mobilization of the median nerve impaired recovery. The tension placed on nerve by subsequent mobilization of flexed joints may also be harmful, causing fibrosis like that seen after traction injury.[49] Mobilization of the proximal nerve end does not appear to be as harmful as mobilization of the distal segment.[118,123] Shortening of the extremity to oppose healthy soft tissues is routinely performed during replantation, but not solely to overcome a nerve gap.

The recent clinical and experimental literature are replete with conflicting opinions on the maximum gap that can be overcome without grafting. Unfortunately, no prospective age-controlled comparisons of gap management techniques are available. Based on personal experience, we use grafts for gaps of 4 cm or greater.

NERVE GRAFTING

In the previous section, we have recommended nerve grafting for gaps of 4 cm or more. Other authors, including Millesi, have recommended grafting for gaps of 2.5 cm or more.[85] Seddon recommended nerve grafting for "large gaps" of nerves.

There are three types of available nerve grafts: heterograft, homograft, and autograft. Heterografts have not been successful. Homografts have enjoyed a limited success, mostly compromised by the immunologic response of the recipient patient. Preserved homografts have been used with some limited success. However, the ultimate fate of the homograft has proved to be an abundance of fibrous tissue, with limited results. Autologous nerve grafts (autografts), on the other hand, preserve the endoneurial structures and contain proliferated Schwann cells that represent an excellent skeleton in which to receive the ingrowing axons.

Historical Review

It is interesting to reexamine the history of nerve grafting, which began in the Listerian era. In November 1866, Lister wrote a letter to his friend, Sir Hector Cameron, about a patient with a tumor of the sciatic nerve. He suggested that after removal of the tumor, it would be worthwhile to form a channel of catgut stitches between the two ends of the nerves so that new nerve tissue might grow down this channel to reinnervate the distal stump. In 1870, Philipeaux and Vulpian performed an experiment in which the lingual nerve was used to bridge a gap in the hypoglossal nerve. In a review of World War I surgery, British surgeons concluded that autogenous grafting was unsuccessful.[13] This effectively set back nerve grafting and retarded progress for approximately 20 years. In 1927 Bunnell published a paper on digital nerve grafting,[20] and in 1942 Sanders reviewed the history of nerve grafting, reported animal experimentation, and prompted a further attempt to use autografts in treatment of patients with large nerve gaps.[110] In 1947 and again in 1963, Seddon reported some measure of success in over 100 patients with nerve grafts.[114,116] The greater successes occurred in children and in the small nerves, such as the digital nerves. Seddon reached an important conclusion: the results of grafting nerve lesions in the digits were far better than secondary suture because the resection of the distal stump could be more generous. This then leads us to the rationale currently employed for nerve grafting.

Millesi, Meissl, and Berger made two important contributions in their experimental work.[87,88] First, the ultimate result of the nerve repair was related to the amount of connective tissue proliferation at the suture site. Inasmuch as epineurium is the primary source of connective tissue at the site of injury to a nerve, they concluded that resection of the epineurium led to less connective tissue (i.e., scarring) at the suture site. Second, these authors concluded that tension at the suture site compromises nerve regeneration and ultimate recovery. This is again related to scar tissue. Tension increases scar tissue and prohibits axonal regeneration. Furthermore, the increased hypertrophied scar tissue due to the tension-ridden nerve juncture causes axonolysis and damage to the already regenerating nerve axons. Millesi, Meissl, and Berger[88] then compared nerve grafting using liberal resection of the damaged ends, epineurectomy, and suture without tension to standard nerve repair with epineurial suture under some tension. They concluded, in this experiment using rabbits, that nerve grafting was better than a suture under tension.

In a second series of experiments, Millesi, Meissl, and Berger[87] transected the sciatic nerves of rabbits, sutured the nerves under normal tension, and then grafted a 5-mm section under normal tension. They found no significant difference in the recovery of the two legs in these animals. They then concluded that under favorable conditions, with no tension, there was no difference between nerve suture and nerve grafting.

Repair Versus Grafting

If one could transform Millesi's experimental data into clinical practice, it might be concluded that a gap in a nerve of 4 cm or more cannot be closed without undue tension and therefore should be grafted. We see gaps of 4 cm in those cases in which nerve tissue has been lost or in secondary cases where the nerve ends have retracted and stuck to adjacent soft tissues. After resection of the neuroma and glioma, the gap is ultimately 4 cm or more and therefore will require a nerve graft. In making the decision to graft, the surgeon should use the operating microscope to examine the cut nerve endings and be absolutely certain that there is a minimum of fibrous tissue and normal fascicular grouping.

We have not seen the situation in which a primary nerve graft should be employed because of wound conditions. However, one might encounter a partially injured nerve in the brachial plexus, such as the lateral cord or a peripheral nerve in the forearm, where there is a significant gap in the injured portion and the normal portion is of normal length. In this unique situation, we could imagine using a primary nerve graft if the conditions are such that one would normally do a primary nerve suture, i.e., those conditions mentioned earlier on page 1320. Thus far in our practice we have not seen an instance where all of these criteria have been met, but we do think it is a theoretical possibility.

Therefore, most if not all nerve grafting will be carried out as a secondary procedure. The surgeon thus has an opportunity to explain to the patient the problem involved and discuss the source of the graft. The appropriate facilities include the operating microscope and a microsurgical team. The surgeon must also study and have a thorough knowledge of the neuroanatomy of the involved peripheral nerve. He must study the charts of Sunderland for the cross-sectional anatomy in the region to be surgically approached. In our experience it has been quite helpful to have Sunderland's charts in the operating room for evaluation after visualization of the cut ends of the nerve. We consider this no reflection on the surgeon's confidence, but rather an indication of one's thoroughness. After the above, careful preparation, the operation should be customized to the individual patient and the individual nerve. Again, we should mention that children will ultimately do far better than adults, and patients over the age of 50 will have limited recovery even with an excellent nerve graft.

Types of Nerve Grafts

There are many types of grafts that can be employed, and a thorough knowledge of all of the types will enable the surgeon to chose the appropriate one for each situation. We prefer different types of grafts in various situations, depending on the size of the recipient nerve, the fascicular structure, and the location in the extremity.

Trunk Graft

The trunk graft uses a whole segment of nerve interposed between the proximal and distal cut ends of the damaged nerve (Fig. 35-5). Trunk grafts have not enjoyed a high success rate because in the revascularization process the center of the trunk graft has become fibrotic and the regenerating axons have been limited in the distal nerve stump. However, Seddon stated that predegeneration may improve this situation. Wallerian degeneration involves intense metabolic activity, but if it has already taken place, as in the predegenerated graft, the metabolic requirements of the degenerated nerve are minimal. In large trunk grafts, such as might be employed for the radial nerve, I do recommend predegenerating the trunk graft, if at all possible. In such a situation the distal sensory branch of the radial nerve is, by definition, already degenerated and makes an ideal graft source. I usually use an already degenerated donor nerve as my graft source in these cases. In an unusual case, I have used a trunk graft from a damaged extremity, predegenerated it by local nerve division, and 4 weeks later taken the distal predegenerated nerve as a graft. This technique has only been used for trunk grafts, however.

In our experience, trunk grafts are used mainly in salvage situations where one is attempting to restore the median nerve and may use the already damaged distal ulnar nerve for recon-

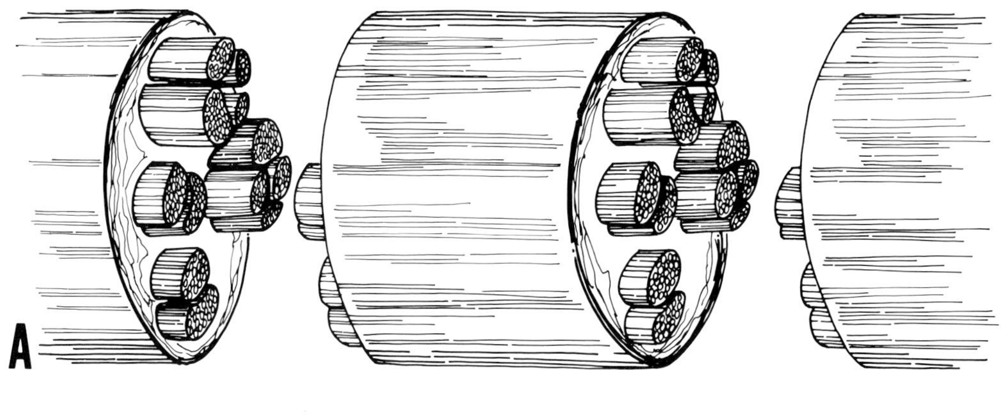

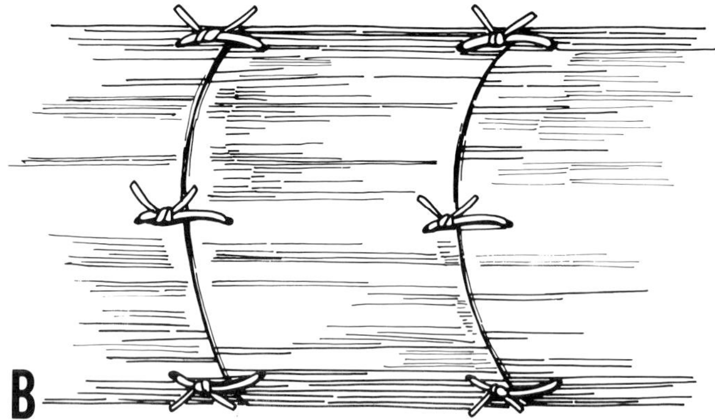

Fig. 35-5. Trunk nerve graft.

stitution of the median nerve. In replacing one or two cords, we have had excellent results using the ulnar nerve as a trunk graft for brachial plexus lesions. One must be careful not to use a trunk graft for reconstruction when sacrificing the distal nerve precludes a more reasonable attempt at total reconstruction. However, in the isolated circumstance of a high median and ulnar nerve lesion, the surgeon may consider sacrificing the predegenerated distal ulnar nerve to graft the median nerve if he or she has decided to concentrate on the median supply to the hand. We have used this approach in hands with the ring and little fingers damaged beyond reconstruction, in which our reconstructive efforts are concentrated on the thumb and index and middle fingers.

Cable Graft

The cable graft is mentioned primarily for historical interest, since other measures have essentially supplanted this technique. A cable was formed by uniting the strands of nerve graft into a unit and then suturing the unit in the gap to the proximal and distal stumps. This has limited success because of the low rate of precise anatomic continuity. However, it is encouraging to note that in Seddon's cases where a cable graft was used for the repair of partial lesions, there was only one failure out of 11 cases. There were also 45 successes out of 53 cases in his later group. He attributed this to many children being included in this group.[114,116]

Pedicle Nerve Graft

When both median and ulnar nerves are damaged, the ulnar nerve may be used as a pedicle graft to repair the median as described by Strange.[124,125] In the first surgical stage, the proximal stumps of median and ulnar nerves are joined to make a "U," and the ulnar nerve is divided far proximally to allow ulnar axons to degenerate while maintaining blood supply to the graft segment. Several months are allowed for median axons to grow through the degenerated ulnar segment, and for the segment to acquire additional blood supply through its juncture with the median nerve. At a second operation the ulnar graft is then swung down, based on its proximal juncture to the median nerve, and joined to the distal median stump. This procedure restores protective sensibility in the median distribution, but two-point discrimination and intrinsic muscle function are not achieved.[42]

Interfascicular Nerve Graft

In spite of the encouraging results reported by Seddon and others, nerve grafting in this country did not enjoy much popularity until the introduction of microneurosurgery and the interfascicular nerve grafting technique as described by Millesi[87] (Fig. 35-6). In using the anatomic principles of groups of fascicles, the interfascicular nerve graft (a better name perhaps is the grouped fascicular nerve graft) employs strands of grafted nerve between groups of fascicles appropriately dissected out and identified. For a successful grouped fascicular nerve graft the following conditions must be met: (1) the wound must be supple, (2) there must be an adequate vascularized bed in which the nerve graft has to lie, (3) the nerve ends must be adequately resected so that there is no scar tissue in the proximal stump, and (4) the nerve ends must be joined by a number of nerve grafts placed in the appropriate anatomic fashion without tension.

A wide exposure is used in this technique, with the tourniquet inflated. The dissection is done from the normal to abnormal tissue, attempting not to disturb the scar tissue in the pathologic site. The whole concept of the operation is to bridge normal nerve to normal nerve tissue. After the stumps are exposed, the operating microscope is employed, and the epineurium is inspected and incised just proximal to the neuroma and the dense scar. The investing epineurium is excised for a distance of approximately 1.5 cm, and then, using the anatomic structure and the operating microscope, one can appropriately map the groups of fascicles and separate these groups in the proximal nerve stump. Each fascicular group is transected at a different level so as not to make a circumferential scar. A similar procedure is done to the distal stump. The entire scarred neuroma and glioma need not be removed, but the nerve grafts must lie in an adequately vascularized bed.

After this dissection, which is tedious and time-consuming, the tourniquet is released and bleeders are electrocoagulated. The arm is then carefully wrapped in a slight compressive dressing while a search for the appropriate donor nerves is done. The sources of nerve graft are discussed in a separate section, but usually cutaneous nerves are used, the sural nerves being the appropriate first choice. After obtaining the donor nerve graft material, these wounds are closed and attention is then redirected to the upper extremity. A map is made of the proximal and distal nerve stumps, depicting the fascicular groups. These groups are then matched according to the maps that are drawn at the operating table, and the nerve graft is interposed between the fascicular groups. Mapping is relatively easy in small defects. However, in large defects (greater than 7 to 10 cm) there can be considerable variation in the fascicular anatomy between the two cut ends, and the best educated guess must be made, according to distribution of the fascicular groups and the different quadrants that might be united with those of the distal stump. Thus, fascicular grouping lessens the margin of error that would be encountered if "pure" fascicular grafting were undertaken. It is important to cut the donor nerve approximately 15 percent longer than the recipient defect to minimize the effective tension and to make the juncture easier. The epineurium must be retracted back from the ends so that it does not become interposed between the cut surfaces of the nerves and nerve grafts. The grafts are then placed between the corresponding fascicular groups. Exact, but loose approximation is used.

One or two 10-0 nylon sutures in each graft are usually sufficient to achieve this union. Hemostasis must be carefully maintained so as not to allow any hematoma between the cut ends of the nerve. Usually the graft on the farthest side from the operator is done first so that one does not disturb the existing grafts that are already in place. After completion of the entire grafting procedure, the wound is very carefully closed so as not to disrupt the grafts. The skin is closed and the limb is immobilized in the position in which the grafts were placed. Nor-

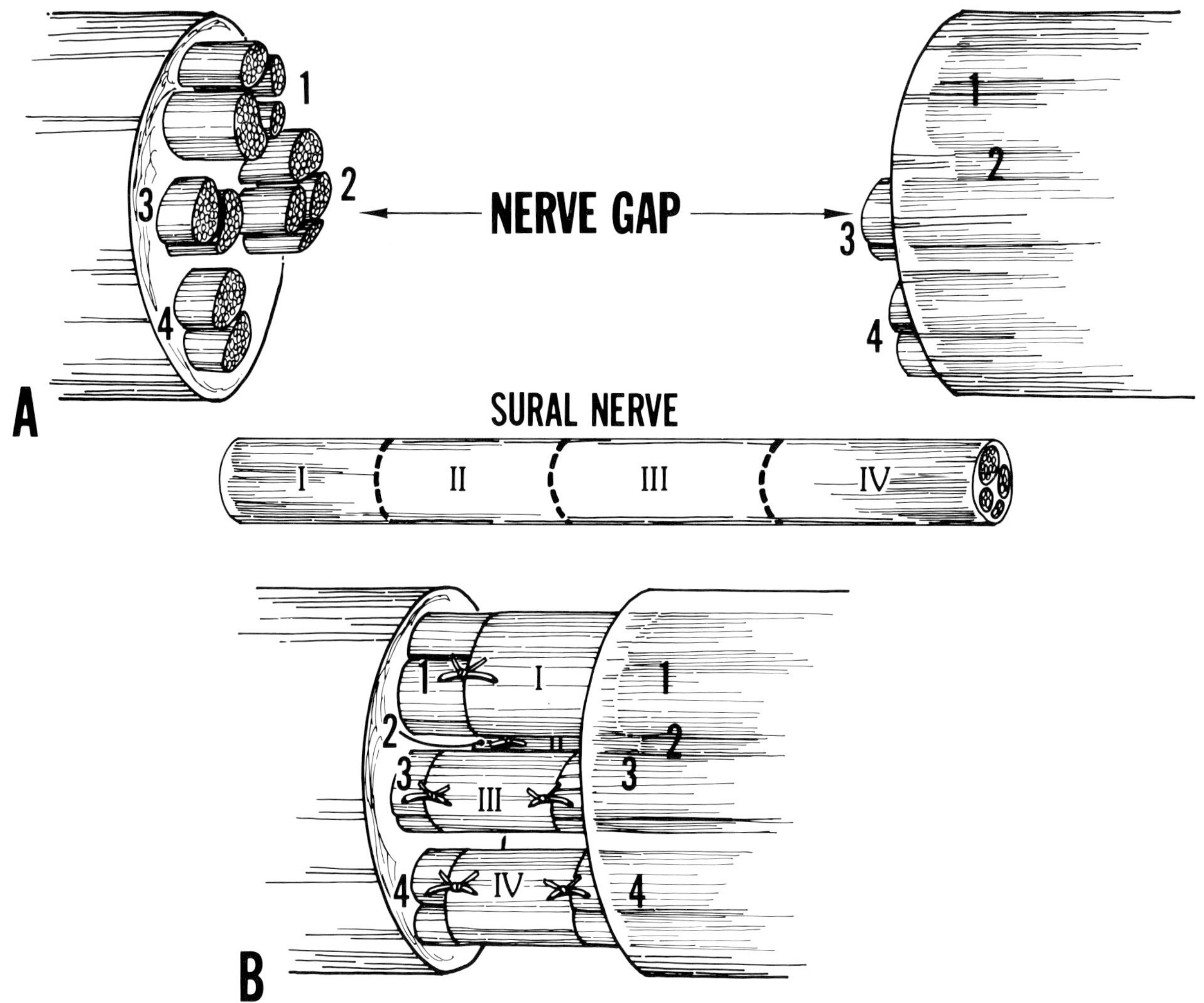

Fig. 35-6. Grouped fascicular (interfascicular) nerve graft.

mally we prefer to have the wrist in neutral position and the elbow in slight flexion. Immobilization is maintained for 10 days, at which time the dressings are removed, the wound is inspected, sutures are removed (if ready), and motion can be begun. Motion, however, is restricted to very gentle motion for another 3 weeks.

The surgeon should expect an advancing Tinel's sign beginning 4 weeks postoperatively, and then subsequently carefully trace the Tinel's sign as it advances through the proximal and distal nerve sutures. In grafts of more than 10 cm, there is sometimes a retardation of axonal regrowth over the second suture line due to scarring, and, if the Tinel's sign does not advance appropriately over the second suture line, a resection of the more distal suture line should be done and primary nerve suture accomplished. I recommend resection of the distal suture site if the Tinel's sign, which had been advancing at the rate of 1 mm/day, ceases progression and is stationary for two return visits over a 2-month period. This is a rare occurrence, but it may salvage a satisfactory reconstruction out of one doomed to failure. Electrical testing is of little use until the Tinel's sign advances to a point where one would normally see motor reinnervation.

A review of Millesi's results with this technique shows that in young patients, below age 30, 60 percent achieved useful motor recovery with defects of 6 cm. Forty percent achieved excellent sensory recovery. The ulnar nerve results showed 50 percent achieving excellent motor recovery and approximately 30 percent achieving excellent sensory recovery. These defects were in the range of 4 to 6 cm. In defects greater than 6 cm, the results tailed off considerably, but there were isolated instances where very useful recovery was obtained from grouped fascicular nerve grafting in long defects. These defects were essentially irreparable by any other means.

Fascicular Nerve Graft

There are few indications for fascicular nerve grafts because the chances of matching corresponding fascicles decrease as the number of fascicles in the nerve increases. However, we have described fascicular nerve grafting in the distal digital nerve beyond the level of the DIP joint.[148] In this series, 11 patients were treated with 12 fascicular nerve grafts at the level of or beyond the terminal trifurcation of the digital nerve. These grafts all extended to a point beyond the DIP joint. All patients had improved sensibility. The technique is depicted in Figure 35-7. The small nerve graft is sutured to the proximal digital-nerve stump and then sutured distally into each individual fascicle of the trifurcated nerve. We have subsequently performed over 20 of these nerve grafts, and the donor site of choice at the present time is the terminal articular branch of the posterior interosseous nerve at the wrist (Fig. 35-8).

Free Vascularized Nerve Graft

Taylor and Ham introduced the free vascularized nerve graft in an attempt to prevent ischemic graft failure.[138] Initial experience with this technique in scarred beds was promising, yet results and indications have remained controversial. Bonney et al[10] reviewed 12 cases of brachial plexus reconstruction with microsurgically revascularized nerve grafts, and could only report an "impression" of improved recovery; Gilbert[39] and Merle et al[84] found no superiority of free vascularized grafting over routine sural grafts.

The many variables of plexus injury and repair make comparison of technique extremely difficult in this area. In the digital nerve, however, evaluation is more straightforward. Rose and Kowalski[109] reported five patients in whom nonvascularized nerve grafts had failed, and who could therefore serve as their own controls. Free vascularized deep peroneal nerve grafts, averaging 6.6 cm in length, restored an average two-point discrimination of 9.5 mm. The authors recommended the procedure for salvage of sensation in the thumb or radial surface of the primary opposing digit. Although free vascularized nerve grafting remains a time consuming, investigational technique, it may be indicated for digital or extremity salvage, especially when graft material is available from an already damaged or amputated part.

Source of Grafts

The source of the donor nerve should be chosen with great care.[135] The sural nerve in the posterior aspect of the lower leg represents the best source of graft material in the majority of series (Fig. 35-9).

In positioning the patient for operation, the posterior aspect of the leg must be accessible to the surgeon. For short grafts where one sural nerve is being used, the semilateral position with support under the shoulder and hip contralateral to the operated hand will give access to the contralateral leg. If both sural nerves must be obtained, it is necessary to place the pa-

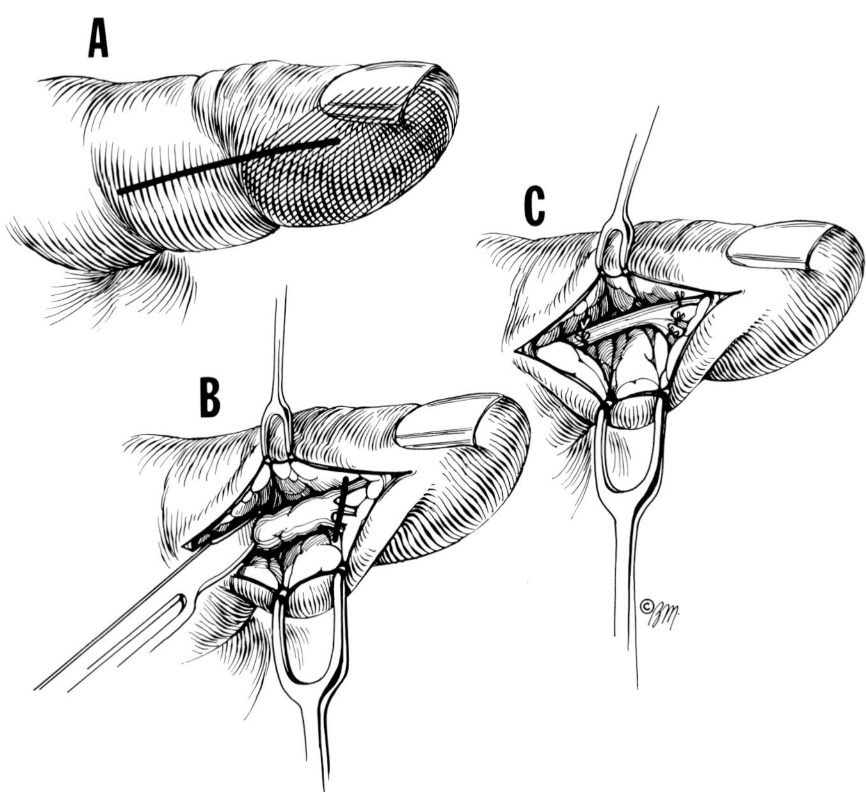

Fig. 35-7. Distal digital fascicular graft. **(A)** Incision line (shaded area indicates insensible region). **(B)** Resection of neuroma. **(C)** Graft to individual terminal fascicles.

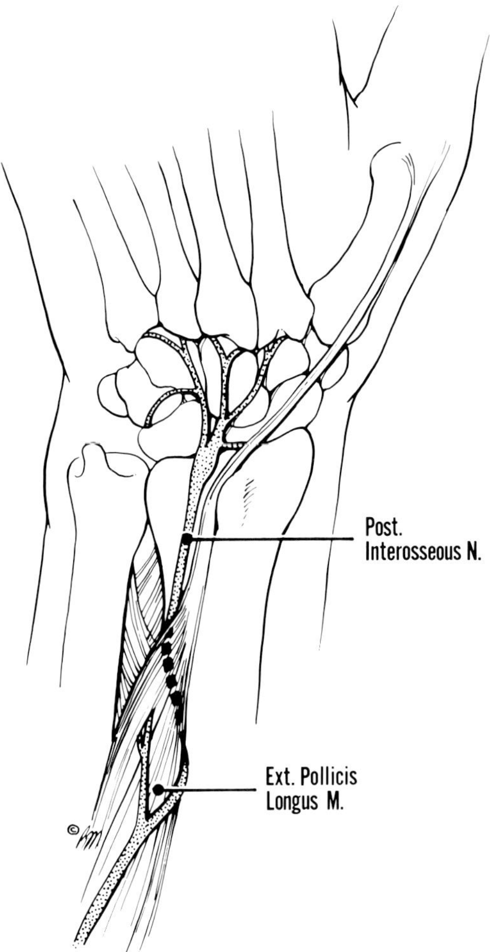

Fig. 35-8. Source of graft—terminal articular branches of posterior interosseous nerve (see text for details).

tient prone, obtain the grafts, and then turn the patient over to the usual position for the operative procedure on the hand. The surgeon, however, must be certain that a graft is feasible before removing the donor nerves. This may require repositioning during the operation.

The sural nerve can be found in the popliteal space just lateral to the lesser saphenous vein proximally, and it lies posterior to the lateral malleolus in the ankle. It may divide in the calf region. It is a little easier to identify the sural nerve distally and trace it proximally, using either a longitudinal or several transverse incisions. Up to 40 cm of graft material can be obtained by this technique. The fasciculi are tightly packed in the interfascicular tissue, which is small in amount, thereby making this an excellent graft source. There are many other cutaneous nerves that can be used.

The medial and lateral antebrachial cutaneous nerves (Fig. 35-10), as well as the distal median and ulnar nerves, have been used for the grafting of digital nerves.[79] It should be noted, however, that these grafts have more interfascicular tissue than the sural nerve, and are thus theoretically a less desirable graft source. The antebrachial cutaneous nerves lie in the subcutaneous tissue adjacent to the basilic (medial) and cephalic (lateral) veins in the proximal forearm. They are obtained through oblique incisions in the proximal forearm using the veins as landmarks.

The terminal branch of the posterior interosseous nerve (see Fig. 35-8) has been used for the most distal digital nerve graft or as a single fascicular strand that can be used to replace one fascicle of the digital nerve. The use of this nerve is limited, but there is no deficit from taking the nerve as it is in articular branch, and, for this reason, it is the prime choice of donor graft for a very small nerve.[28]

The posterior interosseous nerve is found at the wrist level, lying on the interosseous membrane deep to the extensor tendons. As it branches distally, it usually lies just ulnar and deep to the deep pollicis longus tendon and muscle. This nerve is obtained by a longitudinal dorsal wrist incision. After opening the deep fascia, retraction of the extensor tendons reveals the nerve lying on the interosseous membrane. Care should be taken to preserve the extensor retinaculum.

Other cutaneous nerves, such as the lateral and posterior nerves of the thigh, can be used. The greatest amount of interfascicular tissue is found here, and there is considerable separation of the fascicles, limiting the use of these nerves as donors.

The superficial radial nerve is an excellent graft source in that the epineurial tissue is small in amount and the fascicles

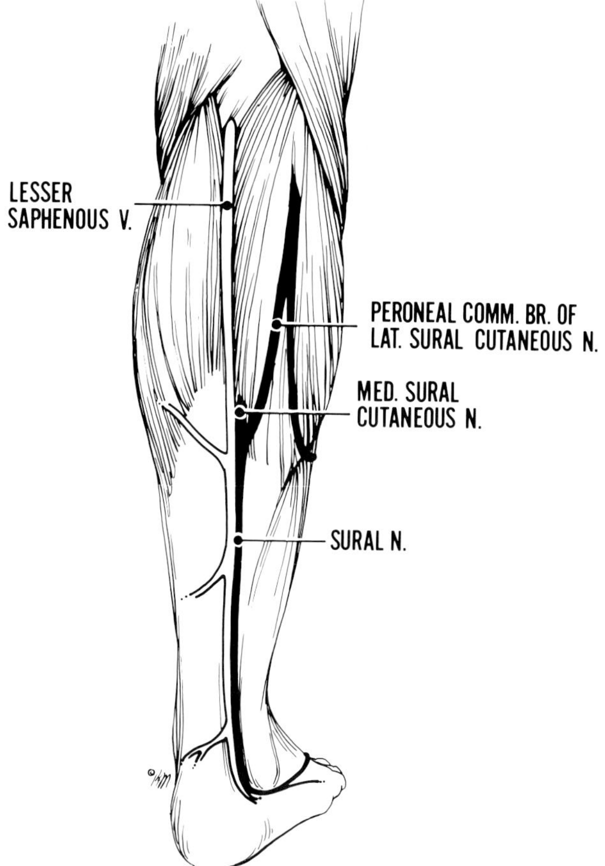

Fig. 35-9. Source of graft—sural nerve (see text for details).

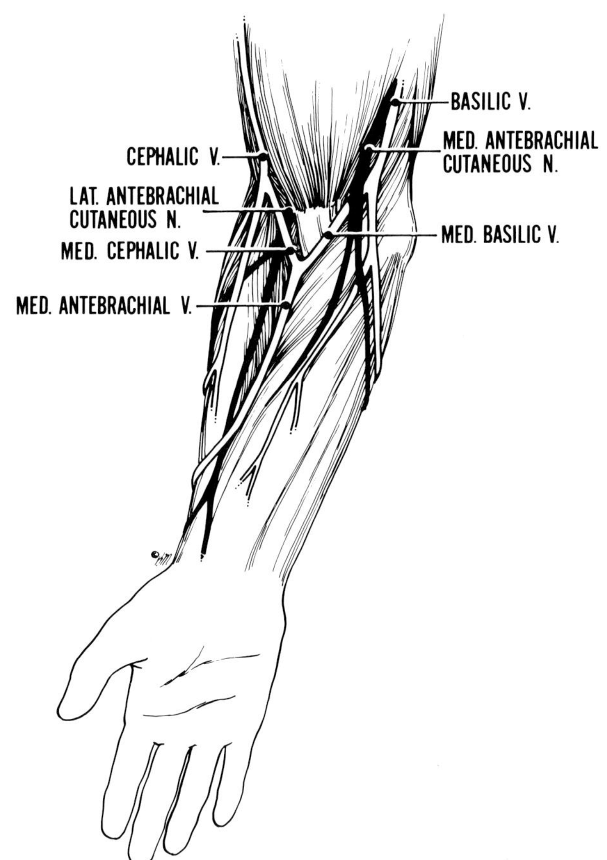

Fig. 35-10. Source of graft—medial and lateral antebrachial cutaneous nerves (see text for details).

are tightly packed. However, the deficit from removing this is significant in the hand, especially in those hands with a concomitant median nerve injury; this nerve should never be taken for a graft in a patient with a median nerve deficit. The ideal use of the superficial radial nerve is in the high radial nerve lesion that requires grafting. It is an excellent choice because the deficit is already present prior to excision of the superficial radial nerve, and this nerve is already predegenerated.

The dorsal branch of the ulnar nerve can similarly be used because one can obtain approximately 15 cm of nerve graft tissue. The deficit of numbness on the dorsum of the hand is not significant in the face of an intact median nerve, and this nerve can similarly be used for the same reasons as the superficial radial nerve to bridge small ulnar nerve defects in the forearm.

Choice of Type of Nerve Graft

The choice of the type of graft depends on the localization of the injury and the preference of the surgeon. In high injuries, we recommend interfascicular, or grouped fascicular, grafting and, in the most distal injuries, fascicular grafting. The donor graft must be chosen with care and the patient must be fully apprised of the deficit that will result from the choice of the donor graft. This is most important, and one of us (E.F.S.W.) has reported a prospective series of 28 nerve grafts in which the patients were questioned before and after the operation.[85] In a high percentage of cases, the patient did not fully understand the deficit that would result, and in a few cases, the deficit was greater than anticipated. A preoperative block of the graft source of the donor graft can be helpful to the surgeon in explaining the ultimate deficit that will occur.

In our opinion, at the present time autogenous grafting is preferable to any other type available.[77] One must be aware of the anatomic structures, the anatomic crossover, and the interfascicular anatomic pattern of the nerve before attempting to bridge a defect with a nerve graft. The nerve graft must be placed in a suitable bed so that vascularization will occur. The surgeon must be aware that tension at the suture line is undesirable and that the interval between injury and grafting should be as short as possible. If return of motor power is to be expected, grafting must be done before a 6-month interval after injury has elapsed. However, protective sensation can be restored after months or even years following injury.

Although there have been some reports on wrapping the suture lines, there are no real clinical indications that this has been beneficial, and at the present time no part of the suture line nor the graft should be wrapped with a foreign material. However, taking all of these considerations into account, we prefer to use a grouped fascicular graft for defects of 4 cm in the median and ulnar nerve and for defects of smaller lengths in the digital nerves.

NEUROMA-IN-CONTINUITY

A neuroma-in-continuity of a major peripheral nerve in the upper extremity presents perhaps the greatest challenge to the managing surgeon. This is because such a lesion may initially be a partial one with sparing of a variable amount of important distal function; or when complete, may in some cases have the potential for spontaneous regeneration and restoration of function; while in other cases, no potential for recovery exists without resection and repair.

The main problem with a neuroma-in-continuity is its unpredictability. The biggest challenge to the treating physician is to utilize all of the available techniques, both surgical and nonsurgical, to arrive at a decision that would accurately predict either recovery without resection and repair or the need for such. It is important to realize that at least 60 percent of nerve injuries, even in civilian practice, do not transect the nerve, but leave it with some degree of continuity.[60] The location of a neuroma-in-continuity in relation to the extremity is another important consideration. A more proximal neuroma-in-continuity will present with a much more mixed distal lesion because of the fascicular arrangement of the proximal nerve; however, in the more distal part of the extremity, a clearer picture of the condition of the nerve may be elicited. Thus, partial lesions of the distal nerves are more likely to damage a fascicle destined for one or more specific distal sites, whereas proximal partial injuries are more likely to damage a cross section of fibers destined for many distal end organs.

Another crucial factor in managing a neuroma-in-continuity is the time element between injury and expected recovery. This is particularly true in the motor system because motor end plates as described earlier in this chapter begin to disintegrate after denervation and have no reinnervation potential after a period of 2 years. The reinnervation potential diminishes dramatically after 9 months. Therefore, it is critical to set time limits for decision making in watching the neuroma-in-continuity because it is very easy to be lulled into a sense of unwarranted optimism watching a portion of the nerve recover and not realizing that perhaps a more important portion of the nerve is *not* recovering. The neuroma-in-continuity can have all levels of axonal injury within the given nerve, including axonal disruption with no hope of regeneration and a physiologic impairment of conduction that has full potential for recovery. To reiterate, when managing a neuroma-in-continuity, the surgeon must take into account the elapsed time from injury and the proposed time of recovery when planning surgery. The total time must not exceed 2 years. This is particularly true in brachial plexus injuries, where recovery could approach 18 months.

Evaluation

The evaluation of a neuroma-in-continuity should include (1) a precise knowledge of the wounding agent, (2) careful and frequent evaluation, (3) the use of Tinel's test, and (4) electrodiagnosis.

Mechanism of Injury

A precise knowledge of the wounding agent is important, and careful examination should be done. Sharp injuries, while likely to lead to transection, sometimes leave the nerve in gross continuity and some of these can recover without resection and suture. Gunshot wounds and crush injuries or nerve contusions due to local open fractures are more likely to recover spontaneously.

Clinical Examination

The necessity for careful and frequent clinical evaluation is paramount to be sure that the nerve is regenerating. I would recommend evaluation at monthly intervals since more frequent evaluation will sometimes cloud the issue by presenting conflicting data. Many times a therapist performing periodic objective sensory and motor evaluation can aid the clinician in this.

Tinel's Test

Tinel's sign is another valuable tool that has been and is still used by many clinicians to signify regeneration. This is a valuable test but only as long as its limitations are kept in mind. Tinel's test is based on the irritability of fine regenerating fibers. Tapping over the course of the nerve where such fibers are present produces paresthesias or tingling in the distribution of the nerves; this signifies regeneration and is a positive sign.[141] Unfortunately such fibers may or may not subsequently increase enough in caliber or gain enough myelination to lead to useful function. A Tinel's sign that is obtained well distal to the injury site tells us that fine fibers have regenerated to that point; its continued progression down the distal course of the nerve would suggest further regeneration, although it does not guarantee functional recovery. A Tinel's sign that cannot be elicited below the injury site 3 to 4 months after injury or suture would mean that not even fine fibers have reached the point being tapped. Thus, the absence of a Tinel's sign distal to the injury becomes an important negative finding that supports the need for exploration.

Electrodiagnosis

Another set of useful diagnostic tools utilizes electrodiagnosis. Electromyography (EMG) tests the innervation of muscles. Signs of denervation, such as fibrillations and denervation potentials, can be seen 2 to 4 weeks after serious injury, the length of interval depending on how far the lesion is from the muscle being tested. If muscles in the distribution of the injured nerve do not show denervational changes, one must make sure that the innervation is not coming from adjacent nerves. With reinput of axons into muscle and some motor endplate reconstruction, the electromyographer finds an increase in insertional activity and a decrease in the number of fibrillations and denervation potentials. If signs of reinnervation in proximal muscles are seen by EMG, they should progress with time into more distal muscles and not remain relegated to one muscle or one set of muscles. However, it should be cautioned that electromyographic evidence of regeneration does not guarantee subsequent useful clinical function because electromyography is a physiologic rather than a functional test. Nonetheless, electromyograms done in a careful and serial fashion can provide valuable information as long as the temporal and interpretive limitations of the test are understood.

Conduction studies are an additional electrodiagnostic aid. However, conduction studies done in the usual fashion are not helpful in the more serious and complete nerve injuries and are mostly used in mild or partial injuries. Nerve action potentials, postulated by Kline,[61,63,65] on the other hand, have been helpful. These are obtained in a noninvasive fashion by stimulating above and below the lesion and then amplifying the response and summing them up by computer. Nerve action potentials of early regeneration can sometimes be recorded. This technique works best for median, ulnar, and some radial nerve lesions, but can be used to stimulate and record from elements distal to the injury where the brachial plexus is involved. This test, along with the other electrical tests, must be used in conjunction with careful clinical observation. No decision should be made exclusively on the presence or absence of a positive noninvasive electrical test. A further electrical test, involving noninvasive evaluation of spinal cord or peripheral nerve–evoked responses, is a useful adjunct to more accurate preoperative delineation of brachial plexus injuries. This technique, popularized by Van Beek,[143] uses the fact that brachial plexus avulsion produces Wallerian degeneration in motor axons only. Some sensory axons are intact because the central cell location is outside the cord. Therefore, a nerve action potential will be transmitted by a sensory axon. Because avulsion has occurred, a spinal cord–evoked response could not be present. All of these electrical aids can be more useful in the operative setting where direct stimulus of the nerve and more accurate recording can be effected.

Surgical Management

If a decision is reached that the state of the neuroma-in-continuity of a given peripheral nerve will not allow sufficient and useful regeneration, then operative intervention becomes necessary. Many times this decision is precipitated by the time factor. The clinician will just not be able to make a total determination even from the clinical and noninvasive studies and will have to make a surgical decision because the available recovery time has elapsed from the time of injury. The patient should be apprised of the various possibilities that may arise at the time of exploration, including neurolysis or resection with either suture repair or nerve grafting of a portion of or the entire nerve.

At surgery, careful proximal and distal exposure of the suspected lesion-in-continuity is essential. Exposure should be generous, and dissection of the lesion itself delayed until both proximal and distal elements have been isolated and identified. Longitudinal blood supply to the nerve should be preserved, but most collaterals can be sacrificed so that a 360-degree exposure of the nerve itself can be obtained. If the neuroma is fusiform, enlargement of up to twice the normal diameter can be compatible with a lesion of the nerve in the Sunderland Grades I–III[130] (Table 35-1). Swelling larger than that favors a Sunderland IV or V lesion. Firmness or hardness suggests a heavy internal scar and total nerve division. In general, the internal architecture of the neuroma is almost always worse than it appears on inspection or palpation. A lateral neuroma suggests partial transection. The injection of saline or other physiologic solutions into lesions-in-continuity in an attempt to delineate fascicles has not proven beneficial because much of the scar preventing regeneration is intrafascicular rather than perineural. We do not advise injecting anything into the nerve to determine the advisability of resection.

After inspection and palpation of the lesion, the nerve can be stimulated both proximal and distal to the lesion to see if muscle function proximal and distal to the lesion can be observed. The standard nerve stimulators in most operating rooms are useful for this technique.[53]

Table 35-1. Sunderland's Grades of Nerve Injury[131]

Grade I
- Interruption of axonal conduction at the site of injury.
- Axonal continuity is preserved.
- There may be segmental demyelinization without Wallerian degeneration.
- This condition is totally reversible.

Grade II
- The axon is severed and the axon fails to survive below the level of injury and for a variable, but short distance proximal to it.
- The endoneurium is preserved.
- Full recovery is expected.

Grade III
- The axon is severed and disintegrated with Wallerian degeneration.
- Endoneurial tube continuity is lost and disorganization of the internal structure of the fascicles occurs (this is the typical traction lesion).
- Recovery is slower and is usually incomplete.

Grade IV
- Total destruction of the internal architecture of the nerve with continuity of the nerve trunk preserved through the epineurium.
- A neuroma forms in this injury.
- Spontaneous recovery can occur, but rarely proceeds to a useful degree.
- This fourth degree injury is an indication for surgical repair of the nerve.

Grade V
- There is loss of continuity of the nerve trunk.
- Surgical repair is mandatory for any useful recovery.

Intraoperative Electrodiagnostic Studies

Intraoperative electrodiagnostic techniques using either nerve action potentials or evoked responses are very helpful.[57,58] The surgeon faced with the need for this very sophisticated technique should either be familiar with the instrumentation and technique or have a working relationship with an electromyographer who can attend at the operative session. While there are some surgeons with particular research interest in this field, most clinical surgeons must maintain a relationship with an electromyographer. The equipment used is the standard, commercially available equipment for electrodiagnosis. A special probe for direct stimulation of the nerve can be modified for existing equipment or by using the probe from an existing nerve stimulator. The electromyographer can assist the surgeon with any modification necessary. In the operating room, there must be a dearth of background electrical activity. Most modern operating rooms are well grounded, but it is best to try the machine in the operating room prior to the clinical situation. Sometimes one operating room in a corner of an operating suite is more conducive to this method of diagnosis than one in the center of the operating suite due to the background electrical activity. The electromyographer can be scheduled to come into the operating room at the appointed time and does not necessarily need to be available during the whole procedure. As the equipment is fairly portable, it can be stored on a cart and be brought readily into the operating room. In our experience, the electromyographer's time is usually no longer than 30 minutes. Kline[60,61,63,65,66] has popularized intraoperative nerve action potential recordings across lesions-in-continuity. Those lesions with flat traces will require resection while those with evoked nerve action potentials need only neurolysis. Kline has been able to do partial repairs because only a portion of the element is regenerating and is responsible for the recorded nerve action potential. In a more distal neuroma-in-continuity, axons may regenerate through a lesion well into the distal stump, and yet be months away from a measurable distal input. For many years, Kline has recorded nerve action potentials across all of these injuries and has reported that this technique is a great aid in decision-making. Therefore, with the lesion exposed, both the stimulating and recording electrodes are placed proximally; if the stimulating and recording system is working correctly, a nerve action potential should be recorded from the proximal stump. In rare circumstances, stretch or lengthy contusions of the nerve extending above the lesion site will make recording of a healthy proximal nerve action potential difficult. Once the nerve action potential is recorded proximally, the recording electrode is moved distally beyond the lesion to see if a nerve action potential can be evoked through the area of injury. If a potential is recorded immediately distal to the neuroma-in-continuity, recording electrodes are moved further down the distal stump to see how far the potential, and presumably, the regenerating fibers of adequate size, have extended. If a nerve action potential cannot be recorded distal to the injury, voltage and amplification are gradually increased until it is difficult to visualize that portion of the trace following the stimulus artifact. Attention should be paid to electrode contact, and blood should be irrigated away from the region of the electrodes. It is generally best to elevate the nerve away from surrounding soft tissue by means of the electrodes, but if need be, the nerve can be stimulated and recorded by isolating short segments on either side of the lesion and placing the electrodes on them.[151]

Van Beek[143] used a technique in which cutaneous EEG electrodes are placed in the midfrontal area for reference, deltoid area for ground, C-4 posterior neck for recording spinal cord–evoked response, and Erb's point for recording peripheral nerve–evoked response. The stimulating electrodes are positioned in the operative field and mechanically held. The wide separation of the intraoperative stimulator electrode and the cutaneously applied recording electrode permits separation between the stimulus artifact and the recording evoked response. The whole nerve, groups of fascicles, or fascicles can be stimulated and the recordings can be made using cutaneous recording electrodes placed at appropriate monitoring sites. In this technique, nerve dissection is minimized. Both measurements of a nerve's compound action potential from a nerve field by direct electrode application or measurement of a response from a far field taking advantage of volume conduction are possible with a computerized system. Van Beek[143] reported that electrically stimulating a nerve during the operation and then recording the evoked response has been useful in approximately 40 percent of his neuroma-in-continuity cases. In his experience the surgical management was altered because of the intraoperative findings.

One of the limitations of this particular technique is that there currently is a lack of definitive criteria to determine the appropriate surgical treatment. Any evoked response across the neuroma seems to mandate neurolysis, and the lack of a response, resection and repair. In Van Beek's[143] series he would not resect nerve segments producing greater than 40 μV evoked response across an injury using direct recording techniques. Using the cutaneous recording technique, normal amplitude ranges between 0.5 and 2.0 μV depending on the nerve and the recording site.

Neurolysis Versus Resection

By using all of the available maneuvers, including inspection, palpation, nerve stimulation, direct recording across the site, and distant recording through a cutaneous electrode, the surgeon can gather much useful information. The ultimate decision on whether to neurolyse or resect the neuroma-in-continuity must be made after distillation of all of the above information and not on one single determination. If a neuroma-in-continuity is large, appears very hard, and has no electrical activity across the area that can be determined, then resection is clearly the treatment of choice. If electrical activity can be discerned and even some muscle contraction noted, then neurolysis is clearly the choice. In the grey area between these two alternatives, all of the factors must be taken into the decision-making process.

Neurolysis

If neurolysis is considered, the nerve must be exposed and, with sufficient magnification, the epineurium carefully opened and resected. All scarred tissue should be removed. Internal dissection of the nerve, however, should be discouraged if there is any danger of fascicular interruption with the surgical technique. Sometimes groups of fascicles can be separated and intrafascicular scar removed. Once done, the local bed of a neurolysed nerve must be evaluated. The scar tissue that will form around the nerve postoperatively as a result of the surgical intervention will sometimes interfere with nerve regeneration. Therefore, if the local muscle bed is not adequate, the use of a local muscle as a bed for an injured nerve or to change the environment of the nerve will allow that nerve to recover with minimal scar tissue.[117,130] This is particularly true if the scarring between the fascia, subcutaneous tissue, and nerves can be eliminated. The nerve, once neurolysed, must regain its normal excursion in the local bed to maintain its ultimate function. In the brachial plexus, a local muscle flap including the pectoral, sternocleidomastoid, and latissimus dorsi can be used to preserve an adequate bed and change the environment from a scarred bed to a more natural environment for the recovering nerve. In the upper arm and forearm, local muscles usually surround the nerve and can be utilized to improve the bed. The ulnar nerve at the elbow would normally be transposed in a submuscular position to improve its bed. Throughout the forearm, the large muscle groups also serve to protect the nerve.

Muscle Flaps for Nerve Coverage

At the level of the wrist, however, there are no muscles covering the nerves, but there are several muscle flaps that can be utilized. The pronator quadratus flap initially described by MacKinnon and Dellon[27] is created by mobilizing the pronator quadratus muscle from the volar aspect of the wrist to cover neuromas-in-continuity of the median or ulnar nerves proximal to the wrist crease. This muscle is a small, flat quadrilateral muscle extending across the volar aspect of the distal radius and ulna. The muscle is supplied by a branch of the volar interosseous artery and nerve, and acts as a pronator of the forearm. However, its removal causes patients to lose pronator ability only when the elbow is markedly flexed or if there is an absence or dysfunction of the pronator teres. The pronator quadratus can be detached from the radius and ulna and elevated to cover either the median or ulnar nerve. More distally, the abductor digiti minimi (ADM) muscle can provide a useful flap to cover neuromas-in-continuity of the ulnar or median nerve distal to the wrist crease and in the region of the carpal canal, as first described by Milward et al.[89] The ADM is a broad, fleshy muscle that arises at the pisiform and ends at a flat tendon inserting at the base of the proximal phalanx of the little finger. It is supplied by a branch of the ulnar nerve and a branch of the ulnar artery and can be mobilized on this neurovascular bundle to cover neuromas-in-continuity throughout the wrist and into the palm. The lumbrical muscle flap described by Wilgis[147] can be used by taking one of the lumbrical muscles on its neurovascular bundle, which arises from the common digital artery and nerve, detaching it from the profundus tendon and using it to cover neuromas-in-continuity of the common and proper digital nerves.

Summary of Surgical Management

When faced with a neuroma-in-continuity the surgeon must develop a time-based protocol for its management. Monthly examinations, with electrical studies interspersed, will aid in the diagnostic management. At critical points the surgeon must make a decision whether operative intervention is necessary. Once this decision is reached, and it frequently is triggered by the time factor—a limit of recovery time—then the surgeon must have a prescribed protocol for treatment during the operation consisting of exposure of the lesion, nerve stimulation, recording techniques, and a clear plan whether neurolysis alone or resection of the neuroma-in-continuity and grafting will be necessary. If resection must be employed, then it is rare that an end-to-end suture can be effected without severe nerve mobilization and flexion of the adjacent joints. One would then resort to nerve grafting techniques as described elsewhere in this chapter.

REHABILITATION OF PATIENTS WITH NERVE REPAIRS

No chapter on the reconstruction of nerve injuries can be complete without a section on rehabilitation and end evaluation of nerve surgery.[155] We think it should be stated at the outset that Onne and others have shown that the ultimate result of nerve suture and/or graft cannot be appropriately evaluated until a period of 3 or possibly 5 years has elapsed.[104] Therefore, the reader should note that most of the series presented in the literature today have had inadequate follow-up.

In the proper evaluation of end results of nerve repair and grafting, the other intact nerves must be anesthetized so that any overlap in sensory or motor input can be eliminated. As an example, sensory contribution of the radial nerve overlaps the tips of the thumb and index finger, often giving false information following median nerve suture. The sensory branch of the radial nerve should be locally anesthetized to allow accurate recording of the median nerve recovery. It is also well known that the ulnar nerve may supply some of the thenar muscles, and therefore objective evaluation of the end results of median nerve recovery should be done with the ulnar nerve blocked. Currently, the most widely accepted method of evaluation of nerve repair is the system devised by Highet[117] (Table 35-2), although this method needs clarification and updating with respect to individual nerves.

The chart shown in Figure 35-11 outlines our recommended 1-year period of rehabilitation. Follow-up should then continue for several more years following nerve suture. Essentially, we can summarize the postoperative care by saying that in the first 3 weeks the repair or graft is protected by plaster splintage and limited motion. In the period between 3 weeks and 3 months, the range of motion gradually increases, taking care not to stretch the repair site. Nerve repairs can be subjected to traction injuries if the suture line is stretched beyond the tensile strength of the nerve. The patient should be examined carefully during this period of time so that secondary deformity is prevented. Prevention may involve the use of external splints, such as a thumb web splint in a median nerve injury or a lumbrical bar in an ulnar nerve injury, to prevent hyperextension of the MP joints and resultant clawhand deformity with stiffness of the PIP joints in flexion. Once the joints are maintained in a supple position, in the period between 3 and 6

Table 35-2. Highet's Method of End Result Evaluation[117]

Motor Recovery	
M0	No contraction
M1	Return of perceptible contraction in the proximal muscles
M2	Return of perceptible contraction in both proximal and distal muscles
M3	Return of function in both proximal and distal muscles of such a degree that all important muscles are sufficiently powerful to act against resistance
M4	Return of function as in Stage 3; in addition, all synergistic and independent movements are possible
M5	Complete recovery
Sensory Recovery	
S0	Absence of sensibility in the autonomous area
S1	Recovery of deep cutaneous pain sensibility within the autonomous area of the nerve
S2	Return of some degree of superficial cutaneous pain and tactile sensibility within the autonomous area of the nerve
S3	Return of superficial cutaneous pain and tactile sensibility throughout the autonomous area, with disappearance of any previous overresponse
S3+	Return of sensibility as in Stage 3; in addition, there is some recovery of two-point discrimination within the autonomous area
S4	Complete recovery

Proximal muscles are defined as extrinsic, and distal as intrinsic muscles in the hand.

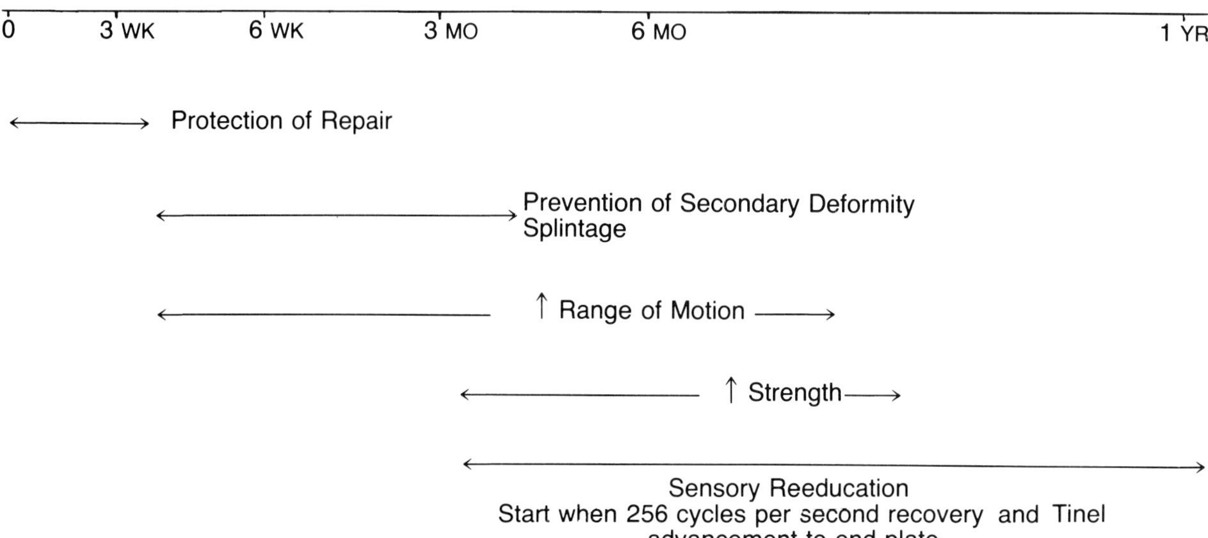

Fig. 35-11. Chart of postoperative rehabilitation of nerve injuries. The goal is to minimize recovery time and maximize functional recovery.

months, the strength of the hand is increased. During this time, the surgeon should be evaluating the nerve repair and studying Tinel's sign. If Tinel's sign does not advance significantly in the period between 3 and 6 months postoperatively, the surgeon must consider redoing the nerve repair or graft. The period of 6 months since the time of injury is critical, as explained earlier in this chapter, because metabolic changes occur both in the muscle and in the proximal nerve cell. Therefore, one must make a decision between 3 and 6 months whether the nerve regeneration is proceeding satisfactorily. If the nerve regeneration is proceeding satisfactorily and advancing Tinel's sign is present, sensory reeducation should be instituted.

Sensory Reeducation

Sensory reeducation was first reported by Dellon, Curtis, and Edgerton when they found near-normal sensation in four adults following nerve repair and intensive sensory retraining.[27-29] This was confirmed by Wynn-Parry and Salter in 1976.[156] Reid reviewed the testing of 150 adult patients with median nerve injury 1 to 5 years postinjury and found that these patients had very poor sensibility.[107] Reeducation was then begun when 256 cycles per second with a tuning fork could be detected at the fingertips. He noticed an improvement in sensibility in all patients using two-point discrimination, point localization, and the Moberg pick-up test as clinical tests. The patients in this study maintained their improvement in two-point discrimination after many years. One woman with a primary repair of her median nerve was found to have two-point discrimination greater than 45 mm 6 months postoperatively. Following 6 weeks of sensory retraining, the two-point discrimination was 11 to 15 mm, and 7 years later the two-point discrimination was 7 mm over the thumb and index finger. This method of sensory retraining is the same spontaneous retraining that a child undergoes following nerve injury. Onne reported excellent recovery of two-point discrimination in children but poor recovery of two-point discrimination in adults.[104] Therefore, we believe that sensory retraining in adults is mandatory following nerve injury. Patients with hyperesthesia or pain cannot be retrained until desensitization is carried out with reduction in the hyperesthesia. After nerve repair one follows Tinel's sign, constant and moving touch, perception of vibration at 30 cycles per second and 256 cycles per second. When 256 cycles per second stimulus is perceived at the fingertips, sensory retraining should be introduced. The method of the training sessions is essentially repetitive use with constant objects. These sessions should last about 10 to 15 minutes, with maximum concentration on the patient's part. The items used are soft objects (such as an eraser of a pencil), various sizes of square, hexagonal, and round objects (such as metal nuts and washers), and the objects used in daily living (such as keys, coins, buttons, and safety pins). Patients must constantly feel these objects, practicing and testing themselves repetitively. We emphasize again that this is a very natural process for the child, but in the adult we must encourage the retraining process. Following repair of a lacerated peripheral nerve, axons regenerate to reinnervate mechanical receptors in the skin. The regrowth is frequently disorderly. The number of nerve endings is not the same as prior to injury, and there is a reduction in the peripheral density of innervation. This altered profile must then be patterned in the brain so that the patient can again decode the information that is being produced by the mechanical receptors in the fingertips.

It is thought that the end-stage of nerve recovery is not reached until approximately 3 to 5 years postinjury. It is our hope that patients will be followed for this 5-year period and that suitable clinical information will be forthcoming. Unfortunately, there are very few reports of clinical series in the literature followed for this length of time. Only with this information will the clinician be able to determine the ultimate results of nerve repair and grafting.

FUTURE CONSIDERATIONS

Nerve Repair

We have reached the limits of nerve suture, a technique introduced in the Middle Ages. Recognition of this fact has generated enthusiasm for maximizing the ability of axons to "find their own way." However, sensory/motor specificity is the only type known to be generated during routine nerve repair with either suture or tubular prostheses.[17] The molecular events that generate specificity in development will have to be identified and duplicated in the adult before we can rely on the axon to find its way to the correct peripheral target. Fortunately, there is still room for mechanical improvements in nerve repair. Group fascicular suture produces fascicular alignment superior to that resulting from epineurial suture, yet is still far from perfect.[71] Experimental techniques for maximizing fascicular alignment result in improved function,[17] modification of these techniques for clinical use may provide incremental improvement in clinical results while awaiting developments at the molecular level. Similarly, pharmacologic[4] and electrical[78] manipulation of regeneration may produce at least modest clinical improvements in the near future.

Nerve Grafting

Allograft nerve, muscle basement membrane, and autologous or inert tubes have recently been used as experimental substitutes for peripheral nerve autograft. Excellent regeneration may now be obtained through nerve allograft if the host is immunosuppressed with Cyclosporin A, maintaining Schwann cell viability.[5] However, the durability of regenerated axons after withdrawal of immunosuppression and subsequent Schwann cell rejection has not been determined. An alternative approach is immediate destruction of the allograft Schwann cells, leaving a hypocellular basement membrane graft.[137]

Muscle basement membrane, autologous vein, and resorbable tubes have been used clinically to bridge digital nerve gaps. Four of 6 adults regained static two-point discrimination (2 pd) of 6 to 14 mm after bridging of 15 to 25 mm gaps with muscle basement membrane.[101] When autologous vein was used, 7 of 9 adults regained static 2 pd of 7 to 12 mm after regeneration across gaps of 23 to 30 mm.[22] When gaps of 15 to 30 mm were enclosed within resorbable tubes, 5 of 11 patients regained moving 2 pd of 3–6 mm (static measurements were not reported), but the remaining 6 regained no 2 pd.[76] In many cases, these results compare favorably with those of autologous nerve grafting. However, experience obtained over short distances in the digital nerve cannot be generalized to greater distances or more complex nerves. Primate axons will cross a gap of up to 3 cm through a variety of prostheses, yet rarely venture further without living Schwann cells. Axons also intermingle when nerve regenerates across a gap.[15] The digital nerve contains an homogenous population of axons destined for a few receptor types, so this intermingling has little functional impact. However, when randomness is imposed upon the multiple axon types within mixed nerve, function is severely impaired.[15,67] The quest for a "bankable" or "off-the-shelf" substitute for autologous nerve graft thus remains in its infancy.

REFERENCES

1. Aird RB, Naffziger HC: The pathology of human striated muscle following denervation. J Neurosurg 10:216–227, 1953
2. Aitken J: The effect of peripheral connexions on the maturation of regenerating nerve fibres. J Anat 83:32–43, 1949
3. Allt G: The Peripheral Nerve. pp. 666–739. Chapman & Hall, London, 1976
4. Badalamente MA, Hurst LC, Paul SB, Stracher A: Enhancement of neuromuscular recovery after nerve repair in primates. J Hand Surg 12B:211–217, 1987
5. Bain JR, Mackinnon SE, Hudson AR, Falk RE, Falk JA, Hunter DA: The peripheral nerve allograft: An assessment of regeneration across nerve allografts in rats immunosuppressed with cyclosporin A. Plast Reconstr Surg 82:1052–1064, 1988
6. Birch R, Raji ARM: Repair of median and ulnar nerves. Primary suture is best. J Bone Joint Surg 73B:154–157, 1991
7. Black MM, Lasek RJ: The use of axonal transport to measure axonal regeneration in rat ventral motor neurons (abstract). Anat Rec 184:360–361, 1976
8. Bolesta MJ, Garrett WE Jr, Ribbeck BM, Glisson RR, Seaber AV, Goldner JL: Immediate and delayed neurorrhaphy in a rabbit model: A functional, histologic, and biochemical comparison. J Hand Surg 13A:352–357, 1988
9. Bondok AA, Sansone FM: Retrograde and transganglionic degeneration of sensory neurons after a peripheral nerve lesion at birth. Exp Neurol 86:322–330, 1984
10. Bonney G, Birch R, Jamieson A, Eames R: Experience with vascularized nerve grafts. Clin Plast Surg 11:137–142, 1984
11. Bora FW: Improved axon regeneration after nerve injury by the pharmacological suppression of neuroma formation. Presented at the 35th Annual Meeting, American Society for Surgery of the Hand. Atlanta, 1980
12. Bowden REM, Gutmann E: Denervation and reinnervation of human voluntary muscle. Brain 67:273–312, 1944
13. Brooks D: The place of nerve grafting in orthopaedic surgery. J Bone Joint Surg 37A:299–305, 1955
14. Brushart TME: Preferential reinnervation of motor nerves by regenerating motor axons. J Neurosci 8:1026–1031, 1988
15. Brushart TM: Topographic specificity of peripheral axon regeneration across enclosed gaps. Soc Neurosc Abstr 16:806, 1990
16. Brushart TM: Preferential motor reinnervation: a sequential double-labeling study. Restor Neurol Neurosc 1:281–287, 1990
17. Brushart TME: The mechanical and humoral control of specificity in nerve repair. pp. 215–230. In Gelberman RH (ed): Operative Nerve Repair and Reconstruction. Philadelphia, JB Lippincott, Philadelphia, 1991
18. Brushart TME: Central course of digital axons within the median nerve of macaca mulatta. J Comp Neurol 311:197–209, 1991
19. Buchthal F, Kühl V: Nerve conduction, tactile sensibility, and the electromyogram after suture or compression of peripheral nerve: a longitudinal study in man. J Neurol Neurosurg Psych 42:436–451, 1979

20. Bunnell S: Surgery of nerves of the hand. Surg Gynecol Obstet 44:145-152, 1927
21. Chauliac GD: On Wounds and Fractures, Brennan WA (trans) Chicago, priv pub, 1923
22. Chiu DTW, Strauch B: A prospective clinical evaluation of autogenous vein grafts used as a nerve conduit for distal sensory nerve defects of 3 cm or less. Plast Reconstr Surg 86:928-934, 1990
23. Chow JA, Van Beek AL, Meyer DL, Johnson MC: Surgical significance of the motor fascicular group of the ulnar nerve in the forearm. J Hand Surg 10A:867-872, 1985
24. Chow JA, Van Beek AL, Bilos ZJ, Meyer DL, Johnson MC: Anatomical basis for repair of ulnar and median nerves in the distal part of the forearm by group fascicular suture and nerve-grafting. J Bone Joint Surg 68A:273-280, 1986
25. Cruikshank W: Experiments on the Nerves, Particularly on Their Reproductions; and on the Spinal Marrow of Living Animals. Philos Trans R Soc Lond 85:177-189, 1795
26. Danielsen N, Lundborg G, Frizell M: Nerve repair and axonal transport: Outgrowth delay and regeneration rate after transection and repair of rabbit hypoglossal nerve. Brain Res 376:125-132, 1986
27. Dellon AL, Mackinnon SE: The pronator quadratus muscle flap. J Hand Surg 9A:423-427, 1984
28. Dellon AL, Seif SS: Anatomic dissections relating the posterior interosseous nerve to the carpus, and the etiology of dorsal wrist ganglion pain. J Hand Surg 3:326-332, 1978
29. Dellon AL, Curtis RM, Edgerton MT: Reeducation of sensation in the hand following nerve injury. J Bone Joint Surg 53A:813, 1971
30. Dellon AL, Curtis RM, Edgerton MT: Evaluating recovery of sensation in the hand following nerve injury. The Johns Hopkins Med J 130:235-243, 1972
31. Dellon AL, Curtis RM, Edgerton MT: Reeducation of sensation in the hand after nerve injury and repair. J Plast Reconstr Surg 53:297, 1974
32. De Medinaceli L, Seaber AV: Experimental nerve reconnection: Importance of initial repair. Microsurgery 10:56-70, 1989
33. Ducker TB, Kempe LG, Hayes GJ: The metabolic background for peripheral nerve surgery. J Neurosurg 30:270-280, 1969
34. Esslen E: Electromyographic findings on two types of misdirection of regenerating axons. Electroencephalogr Clin Neurophysiol 12:738-741, 1960
35. Fawcett JW, Keynes RJ: Peripheral Nerve Regeneration. Annu Rev Neurosci 13:43-60, 1990
36. Forman DS, Wood DK, DeSilva S: Rate of regeneration of sensory axons in transected rat sciatic nerve repaired with epineurial sutures. J Neurol Sci 44:55-59, 1979
37. Galen: Galen on the Affected Parts. Siegel E (trans). S Karger, Basel, Switzerland, 1976
38. Gaul JS: Electrical fascicle identification as an adjunct to nerve repair. J Hand Surg 8:289-296, 1983
39. Gilbert A: Vascularized sural nerve graft. Clin Plast Surg 2:73-77, 1974
40. Grabb WC: Median and ulnar nerve suture. An experimental study comparing primary and secondary repair in monkeys. J Bone Joint Surg 50A:964-972, 1968
41. Grafstein B, McQuarrie IG: Neuronal Plasticity. pp. 155-195. Raven, New York, 1978
42. Greenberg BM, Cuadros CL, Panda M, May JW Jr: St. Clair Strange procedure: Indications, technique, and long-term evaluation. J Hand Surg 13A:928-935, 1988
43. Gruber H, Freilinger G, Holle H, Mandl H: Identification of motor and sensory funiculi in cut nerves and their selective reunion. Br J Plast Surg 29:70-73, 1976
44. Gutmann E: Effect of delay of innervation on recovery of muscle after nerve lesions. J Neurophysiol 11:279-294, 1948
45. Gutmann E, Guttmann L: The effect of galvanic exercise on denervated and reinnervated muscles in rabbit. J Neurol Neurosurg Psychiat 7:7-17, 1944
46. Haighton J: An experimental inquiry concerning the reproduction of nerves. Philos Trans R Soc Lond 85:190-200, 1795
47. Hakstian RW: Funicular orientation by direct stimulation. An aid to peripheral nerve repair. J Bone Joint Surg 50A:1178-1186, 1968
48. Hallin RG: Microneurography in relation to intraneural topography: somatotopic organisation of median nerve fascicles in humans. J Neurol Neurosurg Psych 53:736-744, 1990
49. Highet WB, Holmes W: Traction injuries to the lateral popliteal nerve and traction injuries to peripheral nerves after suture. Br J Surg 30:212-233, 1943
50. Hoffman PN, Cleveland DW, Griffin JW, Landes PW, Cowan NJ, Price DL: Neurofilament gene expression: A major determinant of axonal caliber. Proc Natl Acad Sci USA 84:3472-3476, 1987
51. Horch KW, Lisney SJW: On the number and nature of regenerating myelinated axons after lesions of cutaneous nerves in the cat. J Physiol 313:275-286, 1981
52. Ide C, Tohyama K, Yokota R, Nitatori T, Onodera H: Schwann cell basal lamina and nerve regeneration. Brain Res 288:61-75, 1983
53. Jabaley ME: Electrical nerve stimulation in the awake patient. pp. 241-257. In Gelberman RH (ed): Operative Nerve Repair and Reconstruction. JB Lippincott, Philadelphia, 1991
54. Jabaley ME, Burns JE, Orcutt BA, Bryant WM: Comparison of histologic and functional recovery after peripheral nerve repair. J Hand Surg 1:119-130, 1976
55. Jabaley ME, Wallace WH, Heckler FR: Internal topography of major nerves of the forearm and hand: A current view. J Hand Surg 5:1-18, 1980
56. Jenq C-B, Coggeshall RE: Regeneration of axons in tributary nerves. Brain Res 310:107-121, 1984
57. Jones SJ: Investigation of brachial plexus traction lesions by peripheral and spinal somatosensory evoked potentials. J Neurol Neurosurg Psychiatr 42:107-116, 1979
58. Jones SJ, Parry CB, Landi A: Diagnosis of brachial plexus traction lesions by sensory nerve action potentials and somatosensory evoked potentials. Injury 12(5):376-382, 1981
59. Jurecka W, Ammerer HP, Lassmann H: Regeneration of a transected peripheral nerve; An autoradiographic and electron microscopic study. Acta Neuropathol (Berl) 32:299-312, 1975
60. Kline DG: Early evaluation in peripheral nerve lesions in continuity with a note on nerve recording. Am Surg 34:77, 1968
61. Kline DG: Evaluation of the neuroma in continuity. Ch. 27. In Omer G, Spinner M (eds): Management of Peripheral Nerve Problems. WB Saunders, Philadelphia, 1980
62. Kline DG, Hayes GJ, Morse AS: A comparative study of response of species to peripheral-nerve injury. II. Crush and severance with primary suture. J Neurosurg 21:980-988, 1964
63. Kline DG, Hackett ER: Value of electrophysiologic tests for peripheral nerve neuromas. J Surg Oncol 2:299-310, 1970
64. Kline DG, Hackett ER, Davis GD, Myers MB: Effect of mobilization on the blood supply and regeneration of injured nerves. J Surg Res 12:254-266, 1972
65. Kline DG, Nulsen FE: The neuroma in continuity: Its preoperative and operative management. Surg Clin North Am 52:1189-1209, 1972
66. Kline DG, Hackett ER, Happel LH: Surgery for lesions of the brachial plexus. Arch Neurol 43:170-181, 1986
67. Koerber HR, Seymour AW, Mendell LM: Mismatches between peripheral receptor type and central projections after peripheral nerve regeneration. Neurosci Lett 99:67-72, 1989
68. Krishnamurti A, Kanagasuntheram R, Vij S: Failure of reinner-

vation of Pacinian corpuscle after nerve crush. An electron microscopic study. Acta Neuropath (Berl) 23:338–341, 1973
69. Lang DH, Lister GD, Jevans AW: Histochemical and biochemical aids to nerve repair. pp. 259–271. In Gelberman RH (ed): Operative Nerve Repair and Reconstruction. JB Lippincott, Philadelphia, 1991
70. Langley JN, Anderson HK: The union of different kinds of nerve fibres. J Physiol 31:365–391, 1904
71. Lee KE, Brushart TM: Fascicular Alignment in Epineurial and Group Fascicular Nerve Repairs: a Histologic Study. Presented to the American Society for Reconstructive Microsurgery, Orlando, 1991
72. Lundborg G: The intrinsic vascularization of human peripheral nerves: Structural and functional aspects. J Hand Surg 4:34–41, 1979
73. Lundborg G: Nerve Regeneration and Repair. A review. Acta Orthop Scand 58:145–169, 1987
74. Lundborg G: Nerve Injury and Repair. pp. 32–63. Churchill Livingstone, New York, 1988
75. Lundborg G, Myers R, Powell H: Nerve compression injury and increased endoneurial fluid pressure: "a miniature compartment syndrome." J Neurol Neurosurg Psych 46:1119–1124, 1983
76. Mackinnon SE, Dellon AL: Clinical nerve reconstruction with a bioabsorbable polyglycolic acid tube. Plast Reconstr Surg 85:419–424, 1990
77. Marmor L: Regeneration of peripheral nerves by irradiated homografts. J Bone Joint Surg 46A:383–394, 1964
78. McCaig CD, Rajnicek AM: Electrical fields, nerve growth and nerve regeneration. Exp Physiol 76:473–494, 1991
79. McFarlane RM, Mayer JR: Digital nerve grafts with the lateral antebrachial cutaneous nerve. J Hand Surg 1:169–173, 1976
80. McLellan DL, Swash M: Longitudinal sliding of the median nerve during movements of the upper limb. J Neurol Neuros Phys 39:566–570, 1976
81. McQuarrie I, Idzikowski C: Injuries to Peripheral Nerves. pp. 802–815. In Miller TA, Rowlands BJ (eds): Physiologic Basis of Modern Surgical Care. CV Mosby, St. Louis, 1988
82. McQuarrie IG: Effect of a conditioning lesion on axonal sprout formation at nodes of ranvier. J Comp Neurol 231:239–249, 1985
83. Merle M, Amend P, Cour C, Foucher G, Michon J: Microsurgical Repair of Peripheral Nerve Lesions. Peripheral Nerve Repair and Regeneration 2:17–26, 1986
84. Merle M, Lebreton E, Foucher G: Vascularized nerve grafts: Preliminary results. Presented to the American Society for Reconstructive Microsurgery, Las Vegas, 1985
85. Millesi H: Indication, technique and results of nerve grafting. Handchirurgie, suppl. 2, 1977
86. Millesi H: Peripheral nerve repair: Terminology, questions, and facts. J Reconstr Microsurg 2:21–31, 1985
87. Millesi H, Meissl G, Berger A: The interfascicular nerve-grafting of the median and ulnar nerves. J Bone Joint Surg 54A:727–749, 1972
88. Millesi H, Meissl G, Berger A: Further experience with interfascicular grafting of the median, ulnar and radial nerves. J Bone Joint Surg 58A:209–218, 1976
89. Milward TM, Stott WG, Kleinert HE: The abductor digiti minimi muscle flap. Hand 9:82–85, 1977
90. Mitchell SW: Injuries of Nerves, JB Lippincott, Philadelphia, 1872
91. Moberg E: Methods of examining sensibility of the hand. p. 236. In Flynn JE (ed): Hand Surgery. Williams & Wilkins, Baltimore, 1966
92. Moberg E: Nerve repair in hand surgery—An analysis. Surg Clin North Am 48:985, 1968
93. Morris JH, Hudson AR, Weddell G: A study of degeneration and regeneration in the divided rat sciatic nerve based on electron microscopy. II—The development of the 'regenerating unit'. Z Zellforsch Mikrosk Anat 124:103–130, 1972
94. Muller J: Elements of Physiology. Taylor and Walton, London, 1842
95. Myers RR, Powell HC, Costello ML, Lampert PW, Zweifach BW: Endoneurial fluid pressure: direct measurement with micropipettes. Brain Res 148:510–515, 1978
96. Nakatsuchi Y, Matsui T, Handa Y: Funicular orientation by electrical stimulation and internal neurolysis in peripheral nerve suture. Hand 12:65–74, 1980
97. Nathaniel EJH, Pease DC: Regenerative changes in rat dorsal roots following Wallerian degeneration. J Ultrastruc Res 9:533–549, 1963
98. Nemoto K, Williams HB, Lough J, Chiu RC: The Effects of Electrical Stimulation on Denervated Muscle Using Implantable Electrodes. J Recon Micro 4:251–255, 1988
99. Nicholson OR, Seddon HJ: Nerve repair in civilian practice. Results of treatment of median and ulnar nerve lesions. Br Med J 2:1065–1071, 1957
100. Nix WA, Dahm M: The effect of isometric short-term electrical stimulation on denervated muscle. Muscle Nerve 10:136–143, 1987
101. Norris RW, Glasby MA, Gattuso JM, Bowden REM: Peripheral nerve repair in humans using muscle autografts. A new technique. J Bone Joint Surg 70B:530–533, 1988
102. Ochs S: A Brief History of Nerve Repair and Regeneration. pp. 1–8. In Jewett DL, McCarroll HR (eds): Nerve Repair and Regeneration, CV Mosby, St. Louis, 1980
103. Oester YT, Davis L: Recovery of sensory function. p. 241. In Woodhall B, Beebe GW (eds): Peripheral Nerve Regeneration. Washington, DC, US Government Printing Office, 1956
104. Onne L: Recovery of sensibility and sudomotor activity in the hand after nerve suture. Acta Chir Scand suppl. 300, 1962
105. Paget J: Lectures on Surgical Pathology Delivered at the Royal College of Surgeons of England. Longman, London, 1863
106. Ramon y Cajal S: Degeneration and Regeneration of the Nervous System. May RM (trans) 1928. Reprinted Hafner, New York, 1968
107. Reid RL: Preliminary results of sensibility reeducation following repair of the median nerve. American Society for Surgery of the Hand Newsletter 15, 1977
108. Riley DA, Lang DH: Carbonic anhydrase activity of human peripheral nerves: A possible histochemical aid to nerve repair. J Hand Surg 9A:112–120, 1984
109. Rose EH, Kowalski TA: Restoration of sensibility to anesthetic scarred digits with free vascularized nerve grafts from the dorsum of the foot. J Hand Surg 10A:514–521, 1985
110. Sanders FK: The repair of large gaps in the peripheral nerves. Brain 65:281–337, 1942
111. Sanger JR, Riley DA, Matloub HS, Yousif NJ, Bain JL, Moore GH: Effects of axotomy on the cholinesterase and carbonic anhydrase activities of axons in the proximal and distal stumps of rabbit sciatic nerves: A temporal study. Plast Reconstr Surg 87:726–740, 1991
112. Schady W, Ochoa JL, Torebjörk HE, Chen LS: Peripheral projections of fascicles in the human median nerve. Brain 106:745–760, 1983
113. Schmalbruch H: Motoneuron death after sciatic nerve section in newborn rats. J Comp Neurol 224:252–258, 1984
114. Seddon HJ: The use of autogenous grafts for the repair of large gaps in peripheral nerves. Br J Surg 35:151–167, 1947
115. Seddon HJ: War injuries of peripheral nerves. In wounds of the extremities. Br J Surg War Surgery Suppl 2:325, 1948
116. Seddon HJ: Nerve grafting. J Bone Joint Surg 45B:447–461, 1963

117. Seddon HJ: Surgical Disorders of the Peripheral Nerves. Williams & Wilkins, Baltimore, 1972
118. Seddon HJ, Holmes W: Ischaemic damage in the peripheral stump of a divided nerve. Br J Surg 32:389-391, 1945
119. Seddon HJ, Medawar PB, Smith H: Rate of regeneration of peripheral nerves in man. J Physiol (Lond.) 102:191-215, 1943
120. Shanthaveerappa TR, Bourne GH: Perineural epithelium: A new concept of its role in the integrity of the peripheral nervous system. Science 154:1464-1467, 1966
121. Skene JHP, Jacobson RD, Snipes GJ, McGuire CB, Norden JJ, Freeman JA: A protein induced during nerve growth (GAP-43) is a major component of growth-cone membranes. Science 233:783-786, 1986
122. Spinner M: Injuries to the Major Branches of Peripheral Nerves of the Forearm. 2nd Ed. WB Saunders, Philadelphia, 1978
123. Starkweather RJ, Neviaser RJ, Adams JP, Parsons DB: The effect of devascularization on the regeneration of lacerated peripheral nerves: An experimental study. J Hand Surg 3:163-167, 1978
124. Strange FGStC: An operation for nerve pedicle grafting, preliminary communication. Br J Surg 34:423-425, 1947
125. Strange FGStC: Case report on pedicled nerve graft. Br J Surg 37:331, 1950
126. Sunderland S: The adipose tissue of peripheral nerves. Brain 68:118-122, 1945
127. Sunderland S: The effect of rupture of the perineurium on the contained nerve fibres. Brain 69:149-152, 1946
128. Sunderland S: Capacity of Reinnervated Muscles to Function Efficiently after Prolonged Denervation. Arch Neurol Psych 64:755-771, 1950
129. Sunderland S: The connective tissues of peripheral nerves. Brain 88:841-854, 1965
130. Sunderland S: Nerves and Nerve Injuries. Williams & Wilkins, Baltimore, 1968
131. Sunderland S: Nerves and Nerve Injuries. 2nd Ed. Churchill Livingstone, Edinburgh, 1978
132. Sunderland S: The pros and cons of funicular nerve repair. Founder's Lecture, The American Society for Surgery of the Hand. J Hand Surg 4:201-211, 1979
133. Sunderland S: The anatomy and physiology of nerve injury. Muscle Nerve 13:771-784, 1990
134. Sunderland S, Bradley KC: The cross-sectional area of peripheral nerve trunks devoted to nerve fibres. Brain 72:428-449, 1949
135. Sunderland S, Ray LJ: The selection and use of autografts for bridging gaps in injured nerves. Brain 70:75-92, 1947
136. Sunderland S, Ray LJ: Denervation changes in mammalian striated muscle. J Neurol Neurosurg Psychiat 13:159-177, 1950
137. Tajima K, Tohyama K, Ide C, Abe M: Regeneration through Nerve Allografts in the Cynomolgus Monkey (Macaca fascicularis). J Bone Joint Surg 73A:172-185, 1991
138. Taylor GI, Ham FJ: The free vascularized nerve graft. A further experimental and clinical application of microvascular techniques. Plast Reconstr Surg 57:413-425, 1976
139. Thomas PK: The connective tissue of peripheral nerve: an electron microscope study. J Anat 97:35-44, 1963
140. Thomas PK, Jones DG: The cellular response to nerve injury. 2. Regeneration of the perineurium after nerve section. J Anat 101:45-55, 1967
141. Tinel J: Le signe du "Fourmillement" dans les lesion des nerfs peripheriques. Presse Med 23:388-389, 1915
142. Van Beek A, Glover JL, Zook E: Primary versus delayed-primary neurorrhaphy in rat sciatic nerve. J Surg Res 18:335-339, 1975
143. Van Beek A, Hubble B, Kinkead L, Torros S, Suchy H: Clinical use of nerve stimulation and recording techniques. Plast Reconstr Surg 71:225-238, 1983
144. Vandeput J, Tanner JC, Huypens L: Electro-physiological orientation of the cut ends in primary peripheral nerve repair. Plast Reconstr Surg 44:378-382, 1969
145. Watchmaker GP, Gumucio CA, Crandall RE, Vannier MA, Weeks PM: Fascicular topography of the median nerve: A computer based study to identify branching patterns. J Hand Surg 16A:53-59, 1991
146. West JR: Early History of Mammalian Nerve Regeneration. Neurosci Biobehav Rev 2:27-32, 1978
147. Wilgis EFS: Local muscle flaps in the hand anatomy as related to reconstructive surgery. Bull Hosp Joint Dis 44:552-557, 1984
148. Wilgis EFS, Maxwell GP: Distal digital nerve grafts: Clinical and anatomical studies. J Hand Surg 4:439-443, 1979
149. Wilgis EFS, Murphy R: The significance of longitudinal excursion in peripheral nerves. Hand Clin 2:761-766, 1987
150. Williams HB, Jabaley ME: The importance of internal anatomy of the peripheral nerves to nerve repair in the forearm and hand. Hand Clin 2:689-707, 1986
151. Williams HB, Terzis JK: Single fascicular recordings: An intraoperative diagnostic tool for the management of peripheral nerve lesions. Plast Reconstr Surg 57:562-569, 1976
152. Wise AJ, Topuzlu C, Davis P, Kaye IS: A comparative analysis of macro- and microsurgical neurorrhaphy technics. Am J Surg 117:566-572, 1969
153. Wong WC, Kanagasuntheram R: Early and late effects of median nerve injury on Meissner's and Pacinian corpuscles of the hand of the macaque *(M. fascicularis)*. J Anat 109:135-142, 1971
154. Woodhall B, Nulsen FE, White JC, Davis L: Neurosurgical implications. In Woodhall B, Beebe GW (eds): Peripheral Nerve Regeneration. US Government Printing Office, Washington, DC, 1956
155. Wynn-Parry CB: Diagnosis and aftercare of peripheral-nerve lesions in the upper limb. Founder's Lecture, The American Society for Surgery of the Hand. J Bone Joint Surg 48A:607, 1966
156. Wynn-Parry CB, Salter M: Sensory re-education after median nerve lesions. Hand 8:250-257, 1976
157. Ygge J: Neuronal loss in lumbar dorsal root ganglia after proximal compared to distal sciatic nerve resection: a quantitative study in the rat. Brain Res 478:193-195, 1989
158. Young L, Wray RC, Weeks PM: A randomized prospective comparison of fascicular and epineurial digital nerve repairs. Plast Reconstr Surg 68:89-92, 1981
159. Yunshao H, Shizhen Z: Acetylcholinesterase: A histochemical identification of motor and sensory fascicles in human peripheral nerve and its use during operation. Plast Reconstr Surg 82:125-132, 1988
160. Zachary RB: Results of nerve suture. In Seddon HJ (ed): Peripheral Nerve Injuries. Her Majesty's Stationary Office, London, 1954

36

Entrapment and Compression Neuropathies

William W. Eversmann, Jr.

Entrapment neuropathies of the upper extremity occur in predictable areas, are generally evaluated in a similar manner, and probably have a common pathophysiology. Entrapment neuropathies are nerve injuries. Because the degree of nerve injury is unknown preoperatively or even at the time of surgical release, the prognosis following surgical exploration of an entrapment neuropathy is often uncertain until the patient's clinical response is observed. As a general rule, however, unless an entrapment neuropathy is severe or longstanding, the neuropathy will be relieved by release of the compression on the nerve. The diagnosis of a compression or entrapment neuropathy depends on first demonstrating a neuropathy of the peripheral nerve in the upper extremity and second, on localizing that neuropathy by either electrodiagnosis or physical examination, usually to one of the predictable areas in the upper extremity. The most common methods of identifying a neuropathy are with objective sensory examinations or by demonstrating a nerve conduction deficit along the course of a peripheral nerve.

PATHOPHYSIOLOGY

Since the success of surgical treatment is dependent on an understanding of the pathophysiology of nerve compression, a review of the current concepts of pathophysiology is important in understanding the operative procedures involved in the entrapment neuropathies. There is little doubt that ionic, mechanical, and vascular lesions are all involved in the pathophysiologic mechanism of entrapment neuropathies.[111]

There is a growing body of evidence that tissue pressure plays an important function in the pathophysiologic mechanism, and local experimental compression of the median nerve has been used to simulate the mechanism of tissue pressure. Whether tissue pressure is primary or secondary to ionic, vascular, or mechanical lesions is uncertain, and probably adds to the shroud of confusion that encompasses discussions of the pathophysiologic mechanisms. In recent years, the vascular lesions seem to have become most understandable from the standpoint of the pathophysiologic mechanisms.[224] The vascular anatomy of nerves has been studied since the seventeenth century.[107,108] A segmental vascular supply to the nerve trunk is carried in a mesoneurium, which permits motion and allows changes of position and tension of the nerve with motion of the extremity.[107,108,160] The arcades in the mesoneurium vary with location. The median nerve at the wrist is supplied by the mesoneurium from the volar-ulnar side of the nerve proximal to the transverse carpal ligament, as well as by a mesoneurium from the superficial palmar arch distal to the transverse carpal ligament.[7] The nerve trunk is supplied by this mesoneurium in a regional pattern, the small vessels entering the epineurium of the nerve and immediately dividing into ascending and descending epineurial branches. The epineurial network of vessels forms an anastomotic network that further subdivides into a vascular plexus in the perineurium. The capillary bed within the nerve itself is contained within the fascicles of the nerve so that below the perineurial level of vascular plexus, small end arteries and capillary beds form the remainder of the vascular pattern within the nerve trunks.[107,108]

If there is obstruction of venous return from the nerve by a mechanism as simple as prolonged flexion of the wrist or as complex as a distal radius fracture, venous congestion within the nerve results. Because of this venous congestion within the epineurial and perineurial vascular plexus, there is a generalized slowing of the circulation, not only in the epineurial plexus but also in the intrafascicular tissues. Anoxia of a nerve segment results, which leads to dilatation of the small vessels and capillaries within that segment of the nerve, resulting in endoneurial edema of the tissue.[365] The edema of the nerve segment increases the effect of the original compression, which may have initiated the venous obstruction. If this increased compression or the edema persists for a prolonged period of time, proliferation of fibroblasts within the nerve ensues. This proliferation of fibroblasts eventually leads to scarring within the nerve, further rendering segments of the nerve anoxic because of a barrier of fibroblasts that further inhibits both circulation within the nerve and exchange of vital nutrients between the vascular system and the nerve fibers.

The axioplasmic transport system within an axon combines a system of transport filaments, microtubules, and neurofilaments to transport protein molecules synthesized in the endoplasmic reticulum of the cell body to a location in the axon where they will be chemically active, such as in the wall of the axon or at the terminal endings.[121] Accordingly, protein polypeptides, glycoproteins, glycolipids, catecholamines, and acetylcholinesterase are transported from the cell body along the axon to their active site, using the segmental axonal mitochondria and oxidative phosphorylation to generate the high-energy phosphate necessary for the transport and maintenance of the cell. When a portion of the axon is rendered ischemic with as small a reduction in blood flow as 30 to 50 percent of normal, the reduction in oxidative phosphorylation and production of high-energy phosphate decreases the efficiency of the sodium pump, the axioplasmic transport system, and the integrity of the cell membrane, which will in turn eventually lead to a loss of conduction or transmission along the nerve fiber.[224]

According to studies of various authors, it seems likely that the primary lesion of entrapment neuropathies is vascular compromise of a segment of the axon.[69,111,121,224,365] That segment of the axon rendered ischemic or relatively ischemic through either a change of position, local anatomy, or internal pressure will react not only through a series of vascular mechanisms but, by so doing, will also alter its ionic relationship to its environment and further aggravate the normal internal pressure of the nerve trunk to a degree to account for increased vascular changes and a deterioration of normal function of the nerve trunk. In our studies of intraoperative motor conduction latencies associated with carpal tunnel syndrome, we have suggested that the rapidity of our patients' recovery and restitution of a normal conduction velocity could only be explained by a vascular lesion.[224]

ENTRAPMENT NEUROPATHIES OF THE MEDIAN NERVE

Three distinct entrapment neuropathies of the median nerve have been described. They differ in clinical presentation, physical findings on examination, and surgical treatment. Although there are differentiating points on clinical presentation and examination, the many similarities that these entrapment neuropathies possess often confuse the surgeon, and, as a result, the presentation of any one will usually add at least one of the other two to the differential diagnosis.

Pronator Syndrome

The most proximal entrapment neuropathy of the median nerve, which has been widely studied, is the pronator syndrome.[149] The pronator syndrome presents with pain in the proximal volar surface of the distal arm and forearm, which generally increases with activity. There is reduced sensibility or at least sensory symptoms in the radial three and one-half digits. The wrist flexion test of Phalen is notably negative in this syndrome, and signs are not limited to the deep volar compartment of the forearm, specifically loss of active flexion of the DIP joint of the index finger or the interphalangeal joint of the thumb.

There are four sites of potential compression, all of which produce the signs and symptoms of pronator syndrome. The first of these is compression of the median nerve in the distal third of the humerus beneath a supracondylar process and the ligament of Struthers. The second potential site of compression occurs at the lacertus fibrosus, which courses across the median nerve at the level of the elbow joint. The third site of compression is within the pronator teres muscle, caused either by hypertrophy of the pronator teres muscle or by the aponeurotic fascia on the deep surface of the superficial head or the superficial surface of the deep head of the pronator teres. The final area of potential compression in the pronator syndrome occurs at the arch of the flexor digitorum superficialis muscle as the median nerve passes beneath that muscle to lie immediately deep to and within the muscle fascia of the flexor digitorum superficialis.

Functional testing of the muscles of the proximal forearm may give some indication of the site of compression in pronator syndrome. If symptoms are aggravated by flexion of the elbow against resistance between 120 and 135 degrees flexion, the surgeon must be suspicious of a Struthers' ligament compression. Compression by the lacertus fibrosus will be manifest and aggravated by active flexion of the elbow with the forearm in pronation, and probably only occurs when the median nerve is superficial to and along the lateral edge of the flexor muscle mass where the lacertus fibrosus crosses from the bicipital tendon across the flexor muscle mass (Fig. 36-1).[116,117,137,147,162,178] If the symptoms are increased by resistance to pronation of the forearm, usually combined with flexion of the wrist (to relax the flexor digitorum superficialis), the surgeon should be particularly careful to explore the median nerve as it passes through the pronator teres muscle.[111,138,144,168] If the symptoms of pronator syndrome are aggravated by resisted flexion of the superficialis muscle of the middle finger, the surgeon should be careful to inspect the superficialis arch at the time of exploration.

Electrodiagnostic studies should confirm the clinical diagnosis. In most cases these studies will localize the level of the lesion, will confirm whether the nerve injury is partial or com-

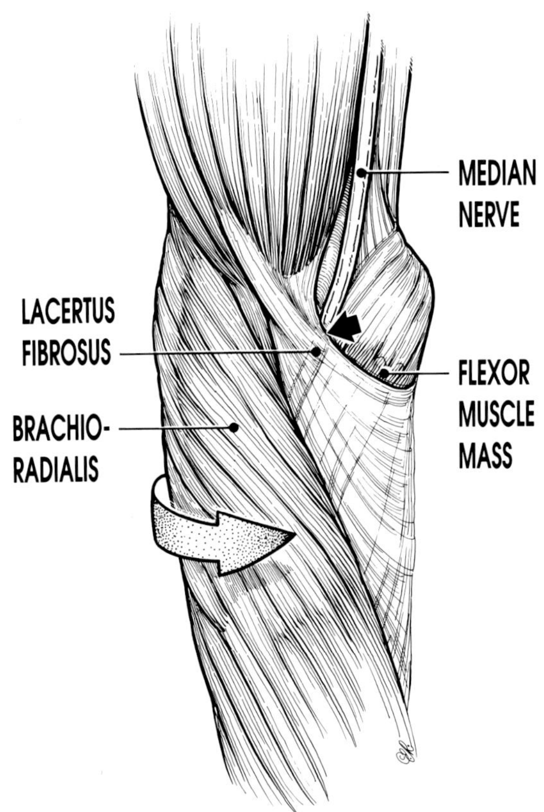

Fig. 36-1. The lacertus fibrosus is tightened with pronation of the forearm *(curved arrow)* as the bicipital tuberosity of the radius passes posteriorly. This tightening of the lacertus fibrosus will compress the median nerve *(solid arrow)* if the nerve does not lie beneath the flexor muscle mass, which itself is often indented by the lacertus fibrosus in pronation.

plete, and in some patients may define a myopathic origin of upper extremity pain. The surgeon should always be aware that nerve conduction velocity determinations are subject to a multitude of variables, including the age of the patient, his temperature, vascular supply of the extremity, regenerating fibers within the nerve, obesity or edema in the extremity, as well as a myriad of technical problems associated with the determination itself. All these factors must be weighed by the surgeon in evaluating the results of electrodiagnostic studies. When the electrodiagnostic studies do not confirm the clinical impression of a pronator syndrome, but the clinical tests for this syndrome continue to implicate the pronator syndrome as the level of compression neuropathy, it is prudent to wait 4 to 6 weeks, at which time repeat electrodiagnostic studies, including nerve conduction velocity and electromyogram, should be repeated. If, on the other hand, the surgeon suspects a pronator syndrome but the clinical signs of this syndrome are absent or questionable, a more proximal lesion, such as a vascular anomaly of the brachial plexus should be considered.

Operative Technique

The operative technique for the release of a pronator syndrome consists of a detailed exploration of the median nerve in the proximal forearm. Although some surgeons prefer to limit the exploration to the suspicious area of the nerve on diagnostic evaluation, operations of limited scope carry with them an inherent risk of failure to recognize more than a single compression, if in fact a single site of compression is isolated.

The exploration for pronator syndrome should begin with an incision at least 5 cm above the elbow joint over the medial neurovascular bundle, zigzagging across the elbow flexion crease to lie midway between the flexor and extensor muscle masses, extending to the midforearm.

A small hook-shaped process of bone, the supracondylar process, may be found 5 cm above the medial epicondyle, projecting anteromedially from the surface of the humerus. This process may form an accessory origin for the pronator teres muscle (Fig. 36-2) through a ligament that was described by Struthers and bears his name.[116,117,178] If the median nerve is entrapped either beneath the supracondylar process or the ligament of Struthers, it is generally accompanied by the brachial artery and veins and lies on the medial aspect of the artery and veins. Following release of the ligament of Struthers, with or without resection of the supracondylar process, the median nerve must be traced distally to the second potential area of

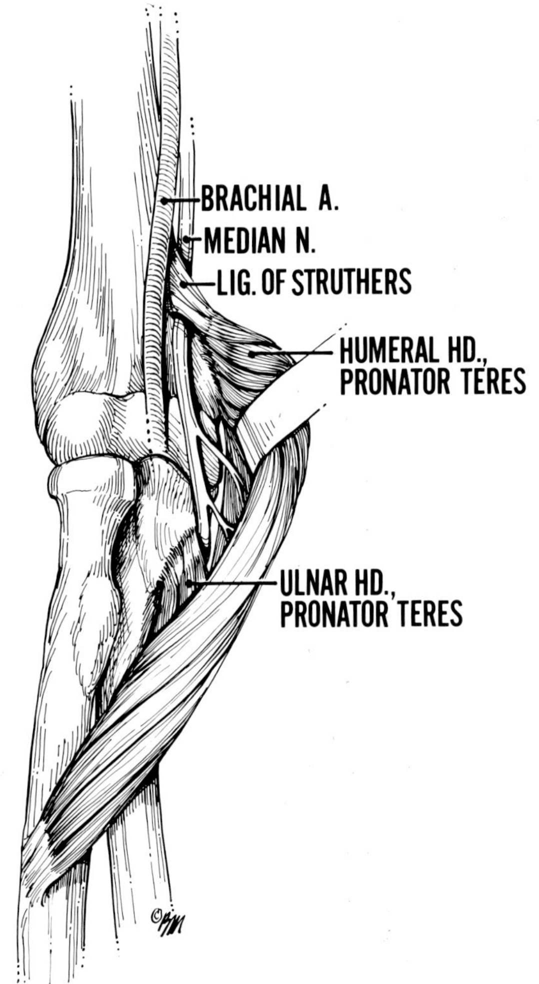

Fig. 36-2. The brachial artery may be superficial to the ligament of Struthers, which forms an accessory origin for the pronator teres.

compression, the fascia of the lacertus fibrosus. Although thickening of the lacertus fibrosus can create a compression neuropathy of the median nerve,[151] it probably only does so when the median nerve lies along the lateral edge and is uncovered by the flexor muscle mass and is, therefore, immediately beneath the lacertus fibrosus. This compression is probably only recognized with the forearm in pronation, which tightens the lacertus fibrosus over the neurovascular bundle and flexor muscle mass. The lacertus fibrosus should be divided routinely during surgery for pronator syndrome. The median nerve is then traced distally as it begins to dive into the pronator muscle.

It is important to recall Henry's admonition that the branches of the median nerve arise from the medial side as the nerve is followed in the proximal forearm.[40] The pronator teres muscle has two heads of origin: the humeral or superficial head arising from the medial epicondyle and the supracondylar ridge; and the ulnar or deep portion arising from the medial side of the coronoid process of the ulna, joining the superficial head at an acute angle. The median nerve enters the forearm between the two heads of the pronator teres.[43] Hypertrophy of the pronator teres muscle, reflections of the muscle fascia forming fibrous bands, and the sharp aponeurotic edge of the deep head of the pronator muscle have all been implicated in compression neuropathies of the median nerve at this level.[111,138,144,168] The operation is continued by exploration of the median nerve as it enters the pronator teres muscle. After the entrance of the nerve into the muscle is inspected, the superficial head of the muscle can be elevated by dissecting the distal insertion of that head from a conjoined tendon with the deep head, which inserts at the midportion of the radius. The superficial head can be elevated, separated along the course of its fibers, and reflected ulnarly in order to explore the median nerve. Elevation of the superficial head of the pronator teres allows the surgeon to see the fourth and last potential compression site of the pronator syndrome, that is, the arch of the superficialis muscle. The flexor digitorum superficialis is the largest muscle of the superficial group in the proximal forearm. The muscle arises from the medial epicondyle of the humerus, joining with a common tendon origin from the ulnar collateral ligament of the elbow joint, and from the intermuscular septum between the ulnar collateral ligament and the remaining muscles of the superficial volar compartment.[37] As the ulnar component of the superficialis joins the radial origin arising from the oblique fibers of the radius emanating from the radial tuberosity, a tendinous aponeurotic arch is formed, under which the median nerve passes. This aponeurotic arch of the superficialis origin constitutes the distal extent of the exploration for entrapment of the median nerve when the patient presents with symptoms and signs of pronator syndrome.

Author's Preferred Method. The author's preferred method of surgical exploration is to begin the exploration of the median nerve 5 cm proximal to the elbow and to trace it distally, taking care to explore all the individual branches to the superficial compartment of muscles. I often isolate a variety of fibrous bands that usually arise beneath the lacertus fibrosus or fascia of the pronator muscle, which will encircle some of the muscular branches of the median nerve as they arise from the medial side of the main trunk. Each of these potential sites of compression must be divided to ensure that a comprehensive release of the median nerve has been accomplished. Preoperative electrodiagnostic findings within the flexor carpi radialis, palmaris longus, flexor digitorum superficialis, or pronator teres do not isolate the area of compression at or above the lacertus fibrosus, since the separate fascial bands affecting individual muscular branches may lead the surgeon away from recognizing a compression neuropathy within the body of the pronator muscle or at the superficialis arch. Therefore, a complete exploration from the area of the ligament of Struthers through the arch of the superficialis is necessary to ensure an adequate release for the pronator syndrome.

Postoperative Management. Since during the closure of the operative wound the superficial head of the pronator teres is either sutured loosely to the tendinous insertion or allowed to lie on the deep head to seek its own level, postoperative care can usually be limited to a soft dressing. A posterior elbow splint may be used for support of the arm during the early postoperative period, positioning the elbow in 45 to 90 degrees flexion. The patient is permitted to begin flexion and extension exercises of the elbow by the fifth postoperative day. If, as a part of the surgical procedure, the entire pronator teres muscle has been detached from its insertion, (which I believe is rarely necessary) the arm should be maintained in some degree of pronation, allowing only flexion and extension exercises of the elbow until tendinous healing of the reattached pronator teres is complete. This immobilization can be accomplished with a Muenster-type cast applied with the forearm in pronation, so that some flexion and extension, but usually not full extension, of the elbow is permitted by the cast.

Anterior Interosseous Syndrome

A compression neuropathy of the anterior interosseous nerve is generally manifested by a vague pain in the proximal forearm that increases with exercise and is relieved with rest. On clinical examination, there is weakness or paralysis of the flexor digitorum profundus of the index finger, the flexor pollicis longus, and the pronator quadratus muscles. The patient will assume an unusual posture of pinch because of loss of function of the profundus to the index finger and the flexor pollicis longus, hyperextending the DIP joint of the index finger and the interphalangeal joint of the thumb.[172] This syndrome characteristically has no sensory symptoms or signs.[177] The diagnosis may be confirmed with electrodiagnostic studies of changes in the electrical pattern in the deep volar compartment muscles.[166] After the diagnosis of an anterior interosseous syndrome is made clinically and the involvement of the deep volar compartment is confirmed electrodiagnostically, surgical exploration of this branch of the median nerve is indicated.[172] If electrodiagnostic studies fail to confirm the diagnosis of anterior interosseous syndrome, the surgeon must consider a higher origin of nerve injury, such as pronator syndrome or vascular anomaly of the brachial plexus, as the cause of symptoms. If these possibilities are excluded, the surgeon should delay exploration of the forearm, and the patient should be restudied electromyographically in 4 to 6 weeks.

Pertinent Anatomy

Although nearly a dozen variations of muscle-tendon units, blood vessels, or enlarged bursae or other tumors have been described as causative of anterior interosseous syndrome, the single common denominator in all these clinical cases has been that the anterior interosseous branch of the median nerve has been compressed in the area of the proximal forearm.[142,143,152,156,164,167,169,170,176,179,181,183,203] Under ordinary circumstances, a detailed exploration of the median nerve, beginning above the anterior interosseous branch and extending into the deep volar compartment, will be sufficient to identify and isolate the area of compression and/or entrapment neuropathy of the anterior interosseous nerve.

Operative Technique

The operation for anterior interosseous syndrome begins as described above for the pronator syndrome, with an incision 5 cm above the elbow joint over the medial neurovascular bundle, zigzagging across the volar elbow crease and continuing to the midforearm between the flexor and extensor muscle masses (Fig. 36-3). The exploration of the median nerve begins proximal to the elbow joint by identifying the median nerve at the level of the elbow and tracing the nerve distally into the

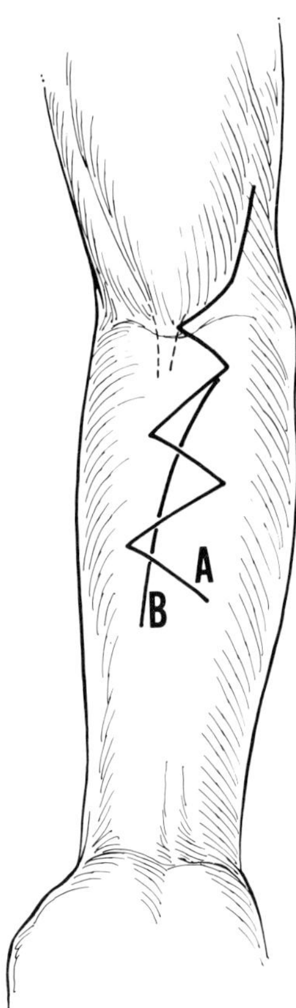

Fig. 36-3. The incision to explore the median and anterior interosseous nerves in the proximal forearm begins at least 5 cm above the elbow flexion crease. Although I prefer the zigzag incision *A*, which offers wider exposure, incision *B* is also adequate.

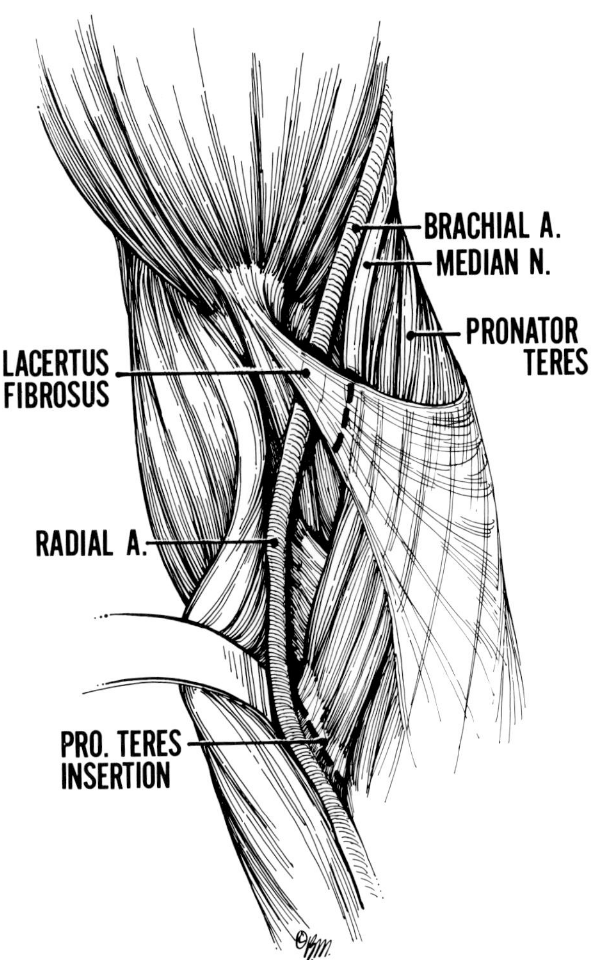

Fig. 36-4. The lacertus fibrosus may act as a compressive band across the flexor muscle mass in pronation; it should be divided with any exploration of the median nerve.

proximal forearm. After the median nerve is isolated medial to the brachial artery and veins, the surgeon can divide the lacertus fibrosus (Fig. 36-4) and trace the nerve distally as it enters the forearm at the level of the pronator teres. The surgeon must be careful to identify those small muscular branches that may have fascial reflections causing isolated compression neuropathies. At the proximal edge of the pronator teres muscle, the superficial head may again need to be elevated, as it was for the pronator syndrome, by detachment of its conjoined tendon insertion at the midportion of the radius and by separation of the muscle fibers of the superficial head from those of the deep head, to expose the median nerve (Fig. 36-5). It may also be necessary to divide the insertion of the deep head of the pronator teres to obtain a satisfactory view of the anterior interosseous nerve as it enters the deep volar compartment beneath the superficialis arch. In rare cases, reflection of the flexor digitorum superficialis muscle origin, as described by Henry in the subcutaneous transfer of the median nerve, may be necessary.[40] In those cases, separation of the origin of the superficialis from its radial border, as well as elevation of the muscle reflecting it ulnarly, will allow the surgeon to see the entire median nerve lying beneath the superficialis arch and within

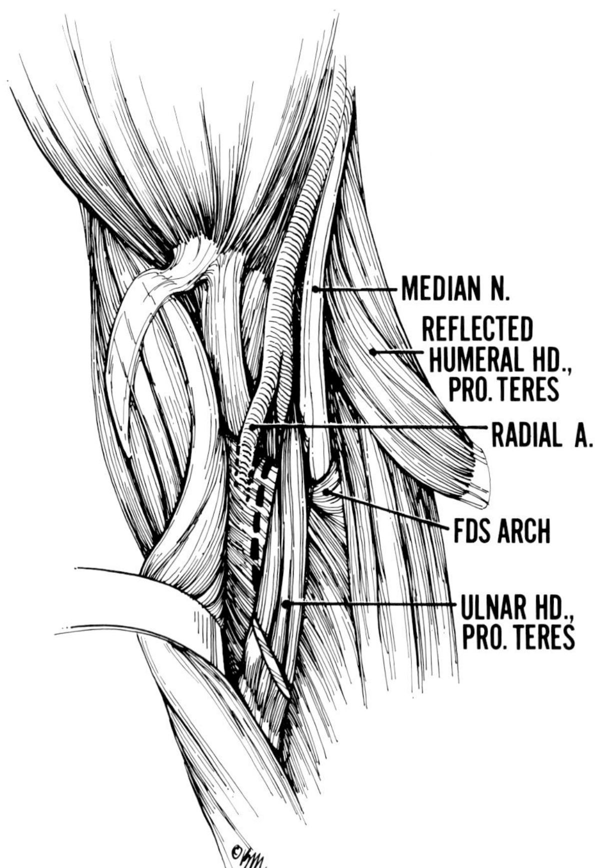

Fig. 36-5. Exposure of the median and anterior interosseous nerves by reflection of the humeral head (superficial head) of the pronator teres also exposes the arch of the superficialis.

the fascia on the deep surface of the superficialis muscle (Fig. 36-6). This exploration deep to the superficialis muscle requires an extensive incision on the volar forearm, extending nearly to the junction of the middle and distal thirds. With this technique, however, the entire median nerve can be explored, and even transposed subcutaneously, placing the superficialis muscle beneath the median nerve but, of course, superficial to the anterior interosseous nerve, and resuturing the pronator teres muscle to its insertion beneath the median nerve as well. The usual findings upon exploration of the anterior interosseous nerve are compression, either by fascial bands on the deep head of the pronator teres or by the tendinous origin of the flexor superficialis, as the nerve separates from the median nerve and comes to lie with a branch of the ulnar artery in the deep volar compartment. Thrombosed or aberrant vessels, as well as enlarged bursae, may also be seen. A variety of aberrant muscles and muscle-tendon units, such as an accessory head of the flexor pollicis longus (Gantzer's muscle[157]), the so-called palmaris profundus,[95] and the flexor carpi radialis brevis,[111] have all been identified as creating a compression neuropathy of the anterior interosseous nerve.

Postoperative Management. The postoperative management following exploration of the anterior interosseous nerve is simplified if the tourniquet is reduced and meticulous hemostasis of the wound is secured. Closure of the subcutaneous tissue and the skin can be accomplished in the usual manner. Most patients are comfortable in a soft dressing supported with a plaster splint for the elbow and wrist, with the wrist in neutral position, the forearm in 45 degrees pronation in order to reduce tension on the pronator teres muscle, particularly if it has been divided and repaired, and the elbow in 45 degrees flexion for comfort. It is important in the early postoperative period that the patient maintain adequate motion of his shoulder and ordinarily flexion and extension of the elbow are begun, by the end of the first week, although pronation and supination of the forearm are usually delayed to allow healing of the pronator teres tendon. Rupture of the repair of the pronator teres tendon has not been a problem; if it should occur, I would not undertake a surgical repair.

Carpal Tunnel Syndrome

Carpal tunnel syndrome is the most common compression neuropathy in the upper extremity. Some authors have attributed the original description of carpal tunnel syndrome to Sir James Paget, who noted the clinical stigmata of the syndrome in 1854.[286] Marie et Foix in 1913 described the pathologic changes of the median nerve.[305] Moersch coined the name of the syndrome in 1938, and Cannon and Love in 1946 described the first series of patients with median nerve compression.[206] In 1947, Brain, Wright, and Wilkerson[200] described six patients who were treated surgically for bilateral carpal tunnel syndrome by surgical release of the transverse carpal ligament. In a series of articles beginning in 1950,[91,330–335] Phalen repeatedly directed the attention of the American medical community to the carpal tunnel syndrome. His contribution to both physicians and surgeons in the recognition and the treatment of carpal tunnel syndrome has been immeasurable.

A variety of symptoms[209,214,242,280,281,361,387] have been associated with carpal tunnel syndrome and a multitude of diseases[27,189,198,208,218,228,245,248,249,258,270,277,278,284,286,290,291,307,308,310,316,324,336,338,343,344,354,364,376,377,379,383] have presented with this syndrome as the presenting symptom complex. The usual symptoms of carpal tunnel syndrome are weakness or clumsiness in the hand, hypesthesia or paresthesias in the distribution of the median nerve, aggravation of the symptoms as the patient uses the hand (especially with grasping), awakening from sleep with numbness in the fingers, and pain in the wrist or distal forearm. Presenting symptoms of shoulder pain or upper arm pain are not uncommon,[209,214,242,281] and proximal migration of pain from the area of the wrist toward the proximal forearm and elbow are relatively common. Although most authors have felt in the past that this syndrome is seen more frequently in females than in males by a ratio of more than 2 to 1, recent reports indicate that the syndrome may be much more common in males than had previously been suggested. Except in selected populations, 50 percent of cases occur in patients between 40 and 60 years of age.[196] Distal lancinating paresthesias in the distribution of the median nerve with percussion of the median nerve at the wrist are suggestive of carpal tunnel syndrome,[363] and reproduction of symptoms with the

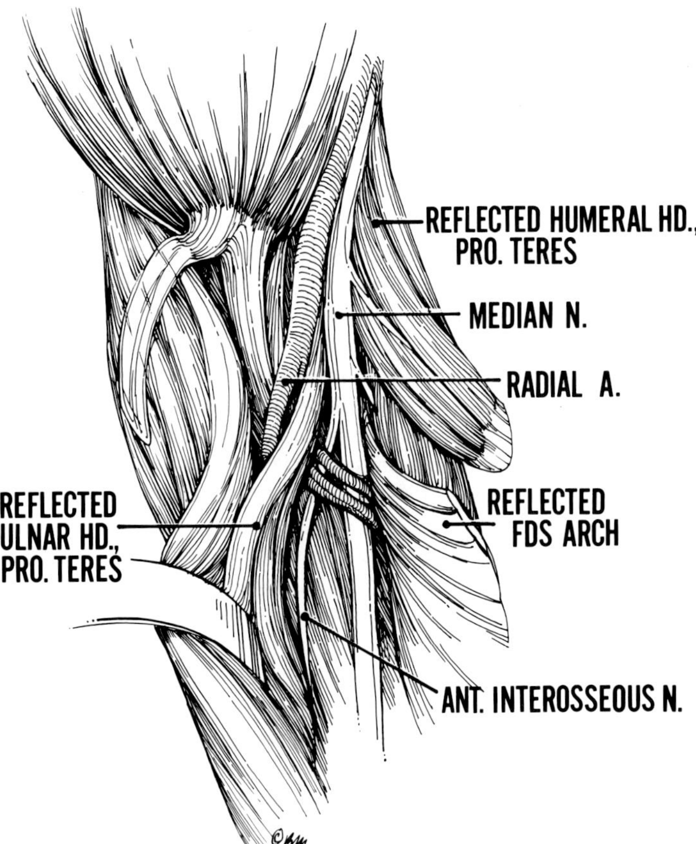

Fig. 36-6. The radial origin of the superficialis muscle is elevated by subperiosteal dissection to expose the deep volar compartment and the anterior interosseous nerve.

wrist flexion test as described by Phalen[331] is generally diagnostic. Symptoms are often relieved by splinting the wrist in a neutral position, taking care that the splint does not lie over the median nerve on the volar surface of the forearm.

Decreased sensibility in the distribution of the median nerve and thenar atrophy are *advanced* signs of this entrapment neuropathy. Although electrodiagnostic studies are widely used to confirm the diagnosis of carpal tunnel syndrome (prolonged motor or sensory conduction latency across the carpal tunnel),[26,68,204,262,273,292,305,315,339,354,370,371] the diagnosis of this syndrome is at least 85 percent certain in the patient with a wrist flexion test that reproduces the symptoms, sensitivity to percussion of the median nerve at the wrist, and objective sensory findings limited to the median nerve distribution. The electromyogram is most useful in those patients in whom the surgeon wishes to differentiate the carpal tunnel syndrome from syndromes of the thoracic outlet and compression syndromes of the lower cervical roots.[315]

The conditions that have been associated with carpal tunnel syndrome include rheumatoid arthritis,[316,356] thyroid imbalance, particularly myxedema,[27,338] acromegaly,[334,385] multiple myeloma,[218] amyloidosis,[286] diabetes mellitus,[286,336] local trauma to the wrist,[184,192,229,274,314] alcoholism, hemophilia,[258,259,277] local tumors such as lipomata or ganglia,[179] hormonal changes associated with menopause,[286,343] pregnancy,[245,284,307] pleonosteosis,[379] gout[248,308,350] and a variety of anatomic anomalies,[95,190,191,195,201,205,266,348] such as aberrant muscles, vascular tumors,[373] and even thrombosis of a persistent median artery[288,309] lying adjacent to the median nerve in the carpal tunnel. Although many anatomic variations have been reported as factors in the carpal tunnel syndrome, there has always been some question about whether such aberrant muscles as the palmaris profundus,[111] anomalous lumbrical muscles,[205,266,348] flexor superficialis muscles,[195,227] or palmaris longus[95,180,181,201] can be a factor in the carpal tunnel syndrome. On the other hand, an enlarged median artery can certainly be a factor in neuritic symptoms of the median nerve. Thrombosis of a persistent median artery[288,309] will precipitate the onset of an acute, extremely painful median neuritis that often requires early surgical care. Carpal tunnel syndrome has been reported in children,[358] presenting as atrophy of the index finger in a juvenile, as described by Lettin.[287] Some authors believe that 60 percent of patients with fractures of the distal radius have at some time during their fracture treatment symptoms of compression of the median nerve in the area of the carpal tunnel. Obviously, not all of these patients require surgical care.

One indication for operative intervention in the carpal tunnel is a failure to respond to conservative therapy. The conservative treatment for median neuritis consists of splinting of the wrist, injection with corticosteroid into the carpal tunnel, and oral nonsteroidal anti-inflammatory medications.

Splinting of the wrist in a neutral position will usually reduce and may even completely relieve the symptoms of carpal tunnel syndrome. I prefer a dorso-ulnar plaster splint across the wrist, positioned so that no portion of the splint lies over the median nerve in the distal forearm or volar aspect of the wrist. The patient will wear the splint during the work day, be splint-free between work and bedtime, and then continue with the splint at night, removing it only upon awakening in the morning. If the patient requires splints on both wrists in the work place, then I have the patient alternate the splints during the day so that he or she is wearing one or the other splint during the entire work day, but each splint is worn only 4 hours of the 8-hour work day. The patient will then wear both splints at night. The patient continues this splinting routine for 6 to 8 weeks, and if symptoms have been completely relieved with the use of the dorso-ulnar gutter splint, the splinting program is continued for approximately another two months. Upon the completion then of 3½ to 4 months of splinting, the splints will gradually be removed, removing the work day splint first and the nighttime splint later over several months. If symptoms recur with removal of the splint after its use for this period of time, the patient is a candidate for operative intervention.

Once popular in the late 1950s and early 1960s[231,243,331,332] injection of corticosteroid into the carpal tunnel has regained popularity in the early 1980s.[239,247,386] The method of injection must be precise and consistent, and there is ample evidence that imprecise placement of the needle, or the use of a needle that is too large, can result in prolonged disability, even permanent injury, to the median nerve. Accordingly, it has been recommended by Wood[386] that needle placement be practiced at the time of carpal tunnel operation, inserting the needle prior to skin incision and then visualizing the actual site of placement after the transverse carpal ligament has been sectioned. Green[247] has suggested the injection of a small amount of local anesthetic to insure correct placement of the needle prior to injection of corticosteroid. In the hands of most skilled surgeons, injection of the carpal tunnel is an effective, though usually transient, therapeutic modality, after which between 65 and 90 percent of patients can be expected to have some recurrence of symptoms that may require carpal tunnel surgical release.

In my opinion, corticosteroid injection into the carpal tunnel[269] is indicated when the entrapment of the median nerve can be predicted to be temporary, such as in pregnancy, or when the patient's activity can be sufficiently modified to anticipate a reduction in stress symptoms at the wrist. In patients with temporary carpal tunnel syndrome, particularly that associated with pregnancy, splinting and an injection of a cortisone preparation combined with a local anesthetic, with care taken to avoid the median nerve, have generally reduced symptoms sufficiently for the patient to complete the pregnancy. Following pregnancy the symptoms of carpal tunnel syndrome usually regress rapidly, certainly over the first 4 to 6 weeks postpartum. Nevertheless, many patients who exhibit signs and symptoms of carpal tunnel syndrome during preg-

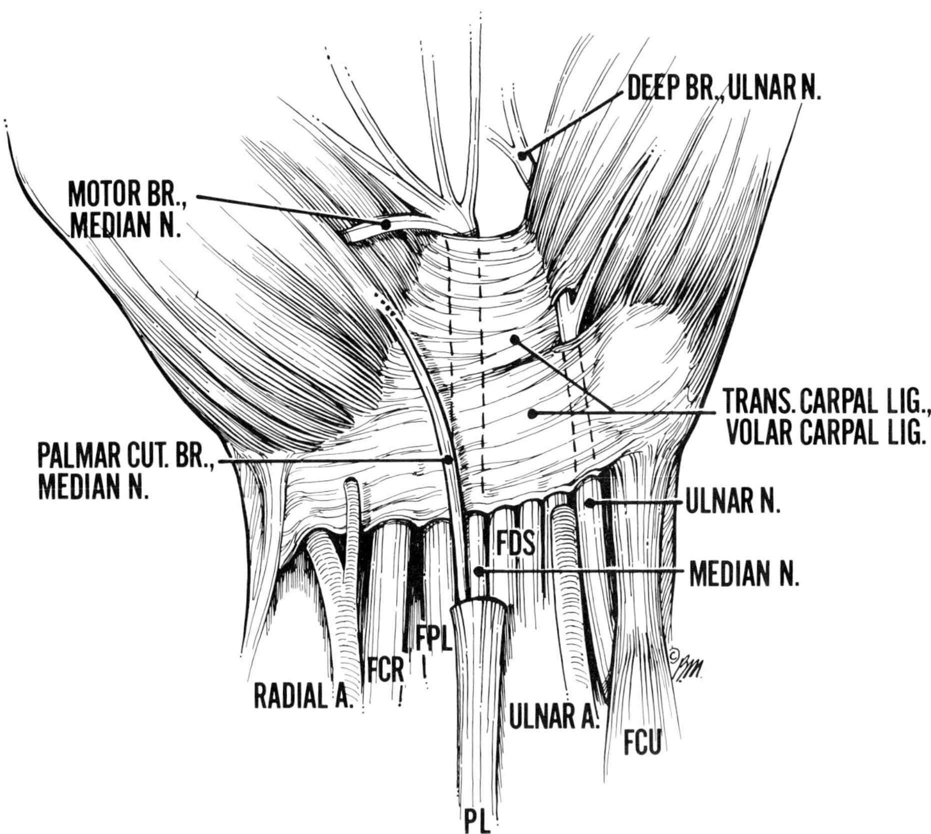

Fig. 36-7. The median nerve and the long flexor tendons transverse the carpal tunnel, lying beneath the transverse carpal ligament.

nancy will have repeated and increasing symptoms during subsequent pregnancies, and will often eventually require surgical release of the transverse carpal ligament either between pregnancies or as they reach the menopausal years.

The repetitive or cumulative trauma syndromes associated with carpal tunnel syndrome that are commonly seen in the work place will normally respond to a combination of conservative treatment consisting of splinting, corticosteroid injection into the carpal tunnel, and change of job activity. If the patient's treatment program does not include a permanent change of job activity, the combination of splinting and injection will provide the patient with only temporary relief of symptoms, and the return to repetitive, stressful activity may very well be accompanied by increasing neuropathy of the median nerve.

Although nonsteroidal anti-inflammatory medications have been prescribed for patients with carpal tunnel syndrome, their effect in the treatment of this condition is uncertain. Presently, I do not use nonsteroidal anti-inflammatory medications as a routine part of conservative treatment of carpal tunnel syndrome.

Pertinent Anatomy

The volar radiocarpal ligament and the volar ligamentous extensions between the carpal bones form the floor of the carpal tunnel. The transverse carpal ligament is a thick fibrous band that arches over the concave surface of the carpal bones, attaching on the radial side to the tuberosity of the scaphoid and a portion of the trapezium and on the ulnar aspect to the pisiform and hook of the hamate. This ligament completes the tunnel through which the long flexor tendons and median nerve pass (Fig. 36-7). The median nerve ordinarily lies superficial, directly beneath the transverse carpal ligament. Of the many anatomic variations that can be associated with carpal tunnel syndrome, none are more important to the surgeon than the variations of the motor branch of the median nerve, which must be protected during the surgical exposure and division of the transverse carpal ligament. Lanz[283] has classified the anatomic variations of the median nerve into four subgroups: (1) variations in the course of the thenar branch of the median nerve, (2) accessory variations of the thenar branch at the distal carpal tunnel, (3) high divisions of the median nerve, and (4) accessory branches proximal to the carpal tunnel. The normal position for the motor branch of the median nerve is the extra ligamentous recurrent course from the median nerve just distal to the transverse carpal ligament, supplying innervation to the thenar muscles (Fig. 36-8). This branching of the median nerve occurs in approximately one-half of cases. The next most common variation of the motor median nerve is the subligamentous branching, in which the recurrent median branch divides from the median nerve beneath the transverse carpal ligament, lies close to the median nerve, and innervates the thenar muscles with a recurrent course distal to the transverse carpal ligament (Fig. 36-9). This subligamentous variation occurs in approximately one-third of cases. The third most common course for the motor branch of the median nerve is transligamentous. In this variation the motor branch of the median nerve divides from the common median nerve beneath the transverse carpal ligament and in its course to the thenar muscles pierces the transverse carpal ligament between 2 and 6 mm from its distal border (Fig. 36-10). This variation, according to Poisel as reported by Lanz,[283] occurs in approximately one out of five patients. The remaining variations in the course of the thenar branch of the median nerve are generally considered to be extremely rare, and yet variations have been reported by numerous authors[195,246,268,302,323,328] (Fig. 36-11).

The second group of variations seen with the motor branch of the median nerve consists of various accessory branches that innervate the thenar muscles. These multiple branches of the median nerve are considered to be rare, but they have been reported occurring distally and coursing parallel to the thenar muscles from the median nerve. High divisions of the median

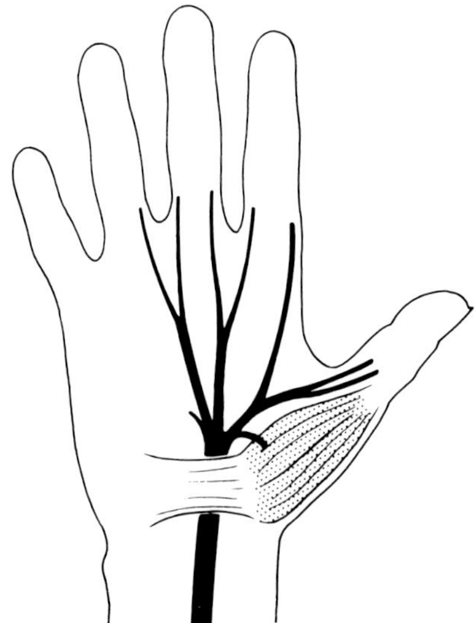

Fig. 36-8. The most common pattern of the motor branch of median nerve is extraligamentous and recurrent. (From Lanz,[283] with permission.)

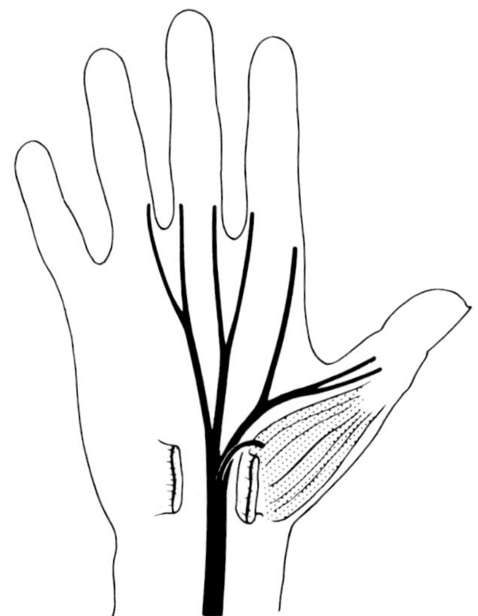

Fig. 36-9. Subligamentous branching of a recurrent median nerve. (From Lanz,[283] with permission.)

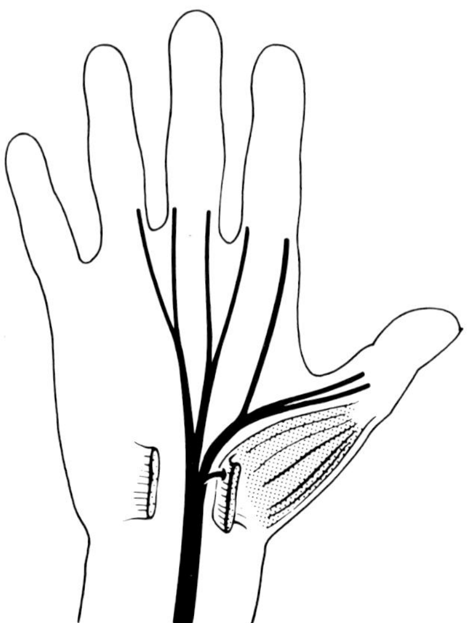

Fig. 36-10. Transligamentous course of the recurrent branch of the median nerve. (From Lanz,[283] with permission.)

nerve in the carpal tunnel are classified in Lanz's Group 3[220,276] (Fig. 36-12). Although these high divisions may arise in the proximal or middle third of the forearm, they generally run parallel to the nerve and are divided from it by a persistent median artery[276] or an aberrant muscle.[348] The median nerve and the motor branch pass deep to the transverse carpal ligament and then divide into the usual multiple branches. In recognizing the possibility of a high division of the median nerve, the careful surgeon will generally have little problem dealing with these variations. The fourth and final classification of anatomic variations of the median nerve at the carpal tunnel includes accessory branches of the median nerve supplying the thenar muscles proximal to the transverse carpal ligament[289,323] (Fig. 36-13). These branches may course superficial to the transverse carpal ligament, arising from the common median nerve proximal to the carpal tunnel and then rejoining the main nerve distal to the ligament prior to again branching from it and supplying motor innervation to the thenar muscles. The transligamentous course of an accessory branch of the median nerve has been reported, as has an ulnar take-off of the accessory transligamentous branch proximal to the carpal tunnel.[283] In addition, I have observed multiple accessory branches of the median nerve passing either proximal and distal to the carpal ligament or transligamentous to supply innervation to the thenar muscles.

In some patients the transverse carpal ligament has a muscular rather than a ligamentous appearance, possibly due to large thenar muscles that extend more ulnarly than normal. The incidence of anomalous motor branches with this anatomic variation is exceptionally high, and recognition of a muscular transverse carpal ligament should immediately alert the surgeon to proceed with extreme caution when transecting the ligament.

Operative Techniques

Although release of the transverse carpal ligament is the basic procedure for the treatment of carpal tunnel syndrome, the approaches to the release of that ligament may vary considerably in the hands of different surgeons. Keeping in mind the many variations that can occur in the motor branch of the median nerve, it seems prudent to design an incision through which the surgeon can protect the branches, even the rare variations, and yet at the same time perform an adequate division of the carpal ligament. A small transverse incision at the base of the palm or in the proximal wrist crease does not allow adequate exploration of the carpal tunnel and endangers the branches of the median nerve, especially those branches that may communicate occasionally with the ulnar nerve at the distal border of the carpal tunnel[283,383] and those variations of the motor branch previously discussed. The surgeon is also

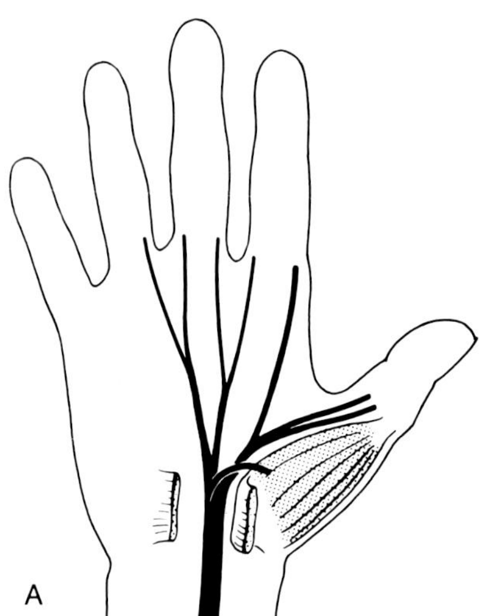

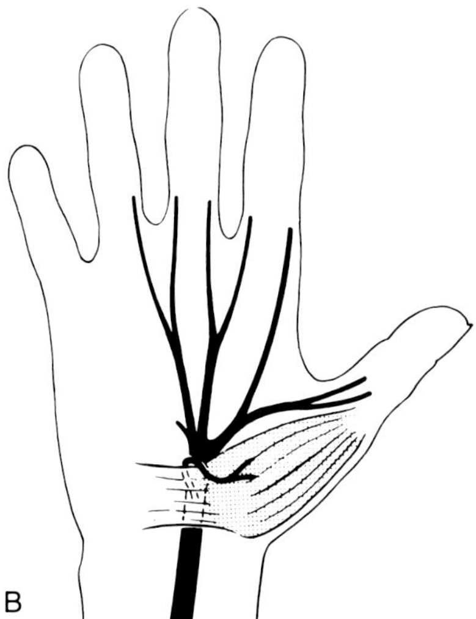

Fig. 36-11. Less common thenar branch variations include **(A)** a branch from the ulnar border of the median nerve and **(B)** a branch lying on top of the transverse carpal ligament. (From Lanz,[283] with permission.)

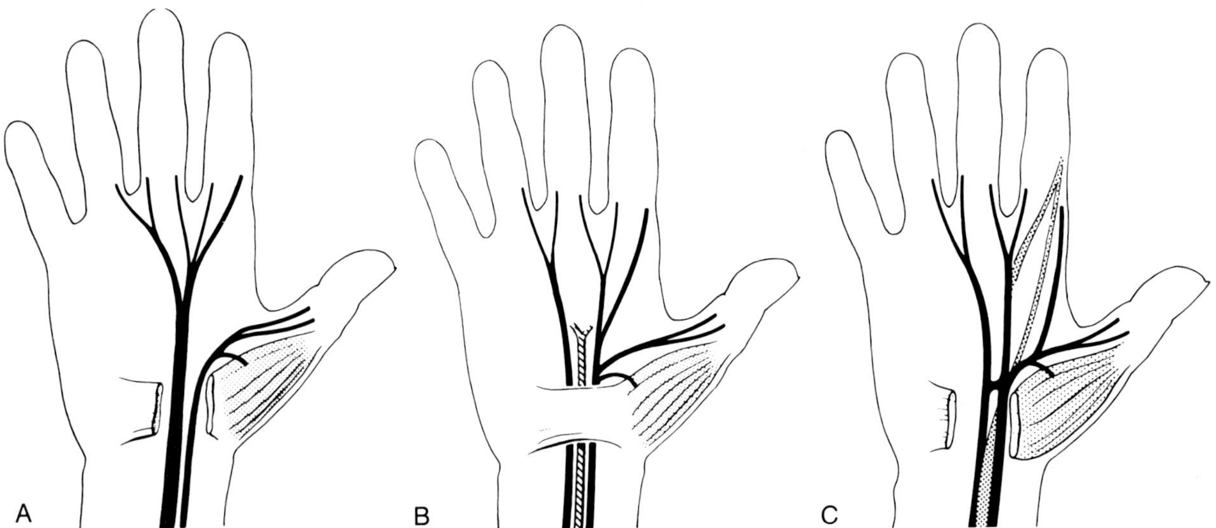

Fig. 36-12. Group III variations of the thenar branch include **(A)** high divisions of the median nerve that may be separated by **(B)** a persistent median artery or **(C)** an aberrant muscle. (From Lanz,[283] with permission.)

more likely to injure the palmar cutaneous branch of the median nerve with the transverse incision in the wrist crease.

A limited approach to the transverse carpal ligament parallel to longitudinal creases at the base of the palm may have some application in exploration of the transverse carpal ligament, but will not identify those motor branches of the median nerve that divide proximal to the transverse carpal ligament, and may jeopardize the more unusual variations that arise in the distal third of the forearm. Several authors[121,207] have pointed out the necessity of avoiding the palmar cutaneous branch of the median nerve in designing an incision to release the transverse carpal ligament. Taleisnik[368] has suggested that an incision over the palm of the hand lie ulnar to the axis of the ring finger at the base of the palm to avoid the medial branch of the palmar cutaneous nerve. Others have emphasized the use of a limited fasciotomy of the distal third of the forearm in the treatment of carpal tunnel syndrome to avoid a constricting band of forearm fascia across the median nerve as it rises from beneath the superficialis muscles or at the wrist flexion crease.

Author's Preferred Method. To accommodate the many anatomic variations and to ensure an adequate release of the median nerve, as well as perform an adequate division of the transverse carpal ligament, I have used an incision that begins distally at the distal border of the transverse carpal ligament and follows the longitudinal crease of the palm, crossing the base of the palm in a zigzag fashion ulnar to the long axis of the ring finger (Fig. 36-14). The incision continues above the proximal wrist crease for approximately 3 cm. Through the proximal portion of this incision, the superficial fascia of the fore-

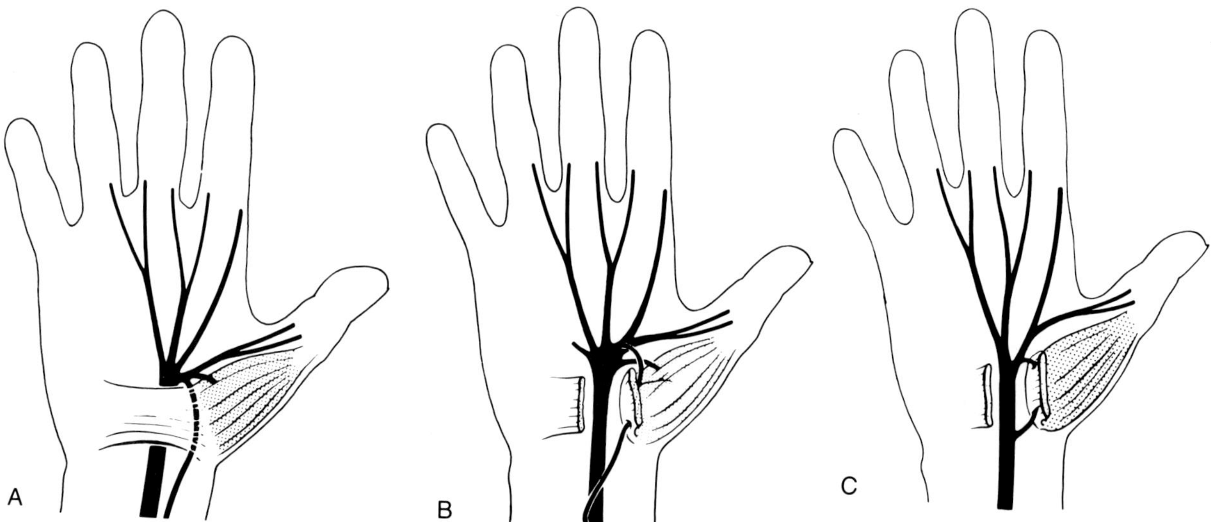

Fig. 36-13. Group IV variations of the thenar branch include those rare instances in which the thenar branch leaves the median nerve proximal to the carpal tunnel. (From Lanz,[283] with permission.)

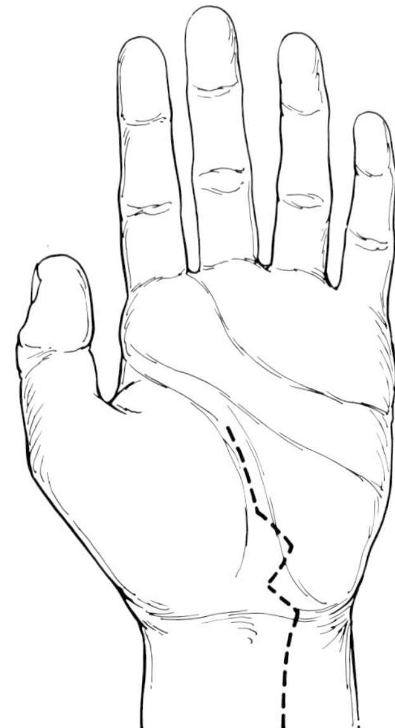

Fig. 36-14. The author's preferred carpal tunnel incision. At the base of the palm the incision is ulnar to the axis of the ring finger.

arm is isolated and divided longitudinally. The ulnar border of the median nerve is identified and a fasciotomy of the distal third of the forearm is performed. By remaining on the ulnar side of the median nerve, often using a hemostat to protect the deep structures, the transverse carpal ligament is divided. The dissection is done in layers, dividing the palmar fascia initially and then extending through the transverse carpal ligament throughout its course.

This exposure and technique allows maximum protection of the median nerve, as well as the tendons of the carpal canal. The transverse carpal ligament is sectioned under direct vision throughout its entire length and those structures on the ulnar side of the incision (that is, the ulnar neurovascular bundle and the superficial vascular arch of the palm) can be seen and protected. This approach at the base of the palm lies ulnar to the axis of the ring finger and is in close proximity to Guyon's canal, which may also be released at the time of carpal tunnel decompression if the surgeon feels that its release is indicated.[500] Because of the increasing association of carpal tunnel syndrome with industrial cumulative trauma disorder, and the common origin of carpal and ulnar tunnel syndromes with repetitive wrist flexion, some surgeons have suggested that the combined release of both carpal and ulnar tunnels in the worker affected by a cumulative trauma disorder associated with median nerve or ulnar nerve compression is the operation of choice to prevent multiple operations and increasing impairment as the result of cumulative trauma.

Following release of the transverse carpal ligament, exploration of the motor branch to identify a transligamentous course of the branch is necessary. If the motor branch of the median nerve passes distal to the transverse carpal ligament, assuming its usual recurrent course to the thenar muscles, no further dissection of the branch is necessary. If, however, a transligamentous course of the motor branch is identified the branch should be freed from its transligamentous passage by further division of the transverse carpal ligament.[111,283] This procedure will eliminate any possibility of compression neuropathy or traction neuropathy at the transligamentous passage as a result of the division of the transverse carpal ligament. If no additional surgery of the median nerve is anticipated (see discussion of internal neurolysis that follows), the skin can be closed, taking care to approximate the skin of the palm anatomically.

Postoperative Management. Postoperative care consists of a period of wrist immobilization from 3 to 14 days, during which time the patient is encouraged to use the hand. Flexion and extension exercises of the fingers and flexion, extension, and rotational exercises of the thumb are encouraged. The usual postoperative course is punctuated with an almost immediate relief of pain and some improvement in the sensibility of the fingers if the patient does not have an axonotmetic or neurotmetic lesion of the median nerve. After the initial and usually dramatic improvement in sensibility, the patient experiences some slight decrease in improvement (about 1 week postoperatively). Improvement will again be realized after this transient partial relapse. The changes in the conduction velocity seem to parallel the patient's clinical response. It has been demonstrated at operation that an immediate improvement in conduction velocity can be anticipated in most cases of carpal tunnel release.[224] In the postoperative period, the conduction velocity, which was prolonged before surgery and returned to a normal range immediately following release of the ligament, rises to some intermediate value at approximately 1 week postoperatively, followed by a gradual return to its normal range within 8 to 12 weeks. Those patients who have a prolonged return of conduction velocity to normal must be anticipated to have a more profound neuropathy, possibly associated with other factors such as diabetes mellitus. Patients with an axonotmesis, of course, can be anticipated to have an advancing Tinel's sign and eventually regain nearly full return of function in the median nerve.

Following carpal tunnel release, swelling at the base of the palm superficial to the carpal tunnel can be expected to persist for 12 to 16 weeks following surgery. During this period of time, and probably concurrent with the swelling, the patient may experience aching pain in the thenar or hypothenar eminences, which has been termed "pillar pain." Heavy activity and gripping will aggravate the pain, which may be accompanied by aching in the distal portion of the forearm or shooting sensations in the distal third of the forearm, which are usually only momentary in duration. Resolution of the swelling at the base of the palm is accompanied by relief of "pillar pain" and distal forearm symptoms.

The return of strength following carpal tunnel release is prolonged. By 6 weeks following surgical release of the deep transverse carpal ligament, patients will usually have only about 50 percent of their preoperative grip strength. As long as the patient is able to exercise and work effectively on increasing grip strength, which should be begun in the second or third postoperative week, by 8 to 10 weeks following carpal tunnel release 75 percent of grip strength will usually be regained. Maximum grip strength and, possibly more importantly, the endurance of grip strength often does not return until 6 months or even longer after surgical release of the carpal tunnel. Perhaps as many as 15 or 20 percent of patients who have had carpal tunnel release will never regain full strength after surgical release of the deep transverse carpal tunnel ligament. Whether this is due to some change in the carpal bone configuration with release of the deep transverse carpal ligament, or to the loss of the pulley mechanism contributed to by the deep transverse carpal tunnel ligament is uncertain. It is probably premature to suggest that grip strength will not ultimately be restored unless the patient has been engaged in an active and vigorous rehabilitation program, has resumed normal activities, and 1 year has elapsed since surgery.

As carpal tunnel syndrome becomes increasingly recognized in the work place as a repetitive trauma or cumulative trauma syndrome, it seems more and more certain that modification of the work environment by redistribution of work mechanics, modification of tools and handles to be more compatible with hand function, and the attention of biomechanical engineering designed to protect the worker will create a focus on the *prevention* of this syndrome, rather than the repeated treatment of the syndrome by release of the deep transverse carpal ligament. An important part of the evaluation of industrial biomechanics will be the evaluation of the employee prior to assumption of a position in the work place, combined with a knowledge of the amount of stress applied to the worker's hands in a particular working environment. It should then be possible, through knowing the stress to which the worker is exposed in doing a specific job and that worker's capacity for stress, to provide a suitable match of the worker's abilities with the job requirement and thereby, hopefully, to reduce the incidence of cumulative trauma or stress-related carpal tunnel syndrome.

Internal Neurolysis

Internal neurolysis or endoneurolysis has been described as an adjunct to the treatment of carpal tunnel syndrome.[215,236] It is known that internal fibrosis of the peripheral nerve will constrict axons and mechanically reduce axoplasmic transport. Internal fibrosis can also reduce blood supply to the axons by producing an unfavorable interface between capillaries and the axon membrane. Internal fibrosis of a peripheral nerve may also act as a barrier to regeneration of axons, and constriction of regenerating axons may reduce recovery of the peripheral nerve. Therefore, I believe this procedure is indicated in those lesions of peripheral nerve in which either some degree of internal fibrosis or constriction by the epineurium can be anticipated to continue to prevent neurologic healing and recovery of peripheral nerve function.

My indications for internal neurolysis in conjunction with release of the carpal tunnel are: (1) atrophy of the thenar muscles, (2) *constant* loss of sensibility in the distribution of the median nerve, (3) deterioration of light touch or two-point discrimination sensibility, (4) severe causalgia confined to the distribution of the median nerve (usually associated with traumatic injuries of the distal radius or carpus), and (5) true neuroma-in-continuity of the median nerve at the time of operation.[215] The latter indication is not apparent until epineurotomy of the nerve is performed in an area of swelling of the median nerve, usually just proximal to the constriction of the transverse carpal ligament. With epineurotomy, the internal fibrosis of the nerve is visualized and internal neurolysis completed.

The risks of internal neurolysis are the destruction of the interfascicular plexus and further vascular damage due to interference of the capillary network within the peripheral nerve segment.[102] These risks have been studied in detail in a primate model by Dellon and MacKinnon,[299] who have shown that with microsurgical technique the increase in scarring and anatomic disruption of the nerve segment is minimal with internal neurolysis. It is, however, true that the end result of any surgical procedure, including internal neurolysis, may be the formation of new scar within the peripheral nerve, and that this new scar may be as detrimental as any other fibrosis.

Because of the marked danger of destruction of the interfascicular plexus, internal neurolysis should be limited to those areas of peripheral nerves where the interfascicular plexus is minimal. Usually these are the more distal areas of the peripheral nerves, such as the median nerve at the wrist or distally, the ulnar nerve at the wrist or distally, and the radial nerve at the elbow and through the supinator muscle. The risks of internal neurolysis are increased in more proximal nerve segments such as the ulnar nerve at the elbow.

Internal neurolysis should not be confused with epineurotomy. The incising of the epineurium, considered by some authors to be a "fasciotomy" of a peripheral nerve, is a much simpler procedure and can be performed with appropriate care at any level of a peripheral nerve.

Also, the procedure of internal neurolysis should not be confused with epineurectomy or removal of the epineurium, which is used by some surgeons to decompress segments of peripheral nerves. Epineurectomy will routinely interfere with the blood supply to a segment of a peripheral nerve by excision of the subepineurial plexus of vessels, which lie on the undersurface of the excised epineurium. Although this procedure may have some place in the dissection of peripheral nerves with internal tumors, in my opinion it has no place in the treatment of entrapment neuropathy.

By relieving scar constriction within the nerve trunk, internal neurolysis effectively decompresses the constricted circulation and constricted fascicles within the segment of the peripheral nerve. In this procedure it is important *not* to breach the perineurium, since dissection of the peripheral nerve at that level will injure the end artery circulation of the axon at the capillary level. One might compare the internal neurolysis procedure to that of epineurotomy, so that if epineurotomy were a fasciotomy of the nerve trunk, internal neurolysis would be a fasciotomy of the fascicles.

The procedure of internal neurolysis must be performed with adequate magnification to allow the interfascicular plexus of nerves to be seen and to protect these vital communications between fascicles. Ordinarily this requires at least 3.5× magnification. I have found that, while learning the procedure, an operating microscope of at least 7× is necessary for the surgeon to perform the procedure and evaluate the dissection. After the procedure is learned, however, most surgeons can perform it using 3.5× loupe magnification. The internal neurolysis procedure is limited to the area of the median nerve that is severely affected and must conform to the indications for the procedure, which have been previously described. If, for example, the indication for the internal neurolysis is atrophy of the thenar muscles, the surgeon should begin the procedure by isolating the motor branch of the median nerve distally and tracing those fascicles contributing to the motor branch through the course of the carpal tunnel. Only those fascicles contributing to the motor branch will then undergo internal neurolysis. Similarly, if a patient has constant loss of sensibility in only the middle finger and intermittent loss of sensibility in the index finger and thumb, only those fascicles contributing to the middle finger need undergo internal neurolysis by tracing the fascicles from distal to proximal through the area of compression.

The procedure is begun by epineurotomy on the radial side of the median nerve at the wrist. The opening of the epineurium should be on the radial side of the median nerve since the segmental circulation of that nerve enters from the ulnar side proximal to the transverse carpal ligament and from the vessels of the superficial arch[107,108,365] distal to the transverse carpal ligament. If small vessels are seen within the nerve itself, the exposure through the epineurium should be to one side or the other of these epineurial vessels. The median nerve should *not* be elevated from its bed of areolar tissue and surrounding peritenon since microcirculation may enter the dorsal aspect of the nerve, and sacrifice of this circulation is contraindicated. Once the epineurium is opened, the fascicles are sighted and gently teased apart using small, sharp-pointed surgical scissors and microsurgical forceps. Separation of the fascicles is performed with care, preserving the interfascicular plexus of nerves. If no intrafascicular scarring is encountered at any point in the dissection, the dissection of the fascicles should be stopped. The wound is closed in the usual fashion for a carpal tunnel release by accurate anatomic approximation of the palmar skin. No deep closure is performed and no interposing tissue is drawn over the median nerve prior to skin closure. Postoperative care following internal neurolysis is the same as for carpal tunnel release. Although I generally splint the wrist in neutral position for 10 days to 2 weeks following internal neurolysis, early, intermittent motion of the wrist in dorsiflexion and palmar flexion out of the splint several times a day may be desirable. The response to the surgery, except in cases of preoperative axonotmesis or neurotmesis of the median nerve, is identical to that seen with carpal tunnel release previously described. The initial response to surgical treatment, the diminution of that response at approximately 1 week postoperatively, and the gradual return of function within the distribution of the median nerve parallel the characteristic findings after simple carpal tunnel release. Based on a review of well over 500 cases of carpal tunnel syndrome, a 10 to 15 percent frequency for the use of the internal neurolysis procedure with carpal tunnel release seems to be constant in a general practice of hand surgery. This figure may be slightly higher if the hand surgeon has an exclusively referral practice, since many of the less severe compressions of the median nerve will be treated by other surgeons.

Endoscopic Carpal Tunnel Release

Since the description by Brain, Wright, and Wilkerson in 1947 of six operatively treated patients with median nerve compression,[200] the open surgical technique for release of the deep transverse carpal ligament has been the treatment of choice for persistent carpal tunnel syndrome unresponsive to nonoperative treatment. However, one disadvantage of this procedure is that most patients have significant tenderness in the surgical incision placed at the midpalmar creases or over the hypothenar eminence. This is especially bothersome in patients who must support their weight on their hands with either crutches or other ambulatory aids. Accordingly, Agee and Chow have independently developed techniques for release of the deep transverse carpal ligament using an endoscopic approach. Agee's technique is done through a small incision just proximal to the wrist flexion crease; that incision is combined with a more distal incision at the mid-palm in the Chow technique.[210,211] The two techniques have many elements in common, yet each technique is an entirely separate entity unto itself and must be learned individually.

Agee Technique. Under tourniquet ischemia and local anesthetic often supplemented with intravenous sedation, a transverse incision is made at the wrist flexion crease (ulnar to the palmaris longus tendon) and a U-shaped flap of fascia is developed at the base of the deep transverse carpal ligament. The ulnar bursa is isolated and the interval between the ulnar bursa and the deep transverse carpal ligament to the level of the hook of the hamate is identified and entered with a special probe. The axis of the ring finger (between the ulnar bursa on the radial side and the ulnar neurovascular bundle and flexor carpi ulnaris tendon on the ulnar side) is the plane used to develop the proper area on the undersurface of the deep transverse carpal ligament for its release. The device developed by Agee, known as the "Inside Job," is then inserted into the developed canal on the deep surface of the deep transverse carpal ligament in alignment with the ring finger. The arthroscope is contained within the device and provides visualization of the undersurface of the deep transverse carpal ligament using the transverse direction of fibrous tissue to identify the ligament. The distal edge of the transverse carpal ligament is identified, and the blade is lifted into cutting position with a trigger on the handle of the device (Fig. 36-15). The instrument is then withdrawn, cutting the deep transverse carpal ligament. Although multiple passes with the device are not recommended, a careful second pass may be required if the ligament is seen through the scope to be incompletely divided.

Problems were encountered with the original device because of difficulty in adequately seeing the blade through the scope. The Agee device was therefore taken off the market for a short time, and trials with a redesigned instrument were begun in April 1992.

Chow Technique. An entry portal is made 1 cm radial and 1 cm proximal to the midpoint of the pisiform, which can be palpated at the ulnar aspect of the wrist.[210,211] The incision is transverse, with its ulnar extent lying along the radial edge of the ulnar neurovascular bundle and flexor carpi ulnaris and extending radially across the ulnar border of the ulnar bursa and contents of the carpal tunnel. A longitudinal incision is made through the fascia, exposing the flexor tendons. The ulnar artery and nerve are protected along the ulnar border of this incision. The flexor tendons are gently retracted radially, and the space between the ulnar neurovascular bundle and the

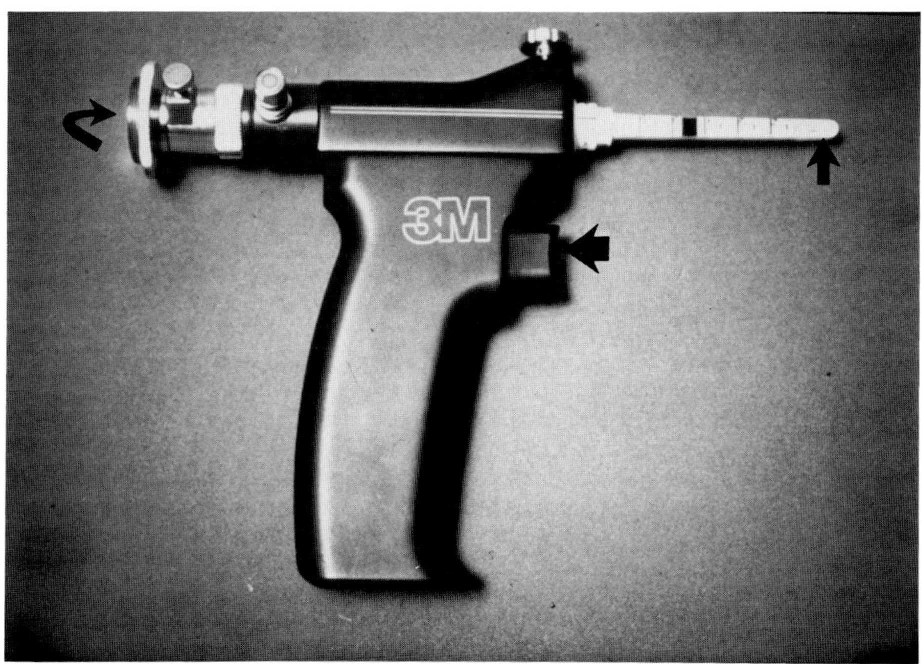

Fig. 36-15. The device developed by Dr. John Agee for endoscopic carpal tunnel release includes a disposable element of white plastic that is inserted into the carpal tunnel to divide the deep transverse carpal ligament. This disposable segment is attached to a pistol grip, the trigger on which *(large arrow)* elevates the scalpel blade on the extreme end of the disposable segment *(small arrow)*. The endoscopic element *(curved arrow)* facing away from the trigger permits the surgeon to visualize the small operative area on the deep surface of the ligament through the endoscope.

flexor tendons is developed with blunt dissectors so that the slotted cannula used in the Chow technique can be guided into the space deep to the transverse carpal ligament while probing toward the hook of the hamate.

The exit portal for the Chow technique in the mid-palm is developed by identifying the point of intersection between a line drawn from the fully abducted thumb across the palm and a straight line from the middle-ring finger web space. The point of intersection of these two lines, generally at a right angle, is then bisected and a transverse incision from the end of that bisector which is proximal and ulnar to the intersection of the defining lines by 1 cm will mark the site of the exit of the cannula and obturator assembly. That exit is facilitated with hyperextension of the wrist as the cannula and obturator assembly is advanced distally toward the exit portal. A small transverse incision allows the cannula to be thrust through the skin, and the hyperextended wrist and hand is now strapped to a hand holder to maintain that position during the division of the deep transverse carpal ligament aided by the arthroscope.

Although Chow initially recommended general endotracheal anesthesia or regional block, presently he recommends the use of a local anesthetic so that the patient's symptoms of neuritis of one or more branches of the ulnar nerve, should they be involved with the obturator, can be appreciated before sectioning the deep transverse carpal ligament. This ligament is sectioned with the aid of the arthroscope and a series of specifically designed knives, which are disposable and designed to be accommodated by the slotted cannula from which the obturator assembly has been withdrawn. The three specially designed knives are not controlled for depth of cut except by their size and their manipulation by the surgeon using arthroscopic control. The arthroscope can be directed from either the proximal or distal end of the slotted cannula, allowing visualization of the cut edges of the transverse carpal ligament from either direction. Following the completion of the procedure, bleeding is assessed, and sensibility in the fingers can be reexamined with the patient under a local anesthetic injected only in the skin of the palm and the skin at the wrist. The wounds are closed in the usual fashion.

The Current Status of Endoscopic Carpal Tunnel Release. Both techniques for endoscopic carpal tunnel release are evolving procedures in the treatment of carpal tunnel syndrome. Major complications from both techniques have been encountered by surgeons properly schooled and instructed in them. Major complications have not been encountered by the surgeons who developed the techniques, probably because of their intensive work in procedure development and their careful understanding of the anatomy of the carpal ligament and its surrounding structures.

Several contraindications to the Chow technique have been suggested. The patient with an extremely stiff wrist is not a good candidate for endoscopic carpal tunnel release by the Chow method. The heavy thick hand with heavily cornified palmar skin is a difficult case in which to use the distal palmar (exit) portal required in this technique. Dupuytren's palmar fibromatosis is a contraindication to the Chow method.

Both techniques for endoscopic carpal tunnel release are designed only to release the transverse carpal ligament, and if the patient requires any additional exploration or surgical intervention such as epineurotomy of the median nerve, ulnar tunnel exploration or release, and/or exploration of the motor branch of either the median or ulnar nerve, a technique other than endoscopy should be used. Because the extent of exploration and the surgical field are limited with endoscopic techniques, the prudent surgeon will complete a more detailed evaluation of the median and ulnar nerve function at the wrist before narrowing the surgical perspective to only the deep transverse carpal ligament. This evaluation may include detailed conduction latencies of the ulnar nerve across the wrist, including a latency to the first dorsal interosseous muscle, so that the nerve conduction latency is known to be normal in the deep branch of ulnar nerve. Because of the importance of the hook of hamate to endoscopic technique as a landmark, the carpal tunnel x-ray that shows the hook of the hamate in profile probably has a unique importance in endoscopic carpal tunnel technique. The preliminary results of endoscopic carpal tunnel release by both techniques are generally good, although major complications such as laceration of the ulnar artery, branch of the median or ulnar nerve, flexor tendon or the median nerve itself have been encountered by one or more surgeons trained in the technique.

Palmar Cutaneous Branch of Median Nerve

The palmar cutaneous branch of the median nerve arises from the median nerve in the distal third of the forearm, passes distally paralleling the median nerve, pierces either the antebrachial fascia, the volar carpal ligament or even the transverse carpal ligament at the wrist, and then divides into medial and lateral branches at the base of the palm (Fig. 36-16). As the palmar cutaneous branch courses superficial and ulnar to the flexor carpi radialis tendon, it enters a short tunnel in the volar carpal ligament or transverse carpal ligament at the end of which it divides into the medial and lateral branches.[43,368] The nerve eventually supplies sensibility to the thenar eminence and the proximal two-fifths of the palm on the radial side. Anatomic variations of the palmar cutaneous branch of the median nerve have included separation from the median nerve at any level in the distal third of the forearm, even at the proximal wrist crease, multiple branches from the median nerve arising at the same or separate levels, and total absence of the palmar cutaneous nerve, in which case a portion of the musculocutaneous nerve (lateral antebrachial cutaneous nerve) and/or the superficial radial nerve will supply sensibility on the radial side of the proximal palm.[43,111,121] Although most lesions of the palmar cutaneous branch of the median nerve are the result of lacerations or iatrogenic injury at the time of surgery,[207] compression neuropathy of the palmar cutaneous branch in its tunnel has been described by Stellbrink.[360] Release of the palmar cutaneous branch of the median nerve in its tunnel at the transverse carpal ligament relieved the patient of his hypesthesias over the thenar eminence.

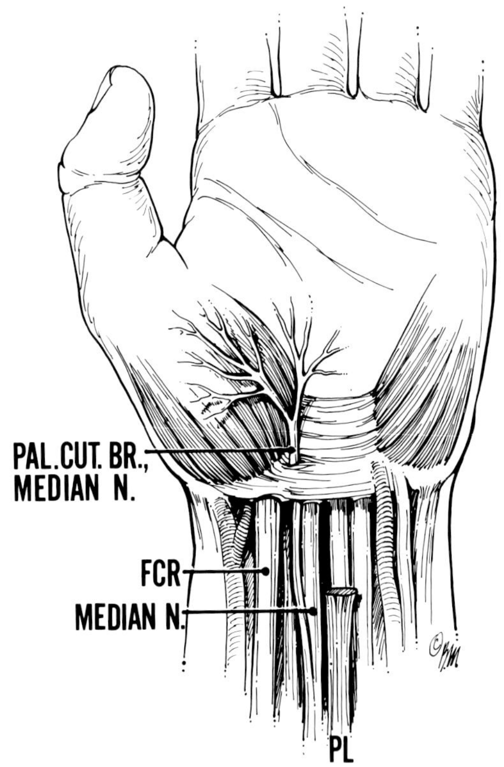

Fig. 36-16. The palmar cutaneous branch of the median nerve may be entrapped as it pierces either the volar carpal or transverse carpal ligament or at the antebrachial fascia.

ENTRAPMENT NEUROPATHIES OF THE ULNAR NERVE

Entrapment neuropathies of the ulnar nerve occur in two areas of the upper extremity. Because of differing clinical presentations, entrapment of the ulnar nerve at the elbow (cubital tunnel syndrome) will rarely be confused with entrapment of the ulnar nerve at the wrist in Guyon's canal (ulnar tunnel syndrome), unless the symptoms are minimal and the physical examination and electrodiagnostic studies are inconclusive.

Ulnar Nerve Entrapment at the Elbow (Cubital Tunnel Syndrome)

Entrapment syndromes of the ulnar nerve near the elbow joint generally present with pain of a lancinating or aching nature on the medial side of the proximal forearm.[421] This pain may migrate proximally or distally into either the arm or forearm. The pain is often accompanied by paresthesias, dysesthesias, or anesthesia in the ulnar one and one-half fingers—the sensory distribution of the ulnar nerve in the hand. Muscle wasting of the ulnar-innervated intrinsic muscles is not uncommon. The entrapment of the ulnar nerve may be localized by a positive percussion test over the ulnar nerve at the elbow, abnormal mobility of the ulnar nerve onto or over the medial epicondyle of the humerus,[398,399] or a positive elbow flexion test with increased numbness in the ulnar one and one-half fingers with full flexion of the elbow and the forearm in supination. Since electrodiagnostic studies[21,24,25,90,127,413] at the elbow are generally expressed as velocity in meters per second rather than as a latency in milliseconds, evaluation of reduced velocities of less than 25 percent are probably not significant and conduction velocities with a reduction across the elbow of greater than 33 percent are always significant. (These percentages are based on our own unpublished studies.) Care must be taken that conduction velocities across the elbow of the ulnar nerve are recorded in a standard position because the flexed elbow position produces less segment-to-segment conduction velocity variation than those obtained with the elbow extended. Similar to other entrapment neuropathies, the use of conduction velocities as a sole indication for surgery is insufficient unless the patient has accompanying clinical findings, such as sensory symptoms and a positive percussion test over the ulnar nerve. The presence of intrinsic muscle wasting is a sign of prolonged compression neuropathy and ordinarily demands early operative intervention. The surgeon should be cautioned about muscle wasting of the intrinsic muscles of the hand in the geriatric patient, since this may be a result of the normal aging process and may not be a manifestation of a compression neuropathy of the ulnar nerve. The presence of fibrillations within the ulnar intrinsic muscles of the hand in such a case is an important sign of neurologic injury.

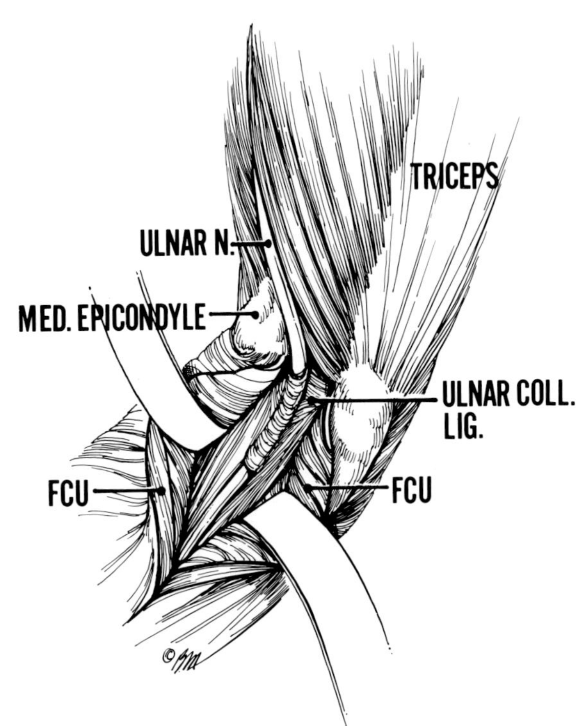

Fig. 36-17. The ulnar nerve lies on the medial head of the triceps muscle, entering the cubital tunnel behind the medial epicondyle and continuing distally beneath the arcade of fascia joining the heads of the flexor carpi ulnaris.

Pertinent Anatomy

The ulnar nerve arises as the continuation and terminal branch of the medial cord of the brachial plexus after the medial cord contributes to the median nerve. At its origin, the ulnar nerve lies medial to the axillary and then the brachial artery as far as the middle third of the humerus. In the middle third of the arm, the ulnar nerve approaches the medial head of the triceps by piercing the medial intermuscular septum and runs along this head of the triceps muscle to the groove between the olecranon and the medial epicondyle of the humerus (Fig. 36-17). The cubital tunnel begins at the so-called ulnar groove just behind the medial epicondyle of the humerus. In the cubital tunnel the ulnar nerve is covered by multiple fascial layers and can be readily palpated coursing behind and beneath the medial epicondyle of the partially flexed elbow. Within the cubital tunnel the ulnar nerve comes to lie beneath the fascial arcade joining the two heads of the flexor carpi ulnaris, passing between these two heads and lying on the anterior or volar surface of the flexor digitorum profundus to the midportion of the forearm.

The anatomy of the cubital tunnel can be divided into three parts: the entrance of the tunnel just posterior to the medial epicondyle, the area of the fascial aponeurosis joining the two heads of the flexor carpi ulnaris, and the muscle bellies of the flexor carpi ulnaris itself. The elliptical, fibroosseous cubital tunnel is bordered laterally by the elbow joint, medially by the heads of the flexor carpi ulnaris origin, and anteriorly, at least at its origin, by the medial epicondyle. Within this canal the ulnar nerve passes from the extensor surface in the arm to the flexor surface in the forearm. Among the suggested causes of entrapment of the ulnar nerve at the elbow[441,442] are the arcade of Struthers[111,117,178]; the anconeus epitrochlearis[111]; the medial head of the triceps[445]; the aponeurosis of the flexor carpai ulnaris; osteophytes, ganglia or lipomata associated with the elbow joint[420,446]; subluxation of the ulnar nerve across the epicondyle[204,392,393,398]; or a combination of these causes, particularly hypertrophy of the medial head of the triceps, which forces the ulnar nerve anteriorly around the medial epicondyle when the triceps contracts. This latter circumstance will produce an ulnar nerve that seems peculiarly subjected to trauma with flexion of the elbow.

Suggested surgical treatment of the cubital tunnel syndrome includes decompression of the ulnar nerve,[449,456] anterior transposition of the ulnar nerve,[393,396,403,428,430,434,442] medial epicondylectomy of the humerus,[402,411,422,424,436] and fascial repairs that prevent subluxation of the nerve. Since subluxation of the ulnar nerve occurs with flexion of the elbow and since fascial repair will create a band across the nerve to prevent its subluxation, it seems theoretically unsound to suggest an operation that might very well cause a compression with the repair. For this reason, although prevention of subluxation seems rational, these procedures have been abandoned and are not even discussed by most authors. The remaining procedures of decompression, transposition, and medial epicondylectomy warrant detailed discussion concerning their use for ulnar nerve entrapment at the elbow.

Operative Techniques

Decompression

The basic operation for ulnar nerve entrapment at the elbow when the compression is by the aponeurosis between the heads of the flexor carpi ulnaris, or the muscle itself, is decompression of the ulnar nerve. The advantages of this operation are (1) simplicity, since the aponeurosis is simply divided over the ulnar nerve; (2) safety, since the ulnar nerve is not disturbed and therefore not robbed of its intrinsic or extrinsic blood supply; and (3) predictability. With this localized compression we can anticipate that the patient will experience immediate relief of paresthesias and dysesthesias and increased sensibility in the short term, if the degree of injury is neurapratic rather than axonotmetic or neurotmetic. Recovery of intrinsic muscles of the hand in the long term will occur with neurapratic and axonotmetic nerve injuries. These results have not been duplicated with anterior transposition. The disadvantage of decompression is the inability to localize the site of compression. If the compression neuropathy is not limited to the aponeurosis or muscle of the flexor carpi ulnaris, the operation will not prove to be sufficient for the patient. The most useful localizing sign of compression is a positive percussion test over the ulnar nerve as the ulnar nerve lies between the superficial and deep heads of the flexor carpi ulnaris. This preoperative finding, combined with the finding at operation of an indentation of the nerve beneath the stout portion of the aponeurosis overlying the heads of the flexor carpi ulnaris (usually with a swelling of the nerve proximal to the site of the compression), is the most reliable indication that the site of compression of the ulnar nerve was indeed localized and can be relieved by decompression.

Decompression begins with an incision from a point midway between the tip of the olecranon and the medial epicondyle of the humerus, extending distally about 6 cm, parallel to the subcutaneous border of the ulna. This incision will normally not cross the small branches of the medial brachial or medial antebrachial cutaneous nerves, but they should be looked for and preserved if encountered. The dissection is deepened through the flexor aponeurosis over the ulnar nerve, taking care to isolate the ulnar nerve in the proximal end of the incision. The aponeurotic band (fibrous arcade of the flexor carpi ulnaris muscle) over the nerve is divided as the nerve is traced distally between the two heads of the muscle. Continuing the fasciotomy of the flexor carpi ulnaris is prudent; I believe that the ulnar nerve should be explored to at least the midportion of the proximal third of the forearm. The branches of the ulnar nerve to the two heads of the flexor carpi ulnaris and to the ulnar half of the profundus are identified, as is the occasional articular branch of the ulnar nerve to the elbow joint. The ulnar nerve is not disturbed in its bed, nor are the accompanying vessels dissected from the nerve. If the typical findings of compression are found within the cubital tunnel and if there is swelling of the nerve proximal to the compression, epineurotomy can be performed to relieve whatever compression may continue from the epineurium. Internal neurolysis of the ulnar nerve at the elbow is unwise, however, because of the rich interfascicular plexus of nerves, a portion of which may be injured with a complete internal neurolysis of the ulnar nerve. Following completion of the release, passive flexion and extension of the elbow should be done to be sure that decompression of the nerve is complete and that the nerve does not now subluxate from its bed, which may cause the patient further problems and necessitate reoperation. If, following the decompression, subluxation of the nerve does occur, anterior transposition or, preferably, medial epicondylectomy should be performed. A skin closure is the only closure necessary after decompression of the ulnar nerve. Postoperative care generally consists of a soft, supporting, well-padded dressing over the elbow; immediate active motion of the elbow in flexion and extension is encouraged.

Anterior Transposition of the Ulnar Nerve

Anterior transposition of the ulnar nerve may be indicated for several syndromes involving compression of the ulnar nerve at the elbow. These indications include subluxation of the ulnar nerve onto or over the medial epicondyle with flexion of the elbow; persistent or progressive valgus deformity, usually secondary to fracture malunion; and a persistently positive elbow flexion test with severe neuritic signs with prolonged flexion of the elbow. It is well known that transposition is used to gain length for repair of the ulnar nerve after laceration. Anterior transposition is also appropriate for those patients in whom a decompression procedure has failed. These patients have usually had a decompression of the ulnar nerve at least 6 and often 12 months or more prior to considering anterior transposition. Although there has been some early improvement following the procedures, the patient's clinical course has not continued to improve, and the symptoms seem now to be aggravated by use of the arm, particularly with repetitive flexion and extension of the elbow. The symptoms improve with careful immobilization of the elbow in a well-padded cast. In such a clinical presentation anterior transposition of the ulnar nerve must be considered.

Some surgeons have used the method of McGowan[434,452] to grade the degree of ulnar neuropathy. In McGowan's first stage (Grade I), the symptoms of ulnar neuropathy are subjective, consisting of minor hypesthesia and paresthesias, whereas in the intermediate stage (Grade II), weakness and wasting of the interossei are found in addition to the hypesthesia. In the final stage (Grade III), marked weakness and wasting of the interossei, adductor pollicis, and hypothenar muscles are combined with complete or partial anesthesia in the ulnar one and one-half fingers. Accordingly, anterior transposition for Grade III and decompression for Grade I and II neuropathy would be appropriate procedures. The degree to which the anterior transposition is performed can vary. The subcutaneous transposition, which gained popularity a few years ago, and the partial or complete submuscular transposition, in which the ulnar nerve is placed parallel to the median nerve as it enters the forearm, have gained wide acceptance as an indicated treatment for cubital tunnel syndrome. The advantage of anterior transposition is that any pathology, visualized or not, will be left behind as the nerve is transposed from the cubital tunnel to its new bed. Tension is removed from the nerve by transposition, and removal of tension may improve blood supply to the nerve. Most authors who transpose to beneath the flexor muscle mass believe that one of the advantages of submuscular transposition is the placement of the nerve in a well-vascularized muscular bed.[393,403,428,444] Learmonth has expanded this concept by showing that nerves usually run in intramuscular beds.[428] The consummate advantage of anterior transposition, according to those authors who favor this procedure, is that the results obtained are better with this procedure than with either decompression or medial epicondylectomy in indicated patients with cubital tunnel syndrome.[393,396,403,430,434,444]

The disadvantages of anterior transposition are that the surgery is more complex than either external decompression or medial epicondylectomy, and that the extensive exposure of the ulnar nerve not only places the branches of the nerve at some risk (especially those to the flexor carpi ulnaris), but also increases the scar in the new bed to which the nerve is transposed. During the transposition the ulnar nerve may be dissociated from its blood supply, which accompanies it. Interference with the medial brachial and medial antebrachial cutaneous nerves is not uncommon during transposition and may produce annoying dysesthesias. Anterior transposition may also create a new site of compression[396,430,444] of the ulnar nerve if the arcade of Struthers, medial intermuscular septum, and flexor muscle mass are not mobilized and/or repaired properly. Another disadvantage of anterior transposition is the more complex postoperative management, consisting of immobilization of the elbow, which may allow cicatrix formation around the ulnar nerve during this period. Finally, some surgeons who do not prefer anterior transposition have indicated that in their patients there seems to be less improvement of motor function of the intrinsic muscles of the hand than with decompression or medial epicondylectomy. To my knowledge, no controlled study to evaluate improvement of motor function in comparable patients treated by different techniques is available to evaluate this objection.

Subcutaneous Transposition. The skin incision for anterior transposition[428] of the ulnar nerve parallels the nerve, curving along the posterior margin of the medial epicondyle to lie 0.5 to 1 cm anterior to the nerve. This incision is desirable to prevent interference with the medial brachial and medial antebrachial cutaneous nerves, a neuroma of which may be distressing to the patient and confusing to the surgeon in the postoperative period. The ulnar nerve is most easily identified immediately behind the medial epicondyle of the humerus. The fascia is thin over the nerve and the nerve can be palpated easily. By lifting the fascia away from the nerve with fine forceps, exposure of the nerve can be safely achieved. Identification of the nerve behind the epicondyle is desirable, since this is an unlikely site of compression by fascia and the area of entrapment can be preserved for detailed examination later during the operation. The ulnar nerve, extending from behind the medial epicondyle, is followed proximally for at least 8 cm. The ulnar nerve lies along the medial head of the triceps, and any encroachment of the muscle on the ulnar nerve,[445] or the appearance of an anomalous muscle, such as the anconeus epitrochlearis,[111] can be identified and its importance in the compression neuropathy evaluated. After the ulnar nerve is traced distally from behind the medial epicondyle, the tight fascia bridging the heads of the flexor carpi ulnaris must be divided with care since this area (i.e., the cubital tunnel) is narrowed and is often the site of the nerve compression.

The exploration distally should be continued to between the heads of the flexor carpi ulnaris, where the arcade and fascia of

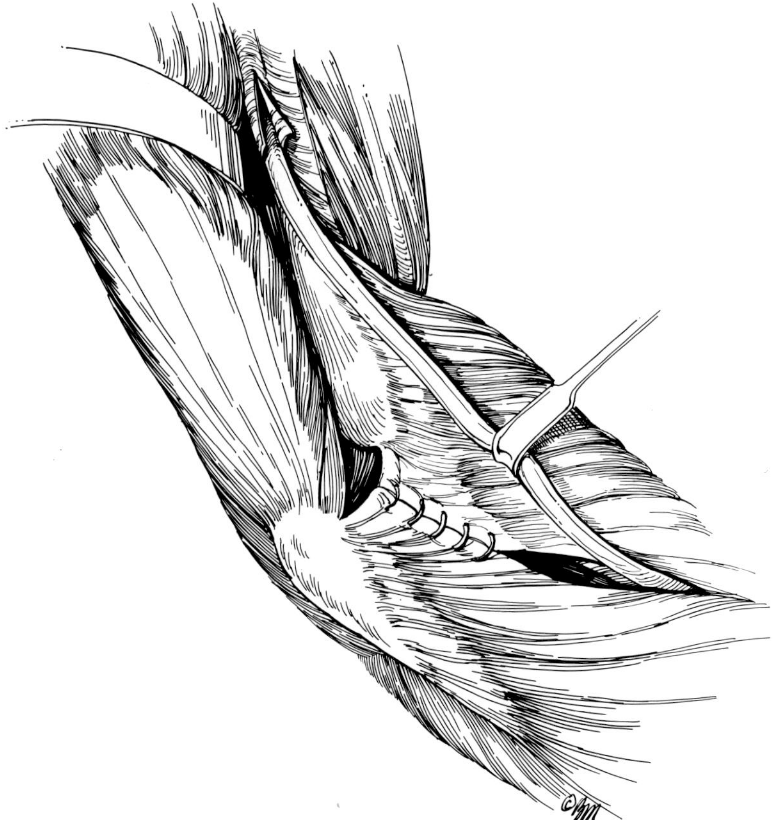

Fig. 36-18. At the completion of a subcutaneous transposition, the arcade of Struthers does not bind the ulnar nerve and there is adequate release of the flexor carpi ulnaris for the ulnar nerve to reenter the forearm.

the flexor carpi ulnaris are divided into the proximal third of the forearm. Care must be taken to protect the muscular branches of the nerve. After the ulnar nerve is exposed from at least 8 cm above the medial epicondyle to between the heads of the flexor carpi ulnaris in the proximal forearm, the surgeon should elevate the nerve from its bed, taking care to include both the arteries and veins accompanying the ulnar nerve in the bulk of tissue to be transposed. After the neurovascular bundle is mobilized, it is transposed anteriorly beneath the elevated skin flap, if a subcutaneous transposition has been chosen (Fig. 36-18). During transposition care must be taken that a new site of constriction is not created proximally by the arcade of Struthers or by the medial intermuscular septum. The medial intermuscular septum can be excised to relieve the ulnar nerve. The third area of concern with subcutaneous transposition is beneath the fascial arcade between the two heads of the flexor carpi ulnaris. If a band has been created, excision of muscle fascia is indicated.[111,396,430,444]

Following subcutaneous transposition, a suture from the anterior skin flap to the medial epicondyle seems advisable to prevent a position change of the transposed ulnar nerve. The skin and subcutaneous tissues are approximated in the usual way.

Submuscular Transposition. If, after mobilization of the neurovascular bundle (Fig. 36-19), the surgeon intends to proceed with a submuscular or partial submuscular transposition, elevation of the flexor muscles from the medial epicondyle is performed. Since the anterior flap of skin and subcutaneous tissue has been reflected anteriorly and the location of the median nerve in the distal third of the brachium is certain, a large hemostat can be directed beneath the flexor muscle mass to elevate the superficial head of the flexor carpi ulnaris with the flexor carpi radialis, palmaris longus, pronator teres, and a portion of the flexor digitorum superficialis. If a partial submuscular transposition is to be performed, a portion of the pronator teres remains unelevated but the other muscles are elevated from their origin on the medial epicondyle. The division of these muscles from the medial epicondyle is performed using sharp dissection, and the muscle origin is reflected distally, preserving the innervation of the superficial head of the flexor carpi ulnaris (Fig. 36-20). If an intermuscular fascial band is encountered between these muscles, it should be excised to allow an uninterrupted bed for the transposed ulnar nerve. Following the formal transposition of the ulnar nerve into the submuscular position, the surgeon must again reexplore the proximal segment of the ulnar nerve to be sure that a fascial band has not encroached upon the nerve. The arcade of Struthers and the medial intermuscular septum should be examined and excised if necessary. Repair of the flexor aponeurosis to the medial epicondyle is undertaken (Fig. 36-21) making sure that a fascial band across the nerve is not created by the repair of the muscles to the medial epicondyle. Rather than closing the fascia over the cubital tunnel, the fasciotomy of the

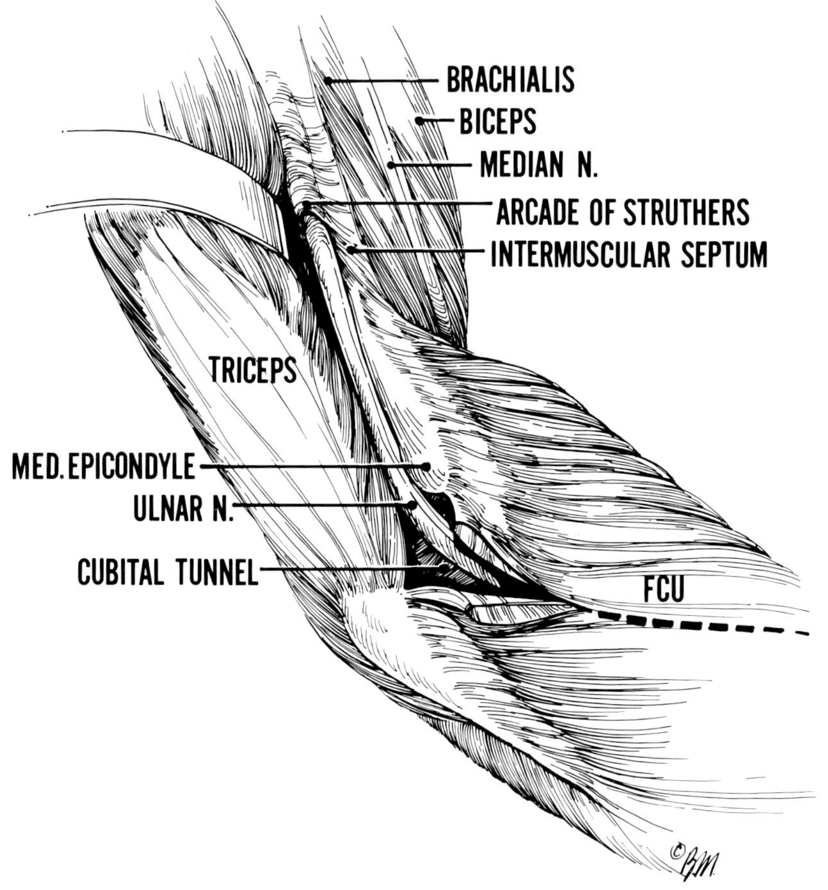

Fig. 36-19. Mobilization of the ulnar nerve and any associated vessels necessitates decompression of the cubital tunnel, fasciotomy of the flexor carpi ulnaris, and dissection along the ulnar nerve, at least 8 cm proximal to the medial epicondyle.

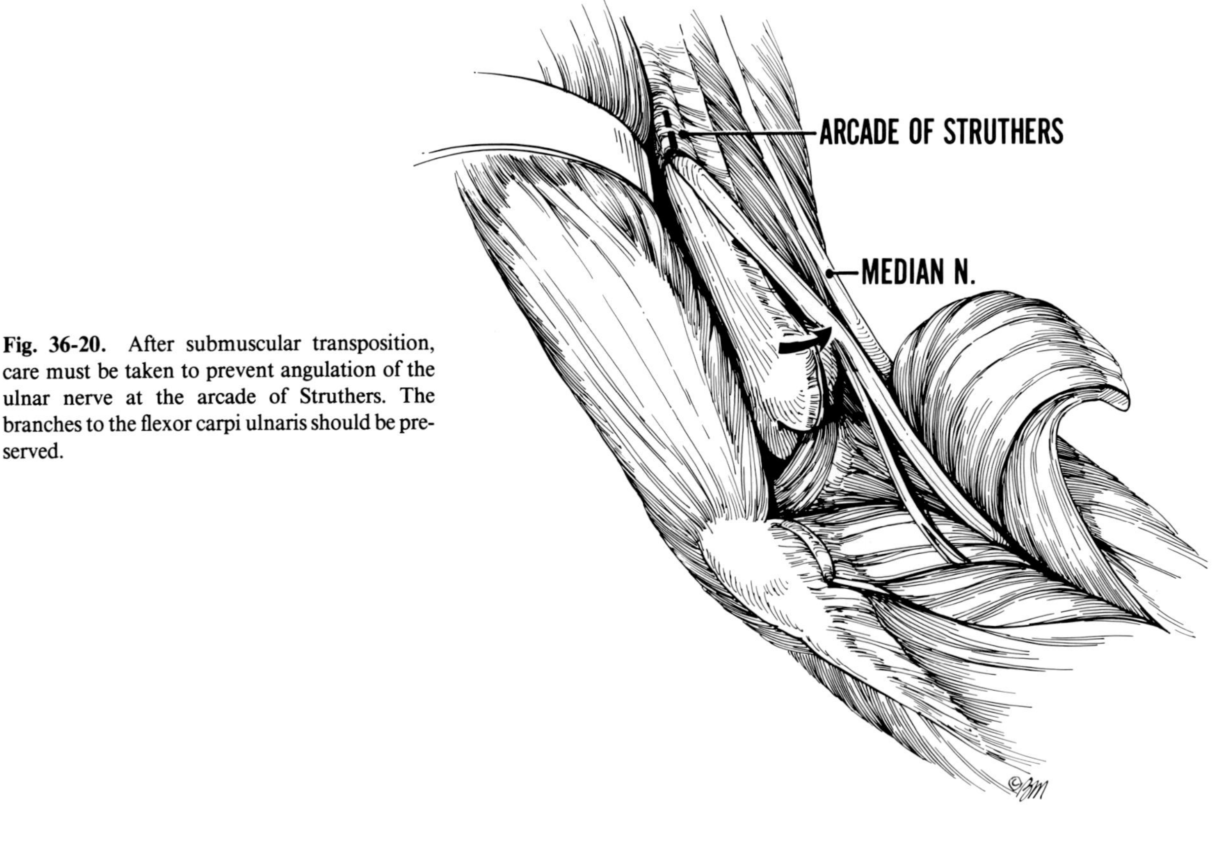

Fig. 36-20. After submuscular transposition, care must be taken to prevent angulation of the ulnar nerve at the arcade of Struthers. The branches to the flexor carpi ulnaris should be preserved.

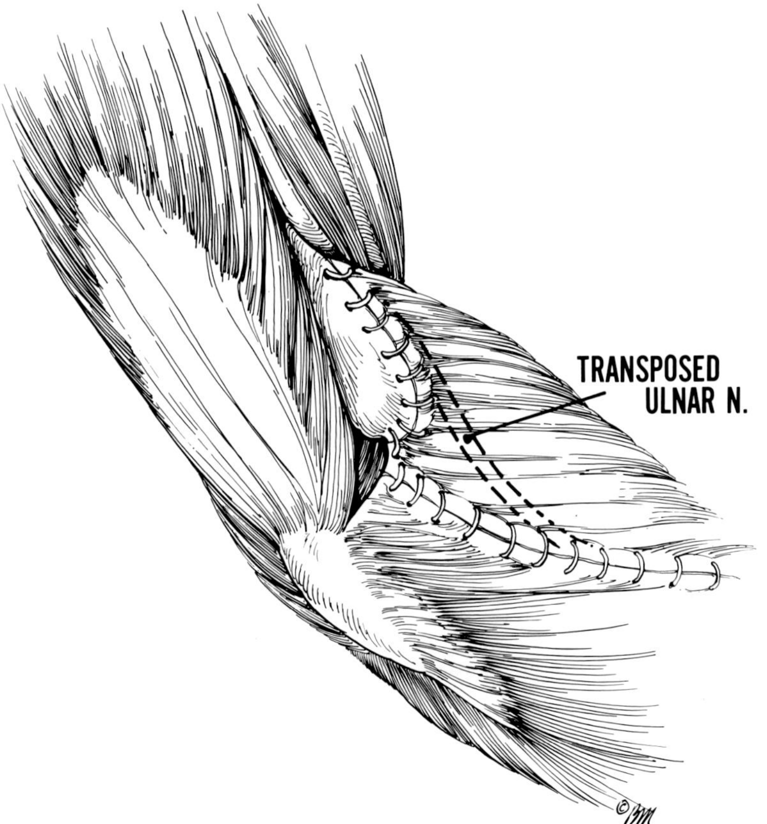

Fig. 36-21. Completion of the submuscular transposition by repair of the flexor muscles to the medial epicondlye.

proximal third of the forearm is allowed to remain open to accommodate additional swelling.

A technique of submuscular transposition by osteotomy of the medial epicondyle has been described,[433] in which the ulnar nerve is transposed through the osteotomy site of the epicondyle to a position lying beneath and within the flexor muscle mass similar to submuscular transposition. This technique seems to this author to be unnecessarily difficult, to not provide the surgeon with the needed exposure to insure that a secondary site of compression is not created, and therefore to offer little benefit to the previously described method of detachment of the flexor muscle origin and reattachment and repair of that origin after transposition of the ulnar nerve.

Postoperative Management. The postoperative management of the patient who has undergone anterior transposition of the ulnar nerve begins with the application of a bulky dressing over the operative site for several days; the dressing should be of sufficient size to provide support and padding for the extremity and the transposed ulnar nerve. A supporting plaster splint across the elbow may be added as long as care is taken that there is *no* pressure over the operative incision or over the transposed nerve that could interfere with the viability of the skin or the recovery of the ulnar nerve. With submuscular transposition, because of the elevation of the flexor origin, it may be advisable to immobilize the elbow and wrist for a few weeks to allow healing of the repaired flexor muscle origin. Following immobilization, gentle exercises are begun, with flexion and extension of both wrist and elbow. These exercises are generally accompanied by some sensation in the distribution of the ulnar nerve, but the exercises can be continued as long as the discomfort is tolerated by the patient.

Medial Epicondylectomy

Over 40 years ago, King and Morgan[424] published their experience with medial epicondylectomy for the treatment of traumatic ulnar neuritis. Their concept was that removal of the medial epicondyle, as one would remove an offending tumor or encroaching foreign body on a nerve, would permit that nerve to find its own optimal position. Although attractive in its simplicity, the concept has not been widely accepted by surgeons, although there have been several favorable studies reported.[402,411,422] The advantage of the procedure is that the nerve is not disturbed during the course of the removal of the medial epicondyle of the humerus. Consequently there is minimal exposure of the nerve, no damage to the proximal muscular branches, and no interference with the blood supply to the nerve. The tension on the nerve as it passes behind the medial epicondyle is removed, and the nerve, by necessity, slides forward and seeks its own position following removal of the restricting epicondyle. The motion possible in the early postoperative period allows the patient to return to normal activity in the shortest possible time. The disadvantage of this procedure includes the loss of the protecting prominence of the medial epicondyle, which may subject the ulnar nerve to repeated direct external trauma. The failure to identify the site of compression of the ulnar nerve is a criticism of this procedure. Since the nerve is not explored during the course of the procedure, one cannot identify a compressive lesion, and the danger of partial or no correction of a compression is a potential disadvantage. However, removal of the epicondyle probably decompresses the nerve at all points implicated in the cubital tunnel syndrome as long as the flexor carpi ulnaris is opened concomitantly. Subluxation of the ulnar nerve following medial epicondylectomy can potentially create a band at the medial intermuscular septum proximally or at the fascia of the flexor carpi ulnaris distally as the nerve seeks its new position. Finally, the detachment of the flexor muscle mass arising from the medial epicondyle, even with provision for their reattachment, and the possibility of injury to the elbow joint if the medial collateral ligaments are detached may be greater disadvantages than other authors have indicated. The indications for this procedure[402,411,422,424,436] have been the occurrence of an ulnar neuropathy at the elbow caused by valgus deformity, nerve displacing callus, and irritating ununited medial epicondyle. Occupational trauma, arthritis of the elbow joint, adhesions, foreign bodies, tumors, blood vessel aberrations, shortening of the nerve after anastomosis for laceration in the forearm, as well as a group of unknown causes account for the rest of the patients in the series reported.[424,436]

A skin incision approximately 8 cm long is made parallel to the ulnar nerve and 1 cm behind the prominence of the medial epicondyle. The center of the incision is at the posterior aspect of the medial epicondyle. The incision is carried to the deep fascia, with care taken to protect any small branches of the medial antebrachial or medial brachial cutaneous nerves that lie over the distal portion of the incision and generally supply the skin over the olecranon prominence below the medial epicondyle. The epicondyle is exposed by sharp, subperiosteal dissection reflecting off the common flexor-pronator origin (Fig. 36-22). The ulnar nerve lies immediately behind the medial epicondyle and should be identified either by palpation or, preferably, under direct vision, since its exposure will ease the ability of the surgeon to protect the nerve during excision of the medial epicondyle. Descriptions of the operation[381,411,424,446] note that there is no need to expose the ulnar nerve or its branches or to disturb its natural bed, since these techniques will result in unwanted scar formation about the nerve. In practice, however, it is safer to expose the nerve, carefully protecting all of the branches, natural bed, and blood supply. After the medial epicondyle and adjacent supracondylar ridge are fully exposed, the entire medial epicondyle and the ridge, or at least a portion of the ridge, are removed using either ronguers, osteotome, or bone saw. A natural guide for the proper plane of the osteotomy is the medial border of the trochlea (Fig. 36-23). By removing the distal portion of the supracondylar ridge, the surgeon will release the intermuscular septum and remove the septum as a possible cause of complications in the postoperative period. The sharp bony edges must be smoothed off posteriorly, but one must not remove so much bone as to enter the elbow joint. If the elbow joint is entered, some elbow stiffness in either flexion or extension in the postoperative period is likely to result. Care should also be taken to leave the collateral ligament intact. Before periosteal closure of the bone surface is done, bone wax may be pressed into the cancellous bone to reduce bleeding. The periosteum that was elevated is closed over the bone surface to reattach the origins of the flexor mus-

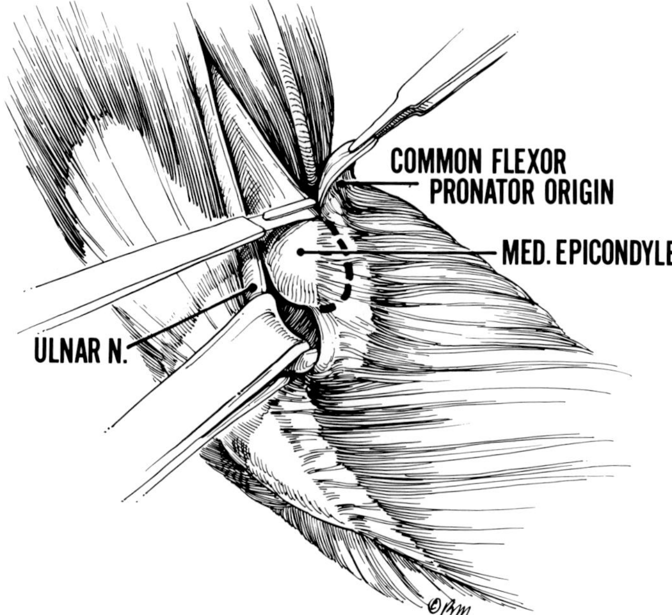

Fig. 36-22. Medial epicondylectomy is begun by protecting the ulnar nerve and elevating the common flexor pronator origin from the medial epicondyle.

cle mass (Fig. 36-24). The skin and subcutaneous tissues are closed in the usual fashion, once again being careful to protect any small branches of the medial brachial or medial antebrachial cutaneous nerves.

Only a soft dressing is required postoperatively, and range of motion exercises of the elbow can be begun within a few days after the operation. Except for the extremes of extension of the elbow, range of motion of the elbow is regained rapidly and even the extremes of extension should be regained within several months.

Author's Preferred Method. Careful preoperative evaluation of the patient with an ulnar entrapment neuropathy at the elbow determines, in my opinion, the selection of the procedure for relief of the neuropathy. If the patient has percussion sensitivity over the ulnar nerve distal to the medial epicondyle in the cubital tunnel, a decompression procedure will be used to relieve the neuritis present at the site of percussion sensitivity. Normally, the decompression will continue between the two heads of the flexor carpi ulnaris. If however, at the time of operation, no site of compression can be localized within the

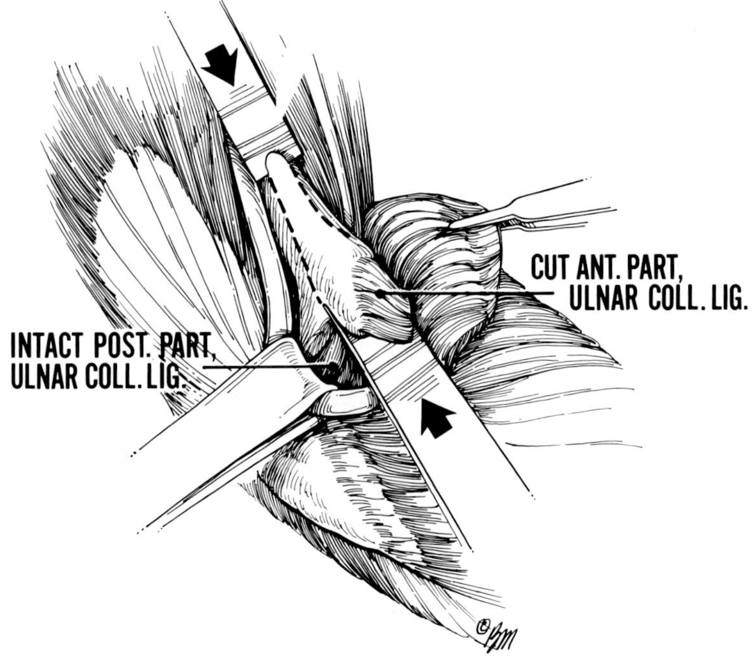

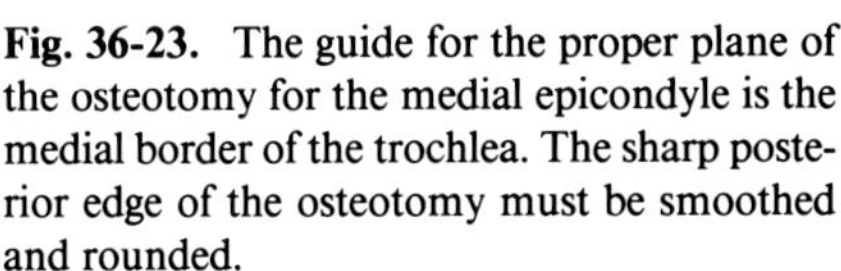
Fig. 36-23. The guide for the proper plane of the osteotomy for the medial epicondyle is the medial border of the trochlea. The sharp posterior edge of the osteotomy must be smoothed and rounded.

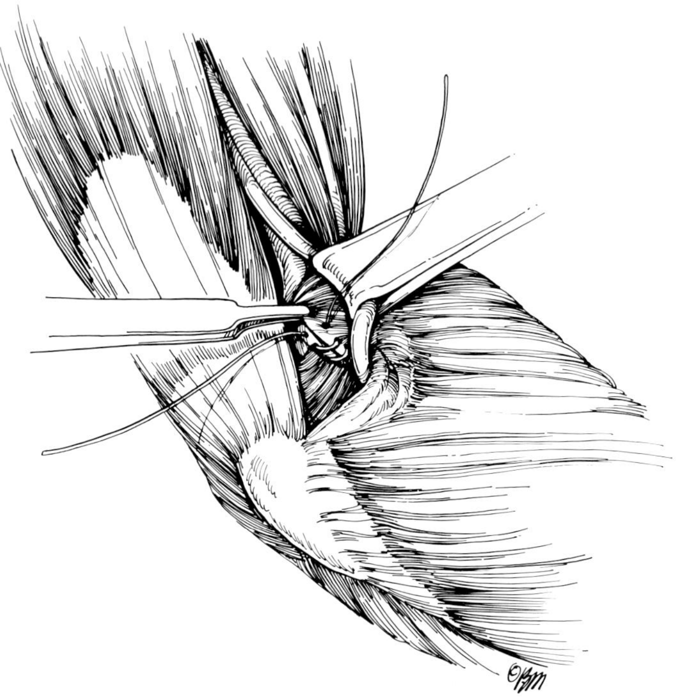

Fig. 36-24. Repair of the flexor-pronator origin to the humerus. After repair of the muscles, the ulnar nerve is allowed to seek its own position, and the arcade of the flexor carpi ulnaris must be opened sufficiently to prevent impingement on the nerve (not shown in the drawing).

cubital tunnel from its entrance behind the medial epicondyle and extending distally between the heads of the flexor carpi ulnaris, I recommend that the operation be continued by performing a medial epicondylectomy and decompression of the ulnar nerve. Decompression of the ulnar nerve combined with medial epicondylectomy has been most effective with my patients in relieving ulnar neuropathy at the elbow. The decompression continues distally between the heads of the flexor carpi ulnaris and proximally for approximately 10 cm proximal to the medial epicondyle. Such a decompression combined with medial epicondylectomy, as has been outlined previously, satisfies many of the criticisms of the medial epicondylectomy procedure. Specifically, the nerve is explored during this procedure, and the medial intermuscular septum is relieved proximally, as is the flexor carpi ulnaris distally. By carrying the exploration of the ulnar nerve 10 cm proximal to the medial epicondyle, the arcade of Struthers, should one exist, can also be decompressed, preventing a secondary neuropathy at the arcade of Struthers. The main criticism of the medial epicondylectomy procedure that remains unanswered with this surgical approach is the loss of the protecting prominence of the medial epicondyle. In a few of my patients—and I would emphasize that this has been less than 10 percent—this has been a minor problem, but has not contributed to increased neuropathy of the ulnar nerve and has not required any secondary treatment, either surgical or orthotic.

Some surgeons have suggested that medial epicondylectomy may weaken flexor-pronator muscle power, but the incidence and severity of this has not been well documented. If measurements are made in the early postoperative period, relative weakness may represent continuing ulnar neuropathy; long-term follow-up studies are needed to resolve this question.

If the patient exhibits subluxation or dislocation of the ulnar nerve, a static or progressive valgus deformity of the elbow, or a positive elbow flexion test reproducing symptoms within 30 seconds of full flexion of the elbow preoperatively, I have found it advisable to proceed with medial epicondylectomy and ulnar nerve decompression as the primary surgical procedure for the relief of ulnar nerve neuropathy. During the course of the operation, I have explored the ulnar nerve from 10 cm proximal to the medial epicondyle to 7 to 8 cm distal to the medial epicondyle, carefully maintaining the tissue contiguous to the ulnar nerve, particularly the vascular structures associated with the nerve.

I prefer medial epicondylectomy decompression over anterior transposition of the ulnar nerve because of the reduced morbidity following operation, improved postoperative results, and earlier return of patients to work.

In the postoperative period, I prefer a soft dressing of sufficient size to support the elbow for the first 4 to 5 days. After the first dressing change, the patient begins range of motion exercises in a light dressing with enough gauze pads to provide some protection of the operative area for an additional week to 10 days. I have not found it necessary to immobilize the flexor muscle repair nor to reattach that repair in a secondary operation in any patient in the last several years.

Symptoms of ulnar neuritis in the early postoperative period are usually associated with wrinkles in or a poorly applied dressing causing direct pressure over the ulnar nerve and the operative site. A simple change in dressing will relieve these symptoms. I have seen one patient who reformed bone at the medial epicondyle in the postoperative period and again became symptomatic approximately 6 months after medial epicondylectomy. Reexcision of the newly formed bone was sufficient to relieve the recurrent symptoms of ulnar neuritis. At the time of reexcision, the ulnar nerve was noted to snap over the new bone exostosis with flexion and extension of the elbow, much as an ulnar nerve might snap over a medial epicondyle as it subluxated from the ulnar groove.

The diagnosis of ulnar neuropathy at the elbow requires two essential determinations by the examining physician and surgeon. The examiner must make the diagnosis of ulnar nerve neuropathy and he must localize that neuropathy to the elbow. In my experience an electrodiagnostic study is extremely helpful in these determinations. The presence of an ulnar neuropathy can be determined by an efficient and complete electrodiagnostic study, usually an electromyogram. An electromyogram that includes studies of the flexor carpi ulnaris, flexor digitorum profundus of the ulnar two fingers, the abductor digiti quinti, the first dorsal interosseous, and the third palmar interosseous generally provides the useful information necessary to confirm an ulnar nerve neuropathy. I would emphasize that the use of the third palmar interosseous is extremely helpful; it seems to be a muscle that is affected very early by the neuropathic process at the elbow. The finding of fibrillations or positive sharp waves in the third palmar interosseous or other ulnarly innervated muscles will confirm the diagnosis of neuropathy in the ulnar nerve.

Localization of the neuropathic process to the area of the elbow may be more difficult electrodiagnostically, and the delay of treatment until the conduction velocity is reduced significantly (30 percent or greater) may lead to an irreversible neuropathic process. I would emphasize that the conduction delay across the elbow in the ulnar nerve is a late sign of cubital tunnel syndrome and may not appear until irreversible damage has been done to the ulnar nerve. As a consequence, the appearance of a conduction delay across the elbow may be a valuable prognostic sign in the evaluation of cubital tunnel syndrome since it may often herald an irreversible lesion. In my experience, the appearance of a significant conduction delay in the ulnar nerve across the elbow has been associated in the postoperative period with a prolonged recovery of ulnar nerve function, if ulnar nerve function recovers at all.

Ulnar Nerve Entrapment in Guyon's Canal (at the Wrist)

Entrapment neuropathy of the ulnar nerve at the wrist may present with a variety of signs and symptoms[463,473,481,490,498,499,502,505,506,510,577] depending on whether the ulnar nerve itself or the superficial or deep branch of the nerve is compressed. An isolated sensory neuropathy or an isolated or even partial motor neuropathy of the deep branch of the ulnar nerve only heralds the anatomic site of compression. The presence of a combined motor and sensory neuropathy of the ulnar nerve indicates that the location of the entrapment[503] is at or proximal to the wrist or in Guyon's canal before the division of the nerve into superficial and deep branches. If there is involvement of the dorsal sensory branch of the ulnar nerve with concomitant involvement of motor and sensory fibers of the ulnar nerve, the site of compression must be at or proximal to the origin of the dorsal branch of the ulnar nerve in the distal third of the forearm. In such cases, the most likely site of compression is in the cubital tunnel.

The confirmed presence of entrapment neuropathy in the region of the wrist, especially if it is progressive, is sufficient indication for operative intervention, except in those few patients where an occupational neuritis with repeated blunt trauma to the hypothenar eminence of the palm might suggest that discontinuance of the blunt trauma would allow resolution of the neuropathic symptoms.[385,464,476,511,515]

Preoperative examination for an ulnar entrapment neuropathy of the wrist includes Allen's test for confirmation of ulnar collateral circulation to the superficial or deep palmar arches. Thrombosis or aneurysm of the ulnar artery or one of its branches can be a cause of ulnar neuropathy, which may be predicted if Allen's test reveals slowed circulation from the ulnar artery (see Chapter 62).

Pertinent Anatomy

Three years following his graduation from medical school, Felix Guyon, in 1861,[470] published a description of the canal at the base of the hypothenar eminence that bears his name. He later concentrated on the urinary tract and became renowned for his operations on the prostate gland.

Joined by the ulnar artery in the midportion of the forearm, the ulnar nerve lying deep to the flexor carpi ulnaris muscle gives off a large dorsal branch in the distal third of the forearm, which passes to the dorsum of the wrist between the flexor carpi ulnaris and the ulna. This dorsal branch eventually divides into two dorsal digital nerves that supply sensation of the ulnar one and one-half fingers. The ulnar nerve continues to the base of the palm and enters Guyon's canal (Fig. 36-25), which is a triangular canal. The roof is formed by the volar carpal ligament, which is blended with the tendinous insertion of the flexor carpi ulnaris into the pisiform bone, and the distal extension of the flexor carpi ulnaris, the pisohamate ligament. The lateral wall is formed by the hook of the hamate and the insertion of the transverse carpal ligament. The medial wall is formed by the fibrous attachments to the pisohamate ligament and the pisiform bone itself.[462,502] The ulnar nerve and artery traverse Guyon's canal. Within the canal, the ulnar nerve bifurcates into the superficial and deep branches; the superficial branch passes distally to the fat pad in the canal; the deep branch, along with a larger branch of the ulnar artery, passes distally and deeply between the origins of the abductor digiti quinti and flexor digiti quinti brevis muscles to supply the deeper interosseous muscles of the hand. There are no tendons or tendon sheaths traversing Guyon's canal as there are in the carpal tunnel, and the roof of this canal is relatively loose and fibrous, rather than rigid and unyielding as is the transverse carpal ligament over the carpal tunnel.

Unlike the carpal tunnel syndrome, in which a majority of patients seem to have an ill-defined onset of the compression neuropathy, compression of the ulnar nerve in Guyon's canal is often associated with an occupational cause, predisposing the nerve to repeated blunt trauma,[457,458,464,511,514] an occult tumorous condition,[468,473,475,478,479,487,489,490,496,501,502,509] particularly a ganglion or lipoma in the region of the ulnar nerve and Guyon's canal, or fractures of the hamate or triangular bone[494,512,515] or ring and little metacarpal bases.[468] Some cases have been attributed to anatomic variations in Guyon's canal.

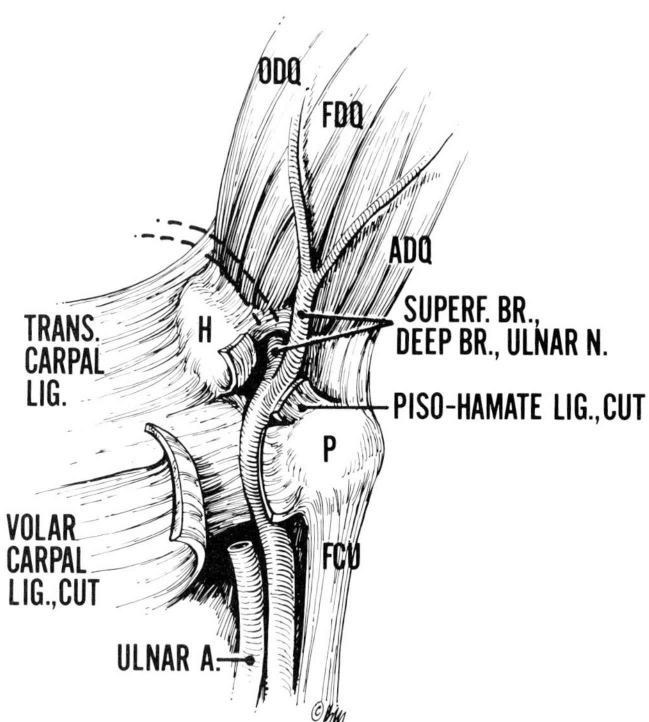

Fig. 36-25. The canal of Guyon with the ulnar nerve traversing from forearm to hand (*H*, hook of hamate; *P*, pisiform).

These reports have been concerned with accessory or anomalous muscles[498,499,505,510] traversing Guyon's canal, arising from the deep fascia of the forearm and passing obliquely through the canal to blend with fibers of the abductor digiti minimi. Anatomic variations in the arrangement of the branches of the ulnar nerve[96,461,464,465,480,484] in the region of the pisiform bone have been described but rarely are the cause of motor or sensory signs. The palmar cutaneous branch of the ulnar nerve,[221] which may arise as far proximally as the middle portion of the forearm, accompanies the ulnar nerve and artery to the hand, perforating the volar carpal ligament and terminating in the skin and at the base of the palm. It may also communicate with the palmar branch of the median nerve. Although recent work has called attention to the presence of this nerve,[221] if the incision to decompress Guyon's canal is not carried ulnarly over the hypothenar eminence, injury to the palmar cutaneous branch of the ulnar nerve will most likely be avoided.

Operative Technique

An incision on the radial border of the flexor carpi ulnaris, beginning several centimeters above the proximal wrist crease and extending in a zigzag fashion across the crease along a line to the ring finger, will provide exposure of Guyon's canal and the ulnar nerve and artery. The ulnar nerve should be isolated above the wrist and traced distally through Guyon's canal by reflecting ulnarly the flexor carpi ulnaris, pisiform bone, and pisohamate ligament. The branches of the ulnar nerve to the hypothenar muscles and the palmaris brevis muscle, as well as the superficial and deep branches of the ulnar nerve, can be identified and preserved with this incision. Just as the palmar cutaneous branch of the median nerve is not exposed during carpal tunnel release, so also is the palmar cutaneous branch of the ulnar nerve not exposed during release of Guyon's canal. Although neuromata of the palmar cutaneous branch of the ulnar nerve have been mentioned as a possible cause of continuing symptoms in the hypothenar eminence,[221] I have not found this to be a problem using the incision described. Since this incision lies near the incision used for carpal tunnel release, when release of Guyon's canal is combined with release of the transverse carpal ligament, a single incision, that for the carpal tunnel, is used. In exploring Guyon's canal at the time of carpal tunnel decompression, the surgeon must be careful to release the band at the proximal wrist flexion crease that may create a new site of compression across the ulnar nerve if neglected.

Postoperative complications peculiar to the release of Guyon's canal are few. Neuroma of the palmar cutaneous branch of the ulnar nerve has been suggested[221] but I have not identified this as a cause of continuing pain at the base of the palm. Failure to release Guyon's canal into the distal third of the forearm can be associated with a continuing entrapment neuropathy in the proximal wrist crease.

COMPRESSION NEUROPATHIES OF THE RADIAL NERVE

Compression neuropathies of the radial nerve occur in predictable areas along the course of the nerve. The lateral intermuscular septum where the radial nerve passes from the posterior to the anterior compartment of the arm is a more common site for compression neuropathy than is generally reported.[543,545] Recorded cases of compression neuropathy relieved surgically[545] at the lateral intermuscular septum are sparse except in those cases associated with major trauma to the arm, particularly in fractures of the humerus.[84,154,531,551,556]

Displaced fractures of the humerus associated with radial nerve palsy are often related to the entrapment of radial nerve at the lateral intermuscular septum of the humerus, and decompression of the nerve at the intermuscular septum with or without internal stabilization of the fractured humerus may be beneficial to the recovery of radial nerve function. The radial nerve seems to be in jeopardy also at the lateral intermuscular septum during open reduction and internal fixation of a fractured humerus, particularly when a plate and screws are applied from the anterolateral approach to the humerus. During the internal fixation of the humeral fracture from the anterolateral approach, the radial nerve should be isolated, protected, and relieved from its entrapment at the lateral intermuscular septum, so that undue tension and neuropathy are not created by the placing of a plate for fixation.

The radial tunnel syndrome,[542,561] a compression neuropathy of the radial nerve from the radial head to the supinator muscle, is the most common entrapment neuropathy of the radial nerve. A patient with this syndrome presents with aching pain in the extensor-supinator muscle mass in the proximal forearm that commonly radiates to the distal arm and distal forearm. If the fascicles of the superficial radial nerve are involved in the entrapment, radiation to the dorsal radial aspect of the hand and dysesthesias and paresthesias in the superficial radial distribution can be found. Two-point discrimination testing of the superficial radial nerve has not been helpful in my patients.

Most authors agree that there are four potential sites of compression within the radial tunnel.[291,560] The first is by fibrous bands lying anterior to the radial head at the entrance to the radial tunnel. The second site occurs at a fan-shaped leash of vessels (the radial recurrent vessels, the so-called leash of Henry), lying across the radial nerve and supplying the brachioradialis and extensor carpi radialis longus muscles. The third potential site of compression occurs at the tendinous margin of the extensor carpi radialis brevis. The fourth and most frequent site is at the arcade of Frohse, which forms a ligamentous band over the deep radial nerve as it enters the supinator muscle.

In my patients, I have observed that the tendinous margin of the extensor carpi radialis brevis and the arcade of Frohse may overlap, forming a scissorlike effect on the deep branch of the radial nerve that may combine to cause the radial tunnel syndrome. I believe that what we actually test with the flexor-pronator test is the combined tightening of the supinator muscle with pronation of the forearm and tightening of the extensor carpi radialis brevis with wrist flexion. At the operating table it is important therefore to recognize this potential combined cause of compression of the radial nerve, and to treat both aspects by not only dividing the arcade of Froshe but also by excision of a portion of the tendinous margin of the extensor carpi radialis brevis. A fifth cause of radial tunnel syndrome has also been described.[568] As the deep branch of the radial nerve passes through the supinator muscle and exits along its distal lateral border, a fascial arcade is often present, lining the superficial head of the supinator muscle just above the existing deep branch of the radial nerve. Because this site has been described as a cause of radial tunnel syndrome, some surgeons release the entire superficial head of the supinator muscle in order to preclude overlooking this area as a cause of continuing compression of the deep branch of the radial nerve.

In some cases the site of compression can be suspected by the physical findings on examination. If the symptoms of radial compression are reproduced by full flexion of the elbow with the forearm in supination and the wrist in neutral postion, the fibrous bands anterior to the radial neck must be suspect. If the symptoms are reproduced with passive pronation of the forearm (elbow at 45 to 90 degrees flexion, wrist in full flexion), particularly if relieved with wrist extension alone, compression by the extensor carpi radialis brevis is likely. When the symptoms are reproduced by isometric active supination from the fully pronated position, compression at the arcade of Frohse is likely.

Electrodiagnostic studies of the radial nerve are helpful if signs of denervation are present on electromyogram. Conduction velocity of the radial nerve across the radial tunnel has not been helpful in my experience.

Since the onset and distribution of pain are similar in the radial tunnel compression and in tennis elbow, these syndromes must be differentiated. Usually the point of maximal tenderness in tennis elbow is over the lateral epicondylar ridge, lateral epicondyle, or radial head, whereas in radial tunnel compression the maximal tenderness is over the supinator muscle, four fingerbreadths distal to the lateral epicondyle. The widely acclaimed, but much less useful, middle finger test (extension of the middle finger against resistance, with the wrist in neutral and the elbow in 45 to 90 degrees) often produces diffuse pain over the extensor muscle mass, which, if localized to the area of maximal tenderness, may be helpful. In the absence of positive findings with the functional tests for radial tunnel syndrome (see above), I have used diagnostic local anesthetic blocks with Xylocaine to differentiate these syndromes. When the instillation of 0.5 to 1 cc of 1 percent Xylocaine four fingerbreadths distal to the lateral epicondyle relieves pain and is accompanied by a deep radial palsy, and a complementary injection more proximal in the region of the lateral epicondyle (usually given on a day after the patient has recovered from the first) does not relieve the patient's symptoms, I have made the diagnosis of radial tunnel compression.

The most distal compression of the radial nerve involves only the superficial (sensory) branch and occurs in the distal third of the forearm. This syndrome, described by Wartenberg[573] in 1932, as "cheiralgia paresthetica," was so named because of its similarity, in Wartenberg's opinion, to meralgia paresthetica of the lateral femoral cutaneous nerve.

Pertinent Anatomy

The radial nerve is a continuation of the posterior cord following separation of the axillary nerve at the inferior border of the glenohumeral joint. It crosses the posterior aspect of the humerus, accompanied by the profunda brachii artery, and reaches the lateral side of the posterior aspect of the arm where it pierces the lateral intermuscular septum at the junction of the middle and distal thirds of the humerus (Fig. 36-26). In the

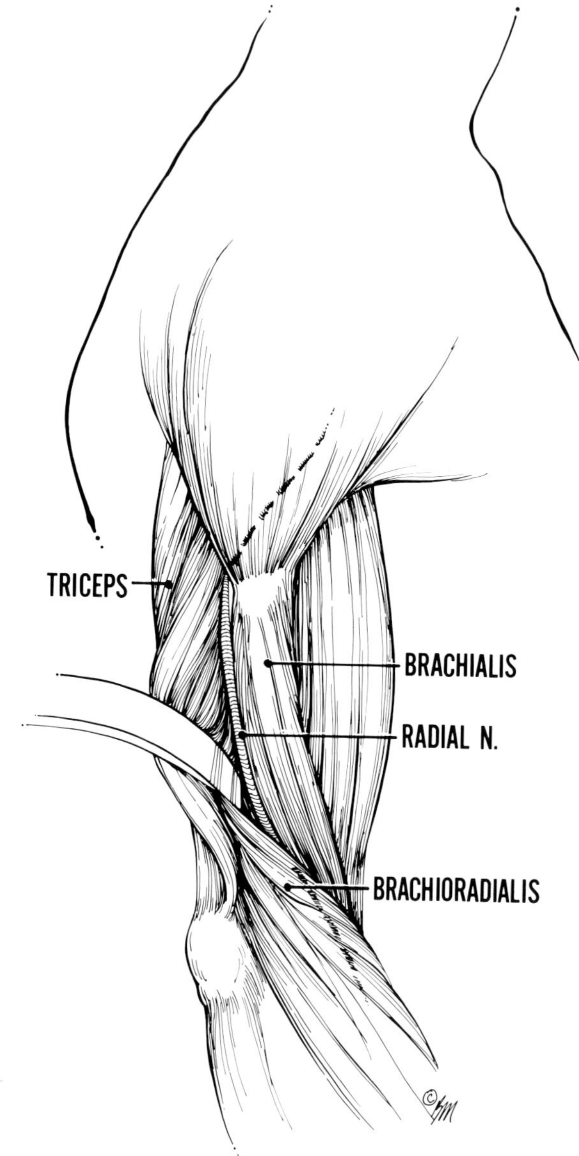

Fig. 36-26. As the radial nerve pierces the lateral intermuscular system, which is the most proximal site of radial nerve compression, the nerve lies between the brachialis and brachioradialis muscles.

anterior compartment, the radial nerve lies between the brachialis and brachioradialis muscles. At the radial head the nerve enters the radial tunnel and then divides into superficial and deep branches. The superficial branch lies beneath the muscle and tendon of the brachioradialis to the distal third of the forearm, where it exits dorsally to supply sensibility on the dorsoradial aspect of the hand. It is well known that sensibility to the dorsoradial aspect of the hand may be overlapped by branches of the musculocutaneous nerve and ulnar nerve in a significant percentage of patients.

The deep branch of the radial nerve within the radial tunnel passes to the dorsolateral aspect of the forearm, around the lateral side of the radius, and between the superficial and deep heads of the supinator muscle, exiting from this muscle at its distal border as multiple muscular branches to the ulnar wrist extensor, the extensor muscles of the fingers, and the extensor and abductor longus muscles of the thumb.

Radial Tunnel Syndrome

Operative Techniques

The basic indication for operation is the persistence of a compression neuropathy that has been documented to be progressive, unrelieved by conservative treatment, and localized by physical examination or electrodiagnostic studies.[267] If a peripheral compression neuropathy is neurapratic and associated with muscular effort, immobilization of the extremity should lead to rather prompt improvement of the neuropathy. If with restitution of muscular effort the neuropathy reappears, surgical decompression of the peripheral nerve is indicated. The basic operation for neuropathies of the radial nerve secondary to entrapment above the level of the radial tunnel is exploration of the radial nerve along its course. Exploration may be carried out either with an incision parallel to the course of the radial nerve or a series of longitudinal incisions, the first lying on the posterior lateral aspect of the distal brachium where the radial nerve can be observed piercing the intermuscular septum, and the second anterior to the lateral intermuscular septum. The longitudinal incisions are preferred to a single incision overlying the course of the radial nerve because the separation of the muscular bundles to expose the nerve is more easily performed through the longitudinal incisions.

Posterior Muscle-Splitting Approach to the Radial Tunnel. Exposure of the radial nerve within the radial tunnel can be accomplished by using either of two surgical approaches. If the compression neuropathy in the radial tunnel is located at the arcade of Frohse, excellent exposure can be provided by a direct approach through the extensor muscles. The muscle bundles are separated distally and the incision is extended proximally, developing the plane between the superficial and deep muscles on the extensor surface to expose the radial nerve as it enters the supinator muscle at the arcade of Frohse (Fig. 36-27). An incision beginning 2 cm from the lateral epicondyle of the humerus and extending distally 7 cm will provide adequate exposure. To develop the interval between the extensor muscles, the dissection is begun in the superficial layer distally, developing the incision from distal to proximal and exposing the supinator muscle and, more proximally, the radial nerve. Exploration of the radial nerve, supinator muscle, arcade of Frohse, and their relationship to each other can be undertaken without difficulty. The advantage of this approach is the limited dissection and, thus, limited morbidity of the patient in the postoperative period. If the compression neuropathy can be localized preoperatively to the arcade of Frohse or to the fascial arcade as the deep branch of the radial nerve exits from the supinator muscle, adequate exposure for the release is possible through this incision. The disadvantage of this approach is the limited anatomic exposure that can be developed through this incision. Inability to localize the lesion to the arcade of Frohse is a contraindication to the use of this limited anatomic approach. The postoperative management after using this approach to the supinator muscle is to splint the wrist for support

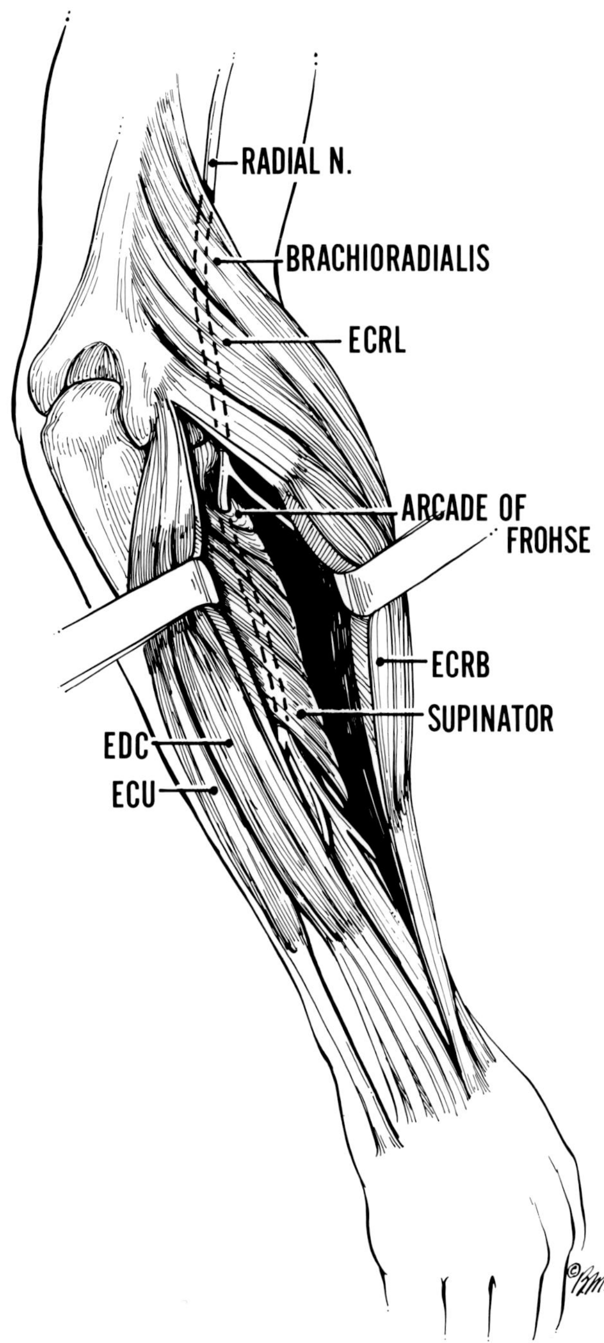

Fig. 36-27. The posterior muscle-splitting approach to the radial tunnel and the arcade of Frohse.

for the early postoperative period, allowing full flexion/extension and pronation/supination by the fourth postoperative day.

Anterolateral Approach to the Radial Tunnel. Since the radial tunnel syndrome[542,561] has been associated with four compressive anatomic lesions, an understanding of these potential lesions (see page 1367) is germane to a discussion of the more generalized approach to decompression of the radial tunnel. In those patients where the entrapment neuropathy of the radial nerve cannot be isolated preoperatively to the arcade of Frohse, a more generalized approach to the radial tunnel will be necessary to identify the site of compression, explore the radial nerve, and release the compressive lesion. Consequently, an anterolateral approach to the radial nerve is advised in these patients (Fig. 36-28). The incision is begun laterally 5 cm above the flexor crease of the elbow and continues across that flexor crease along the ulnar border of the mobile wad. The incision is deepened and the flaps are elevated to the level of the deep fascia of the arm and forearm. The radial nerve is located between the brachioradialis and brachialis muscles, just above the flexor crease of the elbow. It is advisable to trace the radial nerve from this point distally since the first potential lesion, that of the fibrous band lying anterior to the radial head, will be lost if the exploration is begun further distally. The radial recurrent vessels forming a fanlike vascular arcade anteriorly across the radial nerve must be ligated and divided to continue the operation. Since the dissection is generally done with the forearm in supination, it is hard to visualize the potential for compression of the sharp tendinous margin of the extensor carpi radialis brevis unless the surgeon, during the operation, passively pronates the forearm and volarly flexes the wrist. If, during this maneuver, the border of the extensor carpi radialis brevis conforms to an indentation of the radial nerve or if this tendinous margin is otherwise suspected as the cause of the entrapment neuropathy, the fibrous margin should be excised. Finally, the exploration is continued to the arcade of Frohse, where the deep branch dives into the substance of the supinator muscle beneath the arcade. The arcade should be divided with care so that the branch of the radial nerve to the superficial head of the muscle is not also transected during division of the arcade. I have found it desirable to completely divide the superficial head of the supinator muscle as it lies across the deep radial nerve, since the fascial surface on the deep side of this superficial head continues across the nerve for some distance and cannot be adequately explored, except by cutting the superficial head. Complete muscle division also allows exploration of the nerve to the point where the nerve arborizes and leaves the distal margin of the supinator muscle. It seems prudent to free the nerve at the distal margin completely, as well as the proximal arcade, since there can be a fibrous band at the distal margin of the supinator. This exploration can be completed with the forearm in marked pronation and retraction of the superficial layer of extensor muscles laterally to expose the distal border of the supinator.

Postoperative Management. Following completion of the exploration of the radial nerve throughout its course in the radial tunnel, the wound is closed with subcutaneous and skin sutures in the usual fashion. Although I usually provide the patient with a supportive splint for the elbow and forearm, I prefer to begin early motion in pronation and supination of the forearm and flexion and extension of the elbow within 1 week postoperatively. Between therapy sessions, the patient should continue to use the supportive splint for 1 or 2 more weeks, depending on progress following operation.

The postoperative recovery after radial tunnel decompression is generally prolonged when compared to the more common compressive neuropathies of the upper extremity. Ac-

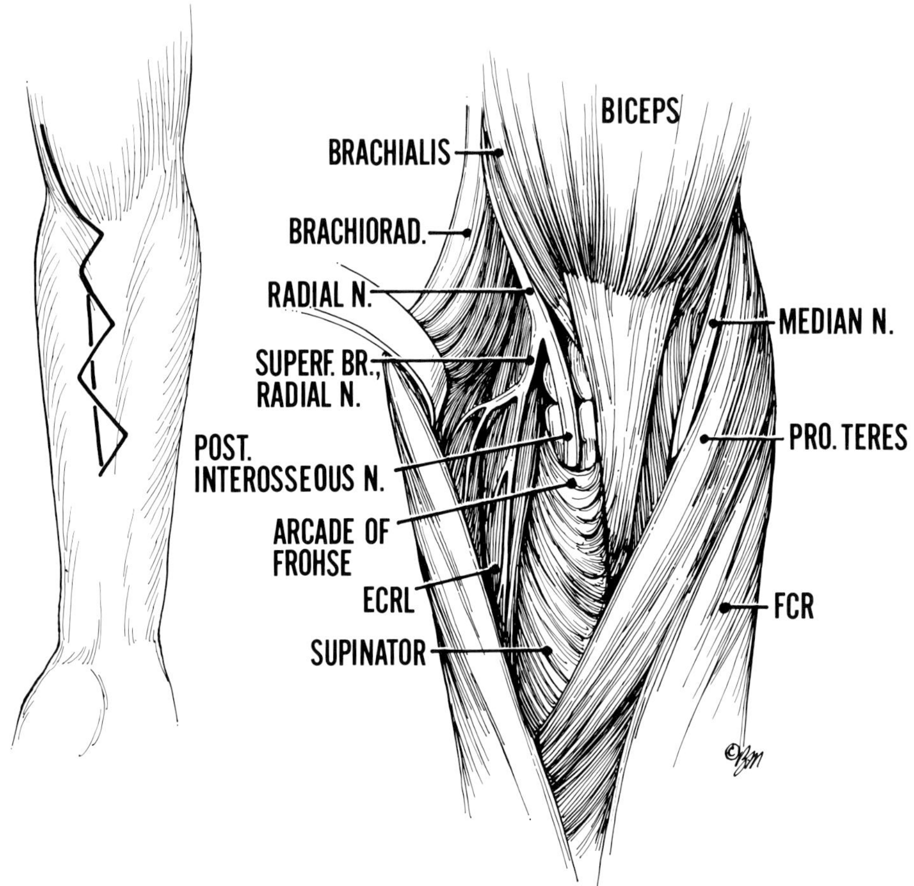

Fig. 36-28. The anterolateral approach to the radial nerve provides the best exposure of the radial tunnel when the compressive lesion cannot be localized to the arcade of Frohse. Although I prefer the zigzag incision for wider exposure, the linear incision is usually adequate.

cordingly, the patient can anticipate an early and definite improvement in symptoms with relief of the dysesthetic pain in the distribution of the radial nerve. Ultimate recovery of the radial nerve, however, seems to be prolonged over a 3- to 4-month period, during which time neurologic recovery of the neuropathy is anticipated.

Author's Preferred Method. Because of its more general applicability to entrapment neuropathies within the radial tunnel, the generalized (anterolateral) approach to the decompression of the tunnel is to be preferred. The ability of the surgeon to evaluate the entire nerve from above the elbow to the distal end of the supinator muscle cannot be overemphasized. Although the incision is less cosmetic than the more limited approach, the completeness of this exploration for neuropathies within the radial tunnel far outweighs the cosmetic disadvantage.

Radial Nerve Compression at the Wrist (Wartenberg's Syndrome)

Wartenberg[573] described an isolated neuritis of the superficial radial nerve (cheiralgia paraesthetica), which still bears his name. The syndrome was described in five patients and was associated with persistent pain on the dorsal radial surface of the distal third of the forearm radiating to the dorsum of the hand, thumb, and index and middle fingers. The location of pain may involve all or part of the distribution of the superficial radial nerve. On examination, there is sensitivity to percussion over the radial nerve within several centimeters of the radial styloid along the dorsal edge of the brachioradialis muscle. The percussion sensitivity radiates to the area of pain and is often associated with numbness. The indication for operative correction is the failure of conservative treatment to relieve the isolated neuritis of the superficial radial nerve.

Isolated neuritis of the superficial radial nerve has been associated with a number of seemingly unrelated causes. Although hemorrhage in the proximal forearm, extrinsic or intrinsic tumors of the radial nerve, and thrombosis of the recurrent radial vessels have been implicated in neuritic syndromes of the superficial radial nerve, injury to the branches of the superficial radial nerve in the distal third of the forearm or dorsum of the wrist are most often iatrogenic or traumatic.[207] The wearing of jewelry, such as elastic watchbands or elastic or tight-fitting bracelets, will produce a neuritis of this nerve, which can be easily relieved with removal of the watchband or bracelet. Anomalies of the muscles along the course of the superficial radial nerve can produce neuritic symptoms associated with numbness and sensitivity to percussion. Some of these muscle anomalies result in tight fascial bands across the nerve, creating an entrapment neuropathy. In those patients in whom the removal of jewelry does not relieve the neuritic symptoms, and immobilization either does not relieve the neuritic symptoms or following reinstitution of active motion the neuritic symptoms promptly reappear, surgical exploration of the superficial radial nerve is indicated.

Dellon and Mackinnon[527,529] have recently reviewed a series of 51 patients with complaints related to entrapment of the superficial radial nerve. Surgical exploration was carried out in 35 hands, and among this group, 49 percent of the patients rated their pain relief as good, but only 37 percent felt that the relief was excellent. It would thus appear, that, as with other affections of the superficial radial nerve, such as iatrogenic and industrial trauma, many of these patients will continue to have persistent dysesthesias, especially aggravated by motion of the wrist.

Pertinent Anatomy

The superficial branch of the radial nerve arises as the distal sensory branch approximately 4 cm distal to the lateral epicondyle of the humerus. The nerve passes distally along the lateral border of the forearm beneath the brachioradialis muscle. During much of its course in the forearm it is accompanied by the radial artery and concomitant vein. At the junction of the middle and distal thirds of the forearm, the superficial radial nerve begins to pass dorsally from beneath the cover of the brachioradialis tendon. The nerve pierces the deep fascia of the distal forearm, divides into two or more branches, and supplies the sensory innervation on the dorsum of the radial side of the hand to the tip of the thumb and to the PIP joints of the index, middle, and possibly the radial half of the ring fingers. An important volar branch innervates a small area at the base of the thumb on the volar aspect of the thenar eminence.

Several important variations of the superficial radial nerve should be noted. The superficial branch of the radial nerve may supply the entire dorsum of the hand, encroaching on the area usually supplied by the ulnar nerve on the dorsum of the ring and little fingers, as well as on the index and middle fingers. Another variation of the superficial radial nerve is its passage superficial rather than deep to the brachioradialis muscle along its course from the proximal third of the forearm to the wrist. The musculocutaneous nerve may innervate the area usually supplied by the superficial radial nerve in varying degrees, even to replace the entire distribution of the superficial radial nerve on the dorsal radial aspect of the hand.

Operative Technique

To accommodate the many variations that have been outlined in the anatomic course of distribution of the superficial radial nerve, the operation should begin on the volar edge of the brachioradialis with an incision extending from the midportion of the lateral surface of the forearm, curving in a serpentine or lazy-S pattern to the dorsoradial aspect of the wrist just distal to the carpometacarpal joints. Through this incision, and by elevating the brachioradialis muscle in the proximal aspect of the incision, the superficial radial nerve can be identified beneath the muscle several centimeters more proximally. The nerve is then traced distally beneath the brachioradialis muscle and can be identified as it begins to pass dorsally and radially in the distal third of the forearm. The distal subcutaneous dissection beneath the incisions is then carefully deepened to identify the brachioradialis tendon and the superficial radial nerve passing dorsal from it in the distal third of the forearm. When entrapped by either the tendinous margin of the brachioradialis, the margin of the extensor carpi radialis longus, or a bridge of superficial fascia of the forearm between these muscles, the entrapment can be relieved by excision of the tendon margin or adjacent fascia. The nerve must be carefully dissected and identified throughout its course to ensure relief of the entrapment. Except when the nerve has been injured and is entrapped in cicatrix or has been partially or completely transected at a previous surgical procedure, I have not identified an entrapment distal to the carpometacarpal joints of the fingers and thumb.

Postoperatively, the skin is closed in a single layer, taking care not to place the sutures so deep as to incarcerate the superficial nerve in the suture line. I prefer to mobilize the wrist as soon as possible to prevent fixed cicatrix formation about the nerve.

THORACIC OUTLET SYNDROME

Thoracic outlet syndrome may present with a variety of vague and confusing symptoms, including pain in the shoulder or supraclavicular fossa, radiating down the extremity in a radicular pattern and often involving the medial border of the arm and forearm. The symptoms are often vague, ill-defined and inconsistent, but may be provoked by a particular activity, such as working overhead, reaching down and behind repetitively, or lying in a particular position (e.g., with the hands overhead, behind the head, or on the side), allowing the symptomatic shoulder to fall away on the upward side.

The common denominator of thoracic outlet syndrome is a vascular and/or neurologic symptom complex related to the subclavian artery and/or the lower trunk of the brachial plexus. Occasionally the middle trunk of the plexus is also involved, thereby involving the seventh cervical root, in addition to the eighth cervical and first thoracic roots. In those cases with middle trunk involvement, the lower trunk is also involved. The vascular lesion may be caused by mechanical compression of the subclavian artery with resultant irritation and spasm of the artery. It may also be neurologic in origin, in which case an endoneuritis of the lower trunk of the brachial plexus creates an irritative lesion of the sympathetic fibers and resultant physiologic susceptibility rather than mechanical compression of the subclavian artery.[121] In either mechanical or neurologic vascular lesions, the subclavian artery is compressed or narrowed, resulting in reduced blood flow to the upper extremity, incipient reduction of the venous outflow if the concomitant subclavian vein is also involved, and relative ischemia of the upper extremity, which may be most marked during provocative muscular tests of the upper limb. The neurologic component of the thoracic outlet syndrome involves a compression neuropathy of the lower trunk of the brachial plexus as it arises from the lower cervical and first thoracic roots, passing superiorly and laterally across the first rib to pass between the scalenus medius muscle posteriorly and the scalenus anterior muscle anteriorly.[1,8,9,61,72,110,133,135] A number of anatomic variations that affect the passage of the neurovascular structures across the first rib may be involved in the neurovascular compression syndrome, including the slope of the first rib,[1] the site of attachment of the anterior scalenus muscles,[8] the size of cross-sectional area of the cleft between the scalenus muscles,[8,133] and variations in the attachment of the scalenus minimus muscle.[110] A common insertion of the anterior and medius scalenus muscles will elevate the vessel and nerve in the passage of the neurovascular structures through the scalene cleft.[121,133] Also, a crescent-type insertion of the anterior scalenus will have a tendency to push the artery and nerve posteriorly and superiorly, making them more susceptible to compression by a sharp tendinous margin of the scalenus medius.[8] A thickening or a prominent suprapleural membrane, also known as Sibson's fascia, may translocate the nerve more posteriorly, making it more susceptible to compression, again by the margin of the scalenus medius.[8]

As with other entrapment syndromes of the upper extremity, thoracic outlet syndrome represents a series of anatomic variations, many of which have specific diagnostic maneuvers to confirm their presence. In Adson's test[1] the patient inhales deeply, holds his breath, elevates his chin, and turns it toward the affected side. If this series of maneuvers reduces or obliterates the radial pulse and/or reproduces the symptoms of the patient's complaint, the scalene muscles, particularly the scalenus anterior, may be the offending agent.

Malalignment of the shoulder, such as from sagging with increasing age, fatigue, ill health, or even poor posture, may narrow the costoclavicular space into which the neurovascular structures pass following the crossing of the scalene cleft. Narrowing of the costoclavicular space and resultant compression in the thoracic outlet may also occur with abnormal cervical ribs,[9,35] fracture calluses of the first rib or clavicle,[31,44] or abnormal posturing of the pectoral girdle, as in the brace syndrome.[61,135] The so-called costoclavicular maneuver, in which the shoulders are drawn downward and backward after which the patient takes a deep breath (with the head and neck in neutral), calls attention to compression in the costoclavicular space in this maneuver reproduces symptoms or obliterates the radial pulse. Many people will have reduced radial pulse with this test; this in itself, without reproducing symptoms, has no clinical significance.

Wright's hyperabduction syndrome[135] is another form of thoracic outlet entrapment, in which neurovascular symptoms in the upper extremities accompany repetitive or long-standing hyperabduction positioning of the pectoral girdle. The posturing assumed by a patient is one in which the arms are above or behind the head with elbows flexed. Wright indicated that two potential sites of entrapment might exist, the first being at the tendon of the pectoralis minor, and the second behind the clavicle, between it and the first rib. Once again, to make the diagnosis of Wright's hyperabduction syndrome, symptoms must be reproduced by this maneuver.

The neurologic signs and symptoms of thoracic outlet syndrome include fullness in the supraclavicular fossa, muscle wasting, atrophy, and weakness. Clumsiness of the hand, particularly apparent in activities of daily living and manipulation of fine objects of the hand, can be seen secondary to weakness or partial paralysis of the intrinsic muscles of the hand or the flexor pollicis longus or flexor digitorum profundus muscles.[67,133] A variety of sensory complaints can be associated with this syndrome. Many of these sensory complaints may be aggravated by cold weather, particularly with vascular involvement, or by carrying objects in the hand or on the shoulder, particularly if those objects displace or reposition the shoulder while being carried. The symptoms are usually increased after a long or tiring day, can be worse at night, and, if the patient sleeps on his side, affect the upper shoulder rather than the shoulder on which the patient sleeps. The shoulder on which the patient sleeps is usually relieved of thoracic outlet symptoms because of the compression of the shoulder and a widening of the costoclavicular space and scalene cleft while in this position. Similarly, elevation of the shoulder relieves the symptoms, and the patient may notice relief as he rests on a table or bar with his shoulders elevated but relaxed while leaning on the elbows. Several authors have noted (but have not explained), that vasomotor changes usually affect the radial side of the hand, specifically the thumb and index finger, rather than the ulnar side of the hand and palm.The vascular signs and symptoms of thoracic outlet syndrome include venous congestion of the upper limb and a bruit or thrill in the supraclavicular fossa, usually more marked with activity of the hand at either eye level or above the head. The symptoms of mild ischemia, particularly during work, may be described by the patient as a tiring or early fatiguing of the hands or arms, and, when dependent, the hand may be congested or bluish in color, possibly turning ischemic or white with elevation, particularly when the elevation is associated by exercise or cold.

Operative Treatment

Operative treatment for thoracic outlet syndrome may vary, depending on the success of localizing the origin of the compression. Although scalenotomies,[8] particularly of the scalenus anterior, have been popular in the past, the relatively frequent failure of this procedure in the treatment of thoracic outlet syndrome has led to the theory that the costoclavicular compression may be the principle mechanism. The correction of this compression syndrome by resection of the first rib has evolved. First rib resection is to be preferred to claviculectomy because decompression of the lower trunk of the brachial plexus as it crosses the first rib with the subclavian vessels is ensured by rib resection. The complications of claviculectomy, particularly those of traction neuritis of the entire brachial plexus, have mitigated against the use of this procedure.

Even though first rib resection is the treatment of choice in thoracic outlet syndrome, the method of removal is disputed. The transaxillary approach[97] has largely replaced the subclavicular, anterior extrapleural, and posterior thoracoplasty approaches, all of which have been used in the past. It should be emphasized that, with resection of the first rib, the attachments of the scalenus muscles are removed and that any cervical rib should be resected at the same operation. This operation results in a thorough removal of the bony structures that may be involved in the compression syndrome at the thoracic outlet, effectively removing the attachment of all of the scalenus muscles (medius, anterior, and minimus) and relieving any incarceration of the neurovascular structures within the scalene cleft at the first rib. As always, the value of this surgical procedure is only as good as the diagnostic procedures, which localize the compression neuropathy, and the skill of the surgeon will be weighed by the preoperative evaluation rather than the intraoperative treatment.

The details of operative procedures for thoracic outlet syndrome are not included in this text as they usually fall outside the purview of most hand surgeons.

CUMULATIVE TRAUMA DISORDERS

Cumulative trauma disorders are a group of health disorders arising from repeated biomechanical stresses to muscles, tendons, ligaments, joints, and secondarily to the nerves of the forearm and hand.[580] Terms such as repetitive motion disorder, occupational overuse syndrome, and repetitive strain injury are synonymous with the more popular term, cumulative trauma disorder.[581,582,586] In the upper extremity distal to the shoulder, the most frequently occurring occupationally induced cumulative trauma disorders are carpal tunnel syndrome, stenosing tenosynovitis of the fingers, stenosing tenosynovitis of the extensor tendon sheath, usually either the first or second dorsal compartments, lateral epicondylitis of the elbow, cubital tunnel syndrome, ulnar tunnel syndrome, and radial tunnel syndrome.[587,600]

Those hazardous conditions that the worker encounters within the work place or a patient encounters outside the work place, which may produce biomechanical stress on the musculoskeletal system, are known as *ergonomic hazards.*[580] Ergonomic hazards can be caused by poor work station design, faulty work methods, improper tools, excessive tool vibration, and unfavorable design characteristics of the job.[593,594,598] A number of unfavorable design characteristics have been isolated, including line speeds that are excessive, increased posture and force requirements, inadequate work/rest ratio, and an excessively high rate of repetition of the work cycle.[589,596,598] These conditions are collectively referred to as *work stressors.* Stressors such as repetitiveness of activity, force requirements, awkwardness of posture, exposure to excessive vibration, and exposure to lower temperatures during the work cycle increase the probability of cumulative trauma disorders.[580]

The term *carpal tunnel syndrome* can be used to designate either a noncumulative trauma disorder or a cumulative trauma disorder resulting from biomechanical stressors previously described. Within the work place, repetitive wrist flexion and extension and continuous use of the fingers with the wrist either extended or more commonly flexed palmarly are the usual hazards associated with this cumulative trauma disorder syndrome.[582,600] The clinical evaluation of the patient and the search for complicating medical conditions in the work-related cumulative trauma disorder are identical to those that are sought for the noncumulative compression neuropathy. The clinical testing of the patient will similarly be identical. The appropriate treatment methods will also be similar, although removal of the ergonomic stressors or ergonomic hazards within a patient's work environment will constitute an additional conservative approach to treatment that can be dependably expected to reduce or reverse the symptom complex experienced by the patient.[600]

In the postoperative period the patient recovering from a cumulative trauma disorder must be carefully evaluated before returning to the work place and reexposure to the ergonomic hazards and repetitive motion activity that may have caused the cumulative trauma disorder.[587,600] A detailed analysis of the job performed by the patient should include the work objective, work standard, work method, design of the work station and equipment, and materials used in the product or function of the work. These details are important in the job analysis decision when the worker returns to the work place.[580,600] Observation of the worker in the work place or videotape documentation of the job and the worker performing it, will aid the surgeon in determining whether or not the postoperative patient can return and be reexposed to the ergonomic hazards. Naturally, elimination or reduction of ergonomic hazards is desirable and in some cases may be necessary to allow return of the injured worker to a previous occupation following surgical treatment.[600]

Since many jobs and many work stations cannot be made free of ergonomic risk, preplacement evaluation of workers before they enter the work place, continued monitoring of workers within the work place using noninvasive techniques,[600] and the comprehensive rehabilitation of postoperative patients before returning to the work place, may be essential components to the safe and successful matching of the worker to the employment.[580]

REFERENCES

General

1. Adson AW: Surgical treatment for symptoms produced by cervical ribs and the scalenus anterior muscle. Surg Gynecol Obstet 85:687, 1947
2. Backhouse KM: Innervation of the hand. Hand 7:107–114, 1975
3. Barber KW Jr, Bianco AJ Jr, Soule EH, MacCarty CS: Benign extraneural soft tissue tumors of the extremities causing compression of nerves. J Bone Joint Surg 44A:98–104, 1962
4. Bateman JE: Trauma to Nerve in Limbs. WB Saunders, Philadelphia, 1962
5. Behse F, Buchthal F, Carlsen F, Knappeis GG: Hereditary neuropathy with liability to pressure palsies: Electrophysiological and histopathological aspect. Brain 95:777–794, 1972
6. Belsole RJ, Lister GD, Kleinert HE: Polyarteritis: A cause of nerve palsy in the extremity. J Hand Surg 3:320–325, 1978
7. Blunt MJ: The vascular anatomy of the median nerve in the forearm and hand. J Anat 93:15, 1959
8. Bonney G: The scalenus medius band. A contribution to the study of the thoracic outlet syndrome. J Bone Joint Surg 47B:268–272, 1965
9. Brannon EW: Cervical rib syndrome. An analysis of nineteen cases and twenty-four operations. J Bone Joint Surg 45A:977–998, 1963

10. Brooks DM: Nerve compression by simple ganglia. J Bone Joint Surg 34B:391-400, 1952
11. Brooks DM: Nerve compression syndromes (editorial). J Bone Joint Surg 45B:445-446, 1963
12. Brown BA: Internal neurolysis in traumatic peripheral nerve lesions in continuity. Surg Clin North Am 52:1167-1175, 1972
13. Chalmers J: Unusual causes of peripheral nerve compression. Hand 10:168-175, 1978
14. Clein LJ: Suprascapular entrapment neuropathy. Neurosurgery 43:337, 1975
15. Cliffton EE: Unusual innervation of the intrinsic muscles of the hand by median and ulnar nerve. Surgery 23:12, 1948
16. Craig WS, Clark JMP: Of peripheral nerve palsies in the newly born. J Obstet Gynecol Br Commonw 65:229-237, 1958
17. Cruz-Martinez A, Barrio M, Perez-Conde MC, Ferrer MT: Electrophysiological aspects of sensory conduction velocity in healthy adults. Ratio between the amplitude of sensory evoked potentials at the wrist on stimulating different fingers in both hands. J Neurol Neurosurg Psychiatry 41:1097-1101, 1978
18. Daube JR: Nerve conduction studies in the thoracic outlet syndrome. Neurology 25:347, 1975
19. Denny-Brown D, Brenner C: Paralysis of nerve induced by direct pressure and by tourniquet. Arch Neurol Psychiatry 51:1-26, 1944
20. Earl CJ, Fullerton PM, Wakefield GS, Schutta HS: Hereditary neuropathy with liability to pressure palsies. A clinical and electrophysiological study of four families. Q J Med 33:481-498, 1964
21. Eisen A: Early diagnosis of ulnar nerve palsy: An electrophysiological study. Neurology 24:256, 1974
22. Eisen A, Schomer D, Melmed C: The application of F-wave measurements in the differentiation of proximal and distal upper limb entrapments. Neurology 27:662-668, 1977
23. Eversmann WW: Compression and entrapment neuropathies of the upper extremity. J Hand Surg 8:759-766, 1983
24. Felsenthal G: Median and ulnar distal motor and sensory latencies in the same normal subject. Arch Phys Med Rehab 58:297, 1977
25. Felsenthal G: Median and ulnar evoked muscle and sensory action potentials. Am J Phys Med 57:167, 1978
26. Felsenthal G: Comparison of evoked potentials in the same hand in normal subjects and in patients with carpal tunnel syndrome. Am J Phys Med 57:228-232, 1978
27. Fincham RW, Cape CA: Neuropathy in myxedema. A study of sensory nerve conduction in the upper extremities. Arch Neurol 19:464, 1968
28. Froshe F, Frankel M: Die Muskeln des menschlichen Armes. pp. 164-175. In Bardeleben's Handbuch der Anatomie des Menschlichen. Fisher, Jena, 1908
29. Furnas DW: Muscle tendon variations in the flexor compartment of the wrist. Plast Reconstr Surg 36:320-324, 1965
30. Gage MP: Scalenus anterior syndrome. Am J Surg 73:252, 1947
31. Gelberman RH, Verdeck WH, Brodhead WT: Supraclavicular nerve entrapment syndrome. J Bone Joint Surg 57A:119, 1975
32. Gilliatt RW: Disorders of peripheral nerve. J R Coll Phys London 1:50, 1966
33. Gilliatt RW, Melville ID, Velate AS, Willison RG: A study of normal nerve action potentials using an averaging technique (barrier grid storage tube). J Neurol Neurosurg Psychiatry 28:191, 1965
34. Gilliatt RW, Ochoa J, Rudge P, Neary D: The cause of nerve damage in acute compression. Trans Am Neurol Assoc 99:71-74, 1974
35. Gilliatt RW, Willison RG, Dietz V, Williams IR: Peripheral nerve conduction in patients with a cervical rib and band. Ann Neurol 4:124, 1978
36. Gilliatt RW, Wilson TG: Ischaemic sensory loss in patients with peripheral nerve lesions. J Neurol Neurosurg Psychiatry 17:104, 1954
37. Goss CM: Anatomy of the Human Body by Henry Gray. 27th Ed. Lea & Febiger, Philadelphia, 1959
38. Gruber W: Ueber die Verbindung des Nervus medianus mit dem Nervus ulnaris am Unterarme des Menschen under Sangethiete. Arch Anat Physiol 37:501-522, 1870
39. Hakstian RW: Funicular orientation by direct stimulation. J Bone Joint Surg 50A:1178-1186, 1968
40. Henry AK: Extensile Exposure. 2nd Ed. Williams & Wilkins, Baltimore, 1970
41. Herbison GJ, Staas WE: Electrical testing: Neuromuscular physiology and clinical application. In Littler JW, Cramer LM, Smith JW (eds): Symposium on Reconstructive Hand Surgery. CV Mosby, St. Louis, 1974
42. Hodes R, Larrabee MG, German W: The human electromyogram in response to nerve stimulation and conduction velocity of motor axons. Arch Neurol Psychiatry 60:340-365, 1948
43. Hollinshead WH: Anatomy for surgeons. The Back and Limbs, 2nd Ed. Vol. 3. Hoeber, New York, 1969
44. Howard FM, Shafer SJ: Injuries to the clavicle with neurovascular complications. A study of fourteen cases. J Bone Joint Surg 47A:1335-1346, 1965
45. Howe JF, Loeser JD, Calvin WH: Mechanosensitivity of dorsal root ganglia and chronically injured axons: A physiological basis for the radicular pain of nerve root compression. Pain 3:25, 1977
46. Hunt JR: The thenar and hypothenar types of neural atrophy of the hand. Am J Med Sci 141:224-241, 1911
47. Hunt JR: Thenar and hypothenar types of neural atrophy of the hand. Br Med J 2:642, 1930
48. Jabaley ME, Wallace WH, Heckler FR: Internal topography of major nerves of the forearm and hand. A current review. J Hand Surg 5:1-18, 1980
49. Johnson EW, Olsen KJ: Clinical value of motor nerve conduction velocity determination. JAMA 172:2030-2035, 1960
50. Kaplan EB: Functional and Surgical Anatomy of the Hand. 2nd Ed. JB Lippincott, Philadelphia, 1965
51. Karpati G, Carpenter S, Eisen AA, Feindel W: Familial multiple peripheral nerve entrapments—an unusual manifestation of a peripheral neuropathy. Trans Am Neurol Assoc 98:267-269, 1973
52. Karpati G, Carpenter S, Eisen AA, Wolfe LS, Feindel W: Multiple peripheral nerve entrapments. Arch Neurol 31:418, 1974
53. Kelso JS, Wallace S, Stelmach G, Weitz G: Sensory and motor impairment in the nerve compression block. Q J Exp Psychol 27:123, 1975
54. Kimura J, Murphy MJ, Varda DI: Electrophysiological study of anomalous innervation of intrinsic hand muscles. Arch Neurol 33:842-844, 1976
55. Kline DG, Hackett ER, May PR: Evaluation of nerve injuries by evoked potentials and electromyography. J Neurosurg 31:128-136, 1969
56. Kline DG, Nulsen FE: The neuroma in continuity. Surg Clin North Am 52:1189-1209, 1972
57. Kopell HP, Thompson WAL: Peripheral Entrapment Neuropathies. Williams & Wilkins, Baltimore, 1963
58. Kuczynski K: Functional micro-anatomy of the peripheral nerve trunks. Hand 6:1-10, 1974
59. Kudrjavcev T: Neurologic complications of thyroid dysfunction. Adv Neurol 19:619, 1978
60. Lahey MD, Aulicino PL: Anomalous muscles associated with compression neuropathies, Orthop Rev 15:19-28, 1986

61. Lain TM: The military brace syndrome: A report of sixteen cases of Erb's palsy occurring in military cadets. J Bone Joint Surg 51A:557–560, 1969
62. Leonard MH: Immediate improvement of sensation on relief of extraneural compression. J Bone Joint Surg 51A:1282–1284, 1969
63. Levine J, Spinner M: Neurolysis in elderly patients. Clin Orthop 80:13–16, 1971
64. Linell EA: The distribution of nerves in the upper limb with reference to variabilities and their clinical significance. J Anat 55:79–112, 1921
65. Lister GD: The Hand, Diagnosis and Indications. Churchill Livingstone, Edinburgh, 1977
66. Littler JW: Principles of reconstructive surgery of the hand. In Converse JM (ed): Reconstructive Plastic Surgery. WB Saunders, Philadelphia, 1964
67. London GW: Normal ulnar nerve conduction velocity across the thoracic outlet: Comparison of two measuring techniques. J Neurol Neurosurg Psychiatry 38:756–760, 1975
68. Ludin HP, Lutschg J, Valsangiacomo F: Comparison of orthodromic and antidromic sensory nerve conduction. 1. Normals and patients with carpal tunnel syndrome. EEG EMG 8:173, 1977
69. Lundborg G: Ischemic nerve injury. Experimental studies on intraneural microvascular pathophysiology and nerve function in a limb subjected to temporary circulatory arrest. Scand J Plast Reconstr Surg (suppl) 6:1–113, 1970
70. Lundborg G, Gelberman RH, Minteer-Convery M, Lee YF, Hargens AR: Median nerve compression in the carpal tunnel—functional response to experimentally induced controlled pressure. J Hand Surg 7:252–259, 1982
71. Marinacci AA: Some unusual causes of pressure neuropathies. Bull Los Angeles Neurol Soc 25:223–231, 1960
72. McIntyre DI: Subcoracoid neurovascular entrapment. Clin Orthop 108:27–30, 1975
73. McRae DL: The significance of abnormalities of the cervical spine. Am J Roentgenol 84:3, 1960
74. Miller R: Observations upon the arrangement of the axillary artery and brachial plexus. Am J Anat 64:143–163, 1939
75. Moldaver J: Tourniquet paralysis syndrome. Arch Surg 68:136, 1954
76. Morrison JT: A palmaris longus muscle with a reversed belly, forming an accessory flexor muscle of the little finger. J Anat Phys 50:324, 1916
77. Murai Y, Anderson I: Studies of sensory conductions: Comparison of latencies of orthodromic and antidromic sensory potentials. J Neurol Neurosurg Psychiatry 38:1187, 1975
78. Nakano KK: The entrapment neuropathies of rheumatoid arthritis. Orthop Clin North Am 6:837, 1975
79. Neary D, Eames RA: The pathology of ulnar nerve compression in man. Neuropathol Appl Neurobiol 1:69–88, 1975
80. Neary D, Ochoa J, Gilliatt RW: Subclinical entrapment neuropathy in man. J Neurol Sci 24:283–298, 1976
81. Nicolle FV, Woolhouse FM: Nerve compression syndromes of the upper limb. J Trauma 5:313–319, 1965
82. Ochoa J: Schwann cell and myelin changes caused by some toxic agents and trauma. Proc R Soc Med 67:131–133, 1974
83. Ochoa J, Fowler TJ, Gilliatt RW: Anatomical changes in peripheral nerves compressed by pneumatic tourniquet. J Anat 113:433–455, 1972
84. Omer GE: Injuries to nerves of the extremity. J Bone Joint Surg 56A:1615–1624, 1974
85. Omer GE, Spinner M: Peripheral nerve testing and suture techniques. pp. 122–143. In AAOS Instructional Course Lectures, Vol. 24. CV Mosby, St. Louis, 1975
86. Paget J: Lectures on Surgical Pathology. 1st Ed. Lindsay & Bakiston, Philadelphia, 1854
87. Pandya NJ: Surgical decompression of nerves in leprosy. An attempt at prevention of deformities. A clinical, electrophysiologic, histopathologic and surgical study. Int J Lepr 46:47, 1978
88. Parks BJ: Postoperative peripheral neuropathies. Surgery 74:348, 1973
89. Parsonage MJ, Turner JWA: Neuralgic amyotrophy. The shoulder-girdle syndrome. Lancet 1:973, 1948
90. Payan J: Electrophysiological localization of ulnar nerve lesions. J Neurol Neurosurg Psychiatry 32:208, 1969
91. Phalen GS, Kendrick JI, Rodriguez JM: Lipomas of the upper extremity. Am J Surg 121:298–306, 1971
92. Rainer WG, Mayer J, Sadler TR Jr, Dirks D: Effect of graded compression on nerve conduction velocity. Arch Surg 107:719, 1973
93. Rank RK, Wakefield AR, Hueston JT: Surgery of Repair as Applied to Hand Injuries. 3rd Ed. Williams & Wilkins, Baltimore, 1968
94. Rask MR: Suprascapular nerve entrapment: A report of two cases treated with suprascapular notch resection. Clin Orthop 123:73–75, 1977
95. Reimann AF, Daseler EH, Anson BJ, Beaton LE: The palmaris longus muscle and tendon. A study of 1600 extremities. Anat Rec 89:495–505, 1944
96. Riche P: Le nerf cubital et las muscles de l'eminence thenar. Bull Mem Soc Anat Paris 5:251–252, 1897
97. Roos D: Transaxillary approach for first rib resection to relieve thoracic outlet syndrome. Ann Surg 163:354, 1966
98. Rowntree T: Anomalous innervation of the hand muscles. J Bone Joint Surg 51B:505–510, 1949
99. Rudge P, Ochoa J, Gilliatt RW: Acute peripheral nerve compression in the baboon. J Neurol Sci 23:403–420, 1974
100. Rydevik B, Lundborg G: Permeability of intraneural microvessels and perineurium following acute, graded experimental nerve compression. Scand J Plast Reconstr Surg 11:179, 1977
101. Rydevik B, Lundborg G, Bagge U: Effects of graded compression on intraneural blood flow. J Hand Surg 6:3–12, 1981
102. Rydevik B, Lundborg G, Nordborg C: Intraneural tissue reactions induced by internal neurolysis. Scand J Plast Reconstr Surg 10:3–8, 1976
103. Seddon HJ: Three types of nerve injury. Brain 66:237–287, 1943
104. Seddon HJ: Surgical Disorders of the Peripheral Nerves. 2nd Ed. Churchill Livingstone, Edinburgh, 1975
105. Simpson JA: Fact and fallacy in measurement of conduction velocity in motor nerves. J Neurol Neurosurg Psychiatry 27:381–385, 1964
106. Smith GE: An account of some rare nerve and muscle anomalies with remarks on their significance. J Anat Physiol 29:84, 1895
107. Smith JW: Factors influencing nerve repair. I. Blood supply to peripheral nerves. Arch Surg 93:335–341, 1966
108. Smith JW: Factors influencing nerve repair. II. Collateral circulation of the peripheral nerves. Arch Surg 93:433–436, 1966
109. Spencer PS, Weinberg HJ, Raine CS, Prineas JW: The perineurial window—a new model of focal demyelination and remyelination. Brain Res 96:323–329, 1975
110. Spinner M: Cryptogenic infraclavicular brachial plexus neuritis (Preliminary report). Bull Hosp Joint Dis 37:98, 1976
111. Spinner M: Injuries to the Major Branches of Peripheral Nerves of the Forearm. 2nd Ed. WB Saunders, Philadelphia, 1978
112. Spinner M, Freundlich BD: An important variation of the palmaris longus. Bull Hosp Joint Dis 28:126, 1967
113. Spinner M, Spencer PS: Nerve compression lesions of the upper extremity. A clinical and experimental review. Clin Orthop 104:46–67, 1974

114. Strain RE, Olson WH: Selective damage of large diameter peripheral nerve fibers by compression. An application of Laplace's law. Exp Neurol 47:68, 1975
115. Straus WL Jr: The phylogeny of the human forearm extensors. Hum Biol 13:23, 203, 1941
116. Struthers J: On a peculiarity of the humerus and humeral artery. Monthly J Med Sci 8:264-267, 1848
117. Struthers J: On some points in the abnormal anatomy of the arm. Br Foreign Medico-Chirurgical Rev 12:523-533, 1854
118. Sunderland S: The intraneural topography of the radial, median and ulnar nerves. Brain 68:243-299, 1945
119. Sunderland S: The innervation of the flexor digitorum profundus and lumbrical muscles. Anat Rec 93:317-321, 1945
120. Sunderland S: Traumatic injuries of peripheral nerves. I. Simple compression injuries of the radial nerve. Brain 68:56-72, 1945
121. Sunderland S: Nerves and Nerve Injuries. Williams & Wilkins, Baltimore, 1968
122. Thomas JE, Lambert EH: Ulnar nerve conduction velocity and H reflex in infants and children. J Appl Physiol 15:1-9, 1960
123. Thomas PK, Sears TA, Gilliatt RW: The range of conduction velocity in normal motor nerve fibers to the small muscles of the hand and foot. J Neurol Neurosurg Psychiatry 22:175-181, 1959
124. Trojaborg W: Prolonged conduction block with axonal degeneration. J Neurol Neurosurg Psychiatry 40:50-57, 1977
125. Turner JWA, Parsonage MJ: Neuralgic amyotrophy (paralytic brachial neuritis.) Lancet 2:209, 1957
126. Upton ARM, McComas AJ: The double crush nerve entrapment syndromes. Lancet 2:359, 1973
127. Wagman IH, Lesse H: Maximum conduction velocities of motor fibers of ulnar nerve in human subject of various ages and sizes. J Neurophysiol 15:235, 1952
128. Watson-Jones R: Primary nerve lesions in injuries of the elbow and wrist. J Bone Joint Surg 12:121, 1930
129. Weir MS: Injuries of Nerves and Their Consequences. JB Lippincott, Philadelphia, 1872
130. White WL, Hanna DC: Troublesome lipomata of the upper extremity. J Bone Joint Surg 44A:1353-1359, 1962
131. Wilbourn AJ, Lambert EH: The forearm median-to-ulnar nerve communication; electrodiagnostic aspects. Neurology 26:368, 1976
132. Williams HB, Terzis JK: Single fascicular recordings: An intraoperative diagnostic tool for the management of peripheral nerve lesions. Plast Reconstr Surg 57:562-569, 1976
133. Williams HT, and Carpenter NH: Surgical treatment of the thoracic outlet compression syndrome. Arch Surg 113:850, 1978
134. Wortis H, Stein MH, Jolliffee N: Fiber dissociation in peripheral neuropathy. Arch Intern Med 69:222, 1942
135. Wright IS: The neurovascular syndrome produced by hyperabduction of the arms. Am Heart J 29:1, 1945

Pronator Syndrome

136. Agnew DH: Bursal tumor producing loss of power of forearm. Am J Med Sci 46:404-405, 1863
137. Barnard LB, McCoy SM: The supracondyloid process of the humerus. J Bone Joint Surg 28:845-850, 1946
138. Beaton LE, Anson BJ: The relation of the median nerve to the pronator teres muscle. Anat Rec 75:23-26, 1939
139. Bell GE Jr, Goldner JL: Compression neuropathy of the median nerve. South Med J 49:966-972, 1956
140. Bucher TPJ: Anterior interosseous nerve syndrome. J Bone Joint Surg 54B:555, 1972
141. Buchthal F, Rosenfalck A, Trojaborg W: Electrophysiological findings in entrapment of the median nerve at wrist and elbow. J Neurol Neurosurg Psychiatry 37:340, 1974
142. Farber JS, Bryan RS: The anterior interosseous nerve syndrome. J Bone Joint Surg 50A:521-523, 1968
143. Fearn CB d'A, Goodfellow JW: Anterior interosseous nerve palsy. J Bone Joint Surg 47B:91-93, 1965
144. Ferner H: Ein Abnormaler verlauf des Nervus medianus vor dem M. pronator teres. Anat Anz 84:151-156, 1937
145. Finelli PF: Anterior interosseous nerve syndrome following cutdown catheterization. Ann Neurol 1:205-206, 1977
146. Gardner-Thorpe C: Anterior interosseous nerve palsy: Spontaneous recovery in two patients. J Neurol Neurosurg Psychiatry 37:1146-1150, 1974
147. Kessel L, Rang M: Supracondylar spur of the humerus. J Bone Joint Surg 48B:765-769, 1966
148. Kiloh LG, Nevin S: Isolated neuritis of the anterior interosseous nerve. Br Med J 1:850-851, 1952
149. Kopell HP, Thompson WAL: Pronator syndrome. N Engl J Med 259:713-715, 1958
150. Krag C: Isolated paralysis of the flexor pollicis longus muscle. An unusual variation of the anterior interosseous nerve syndrome. Case report. Scand J Plast Reconstr Surg 8:250-252, 1974
151. Laha RK, Lunsford D, Dujovny M: Lacertus fibrousus compression of the median nerve. Case report. J Neurosurg 48:838, 1978
152. Lake PA: Anterior interosseous nerve syndrome. J Neurosurg 41:306-309, 1974
153. Leffert RD, Dorfman HD: Antecubital cyst in rheumatoid arthritis. Surgical findings. J Bone Joint Surg 54A:1555-1557, 1972
154. Lipscomb PR, Burleson RJ: Vascular and neural complications in supracondylar fractures of the humerus in children. J Bone Joint Surg 37A:487-492, 1955
155. Macon WL, Futrell JW: Median-nerve neuropathy after percutaneous puncture of the brachial artery in patients receiving anticoagulants. N Engl J Med 288:1396, 1973
156. Maeda K, Miura T, Komada T, Chiba A: Anterior interosseous nerve paralysis. Report of 13 cases and review of Japanese literatures. Hand 9:165-171, 1977
157. Mangani U: Flexor pollicis longus muscle. Its morphology and clinical significance. J Bone Joint Surg 42A:467-470, 1960
158. Mannerfelt L: Median nerve entrapment after dislocation of the elbow. Report of a case. J Bone Joint Surg 50B:152-155, 1968
159. Matev I: A radiological sign of entrapment of the median nerve in the elbow joint after posterior dislocation. J Bone Joint Surg 58B:353-355, 1976
160. McLellan DL, Swash M: Longitudinal sliding of the median nerve during movements of the upper limb. J Neurol Neurosurg Psychiatry 39:566, 1976
161. Mills RH, Mukherjee K, Bassett IB: Anterior interosseous nerve palsy. Br Med J 2:555, 1969
162. Mittal RL, Gupta BR: Median and ulnar nerve palsy: An unusual presentation of the supracondylar process. Report of a case. J Bone Joint Surg 60A:557-558, 1978
163. Morris HH, Peters BH: Pronator syndrome: Clinical and electrophysiological features in seven cases. J Neurol Neurosurg Psychiatry 39:461-464, 1976
164. Nakano KK, Lundergan C, Okihiro MM: Anterior interosseous nerve syndromes. Diagnostic methods and alternative treatments. Arch Neurol 34:477-480, 1977
165. Neundorf B, Kroger M: The anterior interosseous nerve syndrome. J Neurol 213:341, 1976
166. O'Brien MD, Upton ARM: Anterior interosseous nerve syndrome. A case report with neurophysiological investigation. J Neurol Neurosurg Psychiatry 35:531-536, 1972

167. Schmidt H, Eiken O: The anterior interosseous nerve syndrome. Scand J Plast Reconstr Surg 5:53–56, 1971
168. Seyffarth H: Primary myoses in the M. pronator teres as cause of lesion of the N. medianus (the pronator syndrome). Acta Psychiatr Neurol (suppl) 74:251–254, 1951
169. Sharrard WJW: Anterior interosseous neuritis. Report of a case. J Bone Joint Surg 50B:804–805, 1968
170. Smith BH, Herbst BA: Anterior interosseous nerve palsy. Arch Neurol 30:330–331, 1974
171. Solnitzky O: Pronator syndrome: Compression neuropathy of the median nerve at level of pronator teres muscle. Georgetown Med Bull 13:232–238, 1960
172. Spinner M: The functional attitude of the hand afflicted with an anterior interosseous nerve paralysis. Bull Hosp Joint Dis 30:21, 1969
173. Spinner M: The anterior interosseous-nerve syndrome. With special attention to its variations. J Bone Joint Surg 52A:84–94, 1970
174. Spinner M, Schreiber SN: The anterior interosseous-nerve paralysis as a complication of supracondylar fractures in children. J Bone Joint Surg 51A:1584–1590, 1969
175. Steiger RN, Larrick RB, Meyer TL: Median-nerve entrapment following elbow dislocation in children. J Bone Joint Surg 51A:381–385, 1969
176. Stern MB, Rosner LJ, Blinderman EE: Kiloh-Nevin syndrome. Clin Orthop 53:95–98, 1967
177. Stern PJ, Kutz JE: An unusual variant of the anterior interosseous nerve syndrome. J Hand Surg 5:32–34, 1980
178. Struthers J: Anatomical and Physiological Observations. Part I. Sutherland & Knox, Edinburgh, 1854
179. Thomas DF: Kiloh-Nevin syndrome. J Bone Joint Surg 44B:962, 1962
180. Thomsen PB: Processus supracondyloidea humeri with concomitant compression of the median nerve and the ulnar nerve. Acta Orthop Scand 48:391–393, 1977
181. Vichare NA: Spontaneous paralysis of the anterior interosseous nerve. J Bone Joint Surg 50B:806–808, 1968
182. Warren JD: Anterior interosseous nerve palsy as a complication of forearm fractures. J Bone Joint Surg 45B:511–512, 1963
183. Weins E, Lau SCK: The anterior interosseous nerve syndrome. Can J Surg 21:354, 1978

Carpal Tunnel Syndrome

184. Abbott LC, Saunders JB: Injuries of the median nerve in fractures of the lower end of the radius. Surg Gynecol Obstet 57:507, 1933
185. Aiache AE: An early sign of carpal tunnel syndrome. Plast Reconstr Surg 61:130, 1978
186. Amadio PC: Pyridoxine as an adjunct in the treatment of carpal tunnel syndrome. J Hand Surg 10A:237–241, 1985
187. Amadio PC: Carpal tunnel syndrome, pyridoxine, and the work place. J Hand Surg 12A:875–880, 1987
188. Ariyan S, Watson HK: The palmar approach for the visualization and release of the carpal tunnel. An analysis of 429 cases. Plast Reconstr Surg 60:539–547, 1977
189. Arnold AG: The carpal tunnel syndrome in congestive cardiac failure. Postgrad Med J 53:623, 1977
190. Ashby BS: Hypertrophy of the palmaris longus muscle. J Bone Joint Surg 46B:230–232, 1964
191. Backhouse KM, Churchill-Davidson D: Anomalous palmaris longus muscle producing carpal tunnel-like compression. Hand 7:22, 1975
192. Bacorn RW, Kurtze JF: Colles fracture: A study of two thousand cases from the New York State Workmen's Compensation Board. J Bone Joint Surg 35A:643–658, 1953
193. Barfred T, Höjlund AP, Bertheussen K: Median artery in carpal tunnel syndrome. J Hand Surg 10A:864–867, 1985
194. Barfred T, Ipsen T: Congenital carpal tunnel syndrome. J Hand Surg 10A:246–248, 1985
195. Baruch A, Hass A: Anomaly of the median nerve (letter). J Hand Surg 2:331–332, 1977
196. Bendler EM, Greenspun B, Yu J, Erdman WJ: The bilaterality of carpal tunnel syndrome. Arch Phys Med Rehabil 58:362–364, 1977
197. Bleecker ML: Medial surveillance for carpal tunnel syndrome in workers. J Hand Surg 12A:845–848, 1987
198. Blodgett RC Jr, Lipscomb PR, Hill RW: Incidence of hematologic disease in patients with carpal tunnel syndrome. JAMA 182:814, 1962
199. Borgman MF: Carpal tunnel syndrome. Nurse Pract 3:21, 1978
200. Brain WR, Wright AD, Wilkerson M: Spontaneous compression of both median nerves in the carpal tunnel. Six cases treated surgically. Lancet 1:277, 1947
201. Brones MF, Wilgis EFS: Anatomical variations of the palmaris longus, causing carpal tunnel syndrome: Case reports. Plast Reconstr Surg 62:798–800, 1978
202. Brown EZ Jr, Snyder CC: Carpal tunnel syndrome caused by hand injuries. Plast Reconstr Surg 56:41–43, 1975
203. Buchthal F, Rosenfalck A: Sensory conduction from digit to palm and from palm to wrist in the carpal tunnel syndrome. J Neurol Neurosurg Psychiatry 34:243–252, 1971
204. Buchthal F, Rosenfalck A, Trojaborg W: Electrophysiological findings in entrapment of the median nerve at wrist and elbow. J Neurol Neurosurg Psychiatry 37:340, 1974
205. Butler B, Bigley EC: Aberrant index (first) lumbrical tendinous origin associated with carpal tunnel syndrome. A case report. J Bone Joint Surg 53A:160–162, 1971
206. Cannon BW, Love JB: Tardy median palsy: Median neuritis: Median thenar neuritis amenable to surgery. Surgery 20:210, 1946
207. Carroll RE, Green DP: The significance of the palmar cutaneous nerve at the wrist. Clin Orthop 83:24, 1972
208. Champion D: Gouty tenosynovitis and the carpal tunnel syndrome. Med J Aust 1:1030, 1969
209. Cherington M: Proximal pain in the carpal tunnel syndrome. Arch Surg 108:69, 1974
210. Chow JCY: Endoscopic release of the carpal ligament: A new technique for carpal tunnel syndrome. Arthroscopy 5:19–24, 1989
211. Chow JCY: Endoscopic release of the carpal ligament for carpal tunnel syndrome: 22-month clinical result. Arthroscopy 6:288–296, 1990
212. Crow RS: Treatment of the carpal-tunnel syndrome. Br Med J 1:1611–1615, 1960
213. Crymble B: Brachial neuralgia and carpal tunnel syndrome. Br Med J 3:470–471, 1968
214. Cseuz KA, Thomas JE, Lambert EH, Love JG, Lipscomb PR: Long-term results of operation for carpal tunnel syndrome. Mayo Clin Proc 41:232–241, 1966
215. Curtis RM, Eversmann WW: Internal neurolysis as an adjunct to the treatment of the carpal-tunnel syndrome. J Bone Joint Surg 55A:733–740, 1973
216. Das SK, Brown HG: In search of complications in carpal tunnel decompression. Hand 8:243–249, 1976
217. DeLuca FN, Cowen NJ: Median-nerve compression complicating a tendon graft prosthesis. J Bone Joint Surg 57A:553, 1975
218. Doll DC, Weiss RB: Unusual presentations of multiple myeloma. Postgrad Med 61:116–121, 1977

219. Eboth N, Wilson DH: Surgery of the carpal tunnel. Technical note. J Neurosurg 49:316-318, 1978
220. Eiken O, Carstram N, Eddeland A: Anomalous distal branching of the median nerve. Scand J Plast Reconstr Surg 5:149-152, 1971
221. Engber WD, Cmeiner JG: Palmar cutaneous branch of the ulnar nerve. J Hand Surg 5:26-29, 1980
222. Engel J, Zinneman H, Tsur H, Farin I: Carpal tunnel syndrome due to carpal osteophyte. Hand 10:283-284, 1978
223. Entin MA: Carpal tunnel syndrome and its variants. Surg Clin North Am 48:1097-1112, 1968
224. Eversmann WW Jr, Ritsick JA: Intraoperative changes in motor nerve conduction latency in carpal tunnel syndrome. J Hand Surg 3:77-81, 1978
225. Feldman RG, Travers PH, Chirico-Post J, Keyserling WM: Risk assessment in electronic assembly workers: Carpal tunnel syndrome. J Hand Surg 12A:849-855, 1987
226. Fissette J, Onkelinx A, Fandi N: Carpal and Guyon tunnel syndrome in burns at the wrist. J Hand Surg 6:13-15, 1981
227. Floyd T, Burger RS, Sciaroni CA: Bilateral palmaris profundus causing bilateral carpal tunnel syndrome. J Hand Surg 15A:364-366, 1990
228. Folkers K, Ellis J, Watanabe T, Saji S, Kaji M: Biochemical evidence for a deficiency of vitamin B6 in the carpal tunnel syndrome based on a crossover clinical study. Proc Natl Acad Sci USA 75:3410-3412, 1978
229. Folmar RC, Nelson CL, Phalen GS: Ruptures of the flexor tendons in hands of non rheumatoid patients. J Bone Joint Surg 54A:579-584, 1972
230. Foster JB: Hydrocortisone and the carpal tunnel syndrome. Lancet 1:454-456, 1960
231. Freshwater MF, Arons MS: The effect of various adjuncts on the surgical treatment of carpal tunnel syndrome secondary to chronic tenosynovitis. Plast Reconstr Surg 61:93-96, 1978
232. Fuchs PC, Nathan PA, Myers LD: Synovial histology in carpal tunnel syndrome. J Hand Surg 16A:753-758, 1991
233. Fullerton PM: The effect of ischaemia on nerve conduction in the carpal tunnel syndrome. J Neurol Neurosurg Psychiatry 26:385, 1963
234. Gainer JV Jr, Nugent GR: Carpal tunnel syndrome: Report of 430 operations. South Med J 70:325-328, 1977
235. Gardner RC: Confirmed case and diagnosis of pseudocarpal-tunnel (sublimis) syndrome. N Engl J Med 282:858, 1970
236. Gassmann N, Segmuller G, Stanisic M: Carpal tunnel syndrome. Indication, technique and results following epineural and interfascicular neurolysis. Handchirurgie 9:137, 1977
237. Gelberman RH, Aronson D, Weisman MH: Carpal-tunnel syndrome. Results of a prospective trial of steroid injection and splinting. J Bone Joint Surg 62A:1181-1184, 1980
238. Gelberman RH, Hergenroeder PT, Hargens AR, Lundborg GN, Akeson WH: The carpal tunnel syndrome. A study of carpal canal pressures. J Bone Joint Surg 63A:380-383, 1981
239. Gelberman RH, Szabo RM, Williamson RV, Dimick MP: Sensibility testing in peripheral-nerve compression syndromes: An experimental study in humans. J Bone Joint Surg 65A:632-638, 1983
240. Gellman H, Kan D, Gee V, Kuschner SH, Botte MJ: Analysis of pinch and grip strength after carpal tunnel release. J Hand Surg 14A:863-864, 1989
241. Gilliatt RW, Wilson TG: A pneumatic tourniquet test in the carpal-tunnel syndrome. Lancet 2:595, 1953
242. Golding DN: Brachial neuralgia and the carpal tunnel syndrome. Br Med J 3:803, 1968
243. Goodman HV, Foster JB: Effect of local cortico-steroid injection on median nerve conduction in carpal tunnel syndrome. Ann Phys Med 6:287-294, 1962
244. Goodman HV, Gilliatt RW: The effect of treatment on median nerve conduction in patients with the carpal-tunnel syndrome. Ann Phys Med 6:135, 1961
245. Gould JS, Wissinger HA: Carpal tunnel syndrome in pregnancy. South Med J 71:144-145, 1978
246. Graham WP III: Variations of the motor branch of the median nerve at the wrist. Plast Reconstr Surg 51:90-93, 1973
247. Green DP: Diagnostic and therapeutic value of carpal tunnel injection. J Hand Surg 9A:850-854, 1984
248. Green EJ, Dilworth JH, Levitin PM: Tophaceous gout. An unusual cause of bilateral carpal tunnel syndrome. JAMA 237:2747-2748, 1977
249. Grokoest AW, Demartini FE: Systemic disease and the carpal tunnel syndrome. JAMA 155:635, 1954
250. Grundberg AB: Carpal decompression in spite of normal electromyography. J Hand Surg 8:348-349, 1983
251. Grundberg AB, Reagan DS: Compression syndromes in reflex sympathetic dystrophy. J Hand Surg 16A:731-736, 1991
252. Gutmann L: Median-ulnar nerve communications and carpal tunnel syndrome. J Neurol Neurosurg Psychiatry 40:982-986, 1977
253. Guyon MA, Honet JC: Carpal tunnel syndrome or trigger finger associated with neck injury in automobile accidents. Arch Phys Med Rehabil 58:325-327, 1977
254. Harding AE, LeFanu J: Carpal tunnel syndrome related to antebrachial Cimino-Brescia fistula. J Neurol Neurosurg Psychiatry 40:511-513, 1977
255. Harris CM, Tanner E, Goldstein MN, Pettee DS: The surgical treatment of the carpal-tunnel syndrome correlated with preoperative nerve-conduction studies. J Bone Joint Surg 61A:93, 1979
256. Harrison MJ: Lack of evidence of generalized sensory neuropathy in patients with carpal tunnel syndrome. J Neurol Neurosurg Psychiatry 41:957-959, 1978
257. Hart VL, Gaynor V: Roentgenographic study of the carpal canal. J Bone Joint Surg 23:382-383, 1941
258. Hartwell SW Jr, Kurtay M: Carpal tunnel compression caused by hematoma associated with anticoagulant therapy. Report of a case. Cleve Clin Q 33:127, 1966
259. Hayden JW: Median neuropathy in the carpal tunnel caused by spontaneous intraneural hemorrhage. J Bone Joint Surg 46A:1242-1244, 1964
260. Helm PA, Johnson ER, Carlton AM: Peripheral neurological problems in the acute burn patient. Burns 3:123, 1977
261. Holtmann B, Anderson CB: Carpal tunnel syndrome following vascular shunts for hemodialysis. Arch Surg 112:65, 1977
262. Hongell A, Mattsson HS: Neurographic studies before, after, and during operation for median nerve compression in the carpal tunnel syndrome. Scand J Plast Reconstr Surg 5:103, 1971
263. Hunt CM, Abbott K, Robert WH: The median nerve and carpal tunnel syndrome historical features, anatomical basis and clinical experiences. Bull Los Angeles Neurol Soc 25:211, 1960
264. Hunt JR: The neural atrophy of the muscles of the hand without sensory disturbances. A further study of compression neuritis of the thenar branch of the median nerve and the deep palmar branch of the ulnar nerve. Rev Neurol Psychiatry 12:137, 1914
265. Hunt WE, Luckey WT: The carpal tunnel syndrome. Diagnosis and treatment. J Neurosurg 21:178-181, 1964
266. Jabaley ME: Personal observations on the role of the lumbrical muscles in carpal tunnel syndrome. J Hand Surg 3:82-84, 1978
267. Jackson DW, Harkins PD: An aberrant muscle belly of the abductor digiti quinti associated with median nerve paresthesias. Bull Hosp Joint Dis 33:111-115, 1972

268. Johnson RK, Shrewbury MM: Anatomical course of thenar branch of the median nerve—usually in a separate tunnel through the transverse carpal ligament. J Bone Joint Surg 52A:269-273, 1970
269. Jones KG: Carpal tunnel syndrome. J Arkansas Med Soc 75:58, 1978
270. Kaplan H, Clayton M: Carpal tunnel syndrome secondary to Mycobacterium kansasii infection. JAMA 208:1186, 1969
271. Kato H, Ogino T, Nanbu T, Nakamura K: Compression neuropathy of the motor branch of the median nerve caused by palmar ganglion. J Hand Surg 16A:751-752, 1991
272. Katz JN, Stirrat CR: A self-administered hand diagram for the diagnosis of carpal tunnel syndrome. J Hand Surg 15A:360-363, 1990
273. Kemble F: Electrodiagnosis of the carpal tunnel syndrome. J Neurol Neurosurg Psychiatry 31:23, 1968
274. Kendall D: Non-penetrating injuries of the median nerve at the wrist. Brain 73:84, 1950
275. Kenzora JE: Dialysis carpal tunnel syndrome. Orthopedics 1:195, 1978
276. Kessler I: Unusual distribution of the median nerve at the wrist. A case report. Clin Orthop 67:124-126, 1969
277. Khunadorn N, Schlagenhauff RE, Tourbaf K, Papademetriou T: Carpal tunnel syndrome in hemophilia. NY State J Med 77:1314-1315, 1977
278. Klofkorn RW, Steigerwald JC: Carpal tunnel syndrome as the initial manifestation of tuberculosis. Am J Med 60:583, 1976
279. Koenigsberger MR, Moessinger AC: Iatrogenic carpal tunnel syndrome in the newborn infant. J Pediatr 91:443-445, 1977
280. Kremer M, Gilliatt RW, Golding JSR, Wilson TG: Acroparesthesiae in the carpal-tunnel syndrome. Lancet 2:590, 1953
281. Kummel BM, Zazanis GA: Shoulder pain as the presenting complaint in carpal tunnel syndrome. Clin Orthop 92:227-230, 1973
282. Langloh ND, Linscheid RL: Recurrent and unrelieved carpal tunnel syndrome. Clin Orthop 83:41-47, 1972
283. Lanz U: Anatomical variations of the median nerve in the carpal tunnel. J Hand Surg 2:44-53, 1977
284. Layton KB: Acroparesthesia in pregnancy and the carpal tunnel syndrome. Obstet Gynecol 65:823, 1958
285. Lazaro L III: Carpal-tunnel syndrome from an insect sting. J Bone Joint Surg 54A:1095-1096, 1972
286. Leach RE, Odom JA: Systemic causes of the carpal tunnel syndrome. Postgrad Med 44:127-131, 1968
287. Lettin AWF: Carpal tunnel syndrome in childhood. J Bone Joint Surg 47B:556-559, 1965
288. Levy M, Pauker M: Carpal tunnel syndrome due to thrombosed persisting median artery. A case report. Hand 10:65-68, 1978
289. Linburg RM, Albright JA: An anomalous branch of the median nerve. A case report. J Bone Joint Surg 52A:182-183, 1970
290. Linscheid RL, Peterson LFA, Juergens JL: Carpal tunnel syndrome associated with vasospasm. J Bone Joint Surg 49A:1141-1146, 1967
291. Lipscomb PR: Tenosynovitis of the hand and the wrist: Carpal tunnel syndrome, de Quervain's disease, trigger digit. Clin Orthop 13:164-181, 1959
292. Loong SC: The carpal tunnel syndrome: A clinical and electrophysiological study of 250 patients. Proc Aust Assoc Neurol 14:51, 1977
293. Loong SC, Seah SC: Comparison of median and ulnar sensory nerve action potentials in the diagnosis of the carpal tunnel syndrome. J Neurol Neurosurg Psychiatry 34:750, 1971
294. Louis DS, Greene TL, Noellert RC: Complications of carpal tunnel surgery. J Neurosurg 62:352-356, 1985
295. Lourie GM, Levin LS, Toby B, Urbaniak J: Distal rupture of the palmaris longus tendon and fascia as a cause of acute carpal tunnel syndrome. J Hand Surg 15A:367-369, 1990
296. Love JG: Median neuritis; carpal tunnel syndrome; diagnosis and treatment. NC Med J 16:463, 1955
297. MacDonald RI, Lichtman DM, Hanlon JJ, Wilson JN: Complications of surgical release for carpal tunnel syndrome. J Hand Surg 3:70-76, 1978
298. MacDougal B, Weeks PM, Wray RC Jr: Median nerve compression and trigger finger in the mucopolysaccharidoses and related diseases. Plast Reconstr Surg 59:260-263, 1977
299. Mackinnon SE, Dellon AL: An experimental study of treatment methods for chronic nerve compression. In Proceedings of the American Society for Surgery of the Hand. J Hand Surg 11A:759, 1986
300. Mainland D: An uncommon abnormality of the flexor digitorum sublimus muscle. J Anat 62:86-89, 1927
301. Mangani U: Carpal-tunnel syndrome (abstract). J Bone Joint Surg 44A:1036, 1962
302. Mannerfelt L, Hybbinette CH: Important anomaly of the thenar branch of the median nerve. Bull Hosp Joint Dis 33:15-21, 1972
303. Mannerfelt L, Normal O: Attritional ruptures of flexor tendons in rheumatoid arthritis caused by bony spurs in the carpal tunnel. J Bone Joint Surg 51B:270-277, 1969
304. Manske PR: Fracture of the hook of the hamate presenting as carpal tunnel syndrome. Hand 10:181, 1978
305. Marie et Foix P: Atrophie isole de l'eminence thenar d'origine nevritique. Role du ligament annulaire anter ieur de carpe dans la pathogenie de la lesion. Rev Neurol 26:647, 1913
306. Marinacci AA: Comparative value of measurement of nerve conduction velocity and electromyography in diagnosis of carpal tunnel syndrome. Arch Phys Med Rehabil 45:548, 1964
307. Massey EW: Carpal tunnel syndrome in pregnancy. Obstet Gynecol Surg 33:145, 1978
308. Massey EW, O'Brian JT, Georges LB: Carpal tunnel syndrome secondary to carpopedal spasm. Ann Intern Med 88:804-805, 1978
309. Maxwell JA, Keyes JJ, Ketchem LD: Acute carpal tunnel syndrome secondary to thrombosis of a persistent median artery. J Neurosurg 38:774, 1973
310. Mayers LB: Carpal tunnel syndrome secondary to tuberculosis. Arch Neurol 10:426, 1964
311. McCabe SJ, MacKinnon SE, Murray JF: A randomized trial of release versus release plus neurolysis for carpal tunnel syndrome (abstract). J Hand Surg 15A:816-817, 1990
312. McClain EJ, Wissinger HA: The acute carpal tunnel syndrome: Nine case reports. J Trauma 16:75-78, 1976
313. McCormack RM: Carpal-tunnel syndrome. Surg Clin North Am 40:517, 1960
314. Meadoff N: Median nerve injuries in fractures in the region of the wrist. Calif Med 70:252-256, 1949
315. Melvin JL, Schuckmann JA, Lanese RR: Diagnostic specificity of motor and sensory nerve conduction variables in the carpal tunnel syndrome. Arch Phys Med Rehabil 54:69, 1973
316. Michaelis LS: Stenosis of carpal tunnel, compression of median nerve, and flexor tendon sheaths, combines with rheumatoid arthritis elsewhere. Proc R Soc Med 43:414, 1950
317. Moffat JH: Traumatic neuritis of the deep palmar branch of the ulnar nerve. Can Med Assoc J 91:230-231, 1964
318. Muller LH: Anatomical abnormalities of the wrist joint causing neurological symptoms in the hand. J Bone Joint Surg 45B:431, 1963
319. Newman PH: Median nerve compression in the carpal tunnel. Postgrad Med J 24:264, 1948
320. Nissen KI: Etiology of carpal tunnel compression of the median nerve (abstract). J Bone Joint Surg 34B:514, 1952

321. Nissenbaum M, Kleinert HE: Treatment considerations in carpal tunnel syndrome with co-existent Dupuytren's disease. J Hand Surg 5:544–547, 1980
322. Ocker K, Seitz HD: A rare anatomical condition causing carpal tunnel syndrome. Handchirurgie 9:25, 1977
323. Ogden JA: An unusual branch of the median nerve. J Bone Joint Surg 54A:1779–1781, 1972
324. O'Hara LJ, Levin M: Carpal tunnel syndrome and gout. Arch Intern Med 120:180, 1967
325. Okutsu I, Ninomiya S, Hamanaka I, Kuroshima N, Inanami H: Measurement of pressure in the carpal canal before and after endoscopic management of carpal tunnel syndrome. J Bone Joint Surg 71A:679–683, 1989
326. Okutsu I, Ninomiya S, Takatori Y, Ugawa Y: Endoscopic management of carpal tunnel syndrome. Arthroscopy 5:11–18, 1989
327. Paine KWE: The carpal-tunnel syndrome. Can J Surg 6:446, 1963
328. Papathanassiou BT: A variant of the motor branch of the median nerve in the hand. J Bone Joint Surg 50B:156–157, 1968
329. Patrick J: Carpal-tunnel syndrome. Br Med J 1:1377, 1965
330. Phalen GS: Spontaneous compression of the median nerve at the wrist. JAMA 145:1128, 1951
331. Phalen GS: The carpal-tunnel syndrome: Seventeen years' experience in diagnosis and treatment of six hundred fifty-four hands. J Bone Joint Surg 48A:211–228, 1966
332. Phalen GS: Reflections on 21 years' experience with the carpal tunnel syndrome. JAMA 212:1365–1367, 1970
333. Phalen GS: The carpal tunnel syndrome. Clinical evaluation of 598 hands. Clin Orthop 83:29–40, 1972
334. Phalen GS, Gardner WJ, LaLonde AA: Neuropathy of the median nerve due to compression beneath the transverse carpal ligament. J Bone Joint Surg 32A:109–112, 1950
335. Phalen GS, Kendrick JI: Compression neuropathy of median nerve in carpal tunnel. JAMA 164:524, 1957
336. Phillips RS: Carpal tunnel syndrome as manifestation of systemic disease. Ann Rheum Dis 26:59, 1967
337. Posch JL, Marcotte DR: Carpal tunnel syndrome. An analysis of 1201 cases. Orthop Rev 5:25, 1976
338. Purnell DC, Daly DD, Lipscomb PR: Carpal-tunnel syndrome associated with myxedema. Arch Int Med 108:751, 1961
339. Richier HP, Thoden U: Early electroneurographic diagnosis of carpal tunnel syndrome. EEG, EMG 8:187, 1977
340. Richman JA, Gelberman RH, Rydevik BL, Hajek PC, Braun RM, Gylys-Morin VM, Berthoty D: Carpal tunnel syndrome: Morphologic changes after release of the transverse carpal ligament. J Hand Surg 14A:852–857, 1989
341. Rietz KA, Onne L: Analysis of sixty-five operated cases of carpal-tunnel syndrome. Acta Chir Scand 133:443, 1967
342. Robbins H: Anatomical study of the medial nerve in the carpal tunnel and etiologies of the carpal tunnel syndrome. J Bone Joint Surg 45A:953–966, 1963
343. Sabour MS, Fadel HE: The carpal tunnel syndrome—a new complication ascribed to the "Pill." Am J Obstet Gynecol 107:1265, 1970
344. Schiller F, Kolb FO: Carpal tunnel syndrome in acromegaly. Neurology 4:371, 1954
345. Schmitt O, Temme C: Carpal tunnel syndrome in developing pseudarthrosis following isolated fracture of os capitatum. Arch Orthop Trauma Surg 93:25, 1978
346. Schorn D, Hoskinson J, Dickson RA: Bone density and the carpal tunnel syndrome. Hand 10:184–186, 1978
347. Schuind F, Ventura M, Pasteels JL: Idiopathic carpal tunnel syndrome: Histologic study of flexor tendon synovium. J Hand Surg 15A:497–503, 1990
348. Schultz RJ, Endler PM, Huddleston HD: Anomalous median nerve and an anomalous muscle belly of the first lumbrical associated with carpal-tunnel syndrome. J Bone Joint Surg 55A:1744–1746, 1973
349. Seiler JG III, Milek MA, Carpenter GK, Swiontkowski MF: Intraoperative assessment of median nerve blood flow during carpal tunnel release with laser Doppler flowmetry. J Hand Surg 14A:986–991, 1989
350. Seradge H, Seradge E: Median innervated hypothenar muscle: Anomalous branch of median nerve in the carpal tunnel. J Hand Surg 15A:356–359, 1990
351. Seradge H, Seradge E: Piso-triquetral pain syndrome after carpal tunnel release. J Hand Surg 14A:858–862, 1989
352. Shimizu K, Iwasaki R, Hoshikawa H, Yamamuro T: Entrapment neuropathy of the palmar cutaneous branch of the median nerve by the fascia of flexor digitorum superficialis. J Hand Surg 13A:581–583, 1988
353. Silver MA, Gelberman RH, Gellman H, Rhoades CE: Carpal tunnel syndrome: Associated abnormalities in ulnar nerve function and the effect of carpal tunnel release on these abnormalities. J Hand Surg 10A:710–713, 1985
354. Simpson JA: Electrical signs in the diagnosis of carpal tunnel and related syndromes. J Neurol Neurosurg Psychiatry 19:27, 1956
355. Smith EM, Sonstegard DA, Anderson WH Jr: Carpal tunnel syndrome: Contribution of flexor tendons. Arch Phys Med Rehabil 58:379–385, 1977
356. Smukler NM, Patterson JR, Lorenz H, Weiner L: The incidence of the carpal tunnel syndrome in patients with rheumatoid arthritis. Arthritis Rheum 6:298, 1963
357. Spindler HA, Dellon AL: Nerve conduction studies and sensibility testing in carpal tunnel syndrome. J Hand Surg 7:260–263, 1982
358. Starreveld E, Ashenhurst EM: Bilateral carpal tunnel syndrome in childhood. Neurology 25:234, 1975
359. Stein AH Jr: The relation of median nerve compression to Sudeck's syndrome. Surg Gynecol Obstet 115:713–720, 1962
360. Stellbrink G: Compression of the palmar branch of the median nerve by atypical palmaris longus muscle. Handchirurgie 4:155–157, 1972
361. Stephens J, Welch K: Acroparesthesia, a symptom of median nerve compression at the wrist. Arch Surg 73:849, 1956
362. Sterling AP, Eshraghi A, Anderson WV, Habermann ET: Acute carpal tunnel syndrome secondary to a foreign body in the median nerve. Bull Hosp Joint Dis 33:130–134, 1972
363. Stewart JD, Eisen A: Tinel's sign and the carpal tunnel syndrome. Br Med J 2:1125–1126, 1978
364. Stratton CW, Phelps DB, Reller LB: Tuberculoid tenosynovitis and carpal tunnel syndrome caused by mycrobacterium szulgai. Am J Med 65:349–351, 1978
365. Sunderland S: The nerve lesion in the carpal tunnel syndrome. J Neurol Neurosurg Psychiatry 39:615–626, 1976
366. Sutro CJ: Carpal tunnel syndrome caused by calcification in the deep or volar radio-carpal ligament. Bull Hosp Joint Dis 30:23, 1969
367. Szabo RM, Chidgey LK: Stress carpal tunnel pressures in patients with carpal tunnel syndrome and normal patients. J Hand Surg 14A:624–627, 1989
368. Taleisnik J: The palmar cutaneous branch of the median nerve and the approach to the carpal tunnel. An anatomical study. J Bone Joint Surg 55A:1212–1217, 1973
369. Tanzer RC: The carpal-tunnel syndrome. A clinical and anatomical study. J Bone Joint Surg 41A:626–634, 1959
370. Thomas JE, Lambert EH, Cseuz KA: Electrodiagnostic aspects of the carpal tunnel syndrome. Arch Neurol 16:635, 1967

371. Thomas PK: Motor nerve conduction in the carpal tunnel syndrome. Neurology 10:1045, 1960
372. Thomas PK, Fullerton PM: Nerve fibre size in the carpal tunnel syndrome. J Neurol Neurosurg Psychiatry 26:520, 1964
373. Tomkins DG: Median neuropathy in the carpal tunnel caused by tumor-like conditions. J Bone Joint Surg 49A:737–740, 1957
374. Vichare NA: Anomalous muscle belly of the flexor digitorum superficialis. J Bone Joint Surg 52B:757–759, 1970
375. Wainapel SF: Carpal tunnel syndrome letter. Arch Phys Med Rehabil 59:43, 1978
376. Wallace TJ, Cook AW: Carpal tunnel syndrome in pregnancy. Am J Obstet Gynecol 73:1333, 1957
377. Ward LE, Bicker WH, Corbin KB: Median neuritis (carpal tunnel syndrome) caused by gouty tophi. JAMA 167:844, 1958
378. Warren DJ, Otieno LS: Carpal tunnel syndrome in patients on intermittent haemodialysis. Postgrad Med J 51:450, 1975
379. Watson-Jones R: Léri's pleonosteosis, carpal tunnel compression of the median nerve and Morton's metatarsalgia. J Bone Joint Surg 31B:560–571, 1949
380. Werschkul JD: Anomalous course of the recurrent motor branch of the median nerve in a patient with carpal tunnel syndrome. J Neurosurg 47:113–114, 1977
381. Wesser DR, Calostypis F, Hoffman S: The evolutionary significance of an aberrant flexor superficialis muscle in the human palm. J Bone Joint Surg 51A:396–398, 1969
382. Widder S, Shons AR: Carpal tunnel syndrome associated with extra tunnel vascular compression of the median nerve motor branch. J Hand Surg 13A:926–927, 1988
383. Wilson JN: Profiles of the carpal canal. J Bone Joint Surg 36A:127–132, 1954
384. Winkelman NZ, Spinner M: A variant high sensory branch of the median nerve to the third web space. Bull Hosp Joint Dis 34:161–166, 1973
385. Woltman HW: Neuritis associated with acromegaly. Arch Neurol Psychiatry 45:680, 1941
386. Wood MR: Hydrocortisone injections for carpal tunnel syndrome. Hand 12:62–64, 1980
387. Yamaguchi DM, Lipscomb PR, Soule EH: Carpal-tunnel syndrome. Minn Med 48:22, 1965
388. Zachary RB: Thenar palsy due to compression of the median nerve in the carpal tunnel. Surg Gynecol Obstet 81:213, 1945

Cubital Tunnel Syndrome

389. Adson AW: The surgical treatment of progressive ulnar paralysis. Coll Paper Mayo Clin 10:944, 1918
390. Adson AW: Progressive ulnar paralysis. Minn Med 1:455, 1918
391. Apfelberg DB, Larson SJ: Dynamic anatomy of the ulnar nerve at the elbow. Plast Reconstr Surg 51:76–81, 1973
392. Arkin AM: Habitual luxation of the ulnar nerve. J Mt Sinai Hosp 7:208, 1940
393. Broudy AS, Leffert RD, Smith RJ: Technical problems with ulnar nerve transposition at the elbow: Findings and results of reoperation. J Hand Surg 3:85–89, 1978
394. Bryan RS, Lipscomb PR, Svien HJ: Tardy paralysis of the ulnar nerve due to a cyst of the elbow: Report of case. Proc Staff Meeting Mayo Clin 31:473, 1956
395. Burman MA, Sutro CJ: Recurrent luxation of the ulnar nerve by congenital posterior position of the medial epicondyle of the humerus. J Bone Joint Surg 21:958, 1939
396. Campbell JB, Post KD, Morantz RA: A technique for relief of motor and sensory deficits occurring after anterior ulnar transposition. J Neurosurg 40:405–409, 1974
397. Carr JA: Spontaneous ulnar nerve paresis. Br Med J 2:1415, 1957
398. Childress HM: Recurrent ulnar-nerve dislocation at the elbow. J Bone Joint Surg 38A:978–984, 1956
399. Childress HM: Recurrent ulnar-nerve dislocation at the elbow. Clin Orthop 108:168, 1975
400. Clark CB: Compression of the ulnar nerve. Orthop Rev 6:33–38, 1977
401. Clark CB: Cubital tunnel syndrome. JAMA 241:801–802, 1979
402. Craven PR, Green DP: Cubital tunnel syndrome. Treatment by medial epicondylectomy. J Bone Joint Surg 62A:986–989, 1980
403. Curtis BF: Traumatic ulnar neuritis; Transplantation of the nerve. J Nerv Ment Dis 25:480, 1898
404. Dellon AL: Review of treatment results for ulnar nerve entrapment at the elbow. J Hand Surg 14A:688–700, 1989
405. Ekerot L: Postanesthetic ulnar neuropathy at the elbow. Scand J Plast Reconstr Surg 11:225–229, 1977
406. Farquhar-Buzzard E: Some varieties of traumatic and toxic ulnar neuritis. Lancet 1:317, 1922
407. Feindel W, Stratford J: The role of the cubital tunnel in tardy ulnar palsy. Can J Surg 1:287–300, 1958
408. Feindel W, Stratford J: Cubital tunnel compression in tardy ulnar palsy. Can Med Assoc J 78:351–353, 1958
409. Foster RJ, Edshage S: Factors related to the outcome of surgically managed compressive neuropathy at the elbow level. J Hand Surg 6:181–192, 1981
410. Fragiadakis EG, Lamb DW: An unusual cause of ulnar nerve compression. Hand 2:14–16, 1970
411. Froimson AI, Zahrawi F: Treatment of compression neuropathy of the ulnar nerve at the elbow by epicondylectomy and neurolysis. J Hand Surg 5:391–395, 1980
412. Gay JR, Love JG: Diagnosis and treatment of tardy paralysis of the ulnar nerve. Based on a study of 100 cases. J Bone Joint Surg 29:1087–1097, 1947
413. Gilliatt RW, Thomas PK: Changes in nerve conduction with ulnar nerve lesions at the elbow. J Neurol Neurosurg Psychiatry 23:312–320, 1960
414. Goldberg BJ, Light TR, Blair SJ: Ulnar neuropathy at the elbow: Results of medial epicondylectomy. J Hand Surg 14A:182–188, 1989
415. Gurdjian ES: Traumatic ulnar neuritis due to strapping of the elbow and the forearm to the operating table. JAMA 96:944, 1931
416. Hagstrom P: Ulnar nerve compression at the elbow. Results of surgery in 85 cases. Scand J Plast Reconstr Surg 11:59–62, 1977
417. Heithoff SJ, Millender LH, Nalebuff EA, Petruska AJ Jr: Medial epicondylectomy for the treatment of ulnar nerve compression at the elbow. J Hand Surg 15A:22–29, 1990
418. Hirasawa Y, Sawamaura H, Sakakida K: Entrapment neuropathy due to bilateral epitrochleoanconeus muscles: A case report. J Hand Surg 4:181–184, 1979
419. Ho KC, Marmor L: Entrapment of the ulnar nerve at the elbow. Am J Surg 121:355, 1971
420. Hunt JR: Tardy or late paralysis of the ulnar nerve. A form of chronic progressive neuritis developing many years after fracture dislocation of the elbow joint. JAMA 66:11–15, 1916
421. James GGH: Nerve lesions about the elbow. J Bone Joint Surg 38B:589, 1956
422. Jones RE, Gauntt C: Medial epicondylectomy for ulnar nerve compression syndrome at the elbow. Clin Orthop 139:174–178, 1979
423. Kincaid JC, Phillips LH, Daube JR: The evaluation of suspected ulnar neuropathy at the elbow. Arch Neurol 43:44–47, 1986

424. King T, Morgan FP: The treatment of traumatic ulnar neuritis. Mobilization of the ulnar nerve at the elbow by removal of the medial epicondyle and adjacent bone. Aust NZ J Surg 20:33–45, 1950
425. King T, Morgan FP: Late results of removing the medial humeral epicondyle for traumatic ulnar neuritis. J Bone Joint Surg 41B:51–55, 1959
426. Kumar K: Surgical management of leprous ulnar neuritis. Clin Orthop 163:235–242, 1982
427. Kurlan R, Baker P, Miller C, Shoulson E: Severe compression neuropathy following sudden onset of Parkinsonian immobility. Arch Neurol 42:720, 1985
428. Learmonth JR: A technique for transplanting the ulnar nerve. Surg Gynecol Obstet 75:792–793, 1942
429. Leffert RD: Anterior submuscular transposition of the ulnar nerves by the Learmonth technique. J Hand Surg 7:147–155, 1982
430. Lluch AL: Ulnar nerve entrapment after anterior transposition at elbow. NY State J Med 1:75–76, 1975
431. Magee RB, Phalen GS: Tardy ulnar palsy. Am J Surg 78:470, 1949
432. Masear VR, Hill JJ Jr, Cohen SM: Ulnar compression neuropathy secondary to the anconeus epitrochlearis muscle. J Hand Surg 13A:720–724, 1988
433. Mass DP, Silverberg B: Cubital tunnel syndrome: Anterior transposition with epicondylar osteotomy. Orthopedics 9:711–715, 1986
434. McGowan AJ: The results of transposition of the ulnar nerve for traumatic ulnar neuritis. J Bone Joint Surg 32B:293–301, 1950
435. Murakami Y, Komiyama Y: Hypoplasia of the trochlea and the medial epicondyle of the humerus associated with ulnar neuropathy. J Bone Joint Surg 60B:225–227, 1978
436. Neblett C, Ehni G: Medial epicondylectomy for ulnar palsy. J Neurosurg 32:55–62, 1970
437. Osborne G: The surgical treatment of tardy ulnar neuritis. J Bone Joint Surg 39B:782, 1957
438. Osborne GV: Ulnar neuritis. Postgrad Med J 35:392, 1959
439. Osborne GV: Compression neuritis of the ulnar nerve at the elbow. Hand 2:10–16, 1970
440. Panas J: Sur une cause peu connue de paralysie du nerf cubital. Arch Generales che Med 2:5, 1878
441. Pechan J, Julis I: The pressure measurement in the ulnar nerve. A contribution to the pathophysiology of the cubital tunnel syndrome. J Biomech 8:75, 1975
442. Platt H: The pathogenesis and treatment of traumatic neuritis of the ulnar nerve in the postcondylar groove. Br J Surg 13:409–431, 1926
443. Reis ND: Anomalous triceps tendon as a cause for snapping elbow and ulnar neuritis: A case report. J Hand Surg 5:361–362, 1980
444. Richards RL: Traumatic ulnar neuritis. The results of anterior transposition of the ulnar nerve. Edinburgh Med J 52:14–21, 1945
445. Rolfsen L: Snapping triceps tendon with ulnar neuritis. Acta Orthop Scand 41:74–76, 1970
446. Sherren J: Remarks on chronic neuritis of the ulnar nerve due to deformity in the region of the elbow joint. Edinburgh Med J 23:500, 1908
447. Skillern PG Jr: Surgical lesions of the ulnar nerve at the elbow. Surg Clin North Am 2:251, 1922
448. Spinner M, Kaplan EB: The relationship of the ulnar nerve to the medial intermuscular septum in the arm and its clinical significance. Hand 8:239–242, 1976
449. Thomsen PB: Compression neuritis of the ulnar nerve treated with simple decompression. Acta Orthop Scand 48:164–167, 1977
450. Vanderpool DW, Chalmers J, Lamb DW, Whiston TB: Peripheral compression lesions of the ulnar nerve. J Bone Joint Surg 50B:792–803, 1968
451. Wadsworth TG: The cubital tunnel and the external compression syndrome. Anesth Analg 53:303–308, 1974
452. Wadsworth TG: The external compression syndrome of the ulnar nerve at the cubital tunnel. Clin Orthop 124:189–204, 1977
453. Wadsworth TG, Williams JR: Cubital tunnel external compression syndrome. Br Med J 1:662, 1973
454. Wadsworth TG, Williams RM: The cubital tunnel external compression syndrome. Nurs Times 73:1357–1359, 1977
455. Wartenberg R: A sign of ulnar nerve palsy. JAMA 112:1688, 1939
456. Wilson DH, Krout R: Surgery of ulnar neuropathy at the elbow: 16 cases treated by decompression without transposition. Technical note. J Neurosurg 38:780–785, 1973

Ulnar Tunnel Syndrome

457. Bakke JL, Wolff HG: Occupational pressure neuritis of the deep palmar branch of the ulnar nerve. Arch Neurol Psychiatry 60:549–553, 1948
458. Blunden R: Neuritis of deep branch of the ulnar nerve. J Bone Joint Surg 40B:354, 1958
459. Brooks DM: Traumatic ulnar neuritis (editorial). J Bone Joint Surg 32B:291–292, 1950
460. Comtet JJ, Quicot L, Moyen B: Compression of the deep palmar branch of the ulnar nerve by the arch of the adductor pollicis. Hand 10:176–180, 1978
461. Denman EE: An unusual branch of the ulnar nerve in the hand. Hand 9:92–97, 1977
462. Denman EE: The anatomy of the space of Guyon. Hand 10:69–76, 1978
463. Dupont C, Cloutier GE, Prevost Y, Dion MA: Ulnar-tunnel syndrome at the wrist. A report of four cases of ulnar-nerve compression at the wrist. J Bone Joint Surg 47A:757–761, 1965
464. Eckman PB, Perlstein G, Altrocchi PH: Ulnar neuropathy in bicycle riders. Arch Neurol 32:130–131, 1975
465. Fenning JB: Deep ulnar-nerve paralysis resulting from an anatomical abnormality. A case report. J Bone Joint Surg 47A:1381–1385, 1965
466. Fissette J, Onkelinx A, Fandi N: Carpal and Guyon tunnel syndrome in burns at the wrist. J Hand Surg 6:13–15, 1981
467. Freundlich BD, Spinner M: Nerve compression syndrome in derangements of the proximal and distal radioulnar joints. Bull Hosp Joint Dis 19:38–47, 1968
468. Gore DR: Carpometacarpal dislocation producing compression of the deep branch of the ulnar nerve. J Bone Joint Surg 53A:1387–1390, 1971
469. Greene MH, Hadied AM: Bipartate hamulus with ulnar tunnel syndrome—case report and literature review. J Hand Surg 6:605–609, 1981
470. Guyon F: Note sur une disposition anatomique proper á la face antérieure de la région du poignet et non encores décrite par la docteur. Bull Soc Anat Paris. 2nd series. 36:184–186, 1861
471. Harrelson JM, Newman M: Hypertrophy of the flexor carpi ulnaris as a cause of ulnar-nerve compression in the distal part of the forearm. Case report. J Bone Joint Surg 57A:554–555, 1975
472. Harris W: Occupational pressure neuritis of the deep palmar branch of the ulnar nerve. Br Med J 1:98, 1929
473. Hayes CW: Ulnar tunnel syndrome from giant cell tumor of tendon sheath: A case report. J Hand Surg 3:187–188, 1978

474. Hayes JR, Mulholland RC, O'Connor BT: Compression of the deep palmar branch of the ulnar nerve. J Bone Joint Surg 51B:469-472, 1969
475. Howard FM: Ulnar nerve palsy in wrist fractures. J Bone Joint Surg 43A:1197-1201, 1961
476. Hunt JR: Occupation neuritis of the deep palmar branch of the ulnar nerve. A well defined clinical type of professional palsy of the hand. J Nerv Ment Dis 35:673-689, 1908
477. Hunt JR: The neural atrophy of the muscles of the hand without sensory disturbances. A further study of compression neuritis of the thenar branch of the median nerve and the deep palmar branch of the ulnar nerve. Rev Neurol Psychiatry 12:137, 1914
478. Jeffery AK: Compression of the deep palmar branch of the ulnar nerve by an anomalous muscle. J Bone Joint Surg 53B:718-723, 1971
479. Kalisman M, Laborde K, Wolff TW: Ulnar nerve compression secondary to ulnar artery false aneurysm at the Guyon's canal. J Hand Surg 7:137-139, 1982
480. Kaplan EB: Variation of the ulnar nerve at the wrist. Bull Hosp Joint Dis 24:85-88, 1963
481. Kleinert HE, Hayes JR: The ulnar tunnel syndrome. Plast Reconstr Surg 47:21-24, 1971
482. Kuschner SH, Gelberman RH, Jennings C: Ulnar nerve compression at the wrist. J Hand Surg 13A:577-580, 1988
483. Lamb D: Ulnar nerve compression lesions at the wrist and hand. Hand 2:17-18, 1970
484. Lassa R, Shrewbury MM: A variation in the path of the deep motor branch of the ulnar nerve at the wrist. J Bone Joint Surg 57:990-991, 1975
485. Lipscomb PR: Duplication of hypothenar muscles simulating soft-tissue tumor of the hand. J Bone Joint Surg 42A:1058-1061, 1960
486. Magee KR: Neuritis of the deep palmar branch of ulnar nerve. Arch Neurol Psychiatry 73:200-202, 1955
487. Mallet BL, Zilkha KJ: Compression of the ulnar nerve at the wrist by a ganglion. Lancet 1:890, 1955
488. Mannerfelt L: Studies on the hand in ulnar nerve paralysis. A clinical-experimental investigation in normal and anomalous innervation. Acta Orthop Scand suppl. 87:1966
489. McDowell CL, Henceroth WD: Compression of the ulnar nerve in the hand by a ganglion. Report of a case. J Bone Joint Surg 59A:980, 1977
490. McFarland GB, Hoffer MM: Paralysis of the intrinsic muscles of the hand secondary to lipoma in Guyon's canal. J Bone Joint Surg 53A:375-376, 1971
491. McFarlane RM, Mayer JR, Hugill JV: Further observations on the anatomy of the ulnar nerve at the wrist. Hand 8:115-117, 1976
492. Muller LH: Anatomical abnormalities of the wrist joint causing neurological symptoms in the hand. J Bone Joint Surg 45B:431, 1963
493. O'Hara JJ, Stone JH: Ulnar neuropathy at the wrist associated with aberrant flexor carpi ulnaris insertion. J Hand Surg 13A:370-372, 1988
494. Poppi M, Padovani R, Martinelli P, Pozzati E: Fractures of the distal radius with ulnar nerve palsy. J Trauma 18:278-279, 1978
495. Regan PJ, Feldberg L, Bailey BN: Accessory palmaris longus muscle causing ulnar nerve compression at the wrist. J Hand Surg 16A:736-738, 1991
496. Richmond DA: Carpal ganglion with ulnar nerve compression. J Bone Joint Surg 45B:513-515, 1963
497. Russell WR, Whitty CWM: Traumatic neuritis of the deep palmar branch of the ulnar nerve. Lancet 1:828-829, 1947
498. Salgebac S: Ulnar tunnel syndrome caused by anomalous muscles. Case report. Scand J Plast Reconstr Surg 11:255-258, 1977
499. Schjelderup H: Aberrant muscle in the hand causing ulnar nerve compression. J Bone Joint Surg 46B:361, 1964
500. Sedal L, McLeod JG, Walsh JC: Ulnar nerve lesions associated with carpal tunnel syndrome. J Neurol Neurosurg Psychiatry 36:118, 1973
501. Seddon HJ: Carpal ganglion as a cause of paralysis of the deep branch of the ulnar nerve. J Bone Joint Surg 34B:386-390, 1952
502. Shea JD, McClain EJ: Ulnar nerve compression syndromes at and below the wrist. J Bone Joint Surg 51A:1095-1103, 1969
503. Smith RJ: Ulnar nerve compression secondary to ulnar artery false aneurysm at Guyon's canal (letter). J Hand Surg 7:631-632, 1982
504. Stein AH Jr, Morgan HC: Compression of the ulnar nerve at the level of the wrist. Am Prac 13:195-198, 1962
505. Swanson AB, Biddulph SL, Baughman FA Jr, De Groot G: Ulnar nerve compression due to an anomalous muscle in the canal of Guyon. Clin Orthop 83:64-69, 1972
506. Taylor AR: Ulnar nerve compression at the wrist in rheumatoid arthritis. J Bone Joint Surg 56B:142-143, 1974
507. Thurman RT, Jindal P, Wolff TW: Ulnar nerve compression in Guyon's canal caused by calcinosis in scleroderma. J Hand Surg 16A:739-741, 1991
508. Tonkin MA, Lister GD: The palmar brevis profundus. An anomalous muscle associated with ulnar nerve compression at the wrist. J Hand Surg 10A:862-864, 1985
509. Toshima Y, Kimata Y: A case of ganglion causing paralysis of intrinsic muscles innervated by the ulnar nerve. J Bone Joint Surg 43A:153, 1961
510. Turner MS, Caird DM: Anomalous muscles and ulnar nerve compression at the wrist. Hand 9:140-142, 1977
511. Uriburu IJF, Morchio FJ, Marin JC: Compression syndrome of the deep branch of the ulnar nerve. (Piso-hamate hiatus syndrome). J Bone Joint Surg 58A:145-147, 1976
512. Vance RM, Gelberman RH: Acute ulnar neuropathy with fractures at the wrist. J Bone Joint Surg 60A:962-965, 1978
513. Vanderpool DW, Chalmers J, Lamb DW, Whiston TB: Peripheral compression lesions of the ulnar nerve. J Bone Joint Surg 50B:792-803, 1968
514. Worster-Drought C: Pressure neuritis of the deep palmar branch of the ulnar nerve. Br Med J 1:247, 1929
515. Zoega H: Fracture of the lower end of the radius with ulnar nerve palsy. J Bone Joint Surg 48B:514-516, 1966
516. Zook EG, Kucan JO, Guy RJ: Palmar wrist pain caused by ulnar nerve entrapment in the flexor carpi ulnaris tendon. J Hand Surg 13A:732-735, 1988

Radial Nerve Compression Syndromes

517. Austin R: Tardy palsy of the radial nerve from a Monteggia fracture. Injury 7:202-204, 1976
518. Barton NJ: Radial nerve lesions. Hand 5:200-208, 1973
519. Blakemore ME: Posterior interosseous nerve paralysis caused by a lipoma. J R Coll Surg Edinb 24:113, 1979
520. Bowen TL, Stone KH: Posterior interosseous nerve paralysis caused by a ganglion at the elbow. J Bone Joint Surg 48B:774-776, 1966
521. Bryan FS, Miller LS, Panijayanond P: Spontaneous paralysis of the posterior interosseous nerve: A case report and review of the literature. Clin Orthop 80:9-12, 1971
522. Campbell CS, Wulf RF: Lipoma producing a lesion of the deep branch of the radial nerve. J Neurosurg 11:310-311, 1954
523. Capener N: Tennis elbow and posterior interosseous nerve. Br Med J 2:130, 1960
524. Capener N: Posterior interosseous nerve lesions. In Proceedings of the Second Hand Club. J Bone Joint Surg 46B:361, 1964

525. Capener N: The vulnerability of the posterior interosseous nerve of the forearm. A case report and anatomical study. J Bone Joint Surg 48B:770–773, 1966
526. Davies F, Laird M: The supinator muscle and the deep radial (posterior interosseous) nerve. Anat Rec 101:243–250, 1948
527. Dellon AL, Mackinnon SE: Radial sensory nerve entrapment in the forearm. J Hand Surg 11A:199–205, 1986
528. Dharapak C, Nimberg GA: Posterior interosseous nerve compression. Report of a case caused by traumatic aneurysm. Clin Orthop 101:225–228, 1974
529. Ehrlich W, Dellon AL, Mackinnon SE: Cheiralgia paresthetica (Entrapment of the radial sensory nerve). J Hand Surg 11A:196–199, 1986
530. Fuss FK, Wurzl GH: Radial nerve entrapment at the elbow: Surgical anatomy. J Hand Surg 16A:742–747, 1991
531. Garcia A, Maeck BH: Radial nerve injuries in fractures of the shaft of the humerus. Am J Surg 99:625, 1960
532. Gassel MM, Diamantopoulos E: Pattern of conduction times in the distribution of the radial nerve. Neurology 14:222–231, 1964
533. Goldman S, Honet JC, Sobel R, Goldstein AS: Posterior interosseous-nerve palsy in the absence of trauma. Arch Neurol 21:435–441, 1969
534. Hagert CG, Lundborg G, Hansen T: Entrapment of the posterior interosseous nerve. Scand J Plast Reconstr Surg 11:205, 1977
535. Hobhouse N, Heald CB: A case of posterior interosseous paralysis. Br Med J 1:841, 1936
536. Hustead A, Mulder D, MacCarty C: Nontreatment progressive paralysis of the deep radial (posterior interosseous) nerve. Arch Neurol Psychiatry 79:269, 1958
537. Jebsen RH: Motor conduction velocity of distal radial nerve. Arch Phys Med Rehabil 47:12–16, 1966
538. Kruse F Jr: Paralysis of the dorsal interosseous nerve not due to direct trauma. A case showing spontaneous recovery. Neurology 8:307–308, 1958
539. Learmonth JR: A variation in the distribution of the radial branch of the musculo-spiral nerve. J Anat 53:371–372, 1919
540. Lichter RL, Jacobsen T: Tardy palsy of the posterior interosseous nerve with a Monteggia fracture. J Bone Joint Surg 57A:124–125, 1975
541. Linscheid RL: Injuries to radial nerve at wrist. Arch Surg 91:942–946, 1965
542. Lister GD, Belsole RB, Kleinert HE: The radial tunnel syndrome. J Hand Surg 4:52–59, 1979
543. Lotem M, Fried A, Levy M, Solzi P, Najenson T, Nathan H: Radial palsy following muscular effort. A nerve compression syndrome possibly related to a fibrous arch of the lateral head of the triceps. J Bone Joint Surg 53B:500–506, 1971
544. Lubahn JD, Lister GD: Familial radial nerve entrapment syndrome: A case report and literature review. J Hand Surg 8:297–298, 1983
545. Manske PR: Compression of the radial nerve by the triceps muscle. Case report. J Bone Joint Surg 59A:835–836, 1977
546. Marmor L, Lawrence JF, Dubois EL: Posterior interosseous nerve paralysis due to rheumatoid arthritis. J Bone Joint Surg 49A:381–383, 1967
547. Marshall SC, Murray WR: Deep radial nerve palsy associated with rheumatoid arthritis. Clin Orthop 103:157–162, 1974
548. Mayer JH, Mayfield FH: Surgery of the posterior interosseous branch of the radial nerve. Surg Gynecol Obstet 84:979–982, 1947
549. Millender LH, Nalebuff EA, Holdsworth DE: Posterior interosseous nerve syndrome secondary to rheumatoid synovitis. J Bone Joint Surg 55A:753–757, 1973
550. Moon N, Marmor L: Parosteal lipoma of the proximal part of the radius. J Bone Joint Surg 46A:608–614, 1964
551. Morris AH: Irreducible Monteggia lesion with radial-nerve entrapment. J Bone Joint Surg 56A:1744–1746, 1974
552. Moss SH, Switzer HE: Radial tunnel syndrome: A spectrum of clinical presentations. J Hand Surg 8:414–420, 1983
553. Mulholland RC: Non-traumatic progressive paralysis of the posterior interosseous nerve. J Bone Joint Surg 48B:781–785, 1966
554. Nakamichi K, Tachibana S: Radial nerve entrapment by the lateral head of the triceps. J Hand Surg 16A:748–750, 1991
555. Nielsen HO: Posterior interosseous nerve paralysis caused by fibrous band compression at the supinator muscle. A report of four cases. Acta Orthop Scand 47:304–307, 1976
556. Packer JW, Foster RR, Garcia A, Grantham SA: The humeral fracture with radial nerve palsy: Is exploration warranted? Clin Orthop 88:34–38, 1972
557. Popelka S, Vianio K: Entrapment of the posterior interosseous branch of the radial nerve in rheumatoid arthritis. Acta Orthop Scand 45:370–372, 1974
558. Richardson GA, Humphrey MS: Congenital compression of the radial nerve. J Hand Surg 14A:901–903, 1989
559. Richmond DA: Lipoma causing a posterior interosseous nerve lesion. J Bone Joint Surg 35B:83, 1953
560. Riordan DC: Radial nerve paralysis. Orthop Clin North Am 5:283–287, 1974
561. Roles NC, Maudsley RH: Radial tunnel syndrome. Resistant tennis elbow as a nerve entrapment. J Bone Joint Surg 54B:499–508, 1972
562. Salsbury CR: The nerve to the extensor carpi radialis brevis. Br J Surg 26:95–97, 1938
563. Schnitker MT: A technique for transplant of the musculospiral nerve in open reduction of fractures of the mid-shaft of the humerus. J Neurosurg 6:113–117, 1949
564. Sharrard WJW: Posterior interosseous neuritis. J Bone Joint Surg 48B:777–780, 1966
565. Silverstein A: Progressive paralysis of the dorsal interosseous nerve. Report of a case. Arch Neurol Psychiatry 38:885, 1937
566. Spinner M: The arcade of Frohse and its relationship to posterior interosseous nerve paralysis. J Bone Joint Surg 50B:809–812, 1968
567. Spinner M, Freundlich BD, Teicher J: Posterior interosseous nerve palsy as a complication of Monteggia fractures in children. Clin Orthop 58:141, 1968
568. Sponseller PD, Engber WD: Double-entrapment radial tunnel syndrome. J Hand Surg 8:420–423, 1983
569. Stein F, Grabias SL, Deffer PA: Nerve injuries complicating Monteggia lesions. J Bone Joint Surg 53A:1432–1436, 1971
570. Strachan JCH, Ellis BW: Vulnerability of the posterior interosseous nerve during radial head resection. J Bone Joint Surg 53B:320–323, 1971
571. Van Rossum J, Buruma OJS, Kamphuisen HAC, Onvlee GJ: Tennis elbow—a radial tunnel syndrome? J Bone Joint Surg 60B:197–198, 1978
572. Wadsworth TG: Injuries of the capitular (lateral humeral condylar) epiphysis. Clin Orthop 85:127–142, 1972
573. Wartenberg R: Cheiralgia Paraesthetic (Isolierte Neuritis des Ramus superficialis nervi radialis). Z Ges Neurol Psychiatr 141:145–155, 1932
574. Weinberger LM: Non-traumatic paralysis of the dorsal interosseous nerve. Surg Gynecol Obstet 69:358–363, 1939
575. Werner CO: Lateral elbow pain and posterior interosseous nerve entrapment. Acta Orthop Scand suppl. 174:1979
576. Whitely WH, Alpers BJ: Posterior interosseous palsy with spontaneous neuroma formation. Arch Neurol 1:226–229, 1959
577. Wilhelm A: Radialis kompressions syndrome. Hand Chir 8:113, 1976

578. Woltman HW, Learmonth JR: Progressive paralysis of the nervus interosseous dorsalis. Brain 57:25–31, 1934

579. Wu KT, Jordan FR, Eckert C: Lipoma, a cause of paralysis of deep radial (posterior interosseous) nerve. Report of a case and review of the literature. Surg 75:790–795, 1974

Cumulative Trauma Disorders

580. Armstrong TJ: Ergonomics and cumulative trauma disorders of the hand and wrist. pp. 1175–1191. In Hunter JM, Schneider LH, Mackin EJ, Callahan AD, (eds): Rehabilitation of the Hand: Surgery and Therapy. 3rd Ed. CV Mosby, St. Louis, 1990

581. Armstrong TJ, Foulke JA, Joseph BS, Goldstein S: An investigation of cumulative trauma disorders in a poultry processing plant. Am Ind Hyg Assoc J 43:103–116, 1982

582. Armstrong TJ, Radwin RG, Hansen DJ, Kennedy KW: Repetitive trauma disorders: job evaluation and design. Hum Factors 28:325, 1986

583. Birkbeck MQ, Beer TC: Occupation in relation to the carpal tunnel syndrome. Rheumatol Rehab 14:218–221, 1975

584. Brown P: The role of motivation in the recovery of hand. p. 1. In Kasdan J: Occupational Hand and Upper Extremity Injuries and Diseases. Hanley and Belfus, Philadelphia, 1991

585. Browne CD, Nolan BM, Faithfull DK: Occupational repetitive strain injuries: Guidelines for diagnosis and management. Med J Aust 140:329–332, 1984

586. Cannon LJ, Bernacki EJ, Walter SD: Personal and occupational factors associated with carpal tunnel syndrome. J Occup Med 23:255–258, 1981

587. Eversmann WW: Employers' response to occupational disorders. Chapter 6. p. 69. In Millender LH, Louis DS, Simmons BP (eds): Occupational Disorders in the Upper Extremity. Churchill Livingstone, New York, 1991

588. Fine LJ, Silverstein BA, Armstrong TJ, Anderson CA, Sugano DS: Detection of cumulative trauma disorders of upper extremities in the work place. J Occup Med 28:674–678, 1986

589. Finkel ML: The effects of repeated mechanical trauma in the meat industry. Am J Ind Med 8:375, 1985

590. Hadler NM: Occupational illness: The issue of causality. J Occup Med 26:587–593, 1984

591. Hall DT, Bowen DD, Lewiciki RJ, Hall FS: Experiences in Management and Organizational Behavior. 2nd Ed. John Wiley, New York, 1982

592. Ireland DCR: Psychological and physical aspects of occupational arm pain. J Hand Surg 13B:5–10, 1988

593. Iserhagen SJ: Work Injury Prevention and Management. Aspen Publications, Rockville, MD, 1988

594. Liker JK, Joseph BS, Armstrong TJ: From ergonomic theory to practice: organizational factors affecting the utilization of ergonomic knowledge. In Hendrick HW, Brown O Jr (eds): Human Factors on Organizational Design and Management. Elsevier North-Holland, Amsterdam, 1984

595. Mallory M, Bradford H, Freundlich N: An invisible work place hazard gets harder to ignore. pp. 92–93. Business Week, January 30, 1989

596. Margolis W, Kraus JF: The prevalence of carpal tunnel syndrome symptoms in female supermarket checkers. J Occup Med 29:953–956, 1987

597. Masear VR, Hayes JM, Hyde AG: An industrial cause of carpal tunnel syndrome. J Hand Surg 11A:222–227, 1986

598. McKenzie F, Storment J, Van Hook P, Armstrong TJ: A program for control of repetitive trauma disorders associated with hand tool operations in a telecommunications manufacturing facility. Am Ind Hyg Assoc J 46:674–678, 1985

599. Moody L, Arezzo J, Otto D: Screening occupational populations for asymptomatic or early peripheral neuropathy. J Occup Med 28:975–986, 1986

600. Rystrom CM, Eversmann WW Jr: Cumulative trauma intervention in industry: A model program for the upper extremity. pp. 489–505. In Kasdan ML (ed): Occupational Hand & Upper Extremity Injuries & Diseases. Hanley & Belfus, Philadelphia, 1991

37

Neuromas

James H. Herndon

The painful neuroma is a critical problem in the injured hand. A simple hypersensitive neuroma in a finger amputation stump may impair function of the whole hand (Fig. 37-1). Many neuromas remain relatively asymptomatic, but 20 to 30 percent are problematic regardless of what technique of local treatment has been employed.[68]

Neuroma formation, that is, a nodule developing on the severed end of the proximal nerve stump, was first described by Odier in 1811.[69] Wood,[97] Virchow,[93] and Mitchell[63] added further reports of this lesion in the nineteenth century. The nodule forms as a result of injury to the Schwann's cell-endoneurial barrier that confines axons to their endoneurial tubes. Once this barrier is damaged, regenerating axons escape into the surrounding tissue in a disorganized fashion and are accompanied by proliferating fibroblasts, Schwann's cells, and blood vessels.[87]

Many nerve lesions are termed neuromas. In this chapter I discuss only those neuromas in the hand resulting from partial or complete severance of a nerve containing sensory fibers (solely or mixed with motor fibers). Only neuromas containing sensory fibers become painful. Other types of lesions such as Morton's neuroma, pacinian neuroma, acoustic neuroma, and gastric neuroma, and syndromes, such as multiple mucosal neuromas, are not discussed.

ANATOMY

Sunderland[87] has stressed the importance of Schwann's cell and the endoneurium in containing regenerating axons after injury. If this barrier is broken, regenerating axons grow out of the end of the severed nerve in an attempt to reenter their original endoneurial tubes distally to reach the end organs they originally innervated. If the barrier is not broken, regenerating axons remain contained in their original endoneurial tubes and grow distally until they reach their respective end organs.

After axonal continuity has been disrupted by crushing, cutting, or tearing, Wallerian degeneration occurs. After a period of recovery, regrowth of the axons occurs in the proximal portion of the damaged nerve. When these axons reach the end of the endoneurial tube, they escape into a disorganized mass of connective tissue containing fibroblasts, Schwann's cells, macrophages, and capillaries. The axons grow out in many directions and branch irregularly, seeking to restore continuity of the nerve trunk. The growth and direction of the axons are influenced by the barrier of the fibroblasts and Schwann's cells. As a result, axons zigzag through the tissue in a totally disorganized fashion. They branch irregularly and form whorls, spirals, and convolutions (Fig. 37-2). Most are contained in the disorganized mass or nodule of connective tissue that becomes encapsulated. A few escape attempting to reach the distal stump. This nodule at the stump end is called a *neuroma.* With time, progressive fibrosis converts an originally soft nodule into a firm, hard one.[51,84] Recently, myofibroblasts have been identified in neuromas. They increase in the scar tissue from 2 to 6 months after injury and then decrease as the collagen content of the scar increases. Within neuromas the matrix consists of large amounts of glycosaminoglycan compared to minimal amounts of glycosaminoglycan in normal nerves.[2]

In the distal stump, the axons undergo degeneration as well, but since their cell bodies are proximal, they do not regenerate. There is a cellular response in the area of injury with some Schwann's cell and fibroblastic proliferation. However, the response is much less than that in the proximal stump, and without any regenerating axons the nodule that forms is small (always smaller than a neuroma) and is termed a *glioma.*

The size of a neuroma depends on the amount of proliferating connective tissue fibroblasts, Schwann's cells, vessels, and macrophages, but primarily on the number of axons and the extent of axonal ingrowth. Axonal growth is more active the closer the lesion is to the neuron. Therefore, neuromas tend to be larger in nerves injured proximally and smaller when injured peripherally. Also, increased size with more axonal

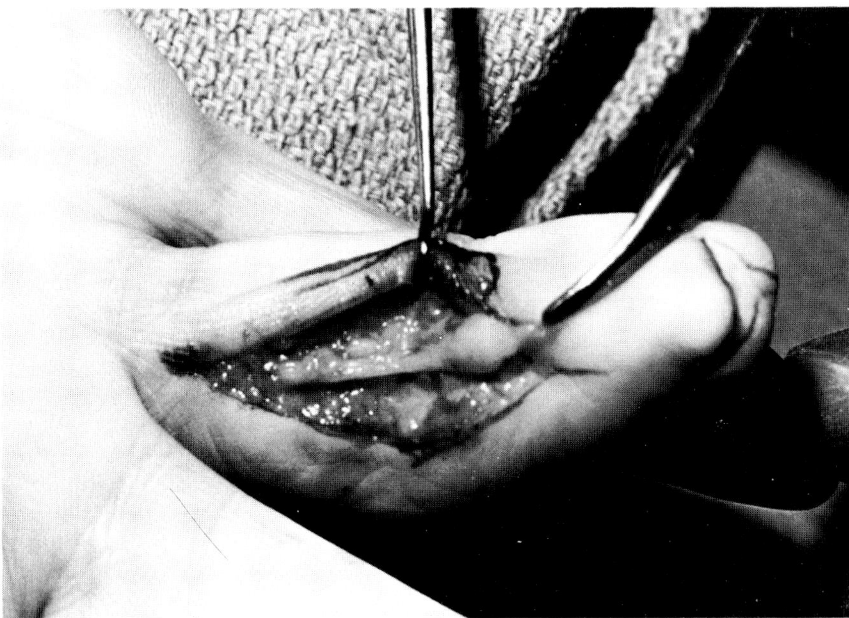

Fig. 37-1. A neuroma at the end of an amputation stump.

growth is seen in nerves with large amounts of connective tissue and small, widely separated funiculi compared to nerves with large, closely packed funiculi. Petropoulos and Stefanko[75] have shown that in dogs the degree of anisomorphism is directly related to the size of the neuroma, that is, there was a marked disarray of all elements compared to smaller neuromas that were isomorphic or had a regular arrangement of all elements. Size and consistency of the neuroma are also affected by the presence of infection or foreign bodies and by repeated irritation such as pressure, friction, or repeated trauma.[8,11,18] Petropoulos and Stefanko have also shown that (in the dog) the blood supply to the nerve stump does not affect neuroma size, but in malnourished animals, the neuromas are always small and atrophic.[75] In addition to these known influences on size, consistency, and symptomatology, other unknown factors exist. For example, a patient with an amputated finger may

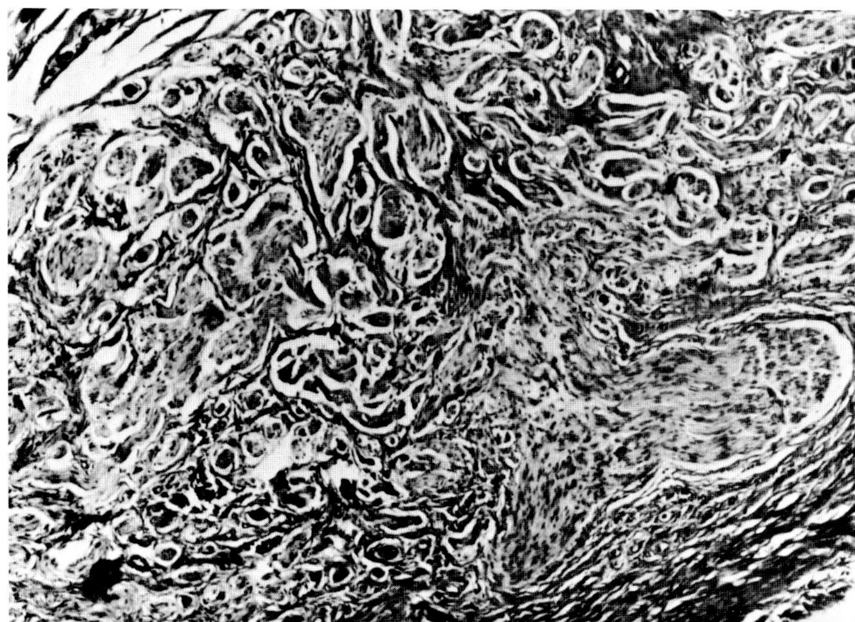

Fig. 37-2. Low-power photomicrograph of a neuroma, demonstrating disorganized tissue composed of axons, fibroblasts, Schwann's cells, and blood vessels.

have a painful neuroma develop in one digital nerve while the other digital nerve remains asymptomatic, even though both received identical primary treatment.

CLASSIFICATION OF NEUROMAS (TABLE 37-1)

Neuromas-in-Continuity

Neuromas-in-continuity are neuromas in a nerve that has not been completely severed. Sunderland described two types: those in which the perineurial sheath is intact and those in which there has been partial division of the nerve.

Spindle Neuromas

Spindle neuromas are swellings or enlargements in an intact nerve secondary to chronic irritation, friction, or pressure. Although they are called neuromas, they are not true neuromas. Histologically, the bulbous area contains increased connective tissue. With repeated continuous trauma, the fibrous tissue proliferates, constricting nerve fibers and interfering with their nutrition. Eventually the swelling becomes a large collagenized mass with fibrotic replacement of the nerve fibers and vessels.[87]

The only exception to this course of events was demonstrated by Spencer, in experiments in which he crushed nerves but kept the perineurium intact. He showed that regenerating axons in such circumstances did grow through the intact perineurium, forming a true neuroma-in-continuity.[84] I am not aware of any examples of this type of neuroma having been reported in humans.

Examples of this type of spindle neuroma are those occurring in Morton's metatarsalgia, the ulnar digital nerve of the thumb in bowler's thumb, the greater occipital nerve where it pierces the trapezius fascia, the lateral femoral cutaneous nerve where it passes beneath the inguinal ligament in meralgia paresthetica, the posterior interosseous nerve on the back of the wrist, the branch of the axillary nerve to the teres minor, and the lateral branch of the deep peroneal where it crosses the tarsal navicular bone.[22,62,65,66,80]

Table 37-1. Classification of Neuromas

I. Neuromas-in-continuity
   A. Spindle neuromas. Lesions in which the perineurium is not broken
   B. Lateral neuromas. Lesions in which the perineurium of some funiculi is broken
   C. Neuromas following nerve repair
II. Neuromas in completely severed nerves
III. Amputation stump neuromas

(Modified from Sunderland,[87] with permission.)

Lateral Neuromas

This type of neuroma occurs when part of the nerve with its perineurium has been injured, and is commonly seen by surgeons dealing with trauma. The size of the neuroma depends on how many funiculi have been damaged and the distance between the severed funiculi. Obviously, the more axons injured, the more will regenerate and therefore the larger the neuroma. Size also depends on the distance between the severed funiculi. For instance, if there is minimal retraction of the ends, the gap is rapidly bridged by proliferating Schwann's cells and fibroblasts, reestablishing the tubes to allow regenerating axons to find their way to their proper distal sheaths and end organs. If the funicular gap is large, this area is not bridged quickly by Schwann's cells and fibroblasts, allowing regenerating axons to escape from their sheaths and thus form a true neuroma on the side of an otherwise intact nerve.

The treatment of lateral neuromas-in-continuity, which can be exceedingly difficult, is discussed in Chapter 35.

Neuromas Following Nerve Repair

Upon inspection of previously repaired severed nerves, the surgeon often finds a neuroma-in-continuity. This does not always happen, but it does occur frequently. Although not proven, funicular repair may decrease the incidence and size of this neuroma by providing end-to-end contact of fascicles, thus minimizing axonal escape. Sunderland has shown that this type of neuroma is more common in severed nerves that contain small, widely separated funiculi, and/or in nerves where the injury has occurred at a level where the cut ends have dissimilar funicular patterns. An example of this would be where a segment of nerve has been excised or destroyed.

Neuromas in Completely Severed Nerves

This is the classic neuroma that surgeons encounter. It forms on the proximal stump of any severed peripheral nerve. Its formation and structure have been discussed earlier under the section on anatomy.

Amputation Stump Neuromas

The neuroma forming at the end of a severed nerve in an amputation stump is the same as the neuroma that forms on the end of a completely severed nerve. There are two important differences, however. In the amputation stump, if the nerve lies near the end of the stump and secondary healing occurs, it is subject to increased fibrosis. It is also subject to repeated trauma from pressure, friction, and concussion, which leads to increased size, edema, fibrosis, and increased sensitivity. In such cases, the neuroma may become so painful that the amputation stump or the whole part becomes useless.

To avoid this problem, the initial treating surgeon should transect the nerve in such a way as to allow it to retract into a bed of healthy soft tissues away from the working surface of the amputation stump. If the tissues are not satisfactory, the end of the nerve should be transferred to an area away from the working surface of the stump, usually dorsally, as is described in the section on relocation of the intact neuroma.

DIAGNOSIS

The diagnosis of a painful neuroma is usually easy to make. Direct tapping over the nerve elicits painful paresthesias. A palpable mass that is tender to touch may be present, and pressure on this mass recreates the patient's symptoms. The pain produced often has a peculiarly intense and unpleasant quality.

In some patients, especially in worker's compensation cases, it may be difficult to determine if the neuroma is indeed the major cause of the patient's pain. In such cases, Green (personal communication) uses differential diagnostic blocks, first with saline and then with lidocaine.

Rarely, one may be fooled by a mass over an intact nerve causing symptoms of a neuroma secondary to pressure on the nerve by the mass. I have had such a case recently of an inclusion cyst overlying one of the terminal branches of the digital nerve in the tip of the finger. The patient presented with classic history and physical findings of a neuroma.

TREATMENT

Sunderland states, "there is no procedure that is completely and consistently successful in preventing neuroma formation."[87] Because of this, the literature is extensive on the subject. Although many different techniques have been described, no universally successful method of treatment has been found. Guttmann and Medawar[42] showed that only destruction of the cell body would inhibit axonal regeneration completely. Any severed nerve will form a neuroma. Probably the best way to minimize neuroma formation is by a careful repair or grafting to allow the regenerating axons the best possible chance to extend into the distal empty funiculi. The debate on the optimal type of repair still persists in the literature, however. Bora, Pleasure, and Didizian[7] have measured the amount of collagen and myelin in the distal portion of severed nerves in rabbits. They found that there was more collagen near the neuroma in the immediate epineurial repair, but 60 percent of the normal myelin production was found in the distal nerve segment compared to 28.3 percent in the immediate perineurial group and less in the delayed groups. In other words, the epineurial repair resulted in more collagen about the periphery of the nerve repair site, whereas the perineurial repair resulted in more internal scarring and therefore less axonal regrowth into the distal segment. I know of no studies comparing the neuroma formation in humans with each of these two types of repair, however. Clinically, Tupper and Booth noted that a well-sealed epineurial repair of a severed nerve rarely results in a painful neuroma.[92]

Nonoperative techniques such as tapping, massage, ultrasound, transcutaneous electrical nerve stimulation[70,94] and other modalities have been tried. I am not aware of any controlled studies to prove their effectiveness, and I therefore believe that operative treatment by repair or translocation to avoid or minimize neuroma formation provides the best likelihood of success. However, I do not believe, as some have suggested, that delay of operative treatment compromises the result.

Resection

Resection of an acutely severed nerve, allowing it to retract back into an area of uninjured soft tissue, is the most commonly preferred treatment of irreparable nerve injuries, especially in amputation stumps.[26] This technique is also used for treatment of a painful neuroma in an area of old injury. Tupper and Booth[92] reported a large series of 316 neuromas treated by simple excisional neurectomy. Injuries were divided into crush, jagged lacerations, and sharp lacerations. They reported that 65 percent of all of these injuries together had satisfactory or excellent results (36.5 percent excellent) from a single resection. Satisfactory or excellent results increased to 78 percent (45 percent excellent) following a second simple neurectomy.

Operative Technique

It is usually easier to first identify the nerve in an area of normal anatomy, isolate the neuroma, and then dissect the nerve free proximally. If it is a terminal branch, it may be helpful to dissect this branch from the main nerve under magnification to avoid any injury to the nerve. The proximal limits of the dissection should be an area of healthy soft tissue, free of scar, where the new nerve end will be well covered and protected. Gentle traction is then applied to the nerve (Fig. 37-3). Excessive traction is avoided to prevent intraneural axonal tears and possible additional neuroma formation. The nerve is then sectioned as far proximally as possible with a sharp knife, scissors, or razor blade, allowing it to retract into the bed of healthy soft tissue.

Crushing

Attempting to suppress axonal regrowth at the end of the severed nerve by crushing the end of the nerve was one of the earliest reported techniques, and it proved to be ineffective in preventing neuroma formation.[52] Stevenson combined the technique of crushing the nerve end with ligating the stump as well.[85]

Multiple Sectioning

Some surgeons believe that if a nerve is sectioned and then repaired at multiple levels proximal to the site of injury, many axons will not find their way back to the original injury site. If they do, the time course will have been sufficiently prolonged so that the end of the nerve will hopefully be covered over with

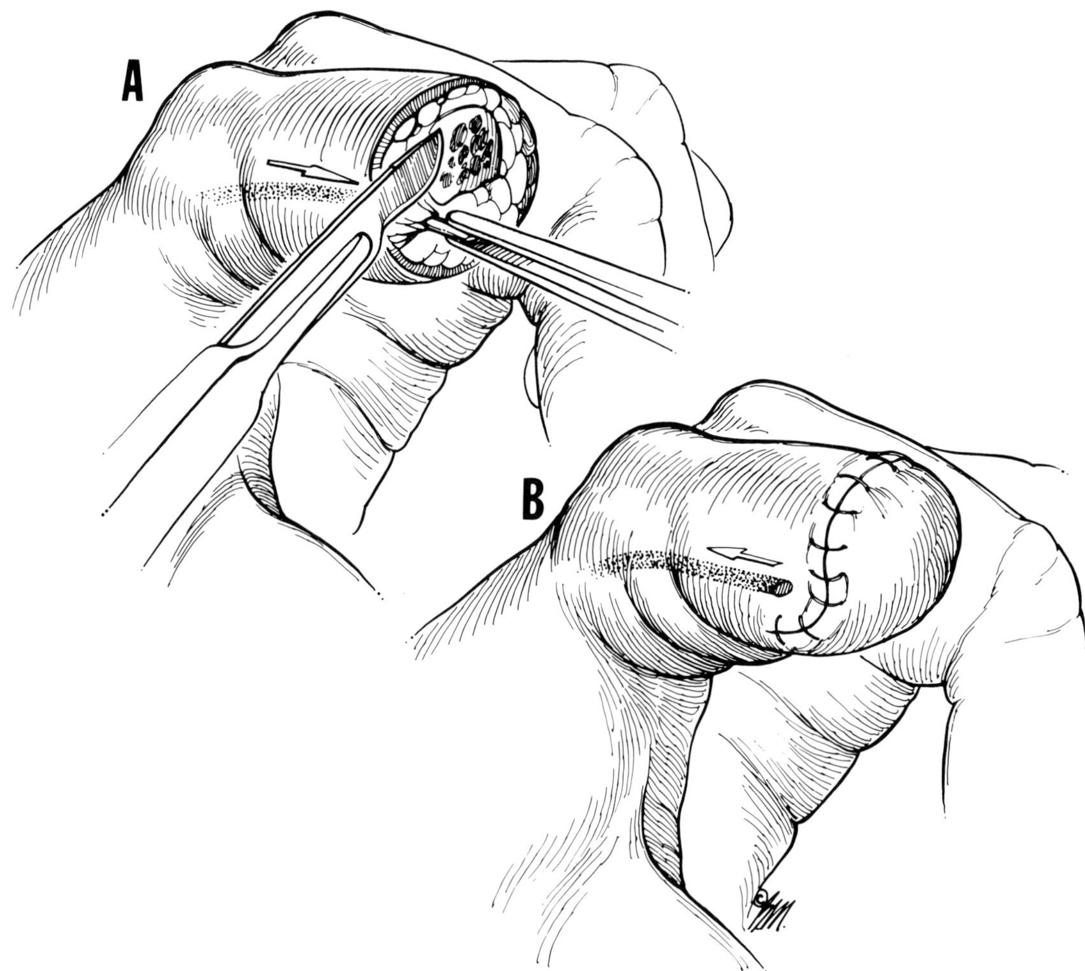

Fig. 37-3. Simple resection of a neuroma. **(A)** The end of the nerve is grasped, pulled gently into the wound, and severed sharply as far proximally as possible. **(B)** The transected nerve end retracts into the proximal normal soft tissues.

scar, thereby impeding neuroma formation. As Sunderland points out, however, this method is not recommended, for it increases neuroma formation at multiple sites, and if the distal endoneurial tubes are closed, neuroma formation is not inhibited, but rather enhanced.[29,58]

Ligation

Ligation of the severed nerve to prevent neuroma formation is controversial. Sunderland believes that the method is of value in limiting neuroma formation.[87] Chavannaz[14] and Jegorow[64] have noted atrophy of the nerve distal to the ligature and reduced volume of the terminal neuroma. The rationale for ligation is to close the funiculi by the suture, thereby preventing axonal regrowth. The technique requires that the ligature be placed around the nerve 5 to 10 cm above the cut end and tied tightly enough to seal the funiculi, but not so tightly as to cut through them. I think this is where the problem arises, for it is probably impossible to secure a ligature around the nerve tightly enough to close the funiculi and not damage the perineurium, with resulting new sites for neuroma formation. Indeed, Petropoulos and Stefanko[74] found terminal neuromas above the ligation site and also reported a neuroma at the nerve end after ligature. The neuroma was smaller, but contained regenerating fibers. Below the ligation, the fibers were nonmedullated, and the authors thought that the nerve fibers had become smaller in order to penetrate the area of the ligature.[74] Other investigators have also found ligation unreliable, experimentally as well as clinically.[15,19,46,48] Ligation has been used in conjunction with other modalities, with mixed success. Such methods have included crushing, injecting the stump with gentian violet, covering the nerve with tannic acid powder and collodion, or the use of gentian violet, formaldehyde, or alcohol as chemical coagulants.[19,46,51,71,85]

Operative Technique

The nerve is dissected free proximally. An area somewhere between 5 and 10 cm above the severed end of the nerve is the site of the ligature. Nonabsorbable material is used. The suture is tied circumferentially around the nerve tightly enough to stop the bleeding, but not so tight as to cut through the nerve. Excess nerve distally may be resected for adequate stump closure (Fig. 37-4).

Radioactive Ligatures

Perl and Whitlock[73] in rats and Gorman, Nold, and King[41] in horses used radioactive phosphate-impregnated chromic ligatures on severed nerves. In rats, axonal regeneration was inhibited by 88 percent. In horses, the neuromas were smaller, but the stumps were more sensitive. Limited use of an injection of a radioactive solution into nerve stumps in patients has produced some favorable results.[73] This is a concept that needs more investigation and may be an area to explore in the future.

Epineurial Closure

Three types of epineurial closure have been described. Chapple drew the epineurium over the end of the sectioned nerve, suturing it closed in an attempt to seal the endoneurial tubes.[13] Corner removed a wedge of the distal nerve in order to close the epineurium. Neuroma formation was not prevented.[17] A combination of crushing and ligation with transposition of the nerve end into muscle was reported by Munro and Mallory[67] Their results were better than those of Chapple or Corner.

Tupper and Booth[92] reported a third method—funiculectomy and epineurial ligation—in 45 neuromas in 28 patients. When this method was used as a primary procedure for a neuroma, 81 percent obtained excellent or satisfactory results (53.1 percent excellent). Three patients had to undergo a second funiculectomy and each showed nerve tissue growing past the ligature site. If a second funiculectomy was done, 87 percent of the patients obtained satisfactory or excellent results. In their hands, this method was better than a simple neurectomy, but they stated that the number of cases was too small to be conclusive.

As with nerve ligation, it is difficult technically to achieve the correct tension on the ligature. In a recent study, Martini and Fromm created an epineural sleeve and sealed it with Histoacryl glue (butyl-2-cyanoacrylate). They compared this method with others, including simple nerve ligation and epineural ligation, and found that the fewest neuromas formed in the glue subset. They reported good results in a clinical trial.[47,59]

Operative Treatment

With the use of a microscope, the nerve is transected proximal to the neuroma. The epineurium is then carefully peeled back over the nerve trunk. Each funiculus is identified and individually sectioned 1 cm proximally. The empty epineurial tube is then doubly ligated with 6-0 nylon (Fig. 37-5). The nerve end is then placed in adjacent healthy tissue.

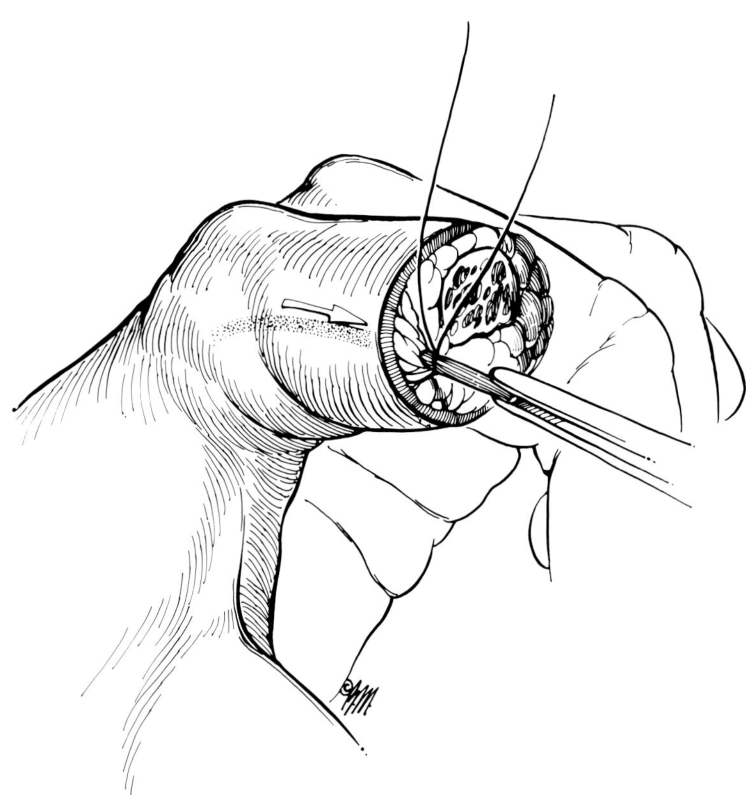

Fig. 37-4. Ligation of a neuroma. The severed nerve end is ligated proximally and the distal portion excised.

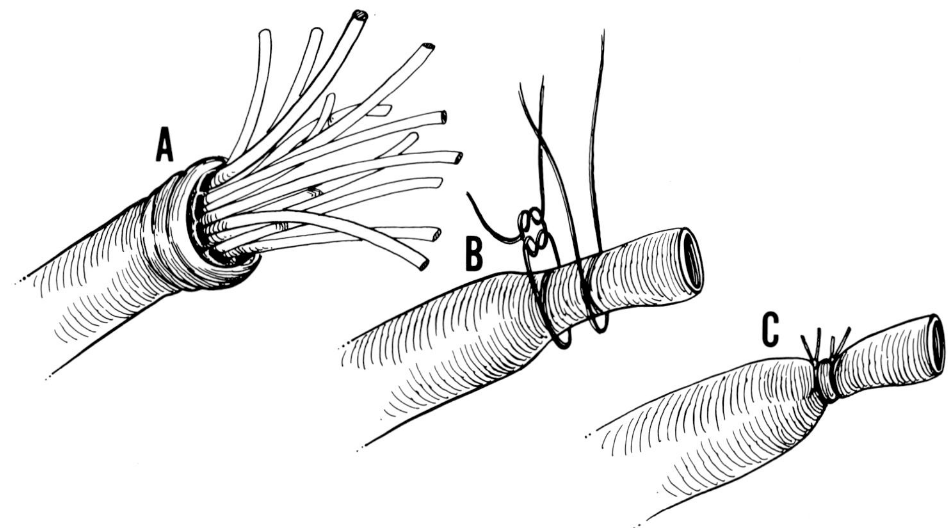

Fig. 37-5. Epineurial closure. **(A)** The epineurium is rolled proximally, exposing the fascicles, which are severed and allowed to retract. **(B)** The epineurium is then pulled distally, forming an empty tube. A double ligature is applied just distal to the severed ends of the fascicles. **(C)** The empty epineurial tube is sealed by the double ligature to prevent axonal outgrowth.

Transposition

In this technique the neuroma is usually excised (in contrast to relocation of the intact neuroma) and the distal portion of the proximal cut end of the nerve is turned back on itself.[14,16] The severed end is placed in an area devoid of scar, essentially similar to resection that allows the cut end to retract into healthy soft tissue. A neuroma still develops at the end of the nerve, but theoretically, there will be less irritation in the new healthy bed. If the nerve is twisted during the procedure, however, small terminal neuromas have been observed in the twisted area.[74] In such cases, the barrier provided by Schwann's cells and endoneurium is disrupted by stretching, and thus the nerve must be handled gently with this technique.

Transposition with Implantation

Implantation of the nerve stump into surrounding tissue has been reported with good success. A requirement for success with this technique appears to be that the central stump of the cut nerve should be dissected out into its longitudinal funiculi, and each of these is implanted into the tissue.[74] The fact that surgeons have implanted the whole nerve stump into surrounding tissue with variable results has possibly led to the relative disfavor of this technique. Tissues used have been the nerve itself, muscle, bone, fascia, and blood vessels, but little is contained in the literature except for the use of the nerve, bone, and muscle. Even with these tissues, the reports are neither conclusive nor comparable.

Implantation into the Same Nerve (Neurocampsis)

Bardenheuer is credited with describing this technique.[74] The cut end of the nerve is implanted into the nerve trunk proximally through an opening made in the epineurium. Petropoulos and Stefanko found that with this technique in dogs a spiral-shaped neuroma was formed that was twice the size of the control neuromas. The neuroma formed was very hypertrophic with prolific regeneration of nerve components.[74] Ashley and Stallings used this end-to-side nerve flap technique successfully in six patients with a 7- to 15-year follow-up. All nerve flaps were transferred beneath a muscle away from scar and pressure sites.[1,47]

Implantation into Muscle

In dogs, Petropoulos and Stefanko dissected out the individual funiculi of the sectioned nerve and implanted each into neighboring muscle tissue.[74] They found no neuroma formation and observed only laminar formations that became lost in the muscle. Dellon et al also recently reported observations that suggest that a classic neuroma does not form when a transected nerve is implanted into muscle.[20] Recently they reported their experience with 78 neuromas in 60 patients with an average follow-up of 31 months. Using this technique, their overall success rate was 82%. However, their results were much worse with digital neuromas, and they advised against using the intrinsic muscle of the hand as a burial site.[21,47]

In humans, I would suspect that even if this technique prevents neuroma formation, it may result in discomfort for the patient because of traction on the nerve end with movement and muscle contraction. Laborde et al abandoned this procedure because of an unacceptably high re-operation rate of 65 percent.[55]

Implantation into Bone

In this method, the nerve end is implanted within the medullary canal of bone.[16,31,83] Boldrey described a technique whereby a suture on the end of the nerve is drawn through a drill hole in bone, securing the amputated nerve stump in the medullary canal. Such a technique has two objectives: (1) to contain the nerve stump in a rigid compartment, thereby restricting neuroma size, and (2) by containing the nerve stump in bone, to protect the neuroma from direct trauma. However, with the nerve fixed in bone, tension on the nerve may result with movement of the extremity. Boldry reported successful use of his technique in one patient, but Munro and Mallory abandoned the procedure.[67] Mass et al recently presented 18 successful results in 20 attempts with this technique.[60] In 11 cases Goldstein and Sturim had excellent or satisfactory results in 10.[38] One additional patient required reoperation because of technical failure when one of two transposed nerves pulled out of the bone. They stressed some important technical details: adequate mobilization of the nerve; no tension on the nerve; avoidance of an excessively acute angle of the nerve as it enters the bone; and no implantation of the nerve just distal to a joint.

Implantation into Another Nerve

Cross union of the terminal ends of two severed nerves in proximity was reported by Langley and Anderson.[56] They demonstrated that axons will not grow into funiculi already containing axons. However, the axons will continue to grow and branch into the epineurial tissue about the funiculi, forming a neuroma-in-continuity. No reports have been found using a funicular repair in such cases. For this procedure to prevent neuroma formation, there must be an even match of funiculi in the two nerves, which is not a likely possibility.

Wood and Mudge described the use of this technique in five patients with painful neuromas after amputations at the wrist or forearm. The median nerve was sutured to the ulnar nerve, and the anterior interosseous to the superficial radial in some cases. They buried these sutured areas beneath muscle and obtained 80 percent to 90 percent reduction in pain.[47,96]

Centrocentral Nerve Union. A new operative procedure, centrocentral nerve union with autogenous transplantation, was described by Gorkisch et al.[40] In this technique two nerves of central origin are sutured together with a simple epineurial repair just as described by Langely and Anderson.[56] In addition however, one of the nerves is severed more proximally, about 10 mm from the epineurial repair. This iatrogenic laceration is also repaired, thus creating an autograft segment. In their 30 patients, only one had complaints suggestive of a neuroma formation. Gonzalez-Darder et al were able to reduce the size of neuroma formation in rats using this technique.[39]

Kon and Bloem reported the use of this technique in 18 patients with 32 digital neuromas. When the neuromas involved both sides of a digit, proper digital nerves were sutured to each other. When only one nerve was involved, the proper digital nerve was sutured to its dorsal branch. Only one patient required re-exploration, and all experienced at least some improvement.[47,53]

Two mechanisms have been suggested as the possible means by which this technique prevents neuroma formation: (1) the proximal axons are removed from the influence of their distal "targets"; and (2) confinement of the proliferative axons and eventual overlapping may increase the intraperineural pressure, which results in a reduction and eventual cessation of protein production and axoplasm flow.[78]

Relocation of Intact Neuroma

In 1967 Littler, realizing that all techniques for management of painful neuromas were subject to the same unknown factors that caused the symptoms in the initial neuroma, developed a new technique.[45] Every effort is made to keep the neuroma intact with its mature encapsulating scar, while transposing it en bloc to an adjacent area free of scar and not subjected to repeated trauma.

A subsequent evaluation of this technique[48] revealed that 82 percent of cases with amputation neuromas and 63 percent of cases with terminal branch neuromas had excellent results and were essentially symptom-free. In the nonamputee group, elimination of the iatrogenic lesions increased the excellent results to 86 percent. Fourteen of the 15 patients with amputations were worker's compensation cases and all but three returned to work. In 28 percent of the neuromas transferred, no sensitivity to percussion could be elicited, and in 73 percent, there was absent to mild sensitivity to direct percussion at the new location. No patient who initially had a successful transfer of the neuroma had recurrent symptoms after prolonged follow-up. Similar long term success with dorsal translocation has been reported by Laborde et al.[55]

Operative Technique

The neuroma with its fibrous capsule is carefully isolated. A proximal area that is free from scar and away from local trauma is selected, preferably deep to a muscle, in a web space, or between the shafts of adjacent metacarpals. A dorsal site is preferable to a palmar location that might lead to pressure on the neuroma with manual activity such as the gripping of tools.

The neuroma-in-continuity with its nerve is then carefully dissected proximally until the neuroma bulb can be transferred to its new location without tension on the nerve. A 5-0 catgut suture is then placed through the capsule (not the neuroma) and tied. Another knot is tied 3 to 4 mm away from the neuroma. The free ends of the suture are then tunneled subcutaneously and passed through the skin proximal to the location selected for the neuroma. This suture is drawn through the skin and tied, maintaining a 3- to 4-mm separation between the dermis and neuroma (Figs. 37-6 and 37-7). The nerve trunk is carefully examined to make certain that no tension or twisting exists along its path. A similar technique is used when the neuroma is buried in muscle. For neuromas in the finger stumps, I prefer to transfer the nerve end into the web space; for neuromas in the palm, the nerve ends are transferred to the dorsum of the hand between the metacarpals.

Coagulation

In an effort to suppress regeneration of axons or to prevent their longitudinal growth by sealing the funicular ends with scar, many investigators have used various types of methods of coagulation of the nerve stump. These include hot water, heat (cauterization), freezing, electrocoagulation, application of chemical coagulants, and radioactive substances.[3,28,29,44,52,57,74]

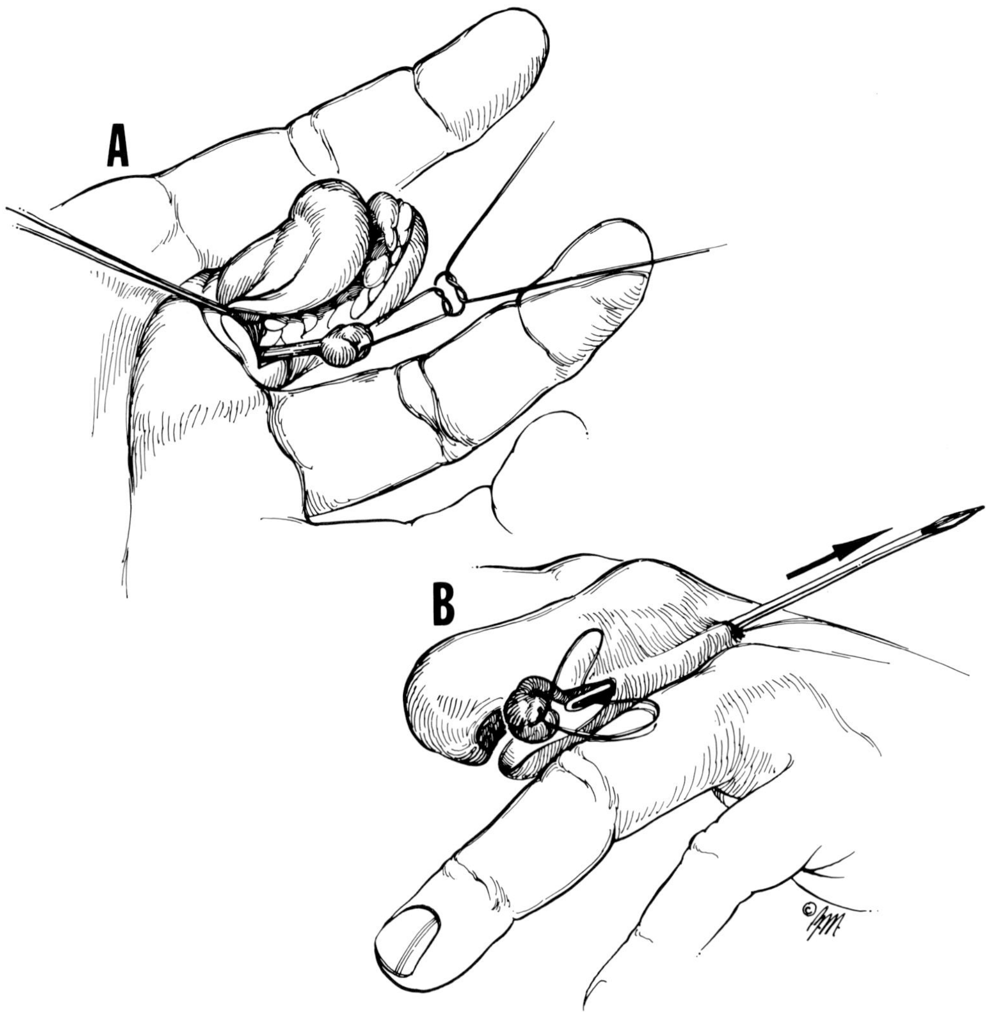

Fig. 37-6. Relocation of an intact neuroma. **(A)** After the neuroma is dissected free, a suture is placed in its capsule. A second knot is tied about 3 to 4 mm from the capsule. **(B)** A tunnel is bluntly dissected in the soft tissues. The neuroma is pulled through the tunnel into an area free from recurrent trauma. The suture is passed through the skin and tied, pulling the second knot up to the dermis.

Physical Methods

Petropoulos and Stefanko studied the use of freezing, cauterization, and electrocoagulation in neuroma formation in dogs.[74] Neuromas did form, but they were smaller than controls. They were typical terminal neuromas of Schwann's type with little perineurial connective tissue proliferation. Others have reported similar findings with only temporary obstruction to regenerating axons.[29]

As Sunderland has pointed out, these methods are generally unsuccessful because it is almost impossible to suppress axonal growth.[87] Holmes and Young[49] and Duncan and Jarvis[25] have shown that in animals, axons have the capacity to regenerate for years. Clinically, this is true in humans as well.

In Italy, Maturo et al have been developing a technique of treating painful amputation neuromas with a CO_2 laser. Twenty-one of their 25 patients had total disappearance of their pain with CO_2 laser beam photocoagulation.[61]

Chemical Methods

Basically, these chemicals are all sclerosing agents. Sunderland has noted that no agent has been shown to effectively suppress all axonal regeneration.[87] These agents create scar tissue at the nerve gaps and may therefore possibly inhibit regrowth of axons into surrounding tissue. The list of agents tried is extensive, including procaine, alcohol, osmic acid, tannic acid, picric acid, chromic acid, hydrochloric acid and pepsin, formaldehyde, iodine, uranium nitrate, gentian violet, phenol, mercuric chloride solution, and nitrogen mustard.[4,5,19,29–32,34,35,42,50,51,71,75–77,79,86]

Sunderland, in his thorough review of the use of these agents, stated that "unfortunately the results of using these chemical agents have been disappointing and the concensus of opinion is that they have no real value in preventing the formation of neuromas."[87] Petropoulos and Stefanko showed that in animals 80 percent alcohol produced the greatest amount of ne-

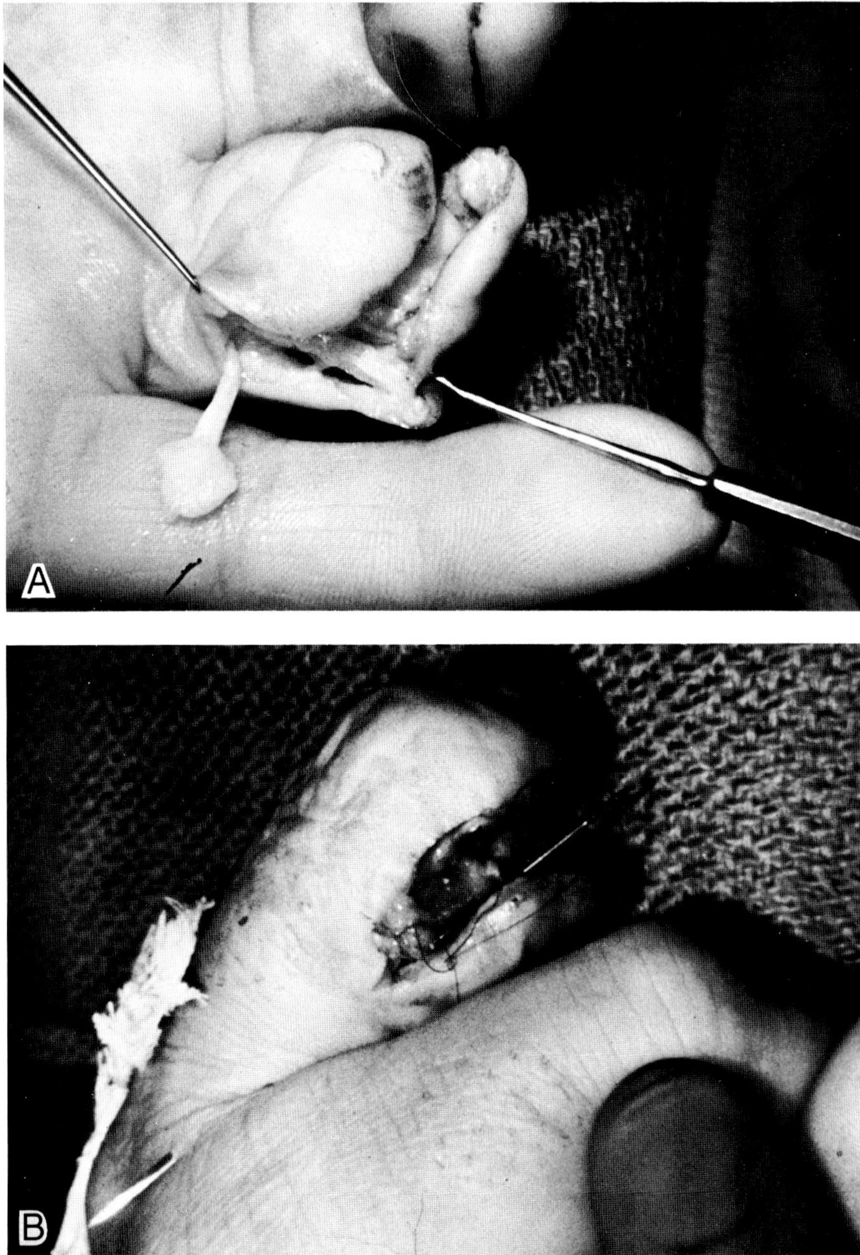

Fig. 37-7. Clinical photographs showing relocation of an intact neuroma. **(A)** The neuroma dissected free. **(B)** Transposition of the neuroma.

crosis of the nerve stump and formaldehyde the least.[75] Their best results were with the use of either local or systemic nitrogen mustard. Often no neuroma was present in these animals. If there was a neuroma, it was small and atrophic, with marked inhibition of Schwann's cell proliferation and minimal scar formation. Guttmann and Medwar in their studies found that formaldehyde and gentian violet were the most effective and alcohol the least effective in inhibiting neuroma formation.[42] Their series was small and the data were not conclusive.

The technique for using these agents locally is to free the distal end of the nerve from all soft tissues. A ligature may or may not be placed proximally (1 to 5 cm). The funiculi are then meticulously dissected apart, and the solution is carefully injected into every individual funiculus. Some investigators also then soak the distal nerve stump in the solution.

Anti-inflammatory Agents (Triamcinolone)

Smith and Gomez injected triamcinolone acetonide into the painful neuroma and surrounding scar tissue in 22 patients.[81] They used either a needle or the Dermo-Jet, injecting the steroid at multiple sites in the deep dermal and subdermal levels. Their rationale was based on the observation that hypertrophic scars and keloids often become soft and flattened after intralesional injection of triamcinolone. Success was obtained in 19 of 34 neuromas so treated, but there was a 29 percent failure rate. This technique worked best in localized digital neuromas and was less successful for deeper neuromas in the palm and wrist.[72,81]

In the rat, some injured sensory fibers ending in an experimental neuroma of the sciatic nerve discharge spontaneously. Corticosteroids have been shown to produce a rapid and prolonged suppression of these discharges, suggesting a membrane action rather than an anti-inflammatory action.[23]

Capping the Nerve End

The divided end of the nerve has been ensheathed in numerous materials in an attempt to diminish neuroma formation. Materials reported include silicone, millipore, gold foil, tantalum, methylmethacrylate, polyethylene, silver, cellophane, Vitallium, glass caps, collodion, Lucite, tin, decalcified bone, fascia, vessel lumen, placental tissue, rubber and plastic femoral artery replacements, dried plasma, and arterial wall tissue.[6,19,27,33,36,37,77,82,88,89,91,95]

Petropoulos and Stefanko[75] showed that in dogs neither tantalum, silver, nor gold inhibited neuroma formation, and, in fact, the neuromas were larger than those in the controls. Other reports are inconclusive, with neuromas continuing to form about the material used. It is difficult to seal the funiculi completely. Poth and Bravo-Fernandez used similar materials plus cellophane, Vitallium, and glass with very unpredictable results.[77] Early success with tantalum was reported by White and Hamlin, but there have been no long-term results reported.[95] Sunderland noted that tantalum does evoke a severe delayed foreign body reaction.[87]

Methylmethacrylate was used by Edds but neuromas continued to form.[27] Collodion has been ineffective. Campbell and colleagues used millipore filters, without success, and it is no longer used.[11]

Silicone Capping

Use of silicone rubber caps over the end of the severed nerve has been more effective than any of the other capping techniques.[6,33,88-90] Swanson, Boeve, and Lumsden reported a series of 18 patients with 38 neuromata.[89] Follow-up averaged 41 months. Fifteen patients had relief of their symptoms, one patient had recurrence of pain and was relieved by recapping, and two patients developed causalgia. Prior to its use in humans, Swanson and colleagues studied the technique in rabbits and demonstrated severed nerves with no neuroma formation. They have shown that several factors are important in inhibiting axonal growth and resultant neuroma formation: (1) the length-to-diameter ratio should be a minimum of 5 : 1, that is, the shorter the cap, the more likely a neuroma will form; and (2) the nerve cap should be only slightly larger than the nerve. It should not fit too loosely, allowing axons to grow back proximally between the cap and the epineurium.

Operative Technique

In Swanson's technique, the first step is to resect the neuroma. A silicone cap slightly larger than the nerve, but not too tight, is chosen (Fig. 37-8). It is trimmed to the appropriate length (5 to 10 times the nerve's diameter). Using a 5-0 nonabsorbable Bunnell-type suture, the cap is secured over the freshly amputated nerve stump (Fig. 37-9). Swanson and colleagues also recommend transfer of the nerve stump to healthy soft tissue if necessary.

Tupper and Booth reported a series of 32 neuromas in 17 patients in whom they used two types of silicone caps.[92] The first was a silicone rubber Ducker-Hayes tube that was passed over the end of the nerve. The proximal portion of the tube was sutured to the epineurium and the distal end was ligated beyond the end of the nerve. In two of these that were reexplored, the cap remained in place, but nerve fibers had grown through the loose proximal opening.

The second type was a Frackelton cap that was fit snugly over the nerve end. Both types of caps became dislodged in six patients. None of the Frackelton caps that were reexplored showed any evidence of funicular escape and neuroma formation. Only 25 percent of their results were excellent. This increased to 31 percent when a second capping was done. If compared to a third simple neurectomy, the results were no different. Tupper and Booth concluded that, in their hands, capping did not improve their results over simple excisional neurectomy.

Soft Tissue Coverage

Brown and Flynn reported four cases of patients with painful neuromas in the hand after multiple operations in whom resection of the scarred area and replacement with abdominal

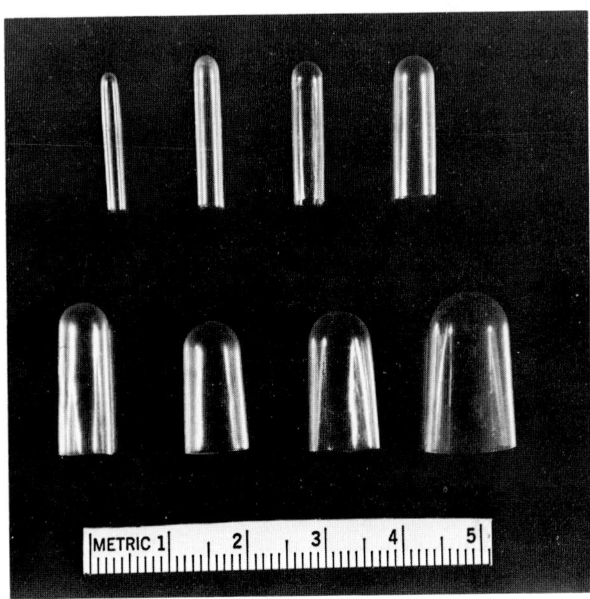

Fig. 37-8. Silicone caps (Swanson design) are available in several sizes. A cap only slightly larger than the diameter of the nerve should be used.

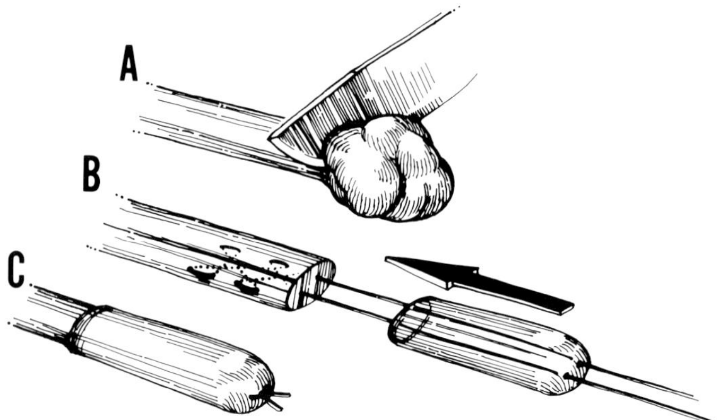

Fig. 37-9. Silicone capping. **(A)** The neuroma is excised. **(B)** A suture is passed through the nerve and the distal end of the silicone cap. **(C)** The silicone cap is pulled over the end of the nerve and secured by tying the suture.

pedicle tissue gave relief of their symptoms.[9] Instead of transferring the nerves to a healthy bed, they moved a healthy bed of tissue to the damaged area. This rather drastic approach represents a possible salvage procedure in patients with scarred tissues in whom other relatively easier methods of treatment have been tried without success.

Author's Preferred Method

The tremendous capacity for axons to regenerate and the many unknown influences resulting in symptomatic neuromas have led to the failure or unpredictability of many of the procedures described in this chapter. Sunderland concluded that silicone capping or ligation combined with the use of a chemical coagulant offers the best chances for success.[87] Petropoulos and Stefanko concluded from their studies that local or systemic nitrogen mustard provided the best results.[75] Swanson, Boeve, and Lumsden prefer silicone capping, and Tupper and Booth obtained better results with resection than with silicone capping.[89,92] Mass et al and Goldstein and Sturim reported good results with transfer of the neuroma into bone.[38,60] The unique concept of centrocentral nerve union described by Gorkisch et al is intriguing, and in selected cases may be potentially very useful.[40] Finally, the CO_2 laser may have a future role in the control of neuroma formation.[61] None of these studies is conclusive, however.

In the management of an amputated nerve end or an irreparable terminal branch laceration, I prefer simple resection, allowing the cut end of the nerve to retract into healthy soft tissues. If the bed is not adequate, I transfer the severed end to another location where local trauma will be minimal. For established neuromas, I prefer relocation of the intact neuroma as described on page 1394. If, however, the distal end of the nerve is present, I would attempt to minimize neuroma formation by resection of the neuroma and repair of the nerve. If too large a gap exists, grafts would be my next choice. Only if the distal portion of the severed nerve were absent or irreparable, would I recommend neuroma relocation. This applies to the commonly encountered neuromas of the superficial branch of radial nerve and the palmar cutaneous branch of median nerve. In case of amputation neuromas, I prefer relocation.

I believe that local nitrogen mustard, local radioactive materials, and silicone capping are all interesting possibilities, and more investigation and clinical use are necessary to find the best method, if one exists. At present, however, I prefer to leave the neuroma intact and transfer it to an area free from local trauma. This is an effective, proven method, even in the difficult, work-injured patient.

REFERENCES

1. Ashley L, Stallings JO: End-to-side nerve flap for treatment of painful neuroma: A 15-year follow-up. J Am Osteopath Assoc 88:621–624, 1988
2. Badalamente MA, Hurst LC, Ellstein J, McDevitt CA: The pathobiology of human neuromas: An electron microscopic and biochemical study. J Hand Surg 10B:49–53, 1985
3. Bate JT: Method of treating nerve ends in amputation stumps. Am J Surg 64:373–374, 1944
4. Benedikt M: Ueber neuralgien und neuralgische Affectionen und deren Behandlung. Klin Z Streitfragen 6:67, 1892
5. Beswerschenko AP: Traumatische Neurome. Entstehungsbedingungen der Neurome und Mittel zur ihren Verhutung. Experimentalle Untersuchungen Zentralbl Chir 56:455, 1929
6. Biddulph SL: The prevention and treatment of painful amputation neuroma. Proceedings of the South African Orthopaedic Association. J Bone Joint Surg 54B:379, 1972
7. Bora FW, Pleasure DE, Didizian NA: A study of nerve regeneration and neuroma formation after nerve suture by various techniques. J Hand Surg 1:138–143, 1976
8. Boyes JH: Bunnell's Surgery of the Hand. p. 426. 3rd Ed. JB Lippincott, Philadelphia, 1956
9. Brown H, Flynn JE: Abdominal pedicle flap for hand neuromas and entrapped nerves. J Bone Joint Surg 55A:575–579, 1973
10. Bunnell S, Boyes JH: Nerve grafts. Am J Surg 44:64–75, 1939
11. Campbell JB, Bassett CAL, Girado JM, Seymour RJ, Rossi JP: Application of mono-molecular filter tubes in bridging gaps in peripheral nerves and for prevention of neuroma formation. A preliminary report. J Neurosurg 13:635, 1956

12. Campbell JB, Bassett CAL, Husby J, Thulin CA, Feringa ER: Microfilter sheaths in peripheral nerve surgery, a laboratory report and preliminary clinical study. J Trauma 1:139-157, 1961
13. Chapple WA: Prevention of nerve bulbs in stumps. Br Med J 1:399, 1918
14. Chavannaz G: A propos de la technique de l'amputation de cuisse. La ligature de nerf grand sciatique. Bull Acad Med 123:123, 1940
15. Cieslak AK, Stout AP: Traumatic and amputation neuromas. Arch Surg 53:646-651, 1946
16. Contini V: Experimental study of amputation neuromas. Arch Ital Chir 56:569-575, 1939
17. Corner EM: The structure, forms and conditions of the ends of divided nerves: With a note on regeneration neuromata. Br J Surg 6:273-278, 1918
18. Davis L, Perret G, Hiller F: Experimental studies in peripheral nerve surgery. Effect of infection on regeneration and functional recovery. Surg Gynecol Obstet 81:302-308, 1945
19. DeCarvalho Pinto VA, Junqueira LCU: A comparative study of the methods for prevention of amputation neuroma. Surg Gynecol Obstet 99:492-496, 1954
20. Dellon AL, Mackinnon SE, Pestronk A: Implantation of sensory nerve into muscle: Preliminary clinical and experimental observations on neuroma formation. Ann Plast Surg 12:30-40, 1984
21. Dellon AL, Mackinnon SE: Treatment of the painful neuroma by neuroma resection and muscle implantation. Plast Reconstr Surg 77:427-436, 1986
22. Devor M, Wall PD: Type of sensory nerve fibre sprouting to form a neuroma. Nature 262:705-707, 1976
23. Devor M, Govrin-Lippmann R, Raber P: Corticosteroids suppress ectopic neural discharge originating in experimental neuromas. Pain 22:127-137, 1985
24. Dobyns JH, O'Brien ET, Linscheid RL, Farrow GM: Bowler's thumb: Diagnosis and treatment. A review of seventeen cases. J Bone Joint Surg 54A:751-755, 1972
25. Duncan D, Jarvis WH: Observations on repeated regeneration of the facial nerve in cats. J Comp Neurol 79:315, 1943
26. Eaton RG: Painful neuromas. pp. 195-202. In Omer GE, Spinner M (eds): Management of Peripheral Nerve Problems. WB Saunders, Philadelphia, 1980
27. Edds MV: Prevention of nerve regeneration and neuroma formation by caps of synthetic resin. J Neurosurg 2:507-509, 1945
28. Erlacher P: Untersuchung und Wiederherstellung der Leitung im peripheren Nerven durch thermische und chemische Mittel. Arch Orthop 23:287, 1924
29. Evans LH, Campbell JB, Pinner-Poole B, Jenny J: Prevention of painful neuromas in horses. J Am Vet Med Assoc 153:313, 1968
30. Fellinger K, Reimer E: Nitrogen Mustard in der Internen Klinik. Wien Klin Wochenschr 61:681-684, 1949
31. Fernandez J: Regeneracao nervosa apos diversos metodos cirgicos visando a prevencao do neuroma de amputacao. Archos Neuropsiquiat 18:341, 1960
32. Foerster O: Therapie der Schussverletzungen der peripheren Nerven. p. 1703. Berlin, 1929
33. Frackelton WH, Teasley JL, Tauras A: Neuromas in the hand treated by nerve transposition and silicone capping. Proceedings of the American Society for Surgery of the Hand. J Bone Joint Surg 53A:813, 1971
34. Fraenkel E: Ueber parenchymatose uberosmimsaure Injektion. Berl Klin Wochenschr 21:234, 1884
35. Frankenthal L: Histologische und experimentelle Untersuchungen über die Wirkungsweise der Injektionstherapie bei Neuralgien, augleich eine histologische Studie über die Nadelstichverletzungen der Nerven. Beitr Klin Chir 143:237, 1928
36. Garrity RW: The use of plastic and rubber tubing in the management of irreparable nerve injuries. Surg Forum 6:517, 1955
37. Gluck T: Ueber Neuroplastik auf dem Wege der Transplantation. Arch Klin Chir 25:606, 1880
38. Goldstein SA, Sturim HS: Intraosseous nerve transposition for treatment of painful neuromas. J Hand Surg 10A:270-274, 1985
39. Gonzalez-Darder J, Baber J, Abell MJ, Mora A: Centrocentral anastomosis in the prevention and treatment of painful terminal neuroma. An Experimental Study in the Rat. J Neurosurg 63:754-758, 1985
40. Gorkisch K, Boese-Landgraf J, Vaubel E: Treatment and prevention of amputation neuromas in hand surgery. Plast Reconstr Surg 73:293-296, 1984
41. Gorman TN, Nold MM, King JM: Use of radioactivity in neurectomy of the horse. Cornell Vet 52:542, 1952
42. Guttmann L, Medawar PB: The chemical inhibition of fibre regeneration and neuroma formation in peripheral nerves. J Neurol Psychiatr 5:130, 1942
43. Hedri A: Zur Behandlung des Nervenquer-schnittes bei Amputationsstumpfen. Munch Med Wochenschr 67:1148, 1920
44. Hedri A: Ein einfaches Verfahren zur Verhutung der Trennungsneurome. Arch Klin Chir 117:842, 1921
45. Herndon JH, Eaton RG, Littler JW: Management of painful neuromas in the hand. J Bone Joint Surg 58A:369-373, 1976
46. Herrmann LG: Painful amputation stumps: Relation to treatment of large mixed nerves at time of amputation. Lyon Chir 52:476, 1956
47. Herndon JH, Hess AV: Neuromas. pp. 1525-1540. In Gelberman RG (ed): Operative Nerve Repair and Reconstruction. JB Lippincott, Philadelphia, 1991
48. Herrmann LG, Gibbs EW: Phantom limb pain: Its relation to treatment of large nerves at time of amputation. Am J Surg 67:168-180, 1945
49. Holmes W, Young JZ: Nerve regeneration after immediate and delayed suture. J Anat 77:63, 1942
50. Huber GC: Injection into Divided Nerve to Prevent Amputation Neuroma. p. 1125. Series Nos. 3 and 4, Medical Dept. of the United States Army in the World War, Vol. 1 (surgery). Government Printing Office, 1920
51. Huber GC, Lewis D: Amputation neuromas. Their development and prevention. Arch Surg 1:85-113, 1920
52. Kirk NT: Amputations: Monograph from Lewis Practice of Surgery, Vol 3. Harper & Row, Hagarstown, MD, 1943
53. Kon M, Bloem JJAM: The treatment of amputation neuromas in fingers with a centrocentral nerve union. Ann Plast Surg 18:506-510, 1987
54. Kreuger H: Ueber Nervenquetschung zur Verhutung schmerzhafter Neurome mach Amputation. Munch Med Wochenschr 63:368, 1916
55. Laborde KJ, Kalisman M, Tsai TM: Results of surgical treatment of painful neuromas of the hand. J Hand Surg 7:190-193, 1982
56. Langley JN, Anderson HK: The union of different kinds of nerve fibres. J Physiol 31:365, 1904
57. Lawen A: Ueber Nervenverisung bei Amputationen. Amputationsneuromen Angiospasmen, Erythromelalgie, seniler Gangren und Ulcus Cruris Varicosum. Beitr Klin Chir 133:405, 1925
58. Leriche R: La Chirurgie de la Douleur. Masson, Paris, 1949
59. Martini A, Fromm B: A new operation for the prevention and treatment of amputation neuromas. J Bone Joint Surg 71B:379-382, 1989
60. Mass DP, Ciano MC, Tortosa R, Newmeyer WL, Kilgore ES Jr: Treatment of painful hand neuromas by their transfer into bone. Plast Reconstr Surg 74:182-185, 1984
61. Maturo L, Del Duce G, Gobbato GP: Painful amputation neuromas: treatment with CO_2 laser (unpublished).
62. Minkow FV, Bassett FH: Bowler's thumb. Clin Orthop 83:115-117, 1972

63. Mitchell SW: Traumatic neuralgia. Section of median nerve. Am J Med Sci 67:2-16, July 1874
64. Molotkow S: Leczenje Ogienstreichlnch Ramneni Perifericzeskich. Nerwow, Leningrad, 1942
65. Morton TG: A peculiar and painful affection of the fourth metatarso-phalangeal articulation. Am J Med Sci 71:37, 1876
66. Mukherjee K, Bassett IB: Meralgia paraesthetica. Br Med J 2(648):55, 1969
67. Munro D, Mallory GK: Elimination of the so-called amputation neuromas of divided peripheral nerves. N Engl J Med 260:358, 1959
68. Nelson AW: The painful neuroma: The regenerating axon versus the epineural sheath. J Surg Res 23:215-221, 1977
69. Odier L: Manual de Medecine Pratique. p. 362. JJ Paschaud, Geneva, 1811
70. Omer GE Jr: Nerve, neuroma, and pain problems related to upper limb amputations. Orthop Clin North Am 12:751-762, 1981
71. Padovani PL: Les douleurs des amputes. Sem Hop Paris 25:817, 1949
72. Pataky PE, Graham WP III, Munger BL: Terminal neuromas treated with triamcinolone acetonide. J Surg Res 14:36-45, 1973
73. Perl JI, Whitlock DG: Use of radioactive colloidal chromic phosphate for prevention of amputation neuroma. J Int Coll Surg 29:77, 1958
74. Petropoulos PC, Stefanko S: Experimental observations on the prevention of neuroma formation. J Surg Res 1:241-248, 1961
75. Petropoulos PC, Stefanko S: Experimental studies of posttraumatic neuromas under various physiologic conditions. J Surg Res 1:235-240, 1961
76. Polley TZ, Brixey AJ Jr: The clinical use of nitrogen mustard. Med Times 79:1-6, 1951
77. Poth EJ, Bravo-Fernandez E: Prevention of neuroma formation by encasement of the severed nerve ends in rigid tubes. Proc Soc Exp Biol Med 56:7-8, 1944
78. Seckel BR: Discussion of treatment and prevention of amputation neuromas in hand surgery. Plast Reconstr Surg 73:297-299, 1984
79. Sicard JA: Traitment des nevrites douloureuses de guerre (causalgie) par l'alcoolisation nerveuse locale. Press Med 24:241, 1916
80. Siegel IM: Bowling thumb neuroma. JAMA 192:263, 1965
81. Smith JR, Gomez NH: Local injection therapy of neuromata of the hand with triamcinolone acetonide. A preliminary study of twenty-two patients. J Bone Joint Surg 52A:71-83, 1970
82. Snow JW: Silastic overlay of troublesome neuromata. Am Soc Surg Hand Corr Newsl 1980:15, 1980
83. Solerio B, Ferrero R: Fixation of nerve stump in bone canal. Minerva Chir 6:640-645, 1951
84. Spencer PS: The traumatic neuroma and proximal stump. Bull Hosp Joint Dis 35:85-102, 1974
85. Stevenson GH: Amputations with special reference to phantom limb sensation. Edinb Med J 57:44, 1950
86. Stookey BP: Surgical and Mechanical Treatment of Peripheral Nerves. WB Saunders, Philadelphia and London, 1922
87. Sunderland S: Nerves and Nerve Injuries, 2nd Ed. Churchill Livingstone, Edinburgh, 1978
88. Swanson AB, Boeve NR, Biddulph SL: Silicone-rubber capping of amputation neuromas. Investigational and clinical experience. Inter-Clin Inf Bull 11:1, 1972
89. Swanson AB, Boeve NR, Lumsden RM: The prevention and treatment of amputation neuromata by silicone capping. J Hand Surg 2:70-78, 1977
90. Synder CC, Knowles RP: Traumatic neuromas (Abstract). J Bone Joint Surg 47A:641, 1965
91. Tauras AP, Frackelton WH: Silicone capping of nerve stumps in the problem of painful neuromas. Surg Forum 18:504, 1967
92. Tupper JW, Booth DM: Treatment of painful neuromas of sensory nerves in the hand: A comparison of traditional and newer methods. J Hand Surg 1:144-151, 1976
93. Virchow R: Die Krankhaften Geschwulste, Vol. 3. A Hirschwald, Berlin, 1863
94. Whipple RR, Unsell RS: Treatment of painful neuromas. Orthop Clin North Am 19:175-185, 1988
95. White JC, Hamlin H: New uses of tantalum in nerve suture, control of neuroma formation and prevention of regeneration after thoracic sympathectomy, illustration of technical procedures. J Neurosurg 2:402-413, 1945
96. Wood VE, Mudge MK: Treatment of neuromas about a major amputation stump. J Hand Surg 12A:302-306, 1987
97. Wood W: Observations on neuromas, with cases and histories of the disease. Trans Med—Chir Soc Edinb 3:68, 1828-1829

38

Radial Nerve Palsy

David P. Green

Loss of radial nerve function in the hand is a significant disability. The patient cannot extend the fingers and thumb and therefore has great difficulty in grasping objects. Perhaps more importantly, the loss of active wrist extension robs the patient of the ability to stabilize the wrist and thumb, further impairing grasp and especially power grip.[31] The tendon transfers to restore function in radial nerve palsy are among the best and most predictable transfers in the upper extremity, but as Riordan[52] has pointed out, "in muscle tendon surgery there is very little hope that errors in technique can be overcome by local adaptation. The success or failure of an operation depends upon the technical competence of the operator and his painstaking after-care." Riordan[53] has also noted that "there is usually only one chance to obtain good restoration of function in such a paralyzed hand."

ANATOMY

Trauma to the upper extremity is such that most injuries of the radial nerve occur distal to the branches to the triceps in the upper arm. For this reason, transfers to restore triceps function are not included in this chapter.

It is imperative that the surgeon make the important distinction between complete radial nerve palsy (excluding the triceps) and posterior interosseous palsy. The radial nerve innervates the BR and ECRL* before it divides into its two terminal branches, the posterior interosseous (motor) and superficial (sensory) branches. Clinically, I believe it is extremely difficult, if not impossible, to determine the integrity of the ECRB in the presence of an intact ECRL, and the presence of the ECRB is variable in posterior interosseous nerve palsy. Usually the ECRB is absent in such cases, although it may be intact. Spinner[58] has noted that the ECRB receives its innervation in the majority of limbs (58 percent) from the superficial radial nerve rather than from the posterior interosseous nerve. In any case, patients with posterior interosseous nerve palsy will have at least one strong radial wrist extensor intact, resulting in radial deviation of the wrist with dorsiflexion, which may be rather marked in some patients (Fig. 38-1). This clinical finding may have significant implications in the choice of appropriate tendon transfers, as discussed later in the chapter.

As it emerges from the supinator about 8 cm distal to the elbow joint, the posterior interosseous nerve splays out into multiple branches, which Spinner[58] has likened to the cauda equina. The difficulty in repairing an untidy laceration of the nerve at this level[48] will often have an important influence on the timing of tendon transfers.

The surgeon who plans to perform transfers for radial nerve palsy must have a profound three-dimensional understanding of the anatomy of the flexor and extensor muscles of the forearm. This is a complex area of anatomy that is difficult to master, and continual review is mandatory. I find that the best sources for augmenting my knowledge of forearm anatomy are actual dissections in the laboratory, Henry's classic book,[27] and the superb atlas of anatomy by McMinn and Hutchings.[37]

REQUIREMENTS IN THE PATIENT WITH RADIAL NERVE PALSY

The patient with irreparable radial nerve palsy needs to be provided with (1) wrist extension, (2) finger (MP joint) extension, and (3) a combination of thumb extension and abduction. The motors available for transfer in a patient with an isolated radial nerve palsy are all the extrinsic muscles innervated by the median and ulnar nerves. This multitude of available motors provides the surgeon with a rather mind-boggling and almost limitless number of possible combinations of

* For simplicity, the abbreviations used throughout this chapter are listed in Table 38-1.

Table 38-1. Abbreviations Used in This Chapter

PT	Pronator teres
FCU	Flexor carpi ulnaris
FCR	Flexor carpi radialis
PL	Palmaris longus
FDP	Flexor digitorum profundus
FDS	Flexor digitorum sublimis (superficialis)
FPL	Flexor pollicis longus
BR	Brachioradialis
ECRL	Extensor carpi radialis longus
ECRB	Extensor carpi radialis brevis
ECU	Extensor carpi ulnaris
APL	Abductor pollicis brevis
EPB	Extensor pollicis brevis
EPL	Extensor pollicis longus
EDC	Extensor digitorum communis
EIP	Extensor indicis proprius
EDM	Extensor digiti minimi
II	Index finger
III	Long finger
IV	Ring finger
V	Small finger

transfers. Indeed, almost every conceivable combination has been tried, and a careful historical review of transfers for radial nerve palsy (see page 1406) will save us from some of the errors of the past.

Unless the patient has a painful neuroma, the sensory part of the radial nerve can usually be ignored. Loss of sensibility on the radial side of the dorsum of the hand is perhaps bothersome but rarely a disability. The patient with a complete radial nerve palsy occasionally will have no demonstrable sensory deficit, because in some patients the superficial branch of radial nerve is absent and its function is preempted by the lateral antebrachial cutaneous nerve.[35,58]

NONOPERATIVE TREATMENT

By far the most important aspects of nonoperative management in the patient with radial nerve palsy are maintenance of full passive range of motion in all joints of the wrist and hand and prevention of contractures, including that of the thumb-index web. In most patients, the constant supervision of a therapist is not required, but the patient himself must be taught very soon after the original nerve injury how to carry out an appropriate exercise program to keep the joints supple. It is the patient's responsibility to do his exercises, and the role of the therapist at this point to teach the patient and to monitor his course to be certain that the exercise program is carried out correctly.

Many types of splints have been described for patients with radial nerve palsy.[4,22,46,62,63] Most of these incorporate some type of dynamic outriggers to extend the fingers and thumb with elastic traction, while allowing full mobility for active flexion. Not all patients with radial nerve palsy need this much elaborate splinting, and each patient's individual needs should dictate the type of splinting used; the same orthosis should not be prescribed for every patient. For example, a telephone operator who wishes to continue working could probably do so with the somewhat cumbersome dynamic splint shown in Figure 38-2. However, an insurance salesman who is more concerned about appearance might be content with only a small, inconspicuous volar cockup wrist splint. In some patients, merely stabilizing the wrist in dorsiflexion will impart remarkably good temporary function. Burkhalter[20] has observed that grip strength may be increased three to five times by simply stabilizing the wrist with a splint. Brand[15] has recommended that if only a wrist splint is worn during the day, the patient should alternate this with a night splint that holds the wrist and fingers in extension. This is because the disturbed balance of the wrist in radial nerve palsy can result in loss of fiber length of the

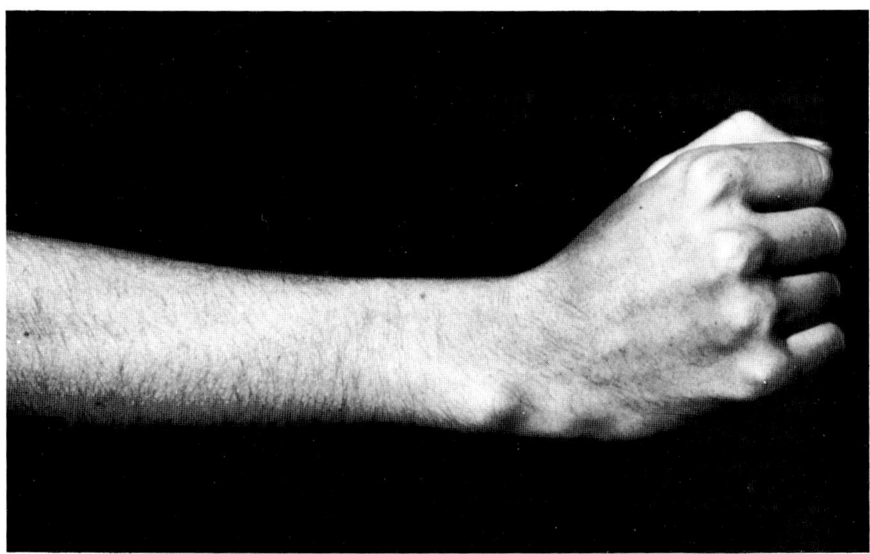

Fig. 38-1. In a patient with posterior interosseous nerve palsy the ECRL is intact, resulting in radial deviation of the wrist in dorsiflexion.

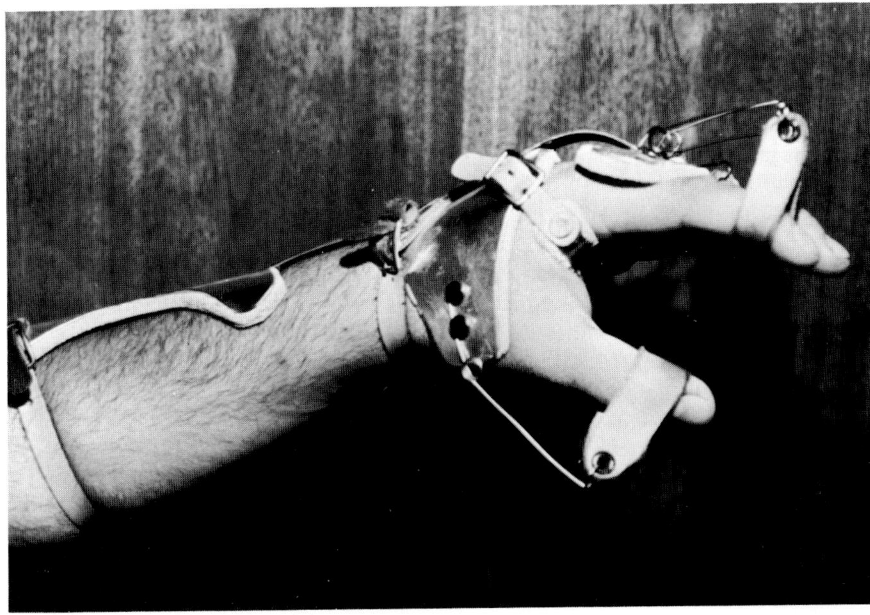

Fig. 38-2. An example of one of the many types of splints designed to provide dynamic extension of the fingers and thumb. Not all patients with radial nerve palsy require this much splinting.

flexor muscles, making it more difficult to achieve normal balance after the final nerve recovery or operation.[15]

Early Transfers ("Internal Splint")

It is perhaps a contraindication in terms to discuss early tendon transfer under nonoperative treatment, but my point is to stress that the concept of early transfers is to provide a temporary "internal splint," and it should not be construed as definitive treatment of the radial nerve palsy.

Burkhalter[20] has claimed that the greatest functional loss in the patient with radial nerve injury is weakness of power grip. Consequently, he has been perhaps the strongest advocate of an early PT to ECRB transfer to eliminate the need for an external splint, and, at the same time, to restore a significant amount of power grip to the patient's hand. In advocating early tendon transfer, Burkhalter has been careful to emphasize what he calls three indications and three important principles. The *indications* are (1) the transfer works as a substitute during ing regrowth of the nerve to eliminate the need for splintage, (2) the transfer works as a helper following reinnervation by aiding the power of a normal muscle to the reinnervated muscles, and (3) the transfer acts as a substitute in cases where the results of nerve repair are statistically poor or in cases where the nerve is irreparable. The important *principles* are: (1) the transfer should not significantly decrease the remaining function in the hand, (2) the transfer should not create a deformity if significant return occurs following nerve repair, and (3) the transfer should be a phasic one or capable of phase conversion.

Burkhalter believes that the PT to ECRB transfer fulfills all of these indications and principles, and he therefore suggests that the operation be done at the time of radial nerve repair or as soon as possible thereafter. The tendon juncture is done end-to-side, and the continuity of ECRB is not disrupted so that it may regain its own function if reinnervation should occur.

I have no personal experience with the use of this transfer as an internal splint, but its use is also supported by Omer[42] and Brand.[13]

OPERATIVE TREATMENT

Principles of Tendon Transfers

The application of certain fundamental principles is essential for successful transfer of muscle tendon units. These important concepts were established by such masters as Mayer,[36] Steindler,[60] and Bunnell[11] and have been reemphasized by Littler,[33] Boyes,[8] Curtis,[23] White,[68] and Brand.[13] They have in fact been repeated so often that their significance may sometimes be obscured by their familiarity, but they remain essential elements in successful tendon transfers.

Correction of Contracture

From the outset in the management of any patient with a peripheral nerve palsy, it is imperative that all joints be kept supple since soft tissue contracture is far easier to prevent than to correct. The essential principle here, of course, is that maximum passive motion of all joints must be present before a tendon transfer is performed, because no tendon transfer can move a stiff joint, and it is impossible for a joint to have more active motion postoperatively than it had passively preoperatively.

Adequate Strength

The tendon chosen as a donor for transfer must be sufficiently strong to perform its new function in its altered position. An appreciation of the relative strengths of the forearm muscles is important to the surgeon in selecting an appropriate motor (Table 38-2). Brand[14,16] has done elaborate anatomic dissections and biomechanical studies in an effort to apply more scientific principles to tendon transfers, and his work should be read by every serious hand surgeon. Brand has noted that work capacity of a muscle is related to volume, and excursion to fiber length.[16] Lieber et al[32] have further noted that the architectural features of individual muscles are highly specialized for function.

Perhaps even more important than the normal strength of a given motor is its current condition, and, in general, a muscle should not be used for transfer unless it can be graded as being at least good (Steindler said 85 percent of normal). If at all possible, I try to avoid using a muscle that has been reinnervated, that is, one that was paralyzed and now has returned to function. Omer[41,43] has noted that a muscle will usually lose one grade of strength (on Highet's clinical scale) following transfer.

Amplitude of Motion

The surgeon must also have some appreciation of the amplitude of tendon excursion for each muscle. Although more precise values of these have been determined,[12,67,70] Boyes[10] suggested the use of the following values for practical purposes.

Wrist flexors and extensors — 33 mm

Finger extensors and EPL — 50 mm

Finger flexors — 70 mm

These numbers have practical significance, since it is obviously impossible for a wrist flexor with an excursion of 33 mm to substitute fully for a finger extensor with an amplitude of 50 mm. Although the *true* amplitude of the tendon cannot be increased, two things can be done to augment its *effective* amplitude. First, a muscle can be converted from monoarticular to biarticular or multiarticular, thereby effectively utilizing the natural tenodesis effect. For example, when the FCU is transferred to the EDC, it is converted to a multiarticular muscle and the *effective* amplitude of the tendon is increased significantly by active volar flexion of the wrist, thereby allowing the transferred wrist flexor to extend the fingers fully (Fig. 38-3). The second factor that can increase amplitude is extensive dissection of the muscle from its surrounding fascial attachments. This is particularly true of the brachioradialis.

Table 38-2. Work Capacity of Forearm Muscles (Boyes[10])

Donor Muscles (Mkg)		Recipient Muscles (Mkg)	
BR	1.9	EPL	0.1
PT	1.2	APL	0.1
FCR	0.8	EPB	0.1
FCU	2.0	EDC	1.7
PL	0.1	EIP	0.5
FDS	4.8	ECRL	1.1
FDP	4.5	ECRB	0.9
FPL	1.2	ECU	1.1

Straight Line of Pull

The pioneers of tendon transfer surgery repeatedly emphasized that the most efficient transfer is one that passes in a direct line from its own origin to the insertion of the tendon being substituted. Although this is not always possible (e.g., in an opponensplasty), it is a desirable goal to seek and is particularly important in the FCU to EDC transfer, which is described later in this chapter.

One Tendon – One Function

It is obvious that a single tendon cannot be expected to do two diametrically opposing actions simultaneously, for example, flex and extend the same joint. It is perhaps not quite so obvious that the effectiveness of a tendon transfer is reduced when it is expected to produce two dissimilar functions even when they are not direct opposites. If a muscle is inserted into two tendons having separate functions, the force and amplitude of the donor tendon will be dissipated and less effective than it would be if it motored only a single tendon.[56] At the very least, if a single tendon is transferred into two separate tendons, the excursion of the two should be the same.[15]

Synergism

There is debate among hand surgeons as to the importance of synergistic motion in the hand, that is, finger flexors acting in concert with wrist extensors and finger extensors with wrist flexors. Littler[33] has been a major advocate of the use of synergistic muscles for transfer whenever possible, and I personally believe it is easier to retrain muscle function after synergistic muscle transfers. A possible exception to this rule is the use of the superficialis (sublimis) tendons, which have more independent cortical control than other muscles in the hand, although I still find it more difficult to retrain the superficialis than synergistic transfers.

Expendable Donor

Removal of a tendon for transfer must not result in unacceptable loss of function; there must be sufficient muscle remaining to substitute for the donor muscle. The classic example of this is the necessity of retaining one strong wrist flexor (PL is not adequate) in any combination of transfers for radial nerve palsy (see page 1406).

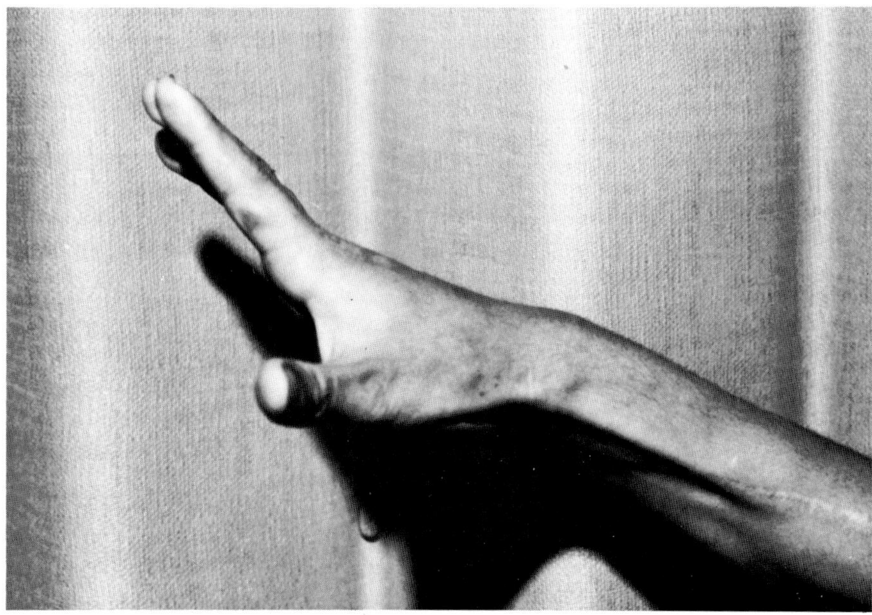

Fig. 38-3. A wrist flexor transferred to the finger extensors does not have sufficient amplitude of excursion to simultaneously extend the wrist and fingers. In this patient following FCU to EDC transfer, note that he uses the tenodesis effect created by active volar flexion of the wrist to enhance the effective excursion of the tendon and thereby achieve excellent active extension of the fingers (compare with Fig. 38-12).

Tissue Equilibrium

The timing of tendon transfers is somewhat controversial, but all authors agree that no transfer should be done until the local tissues are in optimal condition. Steindler's classic expression, "tissue equilibrium" (quoted by Boyes[8]) is a good term; it implies that soft tissue induration is gone, there is no reaction in the wounds, the joints are supple, and the scars are as soft as they are likely to become. To perform tendon transfers or any elective operation before tissue equilibrium has been reached is to invite disaster. If scar tissue remains after maximum recovery has been achieved, the surgeon must consider providing new skin coverage with flaps prior to transfer or else devise transfers that will avoid the scarred areas. Tendon transfers work best when passed between the subcutaneous fat and deep fascial layer; they are not likely to work at all in a pathway of scar. Brand[15] has emphasized the concept of gentle tunnelling, using a blunt-tipped instrument and probing natural tissue planes to find the path of least resistance. When performing tendon transfers, the surgeon should think in terms of trying to minimize scar formation, and skin incisions should be planned so as to place tendon junctures beneath flaps rather than directly beneath incisions.[41]

Timing of Tendon Transfers

The appropriate time to perform transfers for radial nerve palsy is a somewhat controversial subject. As noted previously, several authors[13,15,20,42,48] advocate only a limited transfer (PT to ECRB) almost immediately after injury to act as an internal splint and also to supplement any return in the reinnervated extensor muscles. Brown[19] suggests that it is advisable to proceed with the full component of tendon transfers early when there is a questionable or poor prognosis from the nerve repair. For example, if there is a nerve gap of greater than 4 cm or if there is a large wound or extensive scarring or skin loss over the nerve, he recommends ignoring the nerve and proceeding directly to the tendon transfers. I basically agree with Brown; if the chances of nerve regeneration are poor, there is no point in waiting before doing the transfers. However, if a good repair of the nerve has been accomplished, it is my practice to wait a sufficient period of time before considering transfer. In my opinion, "sufficient time" is determined by using Seddon's[57] figures for nerve regeneration, i.e., approximately 1 mm per day. This means that it may take as long as 5 or 6 months before one sees return in the most proximal muscles (BR and ECRL) following nerve repair in the middle third of the arm (see Fig. 38-13). The remaining muscles should return in orderly progression at the same rate of 1 mm per day (Table 38-3).

To my knowledge, there is little if any popular support for the concept offered by Bevin[5] of never repairing the radial nerve and proceeding directly to tendon transfers. Although he demonstrated impressive differences in disability times (8 weeks after tendon transfers, 7½ months after nerve repair), I believe that most surgeons would agree that the results of radial nerve repair are sufficiently good to warrant routine repair in all cases except perhaps in those identified above by Brown as having a poor prognosis.

There does not appear to be any *upper* time limit as to how

Table 38-3. Distances (cm) from the Distal End of Supinator to the Point of Innervation (Spinner[58])

ECU	1.25
EDC	1.25–1.8
EDM	1.8
APL	5.6
EPB	6.5
EIP	6.8
EPL	7.5

long a delay before transfers are done can be tolerated following nerve injury. Brodman[17] reported successful transfers 24 years after radial nerve injury, despite what he described as "gelatinous degeneration" (i.e., translucent appearance) of the paralyzed tendons at the time of operation.

Historical Review

As with the management of peripheral nerve injuries per se, the development of operative procedures for treatment of irreparable radial nerve palsy mainly evolved during the two world wars. Most of the important articles contributing to our knowledge of transfers for radial nerve palsy are to be found in the immediate post-war years. The tragedies of the wars enabled a few individuals to accumulate a lifetime of experience in a very short period of time. For example, Scuderi[56] reported 45 patients with radial nerve palsy in whom he performed transfers during a 12½ month period.

Sir Robert Jones is credited with being the major innovator of radial nerve transfers, and all the articles in the post–World War I era acknowledge his fundamental contributions. However, the "classic" Jones transfer has been quoted and misquoted so many times in articles and texts that it is worthwhile to review his original articles[28,29] to see exactly what he did advocate. Part of the confusion arises from the fact that Jones did describe at least two slightly different combinations of transfers, as outlined in Table 38-4.

Although the Jones transfers came to be one of the more popular operations for radial nerve palsy, they were by no means universally accepted. Virtually every conceivable combination of transfers for radial nerve palsy has been reported, and the reader interested in this fascinating aspect of medical history is referred to Boyes' superb article,[9] which outlines the multitude of procedures described between 1897 and 1959.

Table 38-4. Jones Transfers

1916[28]
PT to ECRL and ECRB
FCU to EDC III–V
FCR to EIP, EDC II, and EPL
1921[29]
PT to ECRL and ECRB
FCU to EDC III–V
FCR to EIP, EDC II, EPL, EPB, and APL

For the purpose of this discussion, it is important to mention only some of the more important highlights in the development of transfers for radial nerve palsy.

The only part of the classic Jones transfer that has become universally accepted is the use of the PT to provide active wrist extension; however, even this acceptance came relatively recently. Saikku[55] pointed out that at the onset of World War II there were two schools of thought regarding the best method of restoring wrist dorsiflexion in the patient with radial nerve palsy. The British and Americans tended to favor Jones' transfer of the PT to the radial wrist extensors, while the Germans were influenced by the recommendation of Perthes, who advocated a tenodesis or arthrodesis to maintain a dorsiflexed attitude of the wrist. Saikku reviewed a large series comparing the two methods and concluded that the Jones transfer was superior, noting a high failure rate with tenodesis due to loosening. A few authors have favored wrist arthrodesis,[44,60] but most believe that it is important to maintain wrist motion in a patient with radial nerve palsy.[4,8,10,33,49,51,55,71]

The only current controversy regarding the pronator transfer centers around the optimal insertion of the PT[14,15,18,33,38,40,42] (see page 1410).

Major diagreement arises concerning the optimal method of restoring finger extension and thumb extension and abduction. It is clear that Jones advocated transferring both strong wrist flexors (FCU and FCR), a practice apparently not questioned by most of his contemporaries. Although Starr[59] in 1922 was the first to transfer the PL and leave one of the strong wrist flexors intact, his article leads the reader to wonder if he fully appreciated the significance of his contribution. Indeed, it was not until 1946 that Zachary[72] documented and convincingly illustrated the concept that it is desirable to leave one wrist flexor intact. He also showed that the PL is *not* adequate to provide satisfactory wrist flexion if both the FCU and FCR are transferred. Zachary's other contribution was the creation of a standard method of assessing results, which has been modified and used by numerous other authors since 1946.

In 1949, Scuderi[56] refined the PL to rerouted EPL transfer, emphasizing the important principle that function is better when the transfer is done into only one tendon (note in Table 38-4 that by 1921 Jones was suturing the FCR into four tendons with separate functions).

The results of these and other studies gradually evolved into what has been referred to by some as the "standard" set of tendon transfers for radial nerve palsy:

PT to ECRB

FCU to EDC II-V

PL to rerouted EPL

However, the best combination of transfers is still not totally agreed upon. In 1960, Boyes[9] offered a reasonable alternative to the standard set of transfers that seems to have withstood the test of time.[21] Boyes reasoned that the FCU is a more important wrist flexor to preserve than the FCR, because the normal axis of wrist motion is from dorso-radial to volar-ulnar. Brand's extensive biomechanical and clinical studies have led him to the firm conviction that the FCU should *not* be used as a tendon transfer for two reasons[14,15]: (1) FCU is too strong and its excursion too short for transfer to the finger extensors; and (2) its function as the prime ulnar stabilizer of the wrist is too important to sacrifice.

Another reason for not using the FCU set of transfers is that it cannot provide simultaneous wrist dorsiflexion and finger extension. Because the amplitude of the wrist flexors is only about 33 mm and that of the finger extensors is 50 mm, full active extension of the fingers with an FCU or FCR transfer can be achieved only by simultaneous volar flexion of the wrist, relying upon the tenodesis effect of the transfer (Fig. 38-3). Boyes thus concluded that, because of their greater excursion (70 mm), the superficialis (sublimis) tendons would be ideal motors for finger extensors. Yet another reason for his new combination of transfers was to provide more independent control of the thumb and index finger. The combination of transfers he described is as follows:

PT to ECRL and ECRB

FCR to EPB and APL

FDS III to EDC (via interosseous membrane)

FDS IV to EPL and EIP (via interosseous membrane)

Operative Techniques

Although there is almost an infinite number of possible combinations of transfers for radial nerve palsy, I believe it is safe to say that there are three sets of transfers that are currently considered to be the most reasonable alternatives (Table 38-5). Probably the most widely used set of transfers over the past several decades has been that using FCU, although Boyes' combination that utilizes the superficialis tendons for finger extension has also proven to be quite satisfactory. The third combination is that first proposed by Starr[59] in 1922 and more recently described in detail by Brand,[13] which utilizes the FCR instead of the FCU. The operative techniques for these three procedures are described in detail below.

It is of course obvious that in a patient with posterior interosseous palsy the PT transfer is not necessary to restore wrist extension.

Table 38-5. The Best Combinations of Tendon Transfers for Radial Nerve Palsy

FCU transfer
PT to ECRB
FCU to EDC
PL to rerouted EPL
Superficialis transfer (Boyes[9,21])
PT to ECRL and ECRB
FDS III to EDC
FDS IV to EIP and EPL
FCR to APL and EPB
FCR transfer (Starr,[59] Brand,[13] Tsuge[65])
PT to ECRB
FCR to EDC
PL to rerouted EPL

FCU Transfer

Incision #1 (Fig. 38-4) is directed longitudinally over the FCU in the distal half of the forearm. Its distal end is J-shaped, with the transverse extension being long enough to reach the PL tendon. The FCU tendon is transected just proximal to the pisiform and freed up as far proximally as the incision will allow. Separation of this muscle from its particularly dense fascial attachments is facilitated by a special tendon stripper designed by Carroll (Fig. 38-5); however, if this tendon stripper is not available, the dissection of FCU can be done under direct vision by extending incision #1 more proximally. The muscle belly of the FCU is very long, extending usually to within a few centimeters of the insertion of the tendon. I prefer to excise rather generously that part of the muscle belly that is attached to the distal half of the tendon, as this will later facilitate the transfer and cause a less bulky appearance of the muscle in its new position around the ulnar border of the forearm.

Incision #2 begins 2 inches below the medial epicondyle and

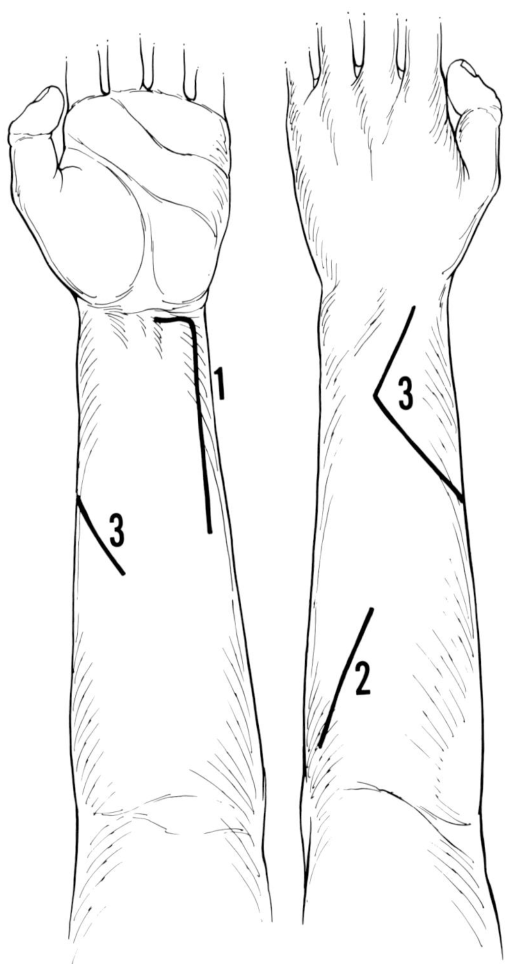

Fig. 38-4. Incisions used in the FCU combination of transfers (see text).

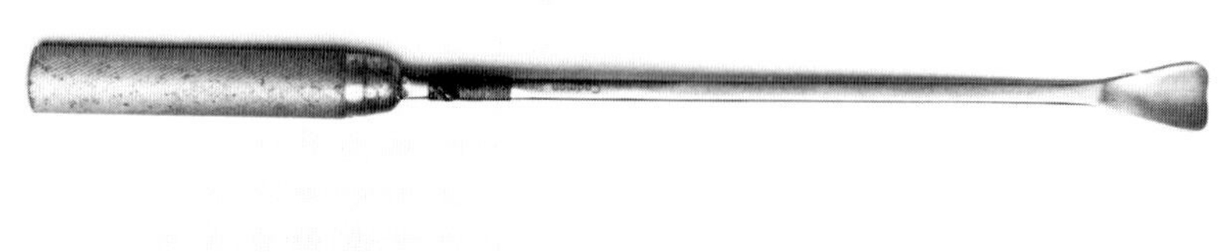

Fig. 38-5. This instrument designed by Carroll facilitates division of the extensive fascial attachments of the muscle belly of FCU.

angles across the dorsum of the proximal forearm, aimed directly toward Lister's tubercle. The deep fascia overlying the FCU muscle belly is *excised* and the remainder of the fascial attachments to the muscle are incised. It is imperative that the FCU be completely freed up so that the entire muscle belly and tendon can be displaced into the proximal wound to redirect the muscle. The limiting factor in the dissection is the innervation of the FCU, which enters the muscle in its proximal 2 inches, and the dissection must not extend this far proximally.

Incision #3 begins on the volar-radial aspect of the midforearm, passes dorsally around the radial border of the forearm in the region of the insertion of the PT, and then angles back on the dorsum of the distal forearm toward Lister's tubercle. The tendon of the PT is identified in the volar aspect of the wound and followed to its insertion on the radius. It is important to free up the insertion with an intact long strip of periosteum in order to ensure that the length will be sufficient for a strong tendon juncture later (Fig. 38-6). Tubiana[66] has emphasized that the PT muscle-tendon unit must be freed up proximally to divide adhesions in order to improve subsequent excursion. The PT muscle and tendon are then passed subcutaneously around the radial border of the forearm, superficial to the BR and ECRL, to be inserted into the ECRB just distal to its musculotendinous junction.

A tendon passer or large Kelly clamp is then passed from the dorsal wound (incision #3) subcutaneously around the ulnar border of the forearm, and the tendon of the FCU is pulled into the dorsal wound (Fig. 38-7). At this point, if there is still excessive bulk of muscle overlying the ulnar border, the FCU muscle belly can be trimmed a bit more. It is imperative that the line of pull of the FCU be as straight as possible from the medial epicondyle to the EDC tendon just proximal to the dorsal retinaculum. If the previous dissection has not freed up all the fascial attachments of FCU, it will be impossible to achieve this important direct pull.

The EPL muscle is then identified in the dorsal wound; it is divided at its musculotendinous junction and rerouted out of Lister's canal toward the volar aspect of the wrist across the anatomic snuffbox (Fig. 38-8). The PL tendon is transected at the wrist, and the muscle-tendon unit is freed up proximally enough to allow a straight line of pull between the PL and the rerouted EPL tendon. The PL tendon is delivered into the dorsal wound in the region of the snuffbox.

A variation in technique recommended by Moberg and Nachemson[39] is to open the dorsal retinaculum to prevent ischemic necrosis of the tendons secondary to postoperative edema. I am not aware of this being a common problem, and I would be concerned about possible bowstringing if the retinaculum were completely cut (which is not mentioned by the authors). Consequently I have not used this modification.

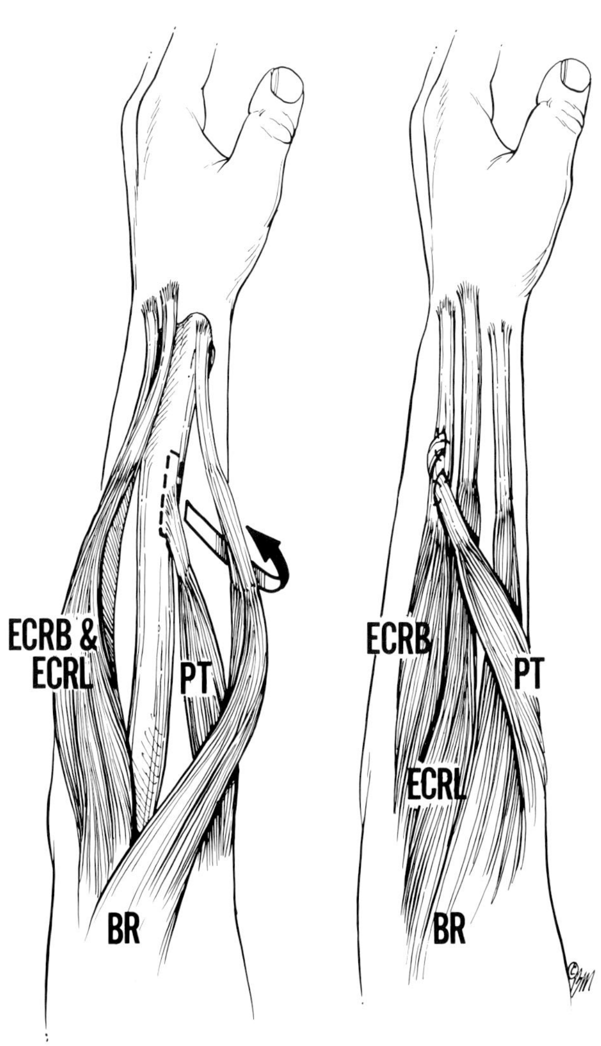

Fig. 38-6. PT to ECRB transfer. It is important to take a strip of periosteum in continuity with the PT insertion to ensure adequate length for the transfer.

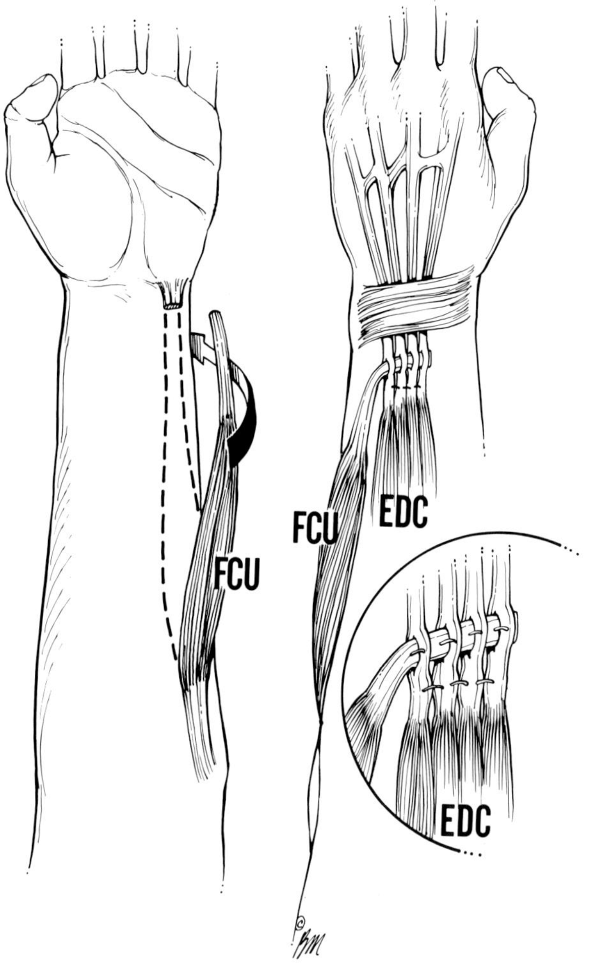

Fig. 38-7. FCU to EDC transfer. The FCU must be freed up extensively to create a direct line of pull from its origin to the new insertion into the EDC tendons just proximal to the dorsal retinaculum. End-to-side juncture is shown here. Moberg and Nachemson[32] have suggested that 4 to 5 cm of the paralyzed EDC tendons be resected proximal to the juncture, allowing an end-to-end suture and a more direct line of pull.

At this point, I prefer to release the tourniquet, establish hemostasis, and close incisions #1 and #2 before doing the final tendon junctures.

Setting the proper tension in the transfers is a somewhat tricky task but is very critical to the outcome of the operation. It is difficult to describe precisely how to adjust tension in tendon transfers, and a certain amount of experience is essential in being able to "feel" the proper tension. In general, however, one should probably err on the side of suturing extensor tendon transfers too tightly rather than too loosely. The tendons must be tight enough to provide full extension of the wrist, fingers, and thumb, yet not so tight as to limit flexion of the digits. I usually suture the PT to ECRB (not including the ECRL) just distal to the musculotendinous junction. The long tongue of periosteum at the end of the PT tendon is woven through the tendon of the ECRB and secured with multiple 4-0 nonabsorbable sutures. (Omer[41] prefers larger [2-0 or 3-0] material.) Even if a tongue of periosteum has been harvested with the PT insertion, I have found that this often provides a rather insecure tendon juncture, and I now routinely reinforce this juncture with a short strip of free tendon graft taken from the ECRL. The transfer is sutured with the PT in maximum tension and the wrist in moderate (45 degrees) dorsiflexion.

The FCU transfer is then sutured. I generally use the technique described by Omer[40] (and depicted in Fig. 38-7), weaving the FCU tendon through the EDC tendons at a 45-degree angle just proximal to the dorsal retinaculum. Moberg and Nachemson[39] have suggested that better results can be achieved if 4 to 5 cm of inactivated EDC muscle-tendon is resected just proximal to the intended site of suture. Although I have not used this technique, it would provide a more direct line of pull since the tendon juncture would be end-to-end rather than end-to-side.[25]

Most authors do not include the EDM in the transfer for fear of creating excessive tension in the small finger. I determine whether to include it by pulling on the EDC tendons with an Allis clamp (proximal to the intended site of juncture); if the small finger extends adequately, the EDM is not included, but

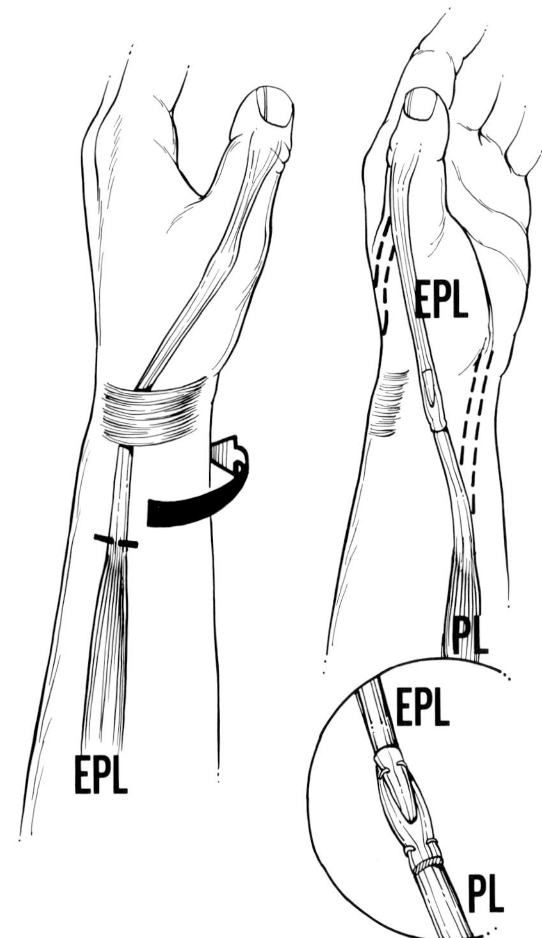

Fig. 38-8. PL to rerouted EPL transfer. By rerouting EPL out of the dorsal retinaculum, the transfer creates a combination of abduction and extension force on the thumb.

if there is an extensor lag in the small finger (signifying an inadequate slip of EDC to the small finger), I include the EDM among the recipient tendons. It is important to suture the FCU tendon into each EDC slip separately and to adjust the tension in the EDC tendons individually so that all four MP joints extend synchronously and evenly. I prefer 4–0 nonabsorbable suture, and the tension I use is with the wrist and MP joints in neutral (0 degrees) and the FCU under maximum tension. A good assistant is very helpful at this point to aid in holding the tension while the tendons are sutured.

Retraction on the distal end of incision #3 will allow the third and final juncture (PL to rerouted EPL) to be made in the region of the anatomic snuffbox superficial to the dorsal retinaculum. The direction of the tendons is essentially in line with the first metacarpal (Fig. 38-9). My preferred tension is with the wrist in neutral and with maximum tension on both the EPL and PL tendons.

The tension must be tested by passively moving the wrist to demonstrate the synergistic action of the new transfer; with the wrist in dorsiflexion, it should be possible to easily flex the fingers completely into the palm, and, with the wrist in volar flexion, the MP joints should pull into full extension but not hyperextension.

Incision #3 is then closed while an assistant stabilizes the position of the wrist and hand to protect the transfers. I prefer to close all three wounds with subcuticular sutures to avoid unattractive crosshatches in the scars.

Postoperative Management

In the operating room, a long arm splint is applied, which immobilizes the forearm in 15 to 30 degrees pronation, the wrist in approximately 45 degrees dorsiflexion, the MP joints in slight (10 to 15 degrees) flexion, and the thumb in maximum extension and abduction. The PIP joints of the fingers are left free. Since limited elbow motion will not cause undue tension on the suture lines, a single sugar tong splint is a satisfactory alternative to the long arm splint. The splint and sutures are removed at 10 to 14 days, and a Munster-type long arm cast is applied in the same position as noted above. The cast is removed at 4 weeks postoperatively, and removable short arm splints to hold the wrist, fingers, and thumb in extension are made, which the patient wears for an additional 2 weeks, removing them only for exercise.

A planned exercise program, begun at 4 weeks, under the guidance of an experienced hand therapist is very beneficial to achieve the optimal results from this procedure. Following these transfers, I find it particularly useful to instruct the patient in synergistic movements. A well-motivated patient should have good control of function by 3 months, although many patients take as long as 6 months to reach maximum recovery.

Potential Problems

Excessive Radial Deviation. Removing the FCU (an important wrist flexor and the only remaining ulnar deviator) from the wrist in a patient with radial nerve palsy may contribute to radial deviation of the hand. This is likely to be further aggravated if the PT is inserted into the ECRL, which Youm et al[70] have shown to be mainly a radial deviator rather than an extensor of the wrist. Even if the transfer is into the more centrally located ECRB, there may be some radial deviation because the ECRB, although more centrally located than the ECRL, still imparts some radial deviation.[13] Also, significant intercommunication between the ECRL and ECRB has been identified by Albright and Linburg.[2] The problem is particularly severe in patients with *posterior interosseous nerve palsy* who have a normally functioning, strong ECRL; in my experi-

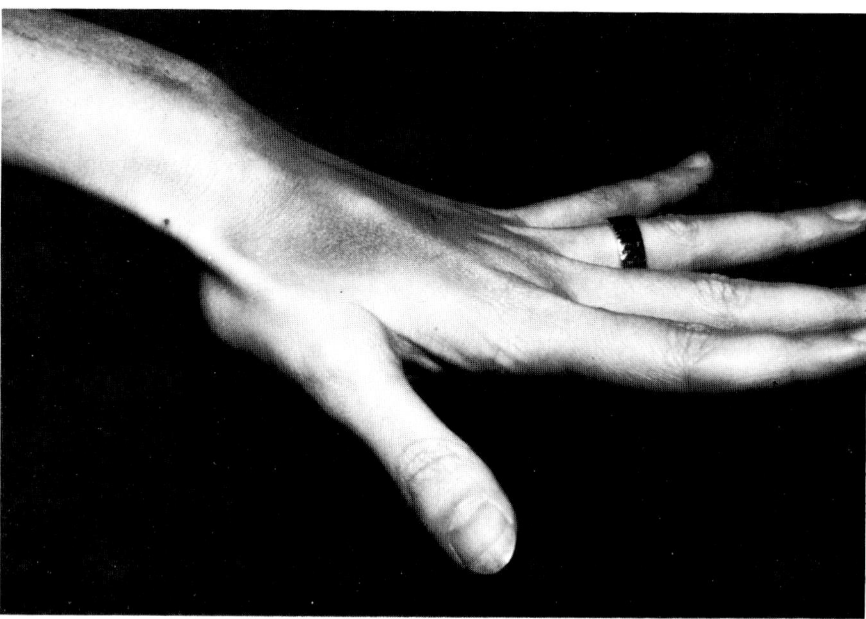

Fig. 38-9. PL to rerouted EPL transfer. Note that the line of pull is essentially in line with the thumb metacarpal.

ence, removing the FCU in these patients can seriously aggravate the radial deviation problem.

Several solutions to the problem have been suggested and are listed below.

Avoidance. If the patient has significant radial deviation preoperatively (e.g., the patient with posterior interosseous nerve palsy), I will not do the FCU transfer. In such cases, I prefer to use Boyes' superficialis transfers or the FCR transfer.

Alter the Insertion. In some patients I have altered the insertion of the radial wrist extensors at the time of PT transfer. The simplest way to do this is to resect the distal 2 to 3 cm of the ECRL tendon and suture the tendon more proximally into the adjacent ECRB, thereby eliminating any possibility of pull through the ECRL insertion. A more radical approach is to shift the distal end of the ECRB into the tendon of the ECU[65] or to include the transposed ECU tendon in the PT to ECRB transfer as suggested by Said.[54] Brand[14] says that this is not a good idea because ECU has a very small moment for extension and such an altered insertion would limit the total extension moment of the PT. His preference is to attach PT to the ECRL and ECRB together proximally, then detach the insertion of ECRL and reinsert it into the base of the fourth metacarpal. Tubiana[66] also prefers to centralize the insertion of the ECRL. In addition to the different moment arms of ECRL and ECRB for wrist extension and radial deviation, he is also concerned about adhesions between the two tendons. Therefore, he sutures PT only to ECRB, but *also* reroutes the insertion of ECRL. The ECRL tendon is divided at its insertion into the base of the second metacarpal, freed up proximally to its musculotendinous junction, rerouted beneath the dorsal retinaculum in the 4th (EDC) compartment, and fixed to the base of the third and fourth metacarpals with sutures and staples (Fig. 38-10).

Absence of the PL. Absence of the PL compromises the FCU set of transfers since it obviously eliminates the important PL to rerouted EPL transfer. In this situation, several authors suggest simply including the EPL into the FCU to EDC transfer, although this significantly limits the abduction component of the transfer's effect on the thumb. Bevin[5] has suggested including all of the thumb extrinsics (EPL, EPB, and APL) in the FCU to EDC transfer, but this seriously violates the one tendon – one function principle. Milford[38] advocated the use of the BR, which is of course possible only in posterior interosseous nerve palsy and not in complete radial nerve palsy. If the BR is used as a transfer, extensive freeing up of the muscle belly is necessary to augment its excursion, and Beasley[4] has commented that the BR is more difficult to reeducate in the rehabilitation program. Tsuge[65] and Goldner[26] have substituted the FDS III or IV for an absent PL.

Not being totally satisfied with any of the above alternatives, I will generally do Boyes' superficialis transfers when the PL is absent.

Bowstringing of the EPL. Tsuge[65] has noted a relatively minor problem of bowstringing of the rerouted EPL tendon across the radial aspect of the wrist. He reported that this may be prevented by hooking the EPL around the insertion of the APL at the time of the tendon transfer. I have no experience with this modification.

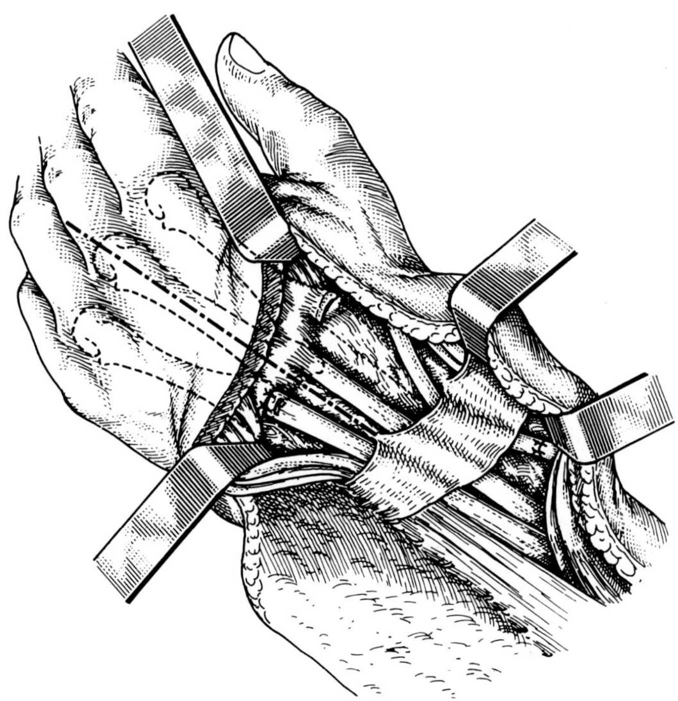

Fig. 38-10. Tubiana's method of re-inserting ECRL into the base of the third and fourth metacarpals (see text for details). (From Tubiana et al,[66] with permission.)

Superficialis Transfer (Boyes[9,21])

Through a long incision on the volar side of the radial aspect of the midforearm, the tendons of PT, ECRL, and ECRB are exposed. The insertion of the PT is removed with a 2- to 3-cm strip of periosteum, and this tendinous portion is interwoven through the ECRB just distal to the musculotendinous junction. As noted on page 1409, the tendon juncture can be reinforced with a short strip of free tendon graft taken from the ECRL if the periosteal strip of PT is not substantial enough to provide secure fixation. In the original descriptions of this transfer,[9,21] PT was sutured to both ECRL and ECRB, but for the reasons noted above, I use only ECRB.

The superficialis (sublimis) tendons of the long and ring fingers are exposed through a transverse incision in the distal palm or through separate transverse incisions at the base of each finger. The tendons are divided proximal to the chiasma, freed up, and delivered into the forearm wound. At a level just proximal to the pronator quadratus, two 1 × 2 cm openings are excised from the interosseous membrane, one on each side of the anterior interosseous artery. Care is taken to protect both the anterior and posterior interosseous vessels. Numerous authors,[1,4] including Boyes,[11] have recommended that the muscle bellies of the transfered muscles be passed through the interosseous space to minimize adhesions. This may necessitate a larger opening in the interosseous membrane than that recommended by Chuinard and colleagues.[21] Others[64] prefer to route the superficialis tendons around the radial and ulnar borders of the forearm, respectively, in an effort to avoid tendon adherence.

A J-shaped incision is then made on the dorsum of the distal forearm; the transverse limb runs from the radial styloid to the ulnar styloid, and the longitudinal limb extends proximally along the ulna. The flexor tendons are passed to the dorsum through the openings in the interosseous membrane, with FDS III routed to the radial side of the profundus mass, between FDP and FPL, and FDS IV to the ulnar side of the profundus muscle mass. Care must be taken to avoid kinking the median nerve as the muscles are passed into the opening. O'Brien (O'Brien ET: personal communication) has noted kinking of the nerve by a band of fascia on the superficialis muscle belly. FDS III is interwoven into the tendons of EIP and EPL, and FDS IV into EDC. The EDM is not included and the recipient tendons are not divided proximal to the tendon juncture. The suture lines are placed proximal to the dorsal retinaculum, which may be narrowed if there is danger of impingement by the tendon junctures.

Reid[48] has described Raffety's technique for setting the tension in this set of transfers. An assistant clenches the patient's fingers and thumb into a fist and brings the wrist into 20 degrees dorsiflexion. This position is maintained until all the transferred tendons are attached to their new insertions under "considerable tension."

Through a transverse incision at the base of the thumb, the FCR tendon is divided and freed up sufficiently to allow it to be turned dorsally and passed through the substance of the APL and EPB tendons, where it is sutured in place. Milford[38] and Omer[43] have stressed the importance of deflating the tourniquet prior to wound closure because of possible damage to the interosseous vessels.

Postoperative Management

Postoperative splints similar to those described on page 1410 are applied and worn for 4 weeks, at which time the sutures are removed and a Thomas splint is worn day and night for the next 2 weeks, except during exercise periods. All external support is then discontinued at 6 weeks postoperatively. The exercise program should emphasize specific control of the superficialis muscles in order to try to take advantage of the greater excursion of these tendons. It should *not* use the tenodesis techniques that are useful after the synergistic (FCU and FCR) transfers.

FCR Transfer (Starr,[59] Brand,[13,14,15] Tsuge[65])

The PT to ECRB transfer, when required, is performed as described previously with the other transfers.

A straight longitudinal incision is made in the distal half of

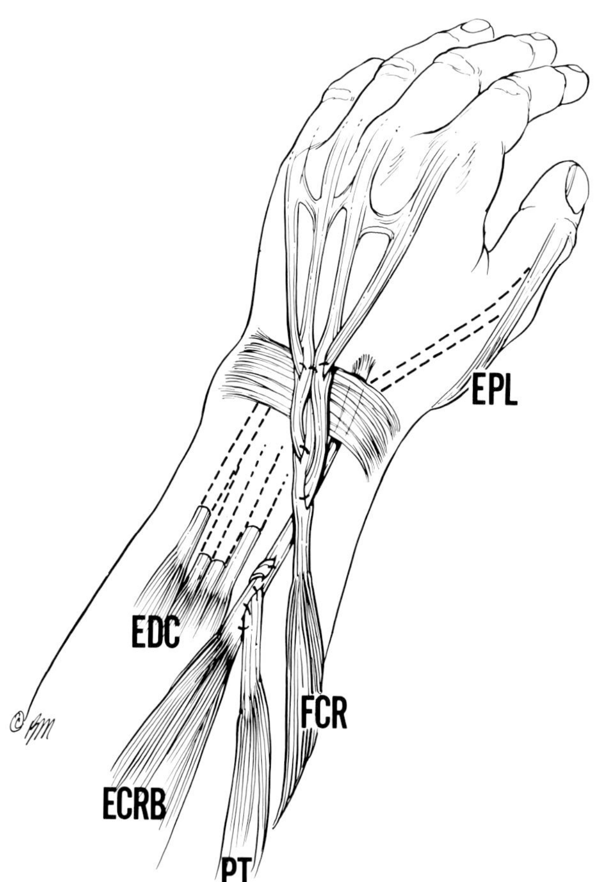

Fig. 38-11. FCR to EDC transfer. Brand[13] suggests that the EDC tendons be transected and transposed superficial to the dorsal retinaculum to create a straight-line end-to-end juncture with the FCR. (Adapted from Brand,[13] with permission.)

the volar radial aspect of the forearm between FCR and PL. Both tendons are identified, transected near their insertions, and freed up to the middle of the forearm to allow re-direction of the tendons to their new insertions. A second longitudinal incision is made on the dorsum, extending from just distal to the dorsal retinaculum to the mid forearm. FCR is passed around the radial border of the forearm through a subcutaneous tunnel, which is created with a blunt-nosed instrument that probes natural tissue planes to find the path of least resistance.[15] The juncture between the FCR and EDC can be made by leaving the EDC in continuity (similar to the FCU transfer depicted in Fig. 38-7), but Brand recommends that the EDC tendons be divided so that a formal end-to-end suture can be done between the FCR and EDC, as shown in Figure 38-11. To avoid the problem of multiple exposed raw tendon ends, Brand suggests burying each cut tendon end. The finger extensor tendons are all tested for extension of the MP joint, and "four good tendons are chosen."[13] These are divided at their musculotendinous junctions, withdrawn distally, superficial to the intact dorsal retinaculum, and redirected to a point over the distal radius where they can meet the FCR tendon in a straight line. They are then retested for effective pull-through at the MP joints in case the change of direction has placed some cross connection under tension. Brand leaves the two best tendons long to join the FCR, suturing the other two to their neighbors more distally. The tendon juncture is done as shown in Figure 38-11, passing the two slips of the EDC into slits in the FCR and burying their ends in a second slit. With the tendons left long, care is taken to ensure appropriate tension on each of the four tendons before making the final cut of the tendons and burying their ends. I would recommend suturing the tendons with the wrist and MP joints in neutral and the FCR tendon under maximum tension. Tsuge[65] has modified the FCR transfer by passing it through the interosseous membrane to obtain a straighter line of pull.

The PL to rerouted EPL transfer is performed as described on page 1408. If the PL is absent, the EPL is joined with the EDC to the FCR transfer.[13] Postoperative management is the same as that described on page 1410.

Author's Preferred Method

I believe it is important for the hand surgeon to be well versed in a least two of the aforementioned transfers, for it is preferable to choose an operation for the individual patient rather than to try to adapt all patients to a single procedure.

In recent years, I have come to prefer the FCR set of transfers for most patients with radial or posterior interosseous nerve palsy. The operation is considerably easier than the FCU set and has the major advantage of leaving the FCU in its very important position as the prime ulnar stabilizer of the wrist.

Boyes' superficialis set of transfers is also an excellent operation and is probably the only way to achieve simultaneous active extension of the wrist and fingers, although in my experience this goal is more likely to be achieved in children than in adults (Fig. 38-12).

The FCU set of transfers is definitely contraindicated in patients with posterior interosseous nerve palsy, and even in complete radial nerve palsy, the FCU transfer may result in some radial deviation of the wrist.

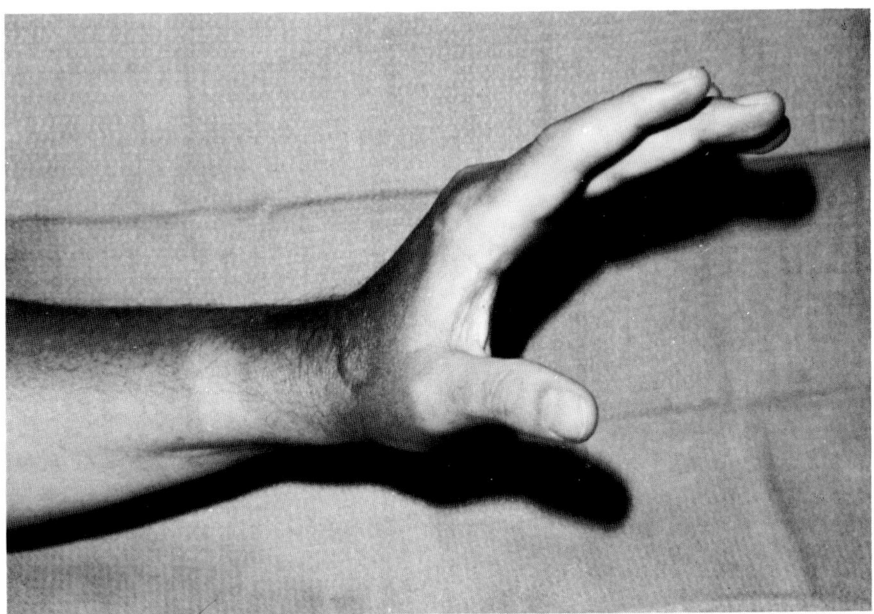

Fig. 38-12. Simultaneous extension of the fingers and wrist is not possible after transfer of a wrist flexor (FCR or FCU) to the finger extensors because of limited tendon excursion. It is possible to achieve this, however, with the Boyes superficialis transfer, as shown in this patient (compare with Fig. 38-3).

RADIAL NERVE PALSY ASSOCIATED WITH FRACTURES OF THE HUMERUS

Few topics generate more heated or emotional discussion in a fracture conference than radial nerve palsy associated with fractures of the humerus. The literature dealing with this topic over the past 40 years serves only to add to the controversy, for one can find at least one article to support virtually any plan of management. It is therefore important to review this entire spectrum of contradictory articles and consider each in its proper context and perspective. An attempt has been made to do that in this section.

The reported incidence of radial nerve palsy associated with humeral fractures has varied from 1.8 to 16 percent,[80-82] although some of these studies were selected or referred series and probably do not reflect an accurate incidence. Using data from a consecutive series of humeral shaft fractures in a major trauma center,[83] the actual incidence is probably less than 10 percent.

There are basically three ways in which radial nerve palsy seen with a humeral shaft fracture can be managed; a discussion of each follows.

Early Exploration of the Nerve

Several authors[76,81,90] have advocated that all radial nerve injuries associated with humeral shaft fractures should be treated with early exploration. They cite the following theoretical advantages to support this position.

1. The status of the nerve (i.e., is it intact, contused, entrapped in the fracture site, impaled on a fragment, or divided?) can be ascertained at the time of injury, thereby facilitating decisions regarding nerve repair or tendon transfers.
2. Stabilization of the fracture by internal fixation protects the radial nerve from further damage.
3. Early operation is technically easier and safer.

Several aspects of these arguments require closer scrutiny. The first question has to do with how many of these patients have a "surgically correctable" lesion. Sim[90] stated that "remediable lesions were encountered too frequently to ignore early exploration," but Kettlekamp et al[79] came to exactly the opposite conclusion after having found *no* surgically correctable lesions in any of the 16 radial nerves that they explored. Sonneveld et al[91] explored 14 cases and found the nerve to be contused in 1 and visibly normal in the other 13.

In a paper published in 1963 that has since been frequently quoted, Holstein and Lewis[78] described a fracture of the distal humerus in which the radial nerve is in particular jeopardy. The proximal spike of this spiral fracture breaks through the lateral cortex of the humerus at or near the point where the nerve is most closely apposed to the bone as it passes through the lateral intermuscular septum from the posterior to the anterior compartment of the arm. Their findings in seven patients with this particular lesion led Holstein and Lewis to the conclusion that early operative intervention was indicated in all such patients. However, a more recent and larger collection of Holstein-Lewis fractures with radial nerve palsy reported by Szalay and Rockwood[93] concluded that early operative treatment is not necessary. Of their 15 patients with this combination of injuries, all 11 who were treated without exploration had complete nerve recovery, and in the 4 patients in whom exploration was carried out, the nerve was found to be in continuity and all had full recovery of nerve function.

Another point regarding early exploration deals with those patients who develop "secondary" radial nerve paralysis in conjunction with a fractured humerus; that is, where the nerve is intact when the patient is first seen and subsequently goes out, usually following fracture reduction. In several articles,[74,76,89] this situation is given as an absolute indication for immediate nerve exploration, although more than one study[73,88] has offered convincing evidence that even secondary radial nerve paralysis can be treated nonoperatively with good expectations for full recovery in most cases.

Finally, the source of the clinical material for each of these studies must be examined. Those who most strongly advocate early exploration based their conclusions on series of patients treated in referral centers (The New York Orthopaedic Hospital[76,81] and the Mayo Clinic[90]), where the percentage of complicated problems and failures from other treatment facilities is unusually high. Sim[74] in fact acknowledged that his series from the Mayo Clinic was difficult to evaluate because most of the patients were referred. Conversely, in those studies drawn from major trauma centers where consecutive series of patients with humeral shaft fractures complicated by radial nerve palsy were evaluated, the authors[73,83,88,93] all agree that nonoperative management of the radial nerve palsy is the treatment of choice.

Exploration at 6 to 8 Weeks If No Return

Shaw and Sakellarides[89] reviewed a series of patients from the Massachusetts General Hospital in 1967 and concluded that the nerve should be explored at 7 to 8 weeks if there is no evidence of return of function. They offered the following reasons for this decision.

1. All patients in their series showed some signs of recovery of nerve function within the first 2 months.
2. An unnecessary operation will be avoided in most patients, in whom spontaneous nerve recovery will occur.
3. There is no interference with fracture healing.
4. The waiting period allows the neuroma to become well delineated and hence to be adequately resected, but is short enough to minimize nerve retraction.

Goldner and Kelley[77] advocated a similar position, but considered the absence of an advancing Tinel's sign to be an important added indication for exploration at 6 to 8 weeks. However, they went on to say that "a longer waiting period could not be criticized, because some of the patients in this group recovered completely without sign of motor recovery for 20 weeks."

Nerve Exploration If No Return After a Longer Waiting Period

Since it is well documented that the *initial* signs of motor recovery may not appear until 4 or 5 months after a radial nerve palsy associated with a fractured humerus, a third option is available. This plan of management is based upon the work of Seddon[85-87] regarding nerve regeneration and is best summarized in the abstract by Szalay and Rockwood.[93] Assuming that a nerve regenerates at the rate of approximately 1 mm a day and adding 30 days as Seddon has suggested,[85] the maximum length of time that *may be required* for motor recovery to *first* manifest itself can easily be calculated by measuring the distance on the x-ray from the fracture site to the point of innervation of the brachioradialis muscle (approximately 2 cm above the lateral epicondyle[87]). In most midshaft humerus fractures, this distance is approximately 90 to 120 mm (Fig. 38-13).

Although EMG evidence of reinervation may precede clinical appearance of motor function by approximately 4 weeks,[84] it may take 4 to 5 months for evidence of function to be seen in the brachioradialis or radial wrist extensors. Therefore, it is altogether logical to wait this long before proceeding with exploration if there is no return of nerve function. The major advantages of this plan of management are: (1) unnecessary operative intervention is avoided in the large majority of patients; (2) most of these patients will regain full recovery of the radial nerve without surgical treatment; and (3) the humerus fracture will usually be healed.

A question that must be raised of course is whether or not the delay in nerve repair for those very few patients in whom neurorrhaphy becomes necessary is excessive and will lessen the chances for good functional recovery. According to Sunderland,[92] a delay of 12 months or even longer is not likely to jeopardize functional motor return following nerve repair, and Seddon[85,87] reported that prognosis for good recovery worsens only after a 12-month delay.

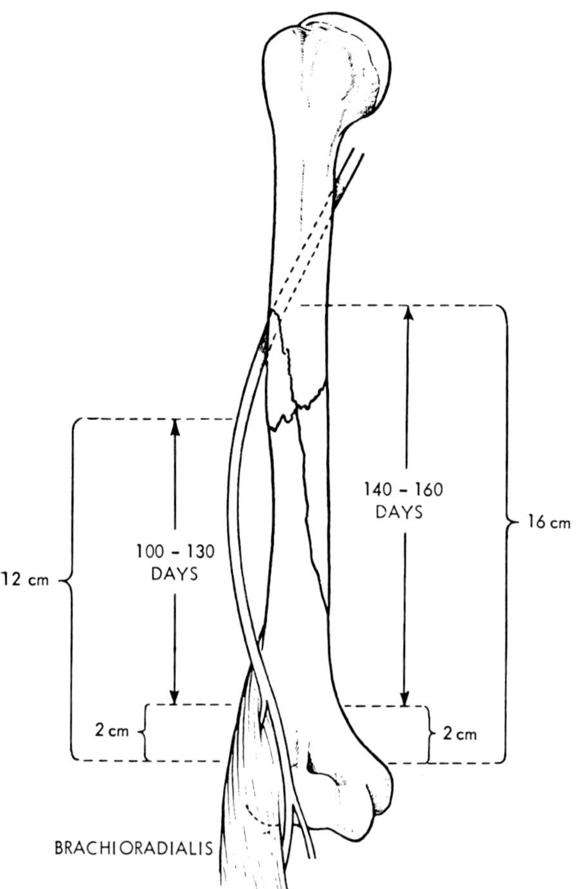

Fig. 38-13. Calculation of the time that must elapse before signs of recovery can be expected after fractures of the shaft of the humerus causing a degenerative lesion of the radial nerve. The information on the left is for a transverse fracture; on the right, for an oblique fracture. (From Seddon,[57] with permission.)

Author's Preferred Method

It has long been my policy to treat most patients with radial nerve palsy associated with humeral shaft fractures nonoperatively, considering exploration of the nerve only after *a realistic* waiting time as outlined in the third option described above and illustrated in Figure 38-13.

There are, however, certain specific indications for early operative treatment of humeral shaft fractures, which in my opinion, include the following: (1) open fractures; (2) fractures in which satisfactory alignment cannot be achieved by closed reduction techniques; and (3) fractures with associated vascu lar injuries. In all such cases, I believe that it is imperative to expose and make visible the radial nerve at the time of operative intervention.

Based upon studies previously cited, I do not consider a secondary nerve radial nerve palsy (i.e., occurring after fracture manipulation), to be *in itself* an absolute indication for early nerve exploration. Rather, I would still rely upon the three indications noted above for early nerve exploration.

Following these indications, it must be acknowledged that there will be a very few patients in whom spontaneous return of function will not occur, but my experience is similar to that of others who have shown that these patients will be so few that routine exploration of all radial nerve injuries is not justified.

Finally, although I favor the third option for management, I find less objection to early exploration than to exploration at 6 to 8 weeks. There may be some valid arguments for early exploration, but in my opinion there is no sound rationale for exploring the nerve at 6 to 8 weeks. If the decision has been made to await spontaneous return of function, I believe that it is only reasonable to wait an *appropriate* period of time.

REFERENCES

1. Adams J, Wood VE: Tendon transfers for irreparable nerve damage in the hand. Orthop Clin North Am 12:403–432, 1981
2. Albright JA, Linburg RM: Common variations of the radial wrist extensors. J Hand Surg 3:134–138, 1978

3. Altman H, Trott RH: Muscle transplantation for paralysis of the radial nerve. J Bone Joint Surg 28:440-446, 1946
4. Beasley RW: Tendon transfers for radial nerve palsy. Orthop Clin North Am 1:439-445, 1970
5. Bevin AG: Early tendon transfer for radial nerve transection. Hand 8:134-136, 1976
6. Billington RW: Tendon transplantation for musculospiral (radial) nerve injury. J Bone Joint Surg 4:538-547, 1922
7. Birch R, St. Clair Strange FG: A new type of peripheral nerve lesion. J Bone Joint Surg 72B:312-313, 1990
8. Boyes JH: Tendon transfers in the hand. In Medicine of Japan in 1959, Proc 15th Gen Assembly Japan Med Cong 5:958-969, 1959
9. Boyes JH: Tendon transfers for radial palsy. Bull Hosp Joint Dis 21:97-105, 1960
10. Boyes JH: Selection of a donor muscle for tendon transfer. Bull Hosp Joint Dis 23:1-4, 1962
11. Boyes JH: Bunnell's Surgery of the Hand. 4th Ed. JB Lippincott, Philadelphia, 1964
12. Brand PW: Biomechanics of tendon transfer. Orthop Clin North Am 5:205-230, 1974
13. Brand PW: Tendon transfers in the forearm. pp. 189-200. In Flynn JE (ed): Hand Surgery. 2nd Ed. Williams & Wilkins, Baltimore, 1975
14. Brand PW: Operations to restore muscle balance to the hand. pp. 127-165. In Clinical Mechanics of the Hand. CV Mosby, St. Louis, 1985
15. Brand PW: Biomechanics of tendon transfer. pp. 190-213. In Lamb DW (ed): The Hand and Upper Limb. Volume 2: The Paralysed Hand. Churchill Livingstone, Edinburgh, 1987
16. Brand PW, Beach RB, Thompson DE: Relative tension and potential excursion of muscles in the forearm and hand. J Hand Surg 6:209-219, 1981
17. Brodman HR: Tendon transfer for old radial nerve paralysis. Arch Surg 76:24-27, 1958
18. Brooks D: Peripheral nerve injuries: Reconstructive techniques. pp. 20-25. In Rob C, Smith R (eds): Operative Surgery. Vol. 8. Butterworth, London, 1969
19. Brown PW: The time factor in surgery of upper-extremity peripheral nerve injury. Clin Orthop 68:14-21, 1970
20. Burkhalter WE: Early tendon transfer in upper extremity peripheral nerve injury. Clin Orthop 104:68-79, 1974
21. Chuinard RG, Boyes JH, Stark HH, Ashworth CR: Tendon transfers for radial nerve palsy: Use of superficialis tendons for digital extension. J Hand Surg 3:560-570, 1978
22. Colditz JC: Splinting for radial nerve palsy. J Hand Therapy 1:18-23, 1987
23. Curtis RM: Fundamental principles of tendon transfer. Orthop Clin North Am 5:231-242, 1974
24. Dunn N: Treatment of lesion of the musculo-spiral nerve in military surgery. Am J Orthop Surg 16:258-265, 1918
25. Entin MA: Restoration of function of paralyzed hand. Surg Clin North Am 44:1049-1059, 1964
26. Goldner JL, Kelley JM: Radial nerve injuries. South Med J 51:873-883, 1958
27. Henry AK: Extensile Exposure. Williams & Wilkins, Baltimore, 1957
28. Jones R: On suture of nerves, and alternative methods of treatment by transplantation of tendon. Br Med J 1:641-643, 1916
29. Jones R: On suture of nerves, and alternative methods of treatment by transplantation of tendon. Br Med J 1:679-682, 1916
30. Jones R: Tendon transplantation in cases of musculospiral injuries not amenable to suture. Am J Surg 35:333-335, 1921
31. Labosky DA, Waggy CA: Apparent weakness of median and ulnar motors in radial nerve palsy. J Hand Surg 11A:528-533, 1986
32. Lieber RL, Fazeli BM, Botte MJ: Architecture of selected wrist flexor and extensor muscles. J Hand Surg 15A:244-250, 1990
33. Littler JW: Restoration of power and stability in the partially paralyzed hand. pp. 3266-3280. In Converse JM (ed): Reconstructive Plastic Surgery. 2nd Ed. WB Saunders, Philadelphia, 1977
34. Luckey CA, McPherson SR: Tendinous reconstruction of the hand following irreparable injury to the peripheral nerves and brachial plexus. J Bone Joint Surg 29:560-581, 1947
35. Mackinnon SE, Dellon AL: The overlap pattern of the lateral antebrachial cutaneous nerve and the superficial branch of the radial nerve. J Hand Surg 10A:522-526, 1985
36. Mayer L: The physiological method of tendon transplantation. Surg Gynecol Obstet 22:182-197, 1916
37. McMinn RMH, Hutchings RT: Color Atlas of Human Anatomy. Year Book Medical, Chicago, 1977
38. Milford LW: Radial nerve palsy. pp. 297-300. In Edmonson AS, Crenshaw AH (eds): Campbell's Operative Orthopaedics. 6th Ed. CV Mosby, St. Louis, 1980
39. Moberg E, Nachemson A: Tendon transfers for defective long extensors of the wrist and fingers. Acta Chir Scand 133:31-34, 1967
40. Omer GE Jr: Evaluation and reconstruction of the forearm and hand after acute traumatic peripheral nerve injuries. J Bone Joint Surg 50A:1454-1478, 1968
41. Omer GE Jr: The technique and timing of tendon transfers. Orthop Clin North Am 5:243-252, 1974
42. Omer GE Jr: Tendon transfers for reconstruction of the forearm and hand following peripheral nerve injuries. pp. 817-846. In Omer GE Jr, Spinner M (eds): Management of Peripheral Nerve Problems. WB Saunders, Philadelphia, 1980
43. Omer GE Jr: Reconstructive procedures for extremities with peripheral nerve defects. Clin Orthop 163:80-91, 1982
44. Parker D: Radial nerve paralysis treated by tendon transplant and arthrodesis of the wrist (abstract). J Bone Joint Surg 45B:626, 1963
45. Parkes AR: Some useful tendon transplants (abstract). J Bone Joint Surg 41B:217, 1959
46. Penner DA: Dorsal splint for radial palsy. Am J Occup Ther 26:46-47, 1972
47. Pulvertaft RG: Techniques in hand surgery (abstract). J Bone Joint Surg 42A:907, 1960
48. Reid RL: Radial Nerve Palsy. Hand Clinics 4:179-185, 1988
49. Riordan DC: Surgery of the paralytic hand. pp. 79-90. In AAOS Instructional Course Lectures, Vol. 16. CV Mosby, St. Louis, 1959
50. Riordan DC: Tendon transfers for nerve paralysis of the hand and wrist. Curr Prac Orthop Surg 2:17-40, 1964
51. Riordan DC: Tendon transfers for median, ulnar or radial nerve palsy (abstract). J Bone Joint Surg 50B:441, 1968
52. Riordan DC: Radial nerve paralysis. Orthop Clin North Am 5:283-287, 1974
53. Riordan DC: Tendon transfers in hand surgery. J Hand Surg 8:748-753, 1983
54. Said GZ: A modified tendon transference for radial nerve paralysis. J Bone Joint Surg 56B:320-322, 1974
55. Saikku LA: Tendon transplantation for radial paralysis. Factors influencing the results of tendon transplantation. Acta Chir Scand 96 suppl. 132:7-100, 1947
56. Scuderi C: Tendon transplants for irreparable radial nerve paralysis. Surg Gynecol Obstet 88:643-651, 1949
57. Seddon H: Surgical Disorders of the Peripheral Nerves. 2nd Ed. p. 31. Churchill Livingstone, Edinburgh, 1975
58. Spinner M: The radial nerve. pp. 28-65. In Injuries to the Major Branches of Peripheral Nerves of the Forearm. WB Saunders, Philadelphia, 1972
59. Starr CL: Army experiences with tendon transference. J Bone Joint Surg 4:3-21, 1922

60. Steindler A: Operative treatment of paralytic conditions of the upper extremity. J Orthop Surg 1:608-624, 1919
61. Stiles HJ: Operative treatment of nerve injuries. Am J Orthop Surg 16:351-363, 1918
62. Thomas FB: A splint for radial (musculospiral) nerve palsy. J Bone Joint Surg 26:602-605, 1944
63. Thomas FB: An improved splint for radial (musculospiral) nerve paralysis. J Bone Joint Surg 33B:272-273, 1951
64. Thomsen M, Rasmussen KB: Tendon transfers for defective long extensors of the wrist and fingers. Scand J Plast Reconstr Surg 3:71-78, 1969
65. Tsuge K, Adachi N: Tendon transfer for extensor palsy of forearm. Hiroshima J Med Sci 18:219-232, 1969
66. Tubiana R, Miller HW IV, Reed S: Restoration of wrist extension after paralysis. Hand Clinics 5:53-67, 1989
67. Wehbé MA, Hunter JM: Flexor tendon gliding in the hand. Part I. In vivo excursions. J Hand Surg 10A:570-574, 1985
68. White WL: Restoration of function and balance of the wrist and hand by tendon transfers. Surg Clin North Am 40:427-459, 1960
69. Wood VE: The extensor carpi radialis intermedius tendon. J Hand Surg 13A:242-245, 1988
70. Youm Y, Thambyrajah K, Flatt AE: Tendon excursion of wrist movers. J Hand Surg 9A:202-209, 1984
71. Young HH, Lowe GH Jr: Tendon transfer operation for irreparable paralysis of the radial nerve. Surg Gynecol Obstet 84:1100-1104, 1947
72. Zachary RB: Tendon transplantation for radial paralysis. Br J Surg 23:358-364, 1946

Radial Nerve Palsy Associated with Fractures of the Humerus

73. Böstman O, Bakalim G, Vainionpää S, Wilppula E, Pätiälä H, Rokkanen P: Radial palsy in shaft fracture of the humerus. Acta Orthop Scand 57:316-319, 1986
74. Duncan DM, Johnson KA, Monkman GR: Fracture of the humerus and radial nerve palsy. Minn Med 57:659-662, 1974
75. Foster RJ, Dixon GL Jr, Bach AW, Appleyard RW, Green TM: Internal fixation of fractures and non-unions of the humeral shaft. J Bone Joint Surg 67A:857-864, 1985
76. Garcia A Jr, Maeck BH: Radial nerve injuries in fractures of the shaft of the humerus. Am J Surg 99:625-627, 1960
77. Goldner JL, Kelley JM: Radial nerve injuries. South Med J 51:873-883, 1958
78. Holstein A, Lewis GB: Fractures of the humerus with radial-nerve paralysis. J Bone Joint Surg 45A:1382-1388, 1963
79. Kettelkamp DB, Alexander H: Clinical review of radial nerve injury. J Trauma 7:424-432, 1967
80. Klenerman L: Fractures of the shaft of the humerus. J Bone Joint Surg 48B:105-111, 1966
81. Packer JW, Foster RR, Garcia A, Grantham SA: The humeral fracture with radial nerve palsy: Is exploration warranted? Clin Orthop 88:34-38, 1972
82. Pennsylvania Orthopedic Society: Fresh midshaft fractures of the humerus in adults: Evaluation of treatment in Pennsylvania during 1952-1956, made by Scientific Research Committee, Pennsylvania Orthopedic Society. Penn Med J 62:848-850, 1959
83. Pollock FH, Drake D, Bovill EG, Day L, Trafton PG: Treatment of radial neuropathy associated with fractures of the humerus. J Bone Joint Surg 63A:239-243, 1981
84. Postacchini F, Morace GB: Fractures of the humerus associated with paralysis of the radial nerve. Ital J Orthop Traumatol 14:455-464, 1988
85. Seddon HJ: Nerve lesions complicating certain closed bone injuries. JAMA 135:691-694, 1947
86. Seddon HJ: The practical value of nerve repair (President's Address). Proc R Soc Med 42:427-436, 1949
87. Seddon HJ: Surgical Disorders of the Peripheral Nerves. 2nd Ed. pp. 242-249. Churchill Livingstone, Edinburgh, 1975
88. Shah JJ, Bhatti NA: Radial nerve paralysis associated with fractures of the humerus. Clin Orthop 172:171-176, 1983
89. Shaw JL, Sakellarides H: Radial-nerve paralysis associated with fractures of the humerus. A review of forty-five cases. J Bone Joint Surg 49A:899-902, 1967
90. Sim FH, Kelly PJ, Henderson ED: Radial-nerve palsy complicating fractures of the humeral shaft (abstract). J Bone Joint Surg 53A:1023-1024, 1971
91. Sonneveld GJ, Patka P, van Mourik JC, Broere G: Treatment of fractures of the shaft of the humerus accompanied by paralysis of the radial nerve. Injury 18:404-406, 1987
92. Sunderland S: Nerves and Nerve Injuries. 2nd Ed. pp. 508-509. Churchill Livingstone, Edinburgh, 1978
93. Szalay EA, Rockwood CA Jr: The Holstein-Lewis fracture revisited. Orthop Trans 7:516, 1983

39

Median Nerve Palsy

William E. Burkhalter

INTRINSIC REPLACEMENT IN MEDIAN NERVE PARALYSIS (RESTORATION OF OPPOSITION)

Median nerve paralysis most frequently is caused by penetrating or perforating wounds of the forearm or wrist area, and less commonly may be secondary to a fracture of the contiguous skeleton along the course of the nerve. In rare instances, the wound may involve only the median nerve. More frequently, however, there is damage to the flexor tendons in lower injuries and damage to the brachial artery in proximal injuries. The motor deficit involves primarily loss of opposition of the thumb in injuries at the level of the wrist or distal forearm, or loss of opposition of the thumb and severe weakness of the extrinsic flexors of the hand in the more proximal injuries. Because of variations of innervation involving primarily the flexor pollicis brevis, unsatisfactory positioning of the thumb following complete median nerve laceration may occur in only 60 to 70 percent of the patients. In other words, 30 to 40 percent of the people with complete median nerve lacerations will not require an opponensplasty regardless of the quality of return following neurorrhaphy.[3,54]

Restoration of opposition of the thumb by tendon transfer is the most commonly employed tendon transfer in the hand. Restoration of opposition (i.e., the development of true pulp-to-pulp pinch between the thumb and index finger or the thumb and index and long fingers) is required only in those patients in whom satisfactory sensibility is likely to be achieved. These patients, then, require precision pinch activities, and true opposition is likely to be required. In patients with limited motor units or poor sensibility, pulp-to-pulp transfer (i.e., restoration of short flexor action) is functionally as important as restoration of true opposition.

Early articles on restoration of opposition of the thumb all dealt with the completely intrinsic-minus thumb. Methods of restoration in these cases were aimed at bringing about short flexor action rather than true opposition of the thumb, as pointed out by Bunnell.[37,38,43,51,55,60] Opposition is a composite of two motions: (1) rotation of the thumb into pronation so that the pulp surfaces of the thumb and index finger face one another, and (2) abduction or lifting of the thumb away from the palm of the hand (palmar abduction). This combination of the two motions is true opposition. In order to render the thumb maximally functional, not only must the thumb be positioned in true opposition, but it must have, in addition, short flexor action so that it can be brought against the fingers with reasonable power through the MP and carpometacarpal joints of the thumb. So-called adductor transfers for power pinch are really not necessary because the adductor pollicis functions as a supinator of the thumb and is a direct antagonist to the pronatory effects that are being restored. A reasonable compromise is a short flexorplasty rather than an adductorplasty (Curtis RM: personal communication). In order to have a maximally functional thumb, the patient should be able to put the thumb into opposition, but also should have short flexor action so that the thumb can be brought against the fingers with power.[63] Without satisfactory function of the short flexor muscles or a short flexor substitute, the extensor pollicis longus becomes the only satisfactory substitute for adductor action. This muscle, through its secondary actions, brings the thumb out of opposition into the supinated position, in addition to bringing about adduction of the first metacarpal.[39] Littler has pointed out that the extensor pollicis longus is the direct antagonist of opposition of the thumb, and although satisfactory opposition may be achieved by any type of opposition transfer, collapse of this opposed position will occur if the extensor pollicis longus is used to substitute for the short flexor adductor group of muscles.[34]

The literature on opposition transfer and the reasons for its failure are most interesting. As pointed out initially by Mayer, the most absolute reason for failure is contracture of the first web space, either the adduction type or the adduction-supination type[40] (Fig. 39-1). In both of these situations, the thumb

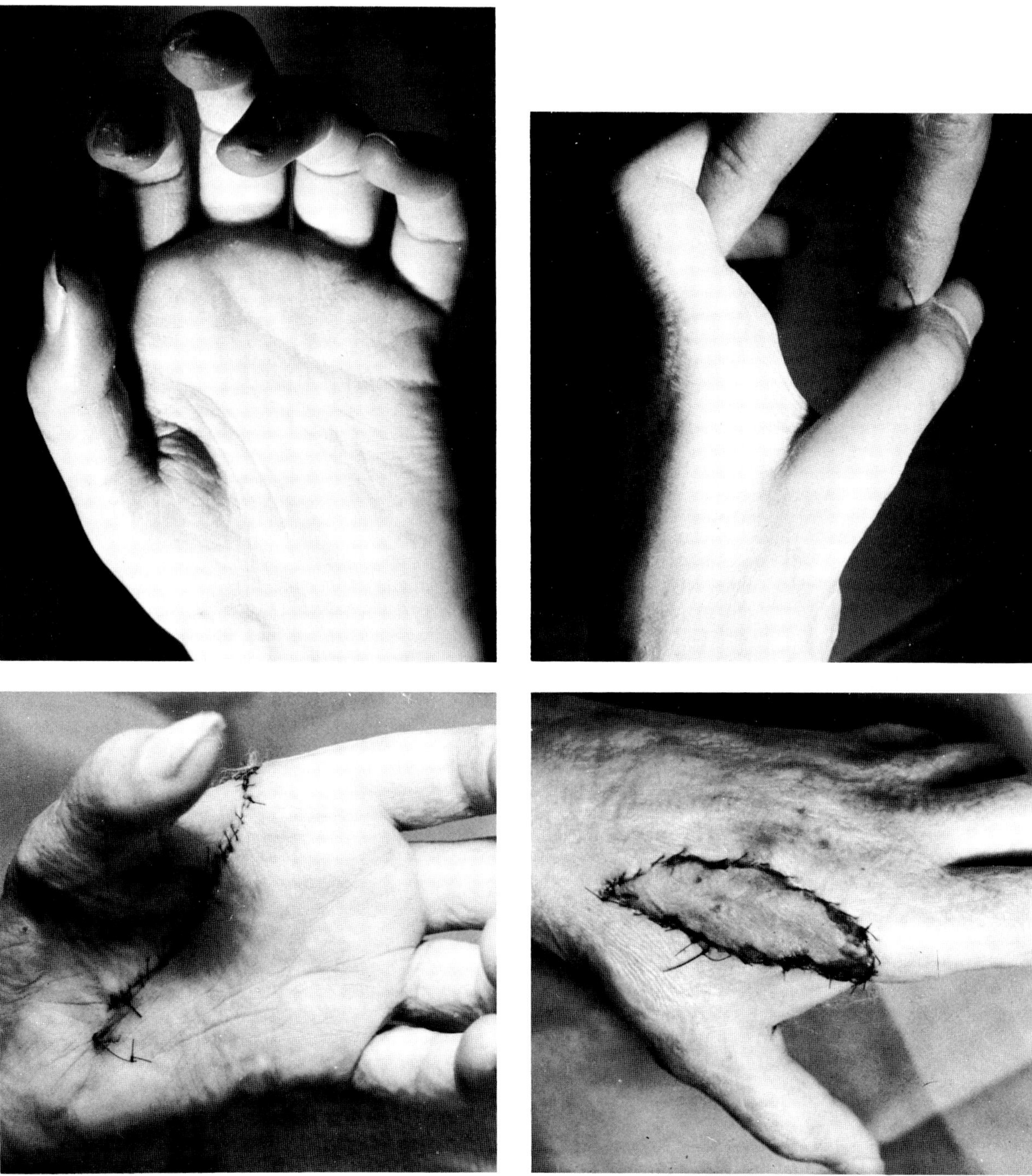

Fig. 39-1. Direct injury to the thenar area, in addition to median nerve laceration, resulted in a significant contracture of the thumb web space, which required release prior to opponensplasty. Position of the thumb was maintained by a threaded Steinmann pin, and a dorsal rotation flap with skin graft allowed good release of the first web space. In certain severe situations, osteotomy of the first metacarpal or excision of the trapezium may be indicated to satisfactorily position the thumb prior to opposition transfer.

cannot really be placed into the fully opposed position passively at the time of transfer. To perform an opponensplasty in the face of a web space contracture indicates either failure to appreciate the problem or to understand what a supination contracture is in terms of rotational deformity in the thumb.[28] If there is a persisting supination contracture, regardless of the motor or pulley used, the operation will bring about only short flexor action without true opposition.[9,21,25,42] If true opposition is to be obtained, the thumb needs to be brought away from the fingers, in addition to being rotated on its long axis into pronation.

Another cause of failure in opposition transfer is inaccurate evaluation of the strength of the individual motor to be used for transfer. If a patient has an isolated laceration of the median nerve, the radial and ulnar innervated musculature should certainly be graded normal or near normal, and we assume that such will be the case. However, in certain disease states or in spotty lesions associated with brachial plexus injury, the motor in question may not have normal strength and, in fact, may not provide sufficient power to position the thumb.[28] Much of our experience in determining individual muscle strength and the basic principles of tendon transfer came from a disease that we no longer see much of—poliomyelitis.

Another area of some concern is the use of reinnervated muscles in an opposition transfer. We are all partial to the use of the flexor digitorum superficialis of the ring finger as the motor for an opponensplasty. In an undamaged state, this muscle tendon unit is an excellent functional transfer and has certainly withstood the test of time.[22,30,33] However, in proximal nerve injury with reinnervation of extrinsic flexors, its use to achieve satisfactory opposition through a transfer should be discouraged. Reinnervated flexor digitorum superficialis muscles lack the strength and certainly the control to bring about satisfactory opposition of the thumb.[3] In summary, then, the two major causes for failure of opposition transfer are the persistence of a contracture, either adduction or adduction-supination, and the use of an inadequate motor for transfer.[1,2]

When choosing a specific type of opposition transfer for an individual patient, I think it is mandatory for the hand surgeon to consider what the situation is that requires the opposition transfer. Is this an isolated peripheral nerve injury or is there associated damage to muscle tendon units and to bone? Is there more than one nerve damaged? What is the level of injury? Has there been direct injury to the soft tissues and perhaps the bone of the thumb itself, in addition to its extrinsics or intrinsics? No single opposition transfer will work for all cases requiring opponensplasty because of the wide variety in patient requirements and associated deficits. In addition to having motors of adequate strength with satisfactory amplitude, a reasonable bed, and tissue equilibrium, the transfer should be expected to do only one other thing and that is to bring about opposition of the thumb. One of the precepts of Steindler[59] and Mayer[40] not often considered is that the deficit created by the transfer should be acceptable to the patient. The use of the abductor digiti minimi for opposition transfer in a high median nerve injury will bring about satisfactory position of the thumb. However, the removal of this muscle tendon unit from the ulnar side of the hand will further compromise the already weakened strength on the flexor side, and I think this would be unacceptable to the patient.

Royle-Thompson Opponensplasty

The most frequently used motor for opponensplasty of the thumb is the flexor digitorum superficialis of either the ring or long finger. The so-called Royle-Thompson opposition transfer uses the motor from the ring finger as described by Royle.[55] Royle, however, used no pulley for the transfer; instead, he passed the motor up the sheath of the flexor pollicis longus and attached the split superficialis tendon to the superficial head of the flexor pollicis brevis and opponens pollicis, respectively. Thompson's modification of this procedure was to use a pulley and a more superficial location of the transfer. The pulley for this procedure is the distal end of the transverse carpal ligament and the ulnar border of the palmar fascia.[62] The route of the transferred digitorum superficialis is subcutaneous across the palm to the area of the thumb MP joint. A dual attachment is made: one through a drill hole in the neck of the first metacarpal, while the other slip of the superficialis is drawn over the MP joint and sutured into the hood mechanism over the proximal phalanx. Three incisions are required for this procedure.

Some thought needs to be given to the removal of the superficialis tendon from the ring finger. Both a persistent flexion contracture of the PIP joint and swan-neck deformity have been reported in as many as 8 percent of the cases in which the superficialis was removed from a finger for a transfer.[29] A volar zigzag or transverse incision is used to cut the dual attachments of the flexor digitorum superficialis in the finger. The distal tags should be long enough so that the volar plate may be reinforced with a few nonabsorbable sutures to these tags. To remove the flexor digitorum superficialis from its insertion into the middle phalanx is to invite a swan-neck deformity. An additional palmar incision will probably be required so that the distal union of the superficialis can be longitudinally opened completely and the flexor digitorum superficialis freed from its loop about the flexor digitorum profundus. The perforation of the flexor digitorum superficialis by the profundus occurs beneath the fibrous (A2) pulley of the proximal phalanx, and it is best to operate distally and proximally to this, leaving the pulley intact.[27,31] This is the usual or classic description of removal of the flexor digitorum superficialis.

An easier method than to operate in the finger is to remove the tendon through an incision in the distal palm only. When using the flexor digitorum superficialis for an opposition transfer, there is adequate tendon length without going into the finger. Generally an incision at the base of the finger will allow opening the flexor tendon sheath between the MP (A1) pulley and the wide proximal phalangeal (A2) pulley. The superficialis begins to divide here and is still located superficial to the profundus. If the superficialis is divided here, the problem with the decussation is avoided and the volar area of the PIP joint is not violated.[45]

At this point another incision is made immediately distal to the carpal tunnel, toward the ulnar side, so that the palmar fascia can be retracted radially. The flexor digitorum superficialis to the ring finger is identified at the distal level of the carpal tunnel. An incision is then made over the dorsum of the MP joint of the thumb and a subcutaneous tunnel is created between the incision in the wrist and the area of the thumb MP joint. The flexor digitorum superficialis is delivered from the finger into the palmar incision and passed subcutaneously across the palm of the hand to the incision on the dorsum of the thumb MP joint. If done in the classic fashion, a drill hole is created through the neck of the first metacarpal and one slip of the superficialis is pulled through this, exiting on the ulnar aspect of the thumb (Fig. 39-2). The second slip of the superficialis is passed superficially over the extensor hood of the MP joint, under the ulnar lateral band of the extensor mechanism

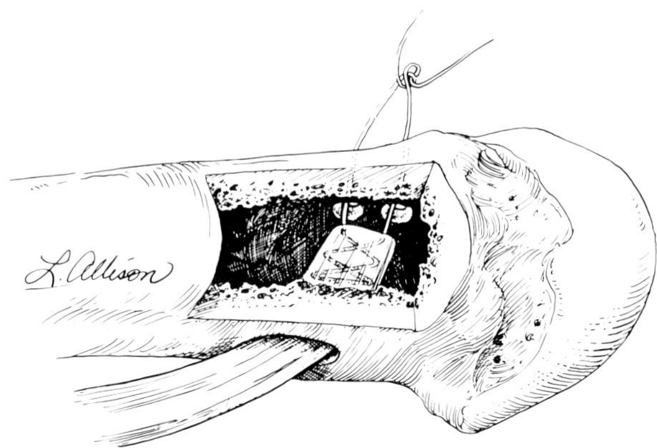

Fig. 39-2. Method of bony attachment of a tendon using internal sutures rather than external pull-out techniques. The opposite cortex from the area of entrance of the tendon is used to anchor the stitch. This, however, does require an incision on the side opposite to the tendon entrance for exposure of the cortex and tying of the suture.

of the thumb, and out through a small transverse incision immediately dorsal to the lateral band. The two ends are then sutured together. Prior to this, the tourniquet should be released and hemostasis obtained. Before suturing the attachment of the transfer, all wounds should be closed, with the exception of the one in the area of the thumb MP joint.

The correct tension is always a major consideration in opposition transfer. In this particular transfer, it is not terribly important because of the enormous amplitude of the flexor digitorum superficialis. However, the tension should be adjusted primarily with the distal attachment in this case. If the reverse is done, no power will be transferred to the extensor pollicis longus or to the proximal phalanx of the thumb, and the transfer will act only on the first metacarpal. Tension is adjusted so that the thumb is in full opposition with the wrist in neutral position. This method of attachment makes the thumb MP joint extremely stable, with some abduction of the joint and some increase in power to the extensor pollicis longus. This transfer courses in line with the fibers of the flexor pollicis brevis superficial head and thus reproduces the action of this muscle. It does not give as wide abduction to the thumb as some other methods, but it is an extremely useful transfer for the completely intrinsic-minus thumb (combined median and ulnar palsy) and in situations with limited motors available for transfer.[26,53]

Classic Bunnell Opponensplasty

With this information as a background, other possible opposition transfers can be considered. In 1938 Bunnell established what have become the standard requirements for restoration of true opposition of the thumb. His precepts were that the transfer should come from the areas of the pisiform to the thumb MP joint subcutaneously. The transfer should have a fixed pulley in the area of the pisiform, the transfer essentially being in line with the fibers of the abductor pollicis brevis. Bunnell's method of attachment distally was through a drill hole on the dorsal ulnar aspect of the proximal phalanx. The transfer thus passed distal to the axis of motion of the MP joint and thereby acted as an MP joint flexor in addition to being a rotator-abductor.[11] This flexion may not be desirable in an operation in which the main function is to position the thumb for use where true short flexor action is already available from other muscles within the hand.

The operative technique of Bunnell is as follows. The method of removal of the superficialis from the ring finger is as described on page 1421. At this point, a word should be said regarding the removal of the flexor digitorum superficialis of the long finger. Removal of this muscle has been done to restore opposition to the thumb, but I believe that this creates too much deficit on the flexor side of the hand. The superficialis to the long finger is an extremely powerful muscle with individual control. I believe that its removal creates an almost unacceptable deficit for the patient in terms of power grip. I suggest that other transfers be used rather than using the superficialis to the long finger. Once the ring finger superficialis is removed, another incision is made proximal to the wrist over the ulnar artery and nerve area. In this fashion the flexor digitorum superficialis to the ring finger can be readily found proximally and the tendon of the flexor carpi ulnaris identified. Three to four centimeters of flexor carpi ulnaris tendon are exposed proximal to the pisiform, and approximately one-half of the flexor carpi ulnaris tendon is divided at this proximal level; that is, a 3- to 4-cm strip of tendon is separated from the remaining portion of the intact flexor carpi ulnaris longitudinally, leaving it attached distally to the pisiform. An incision is then made on the dorsum of the thumb and a subcutaneous tunnel created across the palm from the thumb to the area of the pisiform. The flexor digitorum superficialis of the ring is then delivered into the wrist incision and passed subcutaneously from the pisiform to the thumb incision. The distally based slip of the flexor carpi ulnaris is then sutured to the area of the pisiform to create a fixed loop through which the flexor digitorum superficialis can easily pass passively. Care should be taken not to make this loop too tight, making free motion of the flexor superficialis impossible. It seems much easier to simply loop the flexor digitorum superficialis around the flexor carpi ulnaris prior to its subcutaneous passage across the palm. However, the flexor carpi ulnaris soon becomes ineffective as a pulley, and the transfer then becomes incapable of positioning the thumb.[28] This occurs secondary to proximal migration of the point of direction change of the flexor digitorum superficialis (Fig. 39-3B). Other fixed pulleys in this area that might be used with the flexor digitorum superficialis transfer are the canal of Guyon, immediately radial to the flexor carpi ulnaris,[4] and a window created in the transverse carpal ligament.[58] Also, the slip of flexor carpi ulnaris that was developed to create the pulley loop may instead be sutured to the tendon of the extensor carpi ulnaris close to its attachment to the fifth metacarpal rather than to the pisiform.[56] All of these techniques are valuable and can be selected on the basis of individual preference and local conditions.

The method of attachment distally in the classic Bunnell transfer is through a drill hole in the proximal phalanx on its dorsal ulnar aspect. The tendon is passed subcutaneously across the palm, over the dorsum of the MP joint, but distal to

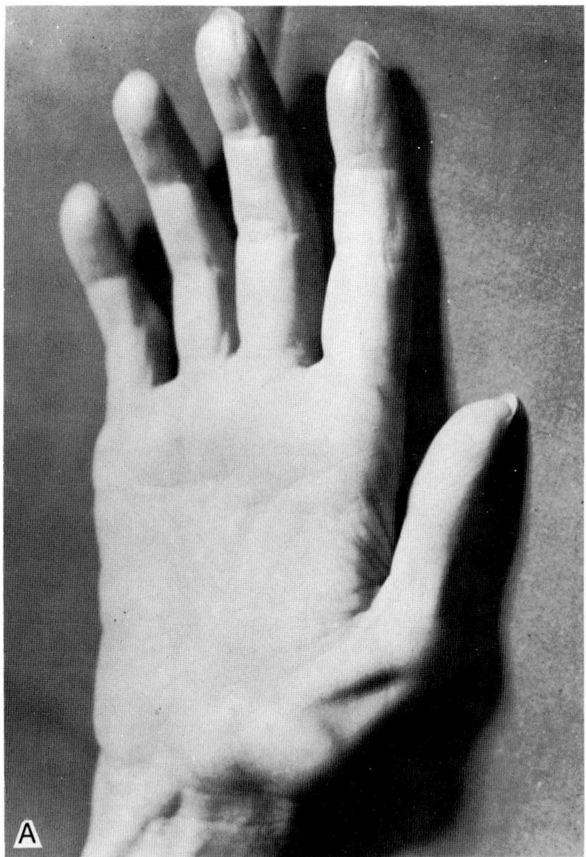

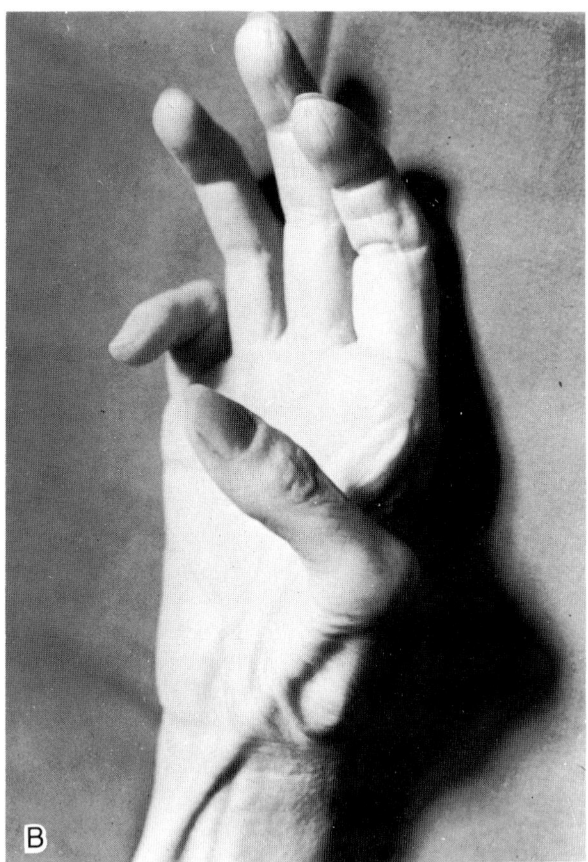

Fig. 39-3. (A&B) A classic Bunnell transfer using the superficialis motor. However, there was no fixed pulley in the area of the pisiform and the transfer was too volar, acting more as a flexor of the MP joint than as a real abductor. Satisfactory opposition needs a fixed pulley at or near the area of the pisiform.

the axis of motion of the joint. A drill hole is created from the dorsal ulnar aspect of the proximal phalanx to the midaxial line radially. This drill hole should be large enough to accommodate at least one slip of the flexor digitorum superficialis. Once the tendon is passed through the drill hole, it may be sutured upon itself, anchored to the periosteum on the radial aspect of the proximal phalanx, or held with a pull-out suture over a dental roll. Tension here is critical. At the completion of the operation, the thumb should rest in full opposition, with the wrist in neutral position.

Methods of Distal Attachment

Prior to discussing other transfers, the methods of distal attachment should be examined in some detail (Fig. 39-4). Both the Bunnell and Royle-Thompson operations use bony attachments. This is probably not necessary and complicates the procedure of opposition transfer unnecessarily. Littler feels that if the function of the abductor pollicis brevis can be duplicated by the opposition transfer, satisfactory function will result. Because of this, the transferred tendon is simply interwoven into the tendon of the abductor pollicis brevis muscle.[34] The Riordan attachment uses interweaving of the transfer into the abductor pollicis brevis tendon, but continuing distally into the hood of the thumb MP joint and to the extensor pollicis longus tendon over the proximal phalanx.[53] This course markedly increases the power of extension of the interphalangeal joint of the thumb. Without a functional flexor pollicis longus, a hyperextension deformity of the interphalangeal joint will likely result with this method of attachment. Brand's method of distal attachment interweaves one slip of the superficialis through the tendon of the abductor pollicis brevis and continues on to the extensor pollicis longus, similiar to Riordan's technique. The other slip, however, comes across the extensor mechanism subcutaneously and is attached to the area of the adductor pollicis. This method brings about considerable stability of the MP joint and is especially indicated in a combined median and ulnar nerve palsy.[4,49]

Phalen and Miller Opponensplasty (Extensor Carpi Ulnaris)

Other methods of distal attachment include the extensor pollicis brevis attachment.[32,50] Bunnell mentioned tenotomy of this muscle tendon unit and the use of the normal attachment of the extensor pollicis brevis as a method of attaching an

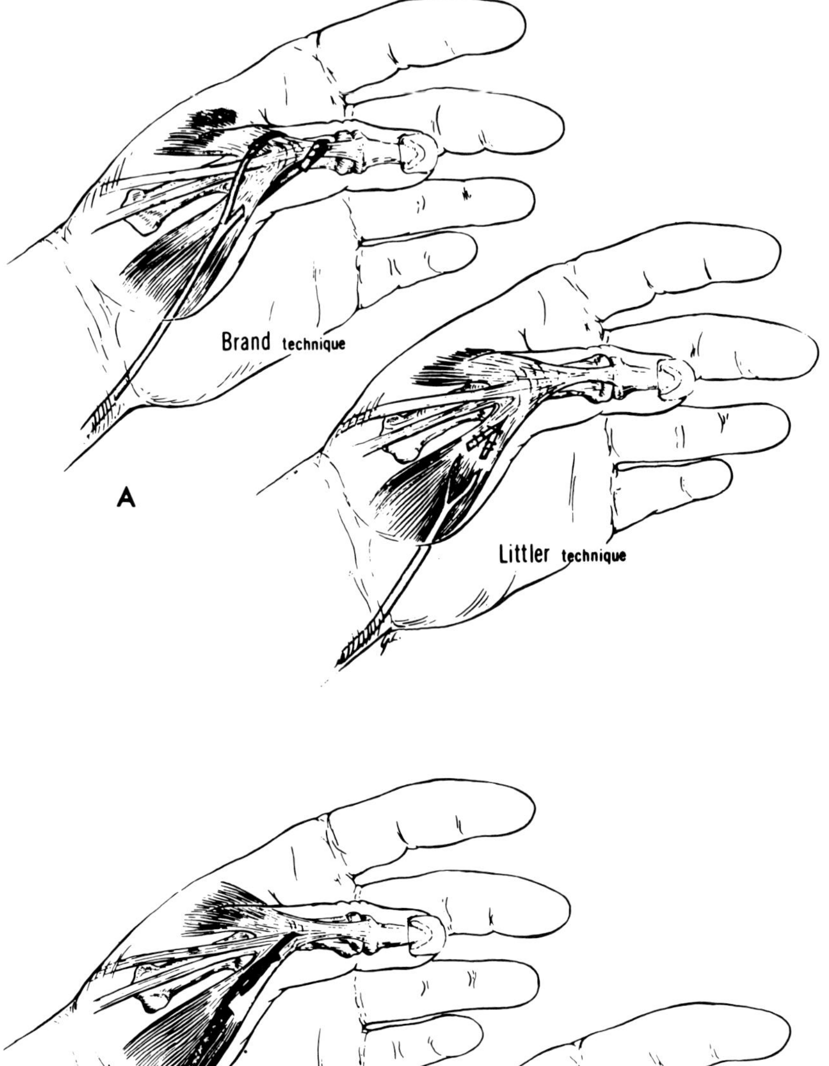

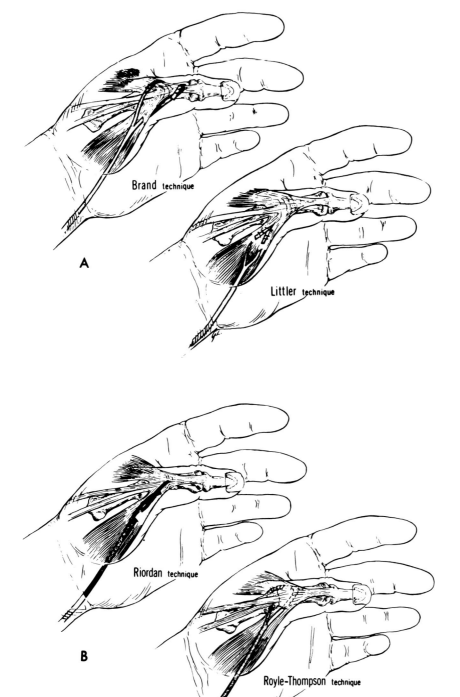

Fig. 39-4. Techniques of distal attachment as described by Brand, Littler, Riordan, and Royle-Thompson. (From Curtis,[19] with permission.)

opposition transfer to the thumb.[11] Using this technique, the extensor pollicis brevis is divided through a short incision at its musculotendinous junction proximal to the first dorsal compartment. An incision in the area of the MP joint is then used to expose the tendon immediately proximal to the MP joint, and the tendon is pulled distally and delivered into the wound. A subcutaneous tunnel is created from its attachment to the proximal phalanx toward the pisiform. Through another incision, the extensor carpi ulnaris is exposed immediately proximal to its attachment into the fifth metacarpal, cut, and freed proximally so that a subcutaneous passage can be made around the ulnar border of the wrist. Depending on the length of the extensor pollicis brevis tendon, the juncture will probably be in the area of the pisiform. This can be a difficult place in which to obtain a gliding tendon junction, but it does emphasize the subcutaneous border of the forearm as the pulley for tendon transfer, bringing about opposition of the thumb.[24] This border is used as a pulley for other transfers, notably the extensor indicis proprius and the extensor digiti minimi opponensplasties. In addition to being an awkward location for a tendon juncture, another problem may develop. The extensor pollicis brevis may slide volarly to the ulnar side of the MP joint so that it no longer acts as an extensor of the joint, acting as a flexor instead. This dorsal instability has been reported to be alleviated by looping the extensor pollicis brevis tendon around the tendon of the extensor pollicis longus prior to its attachment to the motor unit. This seems to provide better stability for the MP joint and prevent the flexion deformity.[31]

Removal of the extensor carpi ulnaris from the wrist to motor an opposition transfer may not be without problems. The extensor carpi ulnaris is primarily an ulnar deviator of the wrist, balancing the radial deviation function of the extensor carpi radialis brevis and extensor carpi radialis longus. Removing the extensor carpi ulnaris for an opposition transfer may result in a radially deviated wrist, especially if the flexor carpi ulnaris is not normal. It would be unwise to remove the extensor carpi ulnaris for a tendon transfer in the presence of a paralyzed or nonfunctional flexor carpi ulnaris muscle tendon unit.[66]

Another combination of motor and distal attachment is the use of the extensor carpi radialis longus as a motor prolonged by the extensor pollicis longus tendon passed around the ulnar border of the wrist.[31] In my opinion, both the extensor carpi ulnaris–extensor pollicis brevis and extensor carpi radialis longus–extensor pollicis longus combination transfers are wasteful of motors that perform useful functions and also place undesirable forces on the MP joint of the thumb. It seems that the distal attachment techniques of Littler, Brand, and Rior-

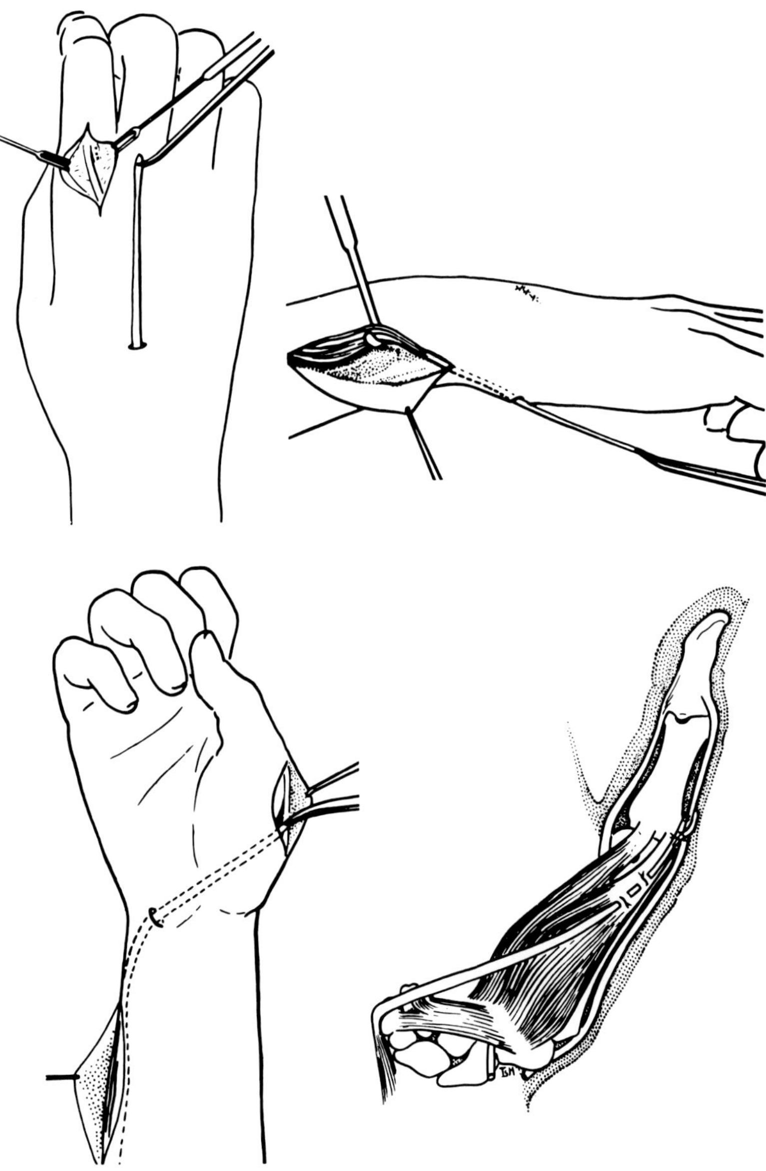

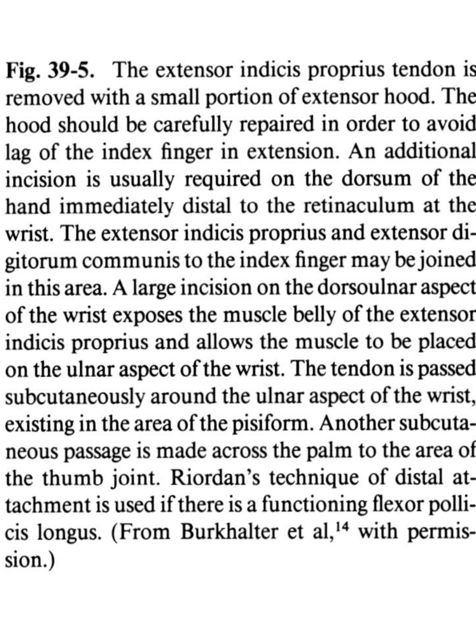

Fig. 39-5. The extensor indicis proprius tendon is removed with a small portion of extensor hood. The hood should be carefully repaired in order to avoid lag of the index finger in extension. An additional incision is usually required on the dorsum of the hand immediately distal to the retinaculum at the wrist. The extensor indicis proprius and extensor digitorum communis to the index finger may be joined in this area. A large incision on the dorsoulnar aspect of the wrist exposes the muscle belly of the extensor indicis proprius and allows the muscle to be placed on the ulnar aspect of the wrist. The tendon is passed subcutaneously around the ulnar aspect of the wrist, existing in the area of the pisiform. Another subcutaneous passage is made across the palm to the area of the thumb joint. Riordan's technique of distal attachment is used if there is a functioning flexor pollicis longus. (From Burkhalter et al,[14] with permission.)

dan all reproduce the function of the abductor pollicis brevis, which is, after all, what the surgeon is trying to restore.

Proprius Extensor Tendon Opponensplasties

Recently both proprius tendon transfers have become popular because of the frequency of damage to muscle tendon units in the distal volar forearm. Both the extensor indicis proprius[12,14] (Fig. 39-5) and the extensor digiti minimi[57,61] (Fig. 39-6) have been described for restoration of opposition. These motors are both available in volar wrist injuries and combined median and ulnar nerve palsies, either high or low, and require only a single muscle tendon unit without a tendon graft. They do not significantly reduce remaining hand function and the techniques of both are very similar. Short incisions are made over the MP joint of either the index or small finger. In the small finger, the presence of an extensor digitorum communis slip from the ring finger should be verified prior to removal of the extensor digiti minimi. Another short incision is made over the base of the fifth metacarpal, and a more extensive exposure is required over the distal forearm along its ulnar aspect. The extensor digiti minimi is brought into the more proximal incision, and a subcutaneous tunnel is created around the ulnar border of the forearm across the palm to the area of the thumb

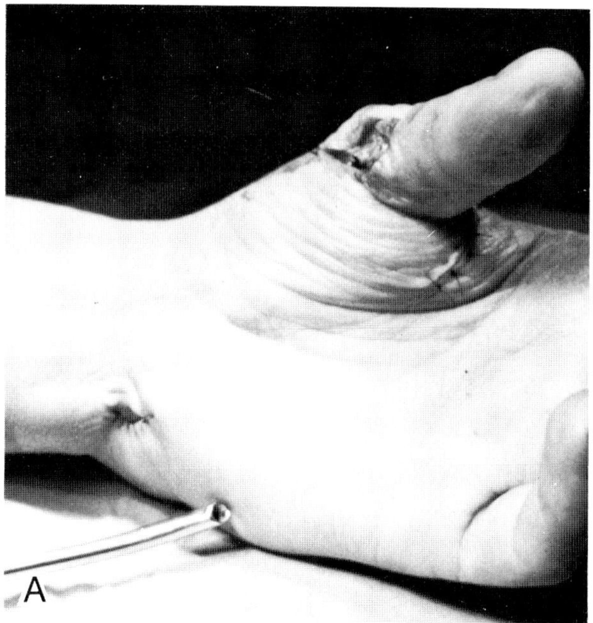

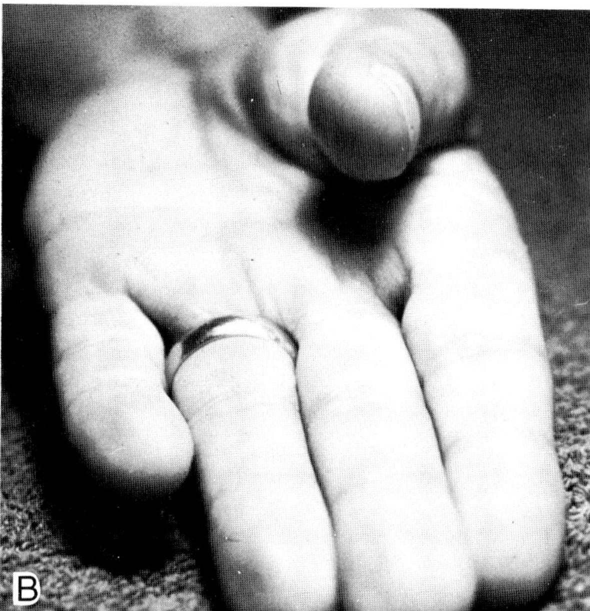

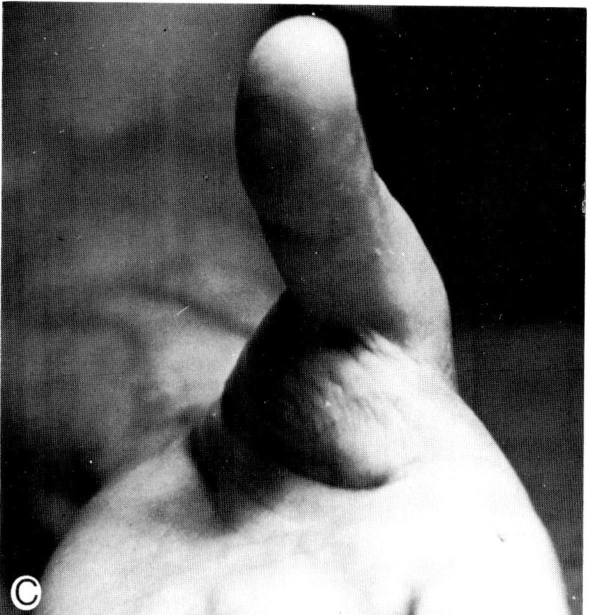

Fig. 39-6. Extensor digiti minimi transfer for opposition of the thumb. Note position at the time of surgery **(A)** and postoperative active abduction and rotation of the thumb **(B&C)** even with an immobile wrist.

MP joint. The method of attachment, as described by Schneider, uses Riordan's technique. As noted previously, the pulley for this transfer is the ulnar aspect of the forearm.[57]

In using the extensor indicis proprius, the tendon is removed along with a small portion of extensor hood. The removal of a portion of the extensor hood allows lengthening of the extensor indicis proprius tendon. The hood excision should taper from the tendon distally into the hood mechanism. This defect in the hood is carefully repaired with interrupted nonabsorbable sutures, an important step in preventing subsequent extensor lag by maintaining normal tension within the hood mechanism.[10]

An additional incision over the dorsum of the hand to separate the extensor indicis from the index communis is frequently required. A larger dorsal ulnar incision is made in the distal forearm. This is used to displace the tendon into the forearm on its ulnar aspect. An additional incision is usually made in the area of the pisiform as well as an incision in the area of the thumb MP joint. The tendon is then passed through the ulnar aspect of the wrist across the MP joint. The attachment is made by Riordan's method, and the pulley again is the ulnar aspect of the forearm.[14]

All of the previously discussed opposition transfers require pulleys, whereas the following one does not.

Palmaris Longus Opponensplasty (Camitz)

A beautifully simple yet effective operation that brings about abduction of the thumb away from the fingers (palmar abduction) is transfer of the palmaris longus to the tendon of the abductor pollicis brevis. The palmaris longus will obviously not reach into the area of the MP joint of the thumb. The muscle tendon unit is prolonged by a strip of palmar fascia as originally described by Camitz[15] (Fig. 39-7). The area of the volar surface of the distal forearm, wrist, and palm are opened as for a generous carpal tunnel release. The palmaris longus tendon is exposed in the wrist, and the palmar skin flaps are elevated to expose the distal palmaris longus in continuity with the palmar fascia. A strip of palmar fascia in continuity with the palmaris longus is then removed. A subcutaneous tunnel is created from the volar surface of the distal forearm to the ten-

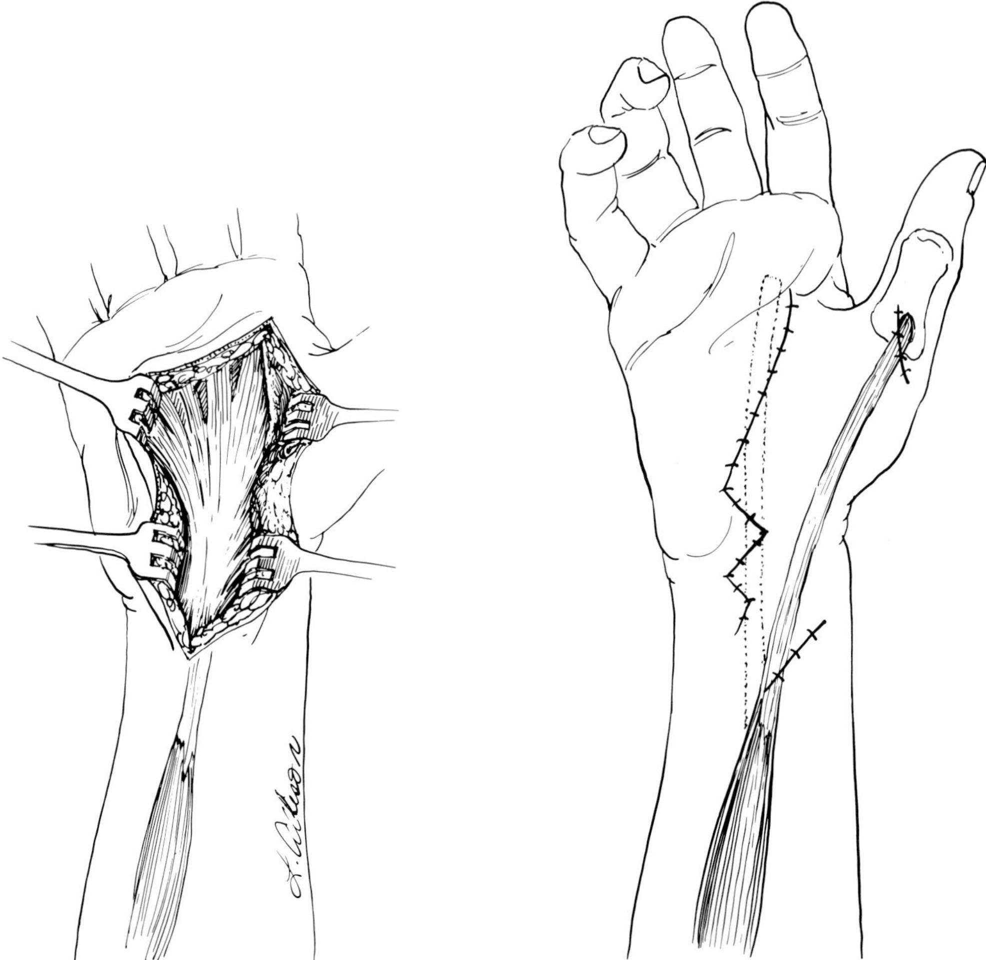

Fig. 39-7. The Camitz transfer in which an elongation of the palmaris longus via the palmar fascia is attached to the area of the abductor pollicis brevis. The subcutaneous tunnel for this transfer runs in a direct line from the wrist to the thumb.

don of the abductor pollicis brevis. The palmar fascia is then pulled into the short incision in the area of the thumb MP joint and sutured into position. The tendon should pull in a straight line from the muscle belly to the thumb MP joint. This transfer does not bring about much in the way of rotation or pronation as the standard transfer, but does result in good palmar abduction of the thumb. The transfer loss is certainly acceptable and the function is reasonable. The transfer has its greatest application in severe carpal tunnel syndromes with thenar paralysis and atrophy (Fig. 39-8). The procedure can be carried out simultaneously with carpal tunnel release.[7,36] Because of the proximity of the palmaris longus to the median nerve, its use in

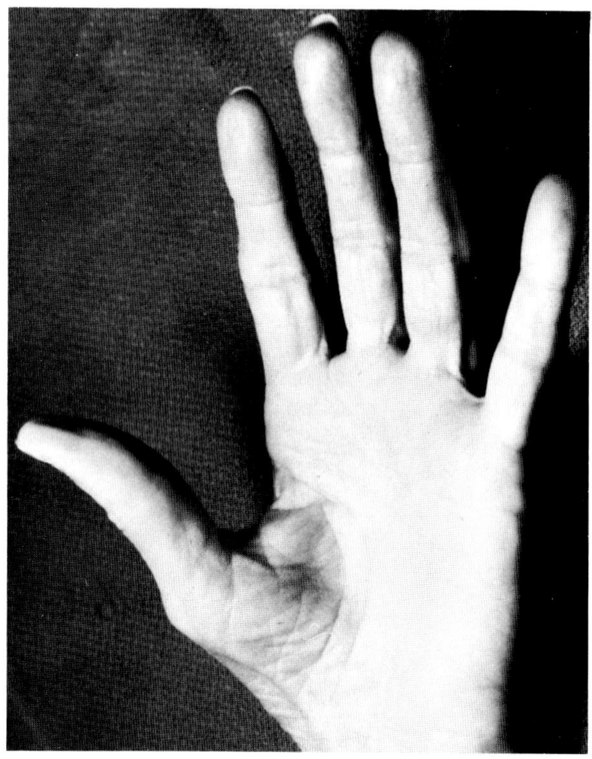

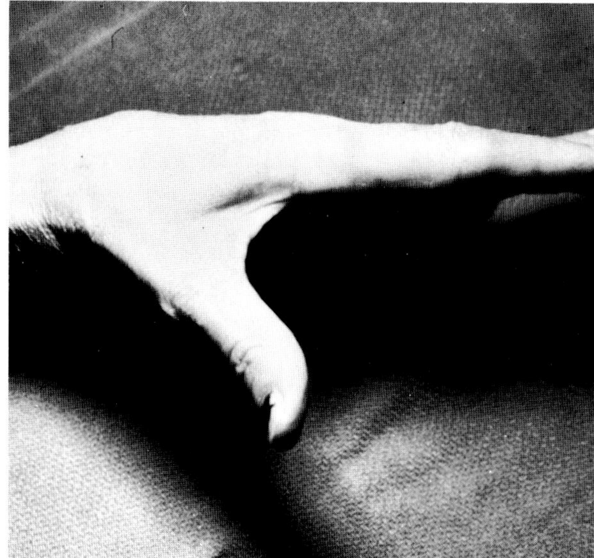

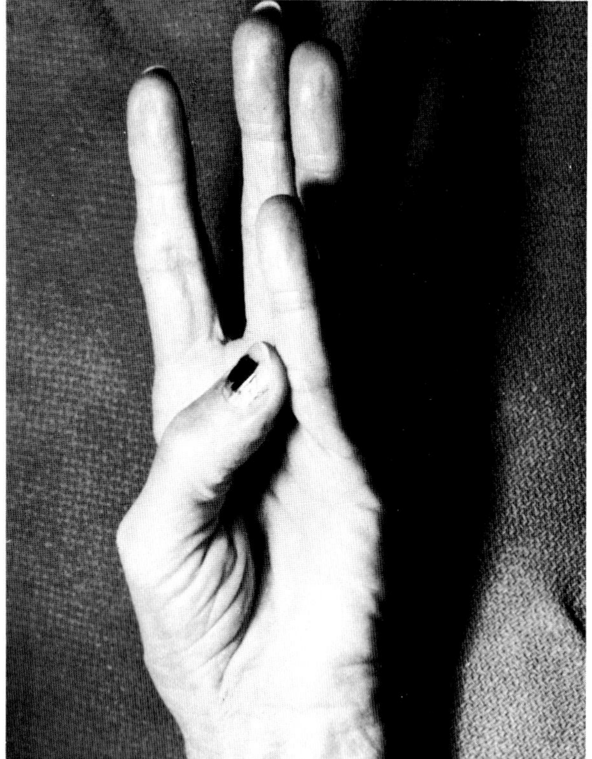

Fig. 39-8. A patient with scapholunate dissociation and long-standing median nerve compression with thenar atrophy, treated at the time of carpal tunnel release by Camitz transfer. There was excellent improvement in abduction of the thumb, but pronation is being supplied by a weak flexor pollicis brevis.

traumatic median nerve injuries at the wrist or distal forearm is limited. Similarly, the palmaris longus is denervated in the more proximal nerve injuries.

Because it brings about only palmar abduction of the thumb, the Camitz transfer is not a true opposition transfer. If the superficial head of the flexor pollicis brevis is innervated by the ulnar nerve, the patient may have satisfactory pronation of the thumb, and adding the Camitz transfer to this may be all that is needed to provide good opposition.

If the transfer is used concomitantly with a carpal tunnel release, as is the usual case, wrist flexion to reduce tension on the opposition transfer may compromise the carpal tunnel release in the postoperative period.

Hypothenar Muscle Opponensplasty (Huber)

Restoration of opposition of the thumb by transfer of an ulnar innervated intrinsic muscle was first described by Huber[27] and later by Nicolaysen,[44] and popularized by Littler and Cooley[35] (Fig. 39-9). The abductor digiti minimi muscle transfer is predicated on the fact that this muscle can survive and function on a thin neurovascular pedicle with almost its entire origin, and certainly its entire insertion, detached. The distal tendon is exposed by a midaxial incision over the proximal phalanx of the small finger ulnarly. The incision continues radially at the level of the distal palmar crease and then immediately radial to the hypothenar bulk. Proximally, the incision curves again ulnarly so as to cross the distal wrist crease. A separate incision is made over the thumb MP joint and a large subcutaneous tunnel created between the thumb area and that area immediately proximal to the pisiform. The flaps are raised and the ulnar digital nerve is carefully identified, elevated, and protected during this operation. The ulnar nerve and artery at the wrist are defined and traced distally until the branches can be seen entering the musculature of the abductor digiti minimi. Only after the neurovascular bundle has been isolated is the attachment of this muscle to the pisiform divided. At this point the muscle is held by its neurovascular pedicle and its attachment to the flexor carpi ulnaris (Fig. 39-10). The muscle is rotated 180 degrees on its long axis, much as one would close a book, and pulled through the subcutaneous tunnel into the thumb area. The distal tendon is then attached to the abductor pollicis brevis tendon only.

In a more recent report,[64] the abductor digiti quinti is not detached from the pisiform and neurovascular structures are not exposed proximally. This limits mobility of this muscle unit proximally and moves the new origin more distally so that it acts more as a short flexor than as a true opponensplasty.

Other Opponensplasties

Another intrinsic opposition replacement, not done frequently in this country, is transfer of the adductor pollicis to the tendon of the superficial head of the flexor pollicis brevis.

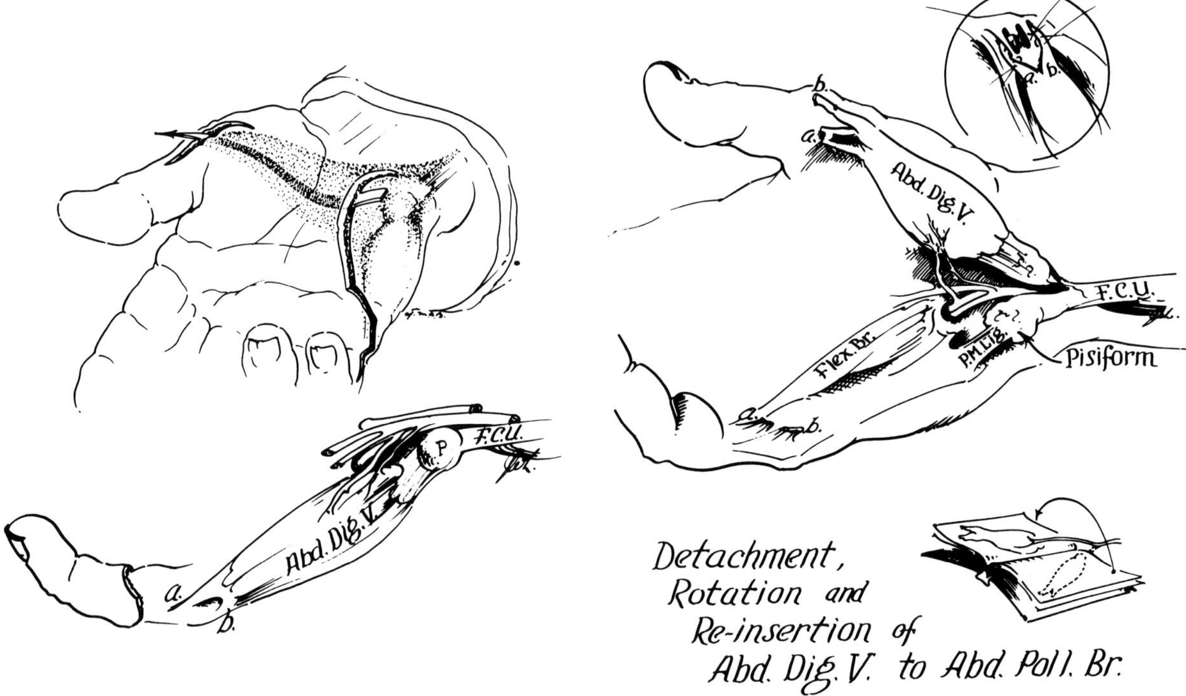

Fig. 39-9. Two incisions are required to expose and transfer the abductor digiti minimi. The neurovascular structures enter the muscle on its deep and radial aspect. The muscle is freed from its fascial attachments to the other hypothenar muscles and from its origin on the pisiform. The origin proximally is the flexor carpi ulnaris (FCU) tendon. The muscle tendon unit is rotated 180 degrees on its long axis and passed between the palmar skin and palmar fascia to the area of the thumb MP joint. The distal attachment is into the tendon of the abductor pollicis brevis muscle. (From Littler and Cooley,[35] with permission.)

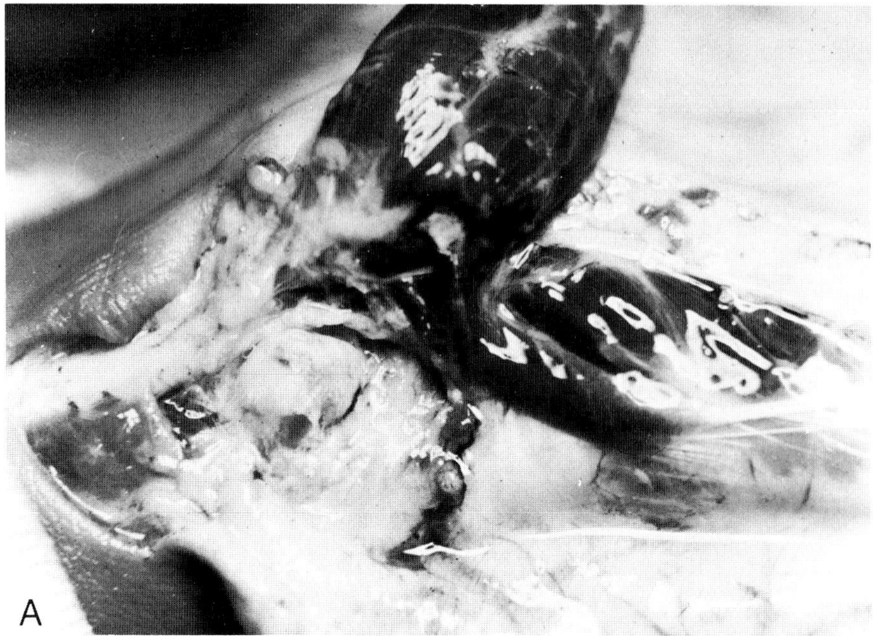

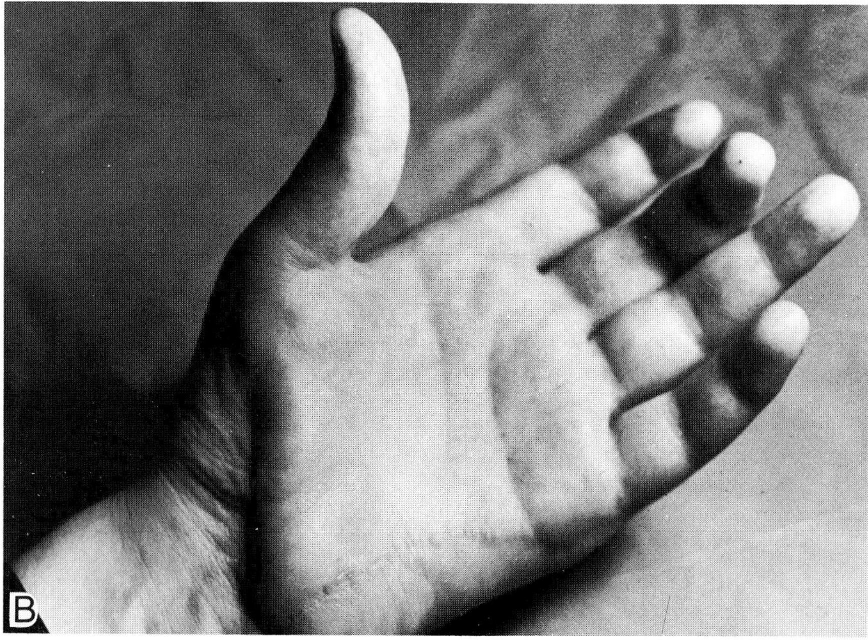

Fig. 39-10. Abductor digiti minimi opponensplasty. **(A)** Freeing of the abductor digiti minimi from the pisiform, leaving as its only remaining attachment the flexor carpi ulnaris, as well as the neurovascular bundle to its base. Satisfactory restoration of function has been achieved **(B&C)**; note that the direction of pull is really from the area of the pisiform in this particular case. *(Figure continues.)*

DeVecchi[20] described this procedure. Orticochea,[48] likewise, described the use of an innervated portion of the flexor pollicis brevis to bring about opposition to the thumb. The adductor pollicis transfer requires an extensive palmar incision, extending from the adductor attachment to the thumb into the palm in the area of the third metacarpal and then proximally toward the thumb. The carpal tunnel should be opened for exposure and protection of the median nerve and its branches. The adductor is released from the thumb, freed from the deep head of the flexor pollicis brevis, brought out from beneath the flexor tendons to the index finger, and passed over the tendons of the index finger, as well as the common neurovascular bundle to the adjacent sides of the index and long fingers. The transfer is then placed superficial to the flexor pollicis longus and attached to the flexor pollicis brevis superficial head only. This transfer restores function of the flexor pollicis brevis and gives some rotation to the thumb but does not bring about true opposition.[47]

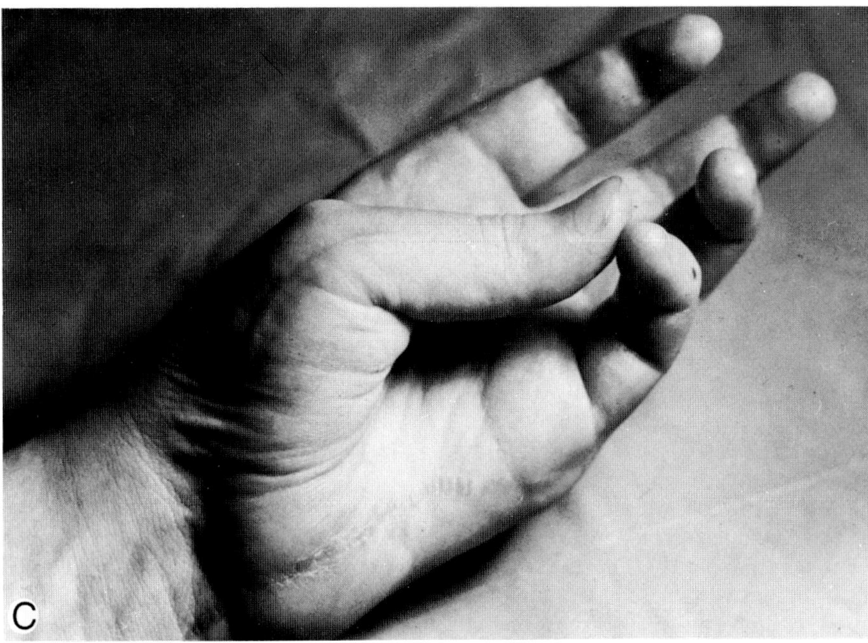

Fig. 39-10 *(Continued).*

Importance of Flexor Pollicis Brevis Power

Opposition of the thumb requires only minimal power to position the thumb for function. To make the thumb maximally functional, however, short flexor action is required in addition to opposition. In most isolated median nerve injuries, the adductor pollicis and at least a portion of the flexor pollicis brevis are functional in addition to the normal extrinsic motors. If short flexor action is present, the thumb may be brought against the fingers with power. Two different motions are required: opposition of the thumb to position the thumb for action, and then short flexor action for power, either prehension or power grip. If both opposition and short flexor action are absent, both functions need to be restored. This will require two transfers or a single transfer to restore short flexor action only, which is a compromise between the two. If a strictly opposition transfer is performed in the absence of short flexor action, two things may occur. As the fingers close against the thumb and power is exerted, the thumb may collapse into supination. The fingers have a supinatory effect on the thumb, and as the thumb attempts to approach the fingers, the opposition transfer relaxes. The pronatory effect of the transfer is lost and collapse occurs. At the same time, because there is no carpometacarpal or MP joint flexor available (short flexor action), the thumb approaches the fingers by the action of the flexor pollicis longus. With this muscle active, the terminal joint flexes initially. As the index finger or index and long fingers contact the flexed interphalangeal joint of the thumb, a crank action is created on the thumb by the fingers, forcing it into supination (Fig. 39-11). In addition to this and in the absence of short flexor action, the only substitute for the adductor pollicis complex is the extensor pollicis longus.[39] The functions of this muscle are supination of the thumb and adduction of the metacarpal and proximal phalanx, and these tend to increase the thumb collapse deformity. Certain opposition transfers provide short flexor power. The Royle-Thompson operation does this by its angle of approach to the thumb, and Bunnell's bony attachment procedure does so by creating MP joint flexion in addition to true opposition.

True opposition transfers with soft tissue distal attachment bring about short flexor action through another method. Those distal attachments that insert into the extensor pollicis longus over the proximal phalanx increase extensor power to the thumb interphalangeal joint. This semiactive tenodesis effect limits passive interphalangeal joint motion of the thumb post-

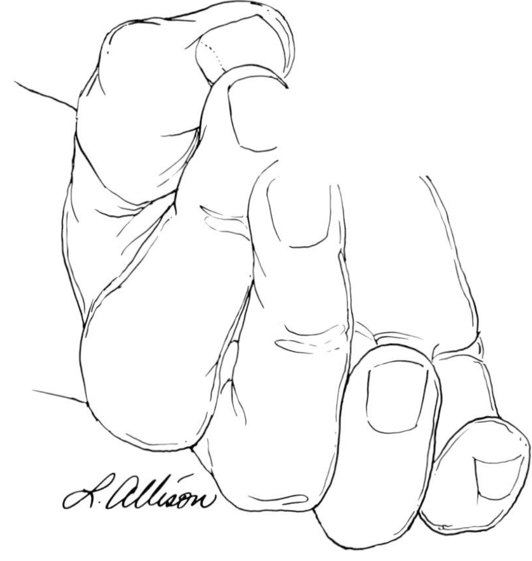

Fig. 39-11. With hyperflexion of the interphalangeal joint, a moment for supination of the thumb occurs if the index finger contacts the thumb with power. Brand calls this the crank-handle effect.

operatively and at the time of surgery, and persists long-term if the opposition motor has satisfactory strength. This limitation of passive interphalangeal joint motion means that when the flexor pollicis longus contracts, all of its excursion is not used up by interphalangeal joint flexion. The remaining excursion is thus available to provide MP and even carpometacarpal flexion. In such a case, short flexor action is achieved by limiting passive flexion of the interphalangeal joint of the thumb.[19] An arthrodesis of the thumb interphalangeal joint would give similar results. In the completely intrinsic-minus thumb in which satisfactory opposition has been obtained, improved function may be achieved by an arthrodesis of the MP joint. This added stability is valuable, but more importantly, the thumb can be hyperpronated so that the pulp of the thumb actually contacts the index finger or the index and long fingers straight on. The fingers then lose their supinatory effect on the thumb. This loss of the supination effect of the thumb can also be appreciated if the MP joint is not arthrodesed in full extension. If the MP joint maintains much flexion, another crank-handle effect for the fingers is created one joint proximally (Fig. 39-12). The fingers working against the thumb with a flexed MP joint force the thumb into supination because of the length of the moment arm. This moment arm actually consists of the entire length of the distal and proximal phalanges of the thumb. Arthrodesis of the MP joint of the thumb in full extension decreases the supinatory or the rotational defect on the thumb by the fingers (Fig. 39-13).

Thumb Extrinsic Opponensplasties

The use of thumb extrinsic muscles that contribute to deformities of the thumb to restore opposition is an attractive concept. To utilize a deforming force and alter its attachment or its muscle-tendon unit approach to the thumb is a concept that stems from the days of poliomyelitis. The two muscle-tendon units that are deforming forces on the thumb with intrinsic muscle paralysis are the flexor pollicis longus and the extensor pollicis longus. Both of these muscles, however, become deforming forces only in the presence of a complete or nearly complete intrinsic-minus thumb. With the absence of short flexor action to the thumb, secondary to injury or disease, overactivity of these two extrinsic muscles occurs. In disease states with progressive paralysis, dual motor tendon transfer to the thumb to provide both opposition and short flexor action is a luxury that cannot be afforded. Obviously, in order to render the thumb maximally functional, one tendon transfer coupled with a joint fusion in the thumb will probably be necessary. Also, in a severely involved hand, true opposition may not be necessary or desirable. Attaining short flexor action alone may render the thumb maximally functional.

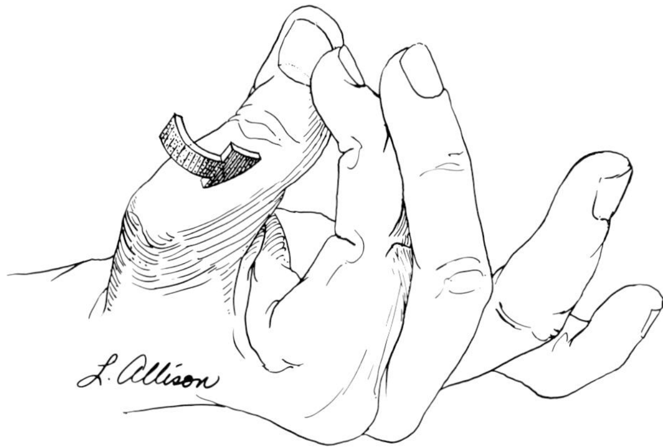

Fig. 39-12. With a flexed thumb MP joint, the index finger exerts a powerful supinatory effect on the thumb. The moment arm is the entire length of the distal and proximal phalanges of the thumb. This is the same crank-handle effect as seen in Figure 39-11, but with an even longer moment arm.

Flexor Pollicis Longus Opponensplasty

One has only to observe the function of the intrinsic-minus thumb to notice the hyperflexed interphalangeal joint and the overactive extensor pollicis longus tendon (Fig. 39-14A,B). Such patients seem to be using both of these extrinsic motors in order to make up for the absence of intrinsic muscles. The hyperflexed interphalangeal joint impairs the pulp of the thumb from properly meeting the index finger in either pulp or key pinch. The fingers tend to strike the nail or the dorsum of the thumb. The flexor pollicis longus has previously been used for an opponensplasty, but classically the routing has been through either the carpal tunnel or its own tendon sheath. Utilizing the flexor pollicis longus tendon with the Thompson pulley or around the ulnar aspect of the flexor carpi ulnaris must be credited to Mangus and Snow.[38] Utilizing the ulnar border of the palmar fascia as a pulley to the rerouted flexor pollicis longus provides short flexor function. Distal attachment of the transferred tendon into the tendon of the abductor pollicis brevis plus arthrodesis of the interphalangeal joint completes the opponensplasty. The flexor pollicis longus now becomes the superficial head of the flexor pollicis brevis. Arthrodesis of the interphalangeal joint in zero degrees allows the pulp of the thumb to meet the fingers correctly. Overactivity of the extensor pollicis longus in this situation tends to disappear. The patient seems to immediately sense without any formal retraining that he now has a functional short flexor muscle and does not need to use the extensor pollicis longus as a secondary adductor (Fig. 39-14C–E). He instead now uses the extensor pollicis longus to clear the thumb away from the fingers and the "new flexor pollicis brevis" in prehension activity. Thus, an overactive thumb extrinsic muscle that had contributed to the deformity has now been rerouted to improve function. In certain long-standing situations, the interphalangeal joint flexion deformity may become fixed. Even in this situation, with adequate excursion and power in the flexor pollicis longus, a satisfactory short flexor can be obtained.

In the case of peripheral nerve disease or spastic paralysis, the flexor pollicis longus may be too weak to utilize as a tendon transfer to improve thumb function. However, a flexion contracture of the interphalangeal joint of the thumb may occur even with a weak flexor pollicis longus. The overactive extensor pollicis longus and the tenodesis action of the flexor pollicis longus with extension and supination of the thumb from the

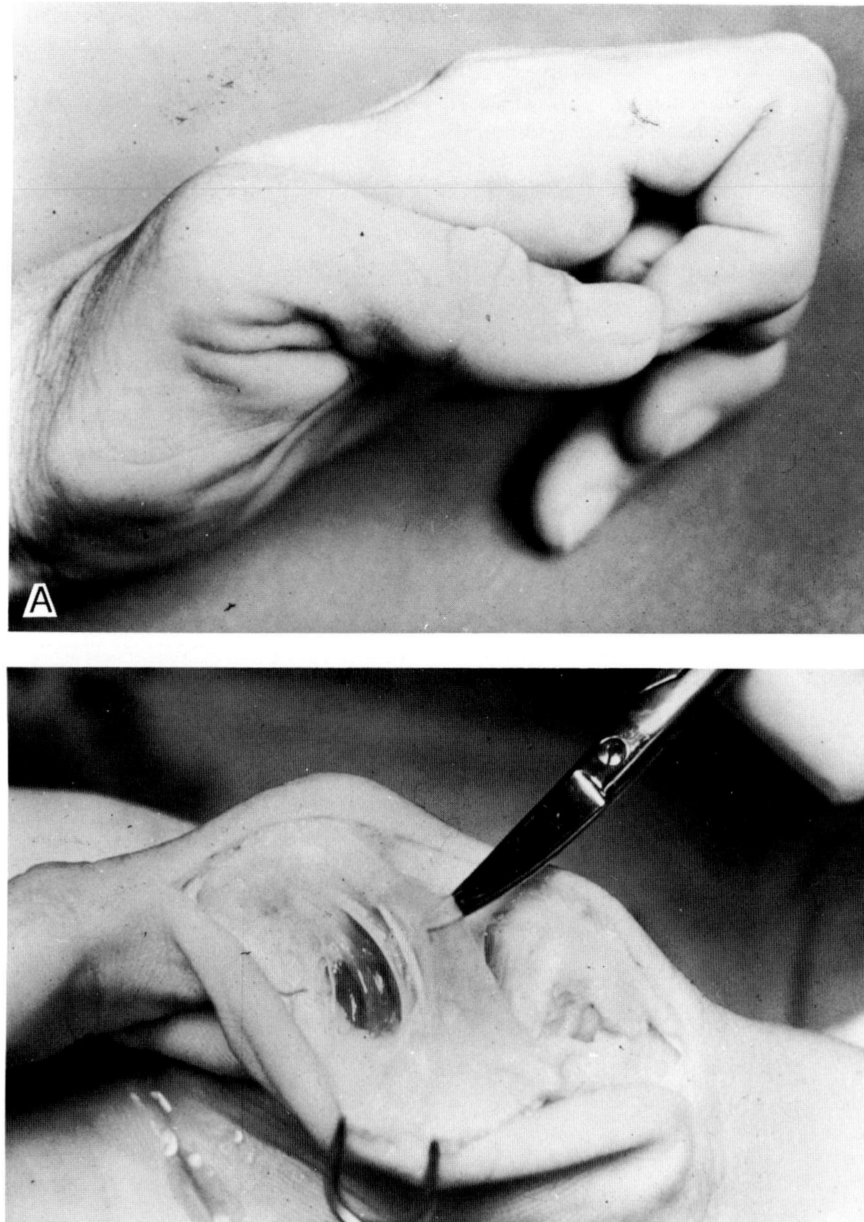

Fig. 39-13. (A&B) A completely intrinsic-minus thumb, in which only a single motor was used to reconstruct thumb function. *(Figure continues.)*

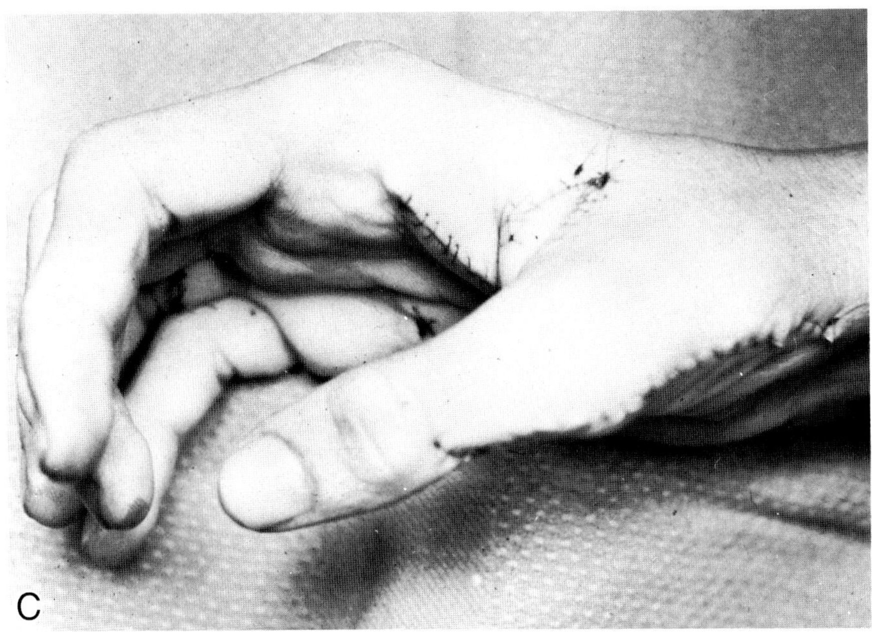

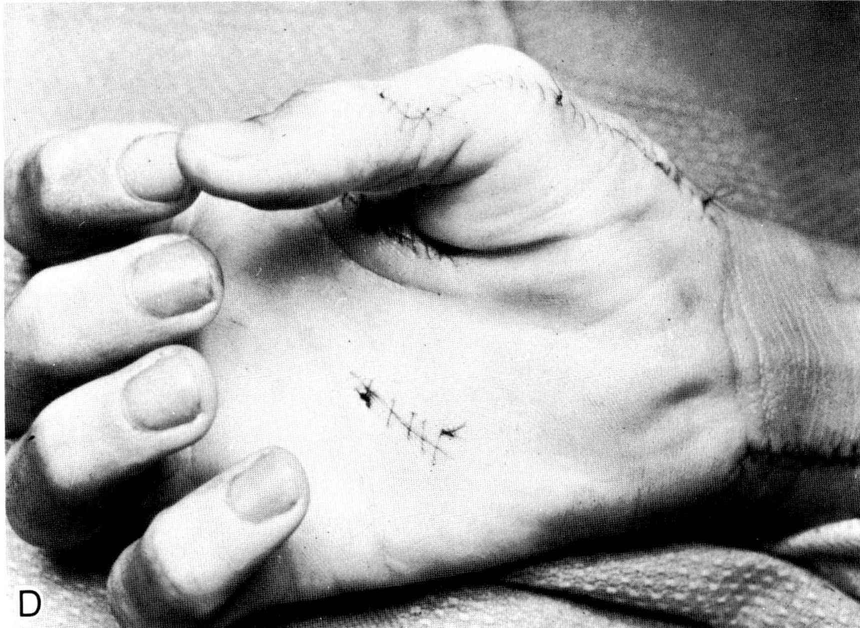

Fig. 39-13 *(Continued).* In spite of adequate release **(C)**, this patient needed either an arthrodesis of the MP joint in full extension or a second transfer for a short flexor-adductor replacement. As the patient attempts to pinch with the thumb against the index finger **(D)**, notice the tremendous crank-handle action that would be exerted on the thumb by the flexing index.

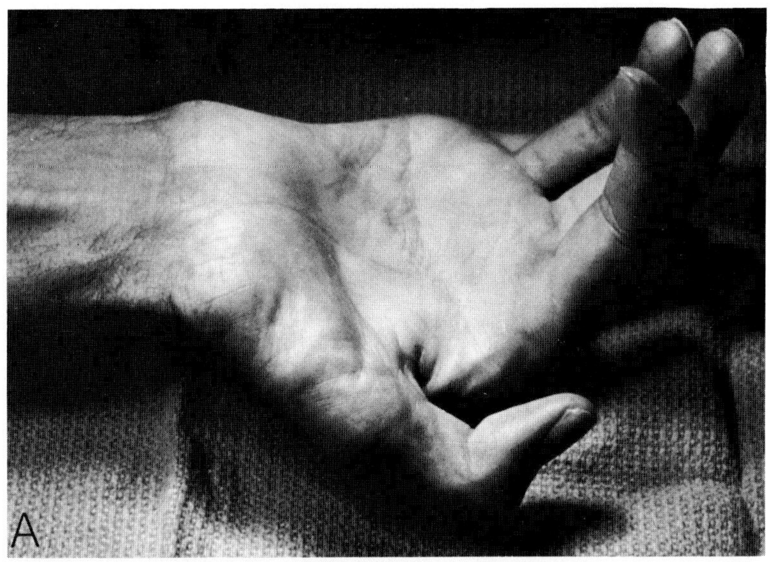

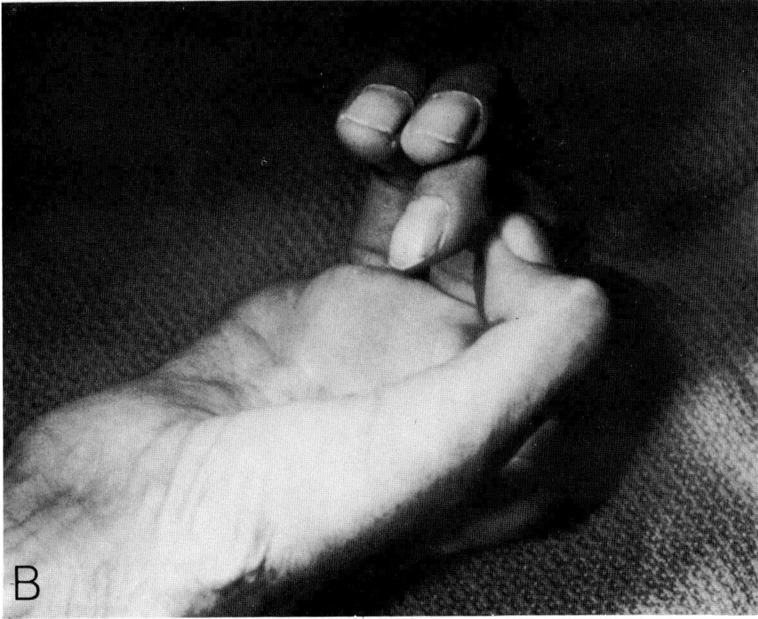

Fig. 39-14. Flexor pollicis longus opponensplasty. This 25-year-old man presented for improvement of hand function with a brachial plexus injury and the equivalent of an intrinsic-minus thumb. In this situation, the extrinsics of the thumb were creating a deformity **(A&B)** and transfer of the flexor pollicis longus with arthrodesis of the interphalangeal joint of the thumb restored much of the activity of the short flexor of the thumb as well as the extensor pollicis longus function. *(Figure continues.)*

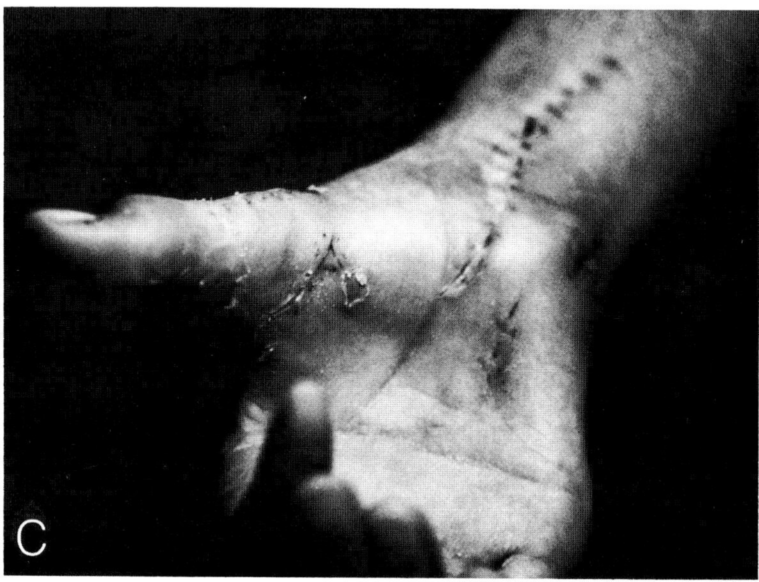

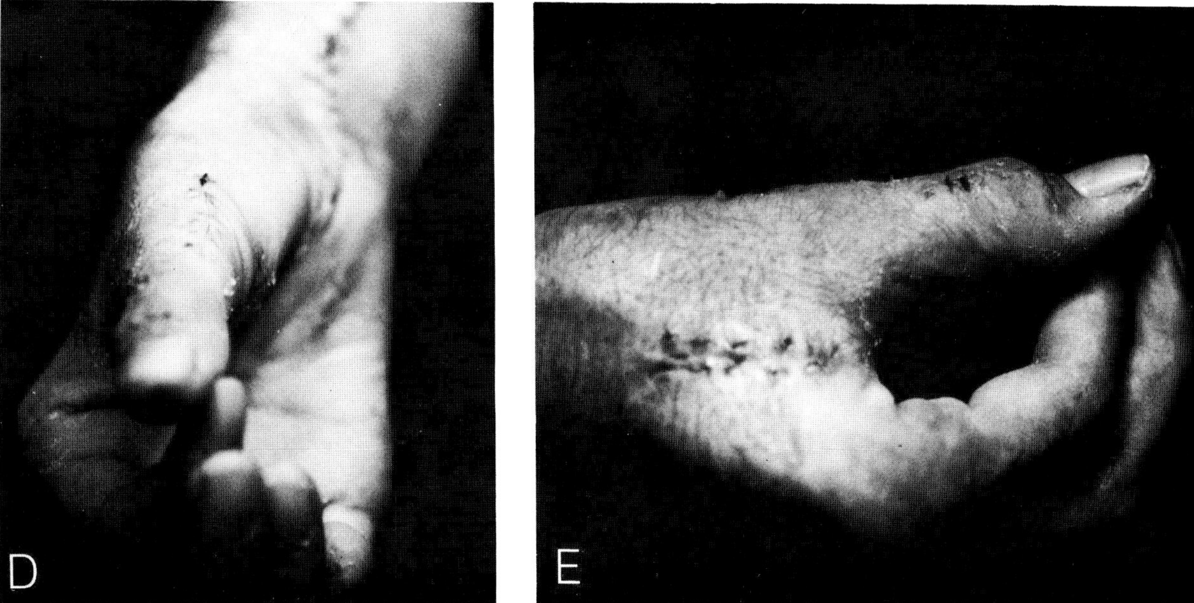

Fig. 39-14 *(Continued).* Immediately upon removal of the cast, the patient's improved thumb function is apparent (**C–E**). The extensor pollicis longus now functions not as an adductor, but as an extensor, and the flexor pollicis longus now functions as a short flexor replacement. The pulley for the flexor pollicis longus was in the area of the pisiform, and the distal attachment was the tendon of the abductor pollicis brevis.

extensor pollicis longus may produce the interphalangeal joint flexion contracture. With a weak flexor pollicis longus and a flexion contracture of the interphalangeal joint of the thumb, only one motor, the extensor pollicis longus, can be causing the deformity. The intrinsic muscles are weak or inactive. The flexor pollicis longus is weak, creating the deformity only by tenodesis. The only functioning motors are the extensor pollicis longus, extensor pollicis brevis, and abductor pollicis longus. All of these are supinators of the thumb. The extensor pollicis longus is also an adductor. Before considering an intermetacarpal bone block to control the thumb, some thought should be given to maintaining thumb mobility by using the only remaining long extrinsic motor, the extensor pollicis longus as described on page 1439. The extensor pollicis longus should, however, only be utilized as an opponensplasty if the patient has active control of this muscle-tendon unit. Using a transferred extensor pollicis longus that is spastic without voluntary control as an opponensplasty will result in a thumb that is always in the way of the fingers. Without voluntary control of the extensor pollicis longus, the abductor pollicis longus by itself cannot clear the thumb from the plane of the fingers during digital flexion.

Operative Technique of Flexor Pollicis Longus Opponensplasty

The distal attachment of the flexor pollicis longus is exposed through a volar zigzag incision, and the tendon is divided at its attachment to the terminal phalanx of the thumb. If there is adherence of the tendon throughout the radial bursa at all, additional, more proximal incisions are required, most commonly at the level of the A1 pulley. At this point, a Y-type incision is made over the dorsum of the interphalangeal joint of the thumb, flaps are developed radially and ulnarly, and the extensor pollicis longus tendon is divided at the level of the joint. The tendon is retracted proximally, the collateral ligaments are incised, and the joint surfaces are exposed. Using rongeurs and a burr, an arthrodesis of the interphalangeal joint is performed using any method of technique and any method of fixation deemed appropriate (see Chapter 4). I prefer to use some type of rigid fixation, either tension band wiring or a screw, because active motion will be begun within 3 or 4 weeks, and good osseous stability is required to allow unrestricted motion of the thumb. I believe that the position of arthrodesis in this situation should be full extension regardless of the method of fixation.

An incision is then made on the radial volar aspect of the wrist, the muscle belly of the flexor pollicis longus is identified in the distal forearm, and the tendon delivered into the proximal wound. Usually the indications for a flexor pollicis longus opponensplasty suggest that there are no functioning ulnar or median intrinsic muscles to the thumb, and this is the reason for the overactivity of the flexor pollicis longus. In a completely intrinsic-minus thumb the only functioning extrinsic muscles (extensor pollicis longus, extensor pollicis brevis, and abductor pollicis longus) are all basically supinators of the thumb. If the flexor pollicis longus is to be used as an opponensplasty, it should have some pronatory effect, not just short flexor action; otherwise the thumb will not rotate enough after the transfer. The pulleys available with this method of opponensplasty are all of those that have been mentioned, including the fixed pulley at the level of the pisiform using a turned back strip of flexor carpi ulnaris; a loop of the tendon around the flexor carpi ulnaris; a window in the carpal tunnel; or the Thompson pulley (i.e., the ulnar border of the palmar fascia at the distal level of the carpal tunnel). The first three pulleys basically provide far more opposition than short flexor action, and in the completely intrinsic-minus thumb are probably not indicated. I believe that the Thompson pulley, which gives more short flexor action but some pronation action, is a far better pulley to use in the completely intrinsic-minus thumb.

An incision for the pulley is then made at the ulnar border of the palmar fascia in line with the ulnar aspect of the ring finger. The flexor tendons can be seen coming from beneath the transverse carpal ligament in the most proximal extent of this incision. A Carroll tendon passer is then passed from distal to proximal, emerging in the proximal incision on the volar radial aspect of the wrist. The flexor pollicis longus tendon is then passed through the depth of the carpal tunnel and brought superficially into the palmar incision. The actual route of the tendon of the flexor pollicis longus should be between the tendons of the flexor digitorum superficialis and those of the flexor digitorum profundus.

An incision is then made in the area of the metacarpophalangeal joint on the dorsoradial aspect of the thumb. It is very important in this type of opponensplasty not to attach the transferred tendon into the tendon of the abductor pollicis brevis. This basically is an abductor of the metacarpophalangeal joint, and such an insertion will only pull the metacarpophalangeal joint into a palmar position with abduction. The goal in this tendon transfer, in addition to providing some pronation and abduction, is to stabilize the metacarpophalangeal joint of the thumb in some flexion. This is the only way to achieve power of the thumb against the fingers. If the transfer is inserted into the abductor pollicis brevis tendon, the thumb will not oppose the fingers with nearly as much power as it will if it is sutured into a more volar position, actually attached to the superficial head of the flexor pollicis brevis. In this way, as the patient uses the single long flexor of the thumb to bring about useful thumb function, he will actually have flexion of the metacarpophalangeal joint with a stable distal joint rather than abduction, which he really does not need. Thus, the reason that the method of distal attachment is slightly different than in other opponensplasties in that what we are really trying to reproduce is short flexor action.

Again using a tunnelling forcep or a Carroll tendon passer, the tendon of the flexor pollicis longus is passed subcutaneously from the palmar incision to the thumb incision. There is so much excursion in the flexor pollicis longus that setting the tension in this transfer is even easier than in the flexor digitorum superficialis opponensplasty. As in other opponensplasties, the thumb should rest in almost the fully opposed position, not to the same extent that it does in the short excursion extensor proprius transfers, but high enough so that the patient has reasonable tension on the muscle-tendon unit when it tries to bring power to either side of the fingers or to the pulp of the fingers. In the patient with this type of severely involved hand, pulp-to-pulp pinch is not as important as pulp of the thumb to side of the index or long fingers.

After release of the tourniquet and hemostasis is established, simple wound closure is accomplished. The wrist is maintained in 30 to 40 degrees volar flexion, with the thumb in full opposition for about 3 to 4 weeks. Following this, rehabilitation is begun with active wrist dorsiflexion, which acts to bring the thumb into full opposition. This is followed by exercises to increase power of the transfer.

The desired end result is basically a single axis thumb, which has lost a lot of the rotation movement that it had with normal intrinsic muscles. This provides a thumb that is able to clear the fingers and still oppose the fingertips as well as the sides of the finger with considerable power. Results of this transfer in my experience have been very good, and there is practially no relearning required with this opponensplasty. I believe that there are distinct advantages to using this transfer in the completely intrinsic-minus thumb, which we have previously

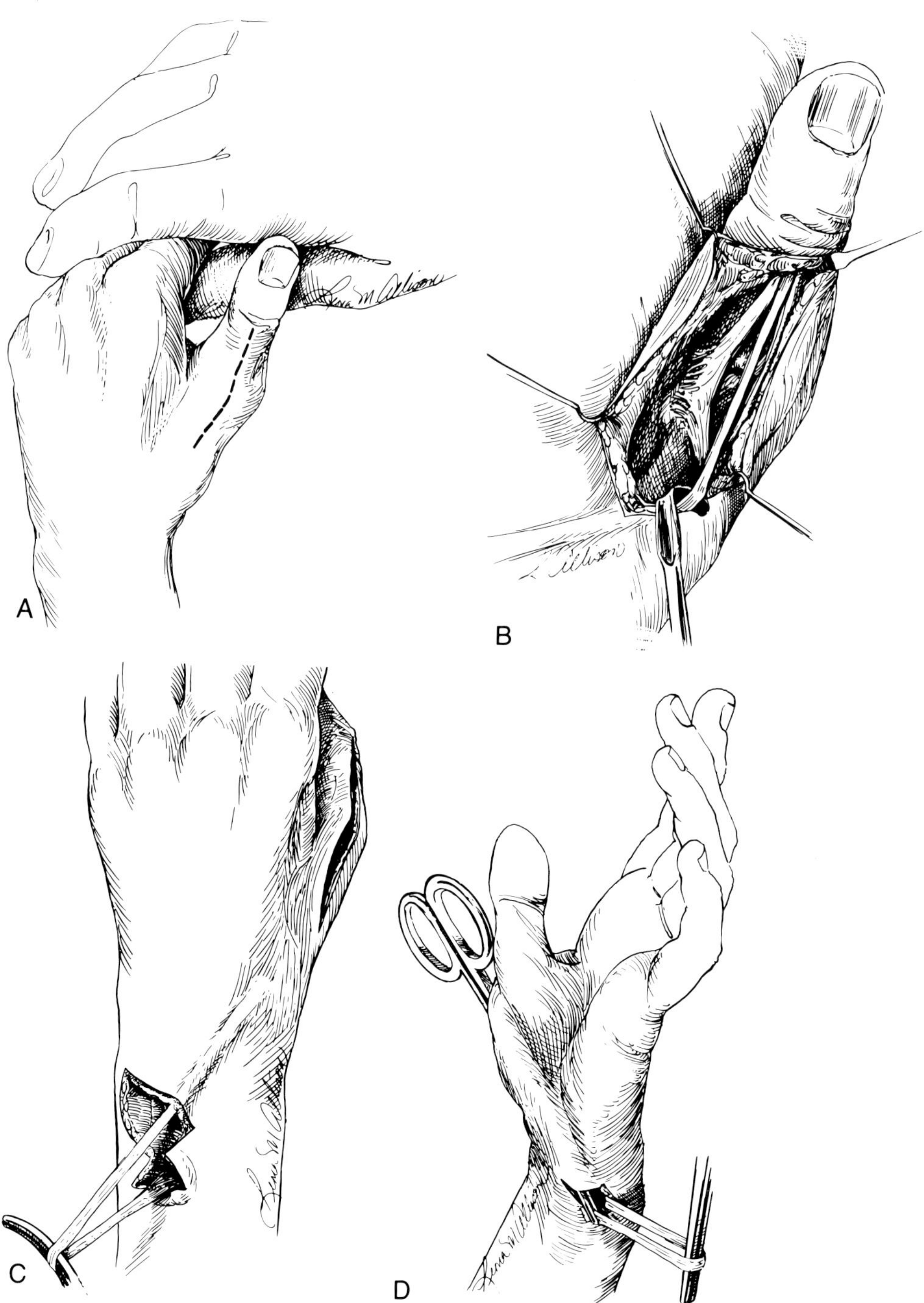

Fig. 39-15. Extensor pollicis longus opponensplasty. The middle portion of the extensor pollicis longus is exposed over the proximal phalanx of the thumb **(A)** and removed in continuity with the main extensor pollicis longus tendon proximal to the MP joint **(B)**. This allows satisfactory length of the transfer. It is then freed up and transferred around the ulnar border of the wrist **(C&D)**. *(Figure continues.)*

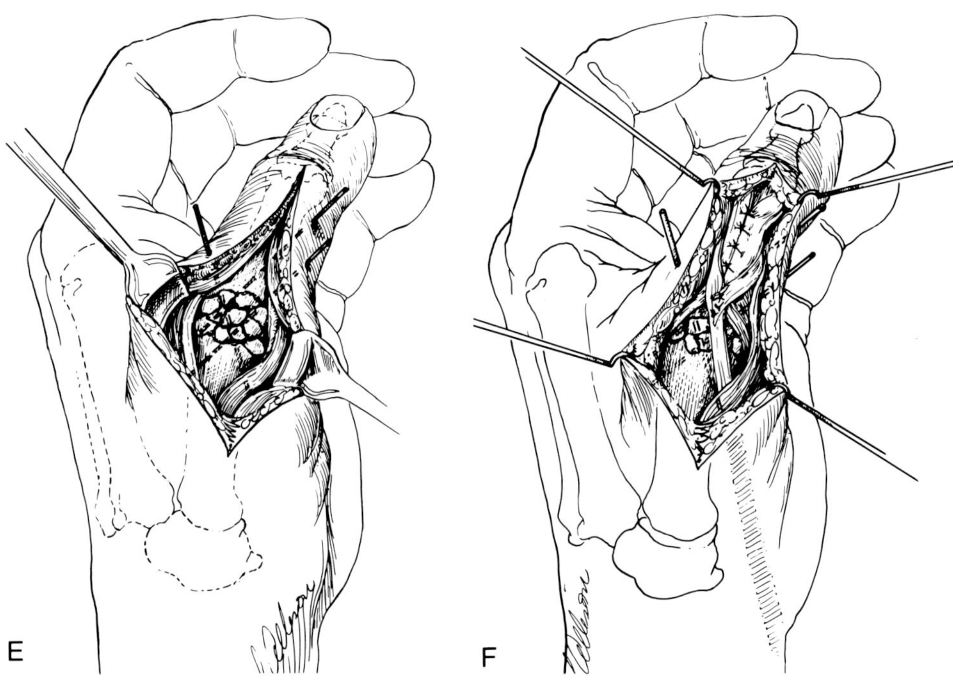

Fig. 39-15 *(Continued).* Following this, an arthrodesis of the thumb MP joint is performed **(E)**. The two lateral bands or the two most lateral portions of the extensor pollicis longus are sutured together and then the transfer is actually sutured into them **(F)**. In addition to arthrodesis of the MP joint, the interphalangeal joint of the thumb should be pinned in extension in order to prevent inadvertent flexion during the healing of this transfer. (From Riley et al,[52] with permission.)

missed because we have felt that opposition is more important than short flexor action.

Extensor Pollicis Longus Opponensplasty

The extensor pollicis longus has been emphasized throughout this discussion as being a direct antagonist to opposition of the thumb. In certain cases in which improvement is not likely to occur following nerve injury, in those cases in which an extended period of time has gone by since the nerve injury, or in those patients who have a paralysis problem based on a progressive disease, some thought should be given to using the extensor pollicis longus as an opposition transfer. With an intrinsic-minus thumb from a median and ulnar nerve paralysis, only supinators and adductors of the thumb are present, and true opposition of the thumb frequently cannot be achieved against these powerful muscles. I have performed a small number of cases of extensor pollicis longus opponensplasty, taking a muscle that is a deforming force in the intrinsic palsied thumb and converting it into a positive force. For this opponensplasty, patients have been selected who are not likely to improve or who are actually likely to get worse because of the associated disease.[52]

Operative Technique of Extensor Pollicis Longus Opponensplasty

The technique of the extensor pollicis longus opponensplasty is as follows (Fig. 39-15). The central portion of the extensor pollicis longus over the proximal phalanx of the thumb is removed in continuity with the extensor pollicis longus tendon over the MP joint through the hood into the middle of the metacarpal area of the thumb. The width of the tendon over the proximal phalanx is approximately one-third of the tendon width that would normally be present. This tendon is then freed from the hood system. A small incision may be necessary over the dorsum of the hand to free it from some adhesions in the area of the third compartment, and a more generous incision is then made on the ulnar aspect of the distal forearm where the muscle belly is identified. The extensor pollicis longus tendon is then pulled into the more ulnar incision proximally. A subcutaneous tunnel is created along the ulnar border of the forearm. A small incision is usually made in the area of the pisiform. The muscle belly is transposed onto the ulnar aspect of the forearm subcutaneously; the tendon is brought out in the area of the pisiform and transferred directly across the palm to the area of the MP joint. All of the patients in whom this operation has been done have had a concomitant arthrodesis of the MP joint of the thumb in full extension and hyperponation. The elongated extensor pollicis longus tendon (i.e., elongated by the intrinsic portion of the tendon) is then interwoven between the two lateral bands that are brought together in the midline and the entire hood is repaired, using this interweaving technique of the transferred extensor pollicis longus and the lateral bands. The interphalangeal joint of the thumb is pinned in full extension at this time. It is most important to make sure that the fixation of the MP joint arthrodesis is secure because active use of this transfer is ideally started within about 4 weeks, at which time the arthrodesis is really not going to be solid. After 4 weeks of immobilization, the patient should be taught to differentiate function of the extensor pollicis longus from function of the abductor pollicis longus. It is most important at the time the transfer is being performed that it is possible for the fingers to actually clear the opposed thumb with the wrist in neutral. No thumb extensor muscle remains, and there is only abductor pollicis longus function available to bring the thumb away so the fingers can close in power grip (Fig. 39-16). The patient is able to clear the thumb for the fingers during power grip activities using this abductor pollicis longus. Our results with this transfer have been most pleasing, and we continue to use it in situations in which the patient is not likely to have any evidence of improvement and has limited motors, or in which the patient's condition is likely to

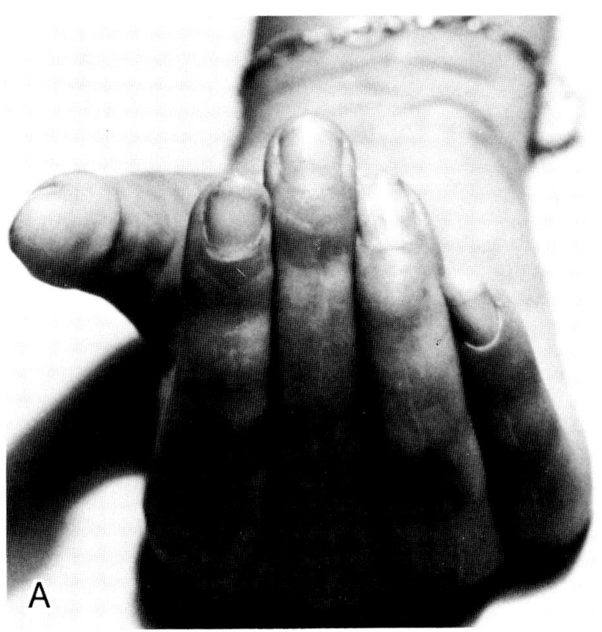

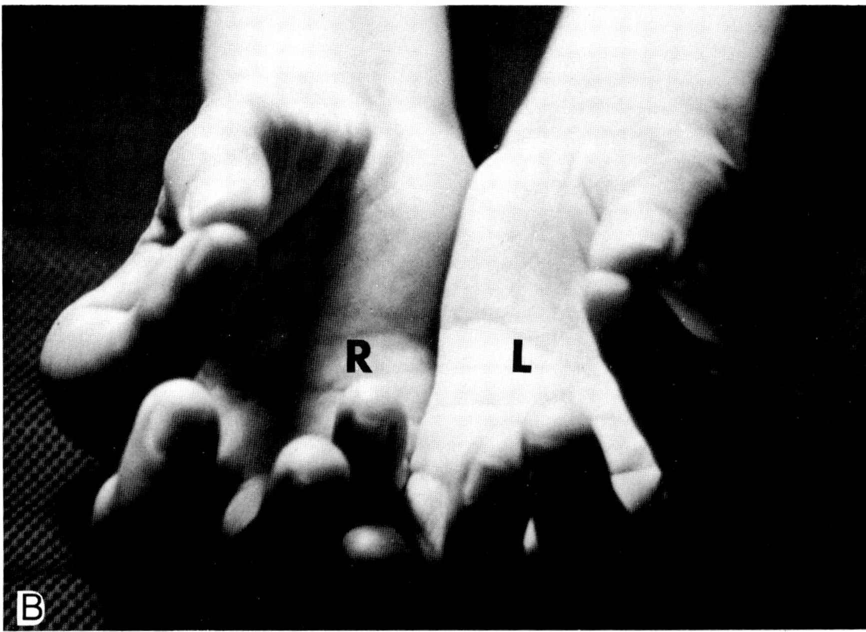

Fig. 39-16. This patient with Charcot-Marie-Tooth disease has undergone arthrodesis of the thumb MP joint as well as an extensor pollicis longus opponensplasty. Note the use of the abductor pollicis longus to move the thumb (**B**) so that power grip is possible as the fingers really clear the thumb. In addition, notice that in the left hand the MP joint has been arthrodesed in hyperpronation whereas in the right it has been done in almost neutral rotation. The crank-handle effect is much less obvious in the left thumb, suggesting that hyperpronation, as well as full extension, is the preferred position of arthrodesis of the thumb MP joint in a patient with combined median and ulnar palsy.

deteriorate, such as in syringomyelia or Charcot-Marie-Tooth disease.[52]

Postoperative Management of Opponensplasty

In general, the postoperative management of opponensplasties is related to whether or not the transfer crosses the wrist joint; if it crosses the wrist joint volarly, the wrist needs to be supported in some way. In most opponensplasties it has been our practice to leave the hand and wrist in a bulky dressing for several days postoperatively and then after this period of time to position the thumb in full opposition for approximately 4 weeks. If the transfer is one of the proprius transfers in which the excursion of the muscle tendon unit is relatively short, it is important that the wrist be placed at about 30 to 35 degrees volar flexion with the thumb in full opposition. If the transferred motor is the superficialis or some other type of transfer that has a considerable range of excursion, merely positioning the thumb in full opposition and the wrist in neutral is generally adequate. If the method of attachment distally involves the extensor pollicis longus over the middle phalanx or the abductor pollicis brevis tendon rather than some type of bony attachment, immobilization of the thumb interphalangeal joint in full extension will probably be required. If not, additional excessive tension will probably be placed on the suture line distally and might result in some attenuation of this attachment. Since at the present time most attachments of the opponensplasty distally use either Riordan's or Brand's method of attachment, certainly interphalangeal joint immobilization should be an integral part of the postoperative management. Since this is a tendon-to-tendon suture, 4 weeks of immobilization is generally adequate. After 4 weeks of immobilization, patients generally regain control very rapidly. Following cast removal in these patients, the emphasis early on should be on rehabilitation to regain wrist motion.

Those transfers that use an ulnar innervated intrinsic muscle (e.g., the abductor digiti minimi to replace a median innervated intrinsic muscle) do not need to be placed in any particular position as far as wrist flexion is concerned, but the thumb should be placed in full opposition.

In most patients, splinting is not required once mobility of the thumb and wrist is started. However, in certain disease states, primarily high median and ulnar nerve palsies or in patients with disease such as Charcot-Marie-Tooth or leprosy, the extensors are so strong and the lack of sensibility may be so profound as to have the patient attenuate his own transfer prior to getting control over the muscle and strengthening of the tendon suture through collagen maturation. In such cases it is important to protect the transfer from overstretching by normal muscles working against the opponensplasty. It has generally been our impression that in such patients who have considerable loss of sensibility in the hand either from disease or injury, prolonged protection of the opponensplasty will be required for up to about 3 months. However, in patients who are less disabled than this and have only an isolated high or low median nerve injury, attenuation of the transfer has not been a major problem and generally these patients do not require immobilization past 4 weeks.

Author's Preferred Method of Opponensplasty

There are many different conditions associated with loss of opposition of the thumb, and there is probably no single opposition transfer that is applicable to all cases in which the thumb is nonfunctional secondary to loss of the abductor pollicis brevis function. Historically, the opposition transfer came about as a substitute primarily in diseased states such as poliomyelitis, in which the thumb usually had complete intrinsic paralysis. However, in present day situations it seems as if more problems with reduced thumb function occur following trauma with or without local injury in the area of the wrist. In these variable circumstances, a single choice of opponensplasty would obviously not be optimal in all cases.[17]

The flexor digitorum superficialis opponensplasty using a fixed pulley in the area of the pisiform, with various methods of attachment in the area of the MP joint of the thumb, has been the standard opponensplasty for years. This is applicable in a low median nerve permanent paralysis without associated tendon injury, and should give excellent thumb function. However, in this type of patient, the intrinsic muscles that bring about short flexor action and adduction of the thumb are functioning, and therefore great strength of opposition is not required. Because of this I generally prefer to use a proprius tendon transfer opponensplasty, either the extensor digiti minimi or the extensor indicis proprius. These muscles with adequate strength and positioning capability allow the use of a muscle that in my opinion is more expendable than the strong flexor digitorum superficialis to the ring finger. There is a significant complication rate associated with superficialis removal from the finger[29,45] and because of this I prefer to use one of the proprius tendons as my primary opponensplasty. Since my experience has been greatest with extensor indicis proprius, I prefer this opponensplasty as my operative procedure in the thumb without tendon injury and with normally functioning, ulnar-innervated intrinsic musculature.

In the case of a high median nerve paralysis or a low median nerve paralysis associated with tendon injury at the level of the wrist, a proprius tendon transfer would be my first choice. In the case of a low injury at the level of the wrist with a median nerve repair, however, often no opponens transfer is indicated. These patients generally regain some function of the abductor pollicis brevis within 6 months and, usually in the case of sharp lacerations, have reasonably good return of function within one year. In these low injuries, contractures can usually be prevented by a short opponens splint, and therefore no internal splint needs to be created by an operative procedure.

My experience with the extensor indicis proprius transfer has been good. The functional defect is acceptable and failures are few. Strength seems to be adequate with ulnar nerve muscles intact, and I continue to be amazed with how well the patients do postoperatively as far as regaining motion with minimal to no rehabilitation.

I think the method of distal attachment should be to the abductor pollicis brevis tendon only. In a high median nerve injury, suturing the distal attachment to the extensor pollicis longus has not been necessary and may result in excessive interphalangeal joint hyperextension, because in patients with a high injury there is no functioning flexor pollicis longus. Therefore, in the patient with an isolated high median nerve injury, I would not use this method of distal attachment, as advocated by Brand or Riordan, unless at the same time I had done some type of transfer to the flexor pollicis longus.

In the patient with a low injury to the median nerve that had required a nerve graft to regain continuity of the nerve, I would again think in terms of the extensor indicis proprius opponensplasty. With deficits involving the ulnar nerve musculature as well, the method of attachment should be to the extensor pollicis longus as well as to the abductor pollicis brevis, as advocated by Riordan and Brand. I believe that this brings about greater rotation of the thumb and limits the interphalangeal joint motion by increasing the tension of the extensor pollicis longus. This high tension then limits passive interphalangeal joint motion so that the excursion of the flexor pollicis longus can provide more proximal control in the MP and carpometacarpal joints of the thumb, rather than just at the interphalangeal joint.

It seems that opposition transfers are functionally much stronger than would be predicted from anatomic studies. In the case of the extensor proprius tendons there are probably at least two reasons for this. One of these is muscle hypertrophy. The extensors have little functional demand placed on them in their normal location as far as strength is concerned. In the new location, however, the demand is increased, and muscle does have the ability to adapt functionally. The second reason is biomechanical. The course of the transferred tendon is from the pisiform subcutaneously across the palm of the hand to the MP area of the thumb. The moments for abduction and pronation of the first metacarpal are greater because of the more superficial location of the transfer as compared with the intact abductor pollicis brevis.[18]

EXTRINSIC REPLACEMENT IN MEDIAN NERVE PARALYSIS

In high median nerve paralysis there is lack of function of the forearm wrist pronator-flexor group with the exception of the flexor carpi ulnaris. Absent muscles include all of the flexor digitorum superficialis, the two radial profundi, and the flexor pollicis longus. Although the radial half of the flexor digitorum profundus is classically denervated, flexion of the long finger is usually complete although considerable weakness of this digit is present. In the index finger only intrinsic flexion is present, and overuse of the intrinsic flexors might bring about intrinsic-plus deformity of the index finger, with loss of passive DIP and PIP flexion. Likewise, the interphalangeal joint of the thumb may develop considerable stiffness secondary to the unopposed action of the extensor pollicis longus and the intrinsic interphalangeal joint extensors. In considering extrinsic replacement, the functions that need to be replaced must be determined. Basically what is desired is flexor power in the index and long fingers, range of motion in the index finger, and range of motion and power in the interphalangeal joint of the thumb. It is certainly desirable to have full finger flexion, but some power is also needed if there is to be minimal likelihood of extrinsic return following nerve graft or nerve repair. The only functions that actually need to be replaced are flexors to the index finger and thumb or to the thumb and index, and long fingers if more power is required. What are the available muscle-tendon units available for transfer? There are really only two or perhaps three. In a high median palsy the brachioradialis and the extensor carpi radialis longus are available and perhaps the extensor carpi ulnaris, if it is not being used for an opposition transfer.[50] Frequently, however, the removal of the extensor carpi ulnaris for transfer brings about a radial deviation deformity of the wrist. Therefore, in general, I think removing this muscle for functions other than an opposition transfer should be discouraged. An alternative to direct transfer for restoration of extrinsic function is side-to-side suture of the functioning flexor digitorum profundi of the ring and small fingers, which are ulnarly innervated, to the denervated portions on the radial side. This adds range of motion to the index finger and perhaps prevents stiffness but does nothing to the extreme weakness on the radial side, which involves both the index and long fingers. Two motors are available for transfer to the flexor pollicis longus: the extensor carpi radialis longus and brachioradialis. The use of these motors provides independent flexion in the interphalangeal joints of the thumb and index finger.

The use of the extensor carpi radialis longus to the flexor digitorum profundus of the index and long fingers is reserved for those patients who need radial side power and are unlikely to obtain significant reinnervation following neurorrhaphy (Fig. 39-17). In order to perform a tendon transfer of new motors to the index finger, or to the index and long fingers and thumb, there must be full range of motion of the wrist or an indifferent result will occur. Similarly, use of the brachioradialis to the flexor pollicis longus requires a full range of wrist motion. The reason for this is explained as follows. The suture line tension between the brachioradialis and the flexor pollicis longus or the extensor carpi radialis longus and the profundus to the index and long fingers is most critical. There is significant disparity in excursion between the flexor digitorum profundus to the index and long fingers (about 50 mm) and the extensor carpi radialis longus (about 30 mm). Therefore, if excessive tension is placed on the transfer, either to the thumb or the index and long fingers, flexion contractures will result. Flexion contractures of the digits on the radial side of the hand reduce hand function considerably because precision activities, which are usually performed by the radial side of the hand, are performed with the interphalangeal joints of both the thumb and fingers in nearly full extension. The tension on this transfer should then be adjusted by the use of a dynamic tenodesis approach (i.e., with synergistic wrist motion). Full volar flexion of the wrist will bring about nearly complete extension of the fingers, and full dorsiflexion of the wrist will allow complete flexion of the fingers. This tenodesis action should be used to adjust the tension of the tendon transfer. Tension for the transfer should be adjusted so that with the wrist at about

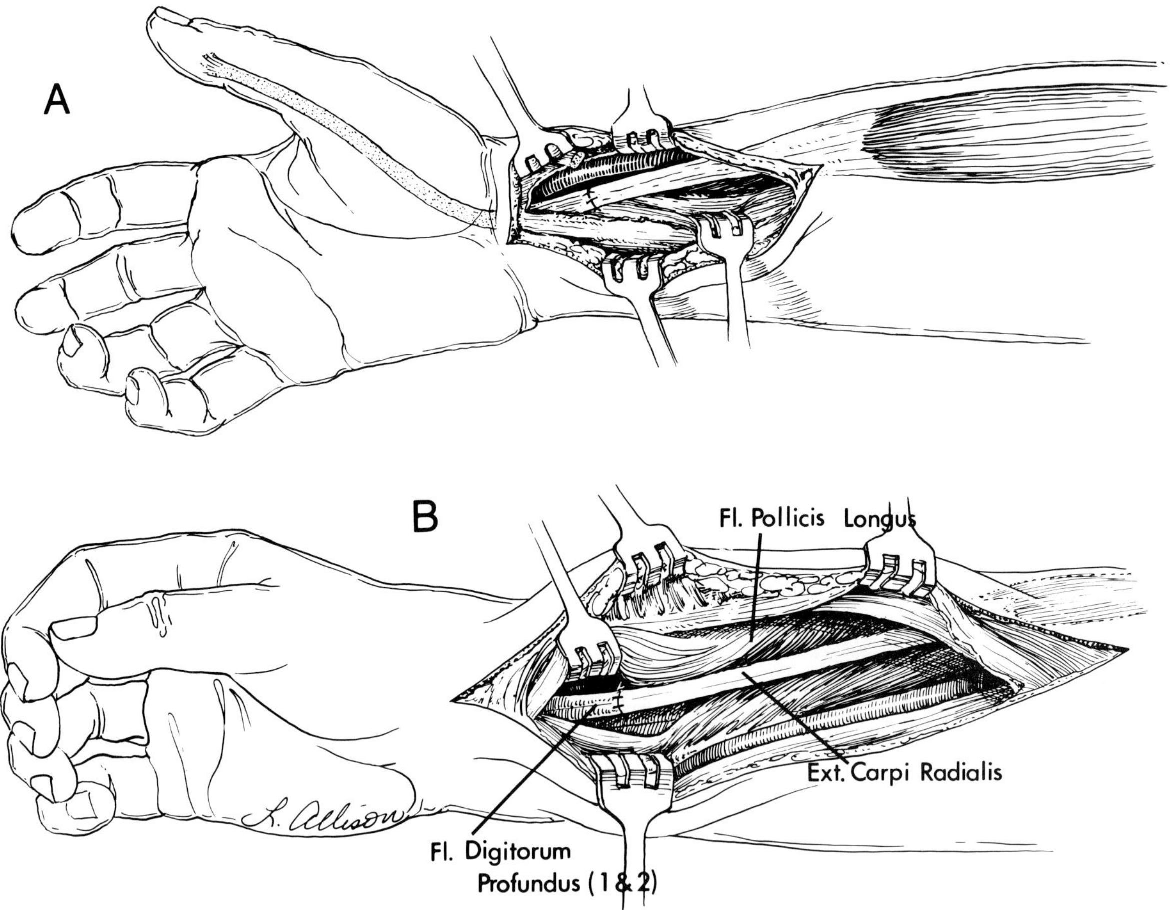

Fig. 39-17. Extrinsic replacement using the brachioradialis to the flexor pollicis longus **(A)** and the extensor carpi radialis longus to the profundi of the index and long fingers **(B)**. In both situations the transfers as shown here are end-to-end. If there is felt to be any chance for extrinsic return following grafting, the transfer should be end-to-side. The end-to-end technique shown here would be used in the patient in whom there is no chance of extrinsic return.

30 degrees volar flexion the fingers come into nearly full extension. With the wrist in 30 to 45 degrees dorsiflexion the fingers should close passively so that the power of the transfer can exert its force with the fingers partially flexed, i.e., the 30 mm of excursion of the extensor carpi radialis longus begins to act when the fingers are almost completely flexed passively by wrist dorsiflexion.

Use of the brachioradialis poses the same problem in terms of excursion, but it must be remembered that the brachioradialis tendon must be freed extensively up to the proximal third of the forearm, well past its musculotendinous junction, in order to develop 30 mm of excursion. Only with this dissection, freeing the tendon widely from the investing fascia of the forearm, is it possible to get 30 mm of excursion in this muscle. The tension then can be adjusted in essentially the same fashion described above for adjusting the tension in the fingers. With the wrist in about 30 degrees volar flexion it should be possible to passively extend all three joints of the thumb completely. This will result in lack of full flexion of the interphalangeal joint by the transfer, but it will essentially stabilize the tip of the thumb and give additional power of flexion to the thumb. As noted previously, most precision pinch activities are performed with the thumb interphalangeal joint in full extension. Therefore, a flexion contracture of this joint at this point can be extremely disabling (Fig. 39-18). If these extrinsic tendon replacements are performed following a nerve repair or nerve graft, the method of attachment should be end-to-side rather than end-to-end. This is true even if considerable time has elapsed since the nerve surgery and all hope of nerve regeneration has been given up. Extremely late recovery is occasionally seen, and because of this, all suture lines should be end-to-side. This type of tendon juncture, of course, allows any subsequent return of power in the reinnervated muscle to augment the transfer.

The primary function of the brachioradialis is elbow flexion, with some supination occurring from a position of full pronation. Its origin is extensive and extends quite far proximally on the humerus. Even if the muscle is extensively freed from the forearm fascia in the proximal forearm prior to transfer, its usefulness remains extremely dependent upon elbow position. With the elbow in full extension, the brachioradialis may provide good thumb interphalangeal joint flexion following its transfer to the flexor pollicis longus. With elbow flexion, however, little power will be transmitted to the interphalangeal

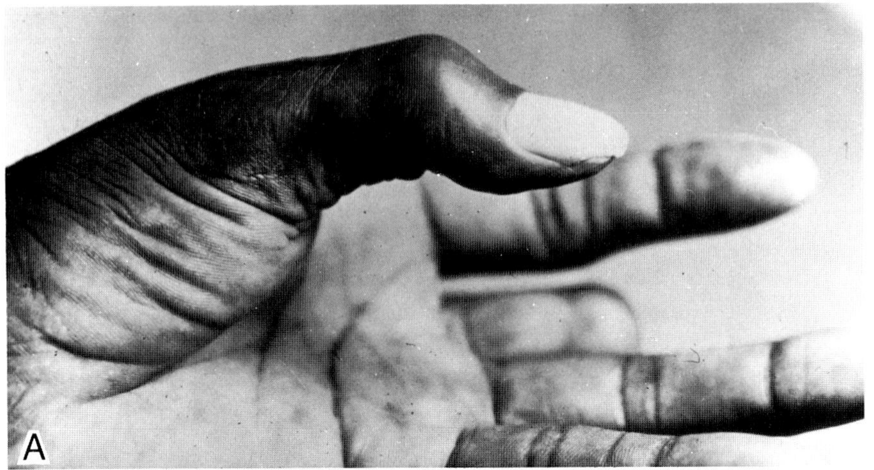

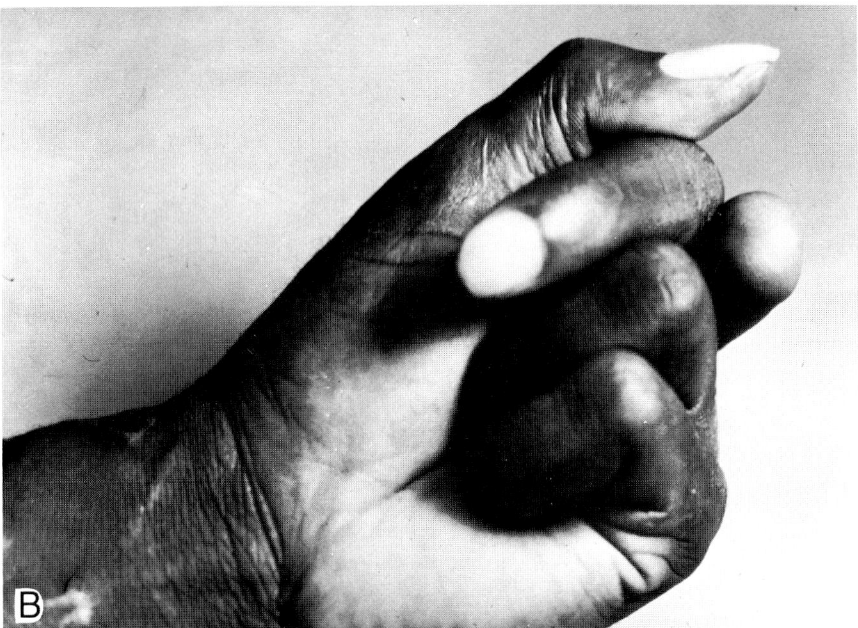

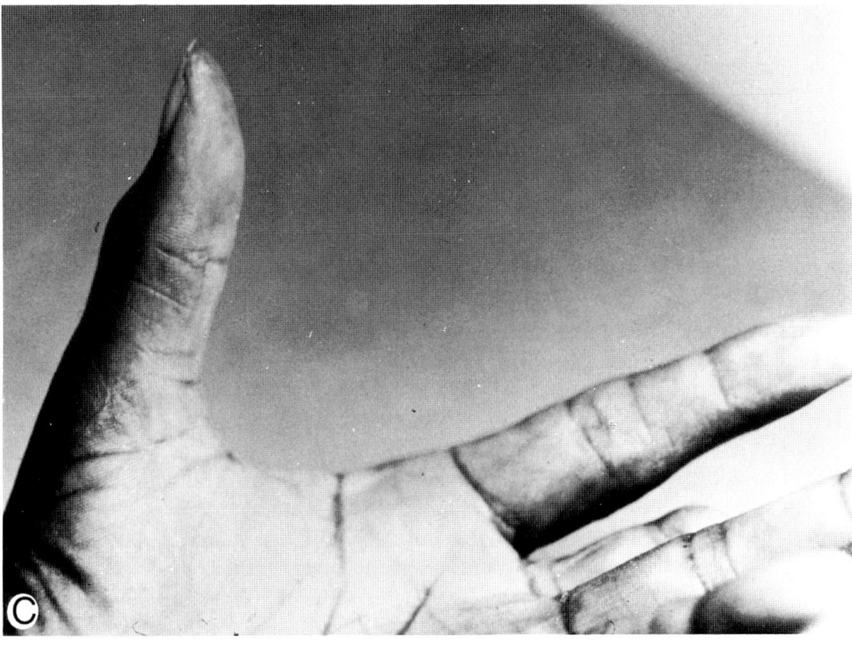

Fig. 39-18. A patient with high median nerve injury in whom the brachioradialis has been transferred to the flexor pollicis longus and the extensor carpi radialis longus to the index finger profundus tendon. There is good power in the flexor pollicis longus, but limited range with the wrist held still. Note the absence of flexion contracture of the index finger and thumb **(C)**.

joint. Our attempts to move the origin distally at the time of transfer have not been successful because of the short vascular branches to the muscle.

Another point to keep in mind when replacing extrinsic function in high median paralysis is the swan-neck deformity. Many patients who have hyperextensible PIP joints will develop swan-neck deformity of the fingers after the onset of median paralysis. This lack of flexor digitorum superficialis function is not always so obvious early on, but with attenuation of the volar support structures of the PIP joint, it may become a functional problem, with locking in extension. In these patients, restoring profundus function to the index and long fingers with tendon transfers will likely accentuate the swan-neck deformity of these digits. There are three methods to avoid the development of this functional problem: (1) the ECRL may be transferred to FDS of the index and long fingers, combined with a tenodesis of the distal joints; (2) arthrodesis of the DIP joints of the index and long may be carried out at the time of the ECRL to FDP transfer; and (3) The FDP tendon can be sutured to the A4 pulley with nonabsorbable suture in each digit at the time of ECRL to FDP transfer. These methods are effective in preventing the swan-neck problem.

TIMING AND SELECTION OF TRANSFERS

Timing

I believe that the selection and timing of transfers performed for both intrinsic and extrinsic paralysis in high median nerve lesions needs some clarification. If a tendon transfer is considered following a neurorrhaphy in the case of a high median nerve laceration, one should expect considerable return in extrinsic flexors. Consequently, probably no tendon transfer is indicated to restore function in the extrinsic flexors of the forearm. On the other hand, if a nerve repair has been performed several months before and no evidence of return has occurred, one should think of doing a transfer that would give additional power rather than just range of motion to the index and long fingers. I think that for all practical purposes, extrinsic replacement for high median nerve palsy is indicated only when nerve grafting is performed. In this case transfers should be performed end-to-side to take advantage of muscle power that may return following the nerve graft. If one elects not to perform extrinsic replacements, maintenance of mobility of the interphalangeal joints of the thumb and index finger will be necessary until recovery occurs. As stated before, because of the difference in amplitude of the muscles transferred, it is most important that the wrist have full range of motion prior to performing any of these short excursion motor transfers.

Regarding further transfers in the upper extremity, I believe that tendon transfers in the upper extremity should be performed as soon after injury and nerve repair as possible to improve overall hand function. Much has been said about the timing of transfers.[4,8,13,46] Transfers should be performed when it is obvious that no further return is going to occur, but this may be as long as several years following neurorrhaphy or grafting. Although there is some controversy regarding this point, I believe that transfers should be performed soon after repair of the nerve. In patients with median nerve palsy, sensory loss may be the most important single deterrent to satisfactory hand function. Even in the presence of sensory loss, however, some function of the hand is possible. Certainly a mobile, opposable thumb that can reach the normal sensible areas of the hand is much more useful than one that cannot be used and cannot even reach the areas of normal sensibility. The functional deficit associated especially with a high median lesion is so profound that I believe all attempts should be made to improve motor function early. Whether this includes just thumb opposition transfer or opposition and extrinsic transfer is frequently dependent on the individual patient, i.e., his requirements for return to work, motivation, need for splintage, and associated injury. I believe that a transfer can work as a substitute during regrowth of the nerve, while at the same time prevent contractures and eliminate the requirement for external splintage. External splintage may severely limit the patient's ability to use the palsied hand, and therefore I believe that the use of an internal splint, that is, the early transfer, is of considerable benefit in the rehabilitation of these patients.[13] If the patient ultimately regains only partial function in the muscles involved, the transfer may act at the same time as a helper. In such cases, the reinnervated muscles may then function with near-normal power. If essentially no return occurs from the neurorrhaphy or nerve graft, the transfer may then act as a permanent substitute. As previously noted, those patients who have significant power in the superficial portion of the flexor pollicis brevis may have a thumb that is maximally functional and will not require an opposition transfer. In my opinion, however, those patients who need an opposition transfer should have it performed soon after neurorrhaphy or grafting.

When asked what muscle substitutes for the abductor pollicis brevis, most physicians quickly respond with the flexor pollicis brevis. This is true, but if the superficial head of this muscle is paralyzed, what works as the substitute? Functional examination of patients with a median nerve palsy reveals that because they are really unable to bring the thumb into opposition, they either substitute by pronation of the forearm or internal rotation and abduction of the shoulder. In picking up an article from a table, the palsied thumb is positioned by the abductor pollicis longus. Therefore, although the thumb index web is open, it is done so not in pronation of the thumb but in supination, because the abductor pollicis longus, extensor pollicis brevis, and extensor pollicis longus are all supinators. To compensate for this supination effect of the substitute musculature, the forearm pronates (Fig. 39-19). Because of lack of good sensibility in the median nerve distribution, the patient has a pattern of use that for all practical purposes is not useful to him. He cannot see the palm of his hand. The real reason for doing an opposition transfer early on after a median nerve paralysis is so that the patient can position his thumb in opposition with the wrist in either supination, neutral, or pronation. Almost all patients will preferentially select either supination or midrotation of the forearm to use the hand; because in these positions the palmar surface of the hand is exposed to the eyes and the patient can then use his eyes to make up for the lack of sensibility in the hand. If, in fact, the patient must use the hand

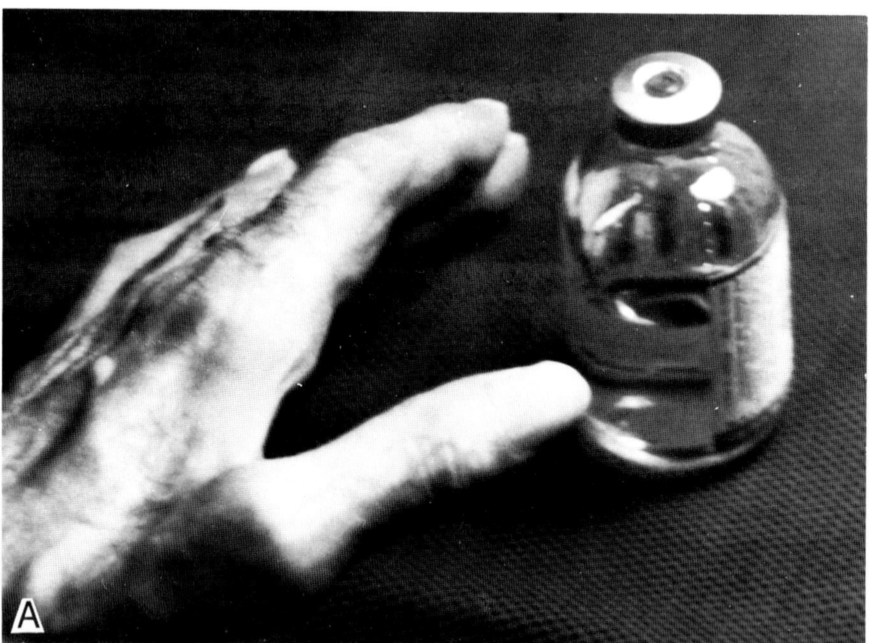

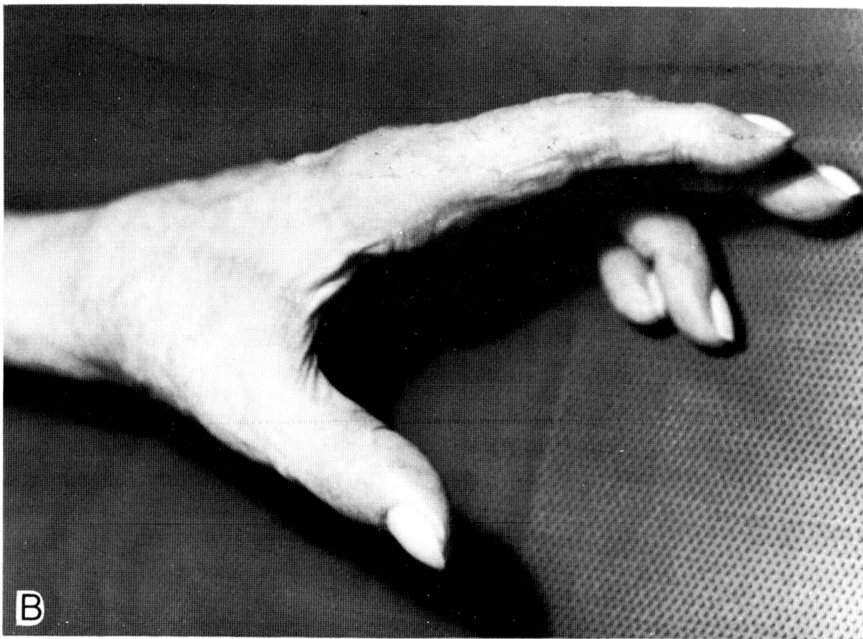

Fig. 39-19. A patient with a brachial plexus injury is shown attempting to pick up a bottle with the hand in full pronation **(A)**. This is a substitute maneuver for an absent abductor pollis brevis or flexor pollicis brevis. Following opponensplasty **(B)**, with the patient's forearm in neutral rotation, it is possible to position the hand for grasp. The patient can see the palmar surface of the hand.

in pronation because of his inability to position the thumb, his eyes are no longer an effective aid in hand use. I would therefore suggest that when thinking of the timing for opponensplasty, the surgeon watch the thumb position when the patient tries to perform activities, such as picking up a glass or change, and note if, in fact, the patient is using his hand in forearm pronation. If so, this patient probably does need an early tendon transfer to restore maximal function in the thumb and hand. If he is able to use the hand to pick up articles and transfer objects from hand to hand with the injured hand in a position other than full pronation, then he is probably not a candidate for early tendon transfer. This is probably because he has an innervated portion of the flexor pollicis brevis, which renders his hand fairly functional.

Selection of Motors

If the decision is made to perform an early tendon transfer to restore opposition of the thumb in a *high* median nerve palsy, what transfer should be used? Obviously, in this case the proprius tendons are the most readily available. These tendons position the thumb well, do not create significant functional deficit by their removal from the hand, and do not require a tendon graft for lengthening. The use of a paralyzed superficialis motored by a functional flexor carpi ulnaris as mentioned by Irwin[28] and Goldner[22] brings about strong opposition of the thumb. This has at least some theoretic objections in that the only remaining wrist flexor is eliminated. Moreover, strong opposition of the thumb is not required as long as there are functioning intrinsic muscles that are capable of acting as a short flexor or short flexor substitute.[18]

To summarize, I would suggest that in a high median nerve injury, the surgeon should think of doing an opposition transfer if pronation of the forearm is a substitute motion used by the patient and that probably one of the proprius tendons is more appropriate for early tendon transfer than anything else. If a neurorrhaphy is possible, I do not think any extrinsic replacement should be used early in the management of the patient. Significant extrinsic power will generally return following a high median nerve neurorrhaphy, and this really does not create a problem. On the other hand, if the patient has required a nerve graft, especially if done late or under unfavorable conditions (e.g., long graft or a poor bed), the anticipated return of function is not likely to be satisfactory. In this patient one may consider doing the extrinsic flexor replacement as previously described; i.e., brachioradialis to flexor pollicis longus and extensor carpi radialis longus to the index and long profundus tendons. All of these transfers, both intrinsic and extrinsic replacements, can be performed at the same time. Since in the postoperative period the wrist is going to be in volar flexion, the thumb can easily be placed in full opposition to release the tension on the brachioradialis transfer to the flexor pollicis longus, as well as reducing the tension on the proprius tendon transfer. This will reduce the tension on the extensor carpi radialis longus transfer to the flexor digitorum profundi.

SUMMARY

All of the significant functional deficits in median nerve injury cannot be restored by tendon transfer. Lack of normal sensibility on the radial aspect of the hand is a real deterrent to hand function. Opposition transfers are many and varied; almost every motor has been used, many pulleys are available, and distal methods of attachment are likewise innumerable. The major reasons for failure to achieve satisfactory opposition of the thumb with a transfer are persistence of a contracture within the thumb (recognized or unrecognized) and the selection of a poor motor. Early opposition transfer (i.e., very soon after neurorrhaphy) should be carried out in those patients who have a pronation attitude of the forearm as a substitute for the nonfunctioning abductor pollicis brevis. Extrinsic replacement probably should be required early only in those patients that have had a nerve graft in less than optimum situations or in those patients in whom, for one reason or another, neurorrhaphy of the median nerve is not considered.

REFERENCES

1. Beasley RW: Principles of tendon transfer. Orthop Clin North Am 1:433–438, 1970
2. Bohr HH: Tendon transposition in paralysis of opposition of the thumb. Acta Chir Scand 105:45, 1953
3. Boswick JA, Stromberg WB: Isolated injury to the median nerve above the elbow. A review of thirteen cases. J Bone Joint Surg 49A:653, 1967
4. Brand PW: The hand in leprosy. p. 279. In Pulverlaft RG (ed): Clinical Surgery of the Hand. Butterworth's, London, 1966
5. Brand PW: Tendon transfer for median and ulnar nerve paralysis. Orthop Clin North Am 1:447–454, 1970
6. Brand PW, Beach RB and Thompson DE: Relative tension and potential excursion of muscles in the forearm and hand. J Hand Surg 6:209–219, 1981
7. Braun RM: Palmaris longus tendon transfer for augmentation of the thenar musculature in low median palsy. J Hand Surg 3:488–491, 1978
8. Brown PW: The time factor in surgery of upper extremity peripheral nerve injury. Clin Orthop 68:14–21, 1970
9. Brown PW: Adduction-flexion contracture of the thumb. Correction with dorsal rotation flap and release of contracture. Clin Orthop 88:161, 1972
10. Browne EZ, Teague MA, Snyder CC: Prevention of extensor lag after indicis proprius tendon transfer. J Hand Surg 4:168–172, 1979
11. Bunnell S: Opposition of the thumb. J Bone Joint Surg 20:269–284, 1938
12. Burkhalter WE: Tendon transfers in median nerve palsy. Orthop Clin North Am 5:271–281, 1974
13. Burkhalter WE: Early tendon transfer in upper extremity peripheral nerve injury. Clin Orthop 104:68–79, 1974
14. Burkhalter WE, Christensen RC, Brown PW: Extensor indicis proprius opponensplasty. J Bone Joint Surg 55A:725–732, 1973
15. Camitz H: Über die Behandlung der Opposition slähmung. Acta Chir Scand 65:77, 1929
16. Chouhy-Aguirre S, Caplan S: Sobre secuelas de lesion alta e irreparable di nervio meidano y cubital y su tratamiento. Prensa Med Argentina 43:2341–2346, 1956
17. Cooney WP: Tendon transfer for median nerve palsy. Hand Clinics 4:155–165, 1988
18. Cooney WP, Linscheid RL, An K: An opposition of the thumb: an anatomic and biomechanical study of tendon transfers. J Hand Surg 9A:777–786, 1984
19. Curtis RM: Opposition of the thumb. Orthop Clin North Am 5:305–321, 1974
20. DeVeechi J: Opposición del pulgar fisiopatologia una nerva operactión transplante del aductor. Bol Soc Cir Uruguay 32:423, 1961
21. Goldner JL, Clippinger FW: Excision of the greater multangular bone as an adjunct to mobilization of the thumb. J Bone Joint Surg 41A:609–625, 1959
22. Goldner JL, Irwin CE: An analysis of paralytic thumb deformities. J Bone Joint Surg 32A:627–639, 1950
23. Groves RJ, Goldner JL: Restoration of strong opposition after median nerve or brachial plexus paralysis. J Bone Joint Surg 57:112–115, 1975

24. Henderson ED: Transfer of wrist extensor and brachioradialis to restore opposition of the thumb. J Bone Joint Surg 44A:513-522, 1962
25. Herrick RT, Lister GD: Control of first web space contracture. Including a review of the literature and a tabulation of opponensplasty techniques. Hand 9:253-264, 1977
26. Hill NA: Restoration of opposition for the paralyzed thumb. Clin Orthop 61:234-249, 1968
27. Huber E: Hilfsoperation bei median Uslähmung. Dtsch Arch Klin Med 136:271, 1921
28. Irwin CE: Transplant to the thumb to restore function of opposition. End results. South Med J 35:257, 1942
29. Jacobs B, Thompson TC: Opposition of the thumb and its restoration. J Bone Joint Surg 42A:1015-1026, 1960
30. Jensen, EG: Restoration of opposition of the thumb. Hand 10:161-167, 1978
31. Kaplan I, Dinner M, Chait L: Use of extensor pollicis longus tendon as a distal extension for an opponens transfer. Plast Reconstr Surg 57:186-189, 1976
32. Kessler I: Transfer of extensor carpi ulnaris to tendon of extensor pollicis brevis for opponensplasty. J Bone Joint Surg 51A:1303-1308, 1969
33. Kirklin JW, Thomas CG: Opponens transplant. An analysis of the method employed and results obtained in 75 cases. Surg Gynecol Obstet 86:213, 1948
34. Littler JW: Tendon transfers and arthrodesis in combined median and ulnar nerve paralysis. J Bone Joint Surg 31A:225-234, 1949
35. Littler JW, Cooley SGE: Opposition of the thumb and its restoration by abductor digiti quinti transfer. J Bone Joint Surg 45A:1389-1396, 1963
36. Littler JW, Li CS: Primary restoration of thumb opposition with median nerve decompression. Plast Reconstr Surg 39:74-75, 1967
37. Makin M: Translocation of the flexor pollicis longus tendon to restore opposition. J Bone Joint Surg 49B:458-461, 1967
38. Mangus DJ: Flexor pollicis longus tendon transfer for restoration of opposition of the thumb. Plast Reconstr Surg 52:155, 1973
39. Mannerfelt L: Structures of the hand in ulnar nerve paralysis. A clinical experimental investigation in normal and anomalies of innervation. Acta Orthop Scand (suppl)87:1966
40. Mayer L: Operative reconstruction of the paralyzed upper extremity. J Bone Joint Surg 21:377, 1939
41. Michelinakis E, Vourexakis H: Tendon transfer for intrinsic muscle paralysis of the thumb in Charcot-Marie Tooth neuropathy. Hand 13:276-278, 1981
42. Mutz SB: Thumb web contracture. Hand 4:236-246, 1972
43. Ney KW: A tendon transplant for intrinsic hand muscle paralysis. Surg Gynecol Obstet 33:342, 1921
44. Nicolaysen J: Transplantation des m. Abductor dig. V. Die Fenlender Oppositions Fehigkeit des Daumens. Dtsch Z Chir 168:133, 1922
45. North ER, Littler JW: Transferring the flexor superficialis tendon: Technical considerations in the prevention of proximal interphalangeal joint disability. J Hand Surg 5:498-501, 1980
46. Omer GE Jr: The technique and timing of tendon transfers. Orthop Clin North Am 5:243-252, 1974
47. Omer GE Jr: Reconstruction of a balanced thumb through tendon transfers. Clin Orthop 195:104-116, 1985
48. Orticochea M: Use of the deep bundle of the flexor pollicis brevis to restore opposition of the thumb. Plast Reconstr Surg 47:220, 1971
49. Palande, DD: Opponensplasty in intrinsic-muscle paralysis of the thumb in leprosy. J Bone Joint Surg 57A:489-493, 1975
50. Phalen GS, Miller RC: Transfer of wrist extensor muscles to restore or reinforce flexion power of the fingers and opposition of the thumb. J Bone Joint Surg 29:993-997, 1947
51. Ramselaar JM: Tendon transfers to restore opposition of the thumb. HE Stefert Kroese NV, Leiden, Holland, 1970
52. Riley WB Jr, Mann RJ, Burkhalter WE: Extensor pollicis longus opponensplasty. J Hand Surg 5:217-220, 1980
53. Riordan DC: Tendon transfers for nerve paralysis of the hand and wrist. Curr Pract Orthop Surg 2:17, 1964
54. Rowntree T: Anomalous innervation of the hand muscles. J Bone Joint Surg 31B:505-510, 1949
55. Royle ND: An operation for paralysis of the intrinsic muscles of the thumb. JAMA 111:612, 1938
56. Sakellarides HT: Modified pulley for opponens tendon transfer. J Bone Joint Surg 52A:178-179, 1970
57. Schneider LH: Opponensplasty using the extensor digiti minimi. J Bone Joint Surg 51A:1297-1302, 1969
58. Snow JW, Fing GH: Use of transverse carpal ligament window for the pulley in tendon transfers for median nerve palsy. Plast Reconstr Surg 48:238, 1971
59. Steindler A: Orthopaedic operations on the hand. JAMA 71:1288, 1918
60. Steindler A: Flexorplasty of the thumb in thenar palsy. Surg Gynecol Obstet 50:1005, 1930
61. Taylor TR: Reconstruction of the hand; a new technique in tenoplasty. Surg Gynecol Obstet 32:237-248, 1921
62. Thompson TC: A modified operation for opponens paralysis. J Bone Joint Surg 24:632-640, 1942
63. Tubiana R, Valentin P: Opposition of the thumb. Surg Clin North Am 48:967, 1968
64. Wissinger HA, Singsen EG: Abductor digiti quinti opponensplasty. J Bone Joint Surg 59A:895-898, 1977
65. Wood VE, Adams J: Complications of opponensplasty with transfer of extensor carpi ulnaris to extensor pollicis brevis. J Hand Surg 9A:699-704, 1984

40

Ulnar Nerve Palsy

George E. Omer, Jr.

Ulnar nerve palsy results in an awkward hand with significant sensibility loss and profound weakness.

CLINICAL PICTURE

There are ten motor and sensory functions lost in ulnar nerve palsy, and it is imperative for the surgeon to understand these deficits before embarking on a reconstructive program.

Motor Loss

1. Loss of flexion of the proximal phalanges of the fingers due to paralysis of the interossei and other intrinsic muscles. If extrinsic muscle function is intact, the ring and little fingers will claw (*Duchenne's sign,* 1867),[29,50] with hyperextension of the proximal phalanges and flexion of the middle and distal phalanges. However, if hyperextension is passively prevented by dorsal pressure, the extensor digitorum communis can extend the middle and distal phalanges (*Bouvier's maneuver,* 1851).[100] An unconscious effort to extend the fingers by tenodesing the extensor tendons with palmar flexion of the wrist only increases the deformity (*André-Thomas sign,* 1917).[50]

   A specific clinical gesture demonstrating ulnar nerve palsy is the "cross your fingers" test.[70] There is inability to cross the flexed long finger dorsally over the index finger, or the index over the long finger, when the palm and fingers are placed on a flat surface.[70] This maneuver tests the first volar interosseous and second dorsal interosseous muscles.[30] A related gesture is the inability to abduct the extended long (middle) finger in radial and ulnar deviation with the hand flat on a surface, which tests the second and third dorsal interossei muscles (*Pitres-Testut sign,* 1925).[30,50]
2. Loss of integration of MP and interphalangeal joint flexion, due to paralysis of the lumbrical muscles to the ring and little fingers.[33] Normal finger flexion is initiated at the MP joint, and then all three finger joints flex simultaneously. In intrinsic paralysis, the MP joint does not flex until interphalangeal joint flexion has been completed. The fingers curl or roll into the palm, and objects are pushed away instead of grasped.
3. Loss of lateral or key pinch of the thumb, due to paralysis of the adductor pollicis muscle, which normally acts as a first metacarpal adductor, a flexor of the thumb MP joint, and an extensor of the thumb interphalangeal joint. Ulnar nerve palsy is obvious when the MP joint of the thumb is hyperextended 10 to 15 degrees with key pinch or gross grip (*Jeanne's sign,* 1915).[16,82]
4. Flattened metacarpal arch (palmar arch) and loss of hypothenar elevation (*Masse's sign,* 1916),[50] due to paralysis of opponens digiti quinti and the decreased range of flexion of the little finger MP joint.[94] These four lost functions above are responsible for the inefficient power grip associated with low (distal) ulnar nerve palsy. Power grip is even weaker in a high (proximal) ulnar nerve palsy.
5. Loss of extrinsic power to the ulnar innervated portion of the flexor digitorum profundus, with inability to flex the distal phalanges of the ring and little fingers (*Pollock's sign,* 1919).[50]
6. Partial loss of wrist flexion, due to paralysis of the flexor carpi ulnaris. The position of the wrist is

significant in power grip, since it is held in neutral.[4] In precision grip, the wrist is dorsiflexed until the thumb lies in line with the radius.

7. Precision grip is impaired in ulnar nerve palsy: loss of active lateral mobility with the fingers in extension, due to paralysis of the interossei and hypothenar muscles.[85,86] Since there is paralysis also of the adductor pollicis muscle, there is inability to bring the tips of the extended digits together into a cone (*Pitres-Testut,* 1925).[50] There is an inability to adduct the extended little finger to the extended ring finger (*Wartenberg's sign,* 1930)[43,50] due to the activity of the extensor digiti minimi, which is unopposed by the paralyzed third palmar interosseous.
8. Loss of distal stability and rotation for tip pinch between the thumb and index finger (*Froment's sign,* 1915)[16,82] (*Bunnell's "O" sign,* 1956),[4,20,50] *(Newspaper sign),* due to paralysis of the first dorsal and second palmar interossei and the adductor pollicis muscles. The thumb interphalangeal joint may flex 80 to 90 degrees as the flexor pollicis longus attempts to hold the object.

   The residual strength for palmar adduction of the thumb (key pinch) may be diminished as much as 77 to 80 percent in ulnar nerve palsy.[50] The impairment for power grip is greater than the loss of power for precise grasp.[4]

Sensory Loss

9. Sensibility function is lost in ulnar nerve palsy over the volar side of the little finger and the ulnar aspect of the volar side of the ring finger.[65,66]
10. In the high (proximal) ulnar nerve palsy, there is additional sensibility loss over the dorso-ulnar aspect of the palm and the dorsal side of the little finger.

Anomalous Innervation Patterns

The ten major functional deficiencies outlined above are found in the patient with the usual innervation pattern for the ulnar nerve. A careful examination of the extremity may demonstrate anomalous innervation patterns: the ulnar nerve always contains axons from the anterior divisions of C8 and T1, but often also contains axons from the anterior division of C7 root. In 5 percent to 10 percent of upper extremities, the motor axons to the flexor carpi ulnaris arise from the C7 root rather than from the C8 and T1 roots;[43] therefore, it is not uncommon to observe a functioning flexor carpi ulnaris with a complete C8 and T1 lesion.

There are several potential anomalous neural patterns of the ulnar nerve in the forearm. The Martin (1763)-Gruber (1870) communication[43,50] occurs adjacent to the ulnar artery in the proximal forearm and is between the median nerve, or its anterior interosseous branch, and the ulnar nerve. There is a 15 percent occurrence of this anomaly, which carries motor axons from the median nerve to the ulnar nerve and on to many of the intrinsic muscles of the hand. There is a second potential communication in the distal forearm between the ulnar nerve and the median nerve that is far less frequent than the Martin-Gruber connection. There is also a communication within the flexor digitorum profundus between the ulnar nerve and the anterior interosseous branch of the median nerve, resulting in potential variations in the innervation of this muscle. The innervation of the flexor digitorum profundus may vary from all ulnar to all median to a completely dual nerve supply.

Riche (1897) and Cannieu (1897) described a potential connection between the motor branch of the ulnar nerve and the recurrent branch of the median nerve in the hand.[43] These anomalous neural patterns occasionally permit a hand to present without deformity even though a complete ulnar palsy is present. For example, the median nerve may innervate all of the lumbricals, and there would be no clawing of the digits. The third lumbrical has dual innervation in 50 percent of upper extremities,[43] and in such a hand, a complete low (distal) ulnar nerve palsy would result in clawing in only the little finger. The first dorsal interosseous is innervated completely or partially by the median nerve in 10 percent of hands and by the radial nerve in 1 percent of hands.[43]

The dorsal cutaneous sensory branch of the ulnar nerve perforates the fascia 6 to 8 cm proximal to the wrist and supplies the dorso-ulnar surface of the hand and the little finger. However, this area can be supplied by the superficial branch of the radial nerve, which will lead to confusion concerning the level of the ulnar nerve lesion.

Diagnostic errors can be avoided with careful voluntary muscle testing, precise evaluation of sensibility and sudomotor activity, anesthetic blocks of intact nerves, and electrodiagnostic studies that include conduction times across selected segments of the ulnar nerve.[59,65,66,68,70]

After complete evaluation of the patient, all possible surgical solutions should be considered. Nerve suture is the basic approach to a nerve palsy,[2] but tendon transfers or joint arthrodeses may be acceptable alternate procedures.[12] Each patient has special problems and reconstruction must be individualized.

TIMING OF TENDON TRANSFERS

Patient evaluation is a major factor in the clinical decision for tendon transfers. The patient must be able to understand what is to be done and be ready to accept the postoperative discipline necessary for rehabilitation. The surgeon should determine whether the patient desires an increased functional performance or cosmetic improvement.

Homeostasis of the involved extremity must be established before elective tendon surgery.[61,73] There should be stable skeletal alignment with near-normal passive motion of joints. Soft tissues should be free of scar contractures and have adequate circulation. Chronic wounds are contraindications to elective surgery. The functional performance expected after tendon transfer should be possible to effect by passive movement before surgery.

An important aspect of initial treatment is the appropriate use of individualized splints, which should be fabricated for each patient and changed whenever indicated.[57,60] Problems in splinting the hand with ulnar nerve palsy are the maintenance of the transverse palmar arch, and adequate lumbrical and thenar stops to maintain the functional position.[52] External splints are sometimes awkward and often interfere with sensory function.

INTERNAL SPLINTS (EARLY TENDON TRANSFERS)

The objectives of selected early tendon transfers are to stimulate sensibility reeducation and to improve the coordination of the residual muscle-tendon units so that they can temporarily substitute for the palsied motors until either they are reinnervated, or the transferred muscle-tendon units become their permanent replacement if the injured nerve does not recover.[22,23,63] A complete reconstructive program with multiple tendon transfers is not indicated for internal splinting; instead, the surgeon should use as few tendon transfers as required to maintain dynamic positions for functional coordination and sensibility reeducation.

Low Ulnar Nerve Palsy "Y" Technique (Omer[5,58,64,71,72])

An isolated tendon transfer cannot restore all of the power requirements in a low ulnar nerve palsy, but a single flexor digitorum superficialis tendon can improve the integration of MP and interphalangeal joint flexion, key pinch for the thumb, and the flattened metacarpal arch. Arthrodesis of the MP joint of the thumb will improve distal stability for tip pinch. The flexor digitorum superficialis tendon of either the ring or long finger is suitable, but the ring finger superficialis is preferable if the ulnar-innervated portion of the flexor digitorum profundus is not paralyzed (Fig. 40-1).

The ring superficialis tendon is exposed through a volar zigzag incision that extends into the palm, and short longitudinal incisions are made over the abductor tubercle of the thumb and the dorsal side of the ring and little fingers at the level of the PIP joint (for dorsal apparatus insertion). There is potential for a residual hyperextension deformity at the PIP joint following release of the superficialis tendon. Therefore, the radial slip of insertion of the superficialis tendon is released proximal to the PIP joint and tenodesed to prevent hyperextension of the joint after completion of the transfer. The ulnar slip of the superficialis tendon is released at its terminal insertion. The flexor sheath should be retained, especially the proximal A1 and A2 pulleys. The flexor digitorum superficialis is first split longitudinally well into the palm, and the ulnar half of the tendon is

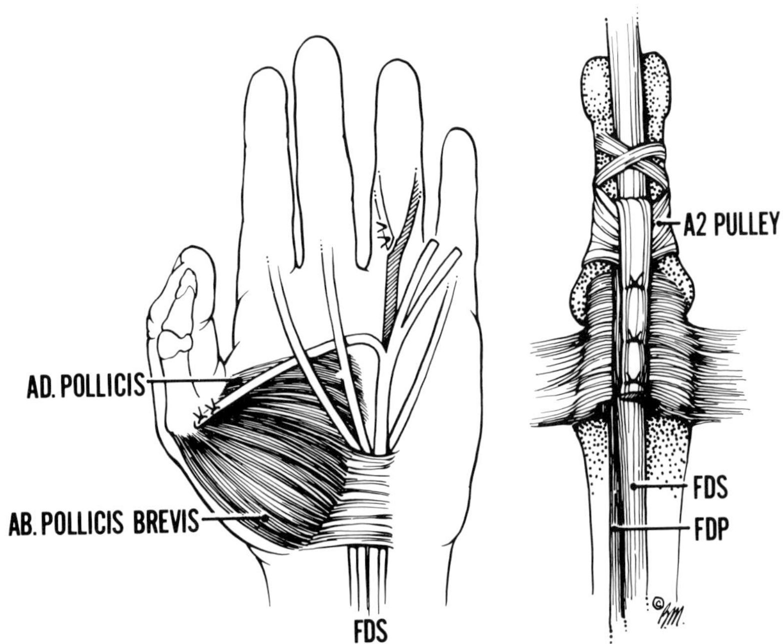

Fig. 40-1. Transfer of the flexor digitorum superficialis *(FDS)* as an "internal splint" for low ulnar nerve palsy. The tendon is detached at the PIP level with tenodesis of the radial half across the joint. The tendon is split into two slips, and the radial half of the tendon passes volar to the adductor pollicis muscle and dorsal to the flexor digitorum profundus *(FDP)* tendons into the insertion of the abductor pollicis brevis. The ulnar half of the tendon is again split into two slips that are directed distally and volar to the deep transverse metacarpal ligament and looped through the A2 annular pulley of the flexor sheath. The result is improved thumb-index pinch, and active flexion returns to the MP joint.

split again into two slips. The two slips of the ulnar half of the tendon are inserted by one of two techniques.

If preoperative testing reveals that the interphalangeal joints cannot be actively extended when the MP joint is stabilized in flexion, the insertion is into the dorsal apparatus. The two slips of the ulnar half of the tendon are directed ulnar to the deep transverse metacarpal ligament and then dorsally to be sutured at the insertion of the central slip of the dorsal apparatus on the middle phalanx of the ring and little fingers. This will correct clawing of these digits. Traction on the transferred tendon slips should flex the MP joints and extend the PIP joint.

A different insertion for the two slips is preferred when increased power for grip is desirable and if the extrinsic extensor will extend the PIP joint with the MP joint stabilized in flexion.[25,46] A longitudinal zigzag incision is made on the volar side of the little finger, in addition to the incision on the volar side of the ring finger. The proximal edges of the flexor sheaths are exposed, and the superficialis slips are passed distally through the flexor sheaths and around the distal edge of the A2 pulley and sutured into place.[28] The A2 pulley has a better moment arm than the A1 pulley.[72] This insertion does not extend the PIP joint, and is similar to dynamic transfers for proximal phalanx flexion.[14,100]

The radial half of the superficialis tendon is directed transversely over the volar surface of the adductor pollicis but dorsal to the flexor tendons and neurovascular structures, and is sutured into the insertion of the abductor pollicis brevis. The pulley for this transfer is the distal edge of the palmar fascia inserted into the third metacarpal.[31] Traction on the transferred half tendon should adduct and pronate the first metacarpal.

The resting tension of the transferred tendon is adjusted at the insertion points while the wrist is in neutral flexion-extension and the hand is supinated into a palm up position. The MP joints of the clawed fingers are placed in 45 degrees flexion, and the PIP joints in zero degrees extension (10 degrees of flexion if tenodesed). The first metacarpal is adducted so that it is parallel with the plane of the second metacarpal in an anterior-posterior projection. This intrinsic-plus position is maintained in plaster immobilization for 4 weeks before active extension is allowed.

Distal stability for tip pinch between the thumb and index finger is improved by arthrodesis of the MP joint of the thumb,[57,60] and is indicated when the patient develops a positive Jeanne's sign following transfer of the flexor digitorum superficialis.[41] The joint is approached through a longitudinal incision on the dorsal side of the thumb. The dorsal apparatus is split between the extensor pollicis longus and brevis tendons. Synovium is excised, and the distal end of the first metacarpal and the proximal end of the proximal phalanx are denuded of soft tissue. The joint surfaces are cut back with a power saw to produce a chevron-shaped mortise, with the point of the chevron directed proximally (Fig. 40-2). The apex of the phalangeal half of the chevron mortise is made perpendicular to the long axis of the proximal phalanx, while that of the metacarpal portion of the chevron is inclined palmarward to obtain the desired angle of flexion for the arthrodesed joint. The desired flexion is 10 to 15 degrees, and the mortise is then stabilized with buried, crossed K-wires. The wires may be removed after bony healing.

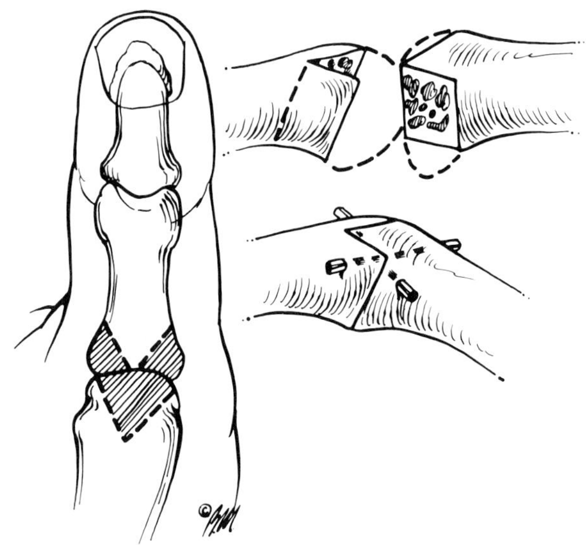

Fig. 40-2. Chevron-shaped mortise for arthrodesis of the MP or PIP joints. The extent of the proximal bone cut on the volar surface determines the amount of flexion. Parallel K-wires may be used for fixation.

This transfer of a single flexor digitorum superficialis tendon and arthrodesis of the thumb MP joint will improve four of the six lost motor functions in a low (distal) ulnar nerve palsy, especially thumb adduction and/or key pinch, (Table 40-1). However, this internal splint transfer does not add strength for proximal phalanx flexion or power grip, which is a major problem in ulnar nerve palsy.[67] Moreover, this transfer decreases grip strength because the superficialis tendon is dissipated into several insertions, while additional strength requires a new muscle-tendon unit in the power train. This transfer should improve the coordination of the residual active muscle-tendon units during the interval between the injury and nerve regeneration, and is not a definitive reconstructive program.

PROXIMAL PHALANX FLEXION

Any surgical procedure that prevents MP joint hyperextension will control the claw deformity initiated by the extrinsic muscles. Brand[9] believes that ulnar nerve palsy will result in a claw deformity in all four fingers, although this may be apparent in the index and middle fingers only during power pinch.

Static Block Techniques (Howard,[20] Mikail,[51] Zancolli[99])

Mikail inserted a bone block on the dorsum of the metacarpal head to prevent hyperextension of the proximal phalanx and reported on six patients followed up to 4 years. Howard suggested a bone slab or wedge from the dorsal side of the metacarpal, which was displaced distalward as a bone block. Arthrodesis has been suggested,[20] but this limits flexion of the fingers into the palm.

Zancolli approaches each MP joint through a volar longitu-

Table 40-1. Internal Splints for Low (Distal) Ulnar Nerve Palsy Using One Primary Tendon (Flexor Digitorum Superficialis)

Needed Function	Internal Splint Transfer	Supplemental Motors
Thumb adduction for key pinch	Radial one-half of flexor digitorum superficialis[58,63,64,72] —long finger	
Proximal phalanx flexion—ring and little fingers; Integration of MP and interphalangeal motion—ring and little finger	Ulnar one-half of flexor digitorum superficialis—split insertion to ring and little fingers[46,47]	
Metacarpal (palmar) transverse arch and adduction for little finger	"Y" insertion of the two halves of the long flexor digitorum superficialis[46,47,71,72]	
Thumb-index tip pinch	Arthrodesis thumb MP joint[58,62,69]	Extensor pollicis brevis to first dorsal interosseous[18]

dinal incision. A short flap with a distal base is cut from the volar plate and drawn proximally and sutured into the metacarpal neck with the joint in 20 degrees flexion.[99] It is necessary to open the A1 pulley of the flexor sheath to incise the flap from the volar plate. The result is a minimal flexion contracture of the MP joint.

Zancolli's procedure has had several modifications (Fig. 40-3). A transverse incision in the distal palmar crease and cutting a triangle into the deep transverse metacarpal ligament on each side of the volar plate flap have provided a better view and a more secure fixation of the flap.[57,60] The excision of a 1.5-cm wide ellipse of palmar skin has been recommended to prevent stretching of the volar plate flap.[15] The advanced volar plate has been inserted into the metacarpal neck and immobilized for a minimum of 6 weeks.[44] Long-term follow-up studies of patients with normally relaxed joint capsules have demonstrated recurrence of clawing.[15]

Bunnell[19,20] performed a flexor pulley advancement as an isolated procedure. Each side of the proximal pulley is split 1.5 to 2.5 cm to the middle of the proximal phalanx. The flexor tendons will then "bowstring," which increases the movement across the MP joint and the power of flexion. The procedure is not effective if there is damage to the extrinsic extensors or the dorsal apparatus of the finger. Fingers often develop ulnar drift when the pulley advancement is carried distal to the A2 pulley.

Static Tenodesis Techniques (Parkes,[75] Riordan[78,80])

Parkes devised a static distal tenodesis by placing a free tendon graft between the radial lateral band of the dorsal apparatus of the finger and the flexor retinaculum (deep transverse metacarpal ligament) in the palm (Fig. 40-4). The tenodesis is sutured with the MP joint in 45 degrees of flexion. The grafts function independently on each finger. I have passed the graft from the dorsal apparatus of the ring finger around the deep transverse metacarpal ligament and on to the dorsal apparatus of the little finger, allowing equivalent tension. Parkes' technique is the most predictable of the static distal tenodeses.

Riordan uses a dorsal approach to expose the extensor carpi radialis longus and the extensor carpi ulnaris tendon. Each tendon is divided longitudinally from its insertion proximally to the juncture of the middle and distal thirds of the forearm. One half of each divided tendon is freed and further split longitudinally. The four tendon slips are left attached at their metacarpal insertion, and the free ends are passed between the metacarpals volar to the deep transverse metacarpal ligament and sutured to the radial lateral bands of the dorsal apparatus. This tenodesis arises distal to the wrist joint, and therefore is a static tenodesis to prevent hyperextension of the MP joint. Only the extensor carpi ulnaris is necessary if only the ring and little fingers are to be tenodesed. The tenodesis are sutured with the wrist in 30 degrees dorsiflexion and the MP joints in 80 degrees flexion.

INTEGRATION OF FINGER FLEXION

The loss of simultaneous MP flexion with interphalangeal extension and flexion prevents the controlled rhythm necessary to hold large and small objects. Most of the tendon transfers designed to improve the synchronous motion of the finger joints found in ulnar palsy attempt to duplicate the lumbrical muscles, and therefore pass volar to the deep transverse metacarpal ligament and insert into the lateral band of the dorsal apparatus.[34,48,86]

Dynamic Tenodesis Techniques (Fowler[34,78])

Fowler developed a wrist-driven active tenodesis by passing two tendon grafts through an opening made in the dorsal retinaculum and passing the four tendon ends through the inter-

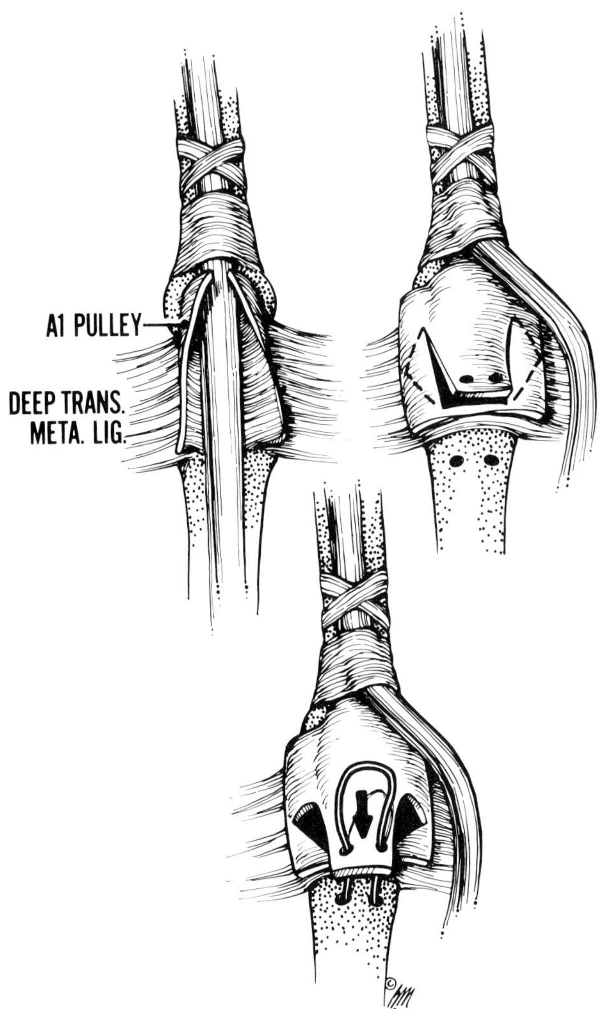

Fig. 40-3. Capsulodesis of the MP joint to control "claw fingers" deformity. The excised triangles extend into the deep transverse metacarpal ligament and allow the volar plate flap to advance proximally to a straight line. The flap is anchored into the metacarpal.

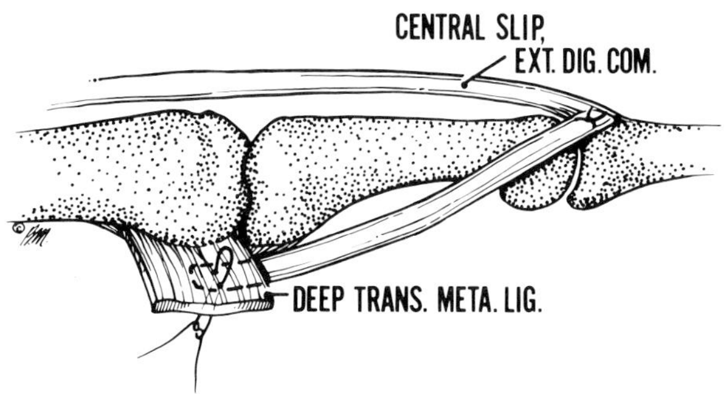

Fig. 40-4. Volar tenodesis to control "claw finger" deformity. A free tendon graft passes from the central slip insertion at the PIP joint through the lumbrical canal to the deep transverse ligament. The tension is adjusted for each individual finger.

metacarpal spaces, then volar to the deep transverse metacarpal ligament, and through the lumbrical canals to the lateral bands of the dorsal apparatus (Fig. 40-5). When the wrist flexes, the tendon grafts are tightened, and active MP flexion with interphalangeal extension is achieved. The tenodeses are sutured with the wrist in 30 degrees dorsiflexion and the MP joints in 80 degrees flexion with the interphalangeal joints in full extension (zero degrees). Tsuge[95] fixes the proximal (high) point of the tenodesis through drill holes in the distal radius to be certain that movements of the wrist act dynamically upon the free tendon graft. I. Kessler (personal communication, April 1980) has used the extensor retinaculum for the proximal part of the tenodesis, but the distal free tendon slips are sutured around the A1 pulley similar to Zancolli's "lasso" procedure. The tendon slips are directed dorsal to volar through the intermetacarpal spaced and sutured with the MP joint in flexion. Extension is blocked at least 3 weeks, but active flexion is continued.

Superficialis Techniques (Riordan,[78-80] Stiles,[92] Bunnell,[7,19] Zancolli[87,99,100])

The Stiles tendon transfer probably was the first tendon transfer performed for intrinsic paralysis. Stiles transferred the superficialis to the extensor digitorum comminus through several tendon slips. Bunnell's modification of Stiles's procedure

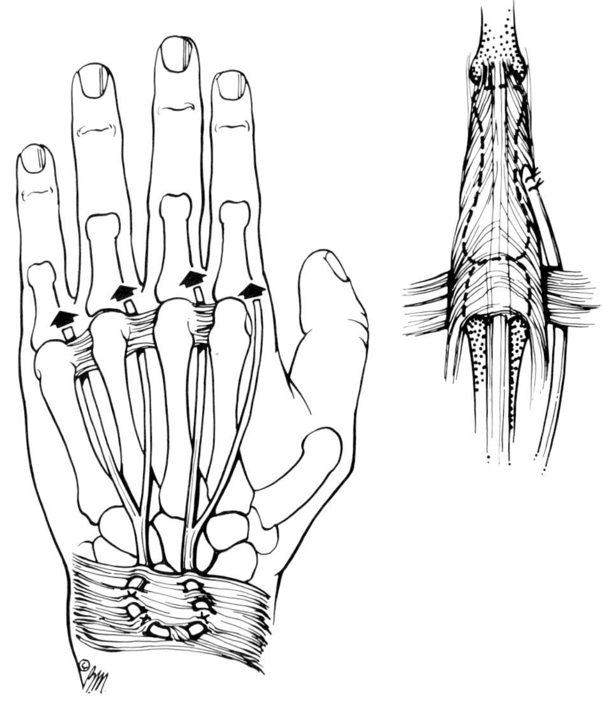

Fig. 40-5. Dynamic dorsal tenodesis to control "claw finger" deformity. The free tendon graft is looped through the extensor retinaculum (dorsal carpal ligament); the slips pass volar to the deep transverse metacarpal ligament and into the lateral bands of the dorsal apparatus.

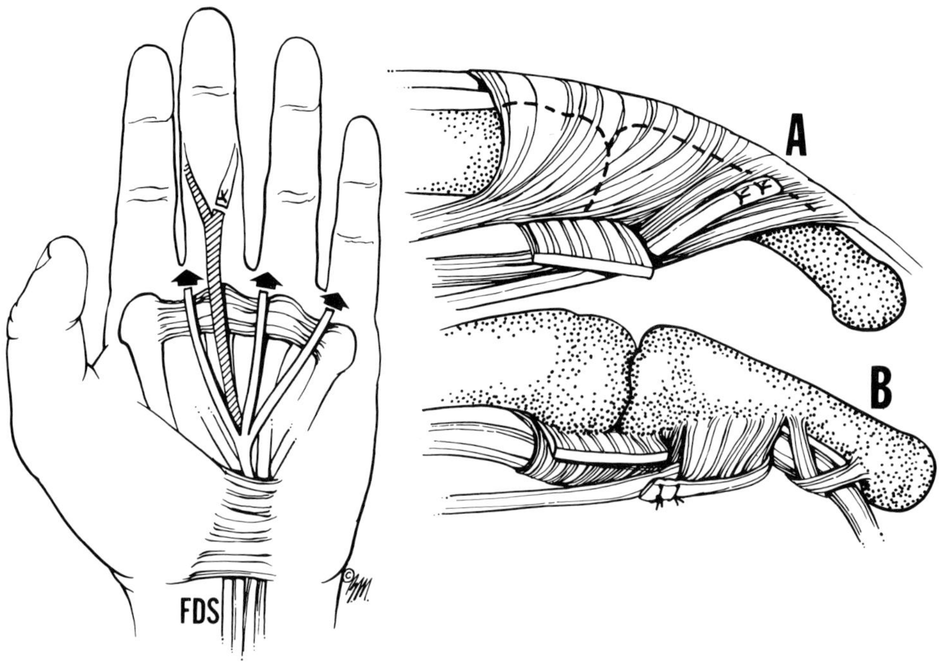

Fig. 40-6. Transfer of a flexor digitorum superficialis *(FDS)* to control "claw-finger" deformity. The tendon is divided into two to four slips, which are passed through the lumbrical canals and volar to the deep transverse metacarpal ligament. The individual slips may be inserted **(A)** into the lateral band of the dorsal apparatus, or **(B)** into the A2 pulley of the flexor sheath. One-half of the distal tendon of the donor superficialis tendon is tenodesed initially across the PIP joint to prevent hyperextension deformity. This transfer does not add power to finger flexion.

transferred the superficialis slips into the intrinsic apparatus to provide both radial and ulnar deviation to each finger. Riordan's modification is the standard technique: The flexor digitorum superficialis of the long finger is split into four slips, and one slip is passed through the lumbrical canal of each finger to be inserted into the radial lateral band of the dorsal apparatus (Fig. 40-6). The slip is sutured with the wrist in 30 degrees palmar flexion, the MP joints in 80 to 90 degrees flexion, and the interphalangeal joints in full extension (zero degrees). A variation in technique is to insert the index slip into the ulnar lateral band of the dorsal apparatus. The procedure should not be used in high (proximal) ulnar nerve palsy unless the index superficialis is used to power the transfer.

Burkhalter[21,25] has recommended attaching the transfer tendon slip directly to the proximal phalanx rather than risking PIP hyperextension with transfer to the lateral band of the lateral band of the dorsal apparatus. Brand's[7] long-term follow-up studies have shown a high incidence of swan-neck deformity, and a flexor tendon sheath insertion may be preferable. The procedure has better long-term results when the tendon slips are sutured under less tension, with the wrist in neutral flexion-extension, the MP joints in 45 to 55 degrees flexion, and the interphalangeal joints in neutral. The operation is not indicated in patients with wrist flexion contracture. It is, however, indicated in those patients whose chief complaint is awkwardness of grip due to lack of synchronous motion of the finger joints.

Zancolli performs the "lasso" procedure through a transverse incision at the level of the distal palmar crease. The proximal pulleys (A1) of the flexor sheaths are exposed, and the flexor digitorum superficialis tendon to be used is sectioned in the finger and divided into two slips. Each tendon slip is retained volar to the deep transverse metacarpal ligament and looped through the A1 proximal pulley and sutured to itself. I use the A2 pulley (Fig. 40-7). I suture the tendon loop with the wrist supinated and flat on the table and the finger in 45 degrees of flexion at the MP joint. Transfers for the little finger should intentionally be tightened in excess of those required for the ring finger. Transfers should be carried to all four fingers because weakness is not limited to the clawing fingers alone.[24,41] A similar procedure utilizing the flexor digitorum superficialis of the ring finger has been performed by Shah.[83] Antia has used the palmaris longus to motor a four-slip graft for lumbrical replacement.[54]

Clinical studies suggest that a finger with intrinsic paralysis cannot give up the flexion activity of the flexor digitorum superficialis. Furthermore, when the superficialis is absent for flexion, it may be too powerful to be used as an extensor. However, if the patient cannot actively extend the interphalangeal joints when the MP joints are stabilized, the superficialis transfer could insert on the central slip at the base of the middle phalanx.[62] If the patient can actively extend the fingers when the proximal phalanx is stabilized, the superficialis transfer could insert into the A2 pulley of the flexor sheath.

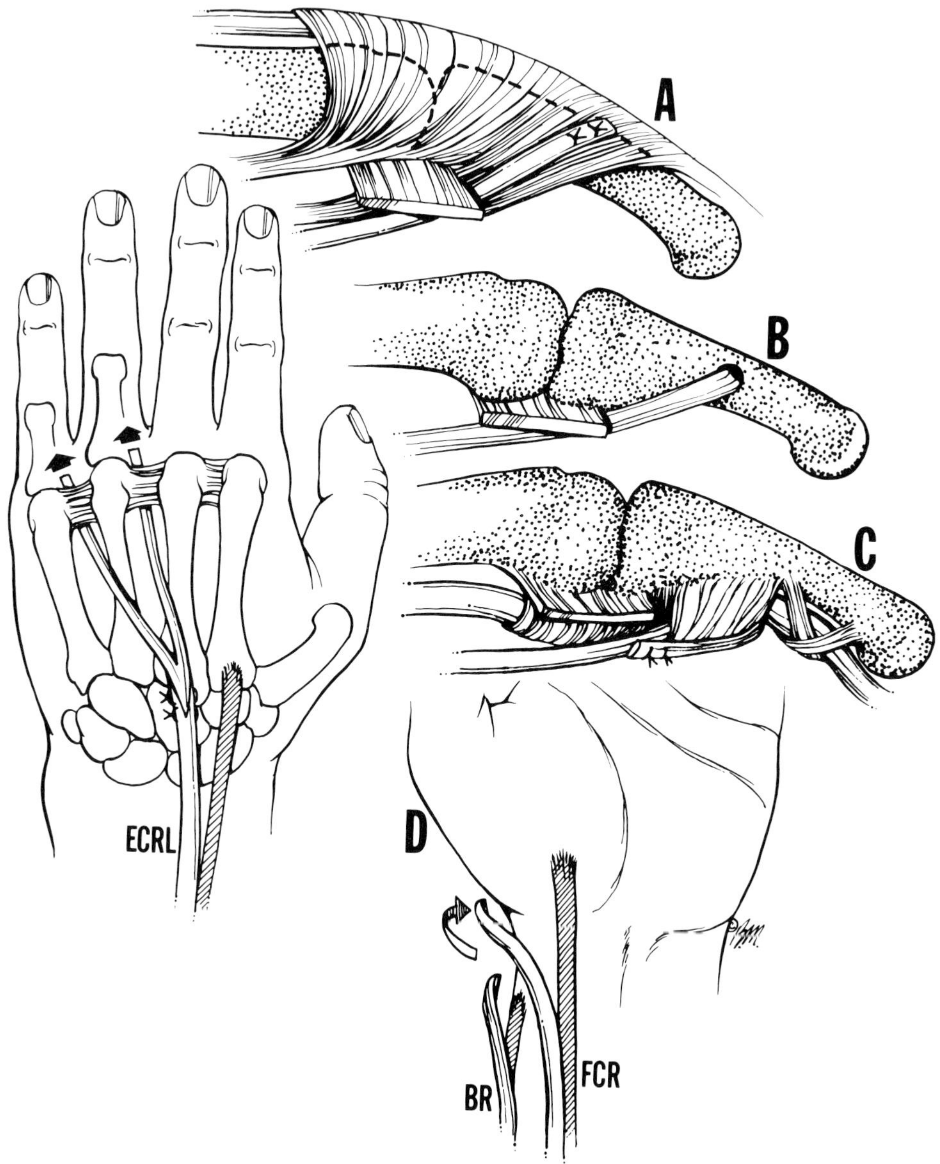

Fig. 40-7. Power flexion of the proximal phalanx can be obtained by utilizing the extensor carpi radialis longus *(ECRL)* or brachioradialis *(BR)*, with a free graft, so that tendon slips pass volar to the deep transverse metacarpal ligament. The insertion of the slips can be either into **(A)** the lateral bands of the dorsal apparatus, **(B)** the bone of the proximal phalanx, or **(C)** the A2 pulley of the flexor sheath. The flexor carpi radialis *(FCR)* may be used instead of the ECRL as the motor **(D)** in patients with palmar flexion deformity.

WRIST LEVEL MOTORS FOR PROXIMAL PHALANX POWER FLEXION AND INTEGRATION OF FINGER FLEXION (BRAND,[6,8] BURKHALTER,[21,25] BROOKS,[14] FOWLER,[32,80] RIORDAN[32,78–80])

The most reliable method to increase power for gross grip is to add an extra muscle-tendon unit to the power-train for flexion of the proximal phalanx. The flexor digitorum superficialis will not increase gross grip power as a transfer. Gross grip power is improved by transferring a wrist extensor or the brachioradialis to flex the MP joints (Fig. 40-7).

Burkhalter and Strait[25] used a free tendon graft, palmaris longus or plantaris, to prolong the extensor carpi radialis longus tendon. The free graft is split into two slips, which are passed through the intermetacarpal spaces between the long and ring fingers and the ring and little fingers. Each tendon slip is passed volar to the deep transverse metacarpal ligament and is attached to the radial aspect of the proximal phalanx of the ring and little fingers. A transverse drill hole is made, into which the tendon slip is inserted and held with a pull-out suture technique. It is important to remove enough intermetacarpal fascia to minimize adhesions of the tendons. Finger extension is not assisted by this transfer.

Postoperative immobilization is continued for 4 weeks, with the wrist maintained in 45 degrees dorsiflexion and the MP joints in 60 degrees flexion. The extensor carpi radialis longus muscle contracts during finger flexion and is easily retrained. The same procedure might utilize the extensor carpi radialis brevis or the brachioradialis as the motor muscle.

Brand has used two techniques that involve wrist extensor muscle-tendon units. The dorsal approach[6] is motored by the extensor carpi radialis brevis (or longus) prolonged by plantaris tendon free grafts. The tendon slips are passed superficial to the dorsal carpal ligament, through the intermetacarpal spaces, and then through the lumbrical canal volar to the deep transverse metacarpal ligament, and attached to the radial lateral bands of the long, ring, and little fingers and the ulnar lateral band of the index finger. Brand noted that a stronger pinch can be obtained by stabilizing the index finger in adduction at the MP joint,[98] and thus a four-tailed (slips) graft could be used in an ulnar nerve palsy.

Brand has modified the dorsal approach by detaching the extensor carpi radialis longus at its insertion and passing it deep to the brachioradialis to the volar side of the forearm 7.5 cm proximal to the wrist.[8] The plantaris or palmaris tendons are used for the free grafts. The lateral bands are identified through dorsoradial incisions over the proximal finger (except the index finger, which has the ulnar lateral band exposed). The tendon slips are directed through the carpal tunnel and distally, volar to the deep transverse metacarpal ligament and into the lateral bands of the dorsal apparatus (Fig. 40-8). The tendons are sutured with the wrist dorsiflexed 45 degrees, the MP joints flexed 70 degrees, and the interphalangeal joints in neutral (zero extension). Potential problems with this procedure include flexion deformity of the wrist secondary to removing a strong wrist extensor, and possible carpal tunnel syndrome secondary to increased tissue in the carpal tunnel.

The original Fowler's technique[32,80] used the extensor indicis proprius tendon and the extensor digiti quinti tendons as direct transfers to the lateral bands of the dorsal apparatus. The technique required excessive tension, and an intrinsic-plus deformity was common. In addition, extension of the little finger was lost if the extensor digiti quinti was the only effective extensor of the little finger. Riordan[78,79,89] modified the procedure by transferring the extensor indicis proprius to the ulnar side of the hand and dividing the tendon into two slips that are passed volar to the deep transverse metacarpal ligament and into the radial lateral bands of the ring and little fingers. The technique is easier than using free tendon grafts. If the median nerve is also involved, a free tendon graft can provide tendon slips for the long and index fingers.

Patients with ulnar palsy often develop wrist palmar flexion deformity resulting from repeated attempts to extend the clawed fingers. Riordan[78,79] transferred the flexor carpi radialis, elongated with a brachioradialis, plantaris, or palmaris free graft. The flexor carpi radialis is passed to the dorsal side of the forearm, and the free tendon slips are passed through the intermetacarpal spaces, then volar to the deep transverse metacarpal ligaments, and into the radial lateral bands of the involved

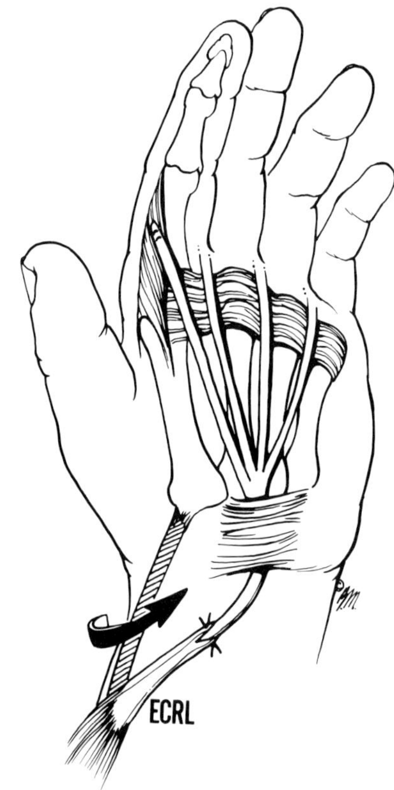

Fig. 40-8. Transfer of the extensor carpi radialis longus *(ECRL)* to control "claw finger" deformity. The ECRL is passed around the radial side of the forearm and extended by a free tendon graft in two to four slips, through the carpal tunnel and volar to the deep transverse metacarpal ligament, into the lateral band of the dorsal apparatus. This transfer adds power to finger flexion.

fingers. The flexor carpi radialis is in phase for interphalangeal extension, and minimal rehabilitation is necessary.

Brooks and Jones[14] described using the flexor carpi radialis or extensor carpi radialis longus prolonged with free toe extensor tendon grafts passed through the carpal tunnel and attached to the A2 pulley of the flexor sheath. Each free graft is sutured back on itself with the wrist held in maximum flexion and the MP joints in neutral position (zero extension). As with the volar route of the Brand transfer, there is risk of median nerve compression with four tendon grafts added to the contents of the carpal canal.[90]

The wrist motor procedures use free grafts. The incidence of absence of the plantaris is about 8 percent, whereas the palmaris longus is absent in approximately 11 to 14 percent. There seems to be no relationship between the absence of the palmaris longus and that of the plantaris. When the plantaris is absent, it is usually absent bilaterally; but when the palmaris longus is absent, its absence is bilateral in 60 percent of cases.[64] Future technology may provide much better assessment: ultrasound has a sensitivity of 95 percent for detecting a plantaris tendon suitable for grafting.[84]

Active (dynamic) flexion of the proximal phalanx does not provide active flexion of the two distal phalanges. In a high (proximal) ulnar nerve palsy, active flexion must be restored to the distal phalanx of the ring and little fingers. Also, active flexion of the proximal phalanx will not ensure extension of the PIP and DIP joints if they are stiff or the extrinsic (EDC) tendons are ineffective. Long-standing ulnar nerve palsy may result in fixed PIP joint flexion contractures of the ring and little fingers, especially in the older patient with "thicker" hands. If the interphalangeal joints are painful and stiff, arthrodesis should be considered.

THUMB-INDEX KEY PINCH AND TIP PINCH

For key pinch the thumb is in adduction and flexion. The adduction force is achieved principally by the adductor pollicis and the radial head of the first dorsal interosseous muscles. To a lesser extent, the extensor pollicis longus and the flexor pollicis longus muscles may contribute.[89] For tip pinch the index finger should be in radial deviation. Biomechanical studies demonstrate 77 to 80 percent loss of power pinch in patients with ulnar nerve palsy.[50]

Thumb Adduction Techniques (Bunnell,[20] Boyes,[5] Goldner,[36,37] Littler,[16,31,33,34,46,47] Smith[88,89])

Thumb adduction may be restored by using a strong wrist motor, the brachioradialis, or several digital tendons. Most tendon transfers for adduction of the thumb provide power pinch only in the range of 25 to 50 percent of normal strength.[16,37,50,88]

Smith released the extensor carpi radialis brevis from its insertion and extended it with a free tendon graft through the second intermetacarpal space. A curved hemostat is tunneled deep (dorsal) to the adductor pollicis and the tendon graft is advanced to the tendon insertion of the adductor pollicis muscle. The transfer should lie dorsal to the dorsal retinaculum to retain its potential for dorsiflexion of the wrist. The graft is adjusted so that the thumb lies just palmar to the index finger when the wrist is in zero degrees of extension.

I believe that the extensor carpi radialis brevis is the best transfer for thumb adduction, but I use a slightly different technique.[69,74] The extensor carpi radialis brevis is sharply released at its insertion and attached to a free tendon graft. The free graft extending the extensor carpi radialis brevis is brought into the palm through the third intermetacarpal space and tunneled superficial (volar) to the adductor pollicis and deep (dorsal) to the flexor tendons and neurovascular structures. The tendon graft is attached to the fascia over the abductor tubercle of the first metacarpal, which improves pronation for pinch[31] (Fig. 40-9). When the wrist is in palmar flexion, the thumb falls into abduction; with the wrist in dorsiflexion, the thumb is drawn firmly against the palm. The average key pinch strength is doubled by this operation.[41,88]

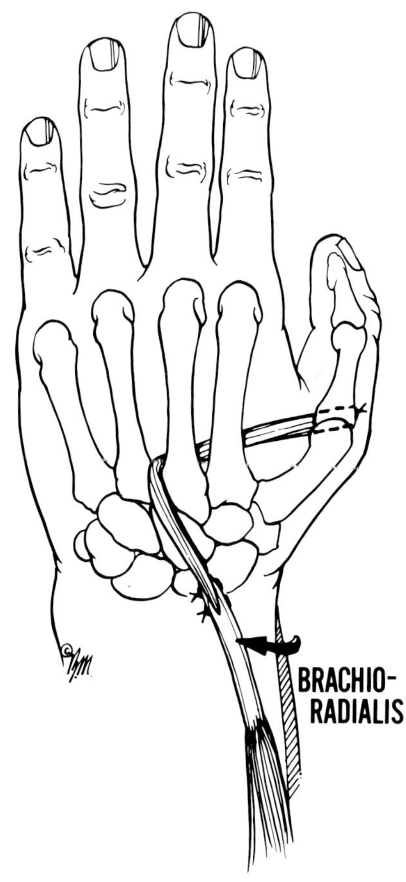

Fig. 40-9. Transfer of the brachioradialis *(BR)* extended with free tendon graft, through the interspace between the third and fourth metacarpals, across the palm volar to the adductor pollicis and dorsal to the finger flexor tendons and neurovascular structures, to insert on the abductor tubercle of the thumb. (The extensor carpi radialis brevis *[ECRB]* can also be used as the motor). This transfer will add power to key pinch, and is preferable to a "volar" transfer (Fig. 40-8).

Boyes has advocated the brachioradialis as the donor muscle because its amplitude of motion is sufficient to allow thumb action whether the wrist is flexed or extended (Fig. 40-9). He also illustrated the extensor carpi ulnaris as the donor muscle.[5] Solonen and Bakalim[91] have used the extensor carpi radialis longus in a similar transfer. All the wrist extensors and the brachioradialis must be elongated with free grafts.

Littler recommended a long or ring flexor digitorum superficialis transfer in those patients with hyperextension deformity of the MP joint of the thumb (Fig. 40-10). The superficialis is detached in the finger, the decussation is split to leave one limb and withdrawn into the palm. [Brown[16] cautioned to leave enough distal tendon to prevent hyperextension (recurvatum) of the PIP joint.] The superficialis tendon is tunneled across the volar surface of the adductor pollicis and sutured to the adductor pollicis tendon at its insertion. Edgerton and Brand[31] recommended an abductor tubercle insertion for improved key pinch. The pulley for this procedure, and one technique that I use,[58,62] is the vertical septum of the palmar fascia attached to the third metacarpal as described by Edgerton and Brand.[31] The thumb and wrist are immobilized for 4 weeks, and then active motion is allowed. Hamlin and Littler[40] reported their results with superficialis transfer and recorded a return of pinch power to 70 percent of the uninvolved hand.

Bunnell's "tendon loop" utilized the extensor digitorum communis to the index finger. The tendon is detached from the index dorsal apparatus and withdrawn to the dorsal carpal ligament. The tendon is elongated with a free tendon graft from the palmaris longus or plantaris, then passed subcutaneously around the ulnar border of the hand and across the palm deep to the flexor tendons, to be inserted into bone on the ulnar side of the base of the proximal phalanx of the thumb at the adductor tubercle. The communis tendon is selected because its muscle is stronger than the extensor indicis proprius. The dorsal apparatus (extensor hood) should be carefully closed to prevent extensor lag of the index finger.[5]

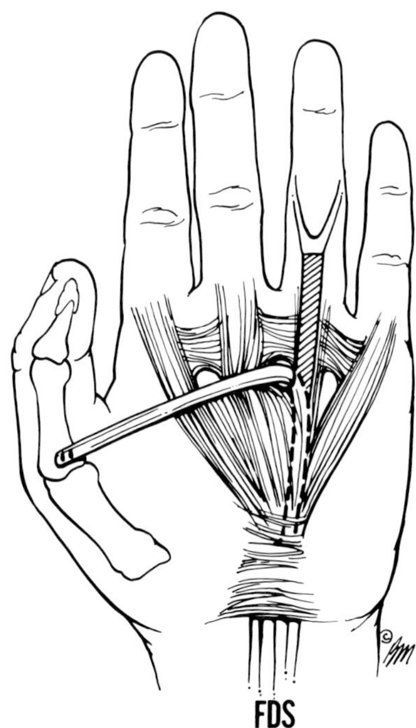

Fig. 40-10. Transfer of flexor digitorum superficialis *(FDS),* through a palmar fascia pulley, to the abductor tubercle of the thumb. This transfer will add power to key pinch, but will further weaken power grasp.

The extensor indicis proprius has also been used as the motor.[16] This more independent tendon is passed volarward between the third and fourth metacarpals and then passed across the transverse muscle belly of the adductor pollicis. The tendon is sutured to the adductor pollicis insertion. Brand[11,31] recommended inserting the transfer into the abductor pollicis brevis tendon as a more functional insertion. Tension is achieved by holding the wrist in zero flexion-extension and the first and second metacarpals parallel to each other in both the lateral and anteroposterior planes. A pull of 2 to 3 kg is exerted on the tendon in this position before sutures are placed.

Goldner[36,37] used the long finger flexor digitorum superficialis, but approached the thumb on the dorsal surface of the hand. The superficialis is withdrawn to the volar side of the wrist. A hole 2 × 3 cm is made in the ulnar side of the pronator quadratus muscle, and the tendon is passed through the interosseous membrane proximal to the wrist joint. The superficialis is passed subcutaneously around the distal end of the extensor carpi ulnaris tendon, which acts as a pulley. The superficialis is then directed under the extensor digitorum communis and other extensor tendons in a line parallel to the extensor pollicis longus. The tendon is sutured into a drill hole on the ulnar aspect of the thumb at the level of the adductor tendon insertion. Immobilization is continued for 3 weeks, maintaining the wrist in 30 degrees palmar flexion, the MP joints in 45 degrees flexion, and the interphalangeal joints in 10 degrees flexion, while the thumb is held about 1 cm away from the index finger.

Index Abduction Techniques (Bunnell,[5,20] Bruner,[18] Graham and Riordan,[39] Hirayama, Atsuta, and Takemitsu,[42] Neviaser, Wilson, and Gardner,[55] Omer[62,71,89])

Neviaser, Wilson, and Gardner recommended the transfer of an accessory slip of the abductor pollicis longus elongated with a free tendon graft—palmaris longus or plantaris—into the tendon of the first dorsal interosseous (Fig. 40-11). The abductor pollicis longus is exposed distal to the first dorsal compartment, and the insertion of its slips are inspected. Only the slip that inserts on the first metacarpal is essential; if there are additional slips, one may be used for the first dorsal interosseous transfer. This transfer does not appreciably increase the force of tip pinch, but it stabilizes the index finger.[89]

Bunnell reported the transfer of the extensor indicis proprius to the tendon of the first dorsal interosseous muscle. The tendon is divided from the index dorsal apparatus and withdrawn at the wrist through a short transverse incision, and passed distally around the radial border of the second metacarpal to insert into the first dorsal interosseous tendon volar to the axis

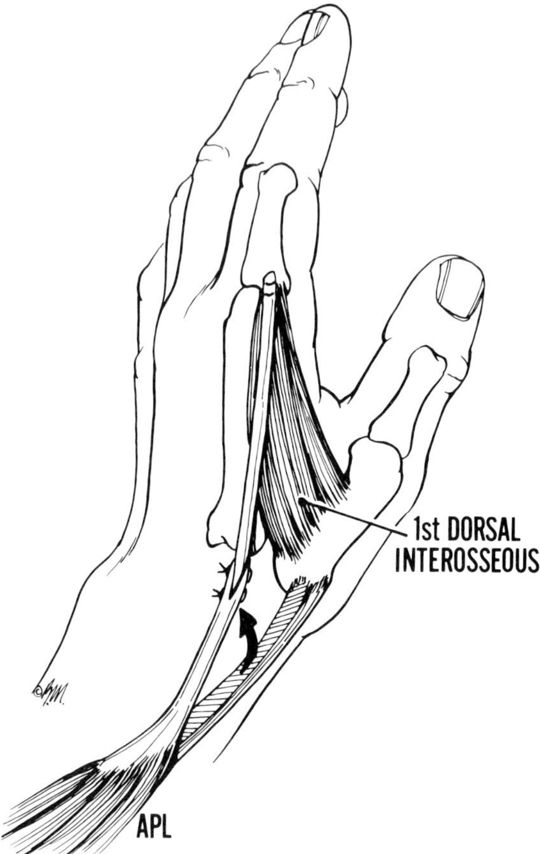

Fig. 40-11. Extension of an accessory slip of the abductor pollicis longus *(APL)*, with a free graft, into the tendon insertion of the first dorsal interosseous. The brachioradialis may be used as an alternative motor.

of motion of the MP joint. The dorsal apparatus should be carefully closed to prevent extension lag of the index finger.[17,54] The transfer must be sutured under considerable tension (2 to 3 kg) for adequate performance.[16] Success is demonstrated by stability during pulp-to-pulp pinch, in that there will be slight flexion of the index MP joint and no adduction of the index finger. Clippinger and Goldner[26,38] believe that this transfer is not a satisfactory procedure, perhaps secondary to a short moment arm and a narrow angle of approach. Solonen and Bakalim[91] improved the approach angle by rerouting the extensor indicis proprius from the wrist around a "dynamic pulley" consisting of the extensor tendons of the thumb. Smith[89] noted that some patients develop a radially deviated (abduction) index finger with this procedure.

I modified Bunnell's transfer by splitting the tendon of the extensor indicis proprius muscle and transferring one slip to the tendon of the first dorsal interosseous muscle and one slip to the tendon of the adductor pollicis muscle. This transfer will not restore strong power pinch, but will stabilize the index finger.

Hirayama and co-workers[42] prolonged the palmaris longus muscle-tendon unit with a strip of palmar fascia and transferred this unit subcutaneously to the dorsum of the hand and distally to the insertion of the first dorsal interosseous. The wrist is immobilized in 10 degrees of dorsiflexion with 30 degrees flexion and 20 degrees abduction of the MP joint of the index finger for 3 weeks. The course of the transposed tendon aligns with the course of the first dorsal interosseous and is rectilinear.[10,12]

Bruner transferred the extensor pollicis brevis to the tendon of the first dorsal interosseous (Fig. 40-12), but Graham and Riordan[39] stated that this tendon is lacking in strength. De Abreu[27] combined transfer of the extensor pollicis brevis tendon to the tendon insertion of the first dorsal interosseous with transfer of the extensor indicis proprius tendon to the tendon insertion of the adductor pollicis muscle as a one-stage procedure. Eyler and Coonrad[26] described a split insertion for a flexor digitorum superficialis transfer, with one-half of the superficialis through the lumbrical canal and the other half subcutaneously toward the dorsal surface.

Graham and Riordan passed a flexor digitorum superficialis, usually from the ring finger, either to bone on the radial side of the proximal phalanx or to the tendon of the first dorsal interosseous. The superficialis is withdrawn at the wrist and directed subcutaneously around the radial aspect of the forearm, over the anatomic snuffbox and the first dorsal interosseous space to the radial aspect of the index finger. Postoperative immobilization includes holding the index finger in abduction and extension with the wrist slightly flexed. At the end of 3 weeks, active motion is permitted.

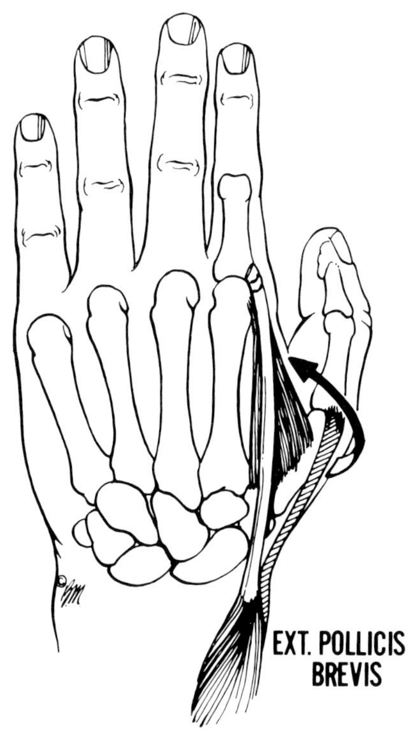

Fig. 40-12. Transfer of the extensor pollicis brevis to the insertion of the first dorsal interosseous to improve index abduction.

Arthrodesis of Thumb Joints (Brand,[9] Brown,[16] Omer,[58,62,69] Tubiana[96])

Brown noted that splinting the ulnar palsied thumb usually increases pinch strength by 1 to 2 kg. The position that I prefer for arthrodesis of the interphalangeal joint of the thumb is 20 to 30 degrees of flexion. Some patients have objected to the loss of motion and considered this a greater problem than the ineffective tip pinch.[41,69] Brown reserved this procedure for patients in whom the interphalangeal joint is noticeably unstable. Tubiana prefers interphalangeal joint arthrodesis to fusion of the MP joint.

I recommend arthrodesis of the MP joint when there is instability in the longitudinal arch of the thumb (see Fig. 40-2). Brand placed the MP joint in 15 degrees flexion, 5 degrees abduction, and 15 degrees pronation. Barden[1] has reported normal active motion of the interphalangeal joint following arthrodesis of the MP joint of the thumb, with correction of Froment's sign.

METACARPAL ARCH RESTORATION AND LITTLE FINGER ABDUCTION

Paralysis of the four dorsal interossei, three volar interossei, and abduction digiti quinti prevents active abduction and adduction of the fingers, with associated instability of the transverse metacarpal arch. It is often emphasized that the wrist must be stable before an operation is performed to reconstruct the hand; therefore, a procedure to improve finger activity must first consider the stability of the transverse metacarpal arch. Instability (flattening) of the transverse metacarpal arch may contribute to recurrent clawing following lumbrical replacement procedures.[77]

Metacarpal Arch Restoration (Bunnell,[5,20] Littler,[46,47] Ranney[76,77])

Bunnell's "tendon-T" operation gives adduction to the thumb and the little finger, while cupping the hand to restore the metacarpal arch. A free tendon graft spans the hand, dorsal to the flexor tendons, from the base of the proximal phalanx of the thumb to the neck of the metacarpal of the little finger. A flexor digitorum superficialis tendon is detached from its insertion and is distally attached by a loop to the center of the free tendon, forming a T. On contraction of the superficialis, the T is converted into a Y, and the metacarpal arch is restored.

Littler transferred a flexor digitorum superficialis but did not use the free tendon graft across the palm. One slip of the superficialis is sutured to the adductor tubercle of the thumb, the other slip to a bony insertion in the base of the proximal phalanx of the little finger.

Ranney depressed the metacarpal arch with a volar transfer of the extensor digiti minimi to the neck of the fifth metacarpal. The extensor digiti minimi is step-cut at its insertion, leaving a strip to be sutured to the extensor digitorum communis. The muscle-tendon unit is withdrawn to the wrist and passed through the forearm between the abductor pollicis longus and the flexor carpi radialis. The extensor digiti minimi tendon then passes subcutaneously in a diagonal course to be sutured to the periosteum of the neck of the fifth metacarpal.

Ahern (personal communication, 1969) has produced an effect similar to that from Ranney's procedure by looping the flexor digitorum superficialis of the little finger around the deep transverse metacarpal ligament between the fourth and fifth metacarpals.

Little Finger Abduction (Blacker, Lister, and Kleinert,[3] Goldner[37])

Blacker, Lister, and Kleinert found that the extensor digiti minimi had the potential to abduct the little finger through its indirect insertion into the abductor tubercle on the proximal phalanx. The balancing force is provided by the third palmar interosseous, which is inactive in ulnar nerve palsy. The problem is corrected with a transfer of the ulnar half of the tendon of the extensor digiti minimi (Fig. 40-13). The ulnar half of the tendon is detached from the dorsal apparatus and dissected proximally to the distal edge of the dorsal carpal ligament (extensor retinaculum). A palmar incision is made that extends obliquely from the distal palmar crease to the proximal digital crease, which will expose the deep transverse metacarpal ligament and the flexor sheath of the little finger. The ulnar half of the extensor digiti minimi is passed between the fourth and fifth metacarpals into the palmar wound. If the little finger is clawed as well as abducted, the tendon slip is inserted into a radially based flap of the flexor tendon sheath just distal to the proximal pulley (Brooks' insertion).[13,14] If the little finger is not clawed, the tendon slip is passed beneath the deep transverse metacarpal ligament and sutured into the phalangeal attachment of the radial collateral ligament of the MP joint of the little finger. The tendon is sutured with the wrist in neutral flexion-extension and the MP joint in 20 degrees flexion. The ring and little fingers are splinted for 4 weeks with the wrist extended and the MP joint flexed. The interphalangeal joints are left free, and motion is encouraged to prevent adhesions of the flexor tendons.

Goldner used the *entire* extensor digiti minimi. The tendon is withdrawn to the level of the dorsal carpal ligament (extensor retinaculum), passed beneath the extensor carpi radialis longus as a pulley, and inserted from the dorsal surface into the oblique fibers of the dorsal apparatus of the little finger or directly into bone. One must be certain that there is a functional slip of the extensor digitorum communis to the little finger prior to removing the entire extensor digiti minimi.

FINGER AND WRIST FLEXION (OMER[57,60,64,71,74])

Brand does not consider the loss of the flexor carpi ulnaris and the ulnar half of the flexor digitorum profundus to be a functional problem; he recommended that tendon transfers

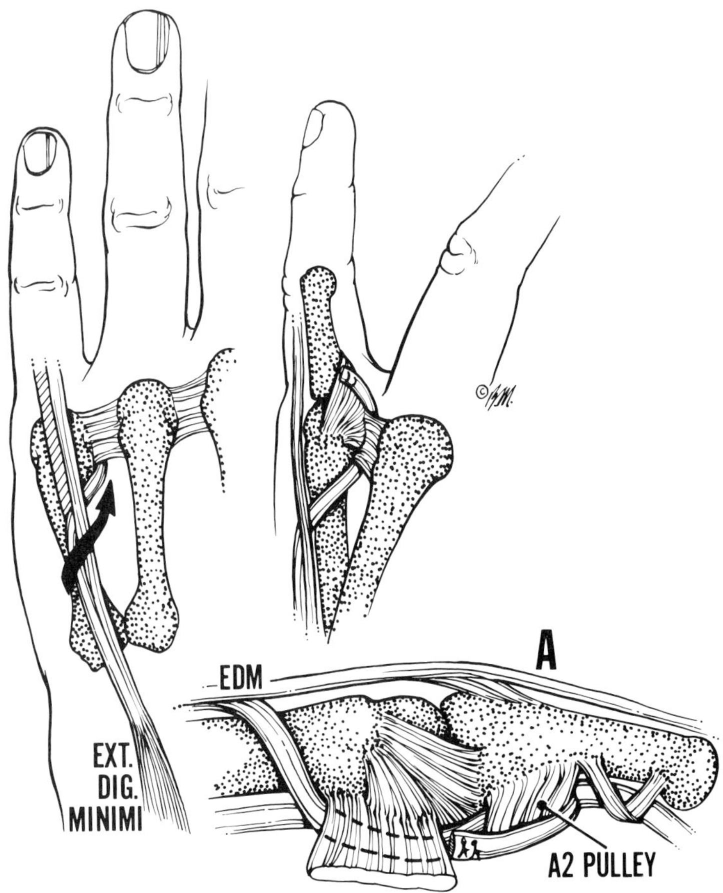

Fig. 40-13. Transfer of the ulnar half of the extensor digiti minimi *(EDM)* to correct persistent abduction of the little finger. The tendon is directed volar to the deep transverse metacarpal ligament and sutured to the phalangeal attachment of the radial collateral ligament of the MP joint of the little finger. **(A)** If the little finger is clawed as well as abducted, the tendon is inserted through the A2 pulley of the flexor sheath.

should not be considered unless there is also median or radial nerve loss[11] (see Chapter 41). However, if there is marked weakness of the ring and little fingers in isolated ulnar nerve paralysis, I attach the profundus tendons cf the ring and little fingers to the profundus tendon of the long finger in the forearm.[57,60,64,71] The index profundus should be left free (Fig. 40-14). The surgeon also should consider tenodesis of the flexor digitorum profundus across the DIP joints of the ring and little fingers.[57,74] Bunnell[20] believed it inadvisable to join the ring and little profundus to the profundus of the long finger because the more long flexors that are working, the more marked should be the clawhand deformity. This has not been my experience, but these patients should also have transfers for proximal phalanx flexion and integration of finger flexion, as well as a procedure to restore the metacarpal arch.

It would be equally useful to transfer the tendon of the flexor carpi radialis to the insertion of the flexor carpi ulnaris in a patient with high ulnar palsy who could perform activities requiring strong wrist flexion. Ulnar deviation is as important for wrist flexion as radial deviation is for wrist extension.

SENSIBILITY

Loss of sensibility for the ulnar border of the hand and loss of proprioception for the little finger are significant functional limitations. Free nerve grafting, vascularized nerve grafts, and free neurovascular cutaneous island flaps are technically demanding and clinically unpredictable. Lewis and coworkers[45,93] performed digital nerve translocation to restore sensation; a functioning digital nerve of median origin is sutured into the nonfunctional ulnar digital nerve of the small finger. These authors reported that 85 percent of their patients obtained sensibility of S3+ or S4 after surgery. Patients who returned to work after surgery rated significantly better than those who did not work.

AUTHOR'S PREFERRED METHODS

Ulnar nerve palsy results in a hand with so many functional problems that there is no "standard" accepted program that is suitable for reconstruction in all patients. Available tendon

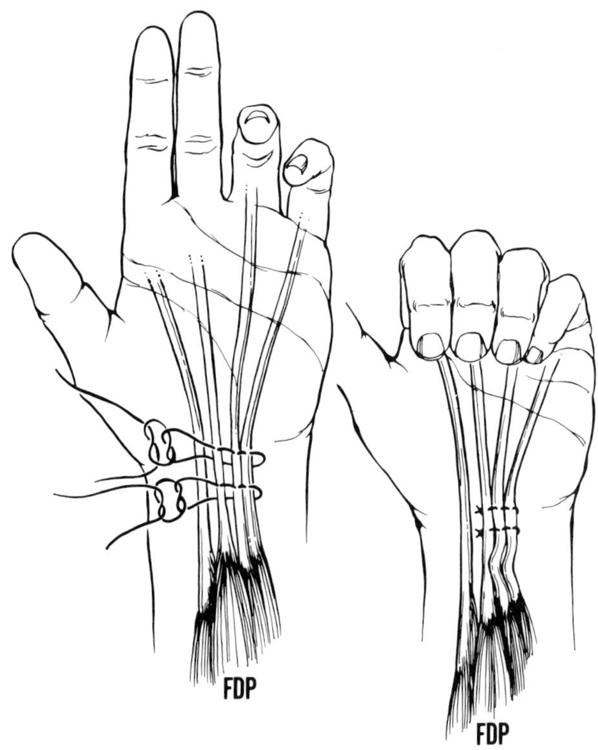

Fig. 40-14. Tenodesis of the profundus tendons of the ring and little fingers to the active flexor digitorum profundus *(FDP)* of the long finger to increase power for gross grip. A double line of sutures is important to prevent "whip-sawing" of the tendons during power grip.

Table 40-2. Author's Preferred Reconstructive Program for Low (Distal) Ulnar Nerve Palsy

Needed Function	Preferred Transfer	Alternate Transfer
Thumb adduction for key pinch	Extensor carpi radialis brevis with free graft between third and fourth metacarpals to abductor tubercle of thumb[88,89]	Flexor digitorum superficialis (long) to abductor tubercle of thumb with palmar fascia as the pulley[46,47]
Proximal phalanx power flexion and integration of MP and interphalangeal motion (clawed fingers)	Extensor carpi radialis longus to all four fingers using four-tailed free graft and flexor sheath insertion[25,64,71,74]	Flexor carpi radialis (if wrist flexion contracture) with four-tailed free graft and flexor sheath insertion[78,79]
Thumb-index tip pinch	Accessory slip of abductor pollicis longus to first dorsal interosseous tendon[55] and arthrodesis of MP joint of thumb[57,60]	Extensor pollicis brevis to first dorsal interosseous tendon[18] (if thumb MP has been fused)
Metacarpal (palmar) transverse arch and adduction for little finger	Extensor digiti minimi transfer volar to the deep transverse metacarpal ligament to the proximal phalanx or dorsal apparatus[3,71] (extensor digitorum comminus to little finger must be effective)[76,77]	Ulnar half of extensor digiti minimi volar to deep transverse metacarpal ligament to radial collateral ligament of MP joint of little finger[3]
Volar sensibility—ring and little fingers	Digital nerve translocation of median nerve origin[45,93]	Free or vascularized nerve graft[53]

Table 40-3. Author's Preferred Reconstructive Program for High (Proximal) Ulnar Nerve Palsy

Needed Function	Preferred Transfer	Alternate Transfers
Thumb adduction for key pinch	Extensor carpi radialis brevis with free graft between third and fourth metacarpals to the abductor tubercle of thumb[88,89] with palmar fascia as pulley	Flexor digitorum superficialis to abductor tubercle of thumb[11,46,47] (long finger superficialis is only candidate)
Proximal phalanx power flexion and integration of MP and interphalangeal motion (clawed fingers)	Extensor carpi radialis longus to all four fingers using four-tailed free graft and flexor sheath (A2 pulley) insertion[25,64,71,74]	Flexor carpi radialis (if wrist flexion contracture) with four-tailed graft and flexor sheath insertion[78,79]
Thumb-index tip pinch	Accessory slip of abductor pollicis longus to first dorsal interosseous tendon and arthrodesis of MP joint of thumb[57,60]	Extensor pollicis brevis to first dorsal interosseous tendon (if thumb MP has been fused)[18]
Metacarpal (palmar) transverse arch and adduction for little finger	Extensor digiti minimi split and ulnar half transferred volar to deep transverse metacarpal ligament to the proximal phalanx or dorsal apparatus[3,71] (extensor digitorum communis to little finger must be effective)[76,77]	If little finger is clawed as well as abducted, insert extensor digiti minimi in A2 pulley of flexor sheath[3,71,76,77]
Distal finger flexion—DIP for ring and little fingers	Flexor digitorum profundus (long) tenodesed to flexor digitorum profundus (ring and little) and tendosesis, DIP joints, ring and little fingers[57,64,71]	
Wrist flexion—ulnar aspect	Flexor carpi radialis to insertion of flexor carpi ulnaris[57]	Palmaris longus to insertion of flexor carpi ulnaris
Volar sensibility—ring and little fingers	Digital nerve translocation of median nerve origin[45,93]	Free or vascularized nerve graft[53]

assets must be invested wisely. For example, the ubiquitous flexor digitorum superficialis has been overused for proximal phalanx flexion, as a substitute for the lumbricals, as a thumb adductor, to restore the metacarpal arch, as an index abductor —yet it provides the only flexor power in the ring and little fingers in a high (proximal) ulnar nerve palsy!

When a precise neurorrhaphy has been performed early in a patient with low (distal) ulnar nerve laceration, the prognosis for reinnervation of palsied muscles has improved during the past decade.[2,35,49,53] In these patients, selected tendon transfers may be performed early as internal splints to support partial function and prevent deformity while awaiting the potential nerve recovery (see Table 40-1).

Patients with a severe extremity injury, a long nerve graft, or a high (proximal) ulnar nerve lesion are all candidates for a complete reconstruction program. The author's preferred transfers, as well as alternative methods, are listed in Tables 40-2 and 40-3. The potential for functional motor action is better than recovery of normal sensibility in the high (proximal) ulnar nerve palsy.

REFERENCES

1. Barden GA: American Society for Surgery of the Hand, Correspondence Club Newsletter 47, 1978
2. Birch R, Raji ARM: Repair of median and ulnar nerves. Primary suture is best. J Bone Joint Surg 73B:154–157, 1991
3. Blacker GJ, Lister GD, Kleinert HE: The abducted little finger in low ulnar nerve palsy. J Hand Surg 1:190–196, 1976
4. Bowden REM, Napier JR: The assessment of hand function after peripheral nerve injuries. J Bone Joint Surg 43B:481–492, 1961
5. Boyes JH: Bunnell's Surgery of the Hand. 4th Ed. p 514. JB Lippincott, Philadelphia, 1964

6. Brand PW: Hand reconstruction in leprosy. p. 117. In British Surgical Practice. Surgical Progress, 1954. Butterworth, London, 1954
7. Brand PW: Paralytic claw hand. With special reference to paralysis in leprosy and treatment by the sublimis transfer of Stiles and Bunnell. J Bone Joint Surg 40B:618–632, 1958
8. Brand PW: Tendon grafting. Illustrated by a new operation for intrinsic paralysis of the fingers. J Bone Joint Surg 43B:444–453, 1961
9. Brand PW: Tendon transfers for median and ulnar nerve paralysis. Orthop Clin North Am 1:447–454, 1970
10. Brand PW: Biomechanics of tendon transfer. Orthop Clin North Am 5:205–230, 1974
11. Brand PW: Tendon transfers in the forearm. pp. 276–293. In Flynn JE (ed): Hand Surgery. 3rd Ed. Williams & Wilkins, Baltimore, 1982
12. Brand PW: Biomechanics of tendon transfer. Hand Clin 4:137–154, 1988
13. Brooks AL: Tendon transfer for intrinsic minus fingers. American Society for Surgery of the Hand, Correspondence Club Newsletter, November 24, 1969
14. Brooks AL, Jones DS: A new intrinsic tendon transfer for the paralytic hand. J Bone Joint Surg 57A:730, 1975
15. Brown PW: Zancolli capsulorrhaphy for ulnar claw hand. Appraisal of forty-four cases. J Bone Joint Surg 52A:868–877, 1970
16. Brown PW: Reconstruction for pinch in ulnar intrinsic palsy. Orthop Clin North Am 5:323–342, 1974
17. Browne EZ Jr, Teague MA, Snyder CC: Prevention of extensor lag after indicis proprius tendon transfer. J Hand Surg 4:168–172, 1979
18. Bruner JM: Tendon transfer to restore abduction of the index finger using the extensor pollicis brevis. Plast Reconstr Surg 3:197–201, 1948
19. Bunnell S: Surgery of the intrinsic muscles of the hand other than those producing opposition of the thumb. J Bone Joint Surg 24:1–31, 1942
20. Bunnell S: Surgery of the Hand. JB Lippincott, Philadelphia, 1944
21. Burkhalter WE: Restoration of power grip in ulnar nerve paralysis. Orthop Clin North Am 5:289–303, 1974
22. Burkhalter WE: Early tendon transfers in upper extremity peripheral nerve injury. Clin Orthop 104:68–79, 1974
23. Burkhalter WE: Tendon transfers as internal splints. pp. 798–804. In Omer GE Jr, Spinner M (eds): Management of Peripheral Nerve Problems. WB Saunders, Philadelphia, 1980
24. Burkhalter WE: Complications of tendon transfer for nerve paralysis of the hand. pp. 50–69. In Boswick JA Jr (ed): Complications in Hand Surgery. WB Saunders, Philadelphia, 1986
25. Burkhalter WE, Strait JL: Metacarpophalangeal flexor replacement for intrinsic-muscle paralysis. J Bone Joint Surg 55A:1667–1676, 1973
26. Clippinger FW, Goldner JL: Tendon transfers as substitutes for paralyzed first dorsal and volar interosseous muscles. Proceedings of the American Society for Surgery of the Hand. J Bone Joint Surg 47A:633, 1965
27. DeAbreu LB: Early restoration of pinch grip after ulnar nerve repair and tendon transfer. J Hand Surg 14B:309–314, 1989
28. Doyle JA, Blythe W: The finger flexor tendon sheath and pulleys: Anatomy and reconstruction. pp. 81–87. In Hunter JM, Schneider LH (eds): AAOS Symposium on Tendon Surgery in the Hand. CV Mosby, St. Louis, 1975
29. Duchenne GB: Physiology of Motion Demonstrated by Electrical Stimulation and Clinical Observation. p. 141. (Translated and edited by Kaplan EB) WB Saunders, Philadelphia, 1959
30. Earle AS, Vlastou C: Crossed fingers and other tests of ulnar nerve motor function. J Hand Surg 5:560–565, 1980
31. Edgerton MT, Brand PW: Restoration of abduction and adduction to the unstable thumb in median and ulnar paralysis. Plast Reconstr Surg 36:150–164, 1965
32. Enna CD, Riordan DC: The Fowler procedure for correction of the paralytic claw hand. Plast Reconstr Surg 52:352–360, 1973
33. Flatt AE: Kinesiology of the Hand. pp. 266–281. AAOS Instr Course Lect, Vol 18. CV Mosby, St. Louis, 1961
34. Fowler SB: Extensor apparatus of the digits (abstract). J Bone Joint Surg 31B:477, 1949
35. Gaul JS Jr: Intrinsic motor recovery—A long-term study of ulnar nerve repair. J Hand Surg 7:502–508, 1982
36. Goldner JL: Replacement of the function of the paralyzed adductor pollicis with the flexor digitorum sublimus—A ten year review. Proceedings of the American Society for Surgery of the Hand. J Bone Joint Surg 49A:583–584, 1967
37. Goldner JL: Tendon transfers for irreparable peripheral nerve injuries of the upper extremity. Orthop Clin North Am 5:343–375, 1974
38. Goldner JL, Irwin CE: An analysis of paralytic thumb deformities. J Bone Joint Surg 32A:627–639, 1950
39. Graham WC, Riordan D: Sublimis transplant to restore abduction of index finger. Plast Reconstr Surg 2:459–462, 1947
40. Hamlin C, Littler JW: Restoration of power pinch. Orthop Trans 3:319–320, 1979
41. Hastings H II, Davidson S: Tendon transfers for ulnar nerve palsy. Evaluation of results and practical treatment considerations. Hand Clinics 4:167–178, 1988
42. Hirayama T, Atsuta Y, Takemitsu Y: Palmaris longus transfer for replacement of the first dorsal interosseous. J Hand Surg 11B:31–34, 1986
43. Kaplan EB, Spinner M: Normal and anomalous innervation patterns in the upper extremity. pp. 75–99. In Omer GE Jr, Spinner M (eds): Management of Peripheral Nerve Problems. WB Saunders, Philadelphia, 1980
44. Leddy JP, Stark HH, Ashworth CR, Boyes JH: Capsulodesis and pulley advancement for the correction of claw finger deformity. J Bone Joint Surg 54A:1465–1471, 1972
45. Lewis RC Jr, Tenny J, Irvine D: The restoration of sensibility by nerve translocation. Bull Hosp Joint Dis Orthop Inst 44:288–296, 1984
46. Littler JW: Tendon transfers and arthrodesis in combined median and ulnar nerve palsies. J Bone Joint Surg 31A:225–234, 1949
47. Littler JW: Restoration of power and stability in the partially paralyzed hand. pp. 1674–1695 In Converse JM: Reconstructive Plastic Surgery, Vol. IV. WB Saunders, Philadelphia, 1964
48. Long C: Intrinsic-extrinsic muscle control of the fingers. Electromyographic studies. J Bone Joint Surg 50A:973–984, 1968
49. Mailander P, Berger A, Schaller E, Ruhe K: Results of primary nerve repair in the upper extremity. Microsurgery 10:147–150, 1989
50. Mannerfelt L: Studies on the hand in ulnar nerve paralysis. A clinical-experimental investigation in normal and anomalous innervation. Acta Orthop Scand (Suppl) 87:89–97, 1966
51. Mikhail IK: Bone block operation for clawhand. Surg Gynecol Obstet 118:1077–1079, 1964
52. Milford L: The Hand. 2nd Ed. pp. 14–27. CV Mosby, St. Louis, 1982
53. Millesi H: Peripheral nerve surgery today: Turning point or continuous development? J Hand Surg 15B:281–287, 1990
54. Moore JR, Weiland AJ, Valdata L: Independent index extension after extensor indicis proprius transfer. J Hand Surg 12A:232–236, 1987

55. Neviaser RJ, Wilson JN, Gardner MM: Abductor pollicis longus transfer for replacement of first dorsal interosseous. J Hand Surg 5:53–57, 1980
56. North ER, Littler JW: Transferring the flexor superficialis tendon: Technical considerations in the prevention of proximal interphalangeal joint disability. J Hand Surg 5:498–501, 1980
57. Omer GE Jr: Evaluation and reconstruction of the forearm and hand after acute traumatic peripheral nerve injuries. J Bone Joint Surg 50A:1454–1478, 1968
58. Omer GE Jr: Restoring power grip in ulnar palsy. Proceedings of the American Society for Surgery of the Hand. J Bone Joint Surg 53A:814, 1971
59. Omer GE Jr: Assessment of peripheral nerve injuries. pp. 1–11. In Cramer LM, Chase RA (eds) Symposium on the Hand (Foundation of the American Society of Plastic and Reconstructive Surgeons, Inc.) Vol. 3. CV Mosby, St. Louis, 1971
60. Omer GE Jr: Evaluation and reconstruction of the forearm and hand after acute traumatic peripheral nerve injuries. pp. 93–119. AAOS Instr. Course Lect, Vol 18J-1. CV Mosby, St. Louis 1973
61. Omer GE Jr: The technique and timing of tendon transfers. Orthop Clin North Am 5:243–252, 1974
62. Omer GE Jr: Tendon transfers in combined nerve lesions. Orthop Clin North Am 5:377–387, 1974
63. Omer GE Jr: Tendon transfers as early internal splints following peripheral nerve injury in the upper extremity. pp. 292–296. In Hunter JM, Schneider LH, Mackin EJ, Bell JA (eds): Rehabilitation of the Hand. CV Mosby, St. Louis, 1978
64. Omer GE Jr: Tendon transfers for reconstruction of the forearm and hand following peripheral nerve injuries. pp. 817–846. In Omer GE Jr, Spinner M (eds): Management of Peripheral Nerve Problems. WB Saunders, Philadelphia, 1980
65. Omer GE Jr: Physical diagnosis of peripheral nerve injuries. Orthop Clin North Am 12:207–228, 1981
66. Omer GE Jr: Methods of assessment of injury and recovery of peripheral nerves. Surg Clin North Am 61:303–319, 1981
67. Omer GE Jr: Early tendon transfers in the rehabilitation of median, radial, and ulnar palsies. Ann Chir Main 1:187–190, 1982
68. Omer GE Jr: Evaluation of the extremity with peripheral nerve injury and timing for nerve suture. pp. 463–486. AAOS Instr Course Lect, Vol. 33. CV Mosby, St. Louis, 1984
69. Omer GE Jr: Reconstruction of a balanced thumb through tendon transfers. Clin Orthop 195:104–116, 1985
70. Omer GE Jr: Acute management of peripheral nerve injuries. Hand Clin 2:193–206, 1986
71. Omer GE Jr: Complications of peripheral nerve injuries, 2nd Ed. pp. 865–908. In Epps CH Jr (ed): Complications in Orthopaedic Surgery. JB Lippincott, Philadelphia, 1986
72. Omer GE Jr: Early tendon transfers as internal splints after nerve injury. pp. 413–418. In Hunter JM, Schneider LH, Mackin EJ (eds): Tendon Surgery in the Hand. CV Mosby, St. Louis, 1987
73. Omer GE, Jr: Timing of tendon transfers in peripheral nerve injury. Hand Clin 4:317–322, 1988
74. Omer GE Jr: The palsied hand. pp. 849–878. In Evarts CM (ed): Surgery of the Musculoskeletal System. 2nd Ed. Churchill Livingstone, New York, 1990
75. Parkes A: Paralytic claw fingers—a graft tenodesis operation. Hand 5:192–199, 1973
76. Ranney DA: Reconstruction of the transverse metacarpal arch in ulnar palsy by transfer of the *extensor digiti minimi*. Plast Reconstr Surg 52:406–412, 1973
77. Ranney DA: The mechanism of arch reversal in the surgically corrected claw hand. Hand 6:266–272, 1974
78. Riordan DC: Tendon transplantations in median-nerve and ulnar-nerve paralysis. J Bone Joint Surg 35A:312–320, 1953
79. Riordan DC: Surgery of the paralytic hand. pp. 79–90. AAOS Instr Course Lect, Vol. 16. CV Mosby, St. Louis, 1959
80. Riordan, DC: Tendon transfers for nerve paralysis of the hand and wrist. Curr Pract Orthop Surg 2:17–40, 1964
81. Riordan DC: Tendon transfers in hand surgery. J Hand Surg 8:748–753, 1983
82. Roullet J: Froment's sign. pp. 37–43. In Michon J, Moberg E (eds): Traumatic Nerve Lesions of the Upper Limb, Group d'Etude de la Main monograph #2. Churchill Livingstone, Edinburgh, 1975
83. Shah A: Correction of ulnar claw hand by a loop of flexor digitorum superficialis motor for lumbrical replacement. J Hand Surg 9B:131–133, 1984
84. Simpson SL, Hertzog MS, Barja RH: The plantaris tendon graft: An ultrasound study. J Hand Surg 16A:708–711, 1991
85. Smith RJ: Balance and kinetics of the fingers under normal and pathological conditions. Clin Orthop 104:92–111, 1974
86. Smith RJ: Intrinsic muscles of the fingers: function, dysfunction, and surgical reconstruction. pp. 200–220. AAOS Instr Course Lect, Vol. 24. CV Mosby, St. Louis, 1975
87. Smith RJ: Surgical treatment of the clawhand. pp. 181–203. In Hunter JM, Schneider LH (eds): AAOS Symposium on Tendon Surgery in the Hand. CV Mosby, St. Louis, 1975
88. Smith RJ: Extensor carpi radialis brevis tendon transfer for thumb adduction—A study of power pinch. J Hand Surg 8:4–15, 1983
89. Smith RJ: Tendon transfers to restore power pinch. pp. 85–102 In Tendon Transfers of the Hand and Forearm. Little, Brown, and Co, Boston, 1987
90. Smith R: Tendon transfers to restore intrinsic muscle function to the fingers. pp. 103–133. In Tendon Transfers of the Hand and Forearm. Little, Brown, and Co, Boston, 1987
91. Solonen KA, Bakalim GE: Restoration of pinch grip in traumatic ulnar palsy. Hand 8:39–44, 1976
92. Stiles HJ, Forrester-Brown MF: Treatment of Injuries of Peripheral Spinal Nerves. p. 166. H. Frowde and Hodder and Stoughton, 1922
93. Stocks GW, Cobb T, Lewis RC Jr: Transfer of sensibility in the hand: A new method to restore sensibility in ulnar nerve palsy with use of microsurgical digital nerve translocation. J Hand Surg 16A:219–226, 1991
94. Sunderland S: The significance of hypothenar elevation in movements of opposition of the thumb. Aust NZ J Surg 13:155–156, 1944
95. Tsuge K: Tendon transfers in median and ulnar nerve paralysis. Hiroshima J Med Sci 16:29–48, 1967
96. Tubiana R: Palliative treatment of paralytic deformities of the thumb. Orthop Clin North Am 4:1141–1160, 1973
97. Tubiana R, Malek R: Paralysis of the intrinsic muscles of the fingers. Surg Clin North Am 48:1139–1148, 1968
98. White WL: Restoration of function and balance of the wrist and hand by tendon transfers. Surg Clin North Am 40:427–459, 1960
99. Zancolli EA: Claw-hand caused by paralysis of the intrinsic muscles. A simple surgical procedure for its correction. J Bone Joint Surg 39A:1076–1080, 1957
100. Zancolli EA: Structural and Dynamic Bases of Hand Surgery, 2nd Ed. pp. 168, 174. JB Lippincott, Philadelphia, 1979

41

Combined Nerve Palsies

George E. Omer, Jr.

When multiple nerves are injured in a single extremity, the functional loss is severe. Circulation is usually impaired, which results in ischemic pain and increased fibrosis. The skeleton may be unstable, with loss of normal joint stability and motion. Muscle-tendon units are often lacerated and sometimes avulsed, increasing the neuromotor impairment, and the resulting scar complicates the technical transfer of remaining intact tendons. Unhealed or chronic wounds are contraindications to elective surgery. As joints stiffen and muscles atrophy, maintaining a mobile extremity without deforming contracture demands persistent therapy and meticulous splinting. The most important aspect of a rehabilitation program is the patient's acceptance of the responsibility and initiative for recovery. Reconstructive procedures should not be undertaken until normal joint motion has been established and skeletal alignment is stable.[53,63]

In addition to the physical condition of the involved extremity, successful tendon transfers depend on the etiology and prognosis of the motor imbalance. The etiology of the motor imbalance is important in predicting the further involvement of additional muscle-tendon units with progressive functional imbalance. The extent of muscle imbalance is usually static after traumatic injury to lower motor neurons, but is often unstable in upper motor neuron problems, such as a series of cerebrovascular accidents. The prognosis for progressive muscle imbalance may be a contraindication for elective surgery.

A major problem in multiple nerve palsy is sensory loss coupled with a loss of position sense and other normal feedback mechanisms.[22,60] Spinal reflex arcs coordinate with the ventral horn motor neurons to produce a pattern of motor function. For each muscle there is an optimal tension at which force and motion are efficient.[10,29,47] In addition, the surgeon must consider the potential for excursion of each muscle in a new position.[8] Abnormal patterns of motor activity enhance the distortion of sensibility that accompanies a peripheral nerve deficit.[64] Sensibility loss is more profound in combined nerve palsies, and motor return rarely passes two major joints distal to the injury.[55] Nerve repairs should be done as soon as clinically appropriate, but other procedures to restore sensibility should be delayed until all indicated tendon transfers have been accomplished and the patient has supple tissues with an established range of motion. Further, precise sensibility requires precise motion.[57]

The motion expected after tendon transfer cannot exceed the passive motion present preoperatively. The preoperative action of the selected motor muscle should be synergistic with the anticipated postoperative action, or at least retrainable by conscious control. Electromyographic studies indicate that a new activity pattern can be developed to correspond with the new mechanical function, but the old activity pattern is not lost.[38,83] Further, the longer the surgeon waits for nerve recovery, the more difficult it is to prevent gradual deformity. Combined nerve palsies are further complicated by the smaller number of motor tendons that are available to stabilize residual function[28,40] or to provide additional function while awaiting potential nerve recovery following neurorrhaphy.[20] Therefore, it is difficult to utilize muscle-tendon units as internal splints to enhance patterns of motion in combined nerve palsies.[59] Muscles with only temporary loss of function, such as a neurapraxia lesion, do not regain normal strength for elective transfer procedures.[44] Previously repaired tendons may be utilized for transfer only under optimal conditions.[21] Poor results in tendon transfers are often related to four factors:[74] less than full passive motion before transfer; adhesions along the course of the transfer; technical failure, such as a juncture disruption; and patient noncompliance. The surgeon should use as few transfers as necessary to meet the objective of balanced performance, because tendon transfers redistribute existing assets rather than creating new ones.

Tendon transfers in combined nerve palsies are more complicated than those in isolated nerve palsy because of complex extremity injuries, poor proprioception, distorted sensibility, weakness of muscles for potential transfer, and the need for multiple operations. Tendon transfers either eliminate deforming forces that produce further imbalances or replace single motions to assist grasp, pinch, or release. Specific composite tissue transplantation is useful in sensory-depleted glabrous skin areas required for precise pinch and grasp, provided precise motor function is available to manipulate the transplanted composite tissue. Tendon or tissue transfers in combined nerve palsies require longer follow-up than isolated nerve palsies to make valid outcome decisions.

LOW MEDIAN-ULNAR NERVE PALSY

This is the most common combined nerve palsy. In late low (distal) median-ulnar palsy the complete loss of palmar sensation and intrinsic motor muscles produces an almost useless claw hand (Fig. 41-1). Reconstruction of the thumb is extremely important,[60] and special effort must be made to prevent adduction contracture of the thumb-index web. Examination demonstrates a flat transverse palmar arch (metacarpal arch), with hyperextension at the MP joints and hyperflexion at the PIP joints. An abducted little finger may be associated with the flat transverse metacarpal arch[17] The patient flexes the wrist to obtain greater finger extension, a functional tenodesis, but with prolonged use this results in a fixed flexion contracture of the wrist[72] (Ahern, GS, personal communication, 1969). The basic requirements for restoration of wrist and hand function are (1) improved key pinch provided by a stronger adductor of the thumb, (2) restored thumb abduction for opposition, (3) strengthened tip pinch between the thumb and index fingers, (4) improved power flexion of the proximal phalanx, (5) restored metacarpal (palmar) transverse arch and correction of the associated abduction deformity of the little finger, and (6) specific sensory area for key or tip pinch.

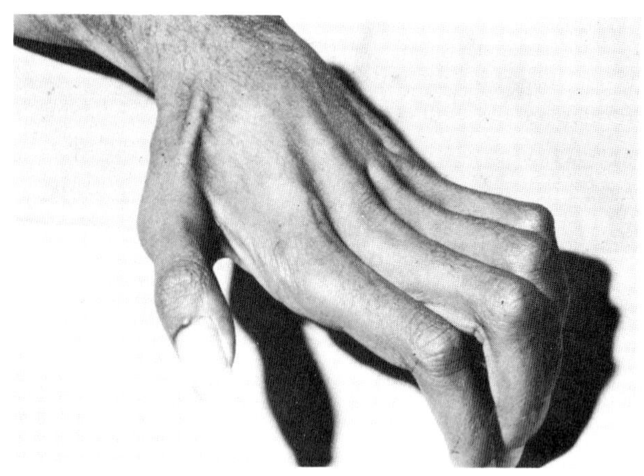

Fig. 41-1. A combined median-ulnar palsy, with intrinsic motor atrophy and atrophy of the volar pulps of the fingers. There is a flat transverse palmar arch and clawing of the fingers. The thumb has developed an adduction contracture.

Additional strength in a palsied power train requires a new muscle-tendon unit, and in combined median-ulnar palsy additional strength must be added by radial innervated muscle-tendon units (Table 41-1).[64] The extensor carpi radialis brevis adductor plasty has been an appropriate transfer. A tendon graft (plantaris or palmaris) is obtained and attached to the distal end of the extensor carpi radialis brevis. The tendon graft

Table 41-1. Combined Low (Distal) Median and Ulnar Palsy

Needed Function	Preferred Transfer	Alternate Transfer
Thumb adduction—key pinch	Extensor carpi radialis brevis with free graft between third and fourth metacarpals, to abductor tubercle of thumb[60,61,76,77]	Flexor digitorum superficialis (long) to abductor tubercle of thumb with palmar fascia and flexor tendons as pulleys[4,33,41,70,79]
Thumb abduction[23,25,60] (opposition)	Extensor indicis proprius around pisiform pulley to insertion of abductor pollics brevis[18,45,58] and extensor pollicis longus tendons[69]	Palmaris longus tendon transfer[11] or Extensor carpi ulnaris with graft[34,39]
Thumb-index tip pinch	Abductor pollicis longus slip to first dorsal interosseous tendon[46] and arthrodesis of thumb MP joint[58]	Extensor pollicis brevis[15,27] or palmaris longus[36] to first dorsal interosseous tendon (thumb MP joint is fused)
Metacarpal (palmar) transverse arch, and adduction for little finger	Extensor digiti minimi to deep transverse metacarpal ligament[1] (extensor digitorum communis to little finger must be active)	Flexor digitorum superficialis of little finger to deep transverse metacarpal ligament between fourth and fifth metacarpals (Ahern, 1969) or Combined as single transfer with thumb adduction transfer[53,58]
Power flexion—proximal phalanx and integration of MP and interphalangeal motion (clawed fingers)	Brachioradialis or extensor carpi radialis longus to all four fingers using four-tailed free graft and flexor sheath insertion (A2 pulley)[5,6,12,19,67,88] or dorsal apparatus	Flexor carpi radialis (if wrist flexion contracture) with four-tailed graft and flexor sheath insertion or dorsal apparatus[69,70,71]
Volar sensibility	Free neurovascular cutaneous island flap[26]	Cross-finger index-to-thumb neurocutaneous flap,[24,30,56] (Superficial radial nerve)

is then passed through the third metacarpal interspace and tunneled just superficial (volar) to the adductor pollicis to the abductor tubercle (tendon) of the thumb. The average key pinch strength is doubled by this operation.[33,76] In addition, the extensor carpi radialis brevis still retains its function as a wrist extensor. Following individualized transfers, the residual loss of sensibility is likely to be a greater functional problem than motor patterns for grasp and pinch.

HIGH MEDIAN-ULNAR NERVE PALSY

The hand will rarely be used for precision activities following this severe injury, even if minimal muscle balance is restored. Atrophy of the finger pulps will discourage both power and precise grip. If the other hand is normal, it is best to direct surgical endeavors toward a key pinch and simple grasp (Table 41-2).

Elbow flexion may be weak due to involvement of the pronator-flexor forearm muscle mass. These muscles initiate flexion against gravity, and are critical if there is weakness of muscles innervated by the musculocutaneous nerve. There is no wrist extensor muscle with adequate amplitude for full flexion of the digits unless the motion is reinforced by active wrist extension. (Fig. 41-2) One disadvantage of brachioradialis transfer to the flexor pollicis longus is that it weakens with elbow flexion. Abduction of the thumb for opposition does not require great strength, and the extensor indicis proprius opponensplasty is adequate; but if needed, the thumb extensor muscles can be rerouted to clear the thumb from the palm[68,82,86] Although there is active thumb extension, the interphalangeal joint may assume a flexed position. This deformity is improved by using Riordan's insertion for opponensplasty (thumb abduction) (see Chapter 39), where the transferred tendon is first sutured to the abductor pollicis brevis tendon and is then extended to be inserted into the long extensor tendon just proximal to the interphalangeal joint.[69,70,71,72,73]

The loss of simultaneous MP flexion with either interphalangeal extension or flexion disrupts the rhythm necessary to grasp large and small objects. There are no available motors to

Table 41-2. Combined High (Proximal) Median and Ulnar Palsy

Needed Function	Preferred Transfer	Alternate Transfer
Thumb adduction—key pinch	Extensor carpi radialis brevis with free graft between third and fourth metacarpals[76,77] to the abductor tubercle of the thumb[60]	Extensor indicis proprius between third and fourth metacarpals[14]
Thumb flexion (IP joint)	Brachioradialis to flexor pollicis longus in forearm[48,51,52]	Tenodesis of flexor pollicis longus distal to MP joint
Thumb abduction (opposition)	Extensor indicis proprius around pisiform pulley[18,45,58,77] to insertion of abductor pollicis brevis (plus) extensor pollicis longus[29]	Extensor carpi ulnaris[34,39] or extensor pollicis longus[68] around pisiform pulley to abductor pollicis brevis (thumb; MP joint is fused and no active flexion at thumb IP joint)
Thumb-index (long) pinch (tip pinch)	Arthrodesis of thumb MP joint (and) abductor pollicis longus slip to first dorsal interosseous tendon[46,54,58]	Extensor pollicis brevis[15,27] or palmaris longus[36] to first dorsal interosseous tendon (and) fusion of thumb MP joint
Finger flexion	Extensor carpi radialis longus to tendons of flexor digitorum profundus[48,52] with tenodesis of DIP joint of three ulnar fingers[7,48]	Biceps brachii extended with flexor carpi radialis tendon to tendons of flexor digitorum profundus[31]
Clawed Fingers—power for flexion of proximal phalanx (and) integration of MP and interphalangeal motion	Tenodesis of all digits with free tendon graft from dorsal carpal ligament volar to deep transverse metacarpal ligament to extensor apparatus[70,71] or from deep transverse metacarpal ligament to extensor apparatus[66]	Capsulodesis of MP volar capsule[85,88] or Arthrodesis of PIP joints[31] or Arthrodesis of MP joints[33]
Metacarpal (palmar) arch and adduction for little finger	Extensor digiti minimi to deep transverse metacarpal ligament[1] (extensor digitorum communis to little finger must be active)	Extensor digiti minimi to radial lateral bands (extensor hood) of the ring and little finger (Fowler-Bunnell)[78]
Wrist flexion		Extensor carpi ulnaris to insertion of flexor carpi ulnaris
Radiovolar sensibility	Superficial radial innervated index fillet flap to palm[49,54,57,58,60] or First dorsal metacarpal artery neurovascular island flap[37,75]	Free vascularized nerve graft[81]

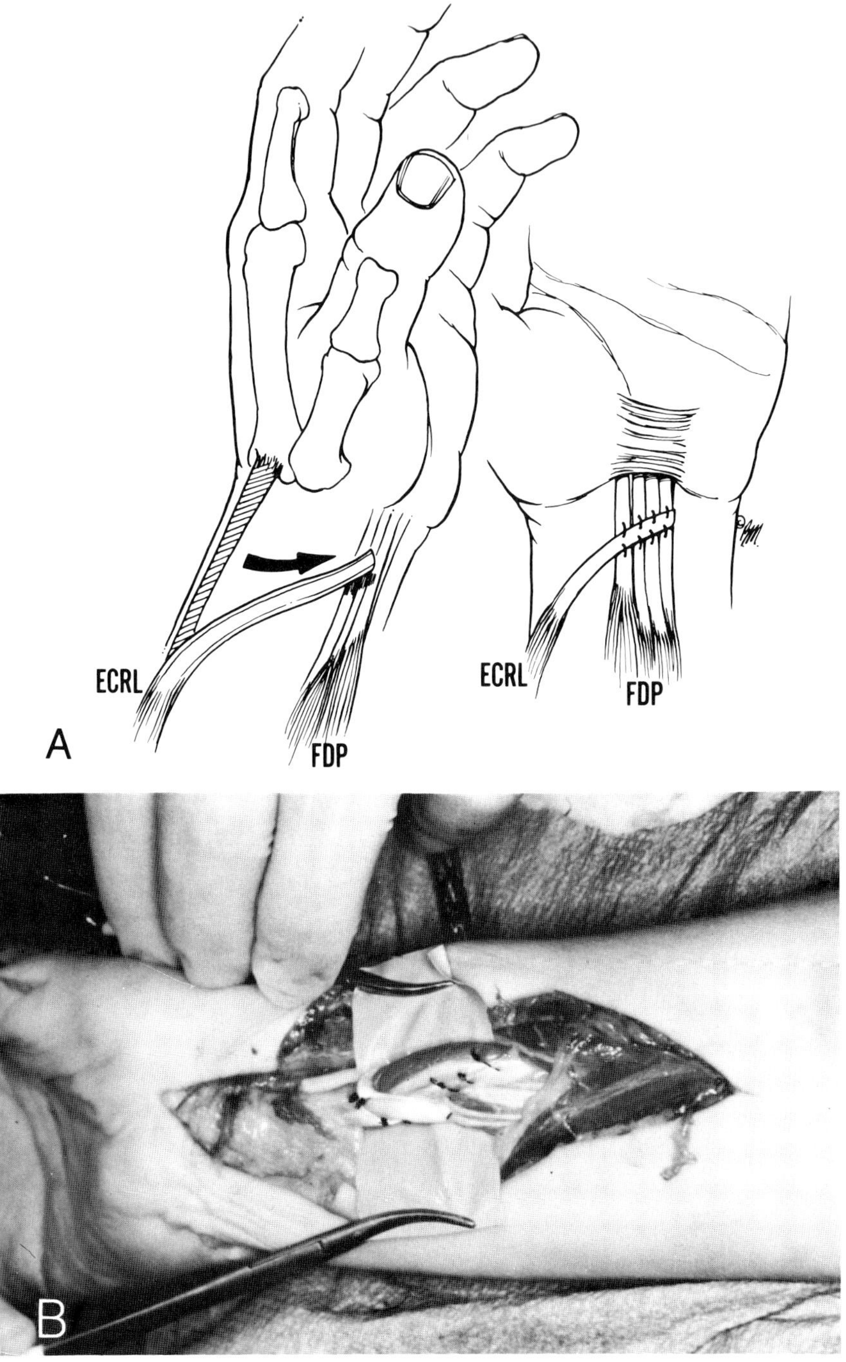

Fig. 41-2. **(A)** Transfer of the extensor carpi radialis longus *(ECRL)* around the radial aspect of the forearm to the tendons of the flexor digitorum profundus *(FDP)* for finger flexion. The tendon juncture should be proximal to the carpal tunnel. The range of finger motion is less than normal because of the comparable limited excursion of the ECRL. **(B)** Intraoperative photograph. The transfer has been sutured well proximal to the transverse carpal ligament.

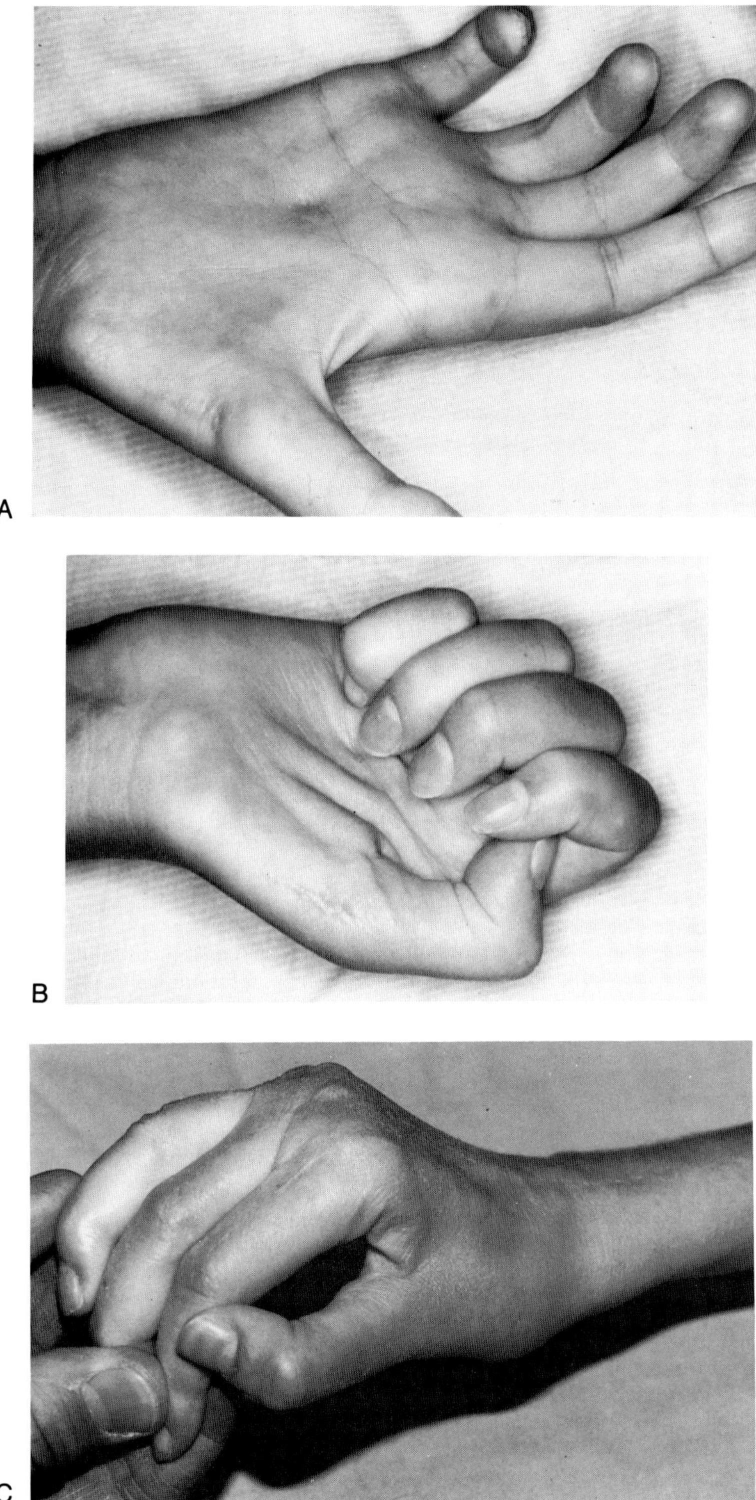

Fig. 41-3. **(A&B)** Range of active motion in a high median-ulnar palsy following reconstruction. The extensor carpi radialis brevis (ECRB), with free graft, provided thumb adduction. The brachioradialis was transferred to the flexor pollicis longus. The extensor carpi radialis longus (ECRL) was passed around the radial aspect of the forearm to the flexor digitorum profundus for finger flexion. The palmaris longus was tenodesed to the abductor pollicis brevis. **(C)** Nine years after injury, intrinsic tenodesis of the index, long, ring, and little fingers was done, using free grafts from the foot. Finger clawing was corrected, but a wrist extension contracture developed with radial deviation of the hand on the wrist. *(Figure continues.)*

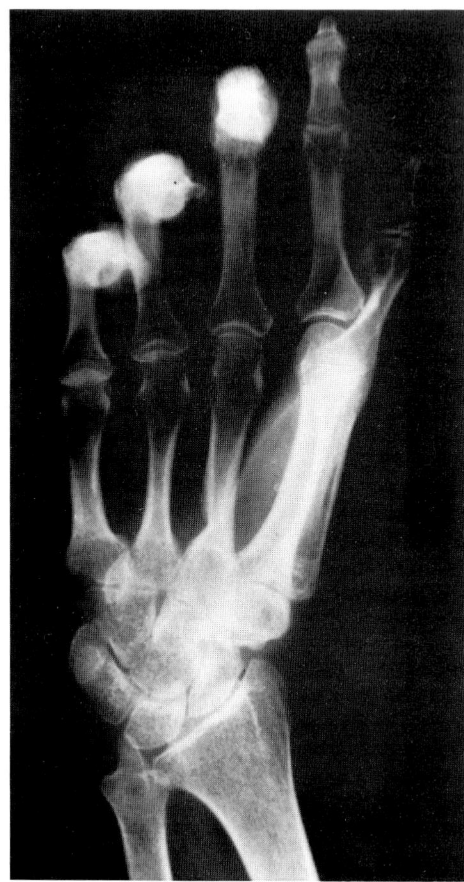

Fig. 41-3 *(Continued).* **(D)** Eleven years after injury, x-rays demonstrated ulnar translocation of the carpus on the radius, loss of thumb-index web space, and a notch in the third metacarpal related probably to the ECRB thumb adduction transfer. There was no improvement in the radial deviation deformity following release of the intrinsic tenodesis and tenolysis of the thumb adductoplasty 12 years after injury.

provide dynamic integration of these motions, so that static techniques must be used. Parkes[66] placed a free tendon graft between the radial lateral band of the dorsal apparatus of the finger and the deep transverse metacarpal ligament. Zancolli[85,88] opens the proximal (A1) pulley of the flexor sheath and a flap is removed from the volar plates (see Chapter 40). Long-term results of the capsulodesis procedure of Zancolli have demonstrated indifferent results in isolated ulnar nerve palsy,[14] but it has been effective in combined palsies.

Before the initial surgical reconstruction it may appear that restoration of intrinsic function will not be necessary. The fingers and the thumb extend fully at the MP joints and may have full extension at the interphalangeal joints despite intrinsic paralysis. The extrinsic extensors can fully extend the interphalangeal joints if they have no antagonists.[78] However, after the first stage of surgery when flexion is restored to the interphalangeal joints, the fingers gradually will assume a clawed position. The common extensors have not been weakened by the procedure to restore flexion; rather, with function retained in the extrinsic extensors and restored to the extrinsic flexors, there is an obvious imbalance of extrinsics over intrinsics.

In time, the wrist will translocate ulnarward on the radius secondary to the concentration of extrinsic forces to the radial side of the hand (Fig. 41-3D) A sequel to the carpal change is a decrease in the thumb-index web space, with loss of ability to grasp larger objects. Perhaps a decade of follow-up study is needed to determine the more appropriate tendon transfer procedures[9]

Sensibility can be transferred to the radiovolar aspect of the hand[2,30,49,54,58] Careful testing of the superficial radial nerve will demonstrate the distal level of sensibility on the dorsum of the index finger. The skeleton of the index finger is removed distal to the proximal third of the second metacarpal. The index ray is excised through a racquet incision at the distal end of good dorsal index sensibility and a longitudinal palmar incision between the second and third metacarpals (see Chapter 3). The insensitive distal skin is discarded. The filleted index finger flap is then fitted into an additional volar defect created for it in the insensitive palmar skin (Fig. 41-4). This broad-based finger flap is innervated by the superficial radial nerve and will provide protective sensibility within the thumb-index web space, which seems to be of benefit in such activities as holding a steering wheel.

An alternative to a sensory island flap is a true neurovascular island flap.[2,37,75] A first dorsal metacarpal artery island flap from the index finger may be used as a neurovascular island flap to resurface the volar tip of the thumb (Fig. 41-5).

HIGH ULNAR-RADIAL NERVE PALSY

These patients retain radiovolar sensibility, and reconstruction is a useful surgical investment to improve function (Table 41-3). Although more than 30 difference procedures are described for isolated radial palsy,[3,43] the combination of ulnar and radial palsy leaves few expendable muscle-tendon units for transfer.

Transfer of the pronator teres to the extensor carpi radialis brevis for wrist extension in a high ulnar-radial nerve palsy results in less radial deviation of the hand than insertion to the extensor carpi radialis longus, and more motion than a yoke insertion to the extensor carpi ulnaris and the extensor carpi radialis longus.[9] Either the long or ring superficialis tendon may be used in low ulnar palsy to improve the integration of MP and interphalangeal joint flexion, key pinch for the thumb, and the flattened metacarpal arch (see Chapter 40), but in a high ulnar palsy, the long superficialis tendon is preferred (Table 41-3) (Fig. 41-6). The superficialis tendon of the little finger is often congenitally absent, or not functionally independent, and therefore should not be used for tendon transfers. The loss of balanced power across the PIP joints caused by removing the superficialis may result ultimately in either a flexion contracture or a swan-neck deformity of these joints. This will occur in some cases in spite of tenodeses of one slip of the superficialis tendon proximal to the PIP joint (see Chapter 39). Since one cannot accurately predict which of these defor-

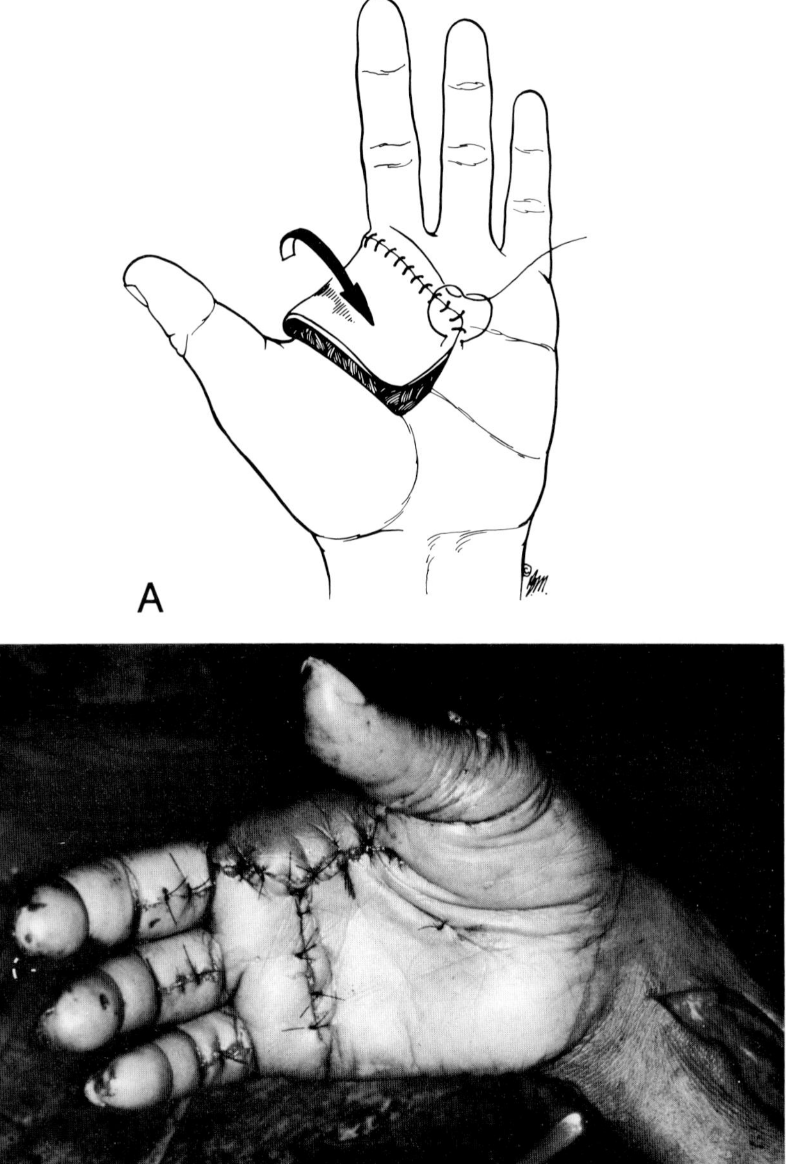

Fig. 41-4. (A) A radial-innervated dorsal skin flap for combined high median-ulnar palsy. The insensitive palmar skin is excised to create space for the fillet flap, which brings radial-innervated skin into the radial side of the palm. **(B)** Intraoperative photograph.

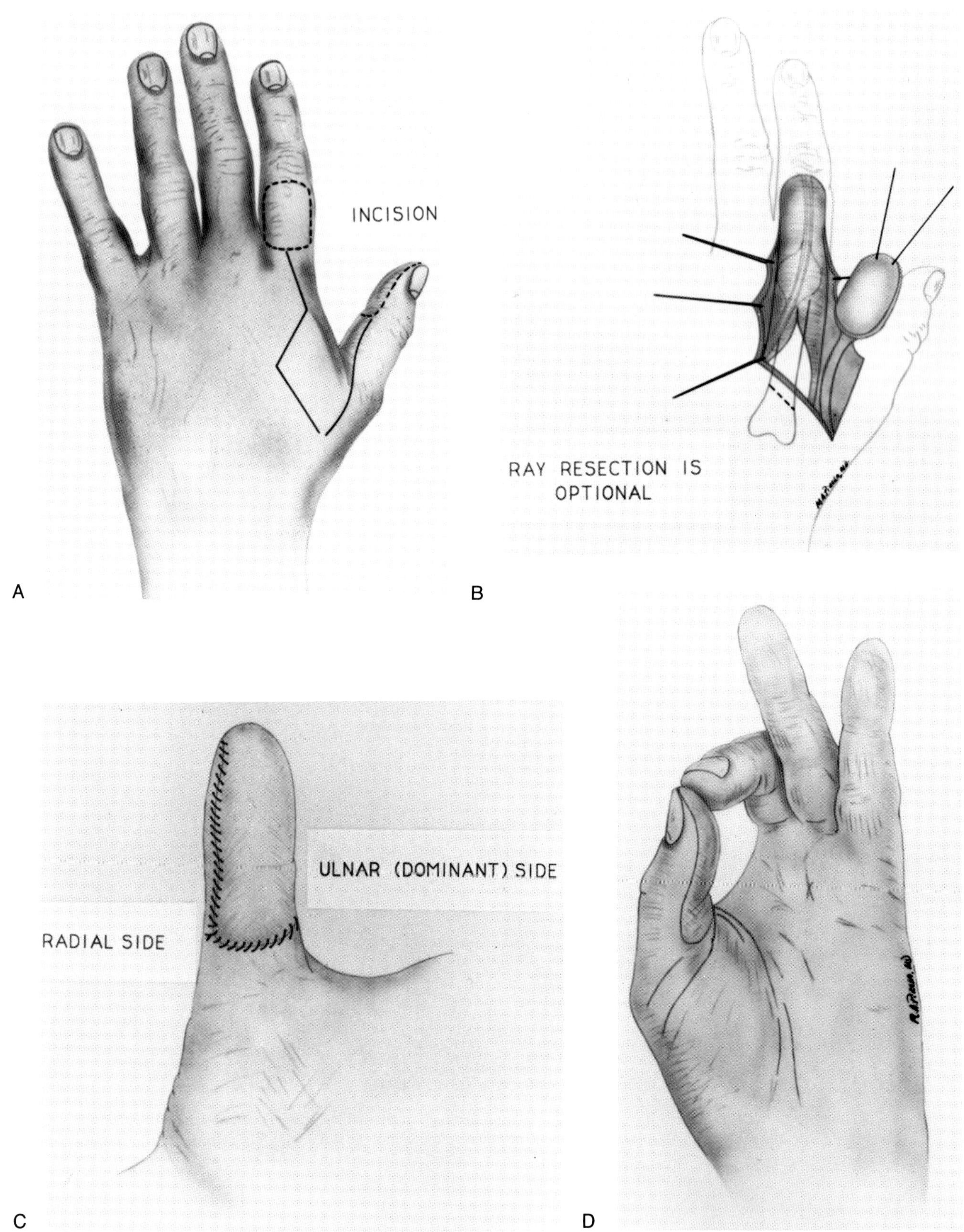

Fig. 41-5. **(A)** Incisions for a radial-innervated neurovascular pedicle flap on the first dorsal metacarpal surface of the index finger between the MP and PIP joints. **(B)** Completed dissection of the first dorsal metacarpal artery neurovascular island flap. The flap is elevated with the neurovascular pedicle. Ray resection is optional. **(C)** Flap in place on the ulnar-palmar surface of the thumb. If the index finger is filleted, a larger flap is available. **(D)** Superficial radial innervated pinch can be obtained. (Courtesy of Miguel Pirela-Cruz, M.D.)

Table 41-3. Combined (High) Ulnar and Radial Palsy

Needed Function	Preferred Transfer	Alternate Transfer
Wrist extension	Pronator teres to extensor carpi radialis brevis[9]	
Thumb adduction-key pinch	One-half flexor digitorum superficialis (long) as split transfer, to abductor tubercle of the thumb[50,54,58]	
Clawed fingers: Metacarpal (palmar transverse arch) (and) Power flexion—proximal phalanx (and) Integration of MP and interphalangeal motion	One-half flexor digitorum superficialis (long) in two slips to A2 pulley as flexor sheath insertion to ring and little fingers[12,50,54,58,88] and, later Arthrodesis of PIP joints, ring and little fingers if unable to fully extend[48,52,54]	Tenodesis with free tendon graft from radial lateral band of dorsal apparatus to deep transverse metacarpal ligament[66] or Capsulodesis of MP volar capsule[58,85,88]
Thumb-index tip pinch	Arthrodesis of thumb MP joint[48,52,54]	
Proximal thumb abduction stability (and) Wrist flexion (radial aspect)	Flexor carpi radialis (yoke insertion) to abductor pollicis longus and extensor pollicis brevis[54,58,61,64]	Tenodesis of abductor pollicis longus to radius[54,58,61,64]
Wrist flexion (ulnar aspect)		Palmaris longus to insertion of flexor carpi ulnaris[61,64]
Finger and thumb extension	Flexor digitorum superficialis (index and ring) through interosseous membrane to extensor digitorum communis and extensor pollicis longus[3]	Palmaris longus to extensor digitorum communis and extensor pollicis longus[71]
Finger flexion (ring and little)	Tenodesis of flexor digitorum profundus of index and long fingers (active motors) to ring and little flexor digitorum profundus[7,84] and Tenodesis of DIP joint of ring and little fingers, using flexor digitorum profundus[48,52]	
Volar sensibility—ring and little fingers	Free vascularized nerve grafts[81]	Free neurovascular cutaneous island flap on pedicles[26]

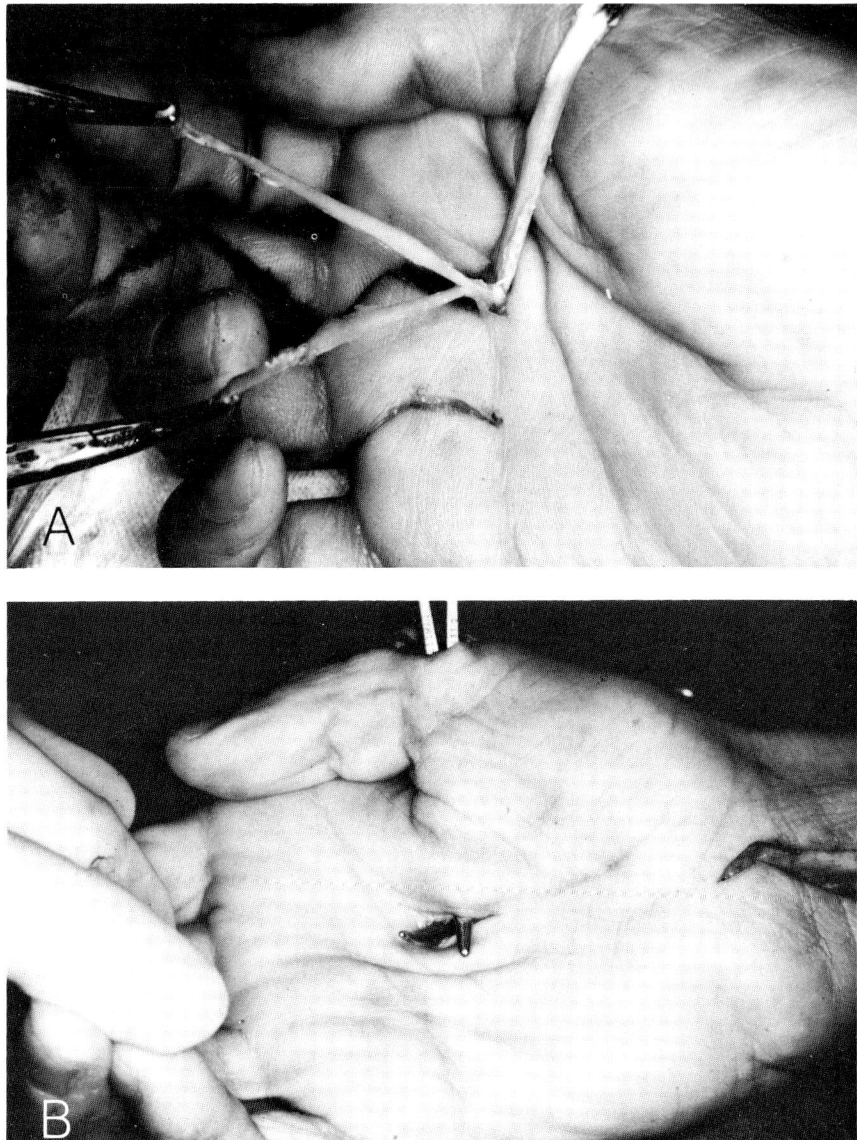

Fig. 41-6. **(A)** The long finger flexor digitorum superficialis as a split transfer. One half of the tendon is separated into two slips, which will be inserted (looped) into the flexor sheaths at the level of the A2 pulleys in the ring and little fingers to correct clawing of those digits. **(B)** The other half of the tendon is passed dorsal to the index flexor sheath, on the volar surface of the adductor pollicis muscle, to be inserted into the tendon insertion of the abductor pollicis brevis.

Table 41-4. Combined High (Proximal) Median and Radial Palsy

Needed Function	Preferred Transfer	Alternate Transfer
Forearm pronation	Biceps brachii tendon rerouting around the radius[65,87]	
Wrist extension and flexion	Radiocarpal arthrodesis[32,80]	
Finger flexion	Tenodesis of flexor digitorum profundus ring and little fingers (active motors) to index and long flexor digitorum profundus[84]	
Finger and thumb extension	Flexor carpi ulnaris to tendons of extensor digitorum communis and extensor pollicis longus[48,52,71]	
Proximal thumb abduction stability	Arthrodesis of thumb MP joint[48,52,58] and Tenodesis of abductor pollicis longus tendon to radius[54]	
Thumb abduction (opposition)		Abductor digiti quiniti to the insertion of the abductor pollicis brevis[42] or Adductor pollicis tendon from adductor tubercle to abductor tubercle[25]
Thumb flexion	Tenodesis of flexor pollicis longus across thumb interphalangeal joint[58]	Biceps brachii extended with flexor carpi radialis tendon to tendon of flexor pollicis longus[31]
Radiovolar sensibility	Free neurovascular cutaneous island flap[49,56]	Free vascularized nerve graft[81] or Neurovascular cutaneous island pedicle from ring finger[49]

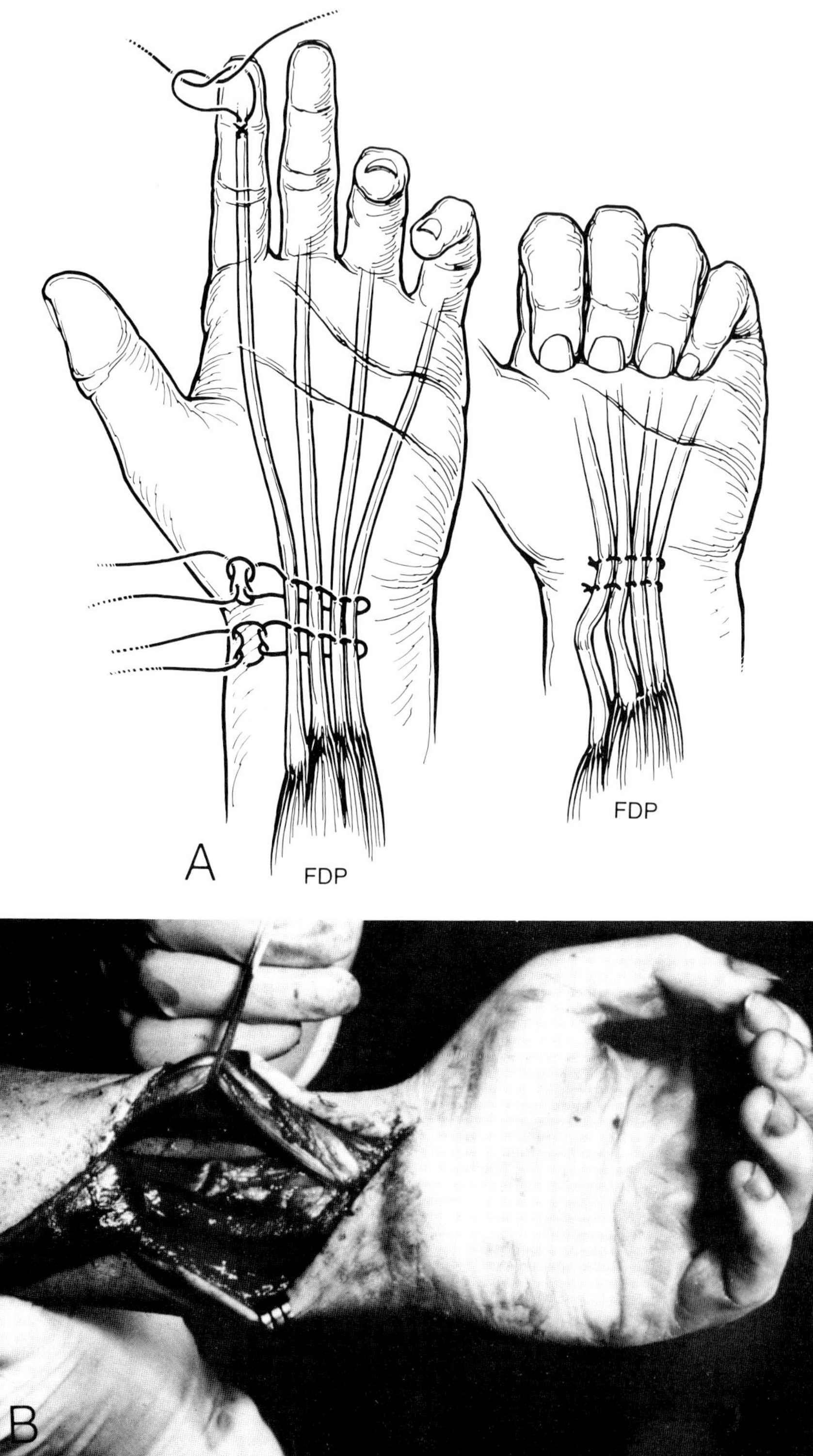

Fig. 41-7. (A) Tenodesis of the denervated index and long finger tendons to the innervated ring and little finger tendons of the flexor digitorum profundus *(FDP)* to provide flexion for all fingers. A double line of sutures is important to prevent "whip sawing" of the tendons with power grip. The index profundus has been tenodesed across the DIP joint to eliminate one joint in the motion train. **(B)** Intraoperative photograph. The finger pulps are in a "straight," rather than oblique, line; i.e., with more tension in the index and long fingers (see text).

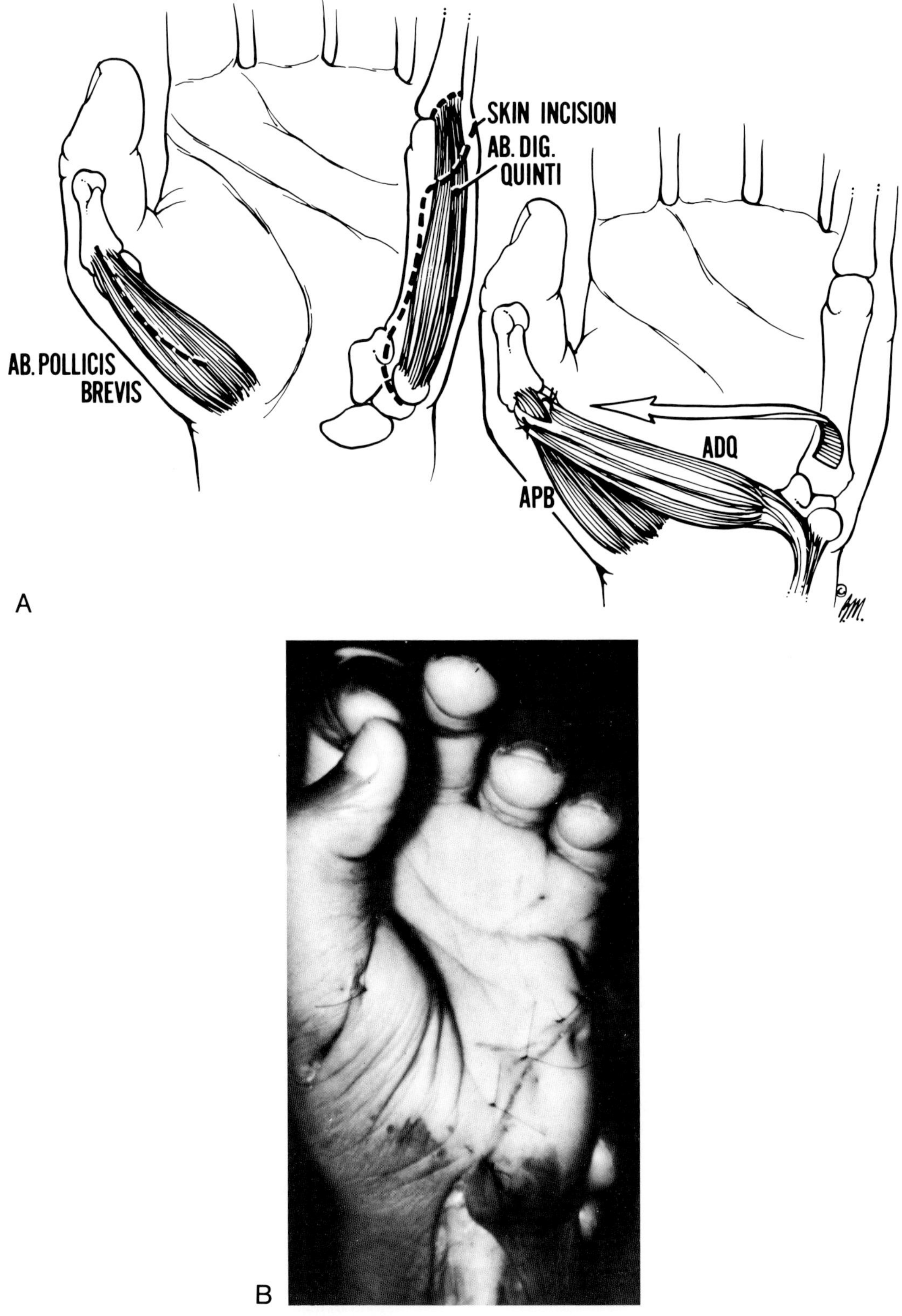

Fig. 41-8. **(A)** Transfer of the abductor digiti quinti *(ADQ)* from its hypothenar position to the thenar area for abduction. Two incisions are made in order to minimize damage to the superficial nerves and the grasping surface of the palm. The muscle is freed from distal to proximal, and then folded over 170 degrees and passed subcutaneously to be inserted into the tendon of the abductor pollicis brevis *(APB)*. **(B)** Intraoperative photograph.

mities may result in an individual patient, I believe that it is preferable to await the onset of deformity before treating it. The most predictable corrective procedure may be arthrodesis of the PIP joint.

HIGH MEDIAN-RADIAL NERVE PALSY

Tendon transfers in this combined nerve lesion will result in a hand that functions only slightly more effectively than a prosthesis.[20] (Table 41-4). All wrist motors are lost except the flexor carpi ulnaris, and radiocarpal (wrist) arthrodesis is indicated. The flexor profundus tendons are sutured side-to-side for ulnar-innervated mass action. (Fig. 41-7). The profundus tendons to the index and long fingers must be under greater tension at the suture line in order to obtain appropriate flexion.

Transfer of the abductor digiti quinti for thumb abduction should not be attempted until the wrist is stabilized and there is normal adduction power for the thumb[20,42] The neurovascular pedicle to the abductor digiti quinti is proximally situated, and the muscle should be freed distally to proximally, then turned like a page in a book to its new position (Fig. 41-8). This muscle has inadequate excursion, but will provide functional thumb opposition. Nonetheless, it is questionable that total hand function is improved, since the little finger, with sensation intact, has now lost its ability for opposition.

SUMMARY

Surgeons concerned with reconstruction of the upper extremity after combined nerve palsies have occurred should be experienced enough to select appropriate procedures based on the individual case. Procedures to restore motor function should be done prior to procedures to improve sensibility, such as a neurovascular island transfer, because precise sensibility requires precise motion. Additional strength requires a new muscle tendon unit in the power train. The anticipated result should be a balanced simplification of functional performance, because surgery will redistribute the few remaining assets rather than create new ones. Highly motivated and skillfull patients create successful surgeons, and the key to success for the surgical techniques is simplicity; complexity invites failure. The specific details of these operative procedures are described in Chapters 38, 39, and 40. Tables 41-1 to 41-4 summarize how these operations might be best used in these complex reconstructive problems.

REFERENCES

1. Blacker GJ, Lister GD, Kleinert HE: The abducted little finger in low ulnar nerve palsy. J Hand Surg 1:190-196, 1976
2. Bralliar F, Horner RL: Sensory cross-finger pedicle graft. J Bone Joint Surg 51A:1264-1268, 1969
3. Boyes JH: Tendon transfers for radial palsy. Bull Hosp Joint Dis 21:97-105, 1959
4. Boyes JH: Bunnell's Surgery of the Hand. 4th Ed. JB Lippincott, Philadelphia, 1964
5. Brand PW: Paralytic claw hand. J Bone Joint Surg 40B:618-632, 1958
6. Brand PW: Tendon grafting. Illustrated by a new operation for intrinsic paralysis of the fingers. J Bone Joint Surg 43B:444-453, 1961
7. Brand PW: Tendon transfers for median and ulnar nerve paralysis. Orthop Clin North Am 1:447-454, 1970
8. Brand PW, Beach RB, Thompson DE: Relative tension and potential excursion of muscles in the forearm and hand. J Hand Surg 6:209-219, 1981
9. Brand PW: Clinical mechanics of the hand, pp. 46-48. CV Mosby, St. Louis, 1985
10. Brand PW: Biomechanics of tendon transfer. Hand Clin 4:137-154, 1988
11. Braun RM: Palmaris longus tendon transfer for augmentation of the thenar musculature in low median palsy. J Hand Surg 3:488-491, 1978
12. Brooks AL, Jones DS: A new intrinsic transfer for the paralytic hand. J Bone Joint Surg 57A:730, 1975
13. Brown PW: The time factor in surgery of upper extremity peripheral nerve injury. Clin Orthop 68:14-21, 1970
14. Brown PW: Reconstruction for pinch in ulnar intrinsic palsy. Orthop Clin North Am, 5:323-342, 1974
15. Bruner JM: Tendon transfer to restore abduction of the index finger using the extensor pollicis brevis. Plast Reconstr Surg 3:197-201, 1948
16. Bunnell S: Opposition of the thumb. J Bone Joint Surg 20:269-284, 1938
17. Burge P: Abducted little finger in low ulnar nerve palsy. J Hand Surg 11B:234-236, 1986
18. Burkhalter WE, Christensen RC, Brown PW: Extensor indicis proprius opponensplasty. J Bone Joint Surg 55A:725-732, 1973
19. Burkhalter WE, Strait JL: Metacarpophalangeal flexor replacement for intrinsic-muscle paralysis. J Bone Joint Surg 55A:1667-1676, 1973
20. Burkhalter WE: Early tendon transfer in upper extremity peripheral nerve injury. Clin Orthop 104:68-79, 1974
21. Chiu H-Y: Use of a previously repaired tendon for tendon transfer. J Hand Surg 12B:185-186, 1987
22. Citron N, Taylor J: Tendon transfer in partially anaesthetic hands. J Hand Surg 12B:14-18, 1987
23. Cooney WP: Tendon transfer for median nerve palsy. Hand Clinics, 4:155-165, 1988
24. Curtis RM: Cross-finger pedicle flap in hand surgery. Am Surg 145:650-655, 1957
25. Curtis RM: Opposition of the thumb. Orthop Clin North Am 5:305-321, 1974
26. Daniel RK, Terzis J, Midgley RD: Restoration of sensation to an anesthetic hand by a free neurovascular flap from the foot. Plast Reconstr Surg 57:275-280, 1976
27. De Abreu LB: Early restoration of pinch grip after ulnar nerve repair and tendon transfer. J Hand Surg 14B:309-314, 1989
28. Eversmann WW, Jr: Tendon transfers for combined nerve injuries. Hand Clinics, 4:187-199, 1988
29. Fleeter TB, Adams JP, Brenner B, Podolsky RJ: A laser diffraction method for measuring muscle sarcomere length in vivo for application to tendon transfers. J Hand Surg 10A:542-546, 1988
30. Gaul JS Jr: Radial-innervated cross finger flap from index to provide sensory pulp to injured thumb. J Bone Joint Surg 51A:1257-1263, 1969
31. Goldner JL: Tendon transfers for irreparable peripheral nerve injuries of the upper extremity. Orthop Clin North Am 5:343-375, 1974

32. Haddad RJ, Riordan DC: Arthrodesis of the wrist. A surgical technique. J Bone Joint Surg 49A:950-954, 1967
33. Hastings H II, Davidson S: Tendon transfers for ulnar nerve palsy. Evaluation of results and practical treatment considerations. Hand Clin 4:167-178, 1988
34. Henderson ED: Transfer of wrist extensors and brachioradialis to restore opposition of the thumb. J Bone Joint Surg 44A:513-522, 1962
35. Hill NA: Restoration of opposition for the paralyzed thumb. Clin Orthop 61:234-240, 1968
36. Hirayama T, Atsuta Y, Takemitsu Y: Palmaris longus transfer for replacement of the first dorsal interosseous. J Hand Surg 11B:84-86, 1986
37. Holevich J: A new method of restoring sensibility to the thumb. J Bone Joint Surg 45B:496-502, 1963
38. Illert M, Trauner M, Weller E, Wiedemann E: Forearm muscles of man can reverse their function after tendon transfers: an electromyographic study. Neurosci Lett 67:129-134, 1986
39. Kessler I: Transfer of the extensor carpi ulnaris to tendon of extensor pollicis brevis for opponensplasty. J Bone Joint Surg 51A:1303-1309, 1969
40. Labosky DA, Waggy CA: Apparent weakness of median and ulnar motors in radial nerve palsy. J Hand Surg 11A:528-533, 1986
41. Littler JW: Tendon transfers and arthrodesis in combined median and ulnar nerve paralysis. J Bone Joint Surg 31A:225-234, 1949
42. Littler JW, Cooley SGE: Opposition of the thumb and its restoration by abductor digiti quinti transfer. J Bone Joint Surg 45A:1389-1396, 1963
43. Moberg E, Nachemson A: Tendon transfers for defective long extensors of the wrist and fingers. Acta Chir Scand, 133:31-34, 1967
44. Moneim MS, Omer GE Jr: Latissimus dorsi muscle transfer for restoration of elbow flexion after brachial plexus disruption. J Hand Surg, 11A:135-139, 1986
45. Moore JR, Weiland AJ, Valdata L: Independent index extension after extensor indicis proprius transfer. J Hand Surg 12A:232-236, 1987
46. Neviaser RJ, Wilson JN, Gardner MM: Abductor pollicis longus transfer for replacement of first dorsal interosseous. J Hand Surg 5:53-57, 1980
47. Omer GE Jr, Vogel JA: Determination of physiological length of a reconstructed muscle-tendon unit through muscle stimulation. J Bone Joint Surg 47A:304-310, 1965
48. Omer GE Jr: Evaluation and reconstruction of the forearm and hand after acute traumatic peripheral nerve injuries. J Bone Joint Surg 50A:1454-1478, 1968
49. Omer GE Jr, Day DJ, Ratcliff H, Lambert P: Neurovascular cutaneous island pedicles for deficient median nerve sensibility. J Bone Joint Surg 52A:1181-1192, 1970
50. Omer GE Jr: Restoring power grip in ulnar palsy. In Proceedings of the American Society for Surgery of the Hand. J Bone Joint Surg 53A:814, 1971
51. Omer GE Jr, Elton RC: Tendon transfers for the nerve injured upper limb. Orthop Rev 1:25-28, 1972
52. Omer GE Jr: Evaluation and reconstruction of the forearm and hand after acute traumatic peripheral nerve injuries. AAOS Instr Course Lect 18,J1:93-119, 1973
53. Omer GE Jr: The technique and timing of tendon transfers. Orthop Clin North Am 5:243-252, 1974
54. Omer GE Jr: Tendon transfers in combined nerve lesions. Orthop Clin North Am 5:377-387, 1974
55. Omer GE Jr: Injuries to nerves of the upper extremity. J Bone Joint Surg 56A:1615-1624, 1974
56. Omer GE Jr: Neurovascular sensory island transplants. In Fredericks S, Brody GS: Neurologic Aspects of Plastic Surgery. Educ Found Amer Soc Plast Reconstr Surg, 17:52-60. CV Mosby, St. Louis, 1978
57. Omer GE Jr, Neurovascular cutaneous island pedicle flaps. pp. 779-790. In Omer GE Jr, Spinner M (eds): Management of Peripheral Nerve Problems. WB Saunders, Philadelphia, 1980
58. Omer GE Jr: Tendon transfers for reconstruction of the forearm and hand following peripheral nerve injuries. pp. 817-846. In Omer GE Jr, Spinner M (eds): Management of Peripheral Nerve Problems. WB Saunders, Philadelphia, 1980
59. Omer GE: Early tendon transfers in the rehabilitation of median, radial, and ulnar palsies. Ann Chir Main 1:187-190, 1982
60. Omer GE Jr: Reconstruction of a balanced thumb through tendon transfers. Clin Orthop 195:104-116, 1985
61. Omer GE Jr: Complications of peripheral nerve injuries. pp. 865-908. In Epps CH (ed): Complications in Orthopaedic Surgery. 2nd Ed. JB Lippincott, Philadelphia, 1986
62. Omer GE Jr: Tendon transfers in radial nerve paralysis, pp. 425-431. In Hunter JM, Schneider LH, Mackin EJ (eds): Tendon Surgery in the Hand. CV Mosby, St. Louis, 1987
63. Omer GE: Timing of tendon transfers in peripheral nerve injury. Hand Clin 4:317-322, 1988
64. Omer GE Jr: The Palsied Hand, pp. 849-878. In Everts CM (ed): Surgery of the Musculoskeletal System. 2nd Ed. Churchill Livingstone, New York, 1990
65. Owings R, Wickstrom J, Perry J, Nickel VL: Biceps brachii rerouting in treatment of paralytic supination contracture of the forearm. J Bone Joint Surg 53A:137-142, 1971
66. Parkes A: Paralytic claw fingers—A graft tenodesis operation. Hand 5:192-199, 1973
67. Peckham PH, Freehafer AA, Keith MW: The influecne of muscle properties in tendon transfer. pp. 310-324. In Brand PW (ed): Clinical Mechanics of the Hand. CV Mosby, St. Louis, 1985
68. Riley WB, Mann RJ, Burkhalter WE: Extensor pollicis longus opponensplasty. J Hand Surg 5:217-220, 1980
69. Riordan DC: Tendon transplantation in median-nerve and ulnar-nerve paralysis. J Bone Joint Surg 35A:312-320, 1953
70. Riordan DC: Surgery of the paralytic hand. pp. 79-90. AAOS Instructional Course Lectures, Vol. 16. CV Mosby, St. Louis, 1959
71. Riordan DC: Tendon transfers for nerve paralysis of the hand and wrist. Curr Pract Orthop Surg 2:17-40, 1964
72. Riordan DC: Tendon transfers in hand surgery. J Hand Surg 8:748-753, 1983
73. Riordan DC: Intrinsic paralysis of the hand. Bull Hosp Joint Disease 44:435-441, 1984
74. Schneider LH: Tendon transfers in muscle and tendon loss. Hand Clinics, 4:267-272, 1988
75. Small JO, Brennen MD: The first dorsal metacarpal artery neurovascular island flap. J Hand Surg 13B:136-145, 1988
76. Smith RJ: Extensor carpi radialis brevis tendon transfer for thumb adduction—A study of power pinch. J Hand Surg 8:4-15, 1983
77. Smith RJ: Tendon transfers to restore power pinch. pp. 86-102. In: Tendon Transfers of the Hand and Forearm. Little, Brown, Boston, 1987
78. Smith RJ: Tendon transfers following injuries about the elbow. pp. 135-150. In: Tendon Transfers of the Hand and Forearm. Little, Brown, Boston, 1987
79. Srinivasan H: Correction of the paralytic claw-thumb by two-tailed transfer of the superficialis tendon through a window in the flexor retinaculum. Plast Reconstr Surg 69:90-95, 1982
80. Stein I: Gill turnabout radial graft for wrist arthrodesis. Surg Gynecol Obstet 106:231-232, 1958
81. Taylor GI: Nerve grafting with simultaneous microvascular reconstruction. Clin Orthop 133:56-70, 1978
82. Tubiana R: Anatomic and physiologic basis for the surgical treat-

ment of paralysis of the hand. J Bone Joint Surg 51A:643–660, 1969
83. Waters RL, Stark LZ, Gubernick I, Bellman H, Barnes G: Electromyographic analysis of brachioradialis to flexor pollicis longus tendon transfer in quadriplegia. J Hand Surg 15A:335–339, 1990
84. White WL: Restoration of function and balance of the wrist and hand by tendon transfers. Surg Clin North Am 40:427–459, 1960
85. Zancolli EA: Claw-hand caused by paralysis of the intrinsic muscles. A simple surgical procedure for its correction. J Bone Joint Surg 39A:1076–1080, 1957
86. Zancolli E: Tendon transfers after ischemic contracture of the forearm. Am J Surg 109:356–360, 1965
87. Zancolli EA: Paralytic supination contracture of the forearm. J Bone Joint Surg 49A:1275–1284, 1967
88. Zancolli EA: Structural and Dynamic Bases of Hand Surgery. 2nd Ed. pp. 174–175. JB Lippincott, Philadelphia, 1979

42

Brachial Plexus

Robert D. Leffert

The treatment of injuries to the brachial plexus is a demanding and difficult area of surgery of the upper extremity. Not only is the anatomy complex and variable, but also the skills required to render comprehensive care cross specialty barriers and require both extensive training and innovative application. Furthermore, the field is by no means static; it continues to evolve as controversies are generated and resolved with the hope of providing better care for these often disastrously impaired patients.

The first report of successful surgery on a traction injury of the brachial plexus appeared in 1900, when William Thornburn of Manchester, England, described improved function in a 16-year-old girl whose plexus had been injured and whose lesion was treated by secondary suture.[169] By 1920, Taylor[165] had accumulated a series of 70 cases of birth palsy treated surgically, and other surgeons had reported their experiences.[129,148] However, the initial enthusiasm for operative treatment, both in obstetric palsy and adult injury, was often engendered by anecdotal reporting and poor documentation, so that by the third decade of this century the tide had turned against direct surgical attack on the plexus.[77] As recently as 1963, Sir Herbert Seddon stated[139]: "Repair of the brachial plexus has proved so disappointing that it should not be done except for the upper trunk."

In practice, surgery on these nerves was largely limited to exploration for prognosis so that peripheral orthopaedic reconstruction or amputation could be performed without delay. By 1973, however, technical improvements in optics, instruments, and suture material revitalized the field with the emergence of microsurgery. Millesi,[107-111] Narakas[118-121] in Lausanne, and Lusskin, Campbell, and Thompson[100] in New York, as well as Alnot,[9,12,13] Allieu,[5,6,8] Sedel,[142,143] Gilbert,[51,52] and Benassy[18] and their colleagues in France reported their experience in surgery of the brachial plexus. A new era of investigation and encouragement had arrived. The contributions of Japanese surgeons to this subject have been particularly interesting and valuable.[61,64,90,114-117,158,161,162,173] The reader is referred to the above-mentioned works, since a detailed presentation of these authors' results is not possible in this brief chapter. In addition, several general discussions of the subject are available for review.[93,95,182] Nevertheless, it should be remembered that each patient must be evaluated individually in terms of the specific techniques that should be employed to restore as much function as possible. It is not sufficient to concentrate on a particular technique for the restoration of function, and to debate whether neurological or peripheral reconstruction is superior or of little use to the patients. They should have the benefit of all existing techniques so that an integrated program can be carried out in their treatment.[19] Generally, this requires that the individual surgeon be well versed in different surgical as well as nonsurgical techniques, and that a team approach be employed.

THE SCOPE OF THE PROBLEM

Although injuries of the brachial plexus can occur under a wide variety of circumstances, they may be considered under the headings listed below.

I. Open injuries of the brachial plexus
II. Closed (traction) injuries of the brachial plexus
  A. Supraclavicular injuries
    1. Supraganglionic
    2. Infraganglionic
  B. Infraclavicular and subclavicular injuries
  C. Combined
  D. Postanesthetic palsy
III. Radiation injury to the brachial plexus
IV. Obstetrical palsy

Open Injuries

Open injuries may be caused by a variety of instruments and missiles. They may be accompanied by life- or limb-threatening vascular injury[123] that, if present, mandates immediate operative exploration. Where there is no vascular injury, direct operative intervention should be determined by the nature of the wound. If caused by a sharp instrument, such as a knife or glass, the assumption may usually be made that whatever nerve deficit exists may be attributed to a division of nerve rather than a contusion or stretch, as might result from a bullet. Operative repair in stab wounds can be done as soon as the patient's condition permits, unless there is a strong likelihood of sepsis. The decision to explore the plexus must be a reasoned one based on the possibility of restoring function. Precisely when such surgery should be done depends on several factors. Since operative exposure, technical requirements, and potential complications require a full and efficient team with potential backups, it is prudent not to start surgery in the middle of the night with a fatigued "skeleton" crew. Assuming there is minimal contamination of the wound, there would be little objection to applying a dressing and proceeding with surgery within 24 hours on an elective basis. Otherwise, I see no objection to closing the wound and waiting for primary healing before doing the exploration and repair. For the primary surgeon who is caring for the patient on an emergency basis, usually in an attempt to arrest hemorrhage or restore vascular perfusion to the limb, and who is not going to be the definitive surgeon for the repair of the neural structures if secondary surgery is to be done at a later date, the best course of action is to tag the divided nerves with marker sutures and to make as detailed a map of the findings as possible. This will avoid the possibility of having the definitive surgery delayed and made much more difficult by the finding of connections between unlike or incorrectly matched nerves. Although this sounds unlikely, I have secondarily explored two such cases in the period of 1 month.

The question of which sharp injuries merit exploration in the absence of vascular injury depends on several factors. The first is whether there is a significant neural deficit that could be expected to benefit from surgical repair (Fig. 42-1). A second is which portions of the plexus have been injured. For example, a patient in whom a very minimal deficit exists might well be expeditiously treated by means of tendon transfer rather than direct surgery on the nerves if the deficit is localized and sensory function is not severely compromised (Fig. 42-2). Furthermore, experience has shown that the upper and intermediate trunks affected by sharp lacerations have a much better prognosis than the lower trunk and its outflow following surgical repair. In the case of children with sharp lacerations, everything that can be repaired should be, since their ability to regenerate and regain function is far superior to that of adults.

A subdivision of open lacerations that presents very severe problems is the chain-saw injury. Unfortunately, these have increased as numbers of unskilled "do-it-yourselfers" have included the chain saw among their tools. The kickback from the chain saw may result in a fatal injury when a ragged laceration of the supraclavicular fossa occurs. In patients who are lucky enough to survive, there is usually extensive damage that involves not only laceration of the nerves, but also, in three cases that I have observed, sufficient traction to produce root avulsion from the spinal cord. If these patients are seen at the time of injury, the nerves should be identified and tagged for later repair unless it is quite clear that avulsion is not a possibility. In the event that it is, myelography should precede secondary exploration. Open wounds of the lower trunk of the brachial plexus are far more likely to be accompanied by vascular injury than those of the upper or intermediate trunks. In addition to their obvious life-threatening nature, they are also liable to further injury of the neural elements during frantic attempts to arrest hemorrhage.

It was formerly believed that gunshot wounds differed from sharp lacerations in terms of the wound mechanism and its effect on nerves. They were rarely initially complete and, if so, usually became partial fairly quickly. The reason this occurred is because of the concussive effect of a bullet, which may have deformed the nerves nearby, thus temporarily interrupting their function. Unfortunately, these old generalizations are based on the relatively low velocity of the projectiles formerly found in both civilian and military weapons. With the evolution of weaponry and the spread of military-type weapons to civilian situations, more high-velocity wounds are seen, and these may involve severe stretch injuries of the nerves that can be just as devastating as direct transsections.

Assuming that there is no significant pulmonary or vascular injury accompanying a bullet wound of the brachial plexus, conservative therapy with local wound care is usually indicated. If no recovery is seen within 3 months, or if there is a major area of neurologic deficit, I believe that they should be explored secondarily.

For patients who develop pain and neurologic dysfunction following the placement of subclavian lines[79] or as a consequence of arteriography,[27,37] the brachial plexus should be explored as soon as there is evidence of increasing local or referred pain or neurologic deficit.

Operative injuries to the brachial plexus and its terminal branches not due to position on the operating table or traction on the limb may occur in operations about the shoulder girdle.[131] If they are realized as resulting from sharp injury, they should be immediately repaired. Unfortunately, their effect is often not appreciated until the patient has awakened from general anesthesia, at which time there may be difficulty in differentiating them from traction lesions due to operative positioning on the operating table. Since the latter injuries usually begin to recover within 6 weeks, it may well be prudent to wait that long to observe what happens before advocating secondary exploration.

For patients who sustain injury to the lower trunk of the brachial plexus during performance of transaxillary first rib resection, the prognosis for recovery of major deficits is extremely poor.[39,71,179] At all times during the course of the surgery, it is most important to have the nerves under direct visualization. The lower trunk is the only part of the plexus that is exposed through this incision, and since it is near the line of section of the rib, it is potentially in harm's way. I have been consulted on several patients who sustained more extensive damage to the plexus with this approach. One such patient had myelographic evidence of multiple root avulsions and a flail-

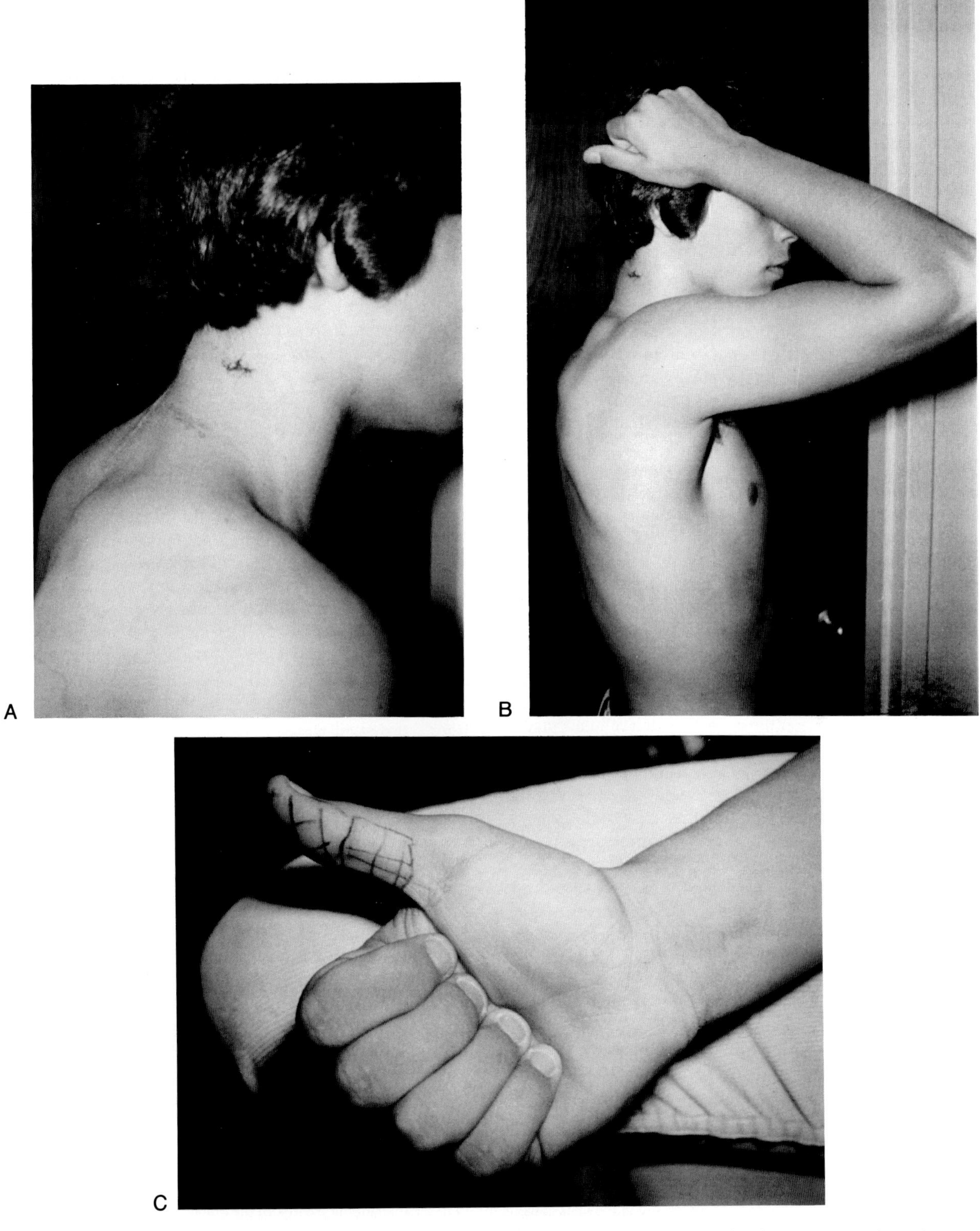

Fig. 42-1. **(A)** This man was referred as an emergency for exploration of a stab wound of his brachial plexus. **(B)** Manual muscle testing disclosed no abnormalities. **(C)** The sole neurologic (sensory) deficit is indicated by the crosshatching on the volar aspect of his thumb. Obviously, there was nothing that could be gained by exploration.

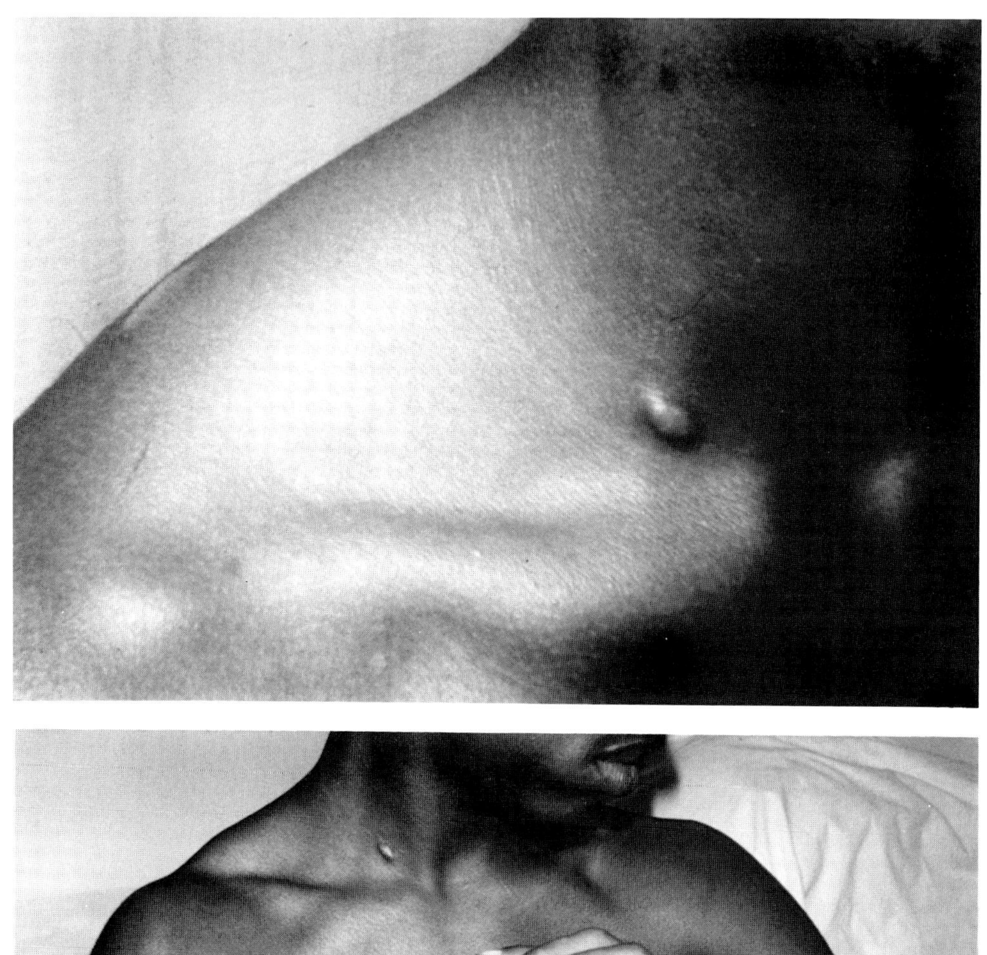

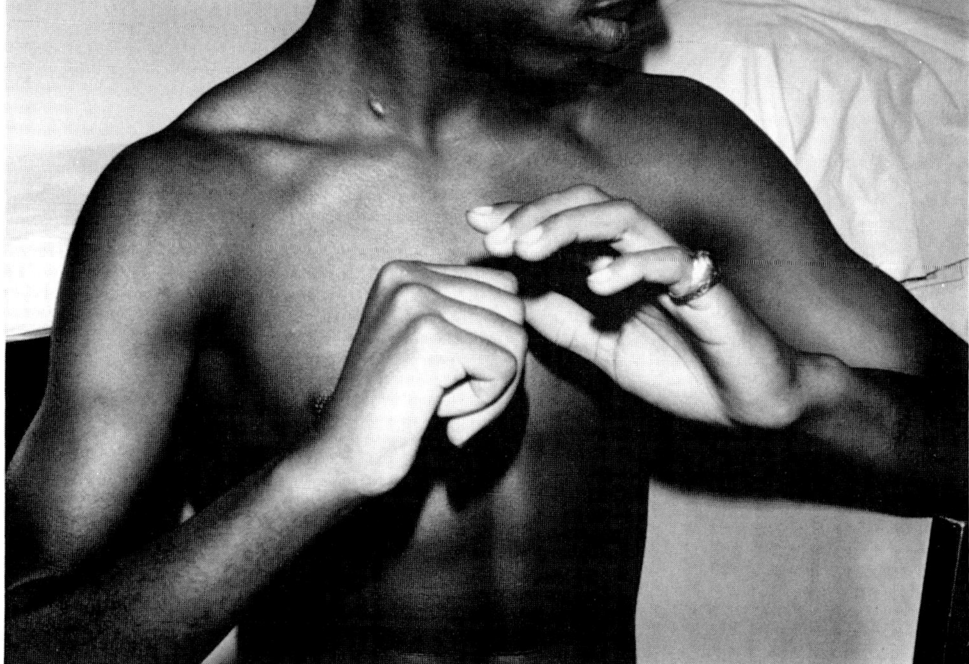

Fig. 42-2. **(A)** A .22-caliber gunshot wound of the neck causing injury to the intermediate trunk of the brachial plexus. **(B)** The functional deficit was paralysis of the finger extensors. *(Figure continues.)*

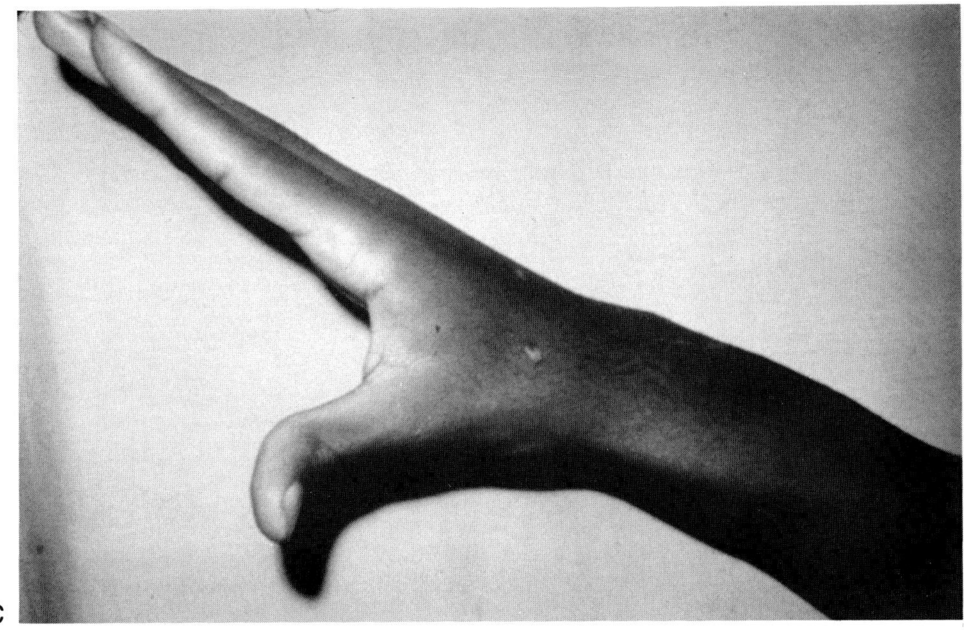

Fig. 42-2 *(Continued).* (C) The result following treatment by transfer of the flexor carpi ulnaris to the finger extensors.

anesthetic arm postoperatively. In these cases the injury was presumably due to excessive traction on the arm, which must be held away from the body in order to do the procedure. For patients with permanent lower trunk palsy, some function may be restored by means of tendon transfers in the hand.

Injury to the long thoracic nerve, resulting in paresis or paralysis of the serratus anterior muscle, is another potential nerve complication of first rib resection in the treatment of thoracic outlet syndrome.[181] The nerve runs just posterior to the middle scalene muscle, and after it crosses the second rib, it proceeds down over the lateral chest wall on the surface of the muscle. It may be divided by a rib shears at the level of first rib, or a traction injury may injure it as the middle scalene is elevated from the rib and retracted. The consequences of permanent serratus palsy are pain and weakness in forward elevation of the arm, and although improvement in function may be achieved by tendon transfer, this complication is best avoided if possible.

Closed Injuries

Supraclavicular Injuries

Most supraclavicular injuries result from falls from motorcycles or from motor vehicle accidents in which the head and shoulder are forcibly separated, causing a variable degree and distribution of stretch on the elements of the plexus.[16,23] Many combinations of injury are possible, depending on the position of the arm, shoulder, and neck at the time of impact[153] (Fig. 42-3). The result is a variety of clinical pictures of motor weakness and sensory loss. In adults these consequences may be generally classified as outlined in Table 42-1, with some allowance for variation in innervation.

Clinical evaluation must be directed toward determination not only of which root levels of the plexus have been damaged, but also whether root avulsion (supraganglionic) or distal rupture (infraganglionic) has occurred. Table 42-2 summarizes the clinical assessment of this aspect of the problem. This information is absolutely essential, since preganglionic or supraganglionic lesions are not directly repairable, although some limited function may be obtained by neurotization techniques,[3,17,56,108,121,122,171,173] which will be discussed below. Those lesions that occur more distally may be repairable, although the functional results of nerve repair and grafting are far from normal in most extensive injuries to the brachial plexus.

It should be categorically stated that all of the methods of evaluation used in the study of brachial plexus injuries are indirect in nature and none of them is totally reliable, although in combination they may achieve a high degree of predictive accuracy. Myelography and electromyography (EMG) are usually delayed for 1 month in patients with a totally flail, anesthetic limb. In the case of myelography done before then, intradural blood clots may obscure detail, and the pseudomeningoceles are not fully formed, although in a severe traction lesion, the dye may be seen to flow out of the spinal canal into the soft tissues of the axilla. EMG examination requires a minimum of 3 weeks for the development of the characteristic fibrillation potentials seen in the presence of denervation.

Patients who have Horner's syndrome, severe pain, fractures of the clavicle or cervical transverse processes, or winged scapulae generally have a poorer prognosis for recovery than those in whom these signs and symptoms are absent. The entity of scapulothoracic dissociation with brachial plexus injury has been recognized as an indicator of root avulsion in addition to vascular injury.[47,83,125] In this situation, a blunt injury to the shoulder girdle results in separation of the scapula from the rib

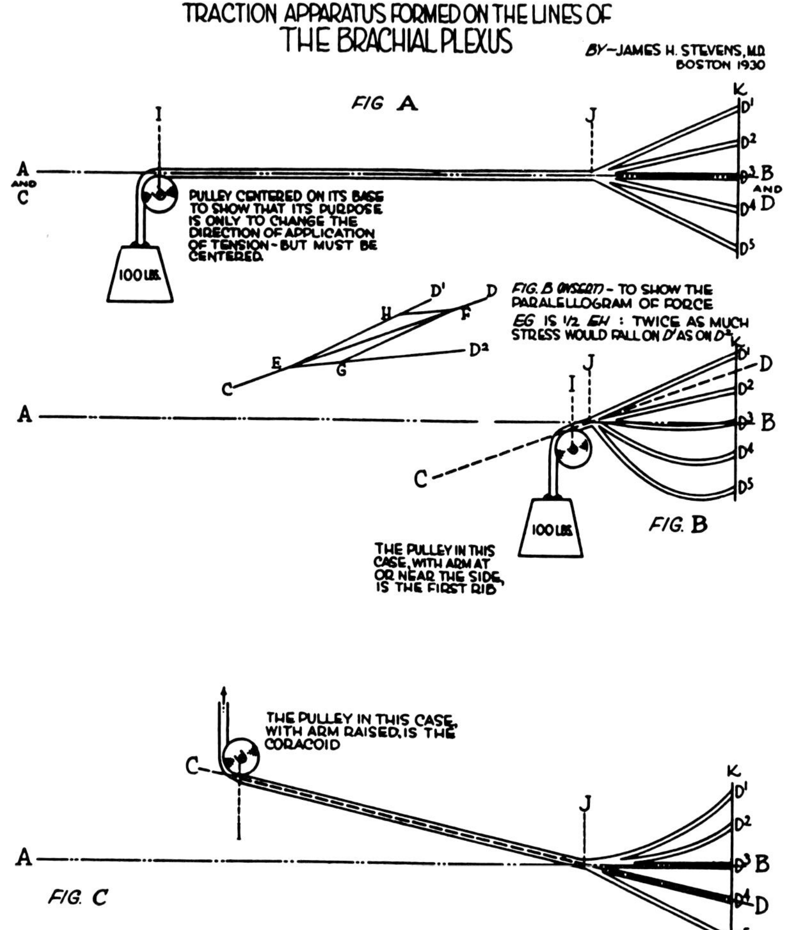

Fig. 42-3. Dr. James Stevens' illustration of traction forces on the brachial plexus. (From Stevens,[153] with permission.)

Table 42-1. Neurologic and Functional Consequences of Brachial Plexus Injury

Roots Involved	Muscles Affected	Functional Loss	Sensory Loss
C5, 6	Deltoid, supraspinatus and infraspinatus, biceps, brachialis, coracobrachialis, brachioradialis, (±) radial wrist extensors, clavicular pectoralis major	Shoulder lateral rotation, abduction and forward flexion, elbow flexion, (±) wrist extension	Thumb and index finger
C5, 6, 7	As above, plus triceps, ECRL and ECRB, FCR, EDC, EPL, EPB, APL	As above, plus elbow, wrist, finger and thumb extensors	As above, plus middle finger
C(7)–8, 1	(EDC, EPL) FDS, FDP, FPL, lumbricals and interossei, thenars and hypothenars	(Finger extension) Finger and thumb flexion, median and ulnar intrinsics	(Middle finger) Little and ring fingers
C5–T1	All of above	All of above	Anesthesia except for medial brachium

(±) = may or may not be present.

Table 42-2. Differentiation of Supra- and Infraganglionic Lesions of the Brachial Plexus

Evaluation Technique	Supraganglionic Lesion	Infraganglionic Lesion
Inspection	Flail arm, winged scapula, Horner's syndrome	Flail arm
Manual muscle testing	Paralysis of serratus anterior, rhomboids, (±) diaphragm, and limb musculature	Paralysis of limb musculature
Sensation	Absent in involved dermatome	Absent in involved dermatome
Tinel's sign	Absent	Present (unless supraganglionic lesions are present at the same level)
Myelography	Traumatic pseudomeningoceles, obliteration of root detail	Normal
EMG	Paravertebral muscle and limb muscle denervation	Limb muscle denervation
Nerve conduction	Motor conduction absent, (±) sensory conduction	Motor and sensory conduction absent
Axon response	Normal. Absent if infraganglionic lesion is present at the same level	Absent

(±) = may or may not be present.

cage. There may be concomitant dislocation of the sternoclavicular or acromioclavicular joints or a displaced fracture of the clavicle (Fig. 42-4). Although this is a rare lesion, it is potentially fatal if the unrecognized rupture of the subclavian artery causes exsanguination. In addition, the incidence of nerve root avulsion is extremely high, and the prognosis for functional recovery is dreadful.[47] An and his colleagues[14] have reported a case of open scapulothoracic dissociation in a child in which the neurovascular structures were intact,[14] but the four cases of closed injury that I have observed in adults have all had no neurologic recovery.

The finding of Horner's syndrome is presumptive evidence of avulsion of the first thoracic nerve root. This is particularly important in the preoperative evaluation of patients who have suffered avulsion injuries of their arms and who are being considered for replantation. Certainly, a patient who has sustained a significant avulsion of the nerve roots supplying such a limb would not be a reasonable candidate.

Although myelography cannot be regarded as absolutely reliable in the demonstration of the avulsion,[67,76] I believe that it still should be done in all cases where that possibility exists. This would include all patients with traction injuries wherein the total distribution of one or more nerve roots is nonfunctional. Large series of patients with brachial plexus injuries have been evaluated with myelography and the results of these studies have then been correlated with the findings at operation.[114,126,134] Although the accuracy of predictability of root avulsion is not the same at all roots, the general level of reliabil-

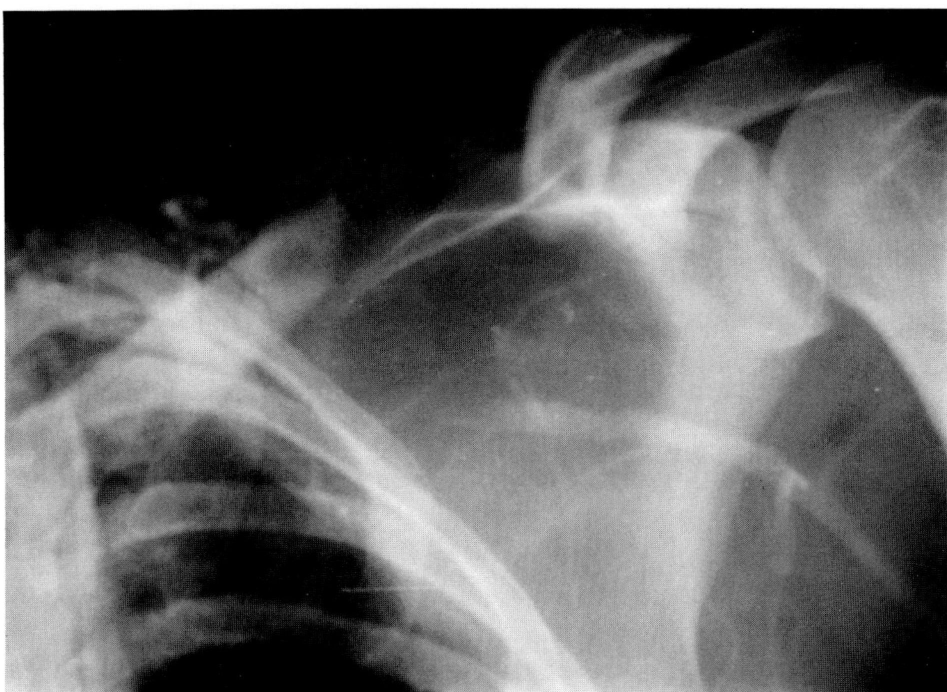

Fig. 42-4. Scapulothoracic dissociation with fracture of the clavicle and arterial transsection.

ity is extremely high, and can be further improved with the use of computed tomography (CT) following the dye study[102,134] (Fig. 42-5). This technique does not demonstrate the status of the extraspinal roots, however, and magnetic resonance imaging (MRI) has been used in an attempt to further refine the anatomic diagnosis.[59] My own limited experience with MRI in this situation has thus far been equivocal, although I believe that as the resolution improves, so will the accuracy and ease of interpretation.

EMG[32] should include needle examination of the posterior cervical musculature to help define root avulsions from distal ruptures of the nerve. As a practical matter, one need not spend long periods of time needling the totally paralyzed limb muscles of a patient with a flail-anesthetic arm, despite the fact that there is no pain associated with this part of the test. What is needed is the information obtained from examination of the cervical paravertebral muscles, serratus, and rhomboids, since these will reflect the status of the intradural nerves and help to define root avulsions. Therefore, it would be preferable to begin the EMG examination with this part of the study despite the fact that there will be discomfort, since if the patient decides to terminate the test thereafter, the important information will have been already obtained.

Sensory nerve action potentials and somatosensory-evoked potentials should be obtained in addition to motor nerve conduction velocity determinations,[25,78,158] since they improve the accuracy of the diagnosis considerably.

The use of intradermal histamine[24] to test axon responses for differentiation of root avulsion versus distal rupture has been discarded since interpretation of the technique may be extremely difficult and there is the potential for histamine allergic response.

Having established the nature of the lesion of the brachial plexus, the surgeon must then map out a treatment algorithm. Since the degree of injury will vary from minor to complete, the needs of the individual patient will vary greatly as well. In general, lesions of the upper trunk have the best prognosis for recovery, since they have the highest incidence of neurapraxias, and the more extensive lesions have the poorest prognosis.[16,24] Fortunately, the practice of "let's wait and see" has given way to aggressive attempts to define the lesion and treat it, since the window of opportunity for neurologic treatment is quite narrow, and most authors now feel that treatment in the first 6 months, if it is to be rendered at all, gives the best prognosis. The specifics of treatment will be discussed under their respective headings in the remainder of this chapter. However, thought must be given to the less spectacular but equally important nonoperative aspects of maintenance of joint mobility, skin integrity, and the psychological well-being of the individual.[95]

Infraclavicular and Subclavicular Injuries

Infraclavicular injuries of the brachial plexus may result from closed skeletal injury in the shoulder girdle, which injures the nerves by local compression or traction. Significant vascular injuries may accompany such fractures and dislocations.[58,156,170] Since the potential excursion of a dislocated humeral head or fragments of a fractured humerus is

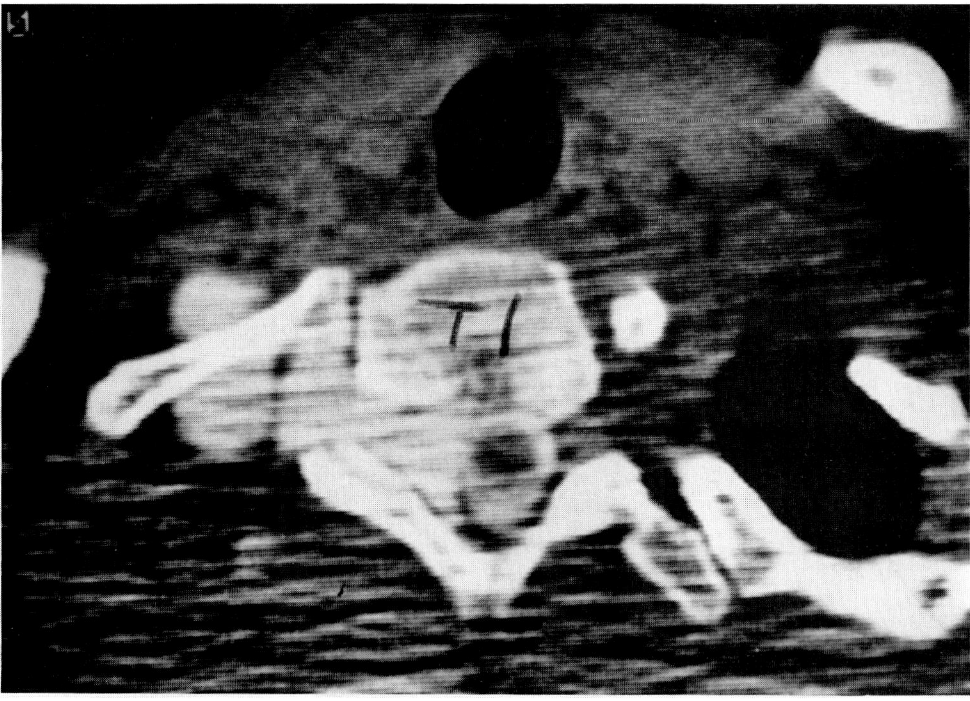

Fig. 42-5. CT myelogram showing pseudomeningocele indicating avulsion of T1 root. Note spinal cord deviation at this level.

considerably limited by soft tissue attachments, the extent of nerve damage is usually less than that found in supraclavicular injuries.[121] Unless there is actual tearing apart of the neural elements by sharp bone fragments or serious vascular injury, these injuries may often be managed conservatively with a good prognosis.[98] However, in patients in whom at 3 to 6 months there is no evidence of recovery from what is thought to be an infraclavicular injury, operative intervention is indicated because the prognosis for recovery of these patients is considerably improved by surgery.[34,121,172] If there is evidence of supraclavicular injury in addition to that below the clavicle, management will be determined by the former, more serious injury. In other words, extensive supraclavicular injuries may extend below the clavicle. In these cases, if surgery is done on the nerves, the infraclavicular plexus and its terminal branches will have to be thoroughly explored. Direct blunt injury to the infraclavicular portions of the plexus may occur in the absence of supraclavicular injury and may produce extensive localized scarring.[157] One of my patients incurred his injury when he ran into a moose on the highway while riding a motorcycle. He had a neurologic deficit localized to the infraclavicular plexus, but had not dislocated his shoulder or sustained any local fractures. Complete exploration of the plexus failed to demonstrate any lesion above the level of the clavicle although the scarring below was quite intense. This was a lesion-in-continuity, so an extensive neurolysis of the infraclavicular plexus was done. Unfortunately, the degree of recovery that he ultimately attained was insufficient to allow him to continue his career as a pianist, although he had adequate function for other activities of daily living. In general, infraclavicular and retroclavicular injuries of the brachial plexus have a considerably better prognosis than supraclavicular injuries.[9]

It should be reemphasized that fresh fractures of the clavicle usually cause extensive supraclavicular traction injuries to the plexus, because they allow even greater excursion than normal between the head and shoulder. Malunion and nonunion of clavicular fractures and those fractures that heal with excessive callus in the retroclavicular space can cause signs and symptoms either of brachial plexus compression or thoracic outlet syndrome, and may require either clavicular osteosynthesis,[80] excision, or resection of the first rib (Fig. 42-6).

Postoperative Brachial Plexus Palsy

Postanesthetic palsy results from injury to the brachial plexus while the patient is undergoing either general or regional anesthesia for the performance of a surgical procedure that is unrelated to the plexus. In the former case, its cause is the patient's position on the operating table and is not directly caused by the surgical manipulation.[75] It is typically due to traction on the plexus of an unconscious and therefore unguarded patient, and usually represents a first degree injury or neurapraxia. As such, the prognosis for recovery is excellent and is often substantially improved by 6 weeks postinjury. Literature reviews in case reports describing this entity usually report the findings in less than 11 cases.[41,44,48] Even patients who initially had total paralysis of the limb postoperatively recovered in less than 11 months. This injury may be prevented in most cases by careful attention to the position of the patient on the operating table, and avoidance of hyperabduction of the arms or excessive lateral flexion of the neck. Shoulder braces applied to the root of the neck of a patient in steep Trendelenberg position are also to be avoided. There are no indications for surgical exploration in these cases unless there is reason to believe that there has been a direct injury to nerves within the operative field.

The persistence of sensory symptoms in the upper limb following brachial plexus anesthetic block is rare[22] although it is possible to injure the nerves directly either by the use of long-bevel needles or repeated probing in order to elicit paresthesias.[145,146] In some cases, intraneural hematoma can result in long-term effects, but these are usually transient, and permanent damage is uncommon unless there has been significant local trauma from needles, contamination of solutions, or an underlying neuropathy.

Radiation Injury to the Brachial Plexus

Radiotherapy for breast cancer has been used with increasing frequency as a modality of treatment because of survival rates comparable with radical surgery in many cases. Although for many years it was considered that nerve tissue was radioresistant,[42] further study revealed that these assumptions were unwarranted.[65] An axonal effect of radiation on peripheral nerves has been demonstrated, ranging from swelling and hyperemia of the nerve to actual degeneration and Schwann cell proliferation.[20] Later effects, which are angiomesenchymal, result in changes in the vasa nervorum, and ultimately obliterate the blood vessels and produce progressive scarring, with ultimate disappearance of the neural elements[186] (Fig.42-7A and B). This is clinically expressed in patients who have had radiation as pain and paresthesias, with ultimate progressive loss of neurologic function. Unfortunately, for patients who have had a near-by malignancy such as breast cancer, the clinician may be hard-pressed to define whether the deficit is due to the effects of radiation or recurrent tumor.[63,92,155,168] Although pain may be found in both groups of patients, it tends to be more severe in patients with malignant plexopathy. The distribution of weakness is not a reliable indicator of the differential diagnosis,[63] although generalized involvement of the plexus seems more common in the radiation group, and lower trunk lesions less common.[112] The presence of a Horner's syndrome is more consistent with neoplastic infiltration than radiation neuropathy.[89,92] Electrodiagnostic findings thought to be specific to patients with radiation neuropathy have been described.[91] Some patients have experienced symptoms immediately following their radiotherapy,[112] while in some clinical series the latent period between the treatment and the onset of the symptoms has been identical with that for patients who have had a recurrence of their tumors.[168] Since the natural history of both radiation neuropathy and neoplastic brachial plexopathy is a progressive loss of neurologic function in most cases, in addition to the question of establishment of the diagnosis, there is the challenge of therapy. The use of CT scanning often may be of value in defining those patients who have tumor, but this is not invariably so, and some of these patients will have to un-

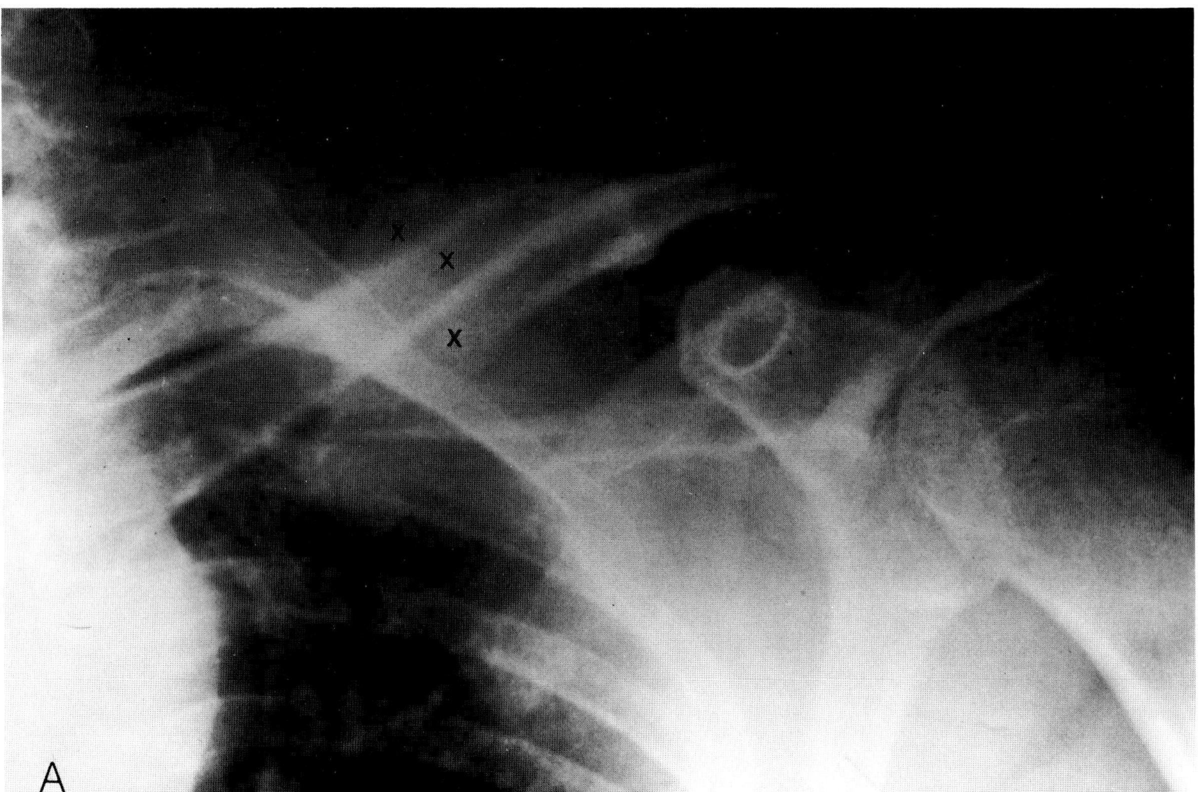

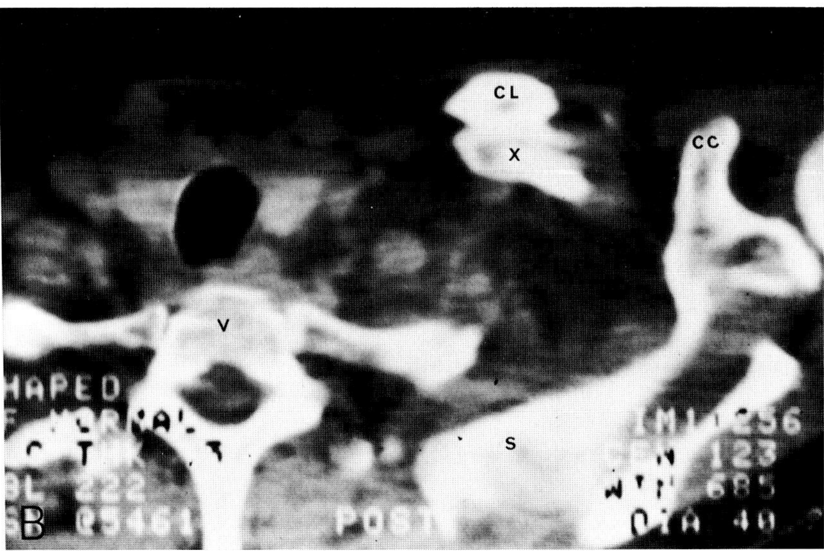

Fig. 42-6. **(A)** Radiographs of the left clavicle of a 42-year-old man 4 months after he sustained a closed midshaft fracture of the clavicle, which was treated with a figure-of-eight harness. He returned to work as a dentist within 2 weeks of his fracture and was asymptomatic until 4 months later when, within a 4-day period, he developed an upper trunk palsy. Note the large amount of callus at the fracture site (indicated by the *X's* above, below and behind the clavicle). **(B)** CT scan of same area. (*V*, vertebral body; *S*, scapula; *CC*, coracoid; *CL*, clavicle; *X*, callus impinging on the brachial plexus.) *(Figure continues.)*

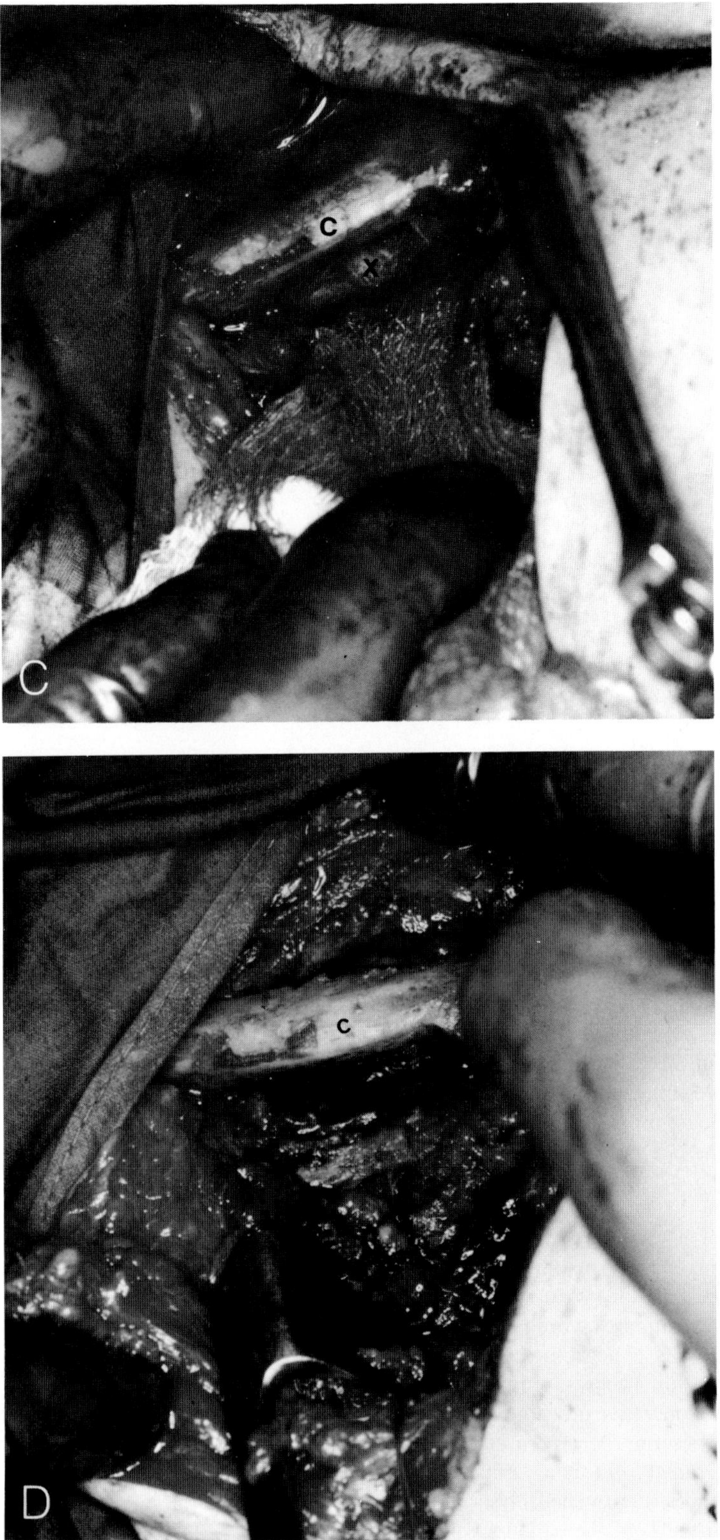

Fig. 42-6 *(Continued).* **(C)** Operative photograph showing the clavicle *(C)* and excess callus *(X)*. **(D)** The subclavian vein has been dissected off the callus, the brachial plexus has been identified and retracted, and the excess bone has been carefully excised from the clavicle *(C)*. Neurologic function returned to normal within 3 weeks of surgery.

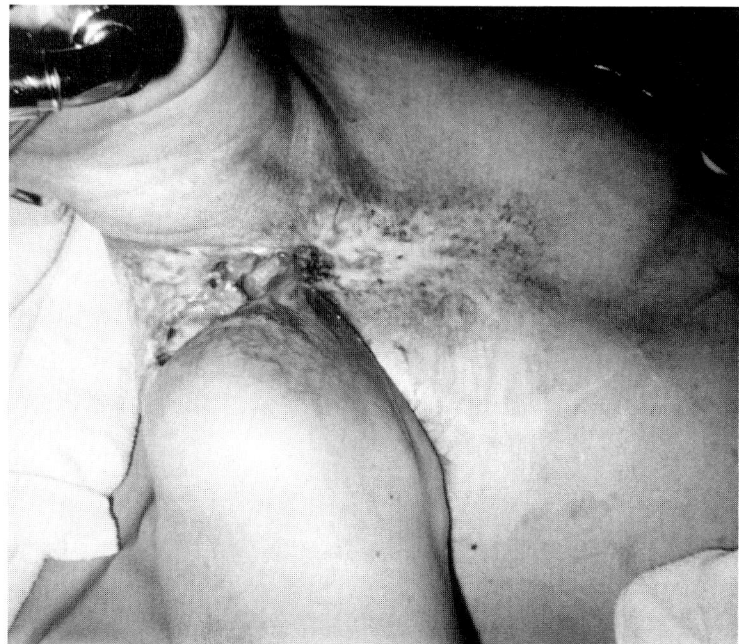
A

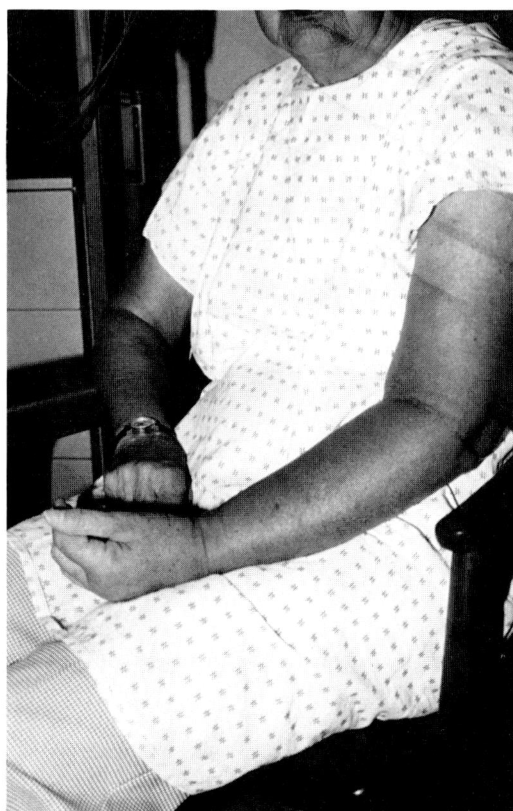
B

Fig. 42-7. **(A)** Radiation burns of skin, bone, and underlying plexus such as this are not seen today with improved therapeutic radiation techniques. **(B)** Marked edema and neurologic loss from radiation for breast cancer. This patient had no superficial skin burns, although the deep tissues of the axilla were indurated.

dergo complete exploration of the plexus in order to settle the issue.[38,175] It should be emphasized that limited explorations are not only inadequate for complete diagnosis, but may be very dangerous, because of the possibility of increased risk of hemorrhage from vessels that have been damaged by radiation.

The treatment of patients presumed to have radiation neuropathy and who are experiencing progression of their symptoms and signs is one that has not been resolved. Unfortunately, there are significant hazards for such operative procedures, as documented by Match.[104] Reports by Brunelli,[30] Ulschmid et al,[174] and LeQuang[99] have described the results of neurolysis accompanied by transplantation of omentum in an attempt to revascularize the plexus damaged by radiation fibrosis. The reported results are favorable with reference to pain and, in occasional cases, to neurologic function as well. Often, the improvement in function was temporary. Because of the hazardous nature of operative procedures in these patients, indications for neurolysis must be very carefully considered. Killer and Hess[86] concluded from their study that radiation plexopathy, with or without surgery (neurolysis and/or omentum transplant), left two-thirds of the patients with severe or total paresis of the arm. However, six of eight of the surgically treated patients, both immediately and in follow-up, seemed to be relieved of their pain. My personal experience has been limited to three cases of neurolysis without free omental grafts, and in these patients, pain relief was temporary and the neurologic deficit was not improved. Obviously, if the entity of radiation-induced brachial plexopathy could be prevented, that would be the best solution, and since its incidence seems to be dose-related,[155] it may well be that this may be an important factor in reducing its incidence. It has been suggested by Powell, Cook, and Parsons[130] that radiation using large doses per fraction is less well tolerated by the brachial plexus than small doses per fraction.*

TECHNIQUE OF OPERATIVE TREATMENT OF THE BRACHIAL PLEXUS

General Considerations and Equipment

Surgeons who treat injuries of the brachial plexus must be prepared to confront the pathologic complexities of the area with a full knowledge of the relevant anatomy. Although numerous treatises on the subject are available for review,[70,72,84,153] it is also mandatory that experience be gained in the anatomy laboratory prior to an actual surgical approach in

* "Doses per fraction" refers to how much of the total treatment dosage is given at each session.

a patient, since it is to be expected that the anatomy will be distorted by the effects of trauma.

The patient's general condition must be adequate to tolerate up to 8 to 10 hours of general anesthesia in the supine, semisitting position. An indwelling urinary catheter should be inserted after the induction of anesthesia and intravenous antibiotics are administered.

Prepping and draping must allow extensile exposure from the neck into the shoulder girdle, chest and arm, as well as access to both legs, should nerve grafts be required. Pneumatic tourniquets are applied to the thighs but are left uninflated until they are needed. The harvesting of sural nerves is clumsy with the patient in this position, and one is tempted to begin the operative procedure by turning the patient to the prone position to facilitate access to the posterior leg, rather than to have to hold it up while harvesting the cutaneous nerves. However, this labor-saving maneuver runs the risk of encountering an unfavorable amount of scarring in the plexus or lack of axons for grafting so that the cutaneous nerves would have been needlessly sacrificed.

An anesthetic technique without total motor paralysis that will allow the use of electrophysiologic monitoring is mandatory. The techniques of somatosensory-evoked potentials are an indispensable aid in the intraoperative evaluation of lesions of the brachial plexus.[78,88,101,154,158] As has been previously stated, although preoperative myelography and electrodiagnostic studies are helpful, they are not infallible, nor is the ability of the surgeon, either by gross inspection or with the use of the operative microscope, to define whether a proximal stump of the nerve is capable of regeneration and whether it retains its central connections. The use of this electrophysiologic equipment requires trained personnel who can work with the surgeon during the course of the procedure. The study of the nerve action potentials in the more distal parts of the plexus can also be extremely valuable.[87]

Blood must be available for use in the event of inadvertent injury to large vessels in the field. Personnel adequate in number and training should be present, depending on local custom and practice. It does not matter what surgical specialties, or combinations thereof, are represented in the operating team, as long as the surgeons are knowledgeable about the anatomic and technical problems that will have to be faced, and can assist or relieve each other to avoid fatigue. The use of either an operating microscope or loupes with magnification of 6× is suggested. Exactly which optical aids are used depends on the experience and preference of the operator. Because of the variable topography and size of the operative field, I use 3.5× and 6× loupes and a fiberoptic headlight for the gross dissection, reserving the operating microscope for the nerve suture if needed.

Surgical Approach

The incision used in most cases is shown in Figure 42-8A. It begins at the midpoint of the posterior border of the sternomastoid muscle and drops to the clavicle. If a strictly vertical incision is used, there is greater danger of producing a hypertrophic scar. This can be minimized by making the incision more obliquely than vertically oriented, and carrying it more medially before curving horizontally beneath the level of the clavicle. It then continues laterally one finger breadth below the clavicle to enter the deltopectoral groove. From here it can be continued down into the arm as necessary (Fig. 42-8B). The platysma muscle is divided in line with the skin incision and preserved for layered closure at the end of the procedure. The external jugular vein will be encountered at this stage of the procedure, running vertically from its termination in the subclavian vein just posterior to the sternomastoid muscle. It is a good landmark for the location of the brachial plexus, which lies between the scalenes directly under it. It is wise to ligate and excise the vein to prevent annoying bleeding during the course of the procedure. The spinal accessory nerve lies relatively superficially on the fascial carpet in the apex of the wound, and it must be protected from harm. The transverse cervical artery and vein cross the plexus in the posterior triangle and must be ligated. The suprascapular vessels are located more inferiorly in the region of the clavicle and they, too, must be found and divided. The omohyoid muscle crosses the plexus obliquely and is divided but tagged for resuture after the nerves have been repaired. The plexus lies between the anterior and middle scalene muscles deep to the fascia, and although it is readily apparent in the dissecting room specimen, in the living patient with a traction injury there may be a solid wall of scarred muscle that makes the precise identification of individual nerves difficult. Fortunately, the phrenic nerve can usually be located by means of a stimulator probe where it crosses the anterior scalene from posterior to anterior as it proceeds distally. Contraction of the diaphragm on stimulation will allow the operator to trace the phrenic nerve upward and ultimately identify C5 and the upper trunk at the level of the intervertebral foramen. Even in the presence of intense scarring, it is usually possible to feel the transverse process of C5 and to better define the root at this level. Electrical stimulation, in addition to evoked potentials, is useful in demonstrating those elements of the plexus that are intact or potentially capable of spontaneous recovery. Therefore, the limb musculature should be palpable, and sterilely draped.

In situations where precise anatomic definition at the level of the roots and trunks is difficult, it is useful to temporarily suspend dissection in the supraclavicular fossa and proceed to the infraclavicular portion of the plexus. This area is readily identifiable by detachment of the pectoralis minor and as much of the pectoralis major from the clavicle as is necessary for exposure. The question of division of the clavicle is to be considered in terms of whether it is possible to gain exposure without osteotomy and the subsequent risk of nonunion. Because the necessary soft tissue dissection virtually skeletonizes the clavicle and its medullary blood supply is meager, the risk of nonunion is very real. The clavicle may be sufficiently raised off the vessels and nerves, usually by placing a bolster pillow beneath the scapula posteriorly, so that it is possible to work beneath it. Retraction on the clavicle and positioning the arm may further facilitate exposure (Fig. 42-9). However, the lower trunk and vessels are dealt with more easily if the clavicle is divided. In those cases where it is necessary, an osteotomy should be done and repair at the end of the procedure should be completed by means of a suitable compression plate.

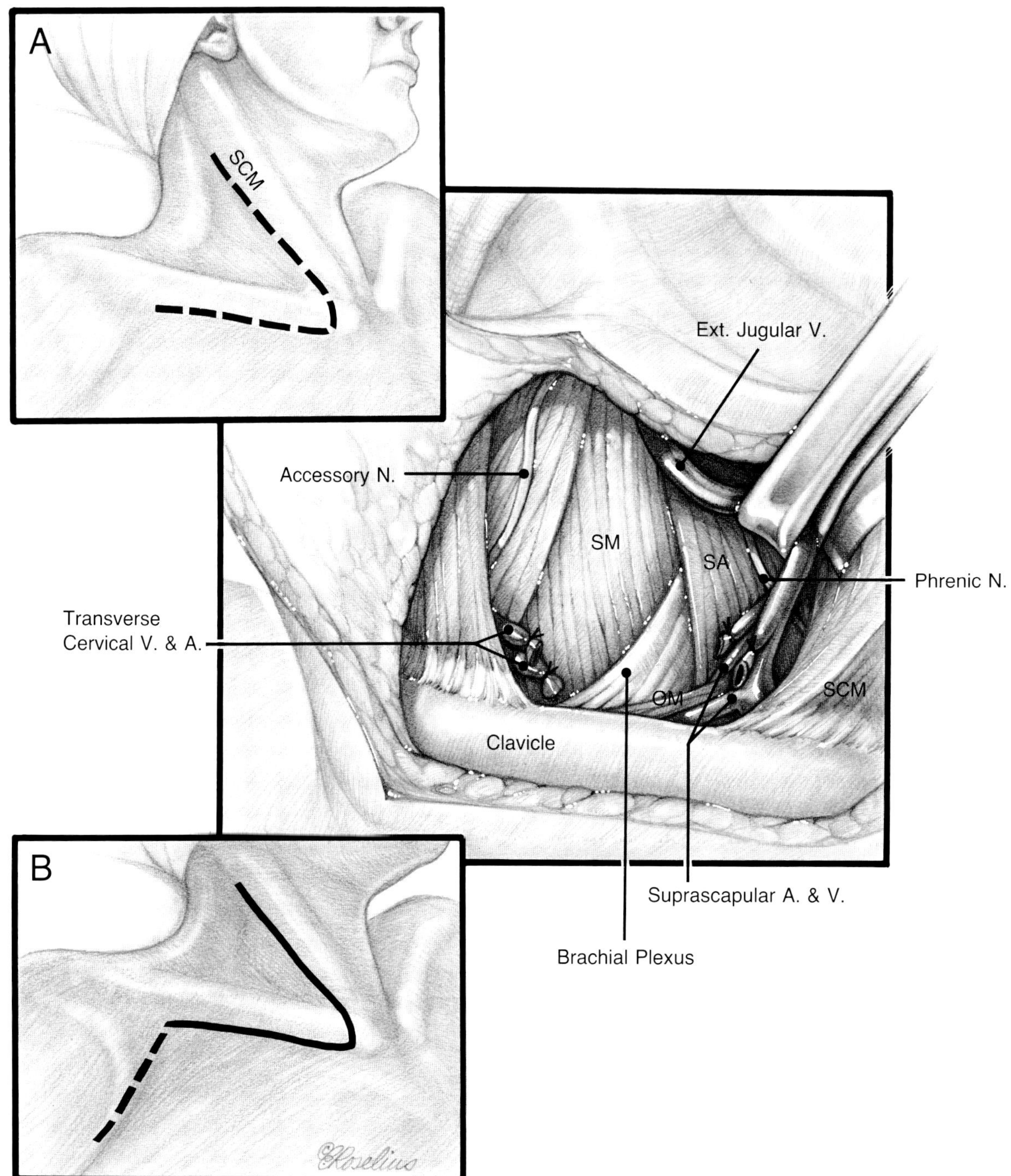

Fig. 42-8. The operative approach to the brachial plexus. The external jugular vein has been retracted rather than excised to show its relationship. Figure **B** shows the extension of the skin incision into the deltopectoral groove.

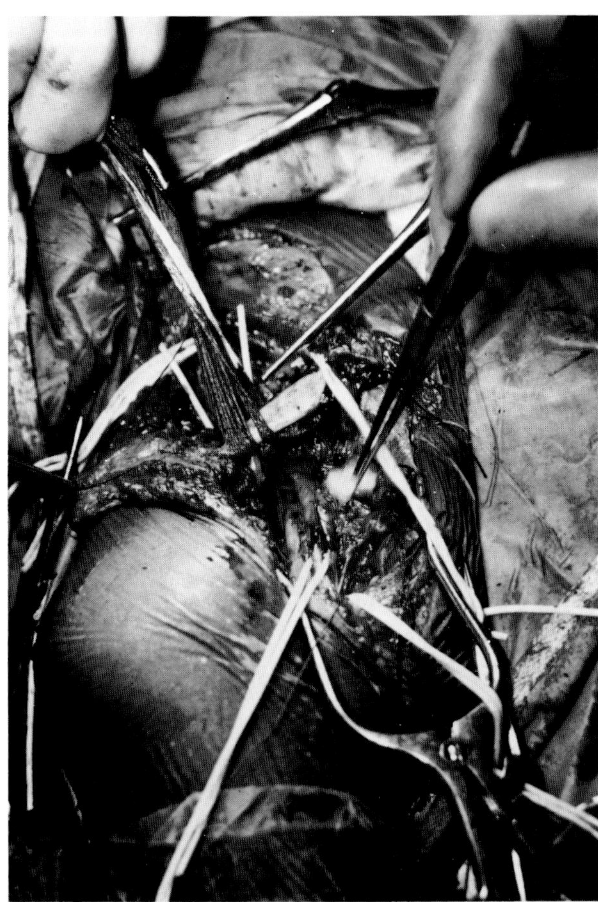

Fig. 42-9. The clavicle is being retracted for exposure. The patient's head is toward the top of the figure, and the neural elements are retracted with small silicone tubes.

Options and Specific Techniques in Neurologic Reconstruction of the Brachial Plexus

Once the elements of the injured plexus have been identified as completely as possible, the surgeon must formulate a plan that can be integrated with what has already been learned by preoperative assessment. In light of the fact that the surgical armamentarium has grown to include many innovative and potentially useful techniques for nerve reconstruction procedures, it is vital that prospective be maintained in the selection of the appropriate one for each individual patient. For the patient with a totally flail-anesthetic arm due to neurotmesis, anything that is recovered will have to come from rejoining nerves. Therefore, in this case nerve repair or grafting will be indispensable. The possibility of such procedures providing even very limited, yet useful, function has reduced the need for amputation of the arm considerably. The provision of alternate sources of axons by means of neurotization operations may make some function attainable even in patients who have suffered complete avulsion of all roots of the plexus. The question that should be asked in each case is what functional result can be anticipated as a consequence of the surgery that is planned, and what real difference will it make to the patient after all is done. Consideration should be given to what could be provided by other means of restoration or peripheral reconstruction using arthrodesis and tendon transfers. Despite the fact that sensibility can only be restored by reconstitution of the nerves, peripheral reconstructions in the hand are more predictable in their ultimate result than central repair of the nerves, and so these factors must be weighed for each case. Finally, if the source of axons for neural reconstruction involves a sacrifice of important function, such as that of the trapezius with use of the spinal accessory nerve in neurotization of the elbow flexors, in my opinion such surgery should not be done in most cases, although I must admit that this is a point of controversy.

Timing

The timing of operative intervention requires emphasis, since a delay of more than 6 months after injury will diminish the chances of functional recovery. It is therefore advantageous to explore these patients prior to that time, which also would minimize scarring and muscle atrophy. For the patient with a completely flail and anesthetic arm, neurologic reconstruction will make the most difference.

Neurolysis

Assuming there has been distal rupture rather than avulsion, the outflow of C5, C6, and C7, the upper and intermediate trunks, can be used as a source of axons for those patients in whom neurotmesis has been demonstrated. For those who are found to have scarring encompassing the neural elements, with neuroma-in-continuity, neurolysis is indicated, and herein the techniques of intraoperative electrophysiologic monitoring are important. For patients with partial lesions-in-continuity, there is a very definite risk of increasing the deficit, especially with internal neurolysis. Allieu and co-workers[5] have emphasized the danger of attempting neurolysis of the upper trunk in a patient who has regained elbow flexion without shoulder abduction, since there is a possibility of losing what has already been recovered. In their series of 14 neurolyses, there were only 2 cases in which recovery absolutely attributed to the neurolysis could be documented. Neurolysis can, in most cases, be external, but should be done with the aid of high magnification and electrophysiologic monitoring.

Nerve Grafting

Because of the nature of traction injuries, direct suture generally is impossible, and gaps must be overcome by means of intercalated grafts of autogenous nerve (Figs. 42-10, 42-11). The choice of donor nerves depends on individual requirements and what can be sacrificed. In the average adult, the sural nerves can yield as much as 35 cm from each leg, and the medial cutaneous nerve of the forearm may be taken in the arm. In cases where there has been documented avulsion of C8

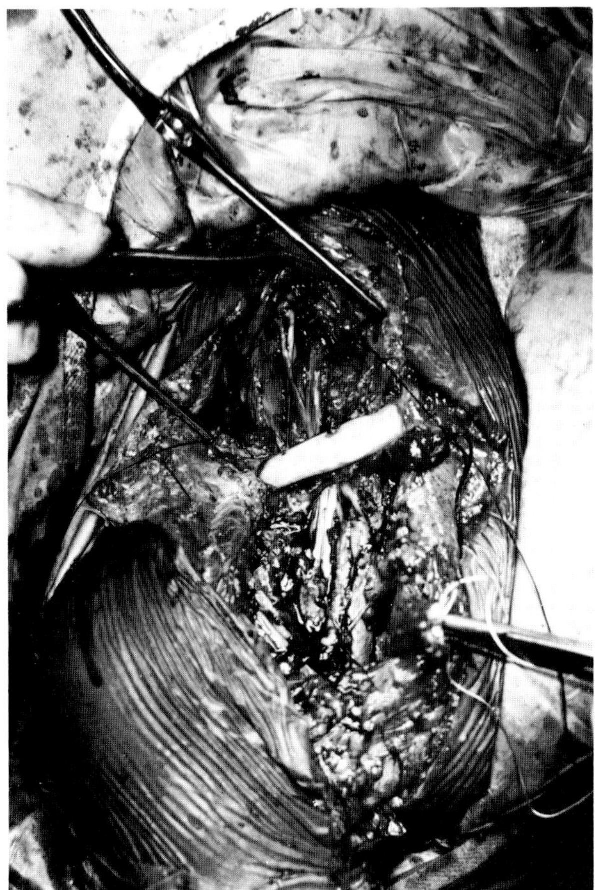

Fig. 42-10. Sural nerve grafts extend from the upper trunk, beneath the clavicle to the lateral cord. In this case, the intervening, scarred plexus was bypassed, not resected.

and T1, the main trunk ulnar nerve may be harvested and used as a graft, although it is usually wise to diminish the diameter of the nerve by stripping out the dorsal sensory branch. The rationale for this maneuver is the necessity for the newly placed graft to survive on the basis of perfusion of nutrients through tissue fluid until such time as a new blood supply can be established. A thick graft has the liability of undergoing central necrosis before this can be accomplished, while it is less likely in a thinner graft or one of multiple strands.

In addition to the usual problems of dealing with a scarred nerve, which require resection of all neuroma prior to grafting, there is a further difficulty found in proximal lesions of the brachial plexus that must be considered. With lesions at the level of the intervertebral foramina or within the scalene muscles, the retrograde effect on parent neurons may be so devastating that the cells may die and the axons disappear from the proximal stumps, making successful repair of any type impossible. This has been well documented by Narakas[119,120] in his consideration of muscle recovery as a function of where in the plexus the suture was done. When grafting is considered feasible and resection of scar from both ends of the neuroma has been accomplished, the length chosen for the grafts should be increased by 15 percent to allow for shrinkage. Usually 9-0 nylon suture is used. Plasma clot may be employed in grafting,[51,141,163] particularly in situations wherein multiple nerves must be reconstructed. This technique is usually combined with a minimal number of sutures to add tensile strength.

As much reconstruction as possible is done if there is adequate root stock, although the lower trunk is rarely successfully grafted in adults and function usually does not return. The results of plexus surgery in numerous large series have been well documented.[5,12,45,61,81,87,106-108,110,111,118-121,127,142,143] In general, the results of neurologic reconstruction by free grafting between the upper trunk and lateral cord or musculocutaneous nerve for restoration of elbow flexion have been that approximately 75 percent of patients regain flexion against gravity and moderate resistance; the strength and function of the best of these grafts is better than anything that can be produced by means of tendon transfer. Unless the outflow of the suprascapular nerve can be reconstituted, useful shoulder function is unlikely even if the deltoid can be recovered, because the absence of active lateral rotation deprives the shoul-

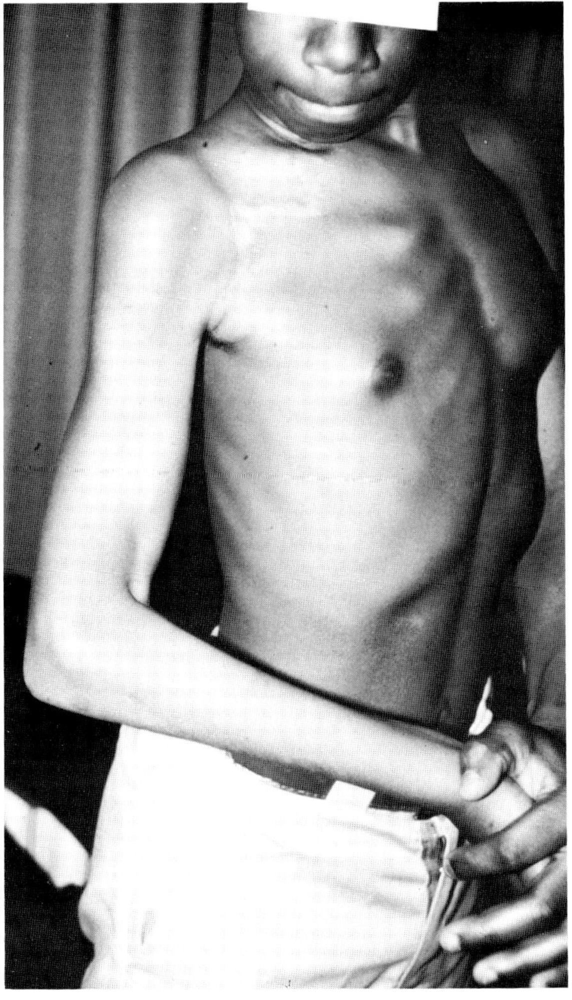

Fig. 42-11. The biceps is able to contract against strong resistance 18 months later.

der of good control and produces the functional equivalent to what might be experienced with a complete traumatic rupture of the rotator cuff. The prognosis for recovery of significant hand function is generally the least favorable and radial nerve function of intermediate character. Narakas stated in 1985 that neurologic reconstruction is worthwhile for about 15 percent of supraclavicular injuries.[121]

The report of the technique of free neurovascular grafting by Taylor and Ham in 1976[166] has generated significant interest in the application of this technique to the brachial plexus.[10,21] Sunderland[159] considers it a controversial procedure of considerable promise that may be applied to situations where a long graft is required and the bed is poorly vascularized or scarred.

For patients with partial function in whom motor control of the hand is intact, but with no good alternatives available for peripheral reconstruction because of paucity of potential motors, consideration should be given to neurologic reconstruction, using the outflow of C5 and C6 distal to the takeoff of the branches supplying the rhomboids and serratus anterior. This, of course, presupposes that there is distal rupture rather than avulsion. The potential for restoration of elbow flexion is favorable in these cases. However, one must weigh those potential gains against the loss of sensibility in the thumb and index finger, if it is intact prior to surgery. Such lesions do exist in partial injury to the upper trunk, and one must be careful not to disconnect the nerves if such is the case (Fig. 42-12A and B).

Neurotization

The question of neurotization is one that has appeal for the patient with a totally flail-anesthetic limb as a result of complete avulsion of the brachial plexus. In 1961 Yeoman and Seddon[183] successfully grafted intercostals 3 and 4 to the musculocutaneous nerve, using the ulnar nerve as a free graft from a forearm amputation specimen.

Following successful neurotization with intercostals, patients initially find that elbow flexion is synchronous with inspiration and may occur involuntarily with coughing or sneezing. However, it is possible to achieve independent action for voluntary elbow flexion. The accumulated experience of Japanese surgeons in this area has been most interesting and intense.[3,81,82,117,149,161,162,171,173] At an international meeting on brachial plexus injuries in Tokyo in 1990, I had the opportunity to personally examine ten of their patients. Three of them had had intercostal grafts to free muscle transfers of gracilis in situations where surgery had been delayed for more than 1 year postinjury. These patients had been operated upon for wrist extension, but secondarily could flex their elbows. The patients that I saw who had had neurotization for elbow flexion had strong elbow flexion, and although they did get a flicker of contraction of the muscles with deep cough, they were able to isolate elbow flexion from respiration. Other workers have contributed their valuable experience with these techniques.[3,45,46,50]

The other nerves that have been used for provision of axons for neurotization of a totally avulsed brachial plexus are the cervical plexus[29] and the spinal accessory nerve.[90] The latter has a significant disadvantage in that if function is lost to the trapezius, it cannot be replaced by any other means, and the possibility of abduction of a shoulder fusion would be impossible if that were an option. Allieu and Cenac reported in 1988[7] on 21 cases of neurotization using the spinal accessory nerve for multiple nerve root avulsions with total paralysis of the upper limb. Two-thirds of their patients achieved at least Grade 3 elbow flexion. They commented that these results are inferior to those obtainable when grafting is performed for distal ruptures of C5 or C6 and considered this neurotization as a second choice. Narakas and Hentz[122] reported an extensive experience for avulsion injuries with neurotization using the long thoracic nerve in 7 cases, the accessory nerve in 30 cases, intercostal nerves in 66 cases, and other nerve transfers within the plexus in 31 cases. They stated that it is possible to obtain good elbow flexion in more than one-half of patients, but only limited shoulder function and no useful finger function was obtained.

The use of the phrenic nerve as a source of axons has been reported upon favorably by Chinese surgeons.[57]

Sunderland has made the comment that because of the great variability in the formation of the brachial plexus and the manner of innervation of the muscles that it supplies, the results of neurotization should be critically examined in light of the possibility that some of the results attributed to neurotization procedures may be the result of spontaneous recovery of alternate pathways. He further advised against the use of the spinal accessory nerve as a donor of axons because of the ptosis of the scapula that is produced and the fact that rotary function of the scapula is lost as well.[159] The reader is referred to Chapter 32 for further discussion of microneural reconstruction techniques.

RECONSTRUCTION OF THE UPPER EXTREMITY IN PATIENTS WITH IRREPARABLE INJURIES

Timing

The timing of peripheral reconstruction, if it is employed, depends on determining that neurologic recovery for a particular muscle or group has plateaued suboptimally, is unlikely, or is impossible. This may be based on either time elapsed since injury or direct knowledge of the status of the nerves. In general, patients more than $1\frac{1}{2}$ years postinjury without evidence of recovery have reached the chronic state where no further recovery is anticipated unless nerve repair has been previously done. In such cases, it may take as long as 18 months postoperatively for recovery of active elbow flexion. For the shoulder, under any circumstances, failure to achieve significant voluntary control at 9 to 12 months usually indicates the permanence of the lesion.

As will no doubt be emphasized in other chapters pertaining to peripheral reconstruction, and particularly tendon transfer of the upper limb for whatever cause of paralysis, the prerequisites of joint mobility, adequate soft tissue cover, and absence of edema must be satisfied (see Chapter 38). In addition, the

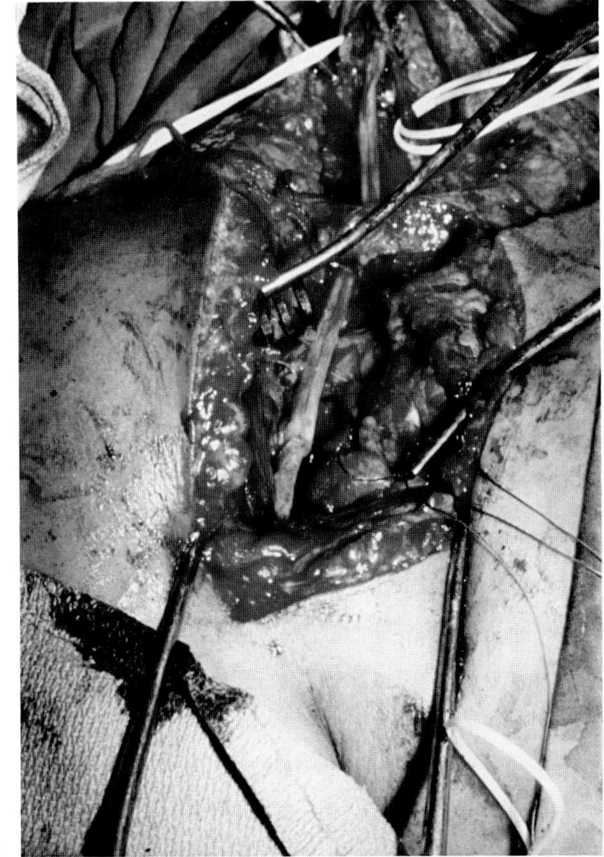

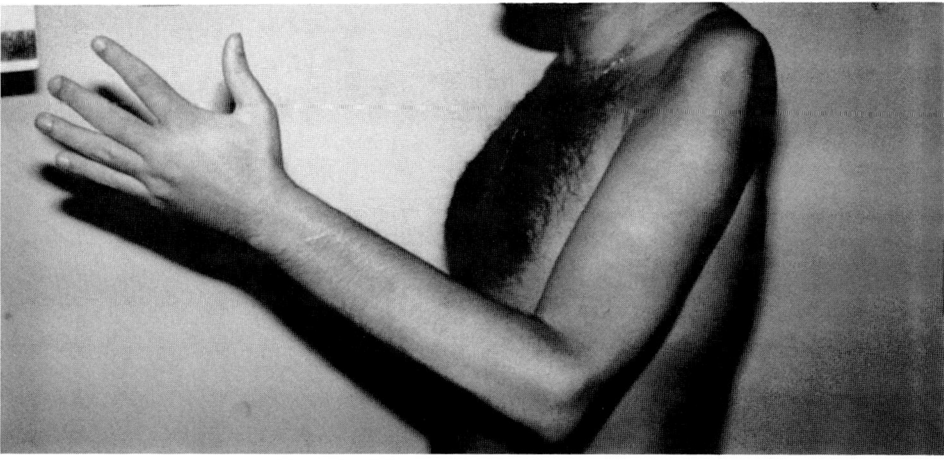

Fig. 42-12. (**A**) Operative exposure of the brachial plexus in a patient with a C5,6,7 traction lesion. There were no good potential motors for restoration of elbow flexion, and sensibility in the thumb and index finger was defective. Sural nerve grafts have been used to bridge the defect between the upper trunk and lateral cord. (**B**) The same patient following reinnervation of elbow flexors and return of protective sensibility to the hand. The shoulder has been fused and tendon transfers have been done for wrist, finger, and thumb extension.

donor muscle must be of adequate strength and amplitude of excursion. Of absolutely vital importance is the cooperation of the patient in whatever program is undertaken. This cannot be assumed under any circumstances, but particularly when there is lack of clarity on the part of any of the participants as to what the ultimate objectives of the program are and what will be required to attain them.

Shoulder Reconstruction

The mobility of the shoulder should be preserved if there is any possibility of providing muscular control by means of multiple tendon transfers.[137] Because of the complex nature of the kinesiology of the normal shoulder, in my opinion it would be naive to assume that all of the muscular functions involved in a motion such as abduction of the arm could be replaced by a single tendon transfer. Nevertheless, Aziz et al[15] reported successful treatment of 27 patients with brachial plexus injury by transfer of the trapezius to the proximal humerus. Preoperatively, all 27 shoulders were subluxated, with an average abduction of 3.5 degrees. Postoperatively, shoulder abduction averaged 45.4 degrees, and subluxation was abolished. All patients were said to be satisfied with their improvement in function. My interpretation of the results of this series would be to compare it with the results of arthrodesis of the shoulder, which corrects the subluxation and generally provides a better active range of motion at the price of having a fused shoulder. I have seen three patients who had had trapezius transfer for brachial plexus injuries. All had trivial active control that would not allow them to reach the horizontal and were seeking improvement in function. Unfortunately, because the trapezius had been interfered with by the unsuccessful transfer, they were not suitable candidates for fusion. It is for this reason that I have not done this transfer.

Since paralysis involves loss of muscles, these are not replaced in the course of tendon transfer; the remaining muscles are merely redistributed in a more efficient way to attempt to augment lost function. Therefore, strength will not be returned to normal, but hopefully, mobility and control of the limb will be enhanced by multiple transfers. In patients who have either suffered partial lesions or experienced partial recovery, it may be possible to use multiple adjacent muscles to augment shoulder control.[74] These procedures must be very carefully and individually planned and executed, as shown by Ober[124] and Harmon.[62] In partial paralysis, for example, if it is working, the posterior deltoid may be rotated anteriorly, and the long heads of the biceps and triceps may be advanced to the acromion with benefit. This maneuver will provide some control of elevation of the arm. Without lateral rotation control, however, the elevated limb will lack rotational stability. The L'Episcopo procedure,[91] in which the insertions of the latissimus dorsi and teres major are transposed posterolaterally to enhance active lateral rotation, is particularly useful in obstetric palsy. In the pediatric population, it is important to verify that the shoulder is not subluxated prior to the transfer.[68] The L'Episcopo procedure can be employed alone when indicated, or in combination with other transfers. Attachment of the transfer may be to bone or to the rotator cuff.[70] The results are significant improvement in function.[97]

For the patient with total loss of shoulder control or in whom transfers are not possible, arthrodesis of the glenohumeral joint is a potential salvage procedure. In order to have maximal control of the shoulder-arm complex, the patient must have preserved at least the function of the serratus anterior and the trapezius. If these scapular motors are deficient, it is preferable to allow the shoulder to remain flail, unless there is persistently painful inferior subluxation of the joint that cannot be controlled by means of an acceptable sling or other appliance.

Arthrodesis of the Shoulder

Over the years that I have been interested in arthrodesis of the shoulder, my preferences for the technique of fusion have evolved as advances in internal fixation have been achieved.[115,132,133,176,180] Historically, fusion of the shoulder was usually done for the control of tuberculous infection or the residua of poliomyelitis. As the former disease became less of a management problem because of antibiotics, the need for avoiding intraarticular fusion techniques disappeared. As polio receded in the industrialized countries of the world, the population of patients to whom fusion was applicable changed as well. Although the method of choice for the treatment of the arthridites has been the maintenance of mobility by means of arthroplasty, fusion is often indicated for the paralytic shoulder where no tendon transfer is practically possible, with the caveats that have been expressed below.

My preferred method for shoulder fusion at the present time is internal fixation with either rigid or pelvic reconstruction plates, using a posterior approach.[94] The patient is placed on the operating table in the lateral decubitus position. The incision extends parallel to and one finger breadth beneath the spine of the scapula. It then continues anterolaterally across the acromion and humeral head to the midlateral line, from which it goes distally along the shaft of the humerus for about 10 cm. Electrocautery is used to traverse the posterior musculature in layers. This method provides an excellent view of the glenohumeral joint and head, as well as the proximal lateral shaft of the humerus. During the entire procedure, the affected arm is supported by a padded bolster from a commercially available abduction splint, which holds it in the intended position for fusion. The shaft of the humerus and the scapula and its vertebral border are palpable within the field and serve as reference landmarks. The position I strive for is approximately 20 to 30 degrees glenohumeral abduction, 30 degrees forward flexion, and 30 to 40 degrees internal rotation, using the lateral aspect of the trunk and the humerus as landmarks.[136] This combination appears to provide the most useful and comfortable function for the fused shoulder.

The glenoid and humeral head are decorticated and shaped for a smooth fit without gaps, usually with broad osteotomes for a planar surface, and internal fixation is used in all cases. Three, four, or five 75- to 85-mm one-half or one-third threaded cancellous screws with washers are drilled through the head. They should penetrate into the relatively more dense subchondral bone of the neck of the glenoid. The acromion may be denuded of soft tissue, partially osteotomized, hinged down, and fixed to the humeral head with an additional screw to serve as an extraarticular site for fusion. A healed fusion is

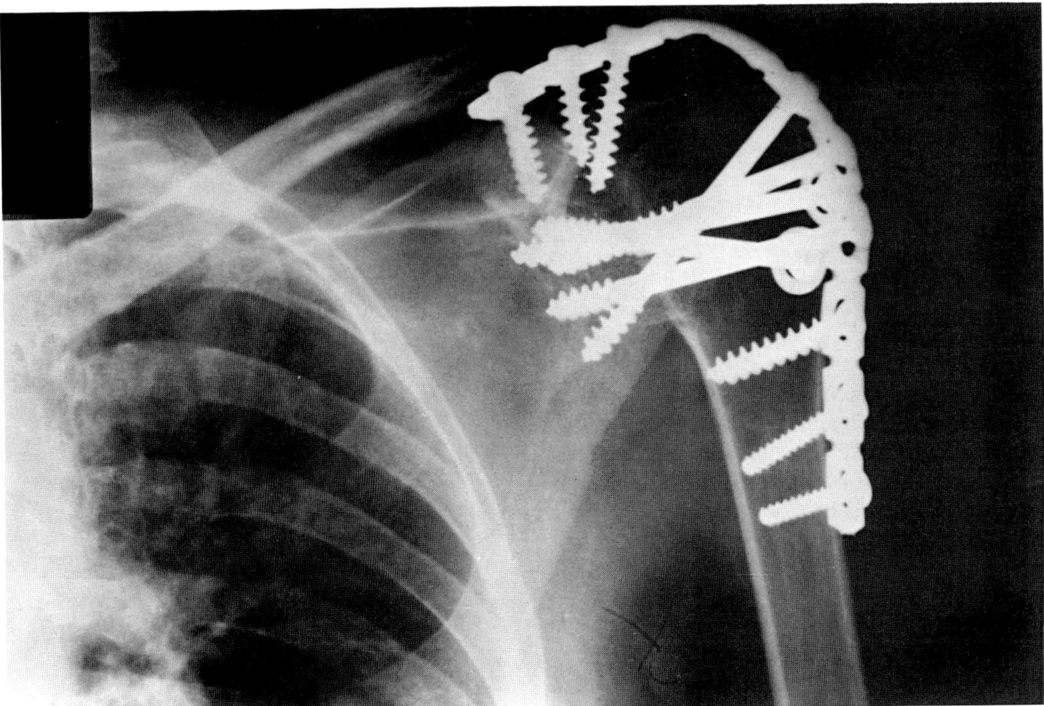

Fig. 42-13. Radiograph of a shoulder fusion using a pelvic reconstruction plate and multiple compression screws.

shown in Figure 42-13. Although one might dispense with it in a trustworthy patient, I employ a spica cast for the first 6 weeks. Since it is difficult to apply in an unconscious patient on the operating table, we defer its application until a few days postoperatively, when the patient can stand comfortably. In the interval, the commercially available bolster splint can be used to safeguard the fusion.

In general, if shoulder fusion is to be one of several staged reconstructive procedures, it should be done as the last operation, except when a pectoralis major transfer is planned to restore elbow flexion.

Restoration of Elbow Flexion

Although surgical reconstruction of the plexus can restore excellent elbow flexion, the predictability of peripheral reconstruction by means of tendon transfer without sacrifice of sensibility in the hand, if it is present, has maintained my preference for it in patients who have partial lesions. Although active control of extension is important, if there is a relative paucity of available motors, flexion is the more important function to regain. A number of useful alternatives are available, but a prerequisite to all methods is a functional arc of passive motion in the elbow.

Steindler Flexorplasty

The procedure that has been used most successfully in more paralytic elbows from any cause is the flexorplasty devised by Arthur Steindler in 1918.[151,152] The flexor-pronator muscles arising from the medial epicondyle are transposed to a more proximal point on the humerus so that their moment for elbow flexion is increased enough to permit active control. Although most patients can flex through a useful range against gravity, it is rare for them to be able to lift more than 5 pounds following such a transfer.[85] Nevertheless, it is a useful operation.[11,31,103] As with all potential candidates for tendon transfer, the preoperative evaluation of the strength of the proposed motors is critical to the success of Steindler flexorplasty or any of its variations. Since the muscles originating from the medial epicondyle of the humerus—the pronator teres, flexor carpi radialis, palmaris longus, flexor carpi ulnaris, and flexor digitorum superficialis—will now serve to flex the elbow in addition to their usual functions, they must have normal or near-normal power to achieve a meaningful result. Patients who already have weak elbow flexion or who can achieve flexion by the so-called Steindler effect preoperatively are most likely to have satisfactory results from surgery. The Steindler effect makes use of contraction of those muscles in a supplementary movement as follows: the patient may achieve elbow flexion by flexing wrist and fingers and pronating the forearm, usually while the arm is forward flexed to the horizontal to eliminate the effect of gravity. Since this is precisely the muscular activity that is enhanced by moving the origins more proximally, it may be used to identify those patients whose muscles are adequate for transfer. Although one may proceed in the absence of a demonstrable Steindler effect, the postoperative result is likely to be barely functional.

The modified technique that I prefer was described by Mayer and Green.[105] The incision (Fig. 42-14A) begins posterior to the medial epicondyle of the humerus and is then directed proximally and anteriorly for 7.5 cm over the distal

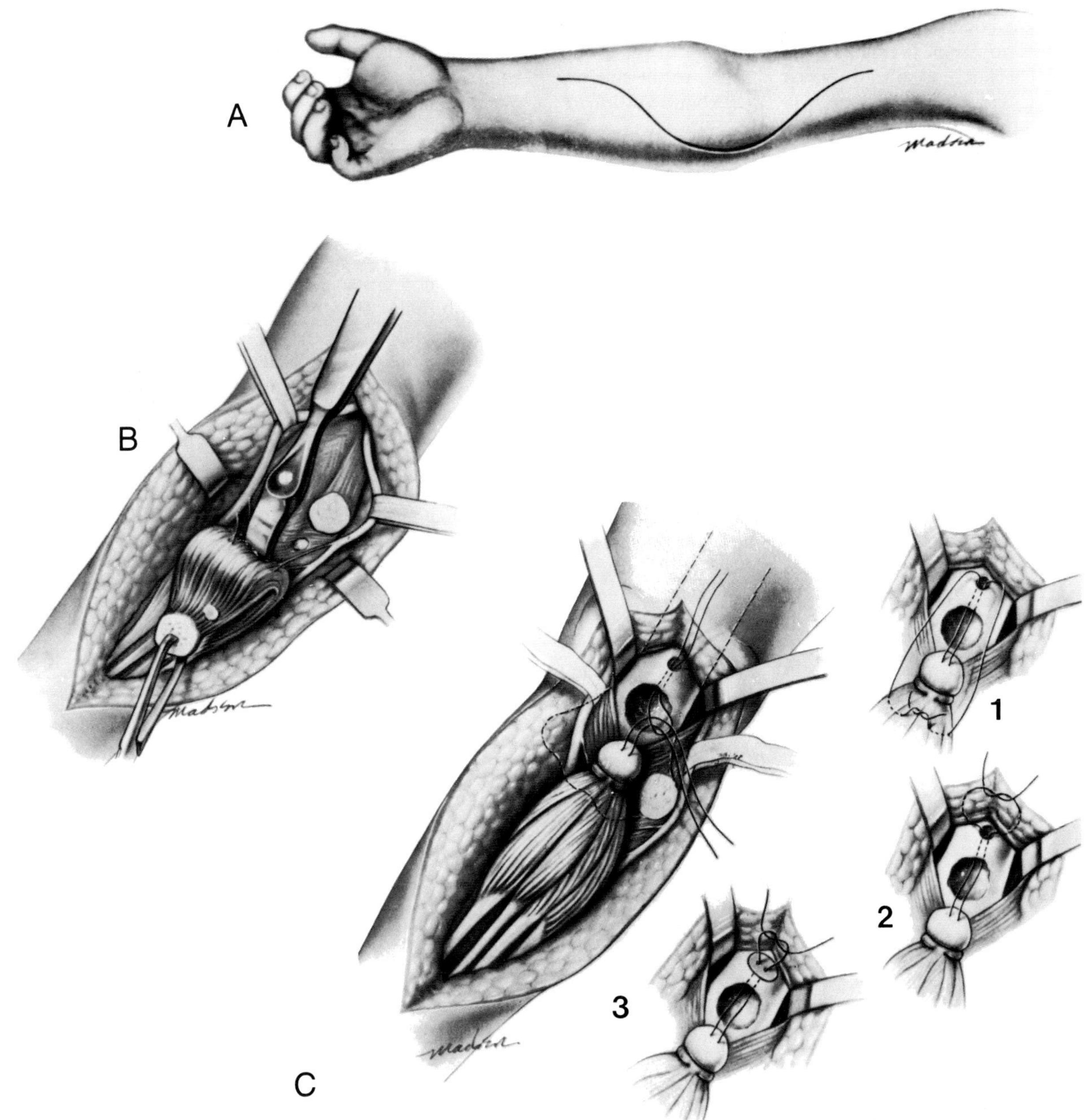

Fig. 42-14. **(A)** Steindler flexorplasty. The skin incision curves gently so that the humerus, the ulnar nerve at the elbow, and the muscles arising from the medial epicondyle are exposed. **(B)** The muscles are stripped from the anterior portion of the elbow joint capsule and ulna. Note the small capsular rent created by the stripping; it should be closed by fine nylon sutures. **(C)** Alternative methods of fixation. That shown in *3*, without the additional button, has proved most satisfactory. (From Mayer and Green,[105] with permission.)

brachium. The incision curves distally over the anterior forearm for 10 cm following the outline of the pronator teres muscle. The skin flap thus formed is retracted gently with the full thickness of subcutaneous tissue, and the incision is then undermined posteriorly to identify the ulnar nerve, which is mobilized from behind the elbow. The articular branch must be sacrificed, but the branches to the flexor carpi ulnaris are preserved and protected as the nerve is mobilized for about 5 cm distal to the elbow. The median nerve is then identified after the fascia over the pronator teres has been incised. The branch of the median nerve to the pronator is usually found on the medial side of the median nerve, 2.5 to 5 cm proximal to the elbow, and it too must be preserved as the nerve is mobilized. The common origin of the pronator and wrist flexor muscles is dissected from above downward and then detached with a fragment of bone from the medial epicondyle using an osteotome (usually 0.5 to 0.75 cm of bone is sufficient) and the muscles are gently retracted while their nerve supply is protected from injury (Fig. 42-14B). Distal stripping of the muscles is continued until, with the elbow acute flexed to 130 degrees, the bone fragment and muscle origin have been advanced 5 to 7 cm proximally. Although in the original Steindler technique the transfer was attached to the medial intermuscular septum and fascia, Mayer used bony fixation to the anterior aspect of the humerus.

The reasons given for this type of attachment are twofold: (1) the attachment to bone is stronger than to fascia; and (2) the more lateral the insertion, the less the pronator effect of the muscles. The original technique had a significant drawback, since with the increased tension on the pronator teres, flexion was usually accompanied by marked pronation of the forearm, a functionally compromised attitude for hand function.

Alternative methods of attachment of the bone and muscle pedicle are shown in Figure 42-14C. The median nerve and brachial artery are retracted gently, and the brachialis is incised so that the humerus can be prepared for receipt of the transfer. I usually use a #5 synthetic suture to ensure retention against the humeral shaft during healing. The distal portion of the wound is closed before the pedicle is secured in its new site and after the tourniquet has been removed and hemostasis has been achieved. The suture of the pedicle to the humerus and soft tissue is then accomplished with the elbow flexed 130 degrees and the forearm supinated. The proximal portion of the wound is then closed and the dressing applied. A posterior plaster splint maintains this position for 4 weeks. Postoperative rehabilitation and muscle reeducation take several months, and no attempt should be made to overcome the last 30 degrees of elbow flexion contracture, since the mechanical advantage in initiation of flexion from a partially flexed position would be lost. For further discussion of this procedure, I would recommend the articles by Segal, Seddon, and Brooks[144] and Kettlekamp and Larson.[85]

Pectoralis Major Transfer

In 1945, Clark[40] devised an ingenious transfer of the sternocostal portion of the pectoralis major muscle for restoration of elbow flexion. This single case report was of a patient who had lost the anterior brachial musculature due to gas gangrene; he had a normal shoulder. The procedure was then adopted for use in patients with paralysis due to either polio or brachial plexus injuries. Many of them had flail shoulders. Consequently, the procedure has not been as popular as it should be because of failure to appreciate several technical points.

The shoulder must either be strong or fused, since with a flail shoulder the power and excursion of the transfer will dissipate in shrugging, adduction, and medial rotation of the humerus, rather than in elbow flexion. The muscle pedicle must be carefully elevated from the chest wall with its nerve and major vessels intact and then routed subcutaneously down the arm to be inserted into the biceps tendon at the elbow (Fig. 42-15). In order to reach the antecubital fossa, the muscle should preserve the fascia from the rectus sheath attached to it so that this tissue, rather than the muscle, is used for the suture. As in the Steindler flexorplasty, the elbow is immobilized in acute flexion by means of a posterior plaster splint with a sling added for 4 weeks. Furthermore, the postoperative power of flexion is

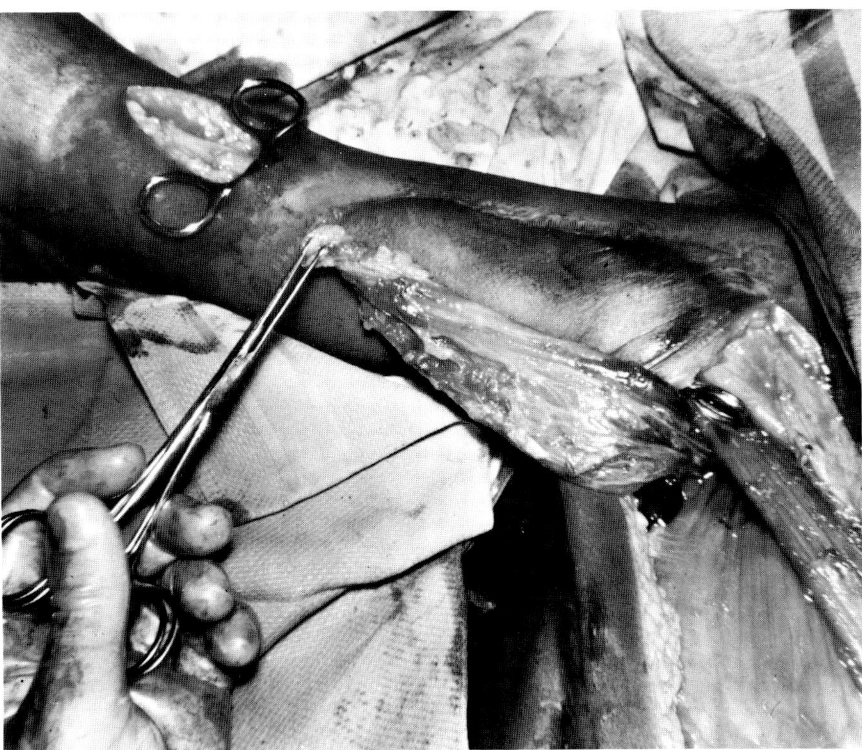

Fig. 42-15. Pectoralis major transfer. The pedicle of pectoralis major, with the nerve and vessels preserved, has been allowed to retract. At resting length, and including the rectus fascia, it just reaches the biceps tendon with the arm adducted.

enhanced if there is some preoperative function and if the arm can be flexed forward to eliminate gravity. In my experience, the functional results of Clark's transfer (Fig. 42-16) have been superior to those of the Steindler operation, so that I reserve the latter procedure for those patients in whom a pectoral transfer is less desirable or impossible. Although the vast majority of my patients with brachial plexus palsy are men, an occasional woman presents with this problem. Thus far, because of the large pectoral incision, I have not done the procedure in a woman. Schottstaedt, Larsen, and Bost,[138] D'Aubigne, Benassy, and Ramadieu[43] and Carroll and Kleinman[36] have proposed modifications of the basic technique aimed at improving the line of pull of the transfer. The Brooks-Seddon pectoral transfer,[28] in which a surgically devascularized biceps brachii is used as the tendon, has not achieved popularity.

Latissimus Dorsi Transfer

As an alternative to the above procedures, the latissimus dorsi, when it is available, may be transferred to the arm as either a replacement for elbow flexion or, less commonly, extension. First proposed by Schottstaedt, Larsen and Bost in 1955,[138] it has also been described in clinical cases by Hovnaninan[73] and Zancolli and Mitre.[185] These authors have reported excellent results. The problem that is often encountered with the use of the latissimus is that it shares the common innervation, C5, 6, 7, with the elbow flexors that are being reinforced, and so it is often not available. Moneim and Omer[113] reported on five brachial plexus injury patients with a latissimus dorsi muscle transfer to restore elbow flexion. The postoperative range of motion and flexion strength were very limited, and evaluation of activities of daily living by a standardized test revealed disappointing results. The authors concluded that this procedure should not be done unless the latissimus dorsi muscle is normal preoperatively. Unfortunately, it rarely is in these patients.

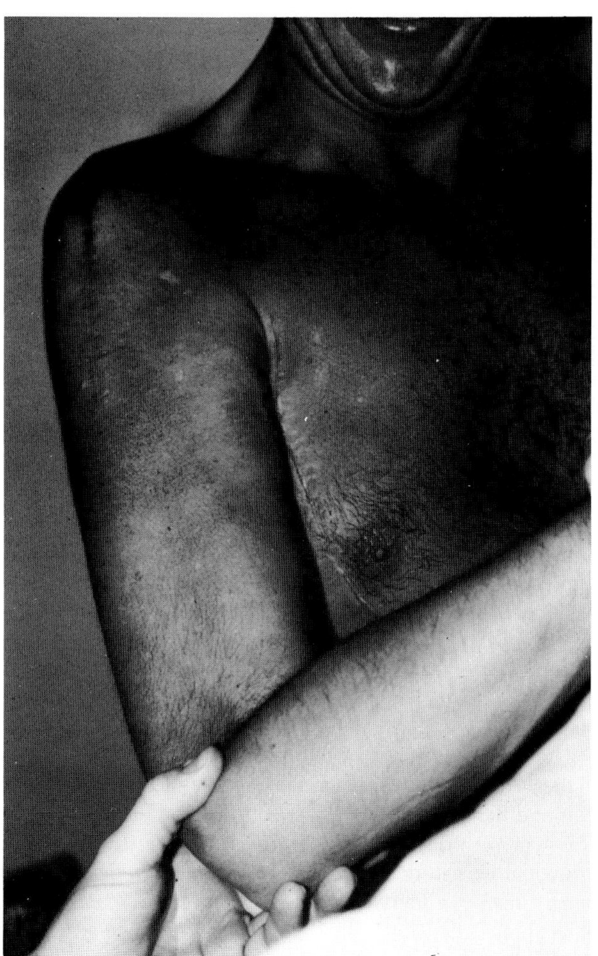

Fig. 42-16. Postoperative appearance of a patient with a Clark's pectoral transfer. Note the bulk of the muscle, which has the ability to support 4.5 kg with comfort.

Triceps Transfer

The triceps transfer, first described by Bunnell[33] and then modified by Carroll and Hill,[35] has been the subject of much controversy and often heated debate. In a patient who has an intact triceps but lacks active elbow flexion, the triceps may be brought forward and attached to the biceps tendon to regain flexion. The entire muscle must be mobilized and detached distally, and, as Carroll has shown, if a tongue of ulnar periosteum is elevated along with muscle, the need for an intercalated fascial graft to the biceps tendon is obviated (Fig. 42-17). There has been little difficulty in achieving postoperative phase conversation[96] and the power and excursion of the transfer are satisfactory.[97] What makes this transfer non grata to many surgeons contemplating reconstruction for elbow flexion is the loss of what they consider the "all-important" triceps. Several of the objections hark back to the polio patients for whom the operation was originally done. Many of these patients had bilateral disease and many walked with crutches. Loss of triceps power in these patients could seriously impair their getting out of chairs or crutch walking. However, the usual patient with a brachial plexus injury has neither of these significant problems. The serious negative factors that remain are as follows: (1) the lack of triceps precludes working with the arm in front of the body or at the horizontal or using the arm as a stabilizer; and (2) although elbow extension can obviously be achieved by the effect of gravity, the smooth action of elbow flexion is materially aided by the presence of an active antagonist; this will, in addition, offset the annoying tendency to otherwise develop a contracture of the unopposed transfer.

Sternocleidomastoid Transfer

The use of the sternocleidomastoid for elbow flexion was first described by Bunnell.[33] Although it can produce excellent elbow flexion, it has the disadvantage of causing an unsightly web in the neck, and occasionally, grotesque manipulations of the face and neck to activate the transfer. These reasons have been sufficient for many surgeons to avoid doing this transfer. I have had the opportunity to observe several cases done by Carroll, and their strength was quite good. Most reconstructive surgeons today regard the procedure as mainly of historic interest.

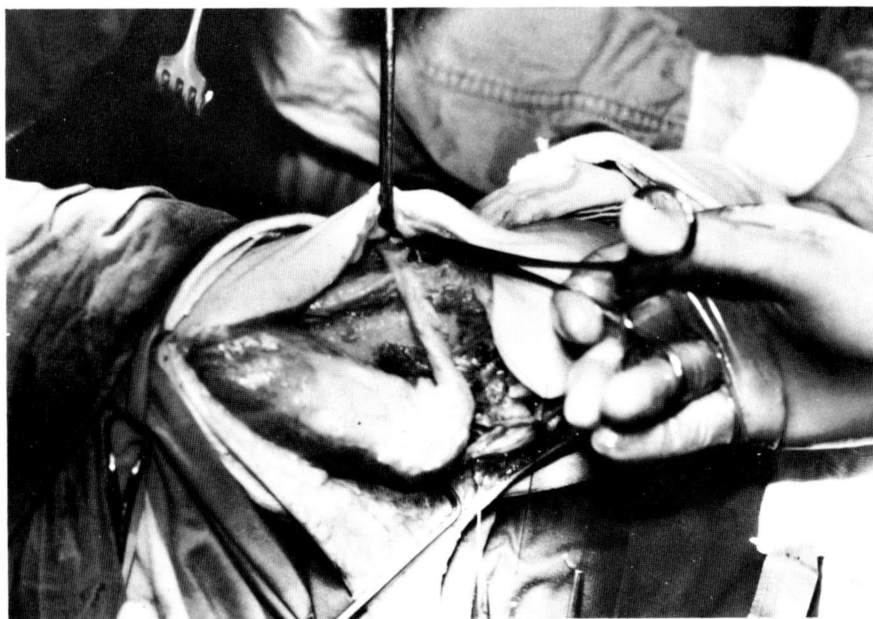

Fig. 42-17. Triceps transfer. The triceps has been elevated from the distal half of the humeral shaft, and the periosteal tongue is being directed subcutaneously and anteriorly to be sutured to the biceps tendon.

Author's Preferred Method

In my experience, the pectoral transfer provides the strongest elbow flexion, assuming that the ipsilateral shoulder is near-normal or is fused so that the power of the muscle is not dissipated in unwanted movements. The Steindler flexorplasty and modifications thereof give active control that tends to be weaker than the pectoral transfer. The triceps transfer is reserved for those situations where no better alternative exists and the patient has unilateral paralysis.

The Wrist

In the reconstruction of an upper extremity weakened by nerve injury, it is desirable to maintain the mobility of the wrist whenever possible, since the functional excursion of all tendons and transfers that cross it is thereby improved. If two tendons of adequate power will not be available for wrist flexion and extension, or if preservation of this motion will make it impossible to adequately reconstruct a functional hand, it is necessary and permissible to arthrodese the wrist. Numerous dependable techniques for achieving solid fusion are available (see Chapter 6). For the paralytic wrist where a subsequent tendon transfer for finger extension is planned, or has already been done, the tendons must be able to glide unimpeded across the joint. In patients who have had wrist fusions done from the dorsal approach, a danger of scarring that will compromise excursion of the finger extensors exists. Both Smith-Petersen[150] and Seddon[140] described fusion using the distal ulna as a bone graft placed across the radiocarpal joint. This requires sacrifice of a normal distal radioulnar joint, and the stability thereby conveyed. It is for this reason that the technique described by Haddad and Riordan[60] is so attractive. Their radial approach uses an iliac graft slotted between the radius and the bases of the second and third metacarpals. It produces an excellent fusion with minimal disturbance to the surrounding structures, and spares the extensor surface the risks of scarring (Fig. 42-18). The Haddad-Riordan fusion remains my preferred technique despite the fact that of 32 such fusions over the past 15 years, I have had three patients who sustained subsequent fractures. All of them were the result of significant trauma that would probably have caused fractures in normal wrists, and two of the three united following closed treatment. The third required a bone graft, which resulted in union. Although the alternative of tenodesis of the wrist tendons is theoretically attractive, my experience with it has been confined to one case to prevent hyperextension, and this, like the two done for opposition of the thumb, stretched out with time and use.[97]

The Hand

The techniques for restoration of active control and stability in the weakened hand of a patient with a brachial plexus injury do not differ from those employed in cases of multiple peripheral nerve injuries. These techniques are discussed in detail in other chapters in this book. However, their application to the hand must be properly timed with reference to reconstruction of the remainder of the limb. It must be modified accordingly if, for example, the same potential motor would be used actively at both ends of the forearm. Whenever possible, the use of the same motor to control multiple functions or joints should be avoided.

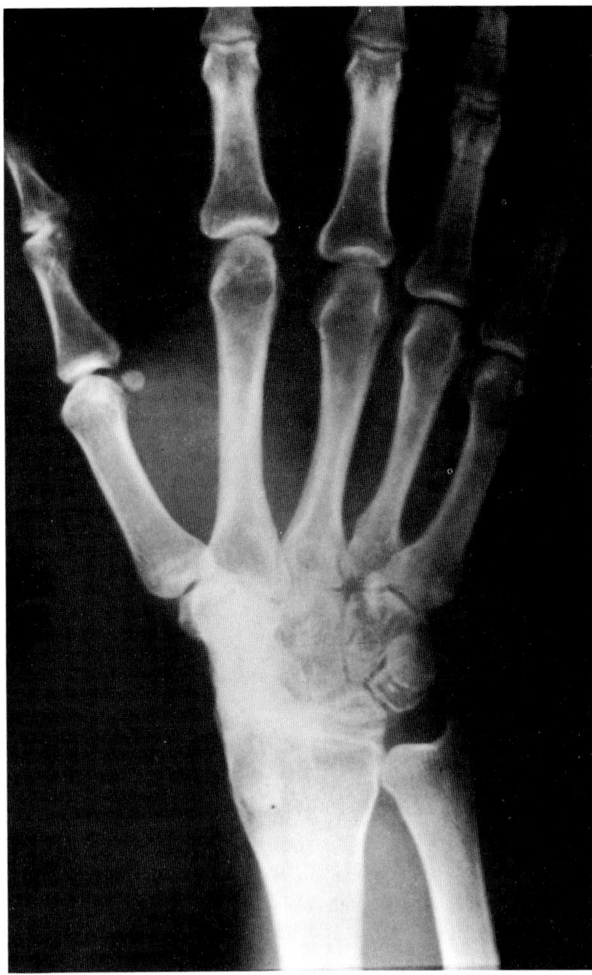

Fig. 42-18. A wrist fused by the Haddad-Riordan technique.

Unless there is significant reason for doing otherwise, the hand should be reconstructed before the remainder of the limb. This is particularly important with reference to the situation in which a shoulder fusion is to be done, since the positioning of such a limb can be extremely awkward once the shoulder is fused.

Personal experience with tendon transfers done in the hands of patients with the residua of brachial plexus injury over a 13-year period was summarized in 1988 by Leffert and Pess.[97] There were 107 transfers done, as follows:

Finger flexion	22
Wrist extension	21
Finger extension	31
Thumb opposition	19
Intrinsics	14

The results are displayed in Figures 42-19 to 42-23. A good result is one in which, postoperatively, the patients had normal or near-normal use of the extremity, good power, and could perform bimanual tasks. As may be seen, the results are very favorable, especially considering the fact that in terms of discrete hand function, one cannot achieve comparable results with neurologic reconstruction for the patient with a supraclavicular traction injury. However, they do not provide sensibility, and ultimately, one must think of employing combinations of techniques, individualized to the particular patient's needs for the most useful result.

The Dilemma of the Flail-Anesthetic Arm

The flail-anesthetic arm that results from neurotmesis of the brachial plexus poses a grave problem, not only for the patient, but for the surgeon as well. Before the resurgence of neurologic reconstruction, there were three general approaches—no active treatment, surgical reconstruction, and amputation. For patients whose deficit, although complete, results from a mixture of root avulsions and distal ruptures, there is now the possibility of attempting some restoration of function by means of neurologic reconstruction. For the patient with total avulsion of the plexus, the possibility of neurotization has already been commented upon (see page 1499). Therefore, while 25 years ago I would have suggested the option of simply placing the insensate upper limb in a sling, for most cases seen in adequate time I now recommend surgical exploration to attempt to repair what can be repaired. Some patients can benefit from functional bracing, which allows use of the limb as an assistive one, without using the hand in contact with objects that are grasped. This is made possible by various adaptive devices or cable-activated hooks. In order for the brace to be effective, however, the shoulder must be locked and there must be some way to achieve elbow flexion. I have found this method of management applicable to a small percentage of patients, limited by the weight and inconvenience of the devices. They do, however, constitute a viable option for some patients.[182]

Surgical reconstruction of the flail-anesthetic arm and hand, consisting of arthrodesis of the shoulder, posterior bone block at the elbow, and various combinations of arthrodeses and tenodeses for the hand and wrist, was advocated by Hendry in 1949[66] and is, in my opinion, most undesirable. It presents the surgical expression of a "very long run for a short slide" in that function is minimal and the insensate limb is vulnerable to fractures and skin breakdown. Although some patients do ask about it, I believe it is contraindicated.

The final solution, that of amputation of the limb, is performed far less frequently today than it was in the past, but must still be considered as a potential rehabilitative procedure for appropriate patients. Fortunately, recent advances in surgical reconstruction of the plexus have diminished the need for amputation. Nevertheless, patients whose limbs become the site of chronic infection, multiple fractures, or nonunions with little or no hope of healing should be advised to have an amputation. If a functional prosthetic fitting is desired, an arthrodesis of the shoulder will be required in those patients who have no shoulder control (Fig. 42-24). As is well known, the incidence of acceptance of upper extremity prostheses and their habitual use after unilateral major amputations is low, and in

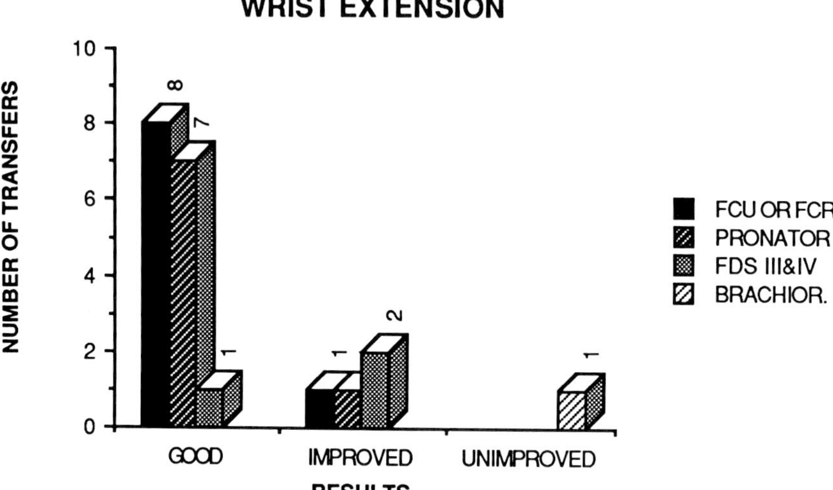

Fig. 42-19. The results of tendon transfers for wrist extension.

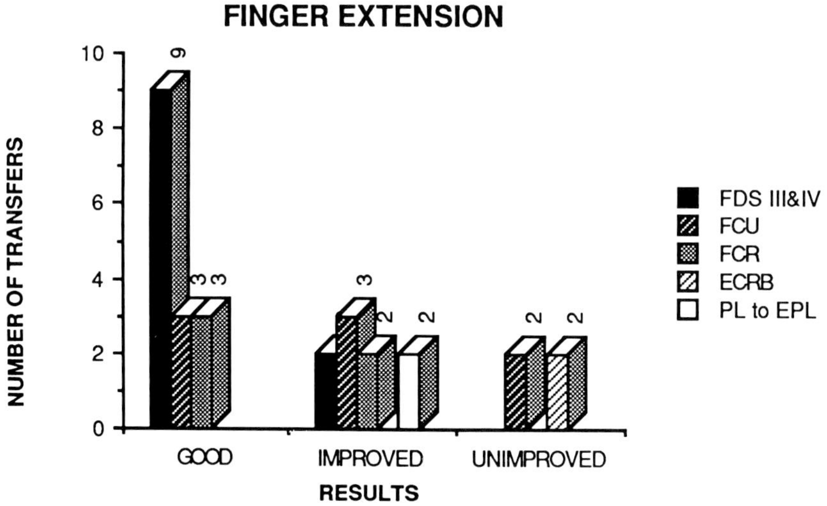

Fig. 42-20. The results of tendon transfers for finger extension.

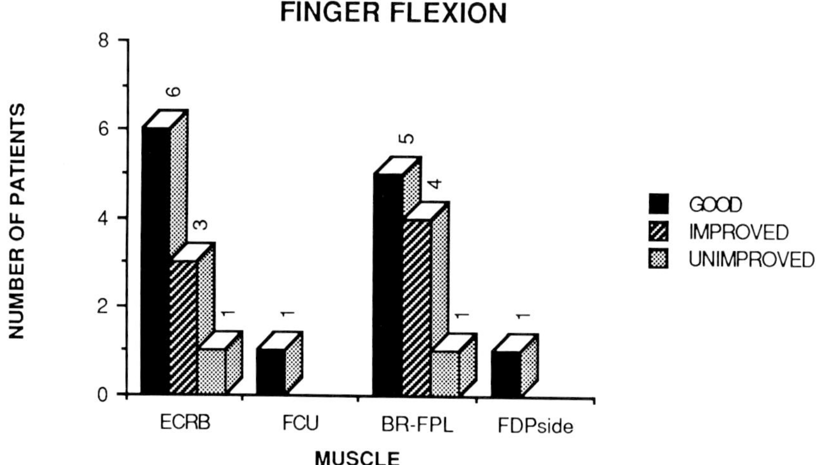

Fig. 42-21. The results of tendon transfer for finger flexion.

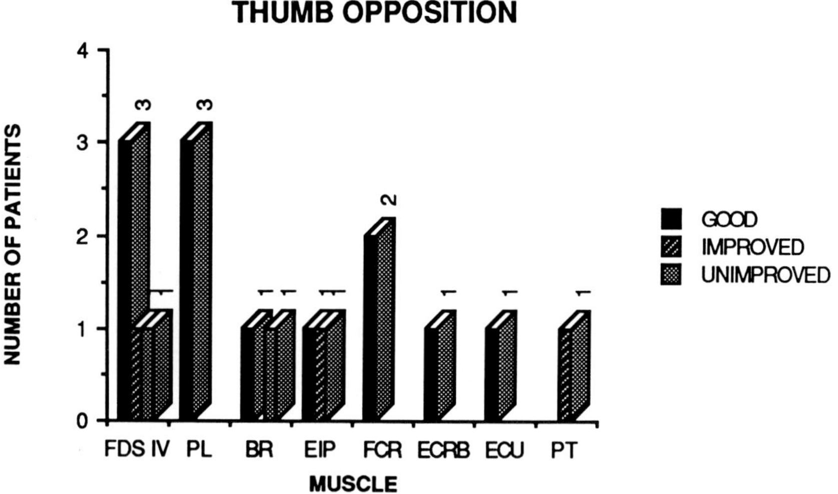

Fig. 42-22. The results of tendon transfer for opposition of the thumb.

brachial plexus injury patients it is even more prejudiced because of sensory loss and the shoulder deficit. For patients who have a contralateral normal limb, the tendency is to use it rather than the prosthesis, and for those seen more than 2 years postinjury, or who have severe phantom pain, the possibility of successful prosthetic fitting is unlikely. Since retention of the elbow, if it has position sense, is an important factor in prosthetic use, all efforts should be expended to amputate below the elbow in these cases, even if the skin sensibility is absent over the potential stump. If elbow proprioception is absent on gross testing, there is no advantage in retaining the joint. The management of the flail-anesthetic arm prior to the renewed interest in neural reconstruction after the middle 1960s was discussed by Yeoman and Seddon on the basis of their extensive experience.[183] However, it should be realized that the newer techniques of neurologic reconstruction and the general feeling in the public at large that "something will come along" have made amputation a much less commonly offered and performed procedure in the treatment of the patient with a major brachial plexus injury.

OBSTETRIC BRACHIAL PLEXUS INJURY (BIRTH PALSY)

Brachial plexus injury sustained by the neonate during difficult delivery has become considerably less common because of modern obstetric management.[1] Nevertheless, such patients

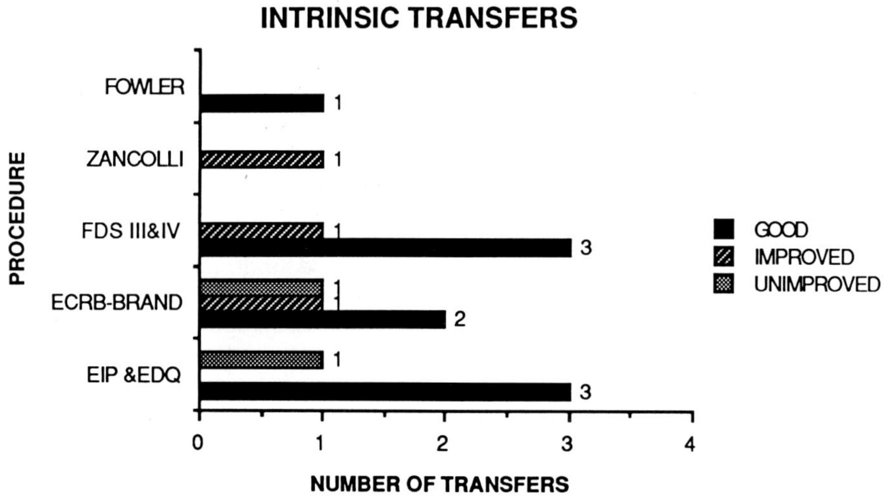

Fig. 42-23. Intrinsic transfers for brachial plexus injuries.

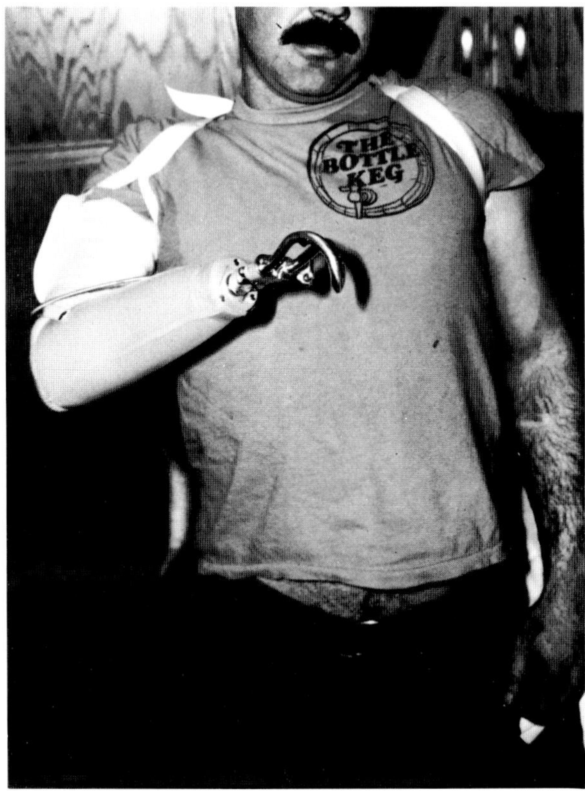

Fig. 42-24. This patient, who initially had a flail-anesthetic arm, regained active elbow flexion by means of a nerve graft from the upper trunk to the lateral cord. A shoulder fusion provided proximal control. Because no recovery was expected or occurred in the hand, the patient elected to undergo forearm amputation and prosthetic fitting. He uses the prosthesis on a regular basis.

are still sporadically seen by pediatricians and orthopaedic surgeons who must manage them through childhood. Growth is a significant factor that can alter form and function in a manner not found in the mature individual who sustains a brachial plexus injury. Specifically, in the growing child, asymmetric muscle forces due to paralysis will be expressed as contractures and bony deformity. These must be anticipated and prevented or treated to diminish their deleterious effects.

The etiology of the nerve injury in obstetric palsy is traction, usually due to fetal malposition, cephalopelvic disproportion, or the use of forceps. The distribution of the lesion is as follows: (1) C5, 6 (Erb's palsy); (2) entire plexus or diffuse partial involvement; and (3) C8, T1 (Klumpke's palsy). This last group is rarely seen in its pure form.

Early diagnosis is aided by a high index of suspicion in those neonates who exhibit asymmetric active upper extremity motion in the presence of a good passive range. Skeletal injuries, such as a fractured clavicle, may result in similar disinclination to move the limb, but they may also accompany brachial plexus injury. Although a clavicle fracture is usually recognizable on x-ray examination, it may be difficult to define other bony injuries that involve the proximal humerus and its epiphysis.

In the neonate or young infant, the lack of ossification in the proximal humeral epiphysis can significantly diminish the ability of the examiner to make a diagnosis of fracture or dislocation on the basis of plain radiographs. White et al[177] advocated arthrography of the infant shoulder as a useful diagnostic procedure in the evaluation of such cases.

Rarely, anterior dislocation may be encountered, and this may be dealt with accordingly, assuming the correct diagnosis has been made.

Early Surgical Exploration

As already stated, during the first two decades of this century, there was considerable enthusiasm for surgical exploration of these obstetric traction injuries.[147,165] Although there were some very good results, there were also intraoperative deaths,[165] and much of the reporting was anecdotal and difficult to interpret. The next 40 years saw a shift to conservatism in the management of neonatal traction injuries parallel to what was being practiced in the adult population; traction injuries were not to be explored.[77] Renewed interest in the surgical approach began with the advances in microsurgical technique as applied to nerve injuries in the 1960s largely due to the efforts of Millesi and Narakas. Relatively cautiously small series of obstetric palsies have been surgically treated by a number of investigators.[4,26,121,128,160,167] The experience of Gilbert in Paris[52,53] has been very extensively analyzed and was originally presented in Tassin's thesis at the University of Paris in 1983.[164] In Tassin's paper, a series of 44 patients were observed prospectively for a 5-year period (1977 through 1982) to provide further data on the natural history of spontaneous recovery of obstetric palsy, and these were compared with the result of the 100 neonates operated upon by Gilbert. Many of these patients were seen almost immediately following birth and were very carefully clinically evaluated. At 3 months, the final evaluation for those infants with residual paralysis consisted of a new manual muscle test, an EMG, and a myelogram. A paralyzed biceps at 3 months was considered the indication for surgery. The operation was performed under general anesthesia with electrophysiologic monitoring to allow for the measurement of somatosensory-evoked potentials intraoperatively. This was found helpful in defining pathology in the presence of traumatic pseudomeningoceles. Tassin's analysis of Gilbert's first 100 cases of surgical reconstruction of the plexus revealed that the timing and quality of recovery were variable and very good for the biceps, with 75 percent of the muscles able to contract to full range against gravity at 2 years, but less good for the deltoid and external rotators. The results were said to be especially good if paralysis was less extensive in the plexus. Tassin concluded that the type of surgical intervention demonstrated by Gilbert improves the prognosis of obstetric paralysis by increasing the number of good shoulders and diminishing the number of very bad ones.

Gilbert's most recent report is of 1,000 patients, seen in the period 1977 to 1987, of whom 241 underwent surgery.[52] On the basis of a very well-organized referral system, he was able to examine many neonates within the first month of birth. Very careful notes were made as to their neurologic deficits. There were 96 patients with lesions of C5, C6, and 81 with deficits of C5,6,7. Sixty-four of the infants had complete loss of brachial plexus function.

If no palpable contraction of the biceps was perceived by 3 months, this was an indication for surgical exploration, which was done without delay. Preoperatively, baseline EMGs were performed, although now Gilbert does not consider them as reliable for determining the indications for surgery, but rather useful in following postoperative recovery. The chest was fluoroscoped to evaluate the movement of the diaphragm. Myelography is no longer done routinely, as compared with his earlier practice.

Gilbert stresses the point that in patients with a flail, anesthetic arm, it is mandatory to explore each root individually. In none of his cases was there complete avulsion of the roots of the plexus as one may occasionally see in adult traction injuries. However, as seen in the adult population, it was the lower roots that were usually avulsed, and distal rupture more often occurred in the upper roots. He states that if three roots are available, the entire plexus should be repaired. Preference is given to the musculocutaneous nerve, the suprascapular nerve, and the lateral root of the median nerve when there are not enough axons to "go around," with the medial root of the median nerve being neurotized by intercostal nerves.

Using the same functional classification as in his previous reports, that of Mallet (Fig. 42-25), the following results were reported for the shoulder at three years,: 81 percent of the C5, 6 group and 76 percent of the C5, 6, 7 group achieved Mallet grade II,III,IV.

For those infants who initially had total paralysis, 22.5 percent achieved grade IV, 42 percent grade III, and 35.5 percent grade II.

In comparison with the "control group" of untreated patients reported by Tassin,[164] this was a strong argument in favor of surgical intervention. In this same group of untreated infants, the recovery in the hand was dismal. Following surgical reconstruction of the nerves, 83 percent had some hand function, and in 30 percent of those who underwent neurotization the function was considered valuable. One-half of the cases experienced partial or complete recovery of intrinsic hand function. This would certainly appear to justify the surgical approach in these cases by surgeons familiar with the techniques.

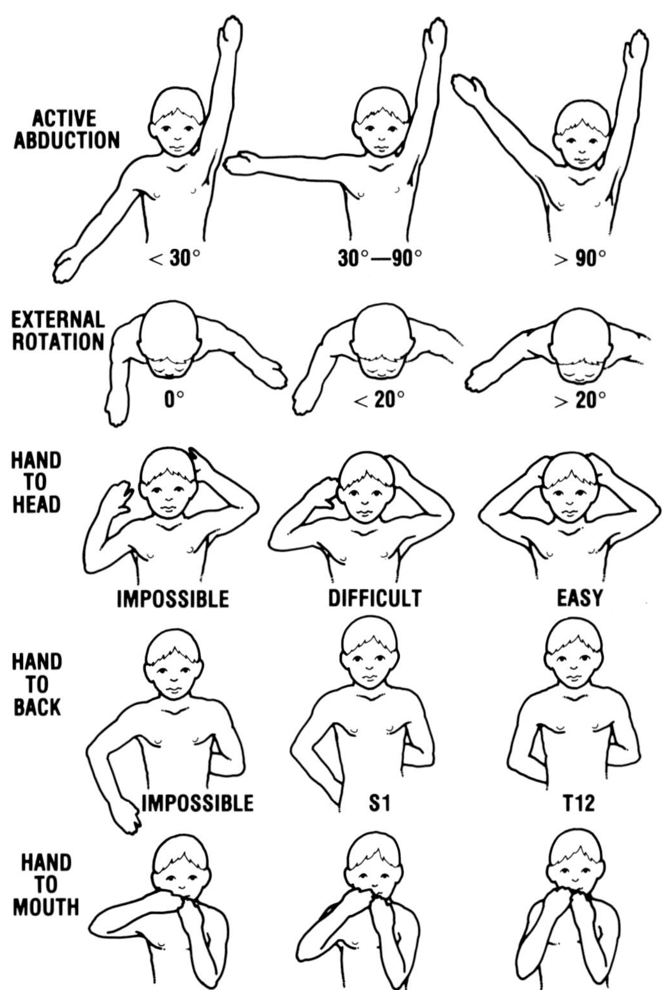

Fig. 42-25. Mallet's functional upper extremity classification. (Adapted from Gilbert et al,[54] with permission.)

Late Reconstruction

For children with partial lesions, use of conservative treatment in the form of range of motion exercises in an attempt to maintain the bimanual character of the child's activities is of greatest importance, since many of the deformities that develop in the growing child can be ameliorated or prevented.

The shoulder will tend to assume an internally rotated and adducted attitude that will require constant vigilance and gentle stretching by those caring for the child. The deficit in those patients who do not respond to treatment or who are neglected will be functionally obvious. Posterior subluxation or dislocation of the glenohumeral joint may be missed, which greatly complicates management. Fixed contractures must be overcome by release of tight anterior structures, using the procedures described by Fairbank[49] and Sever[147] and by active lateral rotation, reinforced by means of tendon transfer if possible. Wickstrom[178] reported that release of the anterior contracture alone was followed by recurrence of the contracture in three of five patients that he followed for 6 years. The procedure of L'Episcopo[91] overcomes this problem by adding a transfer of the latissimus and teres major posterolaterally so that their function is changed from medial to lateral rotation. If the child does not have significant anterior tightness and the problem is lack of lateral rotation control, the procedure may be done through a single posterior incision. However, if there is need for a release, then a long deltopectoral incision may be used either with or without the need for a separate posterior incision, since the procedure may be done all anteriorly. The attachment of the transfer may be to bone or to the rotator cuff.[69] If there is significant incongruity of the glenohumeral joint, osteotomy of the proximal humerus or open reduction of the joint may be required.[135] The evaluation of the glenohumeral joint for the presence of such incongruity can be facilitated by the use of CT scan.[68]

Rotational osteotomy of the humerus has been described for treatment of the loss of lateral rotation due to brachial plexus birth injuries, and the results have been reported as favorable.[55]

Developmental Deformities

The elbow may develop abnormally in a high percentage of children with significant residual weakness of the upper extremity. Aitken's work[2] is particularly valuable when planning management and should be consulted. Aitken studied 107 cases of obstetrical paralysis and found 33 cases of bony deformity of the elbow region, an incidence of 30.8 percent of the series. From his observations, he was able to define the radiographic features of posterior subluxation of the radial head. One can initially observe clubbing of the upper radial metaphysis followed by notching of its anterior aspect and increased ulnar curvature, with posterior displacement of the upper end of the radius. With growth, these changes progress so that by 5 to 8 years of age, the head becomes completely dislocated. Aitken made the point that if the radiographic changes could be identified early, complete dislocation could be prevented by splinting and range of motion exercises. For cases in which the dislocation was established, Aitken had formerly advised operative removal of the radial head. After completion of the investigation described in his article, the operation advised was osteotomy through the proximal third of the ulna, which allowed reposition of the radial axis. Results in 2 cases were encouraging.

Children with obstetrical palsy may have significant and persisting supination contracture of the forearm as a result of muscle imbalance. The problem may be addressed by means of a number of solutions, including osteotomy of the forearm bones. In my opinion, a far more satisfactory solution is the one that was proposed by Zancolli.[184] In this procedure, both the proximal and distal radioulnar joints are released as is the entire interosseous membrane. This allows for passive correction of the deformity. Active pronatory control and maintenance of the correction is achieved by a "Z" lengthening of the distal biceps tendon that allows the segment attached to the radius to be rerouted posterolaterally. Then the tendon is rejoined. The result is that the biceps, formerly a supinator, becomes a pronator. The results of this procedure are generally very good, but there are two caveats. The first is that there is a very real risk of injury to the posterior interosseous nerve both during the release of the interosseous membrane and at the time of tendon transfer about the neck of the radius. The second is failure to appreciate preoperatively the presence of weakness of wrist and finger extension in children who have the forearm chronically supinated because the effect of gravity creates the effect of extension in the absence of active muscle contraction. When the forearm is pronated, this effect is lost, and the child will have a wrist and finger drop. If the weakness is present preoperatively, then the parents must be made aware of it and provisions made for a subsequent transfer to correct this part of the problem.

Psychological Considerations

The forearm and hand of a child with obstetric palsy will often not be used in daily activities. If this is so, or if the patient is embarrassed by the abnormal limb and tends to hide it from view, even the most exquisitely planned and executed surgical reconstruction will be little more than a futile technical exercise. Sometimes the correction of an obvious deformity will have significant psychological benefit for the child, even if the functional benefit is not great. Hence, surgical procedures to be applied to the child or adolescent must be very carefully considered. In general, it is important for the small patient about to undergo a tendon transfer to understand in basic terms what is going to be done, since in this way the cooperation in the postoperative rehabilitation program and the ultimate result will be enhanced. For this reason, I generally delay such surgery until the child is 4 or 5 years of age. On the other hand, if the procedure will make the little patient less different from her schoolmates, then the operation will be of significant benefit from a social point of view and will be even more appreciated.

Finally, growth centers should be spared whenever possible in these paretic limbs that are invariably smaller than their normal counterparts.

REFERENCES

1. Adler JB, Patterson RL: Erb's palsy. Long time results of treatment in eighty-eight cases. J Bone Joint Surg 49A:1052–1064, 1967
2. Aitken J: Deformity of the elbow as a sequel to Erb's obstetrical palsy. J Bone Joint Surg 34B:352–365, 1952
3. Akasaka Y, Hara T, Takahashi M: Restoration of elbow flexion and wrist extension in brachial plexus paralyses by means of free muscle transplantation innervated by intercostal nerve. Ann Chir Main Memb Super 9:341–350, 1990
4. Alanen M, Halonen JP, Katevuo K, Vilkki P: Early surgical exploration and epineural repair in birth brachial palsy. Z Kinderchir 41(6):335–337, 1986
5. Allieu Y: Exploration et traitement direct des lesions nerveuses dans les paralysies traumatiques par elongation du plexus brachial chez l'adulte. Rev Chir Orthop 63:107–122, 1977
6. Allieu Y, Cenac P: Is surgical intervention justifiable for total paralysis secondary to multiple avulsion injuries of the brachial plexus? Hand Clin 4(4):609–618, 1988
7. Allieu Y, Cenac P: Neurotization via the spinal accessory nerve in complete paralysis due to multiple avulsion injuries of the brachial plexus. Clin Orthop 237:67–74, 1988
8. Allieu Y, Clauzel AM, Mekhaldi A, Triki F: Conséquences sur la fonction respiratoire des paralysies du plexus brachial de l'adulte et de leur traitement chirurgical. Rev Chir Orthop 72:455–460, 1986
9. Alnot JY: Traumatic brachial plexus palsy in the adult. Retro- and infraclavicular lesions. Clin Orthop 237:9–16, 1988
10. Alnot JY: The use of ulnar as a vascularized nerve graft in some peculiar conditions and particularly in total palsies of the brachial plexus with C7 C8 D1 avulsions. pp. 637–639. In Brunelli G (ed): Textbook of Microsurgery. Masson, Milano, 1988
11. Alnot JY, Abols Y: Réanimation de la flexion du coude par transferts tendineux dans les paralysies traumatiques du plexus brachial de l'adulte. Apropos de 44 blessés. Rev Chir Orthop 70:313–323, 1984
12. Alnot JY, Augereau B, Frot B: Traitement direct des lesions nerveuses dans les paralysies traumatiques par elongation du plexus brachial chez l'adulte. Chirurgie 103:935–947, 1977
13. Alnot JY, Bayon P: Traumatic paralysis of the brachial plexus. Combined neural and vascular lesions. Chirurgie 112(9):674–679, 1986
14. An HS, Vonderbrink JP, Ebraheim NA, Shiple F, Jackson WT: Open scapulothoracic dissociation with intact neurovascular status in a child. J Orthop Trauma 2(1):36–38, 1988
15. Aziz W, Singer RM, Wolff TW: Transfer of the trapezius for flail shoulder after brachial plexus injury. J Bone Joint Surg 72B:701–704, 1990
16. Barnes R: Traction injuries of the brachial plexus in adults. J Bone Joint Surg 31B:10–16, 1949
17. Battison B, Guizzi P, Vigasio A, Brunelli G: Experimental investigation of cross-nerve transfers relating to repair of brachial plexus avulsion injuries. Microsurgery 11:91–94, 1990
18. Benassy J, Held JP, Bernardeau D, Monteard J: Traumatisms fermes due plexus brachial. Chirurgie 100:374–381, 1973
19. Berger A, Schaller E, Mailänder P: Brachial plexus injuries: An integrated treatment concept. Ann Plast Surg 26(1):70–76, 1991
20. Bergström R: Changes in peripheral nerve tissue after irradiation with high energy protons. Acta Radiologica 58:301–312, 1962
21. Birch R, Dunkerton M, Bonney G, Jamieson AM: Experience with the free vascularized ulnar nerve graft in repair of supraclavicular lesions of the brachial plexus. Clin Orthop 237:96–104, 1988
22. Bonica JJ, Moore DC, Orlov M: Brachial plexus block anesthesia. Am J Surg 78:65–79, 1949
23. Bonney G: Prognosis in traction lesions of the brachial plexus. J Bone Joint Surg 41B:4–35, 1959
24. Bonney G: The value of axon responses in determining the site of lesion in traction injuries of the brachial plexus. Brain 77:588–609, 1954
25. Bonney G, Gilliatt RW: Sensory nerve conduction after traction lesion of the brachial plexus. Proc Roy Soc Med 51:365–367, 1958
26. Boome RS, Kaye JC: Obstetric traction injuries of the brachial plexus: Natural history, indications for surgical repair and results. J Bone Joint Surg 70B:571–576, 1988
27. Braun RM, Newman J, Thacher B: Injury to the brachial plexus as a result of diagnostic arteriography. J Hand Surg 3:90–97, 1978
28. Brooks DM, Seddon HJ: Pectoral transplantation for paralysis of the flexors of the elbow. A new technique. J Bone Joint Surg 41B:36–50, 1959
29. Brunelli G: Neurotization of avulsed roots of the brachial plexus by means of anterior nerves of the cervical plexus. pp. 435–436. In Terzis JK (ed): Microreconstruction of Nerve Injuries. WB Saunders, Philadelphia, 1987
30. Brunelli G: Neurolysis and free microvascular omentum transfer in the treatment of postactinic palsies of the brachial plexus. Int Surg 65:515–519, 1980
31. Bruser P, Noever G: What results can be expected following the biceps replacement operation? An analysis of retrospective data. Handchir Mikrochir Plast Chir 20(4):211–217, 1988
32. Bufalini C, Pescatori G: Posterior cervical electromyography in the diagnosis and prognosis of brachial plexus injuries. J Bone Joint Surg 51B:627–631, 1969
33. Bunnell S: Restoring flexion to the paralytic elbow. J Bone Joint Surg 33A:566–571, 1951
34. Burge P, Rushworth G, Watson N: Patterns of injury to the terminal branches of the brachial plexus. The place for early exploration. J Bone Joint Surg 67B:630–634, 1985
35. Carroll RE, Hill NA: Triceps transfer to restore elbow flexion: A study of 15 patients with paralytic lesions and arthrogryposis. J Bone Joint Surg 52A:239–244, 1970
36. Carroll RE, Kleinman WB: Pectoralis major transplantation to restore elbow flexion to the paralytic limb. J Hand Surg 4:501–507, 1979
37. Carroll SE, Wilkins WW: Two cases of brachial plexus injury following percutaneous arteriograms. Can Med Assoc J 102:861–862, 1970
38. Cascino TL, Kori S, Krol G, Foley KM: CT of the brachial plexus in patients with cancer. Neurology 33:1553–1557, 1983
39. Cherington M, Happer I, Machanic B, Parry L: Surgery for thoracic outlet syndrome may be hazardous to your health. Muscle Nerve 9:632–634, 1986
40. Clark JMP: Reconstruction of biceps brachii by pectoral muscle transplantation. Br J Surg 34:180, 1946
41. Clausen EG: Postoperative ("anesthetic") paralysis of the brachial plexus. A review of the literature and report of nine cases. Surgery 12:933–942, 1942
42. Clemedson CJ, Nelson A: General biology: The adult organism. pp. 95–205. In Errara M (ed): Mechanisms in Radiobiology. Vol. 2. Academic Press, New York, 1960–1961
43. D'Aubigne M, Benassy J, Ramadieu JO: Chirurgie Orthopaedique des Paralysies. pp. 122–139. Masson et Cie, Paris, 1956
44. Dhunér K-G: Nerve injuries following operations: A survey of cases occurring during a six-year period. Anesthesiology 11:289–293, 1950
45. Dolenc VV: Contemporary treatment of peripheral nerve and brachial plexus lesions. Neurosurg Rev 9:149–156, 1986

46. Dolenc VV: Intercostal neurotization of the peripheral nerves in avulsion plexus injuries. Clin Plast Surg 11(1):143-147, 1984
47. Ebraheim NA, An HS, Jackson WT, Pearlstein SR, Burgess A, Tscherne H, Hass N, Kellam J, Wipperman BUJ: Scapulothoracic dissociation. J Bone Joint Surg 70A:428-432, 1988
48. Ewing MR: Postoperative paralysis in the upper extremity. Report of five cases. Lancet 258:99-103, 1950
49. Fairbank HAT: Birth palsy: Subluxation of shoulder-joint in infants and young children. Lancet 1:1217, 1913
50. Friedman AH, Nunley JA II, Goldner RD, Oakes WJ, Goldner JL, Urbaniak JR: Nerve transposition for the restoration of elbow flexion following brachial plexus avulsion injuries. J Neurosurg 72:59-64, 1990
51. Gilbert A: Nerve anastomosis and graft with fibrin glue. pp. 554-556. In Tubiana R (ed): The Hand. Vol. III. WB Saunders, Philadelphia, 1988
52. Gilbert A, Brockman R, Carlioz H: Surgical treatment of brachial plexus birth palsy. Clin Orthop 264:39-47, 1991
53. Gilbert A, Tassin JL: Surgical repair of the brachial plexus in obstetric paralysis. Chirurgie 110:70-75, 1984
54. Gilbert A, Hentz VR, Tassin JL: Brachial plexus reconstruction in obstetric palsy: operative indications and postoperative results. pp 348-364. In Urbaniak JR (ed): Microsurgery for Major Limb Reconstruction. CV Mosby, St. Louis, 1987
55. Goddard NJ, Fixsen JA: Rotation osteotomy of the humerus for birth injuries of the brachial plexus. J Bone Joint Surg 66B:257-259, 1984
56. Gu Y-D, Ma M-K: Nerve transfer for treatment of root avulsion of the brachial plexus: Experimental studies in a rat model. J Reconstr Microsurg 7:15-22, 1991
57. Gu Y-D, Wu M-M, Zhen Y-L, Zhao J-A, Zhang G-M, Chen D-S, Yan J-G, Cheng X-M: Phrenic nerve transfer for brachial plexus motor neurotization. Microsurgery 10:287-289, 1989
58. Gugenheim S, Sanders RJ: Axillary artery rupture caused by shoulder dislocation. Surgery 95:55-58, 1984
59. Gupta RK, Mehta VS, Banerji AK, Jain RK: MR evaluation of brachial plexus injuries. Neuroradiology 31:377-381, 1989
60. Haddad RJ, Riordan DC: Arthrodesis of the wrist. A surgical technique. J Bone Joint Surg 49A:950-954, 1967
61. Hara T: Clinical study of brachial plexus injury. Nippon Seikeigeka Gakkai Zasshi 39(10):959-985, 1966
62. Harmon PH: Surgical reconstruction of the paralytic shoulder by multiple muscle transplantation. J Bone Joint Surg 32A:583-595, 1950
63. Harper CM Jr, Thomas JE, Cascino TL, Litchy WJ: Distinction between neoplastic and radiation-induced brachial plexopathy, with emphasis on the role of EMG. Neurology 39:502-506, 1989
64. Hashimoto T, Mitomo M, Hirabuki N, Miura T, Kawai R, Nakamura H, Kawai H, Ono K, Kozuka T: Nerve root avulsion of birth palsy: Comparison of myelography with CT myelography and somatosensory evoked potential. Radiology 178:841-845, 1991
65. Haymaker W, Lindgren M: Nerve disturbances following exposure to ionizing radiation. pp.388-401. In Vinken PJ, Bruyn GW (eds): Handbook of Clinical Neurology Vol. 7—Diseases of Nerves. Part I. North-Holland Publishing Co., Amsterdam, 1970
66. Hendry AM: The treatment of residual paralysis after brachial plexus injury. J Bone Joint Surg 31B:42-49, 1949
67. Heon M: Myelogram. A questionable aid in diagnosis and prognosis in avulsion of the brachial plexus components by traction injuries. Conn Med J 29:260, 1965
68. Hernandez RJ, Dias L: CT evaluation of the shoulder in children with Erb's palsy. Pediatr Radiol 18:333-336, 1988
69. Hoffer MM, Wickenden R, Roper B: Brachial plexus birth palsies. Results of tendon transfers to the rotator cuff. J Bone Joint Surg 60A:691-695, 1978
70. Hollinshead WH: Anatomy for Surgeons: The Back and Limbs. Vol. 3, Chap. 4. Harper and Rowe, New York, 1969
71. Horowitz SH: Brachial plexus injuries with causalgia resulting from transaxillary rib resection. Arch Surg 120:1189-1191, 1985
72. Hovelacque A: Anatomie des Nerfs Craniens et Radichiens et du System. Grand Sympathique. pp. 385-513. Gaston, Doin et Cie, Paris, 1927
73. Hovnaninan AP: Latissimus dorsi transplantation for loss of flexion or extension at the elbow. A preliminary report of technique. Ann Surg 143:493, 1956
74. Itoh Y, Sasaki T, Ishiguro T, Uchinishi K, Yabe Y, Fukuda H: Transfer of latissimus dorsi to replace a paralysed anterior deltoid. A new technique using an inverted pedicled graft. J Bone Joint Surg 69B:647-651, 1987
75. Jackson L, Keats AS: Mechanism of brachial plexus palsy following anesthesia. Anesthesiology 26:190-194, 1965
76. Jelasic F, Piepgras U: Functional restitution after cervical avulsion injury with 'typical' myelographic findings. Europ Neurol 11:158-163, 1974
77. Jepson PN: Obstetrical paralysis. Ann Surg 91:724-730, 1930
78. Jones SJ, Wynn Parry CB, Landi A: Diagnosis of brachial plexus traction lesions by sensory nerve action potentials and somatosensory evoked potentials. Injury 12:376-382, 1981
79. Joyce DA, Stewart-Wynne EG: Brachial plexopathy complicating central venous catheter insertion. Med J Aust 1:82-83, 1983
80. Jupiter JB, Leffert RD: Non-union of the clavicle: Associated complications and surgical management. J Bone Joint Surg 69A:753-760, 1987
81. Kanaya F, Gonzalez M, Park C-M, Kutz JE, Kleinert HE, Tsai T-M: Improvement in motor function after brachial plexus surgery. J Hand Surg 15A:30-36, 1990
82. Kawai H, Kawabata H, Masada K, Ono K, Yamamoto K, Tsuyuguchi Y, Tada K: Nerve repairs for traumatic brachial plexus palsy with root avulsion. Clin Orthop 237:75-86, 1988
83. Kelbel JM, Jardon OM, Huurman WW: Scapulothoracic dissociation. A case report. Clin Orthop 209:210-214, 1986
84. Kerr AT: The brachial plexus of nerves in man. The variations in its formation and branches. Am J Anat 23:285, 1918
85. Kettlekamp DB, Larson CB: Evaluation of the Steindler flexorplasty. J Bone Joint Surg 45A:513-518, 1963
86. Killer HE, Hess K: Natural history of radiation-induced brachial plexopathy compared with surgically treated patients. J Neurol 237:247-250, 1990
87. Kline DG, Judice DJ: Operative management of selected brachial plexus lesions. J Neurosurg 58:631-649, 1983
88. Kondo M, Matsuda H, Miyawaki Y, Yoshimura M, Shimazu A: A new method of electrodiagnosis during operations on the brachial plexus and peripheral nerve injuries. The value of motor nerve action potentials evoked by trans-skull motor area stimulation. Int Orthop 9:115-121, 1985
89. Kori SH, Foley KM, Posner JB: Brachial plexus lesions in patients with cancer: 100 cases. Neurology 31:45-50, 1981
90. Kotani T, Toshima Y, Matsuda H, Suzuki T: Postoperative results of nerve transposition and brachial plexus injury. Orthop Surg Tokyo 22:963, 1971
91. L'Episcopo JB: Restoration of muscle balance in the treatment of obstetrical paralysis. NY State J Med 39:357-363, 1939
92. Lederman RJ, Wilbourn AJ: Brachial plexopathy: Recurrent cancer or radiation? Neurology 34:1331-1335, 1984
93. Leffert RD: Brachial Plexus Injuries. Churchill Livingstone, New York, 1985
94. Leffert RD (ed): Compression-plate fusion of a flail shoulder. Strategies in Orthopaedic Surgery-Upjohn, Vol. 7. LTI Medica, New Scotland, NY, 1988

95. Leffert RD: Rehabilitation of the patient with a brachial plexus injury. Neurol Clin 5(4):559–568, 1987
96. Leffert RD, Meister M: Patterns of neuromuscular activity following tendon transfer in the upper limb: A preliminary study. J Hand Surg 1:181–189, 1976
97. Leffert RD, Pess GM: Tendon transfers for brachial plexus injury. Hand Clin 4(2):273–288, 1988
98. Leffert RD, Seddon H: Infraclavicular brachial plexus injuries. J Bone Joint Surg 47B:9–22, 1965
99. LeQuang C: Postirradiation lesions of the brachial plexus. Results of surgical treatment. Hand Clin 5(1):23–32, 1989
100. Lusskin R, Campbell JB, Thompson WAL: Post-traumatic lesions of the brachial plexus: Treatment by transclavicular exploration and neurolysis or autograft reconstruction. J Bone Joint Surg 55A:1159–1176, 1973
101. Makachinas T, Ovelmen-Levitt J, Nashold BS Jr: Intraoperative somatosensory evoked potentials. A localizing technique in the DREZ operation. Appl Neurophysiol 51:146–153, 1988
102. Marshall RW, DeSilva RDD: Computerised axial tomography in traction injuries of the brachial plexus. J Bone Joint Surg 68B:734–738, 1986
103. Marshall RW, Williams DH, Birch R, Bonney G: Operations to restore elbow flexion after brachial plexus injuries. J Bone Joint Surg 70B:577–582, 1988
104. Match RM: Radiation-induced brachial plexus paralysis. Arch Surg 110:384–386, 1975
105. Mayer L, Green W: Experiences with the Steindler flexorplasty at the elbow. J Bone Joint Surg 36A:775–789, 1954
106. Meyer RD: Treatment of adult and obstetrical brachial plexus injuries. Orthopedics 9:899–903, 1986
107. Millesi H: Brachial plexus injuries. Nerve grafting. Clin Orthop 237:36–42, 1988
108. Millesi H: Brachial plexus injuries. Management and results. Clin Plast Surg 11(1):115–120, 1984
109. Millesi H: The current state of peripheral nerve surgery in the upper limb. Ann Chir Main 3:18–34, 1984
110. Millesi H: Surgical management of brachial plexus injuries. J Hand Surg 2:367–379, 1977
111. Millesi H, Meissl G, Katzer H: Zur Behandlung der Verletzungen des Plexus Brachialis. Vorchlag einer inegrierten Therapie. Bruns Beitr Klin Chir 220:429, 1973
112. Mondrup K, Olsen NK, Pfeiffer P, Rose C: Clinical and electrodiagnostic findings in breast cancer patients with radiation-induced brachial plexus neuropathy. Acta Neurol Scand 81:153–158, 1990
113. Moneim MS, Omer GE: Latissimus dorsi muscle transfer for restoration of elbow flexion after brachial plexus disruption. J Hand Surg 11A:135–139, 1986
114. Nagano A, Ochiai N, Sugioka H, Hara T, Tsuyama N: Usefulness of myelography in brachial plexus injuries. J Hand Surg 14B:59–64, 1989
115. Nagano A, Okinaga S, Ochiai N, Kurokawa T: Shoulder arthrodesis by external fixation. Clin Orthop 247:97–100, 1989
116. Nagano A, Tsuyama N, Hara T, Sugioka H: Brachial plexus injuries. Prognosis of postganglionic lesions. Arch Orthop Trauma Surg 102:172–178, 1984
117. Nagano A, Tsuyama N, Ochiai N, Hara T, Takahashi M: Direct nerve crossing with the intercostal nerve to treat avulsion injuries of the brachial plexus. J Hand Surg 14A:980–985, 1989
118. Narakas A: Brachial plexus surgery. Orthop Clin North Am 12:303–323, 1981
119. Narakas A: Indications et résultats du traitement chirurgical direct dans les lésions par élongation du plexus brachial. Rev Chir Orthop 63:88–106, 1977
120. Narakas A: The surgical management of brachial plexus injuries. In Daniel RK, Terzis JK (eds): Reconstructive Microsurgery. Vol. 1, Chap. 9. Little, Brown, Boston, 1977
121. Narakas AO: The treatment of brachial plexus injuries. Int Orthop 9:29–36, 1985
122. Narakas AO, Hentz VR: Neurotization in brachial plexus injuries. Indication and results. Clin Orthop 237:43–56, 1988
123. Nelson KG, Jolly PC, Thomas PA: Brachial plexus injuries associated with missile wounds of the chest. A report of nine cases from Viet Nam. J Trauma 8:268–275, 1968
124. Ober FR: Transplantation to improve the function of the shoulder joint and extensor function of the elbow joint. In AAOS Instructional Course Lectures on Reconstructive Surgery, JW Edwards, Ann Arbor, 1944
125. Oreck SL, Burgess A, Levine AM: Traumatic lateral displacement of the scapula: A radiographic sign of neurovascular disruption. J Bone Joint Surg 66A:758–763, 1984
126. Orlandini A, Gualandi GF, Tansini A, Scipione V: Traumatic lesions of the brachial plexus. Evaluation of 144 cases studied using direct cervical myelography and non-ionic contrast media. Radiol Med (Torino) 75:15–19, 1988
127. Pajardi G, Morelli E: Traumatic lesions of the brachial plexus. Microsurgical treatment. J Chir 122:305–309, 1985
128. Piatt JH Jr, Hudson AR, Hoffman HJ: Preliminary experiences with brachial plexus exploration in children: Birth injury and vehicular trauma. Neurosurgery 22:715–723, 1988
129. Platt H: Opening remarks on birth paralysis. J Orthop Surg 2:272, 1920
130. Powell S, Cooke J, Parsons C: Radiation-induced brachial plexus injury: follow-up of two different fractionation schedules. Radiother Oncol 18:213–220, 1990
131. Richards RR, Hudson AR, Bertoia JT, Urbaniak JR, Waddell JP: Injury to the brachial plexus during Putti-Platt and Bristow procedures. A report of eight cases. Am J Sports Med 15:374–380, 1987
132. Richards RR, Waddell JP, Hudson AR: Shoulder arthrodesis for the treatment of brachial plexus palsy. Clin Orthop 198:250–258, 1985
133. Riggins R: Shoulder fusion without external fixation. A preliminary report. J Bone Joint Surg 58A:1007–1008, 1976
134. Roger B, Travers V, Laval-Jeantet M: Imaging of posttraumatic brachial plexus injury. Clin Orthop 237:57–61, 1988
135. Rogers MH: An operation for the correction of deformity due to "obstetrical paralysis". Boston Med Surg J 174:163, 1916
136. Rowe CR: Arthrodesis of the shoulder used in treating painful conditions. Clin Orthop 173:92–96, 1983
137. Saha AK: Surgery of the paralyzed and flail shoulder. Acta Orthop Scan Suppl 97, 1967
138. Schottstaedt ER, Larsen LJ, Bost FC: Complete muscle transposition. J Bone Joint Surg 37A:897–919, 1955
139. Seddon HJ: Nerve grafting. J Bone Joint Surg 45B:447–461, 1963
140. Seddon HJ: Reconstructive surgery of the upper extremity. Poliomyelitis. Second International Poliomyelitis Congress. JB Lippincott, Philadelphia, 1952
141. Seddon HJ, Medawar PB: Fibrin suture of human nerves. Lancet 2:87–88, 1942
142. Sedel L: Repair of severe traction lesions of the brachial plexus. Clin Orthop 237:62–66, 1988
143. Sedel L: Results of surgical repair in brachial plexus injuries. J Bone Joint Surg 64B:54–66, 1982
144. Segal A, Seddon HJ, Brooks DM: Treatment of paralysis of the flexors of the elbow. J Bone Joint Surg 41B:44–50, 1959
145. Selander D, Dhunér K-G, Lundborg G: Peripheral nerve injury due to injection needles used for regional anesthesia. An experi-

mental study of the acute effects of needle point trauma. Acta Anaesth Scand 21:182–188, 1977

146. Selander D, Edshage S, Wolff T: Paresthesiae or no paresthesiae? Nerve lesions after axillary blocks. Acta Anaesth Scand 23:27–33, 1979
147. Sever JW: Obstetric paralysis. Report of eleven hundred cases. JAMA 85:1862–1865, 1925
148. Sharpe W: The operative treatment of brachial plexus paralysis. JAMA 66:876–881, 1916
149. Sibuya M, Homma I, Hara T, Tsuyama N: Expiratory activity in transferred intercostal nerves in brachial plexus injury patients. J Appl Physiol 62(5):1780–1785, 1987
150. Smith-Petersen MN: A new approach to the wrist joint. J Bone Joint Surg 22:122–124, 1940
151. Steindler A: Muscle and tendon transplantation at the elbow. In Thompson JEM (ed): Instructional Course Lectures on Reconstructive Surgery. Vol. 2. AAOS, Chicago, 1944
152. Steindler A: Reconstruction work on hand and forearm. NY State Med J 108:117–119, 1918
153. Stevens JH: Brachial plexus paralysis. pp. 332–381. In Codman EA (ed): The Shoulder. G. Miller & Co., New York, 1934
154. Stober R: Intraoperative function diagnosis in the care of brachial plexus injuries. Handchir Mikrochir Plast Chir 17(1):31–34, 1985
155. Stoll BA, Andrews JT: Radiation-induced peripheral neuropathy. Br Med J 1:834–837, 1966
156. Strecker WB, McAllister JW, Manske PR, Schoenecker PL, Dailey LA: Complete infraclavicular brachial plexus palsy with occlusion of axillary vessels following anterior dislocation of the shoulder joint. J Orthop Trauma 4:121–123, 1990
157. Sturm JT, Perry JF Jr: Brachial plexus injuries from blunt trauma—a harbinger of vascular and thoracic injury. Ann Emerg Med 16:404–406, 1987
158. Sugioka H: Evoked potentials in the investigation of traumatic lesions of the peripheral nerve and the brachial plexus. Clin Orthop 184:85–92, 1984
159. Sunderland S: Nerve Injuries and Their Repair. Churchill Livingstone, Edinburgh, 1991
160. Sztonak L, Warnke JP: Surgical management of perinatal damage of the brachial plexus. Zentralbl Neurochir 48(2):162–167, 1987
161. Tajima T: History, current status, and aspects of hand surgery in Japan. Clin Orthop 184:41–49, 1984
162. Takahashi M: Studies on conversion of motor function in intercostal nerves crossing for complete brachial plexus injuries of root avulsion type. Nippon Seikeigeka Gakkai Zasshi 57(11):1799–1807, 1983
163. Tarlov IM: Autologous plasma clot suture of nerves. Its use in clinical surgery. JAMA 126:741–748, 1944
164. Tassin JL: Paralysies obstetricales du plexus brachial. Evolution spontance, resultats des interventions reparatrices. Thesis, Vol. VII. University of Paris, 1983
165. Taylor AS: Brachial birth palsy and injuries of similar type in adults. Surg Gynecol Obstet 30:494–502, 1920
166. Taylor GI, Ham FJ: The free vascularized nerve graft. A further experimental and clinical application of microvascular techniques. Plast Reconstr Surg 57:413–426, 1976
167. Terzis JK, Liberson WT, Levine R: Our experience in obstetrical brachial plexus palsy. pp. 513–528. In Terzis JK (ed): Microreconstruction of Nerve Injuries. WB Saunders, Philadelphia, 1987
168. Thomas JE, Colby MY Jr: Radiation-induced or metastatic brachial plexopathy? A diagnostic dilemma. JAMA 222:1392–1395, 1972
169. Thornburn W: A clinical lecture on secondary suture of the brachial plexus. Br Med J 1:1073–1075, 1900
170. Tomaszek DE: Combined subclavian artery and brachial plexus injuries from blunt upper-extremity trauma. J Trauma 24:161–163, 1984
171. Tomita Y, Tsai T-M, Burns JT, Karaoguz A, Ogden LL: Intercostal nerve transfer in brachial plexus injuries: An experimental study. Microsurgery 4:95–104, 1983
172. Travlos J, Goldberg I, Boome RS: Brachial plexus lesions associated with dislocated shoulders. J Bone Joint Surg 72B:68–71, 1990
173. Tsuyama N, Hara T: Intercostal nerve transfer in the treatment of brachial plexus injury of root avulsion type. p. 351. In Proc 12th Cong International Soc Orthop Surg Traumatol Exerpta Medica, Amsterdam, 1972
174. Uhlschmid G, Clodius L, Hess K, Smahel J: The treatment of painful infraclavicular brachial plexus paralysis following axillary management and roentgen therapy. Helv Chir Acta 51(6):763–768, 1985
175. Volpin G, Langer R, Stein H: Plexus neuropathy: tumor infiltration or radiation damage. Rofo 152(6):662–666, 1990
176. White JI, Hoffer MM, Lehman M: Arthrodesis of the paralytic shoulder. J Pediatr Orthop 9:684–686, 1989
177. White SJ, Blane CE, DiPietro MA, Kling TFJ, Hensinger RN: Arthrography in evaluation of birth injuries of the shoulder. Can Assoc Radiol J 38(2):113–115, 1987
178. Wickstrom J: Birth injuries of the brachial plexus. Treatment of defects in the shoulder. Clin Orthop 23:187–196, 1962
179. Wilbourn AJ: Thoracic outlet syndrome surgery causing severe brachial plexopathy. Muscle Nerve 11:66–74, 1988
180. Wilde AH, Brems JJ, Boumphrey FRS: Arthrodesis of the shoulder: Current indications and operative technique. Orthop Clin North Am 18(3):463–472, 1987
181. Wood VE, Frykman GK: Winging of the scapula as a complication of first rib resection: A report of six cases. Clin Orthop 149:160–163, 1980
182. Wynn-Parry CB: Update on peripheral nerve injuries. Int Disabil Studies 10:11–20, 1988
183. Yeoman PM, Seddon HJ: Brachial plexus injuries-treatment of the flail arm. J Bone Joint Surg 43B:493–500, 1961
184. Zancolli EL: Paralytic supination contracture of the forearm. J Bone Joint Surg 49A:1275–1284, 1967
185. Zancolli E, Mitre H: Latissimus dorsi transfer to restore elbow flexion. An appraisal of eight cases. J Bone Joint Surg 55A:1265–1275, 1973
186. Zeuke W, Heidrich R: Late paralyses of peripheral nerves after radiotherapy. Psychiatr Neurol Med Psychol (Leipz) 34(6):360–366, 1982

43

Tetraplegia

Charles L. McDowell

PATIENT SELECTION AND CLASSIFICATION

For the surgeon considering operative treatment in a tetraplegic patient, patient selection is the most difficult task to confront. The difficulty lies in the complexity of the physical examination, in which conditions change, especially during the first 12 months after injury, and where spasticity often exists. In addition, there are subjective factors that have a different emphasis in tetraplegic patients than in patients with other conditions. The dramatic change in the patient's life requires a long and arduous psychological adjustment, and some patients fail to adjust sufficiently to handle surgical reconstruction. Other factors to consider include the patient's age, occupation, interests, level of education, learning capacity, economic support, family and agency support, personality type, and understanding of what can and cannot be expected from surgical treatment. Patient selection is not simply a matter of obtaining the objective information and applying a set method of treatment.

Classically, tetraplegic patients have been classified by the cervical spine segment injured by fracture or dislocation, and there has been an assumption that the level of paralysis and sensory loss coincided exactly with the bony injury, producing a precise transverse spinal cord lesion (Fig. 43-1). Careful examination of patients rendered tetraplegic has shown that (1) there is frequently little relationship between the level of the skeletal lesion and the spinal cord lesion, (2) lesions may be asymmetrical, and (3) there may be unusual patterns of sparing of sensory or motor function. Thus a more useful classification had to be developed that used spared functions as its basis. The classification (Table 43-1) used in this chapter was approved by an international group of surgeons working with tetraplegics[30] and modified in 1984 at Giens, France.[31]

Sensory Classification

The sensory classification has two categories: O for ocular or visual afferent input and Cu for cutaneous afferent input. The two-point discrimination test described by Moberg is used to determine cutaneous sensibility. A patient must demonstrate discrimination of 10 mm or less (using the blunt points of a paper clip) to be classified in Group Cu, as it is assumed that the minimum cutaneous sensibility to control grip is 10 mm two-point discrimination. The O (ocular) group depends on vision for afferent information and grip control.

Motor Classification

Muscles are included in the classification of a patient only if they are of at least Grade 4 MRC (Medical Research Council)[32] (Table 43-2). Surgeons disagree as to whether it is possible to distinguish between the function of the extensor carpi radialis longus and the extensor carpi radialis brevis. Some believe that they can test and grade each muscle separately; others do not. Fortunately, both groups agree that the extensor carpi radialis brevis can be assessed best by exposing the tendon at the wrist level under local anesthesia and testing it with weights attached to a sterile pin through the tendon.[4] The patient should be able to lift 3 to 5 pounds of weight for the muscle to be considered classifiable.

Most patients rendered tetraplegic by an injury will fall under the first half of the classification. Moberg pointed out that significantly more high-level cases with more severe paralysis were seen in Scandinavia and the United States than in Argentina. He suggested that the difference might be due to the lower mortality rate in Scandinavia and the United States.[37] If this is true, it means that surgeons in areas with a high survival

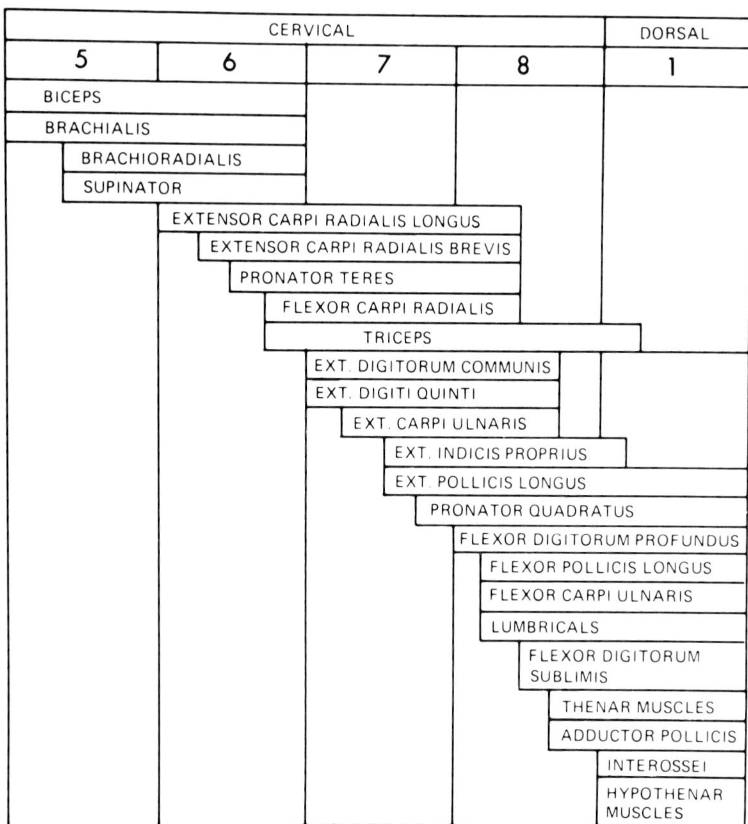

Fig. 43-1. Segmental innervation of muscles of the elbow, forearm, and hand. (From Zancolli,[51] with permission.)

Table 43-1. International Classification for Surgery of the Hand in Tetraplegia (Edinburgh 1978, Modified—Giens 1984)

Sensibility	Motor[a]		Description
O or Cu	Group	Characteristics	Function
	0	No muscle below elbow suitable for transfer	Flexion and supination of the elbow
	1	BR	
	2	ECRL	Extension of the wrist (weak or strong)
	3*	ECRB	Extension of the wrist
	4	PT	Extension and pronation of the wrist
	5	FCR	Flexion of the wrist
	6	Finger extensors	Extrinsic extension of the fingers (partial or complete)
	7	Thumb extensor	Extrinsic extension of the thumb
	8	Partial digital flexors	Extrinsic flexion of the fingers (weak)
	9	Lacks only intrinsics	Extrinsic flexion of the fingers
	X	Exceptions	

[a] BR, brachioradialis; ECRL, extensor carpi radialis longus; ECRB, extensor carpi radialis brevis; PT, pronator teres, FCR, flexor carpi radialis.

* Caution: It is not possible to determine the strength of the ECRB without surgical exposure (see text).

1. This classification does not include the shoulder. It is a guide to the forearm and hand only. Determination of patient suitability for posterior deltoid to triceps transfer or bicepts to triceps transfer is considered separately.
2. The need for triceps reconstruction is stated separately. It may be required in order to make brachioradialis transfers function properly (see text).
3. There is a sensory component to the classification. Afferent input is recorded using the method described by Moberg and precedes the motor classification. Both ocular and cutaneous input should be documented. When vision is the only afferent available the designation is "Occulo" (abbreviated O). Assuming there is 10 mm or less two-point discrimination in the thumb and index finger, the correct classification would be Cu, indicating that the patient has adequate cutaneous sensibility. If two-point discrimination is greater than 10 mm (meaning inadequate cutaneous sensibility), the designation O would precede the motor group (example O 2).
4. Motor grouping assumes that all listed muscles are grade 4 (MRC) or better and a new muscle is added for each group; for example, a Group 3 patient will have BR, ECRL, and ECRB rated at least Grade 4 (MRC).

(Modified from McDowell et al,[31] with permission.)

Table 43-2. Currently Accepted Muscle Grading System First Devised by the British Medical Research Council[32]

0	No contraction
1	Flicker or trace of contraction
2	Active movement with gravity eliminated
3	Active movement against gravity
4	Active movement against gravity and resistance
5	Normal

rate of spinal cord-injured patients will encounter more difficult cases.

Timing of Operative Treatment

Additional guidelines for patient selection, apart from the subjective factors and the patient's classification, are based on information acquired from experience in treating tetraplegic patients. The conference surgeons agreed that serial sensory and muscle testing should be done at about 3-month intervals for at least 1 year after injury before considering operative procedures. Surgical reconstruction should rarely be considered prior to 1 year following spinal cord injury to allow the patient sufficient time to make major psychological adjustments, especially to understand that there is no hope for further recovery. Further delay of reconstruction is indicated if there is evidence of any neurologic recovery; operative treatment is considered only after the motor and sensory improvement has stopped.[18]

Role of Spasticity

Spasticity is a serious consideration in reconstructive surgery for the tetraplegic patient. The degree of spasticity is difficult to evaluate, and its presence may severely compromise results. The conference surgeons agreed that muscles exhibiting uncontrolled spasticity, even though of adequate strength, should not be transferred.[30] Lesser degrees of spasticity constitute a relative contraindication to transfer operations. There are a few situations in which a spastic muscle can be rendered flaccid by neurectomy or tendon release, thus making tenodesis or arthrodesis procedures reasonable possibilities.

Goals of Operative Treatment

Preoperative observation of patients who have enough muscle strength to actively dorsiflex the wrist reveals a tendency to utilize the natural "tenodesis" effect for function; that is, with wrist dorsiflexion, the digital extensor tendons are slack and the digital flexor muscle-tendon units are placed under sufficient tension to cause the thumb to adduct against the side of the index finger and the fingers to flex. This effect should be enhanced whenever possible. Wrist arthrodesis should be avoided because fusion interferes with the pattern of function that the patient has learned to use.

A formerly popular method used to try to obtain grasp in patients with wrist extension only (Groups 2, 3, and 4) had as its goal a three-point "chuck"-type pinch. The operations employed to achieve this included combinations of tendon transfers, tenodesing procedures, and joint fusions.[1,40] The results of such procedures have been judged unacceptable by most surgeons and patients because the thumb and fingers are rendered rigid. Key pinch i.e., thumb to the radial side of the index finger, is easier to accomplish with surgery and is more useful and acceptable to the patient.[36,51] The conference surgeons recommended side pinch (key grip) as a better goal of surgical reconstruction.[30]

DEVELOPMENT OF THE SURGICAL TREATMENT PLAN

Planning of surgical procedures should take into account other needs that may have priority over upper extremity reconstruction. Pressure sores must be cared for, and all scars should be well healed. The patient should be mobilized in a wheelchair so that upper extremity use and training can be optimized. Treatment of other systems, such as urogenital and cardiopulmonary, may take priority. Appropriate expert consultation for these other systems must be sought.

General anesthesia and axillary regional block have been successful in this type of surgery. Few complications have been reported with either method, probably due to the high quality of anesthesia available to the reporting surgeons.[11,39] My preferred method is the axillary regional block. I do not recommend supraclavicular block because of the risk of pneumothorax and/or paralysis of the diaphragm.

Precise muscle and sensory testing should be recorded so that the patient can be properly classified. Both upper extremities should be classified separately, as they may not be the same.

If reconstructive surgery to restore active elbow extension by deltoid-to-triceps transfer is indicated, the transfer should precede other operations. Moberg reasoned that a patient who obtained grasp capability by surgery on the forearm would be frustrated by a deltoid-to-triceps transfer performed later since he would not be able to grasp objects during the prolonged period of elbow immobilization. In addition, an active elbow extensor improves the function of a brachioradialis transfer because it acts as an antagonist.[36]

Only one operation should be performed at a time. This does not mean that small joint fusions or other synergistic procedures should not be combined, but rather that complex operations should be carefully staged. My own experiences indicate that the best outcomes have resulted from the least complex operations. In addition, operations that impair the use of both upper extremities at the same time must be avoided (Zuelzer W: personal communication).

Whether stated or implied by the way they managed their cases, Moberg[37] and House, Gwathmey, and Lundsgaard[19] believe that reconstruction should begin on the dominant extremity if both are classified at the same level. If sparing of function is not symmetrical, reconstruction should begin on the side with better function. I use this approach because some patients, particularly those with significant loss, may be content with reconstruction of only one side. Obviously, if there is inadequate cutaneous sensibility, surgery should be done only on one side as the patient can control the grip visually on only one hand.

At this stage of planning, the surgeon must consider, according to his own experience and judgment, the best functional goals that can be obtained for this patient. Moberg has departed from the priorities established by earlier authors. Prior to his articles, surgeons designed reconstructive procedures that would restore as many lost motor functions as possible. Moberg has emphasized the fact that the hand's function is not simply motor function, but also sensation. He believes that people are very interested in human contact and that hands that are made more rigid by multiple tendon transfers and/or small joint arthrodeses are not well accepted by patients. His concept of the patient's priorities justifies his more conservative approach to surgical reconstruction in cases with few spared muscles.[36]

Contraindications to Operative Treatment

In my experience two factors have had a uniformly adverse effect on results of surgical treatment: spasticity and psychoneurosis. Spasticity that cannot be controlled by the patient is a strong contraindication to surgery. Freehafer, Vonhaam, and Allen[13] and Moberg have stated that some spasticity might be helpful, but judging the degree of spasticity compatible with good results is difficult. In fact, Moberg noted such an error in his poor result group.[35]

Psychoneurosis should be controlled prior to surgery. When the condition was not detected and left untreated, the results of surgery were unsatisfactory from the patient's point of view. Also, psychological problems can interfere significantly with postoperative training.

ELBOW EXTENSION

Elbow extension should be provided in patients whose spinal cord lesion spares the function of the deltoid. This operation has proved useful in patients who are not candidates for any other reconstructive surgery because elbow extension helps the patient stabilize himself in the wheelchair and improves control of self-help devices. It is required where transfer of the brachioradialis is being considered in Group 0 to Group 5 or 6 when the triceps is not innervated. Moberg has shown that active elbow extension improved the function of the transferred brachioradialis. As the brachioradialis is not only a supinator but also an elbow flexor, the deltoid-to-triceps transfer provides an antagonist. Most surgeons agree that the deltoid-to-triceps transfer should be the first operation performed.[30]

Deltoid-to-Triceps Transfer (Moberg)

A curved incision is made along the posterior border of the deltoid muscle, and the muscle is exposed to its insertion on the humerus. The posterior third (spinous portion) of the deltoid origin is separated from the middle or acromial portion distal to the axillary nerve by blunt dissection. The anterior border is dissected free, preserving the fibrous band to the brachialis, if present, which is useful in attaching the graft to the deltoid. The axillary nerve, whose course is about 4 to 5 cm distal to the acromion, must be protected. The posterior portion of the muscle belly is isolated (Fig. 43-2A), and the posterior portion of the insertion is carefully stripped away from the humerus to preserve as much tough tendinous tissue and periosteum as possible. Moberg recommends proximal dissection of the belly to increase the excursion of the muscle to 30 mm. To avoid damage to the axillary nerve, only the superficial aponeurosis is divided at the upper end of the muscle. The tendon of insertion of the triceps into the olecranon is then exposed through a separate curved incision. Tendon grafts to connect the deltoid to the triceps insertion can be obtained from many locations. Moberg prefers the toe extensors to the second, third, and fourth toes, which he obtains through multiple incisions on the dorsum of the foot and anterior surface of the ankle. The additional length required is obtained by adding more small incisions about the ankle or by using a tendon stripper. There should be adequate tendon graft material to make at least three loops at the attachment site.

Next, a tunnel is made between the two incisions on the arm in the plane between subcutaneous fat and the triceps muscle. The tendon grafts are laced into the distal end of the deltoid muscle belly and into the triceps aponeurosis (Fig. 43-2B). The laced tendon grafts are sutured into place with moderate tension while the elbow is held in full extension and the humerus abducted 30 to 40 degrees.

Other variations on Moberg's method of connecting the deltoid to the triceps have been used. The object of the modifications is to improve the strength of the connections and to reduce the time of immobilization. These were reported at the Fourth International Conference on Surgical Rehabilitation of the Upper Limb in Tetraplegia held in Palo Alto, California in May 1991.[26] Gellman uses the tibialis anterior tendon, Lamb uses the extensor carpi radialis longus, Tessier incorporates a woven dacron graft in the repair, and Ejeskar does the operation in two stages. First, he places fascia lata around the deltoid and allows that to heal so that at a second stage, he will have a strong attachment for his tendon grafts to the deltoid.

I prefer Hentz's method[18] of using fascia lata as the interposition graft because of the large contact surface into the triceps tendon insertion and into the muscle belly of the posterior deltoid (Fig. 43-2C). Also, enough length can be obtained to attach the graft to the most distal end of the triceps and even directly to the olecranon if the surgeon wishes. There is not enough experience with any alternative tendon graft method to suggest that these other techniques shorten the time of immobilization and staged rehabilitation described by Moberg. There is enough experience to recommend that the transfer be set relatively tight. Moberg has advanced the triceps insertion

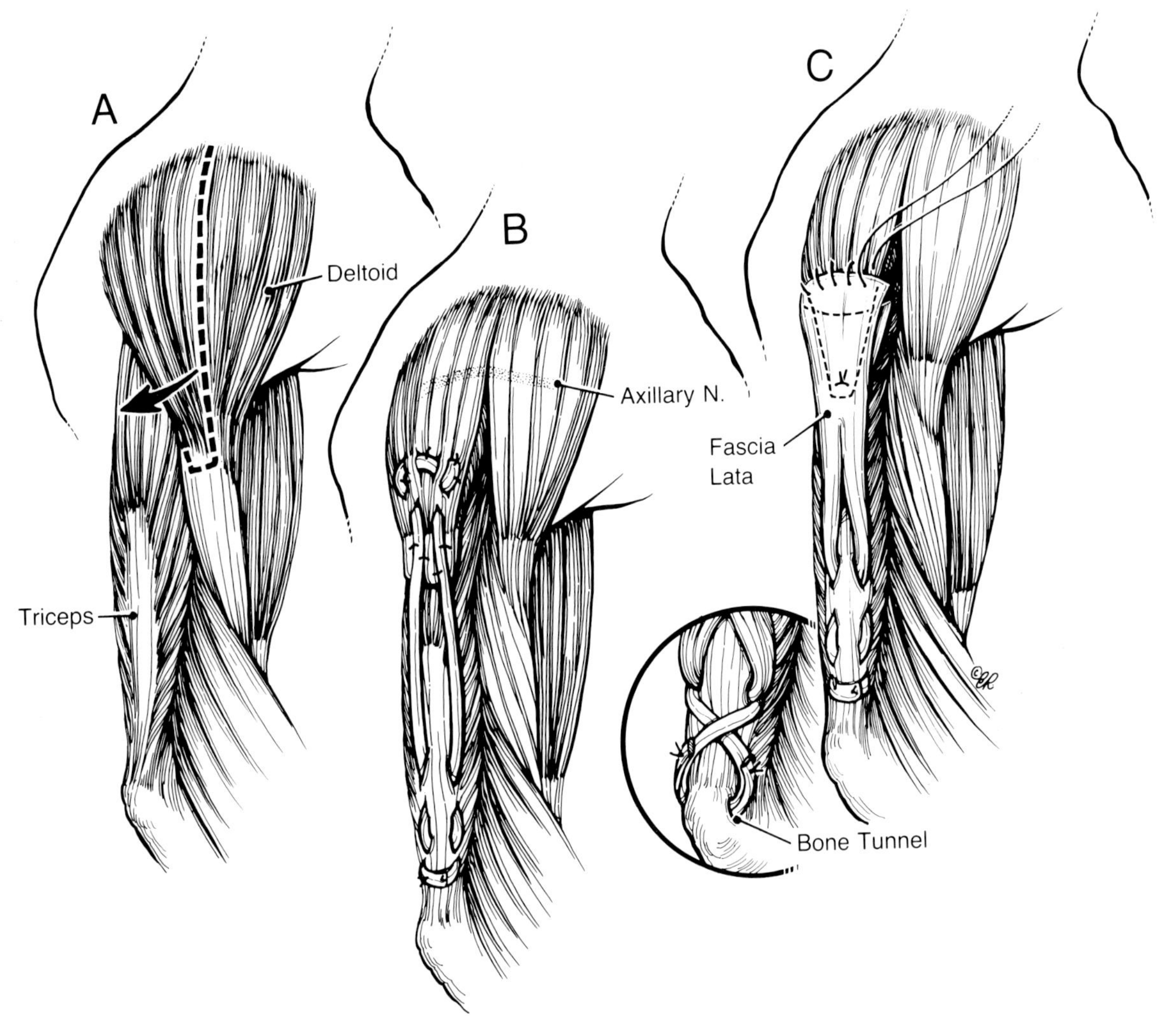

Fig. 43-2. Deltoid-to-triceps transfer (Moberg). **(A)** The posterior border of the muscle belly is isolated, preserving as much of the tendinous insertion as possible. **(B)** Tendon grafts are laced into the distal end of the deltoid muscle belly and triceps aponcurosis. **(C)** Use of fascia lata rather than tendon grafts. Direct insertion into the olecranon through a bone tunnel can also be done with either type of graft.

distalward in some cases where the transfers were too loose (Moberg E: personal communication).

Postoperative Management. A well-padded long arm plaster cylinder is applied to hold the elbow in 10 degrees flexion. The plaster stops just proximal to the wrist. Moberg recommends strapping the cast to the patient's waist until he is able to protect himself to prevent inadvertent stretching of the transfer. Also, he uses a local anesthetic in the deltoid muscle to prevent any inadvertent contraction of the muscle sufficient to rupture or stretch the suture lines during recovery from anesthesia. He administers 20 ml of 1 percent Xylocaine or Carbocaine with 1:200,000 epinephrine. The elbow is immobilized in 10 degrees flexion in the cast for 6 weeks. Gentle active exercises are then done to slowly gain flexion for the next 3 months (at a rate of 5 to 10 degrees flexion per week). For the first 2 months in this phase of rehabilitation, the patient should use a padded night splint designed to hold the elbow in 0 to 10 degrees flexion. The patient may be eager to gain elbow flexion too rapidly, and the surgeon may have to consider the use of a removable splint during part of the day also. Resistive exercises should be delayed until 4 months after surgery.

My patients prefer an elbow brace with a dial-lock hinge that can be used during the stage of progressive elbow flexion beginning at 6 weeks after surgery. It is lighter, cooler, and can be used many times.[18]

FOREARM PRONATION

Pronation is important to patients who have active wrist extension only (Groups 2 and 3). These patients use the automatic or "tenodesis" effect for grasp, but if the hand cannot be pronated, gravity cannot be used to produce palmar flexion and digital extension for release of grasp. Also, those patients using a "tenodesis" brace need pronation for the same reason. Zancolli produces pronation by converting the biceps into a forearm pronator. He reroutes the tendon around the radius in the opposite direction[51] (Fig. 43-3).

PROCEDURES ACCORDING TO CLASSIFICATION

Group 0

Patients whose spinal cord injury level is high enough to be classified under Group 0 may nonetheless be candidates for deltoid-to-triceps transfer for elbow extension. These patients should be considered for orthoses powered by an external source, such as the "CO_2 muscle" or an electric motor. Almost all of these patients can use some assistive devices attached to one hand.

A few patients in Group 0 may have a weak brachioradialis and a weak extensor carpi radialis longus. Tendon transfer may be considered if the surgeon thinks that the brachioradialis is strong enough to transfer to the weak radial wrist extensors and thus achieve sufficient strength to dorsiflex the wrist against resistance. If this is accomplished, the patient may be able to use a wrist-driven flexor hinge splint (Fig. 43-4) or a flexor pollicis longus tenodesis.

Few patients in this group will qualify for transfer. Assessing the strength of the brachioradialis muscle is difficult and requires an experienced examiner. It is best performed by having the patient flex his elbow against resistance, while the examiner evaluates muscle tension by trying to deflect the muscle belly. It is important to remember that the patient will need elbow extension to make good use of a brachioradialis transfer.

It is not likely that a patient in this group will have enough dorsiflexion strength to consider constructing a Moberg-type of simple grip.

Brachioradialis to Radial Wrist Extensor Transfer

Freehafer and Mast have described a useful method of transfer of the brachioradialis to the radial wrist extensors[11,13] (Fig. 43-5). They make an S-shaped or slightly curved incision on the radial side of the forearm near the junction of the proximal and middle thirds. At this site the brachioradialis is on the radial aspect of the forearm, the extensor carpi radialis longus is dorsal and parallel to it, and the extensor carpi radialis brevis is on the ulnar side of the longus. The tendons are exposed by opening their sheaths. The brachioradialis tendon is divided, preserving sufficient length of the proximal stump so that it can be threaded through the tendons of the extensor carpi radialis longus and brevis for a strong tendon juncture. Special care is required to protect the branches of the superficial radial nerve beneath the brachioradialis muscle and tendon. Another critical technical detail is adequate proximal dissection of the brachioradialis muscle belly. It must be mobilized toward the elbow sufficiently to increase its excursion to 3 cm or more.

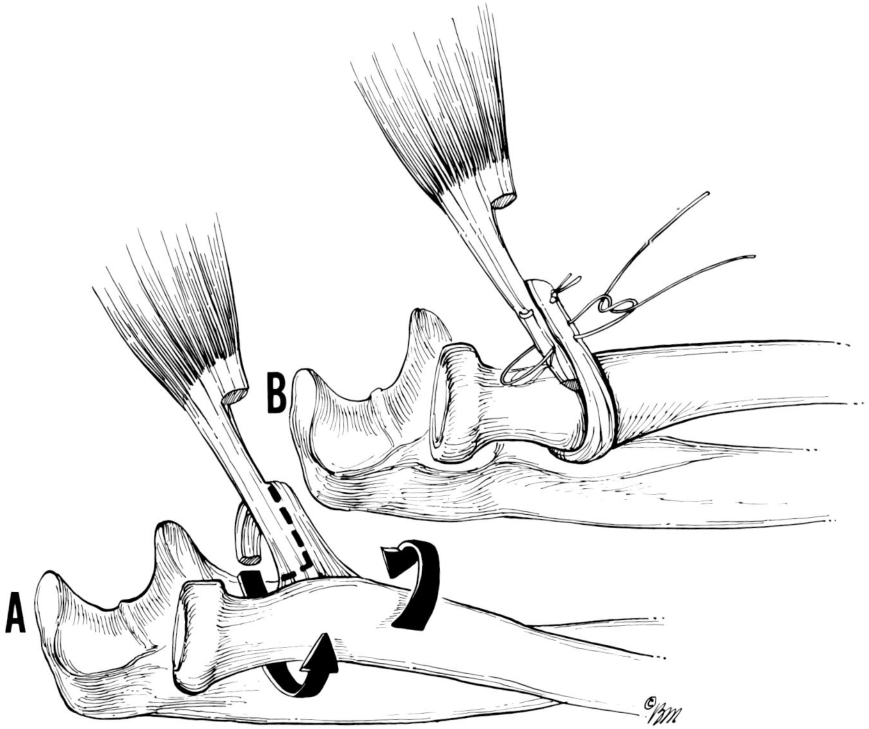

Fig. 43-3. Zancolli's method for rerouting the insertion of the biceps tendon to provide pronation of the forearm. Half of the tendon is passed behind the neck of the radius **(A)**, and then sutured into the remaining biceps tendon **(B)**. (Adapted from Zancolli,[51] with permission.)

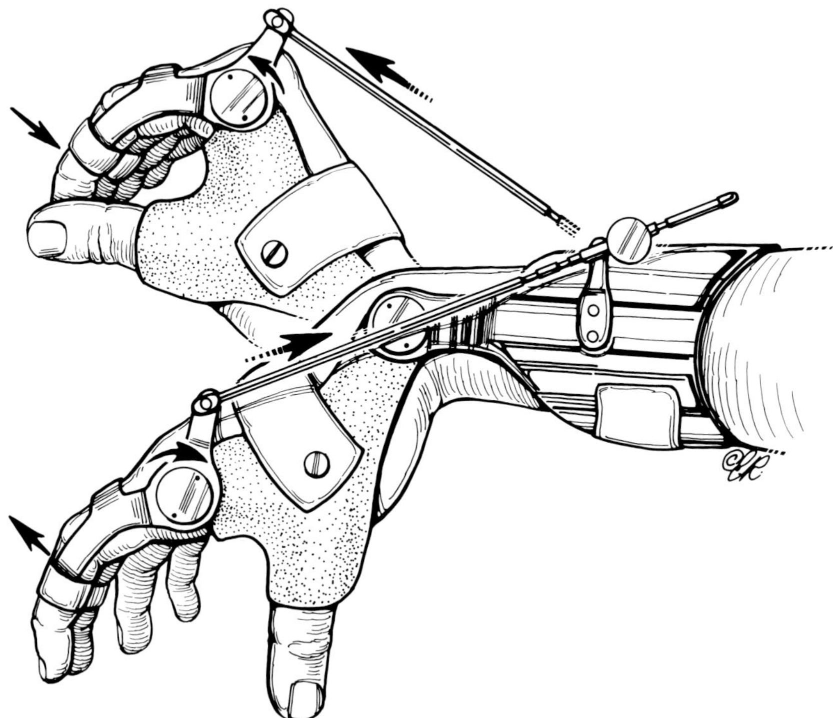

Fig. 43-4. The wrist-driven flexor hinge splint uses the principle of synergistic action. As the wrist is dorsiflexed, the fingers are flexed to bring them into contact with the thumb, which is fixed. As the wrist is volar flexed, the fingers are extended. In patients in Group 0, the splint may be powered by an external source, such as the "CO_2 muscle" or an electric motor. (Courtesy of T. Engen, MD.)

The brachioradialis tendon is passed through a small slit in the two radial wrist extensors, looped back, and sutured to itself. The brachioradialis tendon is also sutured to each of the radial wrist extensors. The tension should be sufficient to hold the wrist in zero degrees, but not so tight that the wrist cannot be fully flexed passively.

Postoperative Management. A long arm cast is applied at operation to hold the elbow in 90 degrees flexion and the wrist in 45 degrees dorsiflexion. The cast is removed at 4 weeks, and the patient is started on active strengthening exercises. A removable splint is worn to support the wrist when the patient is not exercising for an additional 3 weeks.

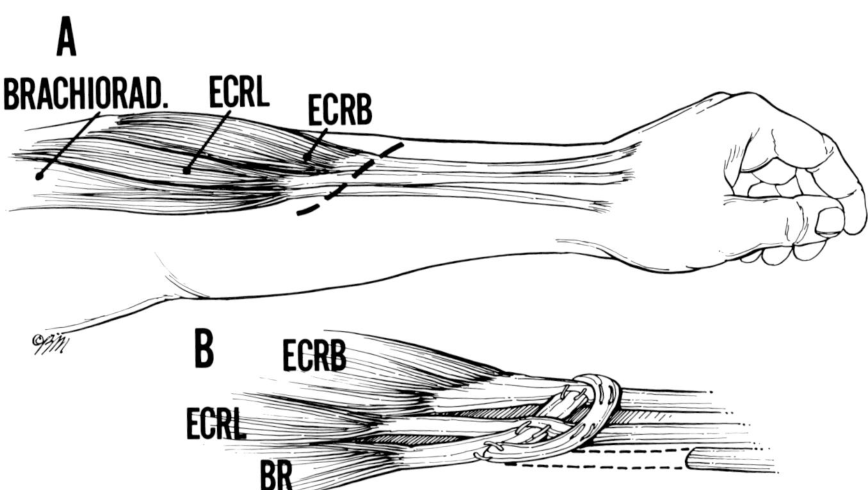

Fig. 43-5. A brachioradialis transfer to extensor carpi radialis longus and extensor carpi radialis brevis. An important technical detail is that the brachioradialis muscle belly must be mobilized completely to the elbow, taking care to protect its nerve supply from the radial nerve.

Group 1

Patients in Group 1 have a strong brachioradialis. Transfer of the brachioradialis to weak or nonfunctioning radial wrist extensors should provide sufficient strength to allow the patient to dorsiflex his wrist against at least 5 pounds of resistance. This is sufficient strength to operate a wrist-driven flexor hinge splint satisfactorily, or to consider a Moberg type of simple hand grip reconstruction to be performed at the same time as the brachioradialis-to-radial wrist extensor transfer is done. As Moberg and others have suggested, the brachioradialis transfer will function better if it has an antagonist. Thus, a deltoid-to-triceps transfer should be done before the brachioradialis is transferred.[30]

The simple hand grip procedure was designed to produce a key grip of thumb-to-radial side of index finger. Moberg[36] believes that the key grip is more useful to the tetraplegic patient. His procedure does not interfere with the interlacing grip used by patients who have no finger motors. The interlacing grip is accomplished by passively weaving a utensil through the fingers. The simple hand grip does not produce a stiff hand, which Moberg believes is unacceptable to the tetraplegic patient because it makes contact with other people less pleasant.[6,37]

The alternative operation is the wrist-driven flexor hinge hand described by Nickel, Perry, and Garrett.[40] Their operation includes making a post of the thumb in an abducted position by arthrodesis of the interphalangeal and MP joints and by insertion of a bone block between the first and second metacarpals. In addition, the interphalangeal joints of the index and long fingers are fused. The profundus tendons of the index and long fingers are tenodesed to the distal radius so that, upon wrist dorsiflexion, the tips of those two fingers are brought into contact with the thumb in a three-point palmar pinch. Their operation has been further modified by Beasley.[1]

In my experience, patient acceptance and functional improvement have been better with a simple hand grip rather than the wrist-driven flexor hinge hand.

Moberg's Simple Hand Grip (Key Pinch) Procedure

Moberg described the simple hand grip reconstruction in six steps (Fig. 43-6).

1. Strong wrist dorsiflexion is a prerequisite, and brachioradialis transfer, if needed, can be done at the same operation. Gravity provides wrist palmar flexion.
2. The annular ligaments of the thumb are released to permit bowstringing of the flexor pollicis longus. This is done through an oblique incision over the flexor surface of the proximal phalanx. The digital nerves and arteries are carefully retracted and the annular ligaments divided. The

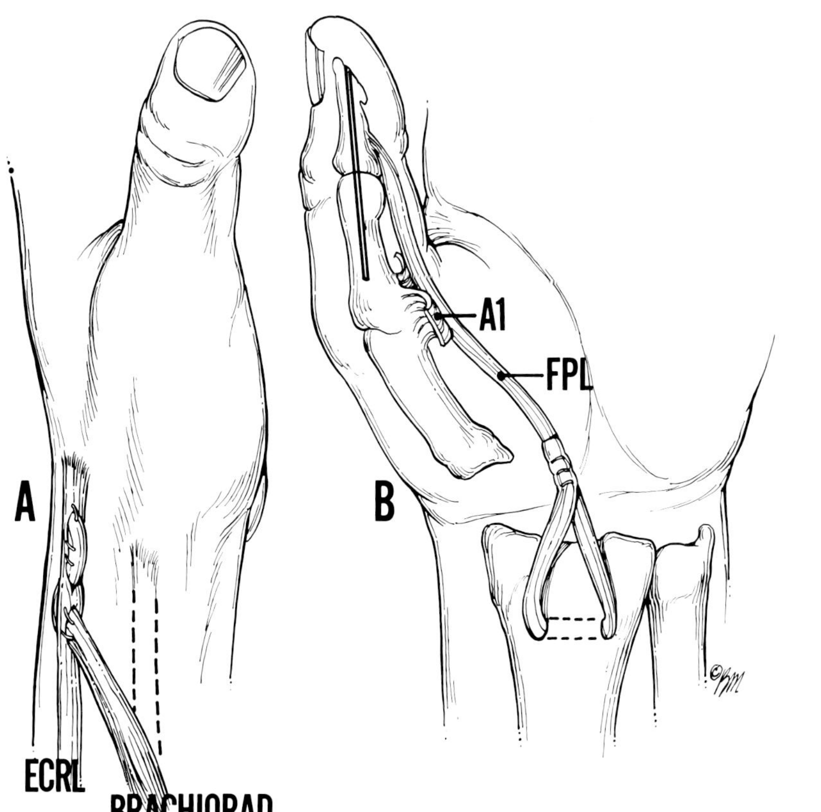

Fig. 43-6. Moberg's operation to create the "simple hand grip" (see text). (From Moberg,[37] with permission.)

results of this phase should be checked by lifting the flexor pollicis longus tendon out of the wound.

3. Release of the annular ligaments will improve the mechanical advantage of the flexor pollicis longus tenodesis to the volar surface of the distal radius. A curved 6- to 7-cm incision is made from the proximal wrist flexion crease along the radial volar side of the forearm. The palmar cutaneous branch of the median nerve should be preserved. The flexor tendons and the median nerve are retracted to expose the flexor pollicis longus tendon. The distal muscle fibers are removed from the tendon, and the tendon is divided 6 to 7 cm proximal to the wrist. An incision is made in the pronator quadratus along its radial border, and the muscle is elevated as a flap toward the ulna. Two holes are made into the metaphysis of the radius and connected, leaving a bridge of cortex between them. The distal stump of the flexor pollicis longus tendon is pulled into the bone through the ulnar hole and out through the radial hole with a wire loop. This wound is then closed temporarily with a single stitch.
4. The surgeon then proceeds to the dorsal tenodesis of the extensor hood mechanism to the metacarpal of the thumb for prevention of hyperflexion of the MP joint. This part of the operation is strongly recommended. A dorsal midline incision is made, the extensor mechanism is displaced, about 3 cm of the periosteum on the dorsum of the metacarpal is scraped, and three or four pairs of holes are made in the cortex. Nonabsorbable sutures are used to compress the extensor mechanism against the scraped periosteum. An arthrodesis of this joint can be used to salvage a failed tenodesis.
5. The thumb interphalangeal joint is fixed with a large threaded K-wire at about zero degrees. The wire should be buried beneath the cortex of the distal phalanx. This can be accomplished by measuring and cutting the pin preoperatively. A slot is made in the blunt end of the pin, which will receive a small screwdriver. At operation the short pin is inserted as far as possible with a drill and driven farther with a screwdriver.
6. Resection or division of the retinaculum over the extensor carpi radialis longus and brevis is done to allow bowstringing and thus improve the mechanical advantage. However, this procedure decreases the amplitude of wrist motion. In a patient with a supination deformity, the tendons may displace to the radial side of the wrist and act as wrist flexors. Finally, the surgeon returns to the forearm where the tenodesis of the flexor pollicis longus is completed. It is attached to itself with a few sutures to make a loop and to test the tension. The thumb should contact the radial side of the index finger with the wrist in neutral.

Since Moberg first reported his simple "key grip" procedure, many of these operations have been done. Hentz, Brown, and Keoshian reviewed their experience in 1983.[18] They agreed that key grip was an achievable functional goal that was well accepted by their patients, but they described a number of complications, which included stretching out of the flexor pollicis longus tenodesis, excessive flexion of the MP joint secondary to stretching of the extensor pollicis longus tenodesis, and frequent breakage of the pin used to fix the thumb interphalangeal joint. My own experience parallels that of Hentz, Brown, and Keoshian. I have accepted their suggestions for modifying the original description by increasing the immobilization time to 4 weeks to try to prevent flexor pollicis longus tenodesis stretching, making a slot in the shaft of the metacarpal for tenodesis of the extensor pollicis longus to try to prevent stretching of that tenodesis, and fusing the thumb interphalangeal joint to try to avoid complications with pin breakage. My experience with the modifications suggested by Hentz and his co-workers[18] has produced a better quality of result.

Brand[2] suggested other modifications, which included avoiding release of the A1 pulley in the thumb and passing the flexor pollicis longus deep to the digital flexor tendons, through Guyon's canal, and on to the radius for tenodesis. He reasoned that the vector produced would provide better thumb adduction and that leaving the A1 pulley intact would reduce the tendency toward thumb MP joint hyperflexion. He also suggested tenodesing the extensor pollicis longus to the radial side of the radius to provide more thumb abduction. A clinical study of Brand's modification showed that the quality of grasp and release was not as good as in the Moberg operation. Reasons proposed[26] were that tenodesing the extensor pollicis longus on the radial side of the radius produces no tension on the tendon upon flexion of the wrist. In addition, passing the flexor pollicis longus around Guyon's canal allows for so much slack in the system that strong wrist dorsiflexion does not produce strong tension (pinch) of the tenodesed flexor pollicis longus.

Postoperative Management. A thumb spica cast is applied with the wrist in slight dorsiflexion to reduce the tension on the brachioradialis transfer, and the thumb is adducted under the fingers to prevent tension at the tenodesis site. Casting is continued for 4 weeks before an active exercise program is started. The program of education in the use of the grip is graduated so that maximum stress on the hand is delayed until 2 months after surgery.

Group 2

This group has active wrist extension because the extensor carpi radialis longus is functioning at MRC Grade 4 or better. In this group the extensor carpi radialis brevis is not functioning or is too weak to change the patient's classification.

Patients in this group can operate a tenodesis splint and are candidates for the simple hand grip reconstruction or any of the other procedures that depend on active wrist extension for some form of automatic grip discussed in Group 1.

The brachioradialis is available for transfer and has been used in a variety of ways. Street and Stambaugh[48] recognized the value of side pinch or "key grip" in 1959 and, in an attempt to increase the strength of pinch, transferred the brachioradialis to the flexor policis longus. Moberg reported four patients with brachioradialis transfer to flexor pollicis longus, and, upon comparison he found the flexor pollicis longus tenodesis to be stronger than the transfer. Also, Moberg used the brachioradialis to open the thumb-index web space to improve the release phase of the grasp-release sequence. He tested the extensor pollicis longus, extensor pollicis brevis, and abductor pollicis longus at surgery to determine which gave the best abduction and then transferred the brachioradialis to that one. He did this operation as a second-stage procedure, following construction of a simple hand grip. He reported that the additional abduction was not as useful to the patient as he had anticipated.[37] House likes to stabilize the thumb carpometacarpal joint with an arthrodesis to assure positioning the thumb in some abduction.[21,52] In selected cases he does transfer the brachioradialis to the flexor pollicis longus.

I do not transfer the brachioradialis in Group 2 patients.

Group 3

As the level of spinal cord injury moves distally, the next muscle innervated is the extensor carpi radialis brevis. Proof of strength of both radial wrist extensors depends on testing by the method of Curtis[4] as described on page 1517. When both radial wrist extensors are stong, one is available for transfer. Most surgeons recommend leaving the extensor carpi radialis brevis in place because its insertion is more central and is a better wrist extensor.[19,27,51]

Patients in Group 3 have strong wrist dorsiflexion and might be content with a flexor hinge splint, but surgical reconstruction should be considered. The surgeon can keep reconstruction simple by performing a simple hand grip procedure or some other tenodesis operation. If a more complex method is selected, the brachioradialis and extensor carpi radialis longus are available for transfer. Zancolli prefers tendon transfers in this group. His procedure is divided into two stages because different positions of immobilization are required for proper healing after each stage.[51]

Zancolli's Two-stage Reconstruction

Stage I

At the first stage, Zancolli's goals are to construct finger and thumb extension tenodeses, prevent or reduce claw deformity with intrinsic tenodeses, and stabilize the thumb by interphalangeal joint fusion. (Capsulodesis of the MP joint is done at the second stage if the joint hyperextends too much for good thumb-to-side-of-index-finger contact.

Zancolli makes an 8- to 10-cm longitudinal incision on the radial side of the forearm and exposes the dorsum of the radius proximal to the extensor retinaculum. A window, large enough to accept the distal stumps of the common extensor tendons (which have been divided just distal to the musculotendinous junction), is made on the dorsum of the radius. Tendon balance is preserved by suturing the distal stumps together. The ends of the sutures are brought through two drill holes made proximal to the window, drawing the tendon stumps snugly into the bone window. The sutures are tied to each other for fixation. Zancolli sets the tension so that the finger MP joints will be extended to zero degrees with the wrist in slight palmar flexion. (In patients in Group 5 who have a functional flexor carpi radialis, he sets the tension in the MP joints with the wrist at zero degrees.)

Zancolli's original description of the procedure utilized a modified Fowler-type intrinsic tenodesis, but he has subsequently described a simpler and more useful method of reducing claw deformity that is called the lasso operation (Fig. 43-7).[51] The operation uses the superficialis to flex the MP joints. In patients with no voluntary flexion of the superficialis, the muscle tone alone can assist. Chevron-shaped incisions are made across the MP joint flexion creases, and the A1 and A2 pulleys are exposed. An incision is made in the A2 pulley distal to the MP jcint. The superficialis tendon is divided through the hole in the A2 pulley. The proximal stump is pulled through the incision in the A2 pulley and it is attached to itself in the form of a loop or "lasso" with side-to-side sutures. Enough tension is applied to produce mild MP joint flexion so that the interphalangeal joints can be extended by the extensor tenodesis when it is activated by wrist palmar flexion.

A strip of the abductor pollicis longus tendon is freed up through the original radial longitudinal incision and is kept small enough to pass it proximally through the tunnel of the extensor pollicis longus around Lister's tubercle and into the window on the dorsum of the radius, where it and the tendon of the extensor pollicis longus are sutured to the bone with wire, as described for the common extensor tendons. This tenodesis will produce thumb extension.

Arthrodesis of the thumb interphalangeal joint is done to prevent hyperflexion of the joint and to facilitate side pinch. I prefer Carroll's technique of small joint fusion (see Chapter 4).

Postoperative Management. Zancolli recommends immobilization for 5 weeks in a cast, with the wrist, thumb, and fingers in extension. He also suggests an additional week of immobilization when the patient has a strong flexor carpi radialis (Group 5). Active extension exercises are then begun; gentle passive exercises are necessary when there is no active flexor carpi radialis. Pins used for fixation of the thumb interphalangeal joint arthrodesis are left in until the fusion is solid at about 8 to 12 weeks.

Stage II

When scar resolution is complete and the preoperative range of motion is restored, the second-stage operation is done. The objective of this operation is to establish some digital flexion.

The same radial lateral incision used in Stage I is reopened to expose the extensor carpi radialis longus and the flexor digitorum profundus tendons. The extensor carpi radialis longus is detached at its insertion and transferred to the flexor digitorum profundus tendons with a side-to-side connection. Tension is set so that the fingers and thumb come together in a lateral pinch with the wrist in about 20 degrees dorsiflexion. The tension is set loosely enough to allow easy release of the fingers during wrist flexion.

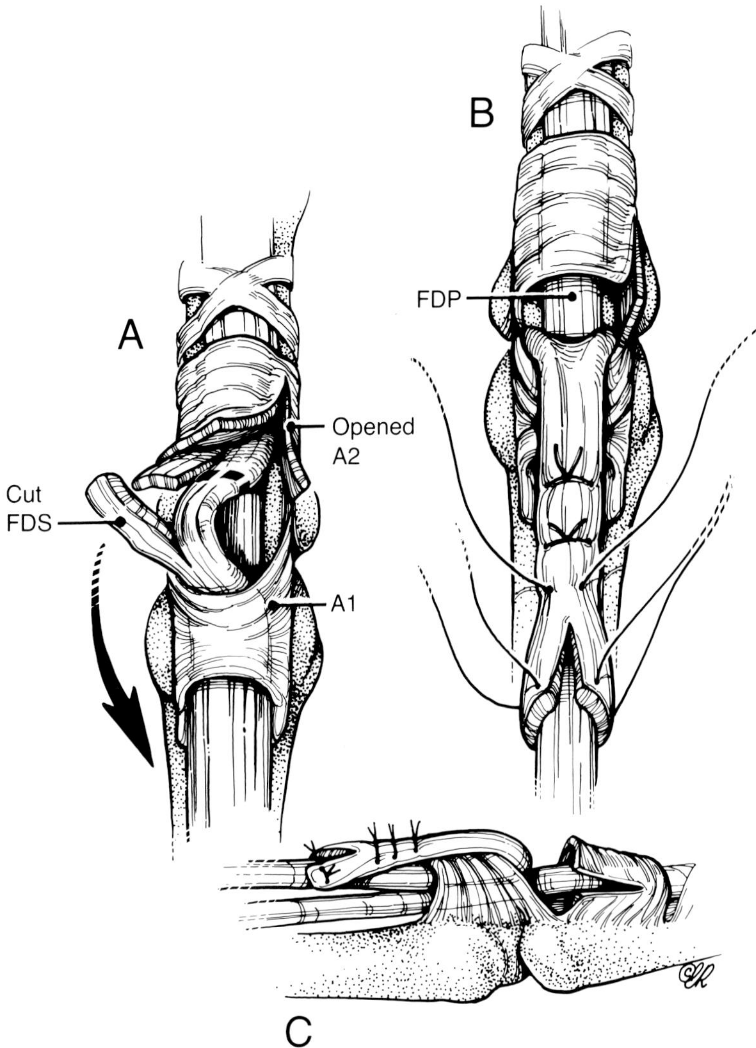

Fig. 43-7. Zancolli's lasso operation can be used to produce some MP joint flexion in Groups 3–9 patients. This facilitates extension of the interphalangeal joints (see text). (Adapted from Zancolli,[51] with permission.)

The brachioradialis is detached from its insertion (leaving a short stump) and dissected well proximally so that maximum excursion can be obtained. The brachioradialis is sutured to the flexor pollicis longus, with tension set to achieve lateral pinch with the wrist in about 20 degrees dorsiflexion (the same as in the extensor carpi radialis longus transfer).

If the thumb MP joint is hyperextended, a capsulodesis should be done. The volar capsule should be fixed to bone. The flexor tendon sheath is exposed through a transverse incision just proximal to the thumb MP joint flexion crease. The sheath is opened and the flexor pollicis longus retracted away from the volar plate. Care should be taken to protect the digital nerves. A longitudinal incision is made in the volar plate to expose the neck of the metacarpal. Two holes are drilled in the bone to receive a nonabsorbable suture. The volar plate is pulled proximally and sutured against the bone. Tension is set with the MP joint in 10 degrees flexion.

Zancolli also constructs a volar tenodesis of the extensor pollicis brevis tendon if the thumb is in excessive extension and lateral pinch is impaired. Through the radial incision, the extensor pollicis brevis tendon is divided as far proximally as possible. The tendon is passed through the flexor carpi radialis tunnel and sutured into the short distal stump of the brachioradialis, which was left in place when it was divided for transfer previously. Tension is set to hold the thumb in complete abduction with the wrist in moderate flexion.

Postoperative Management. Immobilization in a cast for 5 weeks precedes gentle active range of motion exercises.

Group 4

In patients in Group 4 the pronator teres is intact and is available for transfer, but has been used only by Zancolli. The pronator teres is useful in its role as an antagonist to the biceps.

By providing active pronation, it enhances the effect of gravity on the wrist-activated tenodeses. Zancolli has transferred the pronator teres to the flexor carpi radialis to strengthen wrist flexion and further enhance the usefulness of the wrist-activated tenodesis operations.

In patients in this group, I prefer not to transfer the pronator teres to reduce the complexity of the operation. Patients like their ability to control pronation and supination and I believe that preserving this function improves results after tenodesing operations.

In Groups 2, 3, and 4 where the patient has strong wrist extension, Moberg prefers the simpler key grip operation and I agree with his plan with the modifications described.

I reserve the more complex operations for patients in Group 5 and lower where there is also strong wrist flexion and the quality of sensibility is better.

Group 5

The flexor carpi radialis is intact in this group, and the patients have active control of wrist flexion as well as extension. The brachioradialis, extensor carpi radialis longus, and pronator teres muscles are available for transfer. In 1958 Lipscomb, Elkins, and Henderson[27] and in 1971 Lamb and Landry[25] reported transfer of the flexor carpi radialis in this group. The current method favors leaving the flexor carpi radialis in place to preserve wrist control for its beneficial "tenodesis" effect.

The operative plan described by House, Gwathmey, and Lundsgaard[19] conforms to this proposition. These authors leave the extensor carpi radialis brevis and the flexor carpi radialis in place for wrist control and combine extensor tenodeses and tendon transfers to activate the digits in a two-stage operation. House and colleagues call the two stages the *extensor phase* (the wrist is palmar flexed and the digits extend) and *the flexor phase* (the wrist is dorsiflexed to supplement the action of the tendon transfer to the digital flexors). House has been comparing the results of two methods of reconstruction in group 5 patients. The first two-stage method was described in 1976[19] and the second in 1985.[20] His second method uses Zancolli's techniques for thumb stabilization and control of claw deformity of the fingers.[51,52] House concludes in his comparative study that both methods are satisfactory and have slightly different indications.

I prefer his second method because thumb positioning and stabilization is assured if the fusion is successful, and there are less chances for error when balancing transfers to activate the thumb for key pinch. I favor Zancolli's lasso method (Fig. 43-7) of controlling clawing of the fingers because it leaves the hand in a more flexible condition. In addition, it does not prevent extension of the finger MP joints, allowing the patient to open his grasp wide enough to accept larger objects.

House's Two-stage Reconstruction

Extensor Phase

The extensor phase requires either a tenodesis of the common extensor and the extensor pollicis longus to the distal radius or a transfer of the brachioradialis to the common extensors and the extensor pollicis longus for digital extension. The thumb is stabilized by carpometacarpal joint arthrodesis (my preference) or tenodesis of the abductor pollicis longus.

To accomplish either tenodesis or tendon transfer, a gently curved dorsal incision is begun just proximal to Lister's tubercle and is extended in a line convex to the radial side of the forearm for approximately 6 to 8 cm. The branches of the radial nerve must be protected. The skin flap should be dissected far enough to the radial side to expose the insertion of the brachioradialis into the radius if one has chosen the tendon transfer. If the transfer is the method chosen, then the brachioradialis is detached from its insertion into the radius and carefully dissected proximally to detach it from the forearm fascia, which limits its excursion. The brachioradialis is then attached to the extensor pollicis longus and the common extensors to the fingers by passing the distal stump of the brachioradialis through each individual tendon. Tension should be set so that the thumb is in full extension and the MP joints of the fingers are at zero degrees with the wrist in 35 to 40 degrees flexion.

If the choice is to do a tenodesing operation, the extensor pollicis longus and the common extensors are set at the same tension as described for brachioradialis transfer but they are attached to a window made in the distal and dorsal portion of the radius (Fig. 43-8).

Carpometacarpal joint arthrodesis to stabilize the base of the thumb is performed through a transverse or oblique incision at the base of the thumb metacarpal. Care must be taken to identify and protect the multiple branches of the superficial radial

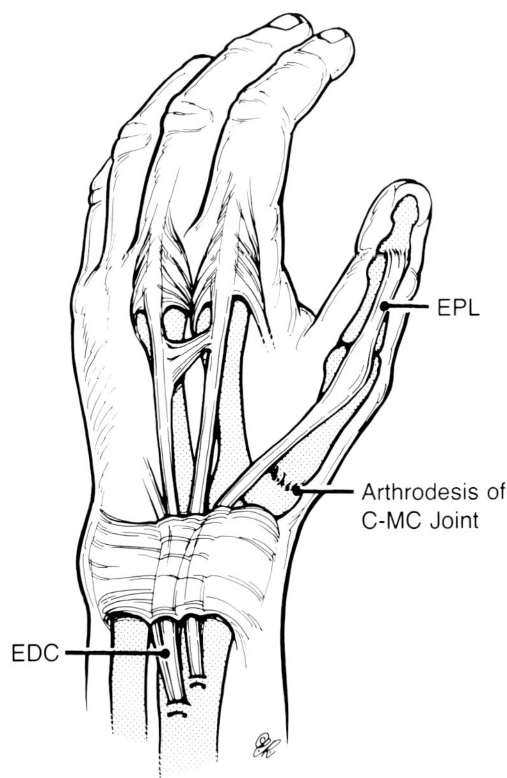

Fig. 43-8. Stage I (extensor phase) of House's two-stage reconstruction for patients in Group 5 (modified—see text). (Adapted from House et al,[19] with permission.)

nerve and the radial artery as it passes dorsal to the capsule of the thumb carpometacarpal joint. The base of the thumb metacarpal and the distal articular surface of the trapezium are removed by osteotomy so that the metacarpal is placed in a position of approximately 40 to 45 degrees palmar abduction, 20 to 25 degrees extension, and 10 to 15 degrees pronation. Either internal or percutaneous fixation is important to increase the chances for union. After carpometacarpal joint fusion some patients may develop a collapse deformity of the thumb, with MP joint hyperextension and IP joint hyperflexion. If that occurs, it can be corrected by arthrodesis of the IP joint or capsulodesis of the MP joint.[20]

Postoperative Management. Postoperative immobilization should hold the wrist in 40 to 45 degrees extension and the cast should include the thumb in the position described above. Immobilization is maintained with a cast or plaster splints for 4 weeks. At this stage, the cast is removed but the thumb carpometacarpal joint arthrodesis should be protected with an orthosis that will still allow wrist flexion and extension and finger flexion and extension for gentle active and passive mobilization. The arthrodesis site at the base of the thumb is protected until there is evidence of solid union.

When the patient has a solid union and passive range of motion is restored so that the tenodesis of the extensor pollicis longus and common extensors is functioning, the second phase can be performed.

Flexor Phase

In the flexor phase, (Fig. 43-9) the available extensor carpi radialis longus and pronator teres are employed for active digital flexion and pinch. All of the transfers are done during one operation. A gently curved incision is made on the flexor surface of the forearm. It should begin distally at the proximal wrist flexion crease and extend proximally about 8 to 10 cm, with the skin flap being convex to the ulnar side. Through this incision, the flexor digitorum profundus and flexor pollicis longus tendons are exposed at and distal to their musculotendinous junctions. Next, the extensor carpi radialis longus is exposed through a small incision over its insertion into the base of the second metacarpal, where it is divided. A portion of the proximal end of the previous (extensor phase) dorsal incision can be used to expose the extensor carpi radialis longus proximal to the bellies of the extensor pollicis brevis and abductor pollicis longus. The tendon is withdrawn into this incision, and the belly is dissected away from its investing fascia to improve its excursion and to create a straight line to its new insertion. It is passed from the proximal dorsal wound through a subcutaneous tunnel around the radial side of the forearm into the volar wound.

The pronator teres is then detached from the radius. A strip of periosteum should be raised distal to its insertion to make the tendon long enough for strong connection to the flexor pollicis longus. A weaving type of juncture is created between the pronator teres and the flexor pollicis longus and between the extensor carpi radialis longus and the profundus tendons to the index, long, ring, and little fingers. Tension is adjusted so that with the wrist in about 30 degrees extension the thumb will touch the radial side of the index finger. To be certain that the tension is not too tight, the wrist should be flexed to check for adequate passive thumb and finger extension by the tenodesis or brachioradialis transfer. In setting the tension at the junction between the extensor carpi radialis longus and the flexor digitorum profundus, one should err on the side of looseness, as it is better too loose than too tight, since when it is too tight, the patient cannot get enough extension to grasp larger objects.

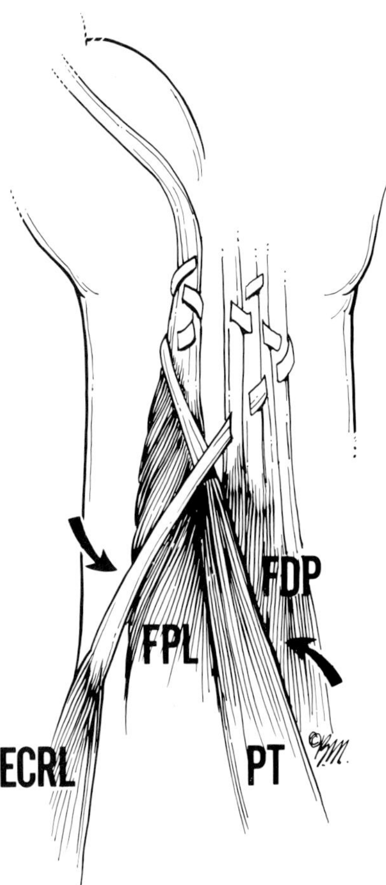

Fig. 43-9. Stage II (flexor phase) of House's two-stage reconstruction for patients in Group 5 (modified—see text). (Adapted from House et al,[19] with permission.)

The final step in the flexor phase is to perform the "lasso" intrinsic transfer (see Fig. 43-7). This part of the procedure can be performed through a single transverse incision across the palm just proximal to the MP joint flexion creases of the fingers. Through this incision, the flexor tendons proximal to the A1 pulley, the A1 pulley, and the proximal portion of the A2 pulley are exposed. The distal portion of the A1 pulley or the proximal portion of the A2 pulley is grasped with a skin hook or other instrument and pulled upon to be certain that it causes flexion of the MP joint. At this site, an L-shaped incision is made in the pulley as depicted in the illustration. Then the superficialis tendon is pulled as far proximal as possible with the PIP joint in flexion, and both tails of the tendon are divided. The two tails are then withdrawn through the L-shaped incision, folded over the intact A1 pulley and sutured to the superficialis proximal to the A1 pulley, thus creating a loop of superficialis tendon around the A1 pulley. Tension is set against the viscoelastic force of the superficialis, as it is paralyzed and will not function actively. Enough tension is applied so that the MP joints extend to 0 degrees when the wrist is flexed to 35 to 40 degrees. If more extension is allowed at the MP joint with the wrist in flexion, the claw deformity will not be ameliorated.

Postoperative Management. The hand is immobilized using plaster splints with the wrist dorsiflexed about 25 degrees and the fingers flexed at the MP joints and gently extended at the interphalangeal joints for about 3 weeks. This should be followed by 4 weeks of graduated active and passive range of motion exercises and muscle reeducation. The patient should not be allowed to push a wheelchair, transfer, or engage in any other activity that causes full wrist dorsiflexion for at least 10 weeks.

Group 6

At this level, the finger extensors are strong, but extensor pollicis longus function is either absent or too weak to extend the thumb adequately. For patients in this group the extensor phase of reconstruction as described for Group 5 is modified. Tenodesis of the common extensors to the radius is not required. The extensor pollicis longus can be sutured to the common extensors so that active extension of the fingers will produce extension of the thumb.

A gently curved incision is made over the distal forearm, beginning proximal to the dorsal retinaculum. The common extensor tendons and the extensor pollicis longus tendon are identified. Peritenon is scraped away from the extensor pollicis longus tendon and the common extensor tendon to the index finger on the adjacent surfaces for about 2 to 3 cm. They are firmly sutured together with three or four horizontal mattress sutures of a nonabsorbable material. If the common extensor tendon to the index finger is small, additional common extensor tendons can be included to produce a strong union. Tension is set with all extensors in the relaxed posture.

Postoperative Management. A short arm cast is applied at operation with the thumb, fingers, and wrist in slight dorsiflexion. The cast is removed in 4 weeks, and the patient begins gentle active extension exercises. Resistance exercises for the thumb and fingers are not allowed until 6 weeks after the operation.

After rehabilitation from this phase is completed, the flexor phase operation is performed as described for Group 5.

Group 7

Patients in this group have a strong extensor pollicis longus, so extensor phase reconstruction is not required. Results following surgery in patients in Groups 6 and 7 are much better than in higher groups because normal extensor function gives the patient more precise control.

Group 8

This group includes all patients who have weak activity of the long flexors. Usually, the long flexors to the ulnar digits (ring and small fingers) are strong and those to the thumb, index, and long fingers are weak.

Flexion of the index and long fingers can be improved or strengthened by connecting all four profundus tendons together. An active motor should be transferred to give independent function of the flexor pollicis longus. Finally, an intrinsic replacement using the "lasso" procedure will ameliorate the tendency toward clawing of the fingers. The thumb can be positioned either by carpometacarpal joint arthrodesis as described with Group 5 or an opponens transfer. I prefer the two-staged reconstruction as described by Zancolli.[52]

Stage I

At the first stage, the profundus tendons are united and a transfer of the brachioradialis to the flexor pollicis longus is done. Both procedures can be done through a gently curved volar incision that should begin near the palmaris longus at the distal wrist flexion crease, making the curve convex to the radial side, and extending to the proximal one-third of the forearm. The palmar cutaneous branch of the median nerve should be protected. The skin should be undermined on the radial side of the forearm sufficiently to expose the brachioradialis for detachment from its insertion and adequate proximal dissection. The median and radial nerves must be protected. The four profundus tendons are exposed by opening the forearm fascia and retracting ulnarward the median nerve with its palmar cutaneous branch and the four superficial tendons. A site in the distal forearm is selected for side-to-side suture of the four profundus tendons. The peritenon is scraped away from the tendons for a distance of 3 cm, and the tendons are sutured together with horizontal mattress sutures using nonabsorbable material. The fingers should be evenly balanced during the connection. Next, the brachioradialis is transferred directly to the flexor pollicis longus and connected by braiding the tendon of the brachioradialis into the tendon of the flexor pollicis longus with the wrist in neutral and the thumb just touching the side of the index finger, with mild tension on the brachioradialis.

Postoperative Management. A thumb spica cast is applied to the fingertips for 4 weeks, with each joint held in about 20 to 30 degrees flexion, the thumb straight at the MP and interphalangeal joints, and the wrist at 30 degrees flexion. Gentle active and passive range of motion and muscle reeducation can begin immediately and should be carried on until a full range of motion is restored.

Stage II

At the second stage, an opponens transfer is used to abduct the thumb, and Zancolli's "lasso" procedure is used to control claw deformity of the fingers. Zancolli recommends transfer of the extensor carpi radialis longus to the flexor digitorum superficialis tendons, to produce active control of the "lasso" intrinsic replacement. The opponens transfer can be motored by the flexor carpi ulnaris, and the palmaris longus can be used as a free tendon graft (if it is not present, a toe extensor or the plantaris tendon may be used) to extend the tendon of the flexor carpi ulnaris to its insertion into the ulnar side of the base of the proximal phalanx of the thumb. The flexor carpi ulnaris is exposed through an L-shaped incision over its insertion, which is split in half for a distance of 3 to 4 cm proximal to its insertion. One-half of the tendon is left attached to the pisiform, and this segment is divided 3 to 4 cm proximal to the insertion. The proximal end of this segment is sutured to the insertion to create a loop. The other half is detached from the pisiform and attached to the proximal end of the free tendon graft using a braiding technique. A subcutaneous tunnel is created from the loop to the MP joint of the thumb. The tendon graft is passed around the loop at the pisiform and through the subcutaneous tunnel to be attached to the tendon of the abductor pollicis brevis at the base of the proximal phalanx. Tension is adjusted so that with the wrist at neutral the thumb pulp will just touch the radial side of the index finger.

The intrinsic replacement procedure is modified as described by Zancolli by transferring the extensor carpi radialis longus tendon to the superficialis tendons in the forearm. Tension on the transfer is set only after the distal portion of the lasso procedure is done at the base of the fingers (see page 1528). Once that portion of the procedure is completed, the union is completed in the forearm. Tension is set so that with the wrist at neutral the MP joints of the fingers are at zero degrees.

Postoperative Management. A thumb spica cast is applied, extending across the MP joints of the fingers so the wrist is fixed at about 30 degrees flexion, the MP joints of the fingers in about 30 degrees flexion, and the thumb in wide abduction and opposition. The cast is removed after 4 weeks, and gentle active motion and muscle reeducation are started. Progression to full active and passive motion should be started 6 weeks after surgery.

This group also includes patients who have Grade 4 MRC strength in all the profundus tendons and the flexor pollicis longus. Because they lack superficialis and intrinsic muscle function only, the reconstruction can be accomplished in a one-stage procedure.

The operation should include an opponens transfer to improve thumb control and the "lasso" operation with an active motor to reduce the claw deformity (intrinsic minus).

Group 9

Patients in Group 9 have functioning superficialis muscles as well as all the other extrinsic flexors and extensors, but do not have intrinsic muscle innervation. In this situation, an opponens transfer is performed as in the second stage for Group 8. The "lasso" operation can be expected to be more effective because the superficialis muscles are under voluntary control in Group 9 patients. The postoperative management is the same as that described for Group 8.

Group X

This group was created so that there would be a place to classify those few patients with unusual levels or amounts of sparing of sensation or muscle innervation. A careful description of the motor and sensory function should be made, and reconstructive procedures will have to be tailored even more carefully for these patients.

REFERENCES

1. Beasly RW: Surgical treatment of hands for C5-C6 tetraplegia. Orthop Clin North Am 14:893–904, 1983
2. Brand PW: Clinical Mechanics of the Hand. CV Mosby, St Louis, 1985
3. Bryan RS: The Moberg deltoid-triceps replacement and key-pinch operations in quadriplegia: Preliminary experiences. Hand 9:207–214, 1977
4. Curtis RM: Tendon transfers in the patient with spinal cord injury. Orthop Clin North Am 5:415–423, 1974
5. DeBenedetti M: Restoration of elbow extension power in the tetraplegic patient using the Moberg technique. J Hand Surg 4:86–89, 1979
6. Dolphin JA: Surgery to the quadriplegic hand: A new operative approach to achieve thumb-finger pinch. In Proceedings of the American Society for Surgery of the Hand. J Bone Joint Surg 52A:1060, 1970
7. Ejeskär A, Dahllöf A: Results of reconstructive surgery in the upper limb of tetraplegic patients. Paraplegia 26:204–208, 1988
8. Flatt AE: An indication for shortening of the thumb. J Bone Joint Surg 46A:1534–1539, 1964
9. Freehafer AA: Flexion and supination deformities of the elbow in tetraplegics. Paraplegia 15:221–225, 1977
10. Freehafer AA, Kelly CM, Peckham HP: Tendon transfer for the restoration of upper limb function after a cervical spinal cord injury. J Hand Surg 9A:887–893, 1984
11. Freehafer AA, Mast WA: Transfer of brachioradialis to improve wrist extension in high spinal-cord injury. J Bone Joint Surg 49A:648–652, 1967
12. Freehafer AA, Peckham PH, Keith MW, Mendelson LS: The brachioradialis: Anatomy, properties, and value for tendon transfer in the tetraplegic. J Hand Surg 13A:99–104, 1988
13. Freehafer AA, Vonhaam E, Allen V: Tendon transfer to improve grasp after injuries of the cervical spinal cord. J Bone Joint Surg 56A:951–959, 1974
14. Friedenberg ZB: Transposition of the biceps brachii for triceps weakness. J Bone Joint Surg 36A:656–658, 1954
15. Grigg P, Finerman GA, Riley LH: Joint-position sense after total hip replacement. J Bone Joint Surg 55A:1016–1025, 1973
16. Hanson RW, Franklin MR: Sexual loss in relation to other functional losses for spinal cord injured males. Arch Phys Med Rehabil 57:291–293, 1976
17. Henderson ED, Lipscomb PR, Elkins EC, Auerback AM, Magness JL: Review of the results of surgical treatment of patients with tetraplegia. J Bone Joint Surg 52A:1059, 1970
18. Hentz VR, Brown M, Keoshian LA: Upper limb reconstruction in quadriplegia: Functional assessment and proposed treatment modifications. J Hand Surg 8:119–131, 1983
19. House JH, Gwathmey FW, Lundsgaard DK: Restoration of strong grasp and lateral pinch in tetraplegia due to cervical spinal cord injury. J Hand Surg 1:152–159, 1976

20. House JH: Reconstruction of the thumb in tetraplegia following spinal cord injury. Clin Orthop 195:117–128, 1985
21. House JH, Shannon MA: Restoration of strong grasp and lateral pinch in tetraplegia: A comparison of two methods of thumb control in each patient. J Hand Surg 10A:22–29, 1985
22. Johnstone BR, Jordan CJ, Buntine JA: A review of surgical rehabilitation of the upper limb in quadriplegia. Paraplegia 26:317–339, 1988
23. Kiwerski J: Recovery of simple hand function in tetraplegia patients following transfer of the musculocutaneous nerve into the median nerve. Paraplegia 20:242–247, 1982
24. Lamb DW, Chan KM: Surgical reconstruction of the upper limb in traumatic tetraplegia: A review of 41 patients. J Bone Joint Surg 65B:291–298, 1983
25. Lamb DW, Landry R: The hand in quadriplegia. Hand 3:31–37, 1971
26. LeClercq C, McDowell CL: Fourth international conference on surgical rehabilitation of the upper limb in tetraplegia. Ann Chir Main Membre Superieur 10:258–260, 1991
27. Lipscomb PR, Elkins EC, Henderson ED: Tendon transfers to restore function of hands in tetraplegia, especially after fracture-dislocation of the sixth cervical vertebra on the seventh. J Bone Joint Surg 40A:1071–1080, 1958
28. Maury M, Guillaumat M, Francois N: Our experience of upper-limb transfers in cases of tetraplegia. Paraplegia 11:245–251, 1973
29. McDowell CL: Tendon transfer to augment wrist extension in the tetraplegic patient. Proc Eighteenth Veterans Administration Spinal Cord Injury Conf 18:78, 1971
30. McDowell CL, Moberg EA, Smith AG: International conference on surgical rehabilitation of the upper limb in tetraplegia. J Hand Surg 4:387–390, 1979
31. McDowell CL, Moberg EA, House JH: The Second International Conference on Surgical Rehabilitation of the Upper Limb in Tetraplegia (Quadriplegia). J Hand Surg 11A:604–608, 1986
32. Medical Research Council: Aids to the investigation of peripheral nerve injuries. War Memorandum No. 7, 2nd Ed. (revised) PL London, His Majesty's Stationary Office, 1943
33. Moberg E: Criticism and study of methods for examining sensibility in the hand. Neurology 12:8–19, 1962
34. Moberg E: Fingers were made before forks. Hand 4:201–206, 1972
35. Moberg E: Surgical treatment for absent single-hand grip and elbow extension in quadriplegia. J Bone Joint Surg 57A:196–206, 1975
36. Moberg E: Reconstruction hand surgery in tetraplegia, stroke and cerebral palsy: Some basic concepts in physiology and neurology. J Hand Surg 1:29–34, 1976
37. Moberg E: The Upper Limb in Tetraplegia. George Thieme, Stuttgart, 1978
38. Moberg E: The present state of surgical rehabilitation of the upper limb in tetraplegia. Paraplegia 25:351–356, 1987
39. Newman JH: The use of the key grip procedure for improving hand function in quadriplegia. Hand 9:215–220, 1977
40. Nickel VL, Perry J, Garrett AL: Development of useful function in the severely paralyzed hand. J Bone Joint Surg 45A:933–952, 1963
41. Norris-Baker C, Stephens M, Rintala D, Willems E: Patient behavior as a predictor of outcomes in spinal cord injury. Arch Phys Med Rehabil 62:602–608, 1981
42. Ober FR, Barr JS: Brachioradialis muscle transposition for triceps weakness. Surg Gynecol Obstet 67:105–107, 1938
43. Omer GE Jr: Evaluation and reconstruction of the forearm and hand after acute traumatic peripheral nerve injuries. J Bone Joint Surg 50A:1454–1478, 1968
44. Peckham PH, Marsolais EB, Mortimer JT: Restoration of key grip and release in the C6 tetraplegic patient through functional electrical stimulation. J Hand Surg 5:462–469, 1980
45. Raczka R, Braun R, Waters RL: Posterior deltoid-to-triceps transfer in quadriplegia. Clin Orthop 187:163–167, 1984
46. Riordan DC: Surgery of the paralytic hand. pp. 79–90. AAOS Instructional Course Lectures. Vol. 16. CV Mosby, St Louis, 1959
47. Smith AG: Early complications of key grip hand surgery for tetraplegia. Paraplegia 19:123–126, 1981
48. Street DM, Stambaugh HD: Finger flexor tenodesis. Clin Orthop 13:155–163, 1959
49. Waters R, Moore KR, Graboff SR, Paris K: Brachioradialis to flexor pollicis longus tendon transfer for active lateral pinch in the tetraplegic. J Hand Surg 10A:385–391, 1985
50. Wilson JN: Providing automatic grasp by flexor tenodesis. J Bone Joint Surg 38A:1019–1024, 1956
51. Zancolli EA: Structural and Dynamic Bases of Hand Surgery. 2nd Ed. pp. 229–262. JB Lippincott, Philadelphia, 1979
52. Zancolli E: Surgery for the quadriplegic hand with active strong wrist extension preserved. A study of 97 cases. Clin Orthop 112:101–113, 1975

44

Open Injuries of the Hand

Paul W. Brown

PRINCIPLES AND PRIORITIES

The Patient

Most severe injuries of the hand are open injuries and how intriguing they are to the surgeon! He is fascinated by the appearance of a laid-open, distorted hand and feels challenged to restore it, or at least to improve it. And so he should be—but he should proceed cautiously lest his fascination lead to surgical myopia with such concentration on the surgical problem that the patient is neglected, leaving him under the care of a surgical mechanic and badly in want of a physician. A broader view must be taken from the very beginning. The patient with an open wound of the hand presents a triple challenge: his welfare, the general nature of his wound, and the specific hand structures that are injured.

Despite the title of this text it should be understood that hand surgeons must not only be surgical technicians, but cognitive physicians who are concerned with the human beings whose diseased or injured hands they are charged to treat. The first priority is to the patient himself; as an injured person and as an injured body. When associated injuries threaten life itself, their immediate management, of course, assumes precedence. When resuscitation is successful and the patient's strength returns, the surgeon must continue to keep in mind this dual consideration of mind and body—this dichotomy of psyche and soma.

With regard to the person, suffice it to say that the wounded hand belongs to a human being who has many fears and questions, and for whom the injury has posed many problems. The hand surgeon is as responsible for assuaging the patient's fears as he is for easing his pain. He must give as much attention to his patient's reaction to the injury as he does to the specific tissues that are damaged. Communication is at least as valuable as penicillin, and technical proficiency, though indispensable, is no substitute for compassion. The patient with an injured hand needs not just a surgical technician, but a physician who is surgically competent.[5,13,17,18,26,27,30,31,47,48,56,70,95,96,102,115,118,124,125,129,131,137,138,139,146,149,150,169,170,175,180]

Multiple Injury

The problem of multiple injuries is always complex as they require a triage, a sorting out and assessment of priorities for treatment. Triage must result in a plan, and the prime planner must be one single physician—one doctor, not a committee of specialists—and that physician must assume primary responsibility for orchestrating what is done to the patient and in what order. Such direction is generally best given by the general surgeon, although any surgical specialist may take command if his particular specialty obviously requires priority. In cases of multiple injury, this is seldom the hand surgeon. When vital organ systems are in jeopardy, the injured hand may be given a low priority for treatment; this may lead to problems of proper surgical timing for the hand, and later, to problems of rehabilitation. This prioritization should not be seen as a struggle for turf, but as an attempt to understand the patient's needs: essential to this is open communication among his attending physicians.

When other injuries or medical conditions preempt the hand surgeon's priorities, he or she must be flexible enough to buy time for the injured hand and must also be able to surrender the ideal treatment for alternative methods that will minimally compromise the end result. If, for instance, skin coverage cannot be done at the best time (i.e., best for the patient's hand, not best for the convenience of the surgeon) because of more pressing surgical priorities, a way must be found to keep the hand supple and well maintained until the next best time is available. Thoracic, abdominal, cardiovascular, intercranial or spinal problems may interfere with or prevent proper timing for debridement and staged surgery of the hand. This, in turn, may lead to other problems and complications. Adaptability to the less than ideal situation is essential and is a measure of the hand surgeon's stature as an experienced physician. Unfortunately, there will be occasions when unavoidable compromise in the treatment of the hand will result in a hand not as good as it might have been if the hand had been the patient's only problem.[130]

Assessment of Injury

History

The essentials of the history are "when," "where," and "how." The "when" indicates the amount of time elapsed and this may determine how the wound is to be managed. The longer contaminants are present, the more entrenched and numerous they become. After 6 hours, closure becomes progressively more dangerous.[39]

The "where" of an injury—the environment in which the injury occurred—may tell something about the type of contamination. Wounds occurring in a relatively clean area, such as the kitchen, may require less attention to debridement and may be closed more safely than those occurring on the battlefield. This parameter of "where" may be deceptive, as even a "clean" area may be laden with all sorts of potential pathogens, such as clostridial spores. Nonetheless, the relative import of "where" must be weighed when assessing the wound and planning treatment.

"How" an injury was incurred will reveal something about the forces expended within the hand and may be a measure of the degree of tissue damage, such as in the distinction between a high and a low-velocity missile wound. It is particularly important to know if there have been crushing forces contributing to the injury, or if materials have been injected under high pressure. Such information may dictate more meticulous exploration and debridement and decompression of closed spaces. It is useful to know what objects and materials caused puncture wounds. Pieces of glass are often hard to find and may not be visible on radiographs, whereas metallic and organic foreign bodies are usually more apparent.

The significance of the injury may also dictate the type of treatment. An on-the-job injury for which all medical expenses will be paid by a third party may allow the salaried patient to opt for more involved salvage procedures than one incurred at home or one incurred by a self-employed or uninsured individual. The circumstances of the injury may affect the patient's reaction to that injury and may determine how well he will cooperate with the surgeon and how well he will participate in treatment, postoperative care, and rehabilitation. Personality, age, dependency, and vocation must also be considered. Attempts to salvage a severed flexor tendon might not be practical for a clerk, but might be mandatory for a musician. A mangled digit with only a 10 percent chance of survival might be better amputated in a self-employed farmer, whereas a young woman might wish every effort made to save the finger regardless of time and expense. The patient with self-inflicted wounds, or one whose life style suggests noncompliance with postoperative recommendations, is generally best served by the simplest and most expedient methods.

Physical Examination

As a prelude to examination of the conscious patient four "C's" must be established: Communication, Confidence, Consent, and Cooperation. Preliminary communication is established by the surgeon's introduction to the patient, explaining who and what the surgeon is. Then, after as complete a history as possible, the surgeon should tell the patient what needs to be done and what is required of the patient. A gentle manner helps. So does a smile. Patients recently injured are in pain and are fearful of more pain. Reassurance, tempered with honesty, helps assure patient assistance in the examination. With Communication comes Confidence. Consent and Cooperation follow in turn. The patient who cooperates allows a much more thorough examination. Further, cooperation makes the examination more pleasant for both patient and physician—or at least less unpleasant. Patient cooperation is predicated on trust in the examiner, and trust is best engendered by the physician's mien and approach.

Examination of the hand should be done whenever possible on a conscious patient, before any anesthesia is given and before a tourniquet is applied. If done in an orderly fashion, with the patient supine and with good lighting, an accurate appraisal of the extent of injury can be obtained in a few minutes. First in importance is circulation. A white hand or digit implies arterial impairment. In dark-skinned patients, the color of the palms and nail beds must be closely observed. A blue, purplish, or dusky color suggests venous stasis and mounting edema. Skin edges and flaps must be scrutinized carefully to assess their vascularity. Grease and dirt may be ground into the skin, making the condition appear worse than it is; aesthetics should not be confused with blood supply.

Bone and joint damage may or may not be apparent on visual and manual examination. Radiographs should be obtained if in doubt—and routinely if the degree of force of the injury has been greater than mild. In carpal injuries, particularly in children, comparative views of the opposite hand are helpful.

Severed extensor tendons should be suspected with dorsal wounds, even if finger extension is possible. Flexor tendon damage is usually apparent when the patient attempts to actively flex his fingers. If he cannot or will not flex a finger, the resting position of the fingers may suggest the damage. The position of "hang-out" is especially valuable in demonstrating flexor tendon in children or in unconscious patients (Figs. 44-1 and 44-2).[39,105]

Nerve injury is frequently missed in emergency room examinations because it is not looked for, but it always becomes apparent later on, when the best opportunity for repair may have been lost. Testing for sensibility must be done before any anesthesia is given. The simplest method is to have the patient

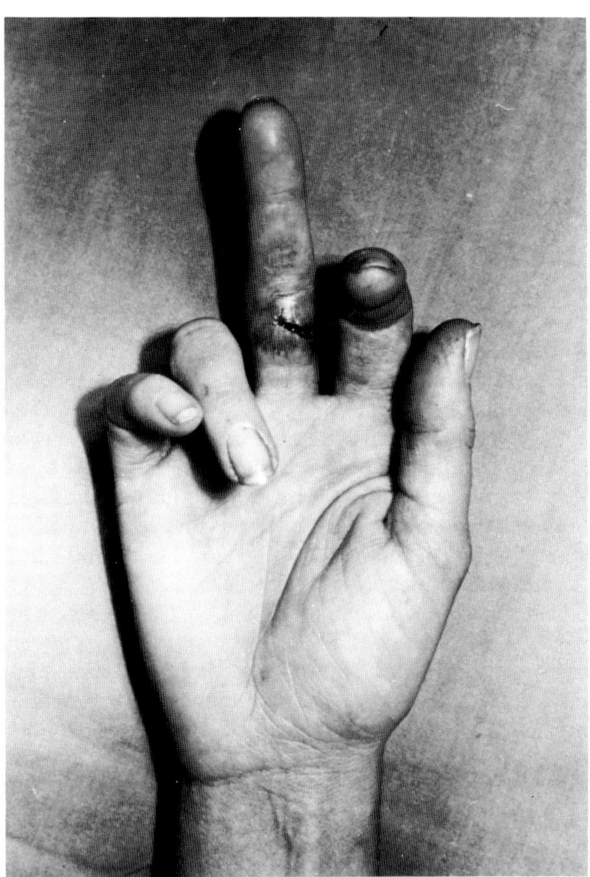

Fig. 44-1. Laceration with a kitchen knife. Flexor digitorum profundus, both slips of flexor digitorum superficialis, and the radial digital nerve were transected 1 hour ago. The position of the middle finger indicates that both tendons are severed. The patient denied sensory loss until his visual field was blocked and sensory examination was repeated.

discriminate between sharp and dull sensation using alternately the point and the head of a pin. This test should be done with the patient's view blocked: if he sees the examination he may report feeling where there is none. Injured patients are frightened, feel vulnerable, and often wish to please the examiner; or they may simply confuse visual with tactile input. If in doubt, a more accurate assessment can be done by using the two ends of a paper clip which has been fashioned to form a horseshoe to test two-point discrimination. Holding the two points about 1 cm apart and moving one or two of the points across the tactile pads of the fingers is a more objective and accurate test of sensibility. Motor nerves are tested by asking the patient to abduct and oppose the thumb and flex the distal finger joints, for median function, to extend fingers, thumb and wrist for radial function, and to spread the extended fingers for ulnar function. A quick check of median and ulnar function may be done by palpating the thenar and first dorsal interosseous muscles as the patient forcibly pinches thumb and index together.[106,131]

Part of the examination is consideration of the patient's complaints of pain. Pain is subjective and dependent on many factors. Seldom can it be accurately evaluated during the initial examination, but extremes, either very severe pain, or the complete lack of it, are significant. Lack of pain may signify nerve damage or psychic problems, whereas agonizing pain, particularly if progressive, may indicate a pressure phenomenon, such as a compartment syndrome.[95]

Blood Flow

Tissue will die without sufficient blood supply; contamination will become infection, and infection will proceed unchecked. The fate of the hand and the outcome of all surgery depend on vascularity. Blood supply has the highest priority (the patient excepted) in the treatment plan, for without it, all else fails.[80,136,154,155,177]

Inadequate blood flow may be primary, that is, impaired ingress due to severed or occluded arteries, or secondary, due to restricted egress resulting from occluded veins, which then results in compartment pressure and edema, which in turn restricts arterial inflow. Severed arteries should be repaired if there are significant areas of avascularity. Blind groping for bleeding vessels in the emergency room is pointless and harm-

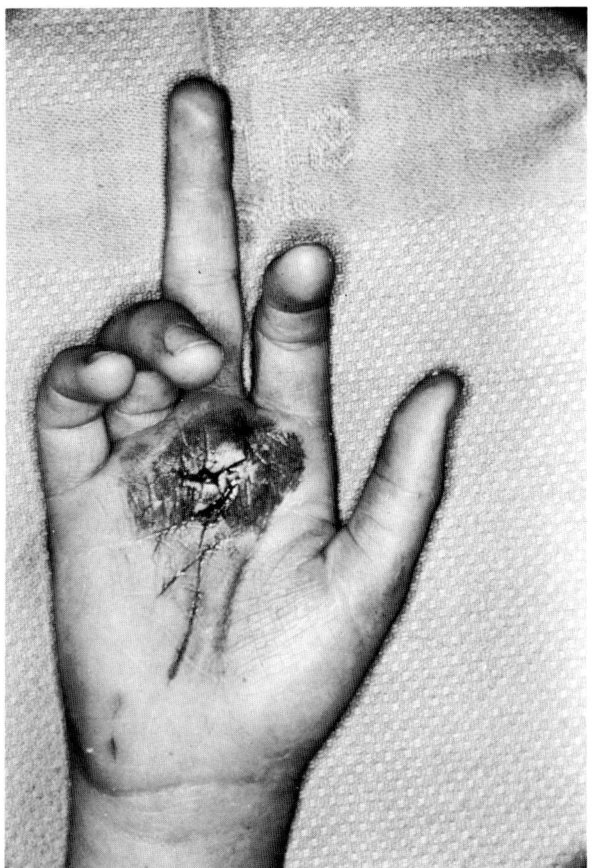

Fig. 44-2. Window pane laceration. Both flexor tendons of the middle finger were severed, as well as the common digital nerve to the third cleft. (From Brown PW: Lacerations of the flexor tendons of the hand. Surg Clin North Am 49:1259, 1969, with permission.)

ful: all bleeding can be controlled with a pressure dressing and elevation until the job can be done in the operating room. Venous repair is seldom required, but decompression of tight spaces—fingers, carpal tunnel, interosseous and thenar spaces, and anterior forearm compartment—may be necessary. Compartment syndromes and progressive edema must be looked for attentively, lest all other problems in the hand become academic.[174]

The Wound Itself

With the patient out of danger and adequate blood flow present, the wound itself must be considered, not simply the specific tissues and structures that have been damaged, but the overall concept of the wound. The term *open wound* is significant in that the mucocutaneous barrier has been violated; not only are the skin and its contents damaged, but bacterial contaminants have been introduced. "Open" implies the threat of infection and the interruption of the healing process. It should also imply that certain urgencies and disciplines are now required that might not be necessary were the skin intact.[27,72,118,119,157-159,195]

Contaminants, as long as they remain simply that, are not harmful. When they begin to proliferate, to colonize, they then assume ascendancy over the body's defenses, and when this happens, the harmless condition of contamination phases over to infection—a pathologic condition. Either the quality or the quantity of bacteria, or a reciprocal combination of the two, may contribute to this. Some bacteria are more virulent than others, but any, in sufficient quantities, may interfere with wound healing. If bacteria exist in quantities of 100,000 or more per gram of tissue, the tissue is infected, or will become so, and will ultimately show some or all of the classic signs of infection (i.e., heat, erythema, induration, pain, and usually purulence).[14,41,74,75,80,85,103,116,153,162-164,167,173]

To prevent contamination from becoming infection, the surgeon must launch a three-pronged attack: he must remove as many bacteria as possible; he must prepare the tissue of the wound to resist the multiplication of the bacteria; and he must attempt to poison the bacteria without damaging the host—in essence, debridement for the first two and antibiotics for the last. It is impossible to sterilize a wound, but cleaning a wound properly will decrease the bacterial count to less than the critical level of 100,000/g, after which the natural defense mechanisms of the body will take care of the rest—providing the next step is properly performed.[22]

This next, important, step is to prepare the contaminated tissues so that they may effectively mobilize the body's defenses. This requires enhancing good blood supply by removing all tissue without supportive blood supply and then stimulating blood flow by allowing free drainage, proper dressings, splinting, active motion, and all of the other effective means of supporting an injured hand in the early postinjury stages. The condition of the contaminated tissue—the environment of the contaminating bacteria—is as influential on subsequent events as the bacteria themselves. Healthy tissue with a good blood supply will actively resist the development of infection.[4,43,116,143]

Debridement

Debridement is the first and most important overt surgical act in treating the open wound. Its purpose is to decrease contamination and to prepare the damaged tissues for healing. If debridement is not well done, infection may develop, tissues will not heal, and all else done surgically will fail.[4,27,85,89,135,199,200,201,204]

Debridement is performed in two ways: by cleansing and by excision. Cleansing—lavage—is best done with sterile saline delivered to the wound in a jet stream that flushes out contaminating bacteria, tissue debris, and foreign material. In a pinch, tap water may be used. A simple, but effective arrangement is a medicine dropper tip attached by tubing to an overhead reservoir. The gravity feed of the saline through the nozzle gives a gentle fluid jet that can be used to explore the entire wound. The pressure head can be varied by lowering or elevating the height of the reservoir. Working the jet through all nooks and crannies of the wound will open up closed planes and spaces and will float out debris and a significant number of bacteria. For large, mangling wounds of the hand, at least 2 liters of fluid should be used. There is no sufficiently convincing evidence that the addition of antibiotics to the lavage solution significantly decreases the chance of infection. Until the point is better proven, antibiotic topical use is not warranted, in my opinion.[147]

Intermittent or pulsating jet lavage from a mechanical pump increases the efficiency of cleansing even further. The force of the jet should be kept low: if too strong it may overly distend spaces with fluid and force debris and bacteria into uncontaminated tissue and tissue planes.[21,39,79,167]

Debridement lavage is seldom popular with emergency and operating room personnel as it is messy, time-consuming, and boring. Support personnel must be made to understand that copious lavage is an effective deterrent to the development of infection.

Surgical debridement, defined by some as wound excision, is as much an art as it is a science. The objective is to remove everything detrimental to wound healing and, at the same time, preserve as much as possible of all tissues useful to hand function or necessary to future reconstructive surgery. There is little that is expendable in the hand: aside from some fat and small amounts of muscle, everything in the hand is necessary for normal function. Conversely, any contaminated or devascularized tissue that is left in the hand may increase the chance of wound breakdown and thereby jeopardize all other tissues in the hand. Compromise is necessary, which is why debridement is an art: later replacement of the structure may be preferable to its retention. Accurate assessment of vascularity is the key to thorough debridement and seldom will a tourniquet be necessary or useful.[22,24]

It has been traditional to excise skin edges of the wound, but this is not necessary unless they are crushed or of questionable viability. It is sometimes impossible to be certain of their condition, as in the tangential distally based flap. It may be preferable to retain this questionable tissue and be prepared to remove it later in redebridement if one has guessed wrong. Bone fragments completely free of soft tissue attachment are usually better removed and replaced later by bone graft if necessary.

Meanwhile the skeletal framework—the architectural integrity of the hand—and the normal lemgth of the fingers can be maintained by K-wires. The initial appearance of battered tendons and nerves can be quite deceptive; they often look damaged beyond repair, but if there is some semblance of continuity their true state of vascularity may not be apparent for several days and often they can be preserved if carefully cleansed and properly dressed.

Extensive hand injuries, particularly the crushed hand, may develop extreme edema, which in turn, may cause increasing pressure and ischemia within restrained spaces. During debridement, potentially tight compartments such as the carpal tunnel should be opened and left open. The surgeon may be reluctant to open spaces not yet contaminated, but decompression is better when done early and can be safely done if lavage is thorough.

The Second Look Concept

A second look and redebridement 3 or 4 days later gives the surgeon the opportunity to remove those pieces of tissue whose viability was questionable initially but now clearly show their nonsalvageable—and dangerous—state. At this time delayed primary repair of tendons and nerves and further skeletal realignment and fixation may be accomplished. On occasion, a third or fourth look may be required. Open wounds require a wide spectrum of surgical timing, ranging from those that can be safely closed immediately to those that should never be closed. Most severe wounds lie somewhere in between those two extremes. The doctrines of "delayed emergency" of Iselin and "staged wound reconstruction" of Burkhalter and colleagues conceive of time as an ally of the surgeon, allowing him to choose the safest and most appropriate time to repair tissue, in contrast to the compulsion to close or cover, wherein time is seen as an opponent. Properly used, time ensures that the disasters of wound breakdown due to premature closure will be avoided.[19,27,34,89,92,137]

Since publication of the previous edition of this text there has been an increasing pressure from government regulators and bureaucrats and third party payers to push physicians to shorten hospital stays, to "expedite treatment," and, in general, to cut corners in the name of "cost effectiveness," but often at the expense of good wound management. This is a short-sighted economy, as the economic cost (to say nothing of the emotional and functional cost) of a wound breakdown due to premature closure is far greater than any saving incurred by closure of a nonacceptant wound.

Indications for Amputation

The severely mangled hand, or parts of it, may clearly be beyond repair (Fig. 44-3). One must be prepared to amputate those parts that would endanger other parts if they were retained. A hand or digit that will have no useful function or that will be grotesque or painful may not serve the patient as well as an amputation would. It is often impossible to predict the outcome, but as long as there is any reasonable hope for useful salvage, the part should be preserved. There are no easy answers for mangled hands in which survival seems marginal: the surgeon must temper optimism with realism. When in doubt, the part should be retained, since it can be removed later if the need becomes obvious; at that time the patient may accept the loss with better grace than if it were done primarily.[24,38]

Skeletal Stability

There are many paradoxes in body kinetics, and none more dramatic than in the hand where a happy marriage of reciprocal opposites—motion versus stability—results in the essentials of useful function. While truly sophisticated function requires the addition of sensibility to this duo, these two basic elements of movement and stability are fundamental to usefulness. They, in turn, dependent as they are on girders, cross members, levers, fulcrums, moments of force, pivots and motors, must have a sound architectural framework. When trauma has disrupted this framework, it must be realigned before the parts can function properly again.

Once the patient is stable and the tissues of the wound cleansed, a golden opportunity awaits the surgeon. In the first few days—or even better, within the first few hours, at the time of debridement—reduction of fractures and correction of distortion are relatively easy (Fig. 44-4). With each passing day, bony displacement becomes progressively more difficult to correct as edema phases over to fibrosis and contracture. Poor reduction, or poor retention of reduction, rapidly becomes malunion, and unreduced joints ankylose as ligaments and capsules congeal and shorten.[128]

Even the most disrupted and mangled hand will usually have bits and pieces of bony scaffolding that can be reassembled. Although gaps and defects may be present here and there, the basic framework must be reassembled if the hand is to function again. Reconstruction is not the term used here, but rather, *reconstitution* (Fig. 44-5). The skin can wait, and so can nerves and tendons: they are only the roof and furnishings of the house, whereas the foundation is basic and one must start with that.[68,126,145,178,184]

The 0.045-inch K-wire has almost universal applicability for the internal stabilization of fractures in the hand. It may be used for intramedullary or oblique transcortical fixation of fractures, or as an internal splint to maintain reduction of joints, or to temporarily prevent joint motion. It may be used as a springy double bayonet (Fig. 44-6) to maintain bone length until a segmental defect can be filled in with bone graft, or it may be used to transfix two or more metacarpals to maintain normal length of the unstable or deficient metacarpal. The K-wire is best inserted with a power drill that can be controlled by one hand, leaving the surgeon's other hand free to stabilize the parts being wired.[23,94]

Traction devices to maintain length or position of damaged digits, though successfully used by some, are hazardous, unwieldy, difficult to maintain, and usually create more problems than they solve.

External splinting for skeletal instability is far less satisfactory than is internal or percutaneous K-wire fixation. The latter allows some active motion in all or most of the hand, whereas the splint impedes the early motion which is so important to rehabilitation of the hand, and is clumsy and

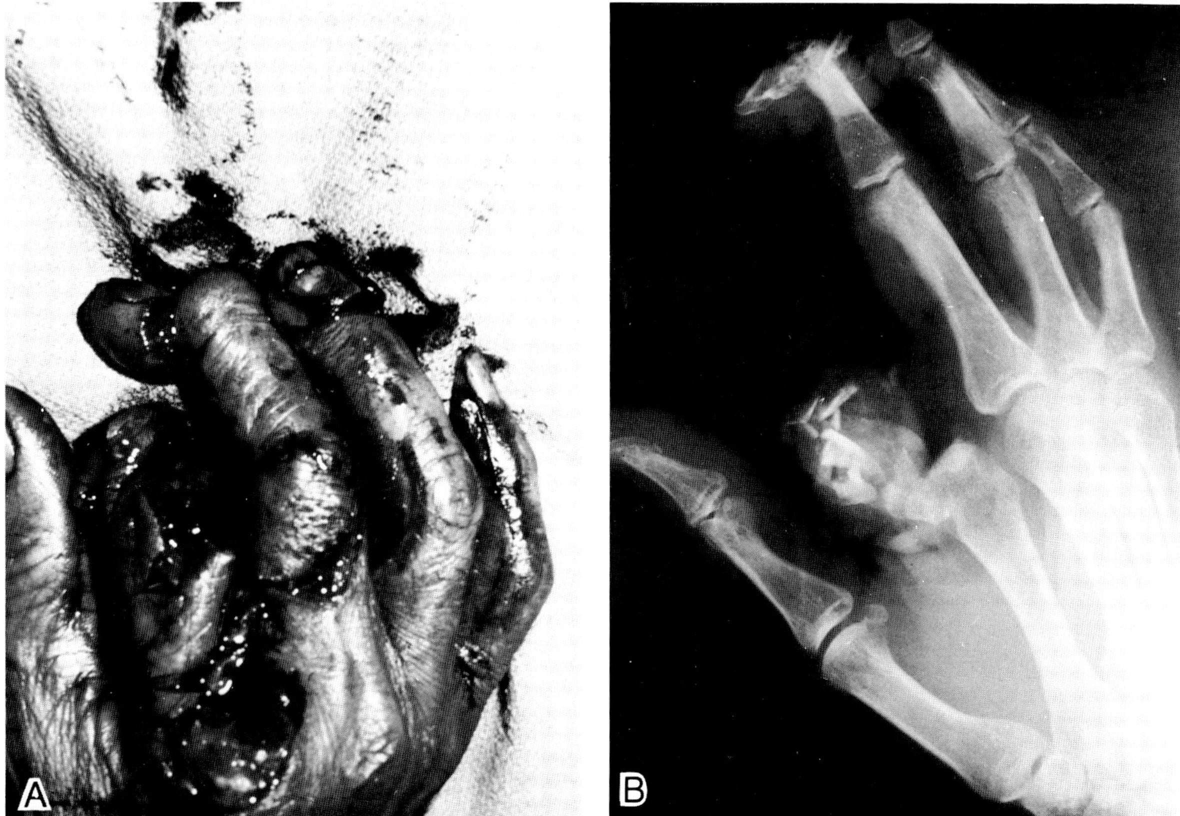

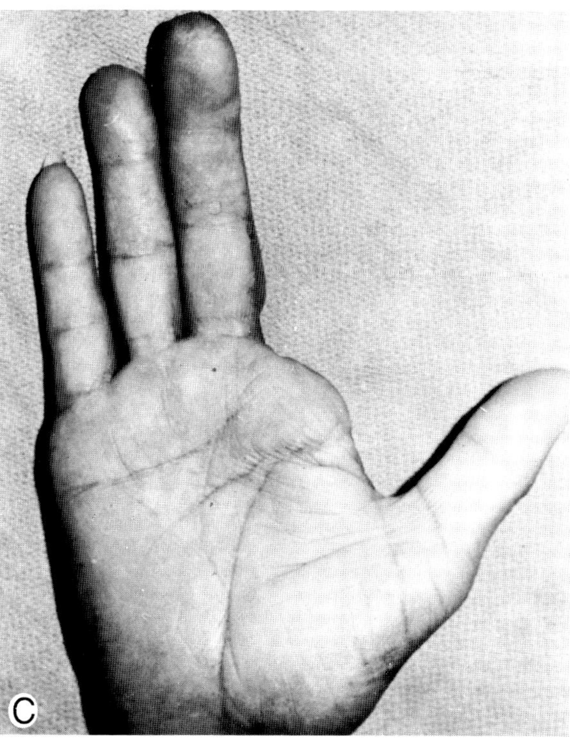

Fig. 44-3. (**A&B**) A manual laborer's hand mangled by a snow blower. Multiple fractures of the index finger phalanges, and multiple injuries of the extensor and flexor tendons and digital nerves and arteries are noted. The index finger is clearly unsalvageable. There is partial amputation of the tips of the middle and ring fingers. (**C**) MP disarticulation allowed prompt healing and early rehabilitation.

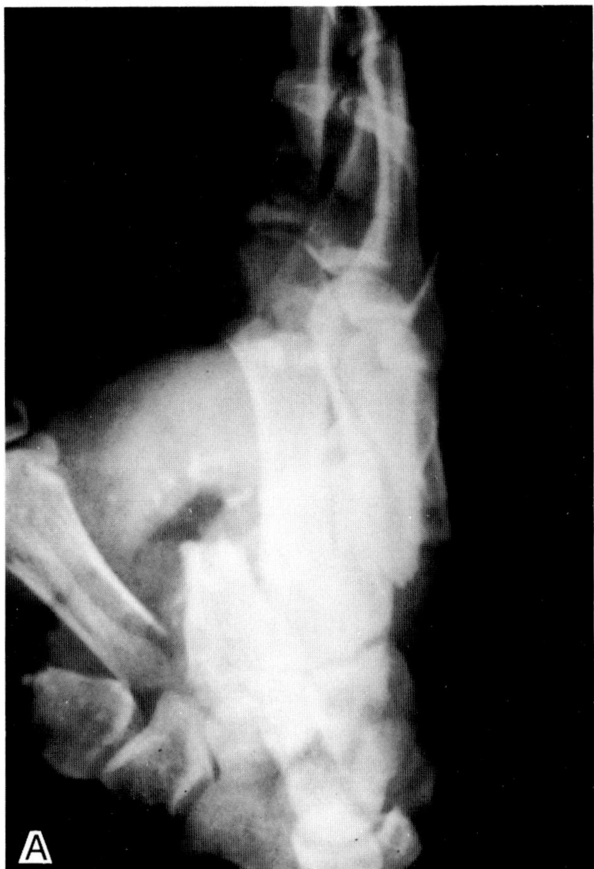

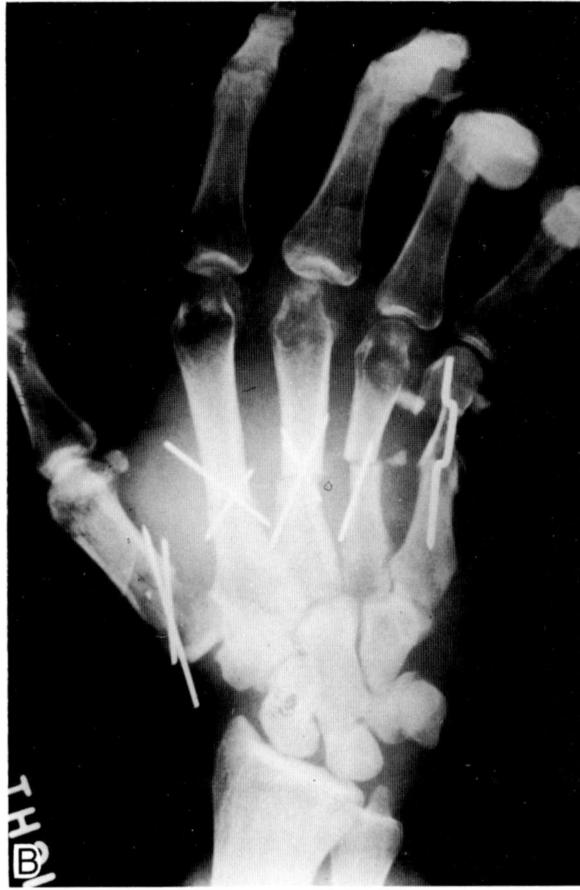

Fig. 44-4. (**A**) Multiple metacarpal fractures from a high-velocity missile. (**B**) Extensive debridement and skeletal fixation. The wounds were closed 2 weeks later, and tendon and nerve reconstruction were carried out 2 months later. (From Brown,[23] with permission.)

often difficult to maintain. The splint may be useful for short periods of time in some types of skin and tendon repairs, but is definitely second best to the K-wire for skeletal problems.[74]

Rigid internal fixation with small metal plates and screws, special bolts and screws, encircling wires, and other orthopaedic gadgetry has had a resurgence of popularity in the past few years. As the hardware and techniques for its use has become more refined, the results of rigid fixation of small bones have improved—which is not to say that it is superior to the use of K-wire fixation. The latter remains the most versatile, and, properly used, has fewer complications. The application of complex hardware often requires excessive tissue exposure and manipulation, the right size or the proper tool always seems to be out of stock, and its removal requires another operation. The complexities of the hardware are proportionate to their complications.[58,94,179,203]

Despite these very real disadvantages, and despite the special training required for their use, there is growing acceptance for the primary application of these devices for open fractures in the hand—often followed by primary closure or coverage. The techniques are demanding and unforgiving: those who use them must be well schooled in their application and in their hazards.[6,46,73]

External skeletal fixation devices have also reappeared on the scene in the past decade or so. They have had a rather unsavory orthopaedic history, but have now been improved to the point where they are more adaptable and useful for the stabilization of long bone and pelvic fractures. They, too, are potentially dangerous, but properly applied they can assist in the reduction of very unstable and complex fractures, and can generally maintain the reduction very well. They also have the questionable advantage of allowing easy access to the wounds overlying the fracture, which may be an invitation to unnecessary poking and prying at the wound. There is not much that the external fixator can accomplish for fractures in the hand that the K-wire cannot, although when expertly used the device can be quite useful in maintaining length of shattered metacarpals. More useful is their application to extremely unstable forearm fractures: the stability they impart may enable the patient to more quickly mobilize his hand than if the forearm were in a cast.[156,171,172]

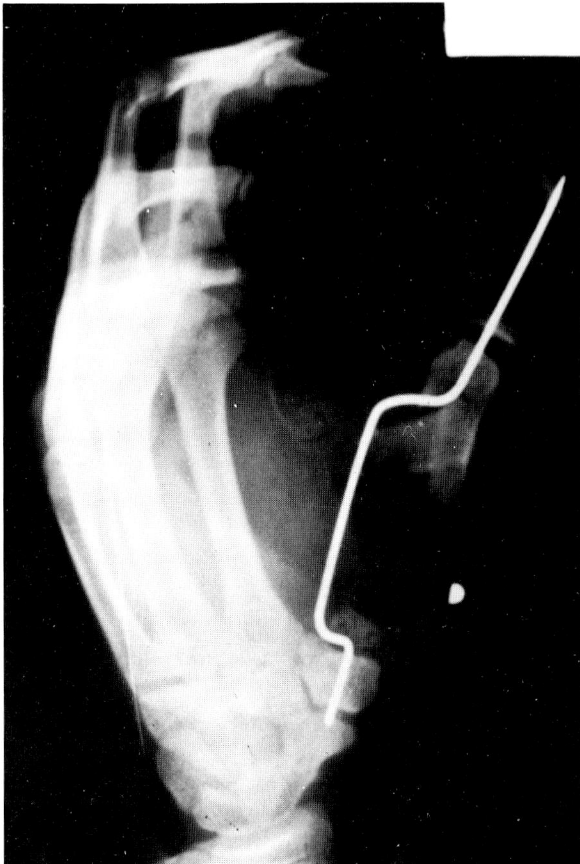

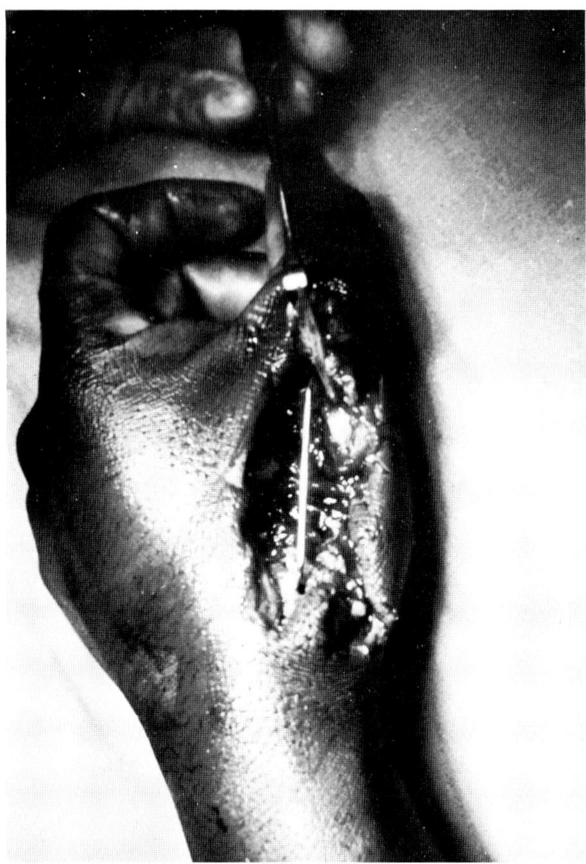

Fig. 44-5. Shotgun muzzle blast injury with avulsion of skin, flexor and extensor tendons, and most of the first metacarpal. After debridement, collapse of the thumb was prevented by a K-wire double bayonet spacer. The wound and K-wire were covered with a dorsal rotation flap 2 weeks later. Bone graft and tendon replacement were done 6 weeks after injury when all wounds were healed.

Deeper Structures

Last priority goes to tendons, nerves, ligaments, articular cartilage, skin, and tissues other than vessels and bone. Open wounds often expose these structures to the outside world, but, contrary to the belief of many surgeons, exposure in itself is not harmful; rather it is the drying out of these structures that may cause irreversible changes. If kept moist by proper dressings, and if adequately supplied with blood, any of these structures will tolerate exposure without harmful effect for varying degrees of time—often many days. If the surgeon is relieved of the compulsion to cover or close exposed tissue prematurely, and if it is possible with equanimity to concentrate on the higher priorities, leaving coverage to a more appropriate time, then more time will be bought to more effectively stage surgical repair and reconstruction. More importantly, by deferring reconstructive work in badly contaminated cases or in hands that may need further debridement, the surgeon greatly decreases the chances of infection. There are no exact criteria for timing. Some tissues and wounds can be safely repaired or covered primarily, whereas repair or coverage of others should be delayed. Each hand, each wound, and each damaged structure must be individually assessed. There is one rule, however, that can be applied to most open injuries: *when in doubt, leave open!*[25,65,123,198]

Skin and Closure

There is no surplus skin in the hand; at least there is little to spare. Dorsal skin can be replaced with reasonably good results but there is no really satisfactory substitute for palmar skin. If skin is damaged beyond repair or is devoid of good blood supply, it must be removed—but every tag, flap, or island that is potentially viable is worthy of strenuous salvage efforts. Where viability is in question, removal can be deferred for a few days. Digits so badly mangled that they must be removed may contribute viable and valuable skin flaps that can be used to replace missing skin in contiguous parts of the hand. Free skin grafts from damaged parts are seldom very successful: only skin still attached to a good blood supply and venous drainage should be used.[121]

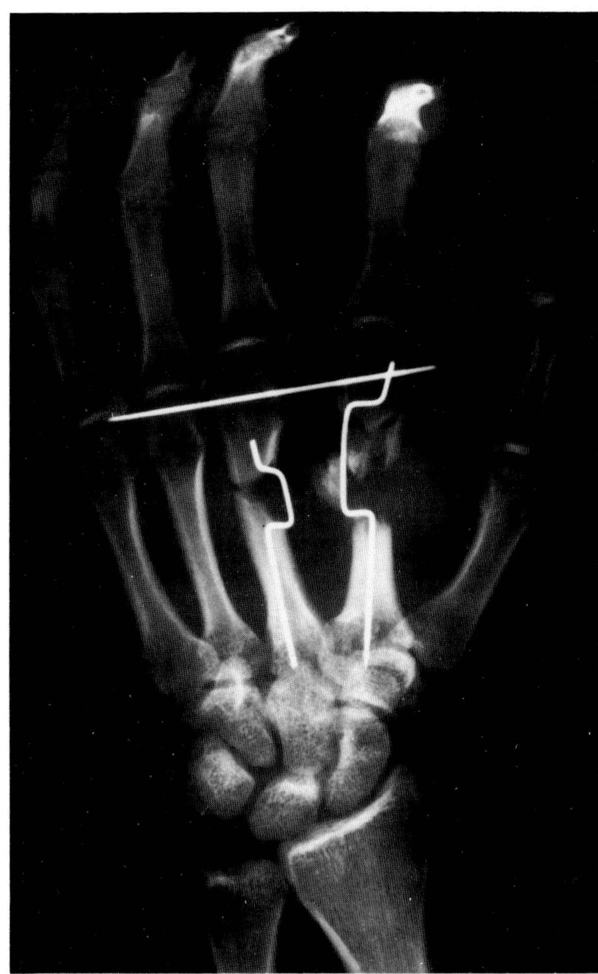

Fig. 44-6. Two months after gunshot wounds with comminution and partial loss of the second and third metacarpals and extensor tendon loss. K-wire spacers and a transverse wire maintain length, preventing shortening until the wound was healed, after which segmental bone grafts were added. (From Jabaley and Peterson,[93] with permission.)

Following debridement, a decision regarding closure or coverage must be made. Certainly it is most desirable to obtain healing by primary intention but there are some wounds that cannot be safely closed primarily: those in which the "golden period" is far exceeded, those in which the degree of contamination is very great, or those in which the adequacy of debridement or of circulation is questionable; healing cannot be imposed on such wounds. To try it is to invite wound breakdown and worse. Many open wounds of the hand may be safely closed and will proceed to orderly healing by *primary intention*. Some should have closure deferred for a few days; if they show no sign of infection they may then be safely closed: this is called *delayed primary closure*. If closure is effected before granulations have formed, that is, within the first week, the wound will still heal by *primary intention*. Wounds with greater contamination, or wounds with tissues of marginal circulation, should be closed secondarily, and a few, such as human bite wounds, should never be closed but instead be allowed to heal by secondary intention. It's worth noting that healing by secondary intention is the *natural* method of wound healing and it evolved long before there were surgeons and surgery.[59,63,66,111,113,202]

The relative advantages and disadvantages of closure must be weighed and many factors carefully assessed. The degree and nature of contamination is important: a wound incurred in the home is less likely to contain as many virulent bacteria as a wound incurred in the barnyard. Time, too, is important; antibiotics have not appreciably changed the principle of the "golden period," they have only extended it a bit. Wounds should not be closed later than about 8 hours postinjury. The state of the contaminated tissue is just as important as the contaminating bacteria. To paraphrase Pasteur: the environment of the microbes is more important than the germs themselves.

Marginally vascular tissues are at higher risk if the skin is closed and the same is true of puncture wounds where contaminants have been introduced deep into spaces and tissues of the hand. If there is a probability of much bleeding or fluid accumulation in the wound, closure will inhibit its free drainage, thereby increasing the risk of infection. Pools of fluid—and this includes hematomas—are avascular and are ideal environments for contaminating bacteria to undergo a metamorphosis from contaminants to pathogens. Contaminants of a wound—and all wounds are contaminated—are opportunistic: it is the surgeon's challenge to deny them conditions which will foster their proliferation—their colonization, which is the basis of infection.[134,164-166]

When the degree of contamination or the extent of vascular impairment is in doubt the wound should be left open. If, by the fourth or fifth day, there is no sign of inflammation, edema, erythema, or pus, the wound can then be closed with a much higher chance of undelayed healing. Although many hand wounds may be closed primarily, more are closed than should be. Those wounds that do not accept closure but go on to infection and breakdown ultimately result in more damage to the hand than the original injury.[191]

Rank and Wakefield's concept of *tidy* and *untidy* wounds is useful in roughly classifying the amount of tissue damage and the degree of contamination. The laceration caused by a knife has relatively little tissue damage, even though important structures may be transected, and usually there are few bacteria in such a wound. This type of wound lends itself well to primary repair, providing all other factors are safely accounted for. The mangled hand from a farm machinery accident or from an explosion may well require a second look and redebridement. Closure of such a wound may jeopardize uneventful healing. Appearance may be deceptive: a hand through which a high-velocity bullet has passed may look quite benign for the first few hours but may have large amounts of devitalized tissue within it, and may later become dangerously edematous.[7,27,152]

When in doubt as to whether to close a wound, a useful middle course is to effect a loose closure with adhesive strips. The strips can be laid on without tension to loosely approximate wound edges and to control distortion of flaps of skin. If there is subsequent edema, the strips will allow the wound to gape, whereas sutures would tend to progressively strangle the

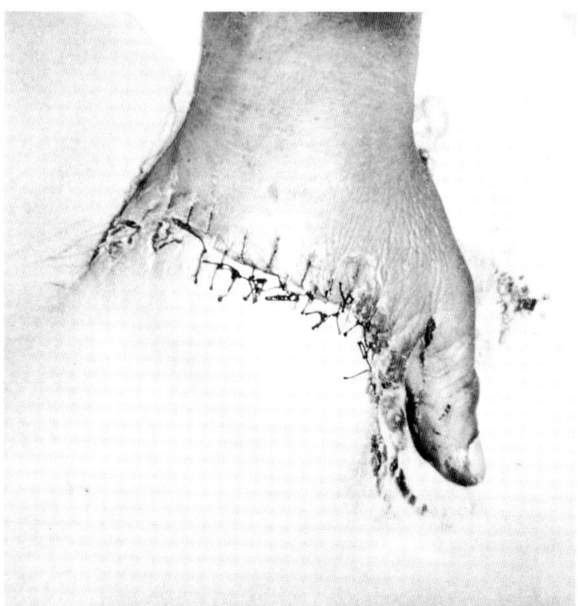

Fig. 44-7. The compulsion to suture. This farmer avulsed four digits in a machine. His surgeon buried the hand in the abdominal wall. When it began to smell bad, some days later, the patient was transferred to another hospital.

skin as tension increased. It should be remembered that any suture under tension creates a small zone of dysvascularity and such a zone may become a small culture medium for its contaminants. It follows, then, that if there are many sutures under tension, there may be many areas of proliferating bacteria.

Charles F. Gregory once said in a lecture: "Primary closure should be based on judgment—plus willingness to take a chance." Reckless surgeons take more chances with their patients than cautious—or thoughtful—ones. There is great pressure on the surgeon and on the emergency room physician to close wounds; pressures from without and pressures from within. The lay public expects wounds to be closed. If emergency room personnel do not understand the principles of wound management, they too may add to the pressure. Pressures from within the surgeon are generated by misconceptions, lack of experience, an erroneous belief that exposed tissue will "get infected," and a compulsion to suture.[12,123,189-191]

Experience in past wars has convincingly demonstrated not only that wounds of the hand may be safely left open, but also that many will do better that way. This knowledge has been acquired at great cost, but as the memory of the last war fades, so too do its lessons, and the old *compulsion to suture* revives and the lessons must be learned all over again in the next war. What a shame that we seem unable to adequately and consistently apply our wartime lessons to our peacetime practice! It

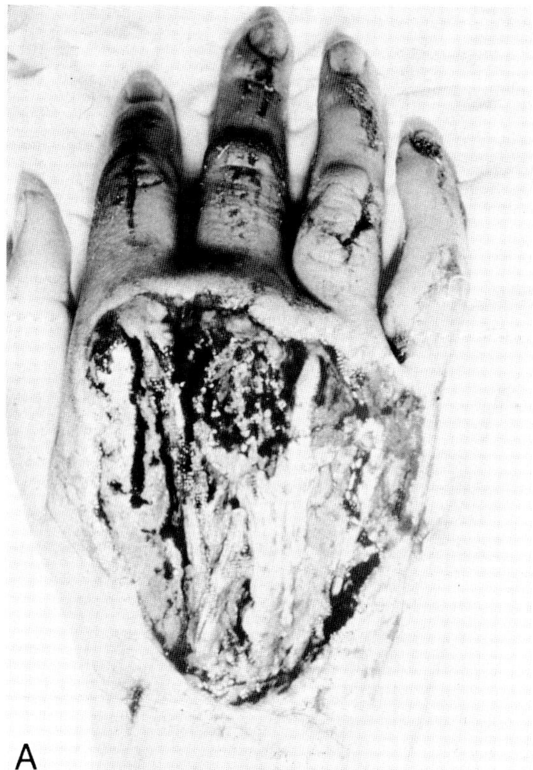

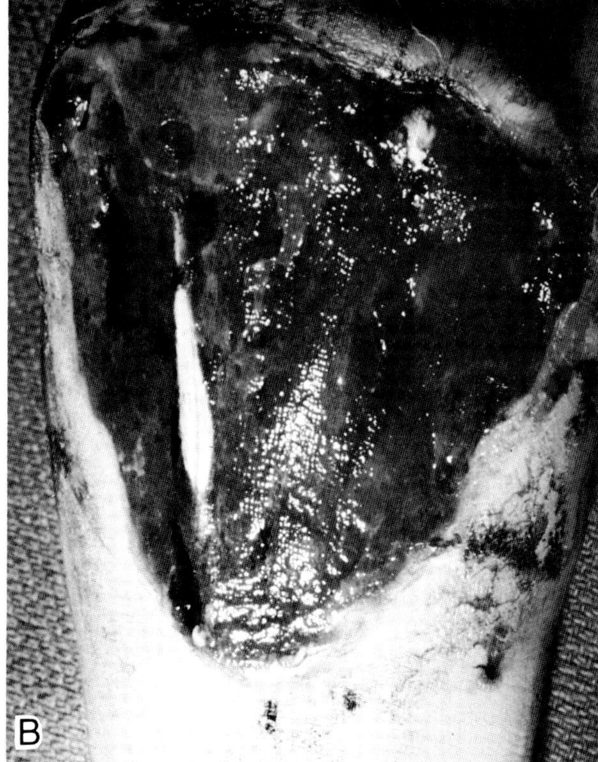

Fig. 44-8. (**A**) An automobile overturned on the hand of this 16-year-old girl, avulsing skin, extensor tendons and joint capsules of the knuckles. A lot of dirt and debris was ground into the wound. Extensive debridement was done, and the wound was covered with fine mesh gauze and compression dressing. Active assisted exercises were started a few days later. (**B**) Thirteen days later. Healthy granulations cover the wound. There is no erythema, induration, edema, pus, or pain. The wound is now an ideal recipient for properly planned skin coverage—in this case, a cross-arm pedicle flap. *(Figure continues.)*

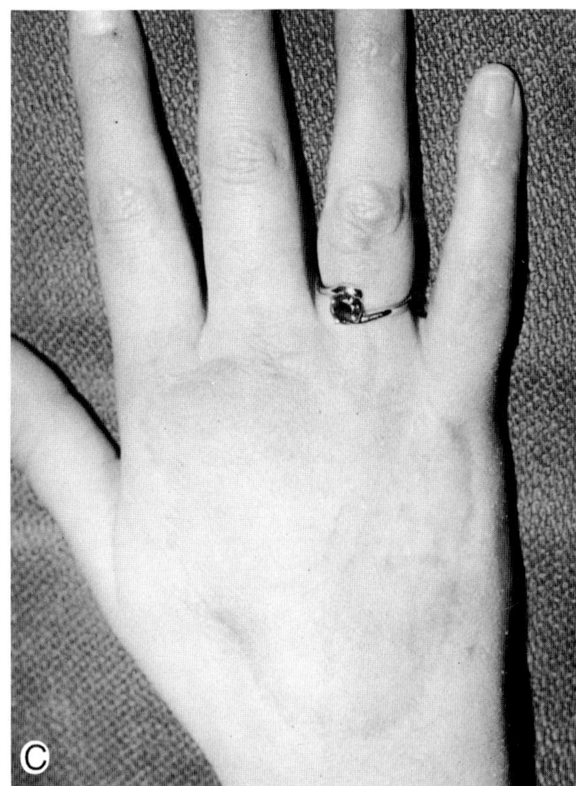

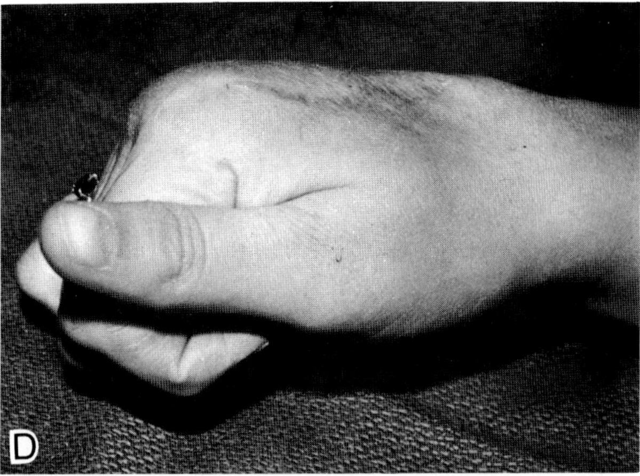

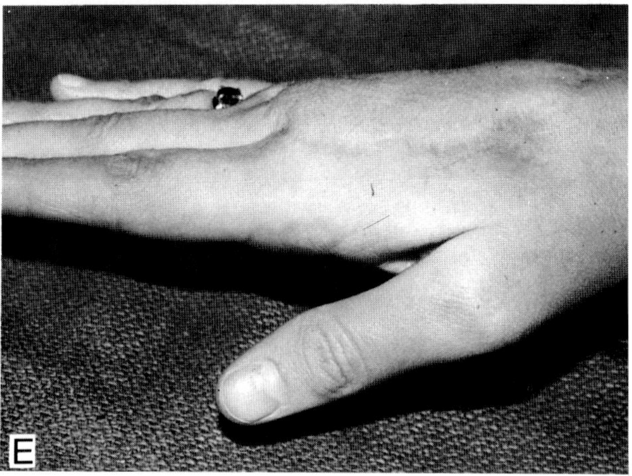

Fig. 44-8. *(Continued).* **(C&D)** The hand 9 months after injury. Three months after detachment of the pedicle flap, four extensor tendon grafts were inserted. Appearance and function compare favorably with results from primary coverage. The delayed transfer of skin decreased the probability of complications and the amount of cicatrix. **(E)** Extensor tendon excursion was excellent beneath the flap on the dorsum of the hand.

has been said that if we do not learn from history we are doomed to repeat our mistakes.[15,33,34,57,111,183,192-195,200-204]

Worse than ill-advised primary closure is the compulsion to cover the avulsed wound with primary skin flaps (Fig. 44-7). When skin transfer—either split- or full-thickness, free or pedicle—is required, the transfer can be done more efficiently and safely by deferring it until one is reasonably certain that infection will not occur and that the tissues appear receptive to coverage. Though widely applied—usually by plastic surgeons and often for the convenience of operating room schedules—it is potentially unsafe and is usually quite unnecessary. Consistently better results will be obtained by delayed skin transfer, when the tissues are receptive to the transfer and when proper attention can be given to planning, operating room availability, and other details (Fig. 44-8).[49,76,107,132]

The development of microsurgical techniques has given us the ability to transfer full-thickness skin, subcutaneous and deeper tissues to wounds and to revascularize them in their new site (see Chapter 28). This exciting addition to our skills offers great promise for dealing with the devastating hand wounds where there has been avulsion of large amounts of skin leaving bone, joints, tendons, nerves and vessels exposed. Such skin transfers are called "microvascular free flaps"—a misleading term, as they are neither free nor are they flaps. Some very impressive results have been demonstrated with this technique; where the transfer has been successful it has facilitated staged reconstruction and rehabilitation of the hand. The costs and complications of such transfer may be considerable. Success depends on a highly skilled team working in a hospital that will consistently give that team all necessary personnel and logistical support; support which few community hospitals can afford. Unless exquisitely well done, such surgery will fail and further jeopardize an already badly damaged hand. Where the highest standards of microvascular surgery—and its postoperative sequellae—cannot be maintained, it is far better to defer closure or coverage until a safer time.[9,10,101,108]

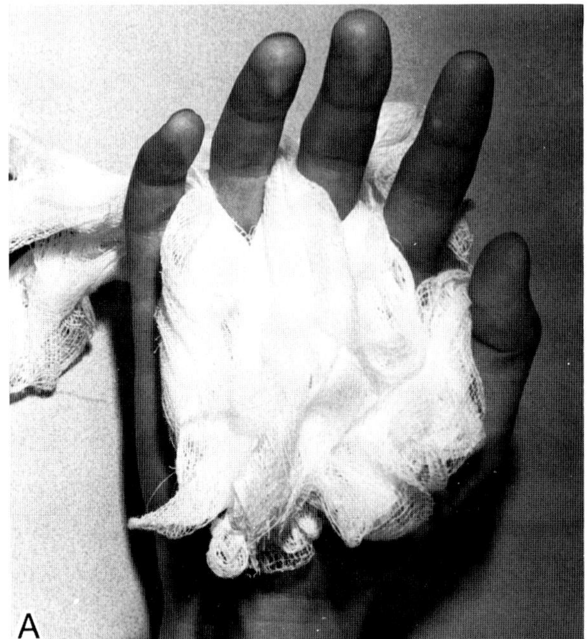

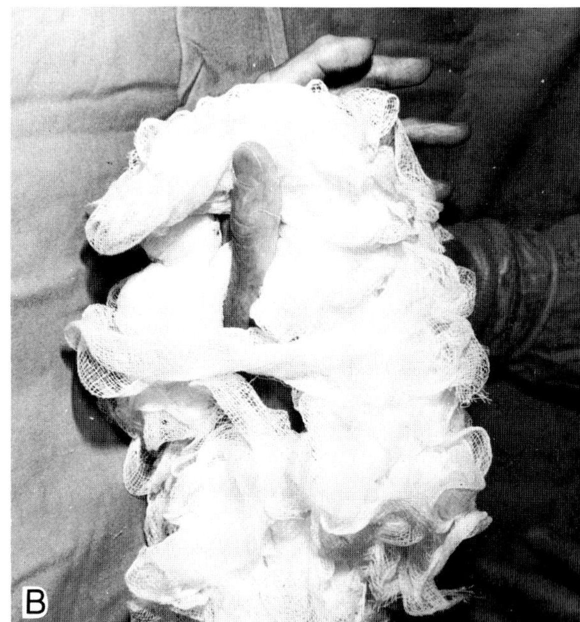

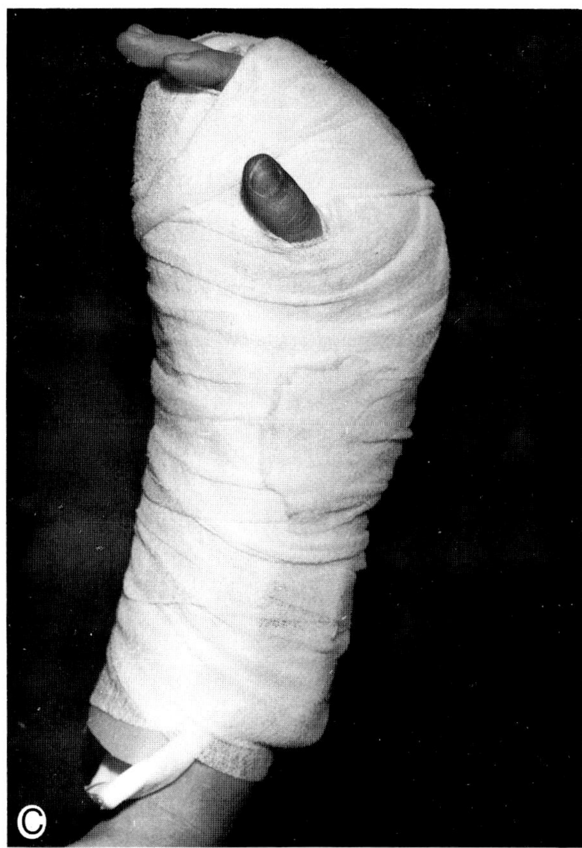

Fig. 44-9. The hand compression dressing. (**A**) The fingers are lightly separated. (**B**) Many fluffed-up surgical sponges. (**C**) Firm, but not tight, uniform compression with the hand in the "position of function." The extremity should now be elevated. (From Brown PW: The hand. pp. 643–686. In Hill GJ III (ed): Outpatient Surgery. 2nd Ed. WB Saunders, Philadelphia, 1980, with permission.)

Dressings

The postdebridement dressing (Fig. 44-9) has several functions: to keep exposed tissues moist, to prevent further contamination, and, importantly, to enhance circulation by the prevention of edema. The wound is covered with fine mesh gauze, lightly impregnated with petrolatum. The fingers are separated by lightly tucking a folded surgical gauze in each finger cleft. A bulky dressing of multiple fluffed-up gauze sponges is then applied from elbow to fingertips while holding the hand and wrist in the position of function: wrist slightly extended, MP and IP joints slightly flexed, thumb abducted and slightly flexed. Dead spaces should be left open: if it seems likely that they will be occluded by tissue flaps, they should be drained with one or more short lengths of 8- or 10-gauge tubing. Packing wounds open is not only unnecessary, but may be harmful, as the packing may block free drainage. The entire dressing is then wrapped with a nonelastic conforming roller gauze bandage. An elastic bandage may be used but is potentially dangerous, as it is deceptively easy to apply it too tightly or to create constricting bands of uneven tension. The entire dressing should apply mild and uniform pressure throughout the hand, wrist, and forearm.

This type of dressing is applicable to most injured hands. It is safe and comfortable and has enough "give" to allow a slight amount of active finger motion, and yet it provides enough stability to make rigid splints unnecessary. If special positions are required, a plaster splint may be molded to either the dorsal or volar side of the dressings. An intrinsic-plus position of flexed MP joints and fully extended interphalangeal joints is desirable where there has been loss of dorsal skin of the hand or fingers, as in the case of severe burns, or where there has been extensive damage to these joints. Immediately following application of the dressing, the extremity should be suspended with the hand held slightly higher than the heart, and this elevation should be maintained until it is certain that edema has either been avoided or controlled. More satisfactory for this elevation than suspending the extremity from the bedframe is to use one of the light plastic foam elevating blocks made especially for this purpose. Such a block enhances mobility of both the extremity and the patient and is better accepted by the patient than suspension[45] (see Chapter 1).

Antibiotics and Tetanus Prophylaxis

Antibiotics are useful adjuncts, but not substitutes, for proper wound care. Overdependence on them to the neglect of meticulous debridement and good tissue management will result in many unnecessary infections. Most open wounds of the hand (or elsewhere) do not require antibiotics: their use should be reserved for wounds where the risk of infection is at least moderate. Such wounds would include bites; deep, penetrating wounds; and mangling or crushing injuries in which the degree of contamination is great or in which debridement has been delayed for more than a few hours. Such wounds should be cultured aerobically and anaerobically at the time of debridement. The appropriate antibiotic can then be selected on the basis of the culture and sensitivity studies. Most hand infections are caused by gram-positive staphylococci and streptococci, although the incidence of infection caused by various gram-negative organisms seems to be steadily increasing as overzealous users of antibiotics create resistant strains. While waiting for the bacteriology laboratory results, hospital patients with severe wounds can be given intravenous methicillin or oxacillin, assuming they have no history of penicillin sensitivity. If gram-negative organisms are cultured and are present in significant numbers a cephalosporin should also be used. Outpatients with high-risk wounds can be started on an oral cephalosporin such as cephradine pending the laboratory reports. Other than in the burn wound, topical antibiotics, or for that matter, any type of locally applied medication, solution, or ointment, have nothing to offer in the treatment of open wounds.[99,144,182]

Tetanus prophylaxis is required for all but the most trivial open wounds of the hand. The guidelines, published by the Committee for Trauma of the American College of Surgeons, should be followed (Fig. 44-10). Particular attention must be given to those patients not previously immunized, those who have not had a booster injection within the past 5 years, and all those with very severe or neglected wounds.[5]

SPECIFIC INJURIES

Abrasions

An abrasion is a split-thickness skin loss in which enough of the deeper layers remain to fully regenerate the lost tissue. Skin loss in which the stratum germinativum has been lost is considered an avulsion.

The tissue loss in an abrasion is not in itself very serious. If abrasions are well cleansed they usually heal quickly, either exposed to air, or under fine mesh gauze overlain by a dry dressing, and without benefit of topical or systemic antibiotics. During the exudative and proliferative phases of wound healing, they become crusted over with a scab, which is an amalgam of precipitated and clotted blood proteins, dead white cells and bacteria. The scab and its underlying bed develop a high bacterial count which then rapidly declines as healing progresses and the scab begins to separate, a process usually lasting 2 to 3 weeks.

The clinical significance of abrasions lies in their association with injury to deeper tissues. During the healing period, the high bacterial count poses a threat to the deeper tissues if they are exposed at the time of injury or during subsequent reparative surgery. Where possible, surgery should be deferred until the abrasion is completely reepithelialized. If this is not possible, the abrasion should be thoroughly scrubbed with a povidone-iodine solution before surgery and the operative wound left open. A delayed primary closure of this wound can be done 3 to 7 days later if the wound appears benign.

Lacerations

The main concern with lacerations is what lies beneath them. Have nerves or tendons been damaged, or have joints been penetrated? One of the most common mistakes made by

Prophylaxis Against Tetanus In Wound Management

General Principles

1
Active immunization against tetanus with tetanus toxoid plays a major role in markedly reducing the incidence of cases of this disease, and the resulting deaths.

2
Recommendations for tetanus prophylaxis are based on 1) the condition of the wound, especially as related to its susceptibility to tetanus, and 2) the patient's immunization history.

3
Regardless of the active immunization status of the patient, all wounds should receive immediate surgical treatment, using meticulous aseptic technique, to remove all devitalized tissue and foreign bodies. Such care is an essential part of prophylaxis against tetanus. (See *A Guide to Initial Therapy of Soft-Tissue Wounds,* American College of Surgeons.)

4 Warning:
The only contraindication to tetanus and diphtheria toxoids for the wounded patient is a history of neurologic or severe hypersensitivity reaction to a previous dose. Local side effects alone do not preclude continued use. If a systemic reaction is suspected to represent allergic hypersensitivity, postpone immunization until appropriate skin testing is performed later. If a contraindication to a tetanus toxoid-containing preparation exists, consider passive immunization against tetanus for a tetanus-prone wound.

Contraindications to pertussis vaccination in infants and children less than seven years old include: a previous adverse reaction after diphtheria and totanus toxoids and pertussis vaccine adsorbed (for pediatric use) (DTP), or single antigen pertussis vaccination; and/or the presence of a neurologic condition characterized by changing developmental or neurologic findings. If such a contraindication to using pertussis vaccine adsorbed (P) exists, diphtheria and tetanus toxoids adsorbed (for pediatric use) (DT) are recommended. Neither a static neurologic condition, such as cerebral palsy, nor a family history of convulsions or other central nervous system disorders is a contraindication to giving vaccines containing the pertussis antigen.

Wound Classification

Clinical Features	Tetanus-Prone Wounds	Nontetanus-Prone Wounds
Age of wound	> 6 hours	≤ 6 hours
Configuration	Stellate wound, avulsion, abrasion	Linear wound
Depth	> 1 cm	≤ 1 cm
Mechanism of injury	Missile, crush, burn, frostbite	Sharp surface (eg, knife, glass)
Signs of infection	Present	Absent
Devitalized tissue	Present	Absent
Contaminants (dirt, feces, soil, saliva, etc.)	Present	Absent
Denervated and/or ischemic tissue	Present	Absent

Fig. 44-10. (From American College of Surgeons: Bulletin, 1987, with permission.)

Immunization Schedule

Verify a history of tetanus immunization from medical records so that appropriate tetanus prophylaxis can be accomplished.

Td: Tetanus and diphtheria toxoids adsorbed (for adult use)
TIG: Tetanus immune globulin (human)

History of Adsorbed Tetanus Toxoid (Doses)	Tetanus-Prone Wounds		Nontetanus-Prone Wounds	
	Td[1]	TIG	Td[1]	TIG
Unknown or fewer than 3	Yes	Yes	Yes	No
3 or more[2]	No[4]	No	No[3]	No

[1]For children less than seven years old: DTP (DT, if pertussis vaccine is contraindicated) is preferable to tetanus toxoid alone. For persons seven years old and older, Td is preferable to tetanus toxoid alone.

[2]If only three doses of fluid toxoid have been received, a fourth dose of toxoid, preferably an adsorbed toxoid, should be given.

[3]Yes, if more than 10 years since last dose.

[4]Yes, if more than five years since last dose. (More frequent boosters are not needed and can accentuate side effects.)

Disposition

Give each patient an appropriate written record describing treatment rendered and providing instructions for follow-up that outline wound care, drug therapy, immunization status, and potential complications. Arrange for completion of active immunization.

Give every wounded patient a wallet-sized card documenting immunization dosage and date received.

For further review of prophylaxis against tetanus, see *A Guide to Prophylaxis Against Tetanus in Wound Management,* available from the American College of Surgeons Trauma Department.

American College of Surgeons
Committee on Trauma
1987

Fig. 44-10. *(Continued)*

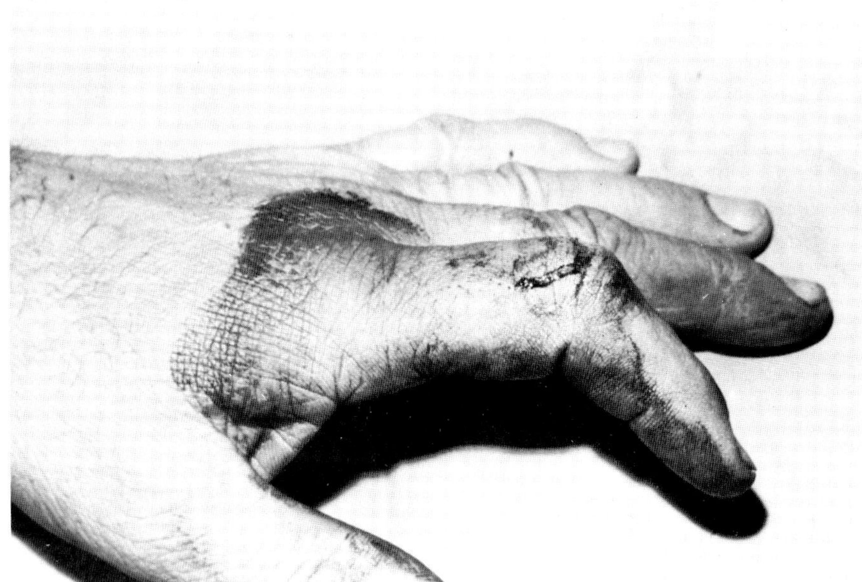

Fig. 44-11. Knife wound. The central slip of the extensor tendon is severed. Repair is needed before the lateral bands migrate volarward, causing boutonnière deformity.

the emergency room physician is to concentrate on suturing the skin and failing to examine adequately for deeper injury. Failure to detect severed flexor tendons or digital nerves under small transverse lacerations through the proximal flexion creases of the fingers, and especially the thumb, is the most common error.

Particularly deceptive is the small laceration over the dorsum of the PIP joint of a finger with a severed central extensor slip underneath (Fig. 44-11). Initially, the patient lacks only about 30 degrees of full active extension of the middle phalanx, but if this is missed, so is the one good opportunity to prevent the insidious development of a boutonniere deformity. Another common, though less serious oversight, is to overlook the severed extensor digitorum communis tendon in a laceration over the MP joint, wherein the patient has lost only 30 or 40 degrees of full extension of the joint.

The laceration — often quite small and not very painful — of a child's midpalm caused by a fall on a broken bottle may look rather innocuous, but deep to it may be found transection of all of the common digital nerves where they spread out from the main trunk of the median nerve (Fig. 44-12).

Lacerations on the volar aspect of the wrist are often accompanied by severed flexor tendons, nerves and vessels in many different combinations. Such injuries often lend themselves well to primary repair of the deep structures. They require careful debridement and thorough examination under ideal circumstances; that is, in the operating room with adequate anesthesia. Seldom is the emergency room an appropriate locale for this. Dorsal wrist lacerations may overlie severed extensor tendons, and careless examination may fail to reveal their injured state, either for the thumb or the other digits.

Lacerations tend to heal themselves very well by secondary intention, and they should be allowed to do so if they are badly

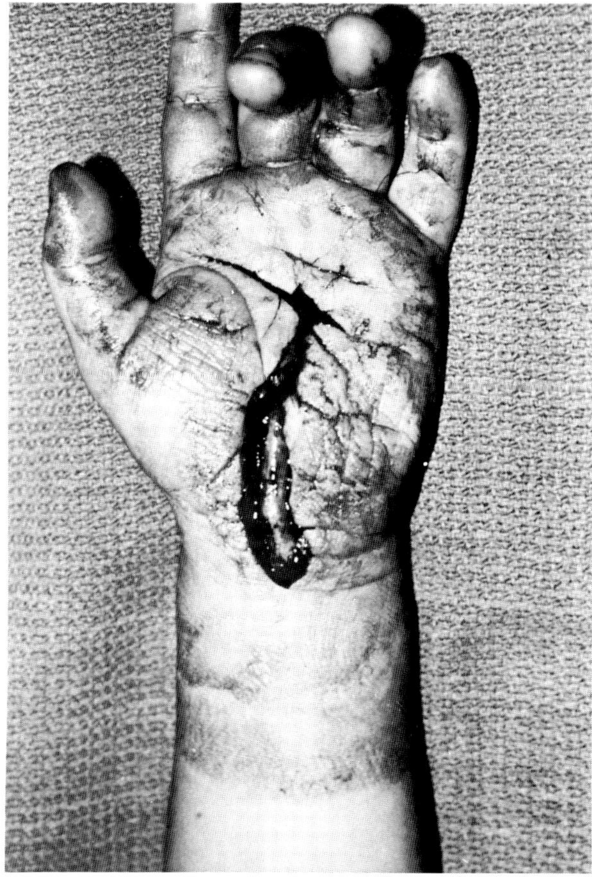

Fig. 44-12. Broken bottle laceration in a 4-year-old child. All branches of the median nerve and both flexor tendons of the index finger are severed. Note "hangout" of the index finger.

contaminated or have been untreated for more than about 8 hours. They do particularly well without benefit of suture if they lie in or parallel to flexion creases or on the dorsum or lateral aspect of the finger. Most lacerations, of course, are sutured primarily, but too often the emphasis is on closure, to the neglect of what lies below.[169]

Crush and Burst

Great pressures applied to the hand shear, compress, and twist tissues, creating havoc in the vascular bed and in the cellular structures of the tissues, causing hemorrhage and the escape of intra- and extracellular fluids into potential spaces and tissue planes. The net result is the formation of hematoma and a progressive edema that in turn leads to the precipitation of proteins, fibrosis and stiffness. Although crush affects all tissues adversely and its sequellae may be irreversible, prompt surgical measures may, nevertheless, salvage much that at first looks hopeless. The fundamental principles of early debridement, decompression, effective dressing, and postoperative elevation are the basics of treatment. Primary reconstructive measures, other than skeletal realignment and stabilization, are seldom advisable, as a weeping tissue base, or one laced with microhemorrhage, offers a poor substrate for satisfactory healing.[69,120]

With such a picture of widespread tissue destruction and its subsequent impairment of blood supply, the crushed hand is particularly vulnerable to the proliferation of contaminating bacteria. It follows then, just as with most other severe injuries, that measures that improve arterial input and venous and lymphatic drainage are the key to healing without infection. Accurate assessment of irreversible ischemia of the intrinsic musculature, fascia and other connective tissue may be impossible in the initial debridement. A second or third look and redebridement are often necessary. Wound culture and careful selection of antibiotics are important as well, but only as an adjunct to the surgical support of tissue vascularity. A corollary to this is that primary closure of an open wound in which crush has been a significant contributor will seriously jeopardize healing, but, perhaps fortunately, closure is often impossible. Postdebridement edema must be expected; any sutures, no matter how loosely placed, may become tight and will then strangle the tissue in which they have been placed.

Crush injuries frequently split the skin with shear and torque forces, or the skin may burst from pressure from within, just as a grape will burst if compressed (Fig. 44-13). The burst finger or palm may result from industrial presses, pistons, and gears, or the dropping of heavy objects on the hand. The burst finger often has a longitudinal rent the length of the flexor surface. The underlying tendons, nerves and vessels may be quite salvageable if the finger is properly managed by avoiding closure under tension; such burst wounds of the skin will usually heal nicely by secondary intention once edema subsides. The burst palm may have masses of muscle extruded from the lateral margins of the hand, or from the thumb web space. Often these muscle masses are viable and should not be removed unless obviously avascular or hopelessly contaminated.[45,88,186]

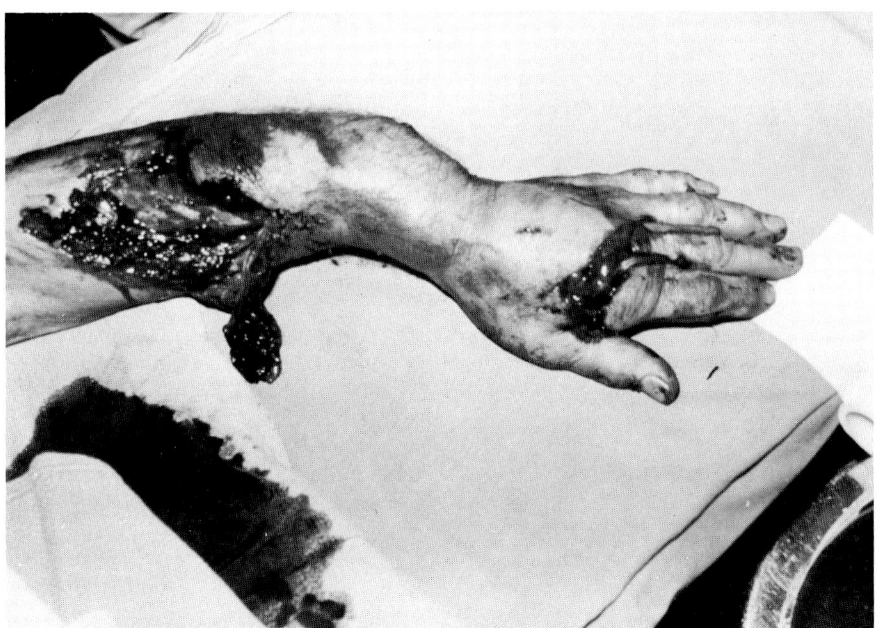

Fig. 44-13. Roller press crush injury with multiple hand and forearm fractures, avulsion of muscles and tendons, and burst injuries of the forearm and hand. Extensive debridement of devascularized tissue and forearm were done. The wounds were left open to be covered with skin grafts 2 weeks later.

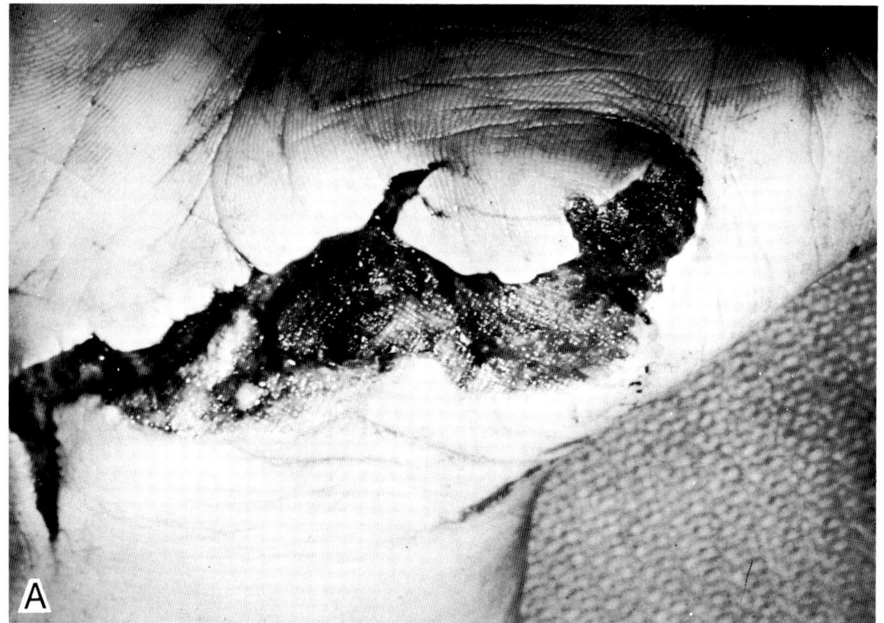

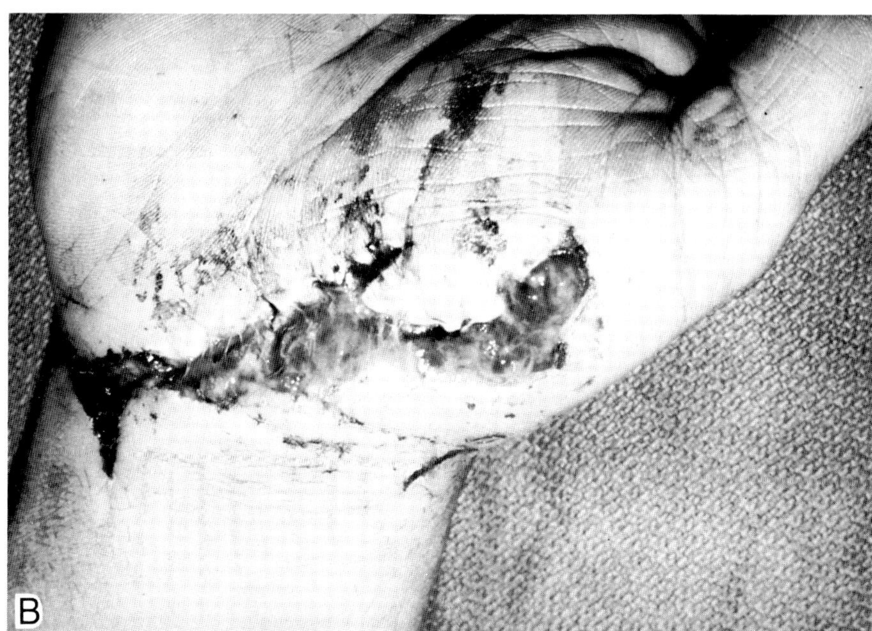

Fig. 44-14. (**A**) Crush, burst, and avulsion of the base of the palm from industrial machinery. The wound was debrided and left open, with compression dressing for several days. Active motion was started at the end of the third day. (**B**) Five days after injury. There is no erythema, induration, pus, or pain. Granulations have appeared earlier than usual. *(Figure continues.)*

Avulsion and Degloving

Parts of the hand that are cut off, torn off, or ground off, either partially or completely, may or may not be suitable for salvage. There are great pressures on the surgeon, from the public and from within, to preserve everything and to reattach all that is detached. The specifics of how and when of amputation management, as well as the principles of skin and other tissue transfer, are covered elsewhere in this text. Other than amputation, most avulsion injuries involve mainly the loss of skin or the creation of distally based flaps of skin. Completely avulsed skin is seldom retrievable, but the distal flap may well be.

Full-thickness skin loss from the dorsum of the hand may leave the underlying extensor tendons relatively unscathed with paratenon intact, or the tendons may be avulsed with the skin, or damaged beyond repair. In the former, split-thickness skin replacement will generally allow satisfactory gliding of the minimally damaged tendon. The time to apply the graft will vary with the degree of contamination, how soon and how well

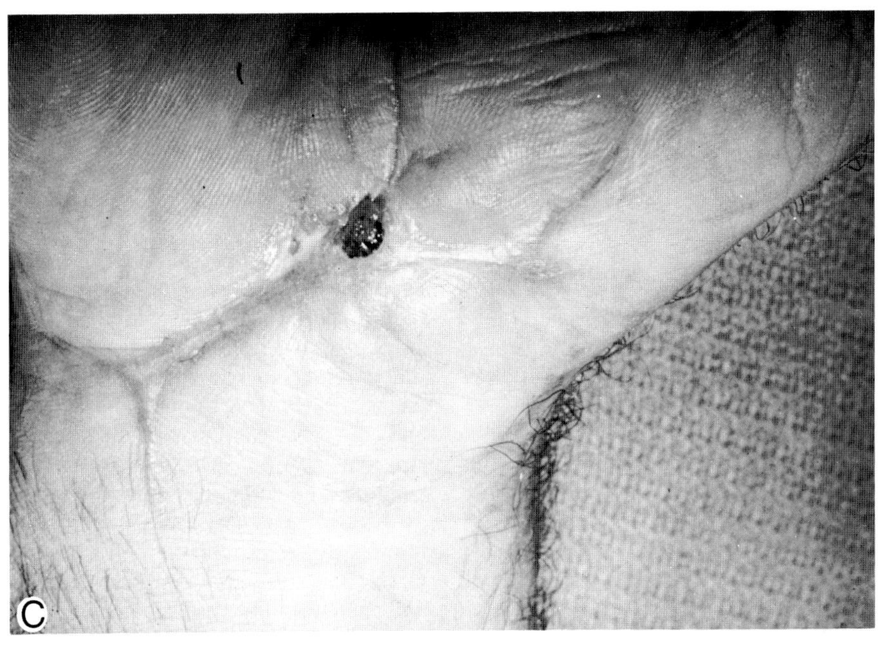

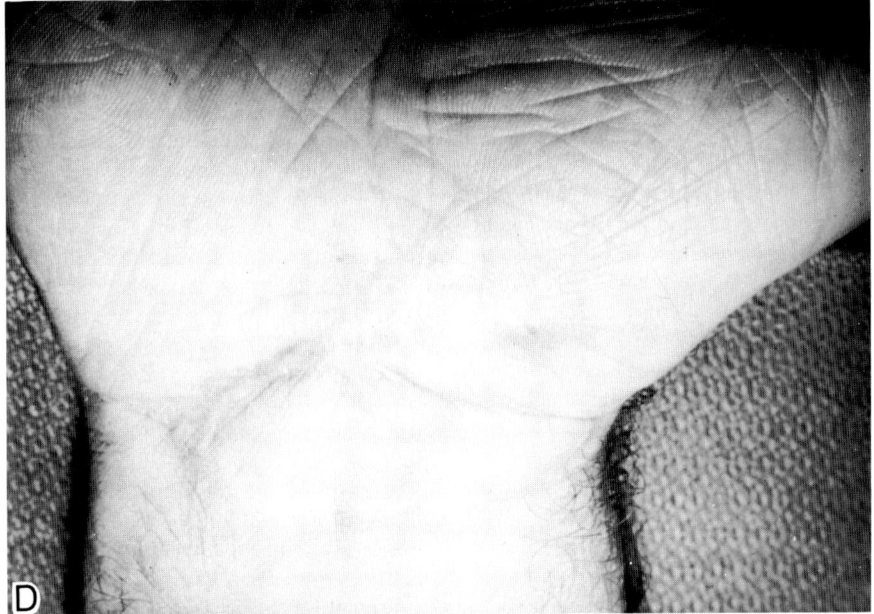

Fig. 44-14 *(Continued).* (**C**) At 6 weeks, the wound has almost completely healed by secondary intention. The patient returned to manual work at 4 weeks. (**D**) Seven weeks after injury, there is normal function and minimal cicatrix.

the debridement is done, and all the other factors bearing on good wound management. Primary skin grafting, immediately after debridement, is not necessary and has all the potential risks (considerable) and gains (minimal) of other forms of primary closure.

If the tendons are avulsed or mangled, their replacement with intercalary tendon grafts, or occasionally by transfer, must be preceded by full-thickness skin replacement, as subdermal fat and areolar tissue will be required to prevent tenodesis. Staged reconstruction in such cases requires careful planning and timing. Wound breakdown and infection, or persistent edema will result in a stiff hand and poor function. Again, primary attention must be paid to the fundamentals of debridement and preparation of the tissue base if uneventful healing is to occur. Premature coverage may create more problems than it solves. The skin flap can be transferred any time in the first 2 or 3 weeks after injury. The ideal time is about the ninth or tenth day, early in the proliferative phase of wound healing, when granulation tissue has just started to appear. In the interim it is important to prevent edema and stiffness with proper dressings, elevation and a combination of active and passive exercises of the digits. The exercise program is particularly important if the avulsion has included the extensor mechanism and capsules of the MP joints.

Full-thickness avulsion of the volar skin of the proximal palm, the "heel of the hand," is often caused by a fall from a motorcycle or bicycle. Skin in this area has an impressive regenerative capacity, and many of these wounds can be allowed to heal by secondary intention (Fig. 44-14). Dressings need not be bulky nor complex; during the healing process the patient should be encouraged to use his hand actively. This appears an unorthodox, even risky, method to the advocates of immediate skin replacement, but I have found that the nature and amount of cicatrix formed compare most favorably with that of successful skin grafts, and compare even more favorably with the scar that results when the skin transfer fails. The healing time is about the same, but with the open method the patient is able to use the hand sooner and is spared additional operations.[42,54]

The vascularity and potential viability of the distally based flap are often difficult to assess (Fig. 44-15). Unless the flap is obviously without hope of survival, the best course is to debride carefully and to replace the flap without benefit (?) of sutures, using adhesive strips instead. Examination of the flap on the third or fourth day will usually reveal whether or not it must be removed or trimmed.

Degloving of a digit, most commonly the ring finger, frequently leaves underlying tendons and joints intact. The problem is generally one of devascularized skin with tearing of the digital vessels and sometimes nerves as well. If the avulsion is complete, with skin completely detached and the finger denuded, skin replacement with either the avulsed skin or by skin graft will not produce a result as functionally or cosmetically satisfactory to the rest of the hand as amputation. Replacement may sometimes succeed where the skin is still attached, or where revascularization is possible, but very careful assessment of the degree of avulsion, the state of the tissues and the patient's individual requirements and wishes must be made before the salvage attempt is made. Microsurgical reanastomosis of both arteries and veins offers promise in some degloving injuries that have hitherto been hopeless, but the functional results have seldom been very good, though the cosmetic results may be more acceptable to some patients than amputation (see Chapter 27).[36,44,67,97,101,109,125,140,161,196]

Amputation

An amputation is the ultimate open wound. Amputations in the hand are covered in Chapter 3, but it is appropriate to give some consideration to the amputation simply as a wound of the hand. The simplest way to treat one is by application of the basic wound care principles already described: debridement, appropriate closure or cover, and early rehabilitation. *For most amputations, for most individuals, in most of the world's medical installations, this simplest course is the best course.* For some types of amputations, in some individuals, in some places, and in some circumstances, reattachment of the severed part may be feasible and may be preferable, but this depends on many factors: the nature of the wound itself, the requirements, wishes and condition of the patient, and the uncompromised availability of competent replantation teams in institutions prepared to give them all the logistical support necessary for this highly specialized surgery. Compromise with these principles will yield compromised results.[26,28,37,104,110,168,176,205]

Machine Mangling

Power machines of industry, farm, and home can cause hand injuries of many types and combinations. Power saws, the whirling blades of automobile radiator fans, lawn mowers and snow blowers, the meshing gears and pulleys, fan belts and rollers of machinery, punch and molding presses, corn pickers and harvesters, meat grinders and shredders, pulverizers, mills, and conveyor belts all make their regular contribution to the emergency room. These moving parts coupled with inattentiveness or human foolishness do great damage: hand parts are avulsed, sliced off, crushed, ground, twisted and lacerated. The injuries are usually complex, with combined elements of contamination, structural disruption, crush, and often thermal and chemical injury as well.[3,29,77,122,127,129,133,168]

The basic fundamentals of treatment apply for these injuries: all repairs must be built on a foundation of the history of the injury, a careful appraisal of the damage, and good overall care of the patient, followed by painstaking debridement. Many of these wounds are highly contaminated with bacteria and foreign particles ground into the tissues: often the history of the injury will tell more of the degree and hazard of contamination than will the appearance of the wound. Industrial accident wounds often appear very dirty due to grease and other lubricants, but grease and grime are far less dangerous than those contaminants that are difficult or impossible to see, such as meat particles, pieces of vegetation, or the myriad of bacteria found in the soil of a lawn or farmland.[20,35,38-40,124,160]

There are often multiple fractures and widespread skeletal disruption and distortion in the mangled hand. The architectural framework of the hand must be reconstituted. Skeletal realignment and stabilization must be accomplished early and the best opportunity for this is during the initial operation. Reduction of dislocations and fractures—reestablishment of the surgical scaffolding—are much easier to accomplish in the freshly injured hand. Satisfactory reduction may be impossible to attain even a few days after the injury.

Premature closure of these complex, heavily contaminated wounds is dangerous; delayed closure, or in some cases, nonclosure, is a safer course. The timing of closure must be predicated on a careful and accurate appraisal of the vascular state of the tissues, the degree of contamination, and the effectiveness of the debridement (Fig. 44-16).

Some of these mangled hands are beyond repair. After careful examination and meticulous debridement, it may still be impossible to determine what will survive and what will be useful. The hand surgeon must walk an uncertain line between realism and optimism. He is obligated to discard all parts that may be detrimental to ultimate hand function, and yet, sometimes seemingly hopelessly damaged tissue will survive the insult of injury. The surgeon must consider the alternatives with every decision he makes; the basic alternative is amputation and he must weigh its advantage against the cost to the

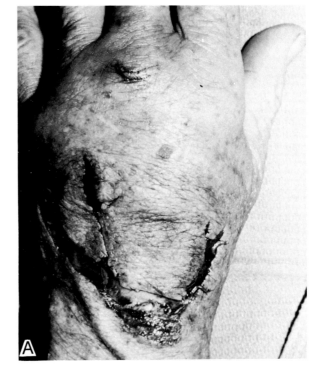

Fig. 44-15. (A) Deceleration on concrete caused this combination of avulsion, abrasion, and a distally based flap. (B) Wound debrided. The flap is held lightly in place with paper strip tapes. (C) Two months later.

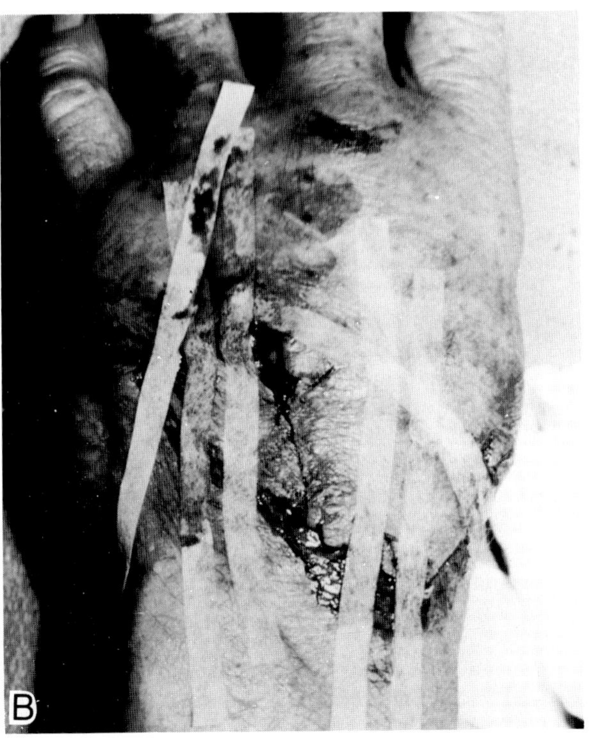

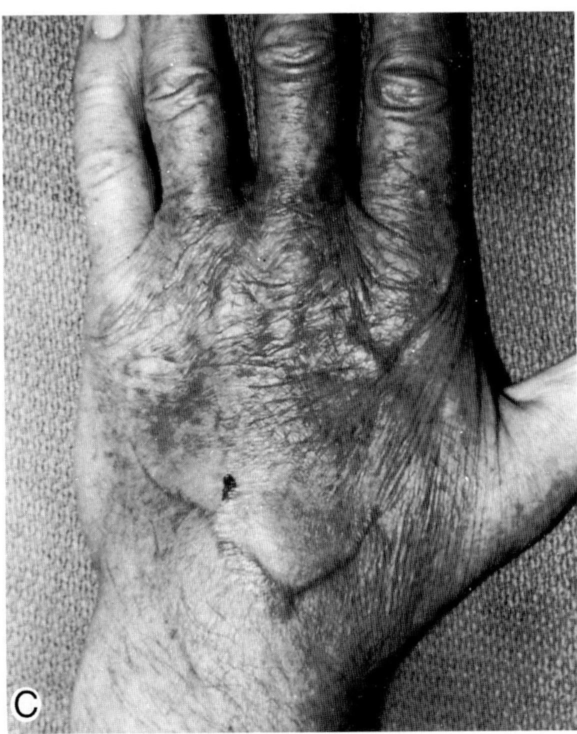

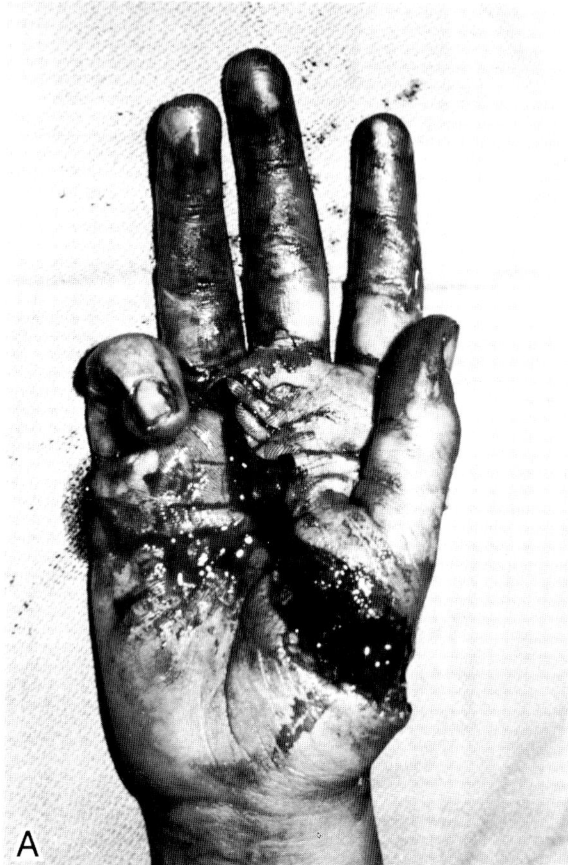

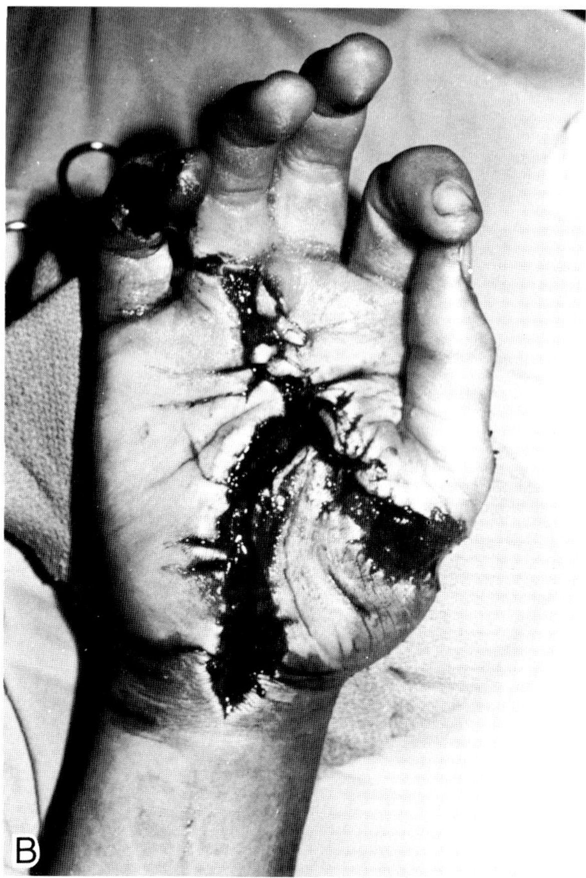

Fig. 44-16. (**A**) The hand of a teenage boy mangled by a power saw. There are comminuted fractures of the first metacarpal; severed extensor and flexor tendons and intrinsic muscles and digital nerves of the thumb; severed flexor tendons and digital nerves of the index, middle and ring fingers; and avulsion of the ulnar border of the small finger. Exploration and debridement were done, the wounds were left open, and no sutures were used. (**B**) On the fourth day, the wound appears benign and ready for delayed primary closure *(Figure continues.)*

patient. Realism may dictate amputation; optimism may counsel retention. Sometimes the outcome is uncertain enough to dictate retention, subject to a second or third look —and consultation with the patient.[24]

Penetration, Injection, and Bites

Sharp instrument penetration, or stab wounds, cause little tissue damage even though important structures may be damaged. The wound is often small and undramatic and frequently causes little discomfort. Careful examination of the hand for tendon, nerve, and artery damage is necessary. Although the wound itself may be of little import, primary repair of these deeper, more important structures is frequently feasible and advisable. Arterial transection or puncture may cause aneurysm or fistula formation that will not be apparent until several days or even months later. It is helpful to know what caused the injury. Wounds from knives or other sharp metal objects seldom need much in the way of exploration or debridement provided a careful examination of hand function has been done prior to anesthesia. Thorough lavage is usually all that is required. If the wounding instrument was glass or an organic material, such as a tree branch or pencil, the wound should probably be explored if there seems a probability that a piece of the material has been left in the depths of the hand.[55]

Penetration of the hand by fluids under pressure, such as paints, lubricants, abrasives, hydraulic fluids, or organic solvents, requires wide surgical opening of the hand, careful lavage, and mechanical debridement. For the first hour or two after injury, these injuries may seem deceptively benign, but rapidly increasing pain and edema then indicate the severity and magnitude of the damage. The management of this type of injury is discussed in Chapter 17.[187]

Bites of carnivores and other animals are mostly penetrating wounds but all have an element of crush proportionate to the size and ferocity of the beast. The animal's teeth carry many types of bacteria deep beneath the skin and deposit them in tissue whose vascularity may have been compromised by crush. Most of these wounds respond well to lavage and nonclosure.[8,197]

Human bites cause more crush and shear, and the extent of

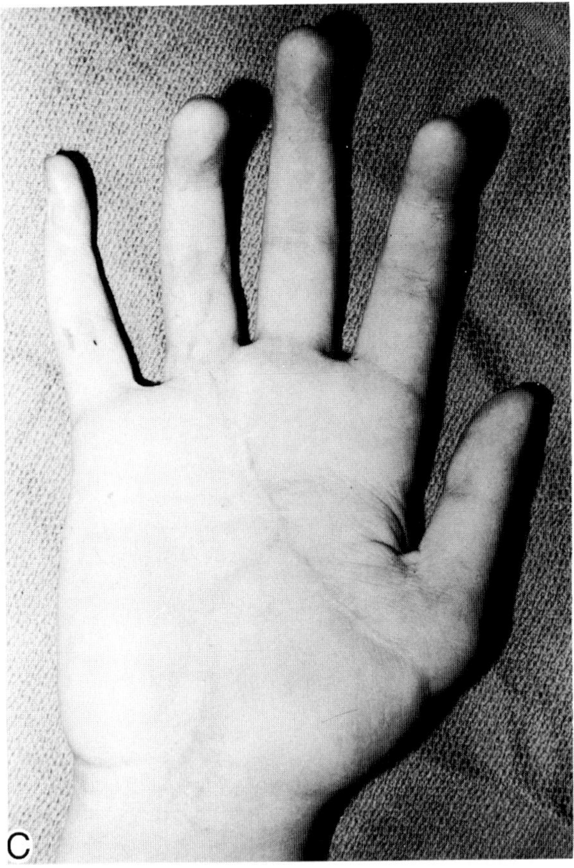

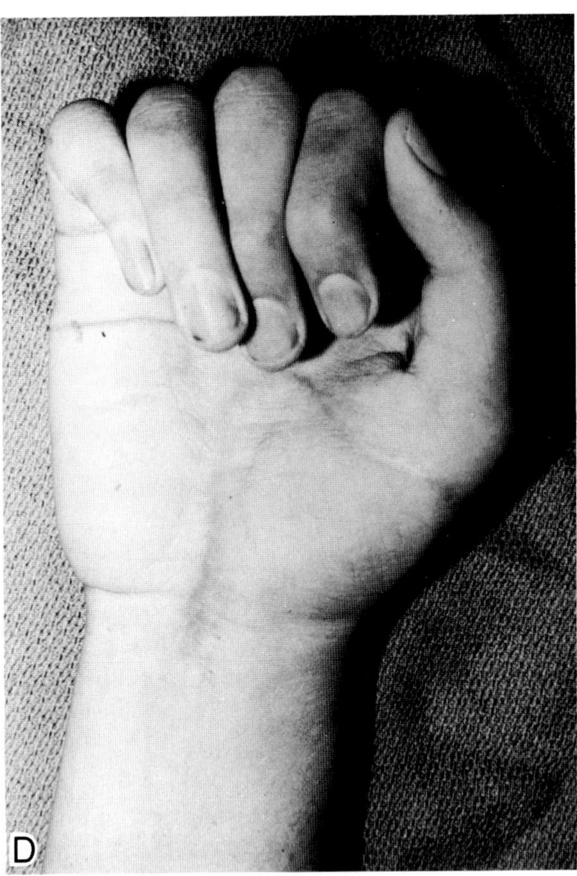

Fig. 44-16 *(Continued).* **(C&D)** Three months after injury and 6 weeks after tendon and nerve grafts. The hand is supple. At 1 year, there was good tendon function and fair sensibility with two-point discrimination to 8 mm.

tissue damage is usually greater than from a dog or cat bite. Furthermore, the microbial flora of human saliva appears to be more varied and virulent than that of the "lower" animals. Careful debridement, copious lavage, nonclosure, and prophylactic antibiotics are all important to their care and will generally allow orderly healing by secondary intention. If the wounds are sutured, not only will they often break down, but the resultant infection may be particularly malignant (often a mixed aerobe-anaerobe type) and may cause widespread tissue destruction and permanent hand impairment.[117,148]

The clenched fist injury incurred by the sharp encounter of a metacarpal head with a human incisor will often open and inoculate an MP joint (Fig. 44-17). If debridement is skimped, or if the wound is closed, pyarthrosis commonly results, followed by articular cartilage degradation, degenerative arthritis, and a stiff, painful, or deformed joint.[50,61,114]

Gunshot Wounds

In evaluating gunshot wounds, it helps to know the type of weapon, and its distance from the patient. Projectiles shot through the hand may be fast or relatively slow, single or multiple, large or small. The surgeon mainly wishes to know how much energy the missile expended within the hand. Since energy equals mass multiplied by velocity squared ($E = MV^2$), the size and weight (M) of the missile is of some importance but its velocity (V) is much more significant. Velocity depends on the type of weapon, the explosive charge, and the distance the projectile has traveled.[15,64,84,87,90]

High-velocity missiles, (those moving faster than 2000 ft/sec) are shot from sporting and military rifles and from machine guns. Most remain in a high-velocity category for a range of several hundred yards. Fragments from artillery shells, bombs, and grenades may sometimes attain high velocities, but their speed (and hence, their destructive energy) usually drops off rapidly within a hundred yards.

Low-velocity missiles come from most .22 caliber weapons and almost all handguns. Shotguns throw a mass of pellets in a spreading pattern for a short distance. Individual shot pellets of buckshot size may retain lethal energy for over 100 yards, but smaller shot pellets of birdshot size lose most of their energy in less than half that distance. Shotgun injuries of the hand are seldom of much consequence beyond a distance of a few yards but most shotgun injuries of the hand are incurred at close range, frequently with the hand held over the muzzle of the gun, and these may be terribly destructive as the compressed wad of shot acts as a single large projectile with considerable

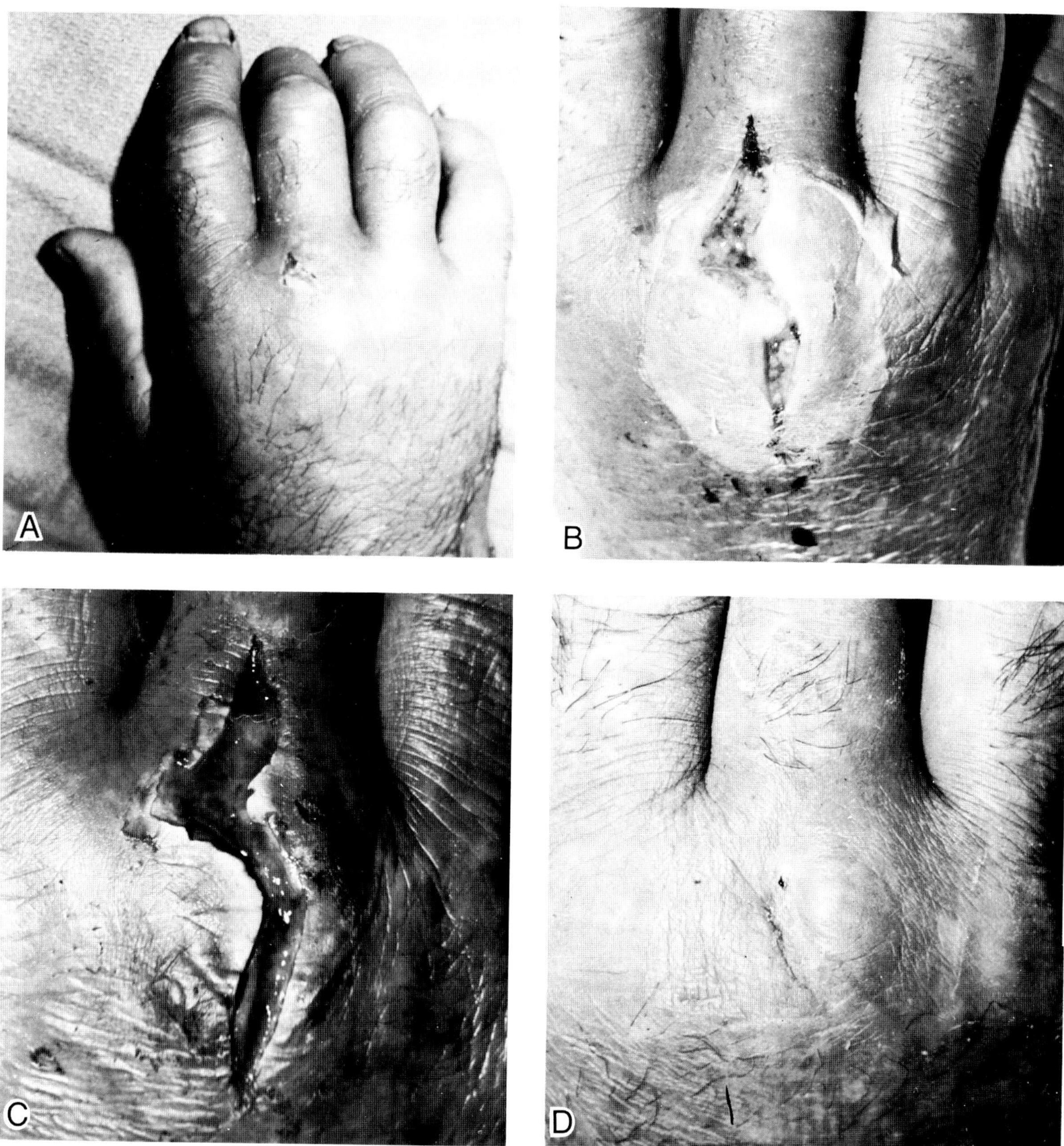

Fig. 44-17. (**A**) A typical clenched fist (human bite) injury with progressive pain and swelling, 4 days after injury. The patient now has active pyarthrosis of the MP joint of the middle finger. In the operating room, the joint was opened widely, debrided of thick pus and torn capsule, and lavaged copiously. No attempt was made to close the joint or wound. Compression dressing, elevation, antibiotics, and early motion were part of the treatment plan. (**B**) Seven days after injury. Pain, erythema, induration, and fever have subsided. Pus is still extruding from the wound as the patient moves the finger. The wound (and the joint) will close spontaneously as the pyarthrosis subsides, and should be allowed to do so. (**C**) Ten days after injury. The joint has closed and the wound is in the proliferative phase of healing. (**D**) Six weeks after injury. The wound is healed, with the joint functional and comfortable.

energy. This shot wad does not begin to disperse until several yards from the muzzle of the gun.[62,188]

The low-velocity missile, from a .22 caliber weapon, or from a .32 or .38 caliber pistol, may fracture a bone or disrupt a joint, but often does surprisingly little damage to a hand. Occasionally a tendon or a nerve may be injured, or a vessel disrupted, but more often the relatively slow-moving bullet tends to deflect these mobile structures rather than transect them. There is usually not much tissue damage, and extensive debridement or decompression is seldom necessary. The entrance wound is small and the exit wound usually only a bit larger. If examination reveals no tendon or nerve damage, and if the hand was not gloved, opening the wound further or exploring its depths is usually not necessary. Through-and-through lavage, fixation of fractures, nonclosure, a bulky dressing, and elevation will suffice. Tetanus prophylaxis is imperative, and a short course of antibiotics is advisable. Active motion should be started early.[1,16,40,62,82,83,180]

High-velocity missile wounds and shotgun blasts at close range are far more serious. Large amounts of tissue are damaged and the requirements for exploration, debridement and decompression are much greater. The assessment of tissue viability is more difficult, and no wounds in this category should be closed primarily. If the missile has struck bone (sometimes it has not) the degree of comminution, distortion, dispersion of bone fragments, and bone loss may be great and skeletal realignment may pose a significant challenge to the surgeon. It is absolutely necessary that the skeletal architecture be reestablished in the primary surgical session; with each succeeding day the task will become more difficult, and after a few days may well be impossible. Segmental defects of bone will require cross-K-wire fixation of fragments to adjacent intact bones or K-wire spacers (K-wires bent into a bayonet configuration) to prevent collapse. Metal plates, screws, and encircling wires are used by some but require much more skill and training in their use than do K-wires. External fixation devices are enjoying an orthopaedic revival; they are occasionally useful in the hand but require a high degree of skill in their application—and even more in their maintenance. For most surgeons, the K-wire is safer, more adaptable, more useful, and more forgiving.

The shotgun charge wad, which may be plastic, felt, or cardboard, should always be looked for in close-range shotgun wounds. The entrance wound of the high-velocity missile is small unless the bullet was tumbling or ricocheting, but the exit wound is usually very large and may avulse great amounts of tissue from the hand or amputate a digit or two. In debriding the high-velocity missile wound, it is advisable for the surgeon to visualize the course of the missile through the hand and to understand that the missile has probably expended great energy within the hand, causing momentary, but extreme distortion, with insult to all tissues within the hand. The high-velocity missile imparts an explosive force to the hand, frequently damaging tissue quite remote from the track of the bullet. Occasionally, though, such a missile will pass cleanly through the hand and expend most of its energy far beyond the hand.[11,35,60,78,90,91,112,141,142]

There is an erroneous tendency to dissociate military from civilian wounds, particularly in the treatment of gunshot wounds of the hand. It is true that there are some differences between the two: military weapons, in general, are more destructive and the wounding environment and degree of contamination are generally worse in military combat than in the civilian milieu, but the degree of destruction, the physiology of wound healing, and the fundamentals of wound care are basically the same. The real difference lies in the surgeon's experience, his prejudices, and his relationship to the patient, and in the pressures to which both patient and surgeon are subjected. These pressures are substantial. The wounded civilian, even though less seriously wounded, makes far greater emotional, economic and vocational demands on the surgeon, and usually the patient's expectations for a good hand are greater than those of the military casualty. The soldier is happy to get out of combat alive, whereas the civilian's injury is often just the beginning of his or her trouble.[2,15,32,51–53,93,183,192–194,199]

Explosion and Blast

Bombs, firecrackers, and other explosive devices may injure hands in many ways. Military high explosive weapons, homemade pipe bombs, dynamite, and blasting caps may tear off a hand or several fingers or blast a hand wide open. There are several elements to the injury: blast effect from the explosion, missile injury from flying debris and container fragments ("shrapnel"), and thermal injury from burning gunpowder, cordite, or other explosive agents. These may cause a complex injury, resulting from any combination of avulsion, laceration, blast, crush, and burns. Contamination with multiple foreign bodies, often driven deep into the tissues of the hand, contributes to the complexities of the injury. Tissue may be torn apart, shredded and impregnated with debris. Tattooing of the skin is common.[185]

The effects of explosives and the direction in which their energy is expended are capricious and unpredictable. An infantry mortar shell is capable of killing large numbers of people within a radius of many yards, yet in some freak accidents the same shell may be detonated in a soldier's hands with only minor injury resulting; or the hands may be mutilated, leaving the rest of the body unscathed. A small, seemingly benign, firecracker, if compressed within the fist, may mangle the hand terribly. The small blasting cap of fulminate of mercury has a very destructive force if contained within the hand, and the same is true of cartridge primers, which are made of similar material. Fireworks, flares, and other pyrotechnic devices also have an explosive force when contained and will add chemical and thermal damage to the injury.

The spectrum of injury from explosive devices is so varied that no specifics for treatment can be given here. The hand surgeon must apply the principles that have been delineated and reiterated throughout this chapter. The plan and course of treatment are based on decision making; logical decisions can only be made by considering all possible courses and choosing the alternative which most closely follows the priorities of surgical principles as applied to the individual patient's needs.[100]

THE ORDER OF PRIORITY FOR OPEN WOUND MANAGEMENT[47,48]

1. The patient as person and body
2. Other injuries; resuscitation
3. History
4. Physical examination
5. Blood supply
6. Debridement
7. Skeletal stability
8. Repair of damaged structures (sometimes)
9. Appropriate timing of closure or coverage

10. Proper dressings and elevation
11. Tetanus prophylaxis and antibiotics
12. Secondary reconstruction
13. Rehabilitation: start as early as possible, preferably while the hand is still in the primary dressing

REFERENCES

1. Adams RW: Small caliber missile blast wounds of the hand. Mechanism and early management. Am J Surg 82:219–226, 1951
2. Allen HA: Hand Injuries in the Mediterranean (North African) Theater of Operations. pp. 79–153. In Bunnell S (ed): Surgery in World War II—Hand Surgery. Office of the Surgeon General, Dept. of the Army, Washington DC, 1955
3. Almdahl SM, Saeboe-Larsen J, Due J Jr: Injuries to the hand inflicted by rotary snowcutters. J Trauma 29:227–228, 1989
4. Altemeier WA: The significance of infection in trauma. Bull Am Coll Surg 57:7–16, February 1972
5. American College of Surgeons, Committee on Trauma: Early Care of the Injured Patient. 2nd Ed. WB Saunders, Philadelphia, 1976
6. Anderson JT, Gustilo RB: Immediate internal fixation in open fractures. Orthop Clin North Am 11:569–578, 1980
7. Ariyan S, Krizek TJ: In defense of the open wound. Arch Surg 111:293–296, 1976
8. Arons MS, Fernando L, Polayes IM: Pasteurella multicida—The major cause of hand infections following domestic animal bites. J Hand Surg 7:47–52, 1982
9. Bailey BN: Skin cover in hand injuries. Injury 2:294–304, 1970
10. Beasley, RW: Principles of soft tissue replacement for the hand. J Hand Surg 8:781–784, 1983
11. Bell, MJ: The management of shotgun wounds. J Trauma 11:522–527, 1971
12. Bennett JE: Skin and soft tissue injuries of the hand in children. Pediatr Clin North Am 22:443–449, 1975
13. Billmire DA, Neale HW, Stern PJ: Acute management of severe hand injuries. Surg Clin North Am 64:683–697, 1984
14. Bornside GH, Bornside BB: Comparison between moist swab and tissue biopsy methods for quantitation of bacteria in experimental incisional wounds. J Trauma 19:103–105, 1979
15. Bowen TE, Bellamy RF (eds): Emergency War Surgery. Second United States Revision of the Emergency War Surgery NATO Handbook. US Dept of Defense. Washington DC, 1988
16. Bowers WH, Preston ET: Low velocity bullet wounds. Contemp Surg 1:57–59, 1973
17. Boyes JH: A philosophy of care of the injured hand. Bull Am Coll Surg 50:341–348, 1965
18. Boyes JH (ed): Bunnell's Surgery of the Hand. 5th Ed. JB Lippincott, Philadelphia, 1970
19. Bragdon RW: Delayed excision in the severely injured hand. Orthop Trans 3:70,1979
20. Brown HC, Williams HB, Woolhouse FM: Principles of salvage in mutilating hand injuries. J Trauma 8:319–332, 1968
21. Brown LL, Shelton HT, Bornside GH, Cohn J Jr: Evaluation of wound irrigation by pulsatile jet and conventional methods. Ann Surg 187:170–173, 1978
22. Brown PW: The prevention of infection in open wounds. Clin Orthop 96:42–50, 1973
23. Brown PW: The management of phalangeal and metacarpal fractures. Surg Clin North Am 53:1393–1437, 1973
24. Brown PW: Sacrifice of the unsatisfactory hand. J Hand Surg 4:417–425, 1979
25. Brown PW: The fate of exposed bone. Am J Surg 137:464–469, 1979
26. Brown PW: The rational selection of treatment for upper extremity amputations. Orthop Clin North Am 12:843–849, 1981
27. Brown PW: Complications following wound care. pp. 314–324. In Boswick JA Jr (ed): Complications in Hand Surgery. WB Saunders, Philadelphia, 1986
28. Brown PW: Complications following amputation of parts of the hand. pp. 197–204. In Boswick JA Jr (ed): Complications in Hand Surgery. WB Saunders, Philadelphia, 1986
29. Bruner JM: Cornpicker injuries of the hand. Plast Reconstr Surg 21:306–314, 1958
30. Bunnell S: Suggestions to improve the early treatment of hand injuries. Bull US Army Med Dept 3:78–82, 1945
31. Bunnell S: The early treatment of hand injuries. J Bone Joint Surg 33A:807, 1951
32. Bunnell S (ed): Hand Surgery in World War II. Office of the Surgeon General, Dept of the Army, Washington DC, 1955
33. Burkhalter WE, Butler B, Metz W, Omer GE Jr: Experience with delayed primary closure of war wounds of the hand in Vietnam. J Bone Joint Surg 50A:945, 1968
34. Burkhalter WE: Care of war injuries of the hand and upper extremity. Report of the War Injury Committee. J Hand Surg 8:810–813, 1983
35. Burkhalter WE: Complex injuries of the hand. pp. 241–257. In Sandzen SC Jr (ed): The Hand and Wrist: Current Management of Complications in Orthopaedics. Williams & Wilkins, Baltimore, 1985
36. Burkhalter WE: Ring avulsion injuries, care of amputated parts, replants, and revascularization. Emerg Med Clin North Am 3:365–371, 1985
37. Burkhalter WE: Fingertip injuries. Emerg Med Clin North Am 3:245–253, 1985
38. Burkhalter WE: Mutilating injuries of the hand. Hand Clin 2:45–68, 1986
39. Burkhalter WE, Brown PW: The Hand. pp. 324–345. In Hill GJ (ed): Outpatient Surgery. 3rd Ed. WB Saunders, Philadelphia, 1988
40. Butler B Jr: Initial management of hand wounds. Milit Med 134:1–7, 1969
41. Cabot H: The doctrine of the prepared soil: A neglected factor in surgical infections. Can Med Assoc J 11:610–614, 1921
42. Carrell A: Cicatrization of wounds. XII. Factors initiating regeneration. J Exp Med 34:425–434, 1921
43. Carrico TJ, Mehrhof AI Jr, Cohen IK: Biology of wound healing. Surg Clin North Am 64:721–733, 1984
44. Carrol RE: Ring injuries in the hand. Clin Orthop 104:175–182, 1974
45. Carter PR: Crush injury of the upper limb: Early and late management. Orthop Clin North Am 14:719–747, 1983
46. Chapman MW: The use of immediate internal fixation in open fractures. Orthop Clin North Am 11:579–591, 1980
47. Chase RA: Surgery of the hand. N Engl J Med 287:1227–1234, 1972
48. Chase RA, Laub DR: The hand: Therapeutic strategy for acute problems. Curr Probl Surg, June 1966
49. Chow JA, Bilos ZJ, Hui P, Hall RF, Seyfer AE, Smith AC: The groin flap in reparative surgery of the hand. Plast Reconstr Surg 77:421–425, 1986
50. Chuinard RG, D'Ambrosia RD: Treatment of human bite infections. Orthop Trans 1:158, 1977
51. Churchill ED: The surgical management of the wounded in the Mediterranean Theater at the time of the fall of Rome. Ann Surg 120:268–283, 1944
52. Cleveland M: Hand injuries in the European Theater of Opera-

tions. pp. 155–184. In Bunnell S (ed): Surgery in World War II—Hand Surgery. Office of the Surgeon General, Dept of the Army, Washington DC, 1955

53. Cleveland M, Manning JG, Stewart WJ: Care of battle casualties and injuries involving bones and joints. J Bone Joint Surg 33A:517, 1951
54. Conolly WB: Spontaneous healing and wound contraction of soft tissues wounds of the hand. Hand 6:26–32, 1974
55. Cutler CW Jr: Injuries of hand by puncture wounds and foreign bodies. Surg Clin North Am 21:485, 1941
56. Cutler CW Jr: The Hand: Its Disabilities and Diseases. WB Saunders, Philadelphia, 1942
57. Cutler CW Jr: Early management of wounds of the hand. Bull US Army Med Dept 85:92–98, 1945
58. Dabezies EJ, Schutte JP: Fixation of metacarpal and phalangeal fractures with miniature plates and screws. J Hand Surg 11A:283–288, 1986
59. de Holl D, Rodeheaver GT, Edgerton MT, Edlich RF: Potentiation of infection by suture closure of dead space. Am J Surg 127:716–720, 1974
60. DeMuth WE Jr, Smith JM: High velocity bullet wounds of muscle and bone: The basis of rational early treatment. J Trauma 6:744–755, 1966
61. Dreyfuss UY, Singer M: Human bites of the hand: A study of 106 patients. J Hand Surg 10A:884–889, 1985
62. Duncan J, Kettelkamp DB: Low velocity gunshot wounds of the hand. Arch Surg 109:395–397, 1974
63. Dunphy JE, VanWinkle W Jr: Repair and Regeneration: The Scientific Basis for Surgical Practice. p. 353. McGraw-Hill, New York, 1968
64. Dziemian AJ, Mendelson JA, Lindsey D: Comparison of the wounding characteristics of some commonly encountered bullets. J Trauma 1:341–353, 1961
65. Edgerton MT: Immediate reconstruction of the injured hand. Surgery 36:329–343, 1954
66. Edlich RF, Rodeheaver GT, Thacker JG, Winn HR, Edgerton MT: Management of soft tissue injury. Clin Plast Surg 4:191–198, 1977
67. Elliot RA, Hoehn JG, Stayman JW: Management of the viable soft tissue cover in degloving injuries. Hand 11:69–71, 1979
68. Elton RC, Bouzard WC: Management of gunshot and fragment wounds of the metacarpus (abstract). J Bone Joint Surg 55A:887, 1973
69. Entin MA: Crushing and avulsing injuries of the hand. Surg Clin North Am 44:1009–1018, 1964
70. Flatt AE: The Care of Minor Hand Injuries. 3rd Ed. CV Mosby, St Louis, 1972
71. Flynn JE: Compound wounds of the hand. Ann Surg 135:500–507, 1952
72. Flynn JE: Acute trauma in the hand. Surg Clin North Am 46:797–812, 1966
73. Freeland AE, Jabaley ME, Burkhalter WE, Chaves AMV: Delayed primary bone grafting in the hand and wrist after traumatic bone loss. J Hand Surg 9A:22–28, 1984
74. Freeland AE: External fixation for skeletal stabilization of severe open fractures of the hand. Clin Orthop 214:93–100, 1987
75. Friedrich PL: Die aeseptische Versorgung frischer Wunden. Arch Klin Chir 57:288–310, 1898
76. Godina M: Early microsurgical reconstruction of complex trauma of the extremities. Plast Reconstr Surg 78:285–292, 1986
77. Gorsche TS, Wood MB: Mutilating corn-picker injuries of the hand. J Hand Surg 13A:423–427, 1989
78. Granberry WM: Gunshot wounds of the hand. Hand 5:220–228, 1973
79. Gross A, Cutright DE, Bhashkar SN: Effectiveness of pulsating water jet lavage in treatment of contaminated crushed wounds. Am J Surg 124:373–377, 1972
80. Gryska PF, Darling RC Jr, Linton RR: Management of acute vascular injuries of the extremities. pp. 84–101. In Adams JP (ed): Current Practices Orthopaedic Surgery, CV Mosby, St. Louis, 1964
81. Hamer ML, Robson MC, Krizek TJ, Southwick WO: Quantitative bacterial analysis of comparative wound irrigations. Ann Surg 181:819–828, 1975
82. Hampton OP Jr: Wounds of the Extremities in Military Surgery. CV Mosby, St. Louis, 1951
83. Hampton OP Jr: The indications for debridement of gunshot (bullet) wounds of the extremities in civilian practice. J Trauma 1:368–372, 1961
84. Harvey EN, McMillen JH, Butler EG, Puckett WO: Mechanism of wounding. pp. 143–235. In Coates JB (ed): Wound Ballistics. Medical Dept, US Army, 1962
85. Haury B, Rodeheaver G, Vensko J, Edgerton MT, Edlich RF: Debridement: An essential component of traumatic wound care. Am J Surg 135:238–242, 1978
86. Heggers JP, Robson MC, Ristroph JD: A rapid method of performing quantitative wound cultures. Milit Med 134:666–667, 1969
87. Hennessy MJ, Banks HH, Leach RD, Quigley TB: Extremity gunshot wound and gunshot fracture in civilian practice. Clin Orthop 114:296–303, 1976
88. Heuston JT: The mechanism and management of the burst finger. Plast Reconstr Surg 39:432, 1967
89. Hoover NW, Ivins JC: Wound debridement. Arch Surg 79:701–710, 1959
90. Hopkinson DAW, Marshall TK: Firearm injuries. Br J Surg 54:344–353, 1967
91. Howland SW, Ritchey SJ: Gunshot wounds in civilian practice. J Bone Joint Surg 53A:47–55, 1971
92. Iselin M: Emergency with delayed operation for wounds of the limbs. J Int Coll Surg 36:374–376, 1961
93. Jabaley ME, Peterson HD: Early treatment of war wounds of the hand and forearm in Vietnam. Ann Surg 177:167–173, 1973
94. Jabaley ME, Freeland AE: Rigid internal fixation in the hand: 104 cases. Plast Reconstr Surg 77:288–298, 1986
95. James JIP: The assessment and management of the injured hand. Hand 2:97–105, 1970
96. Kaplan I: The management of injuries to the hand. Surg Ann 6:283–308, 1974
97. Kay S, Werntz J, Wolff TW: Ring avulsion injuries: Classification and prognosis. J Hand Surg 14A:204–213, 1989
98. Kilgore ES Jr, Graham WP III: The Hand: Surgical and Non-Surgical Management. Lea & Febiger, Philadelphia, 1977
99. Kilgore ES Jr: Hand infections. J Hand Surg 8:723–726, 1983
100. Kleinert HE, Williams DJ: Blast injuries of the hand. J Trauma 2:10–35, 1962
101. Kleinman WB, Dustman JA: Preservation of function following complete degloving injuries to the hand: Use of simultaneous groin flap, random abdominal flap, and partial-thickness skin graft. J Hand Surg 6:82–89, 1981
102. Koch SL: Treatment of hand injuries. N Engl J Med 225:105–109, 1941
103. Krizek TJ, Robson MC: Evolution of quantitative bacteriology in wound management. Am J Surg 130:579–584, 1975
104. Lamon RP, Cicero JJ, Frascone RJ, Hass WF: Open treatment of fingertip amputations. Ann Emerg Med 12:358–360, 1983
105. Lindsay WK: Hand injuries in children. Clin Plast Surg 3:65–75, 1976
106. Lister G: The Hand: Diagnosis and Indications. Churchill Livingstone, Edinburgh, 1977

107. Lister G: Local flaps to the hand. Hand Clin 1:621–640, 1985
108. Lister G, Scheker L: Emergency free flaps to the upper extremity. J Hand Surg 13A:22–28, 1988
109. London PS, Clarke R.: Severe accidental flaying. A plea for initial conservatism. J Bone Joint Surg 41B:658–670, 1959
110. Louis DS, Palmer AK, Burney RE: Open treatment of digital tip injuries. Orthop Trans 3:332, 1979
111. Lowry KF, Curtis GM: Delayed suture in the management of wounds. Analysis of 721 traumatic wounds illustrating the influence of time interval in wound repair. Am J Surg 80:280–287, 1950
112. Luce EA, Griffen WO: Shotgun injuries of the upper extremity. J Trauma 18:487–492, 1978
113. Madden JW: Wound healing: The biological basis of hand surgery. Clin Plast Surg 3:3–11, 1976
114. Mann RJ, Hoffeld TA, Farmer CB: Human bites of the hand: Twenty years of experience. J Hand Surg 2:97–104, 1977
115. Margles, SW: Principles of management of acute hand injuries. Surg Clin North Am 60:665–686, 1980
116. Marshall KA, Edgerton MT, Rodeheaver GT, Magee CM, Edlich RF: Quantitative microbiology: Its application to hand injuries. Am J Surg 131:730–733, 1976
117. Martin LT: Human bites. Guidelines for prompt evaluation and treatment. Postgrad Med 81:221–224, 1987
118. Mason ML: Principles of management of open wounds of the hand. Am J Surg 80:767–771, 1950
119. Mason ML: Treatment of open wounds. Bull Am Coll Surg 42:33–38, 1957
120. Mason ML, Bell JL: The crushed hand. Clin Orthop 13:84–96, 1959
121. Massengill JB: Treatment of skin loss in the hand. Orthop Rev 16:386–393, 1987
122. Maxim ES, Webster FS, Willender DA: The cornpicker hand. J Bone Joint Surg 36A:21–29, 1954
123. McCormack RM: Reconstructive surgery in the immediate care of the severely injured hand. Clin Orthop 13:75–82, 1959
124. McCormack RM: Acute injuries of the hand. pp. 1574–1575. In Converse JM (ed): Reconstructive Plastic Surgery. WB Saunders, Philadelphia, 1974
125. McGregor IA: Degloving injuries. Hand 2:130–133, 1970
126. McLain RF, Steyers C, Stoddard M: Infections in open fractures of the hand. J Hand Surg 16A: 108–117, 1991
127. Melvin PM: Cornpicker injuries of the hand. Arch Surg 104:26–29, 1972
128. Meyer VE, Chiu DT, Beasley RW: The place of internal fixation in surgery of the hand. Clin Plast Surg 1:51–64, 1981
129. Midgley RD, Entin M: Management of mutilating injuries of the hand. Clin Plast Surg 3:99–109, 1976
130. Miles W: Soft tissue trauma. Hand Clin 2:33–43, 1986
131. Milford LW: The Hand. In Crenshaw AH (ed): Campbells' Operative Orthopaedics. 4th Ed. CV Mosby, St Louis, 1963
132. Millard DR Jr, Cooley SGE: A solution to coverage in severe compound dorsal hand injuries. Case Report. Plast Reconstr Surg 49:215–219, 1972
133. Millea TP, Hansen RH: Snowblower injuries to the hand. J Trauma 29:229–233, 1989
134. Moberg E: Emergency Surgery of the Hand. E & S Livingstone, Edinburgh, 1968
135. Morgan MM, Spencer AD, Hershey FB: Debridement of civilian gunshot wounds of soft tissue. J Trauma 1:354–360, 1961
136. Morton JH, Southgate WA, DeWeese JA: Arterial injuries of the extremities. Surg Gynecol Obstet 123:611–627, 1966
137. Newmeyer WL: Primary Care of Hand Injuries. Lea & Febiger, Philadelphia, 1979
138. Newmeyer WL: Problems in primary emergency care of hand injuries. pp. 39–57. In Sandzén SC Jr (ed): The Hand and Wrist: Current Management of Complications in Orthopaedics. Williams & Wilkins, Baltimore, 1985
139. Nicols HM: Manual of Hand Injuries. 2nd Ed. pp. 276–290. Yearbook Medical Publishers, Chicago, 1957
140. Nissenbaum M: Class IIA ring avulsion injuries: an absolute indication for microvascular repair. J Hand Surg 9A:810–815, 1984
141. Omer GE Jr: The early management of gunshot wounds of the extremities. South Dakota J Med 9:340, 1956
142. Paradies LH, Gregory CF: The early treatment of close range gunshot wounds to the extremities. J Bone Joint Surg 48A:425–435, 1966
143. Peacock EE Jr, VanWinkle W Jr: Surgery and Biology of Wound Repair. WB Saunders, Philadelphia, 1970
144. Peacock KC, Hanna DP, Kirkpatrick K, Breidenbach WC, Lister GD, Firrell J: Efficacy of perioperative cefamandole with postoperative cephalexin in the primary outpatient treatment of open wounds of the hand. J Hand Surg 13A:960–964, 1988
145. Peimer CA, Smith RJ, Leffert RD: Distraction-fixation in the primary treatment of metacarpal bone loss. J Hand Surg 6:111–124, 1981
146. Peters CR: Emergency care of the injured hand. Hand Clin 2:507–511, 1986
147. Petty W: Evaluation of the efficacy of topical antimicrobial solutions in reducing bacterial contamination in an experimental wound. Orthop Trans 3:132, 1979
148. Phair IC, Quinton DN: Clenched fist human bite injuries. J Hand Surg 14B:86–87, 1989
149. Pulvertaft RG: Operative surgery series, Vol II. In Rob C, Smith R (eds): The Hand. JB Lippincott, Philadelphia, 1970
150. Pulvertaft RG: Twenty five years of hand surgery. Personal reflections. J Bone Joint Surg 55B:32–55, 1973
151. Raahave D: New technique for quantitative bacteriological sampling of wounds by velvet pads: Clinical sampling trial. J Clin Microbiol 2:277–280, 1975
152. Rank BK, Wakefield AR: Surgery of Repair as Applied to Hand Injuries. 2nd Ed. E & S Livingstone, Edinburgh, 1970
153. Remington JS: The compromised host. Hosp Pract 7:59–70, 1972
154. Rich NM: Vascular trauma in Vietnam. J Cardiovasc Surg 11:368–377, 1970
155. Rich NM, Baugh JH, Hughes CW: Acute arterial injuries in Vietnam: 1000 cases. J Trauma 10:359, 1970
156. Riggs SA, Cooney WP: External fixation of complex hand and wrist fractures. J Trauma 23:332–336, 1983
157. Riordan DC: The primary treatment of acute hand injuries. New Orleans Med Surg J 103:365–371, 1951
158. Riordan DC: Primary treatment of soft tissue injuries of the hand. J La State Med Soc 106:300–304, 1954
159. Riordan DC: Emergency treatment of compound injury of the hand. Am J Orthop 1:30–32, 1958
160. Robinson DC, Hardin CA: Cornpicker injuries. Am J Surg 89:780–783, 1955
161. Robinson DW, Masters FW: Severe avulsion injuries of the extremities including the degloving type. Surg Clin North Am 47:379–388, 1967
162. Robson MC, Duke WF, Krizek TJ: Rapid bacterial screening in the treatment of civilian wounds. J Surg Res 14:426–430, 1973
163. Robson MC, Heggers JP: Bacterial quantification. Milit Med 134:19–24, 1969
164. Robson MC, Heggers JP: Delayed wound closures based on bacterial counts. J Surg Oncol 2:379–383, 1970
165. Robson MC, Krizek TJ, Heggers JP: Biology of surgical infection. Curr Probl Surg, March 1973

166. Robson MC, Lea CE, Dalton JB, Heggers JP: Quantitative bacteriology and delayed wound closures. Surg Forum 19:501-502, 1968
167. Rodeheaver GT, Pettry D, Thacker JG, Edgerton MT, Edlich RF: Wound cleansing by high pressure irrigation. Surg Gynecol Obstet 141:357-362, 1975
168. Rosenthal EA: Treatment of fingertip and nailbed injuries. Orthop Clin North Am 14:675-697, 1983
169. Salisbury RE: Soft tissue injuries of the hand. Hand Clin 2:25-32, 1986
170. Sandzén SC Jr: Treating acute hand and finger injuries. Am Fam Physician 9:74-97, 100-117, 1974
171. Sandzén SC Jr: Complications of external, percutaneous, and internal fixation. pp. 192-205. In Sandzén SC Jr (ed): The Hand and Wrist: Current Management of Complications in Orthopaedics. Williams & Wilkins, Baltimore, 1985
172. Sandzén SC Jr. Complications of the skeletal system of the hand. pp. 107-158. In Sandzén SC Jr (ed): The Hand and Wrist: Current Management of Complications in Orthopaedics. Williams & Wilkins, Baltimore, 1985
173. Saymen DG, Nathan P, Holder IA, Hill EO, MacMillan BG: Infected surface wound: An experimental model and a method for the quantification of bacteria in infected tissues. Appl Microbiol 23:509-514, 1972
174. Scherr DD, Lichti EL, Lambert KL: Tissue-viability assessment with Doppler ultrasonic flow meter in acute injuries of the extremities. J Bone Joint Surg 55A:157-161, 1973
175. Schneewind JH: Surgical emergencies of the hand. Surg Clin North Am 52:203-218, 1972
176. Scott FA: Complications following replantation and revascularization. pp. 205-214. In Boswick JA Jr (ed): Complications in Hand Surgery. WB Saunders, Philadelphia, 1986
177. Spencer FC, Grewe RV: The management of arterial injuries in battle casualties. Ann Surg 141:304-313, 1955
178. Stark HH: Troublesome fractures and dislocations of the hand. p. 130. AAOS Instructional Course Lectures. Vol. 29, CV Mosby, St Louis, 1970
179. Stern PJ, Wieser MJ, Reilly DG: Complications of plate fixation in the hand skeleton. Clin Orthop 214:59-65, 1987
180. Stromberg BV: Management of low velocity gunshot wounds of the hand. South Med J 71:1087-1088, 1978
181. Sturm JT, Cicero JJ: Emergency management of hand injuries. When to repair, when to refer. Postgrad Med 80:97-103, 1986
182. Suprock MD, Hood JM, Lubahn JD: Role of antibiotics in open fractures of the finger. J Hand Surg 15A:761-764, 1990
183. Swanson AB: The treatment of war wounds of the hand. Clin Plast Surg 2:615-626, 1975
184. Swanson TV, Szabo RM, Anderson DD: Open hand fractures: Prognosis and classification. J Hand Surg 16A:101-107, 1991
185. Symonds FC, Garnes NL: Tear gas gun injury of hand. Plast Reconstr Surg 39:175-177, 1967
186. Tajima T: Treatment of open crushing type of industrial injuries of the hand and forearm: Degloving open circumferential, heat press and nail bed injuries. J Trauma 14:995-1011, 1974
187. Thakore HKD: Hand injury with paint-gun. J Hand Surg 10B:124-126, 1985
188. Thoresby FP, Darlow HM: The mechanism of primary infection of bullet wounds. Br J Surg 54:359-361, 1967
189. Tobin GR: Closure of contaminated wounds: Biologic and technical considerations. Surg Clin North Am 64:639-652, 1984
190. Tobin GR: An improved method of delayed primary closure: An aggressive management approach to unfavorable wounds. Surg Clin North Am 64:659-661, 1984
191. Tophoj K, Madsen E: Delayed primary operation for open injuries of the extremities, especially the hand (two-stage treatment). Injury 2:51-54, 1970
192. Trueta, J: Treatment of War Wounds and Fractures. Paul B. Hoeber, New York, 1940
193. Trueta J: The Principles and Practice of War Surgery: With Reference to the Biological Method of the Treatment of War Wounds and Fractures. CV Mosby, St Louis, 1943
194. Trueta J: The treatment of war fractures by the closed method. Clin Orthop 156:8-15, 1981 (Reprint from Proc R Soc Med 33:65, 1939)
195. Upton, J III: Open wounds. In Jupiter JB (ed): Flynn's Hand Surgery, 4th Ed. Williams & Wilkins, Baltimore, 1991
196. Urbaniak JR, Bright DS, Evans JP: Microvascular management of ring avulsion injuries. Orthop Trans 3:306, 1979
197. Van Demark RE Sr, Van Demark RE Jr: Swine bites of the hand. J Hand Surg 16A:136-138, 1991
198. Walker DH: The fate of exposed bone. Reconstr Surg Traumatol 13:141-158, 1972
199. Wangensteen OH, Wangensteen SD: Carl Ryher (1846-1890), great Russian military surgeon: His demonstration of the role of debridement in gunshot wounds and fractures. Surgery 74:641-649, 1973
200. Whelan TJ: Surgical lessons learned and relearned in Vietnam. Surg Ann 7:1-23, 1975
201. Whelan TJ, Burkhalter WE, Gomez A: Management of war wounds. In Welch CE (ed): Advances in Surgery. Vol. 3. Yearbook Medical Publishers, Chicago, 1968
202. Wilson H: Secondary suture of war wounds. A clinical study of 305 secondary closures. Ann Surg 121:152-156, 1945
203. Zimmerman NB, Weiland AJ: Ninety-ninety intraosseous wiring for internal fixation of the digital skeleton. Orthopedics 12:99-104, 1989
204. Ziperman HH: The management of soft tissue missile wounds in war and peace. J Trauma 1:361-367, 1961
205. Zook EG, Doermann A: Management of finger tip trauma. Postgrad Med 83:163-169, 172-176, 1988

45

Combined Injuries

Ueli Büchler
Hill Hastings II

DEFINITIONS

At any given location, injuries of the upper extremity display a broad range of structural and functional complexity. "Relevant structural systems" include bone, joint, extrinsic extensor, extrinsic flexor, intrinsic system, nerve, arterial supply, venous drainage, skin, and nail, as represented in Figure 45-1.

Two main categories of involvement are distinguished:

Isolated Injury

"Isolated injury" involves traumatic damage to a single relevant structural system at one specific location. Examples are a closed fracture, a simple dislocation of a joint, a laceration of the digital flexor tendons without associated neurovascular damage, among others. The association of a nonproblematic injury to the skin is not considered relevant. Therefore, a first-degree open fracture would be included in this category.

Combined Injury

A "combined injury," on the other hand, is defined as a traumatic lesion involving two or more separate, functionally relevant structural systems, at a specific location. Examples include:

a crushing injury of the midhand with a metacarpal fracture, damage to the intrinsic musculature, longitudinal splitting of the extensor tendon, and contusion of the skin

a laceration of the volar aspect of the thumb with partial laceration of the flexor pollicis longus (FPL) and one digital nerve

a power tool injury of the dorsal aspect of the PIP joint with skin defect, extensor tendon laceration, and partial joint damage

a gunshot injury to the forearm with devascularization and multiple structural lesions of bone, muscle, and skin. Amputations are considered to present special states of combined injuries and, therefore, will not be discussed in this chapter.

CHARACTERISTICS OF COMBINED INJURIES

Frequency

Combined injuries comprise about 60 percent of emergencies and roughly 20 percent of post-traumatic secondary reconstructions at our institutions (university-based centers for hand surgery).

Need for Special Skills

Except for sharp lacerations, adequate treatment of combined injuries requires a sophisticated level of hand surgical training with advanced knowledge, technical skills, and experience in skeletal as well as soft tissue reconstruction. A thorough understanding of the modalities of postoperative therapy is called for. Furthermore, the responsible surgeon should master the various methods of secondary reconstruction.

Lack of Treatment Guidelines

While abundant information exists on the treatment of isolated lesions, only a small number of publications have dealt

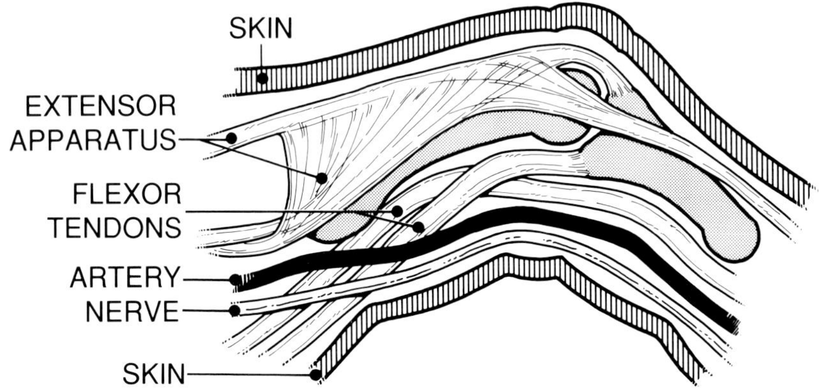

Fig. 45-1. Diagram of relevant structural systems at the proximal phalangeal level of the fingers. Similar schemes may be established for any topographic area and are helpful in understanding the pathophysiology of combined lesions and their management.

with the special consideration of combined injuries of the hand.[1,2,9,13,15-17,21]

Complication Rates

Assessed over a 10-year period, the complication rate was 8 percent for isolated lesions and 17 percent for combined injuries. A better understanding of the treatment requirements of combined injuries during the past 5 years has dropped the respective complication rate to 9 percent in our series.

Number of Procedures

On the average, isolated injuries required 1.32 surgical interventions and combined injuries 2.7 interventions.

Incapacity to Work

The duration of work incapacity was 4.7 times greater in combined than in isolated injuries.

Permanent Disability

As shown in Figure 45-2, permanent disabilities following combined injuries to a given location were more significant than those of isolated lesions. Interestingly, they cover a broad range of the disability scale, which leaves much hope for improvement of results. For other locations of the upper extremity, the numbers would be shifted, but basically similar graphs are expected.

INTERACTIVE RESTRAINTS ON FUNCTIONAL HEALING

The conditions of healing of *isolated injuries* are usually multifactorial, but nevertheless are determined by pathophysiologic factors specific to the affected structural system. It would take special circumstances for other structural systems to become involved. An isolated flexor tendon injury with repair in Zone II, for instance, could become adherent and lead to a fixed flexion contracture of the PIP joint, but this would not normally involve a contracture of the volar capsule of that joint.

In *combined injuries,* the ultimate functional outcome not only relates to the sum of the various lesional components, but also more significantly to the multiple interactions among structural systems involved in the particular pattern of lesion. While an isolated simple extensor tendon laceration in Ver-

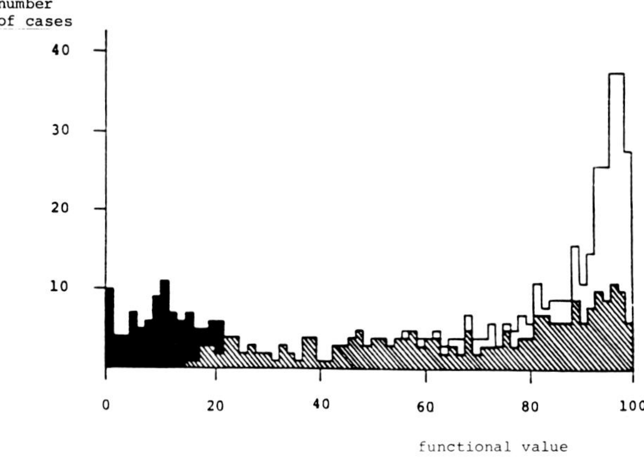

Fig. 45-2. The spectrum of the degree of permanent disability observed in a continuous series of Zone II injuries of the fingers. Isolated lesions are shown in white; combined injuries, including revascularizations and cases with successful replantations are represented with stripes; primary amputations are depicted in black.

Table 45-1. Distribution of Results in Isolated Extensor Tendon Injuries, Isolated Fractures, and Combined Injuries at the Proximal Phalangeal Level of the Finger

	Fair (%)	Good (%)	Excellent (%)
Extensor alone (n = 19)	3	4	93
Fracture alone (n = 25)		8	92
Both together (n = 30)	18	24	58

dan's Zone IV, or an isolated fracture of the proximal phalanx, will each heal with little or no functional deficit, their combination usually leads to marked limitations in the final active range of motion (ROM), as shown in Table 45-1.

For several reasons, interactive functional restraints on healing have not yet been systematically investigated. Clinical data files may not list the full range of complexity encountered in daily practice, and this may make it difficult to grasp specific patterns of combined injuries. In preparing papers on (isolated) injuries of a specific structural system, the material is usually "cleansed" from cases with combined lesions, because —rightfully—these do not seem to belong to the main topic. If combined lesions are nevertheless included in a report, the emphasis remains upon the particular structural system probed.

Clearly, interactive restraints on healing are detrimental to the final functional outcome. They are specific to a particular combination of lesions and relate to a given locus. Scientifically strict examination leads to extremely small sample sizes that are difficult to compare. Nevertheless, previous investigations[4] have demonstrated that the components of the system of motion (bone, joint, muscle, tendon) are tightly interactive, immobilization being the most important single denominator of restraint. An example is given in Table 45-2.

As demonstrated by other authors[8] and verified in our own series, nerve and vascular supply are closely linked, with poor nerve function bearing on the quality of circulation and vice versa. Both systems, however, seem to behave almost independently of the systems of motion.

A third classic example of functional restraints relates to the quality of skin coverage. Flap application, when omitted in cases requiring adequate local revascularization and good surface protection, resulted in significantly higher complication rates and poorer functional outcome.

TYPICAL PATTERNS OF COMBINED INJURIES

In addition to the following typical patterns of combined injuries, a number of other special injuries, each with its own pathophysiology, occur, such as injuries caused by thermal burn, passages of electric current, gunshot cavitations, explosion, and so forth. These all differ widely in their pathophysiology and therefore are necessarily excluded from this discussion. The following are considered "typical patterns," each requiring different management.

Crushing Injuries

Definition

A compressive, crushing force is transmitted to all types of tissue at a given site of injury, leading to contusion, stretching, shearing, and displacement. In contrast to the dorsal or volar combined injuries, crushing lesions are vaguely delineated and may encompass massive contamination, sometimes with foreign body incrustation of tissues. Of the various structural systems, the skin, muscle, vasculature, and bone/joint are affected the most, and their lesions dominate the pathophysiology of this type of trauma, as depicted in Figure 45-3.

Table 45-2. Primary and Final Active Range of Motion in 13 Cases of Volar Combined Injuries to the Proximal Phalanx of the Fingers[a]

	Primary Result				Final Result			
	Poor	Fair	Good	Excellent	Poor	Fair	Good	Excellent
Immediate passive motion[b]	2	1	4	1			7	1
Delayed motion[c]	5				4		1	

[a] Despite the small size of this sample, statistical analysis (Mann-Whitney-U-test) was significant at the $P < .05$ level.

[b] Treated by plating of the fracture, primary flexor tendon repair, and immediate passive mobilization; five of eight digits achieved good or excellent primary results, three fingers were significantly improved by tenolysis.

[c] Treated by nonrigid methods; the flexor tendons were sutured primarily, mobilization was delayed. All five digits had poor ROM results primarily; tenolysis was done in three patients, but improved the results in one case only.

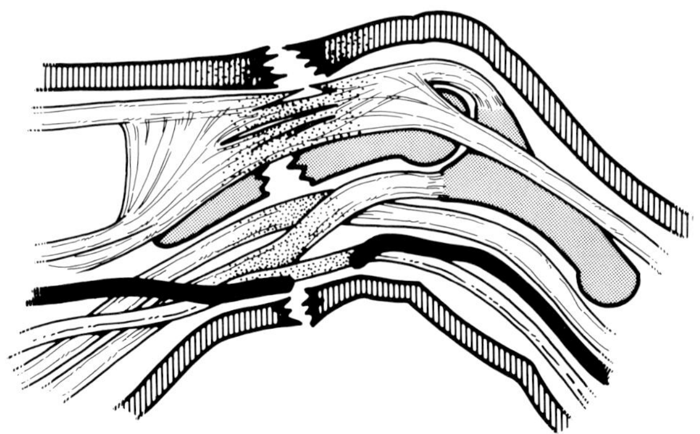

Fig. 45-3. Typical set of lesions inflicted by a crushing injury in Zone II of the finger. Explanations are given in the text.

Bone/Joint

It is important to distinguish the relatively simple and prognostically benign skeletal injuries inflicted by indirect trauma from the problematic bone and/or joint lesions imposed by direct crushing. Diaphysial fractures are usually open, significantly displaced, and grossly unstable. They may be comminuted and then present with multiple, partly devascularized or even extruded fragments; special examples are the problematic palisading fractures of the (proximal) digital phalanges or the two-level (segmental) fractures within the same diaphysis of the forearm bones. In the metaphysis, comminuted fractures usually extend intraarticularly and may be combined with compression of cancellous bone substance, as well as impaction and displacement of articular fragments. Crushing joint injuries involve massive tearing of the capsular and ligamentous apparatus, damage to the cartilage, intraarticular fractures, subluxations or dislocations. At times even a series of skeletal segments is involved. The inherent pathophysiology makes functional skeletal reconstruction a challenge.

Muscle

Tearing of the fascia, crushing and rupture of muscle substance, avulsion from the tendons of origin or insertion, inner overstretching, devascularization, denervation, or a combination thereof may be present to a variable degree. Within an intact fascial sleeve, significant lesions of this kind may go undetected. Even with tears of the fascia, there is an inherent risk of formation of ischemic compartment syndrome.

Tendons

Tendons resist crushing remarkably well and are rarely ruptured, except for avulsion of the tendon of origin or insertion from muscle tissue. Interfascicular tears of the tendon substance, shredding, surface abrasion, and destruction of nutrient pathways are common, however, and explain the enormous tendency of crushed tendons to become adherent.

Vasculature

Especially in conjunction with fractures and/or joint dislocations, significant damage may occur to the arterial and venous vascular tree, leading to critical ischemia or devascularization both locally and at a distance. Usually, the arterial side is more seriously traumatized than the venous network. The main conduits may rupture, suffer subadventitial partial tears, undergo telescopic separation of the components of the vessel wall, sustain insidious avulsion of branches even far away from the main site of injury or undergo other hidden damage to the intima.

Nerves

Unless an avulsion component is superimposed upon a crushing injury, nerves and their branches resist contusion to an astonishing degree, making lesions of more than Sunderland's third degree exceptional.[22]

Skin

The epidermis is contused, stretched, and sometimes torn. The fat of the subcutaneous layer may be compressed peripherally or sheared off. There may be extensive (hidden) skin avulsion along the surface of either the deep or the superficial fascial plane with rupture of septo, fascio and/or musculocutaneous nutrient branches, leading to local ischemia. This pathology makes it difficult (1) to assess the degree and the extent of the skin injury, (2) to judge its survival, and most importantly (3) to predict its revascularization potential when nutritive support is required for the healing of deeper traumatized structures.

Interactive Restraints on Healing

Several pathophysiologic elements threaten functional recovery following crushing trauma:

1. Hidden structural damage (i.e., damage not visible under the operative microscope) may delay or exclude the expected return of function, particularly in nerve injuries.
2. Preserved segments of traumatized tissue displaying decreased circulation may undergo secondary fibrosis or necrosis.
3. Contaminated or hypovital tissue may escape debridement, be buried in the depth of the wound and entail infection, fibrosis, or both, with adverse effect on the capacity for functional healing of adjacent traumatized areas.
4. The crushed segment yields local hypoperfusion detrimental to the functional healing of traumatized structures.
5. Onset of infection is particularly inherent and threatening in crushing injuries.
6. Unless the destabilized skeletal framework is rigidly fixed, passive motion of the dependent joints is difficult to maintain.

7. Crushed tendons have a strong tendency to become adherent if they are not timely and systematically taken through their normal gliding amplitude, which is usually possible only with stable fixation.
8. Crushing injuries are painful and, therefore, interfere with the patient's attempt to comply with the task of early dynamic aftercare.

General Concepts of Treatment

Chances for functional recovery depend upon a multitude of factors. These include the quality of the debridement, the adequacy of prophylaxis against infection, the quality of vascularity, the method of skeletal stabilization, the concept of soft tissue reconstruction (especially with respect to flap coverage), the selection of aftercare modalities, the compliance of the patient, and many others.

Debridement

Tissues that are obviously destroyed, incrusted with dirt, hopelessly devascularized, or massively crushed will undergo later creeping fibrosis. These structures should be removed, regardless of the extent or the depth of the defect created by the debridement. Functionally unessential hypovital tissues should also be eliminated from the wound. On the other hand, important traumatized structures with a potential for functional recovery should be preserved, even if this is doubtful. The problem is that prospectively, it is difficult to delineate between these conditions. A conservative attitude risks ongoing necrosis, infection, delayed healing, dystrophy, excessive scar formation, muscle wasting, inactivity, and progressive loss of function. An aggressive debridement may sacrifice potentially valuable tissue and force one into complex, time-consuming modalities of primary reconstruction. These may be well invested in a young, healthy individual, but may weigh heavily when carried out in a multiply injured or systemically diseased patient. In general terms, we have learned from experience to be generous in the initial debridement and to adopt a concept of extensive primary reconstruction.

Fasciotomy

Closed muscle compartments within reach of the injury and in the dependent devascularized provinces are prophylactically released.

Bone/Joint Stabilization

In crushing injuries, the use of very rigid skeletal stabilization sets the stage for immediate, unimpeded, strong and dynamic aftercare (see below). This, in turn, efficiently limits the inherent adhesiveness of crushed tendons and maintains function of the entire system of motion. "Very rigid skeletal fixation" anticipates three potential problems: (1) the extra load placed upon the site of osteosynthesis by various aftercare modalities when tissue resistance increases (edema formation, inflammation, deposition of fibrin, fibrosis, etc.) or early established contractures are corrected; (2) the risk of avascular necrosis of intercalated fragments; and (3) the eventuality of infection, which mandates maintenance of rigid fixation under adverse conditions. Methods for rigid skeletal stabilization must be based upon established biomechanical principles.[16,20] These may call for primary corticocancellous bone grafting in cases of direct traumatic bone loss, or following the resection of skeletal segments with unrepairable local comminution and/or devascularization. In extraarticular fractures, internal stabilization by plating is currently the method of choice. Intraarticular fractures should be approached by the same stringent concept of firm stabilization. Various methods are available, such as screw fixation, condylar plating, dynamic external fixation,[10] static external or internal fixation, or rarely, primary joint replacement and arthrodesis.

Revascularization

In crushing injuries, three types of ischemia should be distinguished; namely, (1) local ischemia within the traumatized segment, (2) ischemia to the provinces of circulation distal to the site of injury, and (3) a combination thereof. Unless special investigative tools are utilized (such as intra-structural pO_2 measurements), the degree of local ischemia is difficult to assess, and one is forced to rely on the observation of capillary bleeding under the microscope. Local ischemia is the most important determinant of functional healing and complication rates. Segmental vascularity is preserved by limiting surgical dissection and avoiding unessential revascularization-dependent grafts. Adequate debridement and drainage prevents hematoma formation and further embarrassment to the microcirculation that follows with edema or infection induced by retained or contaminated tissues of poor vascularity. Finally, axially-perfused flaps are liberally used to revascularize the affected and surrounding areas.

Distal ischemia is managed by classical methods of revascularization (i.e., by the reconstruction of a sufficient number and an adequate quality of arterial and venous conduits).

Muscle and Tendons

The debridement of massively traumatized musculature may lead to substantial, deep defects (voids) that must be filled with vascularized tissue. One method is to shorten or to narrow the skeletal framework in order to permit direct soft tissue apposition. If this is not justified, pedicled or free muscle or musculocutaneous flaps are ideally suited for filling such large, deep defects. At the same time one may utilize the option of direct motor reconstruction. Ruptured muscle/tendon units, especially if small in number, may immediately be reconstructed by intercalated tendon grafting, tendon transfer, or the interposition of a muscle flap, provided that tendon junctures are made strong enough to sustain early range of motion exercising. Crushed tendons will loose their gliding capacity within a few days unless they are (1) placed in a well vascularized environment, and (2) quickly and frequently mobilized over their entire amplitude (active contraction of the corresponding muscle, passive and active decontraction). Irregularities of tendon surfaces, swelling, fibrinous exudation, and fibroblast activity will build up a significant resistance against ROM exercises; this stresses the need for firm tendon weaves when primary reconstruction is used. In cases with multiple tendon ruptures it may be preferable to delay tendon reconstruction until the wound is completely healed and the capability of full passive ROM definitely established.

Nerves

The degree, depth, and linear extent of the typical crushing/avulsive nerve injury is difficult to assess at the time of injury and, therefore, primary reconstruction is usually not indicated. Exceptions are:

1. Defects of smaller muscle branches close to or within traumatized musculature are immediately reconstructed by interpositional grafting, because it may not be possible to identify the lesion secondarily.
2. Defects of a limited number of sensory branches are treated likewise. Immediate grafting provides for early sensory return. The fact that the number of branches requiring graft reconstruction is limited allows for liberal resection of damaged nerve ends, without greatly increasing the area of donor sensory deficit.
3. Delineated, limited, partial defects of nerve trunks should be grafted immediately, if one anticipates a difficult and extensive secondary intraneural dissection just to recreate the original lesion.
4. With skeletal shortening, direct suture of nerve trunks or branches may be feasible.

Otherwise, lesions in continuity are left unrepaired and placed in a vascular bed. In disruptive lesions, the nerve stumps are placed away from the main wound, marked and secured to adjacent soft tissues with a vessel clip to prevent excessive retraction.

Skin

A temporary loss of epidermal coverage of the hand or other aspects of the upper extremity is not a major problem, as simple (meshed) split or full thickness skin grafting will quickly and reliably establish its healing. The important issue lies in the availability of vascular tissue for (1) filling voids; (2) protection and nourishment of functionally important structures that are exposed; (3) closing portals to inner cavities, such as tendon sheaths or joints; (4) protection and revascularization of bone, tendon, and nerve grafts; and (5) increasing vascularity in cases of segmental local devascularization.[4] Axially supplied musculocutaneous, septocutaneous, and fasciocutaneous flaps are better suited for the task than local random pattern flaps. Whether the flaps carry their own skin or a free skin graft at the recipient site seems unimportant. It is paramount, however, to ensure sufficient pedicle length, ample flap dimensions, and adequate elasticity to accommodate the flap even in extreme positions of motion.

Drainage

Tight closure and sealing of the surface must be avoided, especially when musculature was involved and the wound was contaminated. A great number of passive drains are placed to ensure drainage in a proximal (dependent) direction.

Postoperative Therapy

Prophylactic antibiotics are initiated intraoperatively and continued for 48 to 72 hours. The hand is rested in a position to unload the repaired/reconstructed tendons. Edema, so commonly associated with crushing lesions, is controlled by elevation, slightly compressive dressings, limited administration of crystalloid, and/or low molecular colloidal intravenous fluids. Steroids are occasionally used, under special circumstances, (i.e., massive crush injuries, in which excessive swelling is anticipated). Adequate analgesia is required for the early dynamic aftercare, which must be initiated within 72 hours of injury, before gliding resistance increases. When the skeleton has been rigidly fixed and the tendons are either in continuity, "stably" * reconstructed or left unrepaired, unrestricted active and passive ROM programs are carried out several times daily, even if vascular or nerve grafts have been utilized. This is supplemented by dynamic splinting modalities as required. Muscle strength is maintained and encouraged by active exercise and muscle stimulation. If the initial debridement was doubtful, planned second (and third) look procedures are carried out.

Circulatory deficiency is monitored and immediately addressed, as is secondary necrosis of crushed skin in an area requiring flap coverage. At 8 to 10 weeks, ideally, fracture(s) should be healed, myostatic contracture overcome, passive joint mobility restored, and most of the potential for active motion realized.

Secondary Interventions

Reconstruction requiring temporary immobilization, such as muscle/tendon reconstruction, tendon transfer, nerve grafting, debulking, and others are postponed until the hand may be splinted without risk for late stiffening of the motor systems (about 3 months following the injury). Tertiary procedures, such as tenolysis and capsulotomy are carried out at roughly 6 months.

---

* The term *"stably"* reconstructed tendons refers to a variety of situations. Complete extensor tendon transverse disruptions can be stably reconstructed by the tendon weave technique discussed and illustrated on page 1574. Tendon graft augmentation of extensor repairs allows for postoperative active and passive range of motion therapy. Longitudinal extensor tendon tears that are repaired are also stable enough to allow unrestricted active and passive ROM. Well-repaired flexor tendon disruptions are treated with standard postoperative protocols of passive flexion and active extension.

Volar Combined Injuries

Definition

Volar combined injuries include damage to the palmar skin, the neurovascular elements, the extrinsic flexor system, and the skeletal structures (Figure 45-4). They preserve the extrinsic extensor system, the intrinsic system, the venous outflow, and the dorsal skin.

Sharp lacerations by blade or glass incisions are the most common causes of volar combined injuries. They present with minimal crush and contamination and are rarely violent enough to seriously compromise the integrity of bone and joint. Unless there is a series of closely spaced parallel cuts with compiled local damage, necessitating a more extensive debridement, no tissue defects occur.

Untidy lacerations are frequently inflicted by hand held power tools. Although the wound surface may be ragged and contaminated, it is clearly delineated. (Partial) injury to bone and/or joint is common. One usually deals with limited tissue defects that may preclude direct methods of repair.

Extensive defects, often resulting from industrial injuries, produce the most difficult reconstructive challenges, as one is usually confronted with substantial volar soft tissue loss, devascularization distal to the site of injury, and often widespread segmental devascularization within the area of the defect. Large defects are often encountered involving the flexor system, bone and joint, nerves and skin. Undoubtedly, sizable nerve defects are the most significant feature of this subgroup of volar combined injuries.

Interactive Restraints on Healing

During the healing of volar combined lesions, the components of the motion system that have *not* been directly traumatized (by definition the extrinsic extensor, partly the intrinsic system, and the joints distal to the site of injury) do not automatically retain their functional integrity, as one might hope. In fact, with increasing severity of injury, their performance is increasingly threatened by adhesion formation and joint stiffness. This in turn exerts a large, often definitive, negative restraint on the functional healing capacity of those components of the motion system that needed repair, and ultimately on overall motion performance. Therefore, the preservation of function of the intact structures must receive a very high priority. Rigid osteosynthesis in conjunction with very early, unrestricted mobilization, suppression of edema, and control of pain have been shown to reduce the negative functional restraints. Considering just the requirements of the systems of motion, skeletal shortening should be avoided in the digits, as this would slacken the extrinsic extensor, particularly in Zones III to V. Nerve defects in proximal forearm locations may require bone shortening (see below). A salvage concept of repair must be adopted for the extrinsic flexor system, consisting of either a motion-compatible direct suture, an immediate secure graft,[17] or a delay in favor of secondary reconstruction. Regardless of the method of flexor repair, optimal nutrition of this system must be assured by liberal use of well-vascularized flaps of sufficient dimension and elasticity. Although we hypothesize that associated neurovascular damage might bear on the healing capacity of the systems of motion, this functional restraint has not been proven. There is, however, a relevant interrelation between the quality of arterial circulation and the quality of nerve regeneration. Long-term cold intolerance is decreased with the restoration of adequate axial arterial supply and decent nerve regeneration. Interactive restraints on healing of an associated nerve lesion may occur when axial arterial blood supply is not restored or is secondarily compromised.[3,8]

Interestingly, we were unable to demonstrate a statistically relevant risk for partial or complete dehiscence/separation of standard nerve suture or grafting configurations when adjacent repaired flexor tendons were immediately mobilized, at least not in Zone II.[3] In view of the fundamental impact of nerve supply on the ultimate functional outcome, methods of neurovascular reconstruction must be carefully selected. The nerve repair site may need flap coverage for protection and excellence of nutrition.

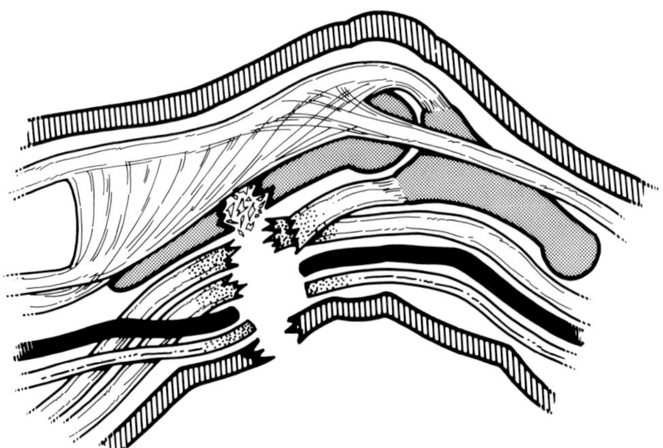

Fig. 45-4. The damaged structures in a volar combined lesion in Zone II of the finger. The volar soft tissues and the phalanx have suffered untidy lacerations with limited defects. The dorsal structures are intact.

General Concepts of Treatment

In **sharp lacerations**, all injured structures are primarily repaired by direct suture.

Untidy lacerations with limited defects require a thorough assessment of the extent of the lesions, particularly with respect to the neurovascular elements in which concealed structural damage may extend a few millimeters beyond the obvious site of injury. A meticulous debridement should be carried out regardless of whether or not grafting or flap procedures may become necessary.

Bone/Joint

Fractures may involve small segmental bone defects. In order to define true anatomic length, it is advisable to obtain x-rays of the contralateral side and to superimpose drawings of the fragments upon a template of the corresponding normal bone. As, per definition, the extensor and (part of) the intrinsic systems are preserved in-continuity, excessive skeletal shortening will result in deficient extension of the dependent joints. Except for the proximal segments of the upper extremity, skeletal shortening will rarely if ever compensate for volar soft tissue defects, as one might hope (Fig. 45-5).

Aside from the need for adequate length restoration of the involved bone segments, it is mandatory to provide rigid skeletal fixation, usually best accomplished by plating. Since the fracture is exposed volarly, a technical difficulty arises with the need for applying the plate according to biomechanical requirements, i.e., to the tension side of bone (usually dorsally). To avoid additional dorsal exposure, one may compromise with a stronger plate applied in the lateral position. For bone defects, compression-resistant segmental bone grafts are used. Because they are not readily revascularized, diaphysial bone grafts from phalanges or metacarpals of amputated adjacent parts should not be used.

Muscles and Tendons

For intrinsic system requirements see under Metacarpal Injuries on page 1579.

Shredded flexor tendon ends must be cut back to (near) normal cross sections. In power tool injuries that create limited segmental defects, it is difficult to determine exactly how much tendon substance is missing; a clue may be obtained by knowing the width of the working blades of the machinery, and by assessing the extent of bone and other soft tissue defects. Provided that mobilization begins very early, there is no added risk to restoration of the flexor system primarily, either by direct suture despite limited gap formation, or by primary grafting. Local requirements as outlined below must be considered, however.

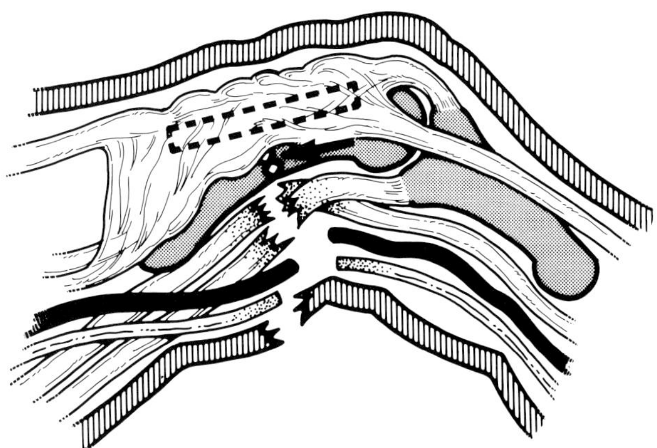

Fig. 45-5. Skeletal shortening is *not* recommended for treating volar combined injuries in Zone II of the finger, because the shortening does not fully compensate the volar soft tissue defect and, moreover, creates redundancy in the extensor apparatus.

Nerves

While damage to the sensory branches and the trunks of the three nerves supplying the hand are readily recognized, it takes a special effort to identify or rule out injuries to the thenar branch of the median nerve, the deep motor branch of the ulnar nerve, and branches to the hypothenar eminence, the deep motor branch of the radial nerve, and other critically important motor nerve branches. Untidy lesions of the proper palmar digital nerves, the common digital nerves of the palm, the motor branches of the median, ulnar, and radial nerves should not be left for secondary reconstruction, because (1) later identification would require a difficult dissection into a scarred area, (2) precious time would be lost for regeneration, and (3) chances for nerve regeneration would not be improved significantly. Efforts to pull small defects of these nerve branches together by direct suture should not be done. Rather, the preferred treatment is with primary interfascicular nerve grafting. This permits unlimited debridement of nerve substance as required, takes tension off the repair site, reduces scar formation, and helps to maintain coaptation under the load of early motion therapy. A prerequisite for primary nerve grafting, however, is the creation of a healthy wound surface with good revascularization capacity.

Controversy exists as to how to deal with small gaps of the major nerve trunks. We favor immediate direct suture if a single 8-0 nylon epineurial suture keeps the nerve ends firmly approximated (with adjacent joints in a neutral position). Maintenance of coaptation of a *completed* repair is tested by placing the extremity in the posture applying the most stress to the sutured nerve(s). If a truncular* nerve gap is present, particularly after the debridement would have necessitated repair under undue tension, secondary nerve reconstruction must be carried out. In the presence of multiple truncular nerve gaps, limited skeletal shortening, either at a fracture site or by osteotomy, should be considered if this would allow for immediate direct nerve repair.

Arterial Lesions

In most volar combined injuries, associated arterial lesions do not endanger survival of the tributary part(s). Nevertheless, it is important to assure axial arterial flow, either by direct suture or interpositional vein grafting, because of the link between the adequacy of perfusion and the quality of nerve regeneration, and because other influences may be applicable (trophic condition, flap survival, potential for local revascularization of grafts, or others).

Skin

Coverage of a volar combined injury with loosely lying, elastic, and well-perfused local skin or flap tissue is essential for the protection and the nutrition of underlying injured structures.

* *Truncular* refers to proximal segments of major nerves prior to significant division.

Should one observe marginal necrosis and/or wound dehiscence, because these basic requirements were not sufficiently met, immediate reintervention and delayed flap coverage are imperative.[6]

Postoperative Therapy

Flexor tendon repair sites are protected by dorsal extension block splinting. Passively supported, active extension exercises are immediately encouraged. Full passive flexion, both isolated and composite for the various dependent joints, are begun within the first 2 days following the injury. Dorsal block splinting is removed for hourly exercises at 4½ weeks and totally discontinued at 5½ weeks. Dynamic extension assist splints may be used after the sixth week. When the outlined treatment concept is followed, secondary procedures are rarely necessary. Delayed nerve grafting should be carried out as soon as the systems of motion have reached their final functional plateau, usually after 8 to 12 weeks. In the presence of adhesions, flexor tenolysis may be rewarding, provided that secondary involvement of the extensor system was minimal, passive joint motion reasonably well preserved, the trophic condition was satisfactory, and the skin quality was right.

Extensive Volar Defects

General Concepts of Treatment

Debridement

The debridement is generally straightforward, as this will not create additional structural gaps but, for the sake of healthy wound margins, merely enlarge preexisting defects to an insignificant degree.

Bone/Joint

Skeletal injuries may extend over more than one segment or present as multi-level lesions. As pointed out previously, reconstruction of nearly normal length of the bony framework by liberal use of intercalated bone grafts is beneficial to the function of the extensor system. With significant joint injuries, primary arthrodesis should be considered, as this will do away with a possibly difficult and problematic joint reconstruction and at the same time reduce the number of tendons to be restored. Again, rigid bone (and graft) fixation favors a safe and timely healing of the skeletal lesions and is indispensable for dynamic aftercare.

Flexor Tendons

Extensive defects in the flexor system preclude direct repair. Within its tendinous portion, immediate grafting may be considered under special circumstances, but it is usually safer to postpone the reconstruction. With massive defects of muscle substance, the ultimate functional detriment is hard to predict; immediate substitution of missing muscle tissue is therefore not generally advised. However, if a pedicled or free muscle or musculocutaneous flap would be indicated for other reasons, its functional capacity should be exploited.

Revascularization

Revascularization of tissues distal to the defect is carried out by well-calibrated interpositional vein grafting of at least one axial arterial conduit, or by the placement of a pedicled or free (composite) flow-through flap. Since surgically interposed vascular conduits bypass the zone of injury, which may well be ischemic on its own, an excellent capillary perfusion pressure to the distal part(s) should be obtained so as to maximize retrograde collateral circulation.

Nerve

For reasons pointed out in the previous section, immediate reconstruction of distal sensory and/or motor nerve branches by interfascicular nerve grafting is advocated; nerve branches contained in pedicled or free neurovascular flaps may serve well as vascularized nerve grafts. Extensive defects of nerve trunks should not be treated initially, because (1) the true extent of such nerve injuries may be difficult to determine even under the operative microscope; (2) the increased risk of early postoperative complications (hematoma, infection, and others) inherent in these injuries might entail the loss of a large mass of precious nerve grafting substance; (3) the conditions for revascularization of conventional nerve grafts may not be ideal even when placed outside their normal anatomic locations in a area of less scarring or brought into contact with flap tissue; and (4) if vascularized nerve grafting is considered, this might be too time-consuming to perform immediately on a critically injured patient. Anticipating the difficulty of secondary identification of truncular nerve stumps within a massively scarred extremity segment, it is advantageous to mark corresponding nerve stumps and their defects with vessel loops of different colors. In multiple truncular nerve gaps of the proximal parts of the upper extremity, the full spectrum of modalities of nerve reconstruction should be considered, including skeletal shortening and direct nerve repair, nerve transfer, free composite flap application, and others.

Skin Defects

Coverage by well-vascularized flaps is necessary to (1) promote wound healing; (2) lower the risk of complications; (3) offset local ischemia; (4) favor revascularization of bone, tendon and/or nerve grafts; (5) fill tissue voids and recontour the profile of the surface; and (6) promote the restitution of lymphatic drainage. Free flaps have become the gold standard of treatment, because they offer a myriad of advantages over conventional flaps. Potential advantages are their unlimited size, their excellent vascularity, their potential for one-step composite tissue reconstruction, and their benefit for postoperative elevation and dynamic aftercare. A warning applies to muscle or musculocutaneous flaps with low resistance flow characteristics: In order to prevent an arterial "steal" phenomenon to conduits used for distal revascularization, it is preferable to perform the anastamoses to unrelated channels of the vascular tree.

Postoperative Therapy

In wounds with gross contamination and/or poor definition of the extent of lesions, an early second look beneath the flap improves the safety of wound control. Range of motion therapy follows the outline given in the previous section, the emphasis being on maintenance of joint and extensor tendon function, while permitting adequate healing of the flexor system in case this was primarily reconstituted.

Secondary Procedures

Secondary procedures are deferred until the systems of motion have reached a functional plateau. Truncular nerve lesions not repaired immediately should be given priority and are preferably reconstructed within 8 to 12 weeks. If the hand is completely denervated, other procedures are better delayed until sensibility has returned to the S1 level.[1] Otherwise, following an additional 6 to 12 weeks, further flexor tendon surgery is carried out (second stage of tendon grafting, muscle reconstruction, tenolysis). A third set of late reconstructions may involve tendon transfers, arthrodeses and/or tenodeses to optimize ultimate motor function. As 1 to 2 incapacitating years may elapse before the final result has been reached, and as it is notoriously difficult to bring the patients back to work after this time, a comprehensive long-term planning of social and professional rehabilitation is particularly important in patients with these types of injuries.

Dorsal Combined Injuries

Definition

Dorsal combined injuries comprise lesions of the dorsal skin, the extensor tendon(s) or extensor apparatus, bone and/or joint, and facultatively, the intrinsic system and the bony insertion of the annular pulley system (Fig. 45-6). The flexor tendons, the volar neurovascular structures, and the volar skin are preserved.

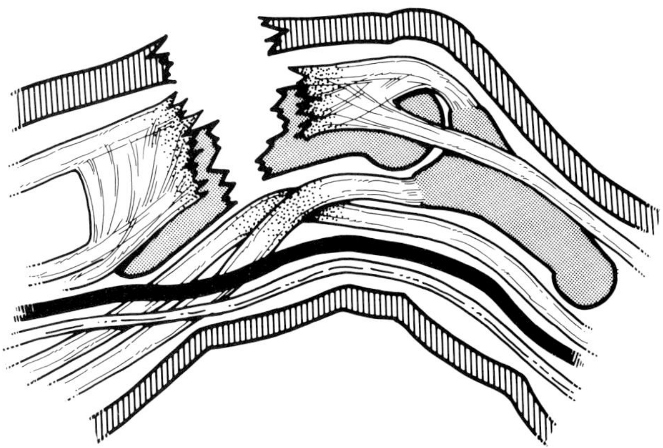

Fig. 45-6. Diagram of a typical dorsal combined injury in Verdan's Zone IV of the finger.

Pure incisive mechanisms of injury (such as knives, scissors, glass) are rarely violent enough to cause serious damage to the skeletal structures. The ordinary dorsal combined injury is inflicted by hand-held or industrial power machinery, such as saws, milling cutters, planers, hoes and others. Depending on the width of the working edges and the action of these tools, more or less extensive tissue defects are created that may be surface dominant, depth dominant, or have a trough-shaped depth involvement. Although ragged, the wound surfaces are usually sharply traumatized, with little hidden damage to adjacent areas. The contamination is generally restricted to the immediate wound surface.

Interactive Restraints on Healing

Within the scenario of a dorsal combined injury, destabilization of the skeletal framework by a fracture or a joint injury entails a serious functional hazard to the flexor system, the intrinsic system, and the joints distal to the site of injury, although per definition, these structures are anatomically intact. Adhesions and contractures of undamaged flexor tendons and dependent joints do occur, particularly if immobilization is required. While these would be benign and would be easily corrected in a simple scenario of injury, their definite negative impact on the functional outcome of complex dorsal combined lesions must not be underestimated. The second interaction relates to the quality of skin coverage. Exposed joints, joint reconstruction sites, fractures, intercalated bone grafts, extensor tendon repair sites, and primary or secondary tendon grafts cannot adequately heal, and may be subject to infection unless excellent local nutrition and protection are provided.

General Concepts of Treatment

Sharply incised dorsal combined injuries are simply treated by direct repair and immobilization.

As outlined above, the components of a dorsal combined injury **incorporating limited or extensive defects** should be addressed with a comprehensive plan of reconstruction, and definitely not with multiple, uncomplementary surgical techniques, even if these are accepted practice in the treatment of identical, but isolated lesions. If a dorsal combined injury was treated by K-wire fixation of the fracture, by delaying the extensor tendon repair and by awaiting the formation of granulation tissue for later split thickness skin grafting, all of which may be reasonable in a different context, a functional fiasco would be inevitable. In the 1970s, we started out with a concept of immediate anatomic reconstruction of all structural systems injured, accepted the need for immobilization during the time of healing, encouraged the return of function with usual methods of postoperative therapy, frequently carried out major secondary tenolysis and capsulotomy procedures, and finally realized that "anatomy now, function later" was not the way to continue. With a clearer understanding of the interactive restraints outlined above, the following concepts are now employed:

Debridement

A very thorough debridement is simple to perform, as usually the wound margins are sharply defined, contamination is limited, and additional structural discontinuity is not created. It may, however, significantly enlarge an existing defect.

Bone/Joint

An extraarticular fracture is stabilized by very rigid methods of osteosynthesis (usually plating), to allow for unimpeded mobilization of the flexor system and of the dependent joints. Very limited skeletal shortening for gaining soft tissue length may be indicated in selected cases, but should not lead to major alteration of flexor system kinetics. A significant bone defect is not closed, but compensated for by interposition of a compact, corticocancellous graft (see Fig. 45-13). With intraarticular fractures, articular defects or joint destruction, a definitive reconstructive procedure is carried out in order to restore framework stability while maintaining a maximum potential of motion (stable internal fixation of an intraarticular fracture, repair or reconstruction of a ligament, osteochondral grafting of a joint surface defect,[13] vascularized joint transfer,[7] prosthetic replacement, arthrodesis with or without intercalated grafting).

Intrinsic System

Defects of the terminal tendons of the abductor pollicis brevis, the adductor pollicis, the first dorsal interosseous, and the abductor digiti quinti are overcome by immediate intercalated tendon grafting with transosseous insertion. Other lesions are left to heal and treated by secondary tendon transfers if needed.

Extensor Mechanism

Two concepts of treatment have evolved with respect to the extrinsic extensor tendon system: In concept #1, the lesion is simply left for secondary reconstruction, and unrestricted active flexion and assisted passive extension exercises are begun immediately. Once the skeletal injury has healed, and once the functional integrity of the flexor tendon system and the dependent joints is definitely "assured," the restoration of continuity to the extensor tendon system (which classically requires some immobilization) will no longer jeopardize the function of the other structural components. Concept #2 uses immediate extensor tendon reconstruction. In order to offset interactive restraints on healing, however, methods of repair compatible with immediate active flexion, passive extension, and assisted active extension are utilized. These comprise the liberal employment of tendon grafts with strong intraosseous insertions and/or sturdy tendon weaves (Fig. 45-7). Repair sites are maximally loaded under vision to assure adequacy of force transmission without dehiscence, and to help select safe modalities of postoperative therapy.

Skin

The skin defect of a dorsal combined injury needs coverage with flap tissue of sufficient dimension (allowing full flexion), elasticity, and excellent vascularity, so as to promote healing of the underlying repair site, especially when bone and/or tendon grafts are used.[4] Tight direct suture or skin grafting is avoided. Unless local flaps suffice, regional axial flaps on their vascular pedicle or free flaps are the gold standard, because they are safe, are independent in size, offer excellent capacity for revascularization, have the potential for venous flow-through reconstruction, and allow systematic elevation.

Postoperative Therapy

Postoperative therapy and secondary interventions: In concept #1, the joints of the hand are rested in full extension and, within 72 hours at the latest, are brought through full passive and then active flexion many times daily to maintain the full arch of motion and to minimize atrophy of the flexor system. Dynamic extension splinting is instituted at an early stage. Secondary reconstruction of the extensor system is carried out when the flap is definitively healed, when a normal trophic condition is reestablished, when free passive joint motion and full active flexion are restored, and when inherent secondary immobilization is no longer likely to compromise the function of the other systems of motion after the third month. When dealing with late defects of the extensor system, one must not necessarily restore original anatomy but also think of using tendon transfers. Debulking of the flap is not safe to carry out simultaneously. Roughly a year following the injury, removal of metal implants, tenolysis/capsulectomy (if necessary) and flap corrections are carried out. In concept #2, postoperative therapy differs in four respects: (1) to keep the motion resistance at a minimum, exercises are begun immediately; (2) active extension is not allowed, except for having the patient hold a position of passively set moderate extension; (3) discriminative flexion (all other joints extended, just PIP flexed; all other joints extended, just MP flexed, etc.) is widely used both passively and actively; (4) composite flexion to more than 70 percent of the arc is not allowed before the third week. If final motion is not satisfactory, tenolysis/capsulotomy procedures are preferably staged, the first intervention being on the extensor side.

Dorsal and Volar Combined Injuries

Definition

Dorsal and volar combined digital injuries include variable degrees of injury to both dorsal and palmar sides of the digit. Although complete amputations represent the extreme example of dorsal and volar combined injury, for obvious reasons

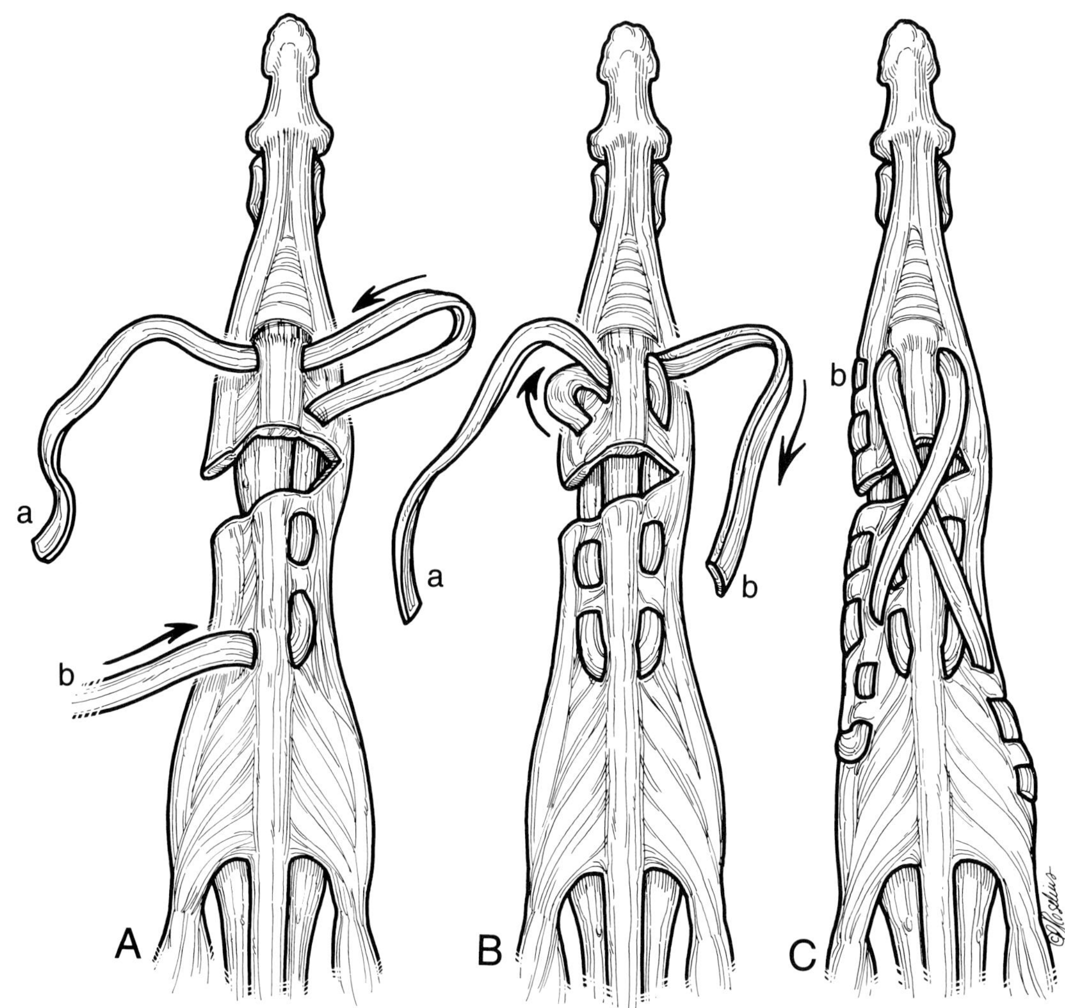

Fig. 45-7. Author's method for primary (or secondary) reconstruction of the extensor apparatus in Zones III to IV of the finger by a tendon graft. The weave is meant to be strong enough for immediate dynamic aftercare.

these will not be covered here. Replantation is discussed in Chapter 27.

Crushing injuries commonly seen in the industrial environment are the most common cause of dorsal and volar combined injuries. Local segmental devascularization is always present, and often distal vascularity is compromised as well. The breadth of segmental injury varies with the type of object or implement causing the crush. Most often, damage on one side of the digit exceeds that on the other.

Untidy lacerations may occur from power tools, such as skill saws or table saws. The extent of dorsal and volar injury depends upon the depth and width of the cutting implement. While distal devascularization is common, the extent of segmental devascularization is usually more limited than in cases caused by crushing mechanism. Partial avulsion or degloving injuries can occur by traction and torsion of the digit by a ring that has been caught suddenly or a glove caught by a rotating power device. In such instances, the extent of segmental devascularization may compare with that seen in crush injuries. The patterns of injury vary greatly.

Extensive defects most often occur from industrial injuries, such as punch presses causing extensive dorsal and volar soft tissue loss, segmental devascularization, and distal devascularization. Large defects in flexor mechanism, bone and joint, and nerve and skin, greatly complicate the assessment of reconstruction potential.

Interactive Restraints on Healing

All components of the system of motion are at risk. By definition, the extrinsic and intrinsic extensor mechanism, as well as the flexor mechanism, are injured either completely or partially. Each system exerts a dramatic negative influence on the healing and functional potential of the other systems. Even when adjacent ligaments and joints are not obviously injured, they invariably become affected by fibrous thickening and arthrofibrosis. Devascularization exerts a highly negative restraint on the functional healing capacity of those components needing repair, as well as adjacent joints that are structurally intact, but often partially injured. Do not underestimate the extent of compromise to the venous and lymphatic system. Edema leads to early fibrosis and limited joint range of motion, and places increased tensile stress on required tendon units with attempted motion. Edema and early fibrosis also place increased forces on fracture repairs. Delayed healing is to be expected, secondary to the segmental devascularization and frequent fracture comminution. For both of these reasons, rigid osteosynthesis is required.

Unless a portion of the system of motion can be preserved, such as passive joint ROM, secondary procedures on the flexor and extensor tendon mechanisms will be difficult, often multiple, and with limited results. Any consideration for secondary extensor or flexor reconstruction will have to be deferred for at least 3 months, as the process of wound healing and achievement of soft tissue homeostasis will be slow. Primary reconstruction of at least one tendon mechanism (flexor or extensor) is essential to isolate later reconstructive procedures to only one side of the digit.

General Concepts of Treatment

The patterns of injury seen in dorsal and volar combined injuries vary greatly. The approaches to treatment, however, are consistent and depend upon whether the injury involves dorsal more significantly than volar tendon structures, volar more than dorsal structures, or equally involves both dorsal and volar tendon structures.

Extrinsic and Intrinsic Extensor Mechanism Disrupted, Flexor Mechanism Injured, But Intact

By definition, all components of the system of motion are at risk. Gliding motion of the flexor mechanism and adjacent joints must be preserved by repair techniques that allow for early ROM; with few exceptions this can be achieved.

Bone/Joint. Fractures may involve segmental bone loss. At least 5 mm of bone shortening can be tolerated by the flexor mechanism; this may facilitate primary repair of the intrinsic and extrinsic extensor mechanism. At the proximal phalangeal level plate fixation is preferred, anticipating significant forces on the bony repair by postoperative edema and ROM therapy. In most instances when the dorsal injury exceeds volar, a dorsal approach and plate application will be favored, as this is biomechanically sound.

Extrinsic and Intrinsic Extensor Mechanism. Shredded tendon must be debrided back to adequate tissue. If bone shortening has been required, primary repair of the extensor mechanism may be possible. More commonly, a significant defect exists, which necessitates either tendon graft reconstruction or tendon transfers.

Nerve Injuries. The treatment of associated nerve injuries is similar to that discussed above under volar combined injuries. In dorsal and combined injuries with the flexor mechanism injured but intact, invariably the digital nerves are in continuity and do not require primary attention. In those rare instances with digital nerve disruption, immediate direct suture is recommended if the segment of injury is limited. When segmental injury is more extensive and sustained by crushing mechanism, delayed reconstruction is advised.

Arterial Lesions. Despite preserved continuity of the flexor mechanism and/or digital nerves, frequently the digital arteries are disrupted. Intraarterial thrombosis or laceration may occur from tenting edges of bony fracture at injury or the acute dislocation that occurs with initial deformity. Arterial reconstruction by direct suture or interpositional vein grafting is advised with the volar dissection limited and dorsal arterial branches from the proper digital branches preserved to proximal and distal dorsal skin.

Skin. The true extent of dorsal skin damage midaxial is often not fully appreciated at injury. Elective incisions may be incorporated within full-thickness areas of dorsal skin loss. When dorsal soft tissue damage is partial thickness, midaxial incisions are preferred. Fracture shortening may allow for adequate skin debridement and primary repair. Dorsal skin closure should allow for full passive interphalangeal joint range of motion. Mid-axial lacerations or extension by incision are left open, anticipating a significant amount of edema postoperatively. This will facilitate wound drainage, allow for swelling, and minimize postoperative pain with ROM.

Postoperative Therapy. The injured but intact flexor mechanisms are protected from adhesions by early range of motion. The extensor mechanism repair is protected by dorsal dynamic extension splinting. As with all dorsal combined injuries, some degree of active extension deficit is to be expected and counteracted by extension splinting between active exercise periods. When the extensor mechanism has been reinforced by tendon graft augmentation, active and passive ROM therapy is allowed. Edema control measures are extremely important, as control of edema will help facilitate early ROM and minimize subsequent fibrosis. This will require several dressing changes each day for at least the first week.

Secondary Interventions. Any secondary procedures will require deferral for at least 3 months, until soft tissue homeostasis has been achieved and maximum early potential achieved. With active and passive flexion deficit, extensor tenolysis and dorsal PIP capsulectomy will improve flexion. Extension deficit is less likely to be improved by extensor tenolysis.

Flexor Mechanism Divided, Extensor Mechanism Intact

Bone/Joint. Rigid osteosynthesis is required. No amount of skeletal shortening can be accepted. This will lead to relative lengthening (redundancy) of the extensor mechanism and result in PIP joint extensor lag and possible subsequent contracture. Interpositional bone grafts are required when significant comminution or segmental defect exists. An additional dorsal surgical incision for skeletal fixation should be avoided. If the dorsal skin and subcutaneous tissue is intact, internal fixation is accomplished by limited exposure and lateral plating.

Intrinsic and Extrinsic Extensor Mechanism. Partial injury to the extensor mechanism may exist either by crush, incomplete tear, or incomplete laceration. In addition, as the injury is more volar than dorsal, usually one lateral side of the digit will be more involved than the other. Partial intrinsic or extrinsic extensor mechanism tears are surgically debrided. No attempt at repair is advised as long as 50 percent of the central extensor mechanism and intrinsic expansion is intact.

Flexor Tendon Mechanism. Treatment is directed as outlined under volar combined digital injuries. Defects up to 5 mm in length distal to the vinculum longum and 10 mm proximal to the vinculum longum are repaired by direct suture. Extensive defects or segmental injuries in the presents of adequate soft tissue coverage are handled by immediate flexor tendon grafting. In the face of impaired segmental vascularity and questionable soft tissue coverage, flexor reconstruction is deferred.

Arterial Lesions. For reasons outlined under Volar Combined Injuries, associated arterial lesions are primarily reconstructed by direct suture or interpositional vein grafting.

Skin. Volar flexor tendon coverage by well-perfused local skin or flap tissue is needed to allow for proper nutrition of the underlying repairs. Mid-axial incisions are most often left open and allowed to heal by secondary intention.

Postoperative Therapy. Flexor tendon repairs are mobilized as described under Volar Combined Injuries. This is initiated within 72 hours. In the future, multiple strand flexor tendon repair techniques may support immediate active ROM therapy.

Flexor and Extensor Mechanisms Divided

Bone/Joint. As in complete amputation, limited skeletal shortening is allowable to gain adequate soft tissue length for extensor and flexor tendon repairs. The method of osteosynthesis utilized will be dependent upon the anticipated postoperative therapy program. Less rigid means of internal fixation may be utilized when early ROM is not anticipated. If reconstruction can be achieved that is adequate enough to allow for active or passive ROM to at least one tendon mechanism, stable osteosynthesis is required.

Intrinsic and Extrinsic Extensor System. Skeletal shortening will usually allow for debridement and appropriate primary repair of the extensor mechanism. Extensive defects of the extensor mechanism as mentioned above will require either tendon graft reconstruction or secondary reconstruction. Tendon repair techniques that require postoperative immobilization will be quite deleterious to the ultimate functional result. The goal in treatment is to reduce the level of injury to one of the former two simpler categories that require significant protection of only one tendon mechanism. This can be achieved by augmenting the extensor tendon repair with a tendon graft that will allow for a postoperative immediate passive ROM program for the repaired flexor mechanism.

Flexor System. Primary flexor tendon repairs are carried out whenever possible. When a segmental gap exists, and the soft tissue bed and intercalary vascularity is adequate, immediate tendon grafting is performed. If primary reconstruction is not possible, secondary reconstruction is accepted, but great importance is placed upon a sturdy extensor reconstruction that will allow for early motion of the injured and divided extensor mechanism and injured adjacent articulations.

REGIONAL PARTICULARITIES

Phalangeal (Digital) Combined Lesions

Crushing Injuries

The small size of individual phalangeal segments and the proximity of adjacent digits predisposes to involvement of two or more phalangeal segments and several adjacent fingers. Clearly, the most precious segments mediating digital motor function are the areas from the MP joints to the bases of the middle phalanges in the fingers. The distal segments of the fingers and the two phalangeal segments of the thumb are not as critical for the ultimate overall function of the hand. Due to the precarious soft tissue sleeve, damage to bone/joint, vasculature, and skin is particularly important in the digits. The debridement is usually straightforward, unless one has to decide on a salvage attempt of an mutilated digit with little hope for survival and functional recovery; if feasible, at least the thumb and three fingers should be reconstructed. Skeletal stabilization may be challenging, especially with the typical palisading diaphyseal fractures (in which segmental replacement by compact grafts is recommended), or with lesions close to but preserving joints (condylar plating). As the extensor aponeurosis yields multiple insertions and does not accommodate length discrepancies, original skeletal proportions should be restored, at least in the proximal phalanx of the finger. Joint injuries often require arthrodesis, arthroplasties being generally unpredictable in combined injuries. Submicroscopic hidden damage to the main vascular conduits is the frustrating difficulty in arterial and venous reconstruction. Chances for survival increase with the use of long interpositional vein grafts; however, they aggravate the relative ischemia within the (bypassed) intercalated traumatized digital segment even if distal revascularization proves successful. Generally, the crushed digital segments of flexor and extensor tendons remain in continuity, except disinsertion of the extensor aponeurosis from the bases of the distal and the middle phalanges and ruptures of the annular pulley system, which should be stably repaired or reconstructed. Nerve injuries are managed as outlined above. Flap coverage is a crucial element in the digital area. In view of unpredictable traumatic damage, side-finger and other homodigital flaps should not be used. Cross-finger flaps may not be available when both adjacent fingers are involved. The retrograde pedicled posterior interosseous flap is a good choice, but does not reach much beyond the PIP joint. Free flaps from the contralateral hand, such as the dmf flap,[6] are advantageous as they may incorporate arterial, vein and nerve grafts and be utilized as flow-through flaps. The concept is summarized in Figure 45-8. (See Chapter 49 for further discussion of choice of flaps.)

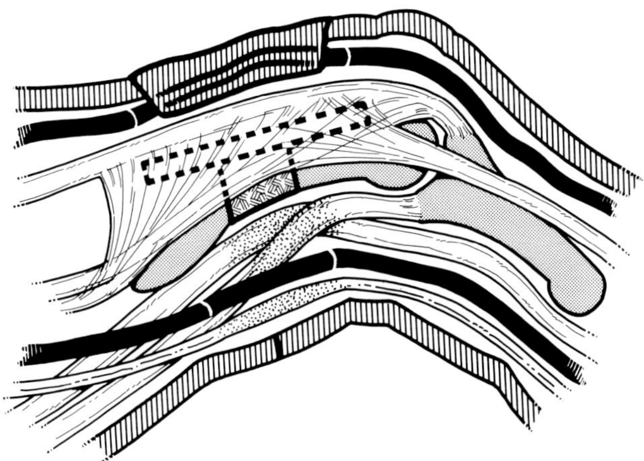

Fig. 45-8. Synopsis of the recommended therapeutic concepts in a Zone II digital crushing injury. A comminuted diaphysial segment is replaced by a corticocancellous bone graft and stabilized by rigid plating to facilitate bone healing, maintain original length of the extensor apparatus, and allow immediate motion. An occluded segment of the arterial system is replaced by a vein graft. No risks are taken with respect to the crushed dorsal skin: this is replaced by a flap designed for flow-through vein reconstruction. In-continuity lesions of the extensor and flexor tendons are "treated" by very early motion therapy.

Volar Combined Digital Injuries

Particularly in Zone II, very untidy lacerations and extensive volar combined injuries represent a serious threat to ultimate digital performance with respect to both motion and sensibility. Therefore, it may be wise to consider primary amputation of one digit in cases where one digit is exclusively or predominantly involved. In addition to the general concept outlined above, the following elements merit special consideration. From the tip of the digit down to the base of the middle phalanx, and from the tip of the thumb to the base of the proximal phalanx, skeletal shortening, with or without fusion of the DIP or the IP joints, may be liberal. Due to the multiple attachments of the extensor mechanism, bone shortening must be limited to less than 0.5 cm in the proximal phalanx, the only exception being complex defects requiring PIP fusion. Flexor tendon defects distal to the vinculum longum of more than about 5 mm should not be closed by direct suture, as this will likely result in tenodesis of the DIP (and possibly the PIP) joint(s) and interfere with the nutrition of the injured tendon. Instead, defects within this zone exceeding tolerable limits should be accepted and dealt with secondarily (Fig. 45-9). At or proximal to the vinculum longum, limited defects of up to 10 mm in length may be closed by direct suture, anticipating increased tension on tendon repair sites with restorative therapy. The strongest possible repair configuration should be used. Multiple strand flexor tendon repair techniques are advised and may in the future prove acceptably tolerant of early protected active flexion exercises. Extensive defects in the flexor system of Zones II to III without significant compromise of the essential annular pulleys may be treated by immediate flexor tendon grafting or tendon transfer, given a low risk of infection, good vascularity and excellent quality soft tissue coverage. For extensive flexor tendon defects aggravated by deficiencies of the annular pulley mechanism, immediate pulley reconstruction, insertion of a Silastic spacer, and provisional attachment of the proximal tendon stumps are advised. No compromise is made regarding closure of volar skin defects, which require flap coverage rather than tight suturing, because postoperative therapy shall entail massive shear forces possibly leading to wound dehiscence, marginal necrosis, infection, and other problems. Unless very small in size, single digital defects should not be closed by randomly perfused homodigital transposition or rotation flaps. Preferably heterodigital neurovascular island flaps, such as the dmf flap[6] which offer excellent vascularity, allow for flow-through distal revascularization and may incorporate vascularized nerve grafts. Pluridigital defects usually require a syndactyly and distant flap coverage (such as retrograde posterior interosseous flap, retrograde fascial radial forearm flap, or free flaps).

Dorsal Combined Digital Injuries

Dorsal combined injuries to the phalanges (and the IP joint) of the thumb may require skeletal reconstruction with arthrodesis of the IP joint, which obviates the need for treating the defect of the extensor tendon. A retrograde posterior interosseous flap can be used for coverage. In the fingers, untidy limited and extensive dorsal combined injuries usually include two or more adjacent digits. In Verdan's Zone I and II lesions, maintenance of DIP function is unimportant, and therefore, skeletal shortening, tenodesis by prolonged pinning or formal arthrodesis of the DIP joint, and flap coverage are performed. Injuries adjacent to the PIP joint with associated injury to the central slip (and the lateral bands) are treated by immediate extensor reconstruction and very early mobilization, provided that the joint is not grossly destabilized. Segmental PIP defects mandate arthrodesis of this joint (either simply, with slight shortening or with the interposition of a solid bone graft[5]), which obviates the need for formal reconstruction of the extensor apparatus. Therapeutic guidelines for Zone IV injuries are presented in Figure 45-10. While the skin loss of a single finger is easily handled by using a reversed cross finger or a dmf flap,[6] pluridigital soft tissue defects must be covered by large, thin, and elastic axial flaps incorporating syndactyly of two or several adjacent fingers. As the axis of the flap will often course transversely over the PIP joint area, such defects may be beyond the reach of retrograde pedicle forearm flaps. The application of a free flap should be considered.

Dorsal and Volar Combined Digital Injuries

Combined dorsal and volar injuries of the thumb very often require arthrodesis of either the metacarpophalangeal (MP) or interphalangeal (IP) joint as a method of handling the skeletal reconstruction. Functional consequences of MP joint arthrodesis are less significant than that of IP joint arthrodesis. Therefore, the decision to fuse the MP joint is more liberally chosen.

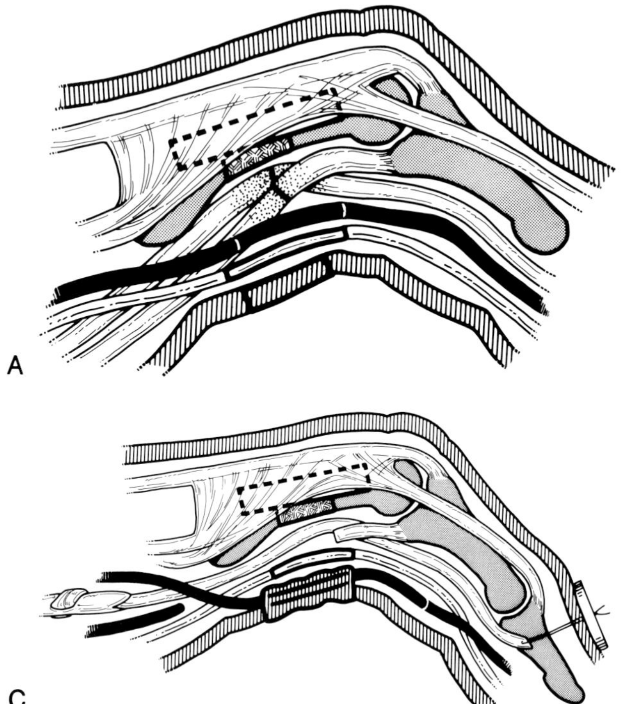

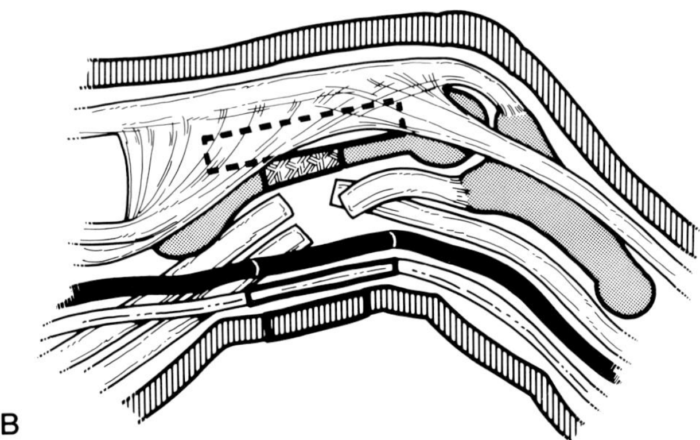

Fig. 45-9. Three concepts for treating volar combined injuries in Zone II of the finger. Near original bone length, skeletal stability, adequate arterial inflow, nerve continuity, and supple skin coverage are always restored, even if primary bone, vein, nerve, or skin grafts are required. The three concepts differ as to the flexor system. In **(A)**, due to very little loss of substance, direct flexor repair is feasible. A more extensive flexor tendon defect is necessarily accepted and left for secondary reconstruction in **(B)**. A radical concept of total primary reconstruction, involving a one-stage tendon graft is applied in **(C)**; note that optimal nutrition is assured by an axial arterial flow-through flap. Regardless of the method for dealing with the flexor tendon lesion, motion is initiated within 72 hours.

Dorsal and volar combined injuries adjacent to the DIP joint are handled by DIP arthrodesis or stabilization of the DIP joint by tenodesis. The functional consequences of accepting little or no DIP motion are limited considering the greater importance of PIP motion, which contributes 85 percent of the total arc of combined DIP and PIP motion.

Extensive soft tissue defects of the distal aspects of the digits are handled by cross finger flap coverage. More proximal soft tissue defects are handled by axial pattern Type 1 or Type 2 dorsal metacarpal flaps;[24] with multiple digit injuries involving distal aspects of digits, shortening the amputation and primary closer to the most severely involved digits might be indicated.

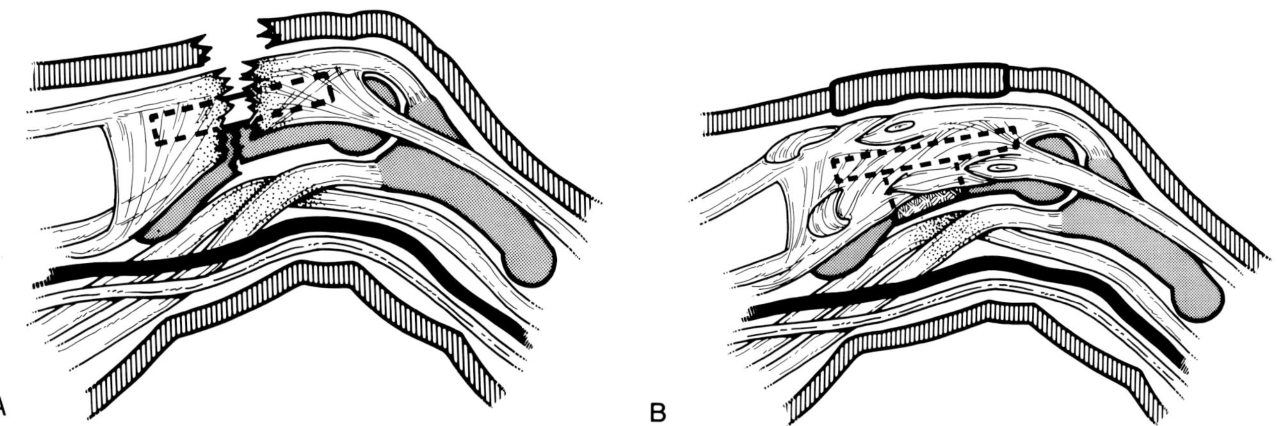

Fig. 45-10. (A&B) Two concepts for treating dorsal combined lesions in Verdan's Zone IV. In **(A)**, slight skeletal shortening was accepted, the fracture stabilized, the extensor tendon left unrepaired, and the skin possibly replaced by flap tissue. The concept shown in **(B)** incorporates rigid reconstruction of near normal skeletal length, "stable" primary extensor tendon reconstruction, and flap coverage. Aftercare is dynamic (early motion) in both cases.

Metacarpal Combined Lesions

Crushing Metacarpal Injuries

The most problematic feature of metacarpal crushing is the involvement of the intrinsic musculature. Fasciotomy and a very thorough debridement are mandatory and often result in massive voids, especially in the depth of the thumb web and the intermetacarpal spaces (Fig. 45-11A–C).

Single or predominant involvement of one ray may warrant primary ray amputation, with various supplemental procedures as possible options: thumb ray replacement by immediate or secondary pollicization, simple deletion of a border finger ray, resection of a central finger ray and immediate ray transfer. The type of osteosynthesis selected is more consequential than in the phalanges. To achieve very rigid skeletal stabilization, massively crushed metacarpal segments need replacement by compression-resistant corticocancellous grafts. With severe joint damage, primary arthrodesis is indicated in the MP joint of the thumb, the carpometacarpal (CMC) joint of the finger rays, and to a lesser degree in the MP joint of the index finger. Fusion of the saddle (CMC) joint of the thumb and the MP joints of the middle and ring fingers is preferably avoided. Revascularization may be challenging because of the variable arterial anatomy in the thumb, frequent disruption of the palmar arches, frequent extensive hidden vascular damage, and a tendency for arterial spasm. It is helpful to release Guyon's canal and the periarterial cages of the palmar aponeurosis, to use extra long vein grafts and to perform end-to-side anastomoses proximally. Primary nerve grafts are liberally employed. As deep voids sometimes coexist with palmar and dorsal skin defects, sophisticated flap designs with up to three components (palmar, buried, volar) may be called for. Prime choices are the posterior interosseous flap, the radial forearm flap, the brachioradialis flap, the lateral arm flap, a very partial latissimus dorsi and serratus anterior bilobed flap, the groin flap and many other pedicled or free flaps (Fig. 45-11D–G).

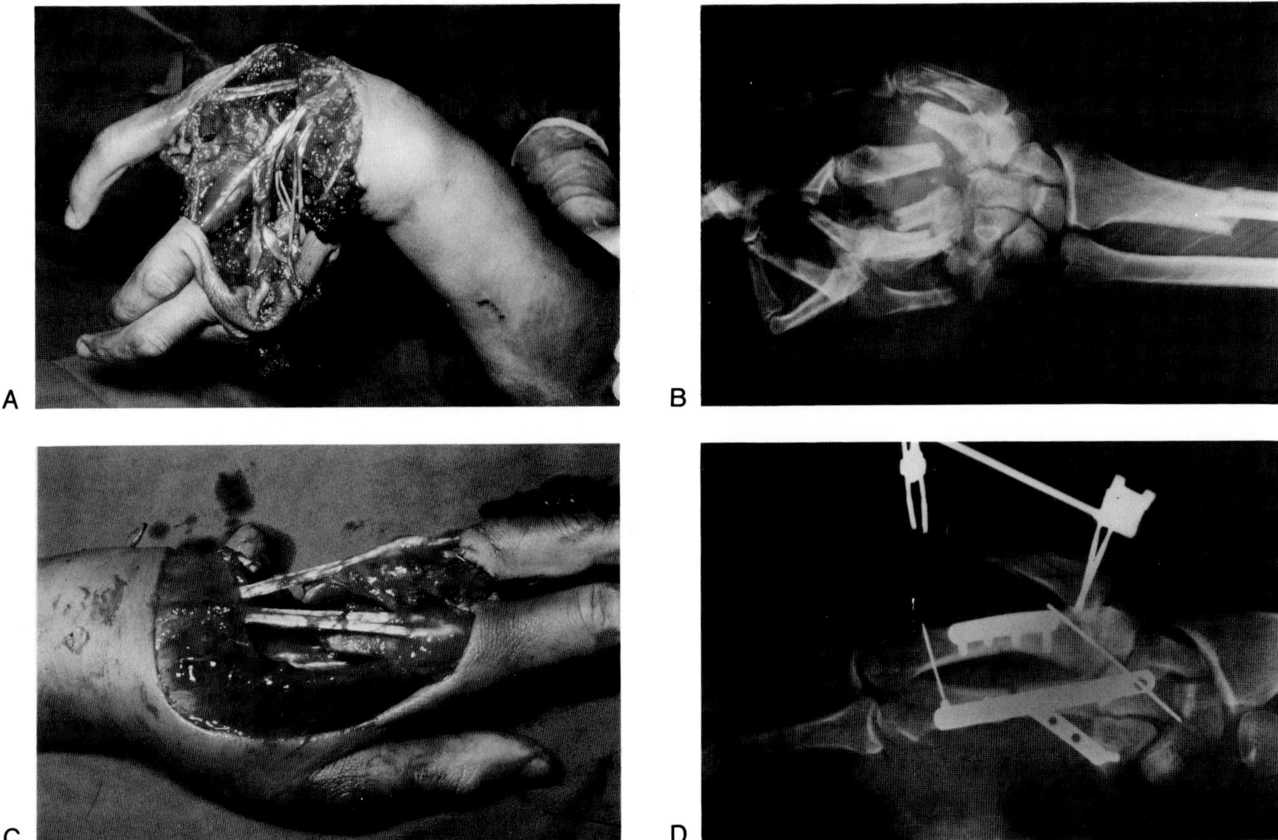

Fig. 45-11. **(A)** Crushing injury of the left midhand with devascularization and severe combined damage to bones, intrinsic muscles, vasculature, and skin; the nerves and tendons remain partly in continuity. **(B)** X-ray reveals multiple displaced fractures at the phalangeal, metacarpal, and forearm level. **(C)** Extensive debridement, including the deletion of two ulnar rays, leads to a clearer understanding of the magnitude of the soft tissue and skeletal defects. **(D)** The thumb ray was stabilized by external fixation. The second metacarpal was plated. The third metacarpal was reconstructed by the interposition of a solid bone graft, carpometacarpal-arthrodesis, and plating. Note the additional obliquely-oriented plate for enhanced fixation of the central ray. *(Figure continues.)*

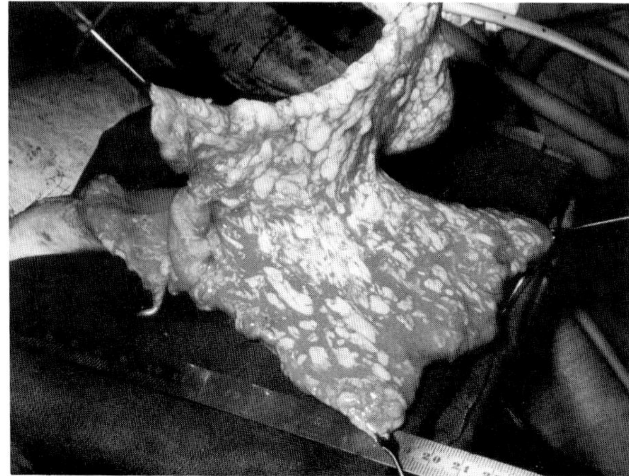

E

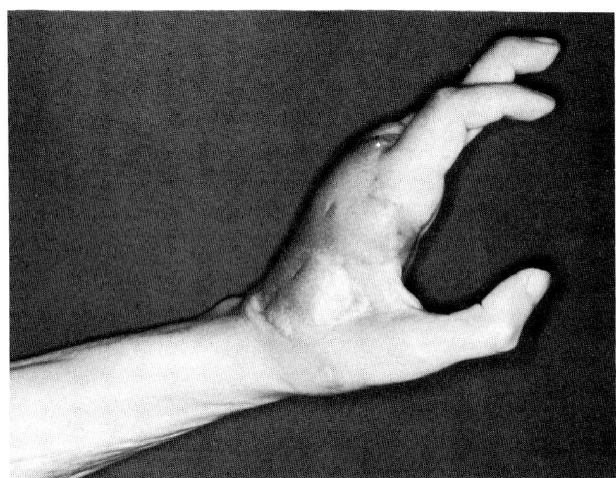

F

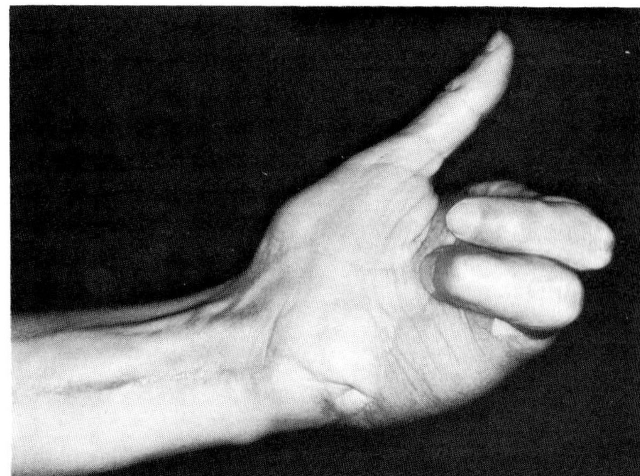

G

Fig. 45-11 *(Continued).* **(E)** Following skeletal stabilization and revascularization, an axial groin flap was split to provide a subcutaneous flap portion for filling the deep defect and a skin flap portion for surface coverage. **(F&G)** Appearance of the hand and finger mobility at 6 months.

Volar Combined Metacarpal Injuries

Reconstruction is planned following the debridement, which may enlarge the extent of untidy lacerations and extensive defects considerably. If this is the only lesion, very extensive defects on the volar aspect of the thumb may mandate primary amputation and secondary pollicization rather than an exotic and often frustrating attempt at reconstruction. Similarly, if a long finger ray is uniquely or predominantly involved, primary ray amputation should be considered. In dealing with skeletal damage to the thumb, there is little hesitation in performing an MP fusion and accepting moderate shortening. In the fingers, MP joint arthrodesis is avoided, particularly in the third and fourth rays, and shortening of more than 1 cm is not accepted unless all finger rays display analogous patterns of injury. Gaps of the flexor tendons less than 1 cm in the thumb and 1.5 cm in the finger are overcome by direct suture. More extensive defects are dealt with secondarily. Smaller defects of the intrinsic system are left without primary reconstruction. Under special circumstances, such as gaps of the terminal tendons of the abductor pollicis brevis, the adductor pollicis, the first dorsal interosseous, and the abductor digiti quinti, intercalated tendon grafting with transosseous insertion may be warranted. Revascularization and nerve reconstruction follow the guidelines discussed previously, with special emphasis on primary reconstruction of the motor branches of the median and ulnar nerves. The retrograde posterior interosseous flap is a first choice selection for coverage of the volar aspect of the thumb, the thumb web, and the palm; with large defects, this is raised in the septo-fascio-subcutaneous modality. An example is shown in Figure 45-12.

Dorsal Combined Metacarpal Injuries

With injuries to the dorsal aspect of the thumb, involvement of the MP joint and adjacent bones frequently necessitates the placement of compact corticocancellous grafts and primary arthrodesis. IP extension is easier to motorize by establishing extensions to the abductor pollicis brevis or the adductor polli-

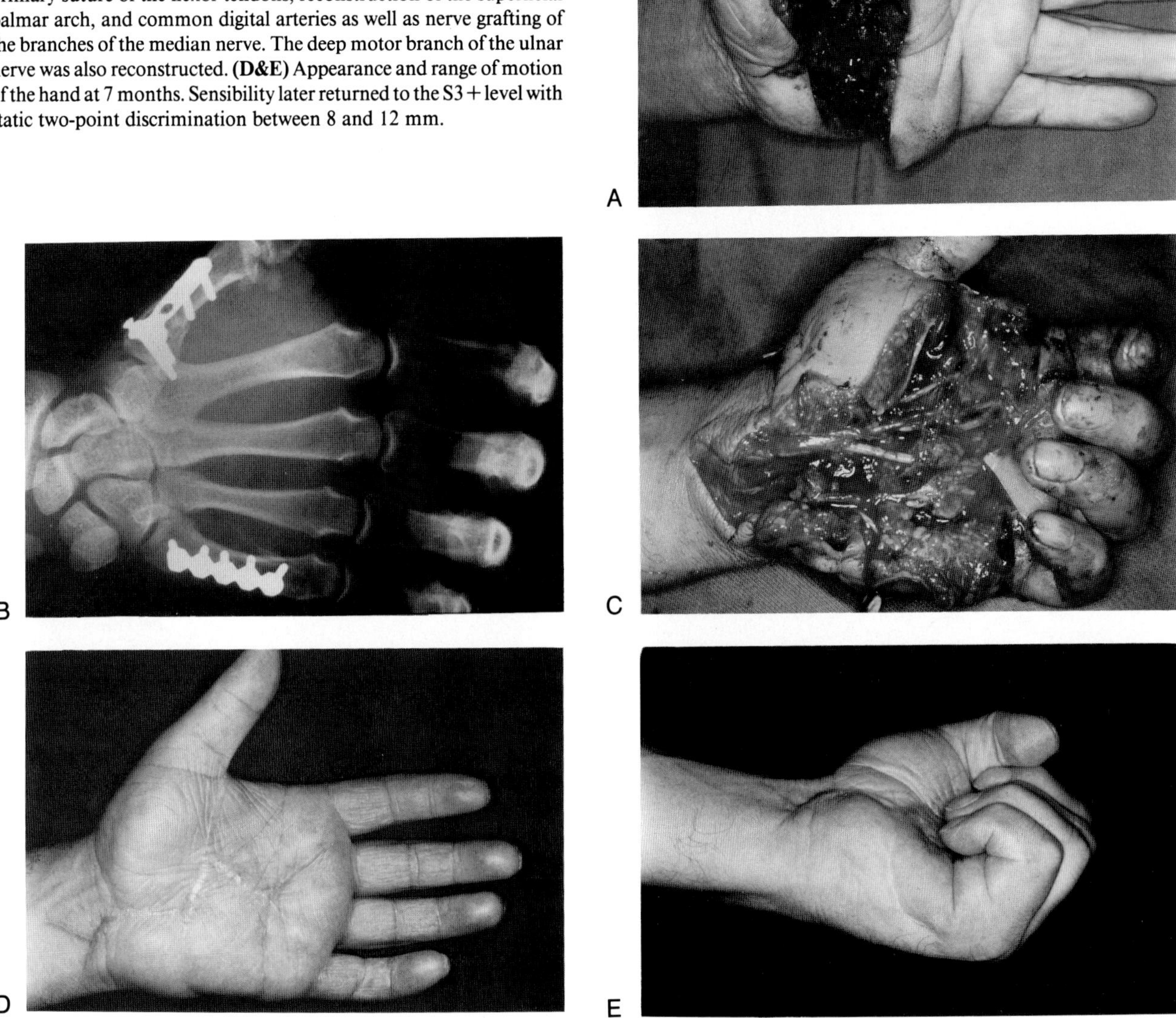

Fig. 45-12. **(A)** A power saw injury with volar combined lesions at the metacarpal level. **(B)** Associated fractures of the first and fifth metacarpals were rigidly fixed with plates. **(C)** An intraoperative view showing primary suture of the flexor tendons, reconstruction of the superficial palmar arch, and common digital arteries as well as nerve grafting of the branches of the median nerve. The deep motor branch of the ulnar nerve was also reconstructed. **(D&E)** Appearance and range of motion of the hand at 7 months. Sensibility later returned to the S3+ level with static two-point discrimination between 8 and 12 mm.

cis than by restoring continuity to the extensor pollicis longus over the skeletal reconstruction site. Excellent coverage is provided by a retrograde posterior interosseous flap. With regard to the long finger metacarpals, the path of dorsal combined injuries is often oblique, both in the frontal and the axial planes. If the injury extends far volarly into the second or the fifth rays and comprises massive injury of the flexor system and the neurovascular structures, primary amputation of that ray may be considered, particularly if elements thereof can be utilized for the reconstruction of less involved rays. Partial defects of the MP joints are amenable to primary osteochondral grafting, either from a deleted MP joint or a metatarsophalangeal joint of the foot.[16] While it is preferable to fuse destroyed MP joints of border finger rays, motion-preserving arthroplasties are preferred in the central digits; we would not hesitate to use a silicone rubber MP prosthesis immediately, even in conjunction with the use of a bone graft for the seating of the stem of the implant (Fig. 45-13). Immediate motion-resistant extensor tendon grafting as described in concept #2 (see p. 1573) is advised. As it is virtually impossible to reconstruct a defect of the sagittal band mechanism, the graft is directly inserted to the dorsal base of the proximal phalanx. Most defects of the metacarpal and/or the MP joint area can be covered either by a retrograde posterior interosseous flap or a radial forearm flap.

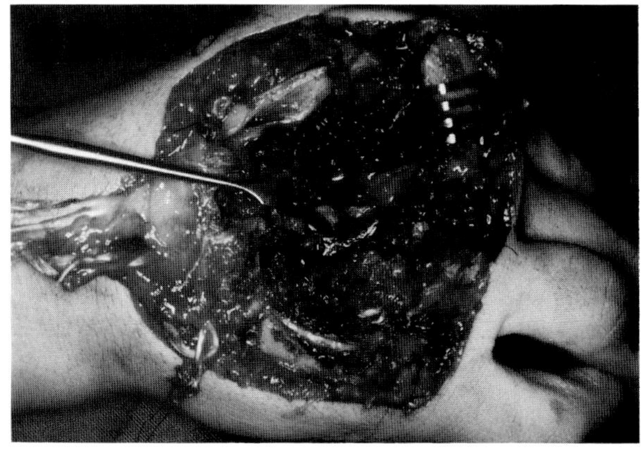

A

Fig. 45-13. **(A)** An industrial accident with an extensive dorsal combined lesion at the metacarpal level, involving defects of the skin, extensor tendons, metacarpals and partly, the intrinsic musculature. **(B)** X-ray demonstrates the extent of the fractures and bone loss in the second through fifth metacarpals. **(C)** The second, third, and fourth metacarpals were reconstructed using solid bone grafts, CMC-fusion, and plating. Note the immediate Swanson Silastic arthroplasty in the fourth MP joint. The fifth ray required simple screw fixation. The extrinsic extensors underwent primary tendon grafting. The skin defect was covered with a groin flap. **(D&E)** The hand, demonstrating finger motion, at 2 years.

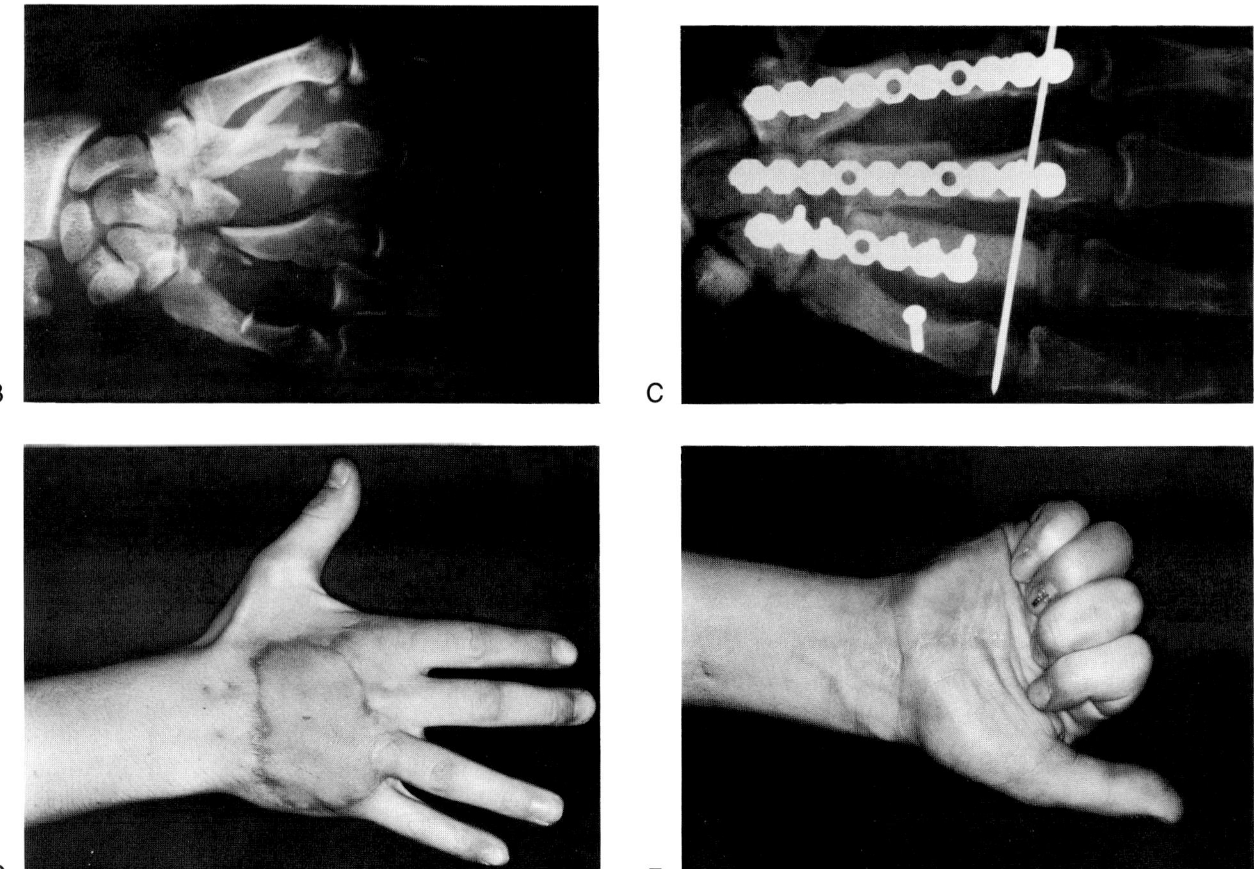

B C D E

Dorsal and Volar Combined Metacarpal Injuries

Dorsal and volar combined metacarpal injuries most commonly occur by direct lacerating trauma as by power saws or grinders. They usually involve multiple metacarpals. Isolated injuries limited to a single ray are less common and usually involve a border ray. When central isolated ray injuries occur, they are usually caused by a dye or stamping type of press. As in both the dorsal and the volar combined injuries, intrinsic musculatures are invariably involved, requiring debridement and resulting in significant dead space. More rigid osteosynthesis is required at the metacarpal level than at the phalangeal level, because of the increased forces at this more proximal level. The risk of joint stiffness at CMC and MP joints is far less significant than at the interphalangeal level. Significant swelling will bring the MP joints into a resting posture of extension, causing a secondary posturing of flexion in the interphalangeal joints. When the most significant injury is to the flexor system, the MP joints can be temporarily pinned in safe position (flexion) allowing early flexor tendon range of motion exercises to the interphalangeal joints.

Skin loss exerts a greater negative functional restraint when the injury is dorsal rather than volar. Palmar defects can often be handled by treatment in an open palm fashion allowing closure by secondary intention. Obvious dorsal soft tissue defects are covered by a retrograde posterior interosseous flap. The greatest difficulty occurs when the dorsal soft tissues of the hand are marginally viable, often raising hope that the coverage is adequate. In such situations second look operations are indicated. The surgeon should be willing to remove poorly oxygenated tissue and replace it with a flap that supplies better blood supply and offers an improved bed for tendon gliding.

Secondary reconstructions are more favorable at the metacarpal level than at the phalangeal level, particularly in cases of extensor reconstruction. When the injury presents large soft tissue coverage requirements, tendon reconstruction can be favorably staged.

Despite debridement of the dysfunctional musculature in dorsal and volar combined metacarpal injuries, subsequent fibrosis frequently leads to intrinsic tightness. This can often be prevented by intrinsic stretching exercises to extend the metacarpophalangeal joints and simultaneously flex the interphalangeal joints, begun as soon as tendon repairs allow. The reconstructive surgeon should be attentive to the potential need to intrinsic releases when there is limited interphalangeal joint flexion.

Combined Lesions Proximal to the Wrist

Crushing Injuries

In the forearm and upper arm, direct skin contusion is frequently more widespread and the shearing/avulsion component usually more pronounced than in more distal injuries. One must pay attention to an insidious *in situ* degloving, which may leave the epidermal layer relatively intact while inflicting serious devascularization to the entire skin sleeve. In order to preserve the major septocutaneous supply lines, additional skin incisions, if needed, are placed between the intermuscular septa. Massive crushing of muscular tissue requires fasciotomy and a liberal, but diligent debridement; this is ideally performed in three to four stages; namely, before revascularization, following restoration of blood flow, and during one or two programmed second look procedures. Unless the duration of ischemia exceeds tolerable limits and requires provisional revascularization (by using bypass shunts), bone/joint fixation precedes other reconstructive steps. Moderate skeletal shortening of 3 to 5 cm is acceptable if this increases the healing potential of the fracture and/or facilitates soft tissue reconstruction. In the forearm, great care is needed to restore accurate comparative lengths of radius and ulna and their correct rotation. If a major diaphysial segment is missing, construction of a one-bone forearm may be a solution. Fractures are usually of the C3 category (AO classification[23]) and call for advanced stabilization techniques. In comminuted intraarticular fractures of the distal radius, immediate wrist fusion is considered, particularly when there is associated carpal disruption and/or major damage to the vulnerable wrist motors. Elbow arthrodesis should be avoided. With critical local and distal ischemia, timely revascularization must be carried out. Long (greater saphenous) vein grafts are used to bridge the crushed/disrupted arterial segment, preferably with an end-to-side anastomosis proximally and an end-to-end repair configuration distally. Mere reconstruction of the ulnar and/or radial arterial axes may not suffice for adequate revascularization of the forearm muscles; it may therefore be crucial to restore continuity to the common, or at least the anterior interosseous artery. Following reestablishment of arterial flow, it is important to quickly control the (usually) profuse bleeding before coagulopathy sets in. At least 30 minutes should be allowed for equilibration of perfusion of the dependent areas before adequacy of venous outflow is assessed and a second debridement of the muscles is undertaken. One should not hesitate to reconstruct a good venous outflow. Nerve lesions are treated as outlined in the general section above. Devascularized avulsed skin is defatted, stabbed for drainage and replaced as full thickness graft in areas in which the underlying tissues are well perfused; in areas with marginal skin vascularity, an ischemic avulsed skin sleeve is simply replaced in the hope of circulatory improvement and survival. Adequate drainage is assured. A second look operation is planned within 72 hours for redebridement of muscles and skin, and a flap is applied to critical areas over which the skin sleeve has not regained sufficient circulation. A pedicled or free (trimmed) latissimus dorsi flap is an excellent selection as it provides good surface coverage, greatly improves local revascularization, and may serve as a functional free muscle transfer in cases of major muscle damage.

Volar Combined Injuries

Except for sharp lacerations that are simply treated by primary repair of all injured structures, pure volar combined injuries at or proximal to the wrist are rare. Moreover, interstructural restraints on healing become less important as one moves more proximally. With limited combined defects, skeletal shortening (either through an existing fracture, a bone defect, a joint defect with arthrodesis, or an elective osteotomy) is liberally performed if this permits the elimination of truncular nerve gaps and allows for direct nerve coaptation. Motor and sensory regenerative capacity being the leading prognostic factor, adverse relative lengthening of the extrinsic extensor system (which may be dealt with secondarily if required) seems less important. In all other instances, skeletal shortening is allowed only if this does not exceed the length adaptation capacity of the extensor system. Extensive single truncular nerve injuries are treated by elective secondary nerve grafting. With arterial injuries, revascularization by intercalated saphenous vein grafting is straightforward but must be quickly established. Fasciotomies, not only on the flexor side, but specifically on all intrinsic compartments of the hand are routinely carried out. Defects of the flexor-pronator mass are handled as outlined in Table 45-3.

When extensive volar defects of the forearm require flap coverage, and the use of a free musculocutaneous transfer (such as a latissimus dorsi flap) is considered, its functional capacity should be exploited by reinnervention. Defects of the flexor aspect of the humerus are treated accordingly. At a later stage, when sensibility has returned to the hand, the primary result may be significantly upgraded by tenolysis, tendon transfers and, perhaps, selected arthrodeses.

Dorsal Combined Injuries

Wrist

With defects limited to the radiocarpal joint, radioscapholunate arthrodesis or proximal row carpectomy should be considered, particularly if the wrist extensors are in continuity. More extensive joint defects require complete arthrodesis. Arthroplasty of the distal radioulnar joint may be required. In view of the close relationship to the extensor compartments, primary tendon reconstruction is usually not indicated. Unless the dorsoulnar aspect of the distal forearm has been injured, retrograde posterior interosseous flap coverage is the first choice; in other instances, a fasciosubcutaneous radial forearm flap may be used.

Distal Forearm

Skeletal injuries are treated as outlined above, but great care is taken to assure correct rotation and respective length of the radius and the ulna. Primary extensor tendon grafting is preferred, particularly if the proximal stumps of the tendons of insertion have retracted deeply into the muscle substance and if the distal tendon weave is located outside the extensor retinaculum. At least the extensor pollicis longus and an index finger extensor tendon should be restored individually; the extensor systems to the other fingers may be replaced conjointly, as independent motion of the third, fourth and fifth fingers is not required. Coverage is best accomplished by a retrograde fasciosubcutaneous radial forearm flap.

Middle and Proximal Forearm

The radius and ulna are anatomically reconstructed and stably plated. The deep motor branch of the radial nerve is formally revised and, in the presence of a surgically correctable defect, is reconstructed with a nerve graft. A defect of the extensor-supinator muscle mass is initially accepted, as there is no possibility of defining the degree, the extent, and the consequence of injuries to the terminal motor nerve branches, and thus of predicting ultimate function of these muscles. Formal flap coverage is not frequently needed, but extensive combined defects may rarely require the application of a free (latissimus dorsi) flap.

SUMMARY

Adequate treatment of "combined injuries" requires an altogether different treatment approach as compared to "isolated injuries." The reconstructive surgeon must be well versed and comfortable in a variety of skeletal and soft tissue reconstructive procedures and recognize the negative interactive restraints posed by varying combination(s) of lesions. Nonoperative and operative treatment regimens that may predictably handle isolated injuries frequently fail when transferred to combined injuries.

By intent, this chapter addresses postoperative therapy in a limited fashion. A responsible surgeon should recognize the

Table 45-3. Treatment of Defects of the Flexor-Pronator Mass

	Tendinous Portion	Muscular Portion
Small gap (less than 2 cm)	Suture under tension	Leave for spontaneous healing
Moderate gap (2–5 cm)	Primary or secondary tendon grafting	Consider flexor-pronator slide and direct coaptation
Extensive (more than 5 cm)	May require primary or secondary free muscle transfer; see text	

importance of carefully orchestrated therapy to insure optimal functional results. Reconstruction can only achieve its full potential when carefully directed by the surgeon and carried through by a highly experienced therapy team. Recognition of the special treatment requirements of combined injuries, honing of surgical judgement and technical skills, with therapy tailored to the specific injury, will substantially decrease complication rates, the number of secondary procedures, and duration of work incapacity.

REFERENCES

1. Blandinskii VF, Komarevtsev VD, Fonareva NV: Restoration of the function of the hand after combined injuries of the flexor tendons, nerves and arteries of the distal part of the forearm in children. Ortop Travmatol Protez 1:7–9, 1989
2. Bongard FS, White GH, Klein SR: Management strategy of complex extremity injuries. Am J Surg 158:151–155, 1989
3. Büchler U: Funktionelle Interaktionen im Heilungsablauf Kombinierter Verletzungen der Hand. These. Univerität Bern, 1988
4. Büchler U: Traumatic soft tissue defects of the extremities. Implications and treatment guidelines. Arch Orthop Trauma Surg 109:321–329, 1990
5. Büchler U, Aiken MA: Arthrodesis of the proximal interphalangeal joint by solid bone grafting and plate fixation in extensive injuries to the dorsal aspect of the finger. J Hand Surg 13A:589–594, 1988
6. Büchler U, Frey HP: The dorsal middle phalangeal finger flap. Handchir Mikrochir Plast Chir 20:239–243, 1988
7. Foucher G: Vascularized joint transfers. pp. 1271–1293. In Green DP (ed): Operative Hand Surgery, 2nd Ed, Churchill Livingstone, New York, 1988
8. Gelberman RH, Urbaniak JR, Bright DS, Levin LS: Digital sensibility following replantation. J Hand Surg 3:313–319, 1978
9. Govenko FS: Combined injuries to the nerves and vessels in children. Zh Vopr Neirokhir 6:12–14, 1989
10. Hastings H II: Unstable metacarpal and phalangeal fracture treatment with screws and plates. Clin Orthop 214:37–52, 1987
11. Hastings H II, Carroll C IV: Treatment of closed articular fractures of the metacarpophalangeal and proximal interphalangeal joints. Hand Clin 4(3):503–527, 1988
12. Hastings H II, Ernst JMJ: Complex articular fractures of the base of the middle phalanx—Treatment by hinged external fixator (abstract). J Hand Surg 13A:306, 1988
13. Herren A, Boulas J, Büchler U: Osteochondral grafting from the 2nd metatarso-phalangeal joint for treating partial defects of the MP joint. (abstract) J Hand Surg (submitted), 1992
14. Mark G, Gautier E: External fixation by complex injuries to the hand. Z Unfallshir-Versicherungsmed-Berufskr 82:86–92, 1989
15. Miguleva I: Primary plastic surgery of flexor tendons and nerves in combined injuries to proximal segments of the fingers. Sov Med 4:50–53, 1988
16. Müller ME, Allgöwer M, Schneider R, Willenegger H (eds): Manual of Internal Fixation. Techniques Recommended by the AO-ASIF Group. pp. 1–107, 134–135, 159–290, 411–426, 453–484. 3rd Ed. Springer-Verlag, New York, 1991
17. Rose EH, Norris MS, Kowalski TA: Microsurgical management of complex fingertip injuries: Comparison to conventional skin grafting. J Reconstr Microsurg 4:89–98, 1988
18. Savage R: In vitro studies of a new method of flexor tendon repair. J Hand Surg 10B:135–141, 1985
19. Savage R, Risitano G: Flexor tendon repair using a "six strand" method of repair and early active mobilisation. J Hand Surg 14B:396–399, 1989
20. Segmüller G: Surgical Stabilization of the Skeleton of the Hand. Williams & Wilkins, Baltimore, 1977
21. Sosoc M, Milicevic S, Budalica M: Treatment of combined injuries of the blood vessels and bones in the extremities. Acta Chir Jugosl 35:261–269, 1988
22. Sunderland S: Nerve Injuries and Their Repair. A Critical Appraisal. pp. 221–232. Churchill Livingstone, Edinburgh, 1991
23. Vlastou C, Earle AS: Beyond replantation: Microsurgical salvage of complex hand injuries. Orthop Rev 16:739–746, 1987
24. Zaidemberg C, Siebert J, Angrigiami C: Colgajo comisural posterior del dorso de la mano. Rev Assoc Argen Orthop Traumatol 53:579–587, 1988

46

Rheumatoid Arthritis in the Hand and Wrist

Paul Feldon
Lewis H. Millender
Edward A. Nalebuff

Significant progress in the reconstruction of the rheumatoid hand has been made over the past two decades. Reconstructive hand surgery has been established as an effective component in the overall management program of the patient with rheumatoid arthritis. Approximately 25 percent of all arthritis surgery is now performed on the hand.[183] However, it should be understood that hand reconstruction does not restore normal function to rheumatoid hands. Pain can be alleviated, severe deformity prevented or corrected, and appearance and function improved; but motion and dexterity still will be limited, and weakness will remain a significant disability.[26,40,62,72,77,113,165,197,213,242,270] Because of the difficulty in consistently restoring or improving function, careful judgment must be used when recommending reconstructive surgery.

The purpose of this chapter is to describe the surgical techniques used to correct rheumatoid hand deformities. However, an understanding of these techniques is only one requirement for the surgeon treating rheumatoid patients. An understanding of the natural history of both the disease and the deformities must be appreciated. In addition, the surgeon must understand the functional needs and limitations of each patient to make appropriate judgments regarding the indications for surgical treatment.[122] By working closely with the rheumatologist, orthopaedic surgeon, and physical and occupational therapists, the hand surgeon will have a clear understanding of the overall treatment program and thereby provide the best care possible for these patients.[42,232]

SURGICAL CONSIDERATIONS IN THE ARTHRITIC PATIENT

The care of the hand affected by rheumatoid arthritis differs in many respects from that of the hand affected by trauma. In the rheumatoid patient, an ongoing process of joint and tendon destruction can persist for many years. Involvement of one joint will affect adjacent joints. Involvement of adjacent joints or recurrent disease can nullify the effects of previous surgery. The manifestations of the disease will vary for each patient. Cooperation between the rheumatologist and the surgeon is essential to provide appropriate surgical recommendations for each individual. The surgeon must understand both the pathophysiology and the natural history of the disease (Fig. 46-1).[24,86,88,125,129,149,254,256,279]

Rheumatoid arthritis is a systemic condition affecting synovial tissue. All deformities, joint destruction, and pathologic anatomy that occur in patients with rheumatoid arthritis are the result of the way in which the diseased and hypertrophied synovial tissue alters its surroundings. Rheumatoid synovium destroys articular cartilage by a poorly understood enzymatic reaction, invades subchondral bone, and stretches the soft tissues that support the involved joint. It also surrounds and invades the flexor and extensor tendons. The result is disruption of the normal architecture of the hand and wrist, and loss of the normal delicate balance of flexor and extensor forces across adjacent joints of the hand-wrist unit.

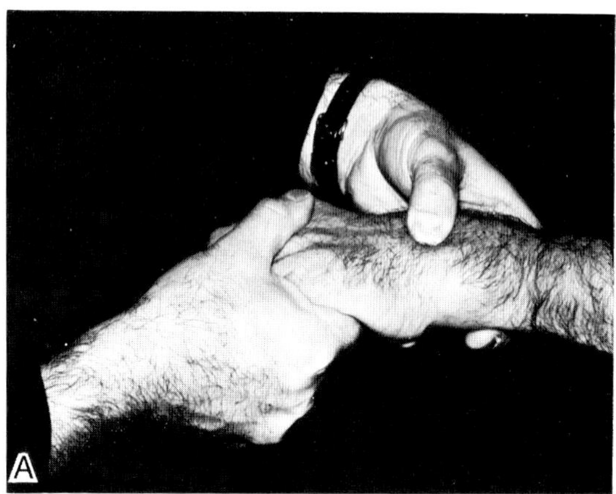

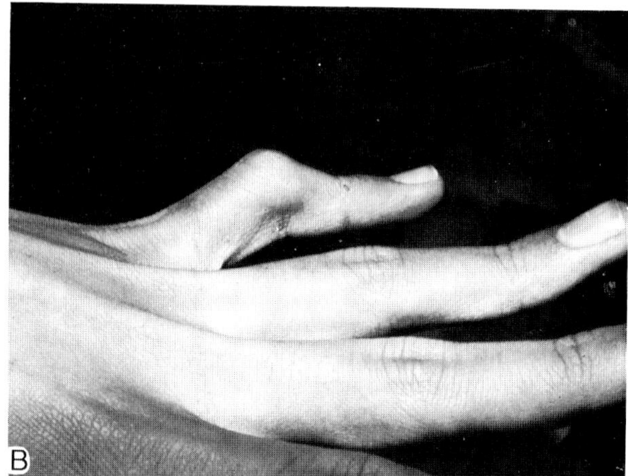

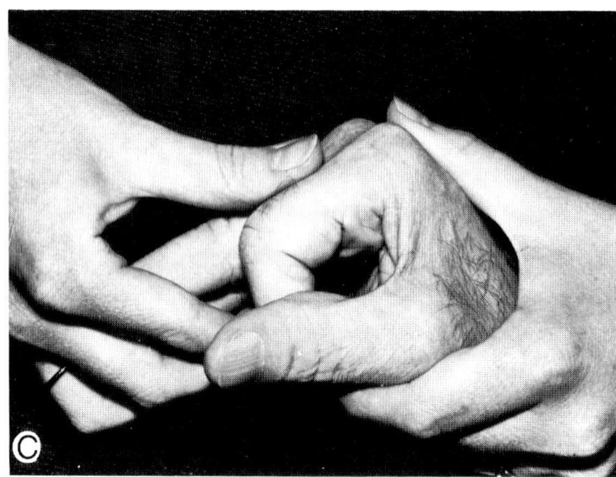

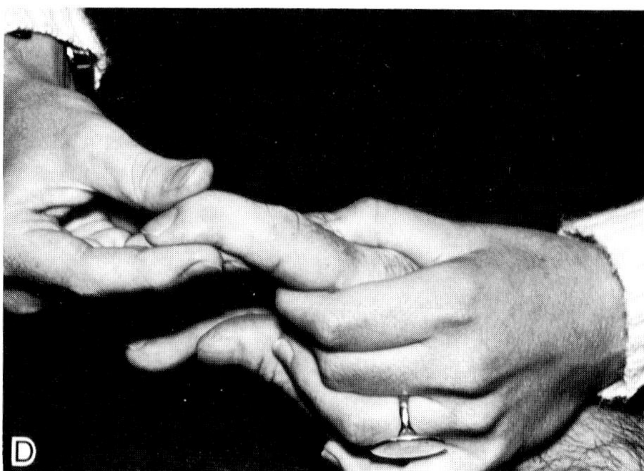

Fig. 46-1. Physical findings in early rheumatoid disease. **(A)** Radiocarpal pain elicited by direct pressure and stress of the wrist joint. **(B)** Early boutonnière deformity for PIP joint synovitis with stretching of the extensor mechanism. **(C&D)** Positive intrinsic muscle tests. **(C)** Notice that when the MP joint is passively flexed the PIP joint has full range of flexion. **(D)** However, when the MP joint is held in extension, intrinsic muscle tightness prevents passive flexion of the PIP joint. (From Millender and Nalebuff,[163] with permission.)

Nearly all of the surgical procedures performed on the rheumatoid hand and wrist fall into one of five groups: (1) synovectomy, (2) tenosynovectomy, (3) tendon surgery, (4) arthroplasty, and (5) arthrodesis.[183]

Judgment in the type and timing of surgical procedures for reconstructing the rheumatoid hand and wrist requires experience. A "cookbook" approach cannot be used. An individual treatment plan must be formulated for each patient based on the status of the hand and the patient's needs, as well as the expertise and experience of the surgeon. The presence of deformity is not, in and of itself, an indication for surgery, as many patients maintain good function in spite of significant deformity. We believe that reconstructive rheumatoid hand surgery is not for the occasional hand surgeon.[36,134,139,230,231]

The surgeon treating the rheumatoid hand must work within the framework of the patient's medical, social, and economic problems. This requires coordination and interaction with the other professionals involved with the patient's care. Good rapport with the patient is essential as the reconstructive program will usually span many months, and often years.

The patient's disease pattern affects the surgical approach in rheumatoid reconstruction. In general, synovectomies are indicated for patients with mild disease controlled by drugs who have persistent synovitis in one or two joints. However, synovectomies are contraindicated in patients with rapidly progressive joint disease. In these patients, frequent observation is required so that reconstructive surgery can be performed prior to the development of severe deformities. Early tenosynovectomy may be required in patients with rapidly progressive desease to prevent tendon rupture.

Better results are possible when reconstruction is performed before severe fixed contractures occur and before significant subluxation or dislocation occurs. After the capsule and supporting ligamentous structures have stretched, the lack of adequate soft tissue support makes the maintenance of joint alignment and function more difficult. Caution must be used when considering reconstructive surgery in patients with mild deformities who are basically healthy and active, but who are frustrated because of their general loss of function. They want to pursue their avocations and/or sports activities, but may not have the strength or endurance to do so. Hand surgery cannot restore full function in these patients and may weaken the hand even further; therefore it is not indicated since it would not produce the desired or expected end result. Such patients need to understand their disease and modify their activities.

Hand surgery also can lead to disappointing results in patients who have significant destruction of multiple joints, but who have minimal pain and who function relatively well in spite of their disease. Many of these patients are older and place fewer demands on their hands. Unless surgery can provide either significant pain relief or a dramatic change in function, the patient's expectations from reconstructive surgery may not be fullfilled.

Patients' expectations from surgery should match the surgeon's goals and anticipated results. They must know that some deformity, especially at the MP joints, is likely to recur following surgery. Nonetheless, Vahvanen[276] reported a high rate of patient satisfaction following reconstructive surgery for rheumatoid disease. There is no substitute for in-depth preoperative discussion between the surgeon and the patient.

MEDICAL CONSIDERATIONS IN THE RHEUMATOID PATIENT

Certain factors should be considered in rheumatoid patients scheduled for hand surgery. A careful preoperative evaluation will alert the surgeon to these, and appropriate consultation can be obtained prior to surgery if needed. Discovering an unexpected condition on the day of surgery that might alter or delay the reconstruction is always disrupting and frustrating.[217]

Cervical spine involvement may be subtle. It is worthwhile to identify instability of the cervical spine preoperatively so that manipulation of the neck during surgery is not a concern if general anesthesia is required. Cervical spine stability should be evaluated clinically as well as radiographically, as there may not be a close correlation between neurologic deficit and radiographic findings. A history of numbness or paresthesias with cervical motion must be heeded.

Tempromandibular (TM) joint involvement may compromise intubation during general anesthesia. The anesthesiologist should be aware of TM involvement so that adequate plans are made for nasotracheal or fiberoptic intubation if these become necessary.

Pulmonary involvement can occur from the disease itself (pulmonary rheumatoid nodules) or as the consequence of antirheumatic therapy with gold or penicillamine.

Felty's syndrome (splenomegaly and neutropenia), while rare, can cause a profound decrease in white blood cell count and thereby increase the susceptibility to infection.

Drug therapy must be taken into account when planning surgery. Systemic steroids and penicillamine can delay wound healing; methotrexate neither impairs this process nor predisposes to infection unless the WBC is low. Methotrexate can alter liver function, which may affect the choice of anesthesia.

Gold, penicillamine, and aspirin can suppress platelet counts. Aspirin affects platelet function for several days, and discontinuing aspirin for several days prior to extensive surgery may be prudent. Nonsteroidal antiinflammatory medication affects platelet aggregation only for several hours. It has been recommended that these drugs be withheld preoperatively for a period equal to five times the dose interval schedule. For example, drugs given four times daily are withheld for 2 days prior to surgery. Those given once daily are withheld for 5 days. These medications can be restarted within 48 hours after surgery.

Every effort should be made to minimize the use of narcotics following surgery. It is easy for patients with chronic pain to become dependent on oral narcotic analgesics. The use of patient-controlled analgesia whereby small amounts of medication are delivered intravenously by pump on demand has been effective in controlling pain and in decreasing the total amount of pain medication used in the postoperative period.

RHEUMATOID VARIANTS

Psoriatic Arthritis

Psoriatic arthritis is a rheumatoid variant that is classified as one of the seronegative spondyloarthropathies along with Reiter's syndrome, ankylosing spondylitis, and the arthritis of inflammatory bowel disease. Approximately 7 percent of patients with psoriasis have some type of inflammatory arthritis.

The pattern of joint involvement in psoriatic arthritis varies widely: 95 percent have peripheral joint involvement; 25 percent have a polyarthritis similar to rheumatoid arthritis; 5 percent have classic DIP joint disease with erosion of the terminal phalanges, DIP joint destruction, nail pitting, and onycolysis. Inflammation of the periosteum, tendons, and tendon insertions may be a factor in the fusiform swelling of digits in this disease, so-called "sausage" swelling. "Pencil-in-cup" joint deformities may be evident on x-rays.[218]

Psoriatic arthritis causes hand deformities similar to those seen in rheumatoid arthritis, yet with several typical differences, aside from usually being associated with psoriatic skin lesions.

In contrast to rheumatoid arthritis, patients with psoriatic arthritis tend to have MP joint extension contractures rather than flexion contractures. Postoperative motion following MP arthroplasty may be limited compared to that usually obtained in rheumatoid patients. If arthroplasties are done, more bone than usual should be resected to allow adequate space for the implant. PIP joint involvement is common and can result in both flexion or extension contractures. Severe fixed flexion deformities are best treated by fusion rather than by arthroplasty. The DIP joints are involved frequently, but rarely need treatment as they tend to fuse spontaneously. Fusiform swelling of the digits (dactylitis psoriatica) may occur, but is treated best by medical means. Tenosynovectomy and other tendon surgery is not often necessary in psoriatic arthritis. Arthritis mutilans, which results in severe loss of bone stock with collapse and shortening of the digit, is not uncommon, and must be treated early and aggressively by joint fusions using iliac crest bone grafts to restore digital length[12,214] (Fig. 46-2).

Systemic Lupus Erythematosus

Systemic lupus erythematosus (SLE) is a multisystem disease in which joint and hand involvement is common.[218] Hand involvement can include symmetrical joint swelling, tenderness, pain with motion, and morning stiffness. Tenosynovitis can occur and may be present without joint involvement. While the deformities may appear similar to those seen in rheumatoid arthritis, ligamentous laxity is the hallmark of this disease rather than joint destruction. If the ligaments and periarticular structures are involved, joint and tendon imbalances occur, but the articular surfaces and joint spaces are preserved. X-rays show deformity, but with normal-appearing joint spaces. The deformities often can be corrected passively, but

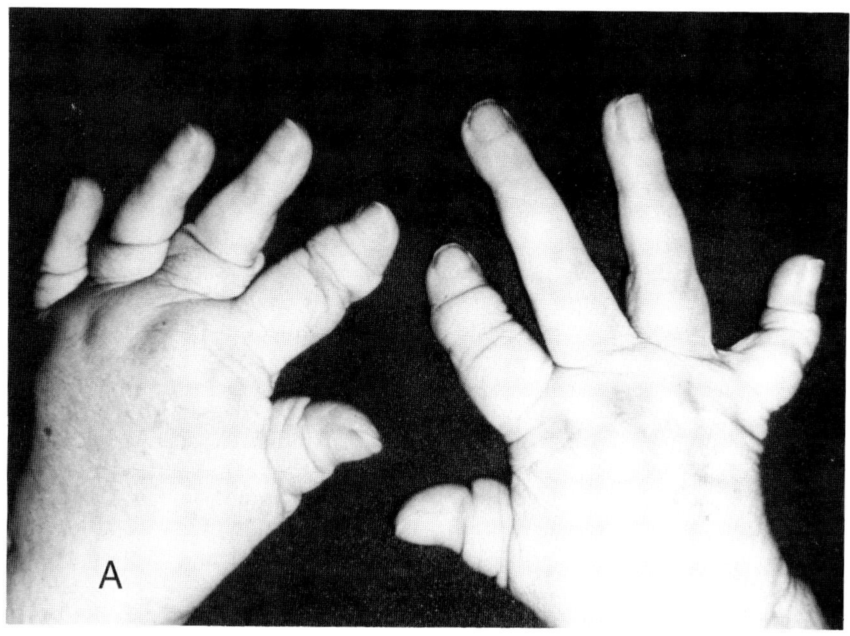

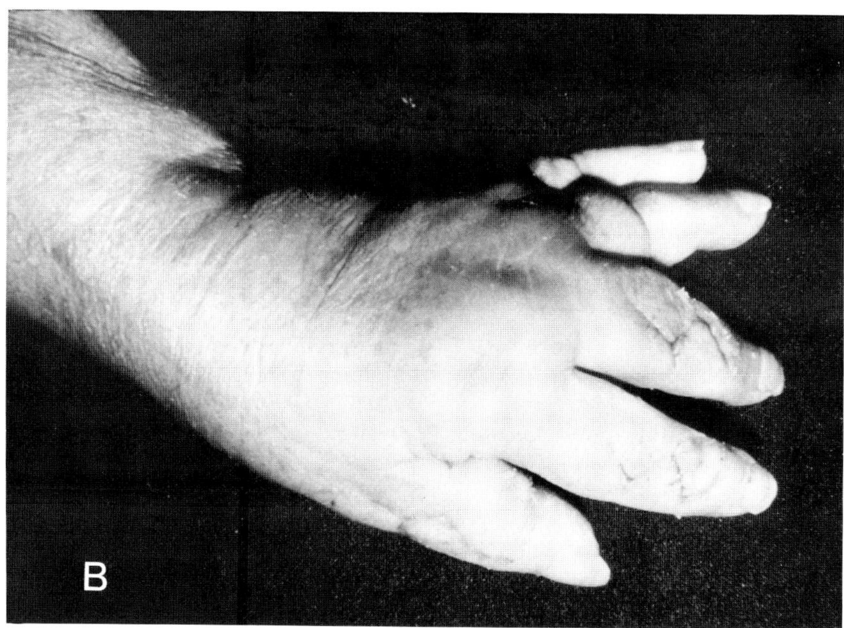

Fig. 46-2. (**A**) Arthritis mutilans with typical "opera-glass" hand deformities. (**B**) Fusions of the interphalangeal joints of the index and middle fingers and of the interphalangeal and metacarpophalangeal joints of the thumb using iliac crest bone grafts to restore pinch function.

attempts to reconstruct the deformities by soft tissue procedures is associated with a frustratingly high recurrence rate. Thus arthroplasties and/or fusions may be necessary even though the joints have been preserved and look uninvolved on x-rays. Surgery in lupus patients should be performed before fixed deformities occur. While not performed frequently in rheumatoid arthritis, arthrodesis of the thumb basal joint may be necessary to control thumb deformities in lupus patients. Soft tissue reconstruction and implant arthroplasties of the basal joint of the thumb are contraindicated, as the deformity is likely to recur with these procedures.[54]

STAGING HAND SURGERY

One of the difficult tasks in rheumatoid surgery is the formulation of a plan for the systematic reconstruction of the hand. Although there are no hard and fast rules, some general principles can be outlined. The priorities for hand surgery in rheumatoid patients are: (1) alleviation of pain, (2) improvement of function, (3) retardation of progression of the disease, and (4) improvement of cosmesis. Appropriate decisions are made more easily if each of these priorities are considered for each patient. Relief of pain is the foremost goal. The indications for surgery to relieve pain are clear and predictable; fusions and arthroplasties accomplish this.

The most difficult decisions regard function and the prevention of progression. Reconstructive surgery is more predictable and preventative surgery is more successful when done early. Function is not synonymous with deformity, and careful evaluation and discussion are needed before surgery to improve function is undertaken.

In general, painful conditions should be alleviated first. Pain may be the most important factor in determining a rheumatoid patient's ability to work. Many patients with severe deformities can work because they are able to adapt to their functional limitations. In contrast, patients with much less deformity but with significant pain are less able to continue gainful employment.[97] A painful wrist or thumb usually will take precedence over dislocated MP joints of the fingers. Acute carpal tunnel syndrome or proliferative dorsal tenosynovitis with a single tendon rupture is allocated high priority to prevent permanent loss of median nerve function or more tendon ruptures (Fig. 46-3).

Mild carpal tunnel syndrome often can be aggravated by any surgical procedure in the hand. Therefore, carpal tunnel release should be considered prior to, or in conjunction with, other surgical procedures on the volar aspect of the wrist.

We usually correct MP joint deformities before treating PIP joint deformities.[176,179,190] Frequently the PIP joint deformity is the result of or is magnified by a primary MP joint deformity. Treating the MP joints first may simplify treatment of the PIP joints. Just restoring MP joint alignment and motion can provide a significant improvement in hand function, even with imperfect PIP joint function. The converse is not necessarily true; reasonable PIP joint motion will do little to improve hand function if the MP joints remain fixed in flexion.[160]

If tendon reconstruction is required in addition to MP joint surgery, we reconstruct the MP joints after the flexor tendons and before the extensor tendons are treated. This facilitates postoperative rehabilitation, as active flexor tendons are a necessity for restoring MP joint motion after arthroplasty, but MP extension can be provided with a dynamic splint, and extensor tendon reconstruction can be done at a second stage without compromising the previous MP joint surgery.[160]

Most patients have bilateral hand problems that require surgical treatment. When similar problems are present bilaterally, we discuss the situation with the patient and allow him to help us decide on which hand to operate first. However, when only one hand is severely disabled, it will take precedence over the other hand. This staging allows the patient to have one hand for his daily needs while the other hand is being rehabilitated following surgery. During the rehabilitation period, the nonoperated hand must perform additional work and this alone may induce a flare of synovitis.

As emphasized by Souter,[234] it is best to begin a reconstructive program with surgical procedures that are predictable in their outcome and effect and to progress in stages to those procedures that are less predictable. Thus, such procedures as wrist stabilization, tenosynovectomy, and distal ulna excision can be performed first, followed by thumb surgery, DIP fusion in the fingers, and MP arthroplasty.

It may be prudent to operate on the less involved hand first, especially in an apprehensive patient. This approach can prevent progressive deformity, provide a better overall result, and allow the patient to assess the potential of further reconstruction. Shoulder and/or elbow reconstruction, if indicated, should be considered prior to hand reconstruction so that rehabilitation of the hand following surgery is not impeded by more proximal problems.

Occasionally, it is necessary to consider hand deformities and upper extremity limitations in view of lower extremity problems. If a painful or deformed hand prevents the use of ambulatory aids such as crutches or walkers, it may be necessary to perform upper extremity surgery before lower extremity surgery.

Hospital use should be maximized so that the total number of admissions (and anesthetics) is reduced. Thus, lower extremity surgery should be coordinated with hand surgery. Frequently, hand surgery and foot surgery can be performed simultaneously by two teams. If appropriate, the patient may be admitted for hand reconstruction, begin hand therapy on the third postoperative day, and undergo hip reconstruction on the sixth or seventh hospital day. When the patient is ready to ambulate following lower extremity surgery, modified walking aids such as platform crutches or walkers are used. The patient's therapy and rehabilitation programs can be well underway by the time of discharge.

In this chapter we have included our philosophy of the management of difficult rheumatoid hand problems. We have tried to summarize the pathology of the deformities and our indications for surgery, as well as the results that can be expected from the procedures. A large reference list has been included, and the reader is encouraged to refer to the original articles by many authors in this field to enhance his understanding of the principles and procedures we describe here.

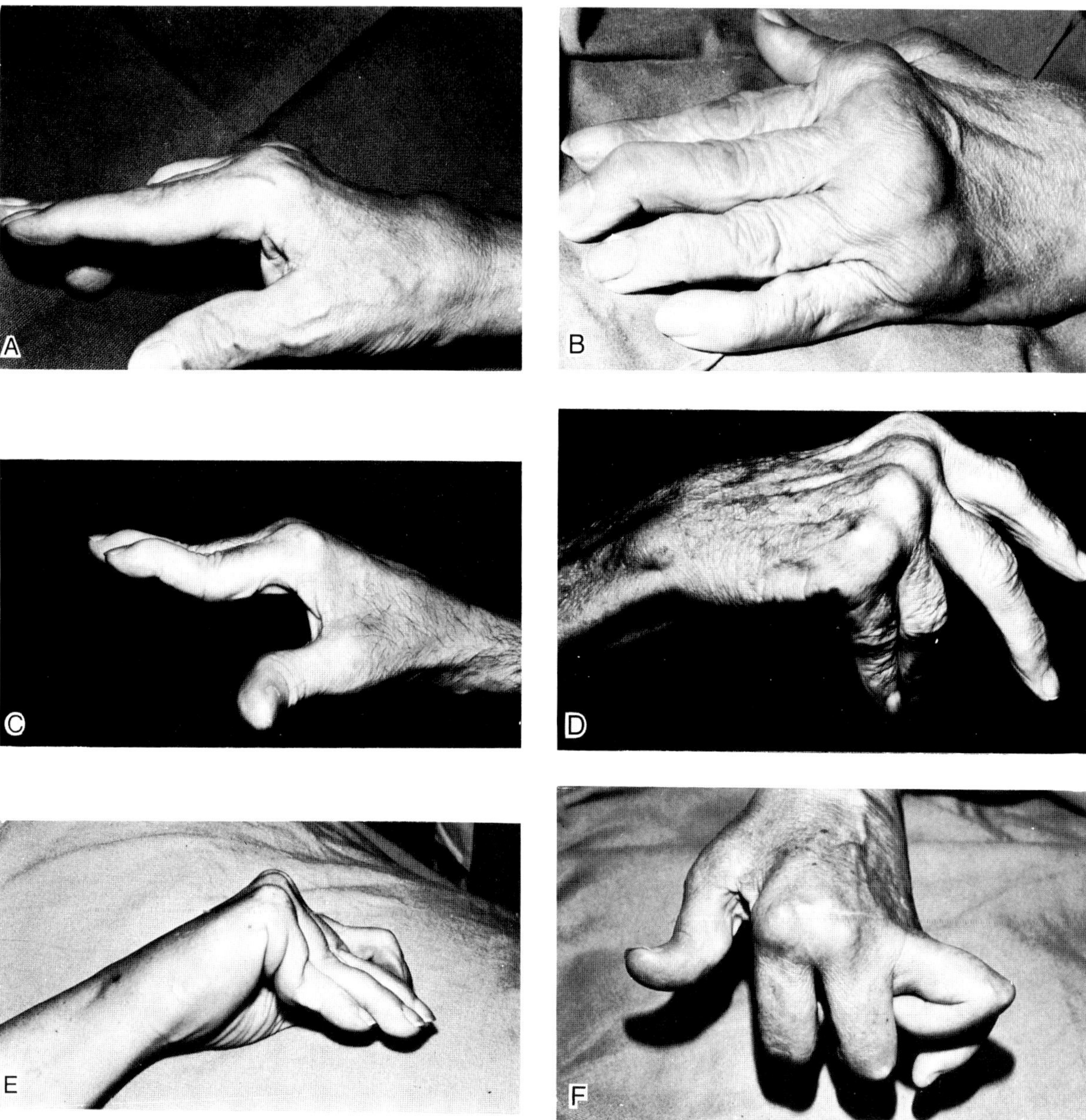

Fig. 46-3. Examples of stages of rheumatoid hand deformities. **(A)** Stage 1: Early MP joint synovitis without deformity. Note early dorsal tenosynovitis. **(B)** Stage 2: Moderate MP joint synovitis without dislocation of the MP joints and without marked bony destruction. **(C)** Stage 2: Early MP joint subluxation with swan-neck deformity. Both of these deformities are correctable passively, and there is no cartilage or bone destruction. The patient is a candidate for intrinsic release, synovectomy, and extensor tendon relocation. **(D)** Stage 3: Classic example of MP joint dislocation without PIP joint involvement. Note absence of wrist joint subluxation and minimal subluxation of the distal ulna. Extensor tendon function is intact. **(E)** Stage 3: Fixed dislocation of the MP joints with secondary swan-neck deformity. Note mallet deformity of the DIP joint in the index finger. **(F)** Stage 4: Severe hand deformity with fixed dislocation of the MP joints and fixed flexion contractures of the PIP joints. The patient has had previous synovectomy. Salvage surgery includes PIP joint arthrodeses and MP joint arthroplasties. (From Millender and Nalebuff,[163] with permission.)

RHEUMATOID NODULES

Subcutaneous nodules are common in rheumatoid arthritis and are seen occasionally in patients with systemic lupus erythematosus. These nodules occur frequently in the olecranon areas (Fig. 46-4A) and on the extensor surfaces of the forearms. They are frequently tender and a source of discomfort to the patient if they are large and/or hard. They can occur on the dorsal aspects of the hand (Fig. 46-4B) where they are unsightly, and/or on the palmar surfaces of the digits where they may interfere with hand function because of pressure sensitivity or compression of digital nerves. They may cause erosion of the overlying skin, and can form a draining sinus from necrosis of the central core of the nodule. Nodules that form in the subcutaneous areas on the volar surfaces of the digits can interfere with function because pressure during grip or pinch causes discomfort.

Symptomatic nodules can be resected. Meticulous hemostasis should be obtained, particularly in the region of the olecranon. The use of a drain usually prevents or minimizes the formation of a postoperative hematoma or seroma. On the palmar surfaces of the digits, care must be taken to protect underlying structures, particularly the neurovascular bundles, and to maintain sufficient skin to allow primary closure. If the wound cannot be closed, skin grafts should be used.

Rheumatoid nodulosis has been described as a separate clin-

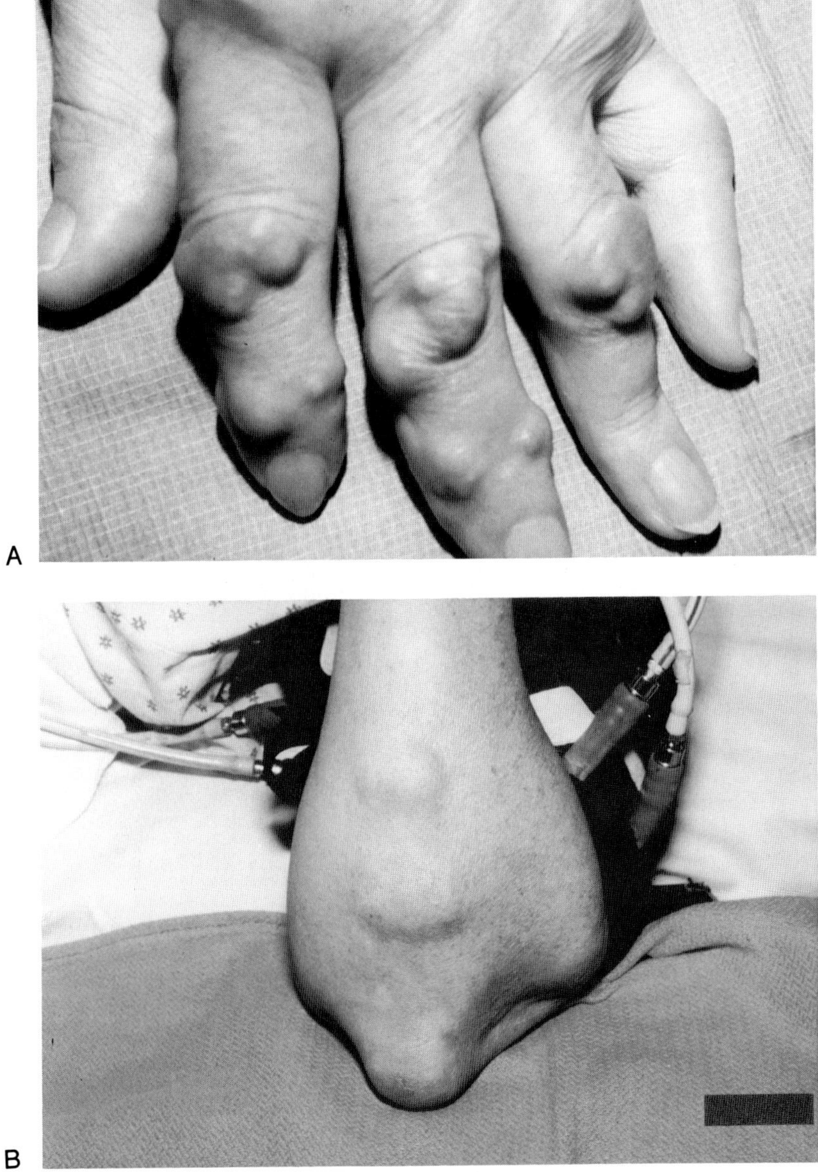

Fig. 46-4. (**A**) Rheumatoid nodulosis on the dorsal aspects of the fingers. (**B**) Rheumatoid nodules on the posterior aspect of the forearm and in the olecranon region can cause considerable discomfort. Resection of these nodules is done through longitudinal incisions.

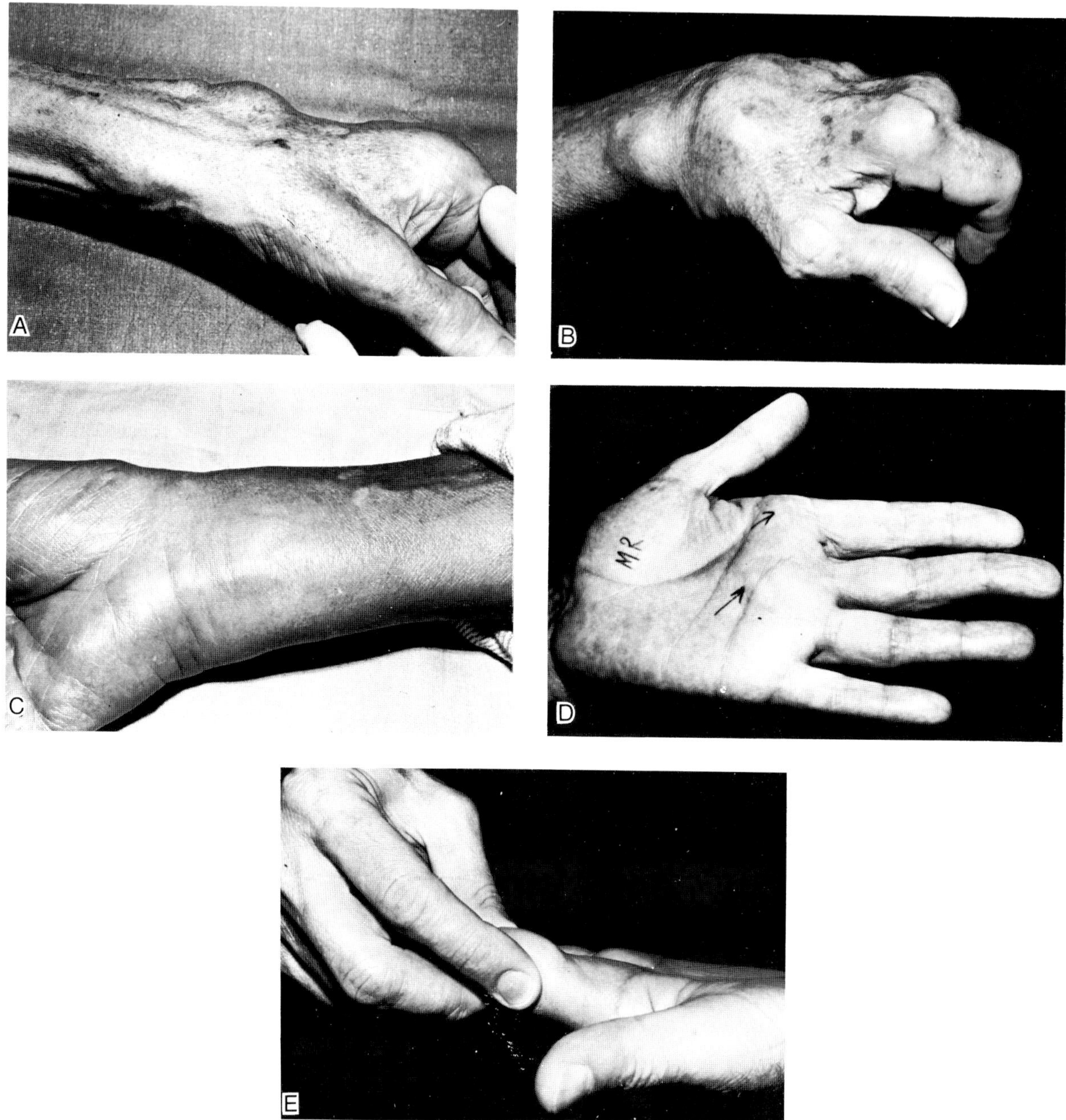

Fig. 46-5. Examples of dorsal (extensor) and flexor tenosynovitis. **(A)** Dorsal tenosynovitis affecting only the extensor digitorum communis compartment. **(B)** More extensive dorsal tenosynovitis affecting multiple extensor tendon compartments. Note bulging along the course of the abductor pollicis longus and extensor pollicis brevis, extensor pollicis longus, and common digital extensors. **(C)** Wrist flexor tenosynovitis. Although there is no bulging, there is volar fullness and loss of normal skin crease marks. **(D)** Palmar flexor tenosynovitis. Flexor nodules are seen over the volar surfaces of the MP joints in the index and long fingers. **(E)** Digital flexor tenosynovitis presenting as volar fullness over the proximal phalanx. (From Millender and Nalebuff,[163] with permission.)

ical entity (rheumatoid variant), and is characterized by multiple subcutaneous nodules usually on the hands and associated with intermittent polyarthralgias, absent or minimal joint involvement, subchondral cystic radiolucencies and a positive rheumatoid factor. Involvement of the hands by prominent subcutaneous nodules, often in clusters, can be extensive. When unsightly, resection of multiple nodules can dramatically improve the appearance of the hand. There is some tendency for these nodules to recur following excision.[80,151]

TENOSYNOVITIS

Rheumatoid arthritis is a disease of the synovium. The synovium-lined sheaths that surround many of the tendons about the hand and wrist can be affected by proliferative synovitis in the same way as are the synovium-lined joint spaces. Tendon sheath involvement is common and may occur months before the symptoms of intraarticular disease are noted.[9,116,118,193]

The three common sites of tendon sheath involvement are the dorsal aspect of the wrist, the volar aspect of the wrist, and the volar aspect of the digits (Fig. 46-5). Rheumatoid tenosynovitis can cause pain, dysfunction of tendons, and, ultimately, tendon rupture following invasion of the tendons by the proliferating synovium. Treatment can relieve pain and, if done before secondary changes have occurred in the surrounding structures and before tendon ruptures have occurred, can prevent both deformity and loss of function. For this reason, dorsal, volar, and digital tenosynovectomy are often the first surgical procedures indicated in rheumatoid patients.[25,111,193,206,240]

Anatomy

On the dorsal aspect of the wrist, the deep fascia thickens to form a band approximately 3 cm in width. This is the dorsal retinaculum, which functions as a pulley for the extensor tendons that run in compartments directly beneath it. Six separate compartments are formed by vertical septa, which run from the volar surface of the retinaculum to the dorsal surface of the radius and ulna. These compartments are referred to numerically. The first (most radial) compartment contains the abductor pollicis longus and extensor pollicis brevis tendons; the second contains the extensor carpi radialis longus and brevis; the third, the extensor pollicis longus; the fourth, the extensor digitorum communis and extensor indicis proprius; the fifth, the extensor digiti quinti; and the sixth, the extensor carpi ulnaris. Each of the tendons within these compartments is surrounded by tenosynovium, which begins just proximal to the proximal edge of the retinaculum and continues distally to the level of the metacarpal bases. The tendons distal to this area are covered by paratenon rather than by tenosynovium.

On the volar aspect of the wrist, the flexor tendons of the fingers and thumb and the median nerve pass into the hand under the transverse carpal ligament (flexor retinaculum). This thick ligament extends across the volar aspect of the carpus attached to four "pillars"—the trapezium and the scaphoid on the radial side of the wrist and the hamate and triquetrum on the ulnar side—to form the roof of the carpal canal. Just before the finger flexors enter the carpal canal, they are surrounded by a common sheath of tenosynovium. The flexor pollicis longus tendon runs in a separate tendon sheath.

The tendon sheaths of the index, middle, and ring fingers extend from midpalm to the DIP joints. The sheaths of the thumb and small finger continue proximally into the carpal tunnel. The flexor tendons within the digits are enclosed in a snug fibroosseous canal that is lined by synovium.

Dorsal (Extensor) Tenosynovitis in the Wrist

Dorsal tenosynovitis is characterized by swelling on the dorsal aspect of the wrist. This may be subtle or massive. It may involve one tendon, a combination of tendons, or all of the tendons in the dorsal compartments. Because the dorsal skin of the wrist and hand is thin and is displaced easily as tenosynovium proliferates, dorsal tenosynovitis usually is obvious and may be the first sign of rheumatoid arthritis. Isolated dorsal tenosynovitis is painless. Because of this, patients tend to ignore the swelling, and tendon rupture frequently is the first manifestation of the condition. When patients with dorsal tenosynovitis complain of pain, one must look for involvement of the radiocarpal or radioulnar joints (Fig. 46-6).

Although early in the disease the synovial tissue remains thin and distends the sheath with fluid, as the disease progresses this tissue thickens and develops a more solid appearance similar to that found within joints affected by advanced rheumatoid arthritis. Small fibrinoid "rice bodies" occasionally fill the tendon sheaths. The hypertrophic synovium adheres to the tendon surfaces and may eventually invade the tendon substance, resulting in weakening and, not infrequently, rupture of the tendon. Occasionally, rheumatoid nodules are found within the tendon substance.

Spontaneous or drug-induced remission of early dorsal tenosynovitis may occur. Rest and/or local injection of a steroid solution also may result in remission. However, if the proliferative synovitis progresses, remission becomes unlikely. The dorsal tenosynovitis becomes unsightly and the risk of tendon rupture increases. For this reason, early dorsal tenosynovectomy is recommended (i.e., if there is no improvement after 4 to 6 months of appropriate medical managment). Although the appearance of the tendons within the compartments affected by tenosynovitis may be poor (as evidenced by fraying), tendon rupture rarely occurs after dorsal tenosynovectomy is performed.[1,10,25,120,164,167,180,206,240]

Dorsal Tenosynovectomy—Operative Technique (Fig. 46-7)

A gently curved, longitudinal incision is made over the dorsal aspect of the wrist just to the ulnar side of the midline. Full-thickness skin flaps, including the subcutaneous tissue, are reflected to expose the underlying extensor retinaculum and deep fascia. The superficial branches of the ulnar and radial nerves remain in the subcutaneous tissue of the flaps and

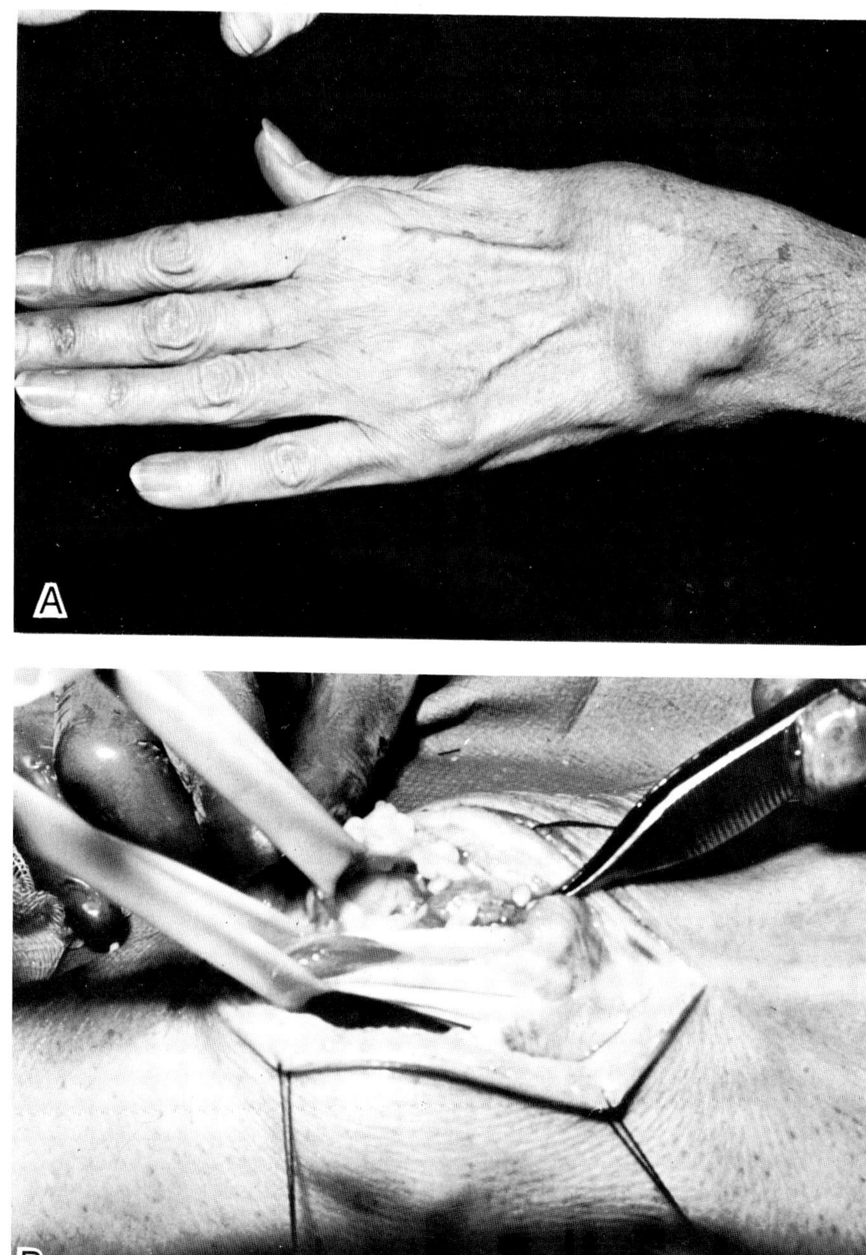

Fig. 46-6. Examples of dorsal tenosynovitis and tendon rupture. **(A)** Dorsal tenosynovitis involving multiple extensor tendon compartments. It is not possible to predict which patients with dorsal tenosynovitis will rupture tendons. **(B)** Dorsal tenosynovitis has been present for 9 months without destruction of extensor tendons. *(Figure continues.)*

thus are protected. Longitudinal veins are preserved if possible, but transverse communicating veins are divided. A longitudinal incision is made through the deep fascia and the extensor retinaculum, entering either into the fourth or sixth extensor compartment. Transverse incisions are made above and below the retinaculum, allowing it to be reflected as a flap. If the retinaculum is incised over the sixth compartment, it is raised as a single, radially based flap; if over the fourth compartment, radially and ulnarly based flaps are elevated. As each extensor compartment is opened, its vertical septum is divided. Care is taken to protect the extensor digiti quinti and extensor pollicis longus tendons, which are contained tightly in their separate compartments. The extensor pollicis longus is particularly at risk as it changes direction distal to Lister's tubercle and crosses the tendons contained in the second dorsal compartment. The first dorsal compartment is not opened unless it is involved significantly. Hypertrophic synovium is removed from each extensor tendon sheath in a systematic manner. The roof of the

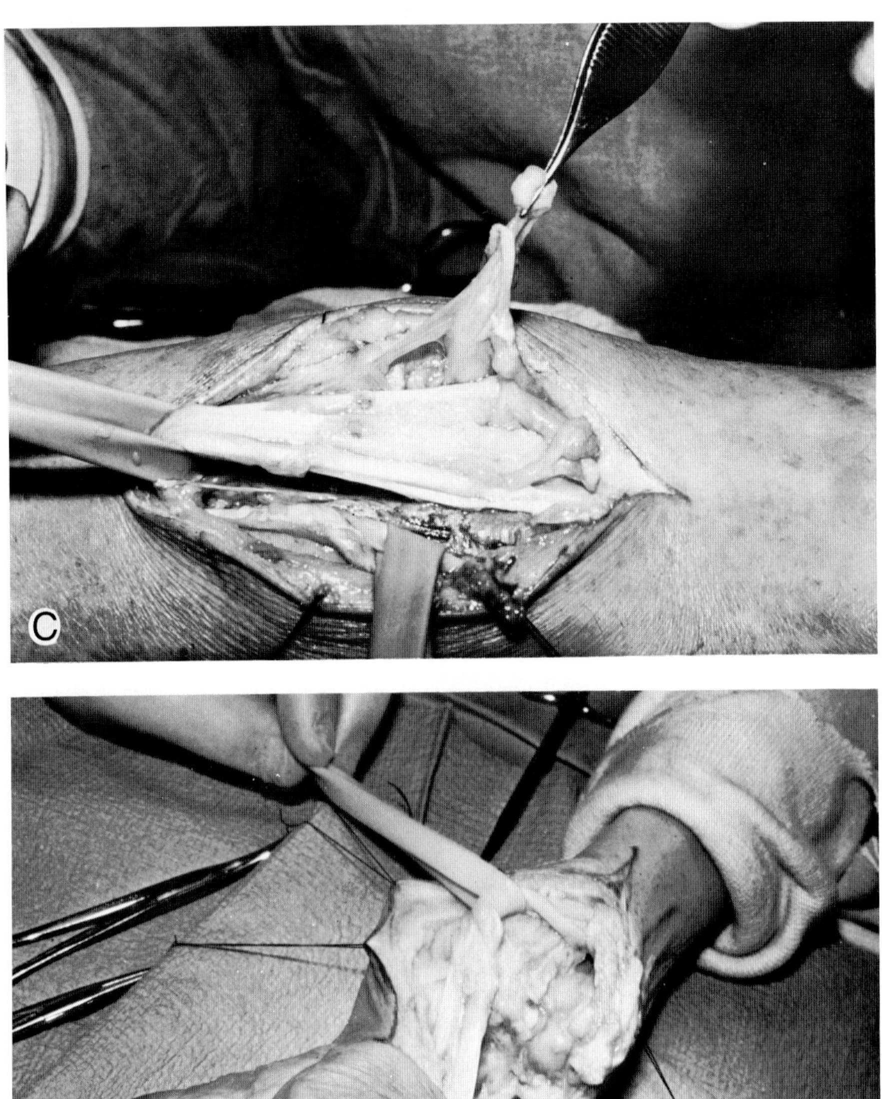

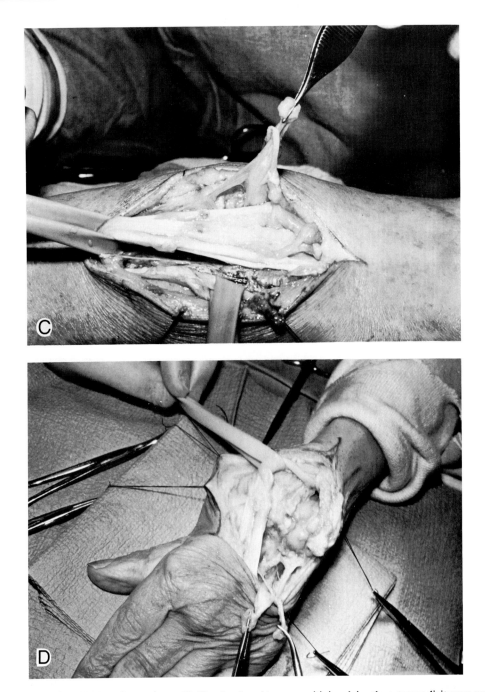

Fig. 46-6 *(Continued).* **(C)** More destructive and infiltrative dorsal tenosynovitis involving the extensor digitorum communis tendons. **(D)** Marked extensor tendon destruction secondary to both infiltrative disease and attrition from subluxation of the wrist. (From Millender and Nalebuff,[164] with permission.)

sheath is opened longitudinally, and the synovium is dissected from the extensor tendons with small scissors. As much of the diseased synovium is removed as possible, although it is sometimes necessary to leave material that is densely adherent to the extensor tendon surface. Frayed areas of the tendons are repaired with interrupted sutures of fine nylon. If an area of tendon appears so attenuated or frayed that tendon rupture appears imminent, the tendon at risk can be sutured to an adjacent extensor tendon above and below the area of damage, or the frayed and attenuated areas can be imbricated. If extensive tendon infiltration is found, similar infiltration may be present in other areas and/or on the contralateral side, and early surgery in these areas should be considered to prevent rupture. A description of the pathologic findings recorded in the operative note is invaluable for future reference.

After a complete tenosynovectomy has been performed, the

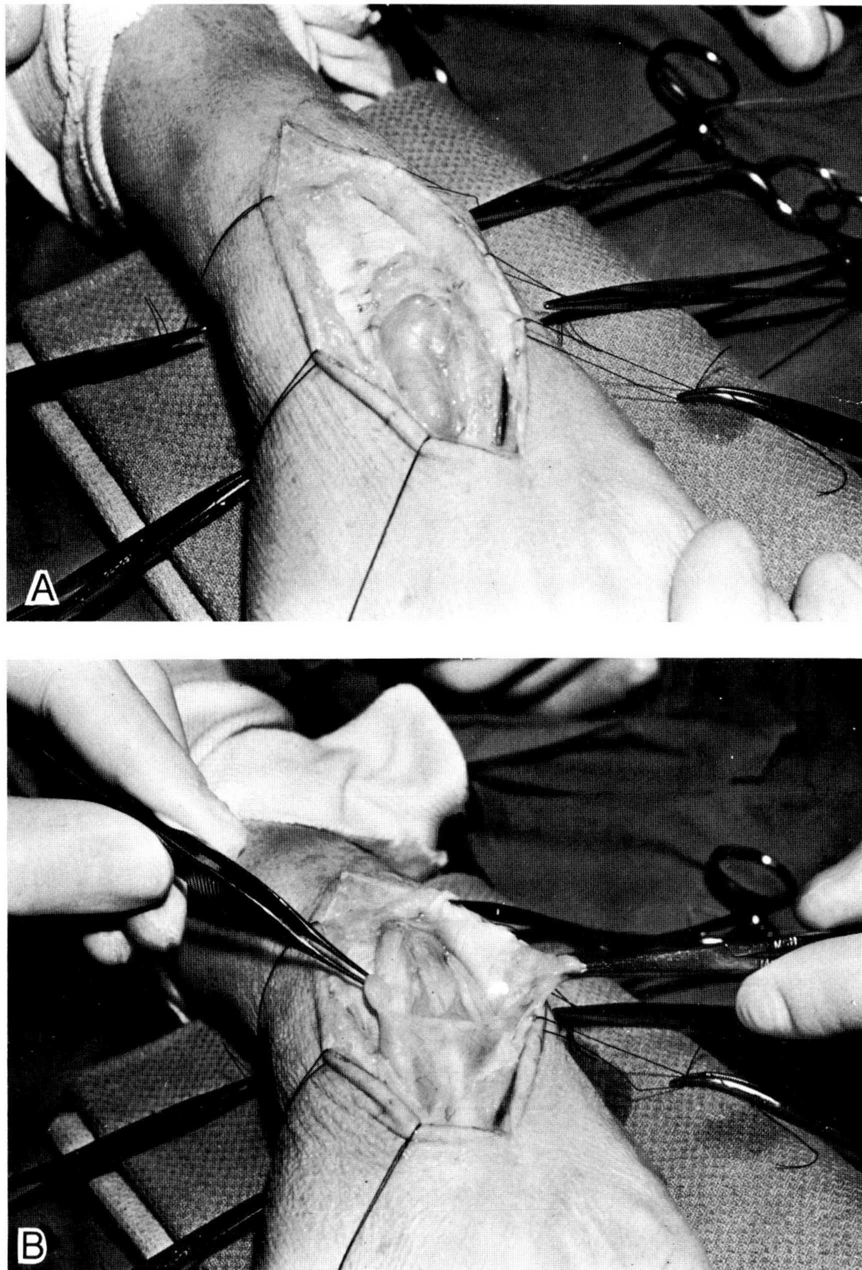

Fig. 46-7. Surgical technique of dorsal tenosynovectomy. **(A)** A slightly curved dorsal incision has been made. The extensor retinaculum and the bulging dorsal tenosynovitis are seen. **(B)** The retinaculum has been incised in the midline and reflected radially and ulnarward. Tenosynovitis is seen surrounding the extensor tendons. *(Figure continues.)*

wrist joint is evaluated. If synovitis is present, the joint is opened and a wrist synovetomy is performed using a small, curved rongeur. The dorsal aspects of the ulna and radius are examined, and any bony spicules, which might cause attrition ruptures, are removed with a rongeur. The distal ulna is resected if it is dislocated and prominent dorsally.

The dorsal retinaculum is passed deep to the extensor tendons and sutured in place to provide a smooth gliding surface beneath the tendons. If bowstringing is anticipated as a potential problem, e.g., in the patient with good dorsiflexion, half of the retinaculum may be retained over the tendons. Studies on the function of the extensor retinaculum suggest that at least a portion of the retinaculum should be retained over the extensor tendons if at all possible.[4] The extensor carpi ulnaris tendon may be stabilized by a narrow segment of the retinaculum.

The tourniquet may be released and bleeding controlled

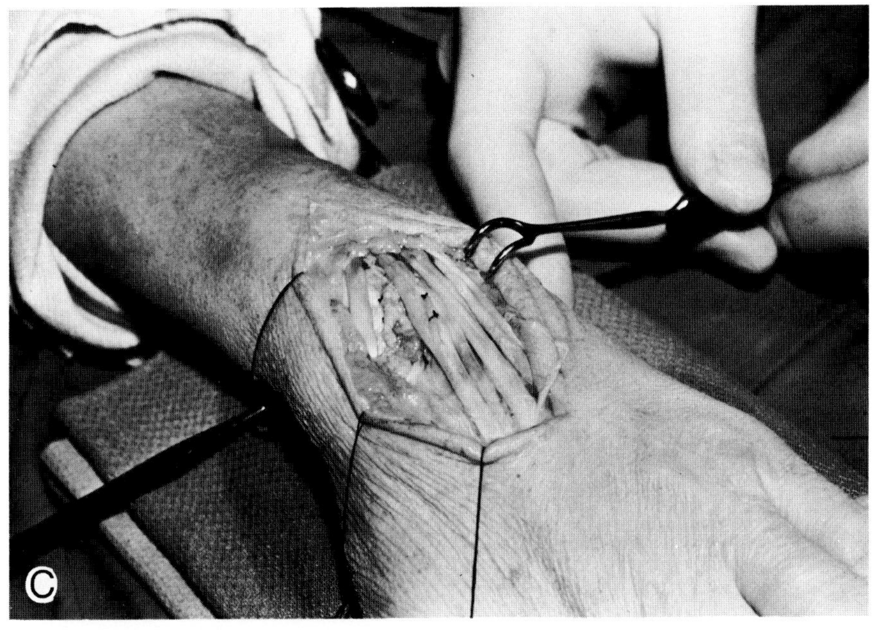

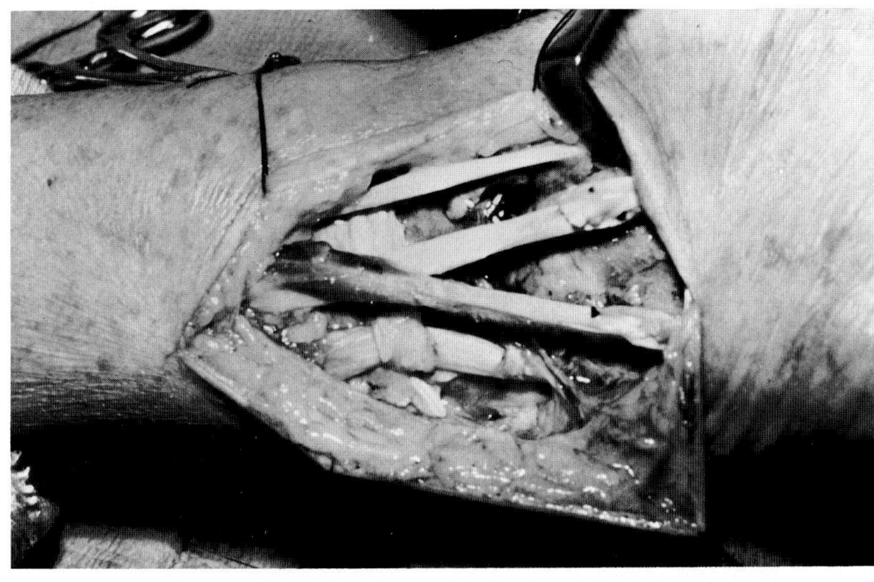

Fig. 46-7 *(Continued).* **(C)** Dorsal tenosynovectomy and retinacular relocation completed. The dorsal retinaculum has been placed deep to the extensor tendons. **(D)** Capsular closure completed and tendon transfer performed. Note extensor carpi ulnaris relocation using a portion of the dorsal retinaculum. *(Figure continues.)*

prior to final closure. If the tourniquet is released and bleeding is minimal, no drain is necessary. However, a small Penrose or suction drain will prevent hematoma formation if the tourniquet is not released. The hand and wrist are immobilized in a bulky conforming dressing and volar plaster splint. The wrist is held in neutral and the fingers are in extension. The drain is removed 24 to 36 hours after surgery.

Dorsal tenosynovectomy can be performed in conjunction with other procedures such as thumb fusion, volar synovectomy, or finger tenosynovectomy. Hand motion is started 24 to 48 hours after surgery. Active extension and flexion are emphasized. Usually motion returns rapidly, but in the patient with a low pain threshold formal hand therapy may be required. The digits should be splinted in extension to prevent extensor lag until active extension is possible. The wrist is supported with a volar splint for 2 weeks following the procedure.

When patients have difficulty regaining active MP joint extension, taping the fingers with the PIP and DIP joints in flexion during active flexion and extension exercise is helpful in improving joint motion. All of the extensor power is concentrated at the MP joint level, and extensor tendon excursion is increased over the areas of surgery (Fig. 46-8).

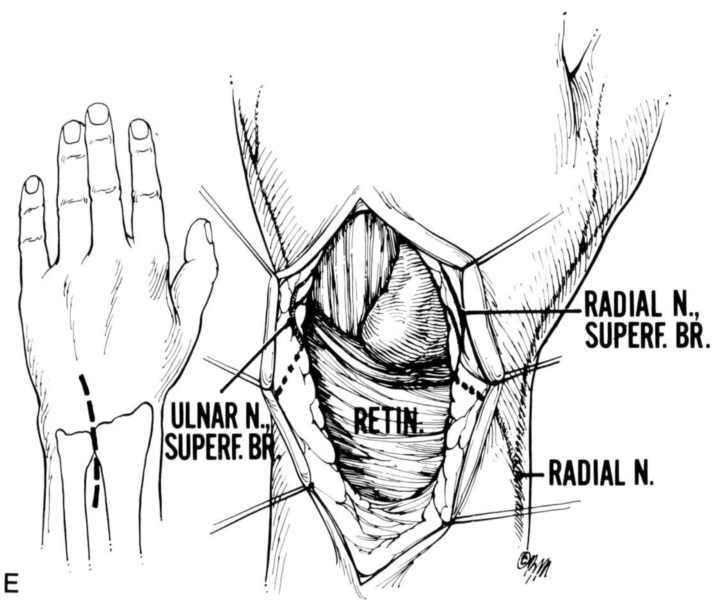

Fig. 46-7 *(Continued).* **(E)** Exposure for dorsal tenosynovectomy. Note superficial branches of radial and ulnar nerves protected in skin flaps. (Figs. **A–C** from Millender and Nalebuff,[164] with permission.)

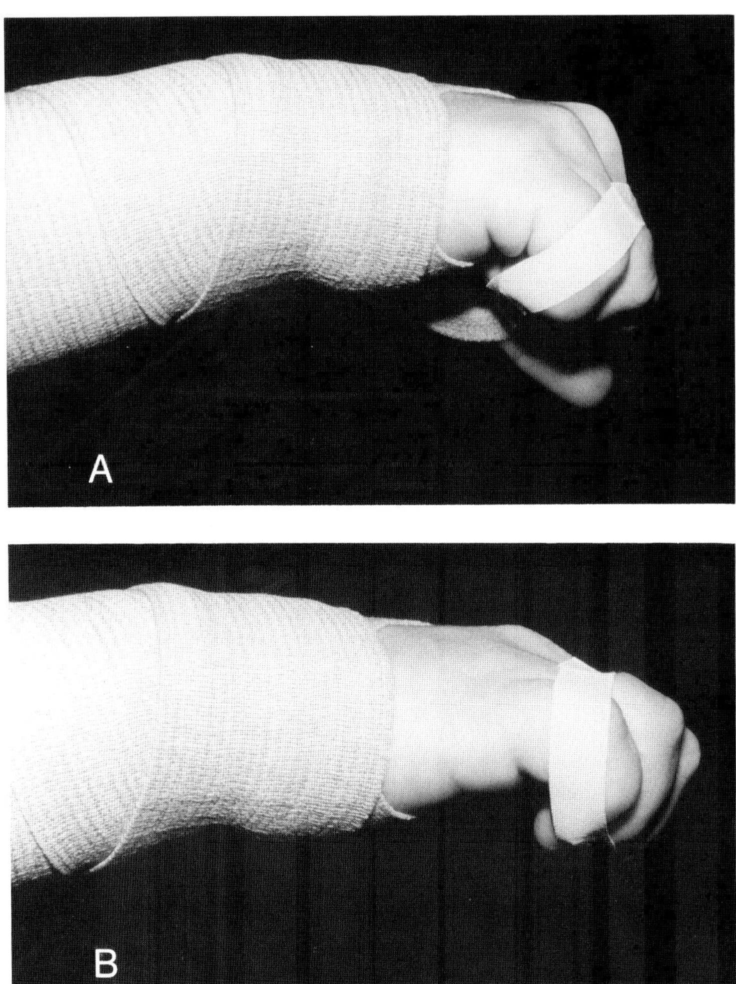

Fig. 46-8. Postoperative MP joint exercises can be done with the PIP and DIP joints taped in flexion. This maximizes extensor tendon excursion as the MP joint moves from flexion **(A)** to extension **(B)**.

Dorsal Tenosynovectomy—Complications

Complications following dorsal tenosynovectomy are infrequent. The most serious complication following dorsal tenosynovectomy is skin necrosis or skin slough. When this occurs, the extensor tendons are exposed and are at risk for rupture or scarring. Hematoma formation under the thin dorsal flaps of rheumatoid patients (especially those on steroids) is the most frequent cause for delayed skin healing. Special care must be taken to prevent hematoma formation. The skin is closed without tension. A layered closure to cover the tendons with subcutaneous tissue sometimes can be done. Occasionally it is useful to put the extensor retinaculum over the tendons to protect them if a skin breakdown occurs. Sutures should not be removed prematurely. If skin slough occurs, the wound can be treated by debridement and coverage with porcine homografts that are reapplied once or twice weekly. The MP joints are splinted in extension until the wound has healed by secondary intention in 2 to 3 weeks (Fig. 46-9). Occasionally, postoperative adhesions may result either in an extensor lag of the MP joints or in loss of active finger flexion. Hand therapy is adjusted to emphasize flexion or extension as necessary. If pain or flexor weakness prevents flexion, passive flexion exercises and dynamic flexion splints are added. If a significant extensor lag develops, a dynamic dorsal extension splint is used. Loss of motion after dorsal tenosynovectomy occurs more often in

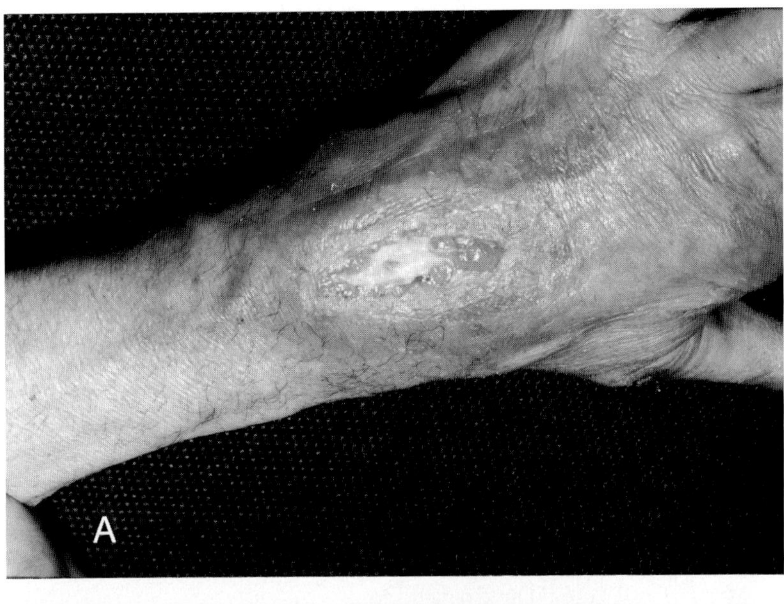

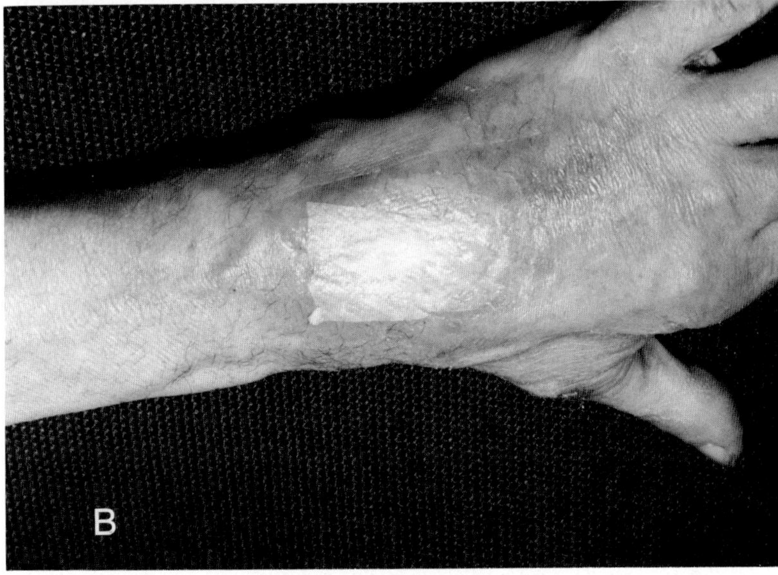

Fig. 46-9. Dorsal skin slough **(A)** is a serious complication and can occur even when a straight incision is used, particularly if the patient is taking systemic (oral) steroids. This slough was treated by debridement and the application of porcine homograft to cover the exposed tendons **(B)** *(Figure continues.)*

those patients whose tendons are found to be in poor condition at the time of surgery, those with multiple joint involvement, and in those with low pain thresholds.

Tenolysis after dorsal tenosynovectomy rarely is necessary. However, if significant impairment of function persists after 6 months of therapy, tenolysis should be considered.

Flexor Tenosynovitis in the Wrist

Whereas swelling on the dorsal aspect of the wrist often is prominent because of the thin skin in the area, hypertrophic synovitis on the volar aspect of the wrist may not be obvious. However, proliferative synovitis of the flexor tendon sheaths occurs commonly and affects the anatomic structures in the area.[33,47,259] Compression of the median nerve may occur, resulting in the symptoms of carpal tunnel syndrome.[11,51,203,272] Restriction of the free-gliding motion of the flexor tendons results in impaired active and passive motion of the fingers.[115]

As in extensor compartmental tenosynovitis, flexor tenosynovitis eventually destroys the outer surfaces of the tendons. The tendons become adherent to one another, and, as synovial tissue invades the tendon substance, tendon ruptures may occur. There may occasionally be complete destruction of the flexor tendons within the confines of the carpal canal.[119]

Although rheumatoid flexor tenosynovitis may respond temporarily to local steroid injection, we believe that early surgical decompression of the carpal canal combined with flexor tenosynovectomy is indicated to prevent permanent damage to the median nerve, which results in pain, numbness, and thenar muscle loss, as well as to preserve independent gliding function of the tendons and to prevent spontaneous rupture.

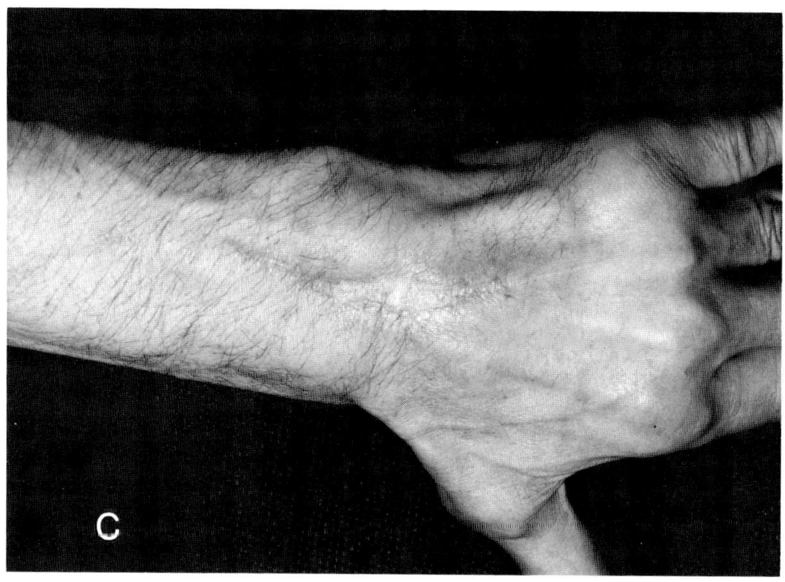

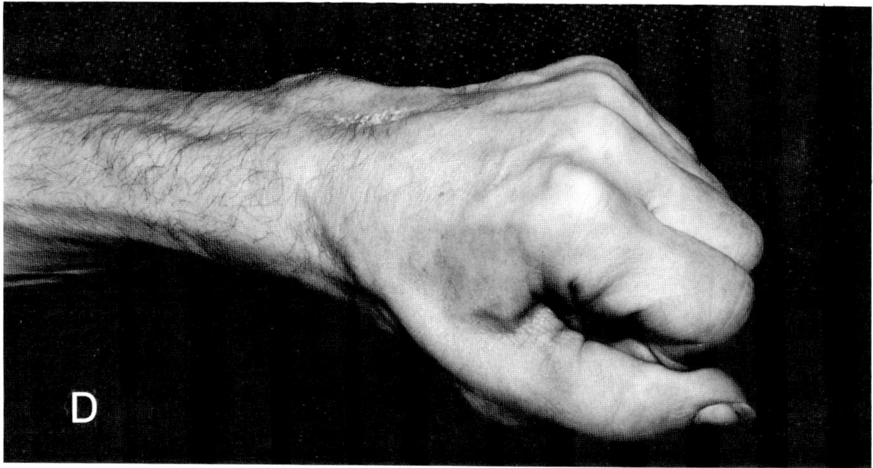

Fig. 46-9 *(Continued).* The MP joints were splinted in extension. Skin closure occurred within 3 weeks (**C**). As expected, active MP joint extension was limited as the result of tendon scarring (**D**).

Flexor Tenosynovectomy (Wrist)—Operative Technique (Fig. 46-10)

An incision is made in the midpalm, parallel to the thenar crease, and is extended proximally, curving ulnarward at the wrist. The incision is extended above the wrist approximately 4 to 5 cm in a zigzag manner. Care should be taken to protect the palmar cutaneous branch of the median nerve at the level of the wrist flexion crease. The deep fascia at the level of the wrist is divided to expose the median nerve. The palmar fascia is incised and separated from the superficial surface of the transverse carpal ligament. The transverse carpal ligament is divided to open the carpal canal.

The median nerve is freed from adherent synovial tissue.

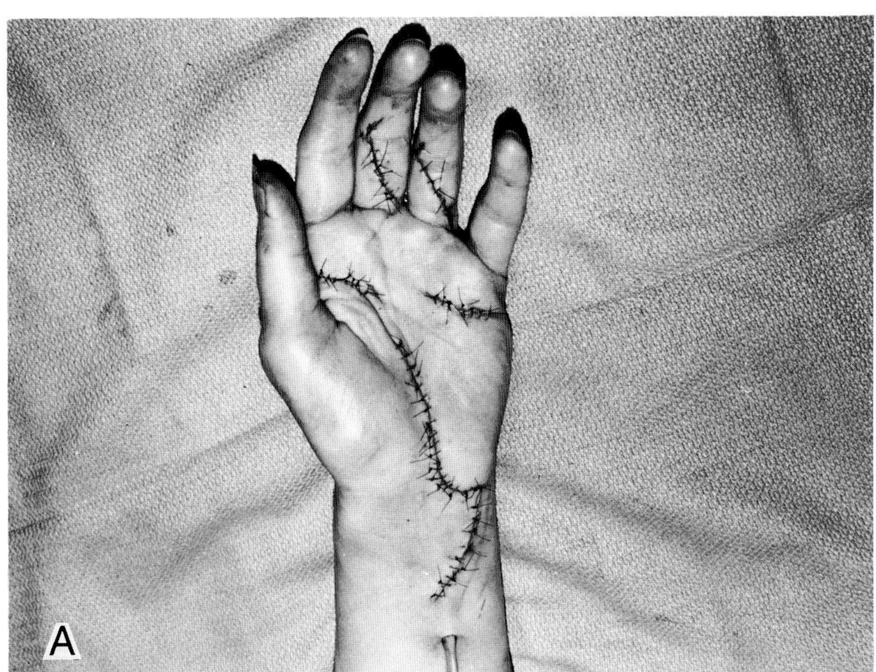

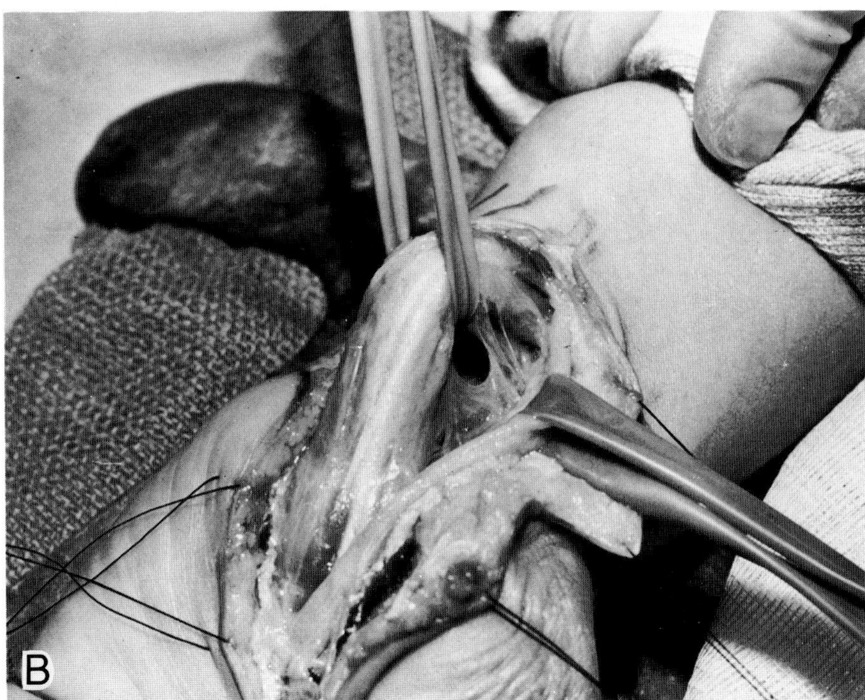

Fig. 46-10. Surgical technique of wrist flexor tenosynovectomy. **(A)** Incisions for wrist, palm, and digital flexor tenosynovectomy. The tube seen emerging from the skin proximal to the incisions is a small Penrose drain, which we prefer over suction catheters for postoperative drainage. **(B)** Flexor tendons exposed at the wrist and elevated into the wound. The median nerve is retracted with a Penrose drain. *(Figure continues.)*

The motor branch of the median nerve is identified and traced into the thenar musculature. If compression of this branch by the fascia of the thenar muscles has occurred, the fascia is divided. The hypertrophic tenosynovium surrounding the flexor tendons is excised, and areas of tendon fraying are repaired as described for the extensor tendons. Occasionally, unsuspected ruptures of the deep flexor tendons may be discovered at this time. If this has occurred and the flexor tendons are functioning by pulling through scar tissue, complete removal of all diseased tissue is not performed. Careful dissection is required when performing an extensive flexor tenosynovectomy, and thought must be given to the consequences of separating each of the deep flexor tendons out of the mass of tenosynovium binding them together. It may be more prudent to separate the superficial flexor tendons and leave the deep flexor tendons in situ, i.e., not separate the flexor digitorum profundus into its four component tendons but merely separate them en masse from their scarred bed.

After tenosynovectomy is performed, the floor of the carpal canal is inspected and palpated. Any bony spicules, particularly over the volar surface of the scaphoid bone, are removed with a rongeur. Exposed bony surfaces are covered by mobiliz-

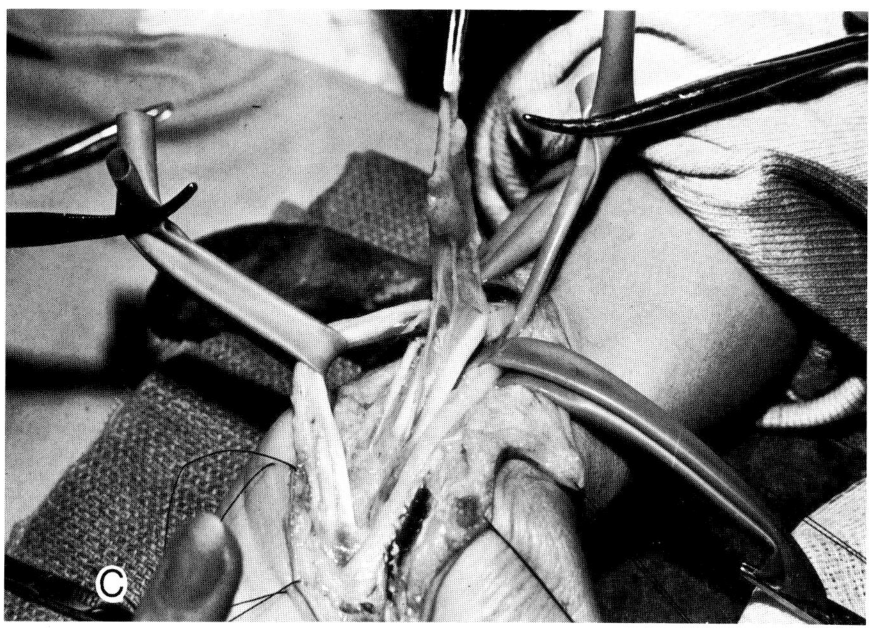

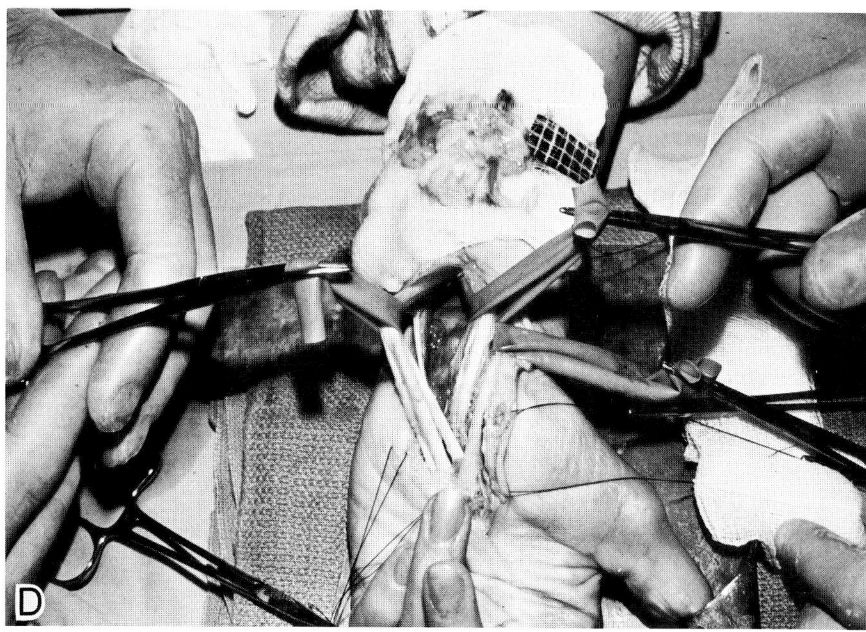

Fig. 46-10 *(Continued).* **(C)** Flexor tenosynovium excised from the flexor tendons. **(D)** Flexor tenosynovectomy completed. The median nerve is retracted to the radial side of the wound. *(Figure continues.)*

ing and suturing local soft tissue.[147] Ertel[63,64] has described a volar rotation flap to close the defect if primary closure is not possible (Fig. 46-11)

Traction is applied to the flexor tendons to check finger motion. Smooth motion of the fingers and thumb should be present. "Catching" signals the presence of tendon nodules in the palm or digits. If smooth motion of the tendons is not present, the involved tendon must be explored as far distally as necessary to remove the nodules. After removal of the nodule, the defect in the tendon is repaired with interrupted fine nylon sutures.

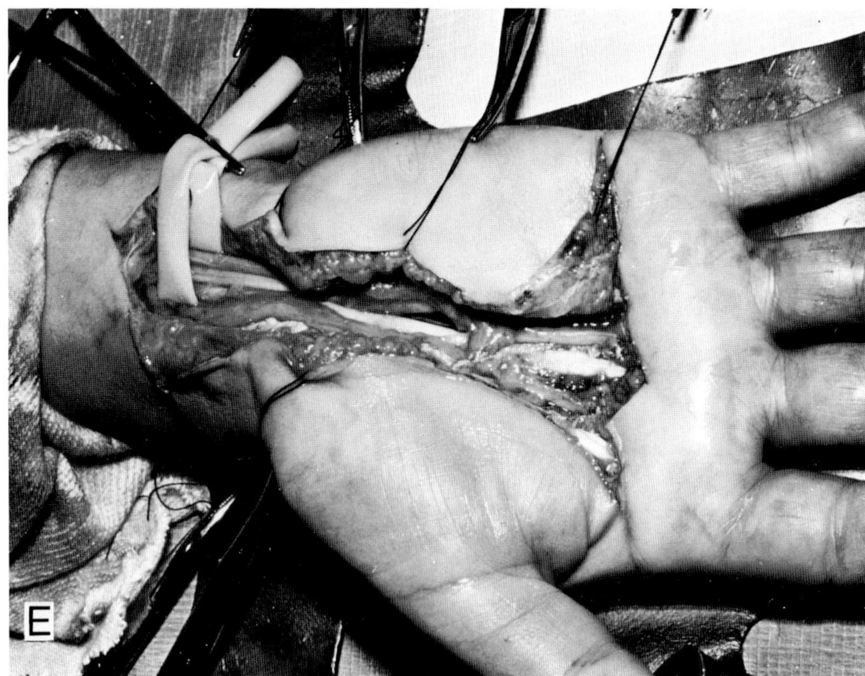

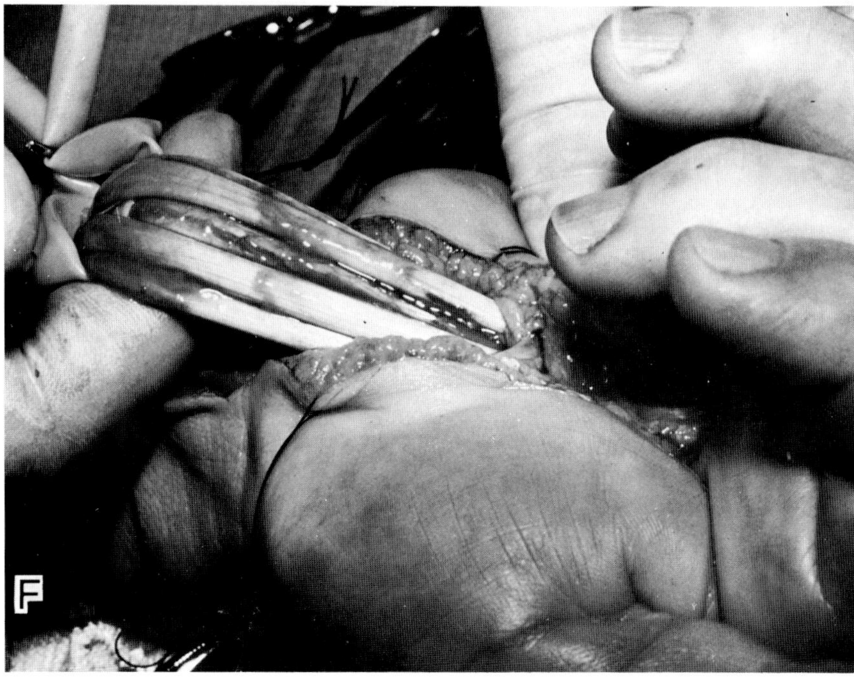

Fig. 46-10 *(Continued).* **(E)** If there is extensive palmar disease, a palmar flap may be raised to provide additional exposure. **(F)** After completion of flexor tenosynovectomy, nearly full tendon excursion is demonstrated. *(Figure continues.)*

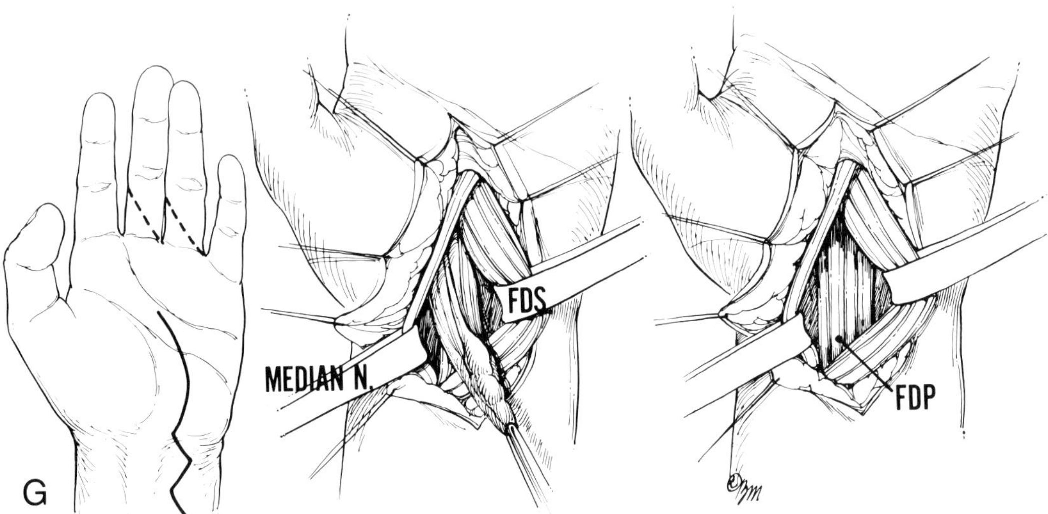

Fig. 46-10 *(Continued).* **(G)** Drawing of the technique. (Figs. A–F from Millender and Nalebuff,[164] with permission.)

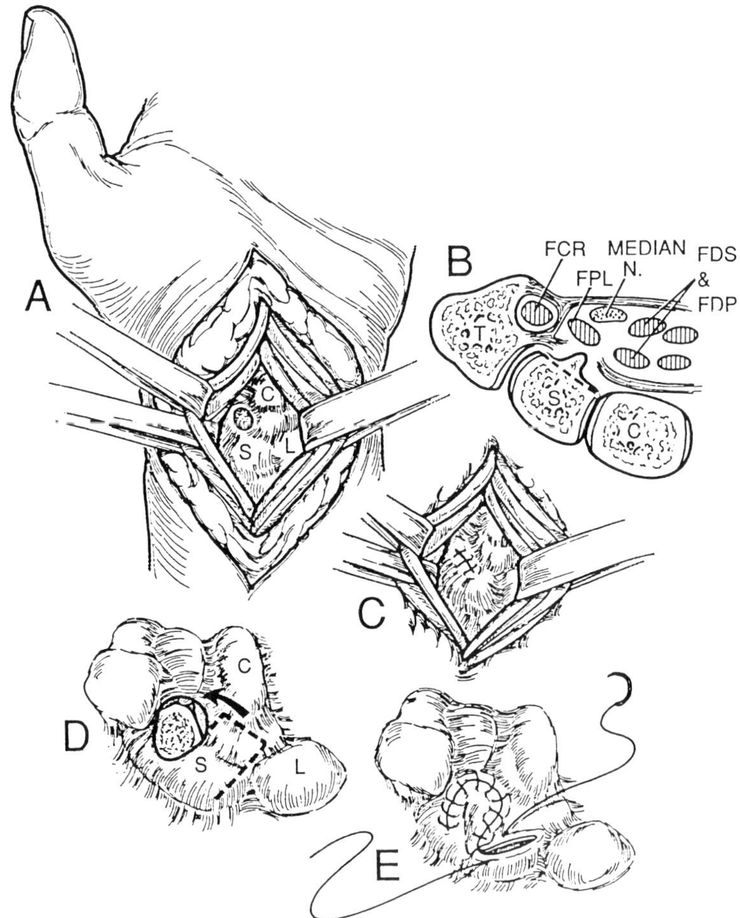

Fig. 46-11. A scaphoid osteophyte can erode through the volar wrist capsule **(A)** resulting in the "Mannerfelt lesion," an attrition rupture of the flexor pollicis longus tendon. **(B)** During a volar tenosynovectomy, the osteophyte is resected and the defect in the capsule closed either primarily **(C)**, or with local rotation flaps of the wrist capsule **(D&E)**.

Flexor Tenosynovitis in the Digits

As described previously, the fibroosseous canal is lined by synovium. This canal is not distensible, and even mild synovial hypertrophy can affect finger function significantly. Discrete rheumatoid nodules can form in one or both flexor tendons within the sheath. Such nodules may occur at different levels. The size of these nodules and their relationship to the annular pulleys will determine the degree of finger dysfunction.[71,95,170,293]

Four clinical patterns of rheumatoid "trigger finger" have been described based on the size and location of the nodules.[177,180] Small, localized areas of disease cause catching of the tendons during flexion. This is Type I triggering, which resembles the triggering that occurs in nonrheumatoid stenosing tenosynovitis. In Type II digital tenosynovitis, flexor tendon nodules are present in the distal palm, which causes the finger to lock as it is flexed. In Type III triggering, a nodule in the flexor profundus tendon in the region of the A2 pulley over the proximal phalanx causes the finger to lock in extension. Type IV flexor tenosynovitis is manifested by generalized tenosynovitis within the fibroosseous canal. There is palpable swelling on the volar aspect of the digit and limitation of motion. Usually, active motion is more restricted than passive motion. This loss of finger motion may result in stiffness of the interphalangeal joints as the periarticular soft tissue structures contract. As the interphalangeal joints become stiff, the diagnosis becomes more difficult, since one cannot differentiate between lack of finger motion because of joint stiffness or restricted excursion of the flexor tendons. Prolonged flexor tenosynovitis within the fibroosseous canal ultimately can result in tendon rupture. Flexor tenosynovectomy and excision of flexor tendon nodules are indicated regardless of the type of tenosynovitis and/or triggering present.[71,111,177,239,293]

Digital Tenosynovectomy—Operative Technique (Fig. 46-12)

We explore the flexor tendon sheaths of rheumatoid patients with digital tenosynovitis through zigzag incisions on the volar aspect of the digits. Such incisions can be extended proximally or distally to provide additional exposure if necessary. The diseased tenosynovium surrounding the tendon is excised. However, the annular pulleys are preserved to prevent bowstringing of the flexor tendons. The pulleys may be narrowed if necessary, but as much pulley as possible is preserved. Nodules within the flexor tendons are excised and the defects closed with fine nylon sutures. After complete tenosynovectomy and nodule excision have been performed, traction is applied to the flexor tendons to confirm smooth gliding. Occasionally, another nodule is present at a different level within the fibroosseous canal and is revealed only after the obvious nodule is excised and flexor tendon excursion is tested. If passive flexion of the finger is greater than the flexion obtained by traction applied to the tendon, additional tenosynovectomy is necessary. The objective of flexor tenosynovectomy is to make active and passive finger flexion equal. Gentle manipulation of stiff joints can be performed to restore passive joint motion at this time. Ferlic and Clayton[71] have recommended excising one slip of the flexor digitorum superficialis tendon to decompress the fibroosseous canal. We do not use this method routinely, but have used it on occasion and prefer it to resecting excessive amounts of annular pulley to allow free excursion of the tendons. On rare occasions, the entire superficial flexor tendon may be excised if it is severely diseased and prevents complete "pull-through" of the profundus tendon.

Postoperatively, finger motion is started early—usually the day following surgery. The patient is taught to stabilize each joint of the operated finger in sequence in order to exercise the superficial and deep flexor tendons independently and thereby avoid adhesions between these two tendons.

TENDON RUPTURES

Tendon ruptures in the hand are common complications of rheumatoid arthritis. The cause and location of these ruptures vary. Attrition ruptures occur as the tendon moves across bone roughened or eroded by chronic synovitis. Attrition ruptures of the extensor tendons occur most frequently at either the distal end of the ulna or at Lister's tubercle, which acts as a bony pulley for the extensor pollicis longus tendon. Attrition ruptures of the flexor tendons occur on the volar aspect of the wrist where they contact the scaphoid. Tendon ruptures also may be caused by direct tendon invasion of rheumatoid tenosynovium, which erodes and weakens the tendon, or by ischemic necrosis from diminished blood supply caused by pressure from proliferative synovium under the dorsal retinaculum, transverse carpal ligament, or flexor tendon pulleys.[56,63,64,119,127,132,147,173,174,181,182,235,277,280]

The treatment options for rheumatoid patients with tendon ruptures are fusions of various joints and tendon transfers. Smith[227] pointed out the significant differences between tendon transfers done in rheumatoid and nonrheumatoid patients. These differences in the rheumatoid patient include the following: (1) the joints to be moved by the transfer may be stiff or unstable; (2) the bed through which the transfer passes may be scarred or irregular, compromising tendon excursion; (3) the tendons to be transferred may have been weakened by ischemia or by tenosynovial invasion; and (4) if the wrist, MP, and/or PIP joints are stiff or deformed, the tenodesis effect of wrist motion or the complementary motion of the MP and PIP joints cannot be relied upon to enhance the performance of the transferred tendons. These factors must be considered carefully when planning tendon transfers to reconstruct rheumatoid tendon ruptures.

Diagnosis

Extensor Tendon Ruptures

Although the correct diagnosis of tendon rupture usually is not difficult, it requires both an observant patient and an informed physician. The sine qua non of tendon rupture is the sudden loss of finger extension or flexion. Tendon ruptures usually are painless and commonly follow trivial hand use or

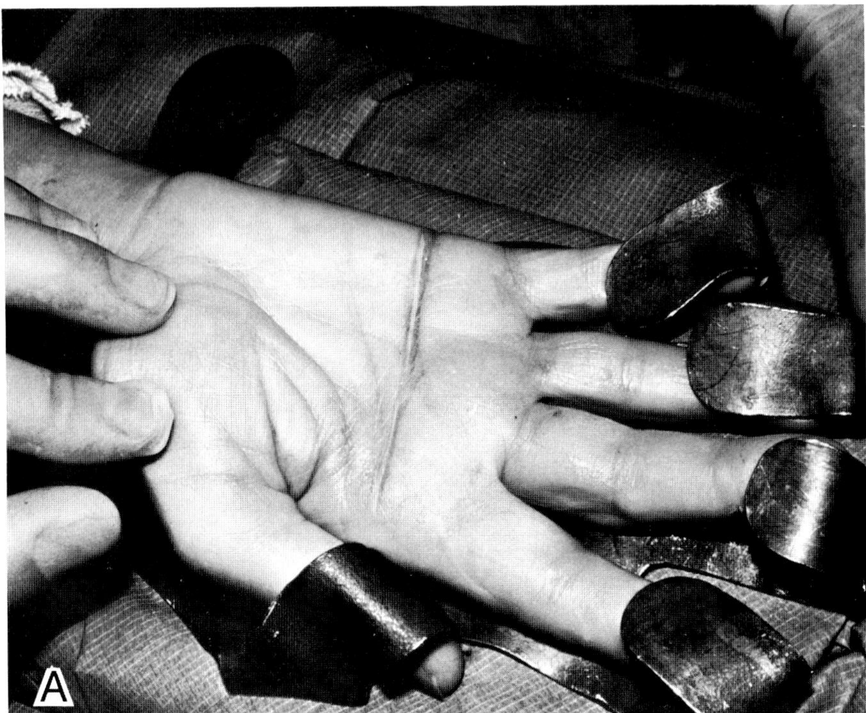

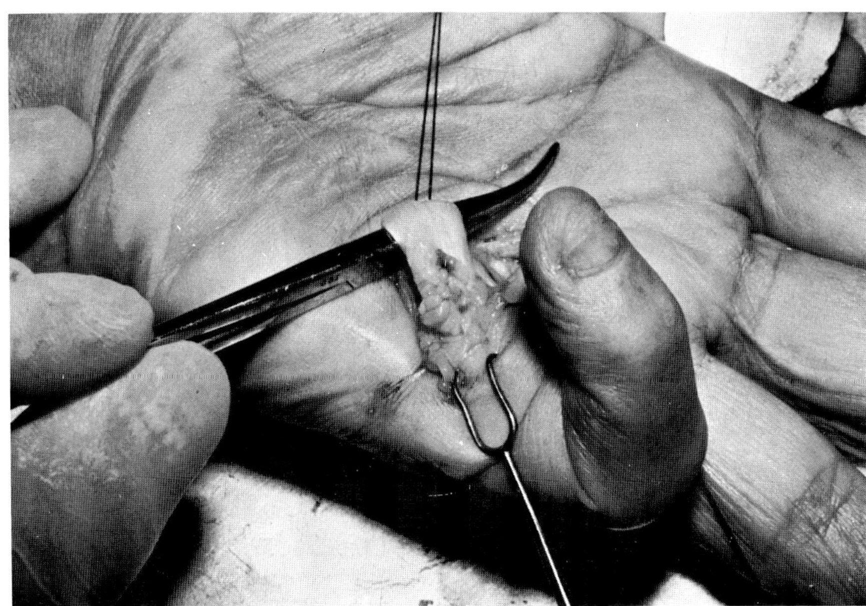

Fig. 46-12. Surgical technique for palmar and digital flexor tenosynovectomy. **(A)** Isolated palmar disease is approached through a transverse palmar incision. **(B&C)** The flexor tendons have been exposed and delivered into the wound, and tenosynovectomy has been performed.*(Figure continues.)*

activity. Rheumatoid patients who become accustomed to frequent variations and limitations of hand function are apt to delay medical attention unless the functional loss following a tendon rupture is obvious to them or is quite significant. Isolated ruptures of the extensor digiti quinti or extensor pollicis longus may cause only limited functional loss and, therefore, may go unrecognized or be overshadowed by more significant deformities.[182]

The factors leading to a single tendon rupture, unless corrected, are often responsible for subsequent ruptures with more significant functional loss. Frequently, after a rupture of the extensor tendon of the small finger, the ring finger extensor will rupture, followed by the long finger extensor and so on (Fig. 46-13). This occurs as the remaining intact tendons shift ulnarward and become abraded over the roughened edges of the distal ulna. Thus, the usual progression of extensor tendon

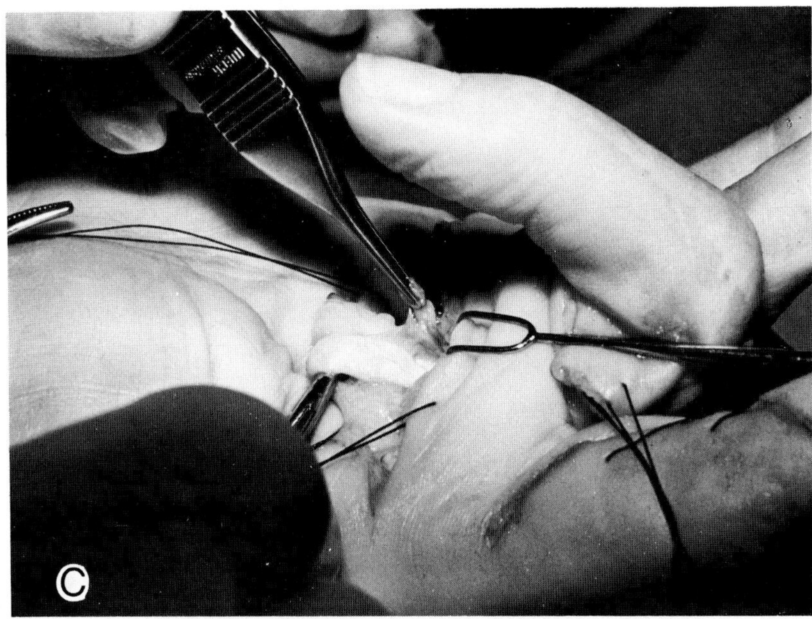

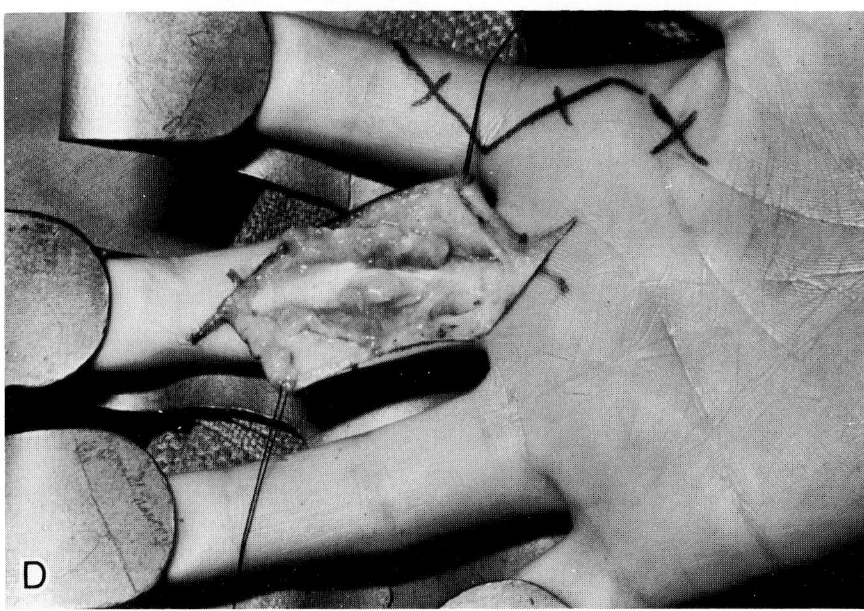

Fig. 46-12 *(Continued).* **(D)** Digital flexor tenosynovitis is exposed by a zigzag incision. *(Figure continues.)*

ruptures is in a radial direction, affecting the index finger last. In our experience, multiple extensor tendon ruptures (especially those that occur in rapid sequence) are the result of attrition as the tendons wear against a bony spicule on the ulnar aspect of the wrists as described by Vaughan-Jackson.[277]

Although the sudden loss of extension of the ring, small, and middle fingers is most likely the result of multiple extensor tendon ruptures, three other conditions occur in rheumatoid arthritis that can mimic tendon rupture and should be excluded before surgery to restore extensor power to the fingers is performed. The most common of these is MP joint dislocation, which results in a flexed and ulnar-deviated position of the finger. The lack of passive MP joint extension and the presence of palpable and/or visible extensor tendons on the dorsal aspect of the hand make the differential diagnosis between the MP joint dislocation and extensor tendon rupture straightforward. The second condition to be excluded is displacement of the extensor tendons into the valleys between the metacarpal heads. When this occurs, extensor force is lost as the tendons now lie volar to the axes of motion of the MP joints. In this condition, the posture of the fingers is similar to that which occurs in cases of multiple extensor tendon ruptures. Differentiation between extensor tendon rupture and displacement of the tendons between the metacarpal heads sometimes can be made if the patient is able to maintain MP joint extension actively after the joints are extended passively. This is not

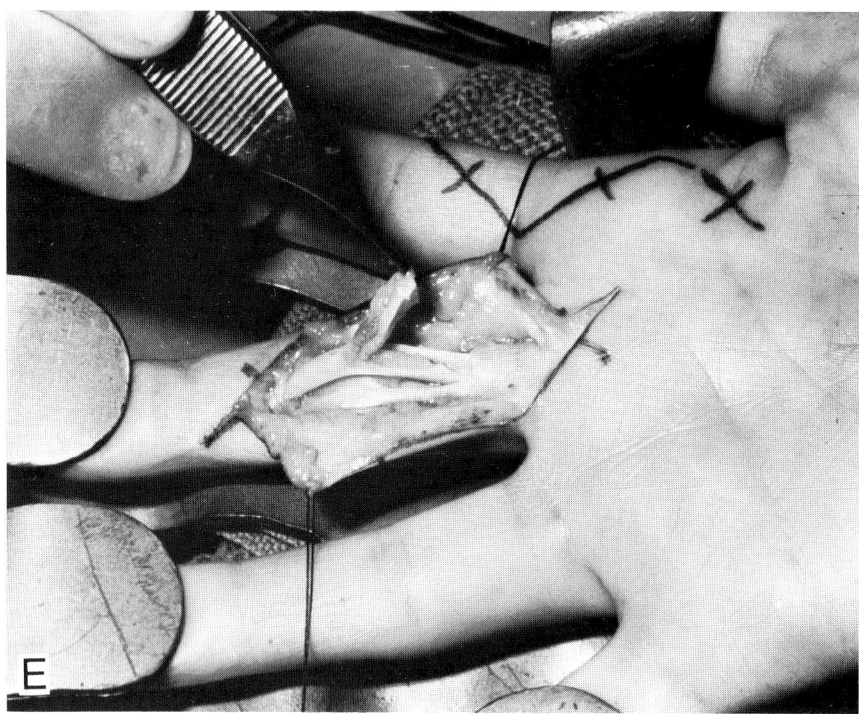

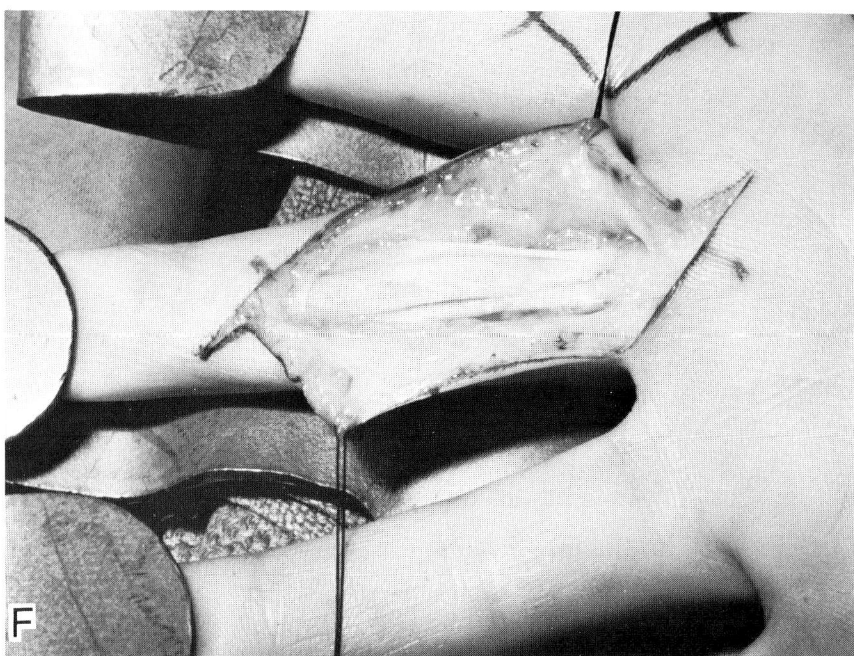

Fig. 46-12 *(Continued).* **(E)** Tenosynovium is excised from the flexor digitorum profundus. Both slips of flexor digitorum superficialis can be seen. **(F)** The flexor digitorum profundus and flexor digitorum superficialis are seen at the completion of flexor tenosynovectomy. *(Figure continues.)*

always the case, and occasionally it is necessary to explore the tendons at the level of the wrist at the time of MP arthroplasty to verify their continuity. The treatment for subluxation of the extensor tendons is relocation over the MP joints with or without MP joint arthroplasty.

The least common, but most difficult condition to diagnose of those simulating multiple extensor tendon rupture is paralysis of the common extensor muscle secondary to posterior interosseous nerve compression.[35,131,148,168,289] Several subtle differences allow tendon rupture to be differentiated from muscle paralysis. Patients with posterior interosseous nerve compression usually demonstrate some radial deviation of the wrist because of paralysis of the extensor carpi ulnaris muscle, in addition to the absence of active finger extension. Soft tissue

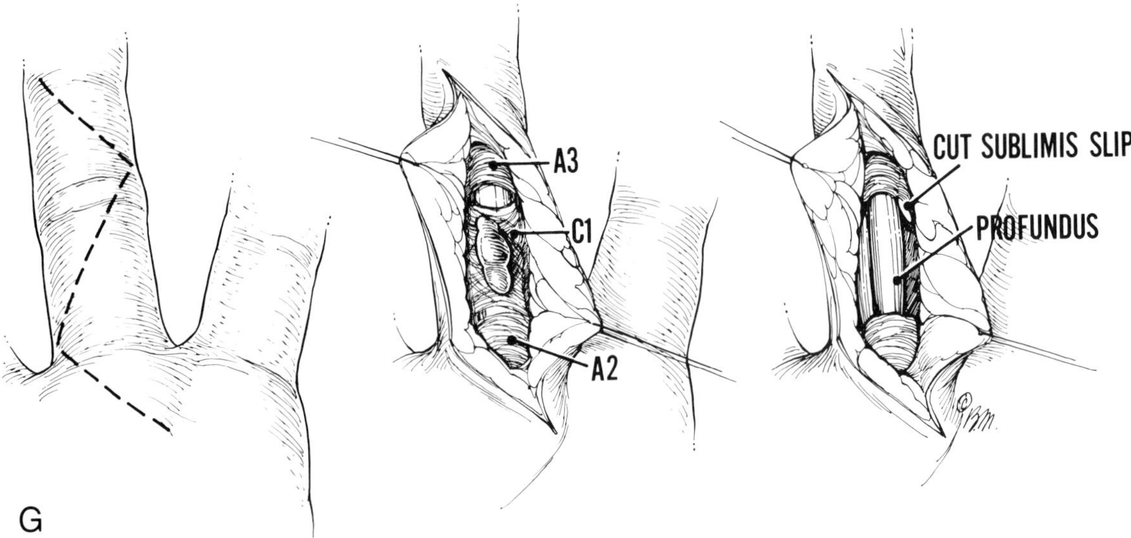

Fig. 46-12 *(Continued).* **(G)** Digital flexor tenosynovectomy. Note the annular pulleys; synovium usually bulges through the thin cruciate pulleys. As much annular pulley as possible is preserved when tenosynovectomy is performed. (Figs. A–F from Millender and Nalebuff,[164] with permission.)

fullness about the elbow signals proliferative synovitis of the radiohumeral and ulnohumeral joints, which can result in compression of the posterior interosseous nerve. In posterior interosseous nerve compression, the extensors of the middle and ring fingers may be weaker than those of the index and small fingers.[227] Thus there will be a greater extensor lag of the middle and ring fingers than of the index and long fingers. In rheumatoid attrition ruptures, the ring and small finger extensors are involved first. The best diagnostic test is the presence or absence of MP joint extension as the wrist is flexed. A positive "tenodesis effect" is found in the paralytic condition because the extensor tendons are in continuity. With tendon rupture, flexion of the wrist usually has no effect on finger extension because the extensor tendons are not in continuity. In addi-

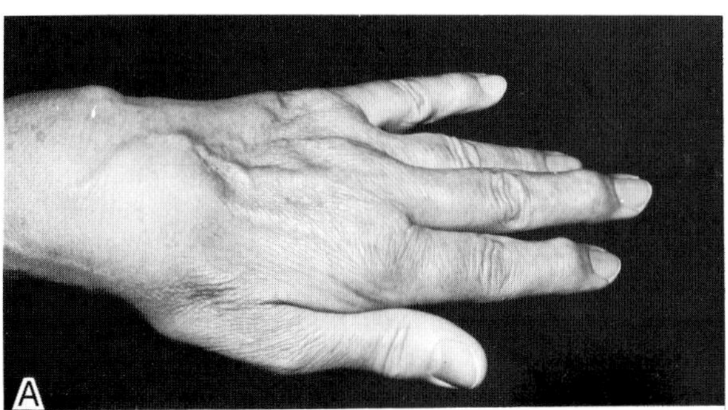

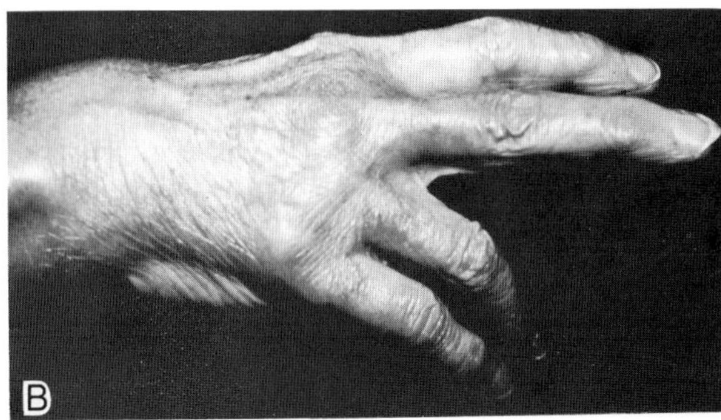

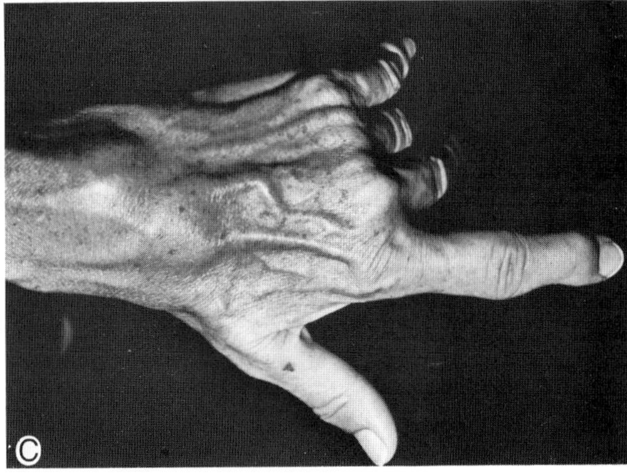

Fig. 46-13. Examples of extensor tendon ruptures. **(A)** Dorsal tenosynovitis and single rupture of the extensor digitorum communis tendon to the ring finger. Note minimal lag associated with single rupture. **(B)** Double rupture of extensor digitorum communis to the ring and small fingers. When two tendons rupture, there is an appreciable extension lag and the disability becomes obvious. **(C)** Triple rupture involving the long, ring, and small fingers. (From Millender and Nalebuff,[164] with permission.)

tion, patients with multiple extensor tendon ruptures usually have dorsal tenosynovitis or a prominent distal ulna, which predisposes to extensor tendon rupture, whereas patients with posterior interosseous nerve compression may have no such findings about the wrist.

Diagnosis

Flexor Tendon Ruptures

Flexor tenosynovitis is not uncommon in rheumatoid arthritis. While carpal tunnel syndrome is the most common manifestation of flexor tenosynovitis at the wrist, weakness, loss of dexterity of the hand, local or radiating pain, and/or discomfort with hand use can occur. Tendon gliding becomes restricted, and progressive loss of active finger flexion ensues. A discrepancy between active and passive finger flexion is characteristic of rheumatoid flexor tenosynovitis. Triggering, locking, loss of the normal finger cascade, and loss of active flexion may occur, particularly with tenosynovitis in the palm or in the fibroosseous canals. Joint stiffness makes concomitant flexor tenosynovitis more difficult to detect. Flexor tendon ruptures occur, but are much less common than extensor tendon ruptures.

Ertel[63,64] found that the presence of inflammatory flexor tenosynovitis adversely affects the outcome of reconstructive surgery. That is, there is less restoration of function after a tendon transfer done for a rupture caused by inflammatory synovitis than after one done for an attrition rupture.

The most common flexor tendon to rupture is the flexor pollicis longus. Patients with this rupture lose active flexion of the interphalangeal joint of the thumb. This occurs when the tendon is eroded by a volar osteophyte on the scaphoid that penetrates the volar wrist capsule.[147] The diagnosis of flexor pollicis longus rupture is not difficult unless there is a fixed hyperextension deformity or stiffness of the interphalangeal joint.

An isolated rupture of the flexor digitorum profundus tendon results in the inability to flex the DIP joint actively.

A condition that mimics flexor profundus tendon ruptures and, in fact, is a precursor to such ruptures is a rheumatoid nodule in the tendon within the fibroosseous canal of the finger. The nodule restricts profundus excursion, and there is loss of active flexion of the DIP joint. This condition is discussed on page 1593.

Rupture of both the superficial and deep flexor tendons causes such obvious functional loss that the diagnosis is straightforward. The patient lacks active PIP and DIP joint motion and can flex the finger only at the MP joint. Of course, passive motion of the finger must be present to conclude that both tendons are ruptured.

After a flexor tendon rupture is recognized, the site of rupture must be determined. Flexor tendon ruptures can occur at the wrist, in the palm, and within the finger. Palpation for fullness (or lack thereof) within the finger can be useful in this regard. Ultimately, surgical exploration is necessary to determine the exact site.

Treatment

Rupture of the Extensor Pollicis Longus

Rupture of the extensor pollicis longus is common in rheumatoid arthritis[56,181,182,198,245] (Fig. 46-14). The functional loss varies, depending upon the functional capacity of the extensor pollicis brevis and on the status of the thumb joints. Although spontaneous rupture of the extensor pollicis longus may cause a "droop" or incomplete extension of the interphalangeal joint of the thumb, more commonly the patient maintains the ability to extend this joint in spite of the rupture. Interphalangeal joint extension is a shared function of the extensor pollicis longus and the intrinsic muscles of the thumb. The intrinsics alone can extend this joint to neutral; the extensor pollicis longus is necessary for IP joint hyperextension. The patient with an extensor pollicis longus rupture loses extension of the MP joint as the extensor pollicis brevis is not strong enough to extend this joint by itself. Occasionally, no deformity occurs at either the MP or interphalangeal joint levels, and the diagnosis often is missed unless a specific test for tendon function is done by asking the patient to extend the thumb with the palm resting on a flat surface while the examiner specifically palpates the tendon of the extensor pollicis longus at the wrist level.

If the tendon is ruptured and the functional loss and/or deformity is significant, extensor pollicis longus function should be restored. The options available include end-to-end repair, tendon graft, or tendon transfer. Although a tendon rupture occasionally can be repaired by end-to-end technique, this is an exception and should not be expected. In general tendon grafts through areas of rheumatoid tissue tend to become adherent. However, a graft used to repair extensor pollicis longus rupture can function satisfactorily. The power and long excursion of the thumb flexor overcomes the adhesions that form on the dorsum. To be effective, however, a proximal motor that is not contracted is required. For this reason, tendon transfers are preferred for the treatment of extensor pollicis longus rupture. The two most commonly used tendons are the extensor indicis proprius and extensor carpi radialis longus. We prefer to use the extensor indicis proprius for several reasons: (1) it can be taken from the index finger at the MP joint level without interfering with the index finger function; (2) in our experience, the patient does not lose independent extension of the index finger as a result of this transfer,[27,286] and (3) we do not like to weaken radial wrist extension, which is very important in maintaining proper wrist alignment.[167,181,182]

Operative Technique

The extensor indicis proprius tendon is identified at the level of the MP joint; it is the most ulnar of the two tendons. It is withdrawn at the wrist through a second transverse incision and passed subcutaneously to the thumb. In the past, we performed an end-to-end or weaving connection of the transferred tendon with the distal stump of the extensor pollicis longus. This was always tedious, and the adjustment of proper tension was difficult once the tendon was sutured. Now, we pass the tendon directly to the MP joint level and weave it into the extensor mechanism. A temporary suture is used to judge ten-

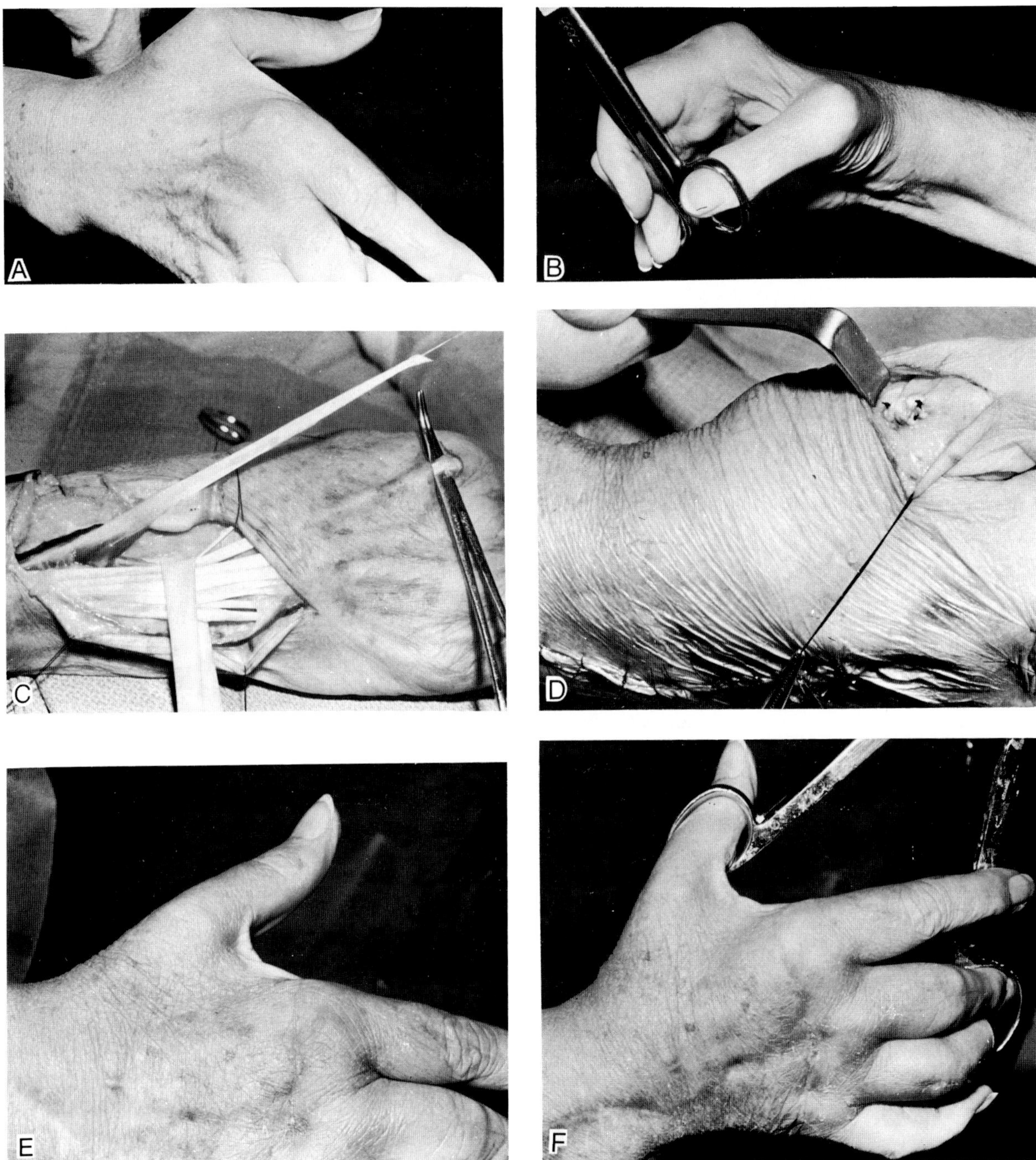

Fig. 46-14. The diagnosis and treatment of extensor pollicis longus tendon rupture. **(A)** The typical posture of an extensor pollicis longus rupture with lack of MP joint extension. The interphalangeal joint is extended by the thumb intrinsic muscles. **(B)** Functional loss using scissors is demonstrated. **(C)** Dorsal tenosynovectomy has been completed. The extensor indicis proprius has been detached from the MP joint of the index finger and withdrawn into the proximal wound. The extensor indicis proprius is identified at the wrist by its distal muscle belly. **(D)** The transfer is woven into the extensor mechanism over the thumb MP joint. **(E&F)** Postoperative improvement in active thumb motion and function. (From Nalebuff,[182] with permission.)

sion. With the correct tension, the thumb will remain in extension when the wrist is flexed. With the wrist extended, passive flexion of the thumb to the small finger pulp should be possible. Weaving of the tendon through the extensor mechanism results in a strong connection and allows us to start motion with confidence after 4 to 5 weeks of immobilization. The result of a properly performed tendon transfer to restore extensor pollicis longus function is usually excellent. If necessary, a dorsal tenosynovectomy and excision of a prominent, dorsally displaced distal ulna are performed at the same time as the extensor indicis proprius transfer.

Rupture of the Finger Extensors

While single tendon ruptures can involve any finger, the small finger is affected most often. The patient demonstrates incomplete extension of the finger at the MP joint level. The amount of extensor lag depends on whether or not both the extensor digiti quinti and the extensor digitorum communis tendons are ruptured. With an isolated extensor digiti quinti rupture, MP joint extension may lag only 30 to 40 degrees. The contribution of the extensor digitorum communis to extension of the small finger is tested by holding the index, middle, and ring finger MP joints in flexion and asking the patient to extend the small finger. An increased extensor lag demonstrates loss of the contribution to extension provided by the extensor digitorum communis. Because of the danger of additional ruptures that complicate treatment, patients in whom the diagnosis of a single tendon rupture has been made are advised to undergo early surgical reconstruction. The surgical treatment of an isolated rupture of any one finger extensor is relatively easy and the functional result usually is excellent.[89,167,181,182,192]

Operative Technique

As stated previously, an end-to-end repair is seldom feasible. We prefer to suture the distal tendon stump to an adjacent extensor tendon. Dorsal tenosynovectomy and removal of any bony spicules from the distal end of the ulna (or ulnar head resection) should be performed at the same time to eliminate the cause of rupture. The dorsal retinaculum should be transferred deep to the extensor tendons to provide a bed for gliding if bone is exposed. This is done before the tendons are reconstructed. Partial transfer of the retinaculum is described in the section on tenosynovectomy. Adjacent tendon suture is particularly easy for an isolated rupture of the middle or ring finger. For example, the distal end of the extensor digitorum communis tendon to the small finger or the extensor digiti quinti is woven through the extensor digitorum communis of the ring finger and sutured. Similarly, the distal end of the ring finger extensor digitorum communis can be transferred to the long finger extensor digitorum communis. If there has not been major loss of tendon substance, an end to end repair can be done. This will cause the other intact tendons to bunch up and appear to be too long. However, the repaired tendon will stretch to match the adjacent intact tendons. Nonabsorbable suture material is used and tension is determined by restoring the appropriate extensor stance (in sequence) to the fingers. The tension must be sufficiently tight so that when the wrist is flexed moderately, the fingers are maintained in complete extension, and when the wrist is extended moderately, the MP joints flex only 20 to 30 degrees.

The use of intravenous regional anesthesia simplifies the task of judging proper tension. After the tendon suture has been completed, the tourniquet can be released. When voluntary muscle control is regained, the patient is asked to extend the fingers. If there is a lag in extension, the tendon tension can be corrected at this time. Skin closure is performed under local infiltration anesthesia if this technique is used.[89,167] If the tourniquet is not released, a drain is used to prevent a subcutaneous hematoma.

Multiple Ruptures of the Extensor Tendons

As additional tendons rupture, the surgical treatment becomes more complicated. With double ruptures of the long and ring finger extensors, it is still possible to use the adjacent suture technique; the stump of the ring finger tendon is attached to the small finger tendon and the stump of the long finger tendon is attached to the index finger tendon. If the extensor digitorum communis to the small finger is not present, the ring finger tendon stump can be sutured to the extensor digiti quinti.

Options and Techniques for Tendon Reconstruction

Double ruptures more frequently involve the ring and small fingers. Although adjacent suture can be performed in some of these patients by connecting both distal tendon stumps to the long finger tendon, there may be difficulty with the small finger. The distal tendon stump of this finger may be so short that it will not reach the ring finger tendon without excessive abduction of the small finger. In this situation, a different method is required, and we use the extensor indicis proprius as a tendon transfer (Fig. 46-15). It is not necessary to divide the tendon as far distally as when it is used for a thumb tendon rupture. Other tendon transfers, such as the extensor carpi ulnaris, have been advocated to restore extension in this situation. However, this wrist extensor is very important in maintaining wrist alignment and power, and we believe that it is best left in its normal position. In addition, it does not have the same excursion as the finger extensors, and its use will result in lack of either full flexion or extension of the small finger. We have used the extensor carpi radialis brevis tendon as a transfer occasionally, with satisfactory, but not excellent results.

As additional extensor tendons rupture, restoring finger extension becomes more difficult. With three or four extensor tendons gone, adjacent suture combined with extensor indicis proprius transfer is no longer sufficient to restore extensor power. In addition, independent and dexterous use of the index finger for pinch and pick-up functions may be lost if the extensor indicis proprius is used for transfer. A donor tendon for transfer that has a strong motor, is expendable, and has the necessary length to reach the distal tendon stump just proximal to the MP joints is needed. The superficial flexor tendons meet

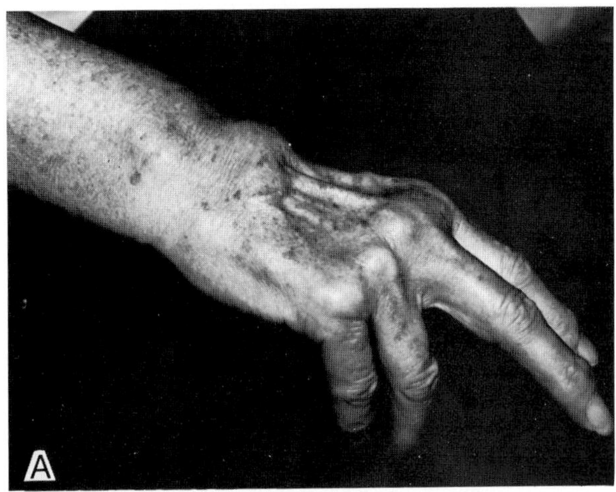

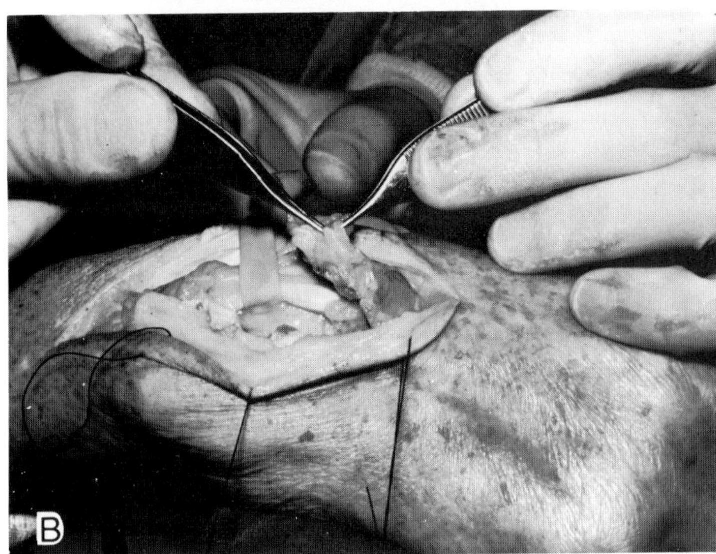

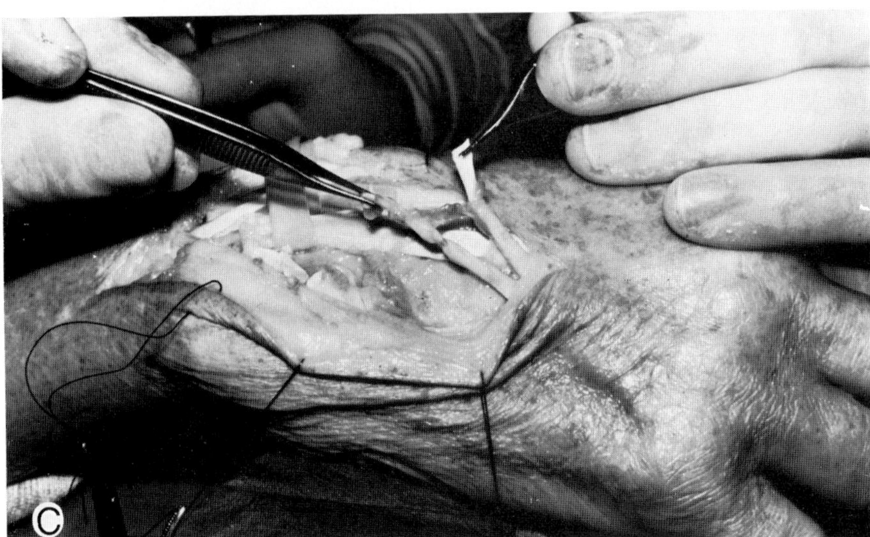

Fig. 46-15. Example of a patient with dorsal tenosynovitis and tendon rupture. **(A)** Dorsal tenosynovitis with double tendon rupture. **(B&C)** Dorsal tenosynovectomy. Note that the tenosynovium is excised prior to tendon transfer. *(Figure continues.)*

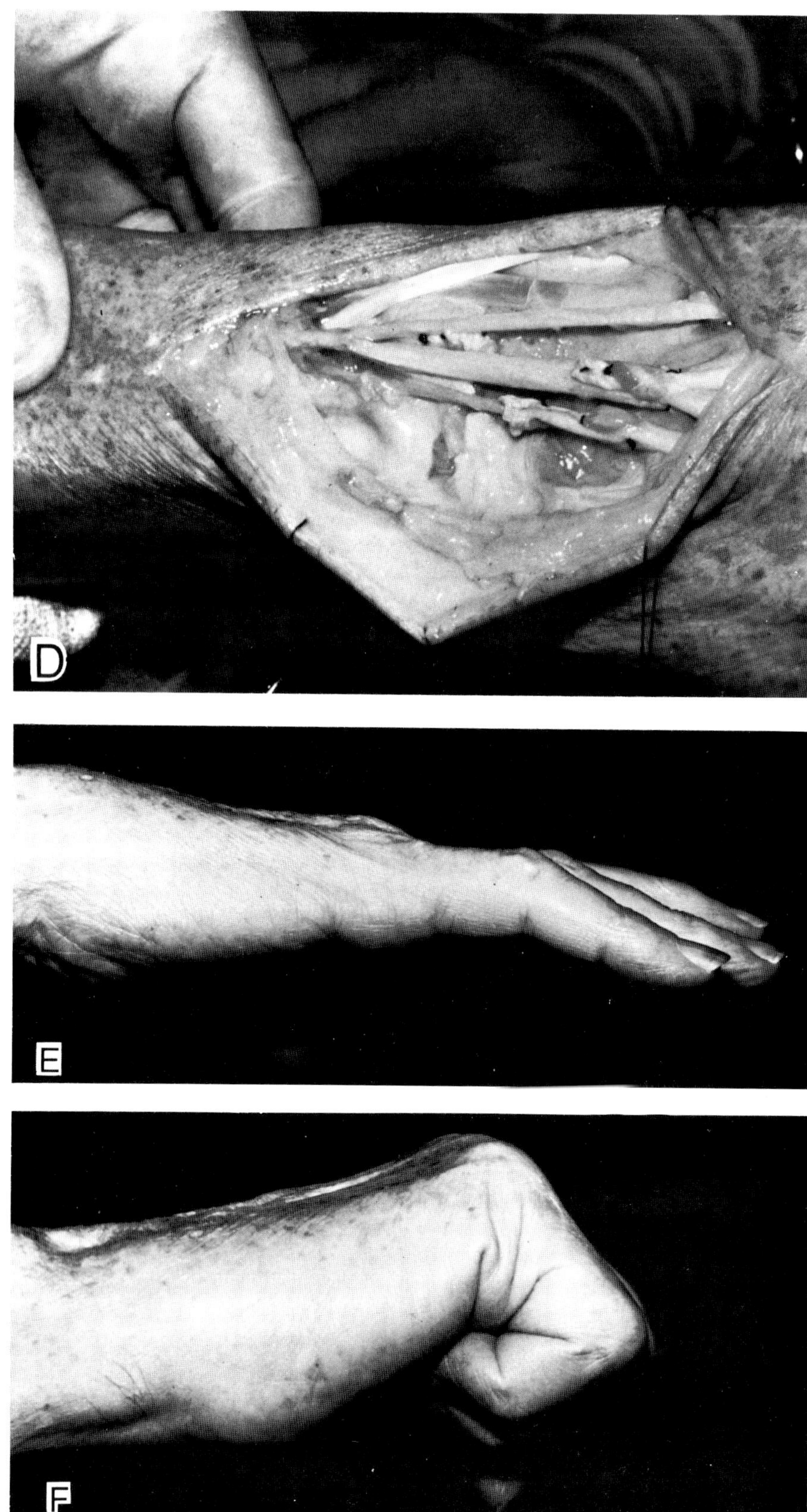

Fig. 46-15 *(Continued).* **(D)** Tendon transfer completed. Extensor indicis proprius has been transferred to the ruptured extensor tendon to the small finger and the ruptured fourth extensor tendon transferred to the intact third extensor tendon. **(E&F)** Restored active range of motion. (From Nalebuff and Millender,[191] with permission.)

these criteria.[192] The flexor digitorum superficialis transfer was advocated first by Boyes[20] for radial nerve plasy. He showed that patients learned to use a former finger flexor as an extensor. In his technique, the transferred tendon was brought through a wide opening in the interosseous membrane to provide a direct route to the site of connection. We prefer this routing of the tendon transfer through the interosseous membrane in patients who have no scarring in the region of the distal forearm and/or wrist. This more direct route of the sublimis tendon provides optimal function of the transfer. A window large enough to allow the muscle belly of the superficialis, rather than just the tendon alone, to be passed into and through the membrane should be made in the interosseous membrane. This will help preserve maximum excursion of the tendon after transfer. (See Chapter 38 for details of the Boyes transfer through the interosseous membrane.)

We have modified Boyes' technique in patients with scarring in the dorsal wrist area, either from previous surgical procedures or from long-standing tendon ruptures. In these patients, we still use the ring sublimis tendon as a motor, but we route the tendon subcutaneously around the radial aspect of the forearm rather than going through the interosseous membrane and the area of scarring. This direction of pull was chosen to eliminate the risk of pulling the fingers into increased ulnar deviation. The technique for the modified transfer is described below (Fig. 46-16).

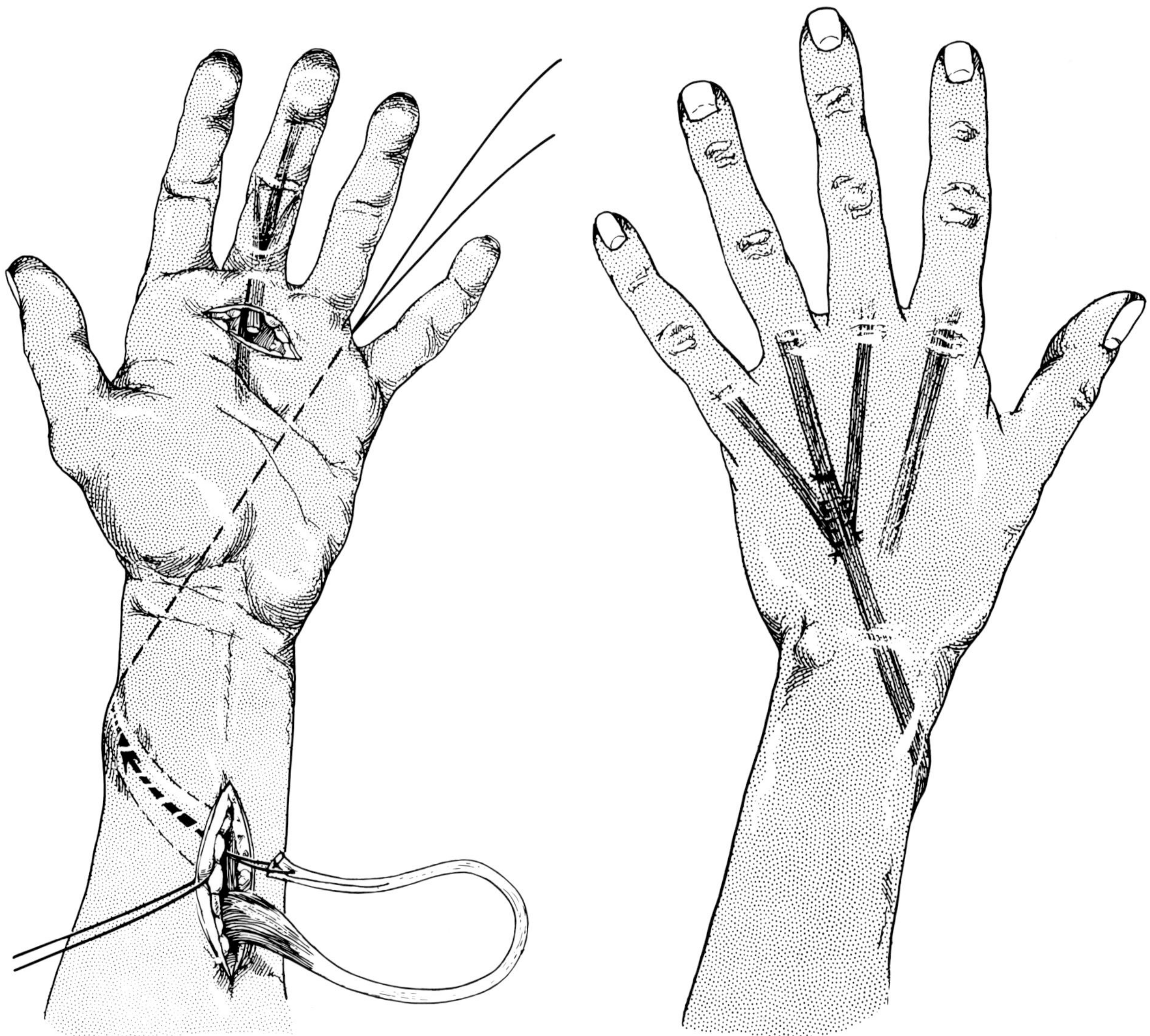

Fig. 46-16. Technique of middle finger sublimis tendon transfer for extensor tendon rupture. An incision is made in the distal palm to divide the sublimis tendon distally. From a second incision on the volar aspect to the ulnar side of the midline, the tendon is passed subcutaneously around the radial aspect of the forearm (deep to the superficial radial nerve) to the dorsal aspect of the hand. In this case, the ruptured middle finger extensor (along with the extensors to small and middle fingers) was sutured to the sublimis tendon transfer rather than to the adjacent index finger extensor. (From Nalebuff and Patel,[192] with permission.)

The transfer is performed through three incisions. A small transverse incision is made in the distal palmar crease, and the tendon is divided after applying proximal traction. This provides enough length to reach the MP joints. A second incision is made on the volar aspect of the forearm. This should be placed ulnar to the midline so that the final transfer will pass deep to the skin incision and thus minimize tendon adherence. The third incision is made on the dorsal aspect of the hand where the transfer is attached to the extensor mechanism of the ring and small fingers. Usually, we suture the middle finger tendon to the adjacent index finger tendon. Care must be taken to route the transferred tendon *deep* to the superficial radial nerve. Otherwise, symptomatic compression of the nerve may occur from the tendon passing over the nerve.

With quadruple tendon ruptures, two superficial flexor tendon transfers are utilized—one to restore extension of the index and middle fingers, the other to restore ring and small finger extension. Again, the judgment of tension is critical. The transfer should be tight enough to have a tenodesis effect as described previously. There is a tendency for the transfer to stretch postoperatively because of the strong flexor pull.

We have utilized the flexor digitorum sublimis transfer in patients who have had a previous wrist fusion. These patients are able to achieve satisfactory extension of the fingers without the benefit of any tenodesis effect.

In patients with multiple tendon ruptures and advanced disease of the thumb MP joint, this joint can be fused and the extensor pollicis longus used as a tendon transfer to the finger extensors.

We have found that primary intercalary or "bridge" grafts can be useful, particularly for triple tendon ruptures. The palmaris longus tendon, or, if the wrist is fused, one of the wrist extensors can be used for the graft. The dorsal wrist incision is extended proximally and the proximal stumps of the ruptured extensor tendons are located and dissected free from scar and adherent soft tissue. The tendon in the best condition is selected for the motor. The bridge graft is inserted between the proximal and distal tendon ends using an interweaving technique. The graft should be put in "tight" as the muscle will gradually stretch postoperatively. Bora[17] reported excellent results (MP joint motion 10 to 75 degrees) in a long-term follow-up study using the palmaris longus as a "loop" tendon graft to bridge the extensor tendon defect following multiple tendon ruptures. The considerations and alternatives for extensor tendon transfers have been summarized by Smith.[227]

In patients with fused wrists, the wrist motors can be utilized to restore finger extension. As noted before, the excursion of these muscles is limited. However, they are valueless with the wrist fused and can be used to extend the fingers without diminishing the power of finger flexion that results when a sublimis transfer is used. We have used both the wrist extensors and flexors to restore finger extension in this situation. The wrist extensors may be of sufficient length for transfer if they are dissected from their insertions on the bases of the metacarpals and the wrist unit is shortened slightly when the radiocarpal joint is prepared for fusion. The wrist flexors frequently are not long enough to reach the ruptured tendon ends, and a supplementary tendon graft is needed. In performing a wrist fusion that is to be followed later at a second stage by tendon transfer for multiple extensor tendon rupture, one or more silicone rubber rods can be inserted at the time of the wrist fusion. This makes the second-stage tendon graft procedure easier and minimizes the risk of postoperative adhesions.

The not infrequent situation of multiple extensor tendon ruptures with associated MP joint disease warrants attention. We do not try to restore finger extension by tendon transfer before restoring joint motion. Unless the MP joints can be extended passively, any transfer will become adherent. Thus, a staged reconstruction usually is necessary. Initially, an MP arthroplasty is done. Postoperatively, dynamic splinting substitutes for the absent extensor tendons. At the second stage, appropriate transfers are done to provide active extensor power. With experience, it is possible to combine the MP joint arthroplasty with a tendon transfer in a single operative procedure. The arthroplasty is done in the routine fashion, following which a flexor digitorum superficialis tendon is brought around the forearm and sutured to the extensor mechanism at the arthroplasty site. The postoperative management of patients with combined arthroplasty and tendon transfers is geared toward protecting the tendon transfer. Therefore, active motion is delayed for 3 weeks. Restoration of complete active motion is not expected in these cases. The results of a combined procedure will fall short when compared with an arthroplasty in the presence of normal tendons or with a tendon transfer in the presence of minimally involved joints.

Rupture of the Flexor Pollicis Longus

The most common flexor tendon to rupture in rheumatoid arthritis is the flexor pollicis longus. It is usually secondary to attrition at the level of the carpal scaphoid bone, and has been referred to as the "Mannerfelt lesion."[147,235] The functional loss is variable. If the patient has a good interphalangeal joint, the loss is apparent. If the MP joint has significant involvement or is fused, the loss of any interphalangeal joint motion results in substantial functional loss. Either terminal joint stability or restoration of active motion must be provided. Even if the interphalangeal joint is fused to provide stable pinch, the volar aspect of the wrist must still be explored. The bony spicule that has disrupted the flexor pollicis longus will affect the tendons of the index finger next and must be removed. One of our patients was found to have ruptures of both the superficial and deep flexor tendons of the index and middle fingers, in addition to the thumb flexor.

Operative Technique (Fig. 46-17)

The volar aspect of the palm and wrist is exposed through a curved incision along the thenar crease and is extended proximally in a zigzag manner. The bony spicule on the ulnar aspect of the scapoid bone, which protrudes into the radial side of the carpal canal, is removed, and the exposed bone is covered by mobilizing adjacent soft tissues.[63,64] Attention then is directed toward restoration of tendon function. The surgical choices include the use of a bridge graft, a standard tendon graft, or a tendon transfer. If both tendon ends can be identified at the wrist level, we prefer to insert a short bridge graft. The palmaris longus is suitable for this, but if it is not present, a slip of the

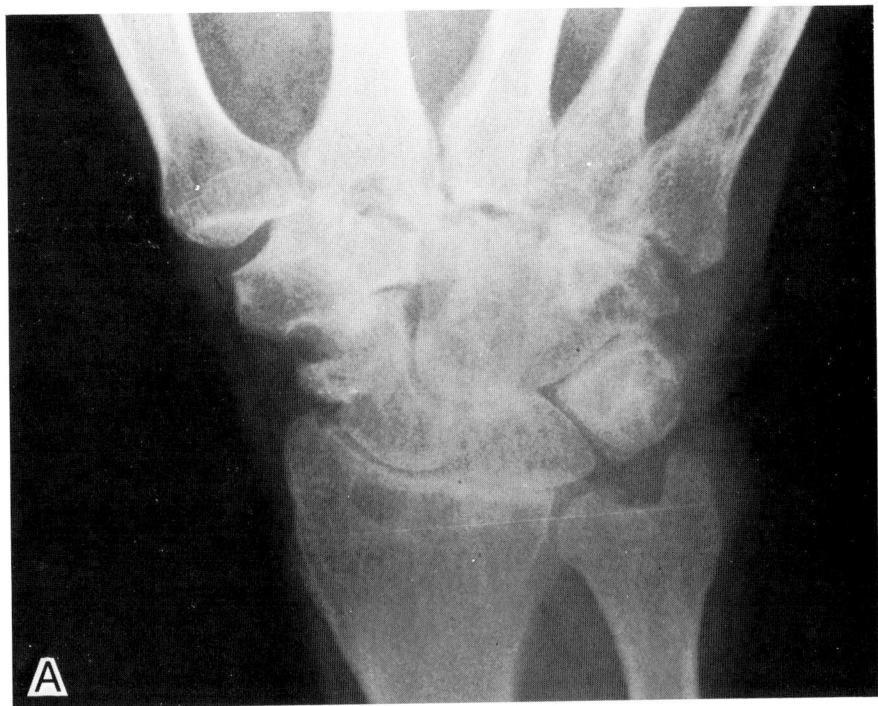

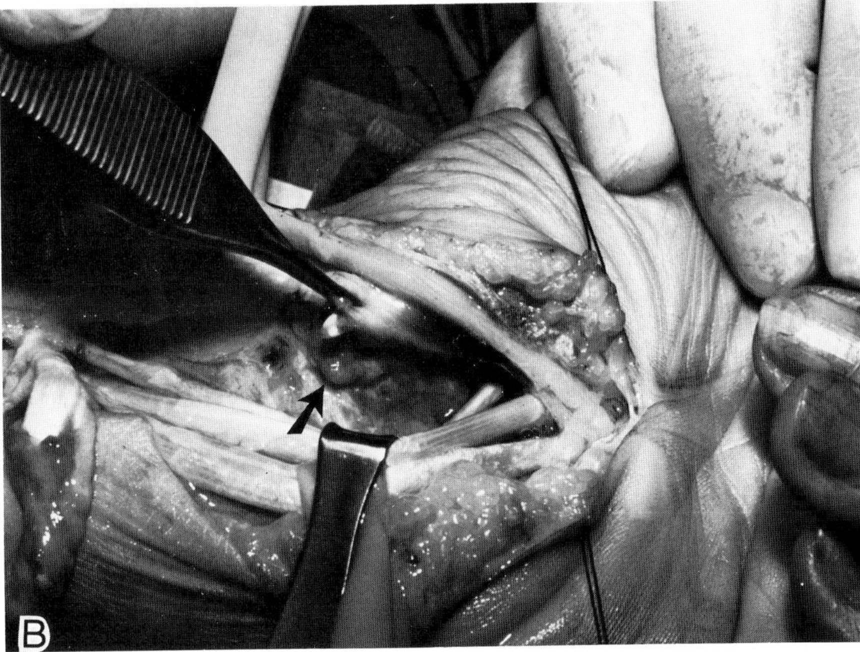

Fig. 46-17. Flexor pollicis longus rupture. **(A)** Radiograph of a patient with ruptured flexor pollicis longus. Note osteophyte of the scaphoid, which caused attrition rupture of the flexor pollicis longus. **(B)** Another patient with a ruptured flexor pollicis longus. Flexor tendons are exposed, and the ruptured flexor pollicis longus is held with forceps. Synovium from the scaphotrapezial joint can be seen *(arrow)*. A sharp spur on the scaphoid can be palpated adjacent to this capsular tear. Note the ruptured proximal tendon and intact finger flexors. *(Figure continues.)*

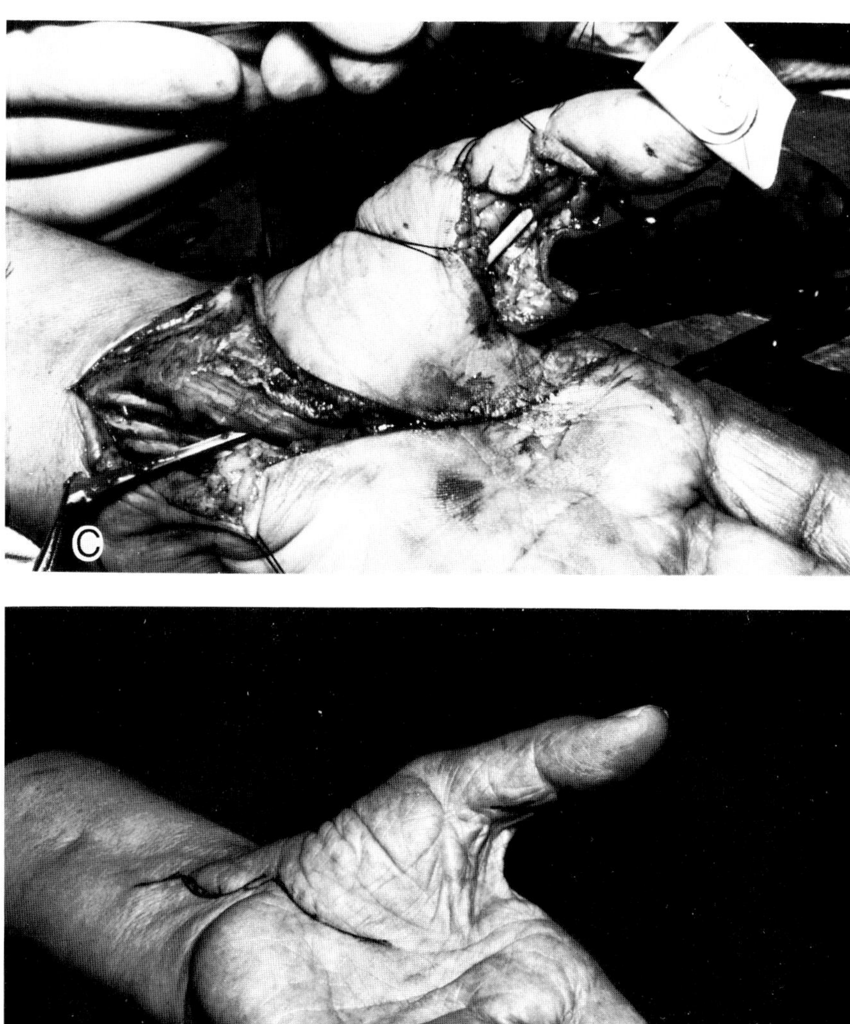

Fig. 46-17 *(Continued).* **(C)** Flexor tendon graft attached by pull-out wire prior to proximal repair. **(D&E)** Range of motion of the interphalangeal joint of the thumb 4 months postoperatively. *(Figure continues.)*

flexor carpi radialis or one of the multiple slips of the abductor pollicis longus can be used. If the distal tendon stump cannot be brought into the wrist incision, we use either a full length tendon graft or transfer a superficial flexor tendon. The superficial flexor is detached in the distal palm and sutured to the volar aspect of the distal phalanx of the thumb with a pull-out suture. A soft rubber catheter or a tendon passer is used to bring the tendon through the sheath and pulley mechanism. The stump of the flexor pollicis longus is elevated and the underlying cortex roughened prior to final attachment of the graft or transfer. A carpal tunnel release and flexor tendon tenosynovectomy usually are performed at the same time.

The thumb and wrist are immobilized in moderate flexion for 3 weeks, following which active motion is started.

Rupture of the Flexor Digitorum Profundus

Rupture of one or more of the deep flexor tendons is not uncommon. If a patient with these ruptures can maintain superficial flexor function (both in range of motion and in strength), the functional loss is minimal. The treatment should match the degree of functional loss. If the distal tendon stump becomes adherent, the patient may lose active flexion but may maintain enough stability of the DIP joint to preclude the need for surgical stabilization.

The most important factor determining the type of treatment is the level of tendon rupture. Flexor tendon ruptures can occur within the finger, at the palm, or at the wrist level. The

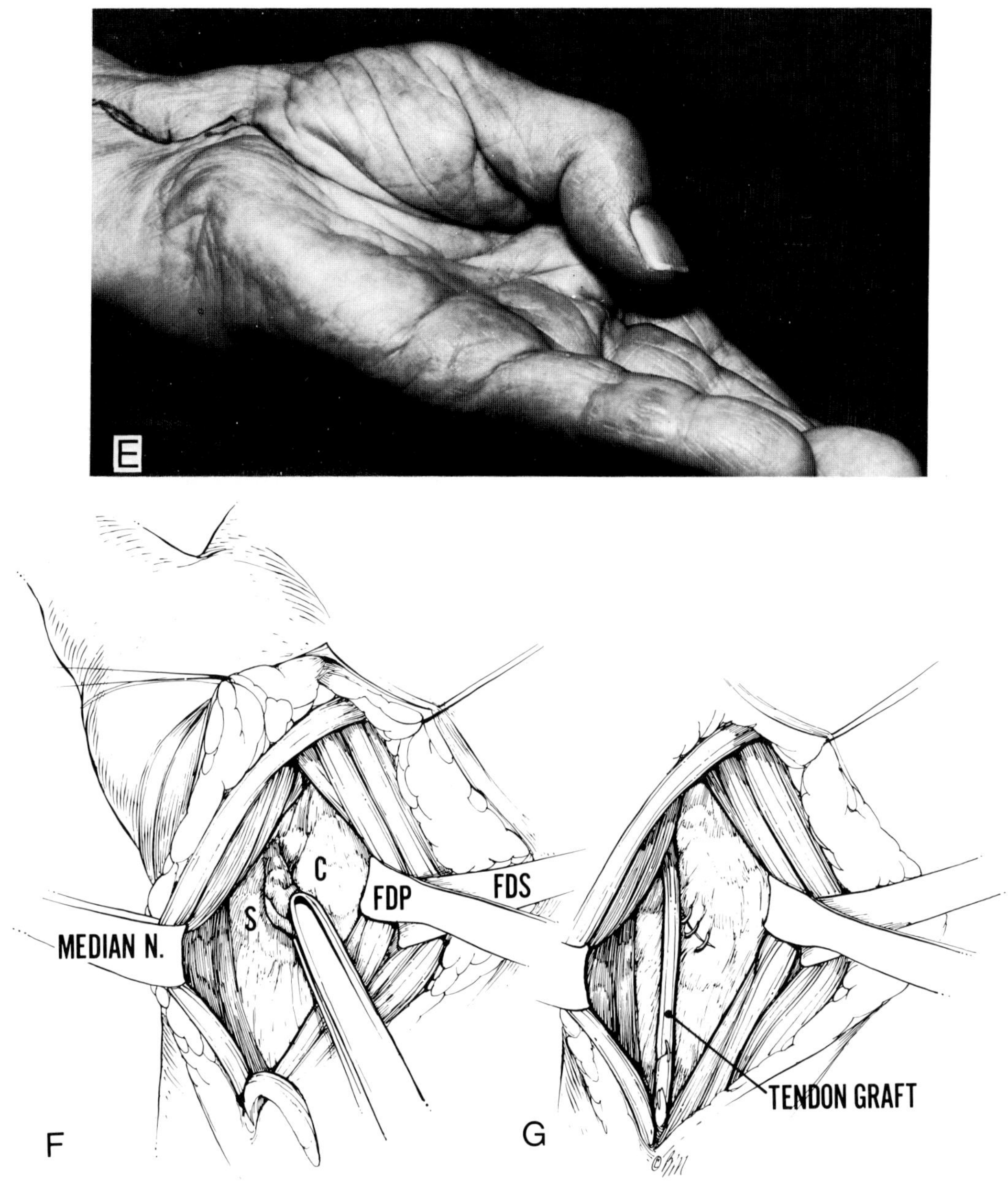

Fig. 46-17 *(Continued).* **(F)** Technique for wrist flexor tenosynovitis associated with flexor pollicis longus rupture. The bulging synovium is removed with a rongeur. The scaphoid osteophyte is removed. A larger volar capsular incision is made if a wrist joint synovectomy is to be performed concurrently (see text). **(G)** The capsular rent is closed and tendon graft is completed. (Figs. A–E from Nalebuff and Millender,[191] with permission.)

palm is the easiest level at which function can be restored. Ruptures in the palm may be less obvious if the ruptured tendon adheres to the adjacent deep flexors. This obscures the diagnosis, as DIP joint flexion is possible with the finger extended and the flexor mass pulls on the distal tendon end through scar tissue, but not when the finger is flexed actively or passively at the PIP joint. This situation can be confused with a flexor tendon nodule that blocks active excursion of the profundus tendon. Clues to the proper diagnosis include the lack of a palpable nodule and an alteration of the resting finger posture with the finger assuming a more extended position than the adjacent fingers.

Flexor tendon ruptures at the palm and wrist levels are treated best by suture of the distal tendon ends to the adjacent intact tendon (Fig. 46-18). This is not possible if the rupture occurs within the fibroosseous canal. In this case, surgery is performed only to remove diseased synovium from the intact superficial flexor, which is now vital to the function of the

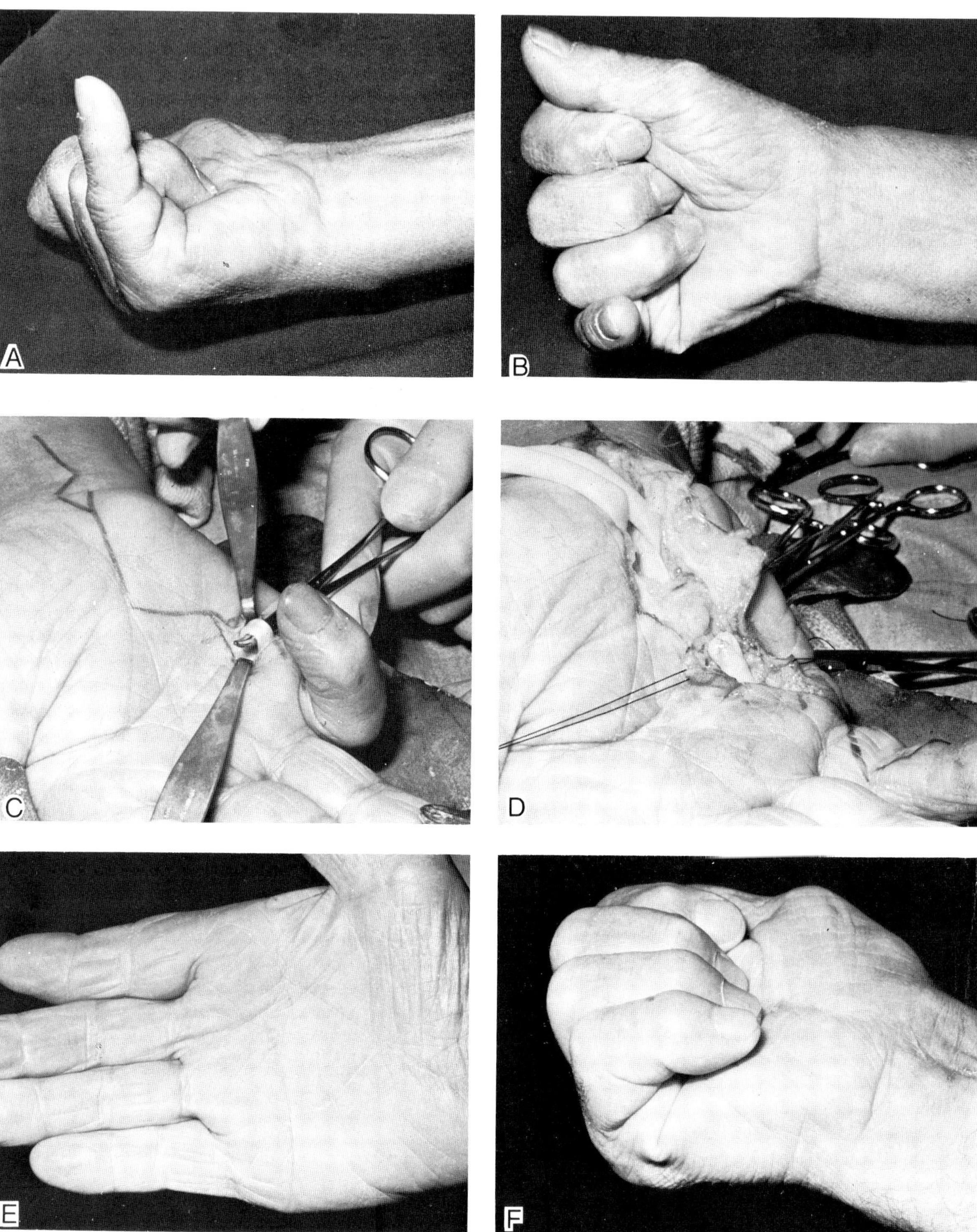

Fig. 46-18. Example of a flexor tendon rupture within the palm treated by suture of the distal tendon stump to the adjacent intact flexor tendon of the ring finger. **(A&B)** Preoperative finger stance. **(C)** Incision at the base of the finger to determine the site of rupture. **(D)** Incision extended proximally and rupture found at the midpalm. **(E&F)** Postoperative function following repair. (From Nalebuff,[182] with permission.)

finger. Caution should be used in considering staged flexor tendon reconstruction of the flexor digitorum profundus through an intact flexor digitorum superficialis. The results with this technique have not been good.[63,64] We prefer to stabilize the DIP joint in these patients rather than to consider a flexor tendon graft through an intact superficialis tendon.

Rupture of the Flexor Digitorum Superficialis

Loss of flexor digitorum superficialis function alone causes no obvious functional loss. In fact, as described previously in the section on tenosynovitis, we occasionally will resect one-half of the superficial flexor in order to restore proper function of the deep flexor tendon. The diagnosis of flexor digitorum superficialis rupture may be made only by careful examination. The treatment should not jeopardize existing tendon function. However, suture to adjacent tendons within the palm or the wrist is feasible. A tenosynovectomy should be done to protect the flexor digitorum profundus tendons.

Rupture of Both Superficial and Deep Finger Flexor Tendons

The loss of both flexor tendons of a finger results in obvious and significant functional loss—the finger "sticks out" from the other fingers and thereby "gets in the way." Restoration of active finger flexion is a goal that is not always possible to achieve. For this reason, it is far better to be aware of early nodular tenosynovitis and to perform a prophylactic tenosynovectomy before tendon rupture occurs. If the ruptures have occured at the wrist, function can be restored by suture to adjacent tendons or by a bridge graft of the profundus tendon with the suture lines placed proximal and distal to the carpal tunnel area. It is not necessary to reconstruct superficial tendon ruptures at the wrist. Therefore an intact portion of a ruptured superficial tendon can be used for bridge grafts to reconstruct ruptured profundus tendons.

If the rupture is in the palm, adjacent suture to a profundus tendon or the transfer of a superficial flexor to the distal profundus stump can be performed.

Within the fibroosseous canal, the same problem encountered in tendon laceration at this level exists, except that the situation is worse. The disease is not localized and the dissection needed for exposure leaves a very poor bed for tendon grafting. In addition, the adjacent joints may have restricted and/or painful motion. In our experience, free flexor tendon grafts have not produced good results in patients with rheumatoid arthritis. Occasionally, if no other alternative is available, we will perform a staged flexor tendon reconstruction using a silicone rubber tendon rod, particularly in younger patients who have minimal joint involvement. The technique is essentially the same as that described for post-traumatic flexor tendon reconstruction (see Chapter 51).

Finally, there are patients for whom, because of advanced age, poor status of the interphalangeal joints, or generalized disease, the wisest choice, with both flexor tendons ruptured within the finger, is to fuse both the PIP and DIP joints in a functional position. In this way, satisfactory function can be restored and pain diminished. Suturing the proximal flexor tendon stumps to the base of the proximal phalanx may augment MP flexor strength if there is free excursion of the flexor tendon proximal to the rupture. Of course, this is a last resort alternative, but it should be given consideration as a method of handling this complicated problem in selected patients.

THE WRIST

The wrist is the keystone of the hand. A painful, unstable, and deformed wrist will impair hand function regardless of the status of the fingers.[77,165] In addition, wrist deformity is a major cause of finger deformity, and, unless wrist alignment is preserved or restored, maintaining correction of finger deformities is difficult, if not impossible.[82,202] An understanding of the pathophysiology of rheumatoid wrist disease is necessary to appreciate the effects of wrist involvement on hand function and finger deformity.[37,149,154,211,212,294]

Natural History of Rheumatoid Wrist Involvement

Rheumatoid synovitis follows predictable patterns. In the wrist, the ulnar styloid, the ulnar head, and the midportion of the scaphoid frequently are the earliest to be involved by rheumatoid synovitis. Progressive synovial proliferation in these areas leads to the various patterns of wrist deformity.

In the ulnar compartment, synovitis stretches the ulnar carpal ligamentous complex and results in changes that Backdahl has called the "caput ulna syndrome."[8] This syndrome is the result of destruction of the ligamentous complex, including the triangular fibrocartilage and ulnar disc, which allows dorsal dislocation of the distal ulna, supination of the carpus on the hand, and volar subluxation of the extensor carpi ulnaris.[50,249,281] The caput ulna syndrome (seen in up to one-third of rheumatoid patients undergoing hand surgery) can result in significant disability. Patients with this syndrome complain of weakness and pain that are aggravated by forearm rotation. Examination of the wrist reveals prominence of the distal ulna, instability of the distal radioulnar joint, limited wrist dorsiflexion, and supination of the carpus on the forearm. As the extensor carpi ulnaris tendon subluxates volarward, normal function of this tendon is diminished, allowing the wrist to deviate radially and setting the stage for attrition ruptures of the ulnar extensor tendons.[280]

Radiocarpal involvement by proliferative synovitis begins beneath the radioscaphocapitate, or "sling," ligament in the region of the deep volar radiocarpal ligament.[258,259] Destruction of these ligaments eventually results in rotatory instability of the scaphoid. In this condition, the scaphoid assumes a volarflexed position. There is secondary loss of carpal height and radial rotation of the carpus and metacarpals on the radius. The combination of rotatory subluxation of the scaphoid, volar subluxation of the ulnar carpus, and dorsal subluxation of the distal ulna produces relative supination of the wrist in relation to the distal forearm. This common pattern of wrist collapse results in imbalance of the extensor tendons, radial shift of the metacarpals, and ulnar deviation of the fingers.[262,264] This deformity is thought to be one of the important factors initiating ulnar deviation of the MP joints, as well as the recurrence of ulnar deviation following MP joint arthroplasty.[202,220,221] (Fig. 46-19).

The untreated, end-stage rheumatoid wrist is dislocated volarward with complete destruction of the carpal bones and complete dissociation of the radioulnar joint. Early surgical treatment can prevent this severe destruction.

Operative Treatment for Rheumatoid Radiocarpal and Radioulnar Joint Deformities

Surgical procedures for the radiocarpal and radioulnar joint are considered either preventive or reconstructive. Preventive procedures include radioulnar joint and radiocarpal joint synovectomy, balancing of wrist extensors, and tenosynovectomy. Reconstructive surgery includes distal ulna excision, distal ulna arthroplasty, reconstruction of the ulnocarpal ligamentous complex, radiocarpal joint arthroplasty, partial wrist fusion, and total wrist arthrodesis.[5,34,41,44,73,75,87,92,96,100,136,146,161,187,196,199,205,210,225,244,262,269,284]

Radiocarpal and Radioulnar Joint Synovectomy — Indications

The indications for wrist joint synovectomy have never been established clearly. There are no studies that demonstrate conclusively that synovectomy will change the natural course of rheumatoid disease. In addition, because the wrist is a multiarticulated complex joint, total synovectomy is impossible. The indications for wrist synovectomy vary among hand surgeons. Lipscomb[137] and others have recommended a several month trial period of conservative therapy prior to synovectomy. Flatt[79] has advocated early synovectomy because of the rapid joint destruction that can occur when active synovitis does not respond to medical therapy. Tajima and Tubiana have found that synovectomy can provide significant pain relief, even in advanced disease. Synovectomy in some cases can thus be an alternative to wrist fusion.

We limit wrist synovectomy to the small group of patients with persistent, painful wrist synovitis and minimal radiographic involvement, who appear to have slowly progressive disease under relatively good medical control and who have been followed for at least 6 months. Wrist splints and intraarticular steroid injections are used in addition to the patient's systemic medical therapy. Synovectomy is recommended if the symptoms persist for 6 to 9 months after instituting the regimen described above and if the radiographs of the wrist have remained unchanged.[164] Shapiro,[224] Thirupathi, Ferlic

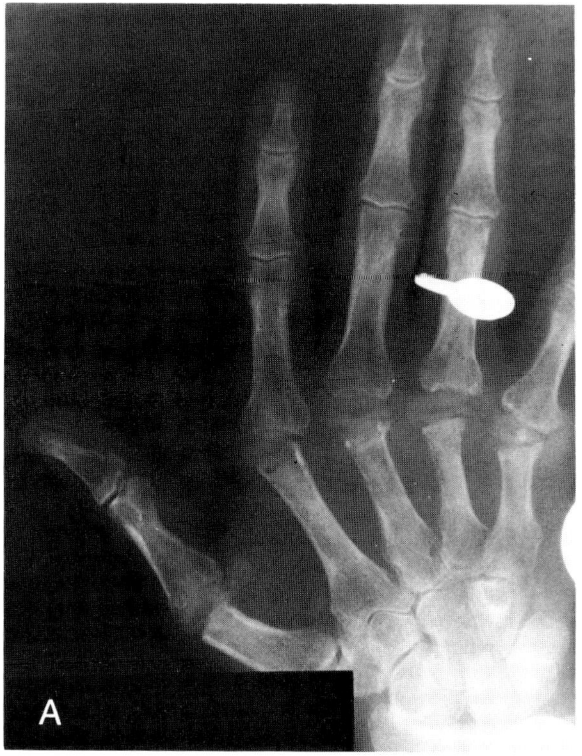

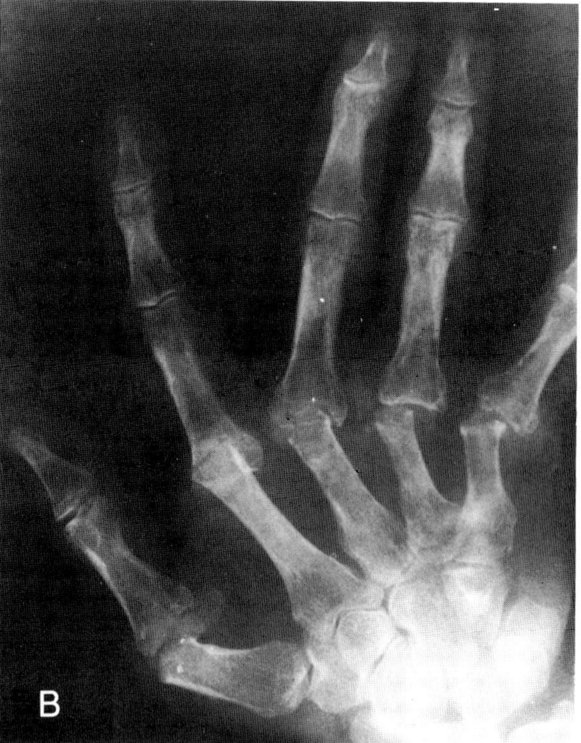

Fig. 46-19. **(A)** A radiograph taken 4 weeks after implant arthroplasties of the MP joints. There is an early collapse deformity of the wrist with vertical rotation of the scaphoid, scapholunate dissociation, and dorsal rotation of the lunate. Note the radial deviation of the metacarpals associated with the wrist collapse, and the reciprocal ulnar deviation of the MP joints. **(B)** Two years after MP arthroplasty increased wrist deformity with ulnar translocation of the carpus and severe recurrent deformity of the MP joints with fracture of the implants has occurred. *(Figure continues.)*

and Clayton,[265] and Brumfeld[28] in separate long-term follow-up reviews of wrist synovectomy found consistent and dramatic relief of pain, and varying loss of wrist motion after wrist synovectomy. Of importance, Shapiro found that grip strength was maintained, not weakened, after synovectomy.

Dorsal Approach for Radiocarpal and Radioulnar Joint Synovectomy— Operative Technique (Fig. 46-20)

The wrist is exposed through a dorsal longitudinal incision that can be midline, slightly radial, or slightly ulnar, depending on the exposure required. An S-shaped, zigzag, or oblique incision should be avoided because of the increased risk of vascular compromise and subsequent skin slough with these incisions. These complications occur most often in patients with thin, atrophic skin and/or in those who are on systemic steroid medication. Care must be taken to preserve the dorsal veins, maintain a thick skin flap, avoid hematoma formation, and perform careful skin closure without tension.

The skin flaps and subcutaneous tissue are dissected from the extensor retinaculum. Care is taken to preserve the dorsal branches of the radial and ulnar nerves. The extensor retinaculum is opened. Flatt and Swanson have recommended entering the sixth extensor compartment and reflecting the entire extensor retinaculum as a radially based flap, releasing each of the dorsal extensor compartments except the first.[77,250] Alternatively, the retinaculum may be opened over the fourth dorsal compartment and reflected as radially and ulnarly based flaps. The terminal branch of the posterior interosseous nerve can be found consistently on the floor of the fourth dorsal compartment, deep to the extensor tendons. This is an articular branch that innervates the wrist joint. It can be resected to partially denervate the wrist joint for pain relief, as described by Buck-Gramcko.[29,52]

A transverse incision is made in the wrist capsule, and a distally based flap is elevated to expose the wrist and intercarpal joints. Synovium usually is seen bulging from the proximal and distal carpal rows. Traction applied to the hand distracts the joints and allows the synovectomy to be performed with a small rongeur. A small, blunt periosteal elevator can be used to provide better exposure within the joint. Periarticular erosions are curetted. If the triangular fibrocartilage is intact, synovium is removed from the area between the triquetrum and the fibrocartilage.

The distal radioulnar joint is exposed through a longitudinal incision proximal to the triangular fibrocartilage. The forearm is rotated to provide exposure as the synovectomy is performed. Bony spurs are removed from the distal ulna, and, again, periarticular erosions are curetted.

After the synovectomy has been completed, the capsular incisions are closed with interrupted nonabsorbable sutures. Closure is performed with the forearm in supination to minimize the tendency for the ulna to subluxate and to allow a

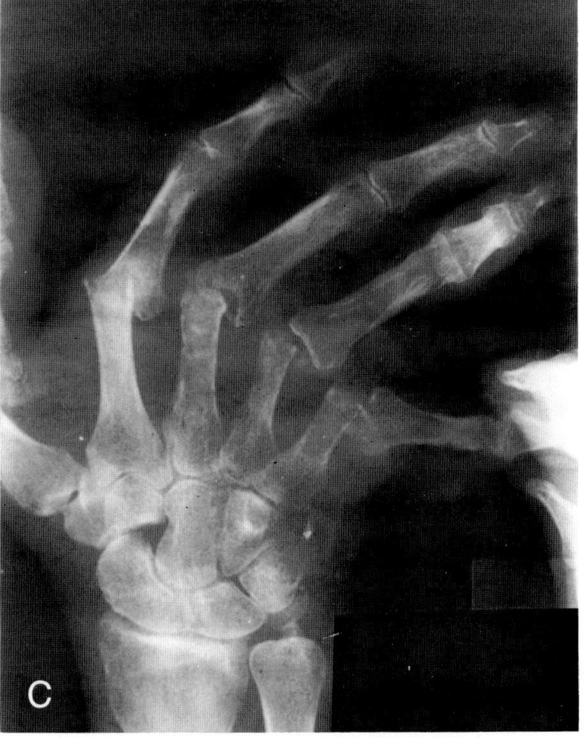

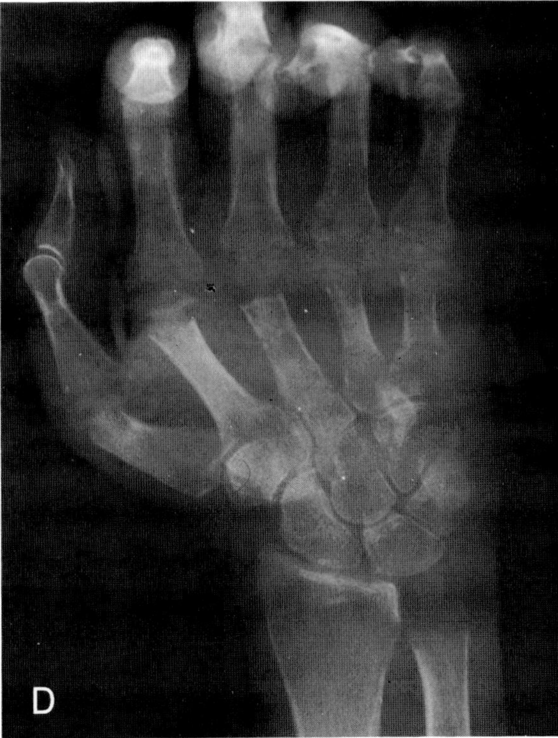

Fig. 46-19 *(Continued).* **(C)** The wrist deformity can be corrected passively. Note that the scapholunate dissociation is corrected as the wrist is held in the neutral position. **(D)** The wrist 4 weeks after reconstruction by resection of the distal ulna, reconstruction of the radioulnar joint and the ruptured extensor carpi ulnaris by tendon graft, and revision of the MP joint implant arthroplasties. Note the improved alignment of the wrist and MP joints.

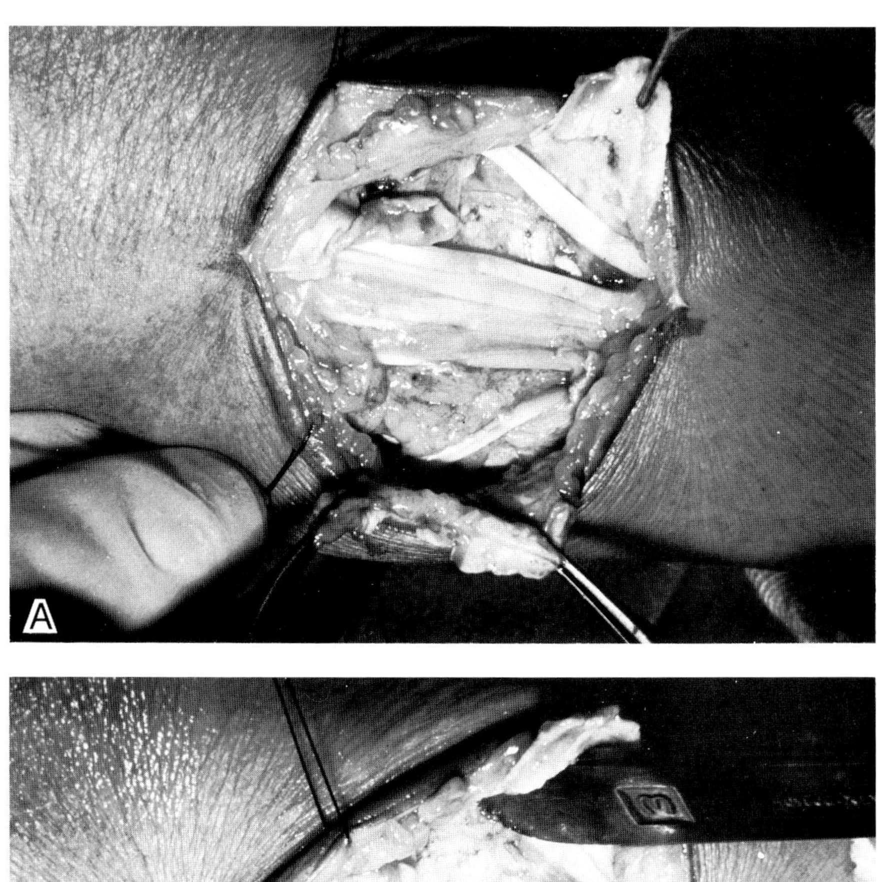

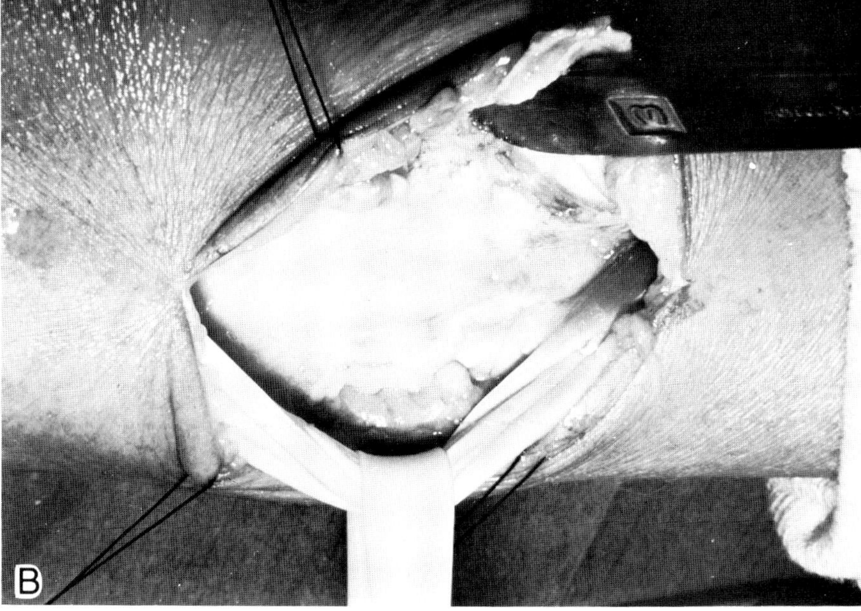

Fig. 46-20. Technique for wrist joint synovectomy. **(A)** The extensor tendons are exposed; dorsal tenosynovectomy has been performed. **(B)** Extensor tendons retracted and wrist capsule exposed. *(Figure continues.)*

tighter closure of the distal radioulnar joint capsule. Tendon rebalancing, dorsal tenosynovectomy, and relocation of the dorsal retinaculum are performed if necessary. The tourniquet may be released at this point and hemostasis obtained. A Penrose or suction drain is placed in the subcutaneous area prior to skin closure.

A bulky compression dressing is applied and the wrist is splinted in neutral. The forearm is held in full supination with sugar-tong splints. The drain is removed in 24 hours. Forearm supination is maintained for approximately 3 weeks. At this time the splints are removed and both forearm and wrist motion are started.

The length of postoperative splinting depends on the degree of wrist ligament laxity present preoperatively and the degree of ligament disruption found at the time of surgery. The greater the laxity, the longer the wrist is splinted postoperatively. Splinting for 4 to 6 weeks may be necessary to allow enough capsular healing to provide stability. We have found that the optimal range of motion after surgery is 30 to 40 degrees flexion and the same range of extension.

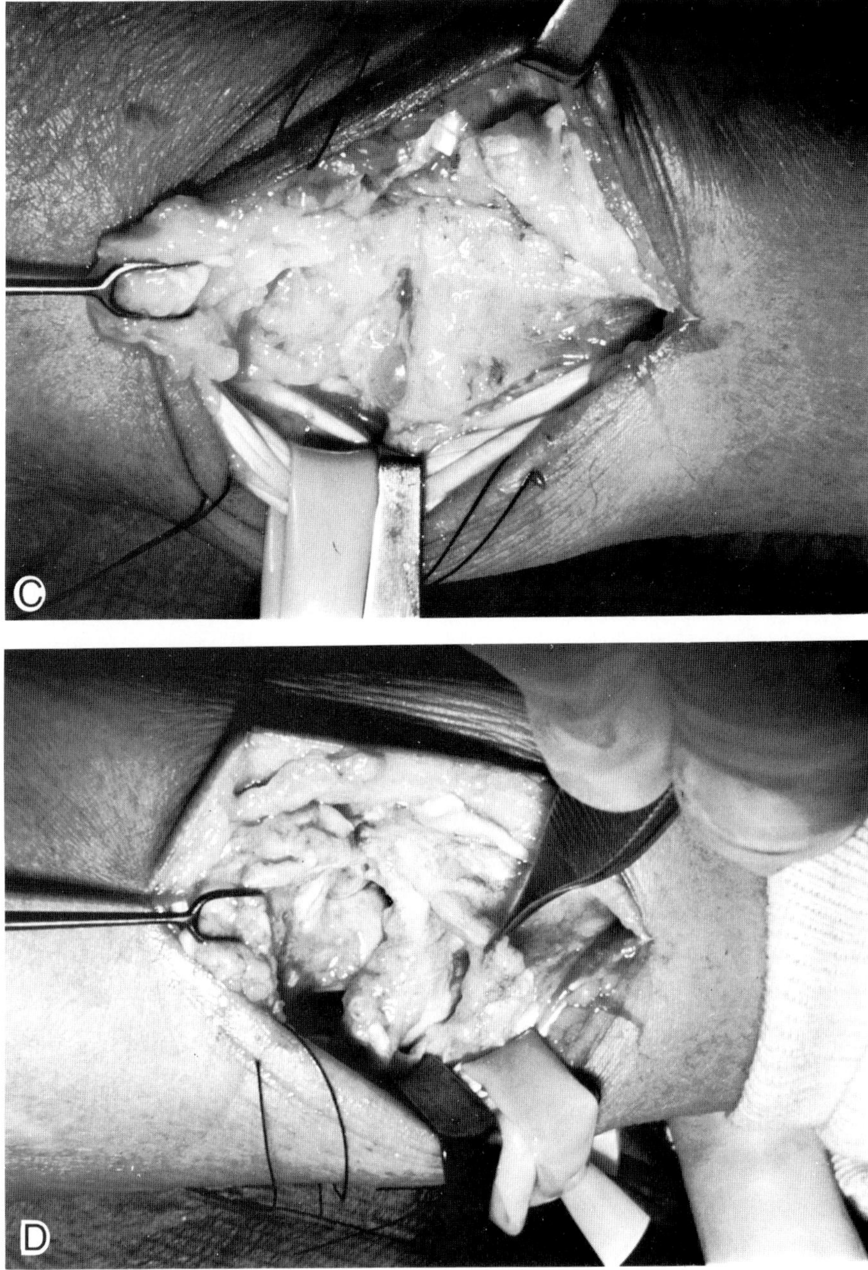

Fig. 46-20 *(Continued).* **(C)** Transverse capsular incision exposes the underlying synovium. **(D)** Proximal and distal carpal rows are exposed and synovectomy is performed with a rongeur. *(Figure continues.)*

Volar Wrist Synovectomy—Operative Technique

A volar wrist synovectomy can be done when a flexor tenosynovectomy is indicated to alleviate median nerve compression or to improve finger motion, or when flexor tendon reconstruction is necessary. Both Straub[244] and Taleisnik[259] have advocated volar wrist synovectomy, in conjunction with wrist flexor tenosynovectomy, to prevent destruction of the deep volar ligaments and secondary rotatory subluxation of the scaphoid.

When present, volar wrist synovitis is manifested by bulging of the volar capsule. The skin incision described for volar tenosynovectomy is used. A transverse incision is made over the bulging volar wrist capsule. Traction is applied to the hand and synovium is removed from the volar portion of the wrist with a rongeur. The volar capsule is closed with interrupted nonabsorbable sutures. The postoperative man-

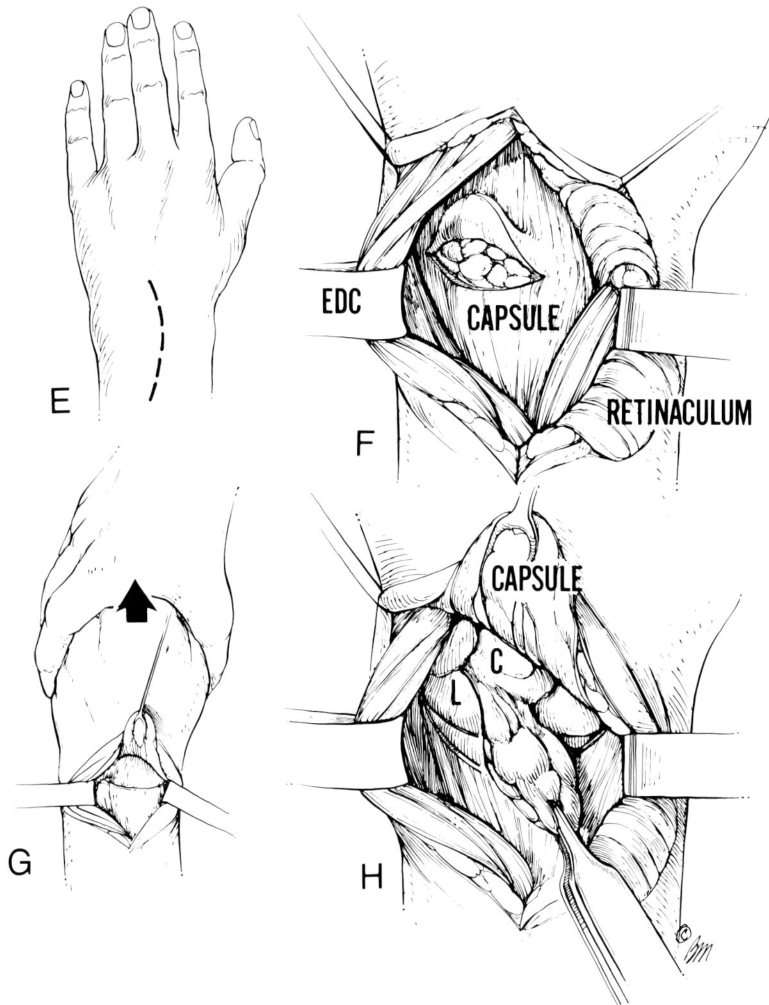

Fig. 46-20 *(Continued).* **(E–H)** Drawing of wrist joint synovectomy technique. Note preservation of capsular flaps for closure.

agement is the same as that described for volar tenosynovectomy.

Distal Ulna Excision and Reconstruction of the Distal Radioulnar Joint Complex

Involvement of the distal radioulnar joint resulting in the caput ulna syndrome is one of the most frequent disabilities in the rheumatoid wrist. For this reason, distal ulna excision and reconstruction of the triangular fibrocartilage and the distal radioulnar joint are performed frequently in the wrist affected by rheumatoid arthritis.

Distal ulna excision was described first by Smith-Peterson and Aufranc for rheumatoid arthritis.[230] It remains our procedure of choice because it is reliable and allows adequate exposure to perform a distal radioulnar joint synovectomy and to reconstruct the triangular fibrocartilage complex. Swanson described distal ulna excision and replacement with a silicone rubber implant.[249–251] The importance of soft tissue reconstruction to correct supination of the carpus and subluxation of the distal ulna has been emphasized by many authors.[8,38,46,49,135,158,172,196,205,208,249,281,288] Destruction of the triangular fibrocartilage ligamentous complex complicates the correction of the supination of the carpus on the distal forearm and the dorsal subluxation of the ulna.

Distal ulna excision for symptoms of the caput ulna syndrome usually is performed in conjunction with dorsal tenosynovectomy and tendon transfer for ruptured extensor tendons or in conjunction with wrist joint synovectomy or wrist joint reconstruction.

Other surgical techniques are available to reconstruct the distal radioulnar joint destroyed by the rheumatoid process. There has been renewed interest in fusion of the distal ulna to the sigmoid notch of the radius with resection of a segment of ulna to allow rotation of forearm (the "Sauve-Kapandji" procedure)[91,264] following reports by Taleisnik[262] and by Hales and Burkhalter.[99] Taleisnik[264] believes that the Sauve-Kapandji procedure is indicated for younger patients with painful distal radioulnar joint dysfunction because it provides stable fixation of the ulnar head, preserves ulnocarpal support, restores forearm rotation, and results in a better cosmetic appearance than does distal ulna resection. He prefers the Sauve-Kapandji procedure to distal ulna resection in patients with impending ulnar translocation not severe enough to warrant radiolunate fusion.

We prefer limited carpal fusion for patients with established or impending ulnar translocation. A segmental osteotomy of the ulna similar to that done in the Sauve-Kapandji procedure occasionally can be used to restore partial forearm rotation in patients with juvenile rheumatoid arthritis who have had spontaneous fusions of the distal radioulnar joint. Bowers[18] has described "hemi-resection" of the distal radioulnar joint with preservation of the ulnar styloid process and interposition of soft tissue between the distal ulna and radius. This procedure preserves the ligaments that arise from the styloid process and support the ulnar side of the carpus (see Chapter 24). Watson[285] has yet another approach to reconstructing the distal radioulnar joint destroyed by rheumatoid arthritis. He uses a resection arthroplasty of the joint that preserves the entire length of the ulna, including the styloid process and the attachments of the triangular fibrocartilage and the joint capsule. This allows rotation throughout the range of forearm motion without contact of the ulna with the radius. All of these procedures have specific advantages and should be considered as alternatives to the standard procedure of distal ulnar resection in selected patients.

Distal Ulna Excision and Reconstruction of the Distal Radioulnar Joint Complex— Operative Technique

The surgical principles of distal ulna excision are important and include the following: (1) limited resection of the distal ulna (2 cm or less) to minimize instability of the remaining ulna, (2) synovectomy of the distal radioulnar joint, (3) correction of carpal supination by suturing the remnant of the triangular fibrocartilage complex to the dorsoulnar corner of the radius, and (4) reconstruction of the dorsal capsule and extensor retinaculum with relocation of the extensor carpi ulnaris from volar to dorsal.

The wrist joint is approached through the dorsal longitudinal wrist incision described previously. The extensor retinaculum is opened. It is usually thin and/or adherent over the capsule of the distal ulna, which makes separation of these two layers difficult. Identification of the volarly subluxated extensor carpi ulnaris also may be difficult. The tendon usually can be palpated on the ulnar aspect of the wrist. Often, tenosynovium is noted bulging in the region of the sixth dorsal compartment. Occasionally, the entire sheath of the sixth compartment is destroyed and the tendon is frayed or ruptured. If the extensor carpi ulnaris has subluxated volarward, it is released and replaced dorsal to the axis of wrist flexion. It can be held in place with a sling of tissue fashioned from the extensor retinaculum.

A longitudinal capsular incision is made over the distal ulna. The capsule and triangular fibrocartilage are reflected from the ulna and preserved. The periosteum of the ulna is elevated, and small bone retractors are placed around the distal ulna. The distal ulna can be sectioned with bone cutter, an osteotome, or a power saw. A towel clip is used to apply traction to the bone fragment when the soft tissue attachments are divided. Approximately 2 cm of bone is resected. If excessive bone is removed, stability of the distal ulna may become a problem.

After the bone is removed, a complete synovectomy of the distal radioulnar joint is performed. Although the triangular fibrocartilage often is destroyed, if it is present, it should be protected during the synovectomy.

Reconstruction of the soft tissue support for both the distal radioulnar joint and the radiocarpal joint is important to correct carpal supination and to stabilize the distal ulna. If the triangular fibrocartilage and the radioulnar ligamentous complex are present, they are sutured tightly to the dorsal and ulnar aspect of the radius.

Various methods have been used to stabilize the distal ulna after resection of the ulnar head. Blatt and Ashworth[15] incised the volar capsule to form a distally based flap. The flap is brought dorsally and fixed to the ulna to reconstitute the ligament (Fig. 46-21).

Linscheid and Dobyns used a different method.[135] A K-wire is used to hold the carpus to the radius in the corrected position. A distally based strip of the extensor carpi ulnaris tendon is detached, woven through the ulnar collateral ligament and any remnants of the triangular fibrocartilage, and sutured to the radius (Fig. 46-22). The dorsal radioulnar capsule is closed tightly, imbricating the tissues when necessary. This is facilitated by supinating the wrist to relocate the ulna. Following this, the extensor retinaculum is relocated deep to the tendons. The position of the extensor carpi ulnaris tendon is corrected if necessary (see below).

O'Donovan, Ruby, and Leslie[132,133,200] used a distally-based slip of extensor carpi ulnaris tendon. The tendon slip is passed through the distal end of the ulna, through a hole made in the dorsal cortex of the ulna, and then is sutured back onto itself.

Breen and Jupiter[23] used a distally-based slip of the flexor carpi ulnaris and a proximally-based slip of the extensor carpi ulnaris to stabilize the distal ulna after ulnar head resection.

A Penrose or suction drain may be placed if the tourniquet is not released. A bulky hand dressing is applied with the wrist and fingers splinted in extension and the forearm in supination. The dressing is changed in 24 hours, at which time the drain is removed. Finger motion is begun immediately. When the fingers are not being exercised, they are splinted in extension until the patient is able to extend them actively.

If the preoperative deformity and/or instability were minimal and if a satisfactory ligamentous reconstruction and tight capsular closure were possible at surgery, short arm splints will provide adequate immobilization postoperatively. Occasionally, a sugar-tong splint to limit forearm motion is useful for pain relief in the first few days after surgery. Gentle forearm motion is allowed gradually as the postoperative pain and swelling decrease. However, if the soft tissue closure was suboptimal, the forearm should be maintained in supination with a long arm splint or cast for 2 to 3 weeks to allow soft tissue healing before forearm motion exercises are started. It is not uncommon to have mild crepitus or a click during forearm

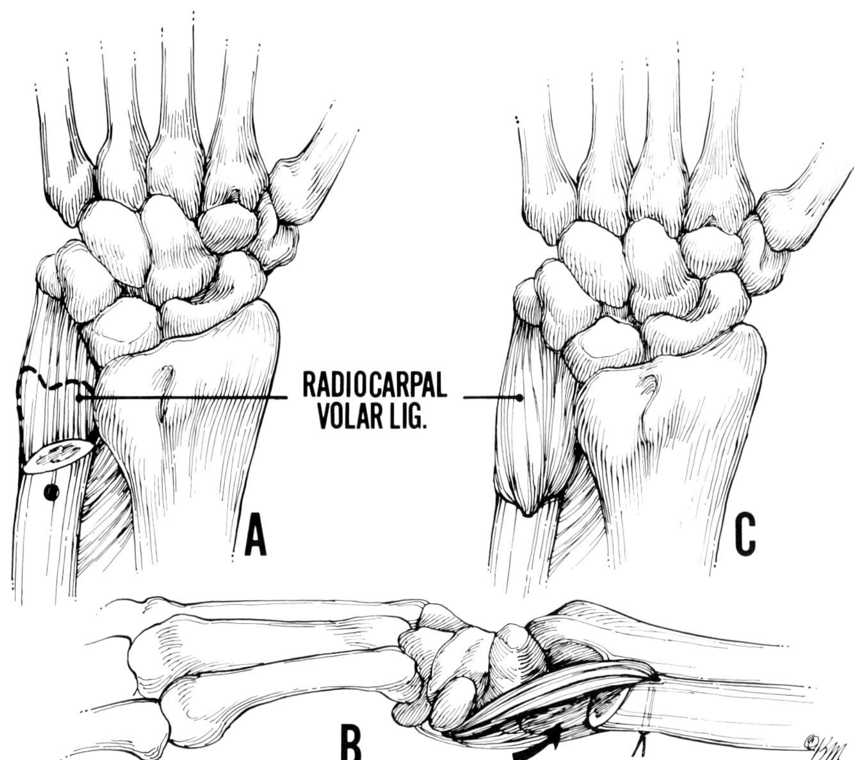

Fig. 46-21. Stabilization of the distal ulna using a flap of volar capsule. **(A)** After distal ulna excision and synovectomy are completed, a distally based flap of volar capsule is reflected. **(B)** The free proximal end is brought dorsalward and sutured to the dorsal cortex of the ulna through drill holes. The flap acts as a volar restraining ligament to prevent dorsal subluxation of the distal ulna. **(C)** Volar flap sutured over the dorsal cortex of the distal ulna.

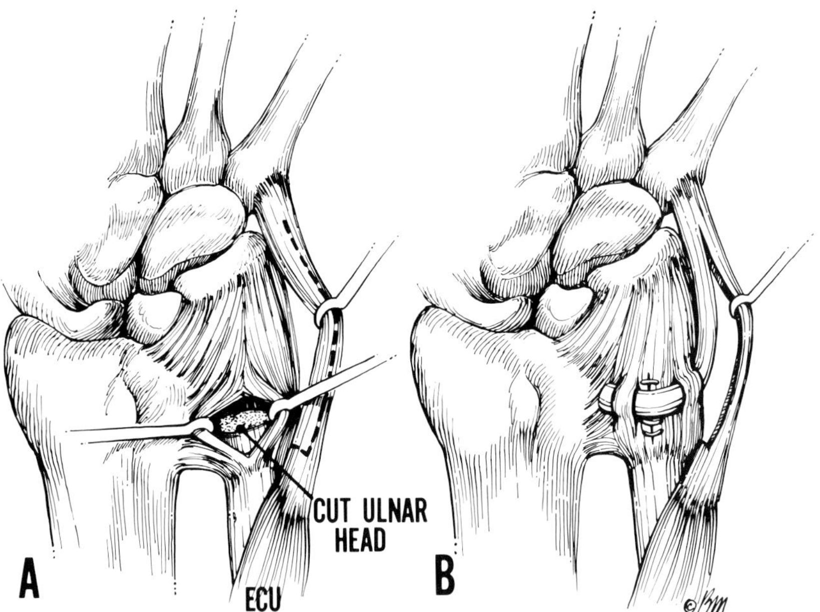

Fig. 46-22. Reconstruction of the distal radioulnar joint following synovectomy and distal ulna excision. **(A)** The dorsal capsule of the distal radioulnar joint is opened longitudinally, a synovectomy is performed, and the distal ulna is excised. (The slip of tendon to be stripped from the extensor carpi ulnaris is shown by the dotted line.) **(B)** A strip of extensor carpi ulnaris is mobilized, passed through the ulnar aspect of the joint capsule, across the dorsal aspect of the joint and sutured to the dorsal capsule over the radius to correct the supination deformity. The radioulnar joint capsule is imbricated to correct the dorsal subluxation of the distal ulna. The dorsal retinaculum can be used to further reinforce the radioulnar joint capsule.

rotation for the first few weeks after motion is started. This usually diminishes gradually and resolves entirely after several months.

Ulnar Head Excision—Complications

The most frequent complication following distal ulna excision is painful forearm rotation. This often will respond to prolonged splinting and a gentle motion exercise program under the direction of a therapist. No surgery is indicated for 3 to 4 months, unless a definite cause for the symptoms is evident. If the symptoms do not remit after several months, and there is instability of the distal ulna on examination, a soft tissue stabilization procedure using the extensor carpi ulnaris to reinforce the distal radioulnar joint capsule can be considered.

We no longer use the Silastic ulnar head implant because of the significant risk of complications, including dislocation of the implant, fracture of the implant stem, bone resorption beneath the collar of the implant, and symptomatic silicone synovitis.

Tendon Transfers to Restore Wrist Balance

A frequent wrist imbalance in rheumatoid arthritis is supination and ulnar translocation of the carpus on the radius. As stated previously, this deformity is associated with the caput ulna syndrome and rotatory instability of the carpus. In the caput ulna syndrome with volar subluxation or dislocation of the extensor carpi ulnaris tendon, there is unopposed radial deviation of the carpus from the pull of the radial wrist extensors. This is exacerbated if there is a concomitant intercarpal dissociation with collapse deformity of the scaphoid.

Clayton has advocated correcting wrist imbalance by transferring the extensor carpi radialis longus to the extensor carpi ulnaris in patients who cannot actively ulnarly deviate the wrist.[19,41,43,44] We have used this transfer in patients with radial deviation of the wrist that is correctable passively. The procedure should be considered in conjunction with wrist joint synovectomy, dorsal tenosynovectomy, and distal ulna excision. However, our indications for this procedure are limited, as most of our patients already have advanced wrist involvement with fixed deformity. In these advanced cases, correction requires major reconstructive surgery (wrist fusion).

Hastings has advocated balancing the wrist by repositioning the extensor carpi ulnaris into its normal dorsal position.[108]

Extensor Carpi Radialis Longus Transfer—Operative Technique

After dorsal tenosynovectomy, distal ulna excision, and ligamentous reconstruction are performed, the extensor carpi radialis longus is divided at the base of the second metacarpal. This can be done through either a separate small incision or the primary surgical incision. The tendon is rerouted dorsal to the finger extensors and sutured into the repositioned extensor carpi ulnaris tendon. At the completion of the transfer, the wrist should maintain a neutral position in the coronal plane (radial and ulnar deviation). The wrist is splinted in the corrected position for 4 weeks prior to beginning exercises.

Extensor Carpi Ulnaris Tendon Repositioning—Operative Technique

During any surgical procedure on the dorsal aspect of the wrist, the extensor carpi ulnaris tendon should be released from its volarly subluxated position and repositioned in its normal dorsal position. If the extensor retinaculum has been reflected radially, a strip of this retinaculum can be split and looped around the extensor carpi ulnaris to hold the tendon dorsal to the axis of wrist flexion. Alternatively, when the retinaculum has been reflected radially and ulnarward, the ulnar portion can be placed deep to the extensor carpi ulnaris and used as a sling to hold the tendon in the corrected position. If there is a tendency for the tendon to subluxate, it can be sutured to the capsule over the dorsal aspect of the carpus.

Reconstruction of the Radiocarpal Joint

The indications for reconstruction of the radiocarpal joint by either arthrodesis or arthroplasty include deformity and instability, which interfere with function, persistent pain unresponsive to conservative therapy, and progressive destruction of the joint seen on radiographic examination.

Historically, arthrodesis has been the reconstructive procedure of choice for the rheumatoid wrist.[31,55,57,124,126,144,188,244] In 1965 Clayton advocated the use of an autogenous bone graft and a Steinmann pin for fixation.[41] In 1971 Mannerfelt described the use of a Rush rod, which was introduced into the third metacarpal and driven across the radius, obviating the need for external fixation.[146] In 1973 we reported a modification of the techniques described by Clayton and Mannerfelt in 60 patients who underwent wrist fusion.[161] All of our patients had relief of pain and improved hand function. Although wrist fusion diminishes pain, wrist motion is lost, which is in itself a disability—especially in patients with stiffness of the opposite wrist (Fig. 46-23).

In the mid-1970s, Swanson developed the silicone rubber wrist arthroplasty for reconstruction of the rheumatoid wrist.[69,250,253] Since that time, it has been the implant used most frequently for wrist arthroplasty. In 1980, we reported our early results in 35 Silastic wrist implant arthroplasties.[92] At that time we concluded that the procedure was preferable to wrist fusion in most patients. In the first edition of this book, we stated that "in patients with persistent pain, relatively good alignment, functional wrist extensors and adequate bone stock, we prefer silicone implant wrist arthroplasty."

In 1986 we reviewed the long-term follow-up (average 5 years) of 71 patients who had undergone wrist arthroplasty with Silastic implants.[22] We found a fracture rate of 20 percent and a failure rate of 25 percent when fractures and revisions for pain and recurrent deformity were combined (Fig. 46-24). Fatti and colleagues[67] reviewed 53 silicone rubber implant arthroplasties and found 90 percent good results in patients followed less than 2.5 years. However, the percentage of good results dropped to 60 percent in those patients followed for more than 2.5 years. Although silicone synovitis has been

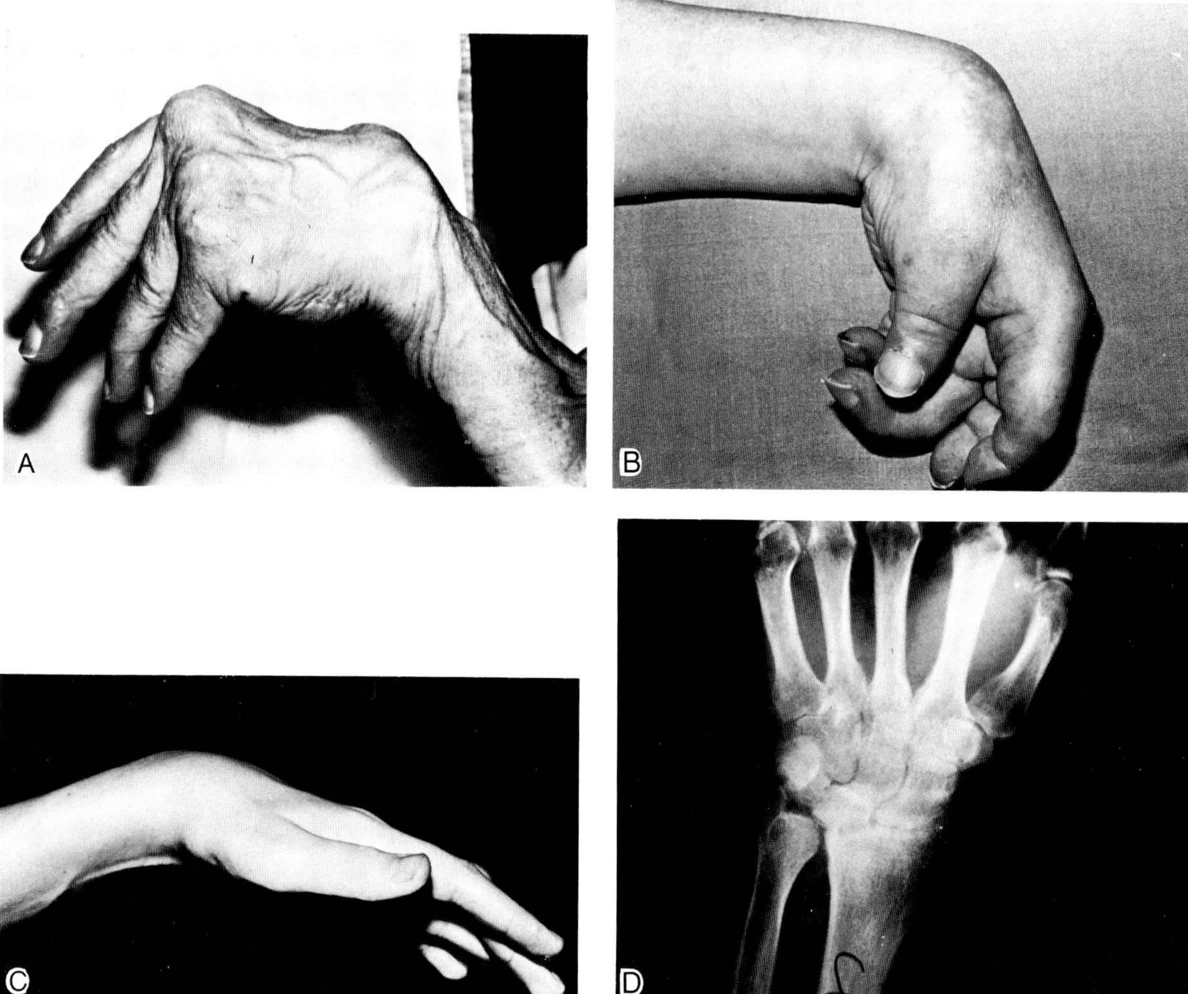

Fig. 46-23. Indications for wrist fusion. **(A)** Wrist subluxation with radiocarpal destruction. **(B)** Severe fixed flexion contracture. **(C)** Less severe, but painful, flexion contracture. **(D)** Satisfactory alignment and stability, but limited and painful motion. (From Millender and Nalebuff,[165] with permission.)

noted following the use of some silicone rubber implants in the hand and wrist,[100,229] this condition has not occurred in our series of wrist arthroplasties. The use of metal grommets may decrease the fracture rate.

Total wrist arthroplasties have been used with inconsistent results.[75,156]

Based on these reports, we have narrowed our indications for Silastic implant wrist arthroplasty. We now limit this procedure to those patients who will have low demand on the wrist after surgery in addition to the previously described criteria of functional wrist range of motion, wrist extensors in good condition, minimal wrist deformity and good bone stock. We feel strongly that bilateral wrist arthroplasties are contraindicated. Those patients who do undergo wrist arthroplasty and require crutches as an ambulatory aid should use only forearm or platform crutches. Patients with arthroplasties should use wrist splints for any activity that will place stress on the wrist. (The operative technique of Silastic wrist arthroplasty is described in Chapter 7.)

Partial wrist fusion has applications in rheumatoid as well as nonrheumatoid wrist disease.[34,136,187,257,261,262,284] Limited wrist fusion is useful in those rheumatoid patients whose disease has destroyed the radiocarpal joints, but has left the midcarpal joints relatively unaffected. Taleisnik has demonstrated the paucity of ligaments in the midcarpal region of the wrist.[260] Since the synovium is concentrated in areas with abundant ligaments, the midcarpal area is the last to become involved, and frequently is preserved even when the radiocarpal joint is not.

The earliest wrist changes in the rheumatoid patient occur as the volar ligaments stabilizing the proximal row are lost, resulting in vertical rotation of the scaphoid, dorsiflexion or volarflexion of the lunate, and/or ulnar translocation of the lunate. These changes can be arrested in their early stages before progressive collapse and joint destruction occurs by fusion of the scaphoid and lunate to the radius. Of course, a destroyed radiocarpal joint can be salvaged by this fusion as well.[136,187] Limited arthrodesis of the involved joints combined with a synovec-

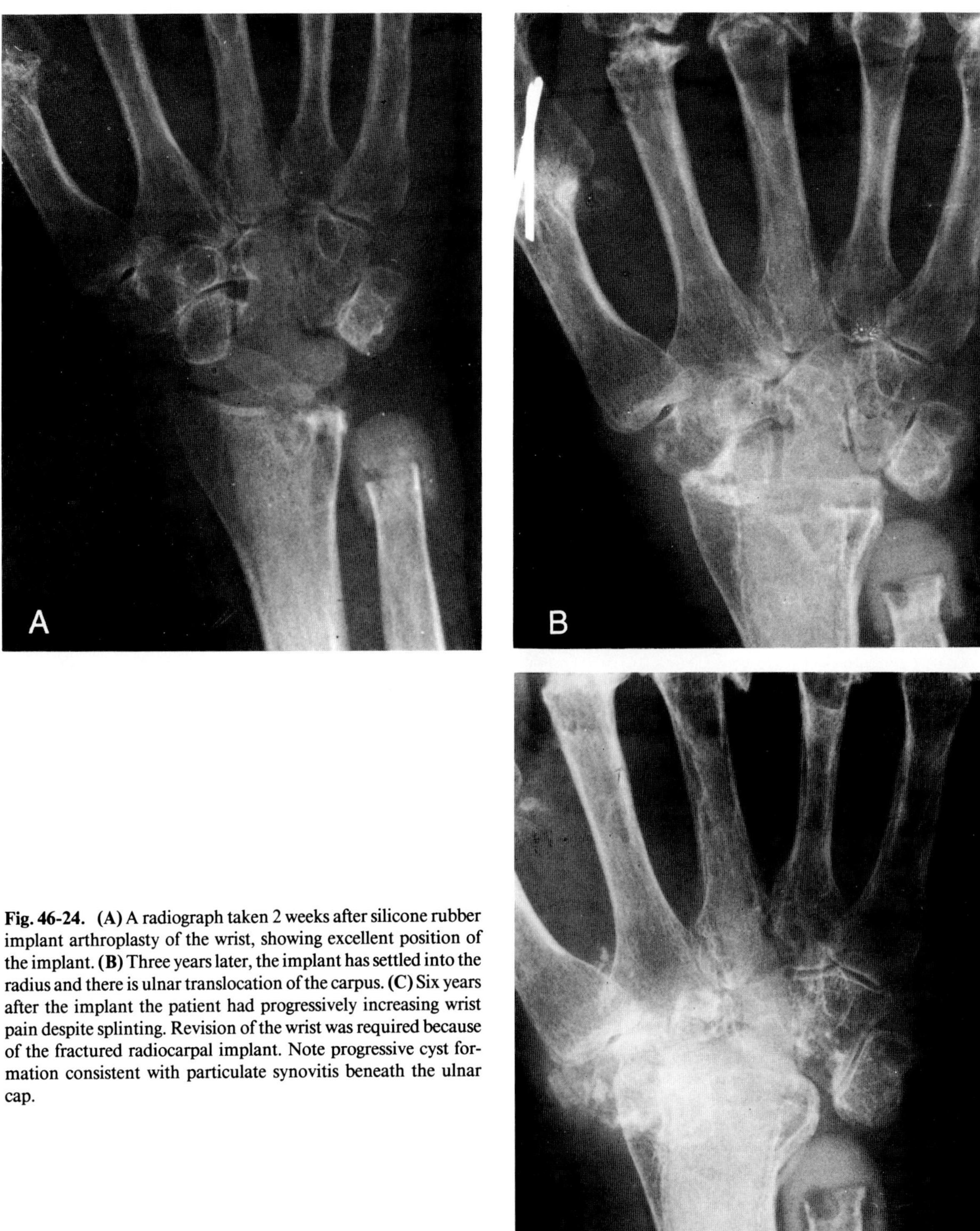

Fig. 46-24. **(A)** A radiograph taken 2 weeks after silicone rubber implant arthroplasty of the wrist, showing excellent position of the implant. **(B)** Three years later, the implant has settled into the radius and there is ulnar translocation of the carpus. **(C)** Six years after the implant the patient had progressively increasing wrist pain despite splinting. Revision of the wrist was required because of the fractured radiocarpal implant. Note progressive cyst formation consistent with particulate synovitis beneath the ulnar cap.

tomy of the less involved joints may relieve pain, yet preserve 25 to 50 percent of wrist motion (Fig. 46-25).

Choice of Operation for the Rheumatoid Wrist

Because of the increased number of surgical options now available for the reconstruction of joints affected by rheumatoid arthritis, preoperative clinical evaluation must be done carefully. After this, a considered recommendation for treatment can be made. Patient education, nonoperative treatment, including splinting and the judicious use of steroid injections, and hand therapy with modification of wrist use patterns all are important.

Distal ulna excision alone may be indicated in the patient whose symptoms are limited to the radioulnar joint and whose radiocarpal joint is stable and functional, even when the radiocarpal joint shows significant destruction on radiographs.[84,85] Distal ulna excision combined with radiocarpal synovectomy can be performed when there is mild to moderate loss of articular cartilage from the radiocarpal joint or early erosive changes within the carpus.

We have found (as have others[224,265]) that synovectomy alone can slow or even prevent progression in some cases. When soft tissue procedures or limited bony procedures are not appropriate, the decision to perform a total wrist arthrodesis or an implant arthroplasty must be made.[282] We have had no experience with total wrist arthroplasty using a metal-plastic prosthesis. (See Chapter 7 for the operative technique of total wrist arthroplasty.)

In summary, our indications for wrist arthroplasty with a Silastic wrist implant have decreased; we favor limited wrist fusions in patients with early collapse patterns of the wrist and in those with destruction limited to the radiocarpal joints. We advise wrist fusion in patients who require radiocarpal reconstruction, but who are likely to place high demand on the wrist after surgery, or who have significant wrist deformity or instability, poor wrist extensor function, or poor bone stock.

Partial Wrist Arthrodesis—Operative Technique

The wrist is exposed as described previously for synovectomy. The proximal and midcarpal rows are identified and a synovectomy is performed using a small rongeur. Articular cartilage is removed from the joints selected for limited fusion. Cancellous bone is exposed by removing or "fish-scaling" the subchondral plate. The contours of the individual carpal bones are preserved to allow apposition of the prepared surfaces. It is

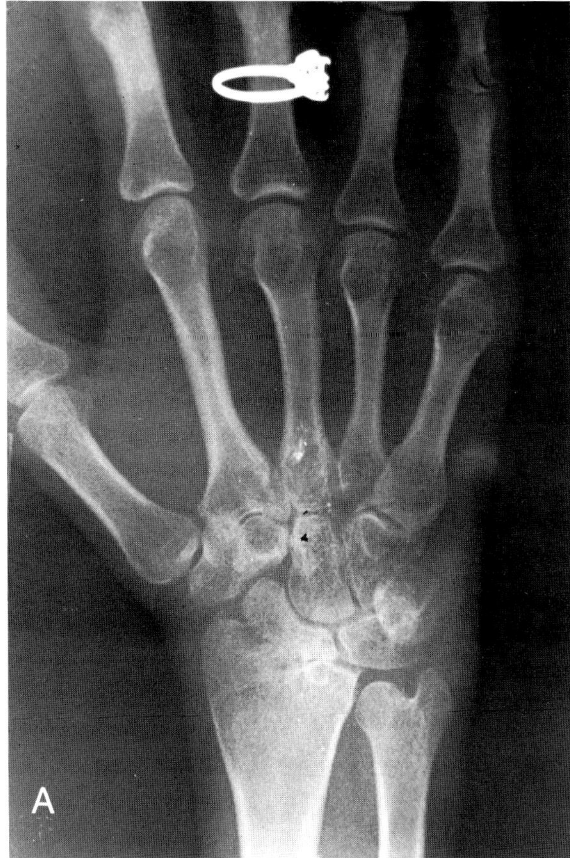

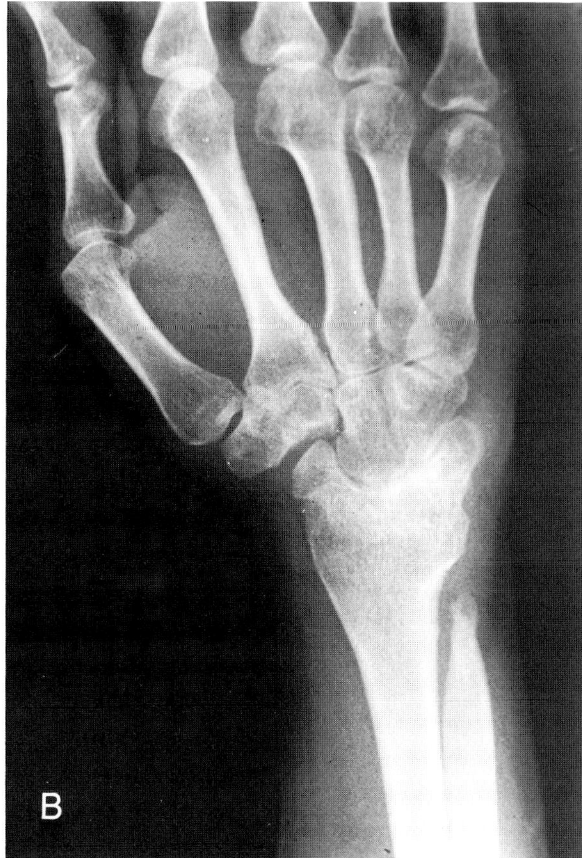

Fig. 46-25. Partial wrist fusion. **(A)** Isolated destruction of the radiocarpal joint and ulnar translocation of the carpus with preservation of the midcarpal joints. **(B)** Correction of wrist alignment with preservation of some wrist motion by partial wrist fusion (radius-scaphoid-lunate).

important to preserve the overall dimensions of the carpus; i.e., the carpal bones should not be "collapsed" onto one another after the cartilage and subchondral are removed. Rather, the resulting space should be filled with bone graft. When a proximal row fusion is performed, we usually fuse the radius, scaphoid, and lunate bones. If the articular surface of the scaphoid is preserved, the fusion may be limited to the radiolunate articulation alone as reported by Chamay[34] and by Linscheid.[136]

If a midcarpal fusion is necessary, we include all of the joints surrounding the capitate.

Autogenous bone graft is used to supplement the fusion site. Cancellous bone is packed between the individual bones to be fused. The distal ulna can be used as bone graft if a distal ulna excision has been performed. Alternatively, bone may be harvested from the distal radius either by removing Lister's tubercle or by making a small window in the dorsal cortex of the distal radius.[152] We prefer internal fixation with multiple 0.045-inch smooth K-wires. These may be cut beneath the skin or be left protruding through the skin. The Shapiro stapling device can be used to augment internal fixation.[223]

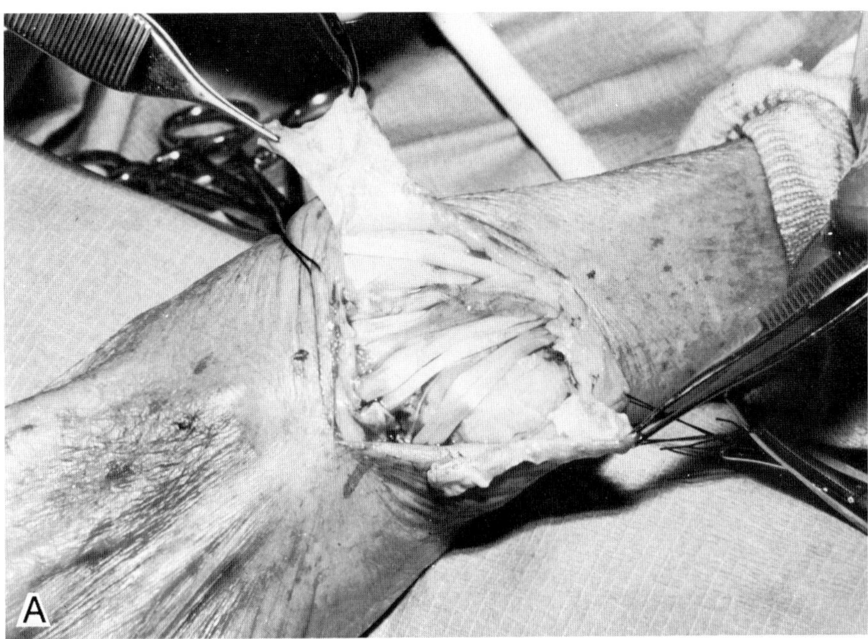

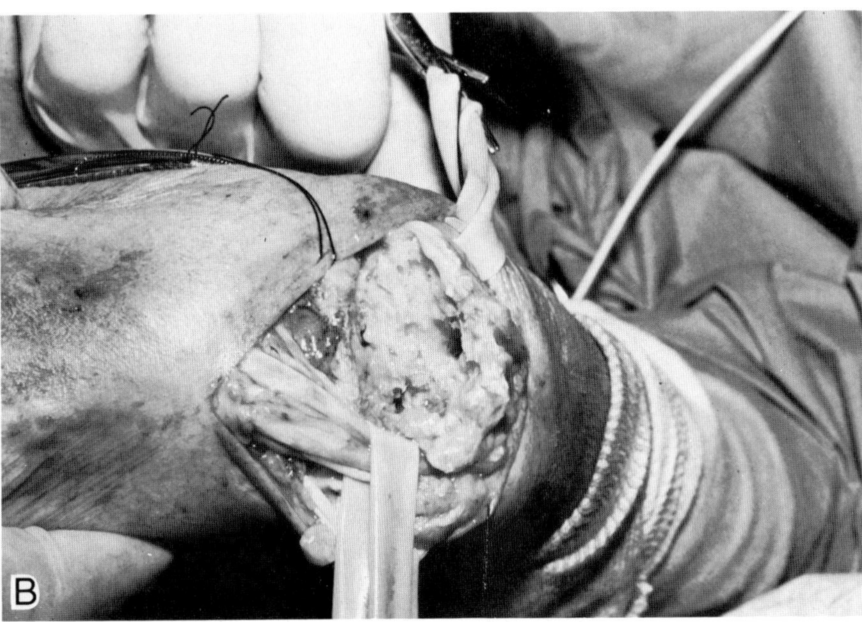

Fig. 46-26. Technique for wrist arthrodesis. **(A)** Slightly curved dorsal incision with the extensor retinaculum reflected and dorsal tenosynovectomy performed. **(B)** Cartilage and sclerotic bone excised and cancellous bone exposed. Note the medullary canal of radius perforated to test the size of the Steinmann pin. *(Figure continues.)*

Postoperatively, the wrist is immobilized in a short arm cast for 4 to 6 weeks, at which time the K-wires are removed. Short arm cast immobilization for an additional 3 to 4 weeks is necessary until there is evidence of solid fusion on radiographs.

We expect to retain 25 to 50 percent normal wrist motion following limited wrist arthrodesis.

Taleisnik[263] has described partial wrist fusion combined with carpal bone implant arthroplasty in selected rheumatoid patients with radiocarpal destruction or ulnar translocation and an unsatisfactory midcarpal articular surface of either the capitate or the scaphoid. If the articular surface of the head of the capitate has been eroded, he excises the proximal pole of the capitate and replaces it with either a Silastic condylar implant or with a soft tissue spacer, such as a rolled-up length of tendon graft ("anchovy"). If the articular surface of the scaphoid is unsatisfactory, but the capitate-lunate articulation has been preserved, he fuses the lunate to the radius and replaces the scaphoid with a Silastic implant. In both procedures, the radiocarpal joint is stabilized and midcarpal motion is maintained.[262]

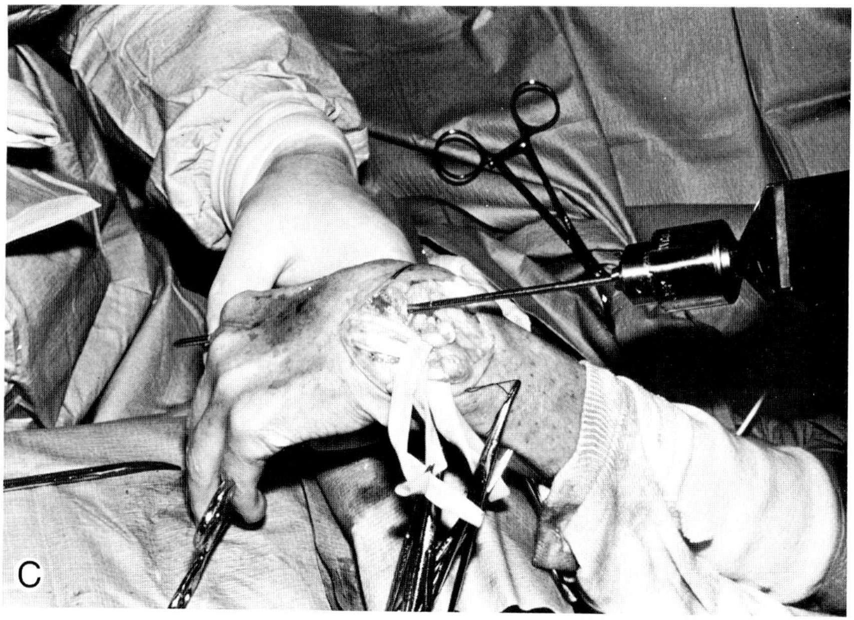

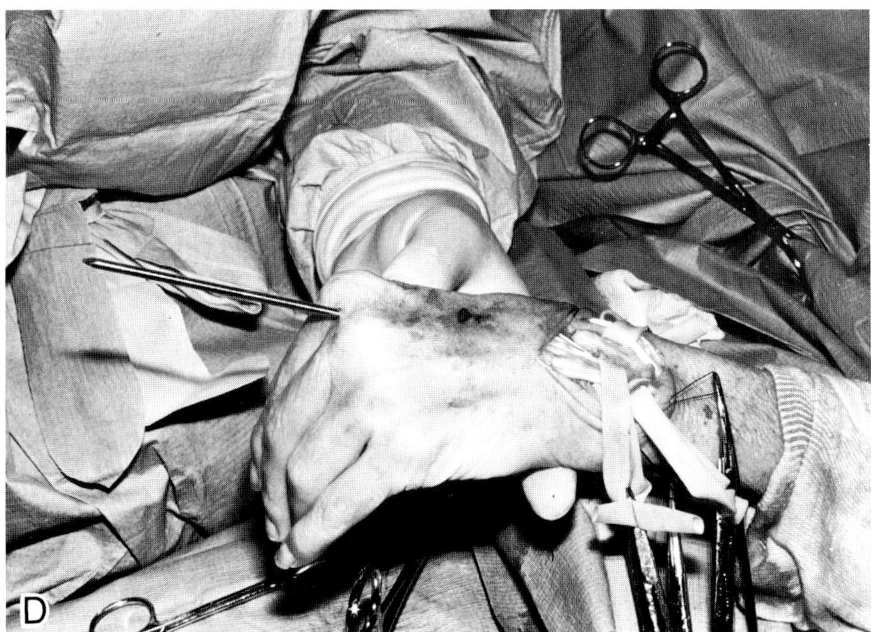

Fig. 46-26 *(Continued).* **(C)** A Steinmann pin introduced into the carpus exits between the second and third metacarpals. **(D)** The Steinmann pin is driven into the radius and countersunk between the second and third metacarpals. *(Figure continues.)*

Wrist Arthrodesis—Operative Technique (Fig. 46-26)

The wrist is exposed through a dorsal longitudinal incision similar to that for the wrist procedures described previously. A dorsal tenosynovectomy and associated procedures are performed. The radiocarpal joint is exposed by elevating a distally-based flap of wrist capsule. The distal ulna is exposed and excised as described previously. The radioulnar capsule and triangular fibrocartilage are preserved for closure later. With traction and moderate flexion, a synovectomy of the radiocarpal joint is performed. The radial collateral ligament is released from the radial styloid, avoiding the abductor pollicis longus and extensor pollicis brevis tendons located in the first dorsal compartment. The cartilage and sclerotic bone are removed from the distal radius and proximal carpal row with a rongeur to provide proper alignment. The amount of bone resected is determined by the degree of deformity and subluxation.

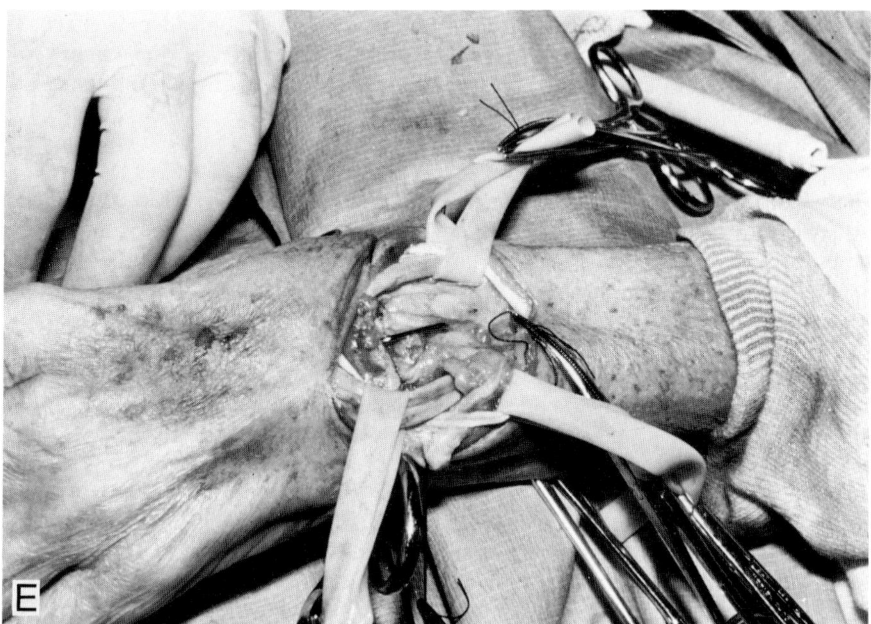

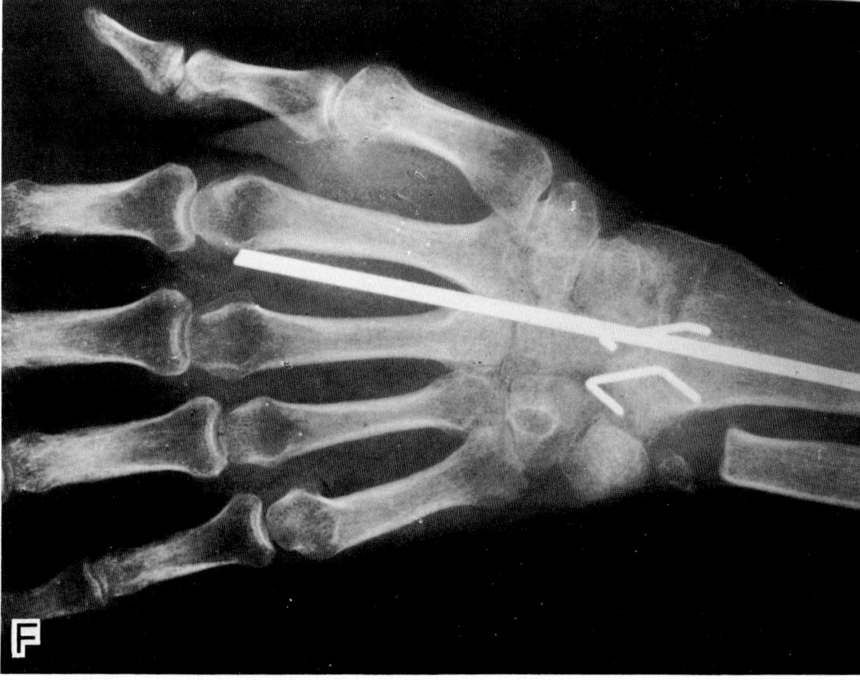

Fig. 46-26 *(Continued).* **(E)** One or two staples are driven across the radiocarpal joint. **(F)** The postoperative radiographic appearance. (From Millender and Nalebuff,[165] with permission.)

In the standard procedure the medullary canal of the radius is perforated with a pointed awl to provide a channel for the Steinmann pin to be used for internal fixation. The largest pin that will fit the medullary canal of the radius is selected. The pin is tapped through the carpus to exit between the second and third or between the third and fourth metacarpals, depending on the alignment between the carpus and radius. The pin should exit between the MP joints. Following this, the pin is tapped with a mallet retrograde into the previously prepared channel in the radius and countersunk approximately 2 cm proximal to the level of MP joints. Cutting the pointed end of the pin with a sterile bolt cutter will minimize the risk of penetrating the cortex as the pin is advanced by tapping it with a mallet. Power should not be used to insert the pin into the radius because of the increased chance of cortex penetration or fracture. Bone chips from the resected segment of the ulna are packed into the radiocarpal joint before the carpus is impacted against the radius. One or two small staples or an obliquely placed K-wire may be used to provide additional fixation of the radiocarpal joint if necessary. The K-wire generally has to be removed later; the staples may remain in permanently.

If there is severe loss of carpal bone stock, the Steinmann pin is introduced into the third metacarpal to provide stability. If the MP joints are dislocated and MP joint arthroplasties are indicated, the rod can be drilled through the distal end of the metacarpal and countersunk proximally, and an MP joint arthroplasty can be performed subsequently. If MP joint arthroplasty is not indicated, the Steinmann pin is introduced into the third metacarpal through a hole in the cortex made just proximal to the collateral ligament. This avoids passing the pin through the interosseous muscles and through the MP joint. Leaving the rod buried in the metacarpal has not caused problems.

This method requires that the wrist be fused in a neutral position, i.e., the metacarpal aligned with the radius. We have found that this is an excellent wrist position for most rheumatoid patients and have utilized this method for patients requiring bilateral wrist fusions. The position of the wrist can be varied only 5 to 10 degrees by adjusting the direction of the pin as it is driven into the radius. The position of the wrist cannot be altered after the rod has been inserted. The single rod, albeit large in diameter, does not provide secure rotatory stability of the carpus to the distal radius.

Feldon uses a modification of the technique described above for wrist fusions in both rheumatoid and nonrheumatoid patients. The wrist is prepared as described previously. Instead of using a single large Steinmann pin, two relatively thin Steinmann pins (3/32 to 7/64-inch diameter) are inserted through the second and third web spaces between the metacarpal bones, across the carpus, and into the medullary canal of the radius. This results in a "stacked-pin" effect in the radius that provides rotational stability as well as anteroposterior and lateral stability, without the need for supplementary internal fixation (Fig. 46-27). The pins are thin enough to be bent after insertion into the radius, allowing final correction and adjustment of the wrist position. Thus, if slightly more dorsiflexion is desired after the rods are in place, the wrist is gently manipulated into the correct position. The use of thinner pins minimizes the potential for compression of the intrinsic muscles of the hand (interossei) by a large rod. Care must be taken to insert the pins through the dorsal portion of the web space to avoid potential damage to the neurovascular structures in the palm. It is sometimes helpful to make a small window in the dorsal cortex of the distal radius. This allows the pins to be guided into the medullary canal of the radius under direct vision. Additional cancellous bone graft may be harvested from the distal radius as well. The pins are cut short beneath the skin in the web spaces and are removed after solid bony union has occurred, usually between 4 to 6 months postoperatively, or if they become symptomatic. However, the pins have been left in situ for many years without adverse effect. The pins are removed under local anesthesia by making a vertical incision in the web space and grasping the pin end with a 10- to 12-inch "diamond-jaw" needle holder.

Solid union has been obtained in more than 30 patients over the past several years. This technique has been used in rheumatoid patients even when carpal bone stock has been minimal. The advantages of this method include ease of hardware insertion and removal, the ability to adjust the position of the wrist at the time of surgery in both the anteroposterior and lateral planes, and stable fixation even with suboptimal bone stock.

Tourniquet release, drainage, and closure are performed as described previously. A bulky dressing and a sugar-tong or long arm splint are used until the first dressing change. After this, only a short arm cast or splint is necessary if the internal fixation is stable and the soft tissue reconstruction of the distal radioulnar joint will allow early forearm rotation. The forearm is held is supination for 2 to 3 weeks if this joint must be protected. Short arm cast or splint immobilization facilitates early motion of the elbow and shoulder, as well as the forearm, and is much easier for patients to tolerate. The patient may walk with platform crutches 7 to 10 days after wrist fusion (Fig. 46-28).

When the single Steinmann pin technique is used, the pin is not removed unless it causes discomfort or migrates. Rarely, the pin migrates distally enough to penetrate the skin. Should this occur, the pin is removed and supplementary external fixation used if appropriate. Reintroduction of a pin that has come through the skin should be avoided because of the risk of infection.

Combined Wrist Arthrodesis and MP Joint Arthroplasty—Operative Technique (Fig. 46-29)

It is not unusual that a patient with severe rheumatoid arthritis will require both wrist fusion and reconstruction of the MP joints. Ordinarily, this would necessitate two separate surgical procedures. However, we have performed both procedures during one operation.[169] This combined procedure is indicated in patients with painful wrists (but without significant wrist deformity) and who are appropriate candidates for MP joint arthroplasty. The single, definite contraindication for this combined procedure is a severely deformed or dislocated wrist that would require extensive exposure to correct the radiocarpal alignment.

A less extensive exposure, without dislocation of the radio-

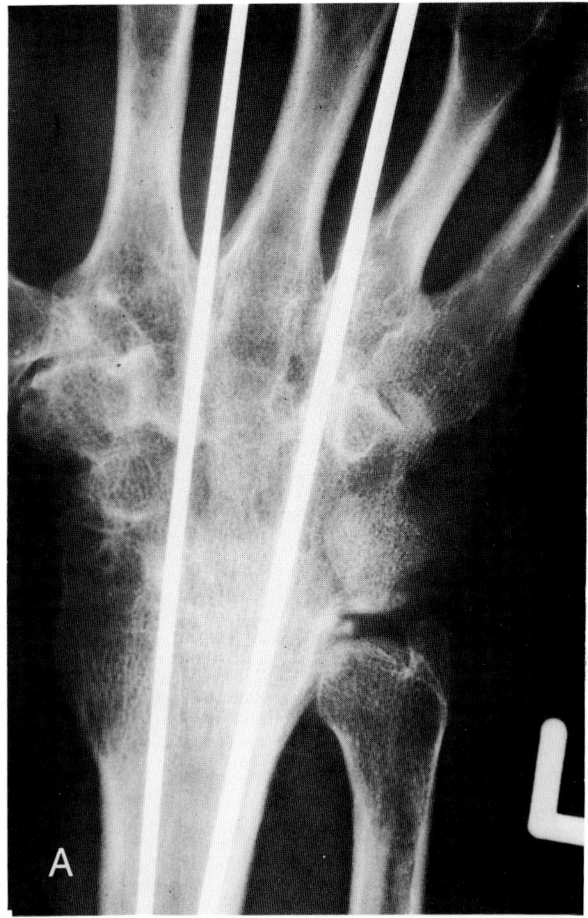

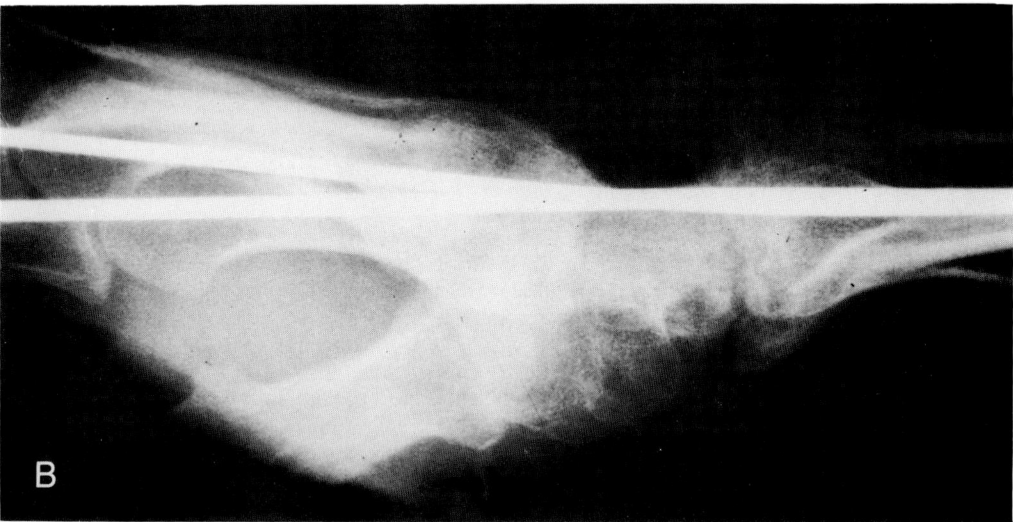

Fig. 46-27. Wrist fusion using dual intermetacarpal-intramedullary Steinmann pins for internal fixation. **(A)** Solid fusion was obtained with the wrist in slight ulnar deviation. **(B)** The wrist is in slight dorsiflexion. The pins are positioned on the dorsal aspect of the wrist to minimize the risk of damage to the soft tissue structures in the palm, and to facilitate placement of the pins in the medullary canal of the radius.

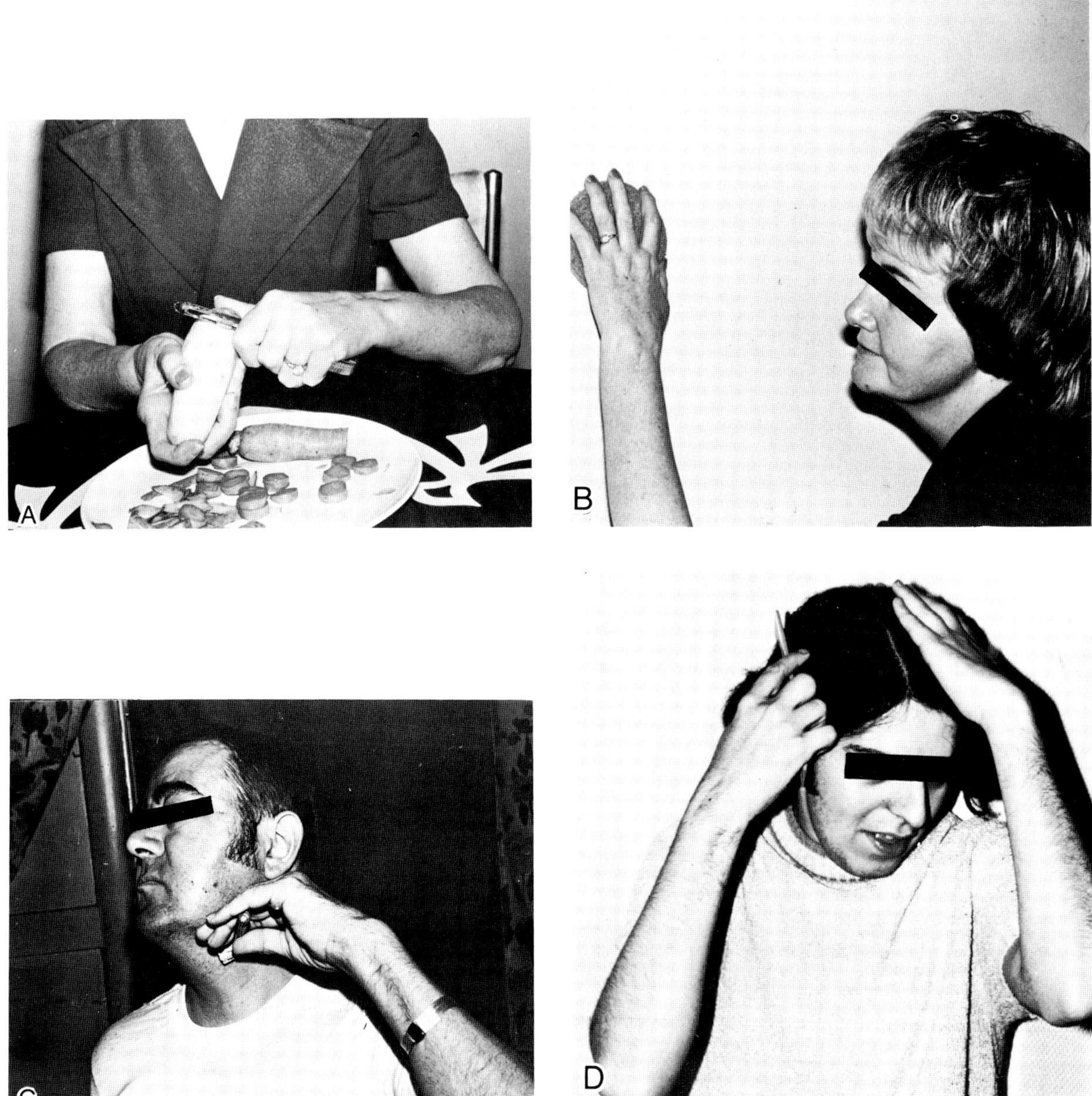

Fig. 46-28. Improved function following wrist fusion. **(A)** Peeling potatoes. **(B)** Adjusting for lack of wrist extension. **(C)** Shaving. **(D)** Substituting elbow flexion for loss of wrist flexion when combing hair. (From Millender and Nalebuff,[165] with permission.)

carpal joint, is used to prepare the wrist for fusion. This allows the MP joint arthroplasty to be performed with minimal risk of excessive postoperative edema and its attendant risk of skin slough and other complications.

The procedure is a modification of the technique for wrist arthrodesis described above. A dorsoulnar skin incision is made, exposing the extensor digiti quinti and, if necessary, the extensor digitorum communis. The distal ulna is excised and a limited dorsal tenosynovectomy is performed. An arthrotomy of the radiocarpal joint is made either through the radioulnar joint capsule or through a separate dorsal radiocarpal capsular incision. Through these incisions, synovectomy, debridement, and preparation of the joint for fusion can be accomplished with a small rongeur. We have found that by removing the cartilage and sclerotic subchondral bone and by softening the distal radius and carpus to form a fusion mass of cancellous bone, solid arthrodesis can be obtained. Preparation is facilitated by applying traction to the hand to distract the joints. If there is moderate flexion or deviation of the radiocarpal joint, alignment can be restored through the limited capsular incision by removing more of the radial styloid and/or carpus with a rongeur. After adequate preparation, the medullary canal of

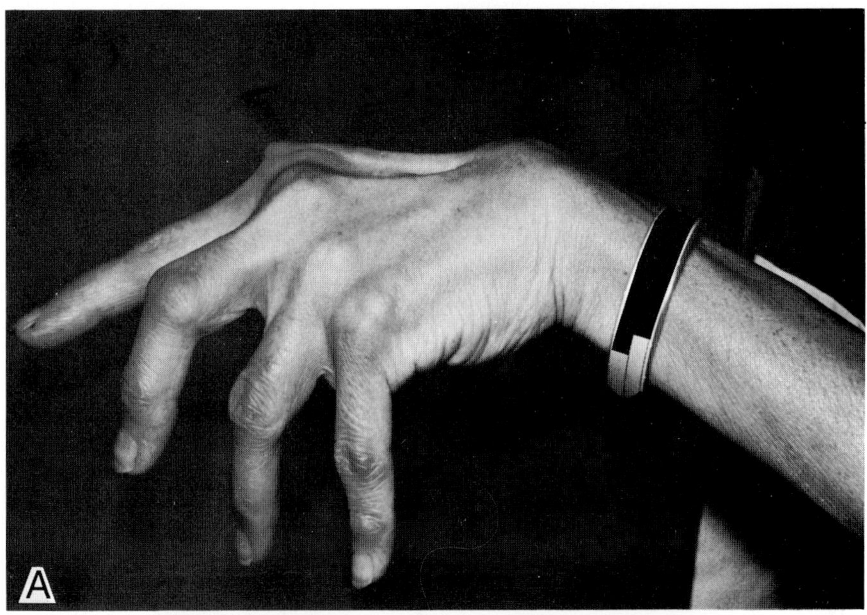

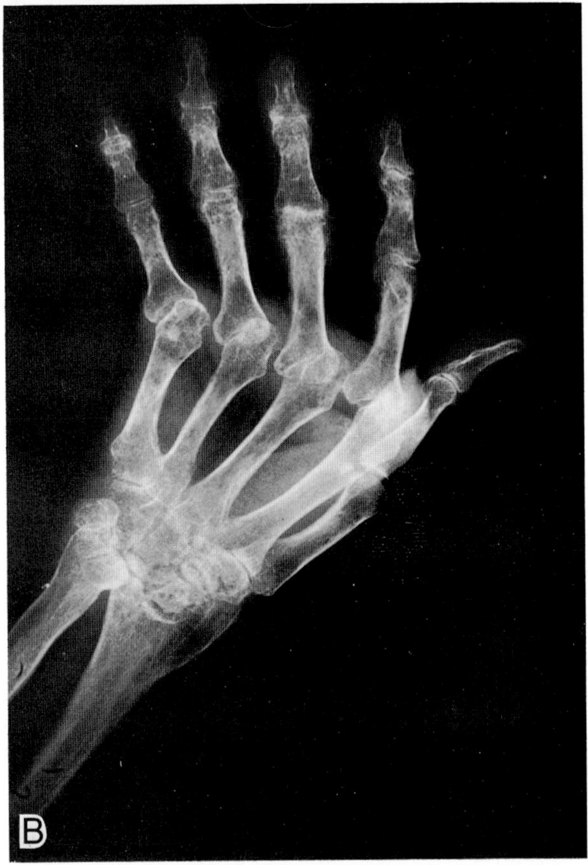

Fig. 46-29. Closed wrist fusion combined with MP joint arthroplasty. **(A)** A patient with a painful wrist and dislocated MP joints. **(B)** Radiograph demonstrates the destroyed wrist joint and dislocated MP joints. *(Figure continues.)*

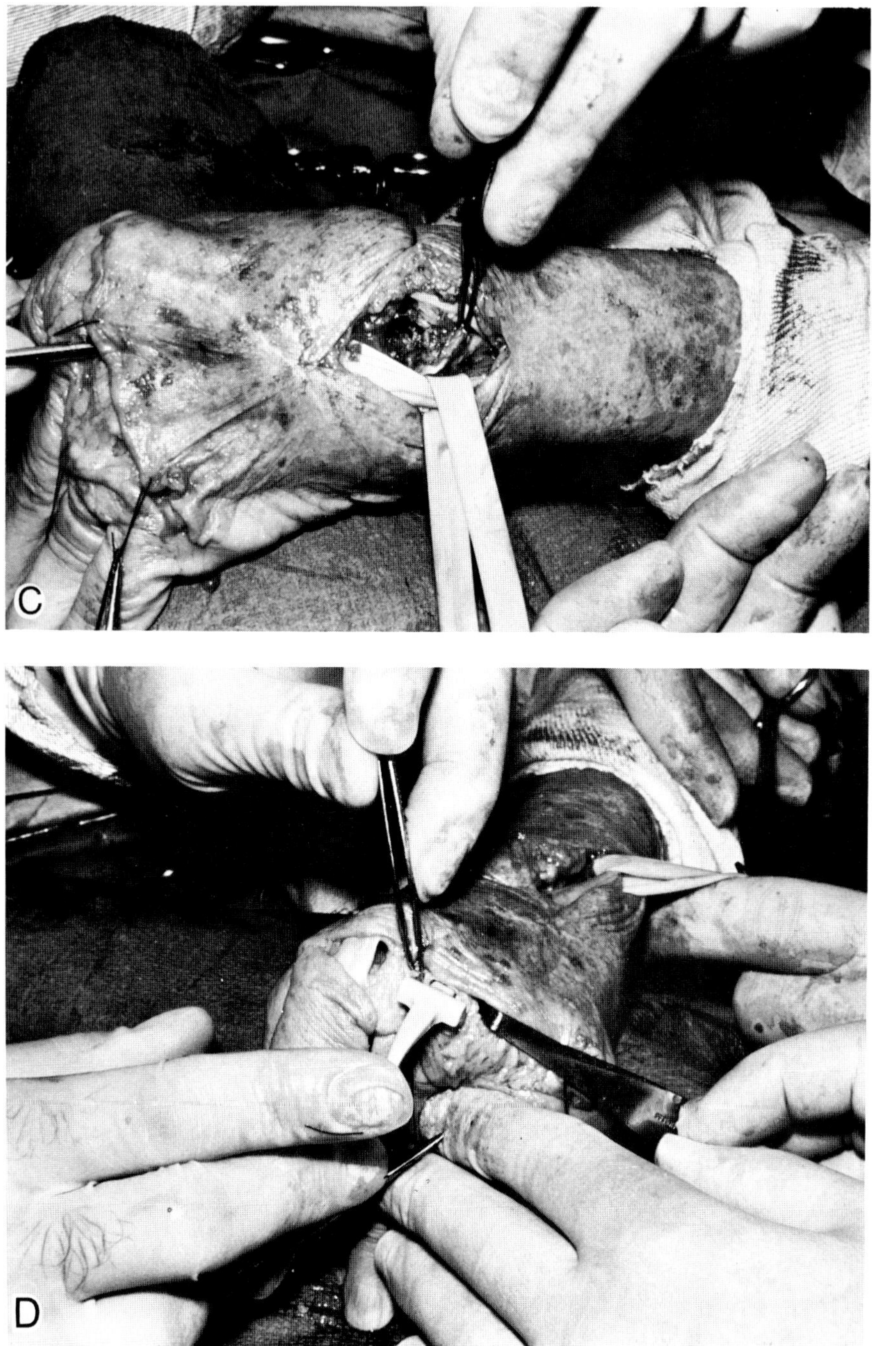

Fig. 46-29 *(Continued).* **(C)** Minimal dorsal tenosynovectomy is performed, the distal ulna is excised, and the distal radius and carpus are crushed with a rongeur to form a fusion mass. The metacarpal heads have been resected and the Steinmann pin has been introduced. **(D)** After the Steinmann pin has been countersunk and a bone plug packed into the metacarpal to prevent distal migration of the Steinmann pin, the implants are introduced. *(Figure continues.)*

the third metacarpal can be aligned with the radius. Following preparation of the wrist, the MP joint arthroplasties are performed using a transverse incision over the metacarpal heads. Prior to introducing the MP joint implant, a large smooth Steinmann pin is introduced into the third metacarpal through the distal end and tapped through the carpus into the radiocarpal joint. The pin is introduced into the medullary canal of the radius under direct vision. Intraoperative radiographs are obtained to confirm appropriate pin position. After the pin has been tapped into the radius, radiocarpal stability is evaluated. A staple across the radiocarpal joint can be used for additional fixation, but it usually is not necessary. The distal end of the

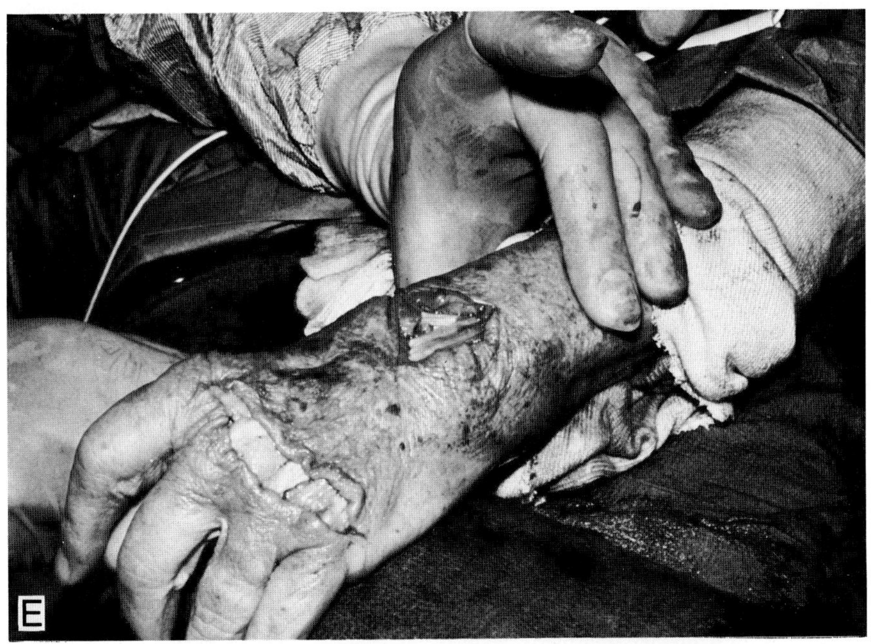

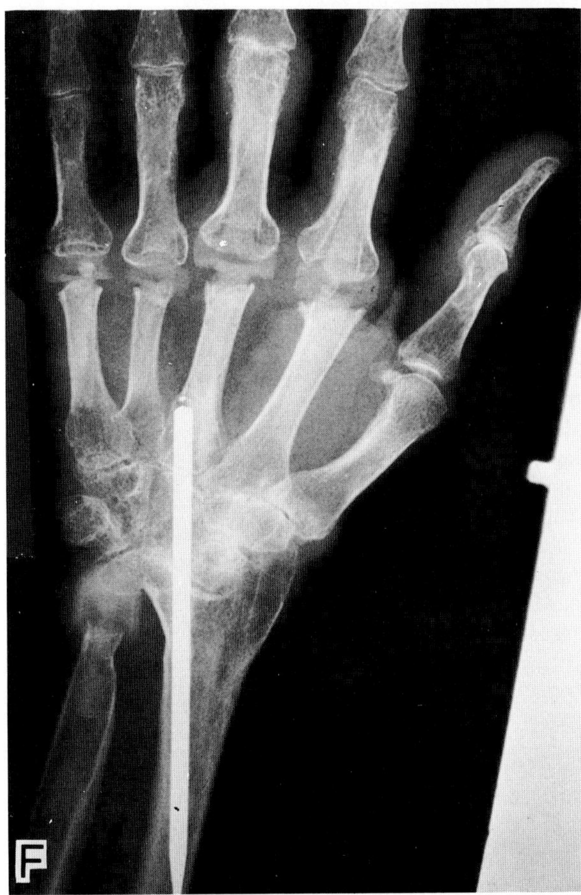

Fig. 46-29 *(Continued).* **(E)** Completed procedure prior to closure. **(F)** Radiographic appearance. Note how far the Steinmann pin has been countersunk in the third metacarpal.

pin is cut and countersunk 3 to 3.5 cm into the metacarpal bone to allow room for the MP joint implant. Care must be taken not to countersink too far so that adequate purchase on the metacarpal is lost. After the pin is countersunk, cancellous bone is tapped into the medullary canal prior to introducing the implant. This assures that the rod will not back out. The MP joint arthroplasties now are completed in the usual manner (see Chapter 7). Routine closure over drains and immobilization in a bulky dressing with a volar plaster splint complete the procedure.

Postoperative management for combined wrist fusion and MP arthroplasty is the same as for MP joint arthroplasty alone. A volar wrist splint is used for 4 to 6 weeks. This splint may be combined with the dynamic splint used for the postoperative management of MP joint arthroplasties or the dynamic splint can be fabricated over a plaster volar wrist splint.

Complications of Wrist Fusion

Complications following wrist fusion were reviewed by Clendenin and Green.[45] The most frequent complication in their series was pseudarthrosis. In our experience, pseudarthrosis occurs infrequently in the rheumatoid patient, usually is asymptomatic, and rarely requires further treatment. Ryu and Watson[215] have described producing a fibrous nonunion intentionally in rheumatoid patients. Other complications occurred rarely, but included deep wound infection, superficial skin necrosis, transient median nerve or superficial radial nerve compression, fracture of the healed fusion, and pin migration.

THE MP JOINTS

The MP joint is the key joint for function of the fingers. Rheumatoid destruction of this joint results in severe deformity and functional loss. MP joints are condylar, allowing motion in two separate planes. Because of this anatomic configuration, their inherent stability is less than that of the interphalangeal joints, and, therefore, they are more vulnerable to the deforming forces present in rheumatoid arthritis.

The causes of deformity of MP joints have been the subject of much debate. There are multiple factors leading to the classic ulnar drift and volar dislocation seen in rheumatoid patients. An understanding of the various factors leading to these deformities is important for the surgeon dealing with these problems.[21,24,68,76,98,103,112,153,228,274,292]

Etiology of Rheumatoid MP Joint Deformities

The deforming forces begin as proliferative synovitis stretches the capsule and ligamentous structures. In the MP joints this proliferation occurs in the recess between the metacarpal head and collateral ligament attachment, resulting in fraying and fragmentation of the collateral ligaments. Flatt believes that loosening of the ligaments markedly decreases the stability of the joint and is one of the early factors leading to progressive deformity.[76] The normal MP joint is stable in full flexion, with little lateral motion possible in this position. However, in the rheumatoid patient the flexed MP joint often can be deviated 45 degrees.

The following factors affect the altered MP joint, ultimately resulting in volar subluxation or dislocation, and ulnar deviation: (1) wrist deformity, (2) flexor and extensor tendon forces, (3) intrinsic muscle imbalance, and (4) the forces of gravity and pinch. Wilson[292] has described the interaction of these forces in detail.

Shapiro[220,221] showed that wrist collapse leads to radial deviation of the metacarpals and, subsequently, to an increased tendency for ulnar deviation of the MP joints affected by the rheumatoid process (see page 1623 and Fig. 46-19). This is an expansion of the intercalary collapse theory of Landsmeer. Pahle and Raunio,[202] Hastings and Evans,[108] and others have confirmed these observations.[228,237,274]

The extrinsic extensor and flexor tendons also affect ulnar drift.[278] In the rheumatoid hand, the extensor tendons often are shifted or even dislocated ulnarward. Selective stretching of the radial side transverse lamina (sagittal band) fibers by synovial proliferation and the normal ulnar shift of the extensor tendons during MP flexion as the fourth and fifth metacarpal bones descend (which may be increased in rheumatoid arthritis by laxity of the fourth and fifth carpometacarpal joints) contribute to this ulnar subluxation.

Flexor tendon forces also contribute to MP joint deformity.[226] Flatt has demonstrated that during pinch there are palmar and ulnar forces in the index and long fingers and a palmar force at the MP joint levels in all four fingers.[77] Stretching of the collateral ligaments of the MP joints, which support the flexor tendon sheath, allows a volar and ulnar shift of the A2 pulley mechanism, which can increase the tendency toward MP joint deformity significantly. The anatomic configuration of the joint and the forces of the intrinsic mechanism contribute to the ulnar deviation tendency.

Operative Treatment of the MP Joint — Indications

Operative procedures for the MP joint are either preventive or reconstructive. The only potentially prophylactic procedure is synovectomy (Fig. 46-30). Reconstructive procedures include soft tissue surgical reconstruction and various types of arthroplasties.

The indications for either synovectomy alone or synovectomy with soft tissue reconstruction are difficult to define because no study has shown definitively that these procedures will affect the natural course of the disease. Although synovectomy is considered by some to arrest the local disease or to slow progression of the disease and allow erosive lesions to heal, recurrence always is possible. Recurrent synovitis may occur as early as several months or as late as many years following the procedure. It is impossible to predetermine those patients that are likely to develop recurrence. In addition, 30 to 50 percent of patients with rheumatoid arthritis will have spontaneous

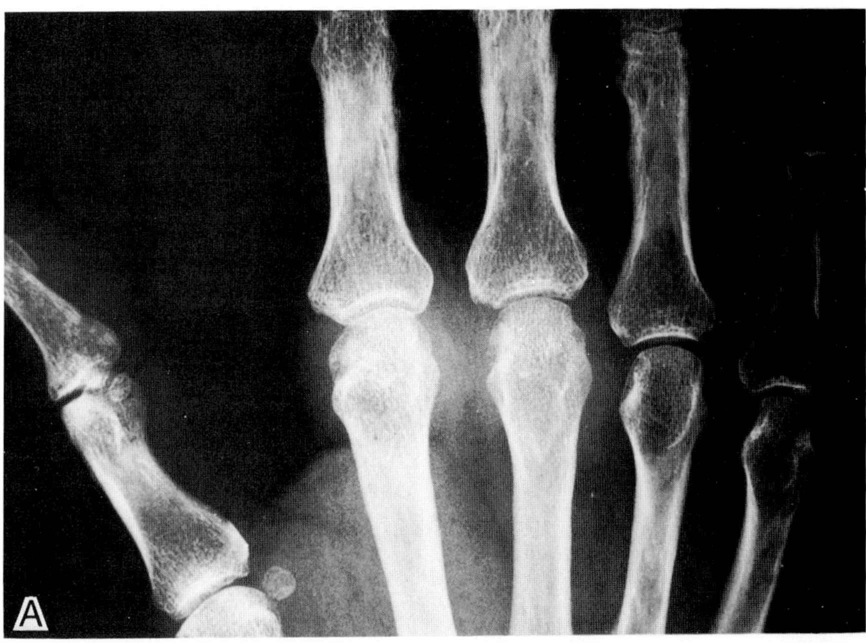

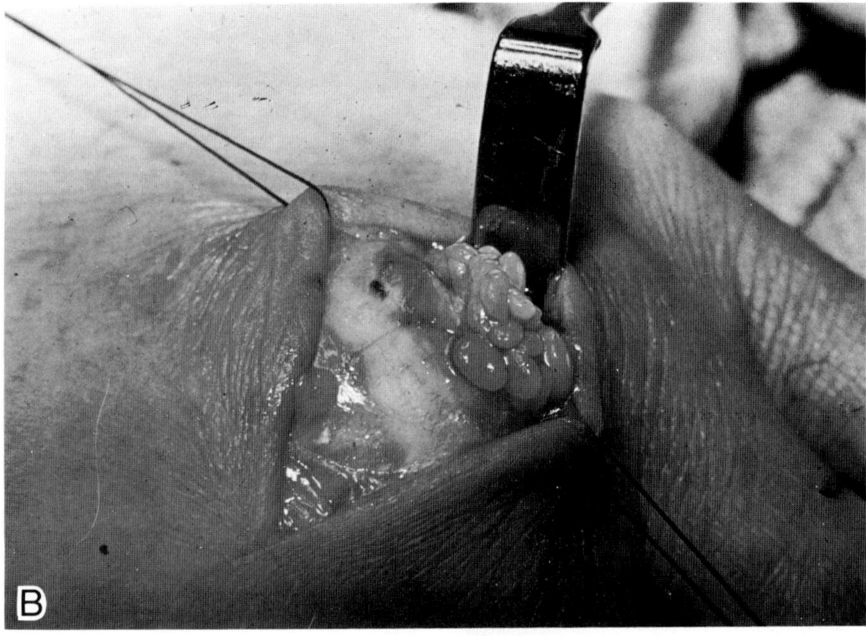

Fig. 46-30. Indications for MP joint synovectomy. **(A)** Radiograph shows minimal cartilage loss, no bony destruction, and no deformity. **(B)** Proliferative synovium bulging dorsally and stretching the extensor mechanism.

remission, thereby making it difficult to evaluate the effectiveness of any preventive surgery.[60,65,171,207,241,275]

Because of the inconclusive results following synovectomy, most rheumatologists and surgeons today take a conservative attitude toward synovectomy of the MP joints. Synovectomy is indicated for the infrequent patient with persistent MP joint synovitis, minimal radiographic changes, and minimal, if any, evidence of deformity. Intermittent, painful synovitis (which is infrequent) is an additional indication for synovectomy. Before considering synovectomy, the patient must have had an adequate trial of conservative therapy, which includes systemic medication, splinting, and up to three local intraarticular steroid injections.[117]

We consider a 6- to 9-month period of conservative therapy necessary before performing synovectomy. Within this time period, some of the patients being considered for the procedure will have a medical remission, and unnecessary surgery will be avoided. Others undergoing conservative therapy will show rapid joint destruction, and these patients would not have a good result from synovectomy. The third group of patients on conservative therapy will continue to have persistent localized synovitis with minimal, if any, deformity and minimal radiographic changes. These patients, we anticipate, will benefit on a long-term basis from synovectomy.

Combined Synovectomy and Soft Tissue Reconstruction

Our indications for combined synovectomy and soft tissue reconstruction to correct deformity are limited because the persistence of multiple deforming forces and the progression of the disease frequently result in recurrence as stated above. Synovectomy with soft tissue reconstruction is considered in a patient who is a candidate for synovectomy, but who, in addition, has early volar subluxation and ulnar drift. If the disease appears to be progressing slowly and the patient is young, soft tissue reconstruction may slow recurrence of the deformity. Occasionally, a patient presents with the inability to extend the MP joint actively because of complete dislocation of the extensor tendons, but can maintain active extension if the MP joints are extended passively. Extensor tendon relocation with synovectomy is indicated for this patient.

We believe that, in view of both the high incidence of recurrence and the alternative of MP arthroplasty, which has proved an effective, predictable, and long-lasting procedure (Fig. 46-31), soft tissue surgery alone is indicated infrequently.[7,16,81,162,176,185,201,246,248,250,273]

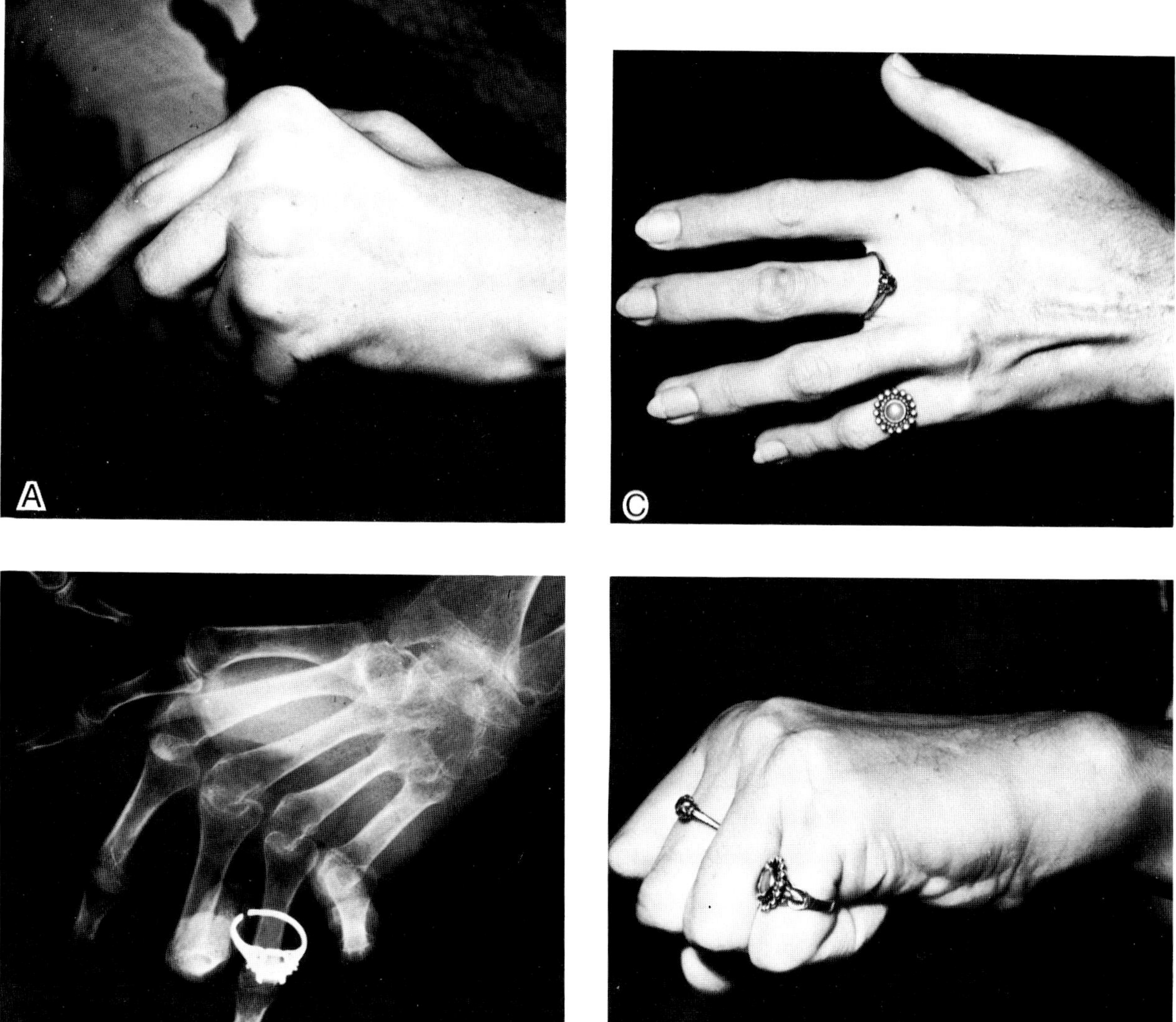

Fig. 46-31. MP joint arthroplasty to improve joint function and appearance of rheumatoid hand deformity. **(A)** Preoperative finger extension. Note MP joint subluxation with associated boutonnière deformity of the middle finger. **(B)** Preoperative radiograph shows advanced wrist involvement in addition to MP and PIP joint deformities. **(C)** Note improved function and appearance of the hand and wrist following combined wrist fusion and MP arthroplasties. **(D)** Postoperative finger flexion. (From Nalebuff and Millender,[191] with permission.)

Contraindications to MP Joint Surgery

There is a group of patients for whom surgery should not be suggested. Although these patients have definite subluxation, ulnar drift, advanced radiographic changes, and a weakened grip, they are usually pain free and have good hand function. While MP joint deformity is present, surgery will not increase their function and would probably weaken their grip. These patients are treated best with night splints and observation every 3 to 4 months. If they maintain satisfactory function, observation should be continued. If they show progressive deformity and dysfunction, they will become candidates for operative treatment.

Operative Techniques for the MP Joint

MP Joint Synovectomy (Fig. 46-32)

MP joint synovectomy on multiple joints is performed through a transverse incision centered over the dorsal aspect of the joints. Synovectomy for a single joint may be performed through a longitudinal incision located just ulnar to the joint. The longitudinal incision also is used when multiple procedures are being performed in one finger, thereby decreasing the risk of excessive swelling. The initial skin incision must not be too deep in order to avoid damage to the extensor tendons that lie immediately beneath the skin. The dorsal veins and nerves

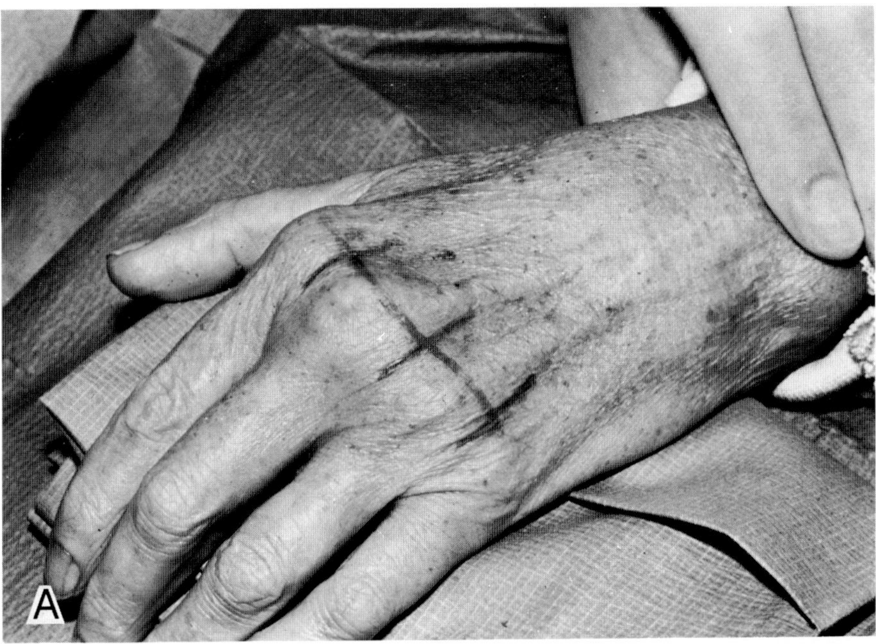

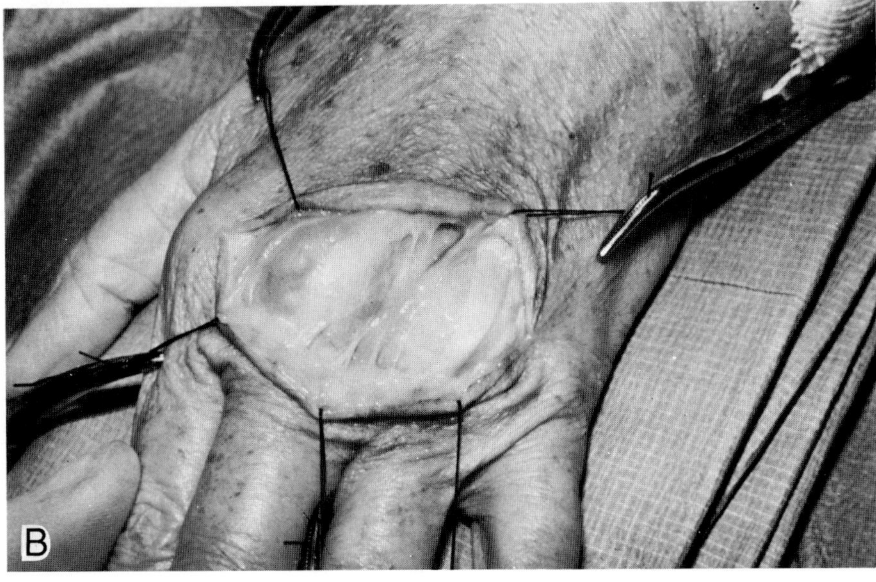

Fig. 46-32. Surgical technique for MP joint synovectomy. **(A)** Transverse incision made over the involved MP joints. **(B)** Bulging synovium has resulted in subluxation of the extensor tendons ulnarward. *(Figure continues.)*

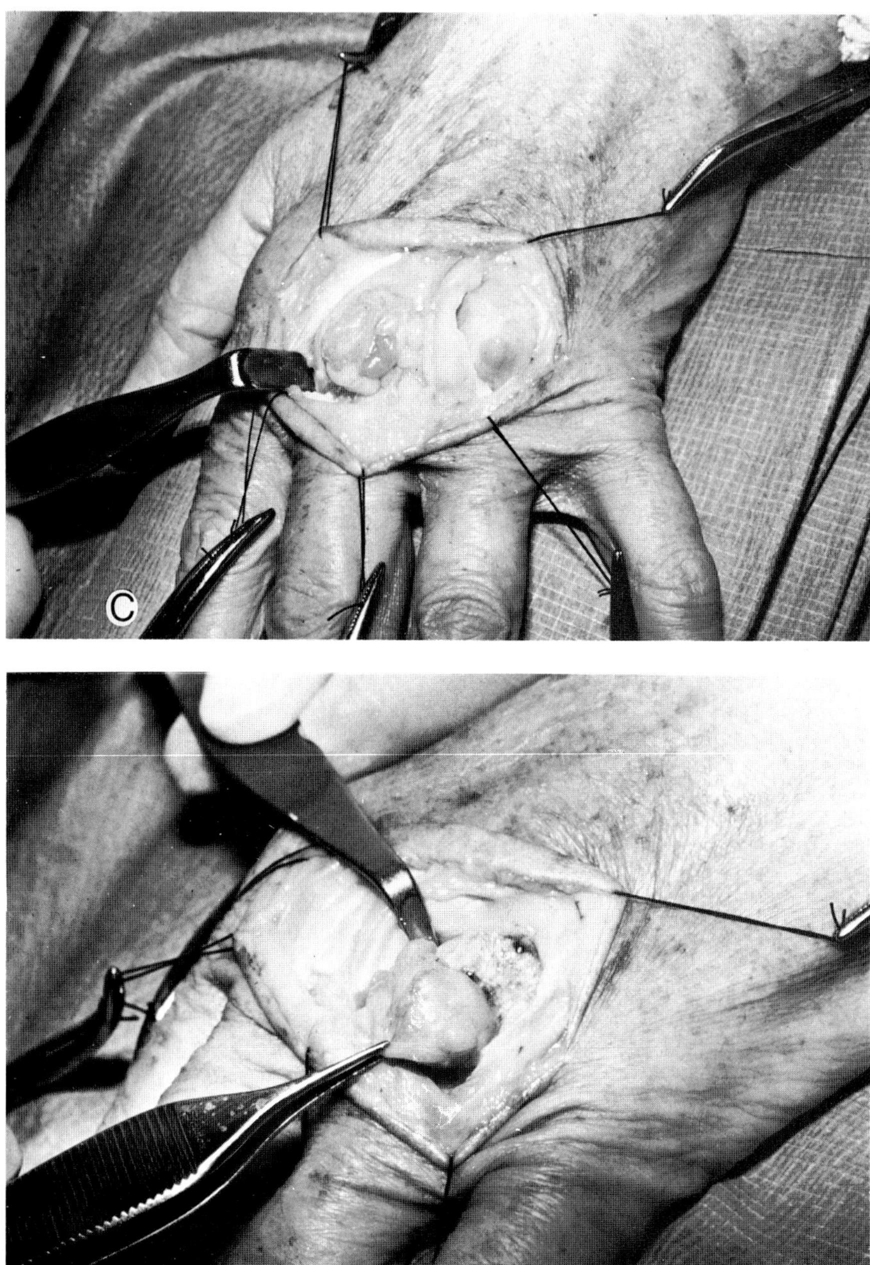

Fig. 46-32 *(Continued).* **(C)** Ulnar transverse fibers and ulnar intrinsic tendons have been released. The extensor tendons are reflected radially, exposing the underlying synovium within the MP joint. **(D)** MP joint synovectomy is performed. *(Figure continues.)*

are located within fat pads in the interdigital spaces. These structures must be protected, as injury to them may result in painful neuromas or dysesthesias and/or increase the risk of postoperative swelling with resultant adherence of the extensor mechanism.[162]

The extensor mechanism is exposed, and the areolar tissue overlying the sagittal bands is separated so that the degree of extensor tendon subluxation to the ulnar side of the joint can be determined. In early cases, there will be minimal subluxation of the tendon and no significant intrinsic tightness. We prefer to expose the joint by making an incision through the ulnar-side sagittal band, volar to and parallel with the extensor tendon. Others enter the joint from the radial side. Swanson has described splitting the extensor mechanism in the middorsal line to avoid damaging either the radial or the ulnar intrinsics. Intrinsic release is performed at this stage, if necessary (see

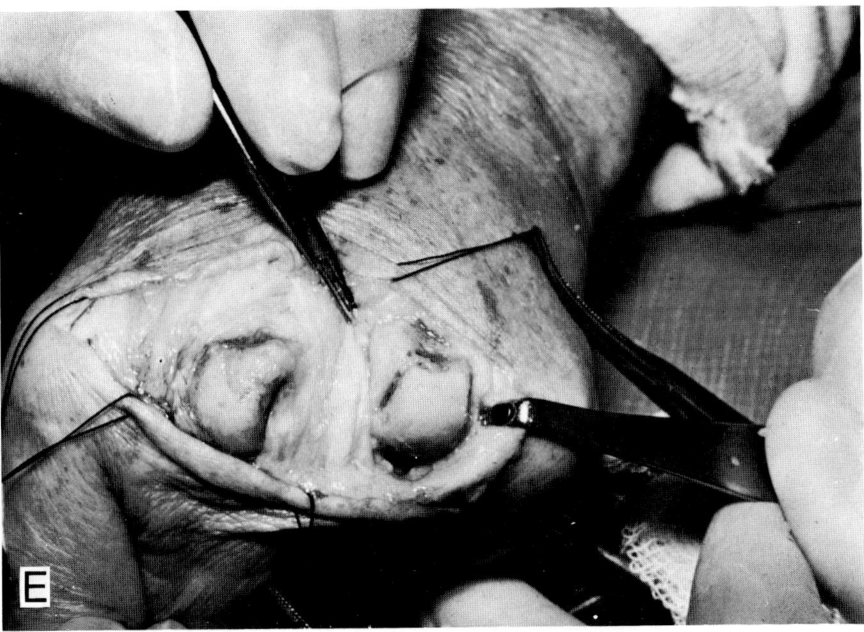

Fig. 46-32 *(Continued).* **(E)** At completion of the MP joint synovectomy, articular cartilage of the metacarpal head is demonstrated. (From Millender and Nalebuff,[164] with permission.)

below). The extensor mechanism is separated from the underlying capsule with small, blunt-tipped scissors. This dissection often is difficult because the capsule has been thinned and disrupted by proliferating synovium that has herniated dorsally or because the capsule is scarred and adherent to the extensor mechanism. The transverse orientation of the fibers of the sagittal bands serves as a guide to the plane between the capsule and extensor mechanism. The extensor mechanism is retracted radially and the joint capsule incised transversely. Bulging synovium is excised by sharp dissection or with a small rongeur. Traction applied to the finger allows easier access to the volar pouch. Synovectomy of the recess between the collateral ligament and metacarpal neck is performed with a small pituitary rongeur or a curette. Cystic areas of the metacarpal head are curetted.

After completing the synovectomy, the extensor mechanism is repositioned. If the mechanism subluxates ulnarward, it must be secured as described on page 1653. No attempt is made to close the dorsal capsule.

The wound is closed over a Penrose or suction drain placed in the subcutaneous area and a bulky conforming dressing is applied.

Active motion is begun 1 to 2 days postoperatively, and a program of dynamic splinting similar to that following MP joint arthroplasty is used for 4 weeks.

Intrinsic Release (Fig. 46-33)

Intrinsic release usually is performed in conjunction with MP joint synovectomy or MP joint arthroplasty, but may be performed as an independent procedure in one or more fingers.[3,101] Either a transverse or longitudinal incision may be used. After the dorsal neurovascular structures have been mobilized and the extensor mechanism has been identified, areolar tissue is freed from the entire ulnar side of the extensor mechanism. The sagittal, transverse, and oblique fibers of the intrinsic mechanism are identified. A longitudinal incision is made in the sagittal band adjacent to the extensor tendon. A curved hemostat is passed beneath the transverse fibers and oblique fibers to exit around the thickened portion of the oblique fibers. These structures are divided, and a section of the oblique fibers may be excised. If a release of the bony attachment is required to obtain adequate position of the MP joint, the proximal portion of the tendon is grasped with a clamp and, using scissors, the tendon attachment into the proximal phalanx is sectioned.

In the small finger, the abductor digiti quinti is a strong ulnar-deforming muscle that must be released. A blunt retractor is used to hold the skin and subcutaneous tissue out of the way. The dorsal branch of the digital nerve of the small finger is protected. The fascial sheath is incised to expose the hypothenar muscles. The abductor digiti quinti is separated from the flexor digiti quinti and is selectively sectioned at its musculotendinous junction. The ulnar neurovascular bundle lies just volar to these muscles and must be protected. Flatt has emphasized the importance of releasing only the abductor digiti quinti without sacrificing the flexor digiti quinti. He has shown that releasing the flexor digiti quinti results in limited MP joint flexion and increased weakness.[77]

Littler[101] has described an alternative method of releasing tight intrinsics. After the intrinsic mechanism is exposed, a triangular portion of the oblique fibers is excised. With this method, the transverse fibers, which act as a yoke to flex the MP joints, are left intact (see Chapter 15).

Flatt[78] has described a modified intrinsic release that he uses for early subluxation of the MP joint or for persistent flexion

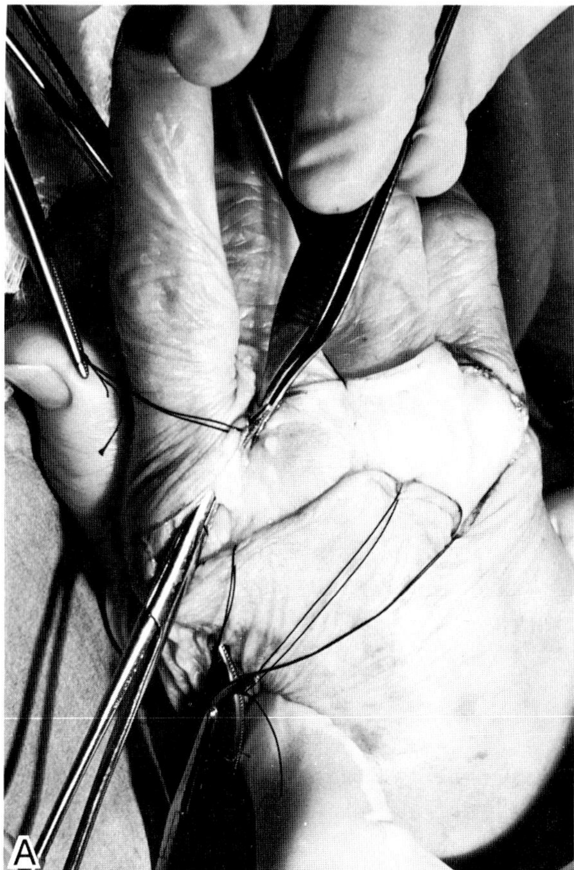

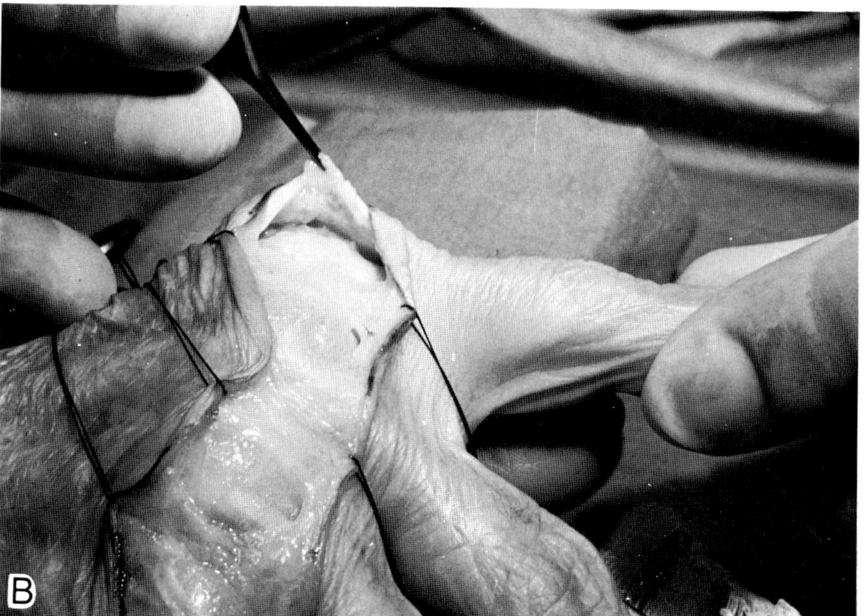

Fig. 46-33. Technique for ulnar intrinsic release and extensor tendon relocation. **(A)** Transverse incision across the MP joints. The ulnar intrinsic tendon is exposed and a hemostat is passed around the transverse and oblique intrinsic fibers prior to their release. **(B)** The extensor mechanism, including the common extensor tendon and radial sagittal and transverse bands, is freed from the underlying capsule. *(Figure continues.)*

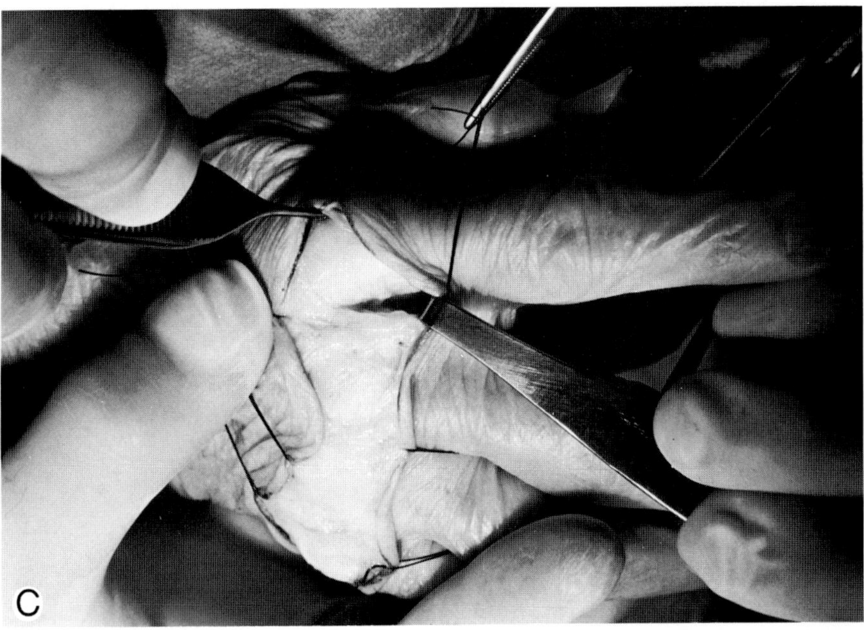

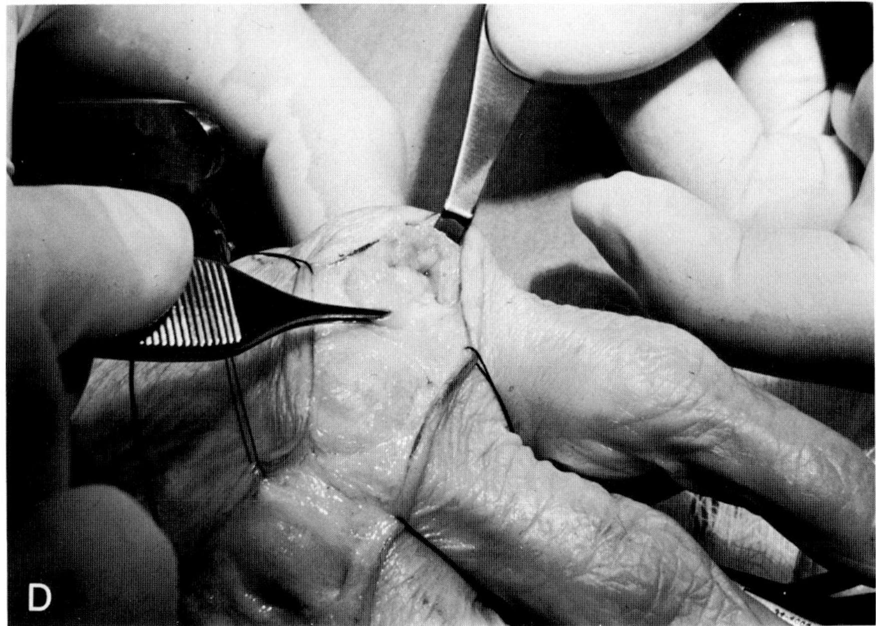

Fig. 46-33 *(Continued).* **(C)** The common extensor tendon and radial sagittal and transverse bands are retracted radially with Adson forceps to expose the capsule of the MP joint. **(D)** The capsule is opened, demonstrating the synovium. *(Figure continues.)*

contracture. He releases that portion of the transverse fibers that aids flexion of the MP joint. If tightness persists after this release, the bony attachment of the intrinsic tendon is released as well.

Crossed Intrinsic Transfer

Straub[242,243] introduced the crossed intrinsic transfer as an additional method to restore finger alignment and prevent recurrent ulnar drift. In principle, the intrinsics are released from the ulnar sides of the index, long, and ring fingers and are transferred to the radial aspect of the adjacent fingers to provide additional radial stability. While we do not use this procedure frequently, Oster and Blair[201] found that it can provide effective long-term correction of ulnar drift.

Crossed intrinsic transfer is performed in conjunction with MP joint synovectomy and soft tissue reconstruction. The intrinsic tendons of the index, long, and ring fingers are exposed as described previously. In Straub's method, the tendon is released from the extensor mechanism over the midportion of

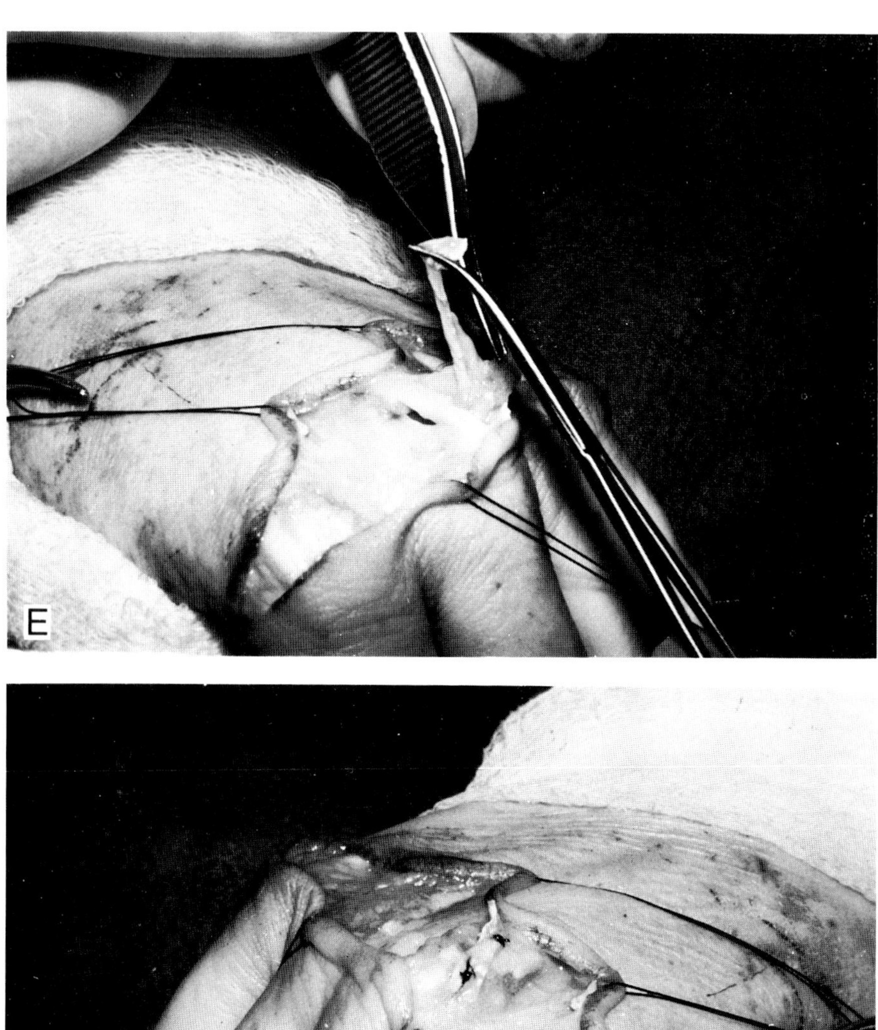

Fig. 46-33 *(Continued).* **(E)** A strip of extensor tendon is split from the ulnar side of the extensor tendon and passed through the underlying joint capsule, and through the radial portion of the extensor mechanism prior to being sutured to itself. **(F)** The tendon strip sutured to itself, centralizing the extensor tendon by attaching it to underlying joint capsule. *(Figure continues.)*

the proximal phalanx and dissected proximally to its musculotendinous junction. The bony attachment is released from the base of the proximal phalanx to allow free excursion of the muscle-tendon unit. Each tendon is transferred to the radial intrinsic mechanism of the adjacent finger. The tendon is woven into the lateral band and sutured.

Flatt[59] believes that the intrinsic transfer performed as described above may cause a swan-neck deformity. He sutures the intrinsic tendon to the radial collateral ligament of the adjacent finger rather than weaving the tendon into the lateral band of the adjacent finger.[59,77]

In Flatt's method, the intrinsic tendons are exposed and released as described above. The extensor expansion is opened on the radial side to expose the collateral ligament. The intrinsic tendon is sutured to the radial collateral ligament at its phalangeal attachment using several interrupted 4–0 sutures. The tension at which the attachment is made is correct if complete finger alignment is restored at the completion of the re-

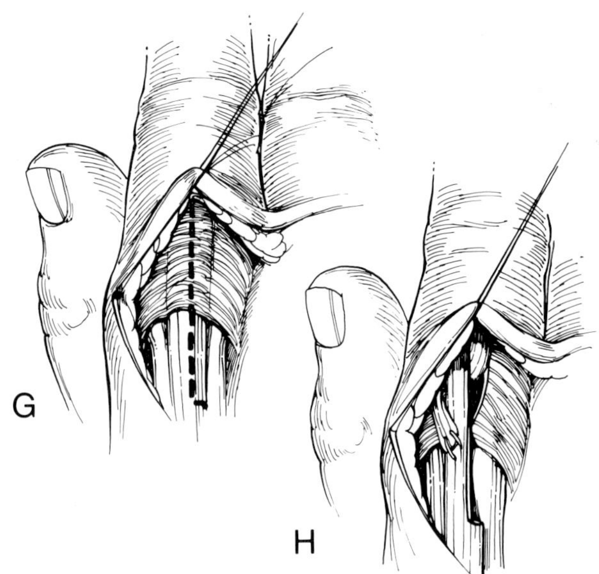

Fig. 46-33 *(Continued).* **(G&H)** Drawing of the tendon relocation technique.

pair. The finger is splinted for 3 weeks before beginning exercises. A dynamic splint is applied then and is used for an additional 3 weeks.

Extensor Tendon Relocation

Realignment of an ulnarly dislocated extensor tendon is necessary to correct deformity, restore extension, and prevent recurrent dislocation. The degree of extensor tendon subluxation will vary from minimal to complete dislocation with the tendon fixed within the intermetacarpal valley. Several different operative techniques have been described to centralize the extensor tendon.[106,159,295]

Longitudinal incisions are used when only one or two fingers are to be done. If all four fingers are to be done, adequate exposure can be obtained through a transverse incision. The subluxated extensor tendon is identified and the sagittal fibers along its ulnar side are incised. A hemostat is placed beneath the transverse and oblique fibers of the intrinsic tendon on the ulnar side, and an intrinsic release is performed. The extensor tendon is dissected free and relocated over the dorsal aspect of the MP joint. The tendon may be maintained in the relocated position by one of three methods.

The simplest but least effective method is to reef the stretched radial sagittal fibers. After the tendon has been relocated, the lax fibers are imbricated with an absorbable 4-0 suture. We use this procedure when there is no tendency for the tendon to resubluxate. However, if there is a tendency for radial deviation of the wrist, which increases the tendency for ulnar subluxation of the tendon, more secure fixation of the tendon must be obtained.

An effective method is that described by Harrison.[102] A 4-cm slip of extensor tendon, 5 mm wide, is detached proximally and freed distally to the distal portion of the MP joint. This is passed through a hole drilled into the dorsal cortex at the base of the proximal phalanx. Zancolli[295] described a method for rebalancing and stabilizing the extensor mechanism by attaching the extensor tendon to the proximal phalanx through drill holes.

We prefer a modification of the Harrison procedure that does not require a hole drilled into the bone. We have found that attachment of the tendon slip described above to the thick capsule at the base of the proximal phalanx is satisfactory. After the tendon slip has been prepared, a transverse incision is made through the capsule on the dorsal aspect of the proximal phalanx. The tendon slip is passed from outside to inside, then out through the capsule and extensor mechanism on the radial side, and finally sutured back to the extensor tendon. This maintains the extensor mechanism in the centralized position. The fingers should be moved through their full range of motion passively after the procedure has been completed to be sure that the tendon stays centralized and does not subluxate either to the ulnar side or to the radial side of the MP joint. Flexion of the MP joint should not be restricted significantly after the tendon has been centralized.

Postoperative Management for Soft Tissue Procedures

At the completion of the surgical procedure, a bulky conforming dressing is used to immobilize the hand with the MP joints in extension and in correct alignment. The drain placed in the subcutaneous area is removed on the first postoperative day and the hand is resplinted. Exercises, supervised by a hand therapist, are begun within the first 3 to 4 days. The fingers are protected during the exercises and are splinted in extension between exercise periods. Exercises are performed three or four times a day. On the fifth to seventh postoperative day, a dynamic splint is fabricated to maintain finger alignment and MP joint extension but also to allow active flexion. This splint is worn during the day, and a plaster "resting" splint is used at night. Both splints are used for 4 to 6 weeks following surgery. Long-term splinting and carefully supervised therapy are important in preventing the postoperative recurrence of deformity.

MP Joint Arthroplasties

These operations are discussed in Chapter 7.

THE PIP JOINTS

PIP Joint Synovectomy

Although synovectomy is performed infrequently at the wrist and MP joints for the reasons discussed previously, the indications for synovectomy of the PIP joint are broader. Progressive PIP joint synovitis that stretches the extensor mechanism will result in a boutonnière deformity that is difficult to reconstruct. The results of PIP joint arthroplasty are less reliable than those of MP joint arthroplasty, and PIP joint fusions are disabling. For these reasons, preservation of PIP joint function is important. In addition, the PIP joint is more stable than the MP joint, and recurrent deformity after synovectomy is less common than after MP joint synovectomy. PIP joint synovectomy has relatively little morbidity. It can be performed on a single joint on an outpatient basis, or in conjunction with other procedures such as tenosynovectomy, MP synovectomy, or MP arthroplasty.[6,60,128,138,140,198,290,291]

PIP Joint Synovectomy— Operative Technique (Fig. 46-34)

The joint is exposed through a slightly curved incision on the dorsal aspect of the finger. A sharply curved flap is avoided to prevent edema within the flap postoperatively. The extensor mechanism is exposed, preserving the longitudinal dorsal veins. The joint is exposed through a longitudinal incision splitting the central slip or through an incision between the lateral band and the central tendon. The location of the capsulotomy is determined by the site of bulging synovium. Hypertrophic synovium is removed by sharp dissection or with a small rongeur. Gentle distal traction of the finger and flexion of the joint will facilitate the synovectomy.

Occasionally, the synovium will bulge laterally. In this case, incising the transverse retinacular ligament and reflecting the lateral band dorsally will expose the synovium bulging through the accessory collateral ligament. A longitudinal incision volar to the collateral ligament allows synovectomy to be performed without injuring the ligament and facilitates the removal of synovium from the volar pouch.

The extensor mechanism is repaired with an absorbable 4–0 suture. A conforming hand dressing is applied with the PIP joint positioned in extension.

Postoperatively, early motion is begun to preserve PIP joint function. Active flexion and extension are started 1 to 2 days following surgery. The joint is splinted in extension, except during exercise periods, for 2 weeks.

FINGER DEFORMITIES

Two finger deformities commonly occur in rheumatoid arthritis: the so-called swan-neck and boutonnière deformities. The former is characterized by PIP joint hyperextension with DIP joint flexion, while the latter is the reverse deformity.

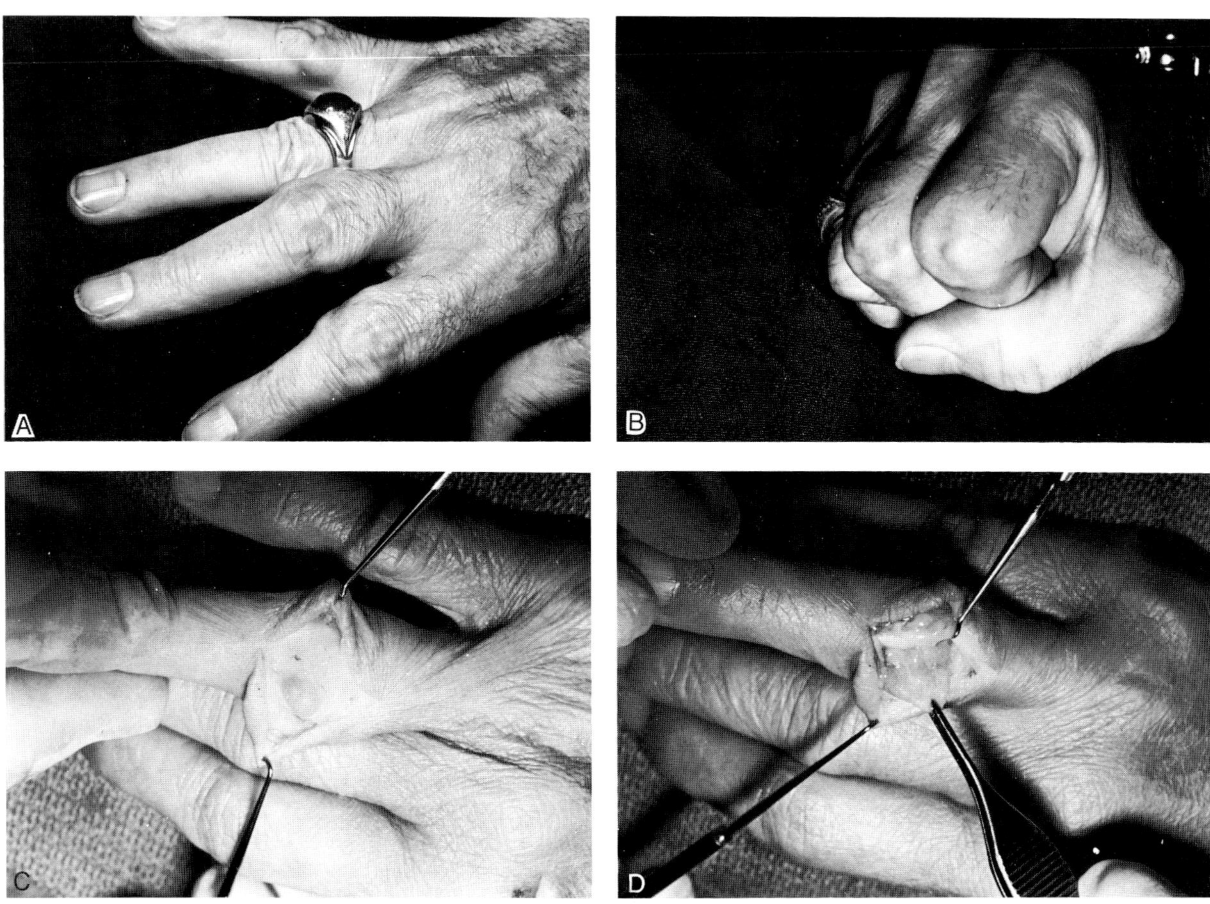

Fig. 46-34. Technique for PIP joint synovectomy. **(A&B)** A patient with PIP joint synovitis in several fingers. **(C)** The extensor mechanism is exposed, demonstrating proliferative synovium bulging between the lateral bands and central slip. **(D)** A longitudinal incision through the stretched extensor mechanism exposes the synovium, which is excised sharply. *(Figure continues.)*

Neither the swan-neck nor the boutonnière deformity is unique to rheumatoid arthritis. Rather, they represent the end result of muscular imbalance caused by the rheumatoid disease. Thus, we occasionally see patients who have both deformities in adjacent fingers of the same hand. Many factors determine the cause of these deformities, as well as the extent of functional loss that they produce[110,128,271,287] This explains the variety of operations recommended to correct these deformities and the diversity of opinion regarding treatment.[13,14,58,61,79,109,157,219]

Swan-neck Deformity

Although all swan-neck deformities have a superficial resemblance to each other, they vary considerably. Careful determination of the type of deformity present is essential for the selection of proper treatment. The significant functional loss associated with this deformity is related directly to the loss of motion at the PIP joint. This may vary from no loss, to partial loss, to almost complete loss of flexion. Patients with almost complete loss of PIP joint flexion can be subdivided further into those with, and those without, preservation of joint space by radiographic examination. We classify these deformities into one of four types, depending on the PIP joint mobility and the condition of the joint surfaces. This classification serves as the basis for our treatment of fingers with swan-neck deformities.[130,179,190,194,222,287]

Type I: PIP Joints Flexible in all Positions

Some rheumatoid patients with swan-neck deformities demonstrate hyperextension of the PIP joint with DIP joint flexion, yet maintain the ability to flex the PIP joint completely. The deformity may originate at either the DIP or PIP joint. At the DIP joint, it starts with stretching or rupture of the terminal extensor tendon attachment, resulting in the so-called mallet deformity. Extensor mechanism imbalance secondary to DIP joint flexion, associated with laxity of the volar plate of the PIP joint, allows the PIP joint to assume a posture of hyperextension. In patients with early deformity, this progression can be observed. However, in the patient who presents with an established deformity, the sequence of events described can be inferred if the DIP joint deformity is more severe than the PIP joint hyperextension.

In other patients, the deformity may originate at the PIP joint, as synovitis stretches out the volar capsule, or if rupture of the superficial flexor tendon removes the force restraining PIP joint hyperextension. In these cases, DIP joint flexion is secondary. Swan-neck deformity originating at the DIP or PIP joint is classified as Type I if full passive motion of the PIP joint is maintained. These patients have only a small functional loss related to the limitation of DIP joint extension. They usually do not have associated MP joint disease.

Treatment of patients with Type I swan-neck deformity is directed at preventing or correcting the PIP joint hyperextension, restoring DIP joint extension, or both. The use of a Silver Ring splint can be helpful in correcting PIP hyperextension while allowing motion[184] (Fig. 46-35). Several surgical procedures can be considered. These include DIP joint fusion, dermadesis (volar to the PIP joint), flexor tenodesis of the PIP joint, and retinacular ligament reconstruction.

Distal Joint (DIP) Fusion

Although correction of the flexion deformity of the DIP joint to restore balance to the finger could be obtained by reattaching the extensor mechanism to restore active control of the

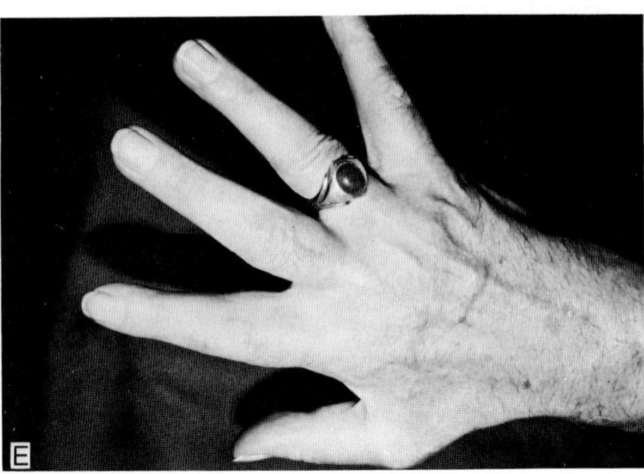

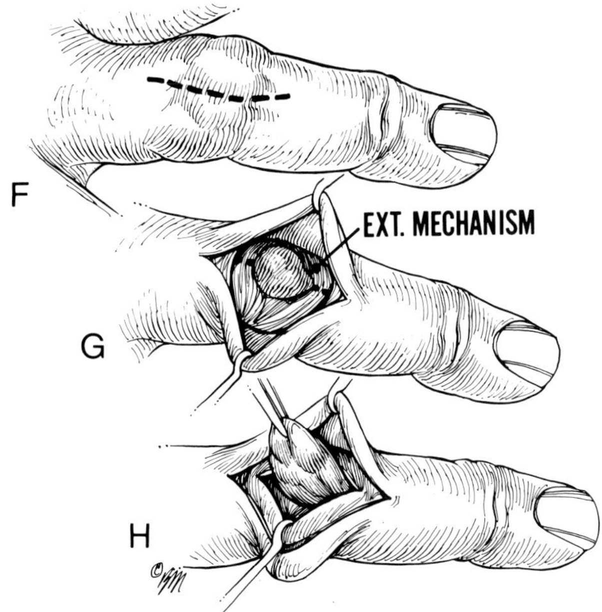

Fig. 46-34 *(Continued).* **(E)** Postoperative picture demonstrates full extension. **(F–H)** Drawing of PIP joint synovectomy technique.

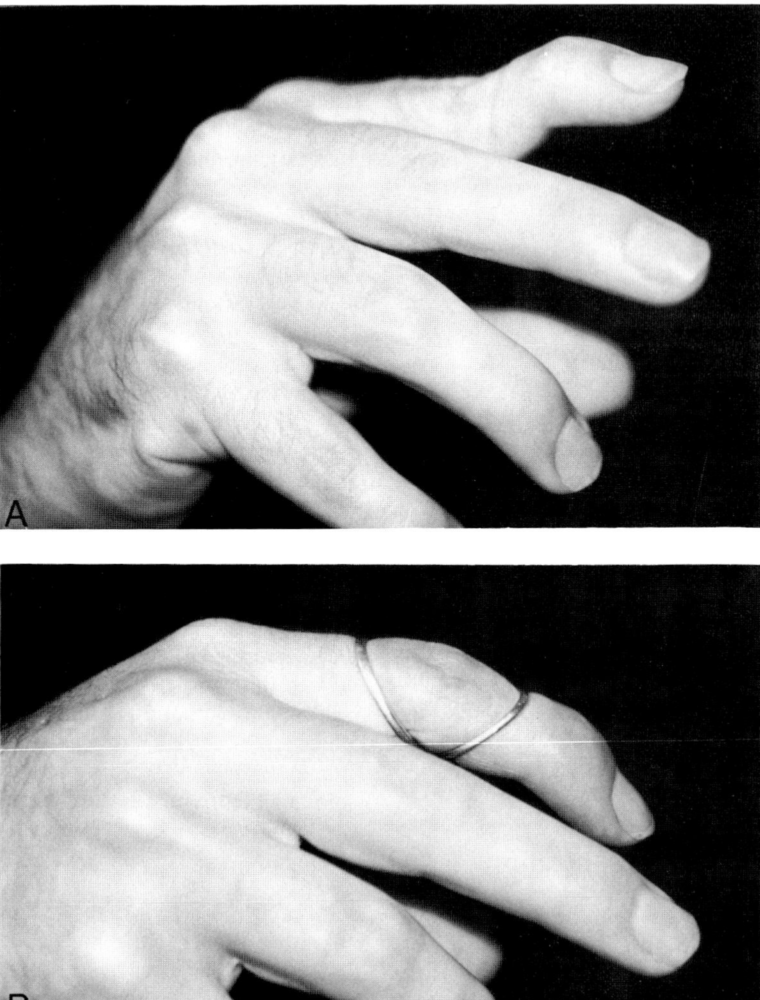

Fig. 46-35. A mild, supple swan-neck deformity (**A**) can be corrected with the Silver Ring splint (**B**).

joint, the reconstructed tendon is subject to the same rheumatoid changes that led to the deformity in the first place. In addition, secondary arthritic changes within the joint may make attempts to restore motion unwise. An alternative treatment is to fuse the DIP joint.[32] We prefer this approach, particularly when the mallet deformity is primary.

We use a dorsal curved skin incision or the "Y" incision described by Swanson.[252] The extensor mechanism is divided transversely. The joint is flexed and the collateral ligaments are divided to improve exposure. The articular cartilage is removed and the bone ends are shaped to provide good bony contact. A longitudinal K-wire is used for internal fixation. To be certain that the wire is introduced into the medullary canal of the middle phalanx, we predrill a small hole in the middle phalanx before passing a slightly larger wire distally through the distal phalanx. This wire should emerge from the pulp just volar to the nail bed. The wire is then passed retrograde across the joint into the predrilled hole in the middle phalanx. Care should be taken not to drill the K-wire too far proximally to avoid damage to the PIP joint. The DIP joint is fixed in neutral position (full extension), our preferred position in the correction of the swan-neck deformity (Fig. 46-36).

The K-wire can be either cut off just below the skin or left exposed. If the wire is left exposed, removal after fusion is easy and the risk of pin tract infection is minimized. However, the finger cannot be immersed in water, and the protruding pin must be covered to prevent injury to the patient and others. Burying the pin under the skin allows washing of the hand, but increases the risk of skin irritation, skin breakdown, and subsequent infection. Usually, we use only one longitudinal K-wire for DIP joints fusions. However, if necessary, an obliquely placed wire is added to control rotation. To facilitate fusion, we commonly add bone grafts to the fusion site. These grafts are essential for patients with extensive erosive changes and significant loss of bony substance.[186] The metacarpal heads removed for implant arthroplasty provide a good source of local bone graft material. External support with a small aluminum splint is advisable for the first 4 to 6 weeks following fusion.

If the pin has been buried, it can be removed in the office after the fusion is solidly healed. Local anesthetic can be in-

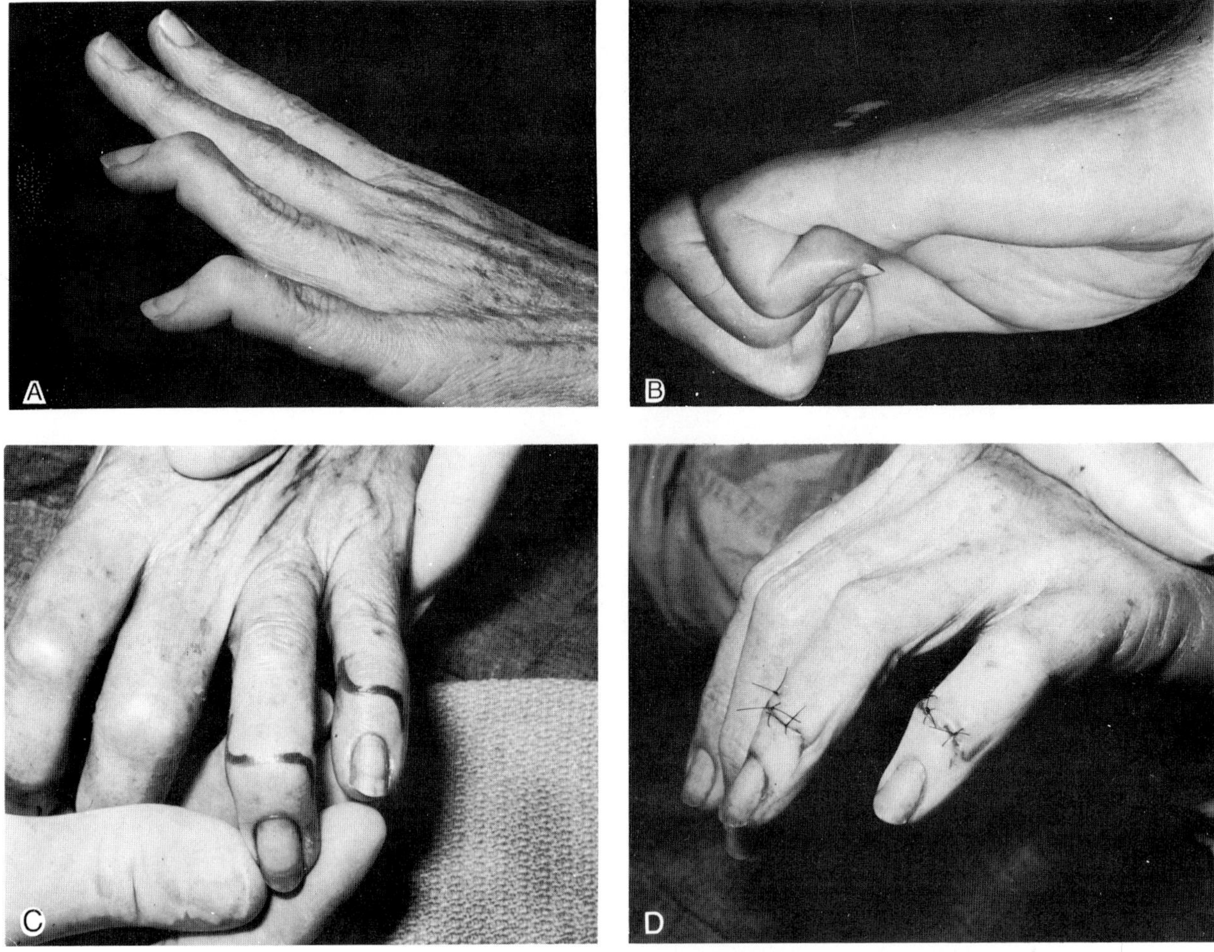

Fig. 46-36. Type I swan-neck deformity with primary defect at the distal joint. **(A)** Note mallet deformity of the distal joint with secondary PIP joint hyperextension. **(B)** The patient demonstrates full flexion of PIP joints. **(C)** One of the incisions used for distal joint fusion. **(D)** Improvement in finger posture following distal joint fusion in extension.

jected directly into the skin and subcutaneous tissue overlying the pin, or a digital block can be given. A stab wound is made over the pin, and the pin is extracted with a needle holder. Occasionally, the pin may migrate proximally so that it is completely or almost completely buried in bone. This will require more extensive dissection to locate and remove the pin, and therefore, should be done in the operating room under optimal conditions that will allow removal of some bone from the distal phalanx to expose the end of the pin.

A Herbert screw also can be used for internal fixation of DIP joint fusions.[66] It provides rigid internal fixation of the fusion and does not need to be removed after the fusion heals. Intramedullary placement assures the preferred straight position of the joint. Relatively rigid fixation provided by the screw precludes the need for prolonged postoperative splinting; 2 to 3 weeks is sufficient.

The Herbert screw has several disadvantages, however. If the screw is inserted incorrectly, the screw threads can damage the germinal matrix of the nail, resulting in nail plate deformity. The distal phalanx must be large enough to accept the trailing threads of the screw. Fixation can be lost if the leading screw threads extend beyond the isthmus of the middle phalanx and toggle in the soft bone of the metaphysis.

We have used the screw more frequently recently, and are pleased with the results when attention is paid to the technical details of inserting the screw (Fig. 46-37).

Surgical Technique—Herbert Screw DIP Joint Fusion. The DIP joint is exposed and the joint surfaces are prepared as described previously. The medullary canal of the middle phalanx is located with a 0.035-inch K-wire. The main (smaller) Herbert drill is used to prepare the canal. The tap is inserted and the canal is tapped through, but not beyond the isthmus. A 0.035-inch K-wire is inserted through the base of the distal phalanx and into the medullary canal. The wire is driven distally to exit on the tip of the finger just below the hyponychium. A transverse stab wound is made where the K-wire exits. The wire is withdrawn and the main drill is inserted through the stab wound, into the tuft of the distal phalanx, and advanced proximally until it emerges at the base of the phalanx. The pilot (larger) drill is inserted through the stab wound and used to enlarge the hole in the tuft. The tap is inserted in the same

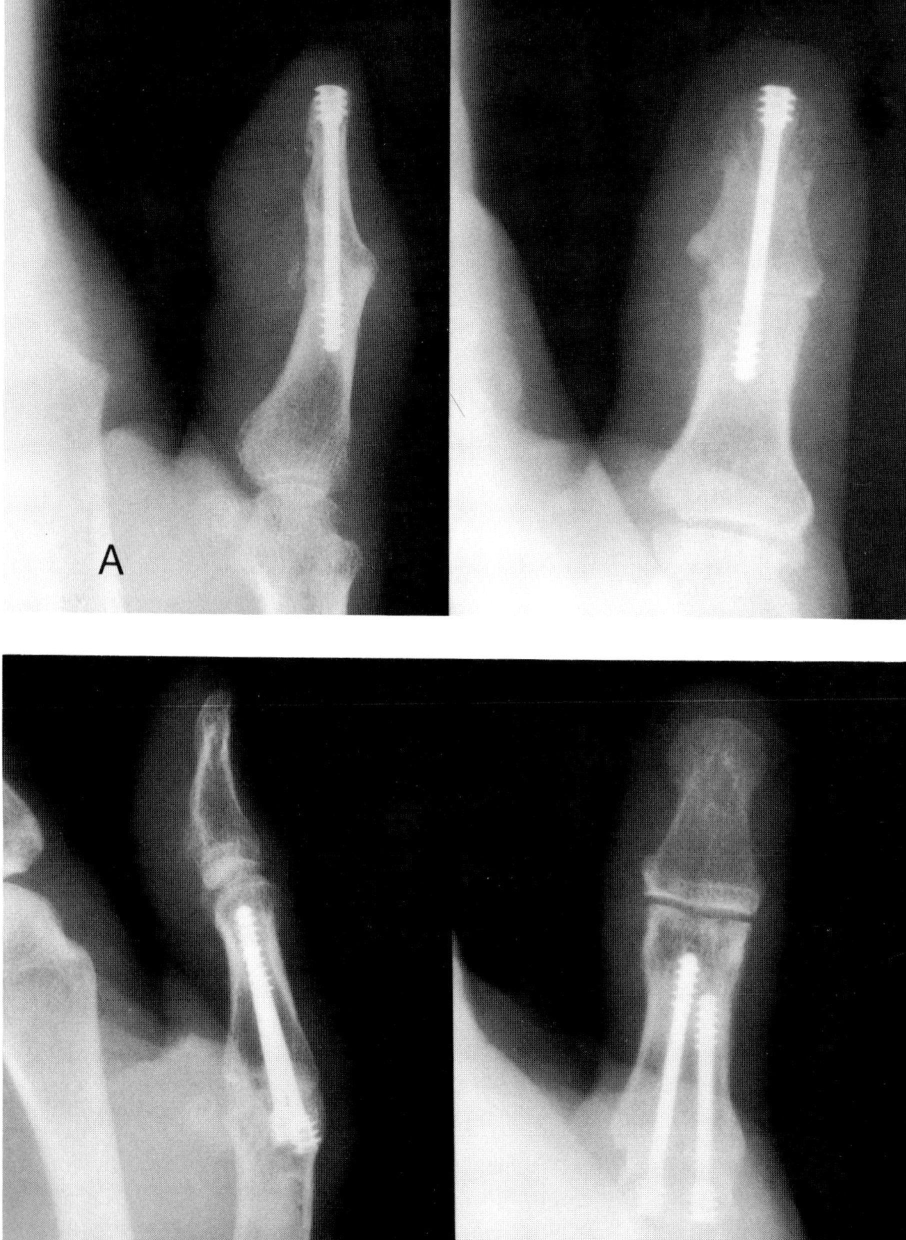

Fig. 46-37. The Herbert screw has provided excellent internal fixation for small joint fusions in rheumatoid patients. A single screw is used for fusion of the thumb IP joint (**A**), while two screws inserted parallel to each other provide rigid fixation of the thumb MP joint (**B**). The leading threads of a screw used to stabilize the DIP joint fusion should extend only into the isthmus of the middle phalanx *(Figure continues.)*

manner. The appropriate length screw is inserted and advanced until it emerges at the base of the distal phalanx. The screw tip is aligned with the hole in the middle phalanx under direct vision and then advanced with the fusion surfaces held tightly together. The trailing threads of the screw are recessed into the tuft. If too long a screw is used, there may be a sudden loss of fixation as the leading thread passes through the isthmus into the softer and wider portion of the phalanx. Rotatory stability can be augmented by inserting a 0.028- or 0.035-inch K-wire parallel to the screw. Intraoperative x-rays should be obtained to confirm proper placement and length of the screw.

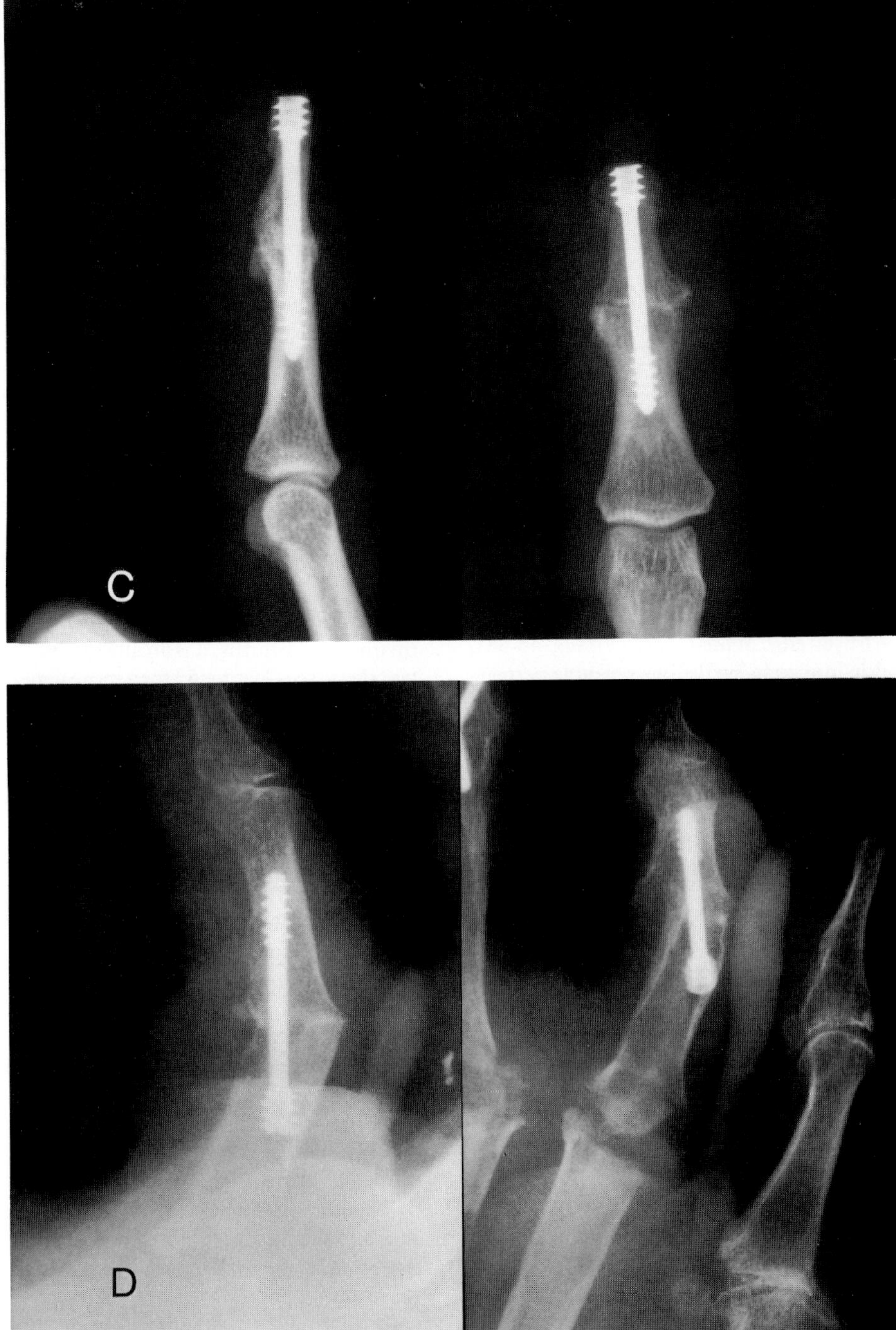

Fig. 46-37 *(Continued).* **(C)** to avoid loss of fixation from toggle of the screw in the softer bone of the metaphysis. MP joint arthroplasties do not preclude the use of the Herbert screw for PIP joint fusions in the rheumatoid patient **(D).**

Dermadesis

Dermadesis[190] is an operative approach that is used occasionally in patients with Type I swan-neck deformities. This procedure attempts to prevent PIP joint hyperextension by creating a skin shortage volarly. An elliptical wedge of skin (4 to 5 mm at its widest point) is removed from the volar aspect of the PIP joint. Care is taken to preserve the venous network just under the skin and to not open or disturb the underlying flexor tendon sheath. The skin is closed with the PIP joint in flexion. This technique is helpful only in mild cases and usually will fail unless it is done in conjunction with other procedures such as DIP joint fusion. When PIP joint hyperextension is primary, we prefer to use a stronger check-rein against hyperextension. Our procedure of choice is flexor tendon tenodesis, using one slip of the flexor digitorum sublimis (superficialis).

Flexor Tendon Tenodesis ("Sublimis Sling")

Patients with PIP joint hyperextension maintain full passive motion but, as the hyperextension increases, begin to develop difficulty in initiating active flexion. These patients require restoration of strong volar support to the joint. We prefer to use a sublimis tendon tenodesis to prevent PIP joint hyperextension. We have found a method of tenodesis similar to that described by Curtis[48] using one slip of superficialis to be useful in correcting rheumatoid swan-neck deformities.

A volar zigzag incision is made over the PIP joint and the flexor tendon sheath is exposed. The thin portions of the sheath on either side of the A3 pulley are excised, preserving the pulley. The flexor tendons are exposed, and care is taken to avoid injury to the vincula passing between the flexor digitorum sublimis to the flexor digitorum profundus tendon. One slip of the superficialis tendon is divided approximately 1.5 cm proximal to the joint. This portion of the superficialis is separated from its corresponding slip but is left attached distally. With the joint in approximately 20 to 30 degrees flexion, the detached slip is fixed proximally to act as a check-rein against extension. The proximal attachment can be made directly into the bone using a pull-out wire or can be made at the thickened margin of the flexor tendon sheath (distal edge of the A2 pulley) (Fig. 46-38).

To attach the tendon into bone, we drill a small hole perpendicular to the shaft of the proximal phalanx. A pull-out wire is used to bring the tendon into the hole and is tied over a button on the dorsum of the finger. A rubber cushion is fabricated from a Penrose drain or a piece of Esmarch bandage and is placed between the skin and button. The attachment to bone is stronger, but is technically more difficult than the attachment to the margin of the fibrous sheath. An easier technique that bears promise is the small Mitek bone anchor which is inserted through a small drill hole and holds a 2-0 or 4-0 suture firmly to the bone. To attach the tendon slip to the sheath, a transverse slit is made in the distal portion of the A2 pulley and the detached tendon slip is passed through this and sutured back onto itself. In both methods, the goal is to create a slight flexion contracture of the PIP joint. For greater purchase, the tendon slip can be attached through or adjacent to the A1 pulley in the distal palm. Postoperatively, the joint is splinted in 30 degrees flexion. We start flexion at 3 weeks to maintain PIP joint function but block hyperextension for at least 6 weeks.

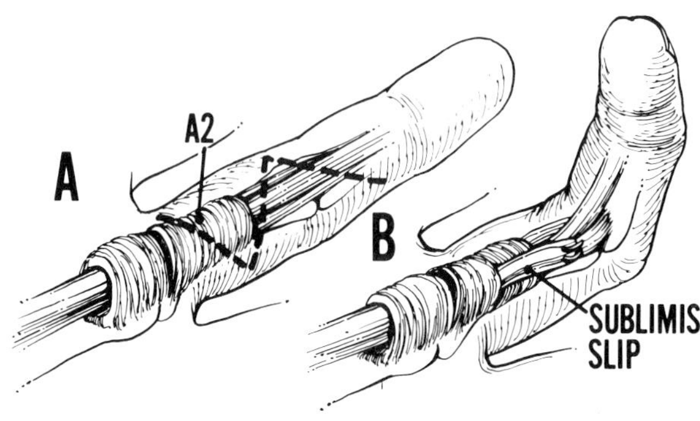

Fig. 46-38. One technique for superficialis tenodesis to correct swan-neck deformity. **(A)** Zigzag incision used to expose the flexor tendon sheath. The incision should be extended far enough proximally to expose the A2 pulley. A tenosynovectomy is performed if necessary. **(B)** A slip of flexor digitorum superficialis (sublimis) is sectioned proximally, passed through a slit in the A2 pulley, and sutured back on itself.

Retinacular Ligament Reconstruction

Littler devised a clever technique to prevent hyperextension while restoring DIP joint extension by reconstructing an oblique retinacular ligament using the ulnar lateral band.[143,268] In this procedure, the ulnar lateral band is freed from the extensor mechanism proximally, but left attached distally. It is passed volar to Cleland's fibers to bring it volar to the axis of PIP joint motion. The band is sutured to the fibrous tendon sheath under enough tension to restore DIP joint extension and prevent PIP hyperextension. In theory, this approach should solve both the DIP and PIP joint problems simultaneously. However, in the rheumatoid patient who has a primary mallet deformity with destruction of the terminal tendon, no amount of tension applied to the relocated lateral band will restore DIP joint extension. Thus, the net result of this procedure will be restriction of PIP joint hyperextension. In rheumatoid arthritis, it is an alternative to dermadesis or flexor tenodesis (see Chapter 53 for a more detailed description of this operation).

Type II: PIP Joint Flexion Limited in Certain Positions

Some rheumatoid patients with swan-neck deformities have restriction of finger flexion only in certain positions. The deformity may appear similar to the Type I deformity. However, on examination, PIP joint flexion is influenced by the position of the MP joint. With the MP joints extended or radially deviated, passive PIP joint flexion is limited. If the MP joint is allowed to flex or deviate ulnarward, PIP joint flexion is increased. In these cases, the swan-neck deformity is secondary to MP joint involvement.

As the MP joints deviate and subluxate and the intrinsics become tight, a secondary swan-neck deformity develops as the result of muscular imbalance. Initially this is supple in most positions and becomes stiff only when the MP joint is in extension and the intrinsics are tightened further. Ultimately, however, the PIP joint becomes stiff regardless of the position of the MP joint.

In these patients, it is not sufficient to restrict PIP joint hyperextension. The intrinsic tightness must be relieved. Any MP joint disorder that initiates or aggravates the muscular imbalance of the finger, i.e., subluxation or deviation, also must be corrected. This is accomplished by intrinsic release in patients with minimally involved MP joints and by combined MP joint arthroplasty and intrinsic release in the others.

Intrinsic Release

Intrinsic muscle release is performed through a dorsoulnar longitudinal incision over the proximal phalanx as described on page 1649. Following this release, PIP joint flexion with the MP joint extended or radially deviated should be improved. Often, we combine intrinsic release with DIP joint fusion or volar dermadesis to correct the PIP joint hyperextension and restore balance.

In patients with associated MP joint disease, MP joint alignment is corrected by implant arthroplasty in addition to intrinsic release. The MP joints are exposed through a transverse incision, and the intrinsic muscle on the ulnar side is released. Although MP joint arthroplasty (Swanson) with resection of the metacarpal heads does lengthen and separate the transected ends of the intrinsic tendon, we prefer to resect the ulnar intrinsic tendon as well to reduce the risk of recurrent intrinsic tightness and ulnar drift of the fingers.

Type III: Limited PIP Joint Flexion in all Positions

In patients with the Type I and II deformities described above, there is only slight to moderate functional loss in spite of the finger deformity. However, patients with marked reduction of PIP joint motion in any position (Type III) have significant loss of hand function, as the ability to grasp objects is reduced greatly. Although it might seem logical to assume that patients with stiff swan-neck deformities have advanced intraarticular changes that require either fusion to bring the finger into a functional position or arthroplasty to restore active motion, radiographic examination often reveals well-preserved joint spaces. In these cases, the structures that restrict passive motion include the extensor mechanism, the collateral ligaments, and the skin. The first step in the surgical reconstruction of the stiff swan-neck deformity is the restoration of passive PIP joint motion. The procedures we use to restore passive motion include joint manipulation, lateral band mobilization, and skin release. Correction of the deformity is delayed until passive motion is restored.

PIP Joint Manipulation

In patients with stiff swan-neck deformities, the soft tissues have contracted about the joint. However, with the patient under anesthesia, it is sometimes possible to obtain 80 to 90 degrees of PIP joint flexion by gentle manipulation. PIP joint manipulation is performed alone rarely; it usually is done in conjunction with intrinsic release, MP arthroplasty, or flexor tenosynovectomy. If the joint is splinted in the flexed position, the tight soft tissues will stretch. After several weeks, the passive motion obtained by manipulation and splinting can be maintained as active motion, provided the flexor tendons have not become adherent. When done in conjunction with MP arthroplasty, temporary K-wire fixation is used to hold the PIP joint in flexion. This concentrates the postoperative exercises on MP joint motion. After 10 days, the pins are removed and therapy is directed to increasing PIP joint motion, using an extension block splint to prevent full extension of the joints. As stated previously, this method has restored 80 to 90 degrees of PIP joint flexion in joints that previously were stiff.

When PIP joint manipulation is performed in conjunction with flexor tenosynovectomy, the joints are not pinned but are splinted in the flexed position postoperatively. Usually, after 24 to 48 hours of splinting, therapy can be initiated using extension block splints. Therapy includes active PIP range of motion exercises with careful splinting in flexion between exercise periods. Initially, exercises are done for 5 minutes, four to six times daily, and increased as pain and endurance allow. Splinting is continued for 2 to 4 weeks, depending on the range of motion obtained. If an extensor lag of the PIP joint develops, extension splinting may be necessary.

Skin Release

The dorsal skin may limit the amount of passive flexion that can be achieved by manipulation. At some point during the manipulation of long-standing fixed deformities into flexion, the dorsal skin blanches. If this is not relieved, skin necrosis occurs directly over the joint.

Dorsal skin tension can be miminized with an oblique incision just distal to the PIP joint, which allows the skin edges to spread. The defect created is the result of skin contracture (not loss) and will close gradually in 2 to 3 weeks. Although initially we used skin grafts to cover these defects, satisfactory healing by secondary intention has convinced us that grafts are not needed. In fact, leaving this portion of the wound open allows drainage and reduces postoperative swelling and pain. It is important that the skin release be distal to the joint so that the extensor mechanism overlying the joint is covered (Fig. 46-39).

Certain precautions must be observed when joint manipulation is performed. Minimal force should be used to bring the PIP joint into flexion. The soft tissues should stretch, not rupture. Fracture of osteopenic bone must be avoided. Therefore, if manipulation is difficult, we proceed to soft tissue release. The procedure we use most often is lateral band mobilization.

Lateral Band Mobilization (Fig. 46-40)

In established swan-neck deformities, the lateral bands are displaced dorsally. Their normal volar shift is lost, and the finger is stiff. We have found that freeing the lateral bands from the central slip using two parallel longitudinal incisions in the extensor mechanism allows the joint to be manipulated gently into full flexion without releasing the collateral ligaments or lengthening the central slip. Full passive flexion often can be achieved by this method. When the procedure is performed under local anesthesia, the shifting of the lateral bands volarward on flexion and relocation dorsally on extension can be observed during active motion.

When we first used this procedure for stiff swan-neck deformities in 1962, our greatest problem was loss of motion following skin closure. Once the skin was sutured, the passive and active motion achieved by the lateral band mobilization was lost. If the skin was allowed to heal before active motion was started, the amount of flexion obtained in the operating room was seldom maintained. We now use a curved dorsal incision with an oblique limb across the middle segment. The proximal portion of the incision is closed with the finger held in flexion. The distal third of the incision usually is left open. The finger is splinted in flexion for 3 to 5 days to stretch the contracted

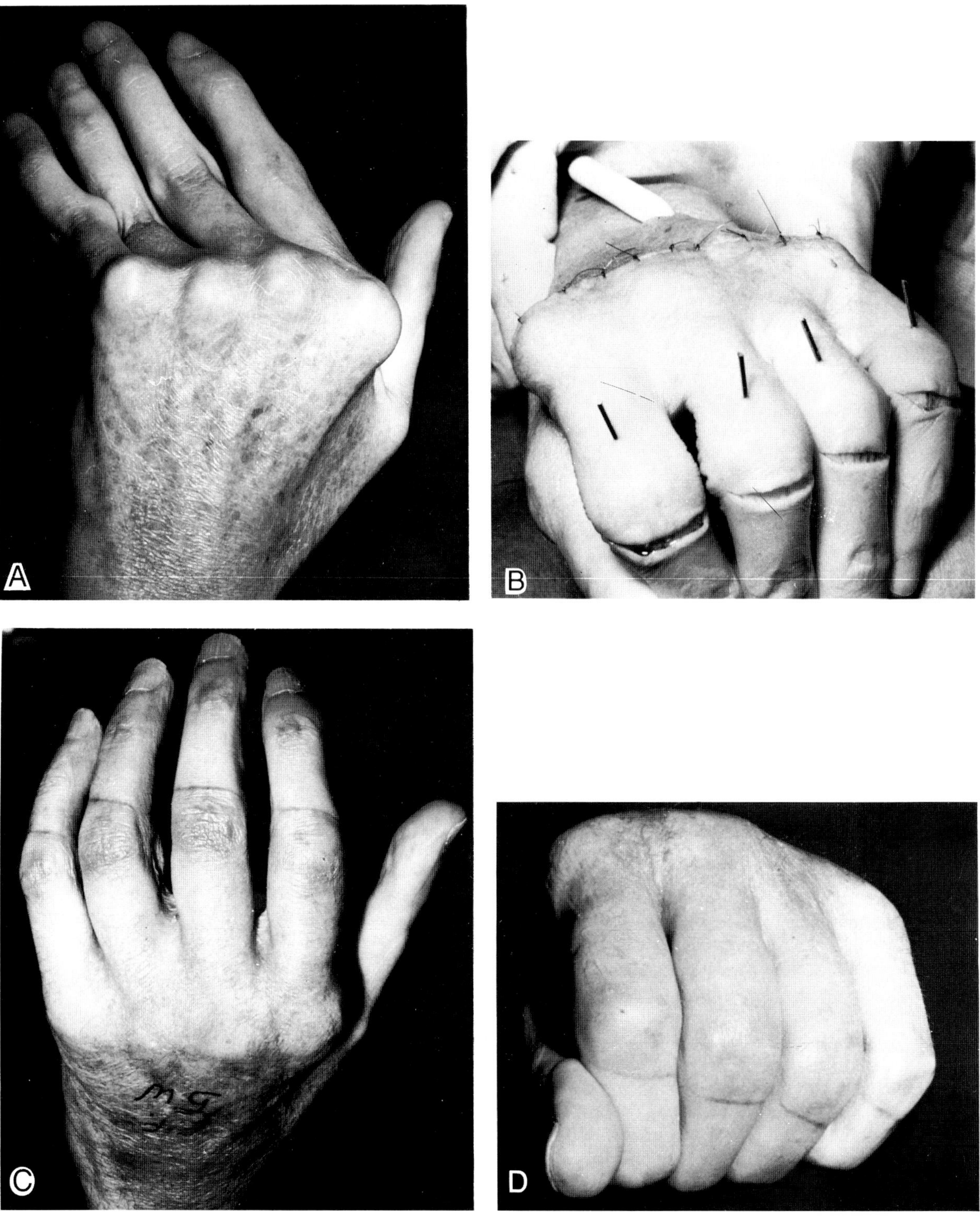

Fig. 46-39. Type III swan-neck deformity treated by PIP joint manipulation, skin release, and MP joint arthroplasty. (**A**) The PIP joints do not flex even with the MP joints in flexion. (**B**) Appearance at surgery following MP arthroplasty, PIP manipulation with K-wire fixation, and skin release. (**C**) Postoperative extension shows improved finger posture. (**D**) Range of flexion achieved postoperatively.

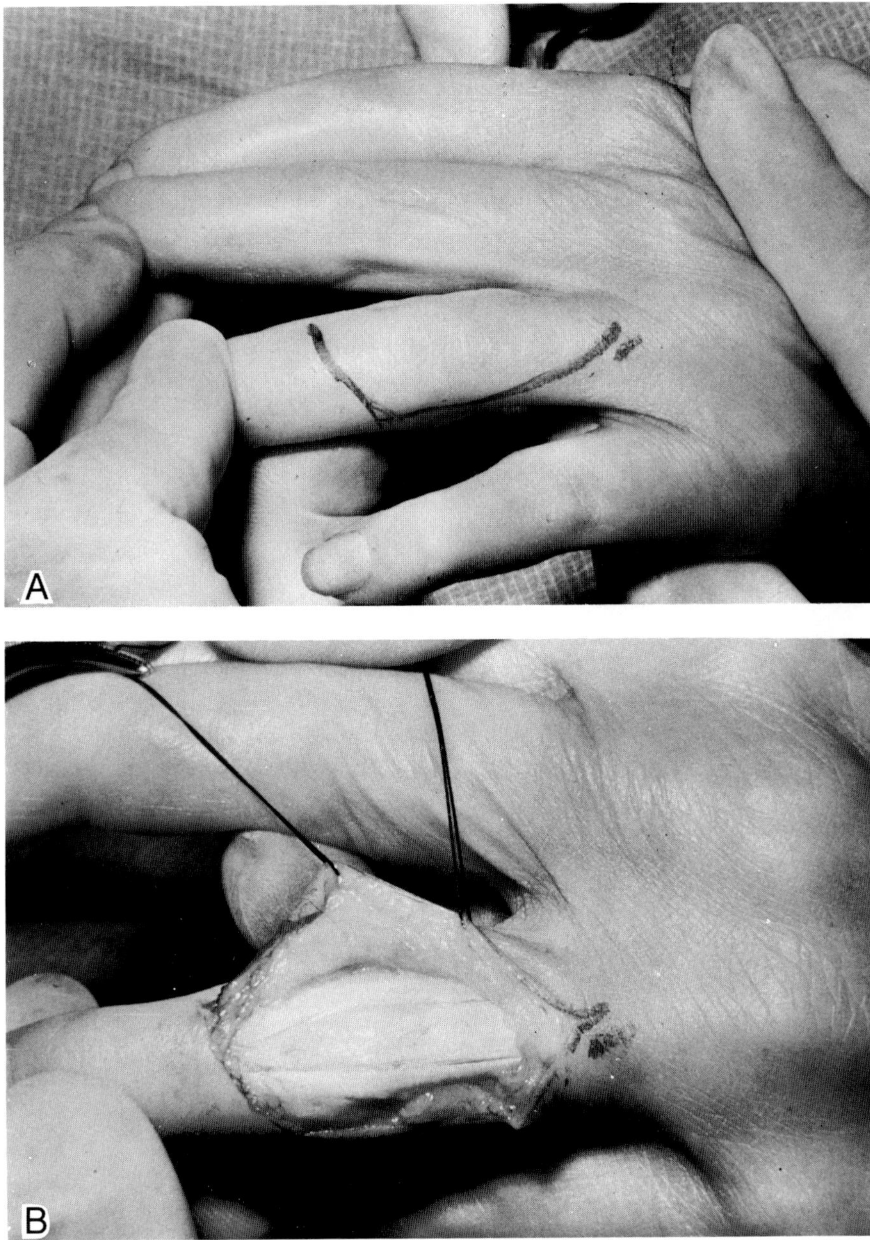

Fig. 46-40. Type III swan-neck deformity treated by lateral band mobilization. **(A)** Incision used to expose the extensor mechanism over the PIP joint. **(B)** Parallel incisions separate the lateral hands from the central slip. *(Figure continues.)*

collateral ligaments. Occasionally, however, it is necessary to release these ligaments, as well as to stepcut lengthen the central slip. A dorsal extension block splint is used to prevent full extension of the PIP joints.[84,184]

Flexor Tenosynovitis Associated with PIP Joint Stiffness

The flexor tendons also must be considered and assessed if optimal results are to be obtained from the procedures described above. Flexor tendon tenosynovitis and secondary flexor tendon adherence are integral etiologic factors of the stiff PIP joint and must be understood in order to provide adequate treatment. Flexor tenosynovitis that limits active PIP joint flexion can result in stiff PIP joints. Conversely, stiff PIP joints, regardless of the cause, will result in adherence of the flexor tendons. In either case, flexor tenosynovectomy or tenolysis must be a consideration in any treatment aimed at the restoration of PIP joint motion.

Adhesions or rupture of the flexors will obviate any passive motion gained by procedures directed at the extensor mechanism or the soft tissues surrounding the joint. However, the preoperative assessment of flexor tendon function is limited if stiff joints are present. For this reason, we now determine the

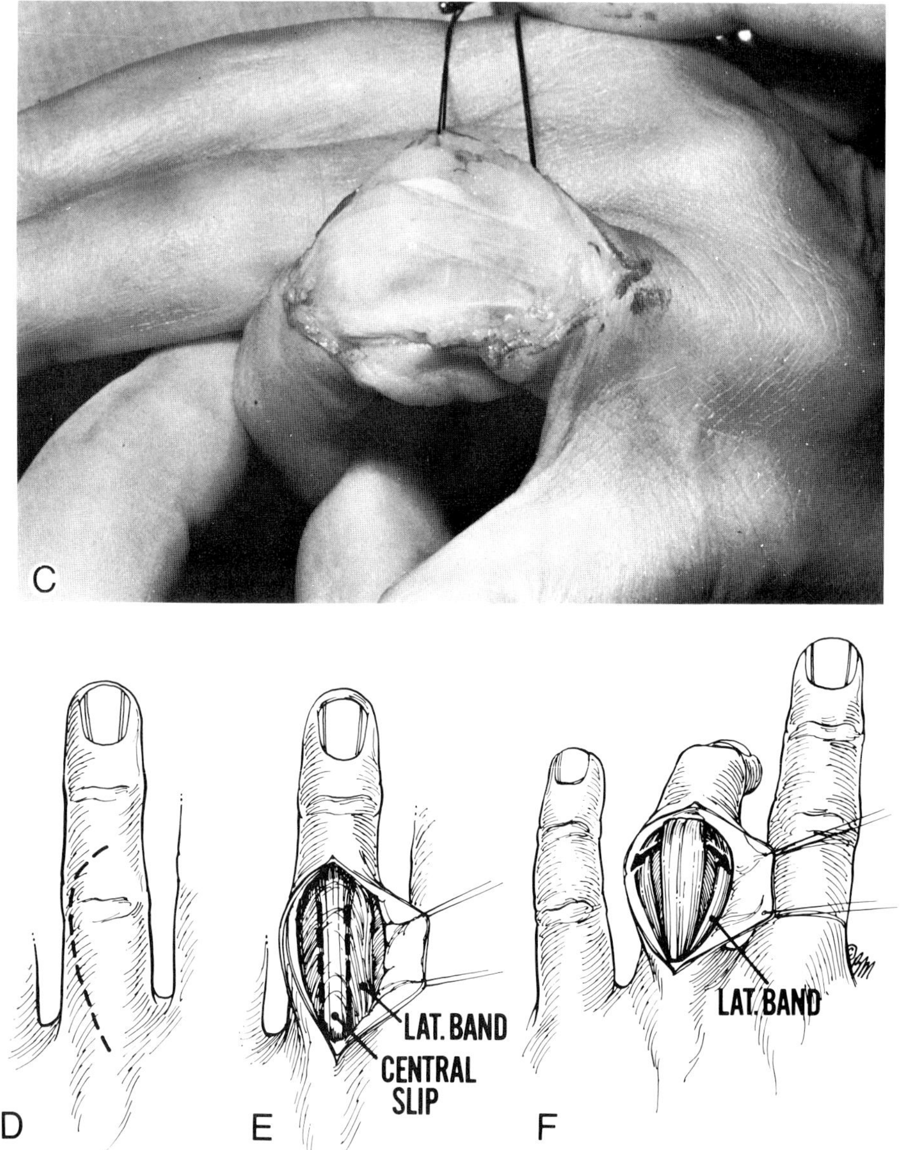

Fig. 46-40 *(Continued).* **(C)** Flexion obtained after manipulation of the PIP joint. Note volar shift of the lateral bands. **(D–F)** Diagrammatic drawing of technique for lateral band mobilization.

status of the flexor tendons in the operating room. If intravenous regional or local anesthesia has been used for either manipulation or lateral band mobilization, the tourniquet is released and the patient is asked to flex the fingers after muscle control has returned. If active motion is not nearly equal to passive motion, anesthesia is reinstituted and the flexor tendons are explored. Adhesions of the tendons are released and rheumatoid nodules within the tendon are removed. If regional block anesthesia has been used, the flexor tendons are exposed in the palm and traction is applied to test flexor tendon excursion. Occasionally, an extensive flexor tenosynovectomy will be required to improve flexor tendon excursion. Postoperatively, supervised splinting and active exercises are important in maintaining the motion gained at the time of surgery (see page 1607).

Type IV: Stiff PIP Joints with Poor Radiographic Appearance

Patients with stiff PIP joints and radiographic evidence of advanced intraarticular changes (Fig. 46-41) require some type of salvage procedure, i.e., fusion or arthroplasty. The factors that must be considered in deciding between these procedures include the fingers involved, the status of adjacent joints, the status of supporting ligamentous structures, and the status of the flexor tendons. We tend to prefer fusion in the index finger where lateral stability is particularly important. The status of adjacent joints also is important. If the MP joints require arthroplasty, we favor fusion at the PIP joint level, although arthroplasty at both levels can be performed with good results. Poor lateral ligamentous support and/or as-

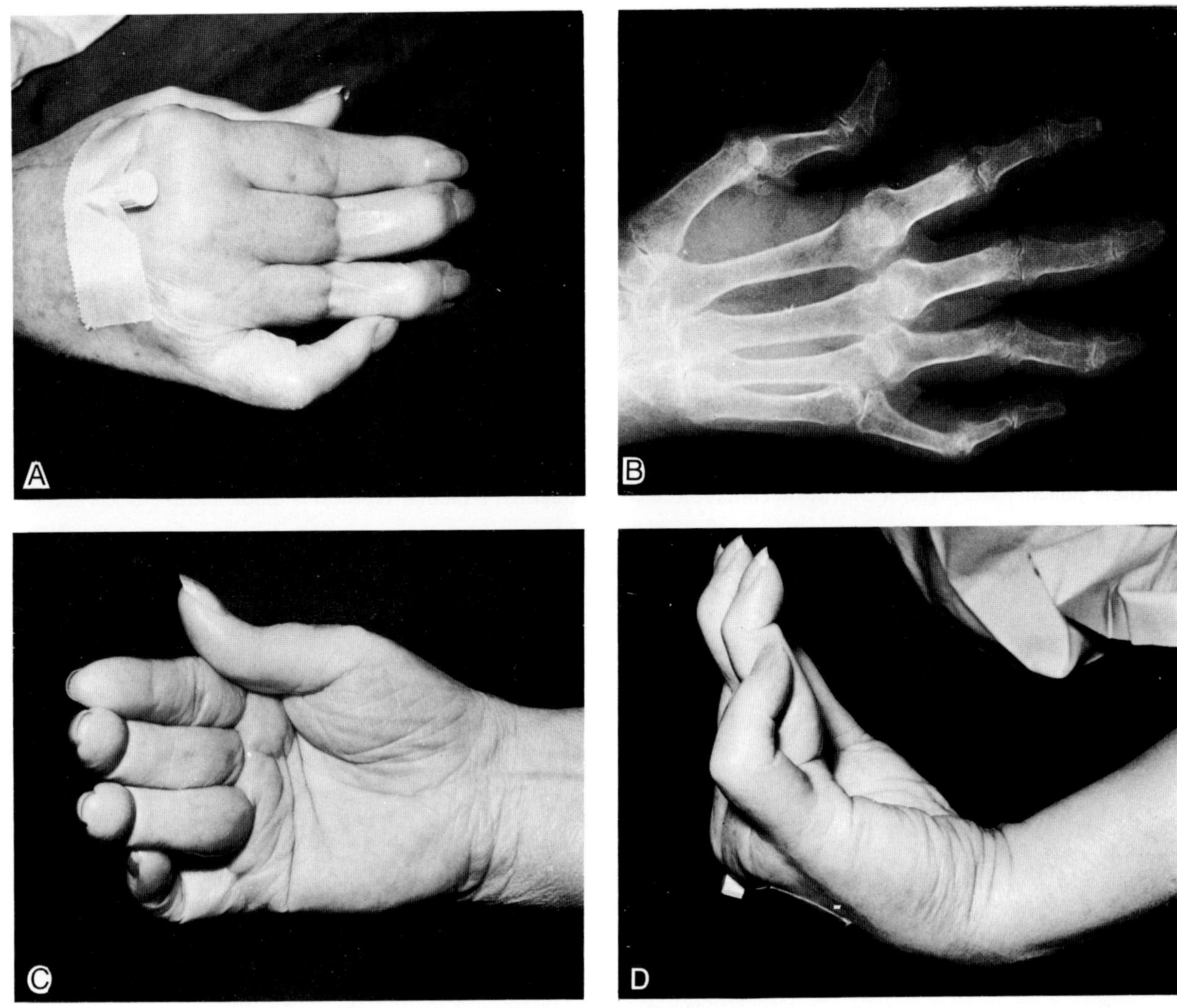

Fig. 46-41. Type IV swan-neck deformity treated by PIP joint arthroplasty. **(A)** Preoperative deformity. **(B)** Radiograph shows severe degeneration of index finger PIP joint and narrowing of other PIP joints. **(C&D)** Lack of PIP flexion during attempted grasp significantly limits hand function. (From Nalebuff and Millender,[190] with permission.)

sociated flexor tendon ruptures also are relative indications for fusion.[93]

PIP Joint Fusion for Swan-neck Deformity

We use a longitudinal skin incision. The extensor mechanism is split in the midline, and the collateral ligaments are detached from the proximal phalanx. The joint is flexed to expose the articular surfaces, which are prepared for fusion by removing the articular cartilage and softening the subchondral bone. At the PIP joint level, we routinely use two crossed K-wires for internal fixation. If the bone stock is adequate and the width of the medullary canal allows, a Herbert screw can be used for internal fixation (see Fig. 46-37). Precise technique is needed to obtain the desired angle of fusion using this method. The position of fusion selected depends on the finger involved and the sex of the patient. In general, the index finger PIP joint is fused in less flexion than that of the middle finger. The degree of flexion is greater in the ring and small fingers to facilitate grip. The amount of flexion chosen ranges from 25 to 45 degrees. In female patients, where cosmesis often is more important than strong grasp, less flexion than the so-called functional position is used. The patient's requirements must be discussed and determined preoperatively. It is helpful to have a small sterile goniometer on the instrument table as it is sometimes difficult to judge the angle of flexion of the PIP joint accurately by eye. Usually the joint is flexed more than is anticipated. Measurement of the angle of flexion after the first pin is inserted will allow correction easily prior to insertion of the final pins.

PIP Joint Arthroplasty

We often perform Swanson implant arthroplasties of the PIP joint for the stiff swan-neck deformity if the adjacent joints, soft tissues, and tendons are in good condition. We prefer arthroplasty, particularly in the ring and small fingers, when restoration of grasp is important.

A curved dorsal incision is used. In our standard technique using the dorsal approach, the extensor mechanism is exposed, split longitudinally in the midline, and reflected to either side of the PIP joint. This allows the tension on the extensor mechanism to be adjusted with a purse-string suture during closure. Nalebuff has modified this approach to avoid damaging the extensor mechanism when this structure is in good condition. The same curved dorsal skin incision is used, but is made slightly longer. An incision in the extensor mechanism is made within the lateral bands. Placing the incision within the substance of the lateral band facilitates closure and maintains the integrity of the transverse retinacular ligament. The subtotal extent of the entire extensor apparatus is moved to one side to expose the PIP joint capsule. The fatty areolar tissue lying between the dorsal periosteum of the phalanges and the extensor tendon is preserved to facilitate tendon gliding postoperatively. The collateral ligaments are divided at their origins on the proximal phalanx and preserved for reattachment following insertion of the implant. The distal end of the proximal phalanx is removed and the medullary canal prepared to accept the stem of the implant. A sufficient amount of bone is removed to relax tension on the contracted extensor mechanism when the implant is inserted to avoid having to lengthen the central slip. The base of the middle phalanx is debrided if necessary, and the articular cartilage and subchondral bone are perforated. The medullary canal is prepared to accept the distal stem of the implant. Closure of the extensor mechanism after insertion of the prosthesis must not be so tight as to prevent full passive flexion of the PIP joint. The central slip may need to be shortened if there is insufficient extension of the PIP joint when tested by either the tenodesis effect during passive wrist motion, or by proximal traction on the extensor mechanism proximal to the PIP joint. Skin closure is done with the joint in slight flexion. If necessary, the distal portion of the wound is left open to avoid excessive skin tension (Fig. 46-42). Frequently, a palmar incision is made and the flexor tendon ex-

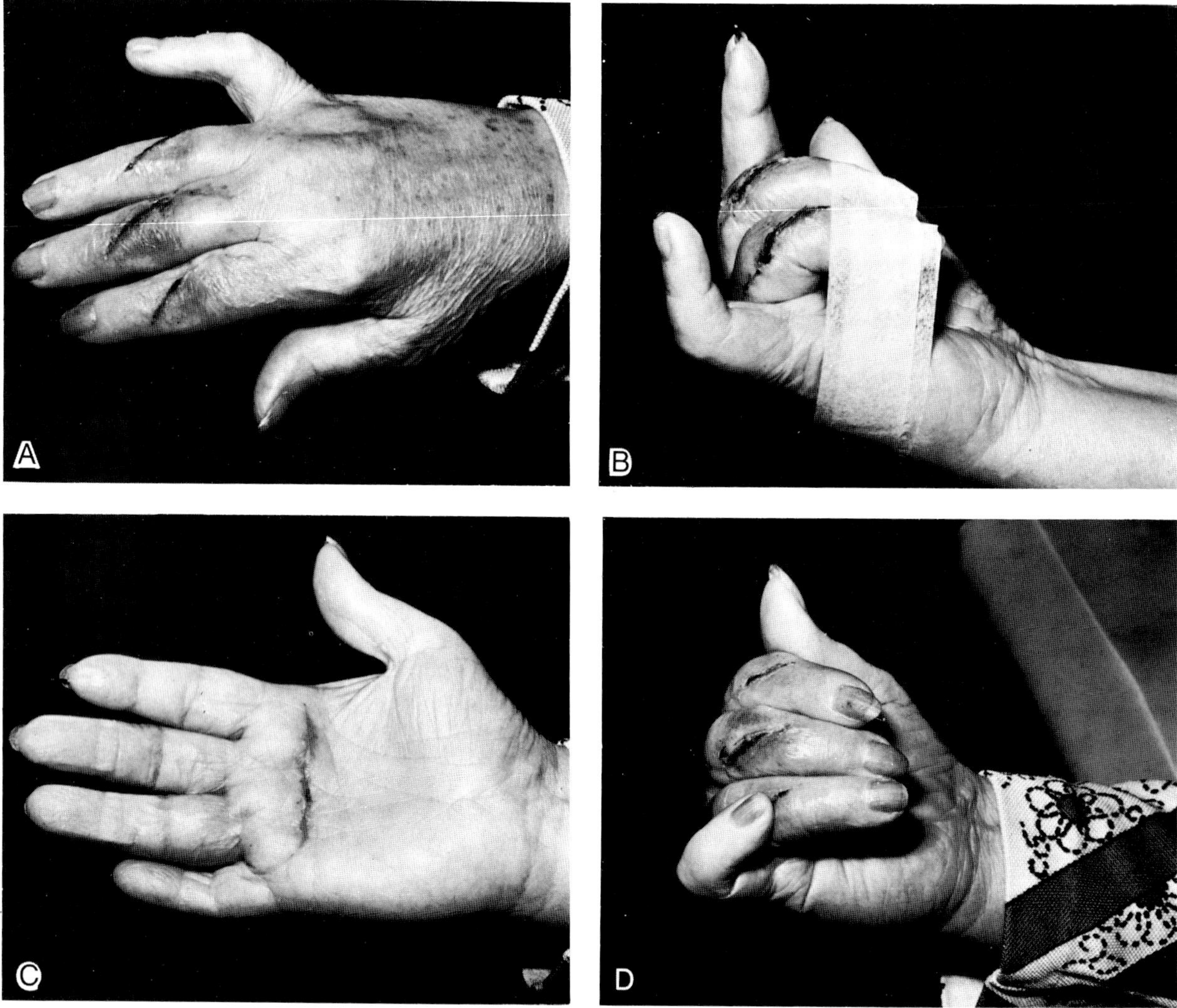

Fig. 46-42. Postoperative appearance of the patient shown in Figure 46-41. **(A)** Improved finger posture. **(B)** Tape used to splint the fingers in flexion during the early postoperative period. **(C)** Postoperative extension. Note the palmar incision used to check flexor tendon function at the time of PIP arthroplasty. **(D)** Active PIP joint flexion. Note healing by secondary intention of the distal portions of the skin incisions left open at surgery. (From Nalebuff and Millender,[190] with permission.)

cursion checked, and a tenolysis performed if needed. Postoperatively, the fingers are splinted in 20 to 30 degrees flexion, and active and gentle passive exercises are begun within several days after operation.

Boutonnière Deformity

Boutonnière deformity occurs frequently in patients with rheumatoid arthritis. Like the swan-neck deformity, it is not specific to this disease and represents an alteration in muscle and tendon balance.[70,141,233,236] The deformity has three components: flexion of the PIP joint, hyperextension of the DIP joint, and hyperextension of the MP joint. While the swan-neck deformity in the rheumatoid patient may originate at any of the finger joints, the boutonnière deformity begins with flexion of the PIP joint. The changes in the adjacent joints are secondary.

Synovial proliferation within the PIP joints stretches the extensor mechanism. As a result, the central slip is unable to maintain full extension of the joint. The lateral bands displace volarward and become fixed in this position. Shortening of the oblique retinacular ligaments results in hyperextension and limited active flexion of the DIP joint. As the flexion deformity of the PIP joint increases, the patient compensates by hyperextending the MP joint. When seen early, the deformities are correctable passively. Later, with fibrosis and contracture of the capsular tissues, the deformity becomes fixed. Functional loss as a result of the boutonnière deformity may remain minimal until the late stages. For this reason, the treatment of early boutonnière deformity should be simple and involve minimal risk. Salvage surgery (fusion or arthroplasty) should be performed only for the severe fixed deformities. Our operative approach to the rheumatoid boutonnière deformity depends on the degree of severity. We classify boutonnière deformities as mild, moderate, or severe on the basis of the degree of flexion of the PIP joint, the presence of passive correctability of this joint, and the status of the PIP joint surfaces.[189]

Stage I: Mild Boutonnière Deformity

In the early stages of the boutonnière deformity there is only a slight lag (10 to 15 degrees) in PIP joint extension. There may be active synovitis of the joint. The DIP joint may or may not be slightly hyperextended. The MP joint usually is normal during this early stage. The extensor lag of the PIP joint can be corrected passively. However, when this is done, there is limited flexion of the DIP joint. Flexion of the DIP joint improves as the PIP joint is flexed. The patient's functional loss is related as much to the lack of full DIP joint flexion as to the lack of PIP extension, but functional impairment is minimal at this stage. Any operative treatment of this mild boutonnière deformity should not jeopardize existing function. We treat the mild boutonnière deformity by extensor tenotomy to improve DIP joint flexion.[53] Dynamic splinting to extend the PIP joint is used postoperatively to restore the balance of the finger. This method does not risk loss of PIP joint flexion. If active PIP joint synovitis is present, we consider either local steroid injection or synovectomy in our treatment plan.

Extensor Tenotomy (Fig. 46-43)

We use a longitudinal incision over the dorsal aspect of the middle phalanx. The extensor mechanism can be divided either obliquely or transversely to allow the DIP joint to flex. Postoperatively, there may be a slight "droop" of the DIP joint, but a significant mallet deformity usually does not develop. This procedure is based on the concept that the oblique retinacular ligament acts to extend the DIP joint. However, the dorsal support provided by the extensor mechanism and joint capsule most likely plays a role in maintaining the normal posture of the joint.

We perform extensor tenotomy under local anesthesia; this allows the alteration of finger stance as well as finger function to be observed at the time of surgery. Occasionally, a significant extensor lag of the DIP joint occurs following the tenotomy. A brief period of postoperative external splinting of this joint usually corrects this problem. If the deformity is not corrected, or if it progresses, the DIP joint can be fused in extension. In most patients, we do not splint the DIP joint postoperatively but encourage active DIP joint flexion with the PIP joint supported by a dynamic, reverse knuckle-bender splint. This is important in restoring proper balance between the two joints.

Stage II: Moderate Boutonnière Deformity

The functional loss of the finger becomes more significant as the flexion deformity of the PIP joint reaches 30 to 40 degrees. Patients usually compensate for this by hyperextending the MP joint. Although there are significant difficulties involved in reconstruction of a fixed moderate boutonnière deformity, we have found that satisfactory correction of the deformity with preservation of active PIP joint flexion can be achieved. All of the procedures described to correct the established boutonnière deformity attempt to restore the extensor power to the PIP joint using local tissue. We do this by shortening the central slip and bringing the lateral bands dorsally. We believe that it is important to combine this procedure with extensor tendon tenotomy at the DIP joint. Unless this is done, there is a risk of restoring PIP extension but markedly limiting DIP flexion. We recommend extensor mechanism reconstruction in patients with moderate progressive deformity if several criteria are met: good dorsal skin, relatively smooth joint surfaces, intact and functioning flexor tendons and, of course, passive correctability of the PIP joint. Flexion deformity at the wrist should be corrected before attempting to restore PIP joint extension. We prefer to reconstruct the PIP joint extensor mechanism prior to, or at the same time as, MP joint arthroplasty, since any residual flexion deformity at the PIP joint has an adverse effect on achieving MP joint flexion after MP joint arthroplasty.

Reconstruction of the Extensor Mechanism for Boutonnière Deformity (Figs. 46-44 and 46-45)

A dorsal longitudinal curved incision is made over the PIP joint. A laterally based skin and subcutaneous flap is elevated to expose the extensor mechanism. This places the skin inci-

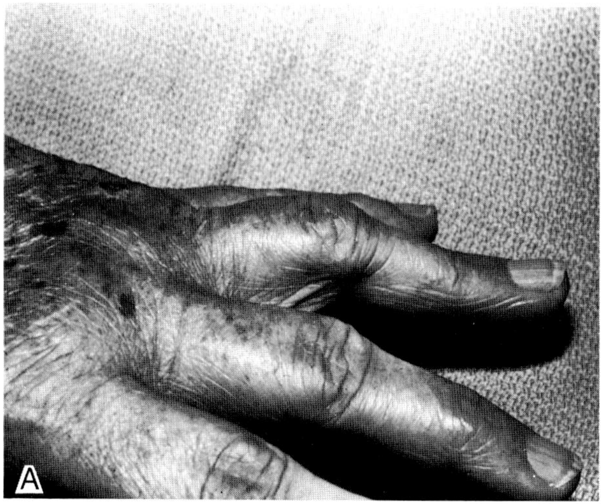

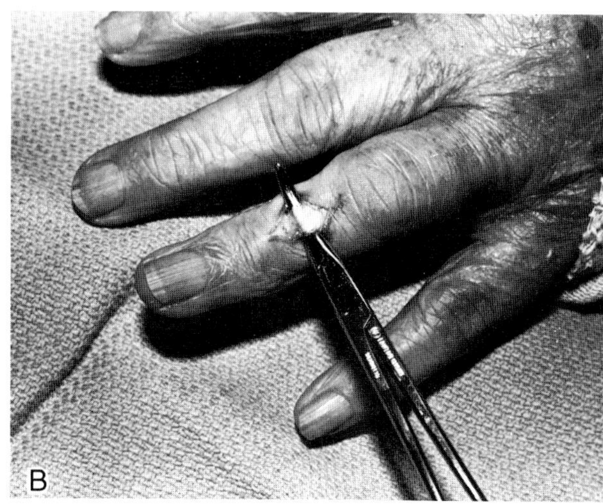

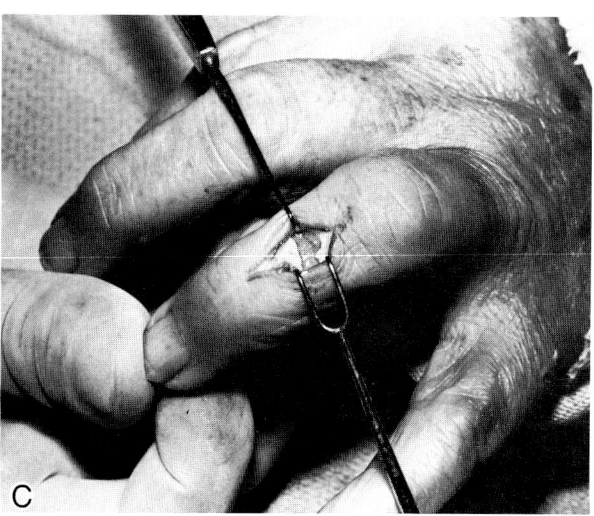

Fig. 46-43. Extensor tenotomy technique for mild boutonnière deformity. **(A)** Preoperative deformity of the ring finger. **(B)** The extensor mechanism is isolated over the middle phalanx through a longitudinal incision. **(C)** Tenotomy of the extensor mechanism can be performed transversely, as shown, or obliquely. Note flexion of the distal joint following tenotomy.

sion away from the site of the extensor tendon repair. The central slip is divided distally, leaving a cuff of tendon attached to the base of the middle phalanx. The central slip is separated from the lateral bands proximally. Inspection of the undersurface of the central slip will show the changes that have occurred from gradual stretching. Approximately $\frac{1}{4}$ inch (6 mm) of the central slip is excised. The remaining portion is reattached to the cuff of the central slip insertion (which was left intact at the base of the middle phalanx) with nonabsorbable sutures. Two longitudinal relaxing incisions are made just volar to the lateral bands. These divide the transverse retinacular ligaments and allow the lateral bands to be brought dorsally. The lateral bands are sutured either to the central slip or to each other. The posture of the finger should be corrected now. However, there is usually increased resistance to passive DIP joint flexion, or even hyperextension of this joint. The extensor mechanism overlying the middle phalanx is divided transversely or obliquely through the distal portion of the incision, allowing the DIP joint to flex. This procedure allows all of the extensor mechanism force to be concentrated at the PIP joint level.

Adjustment of the tension of the central slip is very important. It should be possible to flex the PIP joint passively 70 or 80 degrees after the central slip has been reattached. The strong flexors act to increase the range of flexion after postoperative splinting has been discontinued.

A K-wire is placed across the PIP joint to maintain full extension during the early postoperative period. The DIP joint is left free and active motion of this joint is allowed. After 3 to 4 weeks, the K-wire is removed, and the joint is protected with a reverse knuckle-bender splint during the day and a padded aluminum splint at night for several weeks.

The postoperative program may be modified according to the finger involved and the amount of PIP joint flexion possible after the K-wire is removed. If several fingers are reconstructed simultaneously, we remove the K-wire from the small finger first. In this finger we will accept less correction of PIP joint extension to ensure maximum flexion. The reverse is true for the index finger in which a loss of some flexion is less significant. If necessary, reconstruction of the moderate boutonnière deformity can be performed on all four fingers at the

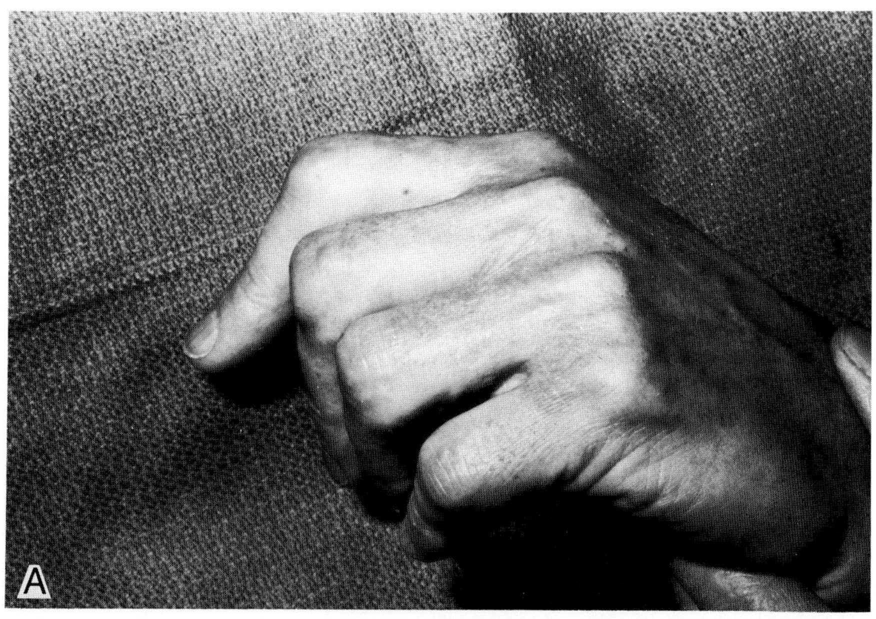

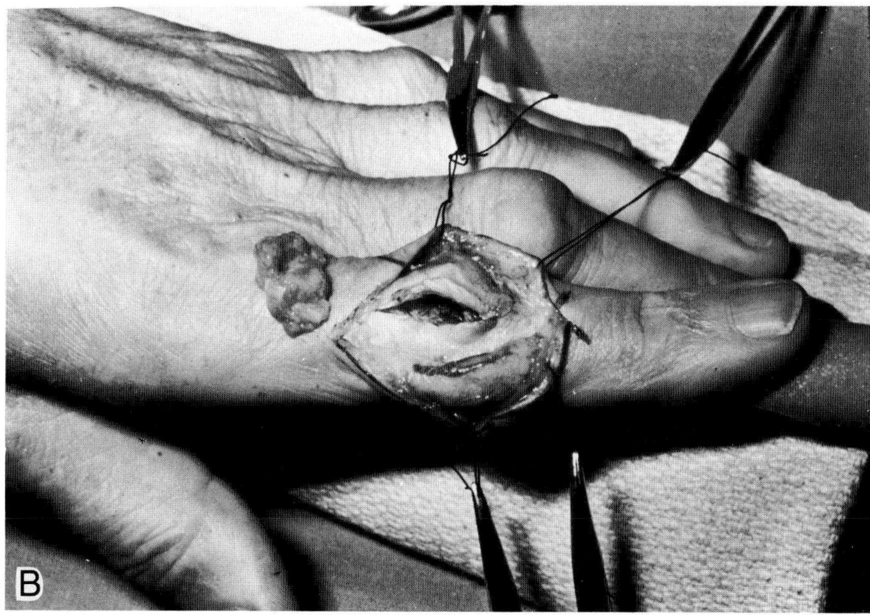

Fig. 46-44. Technique of extensor mechanism reconstruction for boutonnière deformity. **(A)** The patient has moderate boutonnière deformity in all fingers. **(B)** The extensor mechanism is lax following synovectomy. *(Figure continues.)*

same time. In most patients, however, the criteria necessary for this operation are present in only one or two fingers. Limiting the reconstruction to these simplifies the operation as well as the postoperative splinting and exercise program.

Stage III: Severe Boutonnière Deformity

In time, the boutonnière deformity progresses to the point where the PIP joint can no longer be extended passively. No attempt should be made to restore extensor mechanism function unless the joint can be extended passively without excessive force. In this case, restoration of passive motion by dynamic splinting or serial plaster casting is attempted. Occasionally, soft tissue release (dividing the transverse retinacular ligaments and the accessory collateral ligaments) is necessary to restore passive extension. This is combined with extensor mechanism reconstruction. This extensive surgery is not indicated often.

In severe deformities with poor joint surfaces, the alternative treatment is fusion or arthroplasty. Fusion is the standard method used to correct severe fixed flexion deformities in the rheumatoid patient. It is used in patients whose finger extension is so restricted that they are unable to grasp moderate size to large objects.

The position of PIP fusion is chosen to achieve a "functional" position of the involved finger. In the index or middle

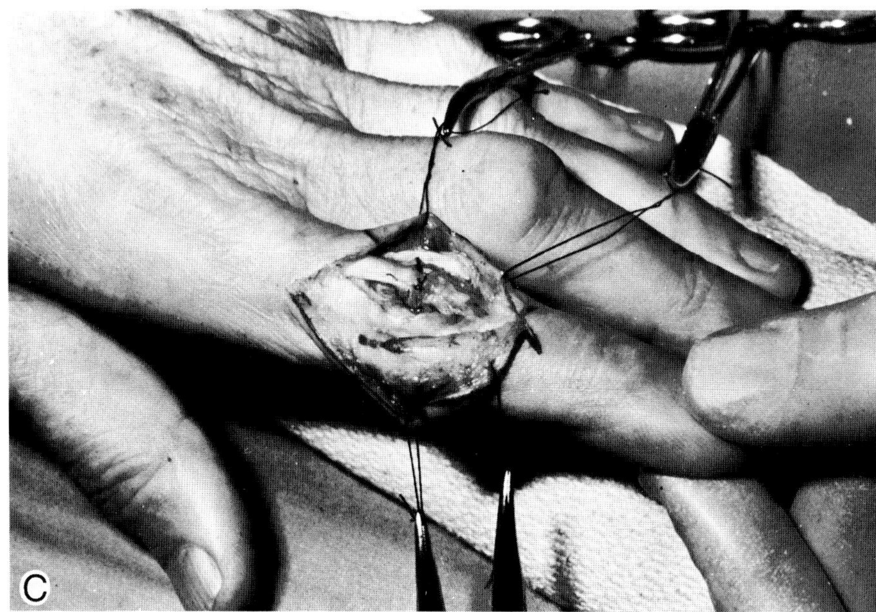

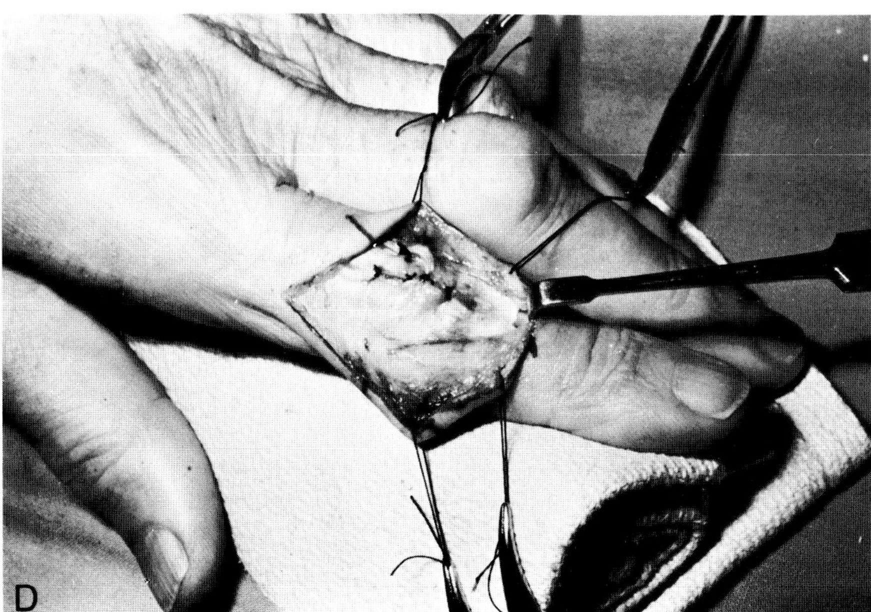

Fig. 46-44 *(Continued).* **(C)** The central slip has been shortened. Note the relaxing incision volar to the lateral band. **(D)** The lateral bands sutured in dorsal position. Note extensor tenotomy over the middle phalanx (at the extreme distal end of the incision).

finger, loss of full flexion is not critical. In patients with severe bilateral boutonnière deformities, we have performed multiple fusions on one hand, leaving the deformities on the other side untreated to maintain the ability to grasp small objects on one side. However, the loss of PIP joint flexion following fusion is compensated, in part, by the gain in MP joint flexion.

PIP Joint Fusion for Boutonnière Deformity

Technically, it is easier to perform PIP joint fusion to correct a fixed flexion deformity than to correct a swan-neck deformity because of the surplus of skin on the dorsal aspect of the finger and the compression of the bone ends that occurs as the joint is straightened. We use either a longitudinal curved incision or, occasionally, a transverse incision over the PIP joint. The extensor mechanism often is nonexistent. The collateral ligaments are divided at their origins on the proximal phalanx. With the finger in maximal flexion, the distal end of the proximal phalanx is removed with an osteotome. The proximal phalanx cut is at a slight angle, directed volarly. The articular cartilage is removed from the base of the middle phalanx, and the subchondral bone is softened with a rongeur. As the finger is straightened, the bone ends are compressed. Bone grafts usually are not needed because of the excellent bone contact.

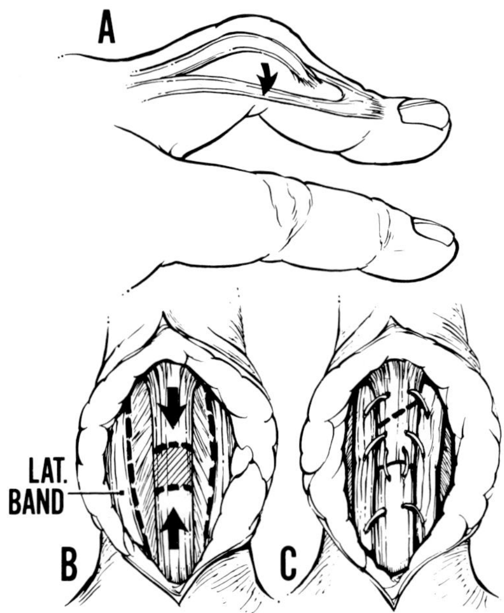

Fig. 46-45. Extensor mechanism reconstruction for boutonnière deformity. **(A)** The arrow shows the fixed volar position of the lateral band. **(B)** Lateral bands mobilized. The portion of the central slip to be excised is shaded. **(C)** The central slip sutured in shortened position and the lateral bands brought dorsalward and sutured to the central slip.

The position of fusion that we choose varies with the finger involved. We prefer 25 degrees flexion for the index finger and gradually increase the flexion to 45 degrees for the small finger. As mentioned previously, confirmation of the desired angle of fusion with a sterile goniometer is suggested. A K-wire is passed longitudinally across the joint (Fig. 46-46) and is supplemented by an obliquely placed wire. These can be cut off flush to the bone and left in place permanently or left protruding through the skin to facilitate removal after fusion has occurred. Again, a Herbert screw may be used as described previously for internal fixation (see Fig. 46-37).[66] External splints are used for the first 4 to 6 weeks until the fusion has started to consolidate. If the MP joints were fixed in hyperextension preoperatively, they are brought into flexion by manipulation, soft tissue release, or arthroplasty.

PIP Joint Arthroplasty for Boutonnière Deformity

PIP joint arthroplasty using a silicone implant is an alternative method for treating the fixed rheumatoid boutonnière deformity. Because the goal of this procedure is to maintain motion, the extensor mechanism must be reconstructed as part of the procedure. This is done by reattaching the central slip to the base of the middle phalanx. Relocation of the lateral bands dorsally is required often as well, to direct all of the extensor force to the PIP joint. Swanson[246,248,250] has shown impressive results with this technique, and we now use it in selected cases.

This approach is particularly appropriate in patients whose deformity involves the ring and small fingers and whose MP joints are flexible, as preservation of PIP motion in these fingers will enhance the ability to grasp. However, we feel that it is not indicated in a very severely flexed PIP joint because of the necessity of resecting excessive bone to provide enough space for the implant.

PIP joint arthroplasty is discussed in more detail in Chapter 7.

THUMB DEFORMITIES

Rheumatoid thumb deformities represent some of the more difficult problems of rheumatoid reconstructive surgery—especially for the surgeon who is unaccustomed to dealing with the rheumatoid hand. In order to evaluate the rheumatoid thumb deformity and to plan appropriate treatment, a clear understanding of the pathophysiology and natural history of these deformities and their resultant clinical disabilities is necessary. The original classification of thumb deformities suggested by Nalebuff included four groups. This classification was revised to include a fifth group. Type I deformity (boutonnière deformity) is the most common, and Type III (swan-neck deformity) is the second most common. Type IV deformity is seen occasionally, and Type II and Type V are more rare. Ratliff[209] has described an additional deformity—interphalangeal and/or MP joint destruction with instability, but without the characteristics of any of the above types.[2,94,121,123,142,150,178,195]

Pathophysiology of Thumb Deformities

Type I Thumb Deformity (Boutonnière Deformity)

Type I deformity is initiated by proliferative MP joint synovitis, which bulges dorsally and results in attenuation of the extensor pollicis brevis tendon insertion, stretching of the extensor hood, and displacement of the extensor pollicis longus tendon ulnarward and volarly. The collateral ligaments are stretched, and intraarticular joint destruction occurs to varying degrees. This loss of dorsal support results in subluxation of the proximal phalanx on the metacarpal and concomitant hyperextension of the interphalangeal joint from the altered pull of both intrinsic muscles and the extensor pollicis longus.

In the early stage, both MP and interphalangeal (IP) joint deformities are correctable passively (Fig. 46-47); however, in time, fixed deformities develop—first of the MP joint alone and later of both the MP and interphalangeal joints.

Indications for Operative Treatment

There are three clinical stages in the development of Type I deformity. Each requires a different type of surgical treatment. In the early stages, there is MP joint subluxation with interphalangeal joint hyperextension, but both joints are correctable passively. Surgical treatment at this stage includes synovectomy of the MP joint and reconstruction of the extensor mechanism. This corrects the MP joint deformity and helps prevent further collapse of the interphalangeal joint, but a review of this

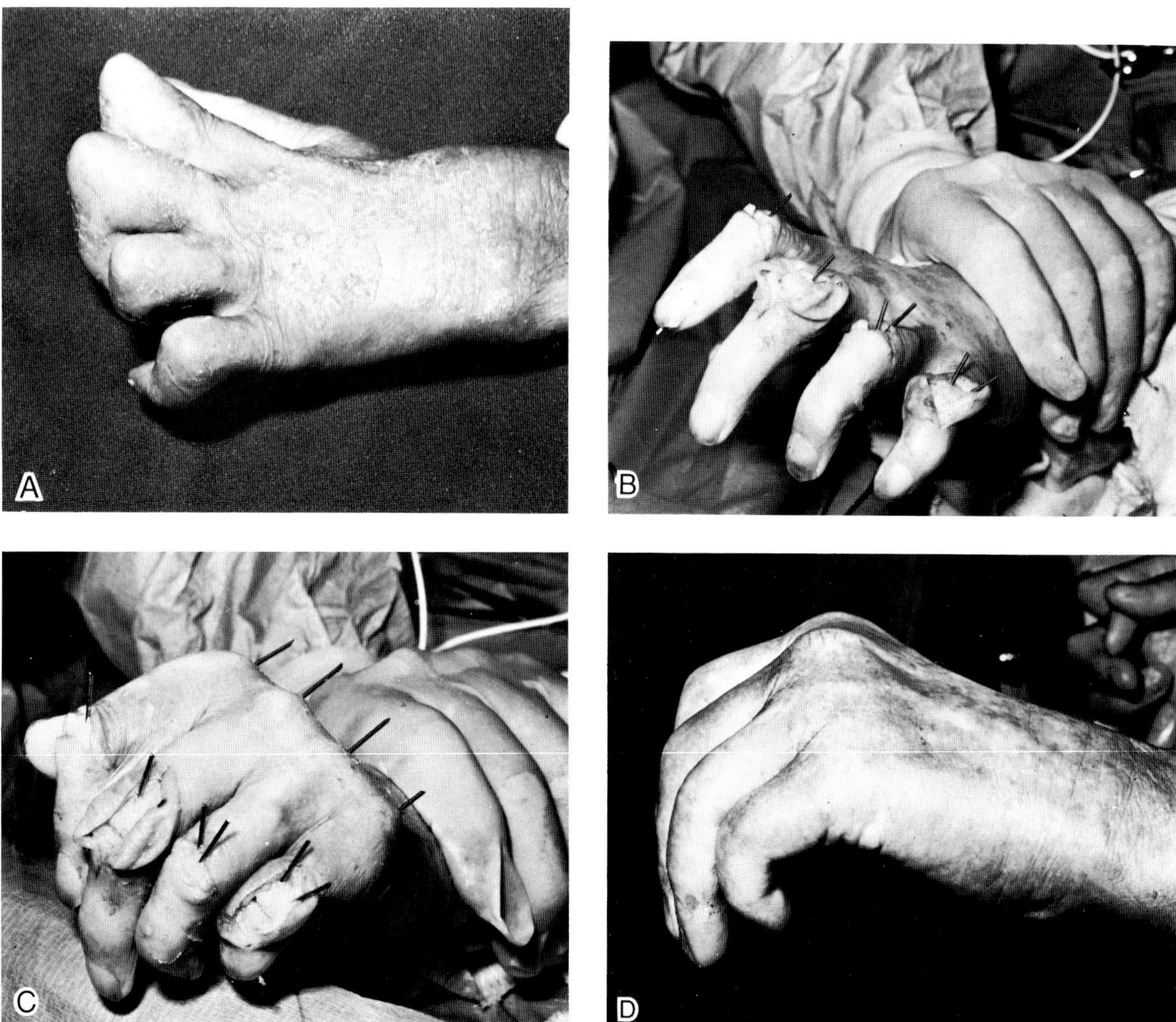

Fig. 46-46. Severe boutonnière deformities treated by PIP fusions. **(A)** Severe fixed flexion contractures of the PIP joints with the MP joints fixed in extension. **(B)** Degree of flexion for fusion increases from the index to small finger. **(C)** MP joints manipulated into flexion and held with K-wires. **(D)** Postoperatively, the finger position is improved and grasp of moderate sized objects is possible. (From Nalebuff and Millender,[189] with permission.)

procedure by Terrono and Millender[266,267] revealed a high late recurrence rate.

In the second stage, a fixed MP joint is present with or without intraarticular joint destruction. The interphalangeal joint deformity is correctable passively. Most patients are seen at this stage. Arthrodesis is recommended for the MP joint if it is totally destroyed and the two adjacent joints are involved minimally. However, if destructive changes are likely to develop at one of the adjacent (carpometacarpal or interphalangeal) joints, MP joint arthroplasty or MP arthroplasty combined with extensor pollicis longus rerouting must be considered. Correction of the deformity at the second stage will prevent the third stage from developing.

The third and most difficult stage is that of both a fixed MP joint flexion deformity and a fixed interphalangeal joint hyperextension deformity. Treatment is dependent on the status of each of the two joints. If the interphalangeal joint is not destroyed and can be released by a dorsal capsulotomy, some degree of IP joint motion can be preserved. If the deformity is too severe, interphalangeal joint arthrodesis is indicated. MP joint surgery will depend on the severity of the deformity, the status of the articular surfaces, and the surgery indicated for the interphalangeal joint. If the interphalangeal joint has been fused, we try to preserve MP joint motion with either synovectomy and extensor pollicis longus rerouting or with silicone implant arthroplasty. However, in the severely deformed or destroyed joints, combined MP and interphalangeal joint fusions sometimes are indicated. Although Ratliff[209] stated that he had never found an indication for arthrodesis of both of these joints, others believe that this is indicated occasionally. If the MP joint is only moderately stiff and has a salvageable joint surface, intrinsic muscle and ligamentous release with recon-

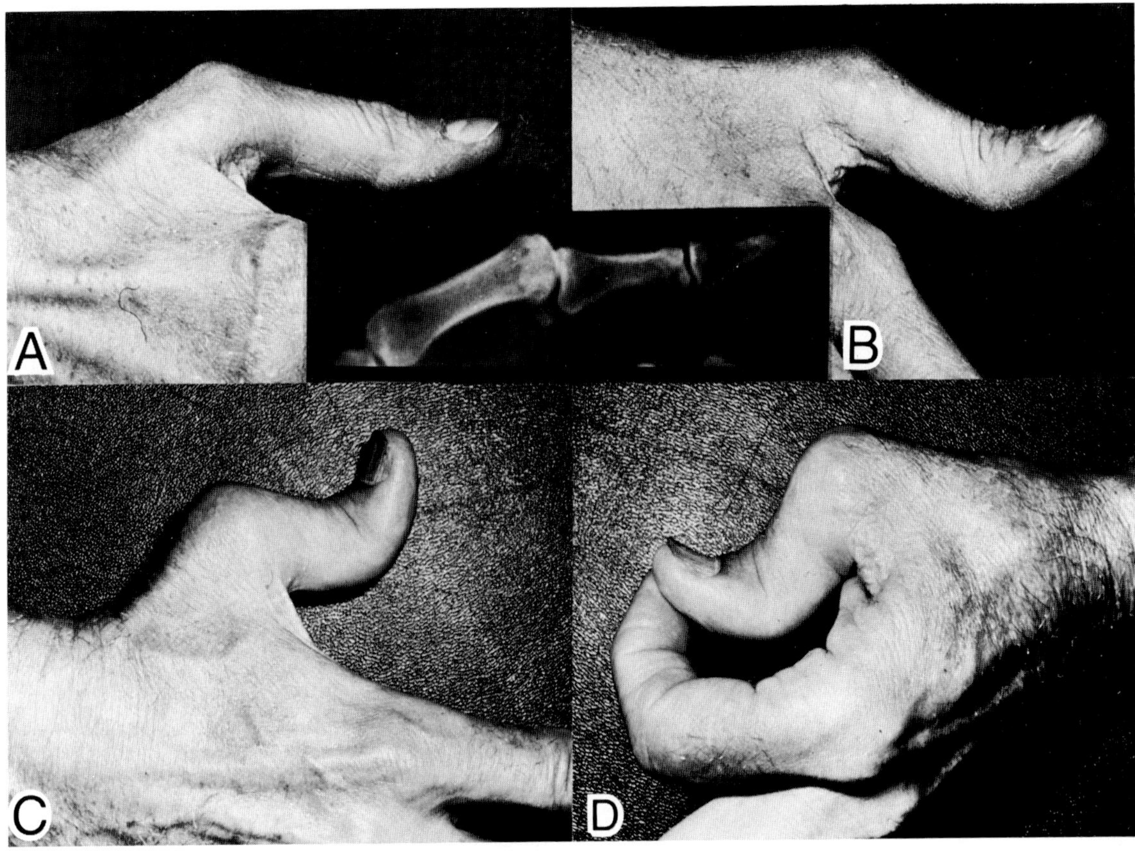

Fig. 46-47. Type I thumb deformity. **(A)** Synovitis of the MP joint stretches the extensor mechanism resulting in MP joint extension lag. Initially the interphalangeal joint is not involved. **(B)** MP joint subluxation with interphalangeal joint hyperextension. As the disease progresses, there is MP joint involvement with cartilage loss and early subluxation. **(C)** Advanced Type I deformity with fixed MP and interphalangeal joint deformity. **(D)** Pinch aggravates the collapse deformity.

struction of the extensor mechanism is indicated. Our most common procedure for the third stage deformity is interphalangeal joint fusion and MP joint arthroplasty (Fig. 46-48).[165,255] We use the hinged Swanson implant designed for the great toe because of its greater strength. The collateral ligaments are tightened during closure and the MP joint is splinted for 4 to 6 weeks after surgery to increase stability of the joint.

Type III Thumb Deformity (Swan-neck Deformity)

The second most common thumb deformity is Type III or swan-neck deformity.[175] This deformity results from disease at the level of the carpometacarpal joint. Synovitis and erosion of the articular surfaces and capsular distension allow dorsal and radial subluxation of the carpometacarpal joint as the thumb is used for grasp. Repeated use may result in complete dislocation of this joint. As the joint subluxates, abduction forces are reduced and adduction contracture of the metacarpal develops (Fig. 46-49). Other reasons for the development of adduction contracture of the first metacarpal have been proposed by various authors. Swanson believes that painful abduction associated with an element of adductor muscle spasm may lead to this deformity.[247] Clayton described contracted adductor muscles preventing abduction of the thumb metacarpal.[39] Vainio postulated that the adduction contracture developed as a result of joint ankylosis and fibrosis.[273,275] Kessler found that neither the adductor muscle nor the first dorsal interosseous muscle ever was contracted, but he did find contracture and shortening of the fascia overlying these muscles.[120] Our experience confirms Kessler's findings.

Hyperextension of the MP joint develops secondary to the metacarpal adduction contracture, if the volar plate is lax. As the patient attempts to open the first web space to grasp, the fixed carpometacarpal joint deformity prevents metacarpal abduction and extension. The extension forces are transmitted to the MP joint, resulting in the hyperextension of this joint. These patients can grasp moderate size objects only by hyperextending the MP joint.

Indications for Operative Treatment

Patients with Type III deformities also are seen in three general stages.

In the first stage, a painful carpometacarpal joint, weak pinch, and various degrees of radiographic carpometacarpal

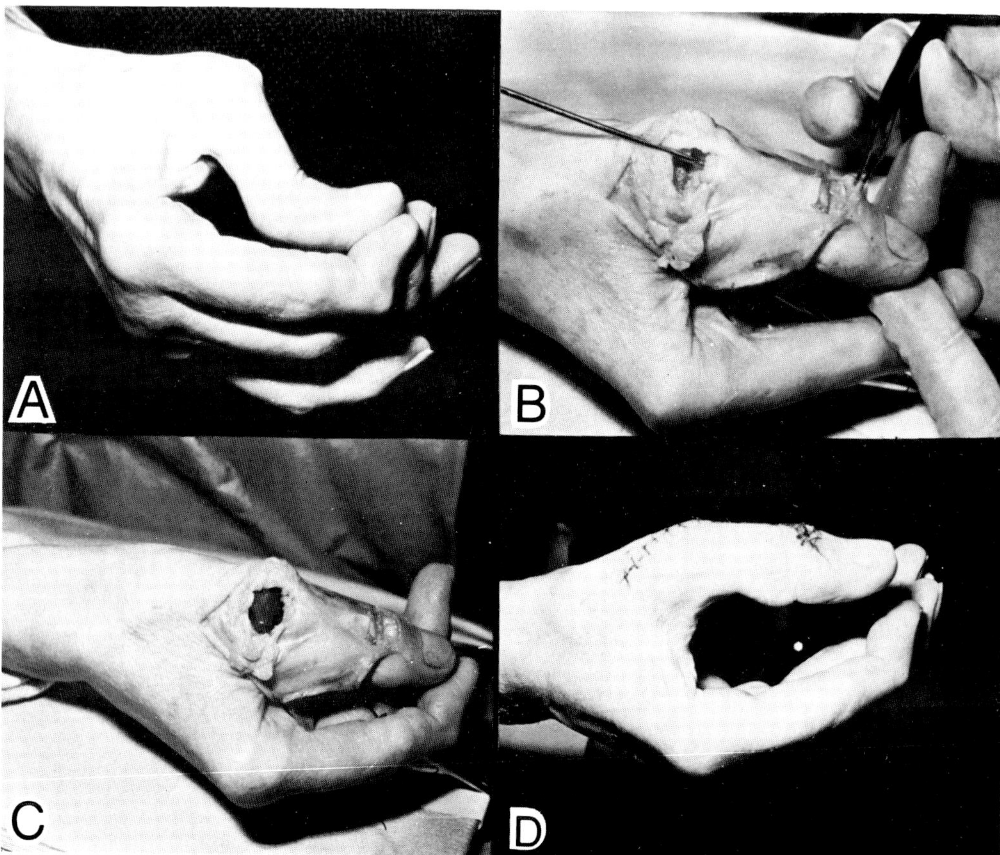

Fig. 46-48. Treatment of advanced Type I deformity. **(A)** Advanced Type I deformity with fixed MP joint and interphalangeal joint deformity. The preferred treatment is MP arthroplasty and interphalangeal joint fusion. **(B)** MP joint prepared for arthroplasty and a longitudinal K-wire inserted across the interphalangeal joint for fusion. **(C)** Silicone implant placed in the MP joint prior to capsular closure. **(D)** Surgical procedure completed with correction of deformity.

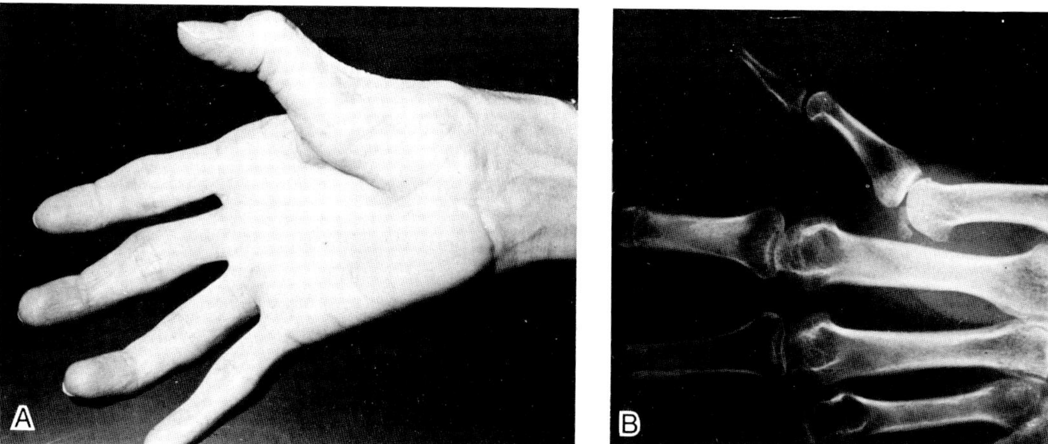

Fig. 46-49. Type III thumb deformity. **(A)** Clinical appearance with carpometacarpal joint subluxation, thumb metacarpal adduction, and secondary MP joint hyperextension. **(B)** Radiograph demonstrates carpometacarpal joint destruction with erosion of the trapezium and metacarpal subluxation.

joint destruction are seen. At this stage there is minimal subluxation, minimal deformity, and no secondary MP joint involvement. Surgical treatment is indicated only for persistent carpometacarpal joint pain after proper conservative therapy has failed. Conservative therapy consists of an adequate trial of systemic medications, 2 to 4 months of splinting, and occasional steriod injections.

The recommended surgical treatment is hemiarthroplasty. Most surgeons believe that total trapezium replacement arthroplasty is contraindicated in the rheumatoid patient because of the high incidence of dislocation associated with poor capsule and bone stock. We are more apt to do a resection arthroplasty rather than an implant arthroplasty. When an implant arthroplasty is done, we use a small concave or convex silicone implant for hemiarthroplasty at this level (see page 1689).

Patients in the second stage show varying degrees of carpometacarpal joint deformity and mild, passively correctable MP joint hyperextension (Fig. 46-50). Unless pain is significant, these patients function quite well, except for weakness of

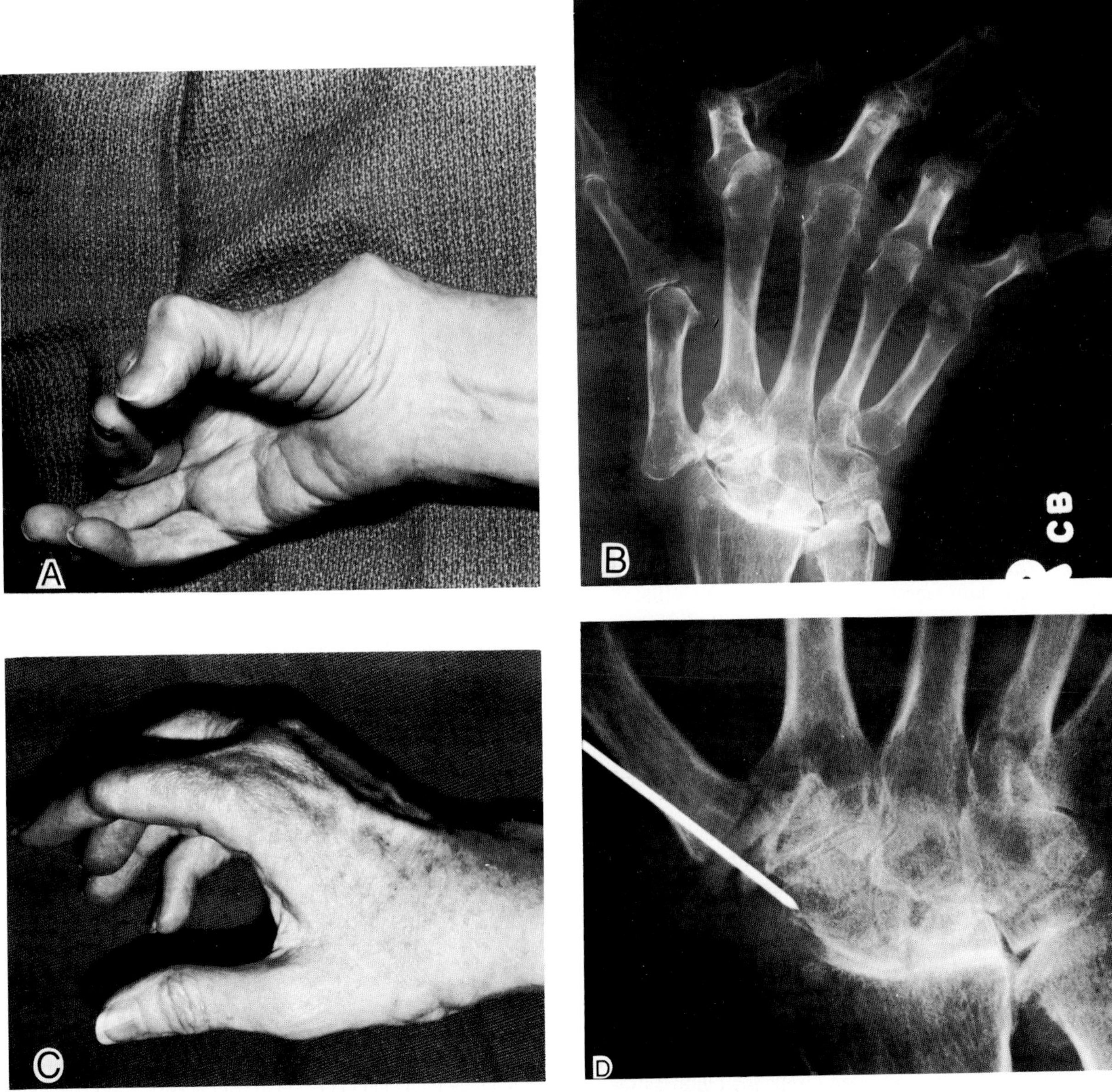

Fig. 46-50. Advanced rheumatoid thumb deformity. **(A)** Dislocated carpometacarpal joint with adduction deformity of the metacarpal and hyperextension deformity of the MP joint. **(B)** Radiograph of the hand. Note collapse deformity of the wrist, dislocation of the MP joints, and lateral dislocation of the index PIP joint. **(C)** After hemiarthroplasty of the carpometacarpal joint and soft tissue reconstruction of the MP joint. **(D)** Radiograph demonstrating hemiarthroplasty with silicone implant. A K-wire is used for temporary implant fixation. (From Nalebuff and Millender,[191] with permission.)

pinch. Our recommended treatment for mild MP joint deformity is implant hemiarthroplasty or resection arthroplasty combined with volar tenodesis of the MP joint. We perform MP joint fusion for advanced deformity or joint destruction.

Advanced Type III deformity includes complete carpometacarpal joint dislocation with a fixed adduction contracture and a fixed hyperextension deformity of the MP joint. These patients have significant disability as a result of the contracted first web space, which prevents grasp of moderate size objects. The zigzag collapse deformity precludes adequate pinch. Carpometacarpal hemiarthroplasty with MP joint fusion is helpful in restoring function to these patients. We have found, as did Kessler, that nearly complete correction of the metacarpal deformity can be obtained by resecting the base of the metacarpal and, if necessary, releasing the deep carpometacarpal ligament. We have found that it is necessary to release the fascia over the first dorsal interosseous muscle only occasionally, and we have never found it necessary to release the adductor muscle. Z-plasty of the skin of the first web space is necessary infrequently as tight skin in rheumatoid patients will stretch after bony and other tissue releases have been performed.[81,90,166]

In a patient with SLE, a CMC joint fusion should be done because of increased ligamentous laxity (see page 1590). Shapiro staples[223] are useful for internal fixation in these fusions.

Type IV Thumb Deformity (Gamekeeper's Deformity)

Type IV deformity is characterized by an abduction deformity of the MP joint with secondary adduction of the thumb metacarpal. This occurs as synovitis of the MP joint stretches the ulnar collateral ligament, resulting in lateral instability of this joint. Secondarily, an adduction contracture of the thumb develops. In some cases, shortening and contracture of the adductor fascia similar to that seen in Type III deformity may occur. The important aspect of Type IV deformity is that there is no primary carpometacarpal joint disease, and, therefore, treatment should be directed to the MP joint.

Indications for Operative Treatment

MP joint synovectomy, collateral ligament reconstruction, and adductor fascia release are performed if these structures are tight.

In the advanced cases either MP joint arthroplasty or MP joint arthrodesis is performed. If fusion is done, it should be accompanied by correction of the adduction contracture. After the MP joint is stabilized, the thenar muscles will function to abduct and oppose the entire thumb ray more effectively and to prevent further adduction of the thumb metacarpal.

Type II Thumb Deformity

Type II deformity, which is seen rarely, is a combination of Type I and III deformities. It consists of MP joint flexion with interphalangeal joint hyperextension and an associated subluxation or dislocation of the carpometacarpal joint. The treatment of this deformity is similar to that for Type I and III deformities.

Type V Thumb Deformity

Type V thumb deformity results from stretching of the MP joint volar plate. The MP joint hyperextends with secondary flexion of the interphalangeal joint as tension on the flexor tendon increases. In contrast to the Type III deformity, the first metacarpal does not assume an adducted position.

Surgical treatment of the Type V thumb deformity is simple; the MP joint is stabilized in flexion, either by volar capsulodesis or by fusion.

Thumb Deformities Secondary to Joint Destruction

Ratliff has described an additional deformity that we see frequently.[209] This is the result of both destruction and instability of the interphalangeal joint and/or the MP joint. Although any type of deformity may develop, lateral deformities are seen frequently at the MP joint and lateral and hyperextension deformities are seen at the interphalangeal joint. These deformities often are the result of the bone destruction and resorption associated with arthritis mutilans. In advanced cases, these cause severe loss of hand function and disability.[186]

Indications for Operative Treatment— Severe Joint Destruction/Arthritis Mutilans

Preventive synovectomy of the interphalangeal or MP joint usually is performed in conjunction with other hand surgery. Synovectomy is so unpredictable in these patients that it is infrequently performed as an isolated procedure. Arthrodesis is the usual procedure of choice for these joints. In patients with arthritis mutilans, arthrodesis should be performed early, before marked bony resorption has occurred. When arthritis mutilans has resulted in marked bone loss, bone grafts will be required to restore or maintain length and to allow fusion to occur.[83,186] Although we have no experience with Harrison-Nicolle "pegs," they may be an alternative in these situations. The "pegs" are polypropylene implants that are utilized as internal splints to stabilize the joint, thereby allowing a bony or fibrous ankylosis to develop around the joint and peg.[102,106]

Operative Techniques for Thumb Reconstruction

Surgery is based on which joint is involved. The classification of deformity by type improves the surgeon's understanding of the problem, but is not important in the overall treatment.

Interphalangeal Joint

The surgical techniques used for reconstruction of the interphalangeal joint are synovectomy, extensor tendon release (for fixed hyperextension deformities), and arthrodesis of the interphalangeal joint.

Synovectomy of the interphalangeal joint may be performed through a dorsal curved or longitudinal incision. Swanson has described a Y incision centered over the interphalangeal joint, which we have found useful.[252] Another incision that we have used is a longitudinal zigzag incision centered over the interphalangeal joint. This protects the terminal branches of the dorsal sensory nerve. After the skin flaps are elevated, the proliferative synovium can be removed from either side of the joint with a small rongeur. A small portion of the extensor mechanism can be detached from the base of the distal phalanx, which, combined with traction on the phalanx, allows easier access to the joint.

Flatt noted that occasionally the major portion of the diseased synovium lies in the volar pouch.[77] In these cases, the synovium may be removed through a midaxial incision on one side of the joint, dividing the accessor collateral ligament. Lipscomb[140] has recommended approaching the joint from the side (the ulnar side in all fingers except the small finger) and releasing the collateral ligament to completely dislocate the joint. The collateral ligament is repaired after a complete synovectomy is performed. The joint is protected with a K-wire for 10 to 12 days prior to beginning motion. We have had no experience with either of these procedures.

After interphalangeal joint synovectomy, the joint is splinted in extension for a few days prior to beginning exercises. The joint should be splinted between exercise periods for 2 weeks to prevent an extensor lag from developing.

Interphalangeal Joint Release

This procedure is performed in conjunction with MP joint fusion or arthroplasty in the moderately severe Type I deformity.

The skin incision utilized is critical, as the dorsal skin is contracted and thereby limits the amount of flexion that can be obtained. Our usual approach uses a lateral incision on either side of the joint. A tenolysis of the extensor mechanism is performed. The dorsal capsule is incised by sliding the blade volar to the extensor mechanism and then rotating it 90 degrees. The dorsal portion of the collateral ligament is released through each incision, and the joint is manipulated into flexion. Usually the joint can be held in 25 to 30 degrees flexion without placing the dorsal skin under undue tension.

Alternatively, a Z-plasty can be used. A longitudinal incision is made over the midportion of the joint. This provides excellent exposure. The release is performed as described above. After the K-wire has been inserted, the incision is converted into a Z-plasty. There rarely is sufficient skin to close the incision completely, and a portion of the wound is left open. This will epithelialize within 10 to 12 days, after which time the K-wire is removed and exercises are started. For several days after the wire is removed, the joint is protected with a plaster or aluminum splint. Occasionally, an extensor lag develops. In these cases, the joint should be splinted in extension to allow the extensor mechanism to contract. Ten to 25 degrees of active joint flexion after these procedures can be expected; a large range of flexion never is obtained.

Interphalangeal Joint Arthrodesis

This is described on page 1657.

MP Joint

Operative procedures for the rheumatoid MP joint include synovectomy, synovectomy with extensor mechanism reconstruction, volar release in conjunction with reconstruction of the extensor mechanism for fixed flexion deformities, arthroplasty, and arthrodesis.[102,104,140,216,238]

Synovectomy of the MP Joint

A slightly curved, longitudinal incision, 3 to 4 cm in length, is made over the MP joint. Radial and ulnar flaps are reflected to expose the extensor mechanism. The sensory branches of the radial nerve must be protected. The joint is exposed by a longitudinal incision between the extensor pollicis longus and extensor pollicis brevis tendons, which are reflected ulnarward and radially, respectively. The synovium bulges dorsally, often having ruptured through the joint capsule. A synovectomy is performed with a small rongeur.

Traction applied to the joint will give additional exposure. Synovium should be removed carefully from the recesses on either side of the collateral ligament attachment to the metacarpal head. Synovitis in this area causes the early bony erosions, which are seen radiographically. A small curette is helpful in entering the tight space between the ligament and the metacarpal head. After synovectomy is completed, the extensor mechanism is closed and the joint splinted in extension. Splinting is continued for 12 to 14 days prior to beginning exercises. In the thumb, MP joint stability is more important than motion, and, therefore, we allow time for adequate soft tissue healing before motion is started.

MP Joint Synovectomy with Extensor Mechanism Reconstruction (Fig. 46-51)

These procedures are indicated for early Type I deformity in which the joint is preserved and subluxation is correctable passively. Nalebuff, Inglis, and Harrison have described separate surgical procedures.[102,114,178]

In each of the methods, the extensor mechanism is exposed as described for synovectomy. The extensor pollicis longus and extensor pollicis brevis tendons are identified. The extensor pollicis brevis usually is attenuated, and the extensor pollicis longus often is displaced ulnarly and volarly.

To perform the extensor pollicis longus rerouting described by Nalebuff, the interval between the extensor pollicis longus and the extensor pollicis brevis is identified. The extensor pollicis longus is transected over the proximal one-third of the proximal phalanx and freed proximally. The attenuated extensor pollicis brevis tendon is dissected from the base of the proximal phalanx and detached from the extensor hood. The joint is approached through a transverse incision in the thin portion of the capsule, leaving the thickened portion of the capsule attached to the base of the proximal phalanx. A transverse incision is made in this thicker capsule distal to the joint, through which the extensor pollicis longus tendon will be passed. A complete synovectomy of the joint is performed. The extensor pollicis longus is passed through the hole in the capsule and pulled back over itself. With the joint held in full extension, the tendon is sutured tightly to itself. The extensor

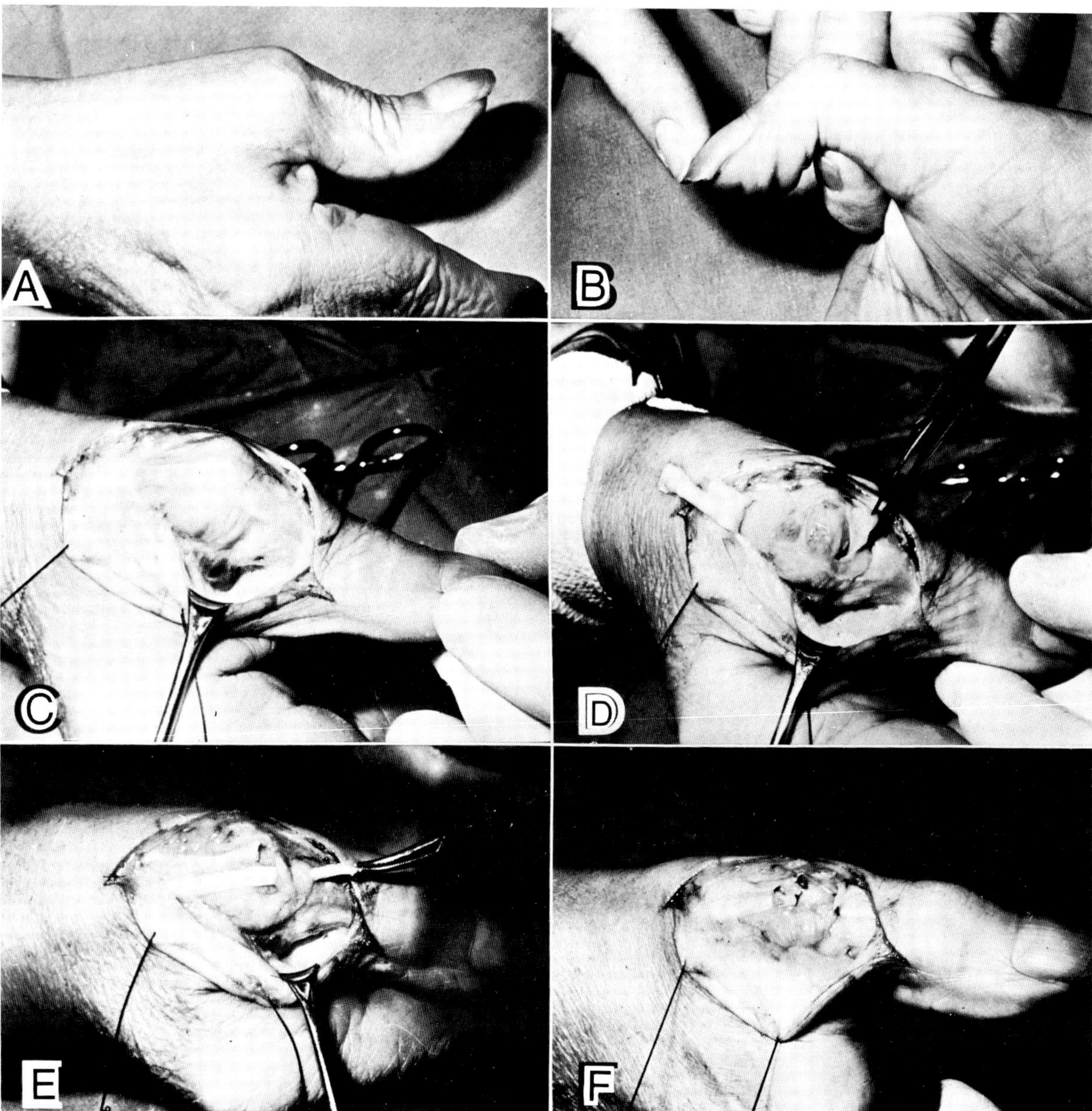

Fig. 46-51. Extensor pollicis longus rerouting for early Type I deformity. **(A)** Type I thumb deformity with MP joint extension lag and interphalangeal joint hyperextension. **(B)** There is full passive extension of the MP joint and flexion of the interphalangeal joint. **(C)** Extensor mechanism exposed demonstrating the stretched extensor pollicis longus and extensor pollicis brevis tendons. **(D)** Extensor pollicis longus and extensor pollicis brevis tendons released. The capsule is exposed and MP joint synovectomy is performed. **(E)** Incision made in the base of the capsule and extensor pollicis longus passed through the capsule. **(F)** Extensor pollicis longus sutured to itself. The extensor pollicis brevis is reconstructed and the deformity is corrected. *(Figure continues.)*

pollicis brevis is pulled distally and sutured into the side of the extensor pollicis longus. Nalebuff has modified his technique for extensor pollicis longus rerouting. He now transects the extensor pollicis longus tendon more proximally and sutures the extensor pollicis brevis tendon to the extensor pollicis longus stump to improve IP joint extension.

The dorsal expansions of the intrinsic tendons on each side of the joint are checked to be sure that they are in their proper position, as they are now the sole extensors of the terminal phalanx. If there is any tendency for these tendons to subluxate volarly, the transverse fibers between the intrinsic tendons over the dorsal aspect of the midportion of the distal phalanx can be tightened to ensure their direct action on the stump of the extensor pollicis longus tendon. An oblique K-wire is used to hold the MP joint in extension.

The thumb is splinted with the interphalangeal joint in extension. Interphalangeal joint flexion and extension exercises are started in a few days. The interphalangeal joint is protected

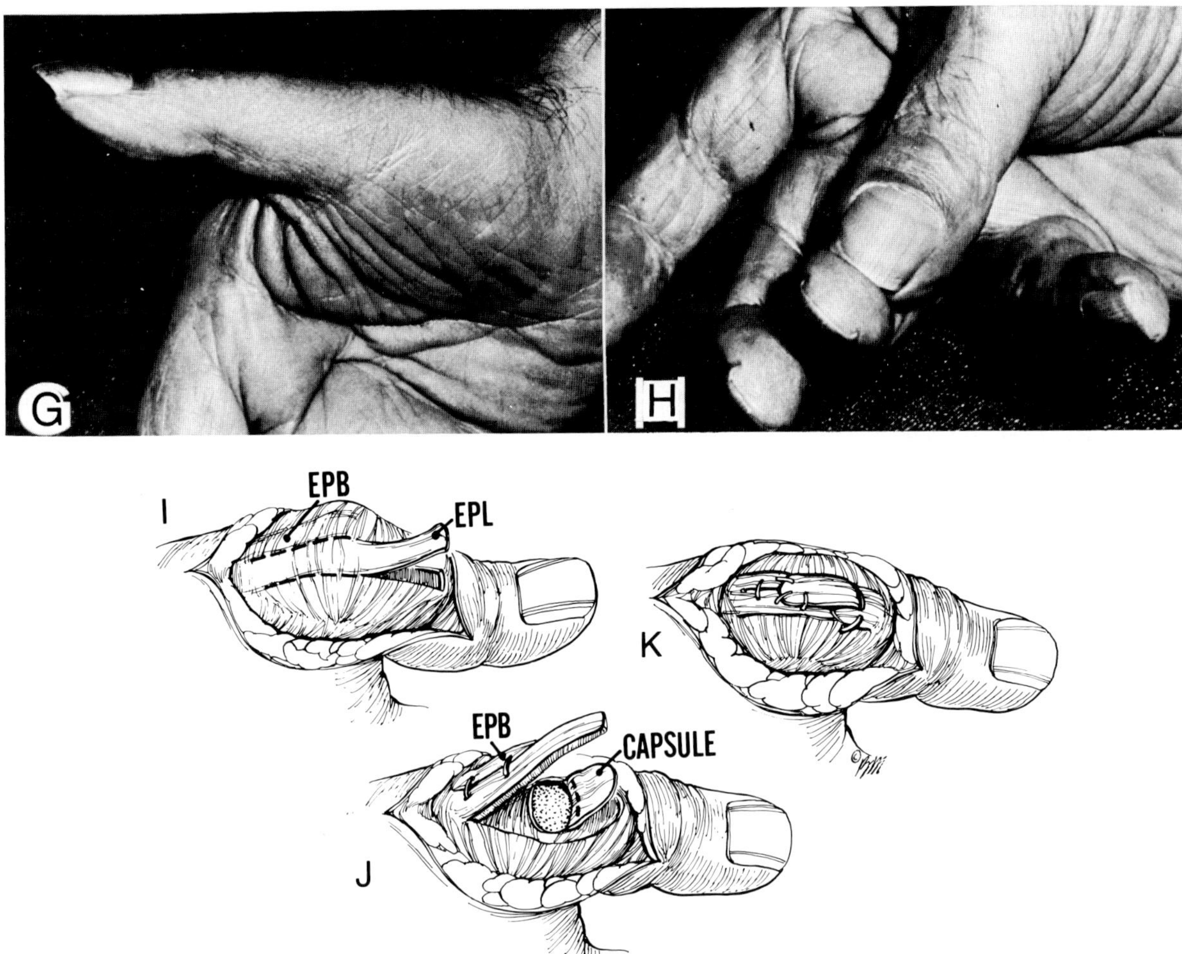

Fig. 46-51 *(Continued).* **(G&H)** Postoperative extension and flexion. **(I)** In the standard method of extensor pollicis longus *(EPL)* rerouting, the extensor pollicis longus tendon is transected between the MP and IP joints and elevated proximally. In Nalebuff's modified technique, the extensor pollicis longus is transected more proximally and the distal stump is sutured to the extensor pollicis brevis *(EPB)* tendon. The proximal stump is passed through the MP joint capsule and sutured back onto itself in both methods **(J&K).**

in extension when not being exercised to prevent an extensor lag. The K-wire across the MP joint is removed in 4 weeks. However, the MP joint is splinted in extension for an additional 1 to 2 weeks to allow complete soft tissue healing. All splinting is discontinued 6 weeks following surgery.

Harrison's[102] procedure for reconstructing the MP joint is similar to the rerouting procedure described above, except that a portion of the extensor pollicis longus is tenodesed to the base of the proximal phalanx by passing the split tendon through a hole in the base of the proximal phalanx and suturing it back to itself. The MP joint is held with a K-wire. The postoperative management is essentially the same as described above.

Inglis[114] splits the extensor mechanism longitudinally between the extensor pollicis longus and extensor pollicis brevis tendons to expose the joint and perform a synovectomy. The abductor pollicis brevis and the adductor pollicis are detached from the extensor hood. These two structures are retracted proximally and laterally. After synovectomy is performed, the extensor pollicis brevis is sutured tightly to the base of the proximal phalanx through a drill hole. The abductor pollicis brevis and adductor pollicis tendons are brought dorsally and attached to the side of the extensor pollicis longus tendon. These three tendons, the abductor pollicis brevis, adductor pollicis, and extensor pollicis longus, now function together as the extensor mechanism.

MP Joint Ligamentous Reconstruction for Type IV Deformity

The skin incision described above is used. The interval between the extensor pollicis longus and extensor pollicis brevis tendons is opened, and the extensor pollicis longus and dorsal expansion of the adductor pollicis are reflected ulnarward. The stretched ulnar collateral ligament is identified. This ligament is detached from the proximal phalanx or metacarpal—whichever end is more attenuated. A synovectomy of the joint is performed. The attenuated portion of the collateral ligament is excised. The freshened end of the collateral ligament is attached to bone using a pull-out suture. The adductor tendon is detached from the base of the proximal phalanx and advanced distally.

The postoperative management is similar to that for the extensor pollicis longus rerouting procedure.

Procedures for Fixed MP Joint Contractures

The procedures performed for fixed MP joint contractures are soft tissue release with extensor reconstruction (in mild to moderate cases) and arthroplasty or arthrodesis (for severe MP joint contractures with extensive cartilage loss). If the deformity is in the range of 25 to 35 degrees and the joint cartilage is involved minimally, soft tissue release may be preferable to arthroplasty or arthrodesis. Flatt[77] has described a procedure that we use in these circumstances.

MP Joint Soft Tissue Release with Extensor Reconstruction. The joint is exposed dorsally. The edges of the extensor mechanism are exposed, and the two winged intrinsic tendons are detached from the extensor pollicis longus distal to the MP joint. This releases the intrinsic tendon from the interphalangeal joint, thereby correcting some of the interphalangeal joint extension contracture. Interphalangeal joint extension now is provided solely by the extensor pollicis longus. If necessary, a dorsal capsulotomy of the interphalangeal joint is done to allow additional interphalangeal joint flexion. The extensor mechanism is freed proximally, releasing the bony attachments to the base of the proximal phalanx on the radial and ulnar sides. This should allow the MP joint to extend. If it cannot be extended, division of the accessory collateral ligament is necessary. Synovectomy is done through the standard dorsal capsular incision. The extensor pollicis brevis is reattached to the proximal phalanx—either to the capsule or to bone. The two winged intrinsic tendons are reattached to the soft tissues around the neck of the metacarpal to provide abduction and adduction of the entire thumb ray.

A K-wire is used to stabilize the MP joint. The postoperative treatment is similar to that described for the extensor mechanism reconstruction of the MP joint on page 1677.

Arthrodesis. The problems with and techniques for arthrodesis of rheumatoid joints differ from those in other clinical conditions and deserve special consideration. In some respects, arthrodesis in these joints is easier than in osteoarthritis or posttraumatic arthritic joints. Exposure is easier because of the laxity of the rheumatoid joint capsule and ligaments, cartilage removal is easier, and, unless there is bony resorption or significant deformity, preparation of subchondral bone and positioning of the bony surfaces prior to pinning are not difficult. Because of these factors, arthrodesis of rheumatoid joints can be performed rapidly, allowing joint fusions to be performed in addition to other major procedures during the allowable period of tourniquet inflation. However, other factors can make arthrodesis of these joints technically difficult. These include marked joint deformity, bone loss, and soft bone that does not afford firm internal fixation by K-wires.

Arthrodesis of Interphalangeal and MP Joints Without Severe Deformity or Bone Loss. Both joints are exposed dorsally, using approaches similar to those for synovectomy. The extensor mechanism and collateral ligaments are divided over the interphalangeal joint, allowing it to be dislocated by hyperflexion. Releasing the collateral ligaments from the metacarpal allows adequate exposure of the MP joint. Cartilage is removed from all surfaces with a rongeur, and soft cancellous bone is exposed over a broad surface. Proximal convex and distal concave surfaces are formed. The surfaces are apposed and checked for firm, stable contact. If MP joint arthroplasty or other arthroplasty has been performed immediately beforehand, the previously resected bone is morselized and packed into the interphalangeal fusion site prior to K-wire insertion. Generally, we fuse the interphalangeal joint in full extension or in very slight flexion. We also rotate the interphalangeal joint into slight pronation, if necessary. An 0.045- or 0.062-inch K-wire is passed distally through the medullary canal of the distal phalanx to exit at the tip, just volar to the nail plate. The exit position of the wire on the fingertip is important. Incorrect placement will damage the nail bed if too dorsal, or will be uncomfortable postoperatively if too volar. With the joint held in the selected position, the wire is drilled proximally into the medullary canal of the proximal phalanx using a power drill. The size of the wire is determined by the softness of the bone and the size of the medullary canal.

After the wire is passed, the bone ends are impacted and stability is checked. If stable, one K-wire is sufficient. If not, an oblique wire is added. The end of the wire is cut and buried deep to the pulp. If the pulp is thin or the wire is cut improperly, wire protrusion and pin tract infection make early wire removal necessary and increase the possibility of nonunion.

A plaster splint is applied after surgery. If the interphalangeal joint alone is fused, an aluminum splint is used to protect the joint for approximately 4 weeks after the sutures are removed.

The MP joint is approached and prepared essentially as described above. However, this joint is transfixed with two crossed K-wires. Although these can be passed retrograde, they are inserted most easily directly across the joint from dorsal and ulnarward on the metacarpal to dorsal and radial on the proximal phalanx and vice versa. The wires should be directed so that they do not exit on the volar surface of the thumb, thereby putting the flexor tendon and/or digital nerves at risk. Dual parallel Herbert screws can be used for internal fixation of MP joint fusions. Inglis[114] recommended fusing the MP joint in 15 degrees flexion, 15 degrees abduction, and 15 degrees internal rotation. We generally agree with this; however, this position is not sacred. If the CMC joint is unstable, the MP joint should be fused in more flexion, up to 25 degrees. It is advisable to measure the position of fusion accurately with a sterile goniometer before the final internal fixation devices are inserted. Intraoperative radiographs also are helpful in confirming the appropriate alignment for fusion.

If, after obtaining stable fixation, the position varies from that described above and is considered suboptimal, the joint can be bent into a better positon if only one small diameter K-wire has been inserted. The second wire is inserted after the position is corrected.

Arthrodesis in Arthritis Mutilans. Loss of bone stock is the major factor that makes fusion in rheumatoid patients difficult. The amount of loss ranges from thinned cortices and absent medullary cancellous bone to severe bone resorption with shortening, as seen in arthritis mutilans.[83,186] Joint exposure may be difficult because of deformity and/or subluxation, and the soft, thin bone may not hold K-wires well. In general, the technique is similar to that used for fusing any rheumatoid joint. However, certain points should be emphasized. Excellent exposure is mandatory. If "pencil-in-cup" deformities are present at the interphalangeal or MP joints, the bones are exposed by excising the capsule from the rim of the bone and the volar plate from the undersurface of the phalanx and by cutting the cartilaginous and cortical rim transversely to obtain a flat surface. After this has been accomplished, the joints can be apposed. However, adequate bone stock must be present. If bone stock is insufficient, cancellous bone from other areas (ie., resected metacarpal heads) is helpful to fill the gap and increase stability (Fig. 46-52). If the metacarpal heads from arthroplasty are devoid of cancellous bone, the cortical bone is crushed and used to fill the cavity. Wires are inserted as described above. A second longitudinal or crossed K-wire may be needed for the interphalangeal joint.

In cases of arthritis mutilans or severe pencil-in-cup deformities with loss of length, bone grafts are important. Shortening is accepted if the joints have fused spontaneously. However, iliac bone blocks often are needed to restore length and to obtain fusion[186] (Fig. 46-53). The joints are exposed and prepared as described above. A bone block from the iliac crest is fashioned, wedged into place, and fixed with longitudinal K-wires. Cancellous bone is packed into the remaining space. These fusions are difficult technically and require 4 to 5 months of immobilization postoperatively.

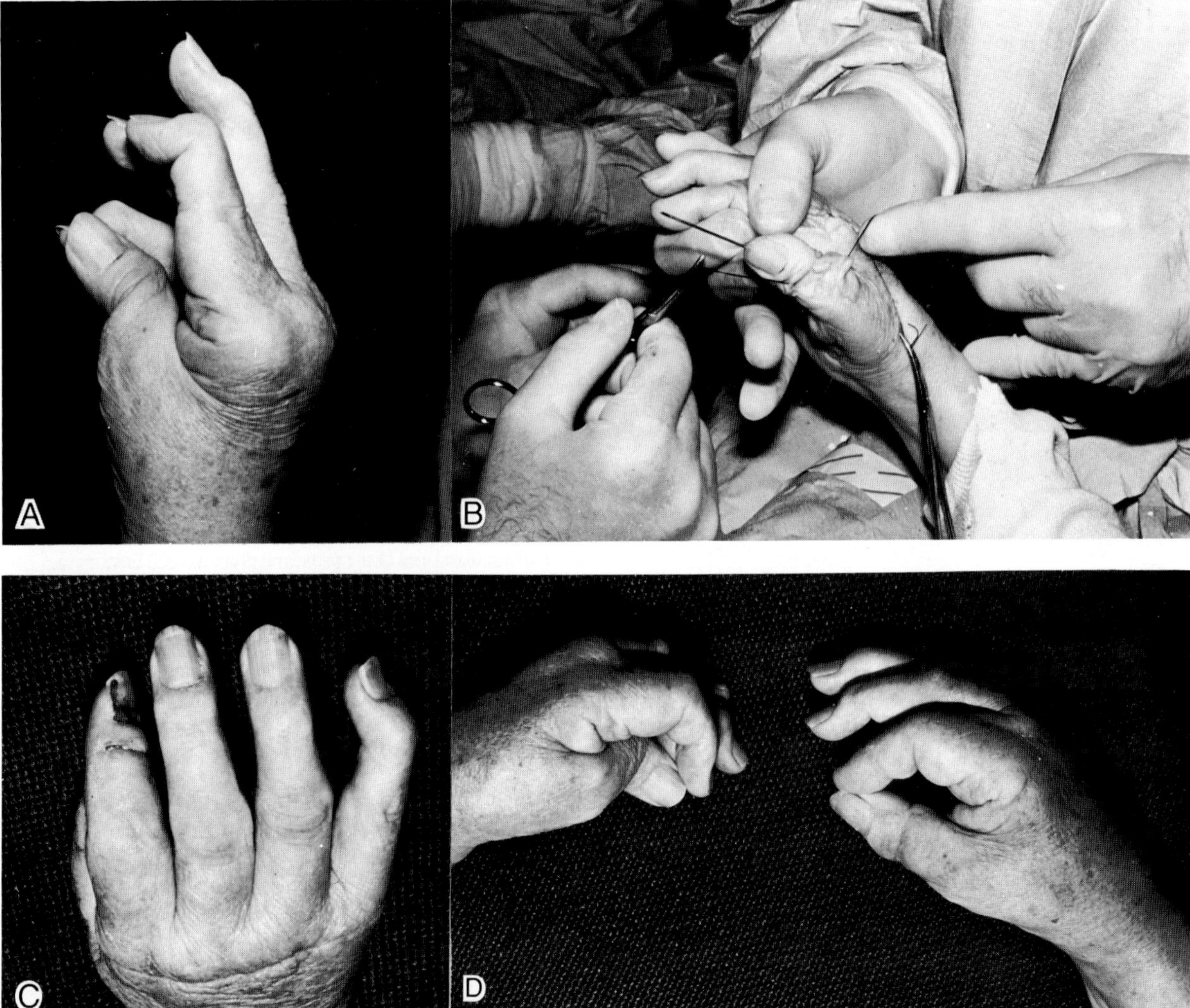

Fig. 46-52. **(A)** Lateral instability of the thumb interphalangeal joint with inability to pinch. Note finger MP joint dislocations and severe mallet deformity of the DIP joint of the index finger. **(B)** Thumb interphalangeal joint fused in exaggerated pronation, using the metacarpal head for a bone block. **(C&D)** Postoperative MP joint arthroplasty with interphalangeal joint thumb fusion and index DIP joint fusion. Note DIP joint fused in exaggerated supination to enable the patient to pulp pinch. Compare the operated with the nonoperated hand. (From Millender and Nalebuff,[165] with permission.)

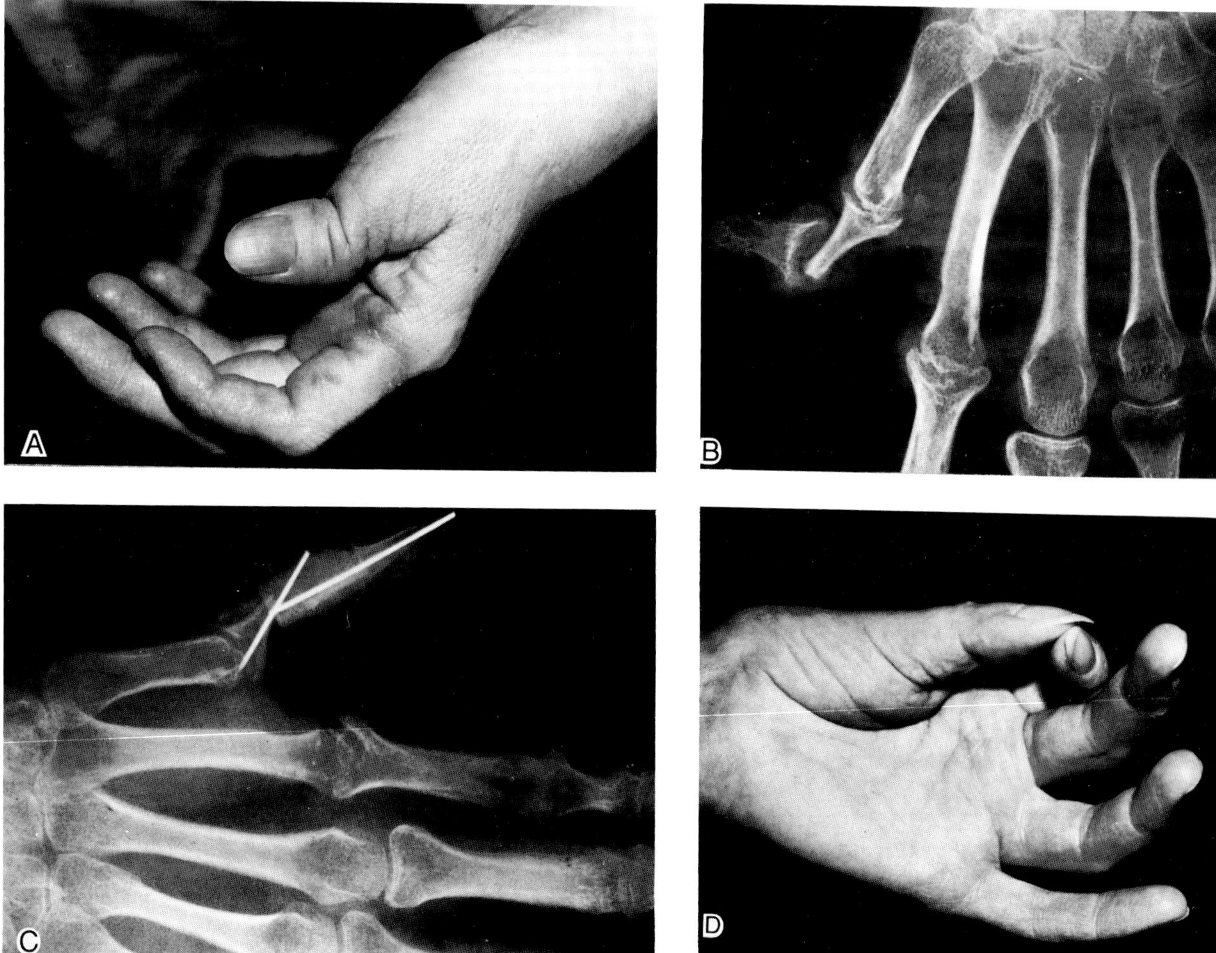

Fig. 46-53. Unstable distal joint of the thumb fused with a bone graft. **(A)** The clinical appearance of the thumb with collapse of the interphalangeal joint. **(B)** Radiograph shows significant absorption of the distal end of the proximal phalanx. **(C)** Postoperative radiograph shows use of bone graft to restore length and facilitate joint fusion. **(D)** Note the stable pulp pinch between the lengthened thumb and index finger. The distal joint is fused in slight flexion. *(Figure continues.)*

Arthrodesis Using Internal Splints. An alternative to formal arthrodesis in cases of arthritis mutilans or severe bone loss is the use of the Harrison peg.[103,106] In some instances of arthritis mutilans, we have used small Swanson MP implants in MP and interphalangeal joints. After these are inserted, K-wires are passed across the joint and implant. External immobilization is used for 10 to 12 weeks. This procedure results in fibrous ankylosis, but does allow some restoration of length with stability of the joint.

Trapeziometacarpal Joint Arthroplasty

The two types of trapeziometacarpal arthroplasty that we use in the rheumatoid patient are hemiarthroplasty and resection arthroplasty.[82,90,165,166,247]

Hemiarthroplasty

A zigzag incision extending from the proximal one-third of the metacarpal along the first extensor compartment is used. The sensory branches of the radial nerve have ramified at this level and must be preserved within the dorsal and volar flaps. Injury to these nerves can cause painful neuromas and dysesthesias along the course of the radial nerve. The radial artery is identified as it passes deep to the abductor pollicis longus and extensor pollicis brevis tendons and is dissected free and retracted. Small branches of the artery that enter the trapeziometacarpal joint are electrocoagulated.

After the radial artery is retracted, the carpometacarpal joint capsule is incised longitudinally and released from the base of the metacarpal. Care is taken to preserve the capsule for later closure. In the loose, subluxated joint, the metacarpal can be

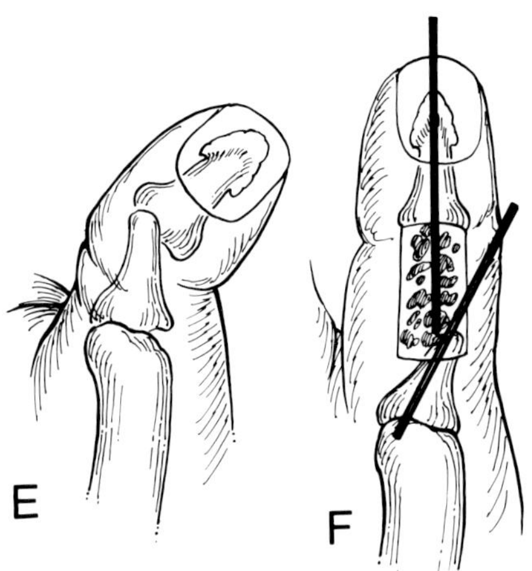

Fig. 46-53 *(Continued).* **(E&F)** Drawing of the interphalangeal joint fusion technique using a bone graft in patients with severe bone loss. (Figs. A–D from Millender,[191] with permission.)

dislocated completely and the entire surface of the metacarpal base visualized. The beveled volar and ulnar surface, which has eroded the dorsal radial facet of the trapezium, can be seen. Enough metacarpal is resected to allow reduction of the dislocation and to provide proper space for the implant.

In stiff, contracted thumbs, resection of the base of the metacarpal is more difficult. After the capsular release, the deep volar carpometacarpal ligament may have to be divided to allow adequate exposure. In addition, partial metacarpal resection may have to be performed before the base can be dislocated into the wound. In each case, enough soft tissue release and bony resection should be done to expose the metacarpal base completely.

In our experience, a formal adductor release rarely is necessary. However, if this is indicated, the fascia over the first dorsal interosseous muscle is incised. The distal limb of the incision can be extended and the skin retracted to allow release of this fascia.

After the metacarpal has been resected, hand-held reamers or power burrs with blunt tips are used to shape the medullary canal to accept the stem of the implant.

Attention now is turned to the trapezium. In joints with

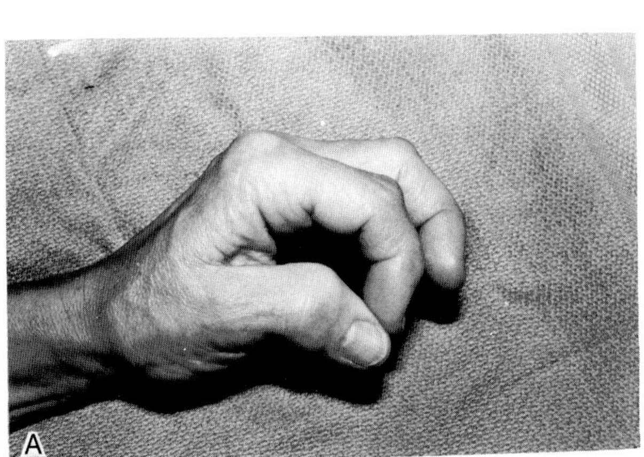

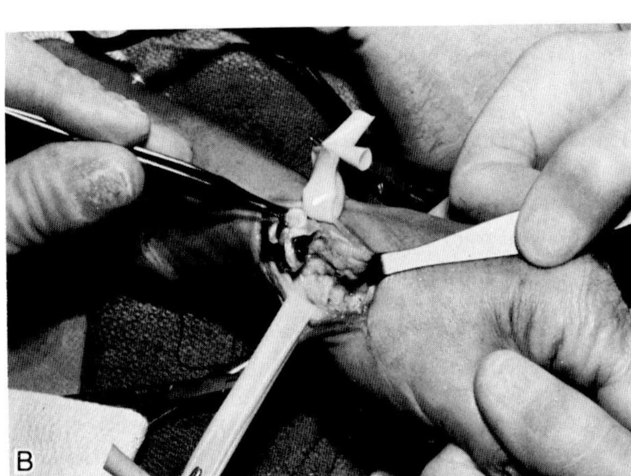

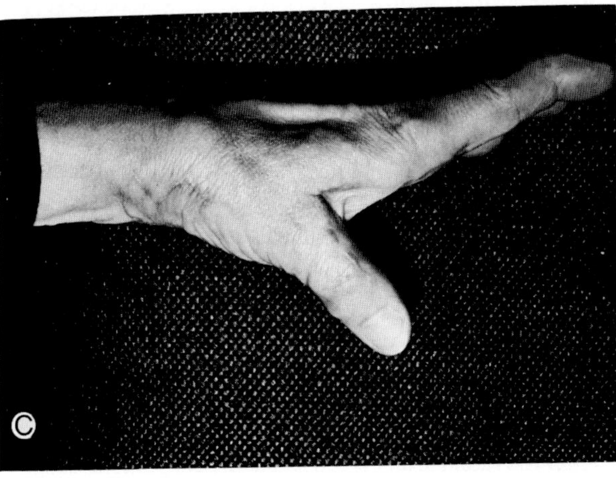

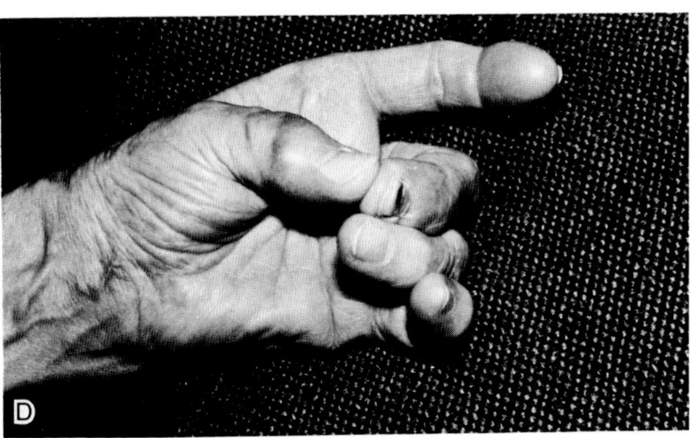

Fig. 46-54. **(A)** Painful, subluxated carpometacarpal joint with associated painful and unstable thumb interphalangeal joint. **(B)** Resection arthroplasty completed and palmaris longus inserted as a spacer. **(C&D)** Postoperative appearance following interpositional palmaris longus arthroplasty combined with interphalangeal joint fusion of the thumb. *(Figure continues.)*

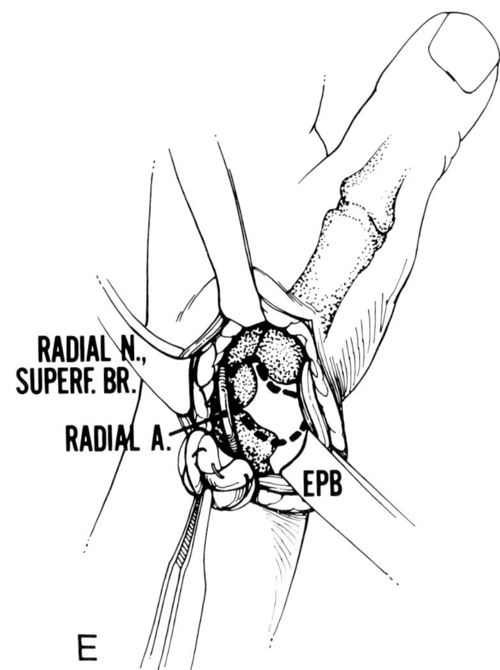

Fig. 46-54 *(Continued).* **(E)** Drawing of carpometacarpal joint resection arthroplasty. Note exposure and protection of the radial nerve and dorsal branch of the radial artery. The extensor pollicis brevis is retracted, and the capsule is preserved for closure over the tendon spacer. The dotted line outlines the excised trapezium. (Figs. A–D from Millender and Nalebuff,[165] with permission.)

minimal subluxation, the trapezium is relatively flat. However, in joints that are subluxated, the dorsoradial surface of the trapezium, and especially the beak of the trapezium, must be excised with a small rongeur to provide a flat surface for the implant. In some cases, a portion of the trapezoid must be removed to allow proper seating of the implant.

The implant that we have used for hemiarthroplasty is the stemmed, concave Swanson great toe implant. A size O is most often the proper size. The implant stem fits into the metacarpal shaft and the base rests on the flat surface of the remodeled trapezium. Swanson has developed a similar implant that has a convex rather than a concave surface. We have tried this implant and have found very little difference in the two designs.

After the implant size has been selected and a trial reduction accomplished, the wound is irrigated and the implant inserted. Because the metacarpal has been shortened, there usually is adequate capsule for closure. A portion of the abductor pollicis longus is used to reinforce the capsule. The abductor pollicis longus should be advanced to ensure adequate postoperative abduction power.

Postoperatively, the thumb is splinted for 3 weeks prior to K-wire removal, following which splinting is continued for 1 to 2 weeks. Exercises are begun at 4 to 5 weeks, and splinting is discontinued after 6 weeks. If a K-wire is not utilized, the thumb must be maintained in a position of abduction to ensure proper seating of the implant and to prevent any tendency toward dislocation.

Other thumb surgery, such as MP joint arthrodesis or interphalangeal joint arthrodesis, can be performed at the same time, if indicated. Hyperextension of the MP joint (as seen in Type III deformity) must be corrected at the time of trapeziometacarpal joint arthroplasty. If there is excessive instability or MP joint destruction. MP joint arthroplasty or arthrodesis should be performed. If there is more than 20 to 30 degrees hyperextension of the MP joint, a volar capsulodesis is indicated to minimize the forces that tend to subluxate the implant.

Resection Arthroplasty

The surgical technique for resection arthroplasty is similar to that for hemiarthroplasty, except that the entire trapezium is excised. After the radial artery has been retracted, a vertical incision is made from the base of the metacarpal over the surface of the trapezium to the scaphotrapezial joint. The capsule is dissected from the trapezium on both the dorsal and volar surfaces. The scaphotrapezial joint is identified and the dissection is extended to this joint. It is easier and safer to remove the trapezium piecemeal with a rongeur than to attempt to remove it in one piece. When the volar surface of the trapezium is removed, care is taken to avoid removing the volar capsule with the bone and to avoid damaging the flexor carpi radialis tendon, which passes through a groove in the trapezium.

The metacarpal is exposed as described for hemiarthroplasty. After the bones have been prepared, a palmaris longus tendon is harvested from the forearm, folded into a small "anchovy," sutured to itself, and packed into the space. The capsule and wound are closed as described previously. Usually a K-wire is not necessary. However, if there is any tendency toward subluxation, a small K-wire may be utilized to prevent collapse of the metacarpal into the space previously occupied by the trapezium. The thumb is splinted in an abducted and opposed position and held for 4 to 5 weeks before exercises are begun. As with hemiarthroplasty, other surgery of the thumb can be performed at the same time if necessary (Fig. 46-54).

While described for the treatment of degenerative arthritis, Burton and Pellegrini's[30,204] ligament reconstruction with tendon interposition arthroplasty (LRTI) can also be useful in the treatment of rheumatoid disease of the thumb CMC joint.

REFERENCES

1. Abernethy PJ, Dennyson WG: Decompression of the extensor tendons at the wrist in rheumatoid arthritis. J Bone Joint Surg 61B:64–68, 1979
2. Achach PC: Deformities of the thumb in the rheumatoid hand. pp. 194–195. In Tubiana R (ed): La Main Rheumatoide. Expansion Scientifique Francaise, Paris, 1969
3. Adamson JE, Horton CE, Crawford HH, Taddeo RJ: The treatment of intrinsic contracture of the rheumatoid hand. Plast Reconstr Surg 42:549–556, 1968
4. Agee JM, Guidera M: Functional significance of the juncturae tendinae in dynamic stabilization of the metacarpophalangeal joints of the fingers. J Hand Surg 5:288, 1980
5. Albright JA, Chase RA: Palmar-shelf arthroplasty of the wrist in

rheumatoid arthritis. A report of nine cases. J Bone Joint Surg 52A:896-906, 1970

6. Ansell BM, Harrison SH, Little H, Thomas B: Synovectomy of proximal interphalangeal joints. Br J Plast Surg 23:380-385, 1970
7. Aptekar RG, Duff IF: Metacarpophalangeal joint surgery in rheumatoid arthritis. Long-term results. Clin Orthop 83:123-127, 1972
8. Backdahl M: The caput ulnae syndrome in rheumatoid arthritis. A study of the morphology, abnormal anatomy and clinical picture. Acta Rheumatol Scand (suppl) 5:1-75, 1963
9. Backhouse KM: Rheumatoid tenosynovial involvement in the hand. Hand 1:7-8, 1969
10. Backhouse KM, Kay AGL, Coomes EN, Kates A: Tendon involvement in the rheumatoid hand. Ann Rheum Dis 30:236-242, 1971
11. Barnes CG, Currey HLF: Carpal tunnel syndrome in rheumatoid arthritis. A clinical and electrodiagnostic survey. Ann Rheum Dis 26:226-233, 1967
12. Belsky MR, Feldon P, Millender LH, Nalebuff EA, Philips C: Hand involvement in psoriatic arthritis. J Hand Surg 7:203-207, 1982
13. Besser MIB: The conservative treatment of the swan-neck deformity in the rheumatoid hand. Hand 10:91-93, 1978
14. Bigelow DR: A surgical solution to the problem swan-neck deformity of rheumatoid arthritis. Clin Orthop 123:89-90, 1977
15. Blatt G, Ashworth CR: Volar capsule transfer for stabilization following resection of the distal end of the ulna. Orthop Trans 3:13-14, 1979
16. Bolton H: Arthroplasty of the metacarpophalangeal joints. Hand 3:131-134, 1971
17. Bora FW Jr, Osterman AL, Thomas VJ, Maitin EC, Polineni S: The treatment of ruptures of multiple extensor tendons at wrist level by a free tendon graft in the rheumatoid patient. J Hand Surg 12A:1038-1040, 1987
18. Bowers WH: Distal radioulnar joint arthroplasty: The hemiresection-interposition technique. J Hand Surg 10A:169-178, 1985
19. Boyce T, Youm Y, Sprague BL, Flatt AE: Clinical and experimental studies on the effect of extensor carpi radialis longus transfer in the rheumatoid hand. J Hand Surg 3:390-394, 1978
20. Boyes JH: Bunnell's Surgery of the Hand. 5th Ed. p. 419. JB Lippincott, Philadelphia, 1970
21. Boyes JH: The role of the intrinsic muscles in rheumatoid deformities. pp. 63-64. In Tubiana R (ed): La Main Rheumatoide. Expansion Scientifique Francaise, Paris, 1969
22. Brase DW, Millender LH: Failure of silicone rubber wrist arthroplasty in rheumatoid arthritis. J Hand Surg 11A:175-183, 1986
23. Breen TF, Jupiter JB: Extensor carpi ulnaris and flexor carpi ulnaris tenodesis of the unstable distal ulna. J Hand Surg 14A:612-617, 1989
24. Brewerton, DA: Pathological anatomy of rheumatoid finger joints. Hand 3:121-124, 1971
25. Brown FE, Brown M-L: Long-term results after tenosynovectomy to treat the rheumatoid hand. J Hand Surg 13A:704-708, 1988
26. Brown PW: Hand surgery in rheumatoid arthritis. Semin Arthritis Rheum 5:327-363, 1976
27. Browne EZ, Teague MA, Snyder CC: Prevention of extensor lag after indicis proprius tendon transfer. J Hand Surg 4:168-172, 1979
28. Brumfield R Jr, Kuschner SH, Gellman H, Liles DN, Van Winckle G: Results of dorsal wrist synovectomies in the rheumatoid hand. J Hand Surg 15A:733-735, 1990
29. Buck-Gramcko D: Denervation of the wrist joint. J Hand Surg 2:54-61, 1977
30. Burton RI, Pellegrini VD Jr: Surgical management of basal joint arthritis of the thumb. Part II. Ligament reconstruction with tendon interposition arthroplasty. J Hand Surg 11A:324-332, 1986
31. Carroll RE, Dick HM: Arthrodesis of the wrist for rheumatoid arthritis. J Bone Joint Surg 53A:1365-1369, 1971
32. Carroll RE, Hill NA: Small joint arthrodesis in hand reconstruction. J Bone Joint Surg 51A:1219-1221, 1969
33. Carvell JE, Mowat AG, Fuller DJ: Trigger wrist phenomenon in rheumatoid arthritis. Hand 15:77-81, 1983
34. Chamay A, Della Santa D, Vilaseca A: Radiolunate arthrodesis, factor of stability for the rheumatoid wrist. Ann Chir Main 2:5-17, 1983
35. Chang LW, Gowans JDC, Granger CV, Millender LH: Entrapment neuropathy of the posterior interosseus nerve. A complication of rheumatoid arthritis. Arthritis Rheum 15:350-352, 1972
36. Clawson DK, Souter WA, Carthum CJ, Hymen ML: Functional assessment of the rheumatoid hand. Clin Orthop 77:203-210, 1971
37. Clawson DK, Convery FR: Surgery in rheumatoid arthritis of the wrist. pp. 135-142. In Cruess RL, Mitchell NS (eds): Surgery of Rheumatoid Arthritis. JB Lippincott, Philadelphia, 1971
38. Clawson MC, Stern PJ: The distal radioulnar joint complex in rheumatoid arthritis: An overview. Hand Clin 7:373-381, 1991
39. Clayton ML: Surgery of the thumb in rheumatoid arthritis. J Bone Joint Surg 44A:1376-1386, 1962
40. Clayton ML: Surgery of the rheumatoid hand. Clin Orthop 36:47-65, 1964
41. Clayton ML: Surgical treatment at the wrist in rheumatoid arthritis. A review of thirty-seven patients. J Bone Joint Surg 47A:741-750, 1965
42. Clayton ML: Historical perspectives on surgery of the rheumatoid hand. Hand Clin 5:111-114, 1989
43. Clayton ML, Ferlic DC: Tendon transfer for radial rotation of the wrist in rheumatoid arthritis. Clin Orthop 100:176-185, 1974
44. Clayton ML, Ferlic DC: The wrist in rheumatoid arthritis. Clin Orthop 106:192-197, 1975
45. Clendenin MB, Green DP: Arthrodesis of the wrist—Complications and their management. J Hand Surg 6:253-257, 1981
46. Cracchiolo A III, Marmor L: Resection of the distal ulna in rheumatoid arthritis. Arthritis Rheum 12:415-422, 1969
47. Craig EV, House JH: Dorsal carpal dislocation and flexor tendon rupture in rheumatoid arthritis: A case report. J Hand Surg 9A:261-264, 1984
48. Curtis R: Sublimis tenodesis. p. 319. In Edmonson AS, Crenshaw AH (eds): Campbell's Operative Orthopaedics. 6th Ed. CV Mosby, St. Louis, 1980
49. Darrach W: Anterior dislocation of the head of the ulna. Ann Surg 56:802-803, 1912
50. Darrach W, Dwight K: Derangement of the inferior radioulnar articulation. Proceedings of the New York Academy of Medicine. Med Rec 87:708, 1915
51. Dell P: Compression of the ulnar nerve at the wrist secondary to a rheumatoid synovial cyst: Case report and review of the literature. J Hand Surg 4:468-473, 1979
52. Dellon AL: Partial dorsal wrist denervation: Resection of the distal posterior interosseous nerve. J Hand Surg 10A:527-533, 1985
53. Dolphin JA: Extensor tenotomy for chronic boutonnière deformity of the finger. Report of two cases. J Bone Joint Surg 47A:161-164, 1965

54. Dray GJ: The hand in systemic lupus erythematosus. Hand Clin 5:145-155, 1989
55. Dupont M, Vainio K: Arthrodesis of the wrist in rheumatoid arthritis. A study of 140 cases. Ann Chir Gynec Fenn 57:513-519, 1968
56. Ehrlich GE, Peterson LT, Sokoloff L, Bunin JJ: Pathogenesis of rupture of extensor tendons at the wrist in rheumatoid arthritis. Arthritis Rheum 2:332-346, 1959
57. Eiken O, Haga T, Salgeback S: Assessment of surgery of the rheumatoid wrist. Scand J Plast Reconstr Surg 9:207-215, 1975
58. Elliott RA Jr: Splints for mallet and boutonniere deformities. Plast Reconstr Surg 52:282-285, 1973
59. Ellison MR, Flatt AE, Kelly KJ: Ulnar drift of the fingers in rheumatoid disease. Treatment by crossed intrinsic tendon transfer. J Bone Joint Surg 53A:1061-1082, 1971
60. Ellison MR, Kelly KJ, Flatt AE: The results of surgical synovectomy of the digital joints in rheumatoid disease. J Bone Joint Surg 53A:1041-1060, 1971
61. Enriquez de Salamanca F: Swan-neck deformity: Mechanism and surgical treatment. Hand 8:215-221, 1976
62. Entin M: Management of early rheumatoid arthritis in the hand. pp. 165-175. In Creuss RL, Mitchell NS (eds): Surgery of Rheumatoid Arthritis. JB Lippincott, Philadelphia, 1971
63. Ertel AN: Flexor tendon ruptures in rheumatoid arthritis. Hand Clin 5:177-190, 1989
64. Ertel AN, Millender LH, Nalebuff E, McKay D, Leslie B: Flexor tendon ruptures in patients with rheumatoid arthritis. J Hand Surg 13A:860-866, 1988
65. Eyring EJ, Longert A, Bass JC: Synovectomy in juvenile rheumatoid arthritis. Indications and short-term results. J Bone Joint Surg 53A:638-651, 1971
66. Faithfull DK, Herbert TJ: Small joint fusions of the hand using the Herbert bone screw. J Hand Surg 9B:167-168, 1984
67. Fatti JF, Palmer AK, Mosher JF: The long-term results of Swanson silicone rubber interpositional wrist arthroplasty. J Hand Surg 11A:166-175, 1986
68. Fearnley GR: Ulnar deviation of the fingers. Ann Rheum Dis 10:126-136, 1951
69. Ferlic DC: Implant arthroplasty of the rheumatoid wrist. Hand Clin 3:169-179, 1987
70. Ferlic DC: Boutonniere deformities in rheumatoid arthritis. Hand Clin 5:215-222, 1989
71. Ferlic DC, Clayton ML: Flexor tenosynovectomy in the rheumatoid finger. J Hand Surg 3:364-367, 1978
72. Ferlic DC, Smyth CJ, Clayton ML: Medical considerations and management of rheumatoid arthritis. J Hand Surg 8:662-666, 1983
73. Fernandez-Palazzi F, Vainio K: Synovectomy of carpal joints in rheumatoid arthritis. A report of 47 cases. Arch Inter Ann Rheum 8:238-258, 1965
74. Figgie MP, Inglis AE, Sobel M, Bohn WW, Fisher DA: Metacarpal-phalangeal joint arthroplasty of the rheumatoid thumb. J Hand Surg 15A:210-216, 1990
75. Figgie MP, Ranawat CS, Inglis AE, Sobel M, Figgie, HE III: Trispherical total wrist arthroplasty in rheumatoid arthritis. J Hand Surg 15A:217-223, 1990
76. Flatt AE: Some pathomechanics of ulnar drift. Plast Reconstr Surg 37:295-303, 1966
77. Flatt AE: The Care of the Rheumatoid Hand. 3rd Ed. CV Mosby, St. Louis, 1974
78. Flatt AE: The arthritic hand. pp 3507-3518. In Converse TM, Littler JW (eds): Plastic and Reconstructive Surgery. 2nd Ed. WB Saunders, Philadelphia, 1977
79. Flatt AE, Ellison MR: Restoration of rheumatoid finger joint function. III. A follow-up note after fourteen years' experience with a metallic-hinge prosthesis. J Bone Joint Surg 54A:1317-1322, 1972
80. Fleisher A, McGrath MH: Rheumatoid nodulosis of the hand. J Hand Surg 9A:404-411, 1984
81. Fowler SB: Arthroplasty of the metacarpophalangeal joint in rheumatoid arthritis. J Bone Joint Surg 44A:1037-1038, 1962
82. Froimson AI: Tendon arthroplasty of the trapeziometacarpal joint. Clin Orthop 70:191-199, 1970
83. Froimson AI: Hand reconstruction in arthritis mutilans. A case report. J Bone Joint Surg 53A:1377-1382, 1971
84. Gainor BJ, Hummel GL: Correction of rheumatoid swan-neck deformity by lateral band mobilization. J Hand Surg 10A:370-376, 1985
85. Gainor BJ, Schaberg J: The rheumatoid wrist after resection of the distal ulna. J Hand Surg 10A:837-844, 1985
86. Garner RW, Mowat AG, Hazleman BL: Wound healing after operations on patients with rheumatoid arthritis. J Bone Joint Surg 55B:134-144, 1973
87. Gellman H, Rankin G, Brumfield R Jr, Chandler D, Williams B: Palmar shelf arthroplasty in the rheumatoid wrist. Results of long-term follow-up. J Bone Joint Surg 71A:223-227, 1989
88. Girzadas D, Shapiro J, Vainio K: Natural course of rheumatoid arthritis of the hand. In Tubiana R (ed): La Main Rheumatoide. Expansion Scientifique Francaise, Paris, 1969
89. Goldner JL: Tendon transfers in rheumatoid arthritis. Orthop Clin North Am 5:425-444, 1974
90. Goldner JL, Clippinger FW: Excision of the greater multangular bone as an adjunct to mobilization of the thumb. J Bone Joint Surg 41A:609-625, 1959
91. Goncalves D: Correction of disorders of the distal radioulnar joint by artificial pseudoarthrosis of the ulna. J Bone Joint Surg 56B:462-464, 1974
92. Goodman MJ, Millender LH, Nalebuff EA, Phillips CA: Arthroplasty of the rheumatoid wrist with silicone rubber: An early evaluation. J Hand Surg 5:114-121, 1980
93. Granowitz S, Vainio K: Proximal interphalangeal joint arthrodesis in rheumatoid arthritis. A follow-up study of 122 operations. Acta Orthop Scand 37:301-310, 1966
94. Grant H: Management of the rheumatoid thumb. pp. 209-212. In Tubiana R (ed): La Main Rheumatoide. Expansion Scientifique Francaise, Paris, 1969
95. Gray RG, Gottlieb NL: Hand flexor tenosynovitis in rheumatoid arthritis. Prevalence, distribution and associated rheumatic features. Arthritis Rheum 20:1003-1008, 1977
96. Haddad RJ, Riordan DC: Arthrodesis of the wrist. A surgical technique. J Bone Joint Surg 49A:950-954, 1967
97. Hagglund KJ, Haley WE, Reveille JD, Alarcón GS: Predicting individual differences in pain and functional impairment among patients with rheumatoid arthitis. Arthritis Rheum 32:851-858, 1989
98. Hakstian RW, Tubiana R: Ulnar deviation of the fingers. The role of joint structure and function. J Bone Joint Surg 49A:299-316, 1967
99. Hales WJ, Burkhalter WE: The three-bone forearm procedure in reconstruction of distal radioulnar abnormalities. J Hand Surg 10A:435, 1985
100. Haloua JP, Collin JP, Schernberg F, Sandre J: Arthroplasty of the rheumatoid wrist with Swanson implant. Long-term results and complications. Ann Chir Main 8:124-134, 1989
101. Harris C Jr, Riordan DC: Intrinsic contracture in the hand and its surgical treatment. J Bone Joint Surg 36A:10-20, 1954
102. Harrison SH: Reconstructive arthroplasty of the metacarpophalangeal joint using the extensor loop operation. Br J Plast Surg 24:307-309, 1971

103. Harrison SH: The Harrison-Nicolle intramedullary peg: Followup study of 100 cases. Hand 6:304–307, 1974
104. Harrison SH: The importance of middle or long finger realignment in ulnar drift. J Hand Surg 1:87–91, 1976
105. Harrison SH, Ansell BM: Surgery of the rheumatoid thumb. Br J Plast Surg 27:242–247, 1974
106. Harrison SH, Nicolle FV: A new intramedullary bone peg for digital arthrodesis. Br J Plast Surg 27:240–241, 1974
107. Harrison SH, Swannell AJ, Ansell BM: Repair of extensor pollicis longus using extensor pollicis brevis in rheumatoid arthritis. Ann Rheum Dis 31:490–492, 1972
108. Hastings DE, Evans JA: Rheumatoid wrist deformities and their relation to ulnar drift. J Bone Joint Surg 57A:930–934, 1975
109. Heywood AWB: Correction of the rheumatoid boutonniere deformity. J Bone Joint Surg 51A:1309–1314, 1969
110. Heywood AWB: The pathogenesis of the rheumatoid swan-neck deformity. Hand 11:176–183, 1979
111. Howard LD Jr: Surgical treatment of rheumatoid tenosynovitis. Am J Surg 89:1163–1168, 1955
112. Hueston JT, Wilson WF: The role of the intrinsic muscles in the production of metacarpophalangeal subluxation in the rheumatoid hand. Plast Reconstr Surg 52:342–345, 1973
113. Inglis AE: Rheumatoid arthritis in the hand. Am J Surg 109:368–374, 1965
114. Inglis AE, Hamlin C, Sengelmann RP, Straub LR: Reconstruction of the metacarpophalangeal joint of the thumb in rheumatoid arthritis. J Bone Joint Surg 54A:704–712, 1972
115. Jackson IT, Paton KC: The extended approach to flexor tendon synovitis in rheumatoid arthritis. Br J Plast Surg 26:122–131, 1973
116. Jacobs JH, Hess EV, Beswick IP: Rheumatoid arthritis presenting as tenosynovitis. J Bone Joint Surg 39B:288–292, 1957
117. Jalava S, Saario R: Treatment of finger joints with local steroids. A double-blind study. Scand J Rheumatol 12:12–14, 1983
118. Kay AGL: Natural history of synovial hypertrophy in the rheumatoid hand. Ann Rheum Dis 30:98–102, 1971
119. Kellgren JH, Ball J: Tendon lesions in rheumatoid arthritis: A clinicopathological study. Ann Rheum Dis 9:48–65, 1950
120. Kessler I: Aetiology and management of adduction contracture of the thumb in rheumatoid arthritis. Hand 5:170–174, 1973
121. Kessler I, Vainio K: Posterior (dorsal) synovectomy for rheumatoid involvement of the hand and wrist. A follow-up study of sixty-six procedures. J Bone Joint Surg 48A:1085–1094, 1966
122. Kinnealey M: The relationship between self concept and hand deformity in rheumatoid arthritis. Am J Occup Ther 24:294–297, 1970
123. Kleinert HE, Frykman G: The wrist and thumb in rheumatoid arthritis. Orthop Clin North Am 4:1085–1096, 1973
124. Kobus RJ, Turner RH: Wrist arthrodesis for treatment of rheumatoid arthritis. J Hand Surg 15A:541–546, 1990
125. Kuczynski K: The synovial structures of the normal and rheumatoid digital joints. Hand 3:41–54, 1971
126. Kulick RG, DeFiore JC, Straub LR, Ranawat CS: Long-term results of dorsal stabilization in the rheumatoid wrist. J Hand Surg 6:272–280, 1981
127. Laine VAI, Vainio KJ: Spontaneous ruptures of tendons in rheumatoid arthritis. Acta Orthop Scand 24:250–257, 1955
128. Laine VAI, Sairanen E, Vainio K: Finger deformities caused by rheumatoid arthritis. J Bone Joint Surg 39A:527–533, 1957
129. Larson A, Dale K, Eek M, Pahle J: Radiographic evaluation of rheumatoid arthritis by standard reference films. J Hand Surg 8:667–669, 1983
130. Leach RE, Baumgard SH: Correction of swan-neck deformity in rheumatoid arthritis. Surg Clin North Am 48:661–686, 1968
131. Leffert RD, Dorfman HD: Antecubital cyst in rheumatoid arthritis—surgical findings. J Bone Joint Surg 54A:1555–1557, 1972
132. Leslie BM: Rheumatoid extensor tendon ruptures. Hand Clin 5:191–202, 1989
133. Leslie BM, Carlson G, Ruby LK: Results of extensor carpi ulnaris tenodesis in the rheumatoid wrist undergoing a distal ulnar excision. J Hand Surg 15A:547–551, 1990
134. Linscheid RL: Surgery for rheumatoid arthritis—Timing and techniques: The upper extremity. J Bone Joint Surg 50A:605–613, 1968
135. Linscheid RL, Dobyns JH: Rheumatoid arthritis of the wrist. Orthop Clin North Am 2:649–665, 1971
136. Linscheid RL, Dobyns JH: Radiolunate arthrodesis. J Hand Surg 10A:821–829, 1985
137. Lipscomb PR: Synovectomy of the wrist for rheumatoid arthritis. JAMA 194:655–659, 1965
138. Lipscomb PR: Is early synovectomy of the small joints of the hand worthwhile? pp. 29–32. In Cramer LM, Chase RA (eds): Symposium on the Hand. Vol 3. CV Mosby, St. Louis, 1971
139. Lipscomb PR: Surgery for rheumatoid arthritis—Timing and techniques: Summary. J Bone Joint Surg 50A:614–617, 1968
140. Lipscomb PR: Synovectomy of the distal two joints of the thumb and fingers in rheumatoid arthritis. J Bone Joint Surg 49A:1135–1140, 1967
141. Littler JW: The prevention and the correction of adduction contracture of the thumb. Clin Orthop 13:182–192, 1959
142. Littler JW: Restoration of the oblique retinacular ligament for correcting hyperextension deformity of the proximal interphalangeal joint. pp. 155–157. In Tubiana R (ed): La Main Rheumatoide. Expansion Scientifique Francaise, Paris, 1969
143. Littler JW, Eaton RG: Redistribution of forces in the correction of the boutonnière deformity. J Bone Joint Surg 49A:1267–1274, 1967
144. Louis DS, Hankin FM, Bowers WH: Capitate-radius arthrodesis: an alternative method of radiocarpal arthrodesis. J Hand Surg 9A:365–369, 1984
145. Mannerfelt LG: Tendon transfers in surgery of the rheumatoid hand. Hand Clin 4:309–316, 1988
146. Mannerfelt L, Malmsten M: Arthodesis of the wrist in rheumatoid arthritis. A technique without external fixation. Scand J Plast Reconstr Surg 5:124–130, 1971
147. Mannerfelt L, Norman O: Attrition ruptures of flexor tendons in rheumatoid arthritis caused by bony spurs in the carpal tunnel. A clinical and radiological study. J Bone Joint Surg 51B:270–277, 1969
148. Marmor L, Lawrence JF, Dubois EL: Posterior interosseous nerve palsy due to rheumatoid arthritis. J Bone Joint Surg 49A:381–383, 1967
149. Martel W, Hayes JT, Duff IF: The pattern of bone erosion in the hand and wrist in rheumatoid arthritis. Radiology 84:204–214, 1965
150. McFarlane RM: Observations on the functional anatomy of the intrinsic muscles of the thumb. J Bone Joint Surg 44A:1073–1088, 1962
151. McGrath MH, Fleischer A: The subcutaneous rheumatoid nodule. Hand Clin 5:127–135, 1989
152. McGrath MH, Watson HK: Late results with local bone graft donor sites in hand surgery. J Hand Surg 6:234–237, 1981
153. McMaster M: The natural history of the rheumatoid metacarpophalangeal joint. J Bone Joint Surg 54B:687–697, 1972
154. McMurtry RY, Youm Y, Flatt AE, Gillespie TE: Kinematics of the wrist. II. Clinical applications. J Bone Joint Surg 60A:955–961, 1978
155. Melone CP Jr, Taras JS: Distal ulna resection, extensor carpi

ulnaris tenodesis, and dorsal synovectomy for the rheumatoid wrist. Hand Clin 7:335-343, 1991
156. Menon J: Total wrist replacement using the modified Volz prosthesis. J Bone Joint Surg 69A:998-1006, 1987
157. Midgley RO: Soft tissue surgery of the rheumatoid hand. pp. 159-163. In Cruess RL, Mitchell NS (eds): Surgery of Rheumatoid Arthritis. JB Lippincott, Philadelphia, 1971
158. Mikic ZD, Helal B: The value of the Darrach procedure in the surgical treatment of rheumatoid arthritis. Clin Orthop 127:175-185, 1977
159. Milford L. The Hand. 2nd Ed. pp. 233-234. CV Mosby, St. Louis, 1982
160. Miller-Breslow A, Millender LH, Feldon PG: Treatment considerations in the complicated rheumatoid hand. Hand Clin 5:279-289, 1989
161. Millender LH, Nalebuff EA: Arthrodesis of the rheumatoid wrist. An evaluation of sixty patients and a description of a different surgical technique. J Bone Joint Surg 55A:1026-1034, 1973
162. Millender LH, Nalebuff EA: Metacarpophalangeal joint arthroplasty utilizing the silicone rubber prosthesis. Orthop Clin North Am 4:349-371, 1973
163. Millender LH, Nalebuff EA: Evaluation and treatment of early rheumatoid hand involvement. Orthop Clin North Am 6:697-708, 1975
164. Millender LH, Nalebuff EA: Preventive surgery—tenosynovectomy and synovectomy. Orthop Clin North Am 6:765-792, 1975
165. Millender LH, Nalebuff EA: Reconstructive surgery in the rheumatoid hand. Orthop Clin North Am 6:709-732, 1975
166. Millender LH, Nalebuff EA, Amadio P, Phillips, C: Interpositional arthroplasty for rheumatoid carpometacarpal joint disease. J Hand Surg 3:533-541, 1978
167. Millender LH, Nalebuff EA, Albin R, Ream JR, Gordon M: Dorsal tenosynovectomy and tendon transfer in the rheumatoid hand. J Bone Joint Surg 56A:601-610, 1974
168. Millender LH, Nalebuff EA, Holdsworth DE: Posterior interosseous nerve syndrome secondary to rheumatoid synovitis. J Bone Joint Surg 55A:753-757, 1973
169. Millender LH, Phillips C: Combined wrist arthrodesis and metacarpophalangeal joint arthroplasty in rheumatoid arthritis. Orthopedics 1:43-48, 1978
170. Millis MB, Millender LH, Nalebuff EA: Stiffness of the proximal interphalangeal joints in rheumatoid arthritis. The role of flexor tenosynovitis. J Bone Joint Surg 58A:801-805, 1976
171. Moberg E: Cartilage lesions. pp. 173-177. In Hijmans W, Paul WD, Herschel H (eds): Early Synovectomy in Rheumatoid Arthritis. Excerpta Medica Foundation, Amsterdam, 1969
172. Moller M: Forty-eight cases of caput ulnae syndrome treated by synovectomy and resection of the distal end of the ulna. Acta Orthop Scand 44:278-282, 1973
173. Moore JR, Valdata L: Tendon ruptures in the rheumatoid hand: Analysis of treatment and functional results in fifty patients. J Hand Surg 10A:433, 1985
174. Moore JR, Weiland AJ, Valdata L: Tendon ruptures in the rheumatoid hand: Analysis of treatment and functional results in 60 patients. J Hand Surg 12A:9-14, 1987
175. Nalebuff EA: Diagnosis, classification and management of rheumatoid thumb deformities. Bull Hosp Joint Dis 29:119-137, 1968
176. Nalebuff EA: Metacarpophalangeal surgery in rheumatoid arthritis. Surg Clin North Am 49:823-832, 1969
177. Nalebuff EA: Nature and management of flexor tendon nodules in the rheumatoid hand. pp. 123-128. In Tubiana R (ed): La Main Rheumatoide. Expansion Scientifique Francaise, Paris, 1969
178. Nalebuff EA: Restoration of balance in the rheumatoid thumb. pp. 197-206. In Turbiana R (ed): La Main Rheumatoide. Expansion Scientifique Francaise, Paris, 1969
179. Nalebuff EA: Surgical treatment of finger deformities in the rheumatoid hand. Surg Clin North Am 49:833-846, 1969
180. Nalebuff EA: Surgical treatment of rheumatoid tenosynovitis in the hand. Surg Clin North Am 49:799-809, 1969
181. Nalebuff EA: Surgical treatment of tendon rupture in the rheumatoid hand. Surg Clin North Am 49:811-822, 1969
182. Nalebuff EA: The recognition and treatment of tendon ruptures in the rheumatoid hand. pp. 255-269. In AAOS Symposium on Tendon Surgery in the Hand. CV Mosby, St. Louis, 1975
183. Nalebuff EA: Rheumatoid hand surgery-update. J Hand Surg 8:678-682, 1983
184. Nalebuff, EA: The rheumatoid swan-neck deformity. Hand Clin 5:203-214, 1989
185. Nalebuff EA: Factors influencing the results of implant surgery in the rheumatoid hand. J Hand Surg 15B:395-403, 1990
186. Nalebuff EA, Garrett J: Opera-glass hand in rheumatoid arthritis. J Hand Surg 1:210-220, 1976
187. Nalebuff EA, Garrod KJ: Present approach to the severely involved rheumatoid wrist. Orthop Clin North Am 15:369-380, 1984
188. Nalebuff EA, Millender LH: Arthrodesis of the rheumatoid wrist. Functional evaluation of a modified technique. Orthop Rev 1:13-18, 1972
189. Nalebuff EA, Millender LH: Surgical treatment of the boutonniere deformity in rheumatoid arthritis. Orthop Clin North Am 6:753-763, 1975
190. Nalebuff EA, Millender LH: Surgical treatment of the swan-neck deformity in rheumatoid arthritis. Orthop Clin North Am 6:733-752, 1975
191. Nalebuff EA, Millender LH: Reconstructive surgery and rehabilitation of the hand. pp. 1900-1920. In Kelly WN, Harris ED, Ruddy S, Sledge CS (eds): Textbook of Rheumatology. WB Saunders, Philadelphia, 1981
192. Nalebuff EA, Patel MR: Flexor digitorum sublimus transfer for multiple extensor tendon ruptures in rheumatoid arthritis. Plast Reconstr Surg 52:530-533, 1973
193. Nalebuff EA, Potter TA: Rheumatoid involvement of tendon and tendon sheaths in the hand. Clin Orthop 59:147-159, 1968
194. Nalebuff EA, Potter TA, Tomaselli R: Surgery of swanneck deformity of the rheumatoid hand: A new approach. Arthritis Rheum 6:289, 1963
195. Napier JR: The form and function of the carpometacarpal joint of the thumb. J Anat 89:362-369, 1955
196. Newman RJ: Excision of the distal ulna in patients with rheumatoid arthritis. J Bone Joint Surg 69B:203-206, 1987
197. Nicolle FV: Recent advances in the management of joint disease in the rheumatoid hand. Hand 5:91-95, 1973
198. Nicolle FV, Holt PJL, Calnan JS: Prophylactic synovectomy of the joints of the rheumatoid hand. Clinical trial with 4-8-year follow up. Ann Rheum Dis 30:476-480, 1971
199. Nylen S, Sollerman C, Haffajee D, Ekelund L: Swanson implant arthroplasty of the wrist in rheumatoid arthritis. J Hand Surg 9B:295-299, 1984
200. O'Donovan TM, Ruby LK: The distal radioulnar joint in rheumatoid arthritis. Hand Clin 5:249-256, 1989
201. Oster LH, Blair WF, Steyers CM, Flatt AE: Crossed intrinsic transfer. J Hand Surg 14A:963-971, 1989
202. Pahle JA, Raunio P: The influence of wrist position on finger deviation in the rheumatoid hand. A clinical and radiological study. J Bone Joint Surg 51B:664-676, 1969
203. Pallis CA, Scott JT: Peripheral neuropathy in rheumatoid arthritis. Br Med J 1:1141-1147, 1965

204. Pellegrini VD Jr, Burton RI: Surgical management of basal joint arthritis of the thumb. Part I. Long-term results of silicone implant arthroplasty. J Hand Surg 11A:309–324, 1986
205. Posner MA, Ambrose L: Excision of the distal ulna in rheumatoid arthritis. Hand Clin 7:383–390, 1991
206. Potter TA, Kuhns JG: Rheumatoid tenosynovitis; Diagnosis and treatment. J Bone Joint Surg 40A:1230–1235, 1958
207. Preston RI: Early synovectomy in rheumatoid arthritis: Introductory paper on the orthopaedic aspects. pp. 44–49. In Hijmans W, Paul WD, Herschel H (eds): Early Synovectomy in Rheumatoid Arthritis. Excerpta Medical Foundation, Amsterdam, 1969
208. Rana NA, Taylor AR: Excision of the distal end of the ulna in rheumatoid arthritis. J Bone Joint Surg 55B:96–105, 1973
209. Ratliff AHC: Deformities of the thumb in rheumatoid arthritis. Hand 3:138–143, 1971
210. Rayan GM, Brentlinger A, Purnell D, Garcia-Moral CA: Functional assessment of bilateral wrist arthrodeses. J Hand Surg 12A:1020–1024, 1987
211. Resnik D: Rheumatoid arthritis of the wrist: Why the ulnar styloid? Radiology 112:29–35, 1974
212. Resnik D, Gmelich JT: Bone fragmentation in the rheumatoid wrist: Radiographic and pathologic considerations. Radiology 114:315–321, 1975
213. Riordan DC, Fowler SB: Surgical treatment of rheumatoid deformities of the hand. J Bone Joint Surg 40A:1431–1432, 1958
214. Rose JH, Belsky MR: Psoriatic arthritis in the hand. Hand Clin 5:137–144, 1989
215. Ryu J, Watson HK, Burgess RC: Rheumatoid wrist reconstruction utilizing a fibrous nonunion and radiocarpal arthrodesis. J Hand Surg 10A:830–836, 1985
216. Salgeback S, Eiken O, Haga T: Surgical treatment of the rheumatoid thumb. Special reference to the metacarpophalangeal joint. Scand J Plast Reconstr Surg 10:153–156, 1976
217. Schneller S: Medical considerations and perioperative care for rheumatoid surgery. Hand Clin 5:115–126, 1989
218. Schumacher HR: Primer on the Rheumatic Diseases. 9th Ed. pp. 1–170. Arthritis Foundation, Atlanta, 1988
219. Scott FA, Boswick JA: Palmar arthroplasty for the treatment of stiff swan-neck deformity. J Hand Surg 8:267–272, 1983
220. Shapiro JS: The etiology of ulnar drift: A new factor. J Bone Joint Surg 50A:634, 1968
221. Shapiro JS: A new factor in the etiology of ulnar drift. Clin Orthop 68:32–43, 1970
222. Shapiro JS: Wrist involvement in rheumatoid swan-neck deformity. J Hand Surg 7:484–491, 1982
223. Shapiro JS: Power staple fixation in hand and wrist surgery: New applications of an old fixation device. J Hand Surg 12A:218–227, 1987
224. Shapiro JS, Rodts T, Labanauskas I, Payne T: Early synovectomy versus late arthroplasty of the rheumatoid wrist: A comparative study. (abstract) J Hand Surg 10A:430, 1985
225. Skoff H: Palmar shelf arthroplasty. A follow-up note. J Bone Joint Surg 70A:1377–1382, 1988
226. Smith EM, Juvinall RC, Bender LF, Pearson JR: Flexor forces and rheumatoid metacarpophalangeal deformities. Clinical implications. JAMA 198:130–134, 1966
227. Smith RJ: Tendon Transfers of the Hand and Forearm. pp. 215–243. Little, Brown, Boston, 1987
228. Smith RJ, Kaplan EB: Rheumatoid deformities at the metacarpophalangeal joints of the fingers. A correlative study of anatomy and pathology. J Bone Joint Surg 49A:31–47, 1967
229. Smith RJ, Atkinson RE, Jupiter JB: Silicone synovitis of the wrist. J Hand Surg 10A:47–60, 1985
230. Smith-Peterson MN, Aufranc OE, Larson CB: Useful surgical procedures for rheumatoid arthritis involving joints of the upper extremity. Arch Surg 46:764–770, 1943
231. Sones DA: Surgery for rheumatoid arthritis—Timing and techniques: General and medical aspects. J Bone Joint Surg 50A:576–586, 1968
232. Sones DA: The medical management of rheumatoid arthritis and the relationship between the rheumatologist and the orthopedic surgeon. Orthop Clin North Am 2:613–621, 1971
233. Souter WA: The problem of boutonniere deformity. Clin Orthop 104:116–133, 1974
234. Souter WA: Planning treatment of the rheumatoid hand. Hand 11:3–16, 1979
235. Spar I: Flexor tendon ruptures in the rheumatoid hand: Bilateral flexor pollicis longus rupture. Clin Orthop 127:186–188, 1977
236. Stack HG: Buttonhole deformity. Hand 3:152–154, 1971
237. Stack HG, Vaughan-Jackson OJ: The zigzag deformity in the rheumatoid hand. Hand 3:62–67, 1971
238. Stanley JK, Smith EJ, Muirhead AG: Arthrodesis of the metacarpo-phalangeal joint of the thumb: A review of 42 cases. J Hand Surg 14B:291–293, 1989
239. Stellbrink G: Trigger finger syndrome in rheumatoid arthritis not caused by flexor tendon nodules. Hand 3:76–79, 1971
240. Stirrat CR: Treatment of tenosynovitis in rheumatoid arthritis. Hand Clin 5:169–175, 1989
241. Strang RFA, Hueston JT: Healing of bony rheumatoid lesions after synovectomy of metacarpophalangeal joints. Med J Aust 1:809, 1965
242. Straub LR: The rheumatoid hand. Clin Orthop 15:127–139, 1959
243. Straub LR: The etiology of finger deformity in the hand affected by rheumatoid arthritis. Bull Hosp Joint Dis 21:322–329, 1960
244. Straub LR, Ranawat CS: The wrist in rheumatoid arthritis. Surgical treatment and results. J Bone Joint Surg 51A:1–20, 1969
245. Straub LR, Wilson EH: Spontaneous rupture of extensor tendons in the hand associated with rheumatoid arthritis. J Bone Joint Surg 38A:1208–1217, 1956
246. Swanson AB: Silicone rubber implants for replacement of arthritic or destroyed joints in the hand. Surg Clin North Am 48:1113–1127, 1968
247. Swanson AB: Disabling arthritis at the base of the thumb. Treatment by resection of the trapezium and flexible (silicone) implant arthroplasty. J Bone Joint Surg 54A:456–471, 1972
248. Swanson AB: Flexible implant arthroplasty for arthritic finger joints. Rationale, technique, and results of treatment. J Bone Joint Surg 54A:435–455, 1972
249. Swanson AB: The ulnar head syndrome and its treatment by implant resection arthroplasty. J Bone Joint Surg 54A:906, 1972
250. Swanson AB: Flexible Implant Resection Arthroplasty in the Hand and Extremities. CV Mosby, St. Louis, 1973
251. Swanson AB: Implant arthroplasty for disabilities of the distal radioulnar joint. Use of a silicone rubber capping implant following resection of the ulnar head. Orthop Clin North Am 4:373–382, 1973
252. Swanson AB: Implant surgery for the joints and tendons in the hand. Continuing medical education course. Grand Rapids, Michigan, Oct 1979
253. Swanson AB, de Groot Swanson G, Maupin BK: Flexible implant arthroplasty of the radiocarpal joint. Surgical technique and long-term study. Clin Orthop 187:94–106, 1984
254. Swanson AB, de Groot Swanson G: Pathogenesis and pathomechanics of rheumatoid deformities in the hand and wrist. Orthop Clin North Am 4:1039–1056, 1973
255. Swanson AB, Herndon JH: Flexible (silicone) implant arthroplasty of the metacarpophalangeal joint of the thumb. J Bone Joint Surg 59A:362–368, 1977

256. Swezey RL: Dynamic factors in deformity of the rheumatoid arthritic hand. Bull Rheum Dis 22:649-659, 1971-1972
257. Taleisnik J: Subtotal arthrodeses of the wrist joint. Clin Orthop 187:81-88, 1984
258. Taleisnik J: The ligaments of the wrist. J Hand Surg 1:110-118, 1976
259. Taleisnik J: Rheumatoid synovitis of the volar compartment of the wrist joint: Its radiological signs and its contribution to wrist and hand deformity. J Hand Surg 4:526-535, 1979
260. Taleisnik J: Wrist: Anatomy, function, and injury. pp. 61-87. In AAOS Instruct Course Lect vol. 27, CV Mosby, St. Louis, 1978
261. Taleisnik J: Rheumatoid arthritis of the wrist. pp. 216-223. In Strickland JW, Steichen JB (eds): Difficult Problems in Hand Surgery. CV Mosby, St. Louis, 1982
262. Taleisnik J: The Wrist. pp. 387-435. Churchill Livingstone, New York, 1985
263. Taleisnik J: Combined radiocarpal arthrodesis and midcarpal (lunocapitate) arthroplasty for treatment of rheumatoid arthritis of the wrist. J Hand Surg 12A:1-8, 1987
264. Taleisnik J: Rheumatoid arthritis of the wrist. Hand Clin 5:257-278, 1989
265. Thirupathi RG, Ferlic DC, Clayton ML: Dorsal wrist synovectomy in rheumatoid arthritis—A long term study. J Hand Surg 8:848-856, 1983
266. Terrono A, Millender L, Nalebuff E: Boutonniere rheumatoid thumb deformity. J Hand Surg 15A:999-1003, 1990
267. Terrono A, Millender L: Surgical treatment of the boutonniere rheumatoid thumb deformity. Hand Clin 5:239-248, 1989
268. Thompson JS, Littler JW, Upton J: The spiral oblique retinacular ligament (SORL). J Hand Surg 3:482-487, 1978
269. Torisu T, Masumi S, Aso K: Utilization of the extensor retinaculum in the radiocarpal joint of rheumatoid wrists. Clin Orthop, 181:179-185, 1983
270. Tubiana R, Achach PC: The place of surgery in the treatment of the rheumatoid hand. pp. 217-218. In Tubiana R (ed): La Main Rheumatoide. Expansion Scientifique Francaise, Paris, 1969
271. Tubiana R, Valentin P: The physiology of the extension of the fingers. Surg Clin North Am 44:907-918, 1964
272. Vainio K: Carpal canal syndrome caused by tenosynovitis. Acta Rheum Scand 4:22-27, 1957
273. Vainio K, Reiman I, Pulkki T: Results of arthroplasty of the metacarpophalangeal joints in rheumatoid arthritis. Reconstr Surg Trauma, 9:1-7, 1967
274. Vainio K, Oka M: Ulnar deviation of the fingers. Ann Rheum Dis 12:122-124, 1953
275. Vainio K: Synovectomies of the hand and wrist in rheumatoid arthritis. p. 11. In Tubiana R (ed): La Main Rheumatoide. Expansion Scientifique Francaise, Paris, 1969
276. Vahvanen V, Viljakka T: Silicone rubber implant arthroplasty of the metacarpophalangeal joint in rheumatoid arthritis: A follow-up study of 32 patients. J Hand Surg 11A:333-339, 1986
277. Vaughan-Jackson OJ: Attrition ruptures of tendons in the rheumatoid hand. J Bone Joint Surg 40A:1431, 1958
278. Vaughan-Jackson OJ: Rheumatoid hand deformities considered in the light of tendon imbalance. I. J Bone Joint Surg 44B:764-775, 1962
279. Vaughan-Jackson OJ: Long term evaluation of the results of the rheumatoid hand. pp. 103-104. In Tubiana R (ed): La Main Rheumatoide. Expansion Scientifique Francaise, Paris, 1969
280. Vaughan-Jackson OJ: Rupture of extensor tendons by attrition at the inferior radioulnar joint. Report of two cases. J Bone Joint Surg 30B:528-530, 1948
281. Vesely DG: The distal radio-ulnar joint. Clin Orthop 51:75-91, 1967
282. Vicar AJ, Burton RI: Surgical management of the rheumatoid wrist. Fusion or arthroplasty. J Hand Surg 10A:430, 1985
283. Vincent KA, Szabo RM, Agee JM: The Sauve-Kapandji procedure for the reconstruction of the rheumatoid distal radioulnar joint (abstract). J Hand Surg 15A:811-812, 1990
284. Watson HK, Goodman ML, Johnson TR: Limited wrist arthrodesis. Part II. Intercarpal and radiocarpal combinations. J Hand Surg 6:223-233, 1981
285. Watson HK, Ryu J, Burgess RC: Matched distal ulnar resection. J Hand Surg 11A:812-817, 1986
286. Weiland AJ, Naiman J: Independent index extension after extensor indicis proprius transfer. J Hand Surg 10A:427, 1985
287. Welsh RP, Hastings DE: Swan-neck deformity in rheumatoid arthritis of the hand. Hand 9:109-116, 1977
288. White RE Jr: Resection of the distal ulna with and without implant arthroplasty in rheumatoid arthritis. J Hand Surg 11A:514-518, 1986
289. White SH, Goodfellow JW, Mowat A: Posterior interosseous nerve palsy in rheumatoid arthritis. J Bone Joint Surg 70B:468-471, 1988
290. Wilde AH, Sawmiller SR: Synovectomy of the proximal interphalangeal joint in rheumatoid arthritis. Cleve Clin Q 36:155-161, 1969
291. Wilde AH: Synovectomy of the proximal interphalangeal joint of the finger in rheumatoid arthritis. J Bone Joint Surg 56A:71-78, 1974
292. Wilson RL, Carlblom ER: The rheumatoid metacarpophalangeal joint. Hand Clin 5:223-237, 1989
293. Wissinger HA: Digital flexor lag in rheumatoid arthritis. Clinical significance and treatment. Plast Reconstr Surg 47:465-468, 1971
294. Youm Y, McMurtry RY, Flatt AE, Gillespie TE: Kinematics of the wrist. I. An experimental study of radial-ulnar deviation and flexion-extension. J Bone Joint Surg 60A:423-431, 1978
295. Zancolli EA: The Structural and Dynamic Bases of Hand Surgery. 2nd Ed. pp. 305-360. JB Lippincott, Philadelphia, 1979

47

Rheumatoid Arthritis in the Elbow

Donald C. Ferlic

EXTRAARTICULAR CONSIDERATIONS

Olecranon Bursae

Rheumatoid elbows are frequently plagued with superficial problems, such as olecranon bursae, which become painful and inflamed. The olecranon bursa does not normally communicate with the elbow joint, but with rheumatoid arthritis it occasionally does, and infection of the joint may present as a draining olecranon bursa. The clinical factor to consider is a bursitis with copious drainage. Bursae tend to recur or drain after excision, although these complications may be minimized by insertion of a drain, excision of the redundant skin, and splinting the elbow in 60 degrees flexion for 2 to 3 weeks following surgery.

Rheumatoid Nodules

Rheumatoid arthritic patients frequently form nodules related to pressure areas. Those about the bony surface of the olecranon may be painful and may ulcerate. Although patients may desire to have these removed, it is important to warn them that these nodules frequently do recur following excision.

Antecubital Cysts

Antecubital cysts in the rheumatoid elbow are similar to Baker's cysts in the knee, and occasionally require excision because of pain or nerve impingement.

Wrist and Shoulder

A relationship exists between elbow and hand and wrist problems and, therefore, when a patient is examined for a hand problem, it is always necessary to consider the elbow as well. Forearm rotation, ulnar nerve problems, and posterior interosseous nerve palsy resulting from elbow synovitis should be kept in mind. A patient with limited forearm rotation may indeed have problems with the distal radioulnar joint, but the rotation may also be limited at the proximal radioulnar joint, which necessitates radial head resection in addition to removal of the distal ulna to restore rotation. Seventy-five percent of our patients who have undergone elbow synovectomy and radial head resection have also had distal ulna resection and synovectomy of the wrist.

Elbow problems are also closely linked to shoulder problems. Good elbow function often compensates for limited shoulder motion.

Posterior Interosseous Nerve Palsy

When a rheumatoid patient presents with an inability to extend the fingers, the pathology may be in the hand, wrist, or elbow, and there may very well be a problem differentiating between posterior interosseous nerve palsy at the elbow,[39](Fig. 47-1) subluxation of the extensor tendons off the MP joints in the hand, or even ruptured extensor tendons at the wrist. This problem can be correctly diagnosed only if one is aware of all these possibilities. A hand with posterior interosseous nerve palsy can often be differentiated by demonstrating a positive tenodesis effect. When the wrist is flexed, the intact extensor tendons should extend the fingers, but if the wrist or MP joints are stiff, the tenodesis effect will not be apparent, and this may present an additional diagnostic problem.

An arthrogram of the elbow may reveal a large antecubital cyst pressing on the posterior interosseous nerve. A steroid injection into the elbow may reslove the inflammation, but synovectomy and nerve decompression may still be necessary.

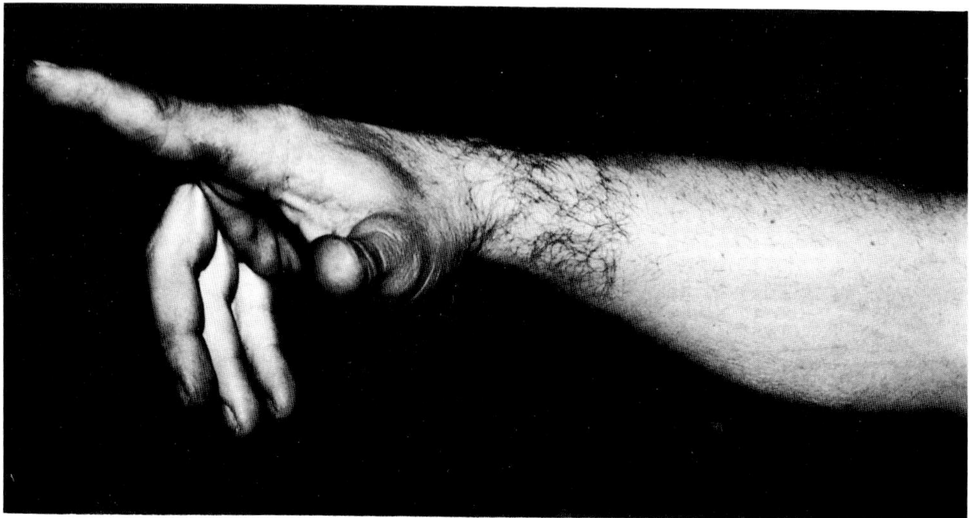

Fig. 47-1. The hand of a patient with posterior interosseous nerve palsy mimics the hand with ruptured extensor tendons at the wrist and the hand with MP joint dislocation, with subluxation of the extensor tendons to the ulnar side of the joints, thereby inhibiting extension of the fingers.

Ulnar Nerve Palsy

The rheumatoid patient may also develop ulnar nerve palsy at the elbow. Bony deformities aggravated by synovitis can lacerate the nerve.[40] The patient may present with numbness and paresthesias in the ulnar nerve distribution in the hand, or just weakness and lack of hand dexterity. This is best treated by decompression and rerouting of the nerve anteriorly (see Chapter 36).

INTRAARTICULAR CONSIDERATIONS

Most large series of patients undergoing surgery for rheumatoid arthritis include relatively few patients having elbow operations, even though the elbow is frequently involved in rheumatoid arthritis. Laine and Vainio[33] found two-thirds of their patients with rheumatoid arthritis to have elbow involvement. Severe elbow problems necessitating surgery arise later in the disease because (1) the onset of elbow symptoms is generally insidious; (2) patients may be unaware of disability until destruction is advanced because range of motion is aided by gravity, which helps to maintain extension, and the activities of daily living help to maintain flexion; (3) loss of pronation is compensated by shoulder motion, and thus the patient is not aware of the elbow problem until shoulder and wrist motion also become limited; and (4) the elbow frequently responds well to conservative measures such as rest, splinting, and analgesics.

Elbow Synovectomy

Elbow synovectomy and debridement was first reported in 1893.[52] Since then, there have been many reports quoting good results.[1,3,10,15,17,27,30,33-35,38,45,51,54,56,59,67,69]

Surgical Approach

Although it is generally agreed upon that this procedure is not necessary in the early stages of rheumatoid arthritis, there is disagreement as to the best surgical approach. Smith-Petersen, Aufranc, and Larson[55] described the basic procedure of radial head excision and synovectomy most widely used today. Inglis, Ranawat, and Straub[27] have advocated a transolecranon approach, by an osteotomy through the midportion of the olecranon process, allowing reflection of the proximal olecranon with the triceps muscle and extensive exposure to the elbow joint. Some[47,69] advocate lateral and medial incisions, while others[1,15,35,38,59] recommend only a lateral incision, except in cases where there are symptoms on the medial side.

Bryan and Morrey[4,44] have advocated a posterior triceps sparing approach (Fig. 47-2). A straight posterior incision is made medial to the midline. The ulnar nerve is identified and protected. It may be transferred anteriorly. The medial aspect of the triceps is elevated from the humerus along the intermuscular septum to the level of the posterior capsule. The superficial fascia of the forearm is incised distally to the periosteum of the medial aspect of the proximal ulna. The periosteum and fascia complex is carefully reflected laterally. The medial part of the complex is the weakest portion of the reflected tissue, so care must be taken to maintain continuity of the triceps mechanism at this point. After release of the triceps from the olecranon, the remaining portion of the triceps mechanism is reflected. The anconeus can be removed subperiosteally from the proximal ulna to expose the radial head. When closing, the triceps is returned to its anatomic location and sutured to the bone, as are the ligaments that have been stripped from the bone.

The transolecranon approach is reported to give good pain relief, but its major disadvantages are potential complications associated with fixation of the bone. Reports on the combined lateral and medial approach[47,68,69] relate postoperative ulnar neuropathy as a complication. I[19,45] favor the lateral approach only. It is safe and simple, and an adequate synovectomy can be carried out on both medial and lateral sides through one lateral incision by subluxating the ulna to obtain medial and posterior exposure.

Indications

Indications for synovectomy and radial head resection are pain, swelling, and reasonable range of motion of the elbow with ARA classification of Stage II or III (Table 47-1). Painful crepitus over the radial head with rotation in an elbow with less crepitus on ulnohumeral motion is the prime indication.

Technique of Elbow Synovectomy

A posterolateral incision extending from the posterior border of the ulna 4 cm distal to the tip of the olecranon to a point 4 cm proximal to the lateral epicondyle of the humerus is made, keeping the forearm pronated to protect the radial nerve (Fig. 47-3). A fascial incision is made along the line between the anconeus and common extensor tendon origins to the triceps tendon posteriorly. The common extensor tendons are detached by sharp dissection from the lateral epicondyle and retracted upward. The radial head is excised, synovectomy carried out, and the ulna subluxated to remove the synovium from the posterior and medial sides. By flexing the elbow, the anterior recess can be cleared, and in extension, the olecranon fossa is similarly exposed. A small double action rongeur is useful for removing the synovium. The coronoid process is partially excised if it limits flexion, and bone from the tip of the olecranon can also be excised if necessary.

A silicone radial head prosthesis may be inserted to prevent proximal migration of the radius, valgus deformity, and to modulate the forces across the elbow. Use of a radial head implant, however, is not accepted by all surgeons. If the radial head does not fit, or if the capitellum is too rough, the implant is omitted.

Walker[65] demonstrated with his biomechanical studies that the amount of force exerted across the elbow joint must reach 9.8 kg before the force is absorbed by the radiohumeral joint. It does not seem that the rheumatoid patient with marked involvement and weakness will achieve such force, but if there is lower extremity involvement, this force is likely to be exceeded with the use of a walker or crutches. In addition, there is a considerable levering effect in the forearm when the elbow is flexed 90 degrees, creating a joint reactive force often magnified at least 20 times. Many rheumatoid patients display a great amount of joint laxity, and the radial head is important in preventing extreme valgus angulation of the elbow,[36] particularly if the medial collateral ligament is unstable. The radial head implant also acts as a spacer and shock absorber to help unload the ulnohumeral joint.

If there is excessive medial pain or ulnar neuropathy, a medial incision is made over the tip of the medial epicondyle 5 cm distal and proximal to the joint. The ulnar nerve is isolated and transposed anteriorly. The muscles originating from the epicondyle are reflected, the capsule incised, and the synovium removed; the important anterior medial collateral ligament is preserved. Care must be taken to avoid injuring the median nerve passing over the anterior aspect of the joint. A bulky dressing with a posterior splint is applied with the elbow at 90 degrees, and active and passive motion is begun in 3 or 4 days.

Controversial Points

The results of synovectomy of the elbow are better than for any other joint. This is probably due to its nonweightbearing status and the decompression effect obtained with radial head excision.

Besides the operative approach, there are other controversies surrounding elbow synovectomy and radial head resection. Whereas most authors believe that the radial head should be routinely excised to achieve good results, Copeland and Taylor[10] stated that results are not influenced by radial head excision. Rymaszewski et al[51] believe that removal of the radial head causes biomechanical changes that can contribute to failure of the procedure.

Another point of controversy is the stage of disease for which this procedure can be effective. We[19,45] have shown through long-term follow-up that the procedure is indicated in ARA Stage II or early Stage III and is less effective in late Stage III or IV. Others[3,10,15,47,59] state that advanced states of destruction do not prejudice results. Brumfield and Resnick[3] reported that although this procedure was not contraindicated in Stage III or IV, little improvement in motion could be anticipated. We found that most of the poor results occurred within 48 months of surgery, while Porter[47] and Rymaszewski[51] showed deteriorating results after 3 years.

The final item of controversy is the use of a radial head prosthesis. We have found no difference between those patients in whom the prosthesis was used and those in whom it was not,[45] but we agree with Bryan and Morrey,[5] who believe that the implant should be limited to the unstable elbow. Swanson,[58] Wadsworth,[64] Mackay,[37] and Rymaszewski,[51] on the other hand, advocate replacing the radial head with a prosthesis if excision is necessary.

We have found a greater incidence of poor results not only in cases with advanced disease stage, but also in those adult patients with juvenile rheumatoid arthritis. The only contraindications to synovectomy and radial head resection are gross joint destruction, instability, and secondary severe stiffness resulting from inflammatory fibrosis.

Elbow Arthroplasty (Without Implant)

For the elbow with more advanced disease, excisional or interpositional arthroplasties have been performed using fascia, dermis, or gelfoam. Excisional arthroplasty for rheumatoid arthritis has been reported by Hurri,[26] Vainio,[62] and Dee.[12] Dee reported six cases with rheumatoid arthritis, all of which were unsatisfactory because of stiffness or instability. Vainio[62] reported on 208 excisional arthroplasties. Fifty-three of these were of the Herbert type, which consists of an extraperiosteal resection of the humeral condyles, the entire olecranon, the coronoid process, and the radial head. The other 155 cases

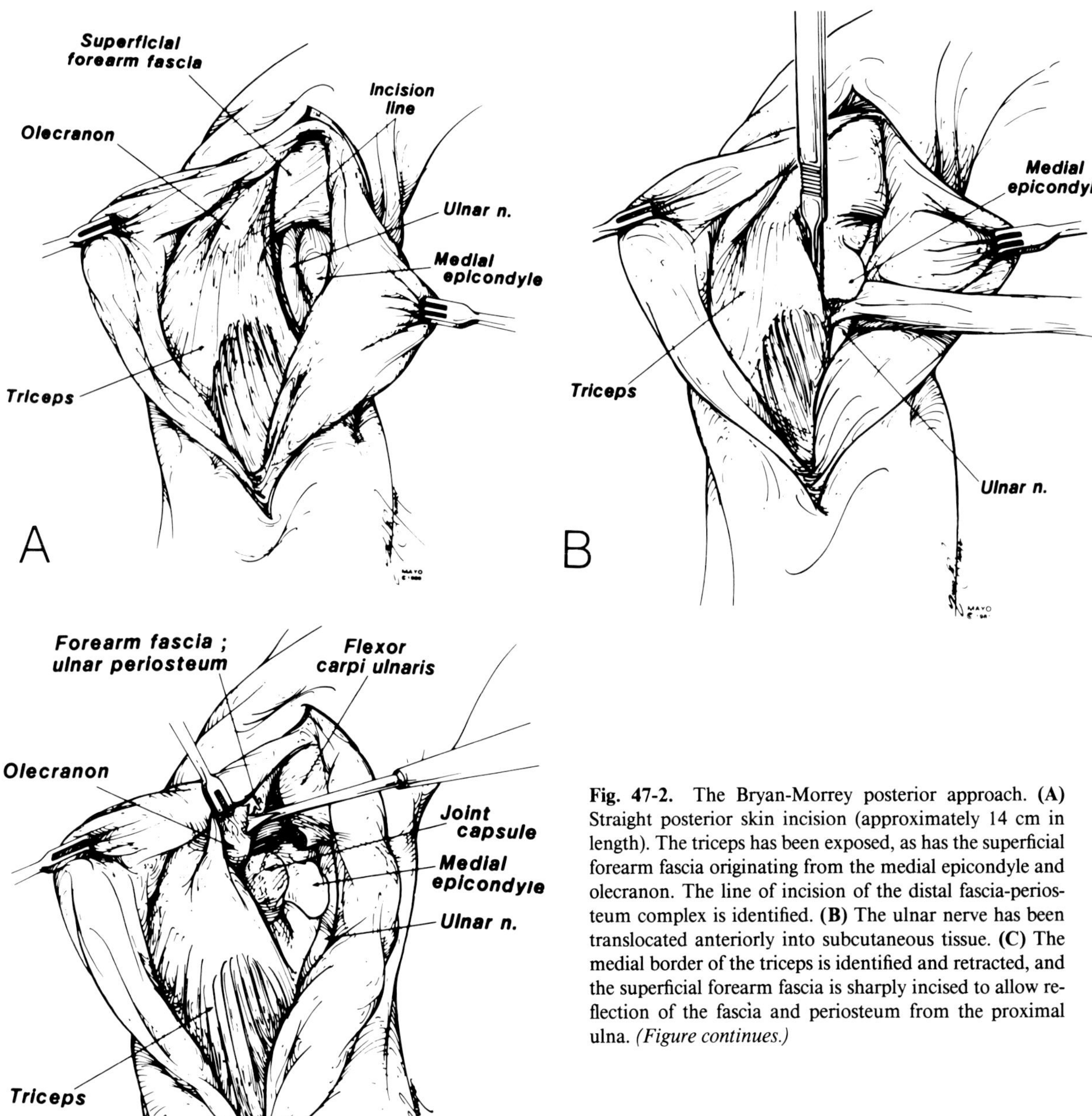

Fig. 47-2. The Bryan-Morrey posterior approach. **(A)** Straight posterior skin incision (approximately 14 cm in length). The triceps has been exposed, as has the superficial forearm fascia originating from the medial epicondyle and olecranon. The line of incision of the distal fascia-periosteum complex is identified. **(B)** The ulnar nerve has been translocated anteriorly into subcutaneous tissue. **(C)** The medial border of the triceps is identified and retracted, and the superficial forearm fascia is sharply incised to allow reflection of the fascia and periosteum from the proximal ulna. *(Figure continues.)*

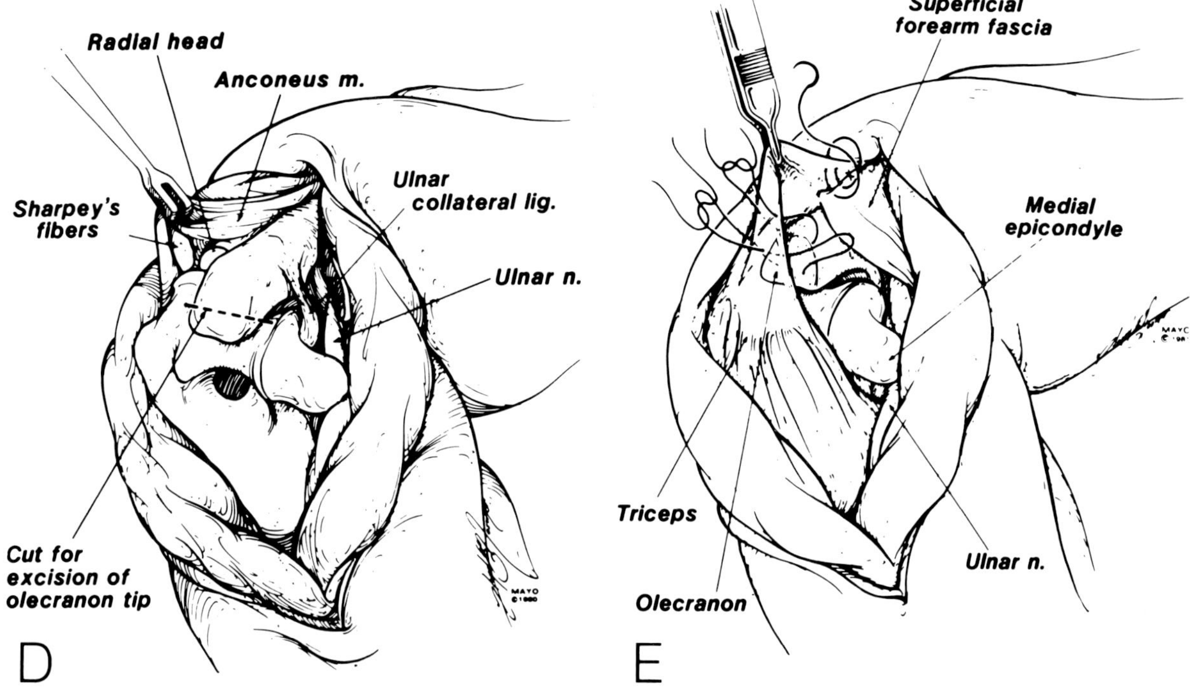

Fig. 47-2 *(Continued).* **(D)** The extensor mechanism has been reflected laterally and the anconeus has been subperiosteally released from the ulna, allowing exposure of the radial head. The junction of the ulna, periosteum, and fascia with the insertion site of Sharpey's fibers is the most tenacious portion of the reflected mechanism. The proximal portion of the olecranon is removed for joint exposure. **(E)** The triceps tendon is reattached to the olecranon by sutures placed through bone. The forearm fascia-periosteum complex is sutured to the margin of the flexor carpi ulnaris. (From Bryan-Morrey,[4] and by permission of Mayo Foundation.)

were the Hoss arthroplasty or its modification, with a free skin graft over the distal end of the humerus. In this arthroplasty, the distal end of the humerus is resected to the shape of a blunt wedge. The mean range of motion was 100 degrees in the Herbert group and 95 degrees in the Hoss group.

Souter,[54] after a literature review, reported that unsatisfactory results with fascial arthroplasty can be as high as 50 percent.[30] Indications for fascial arthroplasty vary from bilateral ankylosis to partial ankylosis with disabling pain.[7,27,35] One theoretical advantage of using an interpositional material instead of simply a resection arthroplasty is reduced bone resorption, but we have not been able to confirm this.

I prefer fascia when performing an interpositional arthro-

Table 47-1. American Rheumatism Association Modified Classification of X-Ray Involvement

Stage I	Osteoporosis
Stage II	Slight subchondral bone or cartilage destruction; osteoporosis
Stage IIIA	Cartilage and bone destruction with joint deformity; joint space not completely lost
Stage IIIB	Total loss of joint space in one view
Stage IV	Total loss of joint space in two views or fibrous or bony ankylosis

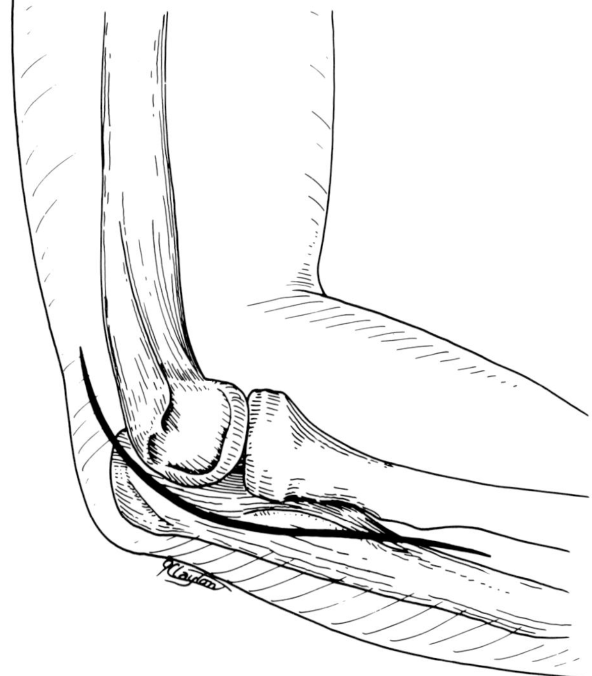

Fig. 47-3. The posterolateral skin incision used for elbow synovectomy extends both proximal and lateral to the radial head.

plasty in a rheumatoid elbow. Indications are a late Stage III or IV elbow with adequate bone stock so that stability is not compromised. The indications for this procedure are much less frequent now that total elbow arthroplasty is available.

Technique of Fascial Arthroplasty

A posterior incision is made just lateral to the elbow midline, extending distally 10 cm, and then curving to the medial side and extending proximally 10 cm (Fig. 47-4). The ulnar nerve is transposed anteriorly, the triceps reflected in a V-fashion (Fig. 47-5), the radial collateral ligament divided, and the joint dislocated. The radial head is excised, the semilunar notch of the olecranon deepened, and the trochlea deepened in such a manner as to provide medial and lateral bony stability (Fig. 47-6). A 5 × 8 cm piece of fascia lata is harvested and sutured over the semilunar notch. The joint is reduced, the collateral ligament sutured, and the wound closed. Bulky dressings and a posterior splint are applied postoperatively, and active and passive motion is begun in 3 or 4 days.

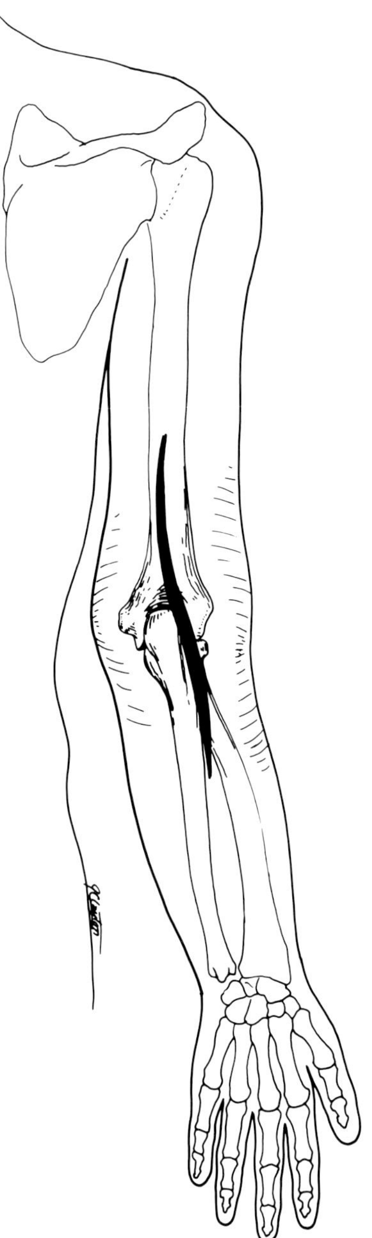

Fig. 47-4. The posterior skin incision used for fascial and implant arthroplasties begins just lateral to the midline, 10 cm distally, curving to the medial side and extending proximally 10 cm.

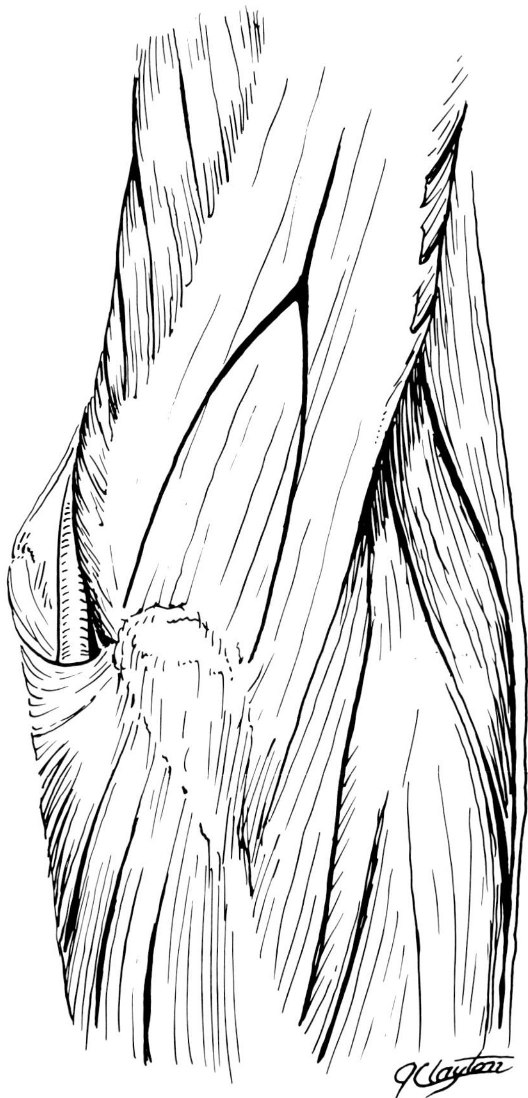

Fig. 47-5. A V-shaped incision is made in the triceps.

We have obtained very favorable results in rheumatoid patients, with a marked decrease in pain and an average range of motion of 100 degrees flexion-extension arc (Fig. 47-7). Failure has been due to further absorption of bone, which some rheumatoid patients exhibit. Instability has been a problem due to the bony configuration of the resected joint and resuturing of the collateral ligament.

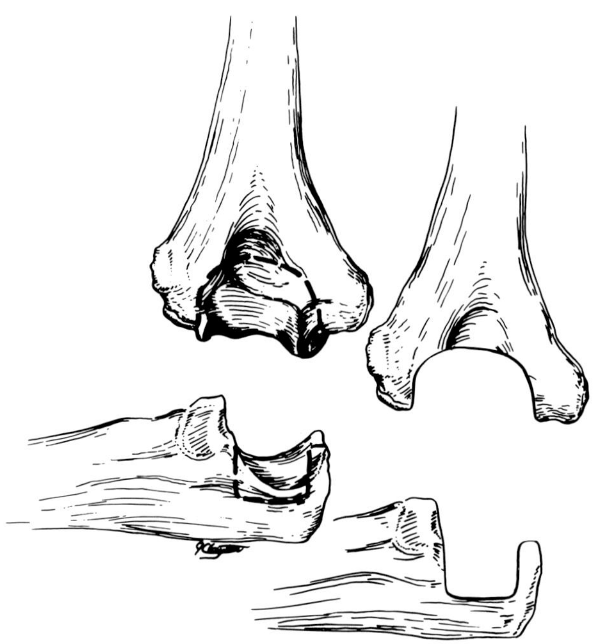

Fig. 47-6. Bone is removed from the semilunar notch of the olecranon and the trochlea so that a stable joint is achieved.

Elbow Arthrodesis

Elbow arthrodesis in the rheumatoid patient is rarely, if ever, indicated. This procedure relieves pain, but markedly interferes with upper extremity function. The single exception may be in an infected or otherwise failed total elbow arthroplasty where there is not enough bone stock for another procedure or where resection arthroplasty is not acceptable.

ELBOW IMPLANT ARTHROPLASTY

Historical Review

There have been numerous reports of implant arthroplasty resulting in high complication rates. Components have frequently been withdrawn from the market for redesign.[13,17]

There are three basic types of elbow replacement (Table 47-2). The constrained hinge is constructed with either metal-to-metal or metal-to-high density polyethylene, through a bushing or a separate polyethylene piece. The semiconstrained elbow is also a hinge, but allows a few degrees of lateral motion. This type was designed to help alleviate some of the loosening problems found with the constrained hinges. The unconstrained elbow consists of separate units of metal-to-high density polyethylene components. Some are designed to be used with a radial head replacement.

In 1971, Peterson and Janes[46] reported on two vitallium mold arthroplasties of the olecranon notch. One was excellent, the other fair.

In 1974, Street and Stevens[57] reported on their use of a metallic distal humeral resurfacing device in 10 patients. Three were for rheumatoid arthritis, and results in two of the three were unsatisfactory. One of the two developed complete elbow ankylosis and a transient ulnar neuropathy. The other was complicated by elbow dislocation, with skin erosion on the medial side. This necessitated removal of the prosthesis, but ankylosis resulted.

Silicone hinge arthroplasty at the elbow has also been tried but was abandoned because of breakage. The results with the rigid hinges have likewise been disappointing. Cooney and Bryan[7] tabulated results on a combination of 111 Schiers, Dee, McKee-Dee, GSB, and Coonrad elbows, with 24 percent showing poor results. Cofield, Morrey, and Bryan[6] tabulated the complications in 346 hinged total elbow replacements of both constrained and semiconstrained types, and found loosening in 13 percent; other complications in their series included 9 percent fracture, 9 percent wound problems, 5 percent infection, 4 percent ankylosis, 6 percent neuropathy, and 2 percent triceps rupture. Twelve required revision.

Coonrad[8] reported on 150 elbows with rheumatoid arthritis done in a multi-center study with 95 percent good results. There were only six failures, four due to loosening and two with infection, although in 12 percent the humeral stems became loose. He concluded that this was a good procedure for rheumatoid arthritis, but not for post-traumatic problems. His original rigid hinge elbow was modified to allow some lateral motion, and the humeral stem was lengthened. The results of this modified prosthesis were even more promising than the earlier model. Coonrad,[9] however, reported two deep infections in 14 elbows, that he personally had to replace.

Inglis and Pellicci[28] reported on 36 semiconstrained elbow replacements followed for a minimum of 2 years and found a 53 percent complication rate, but only one-fourth of the complications affected the outcome. The first 17 in this series were done with a semiconstrained Pritchard-Walker elbow, and the rest with the triaxial prosthesis. There were 22 rheumatoid patients, who did generally better than the post-traumatic group. Of the 19 complications in this group of 36 patients, there were four wound hematomas, two cases of loosening, two fractured humeri, two ulnar neuropathies, two triceps ruptures, two with skin slough, two with broken components, one fractured olecranon, one infection, and one cementophyte.

Brumfield, Volz, and Green[2] reported on the results of two semiconstrained prostheses, the Mayo and AHSC (Volz). These are similar prostheses, with a semiconstrained ulnohumeral articulation and a radial head component. There were 14 patients in each group. All had rheumatoid arthritis except two with osteoarthritis. There was one case of loosening, one in which the humeral ulnar joint dislocated, one superficial infection, and one with ulnar nerve neuropathy. Two patients avulsed the triceps muscle. There were seven cases displaying radiolucency, and three with fracture of the humeral condyle. Generally, pain was decreased or abolished and motion increased. Although this was an encouraging report in 1981, Volz[63] reported in 1985 that he had stopped using the AHSC prosthesis.

In order to decrease the incidence of loosening of the semiconstrained hinged prosthesis and dislocation with the nonhinged prosthesis, Pritchard[48] designed a three-piece nonconstrained surface prosthesis with a radial head. In a group of 13

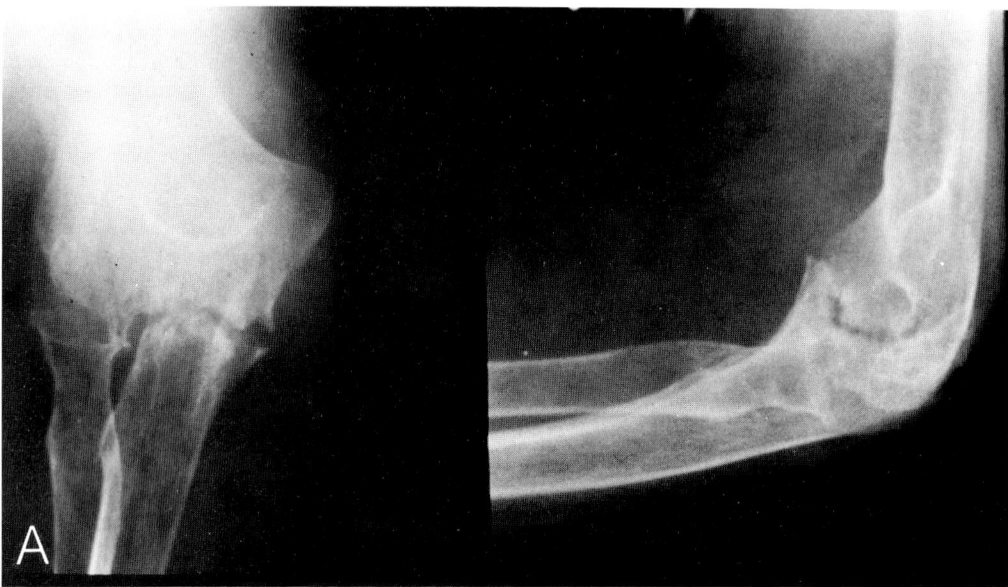

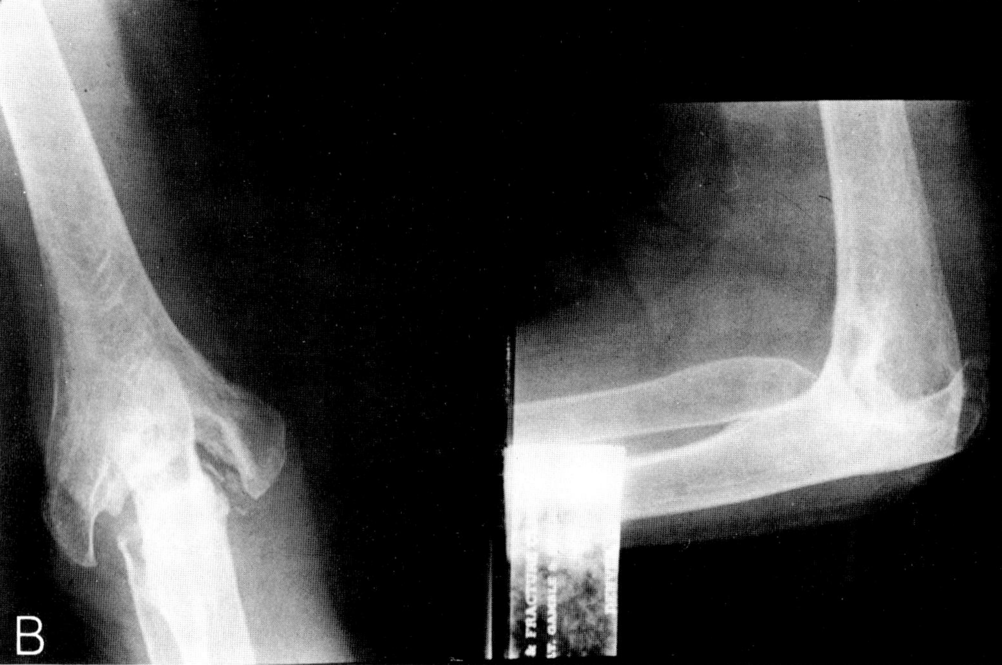

Fig. 47-7. **(A)** Preoperative radiograph of a rheumatoid elbow. **(B)** Postoperative radiograph of an elbow after fascial arthroplasty showing the bone resection and the stable joint.

Table 47-2. Types of Elbow Prostheses

Constrained	Semiconstrained	Nonconstrained
Coonrad I	AHSC (Volz)	Kudo
Schiers	Pritchard-Walker	London
Dee	Pritchard Mark II	Pritchard ERS
GSB	Triaxial	Capitello-condylar (Ewald)
McKee	Coonrad II	Wadsworth
Mazas	Schlein	Cavendish
Stanmore	Silva	Gunston
	St. George-Bucholz	Mayo
	Swanson	Stevens-Street
	Coonrad-Morrey	
	GSB III	
	DEE IV	

elbows (12 rheumatoid arthritis), satisfactory pain relief was achieved and motion increased in all cases. The only complication was a fracture-dislocation of the humeral component in one as a result of a fall. In a later report, Pritchard[49] presented 75 cases from a multicenter study. Although loosening, dislocation, subluxation, triceps rupture, and ulnar nerve problems were noted, he believed that the long-term results were satisfactory.

Gschwend et al[25] modified their original constrained GSB prosthesis to a semiconstrained device and reported on 64 patients with 71 prostheses. They felt that their complication rate was low in comparison with most reports in the world literature and even lower when the long-term complications were considered.

In 1989 Figgie et al[22] reported on total elbow arthroplasty for complete ankylosis of the elbow (19 elbows in 16 patients, including eight with juvenile rheumatoid arthritis and one with rheumatoid arthritis). They used a variety of semiconstrained devices and had 15 excellent or good results. Function improved in all patients, and all had relief of preoperative pain. There was only one failure, this due to infection.

Surgeons at the Mayo Clinic[6,7] obtained satisfactory results in 75 percent of cases with total elbow replacement for rheumatoid arthritis. The rheumatoid patients again showed better results than the patients with post-traumatic arthritis.

The nonconstrained elbows were introduced to alleviate the loosening problem, but these prostheses have also been plagued with a high complication rate. Kudo[32] reported 24 elbow replacements done for rheumatoid arthritis using a resurfacing prosthesis and found 14 excellent and three poor results. Two elbows failed to regain useful motion, one had proximal migration of the humeral component, and one had persistent subluxation with pain and instability.

In 1990 Kudo and Iwano[31] reported on thirty-seven elbows in thirty-six patients. Because of a high incidence of proximal migration of the humeral component they now use a humeral component with an intramedullary stem.

Ewald[16] reported 60 prosthetic replacements for rheumatoid arthritis and found 87 percent good or excellent results. However, he had a 39 percent complication rate with eight requiring revision of the arthroplasty; four for dislocation, two for sepsis, one for loosening, and one for fracture. Five patients experienced recurrent dislocation, and there were five permanent and six transient ulnar nerve palsies. There were three fractures, two of the olecranon and one of the humeral shaft. Three wounds demonstrated some degree of breakdown and skin loss.

In a later report, Ewald[18] used a lateral surgical approach in an attempt to reduce the incidence of soft tissue problems. This group consisted of 54 elbows, with 90 percent good or excellent results. Complications consisted of dislocation in 7 percent, permanent sensory ulnar nerve palsy in 4 percent, and one deep and one superficial wound infection. There were transient ulnar nerve palsies in 14 percent. Thus, the lateral surgical approach did not change the rate of serious complications. Ewald used a cemented radial head prosthesis in eight elbows, but in four of these, there was a radiolucent line at the cement-bone interface of the humeral component as well as the radial head. This compared to only one prosthesis without a radial head implant that had a radiolucent line.

In 1990[53] Simmons, Sullivan, and Ewald presented their follow-up of 312 capitello-condylar arthroplasties followed a minimum of two years. Of these, 91 percent were done for rheumatoid arthritis, 87 percent for juvenile rheumatoid arthritis, and 1 percent for post-traumatic arthritis. Range of motion increased in all planes. Revision surgery was necessary for aseptic loosening in 2 percent and instability in 1 percent. Other complications were deep infection necessitating prosthesis removal (1.5 percent) transient sensory ulnar nerve palsy (16 percent), permanent sensory nerve palsy (5 percent), dislocation (3.5 percent), subluxation-malarticulation (5 percent), and wound problems (8 percent).

Rosenberg and Turner[50] reported on 28 Ewald capitello-condylar arthroplasties for rheumatoid arthritis. Eighty-six percent obtained satisfactory results. There was one failure from loosening, two remote infections, and four cases of dislocation, one of which required additional surgery.

Davis et al[11] reported 30 Ewald elbows for rheumatoid arthritis with excellent pain relief. Two of the 30 developed wound infections, which ultimately required removal of the prosthesis. There were four cases of subluxation, one of which required additional surgery. Three developed ulnar neuropathy, two of which required neurolysis and rerouting of the nerve.

Trancik et al[60] reported on 35 capitello-condylar arthroplasties on 29 patients. Their complication rate was 57 percent with three infections, three dislocations, two intraoperative fractures, nine transient nerve palsies, two postoperative hematomas, and one intraoperative perforation of the ulna. In spite of these problems, pain relief was achieved in all but one patient. There were no unstable elbows.

Weiland et al[66] reported on 40 capitello-condylar arthroplasties in thirty-five patients. Thirty-two had rheumatoid arthritis. Malarticulation or dislocations occurred in ten (29 percent). Two patients developed a deep infection necessitating removal. Seven patients had a transient nerve palsy. The incidence of nerve palsy was reduced when the lateral Kocher approach was adopted.

In spite of these reports, Figgie[20] has stated that the results of triaxial prostheses are as good as total hips, but not as good as total knee arthroplasty.

Judging from these reports, we conclude that elbow replacement should not be performed by the occasional elbow surgeon.

All of our total elbow replacements have been done in rheumatoid patients. Our first four were performed with rigid hinges (three GSB and one Coonrad); the first of these was performed in 1971. We chose the GSB initially because we felt that its small size would preserve bone stock, so that if the device necessitated removal, a stable fascial arthroplasty would still be possible.

These four patients were followed between 22 and 84 months. Two of the elbows are still in excellent condition. Flexion and extension arc is between 104 and 140 degrees, and both have had full forearm rotation. One of the elbows loosened after 6 years and became painful. There was a marked amount of bone resorption and a fracture of the medial humeral pillar. One GSB elbow did well for 7 years before developing a deep wound infection that necessitated operative treatment.

After our initial efforts with the rigid hinges, we[14] started using the nonconstrained resurfacing devices, such as the Ewald (Fig. 47-8), London (Fig. 47-9), and Wadsworth because of the high rate of loosening that has occurred with the original, rigid hinges. Postoperative motion ranged from 95 to 125 degrees of flexion/extension, and 90 to 100 degrees of rotation. Complications, however, have been numerous and quite significant, and because of this, we have limited our use of the nonconstrained elbow to the young rheumatoid patient with a stable joint and adequate bone stock. In all others, we recommend one of the semirigid hinges and have been using the Coonrad-Morrey hinge most often. (Fig. 47-10)

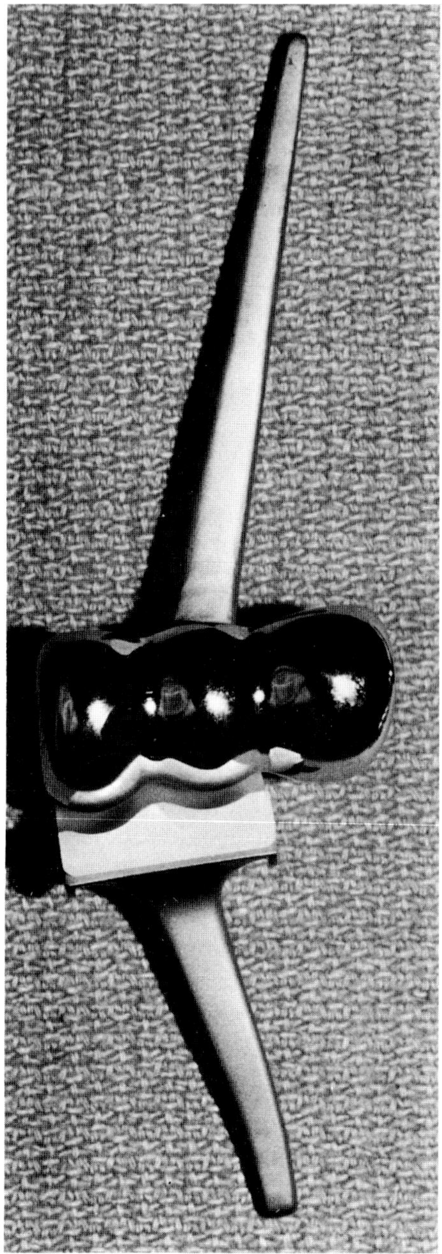

Fig. 47-8. Ewald capitello-condylar elbow replacement.

Indications

The indications for total elbow arthroplasty in the rheumatoid patient are ARA Stage IIIB or IV, significant pain, and adequate condylar bone stock present so that the metal devices are not completely uncovered. The medullary canals of the humerus and ulna must be large enough for the prosthesis to enter. The elbow must be free from infection. There are some rheumatoid elbows in which a prosthesis should not be inserted, specifically those that do not meet the above criteria.

Contraindications

The presence of active sepsis is an absolute contraindication. Surgical revision because of previous sepsis may be necessary, however. Neuropathic joints secondary to diabetes, syringomyelia or other diseases are relative contraindications, as are nutritional deficiencies that might delay prompt healing of the surgical wound. If total elbow arthroplasty is performed in an elbow with existing heterotopic ossification, more ossification may be stimulated, leading to a decreased range of motion.[24]

Technique of Capitello-Condylar (Ewald) Nonconstrained Elbow Arthroplasty

Our technique is similar to that described by Ewald.[18] We prefer the posterior medial Bryan-Morrey (Mayo) approach, but the lateral Kocher approach can also be used.

The patient is placed supine on the table with the elbow across the chest. The ulnar nerve is identified, freed from the

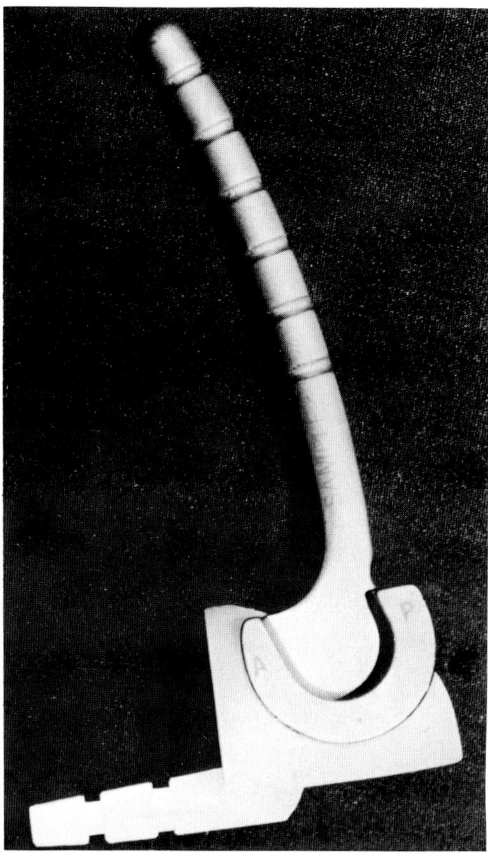

Fig. 47-9. London nonconstrained elbow.

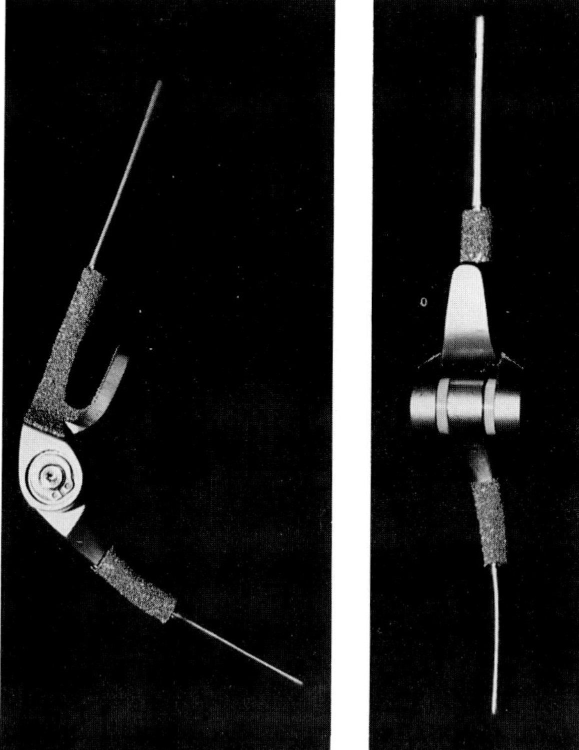

Fig. 47-10. The Morrey-modified Coonrad total elbow prosthesis.

cubital tunnel, and protected. The strong anterior medial collateral ligament is key, and it is preserved (Fig. 47-11A). All structures are released from the lateral epicondyle in such a manner that they can be reattached at the time of closure. The joint is opened on the lateral side, hinging on the intact medial ligaments (Fig. 47-11B).

Synovectomy and joint debridement with removal of scar tissue enhance dislocation of the joint laterally, hinging on the medial capsule. The radial head is excised proximal to the annular ligament (Fig. 47-11C). The deep branch of the radial nerve, although not exposed, is protected by retracting the lateral muscle mass anteriorly with small Bennett retractors. Exposure can be increased by further dissection of the triceps tendon from the tip of the olecranon, taking a thin layer of bone with the tendon. Osteophytes on the margins of the olecranon are debrided. The capitellum and trochlea are debrided back to healthy bone and rounded to fit the humeral component (Fig. 47-11D). Scar tissue is freed from the anterior portion of the distal humerus with an elevator.

In order to properly align the elbow replacement, it is necessary to understand the anatomy of the elbow joint (Figs. 47-12 to 47-14).

The trial humeral component stem is aligned on the shaft centered between the epicondyles, marked with methylene blue, and cut out down to the apex of the olecranon fossa with a rongeur or small saw. An awl is used first to prepare the humerus, followed by a broach and then a larger reamer. The humerus is supported to minimize the possibility of fracture during hand reaming. These humeral component trials have valgus fixation stem angles of 5 degrees, 10 degrees, 15 degrees, and 20 degrees. The 5-degree stem is most commonly used. The remaining portions of both the trochlea and capitellum are debrided anteriorly and posteriorly to allow seating of the metal humeral component on bone. Proper rotational alignment can be achieved by viewing the end of the humerus and using an imaginary line between the center of the capitellum and trochlea as a reference point. This line should bisect the metal humeral component when it is seated on bone.

The awl is directed 18 degrees laterally to penetrate the ulnar canal (Fig. 47-11E). The fixation hole for the ulnar component is progressively enlarged with reamers. To a large extent the ulnar canal is self-aligning for the fixation stem of the ulnar component. In the lateral plane the canal runs at an angle of 55 degrees from the joint line.

The trochlear notch of the ulna is debrided with a rongeur, and a dental burr is used to shape the notch to the metal tray of the ulnar component. This close bony fit is important because it provides rotatory control for the ulnar component.

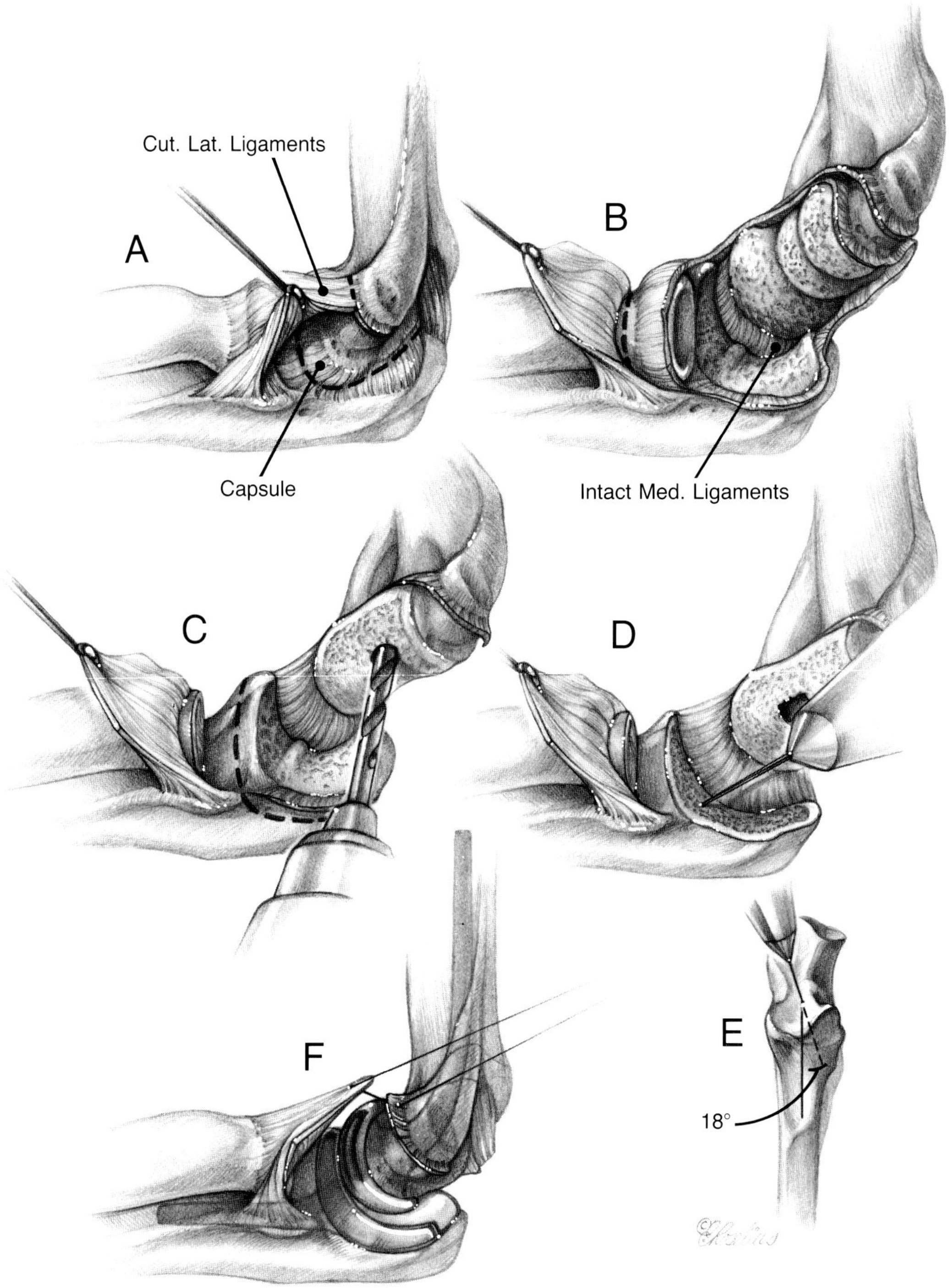

Fig. 47-11. Operative technique for capitello-condylar elbow arthroplasty. **(A)** The lateral ligaments have been cut. It is important to preserve the anterior medial collateral ligament. **(B)** After detaching the lateral ligaments, the elbow is hinged open on the medial ligaments. **(C)** The radial head has been resected, and the medullary canal of the humerus is being prepared to accept the stem of the implant. **(D)** The capitellum and trochlea are debrided back to healthy bone and rounded to fit the humeral component. **(E)** An awl is directed 18 degrees laterally to penetrate the ulnar canal, and the trochlear notch of the ulna is shaped to fit the prosthesis. **(F)** A trial fit of the prosthesis is carried out and then cemented in place.

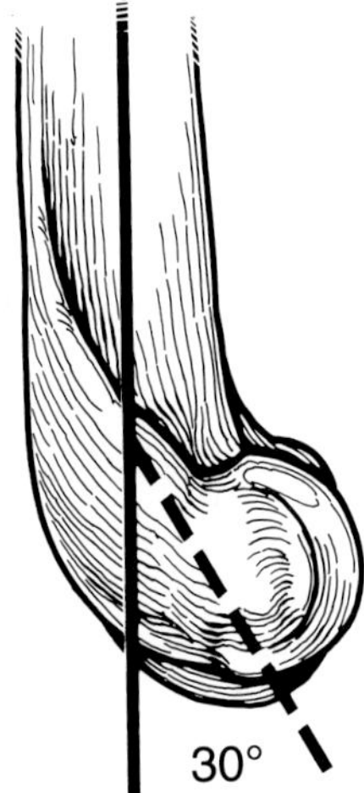

Fig. 47-12. A lateral view of the humerus shows the 30-degree anterior angulation of the articular condyle with respect to the long axis of the humerus. (Adapted from Morrey,[44] and by permission of Mayo Foundation.)

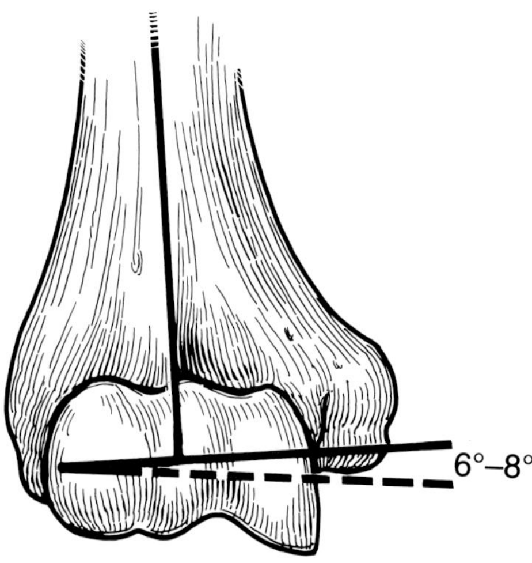

Fig. 47-14. There is approximately 6 to 8 degrees valgus tilt of the distal humeral articulation with respect to the long axis of the humerus. (Adapted from Morrey,[44] and by permission of Mayo Foundation.)

The ulnar component has two fixation stem sizes, thin and regular, and the polyethylene is available in three thicknesses (3, 6, and 9 mm). Also available is a large (15 percent oversized) prosthesis as well. Radiographic templates can assist in size selection.

Trial reduction of the components is performed (Fig. 47-11F). Range of motion, stability, and lack of toggle of the components are checked. A small amount of bone may have to be removed from the olecranon fossa to avoid extension block. No attempt should be made to obtain full extension at surgery unless it existed prior to operation.

If the prosthesis does not track well and dislocates in a rotatory manner, more valgus may have to be provided either by resection of more bone from the capitellum or use of a humeral stem with more valgus. The medial column may also be too tight; if this is the case more bone should be resected from the trochlea of the humerus. Proper soft tissue tension can be checked with the trial components in place and the elbow held in 90 degrees of flexion. The joint surfaces should not separate more than a few millimeters on attempted distraction in 90 degrees of flexion.

Several additional points with regard to technique require

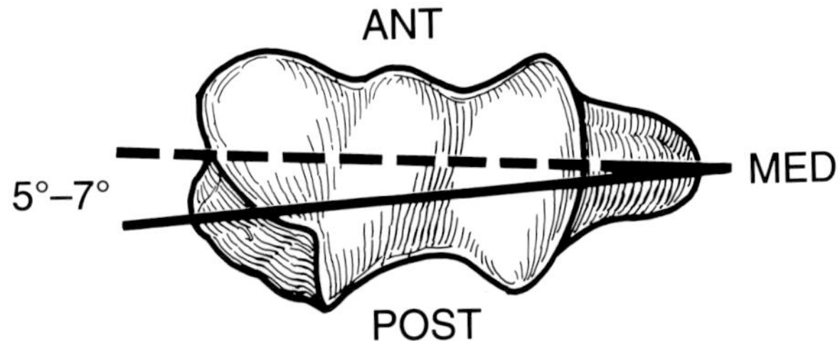

Fig. 47-13. Axial view of the distal humerus demonstrates the 5- to 7-degree internal rotation of the articulation in reference to the line connecting the midportion of the epicondyles. (Adapted from Morrey,[44] and by permission of Mayo Foundation.)

emphasis. It is important to line up the prosthesis with the anterior cortex of the humerus so as to ensure the normal amount of internal rotation. Extraarticular synovial tissue must be debrided from around the medial collateral ligament, where it is always present. If this is not done, the prosthetic fit may be too tight and result in subluxation. To prevent ulnar nerve problems, the elbow should be relocated frequently and the joint should not be translocated ulnarly.

The bone is cleaned with pulsatile lavage, and the medullary canals are blocked with bone removed from the humerus during insertion of the metal component. This added bone will help compress the cement into the bone interstices and restrict the cement to the area of the fixation stems. The bone is packed with dry sponges. Methacrylate is injected into the canals with a syringe and packed by digital pressure. The ulnar component is pressed into place first, followed by the humeral component, on which cement has been added to the under-surface of the trochlea and capitellum. The prostheses are tapped into place, the cement is cleared, and the elbow is held in firm extension to provide force across the joint to drive the methacrylate into bone. Excess cement is removed, and the elbow is dislocated to prevent the ulnar nerve from being burned by curing methacrylate. The ulnar nerve should be protected by a damp sponge. Excess cured cement is then removed. The wound is again irrigated, the tourniquet is deflated, and bleeding points are cauterized. Bleeding can be expected in the lateral extensor mass, branches of the recurrent interosseous artery distally, and the articular branch of the profunda brachii artery proximally.

Closure is in layers, beginning with deep capsular tissue with absorbable interrupted sutures. The next layer to be closed is the anconeus with its fascia to the extensor mass, which includes extensor tendon, lateral collateral ligaments, and extensor muscle fascia. Suction drainage is placed in the radial head space and led out subcutaneously. The muscle fascia, which is continuous with the triceps tendon and expansion, is closed.

Integrity of the deep repair is tested by elbow flexion, and the closure is completed. The subcutaneous tissue is closed, and interrupted nylon skin sutures are used.

A bulky dressing of abdominal pads, sheet wadding, and bias-cut stockinette is used, and a posterior Velcro-fastened splint is applied with the elbow flexed 70 degrees. The suction drain is removed the following day. Range of motion exercises are started 3 to 4 days after the operation, but immobilization may be continued longer if the soft tissue reconstruction is tenuous.

Complications in the Author's Series of Capitello-Condylar (Ewald) Total Elbow Arthroplasties

Eight of 20 Ewald total elbow arthroplasties (40 percent) suffered some type of complication. A total of 12 complications occurred in these eight patients (Table 47-3). There were three cases of postoperative ulnar neuropathy. All totally resolved, but one required anterior transposition of the ulnar nerve. A posterior interosseous neuropathy requiring surgical decompression developed in one patient 4 months following operation.

Skin sloughs developed in two patients. In one, lateral subluxation of the implant developed in the early postoperative period, possibly contributing to this complication. An abdominal pedicle flap was required to obtain skin coverage after two unsuccessful rotational skin flaps were performed. The other skin slough occurred in a patient whose postoperative course was complicated by acute renal failure, gram negative septicemia, and acute cholecystitis requiring a prolonged stay in the intensive care unit. The routine postoperative therapy program was delayed, and upon splint removal, an area of pressure necrosis was noted over the olecranon. Skin coverage was obtained with a rotational skin flap.

In one case, a dislocation with hemarthrosis was noted in the immediate postoperative period. This was treated successfully with open reduction and hematoma drainage, with no further problems in the ensuing 2 years. There have been two cases of implant subluxation. One resolved after 4 weeks of cast immobilization. The other patient is able to control the subluxation by avoiding external rotation of the shoulder, and she desires no further surgery.

Two triceps ruptures occurred, one in the previously mentioned patient with the skin slough. Initial triceps repair was unsuccessful, requiring a second repair with palmaris longus reinforcement (Fig. 47-15). In the other patient, a 70-year-old debilitated patient with rheumatoid arthritis, the triceps ruptured 8 years following total elbow arthroplasty while the patient was using her elbow to get out of a wheelchair. She desires no further surgical treatment.

A deep infection in one patient resulted in the lone clinical failure. This is the same patient who had acute renal failure and a skin slough. Six months after primary wound healing had been obtained, she developed sepsis of the greater trochanteric bursa and ankle. Deep sepsis of her total elbow arthroplasty ensued, presumably of hematogenous origin. This case required permanent removal of the prosthesis for salvage. The

Table 47-3. Complications in the Author's Series of 20 Capitello-Condylar Arthroplasties

Complications	No.
Ulnar neuropathy	3
Posterior interosseous neuropathy	1
Skin slough	2
Dislocation	1
Subluxation	2
Triceps rupture	2
Deep infection	1
Total	12[a]

[a]12 complications occurring in 8 TEA.

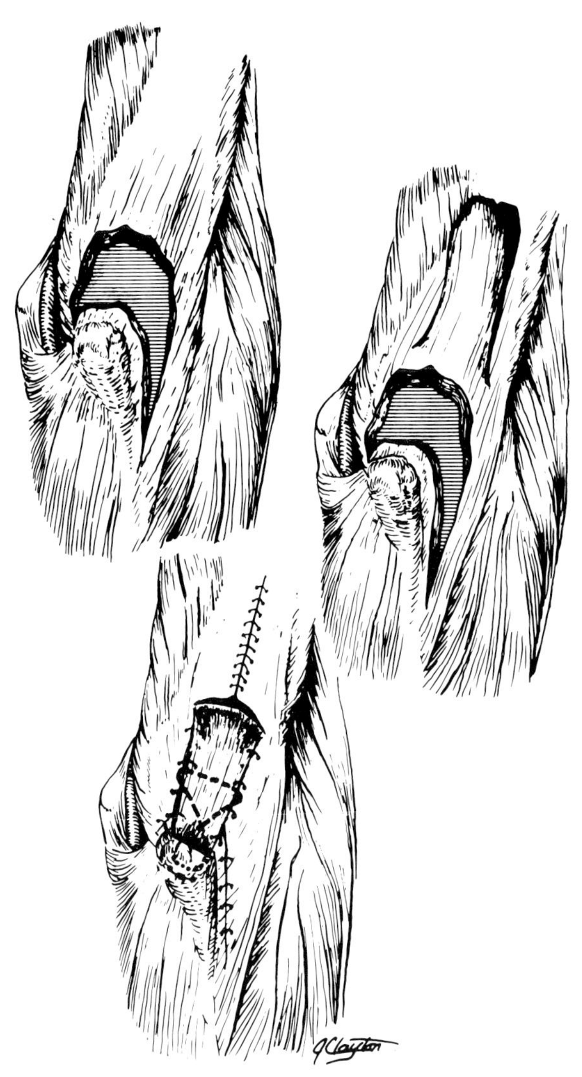

Fig. 47-15. Method of repair of a triceps tendon that has ruptured after total elbow arthroplasty. A tongue of triceps is turned down to bridge the defect.

patient died of sepsis several years after her prosthesis had been removed.

To treat the numerous complications discussed, eleven additional operations were required on five of the patients with total elbow arthroplasties.

Technique of the Hinged Elbow (Morrey-Coonrad) Semiconstrained Arthroplasty

The patient is placed on the table in the lateral decubitus position. A sterile arm tourniquet is used. Either the posteromedial Mayo approach or the lateral Kocher approach is used. If the lateral approach is chosen, the triceps is dissected off the olecranon with a thin layer of bone so that the entire triceps mechanism is kept intact and reflected medially. (Wolfe and Ranawat[70] suggested using an osteoanconeus flap for exposure.) The ulnar nerve is decompressed and gently retracted. The joint is opened either medially or on the lateral side. A synovectomy and joint debridement is carried out and the ulna is dislocated. The radial head is excised proximal to the annular ligament. One centimeter of the tip of the olecranon is excised. The midportion of the trochlea is removed to allow the medullary canal of the humerus to be identified. A power burr is used to locate and start the entrance to the medullary canal of the humerus through the olecranon fossa. The canal is then enlarged with a twist reamer and a rasp. The trochlea is removed using the cutting block or the trial prosthesis as a guide. Most of the hinged prosthesis, including the Coonrad, come in different sizes and different stem lengths. Preoperative study of the x-rays with the template overlays is helpful in determining proper size. The limiting factor usually is the size of the distal humerus or proximal ulna, not the size of the medullary canals. It is usually not necessary to have longer than a 4- to 6-inch humeral stem unless a revision is being done. Another reason to keep the stem lengths short in the rheumatoid patient is that a shoulder replacement may be needed in the future, and enough room must be left in the humerus to accomodate the stem of the humeral head prosthesis. Care needs to be taken so as not to fracture either supracondylar column, which can be quite thin after removal of the relatively large amount of bone that is necessary for fitting of the humeral component. If a fracture does occur, it should be fixed with K-wires or other internal fixation devices.

The trial component is inserted, and care should be taken to ensure that the axis of rotation is aligned to the normal axis of the humerus. This means that the hinge will probably be covered by the condyles unless there has been an excessive amount of erosion, bone has been previously resected, or there is an ununited fracture.

The ulna is then prepared with rasps, burrs, and reamers. The medullary canal of the ulna is located with a short Rush pin and is progressively enlarged with reamers. The surgeon must be aware that the shaft of the ulna is angled a few degrees lateral to the articulation to prevent penetration of the cortex (see Fig. 47-11E). The center of the ulnar prosthesis should lie midway between the proximal and distal borders of the sigmoid notch. Bone is removed from the sigmoid notch as needed to ensure appropriate seating of the component. It is desirable to have all the metallic beads on the surface of the prosthesis covered with bone.

If the Morrey-modified-Coonrad implant is used, a bone graft from the resected trochlea is shaped to fit beneath the anterior flange.

A trial reduction is then carried out. It may be necessary to remove more bone from the olecranon tip to gain more extension or from the coronoid to obtain more flexion. When the motion and alignment are satisfactory, bone plugs made from the resected bone are inserted in the medullary canals so that cement does not go more than 1 cm beyond the ends of the prosthesis. The canals are cleaned with pulsatile lavage and dried thoroughly with a sponge.

The components are assembled, cement is injected into the canals and the prosthesis inserted. If desired, the components may be cemented separately; if this is done, the ulnar component must be cemented in first because if the humerus is inserted first it will not be possible to correct the two halves. The excess cement is removed, taking care to cover with cement any beads that are not already covered with bone. The cement is left to harden and the area inspected for excess cement. Range of motion is checked.

The tourniquet is deflated. Hemostasis is established. A suction drain is placed. The capsule and ligaments are reapproximated, but ligamentous stability is not necessary, as this is provided by the joint itself. The triceps mechanism is replaced and sutured to the medial fascia and to bone through drill holes if necessary. The ulnar nerve is transposed anteriorly in the subcutaneous layer. The wound is closed. A bulky dressing is applied with the elbow in 70 degrees of flexion.

Postoperatively, protected motion may be started after the third to fifth day. However, leaving the elbow splinted for 2 or 3 weeks will not interfere with the final motion obtained and may be necessary if the triceps has been disrupted or if there is some question about wound healing.

Concomitant Shoulder Joint Replacement

What of the patient that is in need of a shoulder replacement in the same extremity as the elbow? Friedman and Ewald[23] found no contraindication to operating on one joint when the other had a fixed deformity. The results of an arthroplasty of either the shoulder or the elbow with respect to motion, pain, and function were not found to be compromised when the two arthroplasties were performed in the same extremity. When both the shoulder and the elbow are involved, the joint that causes the most pain and disability should be operated on first. If both joints appear to be equally involved, they recommended that the elbow be operated on first, as this results in greater functional improvement and allows a longer interval between arthroplasties. I believe, however, that the shoulder should be done first if both joints are equally involved because there are fewer serious complications with a shoulder replacement. Also, we have found that after a shoulder has become pain-free following an arthroplasty, the affected elbow can be protected enough so that the patient may not feel the need for an elbow arthroplasty.

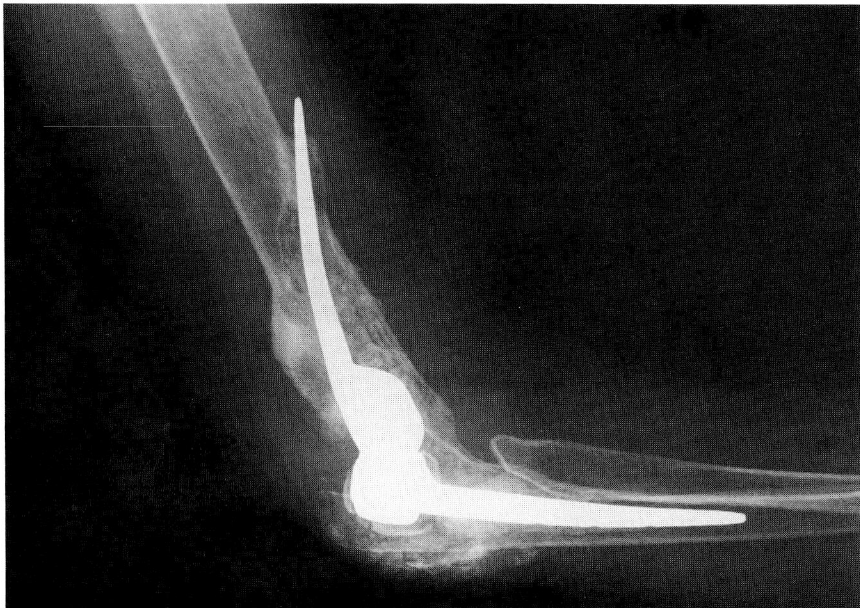

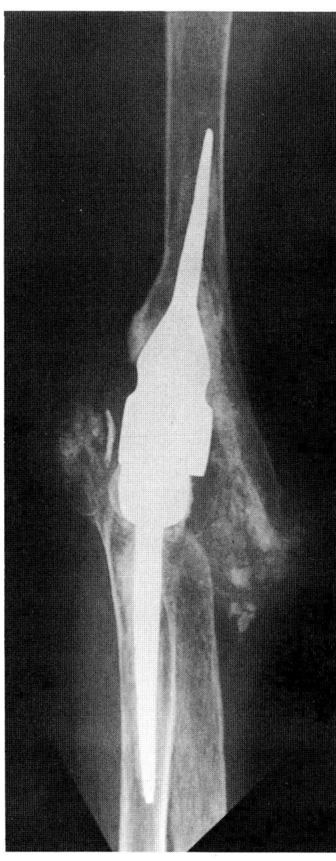

A B

Fig. 47-16. **(A&B)** Thirteen years post-GSB arthroplasty showing aseptic loosening, erosion, and marked bone destruction. *(Figure continues.)*

Salvage of the Failed Elbow Arthroplasty

Of all major total joint replacements, the elbow has shown the highest complication rate. In the case of infection, Morrey and Bryan[42] found that a resection arthroplasty was necessary in 10 of 14 elbows in order to control the infection. In one, the elbow was salvaged by early debridement. In two, a new implant was reinserted after removal of the first prosthesis and control of infection. The last patient had had a paretic upper extremity following a cerebral vascular accident and her extremity was amputated. In case of failure, a reasonable back-up plan for salvage must be available.[13,29,41]

In the case of aseptic failure of a stemmed prosthesis with good bone stock, the old prosthesis can be removed and a new one reimplanted. In the case where there is severe bone loss, a two-stage procedure may be necessary: bone graft followed 6 months later by insertion of a new prosthesis.

In a more recent report[43] the same authors reported 33 revisions. Of these, 22 were in rheumatoid patients. Three of the revised elbows became infected—two of these in rheumatoid elbows. Only 13 of these 33 elbows were not associated with at least one complication. Twelve complications occurred in 10 patients who had rheumatoid arthritis. The selection of the implant chosen for revision in the earlier cases depended on whether or not any components were solid and could be left in place. Since 1981 the Coonrad-Morrey device has been used exclusively, and some of the revisions using this device failed. Eight (23 percent) of the revised components became loose in seven of 30 elbows that had not become infected.

Figgie et al[21] reported on 10 elbow arthroplasties that failed. Six of these were for dislocation following failure of the bearing mechanism. In each case, the humeral and/or ulnar center of rotation had been malaligned. An additional four elbows were revised for component loosening and one for malalignment. Two of these failed, one because of sepsis.

In the case where it is unwise or impossible to reinsert a prosthesis, resection arthroplasty is usually performed. In doing this the following points are useful in obtaining stability: (1) transfer the flexor and extensor muscles proximally; (2) insert a triceps flap between the bone ends; (3) advance the distal triceps; and (4) notch the bone to enhance stability if enough bone stock remains. An arthrodesis may be indicated, but it is very difficult because of lack of bone stock. Lastly, an allograft may be considered.

Urbaniak[61] presented 10 cases of allografts of the elbow, although none were done in rheumatoid patients. Complications included nonunion or delayed union in two patients,

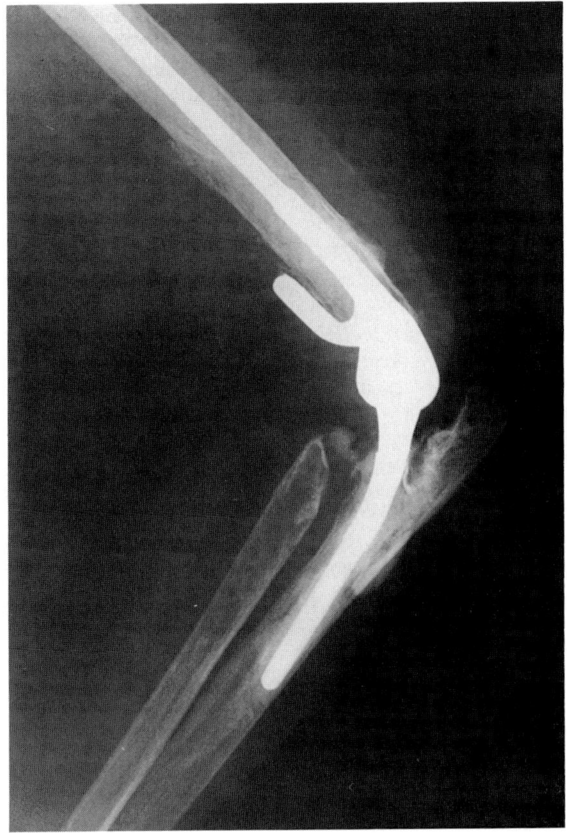

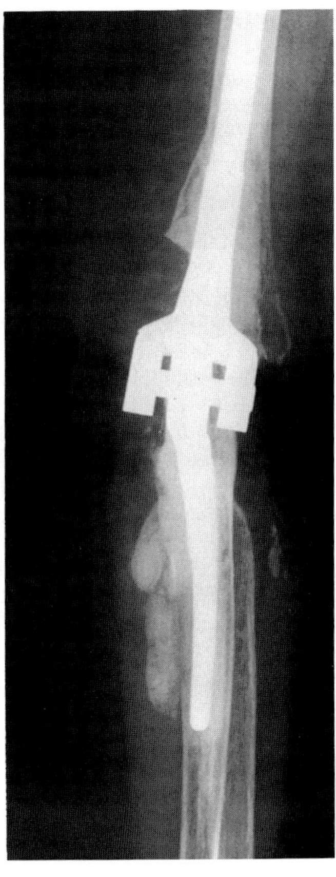

Fig. 47-16 *(Continued).* **(C&D)** Revision with a Morrey-Coonrad elbow.

joint instability in two, and radial palsy and graft resorption in one each. Significant joint deterioration was noted at 2 years. His indications for this procedure are patients who are too young or who have insufficient bone stock for conventional implant arthroplasty, or those who refuse elbow arthrodesis.

Failure of an unstemmed prosthesis is easier to reconstruct. This can be achieved by tissue interpositional arthroplasty, insertion of a stemmed prosthesis, or fusion.

Revision for aseptic loosening or dislocation is best handled by removing the components and inserting one of the constrained prostheses. (Fig. 47-16) The Morrey-modified-Coonrad has been useful in these cases. Reconstruction of the soft tissue restraints for dislocation has not been reliable. Dislocation or subluxation is apt to be due to malalignment, and regardless of the type of prosthesis used for revision, the axis of motion needs to be corrected.

There have been many complications and failures with total elbow replacement, and there will be more as time passes. Future design modifications may be useful; smaller components that save bone stock may be helpful so that in case of failure, stability can be maintained. Alternatives to cement fixation may also be useful. The goal should be a biological implant, such as an allograft, but the ultimate goal, of course, is eradication of the disease itself.

REFERENCES

1. Anderson LD, Heppenstall M: Synovectomy of the elbow and excision of the radial head in rheumatoid arthritis. In Cruess RL, Mitchel NS (eds): Surgery of Rheumatoid Arthritis. JB Lippincott, Philadelphia, 1971
2. Brumfield RH Jr, Volz RG, Green JF: Total elbow arthroplasty: A clinical review of 30 cases employing the Mayo and AHSC prostheses. Clin Orthop 158:137–141, 1981
3. Brumfield RH, Resnick CT: Synovectomy of the elbow in rheumatoid arthritis. J Bone Joint Surg 67A:16–20, 1985
4. Bryan RS, Morrey BF: Extensive posterior exposure of the elbow: A triceps-sparing approach. Clin Orthop 166:188–192, 1982
5. Bryan RS, Morrey BF: Rheumatoid arthritis of the elbow. In Evarts CMc (ed): Surgery of the Musculoskeletal System. Vol. 2, Section 3, Churchill Livingstone, New York, 1983
6. Cofield RH, Morrey EF, Bryan RS: Total shoulder and total elbow arthroplasties: The current state of development. Part 2. JCE Orthop 7(1):17, 1979
7. Cooney WP III, Bryan RS: Rheumatoid arthritis in the upper extremity. Treatment of the elbow and shoulder joints. pp. 247–262, AAOS Instructional Course Lectures. Vol. 28. CV Mosby, St Louis, 1979
8. Coonrad RP: Results with the Coonrad total elbow arthroplasty. Presented to the Piedmont Orthopaedic Society. Boca Raton, May 1980

9. Coonrad RP: Infection in total elbow arthroplasties. American Soc for Surg of the Hand Correspondence Letter, April 1, 1981
10. Copeland SA, Taylor JG: Synovectomy of the elbow in rheumatoid arthritis. The place of excision of the head of the radius. J Bone Joint Surg 61B:69–73, 1979
11. Davis RF, Weiland AJ, Hungerford DS, Moore JR, Volenec-Dowling S. Non-constrained total elbow replacement. Orthop Trans 6:341–342, 1982
12. Dee R: Total replacement of the elbow joint. Orthop Clin North Am 4:415–433, 1973
13. Dee R: Reconstructive surgery following total elbow endoprosthesis. Clin Orthop 170:196–201, 1982
14. Dennis DA, Clayton ML, Ferlic DC, Stringer EA, Bramlett KW: Capitello-condylar total elbow arthroplasty for rheumatoid arthritis. J Arthroplasty (suppl)5:S83–S88, 1990
15. Eichenblat M, Hass A, Kessler I: Synovectomy of the elbow in rheumatoid arthritis. J Bone Joint Surg 64A:1074–1078, 1982
16. Ewald FC, Scheinberg RD, Poss R, Thomas WH, Scott RD, Sledge CB: Capitello condylar total elbow arthroplasty. J Bone Joint Surg 62A:1259–1263, 1980
17. Ewald FC: Reconstructive surgery and rehabilitation of the elbow. pp. 1921–1943. In Kelley WN, Harris ED, Ruddy S, Sledge CB (eds): Textbook of Rheumatology. WB Saunders, Philadelphia, 1981
18. Ewald FC, Jacobs MA: Total elbow arthroplasty. Clin Orthop 182:137–142, 1984
19. Ferlic DC, Patchett CE, Clayton ML: Elbow synovectomy in rheumatoid arthritis. Long term results. Clin Orthop 220:119–125, 1987
20. Figgie HE III: Current concepts in total elbow arthroplasty. AAOS Summer Institute, Chicago, IL, Sept 1989
21. Figgie HE III, Inglis AE, Ranawat CS, Rosenberg GM: Results of total elbow arthroplasty as a salvage procedure for failed elbow reconstructive operations. Clin Orthop 219:185–193, 1987
22. Figgie MP, Inglis AE, Mow CS, Figgie HE III: Total elbow arthroplasty for complete ankylosis of the elbow. J Bone Joint Surg 71A:513–520, 1989
23. Friedman RJ, Ewald FC: Arthroplasty of the ipsilateral shoulder and elbow in patients who have rheumatoid arthritis. J Bone Joint Surg 69A:661–666, 1987
24. Goldberg VM, Figgie HE III, Inglis AE, and Figgie MP: Current concepts review. Total elbow arthroplasty. J Bone Joint Surg 70A:778–783, 1988
25. Gschwend N, Loehr J, Ivosevic-Radovanovic D, Scheier H, Munzinger U: Semiconstrained elbow prostheses with special reference to the GSB III prosthesis. Clin Orthop 232:104–111, 1988
26. Hurri L, Pulkki T, Vainio K: Arthroplasty of the elbow in rheumatoid arthritis. Acta Chir Scand 127:459, 1964
27. Inglis AE, Ranawat CS, Straub LR: Synovectomy and debridement of the elbow in rheumatoid arthritis. J Bone Joint Surg 53A:652–662, 1971
28. Inglis AE, Pellicci PM: Total elbow replacement. J Bone Joint Surg 62A:1252–1258, 1980
29. Inglis AE: Revision surgery following a failed total elbow arthroplasty. Clin Orthop 170:213–218, 1982
30. Knight RA, Van Zandt IL: Arthroplasty of the elbow: An end result study. J Bone Joint Surg 34A:610–618, 1952
31. Kudo H, Iwano K: Total elbow arthroplasty with a nonconstrained surface replacement prosthesis in patients who have rheumatoid arthritis. A long-term follow-up study. J Bone Joint Surg 72A:355–362, 1990
32. Kudo H, Iwano K, Watanabe S: Total replacement of the rheumatoid elbow with a hingeless prosthesis. J Bone Joint Surg 62A:277–285, 1980
33. Laine V, Vainio K: The elbow in rheumatoid arthritis. p. 112. In Hijmans WDP, Herschel H (eds): Early Synovectomy in Rheumatoid Arthritis. Proceedings of the Symposium on Early Synovectomy in Rheumatoid Arthritis, Amsterdam, April 12–15, 1967. Excerpta Medica Foundation, Amsterdam, 1969
34. Lanyi V, Preston R, McEwen C: Synovectomy in rheumatoid arthritis. NY State J Med 68:3135–3137, 1968
35. Linscheid RL: Surgery for rheumatoid arthritis—Timing and techniques. The upper extremity. J Bone Joint Surg 50A:605–613, 1968
36. London JT, Brumfield RH, Ferlic DC, Morrey BF, Volz RG: Symposium: Total elbow arthroplasty. Contemp Orthop 3:541, 1981
37. MacKay I, Fitzgerald B, Miller JH: Silastic radial head prosthesis in rheumatoid arthritis. Acta Orthop Scand 53:63–66, 1982
38. Marmar L: Surgery of the rheumatoid elbow. Follow up study on synovectomy combined with radial head excision. J Bone Joint Surg 54A:573–578, 1972
39. Millender LH, Nalebuff EA, Holdsworth DE: Posterior interosseous-nerve syndrome secondary to rheumatoid synovitis. J Bone Joint Surg 55A:753–757, 1973
40. Moore JR, Weiland AJ: Bilateral attritional rupture of the ulnar nerve at the elbow. J Hand Surg 5:358–360, 1980
41. Morrey BF, Bryan RS: Complications of total elbow arthroplasty. Clin Orthop 170:204–212, 1982
42. Morrey BF, Bryan RS: Infection after total elbow arthroplasty. J Bone Joint Surg 65A:330–338, 1983
43. Morrey BF, Bryan RS: Revision total elbow arthroplasty. J Bone Joint Surg, 69A:523–532, 1987
44. Morrey BF: The Elbow and Its Disorders. WB Saunders, Philadelphia, 1985
45. Patchett C, Ferlic DC, Clayton ML: Elbow synovectomy in rheumatoid arthritis. Long-term results. Arth Rheum 28(4)Suppl:S37, 1985
46. Peterson LFA, Janes JM: Surgery of the rheumatoid elbow. Orthop Clin North Am 2(3):667–677, 1971
47. Porter BB, Richardson C, Vainio K: Rheumatoid arthritis of the elbow. The results of synovectomy. J Bone Joint Surg 56B:427–437, 1974
48. Pritchard RW: Anatomic surface elbow arthroplasty. A preliminary report. Clin Orthop 179:223–230, 1983
49. Pritchard RW: Personal experience using a three piece surface elbow replacement. AAOS Summer Institute, Course Syllabus, Chicago, IL, Sept 1989
50. Rosenberg GM, Turner RH: Nonconstrained total elbow arthroplasty. Clin Orthop 187:154–162, 1984
51. Rymaszewski LA, Mackay I, Amis AA, Miller JH: Long-term effects of excision of the radial head in rheumatoid arthritis. J Bone Joint Surg 66B:109–113, 1984
52. Schuller M: Chirurgische mittheilungen uber die chronisch. Rheumatishen gelerkentzundungen. Arch Klin Chir 45:153, 1893
53. Simmons ED, Sullivan JA, Ewald FC: Long-term review of the capitello-condylar total elbow replacement. Orthop Trans 14:256, 1990
54. Souter WA: Arthroplasty of the elbow, with particular reference to metallic hinge arthroplasty in rheumatoid patients. Orthop Clin North Am 4:395–413, 1973
55. Smith-Petersen MN, Aufranc OE, Larson CB: Useful surgical procedures for rheumatoid arthritis involving joints of the upper extremity. Arch Surg 46:764–770, 1943
56. Straub LR: Surgical rehabilitation of the hand and upper extremity in rheumatoid arthritis. Bull Rheum Dis 12:265–268, 1962 1962
57. Street DM, Stevens PS: A humeral replacement prosthesis for the elbow. Results in ten elbows. J Bone Joint Surg 56A:1147–1158, 1974

58. Swanson AB: Flexible Implant Resection Arthroplasty in the Hand and Extremity. p. 275. CV Mosby, St Louis, 1973
59. Torgerson WR, Leach RE: Synovectomy of the elbow in rheumatoid arthritis. A report of five cases. J Bone Joint Surg 52A:371–375, 1970
60. Trancik T, Wilde AH, and Borden LS: Capitello-condylar total elbow arthroplasty. Two- to eight-year experience. Clin Orthop 223:175–180, 1987
61. Urbaniak JR, Black KE, Sehayik R: Cadaveric elbow allografts—Six years experience. Orthop Trans 8:488, 1984
62. Vainio K: Surgery of rheumatoid arthritis. Surg Ann 6:309–335, 1974
63. Volz RE: Total elbow arthroplasty, current states. Presented to the Annual Meeting of the American Shoulder and Elbow Surgeons, Las Vegas, January 1985
64. Wadsworth TG: The Elbow. Churchill Livingstone, New York, 1982
65. Walker PS: Human Joints and Their Artificial Replacements. pp. 190–195. Charles C Thomas, Springfield, IL, 1978
66. Weiland AJ, Weiss A-PC, Wills RP, and Moore JR: Capitello condylar total elbow replacement. A long-term follow-up study. J Bone Joint Surg 71A:217–222, 1989
67. Wilkinson MC, Lowry JH: Synovectomy for rheumatoid arthritis. J Bone Joint Surg 47B:482–488, 1965
68. Wilson DW: Synovectomy of the elbow for rheumatoid arthritis. Proc Roy Soc Med 64(1):264–266, 1971
69. Wilson DW, Arden GP, Ansell BM: Synovectomy of the elbow in rheumatoid arthritis. J Bone Joint Surg 55B:106–111, 1973
70. Wolfe SW, Ranawat CS: The osteo-anconeous flap. An approach for total elbow arthroplasty. J Bone Joint Surg 72A:684–688, 1990

48

Skin Grafts

Earl Z. Browne, Jr.

Skin, the largest organ of the body, serves a vital function in many ways. It not only functions as a semipermeable membrane and a barrier to undesirable substances, but also contributes to homeostasis through temperature regulation and sensibility. This latter function—perception of stimuli—is most important in the hand, especially in the palmar half.

All skin is composed of a thick layer of dermis covered by epidermis. The epidermis comprises only about 5 percent of the thickness of the skin, and thickness varies considerably.[5,73] The quality of skin depends to a great extent on the epidermal appendages contained in the dermis, which also vary a great deal from area to area. This is especially true for the skin of the palmar and plantar areas, which contains no hair or sebaceous glands but is the almost exclusive domain of Meissner's and Vater-Pacini sensory end organs.[50] It is reasonable to think of the epidermis as the barrier and the dermis as the functional portion of the skin.

One must also consider the hand as an organ and think of the skin as an envelope enclosing a multitude of tendons, nerves, vessels, bones, and joints. In order for the hand to function properly, this skin envelope must be elastic and nonadherent, contain as many of the appropriate appendages as possible, and be large enough to allow freedom of motion. The palm skin must also be thick enough to withstand pressure and friction caused by grasp and pinch.

When considering the replacement of hand skin, as is done in skin grafting, one must keep these principles in mind. It is convenient to divide the hand into dorsal and volar surfaces, each having different basic requisites. Dorsal skin must be thinner, more elastic, loose enough to not restrict flexion, and serve as a barrier to cover tendons and joints. Volar skin must be thicker and tougher, while still being loose and elastic enough to allow motion, but above all, it must retain its function of sensibility. It is usually possible to replace dorsal skin by grafting; this is often not possible with volar skin.

HISTOLOGY OF SKIN

Figures 48-1 and 48-2 depict the major differences between dorsal and palmar hand skin. Common to both is the irregularity of the border between the basal layer of the epidermis and the dermis, forming the dermal papillae and the epidermal rete ridges. Both also contain intraepidermal nerve endings terminating in Merkel's cell neurite complexes and sweat ducts extending out from glands located in the base of the dermis and subcutaneous fat.[58] Although not shown in Figures 48-1 and 48-2, a network of blood vessels and sensory and autonomic nerve fibers in the dermis is shared by all skin.

Figure 48-1 represents dorsal hand skin, which is similar to skin found anywhere else on the body. The basal layer of the epidermis is continuous with the hair sheath and sebaceous glands. Hair follicles lie at different depths and are surrounded by a network of fine nerve endings.

Figure 48-2 depicts the palmar hand skin. The papillae and ridges are deeper and the keratin layer is considerably thicker than those of the dorsal hand skin. Most significant, however, are the absence of the pilosebaceous structures and the presence of the specialized encapsulated nerve endings. Meissner's corpuscles are present in dermal papillae, and Vater-Pacini corpuscles are present in the deep dermis. These latter structures are also found along nerve trunks, joints, and other areas, but exist in the skin almost exclusively in digits and genital areas.

SUBSTITUTION BY SKIN GRAFTS

Since it is similar to the skin of most areas, dorsal hand skin can be adequately replaced by skin grafts. When a split-thickness graft is removed, healing of the donor area occurs by epithelialization from hair follicles and very little dermal re-

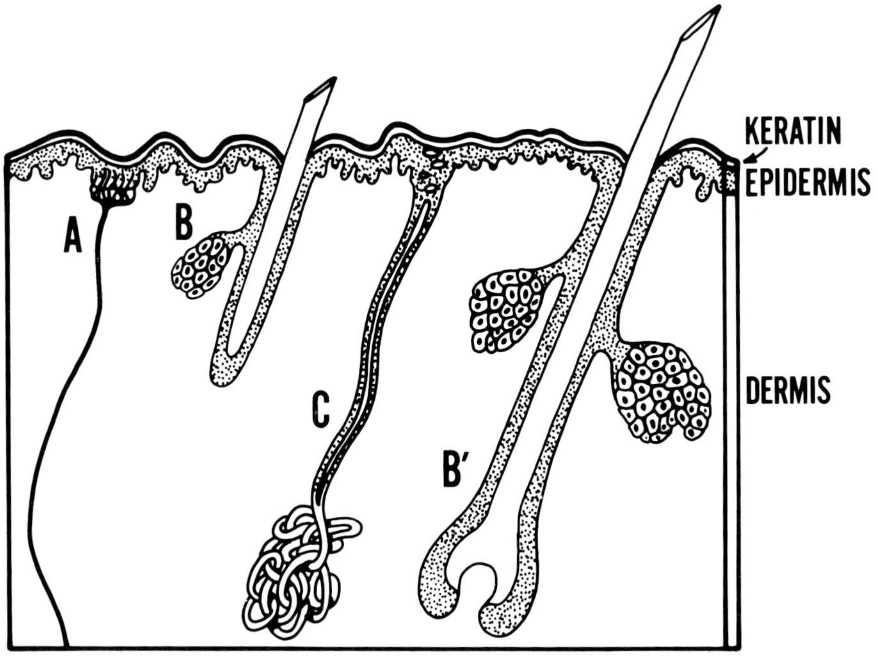

Fig. 48-1. Dorsal hand skin is similar to skin of the rest of the body, having hair and sebaceous glands. **(A)** Merkel's cell neurite complex; **(B)** hair follicle and sebaceous apparatus; **(B′)** sweat gland.

generation occurs. The deeper the graft, the better the quality of the skin, but the less there is left behind at the donor site to heal.[6,69] Also, a deeper graft increases the chance of reinnervation of Merkel's complexes and restoration of sensibility in the recipient site.[2,33]

No matter how thick the graft is, however, palmar skin cannot be fully substituted by ordinary grafts, since there will be an absence of the special dermal neural mechanoreceptors. Only glabrous skin will provide these, and there is unfortunately not much available for grafting.[55] Thick grafts will transfer hair follicles, however, resulting in unwanted hair growth on palmar surfaces.[75] In addition to poor return of sensibility, grafts

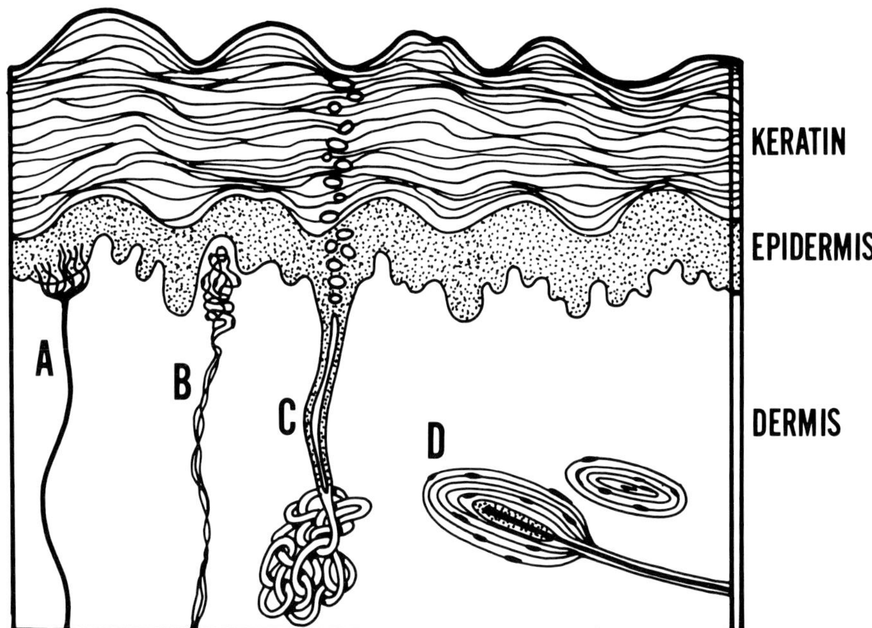

Fig. 48-2. Palmar hand skin. There are no pilosebaceous structures present. Meissner's and Pacinian corpuscles exist almost exclusively here. **(A)** Merkel's cell neurite complex; **(B)** Meissner's corpuscle; **(C)** sweat gland; **(D)** Vater-Pacini corpuscle.

on palmar areas do not provide the padding of subcutaneous tissue often necessary to cover tendons and nerves. In general, palmar grafts should be considered a compromise, and are usually only indicated in release of flexion contractures in areas not requiring critical sensibility.

RESPONSE TO INJURY

Any injury that results in the loss of a full-thickness segment of skin initiates the process of wound contraction.[1,3,28,61] Although beneficial in helping to minimize defects in other parts of the body, this process of gradual shrinking in of the wound edges can be disastrous in hand wounds (Fig. 48-3). It appears that fibroblasts migrate into the base of the wound and differentiate into so-called myofibroblasts.[36,61] These cells appear to have the ability to contract, and the network of these cells and collagen fibers that forms in the base of the wound is responsible for pulling the wound edges together.[35,54] It has been shown that contraction can be temporarily halted by treatment of the wound with smooth muscle relaxants.[59] This process is not altered by epithelialization and appears to continue unchecked until the tension in the wound equals the tension in the stretched skin.[7,67] Once the contraction process has begun, it is not altered to any extent by split-thickness skin grafting.[27,32,68]

In a series of experiments by Stone and Madden, wounds in animals were treated with immediate grafting, delayed grafting, and immediate and delayed grafting with splinting.[74] They concluded that immediate grafting with split-thickness skin did not significantly affect wound contraction. However, immediate grafting and splinting with a compressive dressing for 7 days did significantly inhibit wound contraction. On the other hand, delayed grafting had no effect on wound contraction, no matter what adjunct therapy was used. Splinting, although effective with immediate grafting, was ineffective in preventing contraction when used with the delayed grafts.

It is generally believed that the condition of the wound is the main determinant in the result of skin grafting.[25] Even full-thickness skin grafts can be found to contract if wound contraction has already begun.[4,32,68] Rudolph has found that application of split-thickness skin does not seem to have as much effect on the differentiation of the fibroblasts into the myofibroblast as a full-thickness graft.[66] He has shown in animal experiments that wounds mature much more rapidly after application of full-thickness grafts than split-thickness.

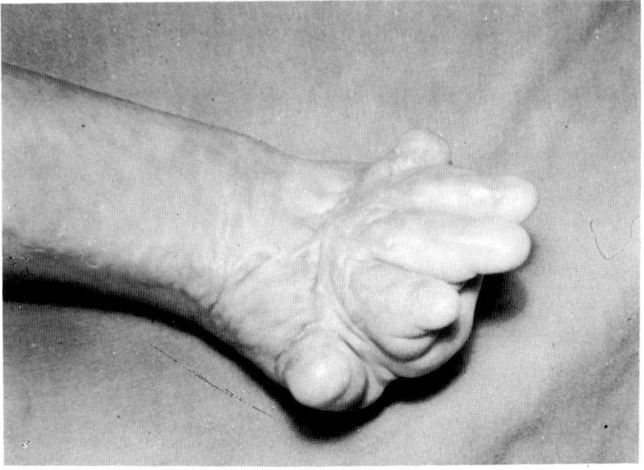

Fig. 48-3. End result of uninhibited wound contraction of the dorsum of the hand.

EFFECT OF INFECTION ON WOUND HEALING

A great deal of bacteria is normally present in skin. It has been estimated that about one thousand (10^3) organisms per gram of tissue are normally present in hair follicles and crevices and recesses of the skin. This number of organisms does not seem to be significant in affecting wound healing.[48] However, when contamination of the wound takes place, much higher levels are present. Surface bacteria, which can be easily removed, do not appear to be important in skin grafting if the wound is carefully prepared prior to operation. On the other hand, penetration of the bed of the wound is of great significance.[51] It has been established that 10^5 organisms per gram of tissue is a fairly critical level of contamination.[43] Wounds that contain fewer organisms than this do not commonly become infected. In a series of skin grafts applied to contaminated wounds, Krizek, Robson, and Kho have shown that no matter what technique was used to prepare the bed of the wound for grafting, a bacterial count of greater than 10^5 organisms resulted in a successful skin graft take of only 19 percent.[48] If the count was fewer than 10^5, however, there was a 94 percent successful take.

VASCULARITY OF THE WOUND

After application of a skin graft to the wound, the graft first survives in a precarious fashion, apparently nourished by transudate from the wound. This has been referred to as "plasmatic circulation."[24] It is imperative that the graft become vascularized for ultimate survival, however, and anything that acts as a barrier to this process will cause loss of the graft.[8,19,20] The most potent of all barriers is blood, and hematoma will kill a graft even in the absence of infection.[26]

The actual process of vascularization is not altogether clear, but it is certain that this process must begin within a few days if the graft is to survive.[10-12] Whether or not coaptation of the cut vessels in the graft to the vessels in their recipient bed (the process of inosculation) occurs to any extent is disputed.[23] It appears that the more important process is the ingrowth of capillary buds into the skin graft from the edges of the wound and, more importantly, from the bed of the wound.[8,21,22] For this process to take place, there must be a vascularized bed containing the necessary fine network of capillaries from which budding will take place. Grafts will not take on denuded bone or tendon, and they are not satisfactory coverage for vital structures.

TIMING OF GRAFTING

From the previous discussion, it is obvious that grafting the wound as soon as it is clean enough and after the fine network of vessels has been established is ideal (Fig. 48-4). In this way, contamination of the wound and establishment of a large milieu of myofibroblasts are avoided. In general, immediate debridement and grafting are often possible, and no more than 2 or 3 days should be allowed to pass for the purpose of establishment of a good bed. The principle of allowing a healthy bed of granulation to develop is no longer considered correct, and it should be replaced with the concept of early grafting (Fig. 48-5).

Bacterial Content Determination

If it appears that the wound may be infected, then determination of the bacterial content is necessary. Rather than rely on a wound swab to determine the presence of bacteria, which may yield a false positive, it is important to know whether or not the bed of the wound has become colonized with pathogenic bacteria. A useful method of determining this is by performing a wound biopsy. In order to do this, the surface of the wound is cleaned to prevent contamination, and a segment of tissue weighing about 1 g is removed. This can be done conveniently with a punch biopsy. A colony count culture can be obtained from the biopsy material, or a more rapid determination can be made by crushing the tissue and examining it mi-

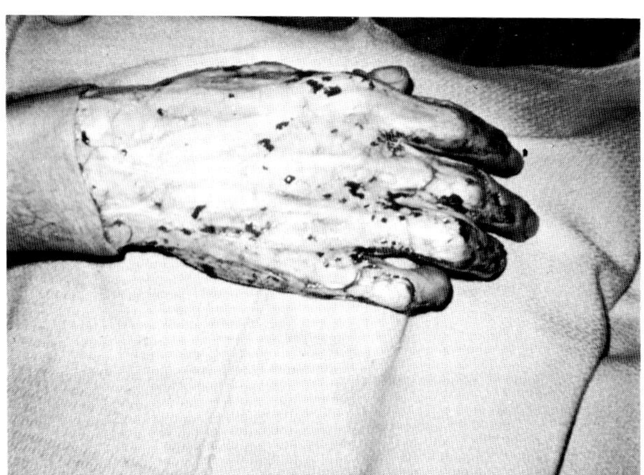

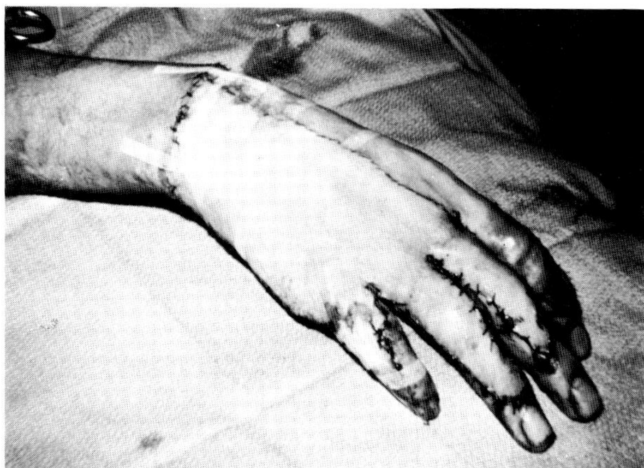

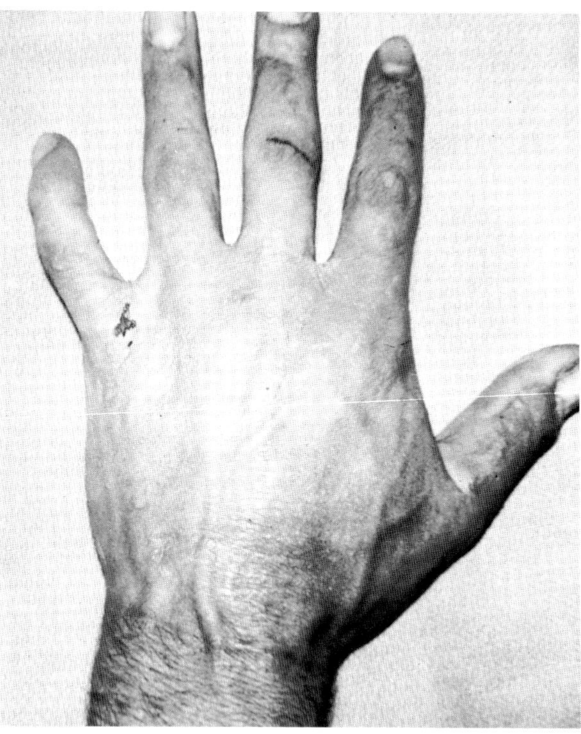

Fig. 48-4. Expected result of immediate grafting and splinting in resurfacing a hypertrophic burn scar of the dorsum of the hand.

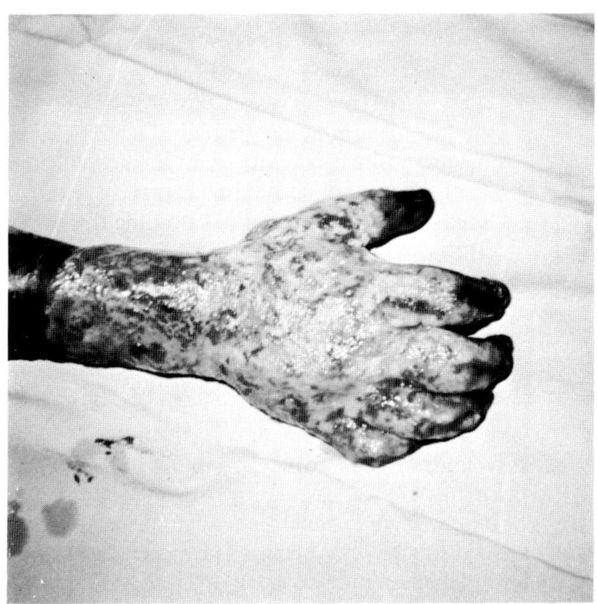

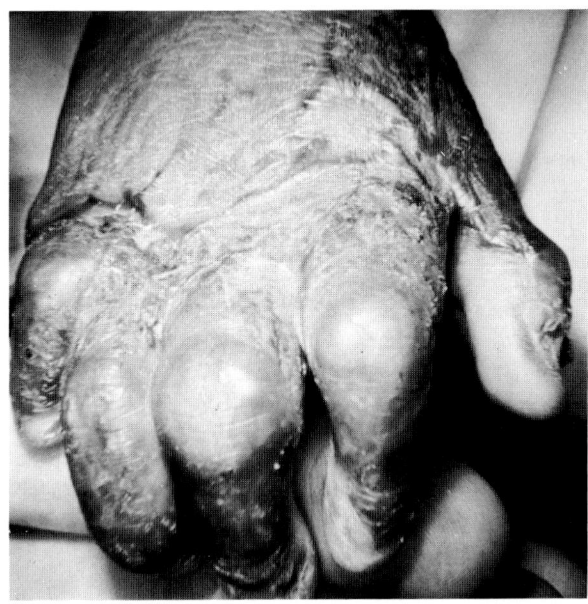

Fig. 48-5. Expected result of grafting a bed of exuberant "granulation tissue." In reality, this is a chronically infected mass of fibrotic tissue. Poor take of the graft occurs, and wound contraction progresses to contracture, as in this patient.

croscopically. It has been said that a bacterial presence greater than 1 per high power field roughly corresponds to a critical level of 10^5 organisms.[48]

Temporary Storage of Skin Grafts

There are times when the wound may not seem to be ideal to receive a graft, because of either infection, bleeding, or poor vascularity. It is often convenient to remove skin from the donor site at the time of operation for wound preparation, in order to avoid another anesthetic and operation. In this way, the skin can be stored while the wound is being prepared by soaks or periodic bedside debridement to reach an ideal state.

There are very convenient methods for storing such skin grafts if they are removed. One is simply to replace the skin on the donor site from which it was removed. The graft will begin to take, and will remain well-nourished and viable. If this technique is used, it is necessary to remove the graft before significant tensile strength has occurred. This may be done by injecting a saline and local anesthetic solution between the graft and the donor site, and the graft can be placed on the recipient site at the bedside.[77]

Another technique is to store the skin graft in tissue culture medium during this interval. The common practice is to wrap the skin graft in a saline-soaked sponge and store it in the refrigerator. This is effective for a few days, but seldom can the graft remain viable more than a week. It has been shown that by storing the graft in tissue culture medium with various additives the viability of the graft can be markedly prolonged. Hurst et al[45] have demonstrated that the use of McCoy's 5-A medium containing amino acids and vitamins can allow skin grafts to be stored successfully for up to 30 days.[50] The method of preparing the medium and storage of the grafts is described in detail in their article. It has been my experience that this is an excellent method for 10 days to 2 weeks, but after that time the quality of the skin does not seem to be as good as the quality of a freshly harvested graft.

TYPES OF GRAFTS

Although it is true that full-thickness grafts afford better protection, hold up better, establish better sensibility, contain more epidermal appendages, and contract less than split-thickness grafts, thick grafts are not always desirable. There are several disadvantages to thick grafts.

Full-thickness grafts do not take as readily as split grafts. It is generally accepted that this is due to the greater distance through which the capillary buds must migrate to reach the cellular layer of the skin, thus affecting survival.[19-21] The full-thickness graft requires a much better bed on which to be placed, and the graft is much more prone to infection.

In addition, the availability of skin must be considered. It is not always possible to sacrifice enough skin to afford the luxury of full-thickness grafting, and split-thickness grafts must often be substituted. In general, full-thickness grafts should only be used in situations where the quality of the skin and the tendency to less contracture are crucial. As a rule, these conditions are only necessary on palmar skin grafts, and the greater level of return of sensibility is an added bonus under these circumstances. Dorsal wounds can generally be treated very adequately with intermediate split-thickness grafts.

Skin Thickness

When determining the thickness of a graft to be removed, the skin thickness of the donor area must be considered. Epidermis and dermis vary according to age and sex, as well as location.[5] It is said that the epidermis ranges from 20 to 1400 μ in thickness, and the dermis from 400 to 2500 μ.[73] When considering donor sites, however, there is only a practical range of 25 to 80 μ of epidermis, and 500 to 1800 μ of dermis. In relation to dermatome settings, these values translate to 0.001 to 0.003 inch of epidermis and 0.020 to 0.070 inch of dermis.

In donor areas, in general, the epidermis is quite thin in infants and reaches a maximum thickness at puberty, becoming thinner with age until it becomes almost as thin in old age as it was during childhood. There is very little difference in epidermis thickness between sexes. The dermis, however, remains relatively thin in youth, reaching its maximum thickness at about the fourth decade, then subsequently becoming thin again in old age. There is a marked difference between sexes, with male dermis being significantly thicker than that of female.

The skin of the trunk and dorsal and lateral surfaces of the extremities are the thickest areas. Skin thickness may range from 0.020 to 0.025 inch in a small child to 0.100 inch on the anterior abdomen of an adult male. In general, most donor sites cannot be expected to be much thicker than about 0.060 inch in a male and about 0.040 inch in a female.

Split-Thickness Grafting

Historical Perspective

There are several names commonly associated with skin grafts.[65] Although Reverdin was not the first to successfully perform grafting, in 1872 he drew attention to the technique by successfully performing small pinch grafts, primarily of the epidermis, measuring 1 to 2 mm in diameter.[64] In 1874 Thiersch extended the use of this type of graft using large sheets of thin skin grafts to cover wounds.[76] These grafts were generally somewhat thicker than the Reverdin grafts. The term "intermediate split-thickness graft" was first applied by Blair and Brown in 1929.[13] The full-thickness graft is generally thought of as a Wolfe graft, even though his work in 1875 was not the first of its type.

Choice of Donor Sites

It must be remembered that the removal of a skin graft is a morbid procedure. Although regeneration of the epidermis will occur, it appears that the loss of the dermis is irretrievable.[69] The thicker the skin graft, the poorer the quality of the donor site after healing. Therefore, the thickness of the desired graft must, to a certain extent, determine the location of the donor site. The thicker portions of the body, such as the posterolateral aspects of the trunk and thighs, afford the best chance of good healing when a thick graft is desired.[5] The thinner areas, such as the inner aspect of the thigh, are generally unsuitable for donor sites (unless they are absolutely necessary) due to the poor quality of healing of the donor site and the tendency of the skin graft to hyperpigment in its new area.[52,57]

So that morbidity and subsequent scarring are prevented, a reasonable guideline for graft thickness is offered in Table 48-1.

Table 48-1. Guidelines for Appropriate Thickness of Skin Grafts

Infants	Never over 0.008 inch
Prepubertal children	If necessarily greater than 0.010 inch, remove from lower abdomen or buttocks
Adult males	0.015 inch from thighs, 0.018 inch from abdomen or buttocks
Adult females	Try never to use inner thigh; if greater than 0.015 inch, use lower abdomen
Elderly adults	Treat like children's skin

Most wounds are best covered by grafts of approximately 0.015 inch thickness. These are generally considered to be grafts of intermediate thickness, although this term was originally applied to grafts removing 25 to 75 percent of the skin thickness.[13] Thinner grafts of 0.010 to 0.012 inch may be best for wounds where graft survival is at risk. Grafts greater than 0.018 inch are seldom indicated, because of donor site morbidity. If thicker skin is desired, it is best to use a full-thickness graft.

If possible, a graft should be taken from an area that is easy to care for during the healing process. No one likes to have to lie or sit on a donor site, and donor areas that cross intertriginous areas are very unsuitable, due to the constant cracking and subsequent drainage with motion of the area. In women and children, it is desirable to remove the graft from the lateral aspect of the upper thigh or buttocks, or perhaps the lower portion of the abdomen, so that the donor site can subsequently be covered by a bathing suit or some other article of clothing. It is important to remember that the thicker the skin graft, the more hair follicles transferred in the graft; thus, whenever possible, a relatively hairless area should be selected as a donor site for the hand.[77]

Free-Hand Grafts

Pinch or Reverdin grafts are almost never used in hand surgery. In the instance where a very small defect is present, however, a pinch graft can be taken by raising up an area of anesthetized skin with a skin hook. It is very convenient to anesthetize the skin with an intradermal injection of lidocaine for this purpose. This not only affords anesthesia, but thickens the skin so that a tangential cut will remove relatively more epidermis and minimize the effect of removing a divot. A piece 1 to 2 mm in diameter can then be removed using a #15 knife blade. Most wounds of this size will heal by themselves as rapidly as a graft will take, and grafting such small wounds is rarely if ever indicated. The method of grafting by multiple pinches has been replaced by mesh grafting.

A larger piece of skin can be removed with a #10 knife blade by dissecting superficially just under the surface of the skin. It is convenient to make a very shallow incision in the skin that has been distended with intradermal lidocaine prior to beginning the tangential dissection. In this way, the appropriate depth

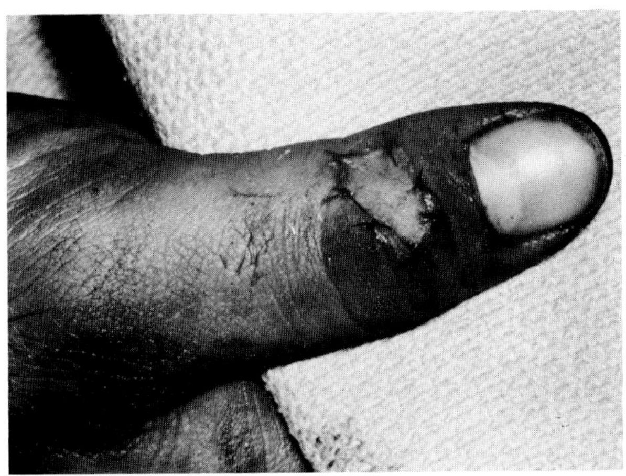

Fig. 48-6. A free-hand graft used to replace a small area of dorsal skin avulsion.

and width of the graft can be selected. The blade is then placed into the depth of the incision, and with a back and forth sawing action, parallel to the skin, the desired size of graft can be removed. It is possible to remove a reasonably uniform piece of skin up to about the size of a dime using this technique (Fig. 48-6).

A much more satisfactory method of free-hand grafting is made possible by the use of the Webster skin graft knife. This is a metal handle containing a groove into which a single edged Weck blade is inserted. The instrument can be used in the same fashion as the knife blade and handle, but it is possible to remove a much larger piece of skin. This is dependent on a number of factors, including the width and sharpness of the blade, as well as the ease of using the handle.

A modification of this knife is known as the Goulian knife set.[39] There are a number of depth gauges available that can be fitted over the blade (Fig. 48-7). These gauges vary in thickness, from 0.004 to 0.030 inch. By placing the gauge next to the skin, the appropriate depth and angle of cut are automatically established. A strip of skin 2 cm or so in width can easily be removed, and with practice a long strip can be taken (Fig. 48-8). This instrument has the advantage of removing a strip of skin of uniform thickness.

Although it is very convenient to remove skin from the upper inner forearm since it is in the operative field, this is, in practice, a very poor procedure. The skin of the forearm is relatively thin in this area,[73] and often the scar is less than satisfactory. These scars are very obvious to both the patient and the casual observer, and many times women will complain more of the donor site scar than of the recipient area. It is preferable to remove these grafts from areas of thicker skin, where the scar will not be so readily apparent.

Types of Dermatomes

Brown Dermatome

This instrument was the first automatic dermatome to be developed and is available in both electric and air-driven models.[9] The Brown dermatome has the advantage of rapid removal of large pieces of skin graft. The instrument is fitted with a disposable blade and has knobs for adjusting both the width and the thickness of the desired piece of skin. The depth gauge on the top left-hand side of the front of the machine should be opened fully. Next, the blade is set down inside the instrument, fitting the three holes in the blade over the corresponding projections on the machine, sliding the blade down, and fastening it securely (Fig. 48-9). The thickness is set using the depth gauge, measured in thousandths of an inch. It is important to recognize that this gauge is not entirely accurate as a rule, and the space between the edge of the blade and the leading edge of the dermatome should be visually inspected to make sure that it is satisfactory. If desired, this depth can be measured with shims of predetermined thicknesses. A simple method of estimating the thickness of the graft is done by the use of a #15 scalpel blade. The bevel of the blade is placed in the gap between the dermatome and its blade. It is estimated that if only the very sharp edge of the blade can fit in this space that this is about ten thousandths of an inch (0.010 in). If, however,

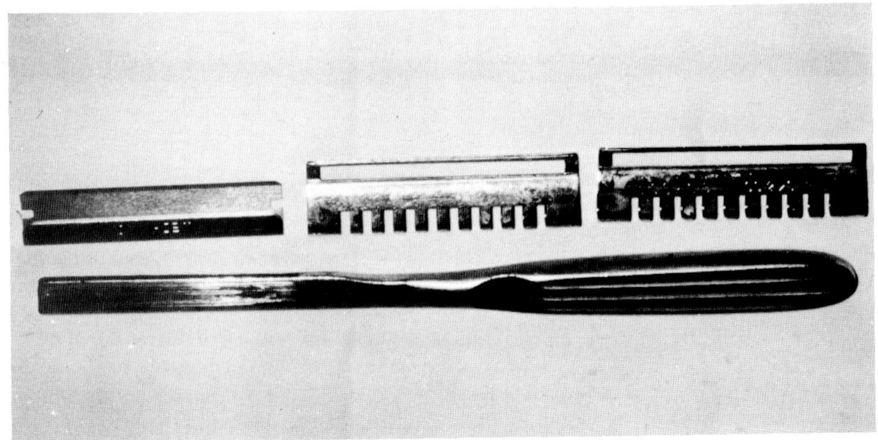

Fig. 48-7. The Goulian skin graft knife set before assembly. Depth gauges of many thickness are available, making it possible to remove a graft of uniform thickness.

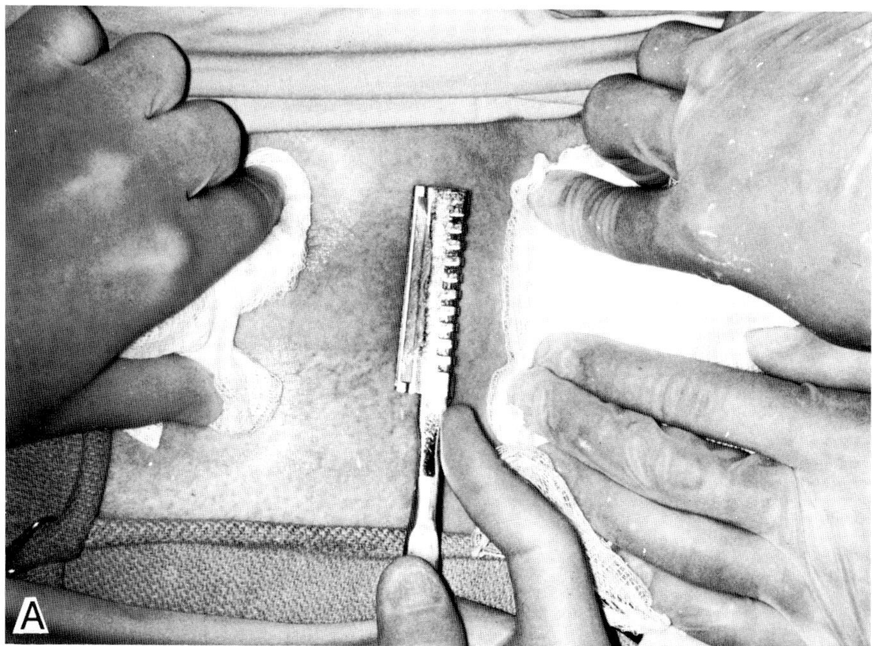

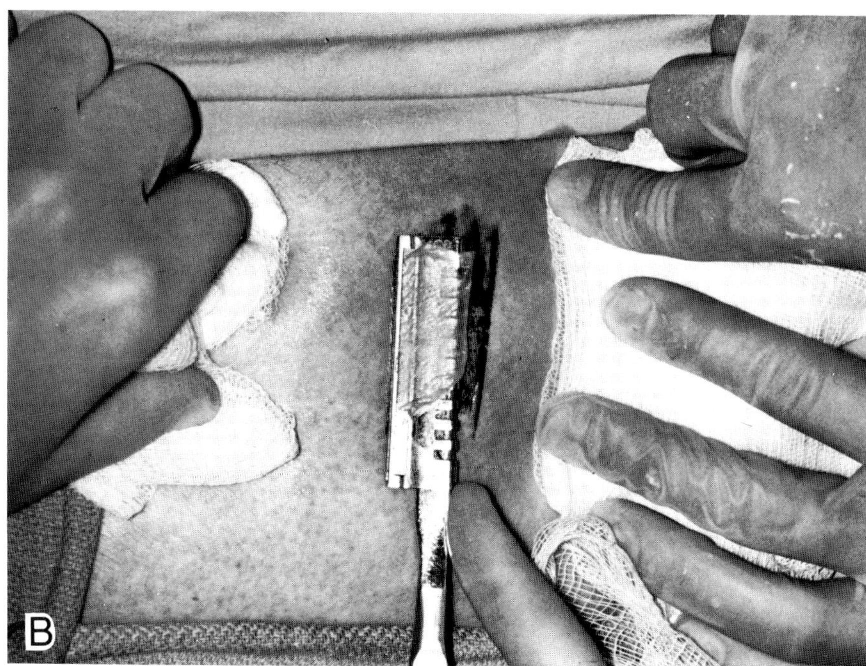

Fig. 48-8. (A) Goulian dermatome placed with the depth gauge next to skin. **(B)** A strip of skin removed with back and forth sawing action.

the entire thickness of the blade just barely passes through the space, then it is approximately fifteen thousandths of an inch (0.015 in).[66]

The donor site may be prepared in whatever fashion desired, but it is important not to leave a sticky solution on the skin, as this will interfere with the sliding of the dermatome, causing an uneven thickness of the graft. One satisfactory method is to cleanse the skin with Betadine solution and remove all of the solution with alcohol. Both the skin and the undersurface of the dermatome are lightly lubricated with mineral oil. After connecting the dermatome to the appropriate power source, the instrument is applied with the undersurface flat on the skin. Care must be taken not to dig the blade into the skin as this can cause the machine to cut too deeply on the edges. Too much forward tilting of the dermatome and heavy pressure can cause the machine to skip, thus resulting in an uneven texture of the

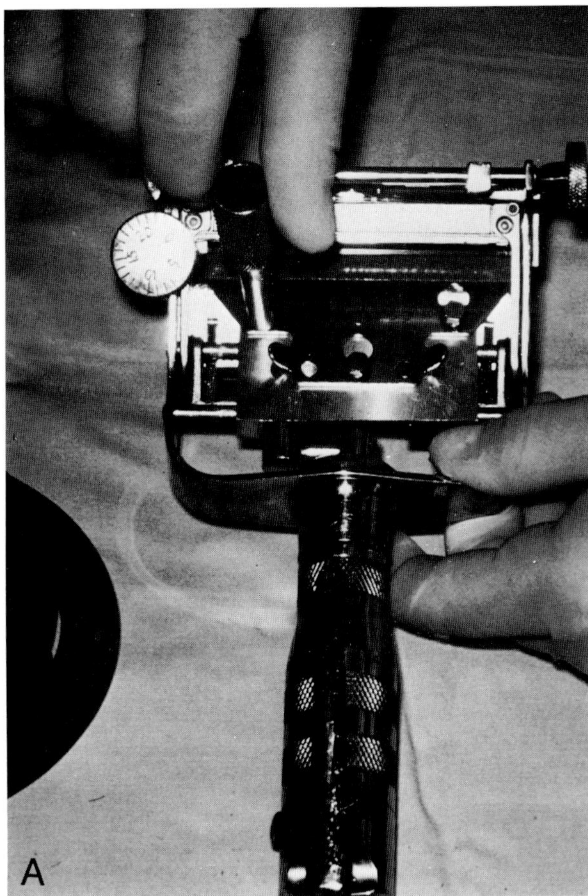

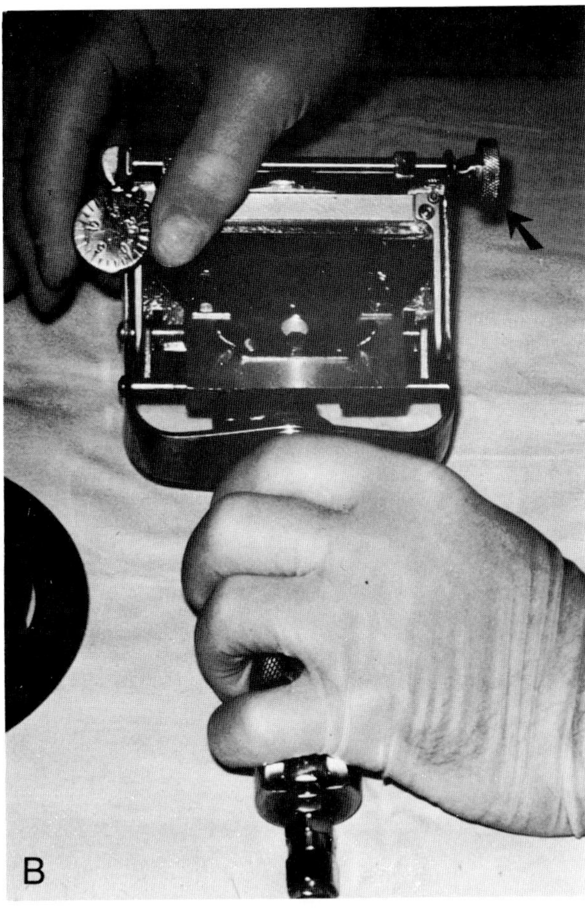

Fig. 48-9. The Brown dermatome. **(A)** The blade is fitted in position and securely tightened. **(B)** Skin graft depth is adjusted by the knob on the left, and graft width is adjusted by the knob on the right *(arrow)*.

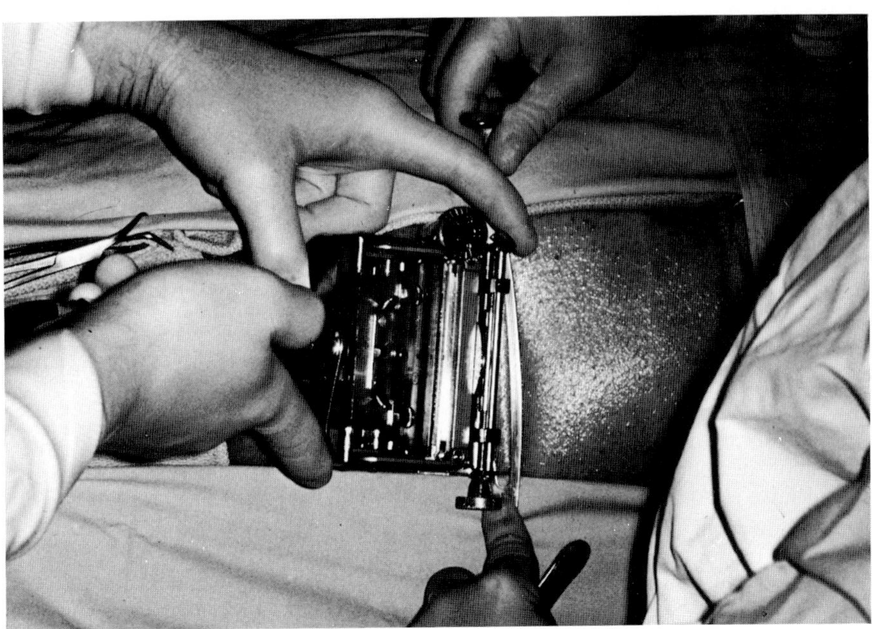

Fig. 48-10. Traction is held in front of the dermatome with a flat object as the instrument is advanced. Countertraction is maintained behind the advance.

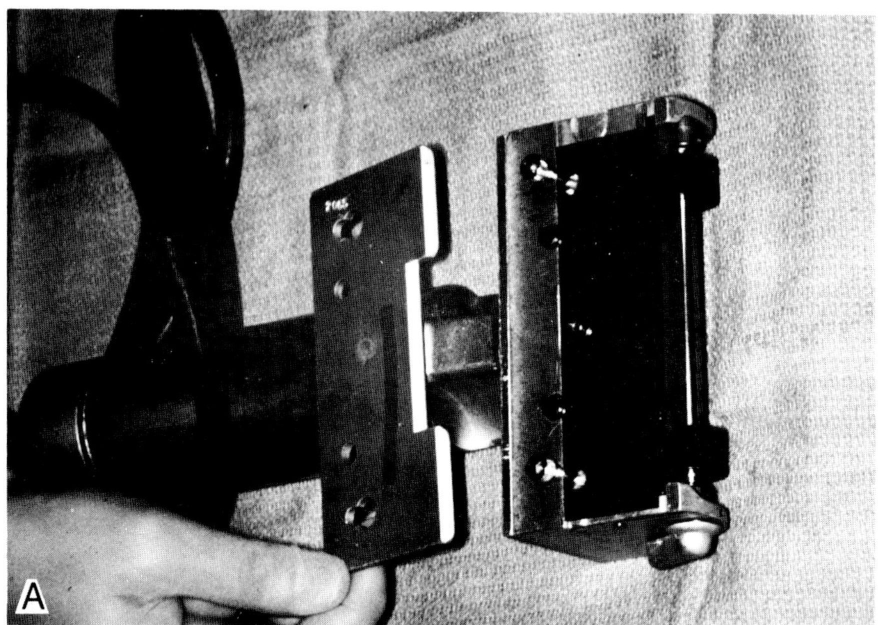

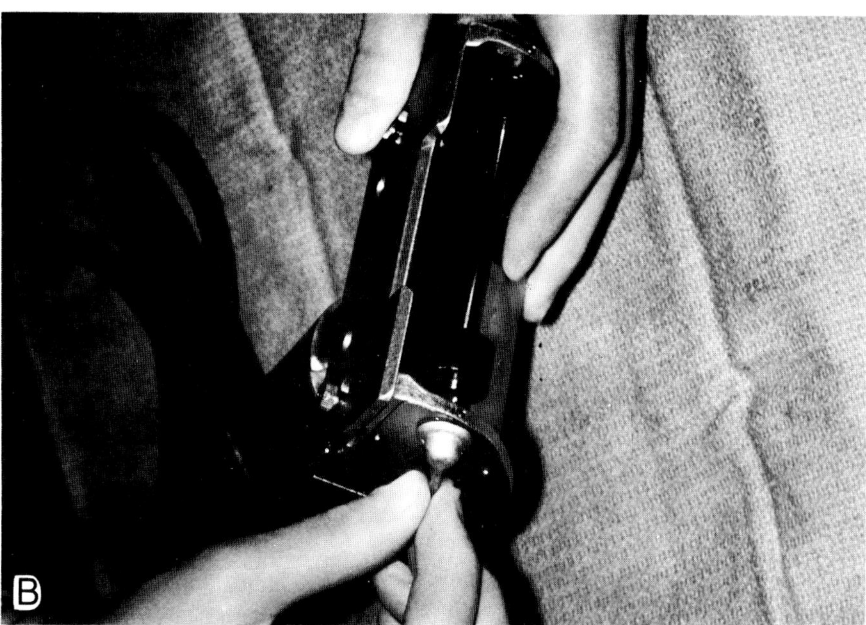

Fig. 48-11. The Padgett electric dermatome. The width is determined by plate selection **(A)**, and the depth is determined by gauge adjustment **(B)**.

graft. There is also a tendency toward irregularities in the graft because of the ridges present on the undersurface of the instrument. An assistant should hold traction on the skin in the direction in which the dermatome will be advanced. This can be done effectively by using a tongue blade or flat retractor (Fig. 48-10). The surgeon then holds countertraction behind the machine with the other hand. The cutting action is begun by depressing the lever on the handle, and the dermatome is advanced slowly, avoiding skips and jumps. If possible, an assistant can grasp the edge of the skin that will slide up into the dermatome above the blade and hold this in the air as the cutting action commences. It can then be determined whether or not the graft is of proper thickness and width, and appropriate adjustments can be made. When a piece of skin of appropriate size has been removed, the dermatome is raised upward off the surface of the donor area, thus separating the graft from the donor site. If more than one piece of skin is to be removed, care should be taken to avoid having blood draining down on the second donor area, and the undersurface of the dermatome should be cleaned in order to prevent skipping.

Padgett Electric Dermatome

This dermatome is also motorized and uses a disposable blade with a cutting action similar to that of the Brown dermatome. There is a variable depth gauge on the side of this instrument that is generally more accurate than the one on the Brown dermatome. There are three plates that determine the width of the graft. After determination of the desired width, the blade is fitted on the machine and the appropriate plate is placed over the two screws and screwed down tightly (Fig. 48-11). To put the blade on, it is necessary to first slip the base of the blade under the two projecting metal pieces and snap it down so that the hole in the blade fits onto the projection of the drive shaft. The appropriate thickness of the graft is selected by moving the blade up and down, using the depth gauge on the side of the machine.

The skin is prepared in the same fashion as that described for the Brown dermatome. The dermatome is placed flat on the donor site and traction is held behind the dermatome. It is not necessary to stretch the skin in the direction in which the dermatome will be advanced (Fig. 48-12). It is very easy to remove a piece of skin with this dermatome, and very minimal pres-

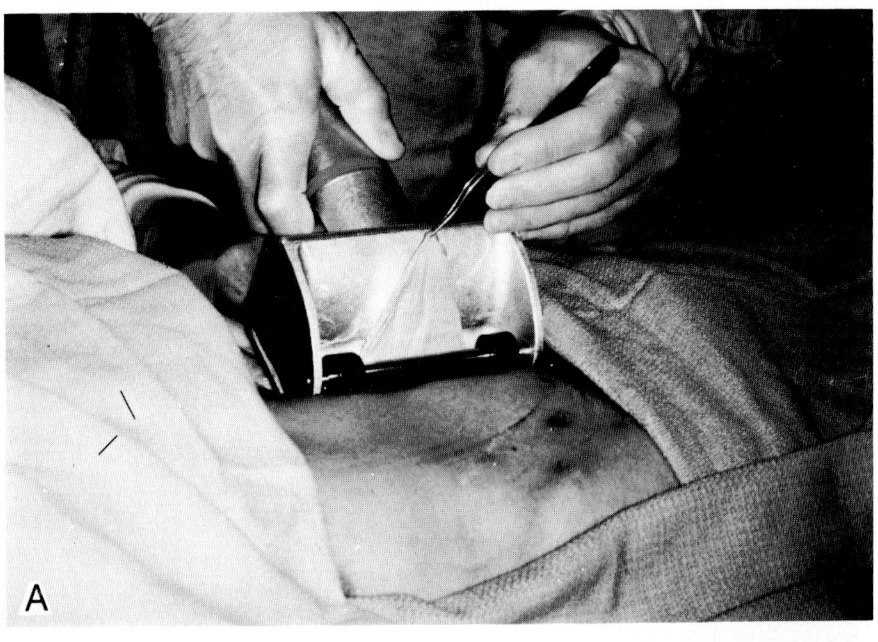

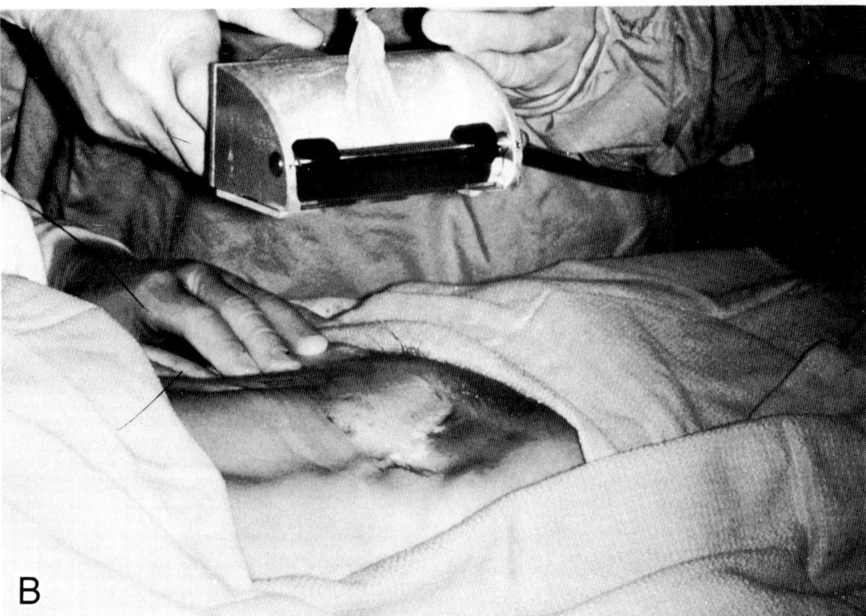

Fig. 48-12. As the dermatome is advanced, traction behind the machine is maintained. The graft is lifted by the surgeon **(A)** and severed simply by lifting upward **(B)**.

sure should be exerted on the donor area. A common mistake is to dig the edges of the dermatome into the skin and press too hard, creating an improper cutting angle. As the dermatome is advanced, the skin may be lifted up to check the thickness, if desired. This is not necessary, however, and in general, a very uniform piece of skin is removed using this dermatome.

Zimmer Air Dermatome

A similar instrument has recently been produced by Zimmer, and is used in the same fashion as the Padgett electric (Fig. 48-13). A special disposable blade is made to fit the dermatome and snaps easily onto the reciprocating post. The width gauges are then fitted in place and screwed down in the same fashion. As seen in Figure 48-14, there are four fixed widths; the most narrow one is very useful for taking small grafts such as would be placed on one finger, or filling the defect made by a cross-finger flap, etc. Unfortunately, the largest one is a little too wide to fit into the standard skin mesher, but a graft that wide is rarely required for hand surgery, anyway. The thickness of the graft is adjusted by a gauge on the side of the instrument in the same fashion as the Padgett dermatome, and the technique of skin harvest is identical.

Although this is a comparable instrument to the Padgett, there are some advantages.

Since it is air driven, the handle is smaller and lighter, making its use a little more effortless. Also, it can be autoclaved repeatedly, making it available for more than one case in a day. We have found it best to gas sterilize the Padgett in order to minimize the repair rate. Although I still frequently use the Padgett, I have grown to like the Zimmer instrument, and use it preferentially over all other dermatomes.

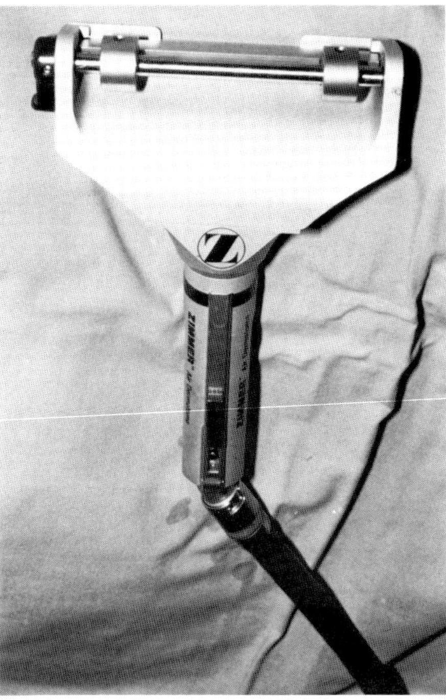

Fig. 48-13. The Zimmer air dermatome assembled for use. The adjusting gauge is on the left side.

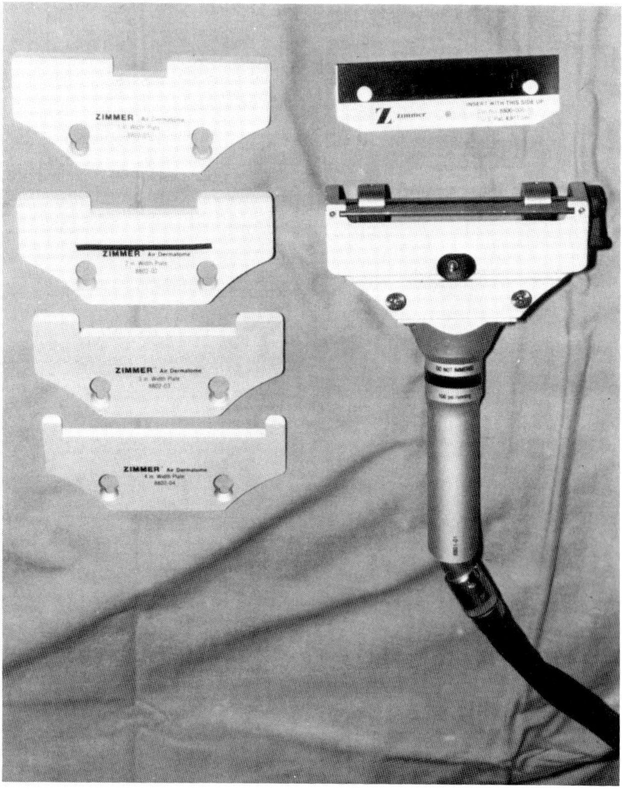

Fig. 48-14. The undersurface of the Zimmer air dermatome, showing the disposable blade, which is fitted over a reciprocating post and covered by plate to select the desired graft width.

Davol Dermatome

The Davol dermatome is a disposable head that is fitted onto a motorized handle similar to that of an electric toothbrush (Fig. 48-15). There is a sterile pastic bag into which the toothbrush handle is dropped, and the bag is sealed with a twist tie. The head is fitted onto the handle, taking care to align the dot on the head with the dot on the handle. The blade is then powered by turning the handle on with the switch on the side of the handle. Skin is removed in a fashion similar to the procedure with the Brown and Padgett dermatomes.

The head is preset at 0.015 inch, and the width is constant at about 2 cm. Although the depth of the blade cannot be varied, it is possible to remove a thinner piece of skin by pressing the blade down lightly. It is also possible to accomplish the same effect by distending the skin with an intradermal injection of local anesthetic.

The advantage of this dermatome is that it allows removal of a small piece of skin with a minimal amount of trouble in setting up instruments. It also has the dubious advantage of disposability, but it is necessary to keep the battery handle charged. One must be careful to examine the blade before using the instrument as sometimes this can be crooked, causing the blade to cut much deeper on one side than on the other. This problem is easily avoided by centering the blade before using it.

It is also possible to cut too deeply, especially along the edges

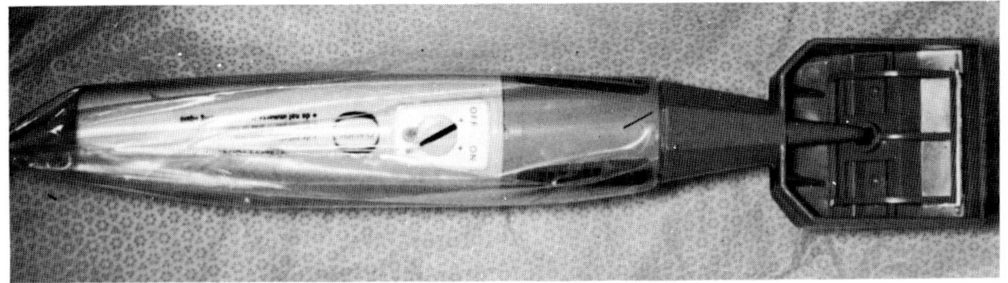

Fig. 48-15. The Davol dermatome. Disposable head fitted onto the toothbrush handle.

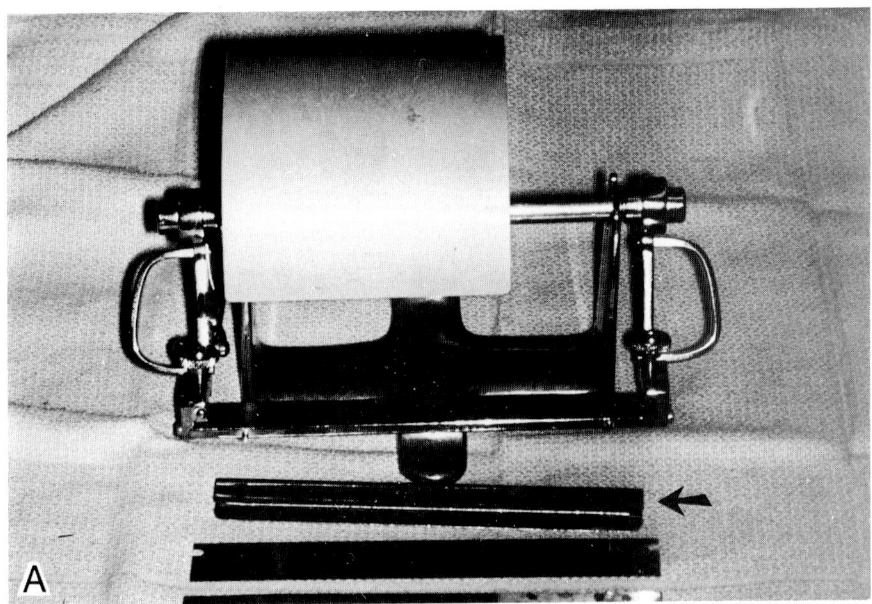

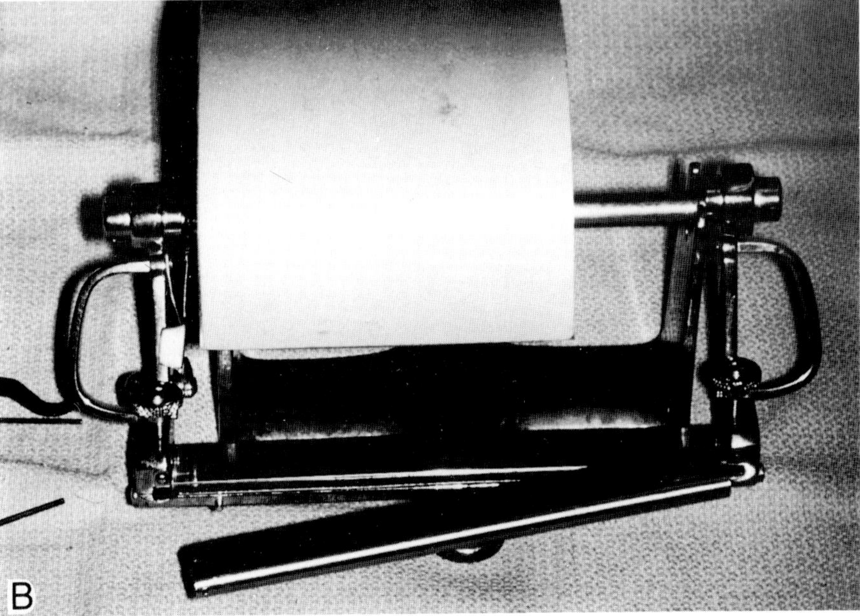

Fig. 48-16. The Padgett drum dermatome **(A)**. The shim *(arrow)* is first placed in the handle, followed by the blade, and secured by the guard **(B)**.

of the blade, if the machine is pressed down too hard into the skin with an acute angle. It is important not to expect too much from this instrument, and it should not be used to obtain large or thick pieces of skin.

Drum Dermatomes

There are two types of drum dermatomes, which are manual but do allow the surgeon to remove a large piece of skin of variable depth and width. These are the Padgett (Fig. 48-16) and the Reese. These instruments depend on the use of glue or a specially designed tape that causes the skin to stick to the surface of the drum so that the cutting blade can slide back and forth removing a piece of skin that remains adherent to the drum.[63] Since the advent of the good power-driven dermatomes, the drum dermatomes are probably of more historic interest than of practical value. They do offer one outstanding advantage under certain circumstances, however, in that a piece of skin can be removed from any region of the body, even in areas that are ordinarily very difficult to remove grafts from, such as over the rib cage. It is almost impossible to remove a good piece of skin from this area using the motor-driven der-

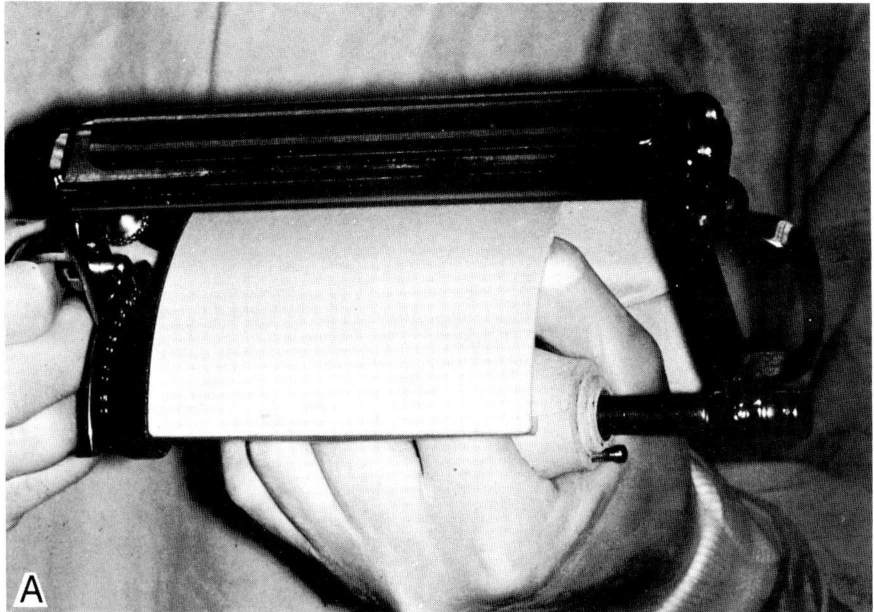

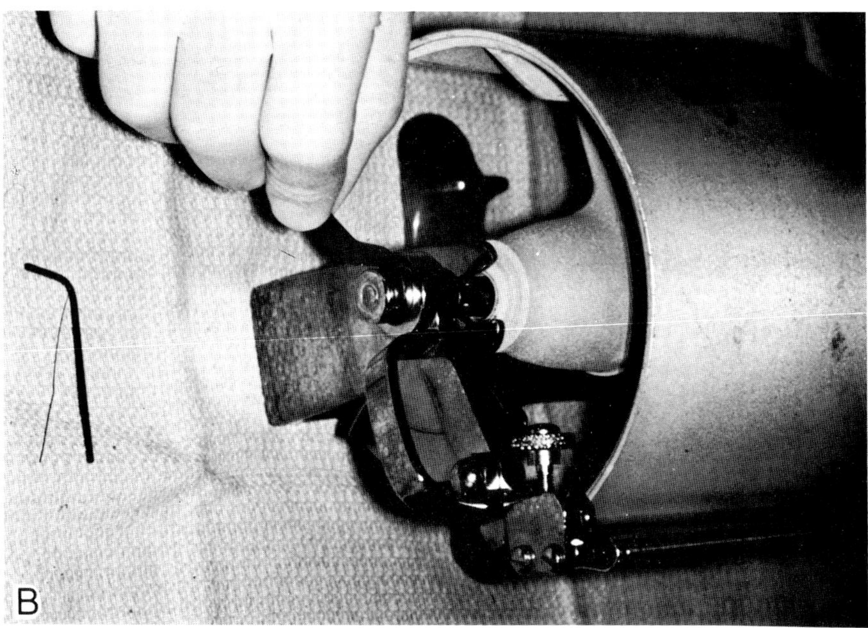

Fig. 48-17. **(A)** Depth must be determined by sight as well as by markings on the gauge. **(B)** Unevenness may be corrected by adjusting the cam.

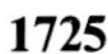

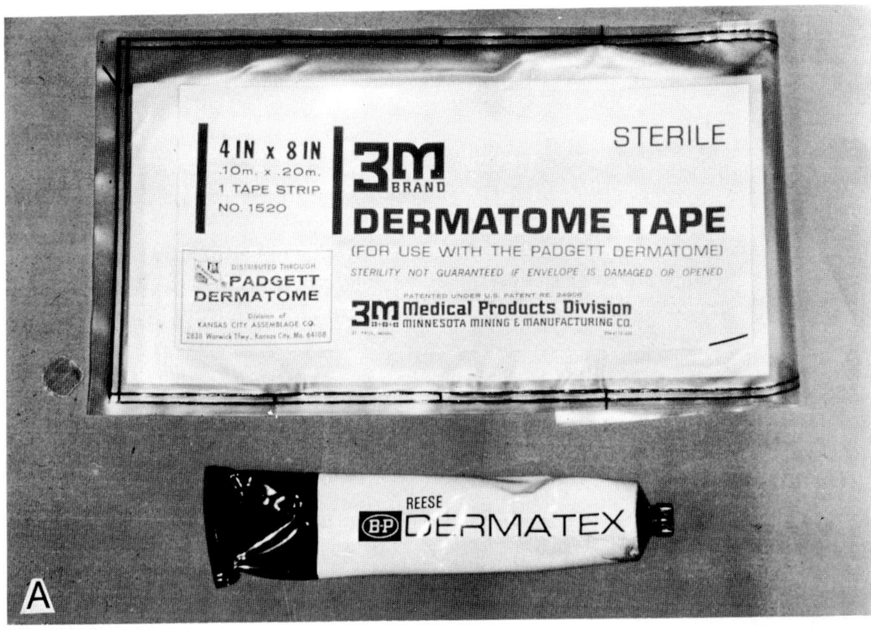

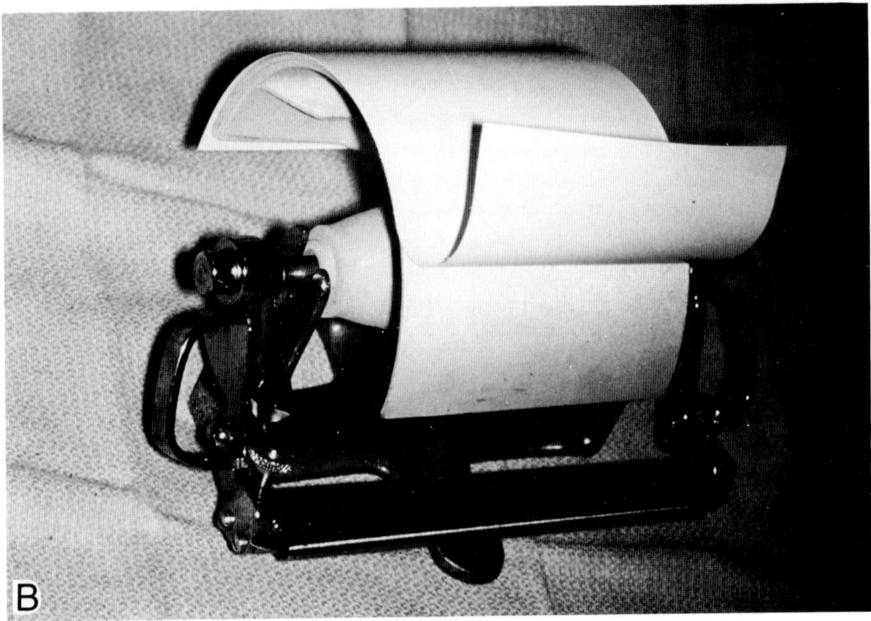

Fig. 48-18. **(A)** Either glue or a special tape may be used to make the skin stick to the drum. **(B)** Adhesive backing is present on both sides of the tape.

matomes. However, a very satisfactory piece of skin of uniform thickness can be removed from virtually any part of the body with the drum, since it lifts the skin to be cut in the air rather than pressing it down over an uneven surface.

The Padgett dermatome is assembled, after placing the dermatome on its stand, by slipping the little knob on the side of the dermatome into the hole on the stand. It is *imperative* that the knife blade never be placed into this dermatome unless the machine is stabilized! Very severe injuries, such as tendon and nerve lacerations, have been sustained by surgeons who have allowed the blade to flip around while holding the drum. When the dermatome is being used, the operator must always make sure that one hand is kept inside the drum, and the other hand on the handle.

A disposable shim is first placed into the blade holder after loosening the turn bolts (Fig. 48-16). Next, the blade is placed in the handle and the guard is slipped over to hold the blade flush with the handle. The thickness of the graft is determined by moving the handle closer or further away from the drum as desired by pushing on the depth gauge with the thumb (Fig. 48-17). This activates a cam, and if the sides are unequal, this can be adjusted by using the tool provided with the dermatome

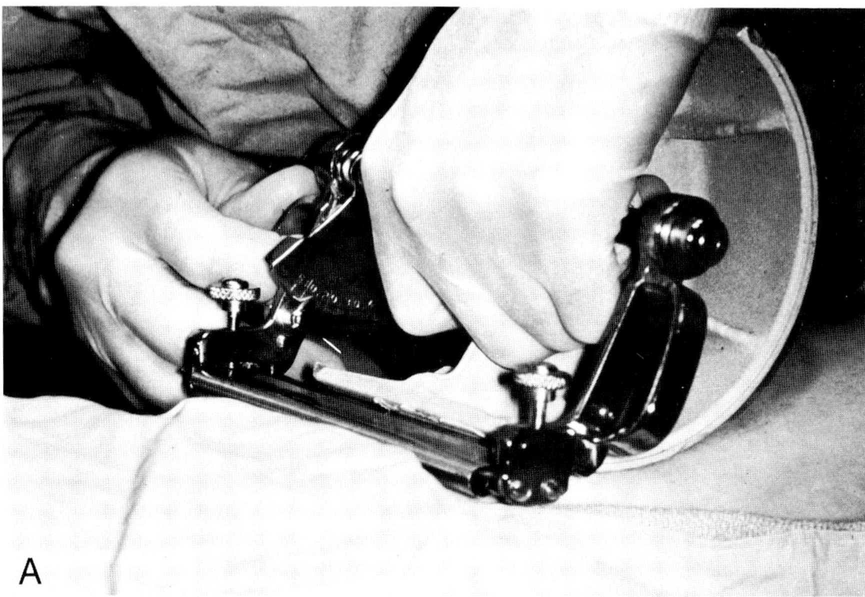

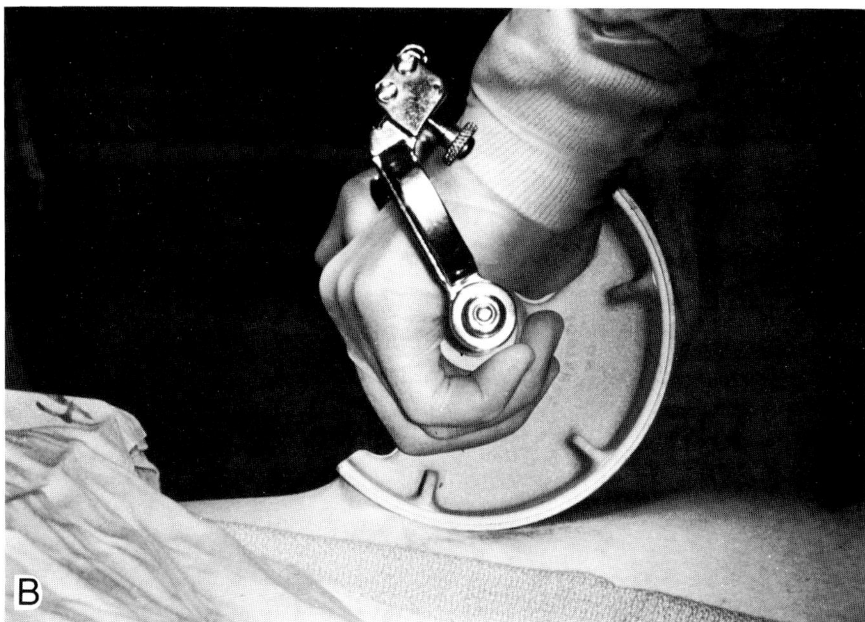

Fig. 48-19. The correct method of cutting with a drum dermatome. **(A)** After sticking the leading edge, **(B&C)** forward pressure is maintained with the base of the hand so that the skin rolls up instead of pulling loose from the drum. *(Figure continues.)*

after loosening the little set screws on the ends of the handle. The thickness must be determined by looking at the space between the ends of the blade and the drum, as the marks on the depth gauge are often only a relative indication of thickness.

The skin is prepared using any antiseptic agent desired, but this must all be carefully removed with water or alcohol, and the skin must be defatted very carefully with a solvent such as acetone. If this is not done, the drum will not stick to the skin and the dermatome will not work.

Either a glue or a special tape can be used with this dermatome (Fig. 48-18). If glue is selected, a very thin solution of the glue must be painted on the donor site and another thin layer on the surface of the drum. It is much easier to use the Dermatape, in which case no glue is necessary. The tape is placed on the surface of the drum after removing one backing, and is smoothed down while the other backing is removed.

The leading edge of the drum is then pushed down firmly onto the surface of the skin, and by using the base of the hand with a forward pushing action, the edge of the skin is rolled up to be presented for cutting. It is important not to merely tilt the hand back, as this will cause the skin to pull loose from the drum (Fig. 48-19). The handle is then rotated forward, and by moving it back and forth, the skin is cut loose. It is very easy to

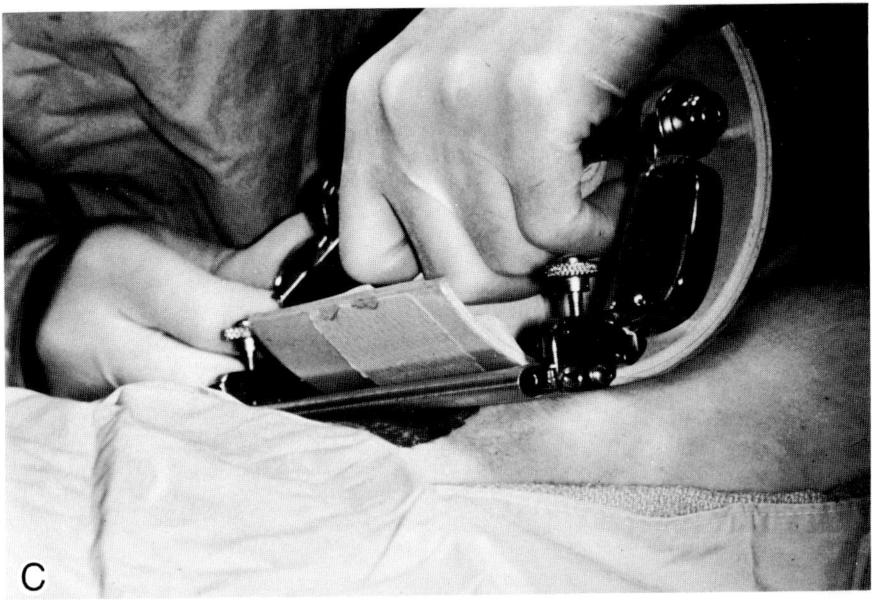

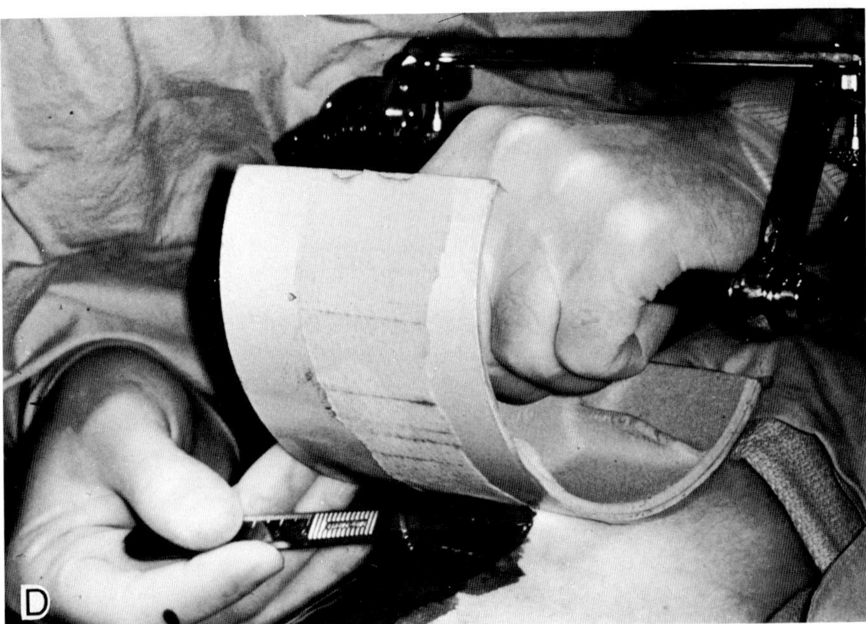

Fig. 48-19 *(Continued).* **(D)** The skin is severed with a scalpel.

cause a full-thickness cut on the edges of the dermatome unless one is very cautious, and the drum must be kept level so that one edge will not dig further than the other. After the drum has been tilted about halfway, it is convenient to change the position of the hand so that further cutting can be done. The cutting should be started with the hand pronated and then changed to supination, which by flexing the wrist allows further rotation of the drum to obtain a longer piece of skin. The surgeon must stop cutting while changing the position of his hand. Upon completion of the cut, the edge of the donor site should be divided with a scalpel and the instrument replaced on its stand. The skin is then pulled loose from the Dermatape.

If glue is used, it should always be diluted with a solvent to prevent excess glue from staying on the surface of the skin and sticking the graft together, making it very unmanageable. If more than one piece of skin is to be removed with this dermatome, it is imperative that all blood be removed from the surface of the instrument and from the second donor site, as the tape will never stick unless the skin is very clean and dry.

Mesh Grafting

There are times when the condition of the wound cannot be made optimal for grafting. The risk of infection or hematoma may be so great that the chances of survival of a sheet of auto-

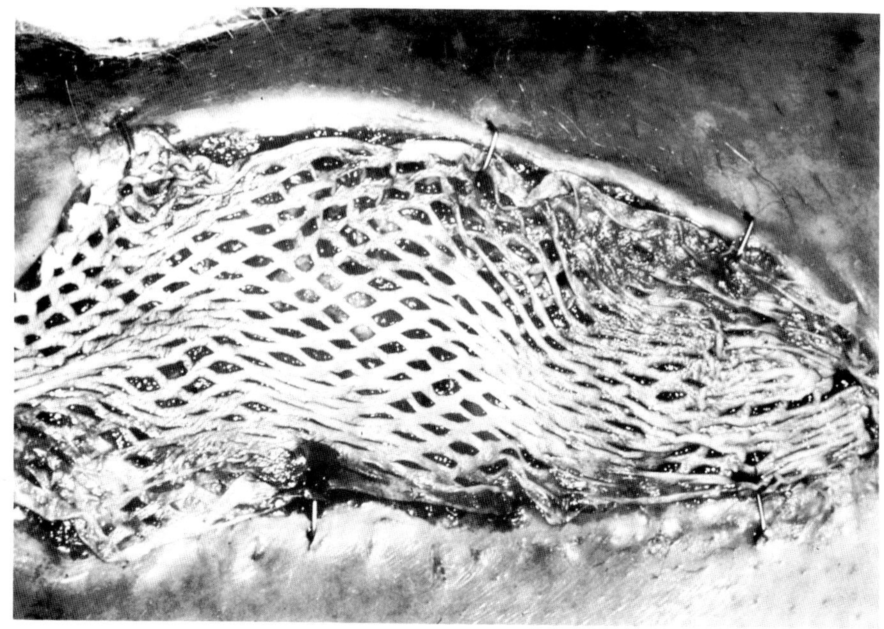

Fig. 48-20. Meshed skin in place on suboptimal wound.

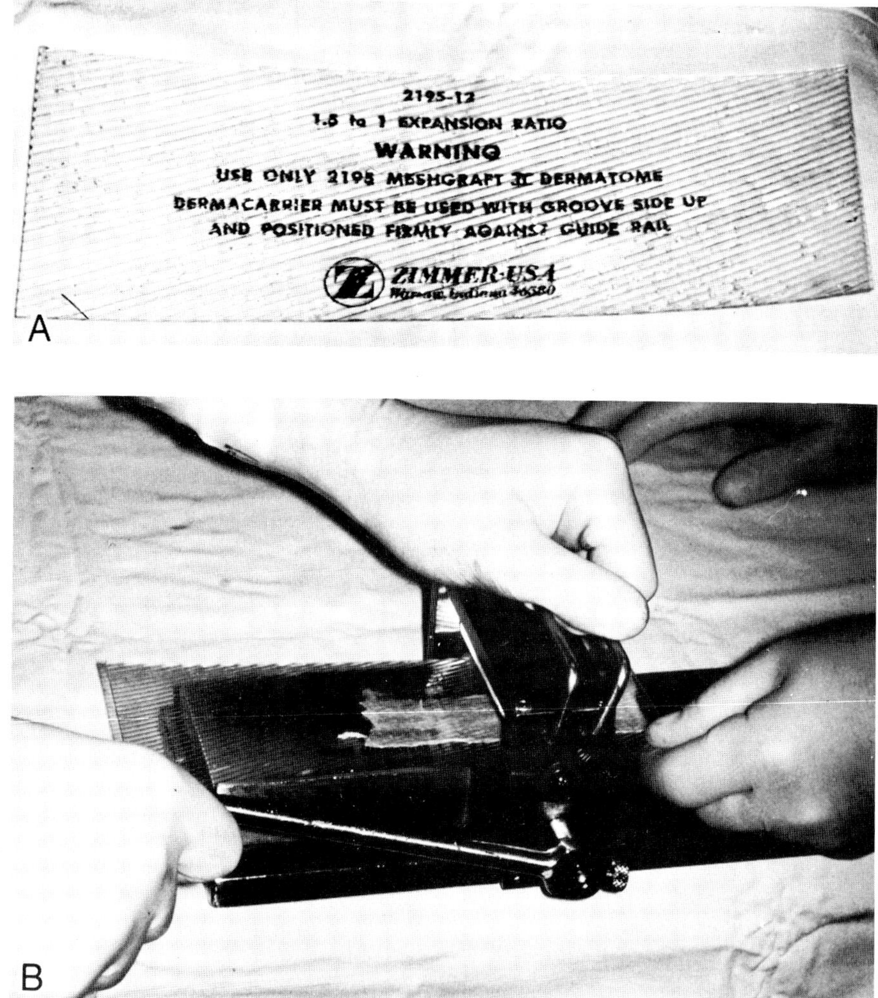

Fig. 48-21. Skin mesher. Skin is placed on the special carrier **(A)** and passed through the cutting blades by turning the crank **(B)**.

graft would be small. In these instances, it is often wise to use a piece of skin that has been meshed so that many perforations are present through which blood or exudate may escape.[53,71] An instrument has been devised that will automatically make these perforations. The skin can then be expanded so that the interstices will allow drainage and then rapidly become epithelialized (Fig. 48-20). This method of grafting has wide application in the treatment of burns and large, contaminated wounds.[38,45,53]

It must be remembered, however, that only the portion of the wound that has skin applied to it is being grafted, and the interstices of the mesh are being left open and allowed to epithelialize. The quality of the graft will obviously not be as good as a sheet of skin, and the tendency toward contraction and poor cosmetic results will be greater. If meshed grafts of this nature are placed over flexion creases, then joint contractures are apt to occur.[18] These factors can be limited somewhat by compression, and it is imperative to treat wounds grafted in this fashion with long-term compression, such as can be obtained by use of the Jobst pressure glove. I feel that because of contraction and poor cosmetic results, the use of mesh grafting has very little place in hand surgery, except in instances where the hand wounds are only part of a larger overall injury that produces a large, contamined wound. It is sometimes convenient to use a mesh graft as a "temporary" biologic dressing, however, when one realizes that the coverage obtained by this graft is intended as only temporary, until a later resurfacing procedure can be done as part of reconstruction.

Preparation of a Meshed Graft

A split-thickness graft should be removed using any desired dermatome. The graft is then spread out onto the surface of a plastic carrier, which is provided with the dermatome (Fig. 48-21). It is desirable to remove a relatively thin graft for the purpose of meshing, since not only will the graft probably be vascularized more readily, but a thick graft tends to curl up on the carrier, making it very difficult to feed into the machine for proper meshing. Grafts of approximately 0.012 inch are appropriate for this kind of application. After the graft has been carefully spread out onto the surface of the carrier, it is then fed into the lower end of the machine and run through the mesh by using the hand crank. There are carriers with cuts of different sizes allowing expansion of varying degree, but I recommend never using a mesh greater than the smallest expansion ratio size of 1.5 to 1 for hand surgery.

An alternate method of meshing skin grafts is one that provides multiple holes for drainage, but does not allow for expansion. Instead of placing the graft on the mesh card and feeding it through the mesher in the usual fashion, the mesh card can be divided into sections, and these pieces are then placed side by side rather than end on end. If the graft is then placed on these lined-up pieces of mesh card the result is the skin passing through the mesher at a 90-degree angle from the direction that it would ordinarily go through (Fig. 48-22). This makes a multitude of little punctate holes rather than slits, and when this is placed on the wound there are multiple very fine drainage holes present but minimal if any expansion (Fig. 48-23). Skin meshed in this fashion is not as effective when placed on the suboptimal wound, but the cosmetic effect is probably superior. It is absolutely critical that the card be fed through the mesher with the grooved side up, however. If the skin is inadvertently placed on the wrong side of the mesh card and then passed through the dermatome, the result will be multiple strands of spaghetti. Skin meshed in this fashion is probably a better graft to place over flexion creases to minimize contraction.

Full-Thickness Grafts

Full-thickness grafts transfer all of the skin appendages and nerve endings except those sweat glands located in the subcutaneous tissue and some of the Vater-Pacini corpuscles of palmar and plantar skin.[50] This thickness is an advantage for the restoration of sensibility and quality of coverage. These grafts must always be taken from relatively hairless areas to minimize subsequent hair growth in the recipient area. Good donor sites for this type of skin are in the lower and lateral abdominal areas. It is possible to obtain good quality, relatively hairless skin here, and the area is loose enough to allow a large piece of skin to be removed with no subsequent defect after wound closure.[67] Smaller pieces can be removed from the extremity being operated on, and this is often very convenient, since the area has been prepared along with the operative site. Recommended areas for donor sites are in the volar wrist crease (Fig. 48-24) and the medial aspect of the antecubital fossa. It is possible to make transverse excision of skin that will provide good skin and minimal donor-area scarring.

Almost all full-thickness grafts will be placed on the palmar aspect of the hand; thus the surgeon must remember that there is a marked difference in pigmentation of the palmar skin in black patients, and the donor sites just mentioned should be avoided if possible. Whenever possible, the plantar skin of the instep should be used in order to obtain a color match.[56] This has the added advantage of transferring skin of a more similar nature, containing Meissner's corpuscles, thereby restoring better sensibility in addition to color match. In instances where sensibility is critical, such as in the fingertips, a fairly large piece of "fingerprint" skin can be obtained from the hypothenar area (Fig. 48-25). Removal of a piece of skin in this area will cause some tightness and "dog-ears," but this will flatten out considerably in time.

Technique of Obtaining a Full-Thickness Graft

After the appropriate size has been determined, an ovoid of skin is excised from the predetermined area with the axis in the direction of minimal tension. The wound is then closed in standard fashion, undermining the edges as necessary to achieve approximation. Since there will be a moderate amount of tension on the edges, it is probably best to close the wound with buried subdermal sutures and a subcuticular suture in order to minimize the crosshatching that might occur with ordinary cutaneous sutures. The wound can then be dressed with Steri-strips only.

It is necessary to remove all fat and subcutaneous tissue from the undersurface of the graft, as this will otherwise act as a

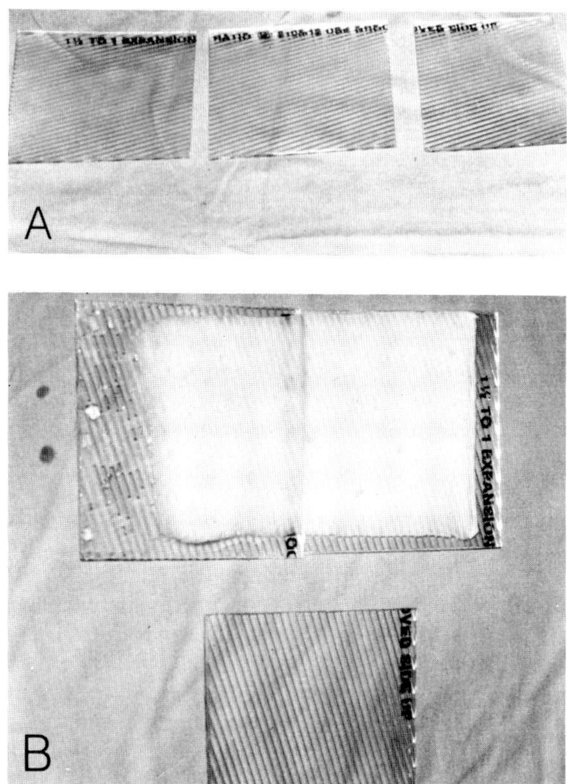

Fig. 48-22. Method of dividing (A) and realigning (B) a mesh card in order to pass it through the mesher at a 90-degree angle from the usual orientation.

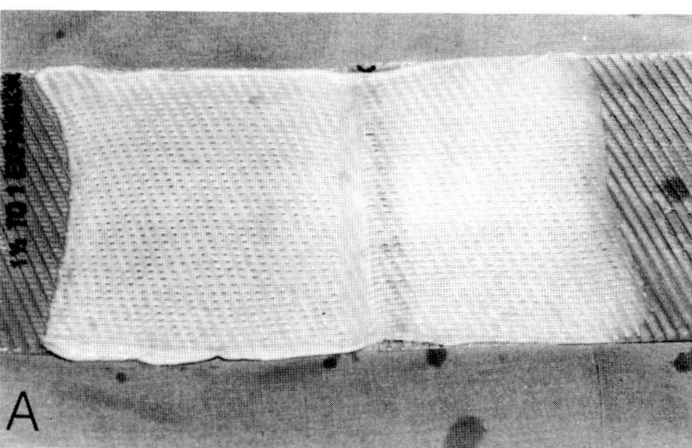

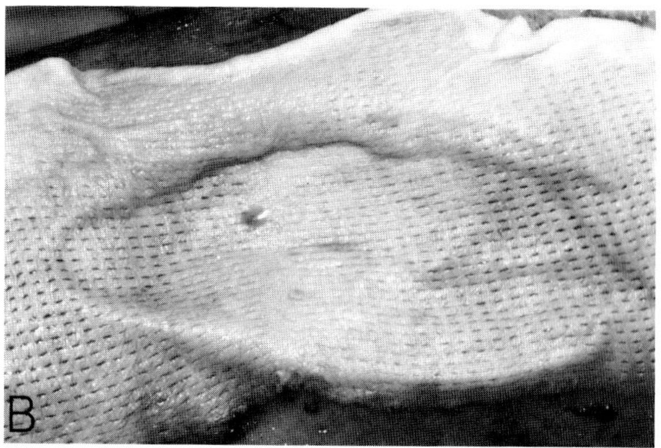

Fig. 48-23. When the skin is passed through the mesher in this fashion, multiple small drainage holes are created (A), but expansion is then minimal (B).

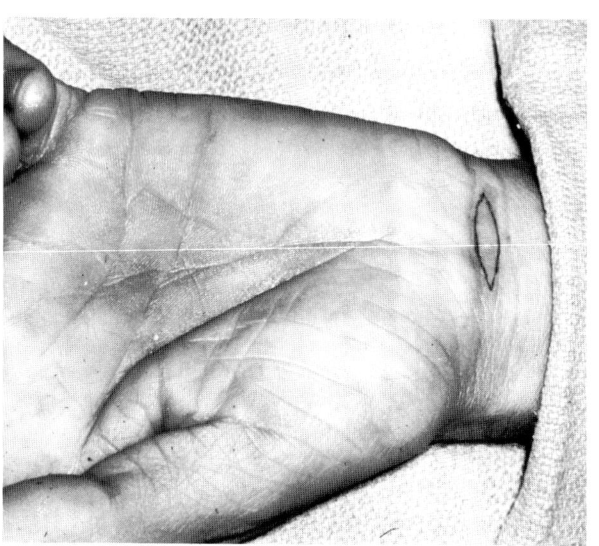

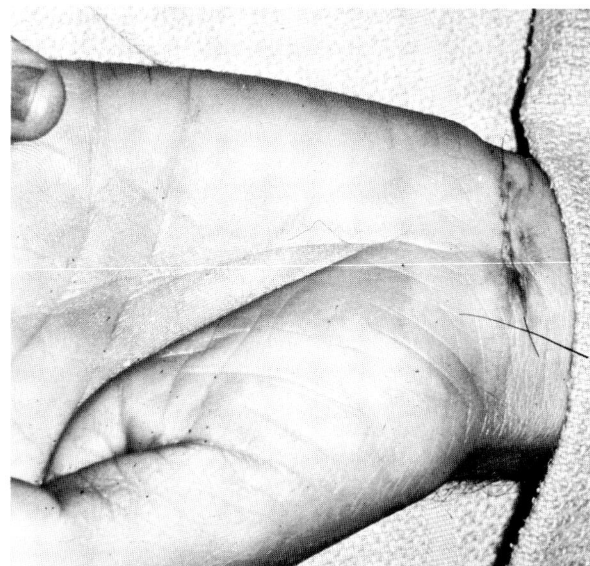

Fig. 48-24. Removal of a full-thickness graft from the wrist crease area, resulting in minimal donor deformity.

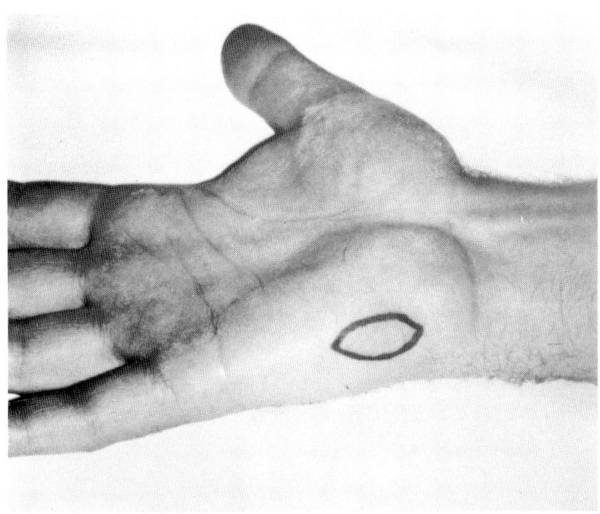

Fig. 48-25. The hypothenar donor area provides a source of "fingerprint" skin.

barrier preventing vascularization. If desired, this can be done at the time of removal of the graft by very carefully excising only the skin, lifting the skin off of its bed of subcutaneous tissue by dissecting sharply with a scalpel in the subdermal plane. This is time-consuming and tedious, however, and in instances where a relatively large graft is removed, the subcutaneous tissue that is left behind will make it difficult to close the wound. This is especially true in little children in whom congenital anomalies are being corrected, and it is necessary to excise the subcutaneous tissue in order to facilitate wound closure.

A much easier method of de-fatting the graft is to simply excise the skin and subcutaneous tissue in one block, thus allowing easy wound closure. The fat can then be quickly removed from the undersurface of the skin with a pair of fine, sharp-pointed scissors. This is facilitated by placing small mosquito hemostats on the very tips at each end of the graft and draping the skin over a finger or the thumb, keeping tension on both hemostats (Fig. 48-26). If some tension is maintained, it is very easy to snip away the fat in this fashion.

If more than one piece is needed, as would be necessary if several contractures were being released, it is sometimes difficult to determine exactly how much skin will be required. It is particularly frustrating to go through all the time and trouble to remove a piece of skin and close the wound, only to find out that one does not have enough skin to adequately fill the defect. Templates can easily be made using the paper in which gloves are wrapped. If a piece of the glove paper is pressed into the depth of the defect before the tourniquet is released, there is usually enough blood and fluid present to stain the paper so that the appropriate shape can be cut out. It should then be fitted into the defect to make sure that it is the appropriate size. When there is more than one template, they can be put together appropriately so that one large template can be excised which will contain enough skin to fill all the defects (Fig. 48-27). The resultant large piece of skin can then be used to fill the defects one at a time by sewing one edge of the graft into the largest defect and trimming it to fit, and repeating this process for all of the subsequent defects. In order to save time, the templates can be marked on the surface of the piece of skin to be removed prior to raising it, and then as soon as the graft is available it can be cut into sections and each piece can be sewn in simultaneously. Invariably, it seems that this method produces one piece of skin that is a little too small and another

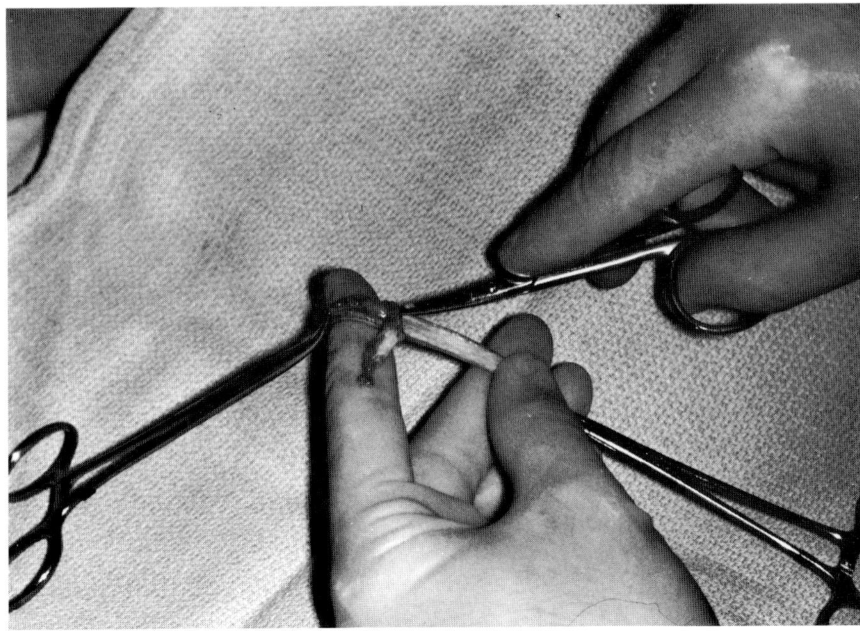

Fig. 48-26. Technique of removal of subcutaneous tissue from the undersurface of a full-thickness graft.

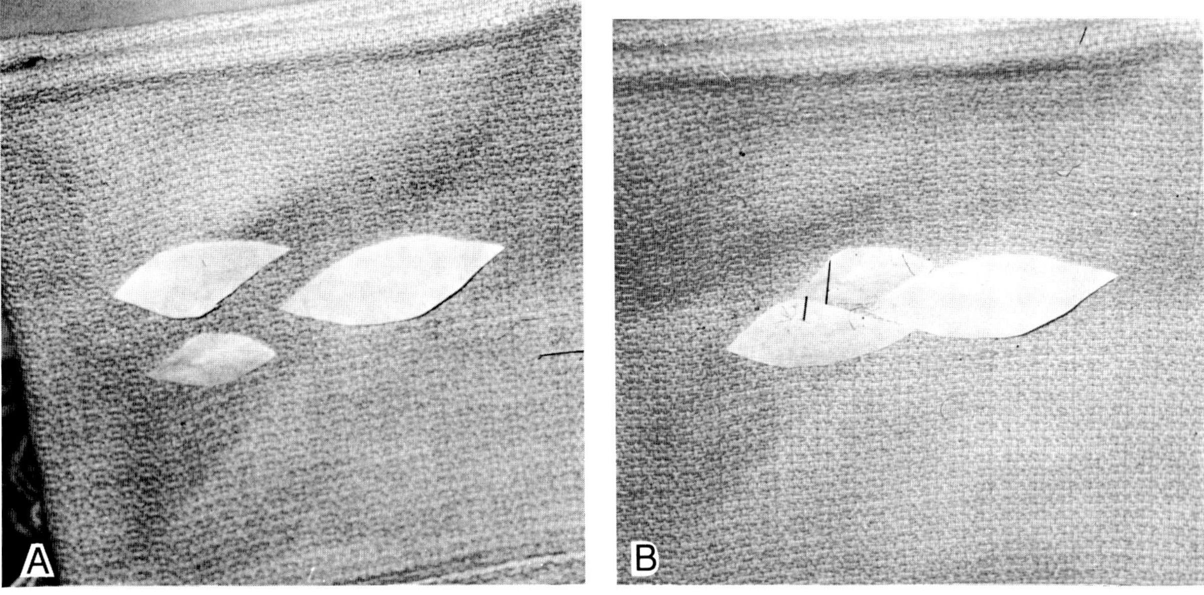

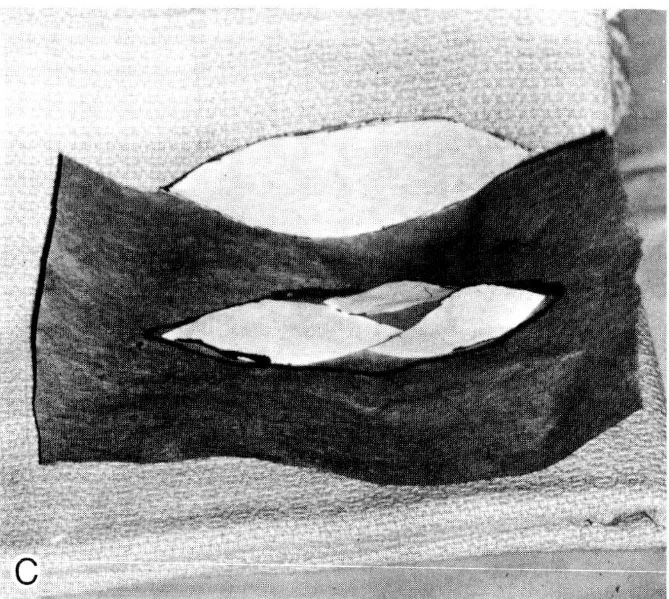

Fig. 48-27. Method of determining adequacy of skin to fill multiple defects. A template is made of each defect (**A**) and combined (**B**) to form one template large enough to provide sufficient skin (**C**).

piece that is a little too big, however, so the more tedious method of cutting and sewing the grafts a little bit at a time is probably safer.

If grafting is to be done for release of contracture, it should always be remembered that the cardinal principle of contracture release is recreating the original defect before attempting to fill up the hole.[21]

Choice of Graft

As previously indicated, a thicker graft contracts less, holds up better, and regains better sensibility than a thinner one does. In general, split-thickness grafts should not be used on palmar surfaces of the skin unless there is no other choice, or the coverage is considered to be temporary, with secondary resurfacing to be followed at a later date. If split-thickness grafts are to be used, they should be relatively thick and long-term compression with a Jobst glove should be used. Except in dire circumstances, placing a meshed graft on the palmar surface of the hand is probably never indicated.

Full-thickness grafts are seldom indicated on the dorsal surface of the hand. The need for coverage is not as critical on the dorsum, and split-thickness grafts are generally satisfactory. In addition, the convexity of the dorsum and the subsequent greater tension on the wound edges with motion in the postoperative period appear to allow split grafts to be used with less contraction than would be the case on the concave palmar aspect. The general rule is that a sheet of graft of good quality skin approximately 0.015-inch thick, if placed on a well-vascularized bed early in the evolution of the wound, will heal so well that it is difficult for the casual observer to know that a graft has been done (see Fig. 48-4). If the bed is not ideal, it makes no difference what kind of graft is used, as the result will always be less than satisfactory (see Fig. 48-5). Bare tendon, bone denuded of periosteum, and nerves and vessels bowstringing in the wound should never be grafted; in such instances, coverage should be obtained by the use of a flap[21] (see Chapter 49).

Preparation of the Recipient Site

The recipient bed should be debrided so that all necrotic material and granulation tissue are removed. The bed of the wound should contain only a fine lacy network of capillaries. Often, after debridement of a wound or removal of a thick scar for resurfacing purposes, it is not possible to obtain an adequate bed for grafting. If it is not possible to obtain adequate hemostasis by coagulating bleeding points after release of the tourniquet, it is best to reinflate the tourniquet, wash away all the blood with saline, and dress the wound with fine mesh gauze and a dressing that will afford light compression and splinting before releasing the tourniquet again. If desired, rubber catheters can be incorporated into the dressing just above the fine mesh gauze so that antibiotic solutions can be instilled periodically to keep the dressing and the wound moist. After waiting 48 to 72 hours, the dressings can be removed while irrigating copiously, and healthy tissue with a fine network of blood vessels will be found.

Filling the Defect with the Graft

In general, a graft on a convex surface can be placed on the wound with normal tension and held in place in whatever fashion is desired. The convexity will tend to hold the graft in place, and by securing it to the edges of the defect, the tendency toward shearing will be minimal. One must always remember that the secret to grafting is the amount of dermis that is placed into the wound and that it is a mistake to stretch a graft tightly to cause compression of the wound. This will result in less dermis being grafted, thereby yielding a poorer result. The graft itself will not cause pressure on the bed, as any amount of fluid will easily lift the graft up no matter how tightly it is stretched. Compression must come from external dressings. Any blood present under the graft should be irrigated out with saline (Fig. 48-28).

Grafts on the dorsum of the hand may be sutured in place with nylon sutures, and it is very quick and convenient to use skin staples.[15] This is especially true when mesh graft is being used. After closure is completed, the graft is covered with a compressive dressing and splint (Fig. 48-29). If infection is a concern, a material that is permeable to saline should be used so that irrigation of an antibiotic solution through a catheter can be accomplished. This is essential in the use of a meshed graft, since the graft has a tendency to dry out. The take will be much better if the graft is kept moist by periodic saline instillations.[41]

If infection is not judged to be a problem, it is preferable to cover the wound with a type of gauze that will not stick to the skin graft and pull it off at the time of dressing change. One excellent material for this use is scarlet red gauze (Fig. 48-30). This material, often called "magic red" by its devotees, is a messy substance that stains red on contact. Its superiority lies in the beeswax and other greasy substances in the base, and it makes an excellent dressing when covered with cotton balls that have been saturated in saline. This can be fitted over the wound to the desired shape and depth and then covered with a dressing and splint.

Grafts placed on a concave surface must always be held securely in place. They will have the natural tendency to float up off the wound as serum collects under them. One excellent method of preventing this is the use of a bolus or tie-over dressing. In this technique, grafts are placed into the concavity and sutured around the edges with strands of suture that are left long (Fig. 48-31). After completion of suturing, the graft is covered with scarlet red or a similar gauze and the concavity is filled with wet cotton. The ends of the sutures are then tied over the dressing to make a package that will hold the graft in place, preventing shearing, minimizing serous accumulation, and hopefully causing some pressure on the base of the wound. This is an especially good dressing for a full-thickness graft.

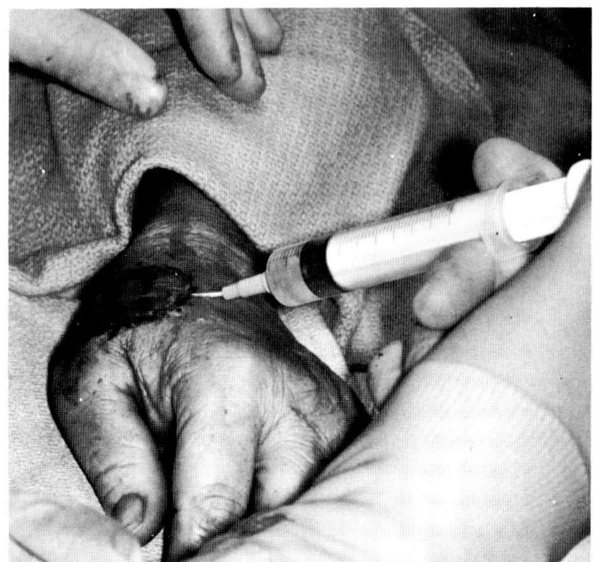

Fig. 48-28. All blood must be irrigated out from beneath a graft. This can be done with saline, using a syringe and flexible catheter.

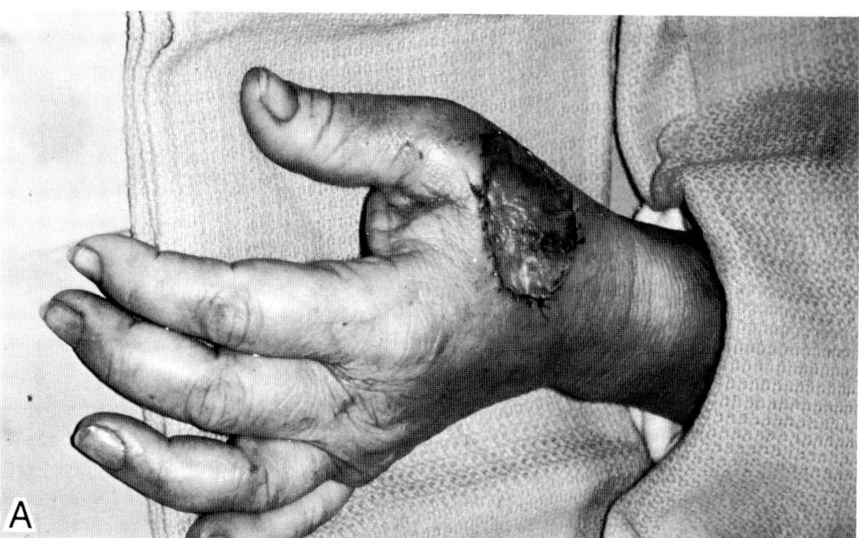

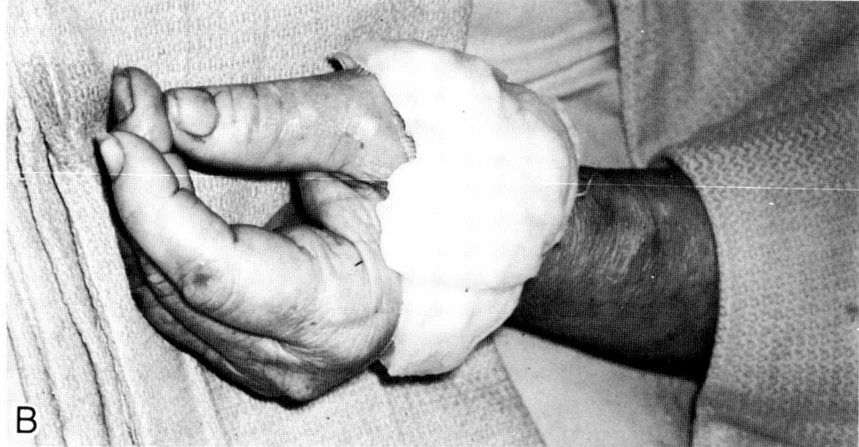

Fig. 48-29. Grafts on a convex surface **(A)** will tend to stay in place with minimal shearing force. A compressive dressing **(B)** and splint are sufficient.

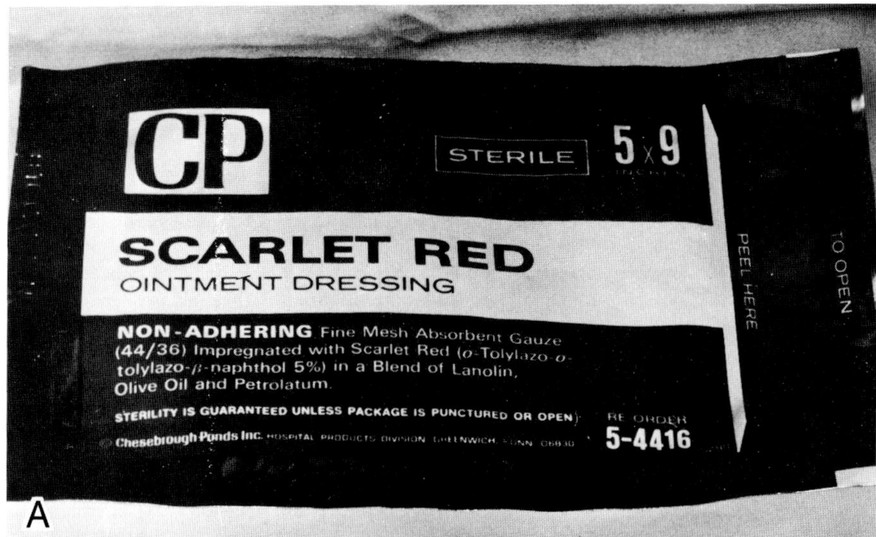

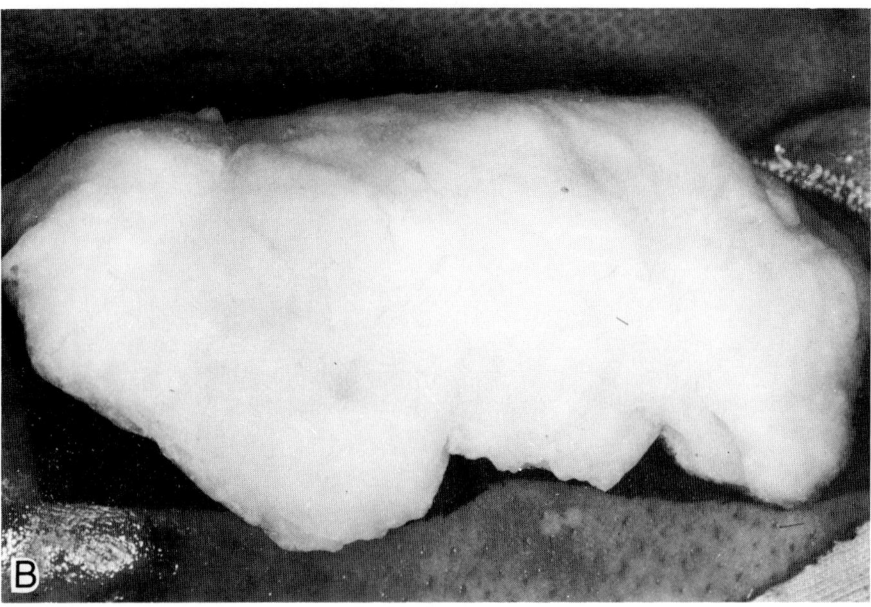

Fig. 48-30. Scarlet red gauze **(A)** covered by wet cotton balls **(B)** makes a nice compression dresssing that does not stick to the graft during dressing change. It is occlusive, however, and should not be used if there is risk of infection.

This bolus dressing can be used anywhere desired, but its use is difficult on a convex surface since the sutures tend to pull the graft up from the edges of the defect.

Postoperative Care

There are two schools of thought in caring for skin grafts.[16,17,21,27,49,62,67] Some surgeons like to look at the grafts within 24 hours so that if a hematoma is present it can be evacuated. The other school says that doing this might disturb the graft that is getting along well, and that a hematoma could be stirred up at that time. In addition, it is almost never possible to put on as good a dressing as the one put on at the time of operation.

My feeling is that one must consider the risk of hematoma and infection. If it is anticipated that either of these might be a problem, the dressing should be removed at 24 hours and the wound inspected periodically. If fluid collects under the graft, this should be evacuated by stabbing the graft with a #11 knife blade and gently rolling the graft with a cotton tip applicator in order to remove the fluid. Care should be taken to roll and not rub, since rubbing can cause shearing of the graft from the bed.

If there is really no reason to suspect that either of these problems will arise, the wound can be followed along just as any other wound would be. As long as there is no drainage, foul

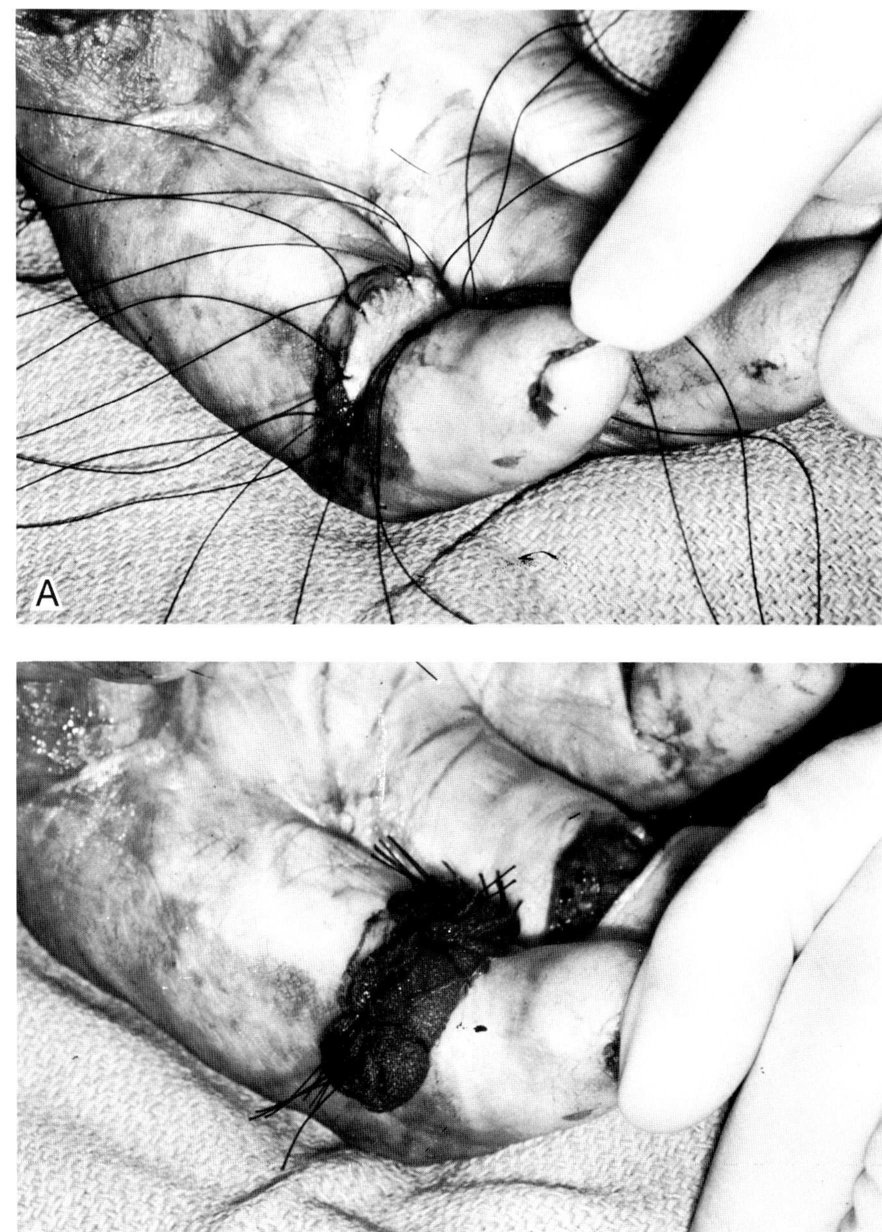

Fig. 48-31. A full-thickness graft in a concave surface being held into the depth of the defect by a tie-over dressing. Ends of the sutures are left long **(A)** and tied together over a bolus of gauze and cotton **(B)**.

smell, fever, or other cause for concern, the splint and dressing can be left undisturbed for 7 to 10 days. After this, the dressing can be removed, and if healing appears to be satisfactory, early guarded motion may begin.

It must be remembered that a skin graft is just like any other wound; that is, there is very little tensile strength present until enough collagen deposition has occurred to cause the wound to be strong. Therefore, even though the graft may be well vascularized at this stage, it will be very prone to injury due to shearing forces for another 10 days. If blisters develop, motion should be stopped and grafts should be adequately protected for a few more days. Usually, the grafts are adherent enough to allow the application of Jobst gloves about 10 to 14 days after the initial procedure.

Small areas of graft loss several millimeters in diameter will generally fill in satisfactorily without excessive scarring, especially if compression with a Jobst support is used.[37] Larger areas of loss should be debrided and regrafted. After the take is judged to be satisfactory, the grafts should be kept lubricated with a moisturizing lotion or a cream.

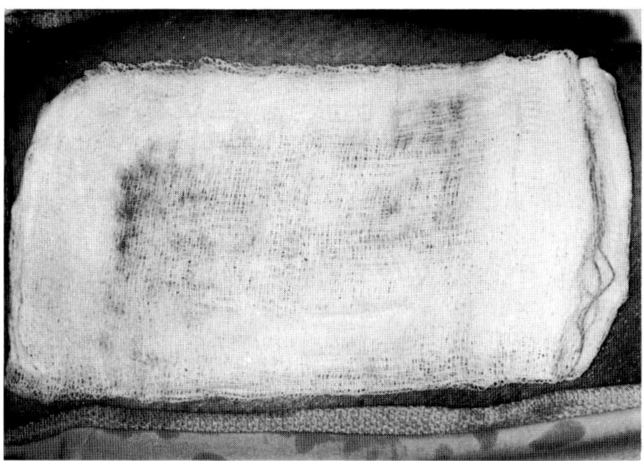
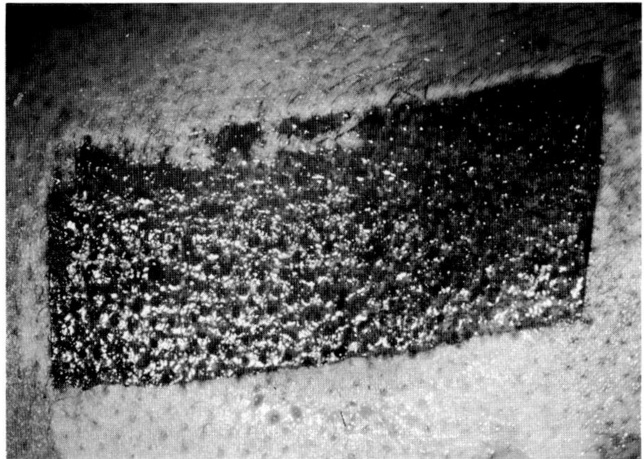

Fig. 48-32. If the donor site is treated by the open air method, the wound must be dried out before the patient leaves the operating table. This can be done by causing vasoconstriction with lidocaine with 1:200,000 epinephrine and keeping the wound dabbed dry until a thin fibrin layer forms.

Care of the Donor Site

Full-thickness sites require no special care and should be treated like any other wound. Split-thickness grafts, however, are a very morbid event, and the patient should be told before grafting that the donor site will probably cause a great deal more discomfort than the grafted area.

A donor site is just like a skinned knee. The sooner it dries out and forms a scab, the quicker it will become asymptomatic. This obviously is a factor of depth, as a thinner graft will heal much more rapidly than a thick graft. If a thin scab forms on the surface of the donor site, it will generally separate in about 14 days.

There are probably hundreds of ways of treating donor sites, involving application of every known kind of dressing or medication.[40,42,47,69] The longer it takes for the wound to become dry and the thicker the resultant eschar, however, the more morbidity the patient will suffer. I have tried almost all the methods and recommend the immediate open-exposure technique. It is imperative, however, that the wound be absolutely dry before the patient is removed from the operating table for this to work.

Immediately after removal of the skin graft, the donor areas should be covered with a sponge saturated in lidocaine containing 1:200,000 epinephrine (Fig. 48-32). This should be left undisturbed for 10 minutes or so until active bleeding has stopped. The gauze should then be carefully removed and another gauze containing the local anesthetic should be applied if there is any more oozing. Instead of using the epinephrine solution, topical thrombin concentration of 5000 units diluted in 5 ml of isotonic saline can be applied to the donor site, and then reapplied in a few minutes until all bleeding stops. This is just as effective and probably quicker, but the thrombin costs

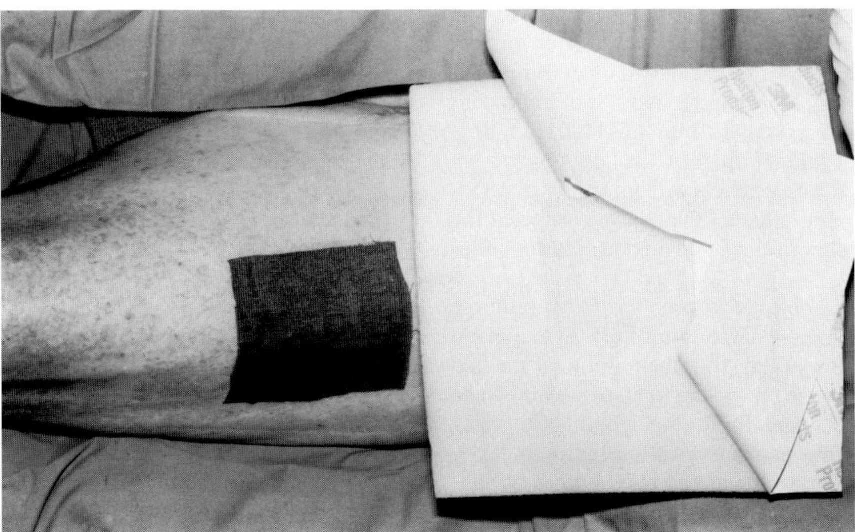

Fig. 48-33. The donor site has been covered with scarlet red gauze, which will be covered in turn by Reston foam. A square section of the adhesive surface has been removed to facilitate drainage.

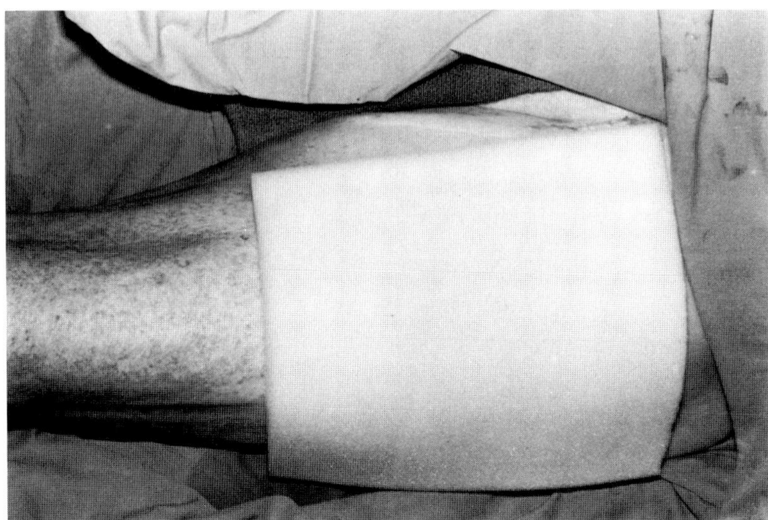

Fig. 48-34. Reston foam stuck in place on a leg, covering the donor site.

considerably more than the local anesthetic. A member of the operating team should be entrusted with the care of the donor site during the operation so that after the second gauze is removed, the wound will be completely dry and kept so by dabbing it with gauze. If a thin fibrin deposit is present over the surface of the wound and there is no bleeding at the completion of the procedure, the donor site will dry out very rapidly and the patient will suffer very little postoperative pain. The patient or his family can be supplied with gauze to keep dabbing at the donor site so that it can remain dry; periodic heat from a gooseneck lamp may help. If a thick bloody eschar is prevented, the wound will generally be quite dry within 24 hours and there will be very little discomfort with walking after 2 or 3 days.

The use of synthetic semipermeable membranes, such as Opsite, has become very popular, primarily because the pain is markedly reduced when the wound is covered and allowed to remain moist.[32-35] In this instance, the donor site is dried as much as possible, and the material is stretched over the raw area and tacked down to the intact skin. Although this is very effective in relieving pain, the wound remains moist and continues to ooze, and it is necessary to drain this fluid from time to time to prevent a coagulum from forming. I personally have had a number of very sad experiences with infections developing under the Opsite, and a few of these have converted the donor site into a very slow healing, and on one occasion, nonhealing wound.

Scarlet red gauze has objectively been shown to promote epithelialization.[38] Treatment of the donor site with scarlet red gauze results in excellent healing, but the traditional method that has been used of leaving the gauze open to the air can be quite painful. A very useful modification can be made by using scarlet red to produce the same moist, warm environment created by synthetic semipermeable membranes. First the donor bed must be made as dry as possible (as described in the text earlier). Just before ending the operation, the wound is covered with scarlet red gauze and that in turn covered with a polyurethane foam dressing (Fig. 48-33). 3M Corporation makes a very convenient product for this purpose, Reston foam, which can be gas sterilized. It comes in sheets with an excellent adhesive on one side, covered with a paper backing. The first step is to cut off a square of both paper and adhesive the same size as the donor site (as shown in Fig. 48-33) in order to allow fluid to ooze through, rather than collect under the gauze. Then all the paper backing is peeled off and the foam is stuck onto the skin surrounding the donor site (Fig. 48-34). The foam will absorb the oozing fluid and allow it to evaporate, but the remaining protein constituents on top of the greasy gauze will make the dressing semi-occlusive. The bed will dry out, the gauze will adhere, and epithelialization will take place underneath. One must take care to wash off any antiseptic solution from the skin surrounding the donor site, and to de-fat the area by washing carefully with alcohol before applying the foam. If that is done, the foam sticks beautifully to the skin and stays in place until the wound is healed, so that everything can be peeled off together. The foam acts as a cushion for clothing and the bed, and the donor site is almost totally pain free. Although I personally would want the open air technique used on me if I had a skin graft done, most people would not want to put up with it, so this technique has become my most frequent dressing.

REFERENCES

1. Abercrombie M, James DW, Newcombe JF: Wound contraction in rabbit skin. Studied by splinting the wound edges. J Anat 94:170–182, 1960
2. Adeymo O, Wyburn GM: Innervation of skin grafts. Transplant Bull 4:152–153, 1957
3. Ariyan S, Enriquez R, Krizek TJ: Wound contraction and fibrocontractive disorders. Arch Surg 113:1034–1046, 1978
4. Baran NK, Horton CE: Growth of skin grafts, flaps and scars in young minipigs. Plast Reconstr Surg 50:487–496, 1972
5. Barker DE: Skin thickness in the human. Plast Reconstr Surg 7:115–116, 1951

6. Barnett AB, Ott R, Laub DR: Failure of healing of split skin graft donor sites in anhidrotic ectodermal dysplasia. Plast Reconstr Surg 64:97-100, 1979
7. Bauer PS, Larson DL, Stacey TR: The observation of myofibroblasts in hypertrophic scars. Surg Gynecol Obstet 141:22-26, 1975
8. Bellman S, Velander E, Frank HA, Lambert PB: Survival of arteries in experimental full thickness skin autografts. Transplantation 2:167-174, 1964
9. Bennett JE, Miller SR: Evolution of the electrodermatome. Plast Reconstr Surg 45:131-134, 1970
10. Birch J, Branemark PI: The vascularization of a free full thickness skin graft. I. A vital microscopic study. Scand J Plast Reconstr Surg 3:1-10, 1969
11. Birch J, Branemark PI, Lundskog J: The vascularization of a free full thickness skin graft. II. A microangiographic study. Scand J Plast Reconstr Surg 3:11-17, 1969
12. Birch J, Branemark PI, Nilsson K: The vascularization of a free full thickness skin graft. III. An infrared thermographic study. Scand J Plast Reconstr Surg 3:18-22, 1969
13. Blair VP, Brown JB: Use and uses of large split skin grafts of intermediate thickness. Surg Gynecol Obstet 49:82-97, 1929
14. Briggaman RA, Wheeler CE: Epidermal-dermal interactions in adult human skin: Role of dermis in epidermal maintenance. J Invest Dermatol 51:454-465, 1968
15. Brody GS, Mackby LF: Rapid application of skin grafts. Arch Surg 112:855-856, 1977
16. Brown JB, McDowell F: Massive repairs of burns with thick split skin grafts. Ann Surg 115:658-674, 1942
17. Brown JB, McDowell F: Skin Grafting. 3rd Ed. JB Lippincott, Philadelphia, 1958
18. Browne EZ: Complications of skin grafts and pedicle flaps. Hand Clinics 2:353-359, 1986
19. Castermans A: Vascularization of skin grafts. Transplant Bull 4:153-154, 1957
20. Clemmesen T: The early circulation in split-skin grafts. Restoration of blood supply to split-skin autografts. Acta Chir Scand 127:1-8, 1964
21. Converse JM, McCarthy JG, Brauer RO, Ballantyne DL: Transplantation of skin: Grafts and flaps. pp. 152-239. In Converse JM (ed): Reconstructive Plastic Surgery. 2nd Ed. WB Saunders, Philadelphia, 1977
22. Converse JM, Rapaport FT: The vascularization of skin autografts and homografts: An experimental study in man. Ann Surg 143:306-315, 1956
23. Converse JM, Smahel J, Ballantyne DL, Harper AD: Innosculation of vessels of skin graft and host bed: A fortuitous encounter. Br J Plast Surg 28:274-282, 1975
24. Converse JM, Uhlschmid GK, Ballantyne DL: "Plasmatic circulation" in skin grafts. Plast Reconstr Surg 43:495-499, 1969
25. Corps BVM: The effect of graft thickness, donor site and graft bed on graft shrinkage in the hooded rat. Br J Plast Surg 22:125-133, 1969
26. Creech BJ, DeVito RV, Eade GG: Viability of split skin grafts from pigs following incubation on autologous blood or serum for various periods. Plast Reconstr Surg 51:572-574, 1973
27. Cronin TD: The use of a molded splint to prevent contracture after split skin grafting on the neck. Plast Reconstr Surg 27:7-18, 1961
28. Cuthbertson AM: Contraction of full thickness skin wounds in the rat. Surg Gynecol Obstet 108:421-432, 1959
29. Das SK, Munro IR: Painless wettable split-skin graft donor site dressings. Ann Plast Surg 7:48-53, 1981
30. Dellon AL: Two point discrimination and Meissner corpuscles. Plast Reconstr Surg 60:270-271, 1977
31. Dinner MI, Peters CR, Sherer J: Use of semipermeable polyurethane membrane as a dressing for split skin graft donor sites. Plast Reconstr Surg 64:112-114, 1979
32. Donoff RB, Grillo HC: The effects of skin grafting on healing open wounds in rabbits. J Surg Res 19:163-167, 1975
33. Fitzgerald MJT, Martin F, Paletta FX: Innervation of skin grafts. Surg Gynecol Obstet 124:808-812, 1967
34. Fodor PB: Scarlet red. Ann Plast Surg 4:45-47, 1980
35. Gabbiani G, Hirschel BJ, Ryan GB, Statkov PR, Majno G: Granulation tissue as a contractile organ. A study of structure and function. J Exp Med 135:719-734, 1972
36. Gabbiani G, Majno G: Dupuytren's contracture: Fibroblast contraction? An ultrastructural study. Am J Pathol 66:131-138, 1972
37. Gingrass P, Grabb WC, Gingrass RP: Rat skin autografts over Silastic implants:A study of the bridging phenomenon. Plast Reconstr Surg 55:65-70, 1975
38. Golden GT, Power CG, Skinner JR, Fox JW, Hiebert JM, Edgerton MT, Edlich RF: A technic of lower extremity mesh grafting with early ambulation. Am J Surg 133:646-647, 1977
39. Goulian D: A new economical dermatome. Plast Reconstr Surg 42:85-86, 1968
40. Hagstrom WJ, Landa SJF, Elstrom JA, Stuteville OH, Beers MD: The use of a hemostatic agent as a definitive dressing in the management of the donor sites in partial thickness skin grafting. Plast Reconstr Surg 39:628-632, 1967
41. Hagstrom WJ, Nassos TP, Boswick JA, Stuteville OH: The importance of occlusive dressings in the treatment of mesh skin grafts. Plast Reconstr Surg 38:137-141, 1966
42. Harris DR, Filarsky SA, Hector RE: The effect of Silastic sheet dressings on the healing of spilt skin donor sites. Plast Reconstr Surg 52:189-190, 1973
43. Heggars JP, Robson MC, Ristroph JD: A rapid method of performing quantitative wound cultures. Milit Med 134:666-667, 1969
44. Horch KW, Tuckett RP, Burgess PR: A key to the classification of cutaneous mechanoreceptors. J Invest Dermatol 69:75-82, 1977
45. Hurst LN, Brown DH, Murray KA: Prolonged life and improved quality for stored skin grafts. Plast Reconstr Surg 73:105-109, 1984
46. Jackson DM, Stone PA: Tangential excision and grafting of burns. Br J Plast Surg 25:416-426, 1972
47. Koonin AJ, Melmed EP: Painless donor sites. S Afr Med J 47:2241-2242, 1973
48. Krizek TJ, Robson MC, Kho E: Bacterial growth and skin graft survival. Surg Forum 18:518-519, 1967
49. Lehman JA, Saddawi N: Delayed open skin grafting. Br J Plast Surg 28:46-48, 1975
50. Lever WF: Histology of the skin. pp. 9-45. In Lever WF, Shaumburg-Lever G (eds): Histopathology of the Skin. 5th Ed. JB Lippincott, Philadelphia, 1975
51. Levine NS, Lindberg RB, Mason AD, Pruitt BA: The quantitative swab culture and smear: A quick, simple method for determining the number of viable aerobic bacteria on open wounds. J Trauma 16:89-94, 1976
52. Lopez-Mas J, Ortiz-Monasterio F, Viale de Gonzalez M, Olmedo A: Skin graft pigmentation. A new approach to prevention. Plast Reconstr Surg 49:18-21, 1972
53. MacMillan BG: The use of mesh grafting in treating burns. Surg Clin North Am 50:1347-1359, 1970
54. Madden JW: On the "contractile fibroblast." Plast Reconstr Surg 52:291-292, 1973
55. Maquieira NO: An innervated full-thickness skin graft to restore sensibility to fingertips and heels. Plast Reconstr Surg 53:568-575, 1974
56. Micks JE, Wilson JN: Full-thickness sole skin grafts for resurfacing the hand. J Bone Joint Surg 49A:1128-1134, 1967

57. Mir y Mir L: The problem of pigmentation in the cutaneous graft. Br J Plast Surg 14:303-307, 1961
58. Montagna W: Morphology of cutaneous sensory receptors. J Invest Dermatol 69:4-7, 1977
59. Morton D, Madden JW, Peacock EE: Effect of a local smooth muscle antagonist on wound contraction. Surg Forum 23:511-512, 1972
60. Nakayama Y, Chuang YM: A scalpel blade as a substitute for calibrator of the dermatome. Plast Reconstr Surg 72:405-407, 1983
61. Peacock EE, Van Winkle W: Wound Repair. 2nd Ed. WB Saunders, Philadelphia, 1976
62. Polk HC: Adherence of thin skin grafts. Surg Forum 17:487-489, 1966
63. Reese JD: Dermatape: A new method for management of split skin grafts. Plast Reconstr Surg 1:98-105, 1946
64. Reverdin JL: De la Greffe epidermique. Arch Gen Med 19:276, 555, 703, 1972
65. Rogers BO: Historical development of free skin grafting. Surg Clin North Am 39:289-311, 1959
66. Rudolph R: Inhibition of myofibroblasts by skin grafts. Plast Reconstr Surg 63:473-480, 1979
67. Rudolph R, Fisher JC, Ninnemann JL: Skin Grafting. Little, Brown, Boston, 1979
68. Rudolph R, Suzuki M, Guber S, Woodward M: Control of contractile fibroblasts by skin grafts. Surg Forum 28:524-525, 1977
69. Sawhney CP, Subbaraju GV, Chakravarti RN: Healing of donor sites of split skin graft. Br J Plat Reconstr Surg 22:359-364, 1969
70. Shepard GH: The storage of split skin grafts on their donor sites. Clinical and experimental study. Plast Reconstr Surg 49:115-122, 1972
71. Smahel J, Ganzoni N: Experiments with mesh grafts. Acta Chir Plast (Prague) 14:90-99, 1972
72. Smith DJ, Hughes CE: Application of topical thrombin for skin graft donor sites. Plast Reconstr Surg 69:1028-1029, 1982
73. Southwood WFW: The thickness of the skin. Plast Reconstr Surg 15:423-429, 1955
74. Stone PA, Madden JW: Effect of primary and delayed skin grafting on wound contraction. Surg Forum 25:41-44, 1974
75. Terzis JK: Functional aspects of reinnervation of free skin grafts. Plast Reconstr Surg 58:142-156, 1976
76. Thiersch C: Über Hautverplanzung. Verh Dtsch Ges Chir 15:17, 1886
77. Vecchione TR: Hair growth as a late sequela in skin grafts from the groin. Br J Plast Surg 30:52-53, 1977
78. Wolfe JR: A new method of performing plastic operations. Br Med J 2:360, 1875

49

Skin Flaps

Graham D. Lister

Healing by secondary intention involves significant scar formation. Since scar limits the motion that is essential for function in many areas of the upper extremity, every effort must be made to achieve primary wound healing. Skin defects that are the result of injury or surgery should therefore be closed directly or covered with imported skin. In certain situations free skin grafts will suffice. In others, free grafts may not "take" or may, by their necessary adhesion to underlying tissue, be unsuitable. "Take" of a skin graft requires that the bed on which it is placed have a blood supply adequate to revascularize the free graft. This blood supply is not present when bare bone, cartilage, or tendon is exposed in the wound. "Take" requires firm adhesion of the graft. This is not acceptable when further surgery is planned beneath the new skin cover, for example, when tendon grafts will be necessary after a road surface avulsion of the dorsum of the hand. It is also not suitable where the firm adhesion of the graft prevents mobility of the skin envelope over underlying structures, for example where a graft on a finger tip is adherent to bone. Shear forces applied in daily use will cause intermittent avascularity of the skin and eventual breakdown. A similar mechanism of breakdown may occur when grafts have been placed over the convex aspect of joints. Flexion renders the graft taut and avascular. That allied with normal trauma results in ulceration. To a degree that is inversely proportional to its content of dermis, a free skin graft will contract during the 6 months after its application to the extent that its location permits. Thus on the dorsum of the hand, which is subjected to repeated stretching by normal use, less contracture will occur than on the flexion aspect of a joint. In the latter location only full-thickness grafts with perfect take are suitable. In any of the circumstances outlined above where free grafts do not provide the best skin, flap cover is indicated.

TYPES OF FLAPS

A flap is skin with a varying amount of underlying tissue that is used to cover a defect and that receives its blood supply from a source other than the tissue on which it is laid. That part of the flap that provides the blood supply is termed the "pedicle." The term "pedicle flap" is tautologous, as all flaps have pedicles. Table 49-1 lists the various flaps discussed in this chapter.

Random-Pattern Flaps

The manner in which the skin receives its blood supply has been studied by many anatomists, notably Tomsa, Spalteholz, Manchot, and Salmon.[327] In recent years, Lamberty[176] has again described angiotomes in the upper limb, these being areas of skin with a known single arterial supply. The constancy of these arteries has been confirmed by Doppler studies in patients[325] and volunteers.[126] Taylor[324] has studied the "venosomes" and reported that venous territories correspond closely to recognized areas of arterial supply. Pearl[251,252] has shown that this supply may be present in four vascular layers or strata—subdermal, subcutaneous,[202] fascial, and muscular. The blood supply of a flap may come, not from a single arteriovenous pedicle, but from the many minute vessels of the subdermal or subcutaneous plexus. Such a flap is termed "random pattern."[218] Although the shape of the flap need not be quadrilateral, it is usually conceived as such and it is raised by incising three of the four sides. The fourth constitutes the pedicle, or "base" of the flap. The side opposite the base is called the "free margin." Since the adequacy of the subdermal plexus varies from location to location, the area of skin that can be sup-

Table 49-1. Types of Flaps Discussed in this Chapter

	Random	Axial
Local	Transposition	Axial flag FDMA SDMA Reversed dorsal metacarpal
	Rotation	
	Advancement—rectangular	Advancement—V-Y (Moberg)
Regional	Cross-finger Thenar	Neurovascular island Fillet Scapular Forearm Reversed PIA Latissimus
Distant	Infraclavicular Cross-arm	Groin

ported by the vessels of the pedicle also varies. As a general rule, a random-pattern flap with a length not exceeding the width of the pedicle, in other words a rhomboid, is considered to be reliable with respect to blood supply. This is the "one-to-one" (1:1) rule. It does not always apply. For example, it is too cautious for the face and too bold for the foot. Observation of the rule and the need to protect the pedicle from undue distortion that would impair blood flow through the subdermal plexus clearly limit the range of applications for the random-pattern flap. This rather inadequate blood supply of the random-pattern flap may be enhanced by a "delay" procedure.[87,216,332] In a delay, the margins of the flap are incised and the flap raised, but it is then sutured back into its bed. The flap is only transferred some time later, at which point it is more robust and better vascularized. The optimum delay has been shown to be around 10 days. During that time both arteries and veins that were random become enlarged and oriented parallel to the axis of the pedicle. They are therefore more able to support the flap when it is transferred.

Axial-Pattern Flaps

Where a flap receives its blood supply from a single, constant vessel, it is termed "axial pattern." Such a single vessel is materially larger than those of the subdermal plexus. For example, the superficial circumflex iliac artery that supplies the groin flap (see page 1803) has an average diameter of 2 mm, or five times that of the largest subdermal vessel. While Poiseuille's law of flow in rigid tubes cannot be applied precisely to blood vessels, it indicates that flow would be approximately 625 times greater through the axial vessel of the groin flap than through a subdermal vessel. The area of skin supplied by such an axial vessel is termed a "vascular territory."

Where the vascular territories of two axial pedicles meet is termed a "watershed," and the small arteries that cross it, "choke vessels." In these areas veins have no valves and can be said to allow blood to "oscillate" between territories. Occlusion of one of the two pedicles results in a shift of the watershed toward the occlusion, extending the vascular territory of the other, open pedicle. In raising an axial-pattern flap, it is safe to increase the length of the flap beyond the known vascular territory by that amount which would constitute a random-pattern flap. That is, a safe axial-pattern flap equals the vascular territory plus a 1:1 extension.

The vessel of an axial-pattern flap may be purely cutaneous (Fig. 49-1A), supplying skin alone and proceeding directly to it. The superficial circumflex iliac artery to the groin flap is such a vessel. In reaching its cutaneous territory, the axial vessel may first supply fascia (Fig. 49-1B). In such circumstances, the vessel commonly reaches the fascia by running in an intermuscular septum. Since this is attached to bone, a segment of bone may be taken with skin and be vascularized by the same pedicle. Axial flaps whose vessels first pass through fascia are termed "fasciocutaneous." As with the musculocutaneous flap, fascia may be transferred without skin, but not skin without fascia. Such a flap is the lateral arm flap supplied by the posterior radial collateral artery. The axial vessel may first supply muscle (Fig. 49-1C). The secondary vessels to the overlying skin are multiple,[27] so that the muscle must be taken with the skin to ensure survival of the skin, but may itself be transferred

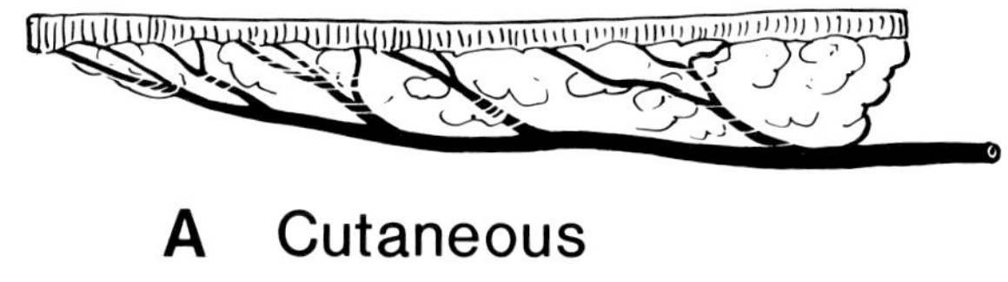

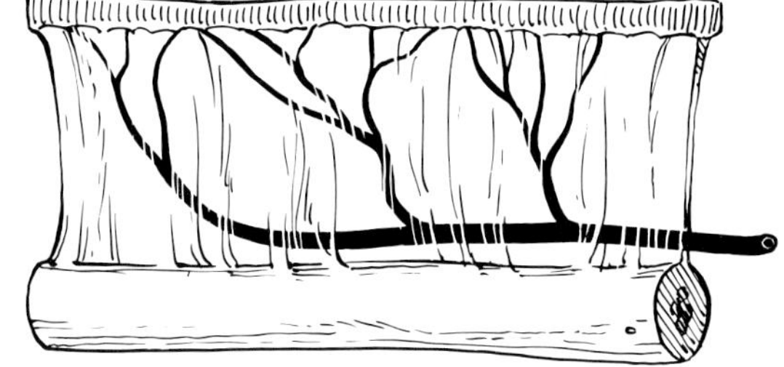

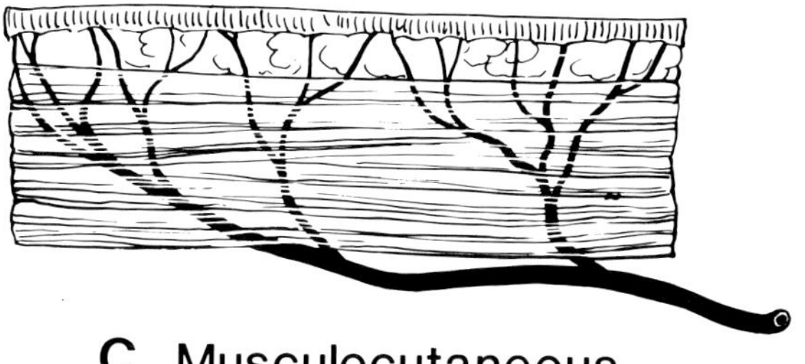

Fig. 49-1. Axial pattern flaps are either cutaneous, fasciocutaneous, or musculocutaneous depending upon the source of the major portion of their blood supply. Fasciocutaneous vessels commonly run in intermuscular septa and therefore supply the periosteum of underlying bone. The flap can be taken with a segment of that bone where necessary.

without skin. Such flaps have been called "musculocutaneous," "myocutaneous," and "myodermal." An example is the latissimus dorsi flap, supplied by the thoracodorsal artery.

Axial-pattern flaps clearly have several advantages over the random pattern. The 1 : 1 ratio can be disregarded. Axial flaps with a much larger ratio will have a blood supply superior to that of random flaps. It has been shown experimentally that axial-pattern flaps resist infection better than random.[253] Because flaps can be made longer, they can cover a larger primary defect. In addition, the flap tissue adjacent to the pedicle need not be applied to the defect, permitting much more freedom of movement of the part to which the flap is attached. This "bridge segment" between the primary and secondary defects may be sutured free edge to free edge, creating a tube that closes off all exposed subcutaneous tissue—a "tube pedicle." A further advantage of the axial-pattern flap is that the pedicle can be made much narrower, even to the point of reducing it to the (neuro)arteriovenous bundle itself, in which event it is called an "island" or "kite" flap. This permits much more movement of the flap than is possible with a wide skin pedicle. Finally, with the advent of reliable microvascular technology, the pedicle can be divided and anastomosed to vessels adjacent to the primary defect—the so-called "free flap." The disadvantage of the axial-pattern flap is that its vascular pedicle must always be preserved at the time of raising; it cannot at that first stage, therefore, be thinned to the same degree as a random-pattern flap that depends on the subdermal vessels. The vascular advantages of the axial flap are all lost when the pedicle is divided. Indeed, in those instances in which skin from the bridge segment is to be used on an area adjacent to the primary defect, it is prudent to divide the artery in the pedicle 1 week before complete detachment. This constitutes a delay of sorts, as it promotes increased blood flow across the wound of inset into the primary defect.

Staging of Flaps

Flaps that come from skin adjacent to the primary defect are called "local." They require only one operative procedure for their completion. Flaps that come from elsewhere on the limb and commonly require two stages are called "regional." Those from other parts of the body are dubbed "distant." With the exception of free flaps, all distant flaps require at least two stages. In the first, the flap is "raised" and "applied," "attached," or "inset." In the second, the pedicle is divided and the free margins "inset." This commonly requires the excision of fibrous tissue that has formed between the base of the flap and the primary defect to permit a smooth closure. In certain instances where the blood supply is doubtful after division of the pedicle, the final inset may be left until a third stage. All three categories of flap—local, regional, and distant—have both random and axial pattern varieties.

The wound to which a flap is to be applied is called the "primary defect" or "recipient site." This may be simply the wound created by trauma. However, this is rare, for the skin margins are rarely perfect in such a case. It is usually necessary to excise the wound edges to healthy skin. Similarly, it is important in creating the primary defect in secondary reconstruction that all scarred skin be excised so that the flap will be sutured to healthy margins. A "pattern" of this final primary defect should be taken for future use. This is easily done by marking the margins with ink and taking an imprint of this with a pliable, nonporous material (e.g., a piece of Esmarch bandage), the surface of which has been moistened with alcohol (see Fig. 49-42A). The wound from which the flap is taken is termed the "secondary defect." The secondary defect may be closed directly, as in a groin flap, or may require application of a skin graft, as in a cross-finger flap. The region from which a skin graft is taken is called the "donor site."

Raising a Flap

Between the vascular strata defined above—subdermis, subcutaneous tissue, fascia, and muscle—lie relatively avascular planes. It is in these planes that the dissection of the elected flap should proceed. It is evident that, in order to attain these planes, it is necessary to cut through the vessels of the more superficial strata. Thus, in raising a fascial flap, one must first incise the subdermal and subcutaneous plexus and then the fascia. Only when the surgeon has cut through the peripheral ramifications of the vessels from which the flap obtains its blood supply is he in the correct plane. To be one plane too superficial results in division of the vessel, or branches of the vessel, supplying the flap. To be one plane too deep results in a time-consuming, often bloody, and entirely unnecessary struggle.

Applied tension plays a major role in flap dissection. Once the marginal incision has been carried down to the correct plane for dissection, skin hooks or stay sutures should be applied to the corners of the flap. Firm upward traction away from the bed will display the plane for dissection. Often this contains only loose areolar tissue that can be stroked away with a knife. Care must be taken not to create a "cave" beneath the flap; that is, a central recess between two marginal pillars of unincised skin, muscle or fascia. No tension can be applied to the tissues in such a cave, and dissection therein may result in damage to the pedicle. Rather, the marginal pillars should be incised progressively in such a way as to avoid caves and permit tension to be applied evenly, thereby protecting the pedicle. Tension on a flap lifts the pedicle off the floor of the secondary defect, on which the knife is dissecting, into the roof formed by the inclined vascular stratum. If dissection proceeds far enough, a point will be reached where the pedicle emerges through the floor to gain the roof. At that point the surgeon decides whether he needs to proceed. To do so will require dissection of the pedicle. All progress thus far is best made with a scalpel. A scalpel is the instrument of choice both to incise the vascular strata and to dissect the planes, provided only that appropriate tension can be applied to the tissues. Cutting with a knife is a result of two opposing forces: the pressure applied to the knife and the resistance offered by the tissues. The traction applied to a flap produces, and varies, that resistance. It therefore plays a primary role in determining which tissue is cut and which is not. This is why the blade must always be equally sharp, and why the assistant who holds the flap must do so at

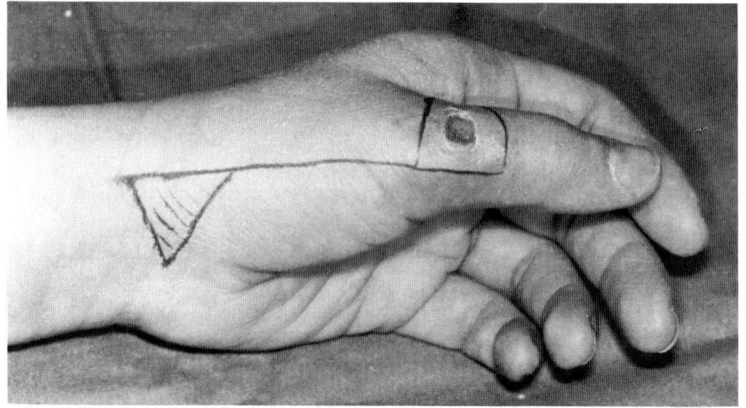

A

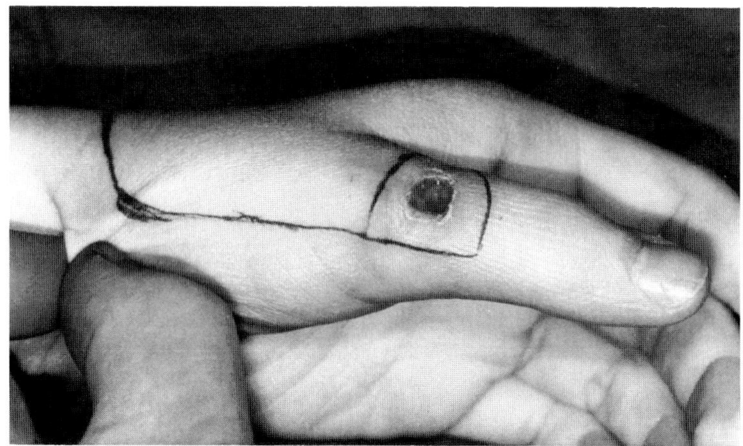

B

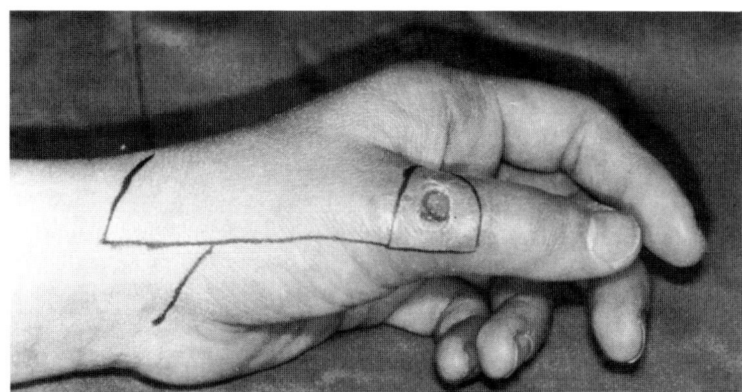

C

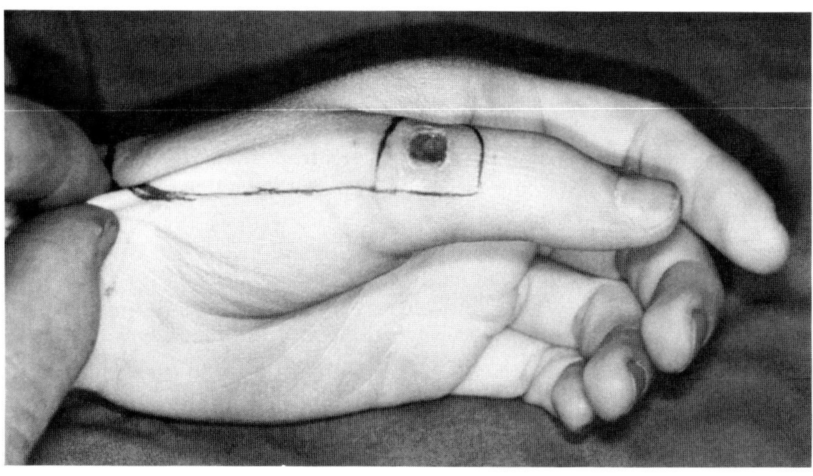

D

Fig. 49-2. Testing for maximum extensibility in choosing the best area from which to obtain tissue to close the ulcer on the dorsal aspect of the thumb. **(A&B)** The use of the Burow's triangle with a sliding transposition flap would require tissue to be available in the longitudinal axis on the palmar surface of the wrist. **(C&D)** If it were elected to use a Z-plasty to advance the tissue by the lengthening of the central limb, then tissue would need to be available around the circumference of the wrist, since lengthening of the central limb requires shortening of the transverse axis. *(Figure continues.)*

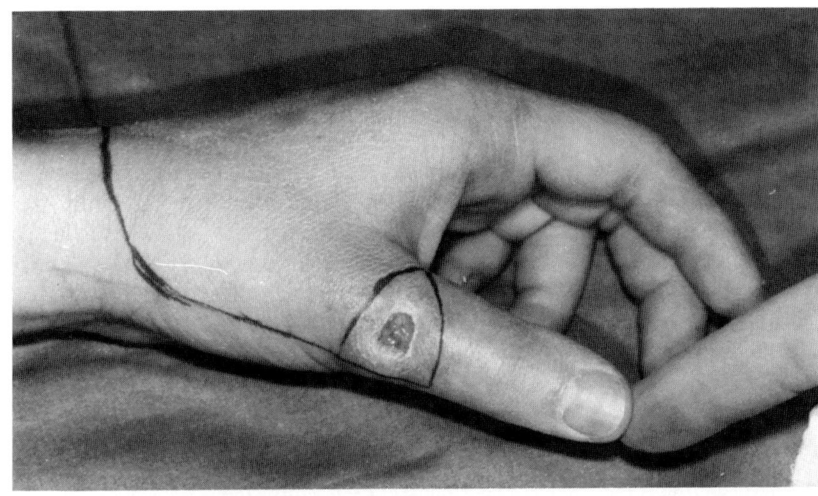
E

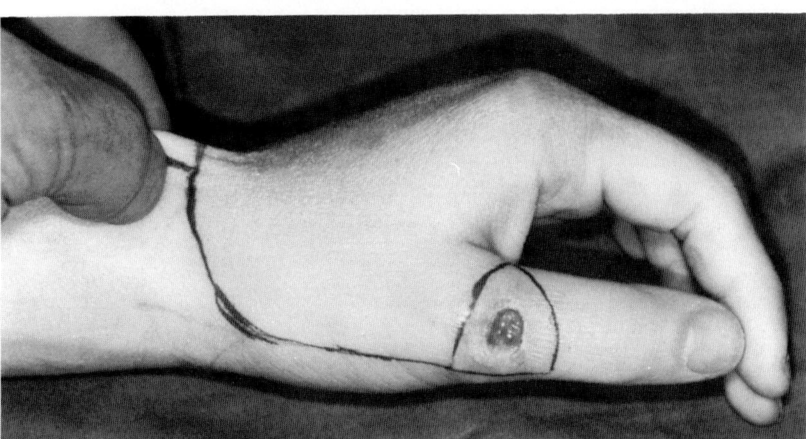
F

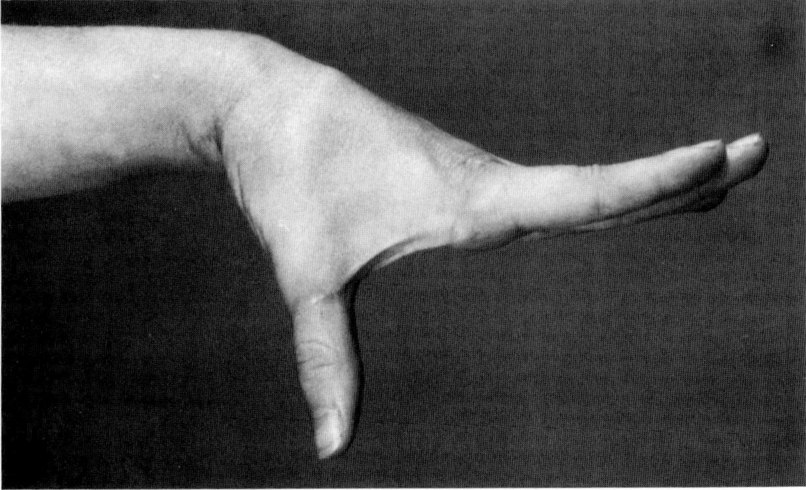
G

Fig. 49-2 *(Continued).* **(E&F)** If a rotation flap were selected then tissue would be required on the opposite aspect of the rotation flap from the defect; that is in the circumference of the wrist on its dorsal aspect. **(G)** A rotation flap was selected and satisfactory healing achieved.

the tension first applied by the surgeon. If he cannot do so, the surgeon must apply the necessary tension by grasping and lifting surrounding tissues with dissecting forceps as he proceeds.

Scissors provide both the pressure and the resistance required to cut tissue. They are required where the surgeon cannot efficiently control the relationship between tissue tension and knife pressure. When scissors are introduced closed into the tissues and then opened under gentle pressure to clear planes, they can be both precise and innocuous. They create and enter "caves," defining structures to be preserved and those to be divided. When scissors are introduced open and then closed to cut, they are less precise than a knife and can do harm in the hands of the most experienced. It is therefore important when using scissors to cut that the surgeon see both surfaces of the tissue to be divided so that he is confident what tissues are included between the jaws of the scissors. This often requires that closed-to-open scissor dissection proceed until the instrument can be seen through the tissue to be cut. Such scissor dissection is required as a vascular pedicle is mobilized. Although it has been shown that metal clips are not secure and that bipolar coagulation may harm the pedicle,[276] both are routinely employed in dissecting the pedicle. The clips must be applied with sufficient force to ensure that they will not slip. The coagulation must be of adequate temperature and the pedicle (i.e., the main vessel) should be insulated by holding the branch with smooth forceps between the pedicle and the point of coagulation.

LOCAL FLAPS

Since they are of identical or similar qualities to the skin lost, local flaps are the most desirable means of providing cover for a defect.[185] They are, however, severely limited in their availability. This is because there is relatively little skin on the hand and because much of it must remain inviolate to preserve function. The skin of the webs, for example, should never be used for flaps, nor should areas of daily contact. Some skin, such as that of the palm, will not move to the extent necessary for most local flap design. The surgeon must carefully weigh these considerations in selecting a flap. "Lines of maximum extensibility"[187] around which the flap should be planned should be selected by pinching the skin (Fig. 49-2A–G). These are the lines along which skin is most available, and therefore pinches up more easily. This should be done with the hand in various positions to ensure that function will not be impaired. For example, the skin of the dorsum appears superfluous in extension, but not in flexion.

There are three groups of local flap: "transposition," "rotation," and "advancement." In the advancement flap the pedicle is that side of the flap opposite the primary defect. In transposition and rotation designs the flap moves laterally relative to the pedicle to cover the defect. These two differ in that the transposition flap leaves a secondary defect that is closed either directly or by application of new skin cover, while the rotation flap leaves no secondary defect, the flap skin being stretched to close the primary defect. This is achieved by "differential suturing" in which a slightly smaller amount of the flap edge than of the edge of the bed is included between each two adjacent sutures, thereby advancing the flap. Transposition and advancement flaps may be random or axial pattern in design. The vascular basis of the axial pattern may be simply a subcutaneous pedicle rich in small vessels[81] or, more reliably, a single known vessel. The advantage of the axial pattern, apart from its potentially larger area and greater reliability due to superior circulation, is the fact that its pedicle can be reduced to the vessels alone, giving greater mobility. In the advancement flap this simply permits more advancement, a gain that can be measured in millimeters. In the axial-pattern transposition flap, however, the gain in mobility is limited only by the length of pedicle that can be developed. The longer the pedicle, the more the flap becomes a vascular island flap rather than a simple transposition. The distinction between a long axial transposition flap and a vascular island is arbitrary. For the purposes of this chapter, a flap has been classified as a vascular island when the pedicle is the proper digital artery or larger.

Transposition Flaps

Random Pattern

The theory behind transposition flaps has been analyzed in some detail.[186] There are two basic types of random-pattern transposition flap.

Type I — Transposition Leaving a Secondary Defect Requiring Skin Cover

The basic design of this first type and the problems likely to be encountered in its use can be illustrated by using an equilateral model (Fig. 49-3). The first step in planning such a flap is to triangulate the primary defect, either in fact or conceptually. In the equilateral model (FLA in Fig. 49-3[1]), one side of the defect is extended by its own length (to P). From the end of that extension, another line of equal length (PS) is drawn parallel to the nearest side (AF) of the primary defect. The end of that line (S) is the most important in the whole design and is called the *pivot point.* As the flap is raised and transposed, it is this point around which the flap moves into the primary defect. By measuring from the pivot point to the far corner of the defect (S to L) and then to the diagonally opposite corner of the flap (S to A), one determines the amount by which the flap must stretch to cover the defect. The latter dimension (SA) is consequently called the *critical line.* In the simple equilateral model the critical line would have to stretch by 75 percent of its original length to achieve closure of the primary defect (Fig. 49-3[2]), which is beyond the physical capabilities of normal skin.[178] Several solutions are available.

A Wider Flap. If the length of the first line drawn (AP) is doubled, the stretch required in the critical line of the resultant flap becomes 50 percent. If it is made three times longer, the stretch becomes 33 percent (Fig. 49-3[3] and 3[4]); four times, 25 percent; five times, 16 percent. It follows that to avoid vascular embarrassment due to excessive tension, flaps should be made as wide as local tissues will permit.

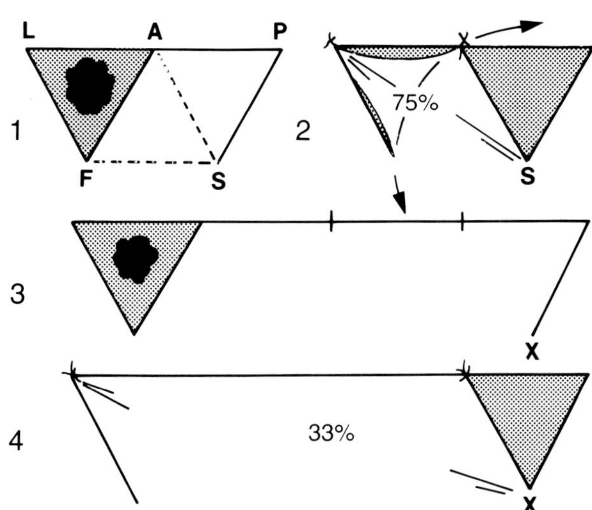

Fig. 49-3. Transposition flap. In this equilateral model *(1)* all lines are equal in length. *S* is the pivot point and *SA* the critical line, since this is the skin that will have to stretch as the flap is transposed *(2)* into the primary defect. The lengthening on the critical line in an equilateral design is 75 percent. One device to reduce the stretch on the critical line is to make the flap wider. If as here the flap is three times as wide *(3)*, the stretch required in the critical line *(4)* is 33 percent. (Modified from Lister,[185] with permission.)

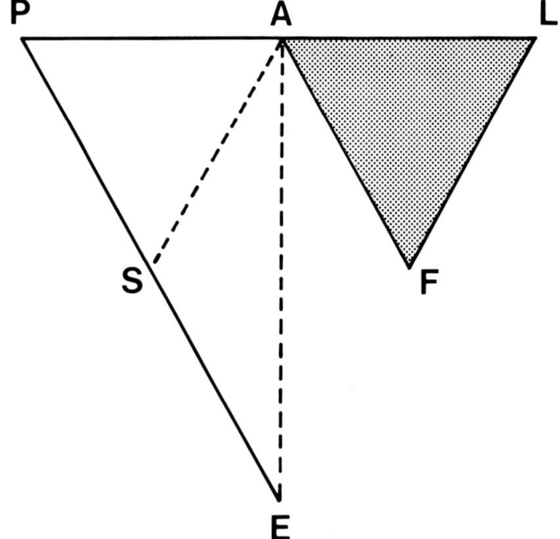

Fig. 49-4. Extension cut. An extension cut has been made here from *S* to *E* of the same length as all other lines in this design. The resultant stretch required in the critical line, now *EA*, is 16 percent. (Modified from Lister,[185] with permission.)

A Longer Flap Design. Lengthening FA and SP (in Fig. 49-3[1]) to move the free margin of the flap (AP) further from the base will lengthen the critical line and thereby decrease tension after transposition. However, there are two adverse effects. First, the design exceeds the length/breadth ratio of 1 : 1, thereby jeopardizing the circulation of the flap. Second, the flap does not "fit" well since the edges to be sutured (FL to FA) are now of differing lengths, creating a "dog-ear" at F. (Whenever an open angle of skin is closed, a standing cone or dog-ear is created.[181])

An Extension Cut. If the second cut of the flap is extended (to E in Fig. 49-4), thereby shifting the pivot point, the critical line is lengthened. If the cut is lengthened by a distance equal to all other cuts in the equilateral model (SE in Fig. 49-4), the stretch necessary in the critical line becomes only 16 percent.

A Back Cut. The pivot point can be moved closer to the primary defect by incising toward its apex, thereby reducing the stretch required in the critical line. This incision (SB in Fig. 49-5) toward the primary defect is a back cut.

Both extension and back cuts can be planned, or used extemporaneously when a flap is clearly under tension. They are, therefore, valuable maneuvers. Both, however, transgress the 1 : 1 length/breadth ratio. The impairment of blood supply can be reduced by incising through skin alone, leaving the subdermal plexus intact. In any event it should be understood that the release of undue tension sufficient to impair blood flow in a particular flap[308] should *always* take precedence over slavish adherence to a general rule, such as the length/breadth ratio (Fig. 49-6).

Type II—Transposition with Direct Closure of the Secondary Defect

In this second variety of transposition flap, the flap passes across a "promontory" of normal, undisturbed skin (RMI in Fig. 49-7) to gain the primary defect. If the secondary defect is then covered with imported skin, the same rules apply as in the first variety, with the pivot point and the critical line playing identical roles as above. If, however, the secondary defect is closed directly, other factors become important. The pivot point of such a flap must be sutured to the tip of the promontory between the primary and secondary defects. To achieve this, either the pivot point or the promontory, or both, must move. The key to the planning of such a flap is to ensure that such approximation is possible. In this design of transposition flap little or no stretch occurs in the flap itself. The critical line

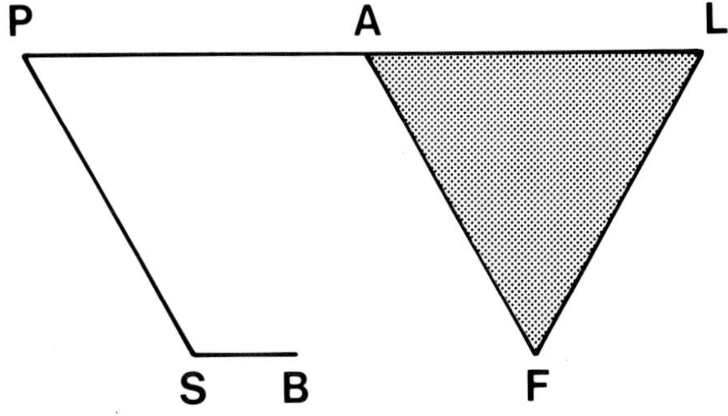

Fig. 49-5. Back-cut. By moving the pivot point *S* toward the primary defect by the incision *SB*, the stretch on the critical line is progressively reduced. This back-cut also reduces the circulation to this random pattern flap. (Modified from Lister,[185] with permission.)

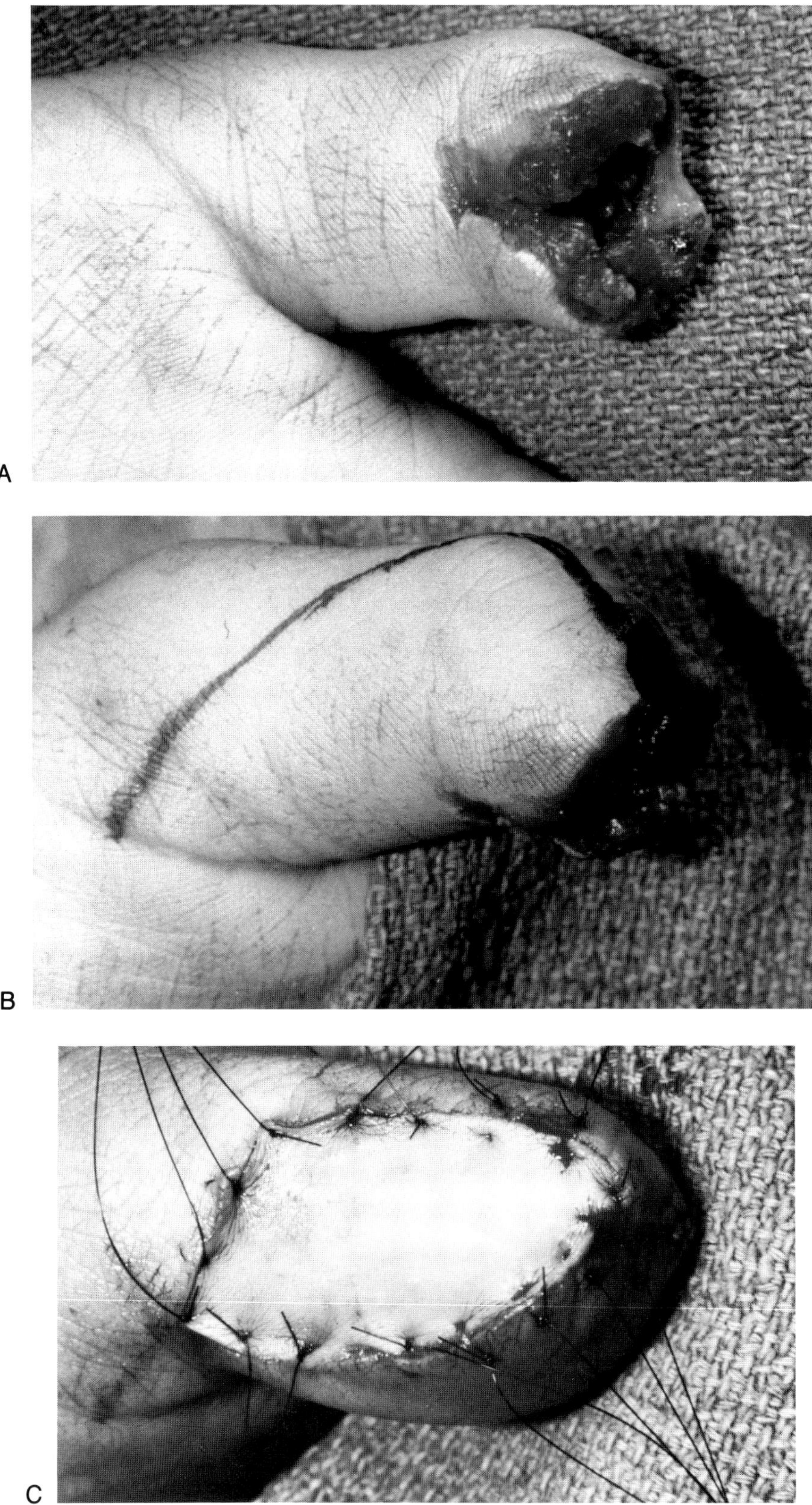

Fig. 49-6. Transposition flap. **(A)** The defect on the palmar aspect of the thumb is naturally triangular in shape. **(B)** The distal margin of the triangle is extended on to the dorsoradial aspect of the thumb and the transposition flap designed. It would be almost equilateral in design if the second incision marked had been stopped at its midpoint. Such a flap would not have transposed and the incision was therefore continued with an extension cut down to the metacarpophalangeal crease. **(C)** After transposition, the secondary defect is covered with a split-thickness skin graft. *(Figure continues.)*

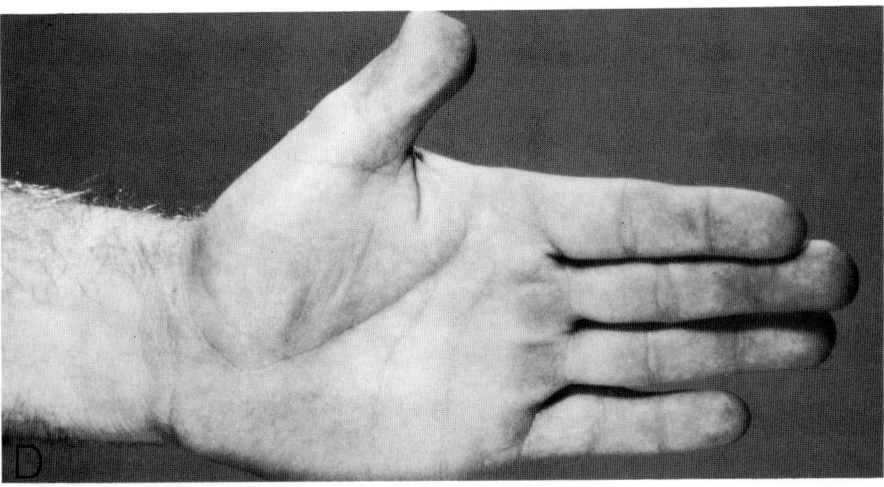

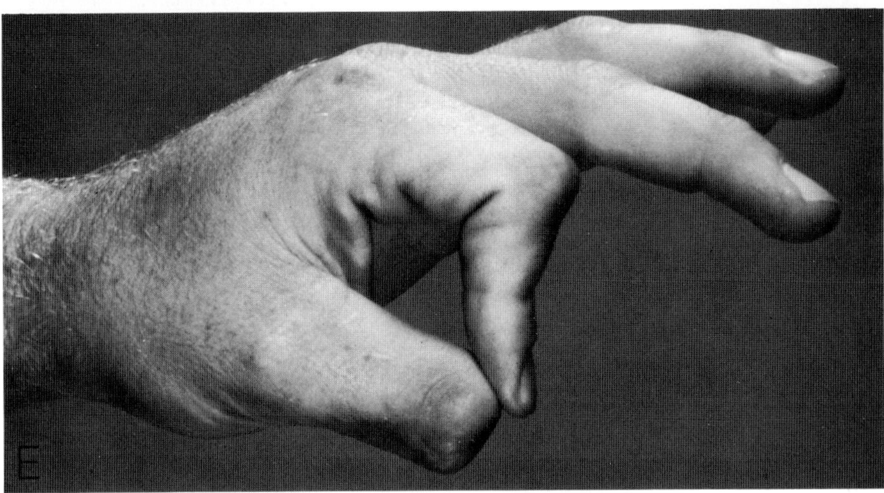

Fig. 49-6 *(Continued).* **(D&E)** The result.

is of no consequence. The most disciplined and geometric examples of this second type of transposition flap are the flaps of Limberg and Dufourmentel.[187] In both, the original defect is rhomboid in shape and therefore equilateral. The transverse diagonal of the Limberg flap defect is equal to any of its sides. To create the flap, the transverse diagonal (HM in Fig. 49-7[1]) is produced in either direction by an equal distance (MI). The second side of the transposition flap (ID) is then drawn parallel to either of the two sides of the primary defect (MO or MR), with which the last line is in contact. It follows that there are four potential sites where the flap can be created for this single defect. Unlike that of the Limberg, the transverse diagonal of the defect for the Dufourmentel flap can be of any length. To design the flap, both the transverse diagonal and one or the other of the adjacent sides are produced (GT to G′ and NT to N′ in Fig. 49-7[3]). The resulting angle between these lines is bisected by the first side of the flap (TX), which is equal in length to any one of the sides of the basic design. From its end the second side of the transposition flap (XC) is drawn parallel to the longitudinal axis of the defect (UN) and of equal length to the first side. As with the Limberg, there are four possible flaps for each defect. In both the Limberg and Dufourmentel designs the surgeon has two choices to make. The first is to choose the orientation of the defect, if it is to be created by excision. This may be determined by the shape of the lesion, for appropriate tumor clearance should be taken while discarding as little normal skin as possible. The second is to choose between the four flaps available for that defect. One or more may not be available because the skin is unsatisfactory or because it is of functional importance. Otherwise, the surgeon should select the flap that permits the most easy approximation of the pivot point to the promontory (D to M in Fig. 49-7[1] and C to T in Fig. 49-7[3]). This selection can be made by simply pinching the skin to find the line of maximum extensibility. If the primary defect is to be created by the surgeon, the flap can be planned in reverse by placing both the pivot point and the tip of the promontory on that line. Once the flap has been raised, approximation of the pivot point to the promontory both places the flap in position and closes the secondary defect.

All random-pattern transposition flaps are variants of one of these two basic designs or a combination of the two. In the first, there is little local skin to spare and the elasticity of the skin

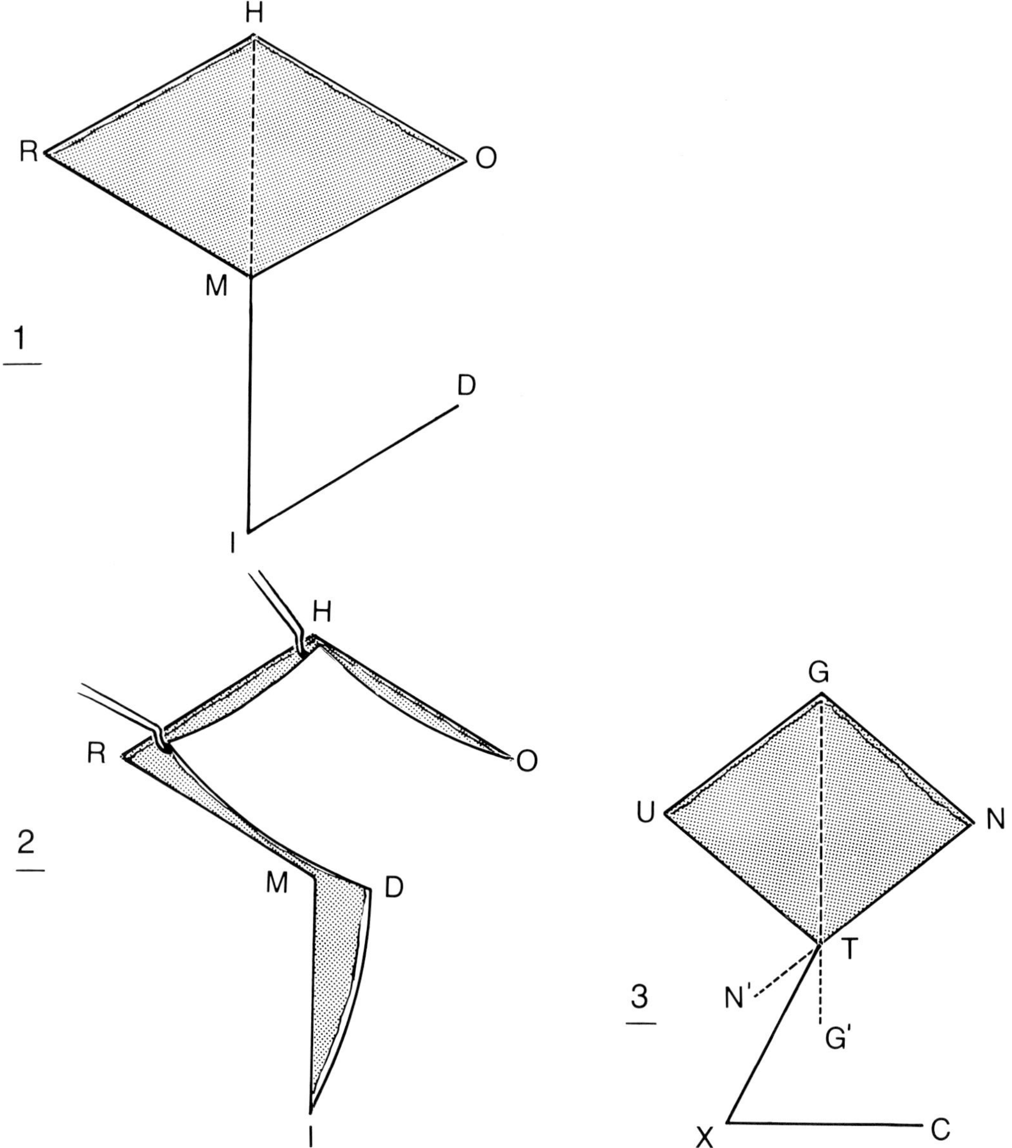

Fig. 49-7. Rhomboid flap design. **(1)** In the Limberg design, all dimensions of the rhomboid that form the primary defect HOMR are equal, including the transverse diagonal *HM*. This has been extended by the same length to *I* and the line *ID* drawn parallel to *MO*. **(2)** The flap is transposed by moving the pivot point *D* to the promontory *M*. If this can be achieved, the flap will fit. **(3)** In the Dufourmentel flap, the transverse diagonal can be of any length. The transverse diagonal *GT* and one of the adjacent sides *NT* are extended to *G′* and *N′* respectively. The angle that they so form is bisected by a line of equal length to one of the sides of the primary defect *TX*. *XC* is then drawn parallel to the longitudinal diameter diagonal *UN*. Transposition is performed by approximating the pivot point *C* to the promontory *T*. (Modified from Lister,[185] with permission.)

along the critical line is important. In the second, slack skin allows movement of the pivot point to the promontory and little stretch of the flap is required. In many flaps, both elasticity and movement of the pivot point play a role.

Variants of Type I

The Gibraiel flap,[109] described previously as a simple rotation flap, is a pure variant of the Type I transposition flap, and is so presented by the original author, moving as it does skin from the lateral aspect of the digit to the flexor surface. There is little or no movement of the pivot point and a full-thickness graft is applied to the secondary defect. In the "sliding" flap described by Smith[299] to cover the dorsal aspect of the PIP joint the defect is not triangulated. Rather, the apex (F in Fig. 49-3) is left curvilinear so that the resultant dog-ear permits movement of the joint.

The "cocked-hat" flap,[18] attributed to Gillies,[268] is a more complex variant used to lengthen the thumb (see also Chapter 57). A dorsal transverse incision at the base of the shortened thumb permits dissection of the skin cover of the entire thumb on a palmar pedicle. The flap is transposed on this pedicle, a bone graft of the maximum length that the flap will accommodate is inserted, and a skin graft is placed on the secondary defect. (This is not an advancement flap, since the pedicle is not on the opposite side of the flap from the defect, and movement is achieved by pivoting around the pedicle and not by stretching or elongating it.)

Variants of Type II

Z-Plasty. The Z-plasty is a form of Type II flap in which the flap and the promontory of skin form the two transposition flaps.[102] Conversely, the rhomboid flap may be considered as a specialized Z-plasty, with the Z being formed by the sides of the triangular flap and one contiguous side of the primary defect (for example RMID in Fig. 49-7[1]). The sides of a standard—stereometric as opposed to planimetric[273]—Z-plasty should always be of equal length, but the angles vary according to the needs of the situation and the local skin topography. The angles of the design may also differ one from the other. As the angles increase, so does the lengthening that occurs along the line of the central limb of the design when the flaps are transposed.[161] The commonly used 60-degree Z-plasty theoretically results in 75 percent lengthening along the line of the central limb (Fig. 49-8). The skin that is introduced into the line of the central limb is derived from the transverse axis of that line. Said another way, skin must be available lateral to the central limb before a Z-plasty can be employed. If sufficient skin is not present for one large Z-plasty, multiple Z-plasties can be used in series (Fig. 49-9), for the longitudinal gain is aggregate, whereas the transverse loss is not. The following are important points in technique (Fig. 49-10):

1. The angles and limbs should be measured with a ruler and protractor (Fig. 49-10A and B). When this is not done mistakes are made, the most common being to cut the angles at 45 degrees believing them to be 60 degrees.
2. The incisions of the Z-plasty should be cut and tested in sequence (Fig. 49-10C and D).

First, the central limb and one side limb should be incised. The flap so created should be raised and carried across the central limb with a skin hook. If the side limb cut on the flap can be brought by at least half its length across the central limb (Fig. 49-10D), there is sufficient tissue transversely and the

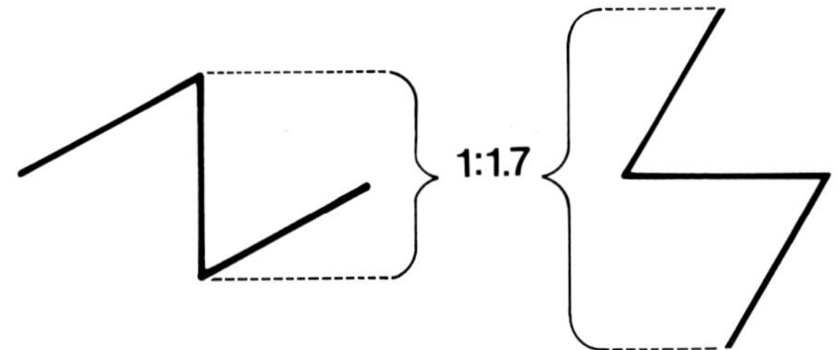

Fig. 49-8. Standard 60-degree Z-plasty. Here all limbs of the Z-plasty are of equal length and the angles between the limbs are 60 degrees. When the flaps are transposed, the lengthening that is achieved along the line of the central limb is some 70 to 75 percent of its original length.

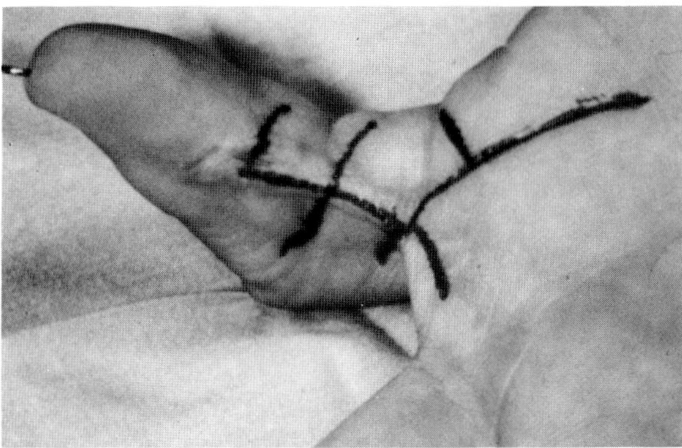

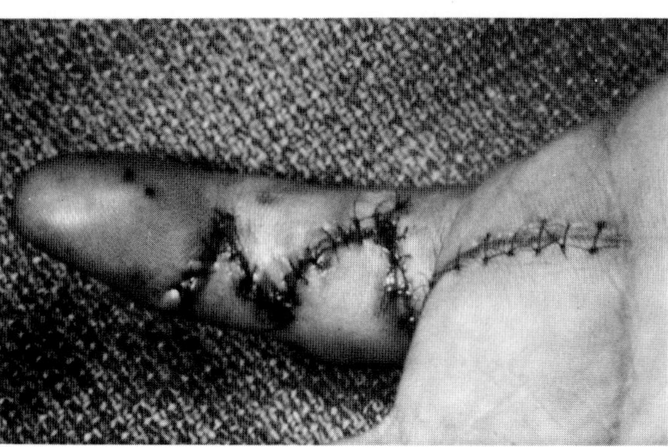

Fig. 49-9. Multiple Z-plasty. Considerable lengthening is required in this scar, and therefore three Z-plasties have been planned in series. The resultant lengthening will be along the line of the central limb. The shortening will be one-third of that lengthening and be distributed evenly along the transverse axes of the three Z-plasties. In the second figure it is seen that only two of the Z-plasties were cut on the finger and the necessary lengthening was achieved. (Modified from Lister,[185] with permission.)

design was well chosen (Fig. 49-10E). If it goes further, a larger Z-plasty would work if more lengthening is required. Such a larger design can be made simply by lengthening both initial cuts and testing again. If this first flap can be carried less than half way across the central limb, the design was too ambitious and must be modified. Since only two limbs have been cut, this modification can be done relatively easily by shortening both the proposed central limb and the as yet uncut second side limb. The excessively long first side limb is simply shortened with one or two stitches.

Four-Flap Z-Plasty. In order to gain greater lengthening along the central limb, the angles of the Z-plasty may be increased. When 120-degree Z-plasty flaps are transposed, the resultant central limb lengthening is theoretically 164 percent. However, flaps with angles much over 60 degrees are difficult to transpose: the pivot points cannot be brought to meet the promontories. This difficulty can be overcome by dividing each flap into two (Fig. 49-11). For example, in the split 120-degree Z-plasty described seventy-five years ago by Limberg,[181] four 60-degree flaps are created. Once again, the design is best created by repeatedly using a ruler and protractor or, better still, calipers set to the same length, nine times in all. Such

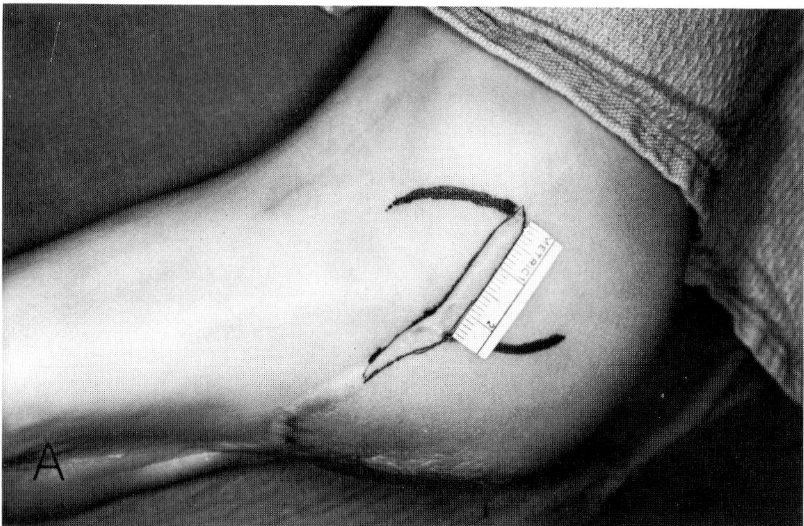

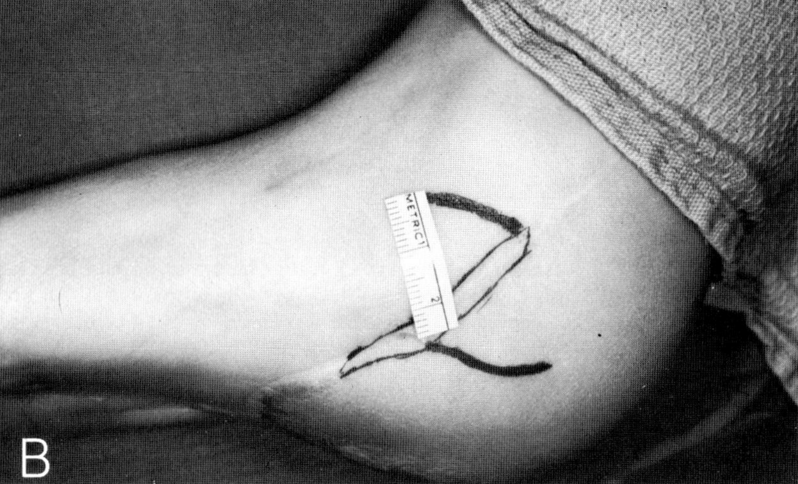

Fig. 49-10. In designing this 60-degree Z-plasty, all measurements are equal; that is, the initial central limb of the "Z" **(A)** is the same length as each of the side limbs, but is also the distance **(B)** between the tip of one of the side limbs and the end of the central limb from which the other side limb originates. This will create a 60-degree Z-plasty. *(Figure continues.)*

four-flap Z-plasties are applicable only in very acute contractures, often in the first web. The angle at which the dorsal skin meets the palmar at the web—the ridge angle—must not exceed 30 degrees or the flaps will not move sufficiently.

Other Types. Further combinations and extensions of the Type II design include the two- and three-flap rhomboid,[141] the double-Z rhomboid,[60,62] and the interdigital butterfly flap.[289] The latter consists of two opposed Z-plasties with a small intervening Y-V advancement flap. The "butterfly" is related to the "seagull," [302] also described for web release.

Departing from the rigid discipline of geometric design but adhering to the same principles, free-hand transposition flaps of random pattern design in which the secondary defect is closed directly are also of Type II. Such are the flaps designed in a digit to be transposed from dorsal or lateral to palmar as described by Green and Dominguez[118] and by Ogunro.[244] These may be employed to close defects caused by either injury or surgical release of scar contractures. Because it is possible to bring the pivot point to the promontory tip, there is little or no tension on the flap itself.

Flaps with Both Type I and Type II Features

In these flaps, some movement of the pivot point occurs but there is insufficient skin available to allow complete closure of the secondary defect, which itself requires imported skin cover. For this reason, the flap is stretched to reach the primary defect, and measurement of the critical line as it is before and as it would be after transposition remains an important part of the planning of the flap. The potential movement of the pivot point and the resultant reduction in the stretch required of the critical line can be assessed by applying traction to a skin hook impaled in the proposed location of the pivot point.

Flaps of this group include flaps from the dorsum of the digit to the palmar surface used in releasing Dupuytren's contracture[123]; flaps from the lateral aspect of the digit to resurface the dorsal aspect of the PIP joint following burns—this flap has been described by Lueders and Shapiro[196] as a rotation flap, which it is not by the definition stated earlier; and flaps used in release of adduction contractures of the first web space and derived from the dorsum of the index finger[306] and the dorsum of the thumb.[280,315] In both the latter two designs the first web is

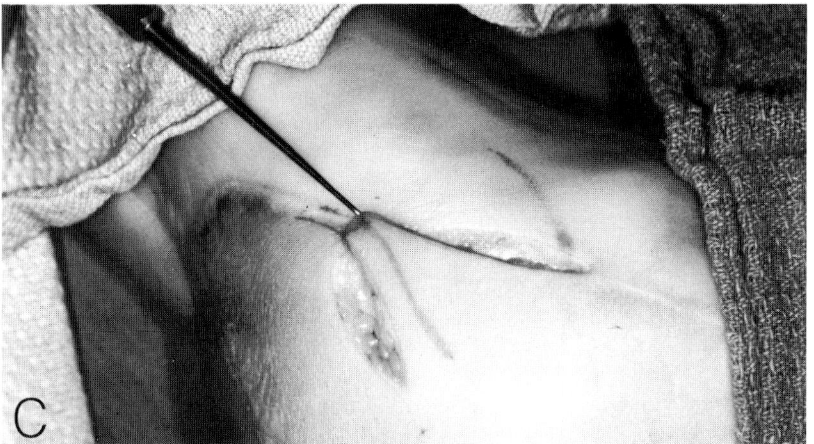

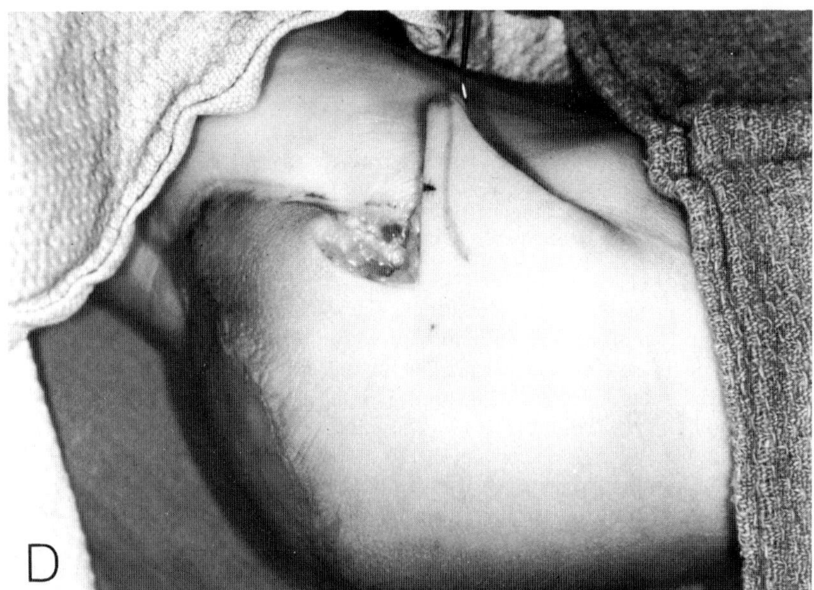

Fig. 49-10 *(Continued).* **(C)** The first flap has been cut and *(D)* is transposed across the central limb. The center point of the side limb has been marked with a tick on its margin. It can be seen that this can be carried with comfort well across the central limb. The initial design is therefore satisfactory and can even be made larger if wished. **(E)** The flaps are transposed and sutured into position without problems.

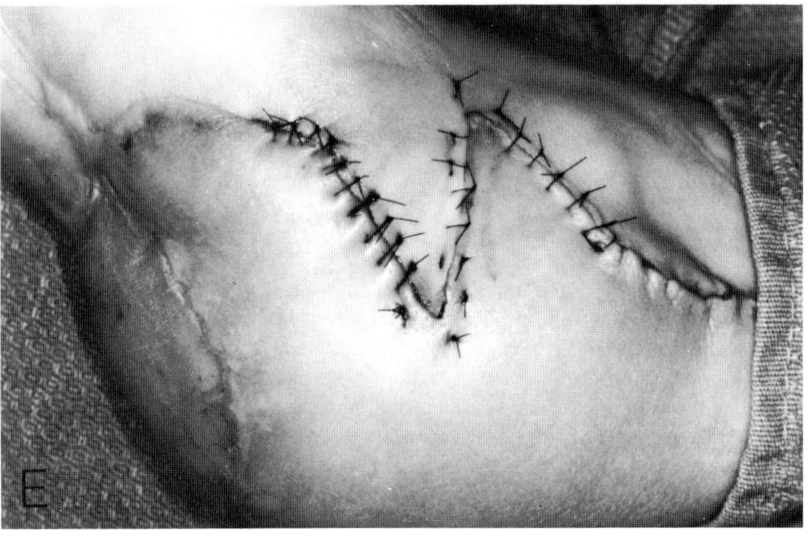

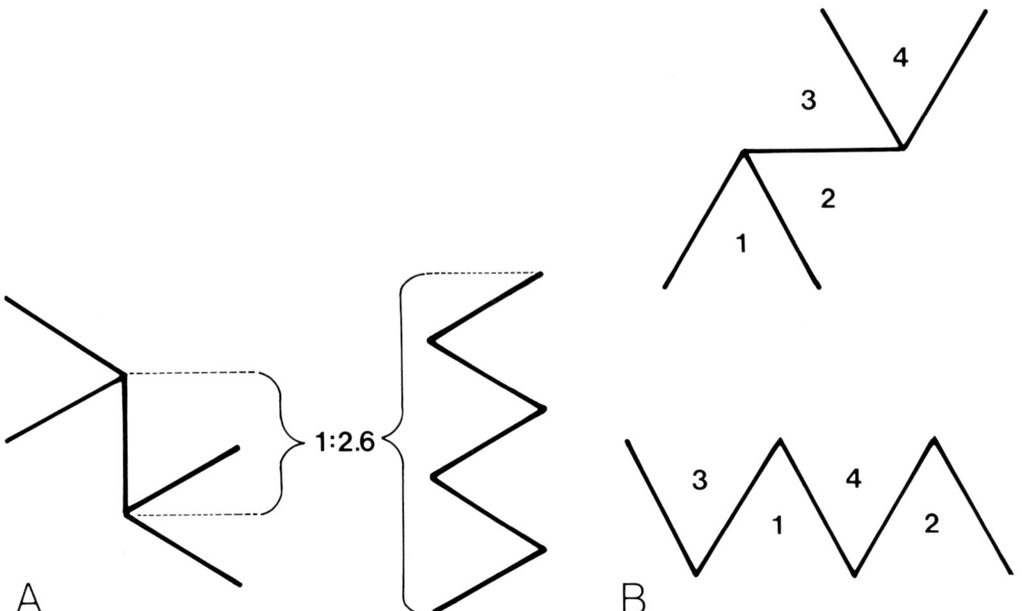

Fig. 49-11. Four-flap Z-plasty. **(A)** In the four-flap Z-plasty, all measurements are equal, that is, each limb of the design is of equal length but so also are the distances between any two adjacent points in the design. When the flaps are transposed, the two 120-degree angles are closed. As a result, the distance between the points at either end of the initial central limb is some 264 percent of its original length. **(B)** The transposition that is achieved is shown by numbering the flaps. It will be seen that the two 120-degree angles are closed, putting *2* in the right hand incision and *3* in the left hand incision, and interdigitating flaps *1* and *4*.

released through a single incision traversing the web and continuing around on to the dorsum of the web to run just to the radial side of the second metacarpal. The pivot point of the proposed flap is then selected: in the thumb on the radial side just proximal to the MP joint (Fig. 49-12); on the index finger to the ulnar side of the neck of the second metacarpal (Fig. 49-13A–D). Moving the pivot point with a hook as described above, the length of the critical line as it will be after transposition is then measured from the pivot point to the proximal, palmar end of the releasing incision. In so doing, care must be taken to follow the edge of the wound in the web and to not go directly across the defect dorsal to palmar. This length is then transferred to the donor digit. If that length cannot be accommodated because the digit proximal to the nailbed is too short, then the distance by which it fails is the amount by which the flap will have to stretch. Devices such as the back-cut and extension cut can be employed as described for Type I.

Types I and II Used in Combination

Two combinations have been described to resurface the stump of an amputated thumb. Argamaso[7] employed a radially based Type I transposition and covered the defect with a transposition flap from the dorsum of the index finger as described above. Winspur[343] used an ulnar-based transposition advancement, preserving both neurovascular bundles. He moved the tissue and deepened the first web space by a simple Z-plasty designed with the central limb along the margin of the web.

Axial Pattern

Vessels that serve to enhance the vascularity of transposition flaps have been isolated at the level of the distal and proximal phalanges. Dorsal digital branches of the digital artery and nerve at the level of the distal phalanx were first described by Holevich.[137] They form the pedicle for dorsolateral flaps transposed to cover digital pulp defects as described by Flint and Harrison,[90] Lesavoy,[179] and notably Joshi.[151-154] Pho[257] demonstrated similar vessels arising from the radial digital artery of the thumb and employed flaps based on those vessels and the radial digital nerve and artery to resurface the pulp of the thumb. He states that skin can be taken from the MP joint out to within millimeters of the nailfold, but advises that a skin bridge be retained until tourniquet release demonstrates satisfactory flow.

In 1973, both Vilain[338] and Iselin[143] described a flag flap raised on the dorsum of the middle phalanx and so called because the pedicle, narrowed by a generous back-cut, was further mobilized by parallel incisions resembling the pole of the flag. No arterial pedicle was described for this flap and the author has no experience with it.

The skin of the dorsum of the proximal phalanx, especially of the index and middle fingers, has been shown to receive axial flow from the branches of the first and second dorsal metacarpal arteries, vessels which are present in 90 percent and 97 percent of hands, respectively.[80] Both of these vessels arise from the radial artery or its communications with the dorsal carpal arch, the posterior interosseous artery, the deep palmar arch, and the ulnar digital artery of the thumb. Stated more

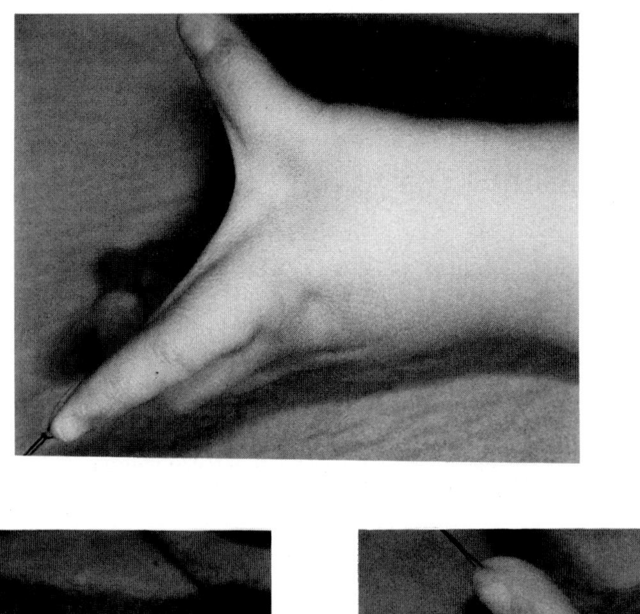

A

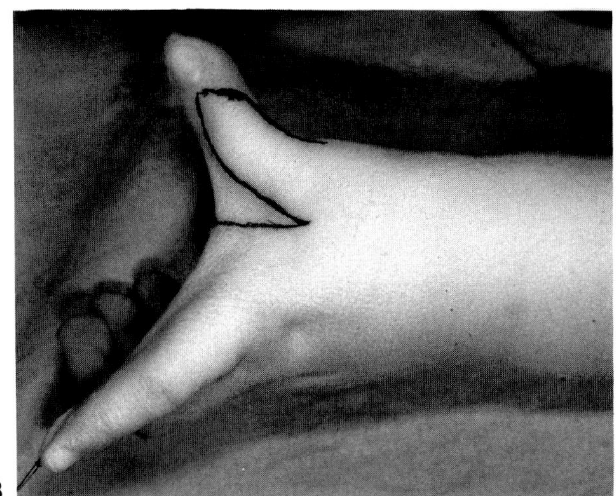

B

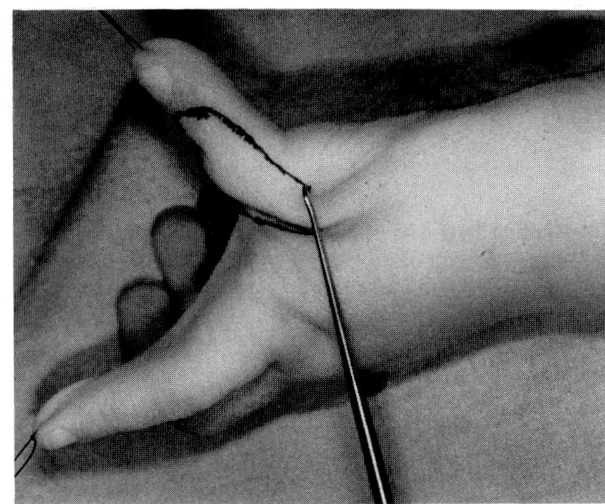

C

Fig. 49-12. Transposition flap from the dorsum of the thumb. **(A)** In releasing an arthrogrypotic first web space contracture, it is planned **(B)** to incise down the center point of the web both dorsally and on the palmar aspect, where the incision will be carried across the palmar aspect of the MP joint to release the flexion contracture of the thumb. **(C)** By moving the pivot point with a hook and measuring from this point to the far side of the flexion surface of the thumb (that is, the end of the planned releasing incision—see **E**), and then measuring from the pivot point to the tip of the flap, it can be appreciated that some, but not much, stretch will be required in the flap. *(Figure continues.)*

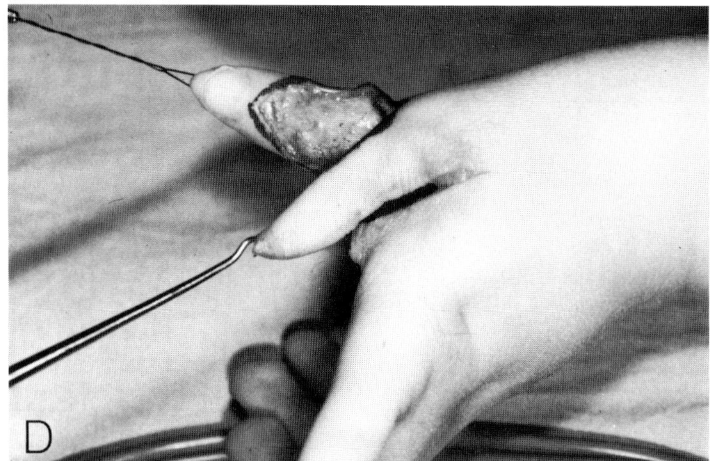

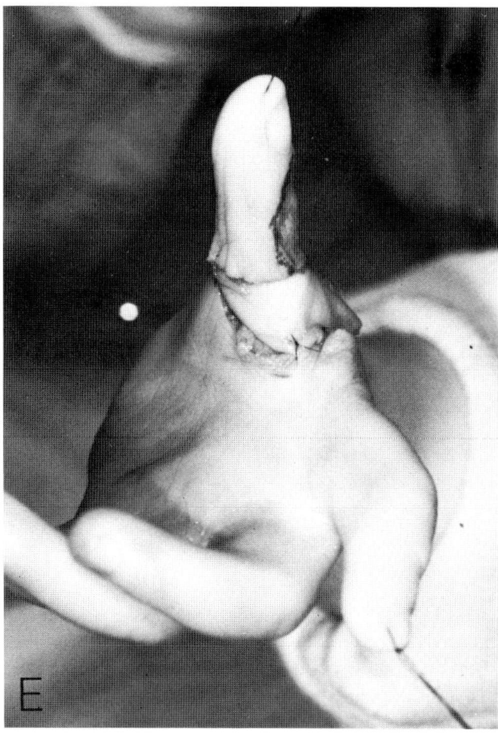

Fig. 49-12 *(Continued).* **(D)** The flap is raised and **(E)** transposed into position, widening the web space and also covering the release of the flexion contracture. The secondary defect is covered with a full-thickness skin graft.

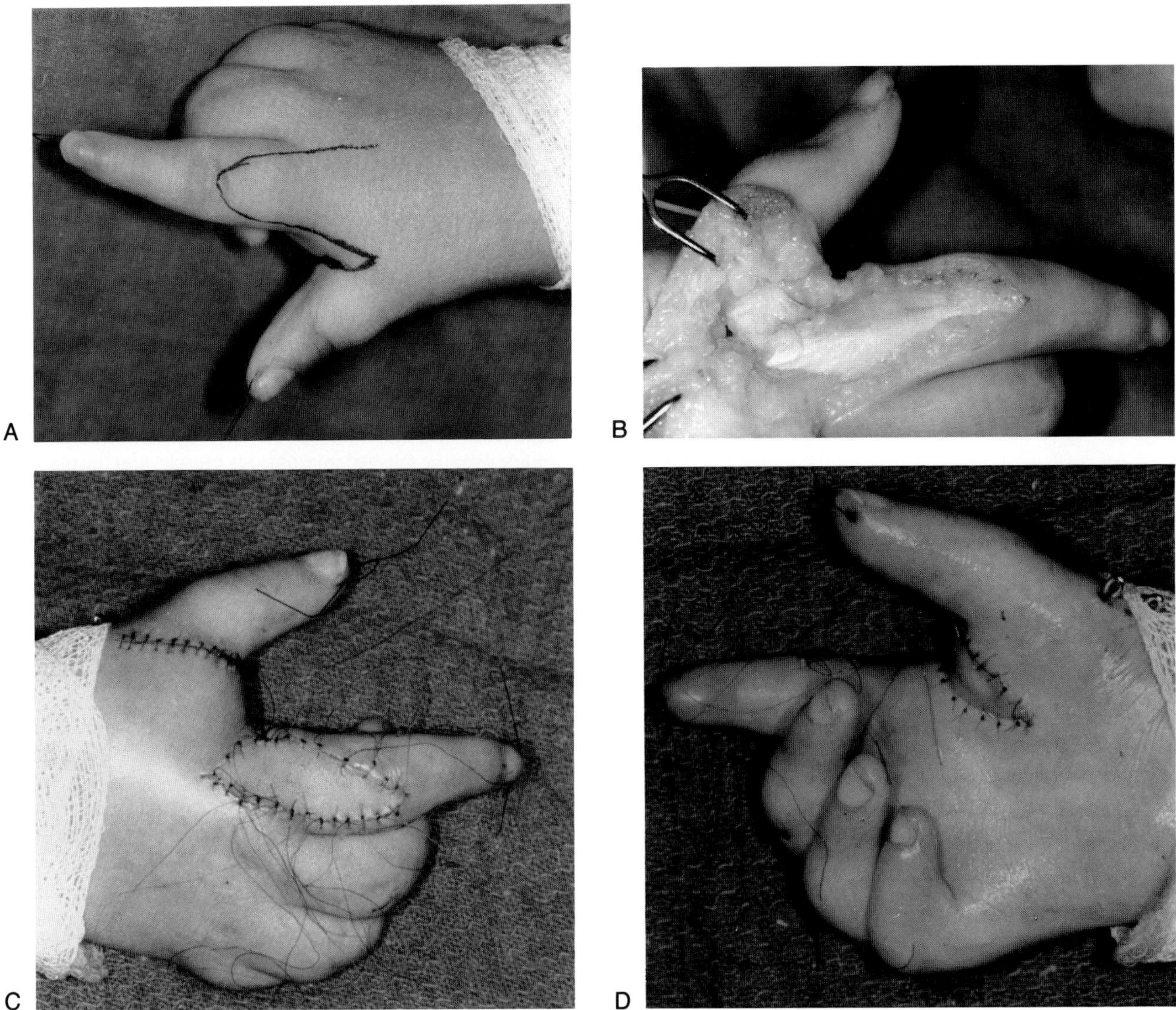

Fig. 49-13. Transposition flap from the index finger. **(A)** The flap is drawn out in combination with releasing the first web space in a patient with arthrogryposis. **(B)** Incision and raising of the flap reveals tight bands in the first web space, which are released. **(C)** The flap has been transposed and a thick split-thickness skin graft applied to the secondary defect. **(D)** The thumb has been pinned in abduction and the flap can be seen to reach to the level of the superficial palmar arch.

simply, both vessels arise from arteries around the base of the second metacarpal. They pursue courses either immediately above or immediately below the fascia of the interosseous muscles. At the web space, the second dorsal metacarpal artery has a constant anastomosis with the palmar metacarpal artery, which is doubly significant in flap design, for this vessel must be divided if a longer arc of rotation is to be achieved on a proximally based flap, while it also serves as the axial vessel of reversed dorsal metacarpal flaps.[203,261] According to the dissections of Johnson and Cohen,[145] the branches of these vessels supply the dorsal skin no further than the proximal interphalangeal joint. The venous drainage of these flaps is excellent, being through either end of the proximal venous arcade, which is of very large caliber[232] (Fig. 49-14). These dorsal vessels form the axial basis of four distinct flaps—the "axial flag flap," the first dorsal metacarpal artery (FDMA) flap, the second dorsal metacarpal artery (SDMA) flap and the reversed dorsal metacarpal flap. Those proximally based can readily transfer sensibility by incorporating the branches of the radial nerve to the dorsal skin.

Axial Flag Flap[186]

This simple flap requires no pedicle dissection, for it is based on the web space of the donor finger. As the dorsal metacarpal artery has been shown to be reliably present in the second interspace, and less so in the others, all but two axial flag flaps in my personal series have been based on that space and raised from either the index or the middle finger. Because the pedicle need be only as wide as the vessels, the mobility in this flap is its

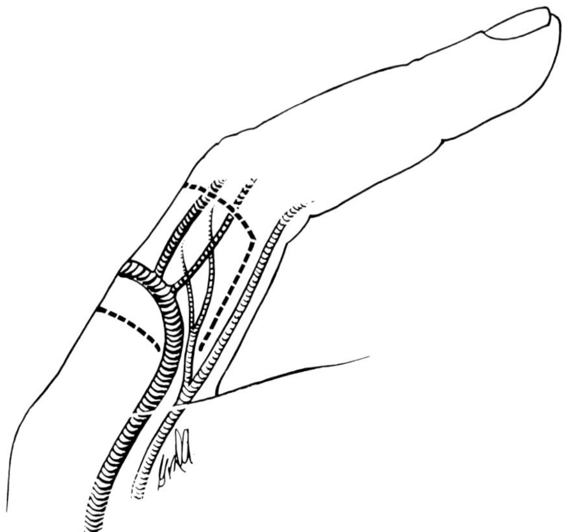

Fig. 49-14. Axial flag flap. The axial flag flap receives its blood supply from a dorsal digital artery that originates either from the proper digital artery to that finger or from an extension of the dorsal metacarpal artery. Drainage is through the proximal venous arcade to the web space veins. (Modified from Lister,[185] with permission.)

single major advantage. From the dorsum of the middle finger, for example, it can be rotated to cover the dorsum of either the proximal phalanx of the index or the metacarpophalangeal joint of either index or middle (Fig. 49-15A). It can also, by being passed through the web space, cover the palmar surface of either proximal phalanx or either metacarpophalangeal joint (Fig. 49-15B). Before commencing elevation of the flap, the presence of the vessel can be confirmed by Doppler examination.[126] As with the cross-finger flap the entire skin of the dorsum of the selected proximal phalanx is raised (Fig. 49-16), from midlateral line to midlateral line, and from the proximal extension crease of the proximal interphalangeal joint distally to the level of the free margin of the web proximally. As with all random flaps the plane of dissection is beneath the subcutaneous vascular stratum, leaving the loose paratenon on the extensor hood.

Dorsal Metacarpal Artery Flaps (FDMA,[80,91,262,296] SDMA[79])

These flaps are dissected from distal to proximal. The skin of the dorsum of the selected proximal phalanx is lifted as an island from the paratenon of the extensor tendon. An incision is made over the selected interosseous muscle, and the margins are elevated as thin, subdermal flaps, until it is felt that sufficient veins for drainage have been exposed. The fascia of the interosseous muscle is raised from the underlying muscle. In the SDMA flap, the base of which lies at the point of divergence of the extensors to index and middle, the fascia can only be raised out as far as the web space, at which point the anastomosis with the palmar interosseous must be defined and ligated, to permit a full arc of rotation. This pedicle contains, undissected, the metacarpal artery, veins and branches of the radial nerve. The flap can then be transposed to cover defects of the thumb, first web space, and as far to the ulnar side of the hand as the head of the fifth metacarpal.

The reversed[203,261] dorsal metacarpal flap is raised in similar fashion but from the dorsal skin of the hand, using the com-

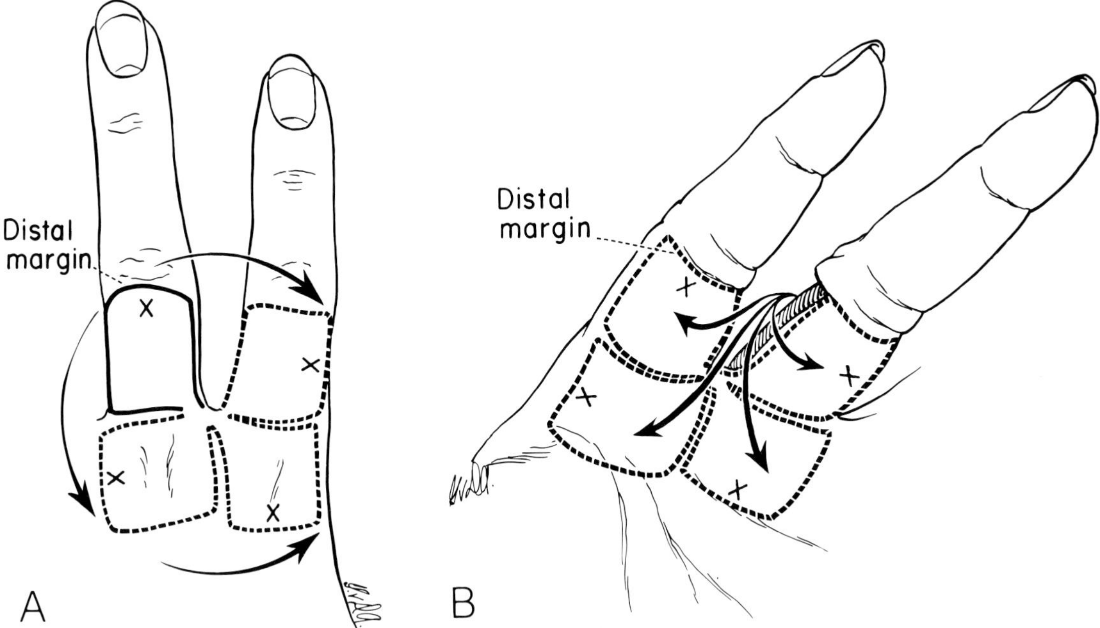

Fig. 49-15. **(A)** An axial flag flap raised on the dorsum of the middle finger can be rotated to cover defects on the proximal phalanx of the index finger or over the MP joint of either of those two digits. **(B)** By carrying the flap through the web space, it can reach defects on the palmar surface of the MP joint of either the index or middle fingers. (Modified from Lister,[185] with permission.)

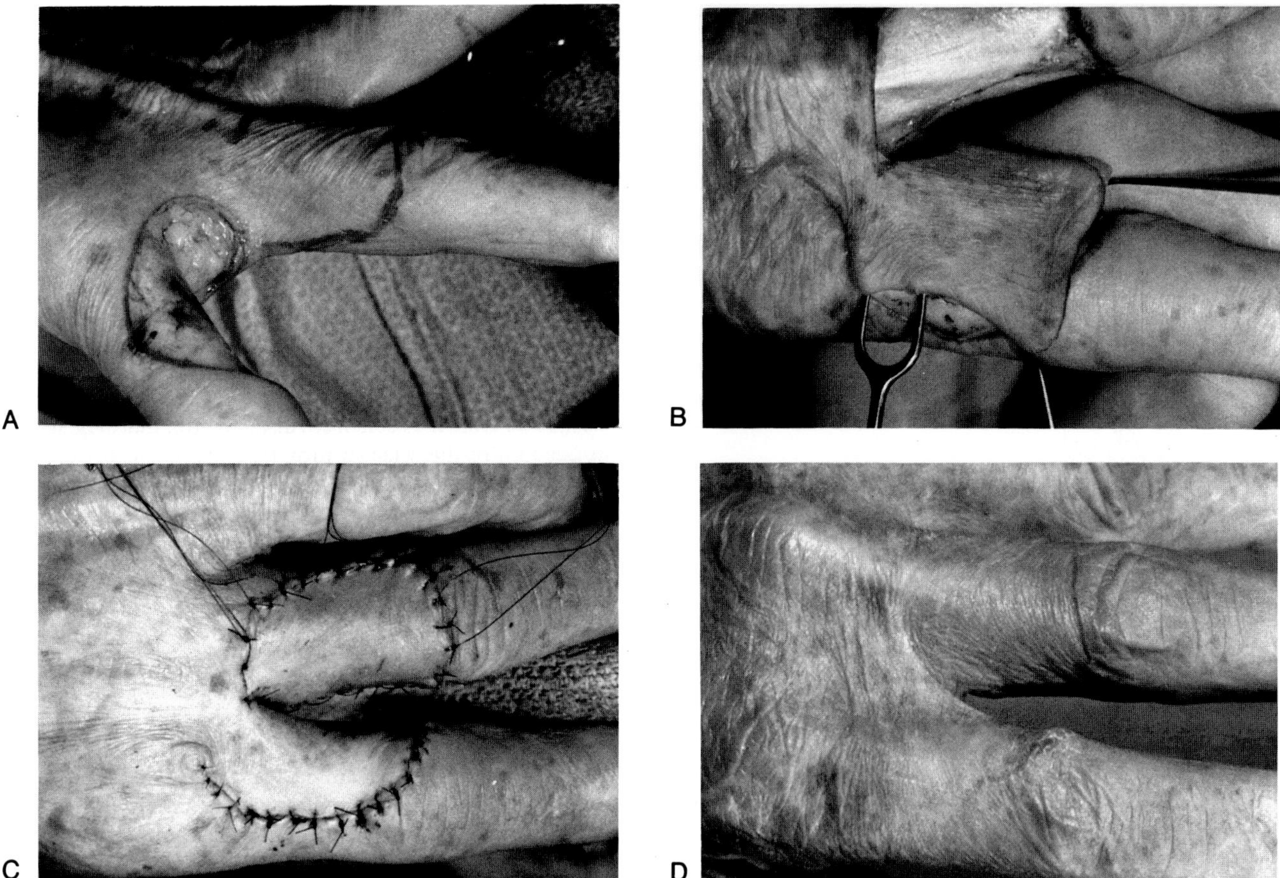

Fig. 49-16. Axial flag flap. **(A)** After resection of a squamous cell carcinoma that was adherent to the underlying digital nerve, and after nerve grafting, cover of a defect on the dorsal and ulnar aspect of the index finger is achieved by use of an axial flag flap. The pedicle is left relatively wide but it can be reduced down to the vessels alone, as shown in Figure 49-49. **(B)** The flap transposes with ease. **(C)** The secondary defect is covered with a full-thickness skin graft. **(D)** The result.

munication between dorsal and palmar metacarpal arteries as the axial vessel. This flap can evidently go no further in the finger than can the axial flag flap, but is a useful alternative when that flap is not available.

A similar flap, but with the pedicle based more distally, has been described[170,173] for repair of fingertip injuries. Flow depends upon the integrity of the palmar digital arch that lies beneath the palmar plate and drainage upon retrograde flow in the fine veins around the artery. It has the advantage of confining the reconstruction to the injured finger.

Rotation Flaps

All rotation flaps are random pattern. As with the basic transposition flap, the surgeon should commence the design for a rotation flap by triangulating the primary defect. Unlike the two basic designs of transposition flap, there is nothing geometric to the rotation flap. The base of the defect—that side opposite the angle which is to be closed—is extended in the direction from which the surgeon has determined tissue is available. The line is continued in a gentle curve until the surgeon deems that, by differentially suturing the wound, the flap can be advanced to cover the defect. This is very arbitrary and therefore requires experience; however, there are some general rules that help.

First, the flap should be made as large as is reasonably possible. Not only does this provide more tissue to stretch into the defect but it also makes the differential suturing easier, more even, and therefore more acceptable esthetically. As one plastic surgery teacher was wont to say, "Think of a flap and then double it." Second, the availability of tissue should be checked in that area where two further devices may relax a tight flap. This area is at the end of the flap incision and on the side of the incision opposite to the primary defect. It can be called the "critical area" (and is that surrounding 2X in Fig. 49-17). If skin is available there and the simple rotation flap does not move adequately, one of two steps can be taken. A back cut can be made on the flap side of the incision at its far end and at right angles to it (Fig. 49-17). The back-cut is opened fully, that is, to 180 degrees, and sutured to the "critical area" previously shown to have some loose skin. By opening the back-cut thus, the length of that side of the rotation flap has been increased by

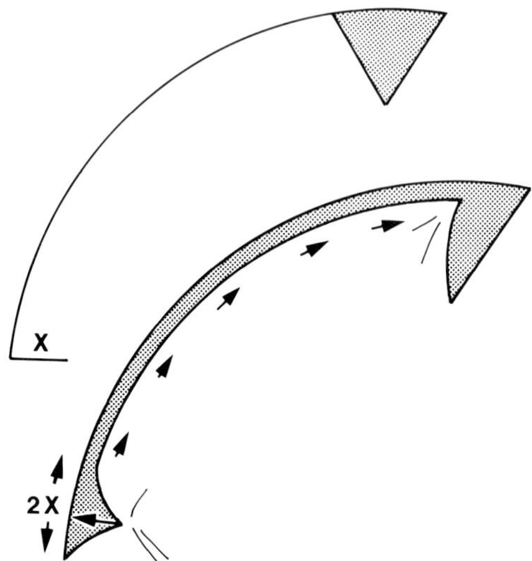

Fig. 49-17. Rotation flap. The primary defect is triangulated and necessary gain is achieved by differential suturing of the two flap margins. Where the gain achieved is insufficient and there is skin available in the "critical area," that is, the area under *2X*, a back-cut *X* may be cut that will lengthen the margin of the flap. (Modified from Lister,[185] with permission.)

twice the length of the back-cut. It follows that, if the back-cut is made half the length of the base of the triangle that is the primary defect, no differential suturing will be required to close the defect. This is attractive, but the surgeon must remember two things—the back-cut reduces flap circulation as it is directed across the pedicle, and tissue must be available in the critical area to advance into the back-cut. The alternate step is the use of a Burow's triangle (Fig. 49-18). A Burow's triangle is normal skin that is excised to facilitate movement of a flap. In this circumstance of a rotation flap, the triangle is excised from the critical area. Closure of the triangular defect moves the rotation flap toward the primary defect. If the Burow's triangle is made as large as the primary defect, no differential suturing or stretching is necessary. Two rotation flaps, one concave and the other convex, are moved equal distances in opposite directions.

A final solution to problems that arise in moving a rotation flap is to incise a generous back-cut and skin graft the resultant defect, that is, convert it to a Type I transposition flap.

Multiple rotation flaps are uncommon, but have been described to move skin from the dorsum of the wrist into the first web space.[89]

Advancement Flaps

In an advancement flap, the leading edge of the flap is drawn directly away from its vascular base to cover the primary defect. In the simplest design, the primary defect is considered as a rectangle. The two short sides of the rectangle are produced as the lateral incisions of the advancement flap until the surgeon deems that, by differential suturing, the flap can be advanced into the defect. A simple advancement flap for use in thumb tip amputation was described by Moberg[229] (Fig. 49-19). (See also Chapter 57.) This is reserved for amputations through the distal phalanx, since flexion of the interphalangeal joint may be required to assist in closure of the defect. The two parallel incisions to create the flap are made just dorsal to the two neurovascular bundles of the thumb, which are carefully preserved throughout dissection. The flap is then elevated from the flexor tendon sheath. Since the bundles are included in the flap, there is theoretically no limit to the length of the flap, but customarily the base is placed at the MP joint skin flexion crease. If difficulty is encountered in advancing the flap over the thumb tip, four tactics are available. First, the interphalangeal joint can be flexed, and if necessary pinned in flexion, thus moving the primary defect into the flap. This procedure may cause fears of later problems with extension, but they are unfounded unless the joint is arthritic or has been injured. Second, the lateral incisions can be extended toward the palm, yielding a greater length over which skin can be advanced. The defects on either aspect of the base can then be closed with two small rotation flaps.[64] Third, two Burow's triangles can be excised to assist in advancement, one from either side of the base of the flap, provided of course that tissue is available (Fig. 49-20). Fourth, as there are two vascular bundles in the base of the flap, the skin of the base can be incised to create an island (Fig. 49-21). A full-thickness graft is applied to the secondary defect overlying the neurovascular bundles and tendon sheath. Posner and Smith[258] reported 22 Moberg advancement flaps with no slough or flexion contracture and normal two-point discrimination. This advancement is perfectly safe in the thumb, for the dorsum is well-perfused by dorsal branches from the radial artery. A similar procedure has been reported in the finger,[243,303] but greater care must be exercised here or loss of the dorsal skin may result (see Fig. 5-24 in Beasley[22]). Macht and Watson[197] reported 69 cases with no skin necrosis either palmar or dorsal, two-point discrimination within 2 mm of normal, and a maximum flexion deficit of 5 degrees. However, they emphasized the importance of maintaining the dorsal branches of the proper digital arteries. Increased padding of the pulp with a free dermal graft placed beneath the palmar advancement flap has been advocated by Arons.[9]

V-Y Advancement

Commonly used to repair fingertip amputations, the V-Y advancement may be single midline or double lateral. Which is used, and indeed whether the technique is appropriate at all, is determined by examining the primary defect. First, is bone exposed? If not, then probably a skin graft would suffice. Second, is there at least one half of the nailbed remaining and is that nailbed supported by bone? If not, then consideration should be given to ablation of the nailbed and revision of the amputation. Third, what is the angle of the amputation (Fig. 49-22)? If more tissue has been lost from the palmar than from the dorsal surface (Fig. 49-22C), then a local palmar flap is unlikely to provide the necessary cover and a cross-finger or thenar flap is required. If the loss is equal (Fig. 49-22A), or greater on the dorsal aspect (Fig. 49-22B), then a V-Y flap can be used provided the skin from which it comes is not also damaged. Whether a single midline or double lateral is used

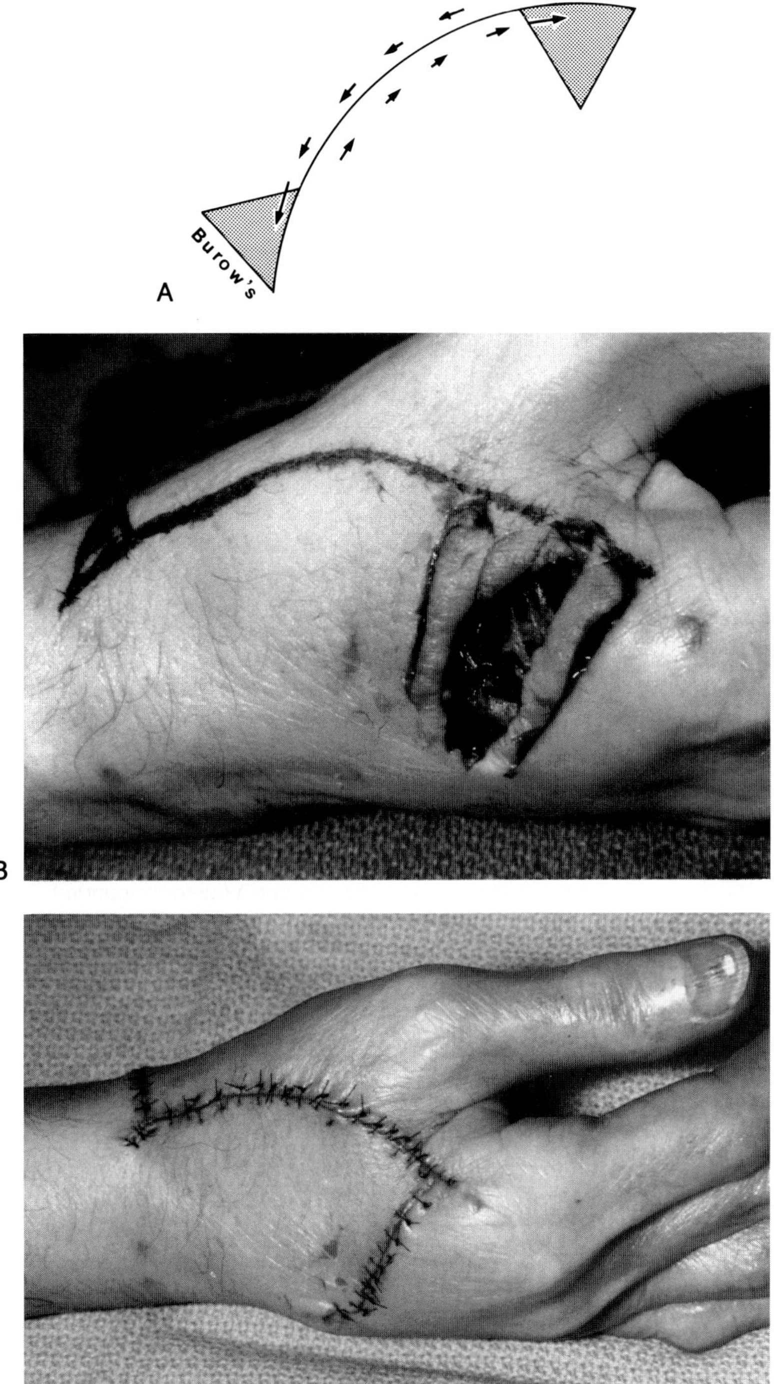

Fig. 49-18. **(A)** Another device for assisting in movement of a rotation flap is to excise the critical area as a Burow's triangle and thereby rotate both the flap and the adjacent skin. **(B)** Here an irregular saw injury to the dorsum of the hand has created a skin loss that has been triangulated. A rotation flap was designed and a Burow's triangle excised over the region of the snuffbox. **(C)** The flap in place. (Fig. A modified from Lister,[185] with permission.)

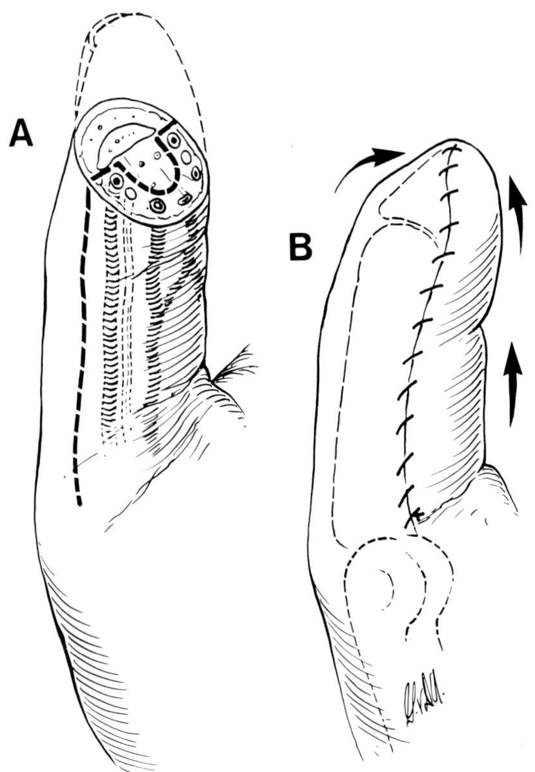

Fig. 49-19. Moberg advancement flap. **(A)** Most useful for amputations distal to the thumb interphalangeal joint, the Moberg advancement flap is composed of the entire palmar skin of the thumb, including the neurovascular bundles. **(B)** Flexion of the interphalangeal joint assists in coverage of the defect by the advancement flap. (Modified from Lister,[185] with permission.)

depends upon whether there is more skin in the midline or laterally.

There are three facts to remember if a V-Y flap is to be raised successfully.[341] First, more problems arise through inadequate mobilization than excessive—the flap should advance easily into position (Fig. 49-23). Second, only nerves and vessels need be kept intact.[25] Third, the nerves and vessels in the pulp are slender, elastic, and will not resist appreciably the movement of the flap; a corollary of this rule is that any tissue that does offer firm resistance can be divided with impunity. The apex of the "V" in a single midline advancement[12,330] for most fingertip amputations worthy of reconstruction (i.e., at, or distal to, the midportion of the nail) should be at the distal digital crease. In the rare case where length is deemed sufficiently important to justify a V-Y advancement in more proximal amputations, the apex can be placed more proximally. The base of the triangle, which lies on the free distal margin, should be as wide as the nailbed, but no wider or the tip will have a flattened appearance. The incisions are made through the skin with a knife, carrying it to bone at either end of the base where there are periosteal attachments but no vessels. These periosteal attachments should be divided. Using tenotomy scissors, the deep surface of the flap is freed completely from the underlying tendon sheath as far as its apex. The skin and subcutaneous tissue some 6 or 7 mm on either aspect of the apex is incised down to the sheath. With skin hooks on one lateral margin of the flap distracting the flap away from the digit (Fig. 49-23A), the lateral subcutaneous tissues that contain the pedicle of the flap are spread apart with curved ring-handled microscissors. Using loupe magnification, any restraining bands are accurately defined and divided, remembering that nerves and vessels will not resist gentle traction.[291]

(An anatomical point should be made here. The veins that accompany the artery of the digital neurovascular bundle are at different levels and of differing, smaller caliber. Therefore, in dissecting a neurovascular bundle for any form of island flap in the digit no attempt should ever be made to define the artery and nerve independently, for such skeletonization will serve only to damage the veins and thereby seriously impair flap drainage.)

The procedure is repeated on the other lateral margin. The flap should then advance easily into place (Fig. 49-23B and C). If it does not, and firm resistance is encountered, one of the fibrous septa must still be intact. It must be sought out and divided. This process is repeated until the flap moves easily. The dissection required to achieve this mobilization is impressive and causes some concern, even to the experienced. If the flap still does not reach the nailbed when all septa have been divided, it is probable that the angle of amputation was such that more palmar skin was lost than had been appreciated. In that event, one *must not* be tempted to remove any of the bony support of the nailbed, for a hooked or beaked nail will result. Rather, the flap should be advanced as far as possible to cover the bone and a split-thickness skin graft applied to the raw edge of the flap. Closure of the flap should be commenced at the apex, creating the vertical stem of the Y and so advancing the flap. Like the inset of other neurovascular island flaps, this can be done with the tourniquet inflated, for no cautery should be brought near the pedicles of the flap after its release. On completion and after tourniquet release, color usually returns to the flap. If it does not, time and warmth in the form of hot packs should be permitted to play their valuable role for 20 timed minutes. If there is still inadequate flow, the most distal su-

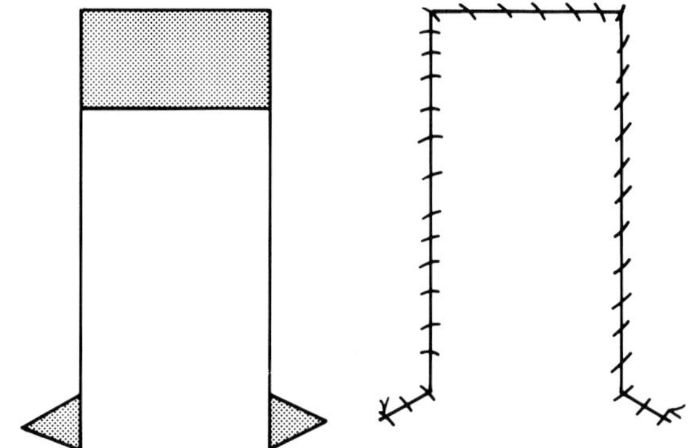

Fig. 49-20. Advancement flap. If a defect can be considered as a rectangle, an advancement flap can be designed by extending the two short sides of the rectangle. The advancement movement can be assisted also by excision of two Burow's triangles on the outer aspect of the design. (Modified from Lister,[185] with permission.)

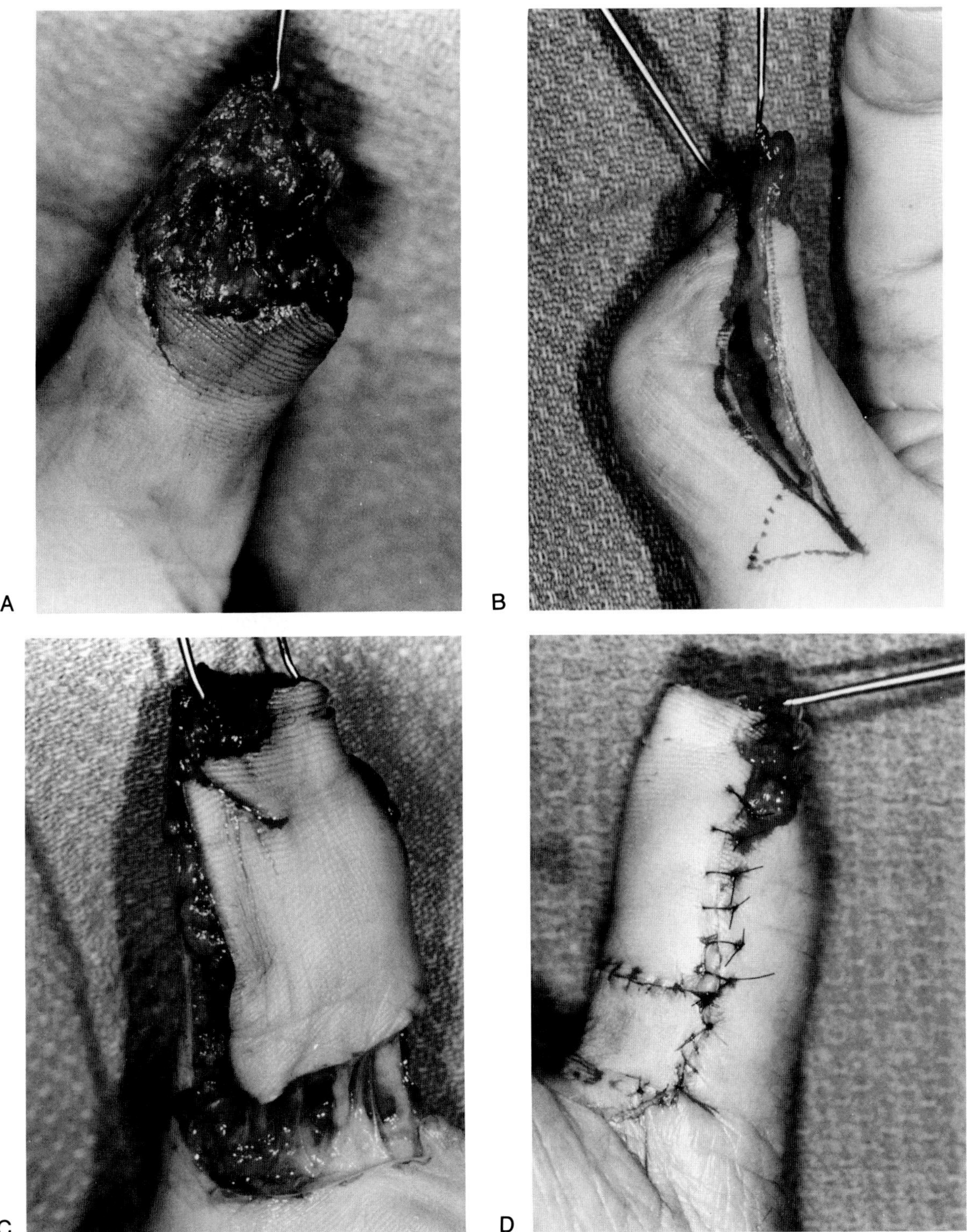

Fig. 49-21. **(A)** A full-thickness defect of the thumb is to be closed by a Moberg advancement flap. **(B)** When the flap is mobilized and the thumb flexed fully it is seen that the flap will cover the defect, but only with some tension (note that a potential Burow's triangle has been marked out at the base of the flap). **(C)** To release the tension, the flap has been divided across its base and the neurovascular bundles carefully preserved. **(D)** The flap has been sutured in place and the secondary defect covered with a full-thickness skin graft.

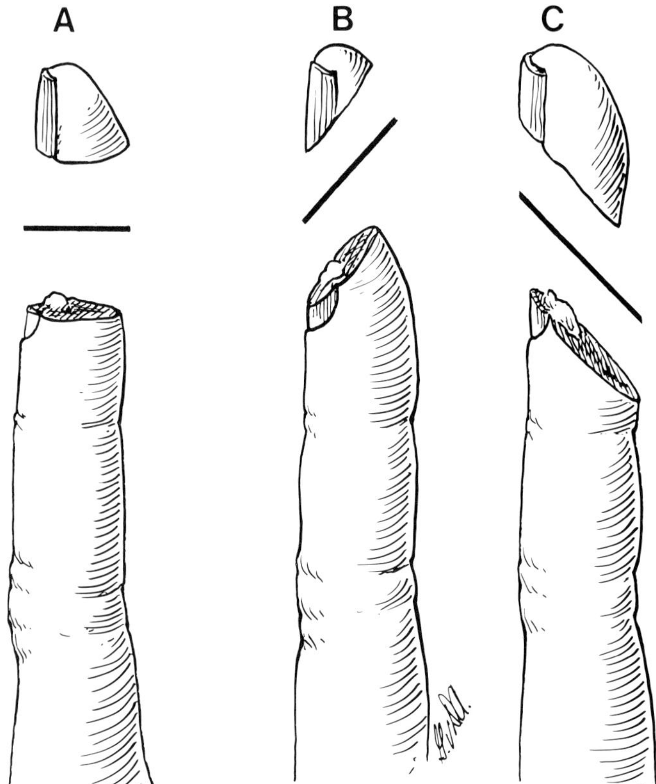

Fig. 49-22. Suitability for coverage with local flaps is determined by looking at the angle of amputation. Amputations that are transverse **(A)** or have more dorsal loss **(B)** can be treated by local flaps. Where the loss is more palmar **(C)**, palmar flaps have been described (see text) but regional flaps are more reliable. (Modified from Lister GD: The Hand: Diagnosis and Indications. 2nd Ed., Churchill Livingstone, Edinburgh, 1984, with permission.)

ture(s) in the vertical limb of the Y should be released, which usually produces the desired effect.

While more palmar loss than dorsal usually contraindicates such palmar V-Y advancement flaps, Furlow[101] has shown good results with V-Y "cup" flaps. He sutures the two distal angles of the triangle together after mobilizing the flap, which forms a cup that fits over the tip.

The lateral or Kutler[172] V-Y advancement flap[98,291] (Fig. 49-24) is raised in identical fashion to the midline V-Y with the exception that there is only one neurovascular bundle to be protected in each flap. Oblique V-Y advancement flaps have also been described.[336] V-Y flaps need not be based on a single known pedicle such as the proper digital artery and nerve. They can be raised on a pedicle of subcutaneous tissue, relying on random vessels contained therein. In such flaps the pedicle is made as wide as possible. Such V-Y flaps have been described for closure of defects and release of contractures.[241]

Regional Flaps

Regional flaps derive from tissues not immediately adjacent to the primary defect but from its vicinity. Thus most regional flaps in the hand are raised from another part of the hand. They are both random and axial pattern with respect to their blood supply. In regional flaps the merit of the axial design is very apparent, for all require only one surgical procedure, whereas regional flaps of random design all require at least two. At the first operation the flap is raised and applied to the primary defect. At the second the pedicle is divided and inset.

Random-Pattern Regional Flaps

The cross-finger and thenar flaps are random-pattern regional flaps. Both are used in the repair of fingertip defects, in particular those with bone exposed and with more loss of palmar tissue than dorsal. The choice between the two is dictated for many surgeons by the sex and age of the patient. For them, the thenar flap is reserved for the young female, since it often requires somewhat more flexion of the injured finger than does the cross-finger and therefore carries a greater theoretical risk of persistent joint contracture. The joints in such a patient are likely to be more supple than in her older male counterpart and she is also more likely to find unacceptable the secondary defect resulting from a cross-finger flap. While the thenar flap is used solely for fingertip injuries, the cross-finger flap and its variants are used also for defects of the dorsal and palmar aspects of all digits.

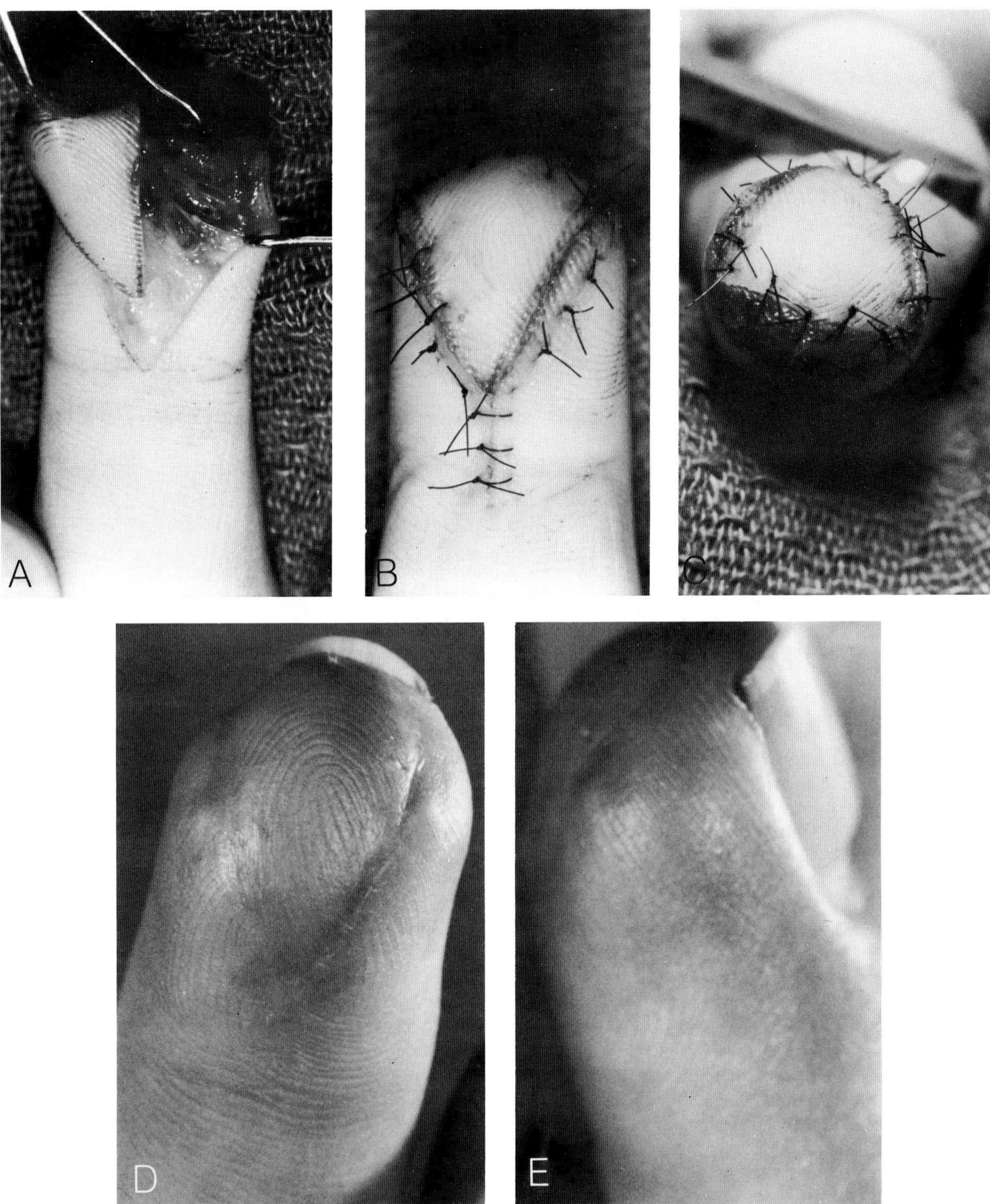

Fig. 49-23. V-Y Advancement. **(A)** The mobilization required down to the vessels of the flap can be seen. The movement achieved by this mobilization is sufficient to permit easy suture **(B)** over the amputation **(C)**. **(D&E)** The result at an early stage.

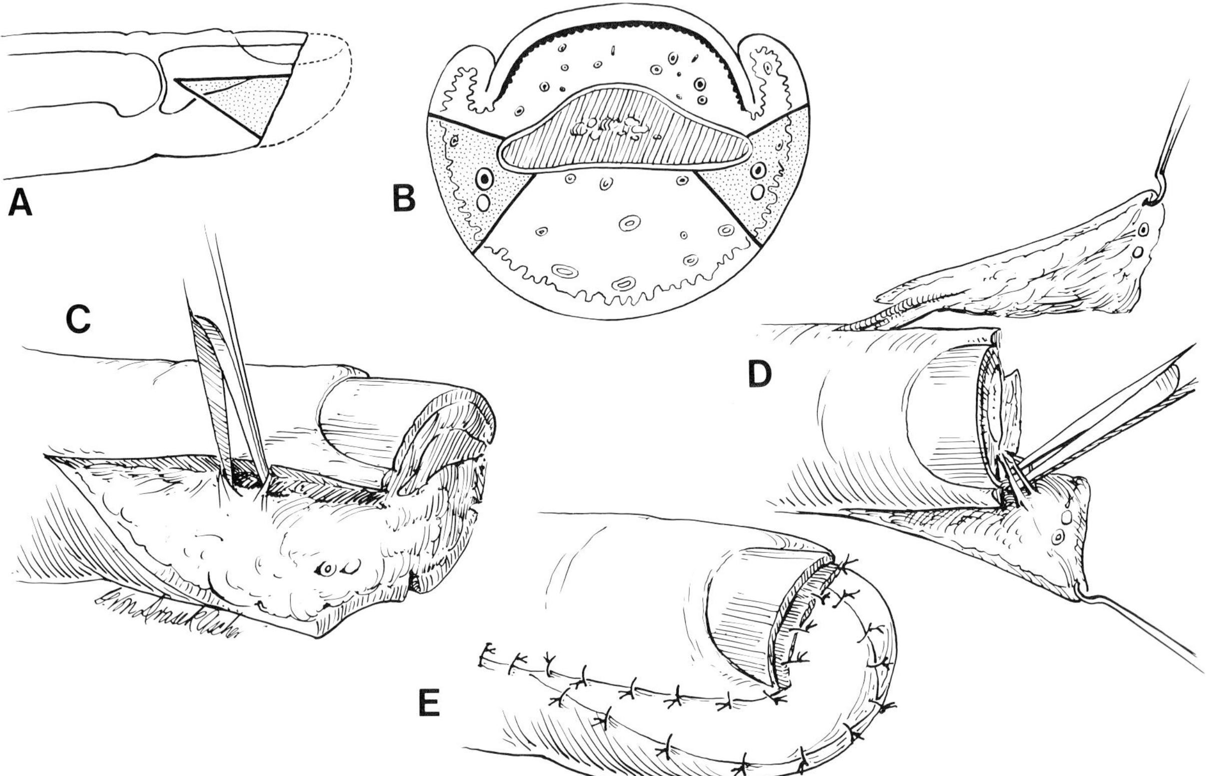

Fig. 49-24. Kutler double lateral V-Y advancements. **(A)** The advancement flaps are designed over the neurovascular pedicles and carried right down to bone **(B)**. The fibrous septa are defined and **(C)** divided, permitting free mobilization **(D)** on the neurovascular pedicles alone. The flaps then advance readily to the midline **(E)**.

Cross-Finger Flap

While the cross-finger flap has several variants that are outlined below, the basic design is for loss of palmar digital tissue and is fashioned on the dorsal aspect of the middle phalanx of the adjacent finger.[157] For pulp loss, the middle is used for the index but otherwise the donor finger is that radial to the injured one. Flaps to and from the thumb are discussed below. The cross-finger flap can be tailored to fit a pattern of the primary defect. It has been recommended, however, that the primary defect be squared off[168] and that the largest flap available from the dorsal aspect of the middle phalanx be raised in all cases. The merits of this approach are that the vascularity of the flap is assured and the secondary defect once healed is perhaps less conspicuous. The disadvantage is that one would excise normal skin from the injured digit. A compromise is chosen, in which the full flap is raised but is then tailored to the primary defect. That margin of the defect which is adjacent to the donor finger is designated "the hinge" (AB in Fig. 49-25A). It corresponds closely to the base of the flap, which is also called a hinge (A′B′ in Fig. 49-25B). It is similar to the pivot point of transposition flaps in that it is a fixed reference around which tissues move. It differs in that it is a line rather than a point. A pattern of the primary defect is made and turned through 180 degrees around the hinge and applied to the dorsum of the donor finger. By adjusting the position of the hinge the necessary flap can be derived entirely from the skin of the dorsum of the middle phalanx. The flap to be raised is then outlined to include not only the necessary flap but also all of the skin of the dorsum of the middle phalanx, from midlateral line to midlateral line and from the proximal extension crease of the DIP joint to the distal extension crease of the PIP joint. In marking the hinge it should be recalled that in all random-pattern flaps the direction that they face can be altered by extension cuts (see Fig. 49-41). Thus, in the cross-finger flap a proximal transverse incision that extends more palmar than the distal transverse incision will cause the deep surface of the flap to face proximally; one in which the distal cut extends more palmar will face distally. The former is more often required, causing the flap to fit well to an amputation stump (Fig. 49-26). The latter is needed only in longer, more palmar defects where considerable flexion of the injured finger is necessary. The flap margins are incised. Immediately beneath the skin multiple longitudinal veins will be encountered. These should be coagulated and cut in order to reach the correct plane, which lies immediately superficial to the extensor tendon. Once the veins are divided, the flap is raised with ease, since only loose areolar tissue lies in the plane of dissection. The flap is hinged away from the donor site and applied to the primary defect to check the fit. If the pedicle is kinked to reach the defect, this can often be eliminated by extending either the proximal or distal transverse cut of the flap. Where the flap does not fold easily away from the donor finger, Cleland's ligament may be restraining it. The ligament can be incised to permit easier folding of the

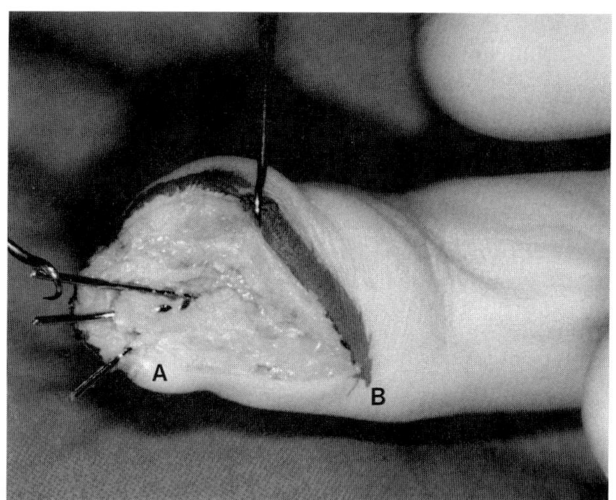

A

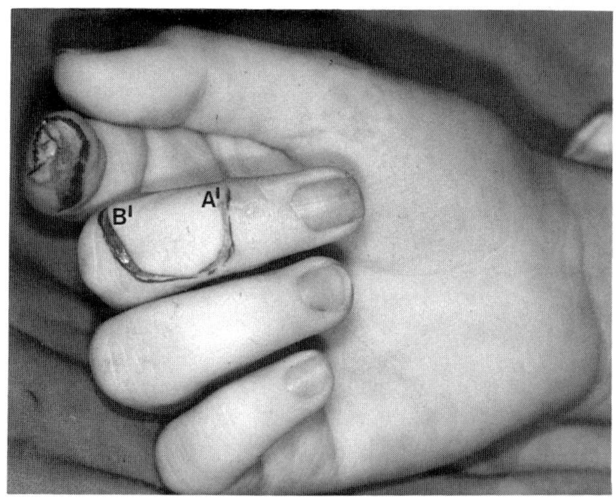

B

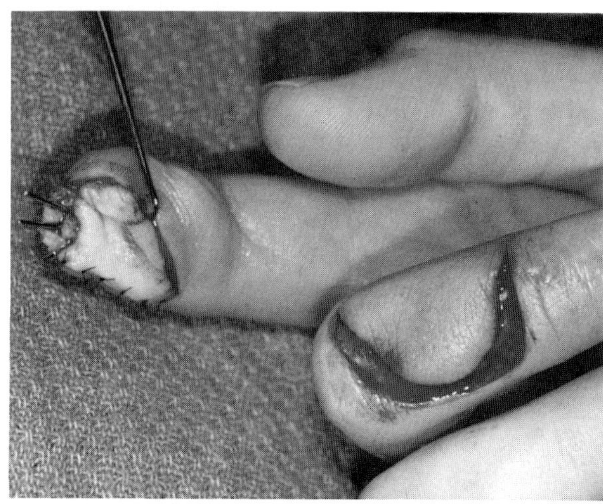

C

Fig. 49-25. Cross-finger flap. **(A)** The primary defect has been created in an attempt to release a severely hooked nail that the patient wishes to keep. The "hinge" of the primary defect is marked *"AB"*. **(B)** The cross-finger flap has been raised from the dorsum of the adjacent middle finger. Its hinge is marked *"A′ B′ "* **(C)** The full-thickness skin flap is sewn initially to the hinge of the primary defect. *(Figure continues.)*

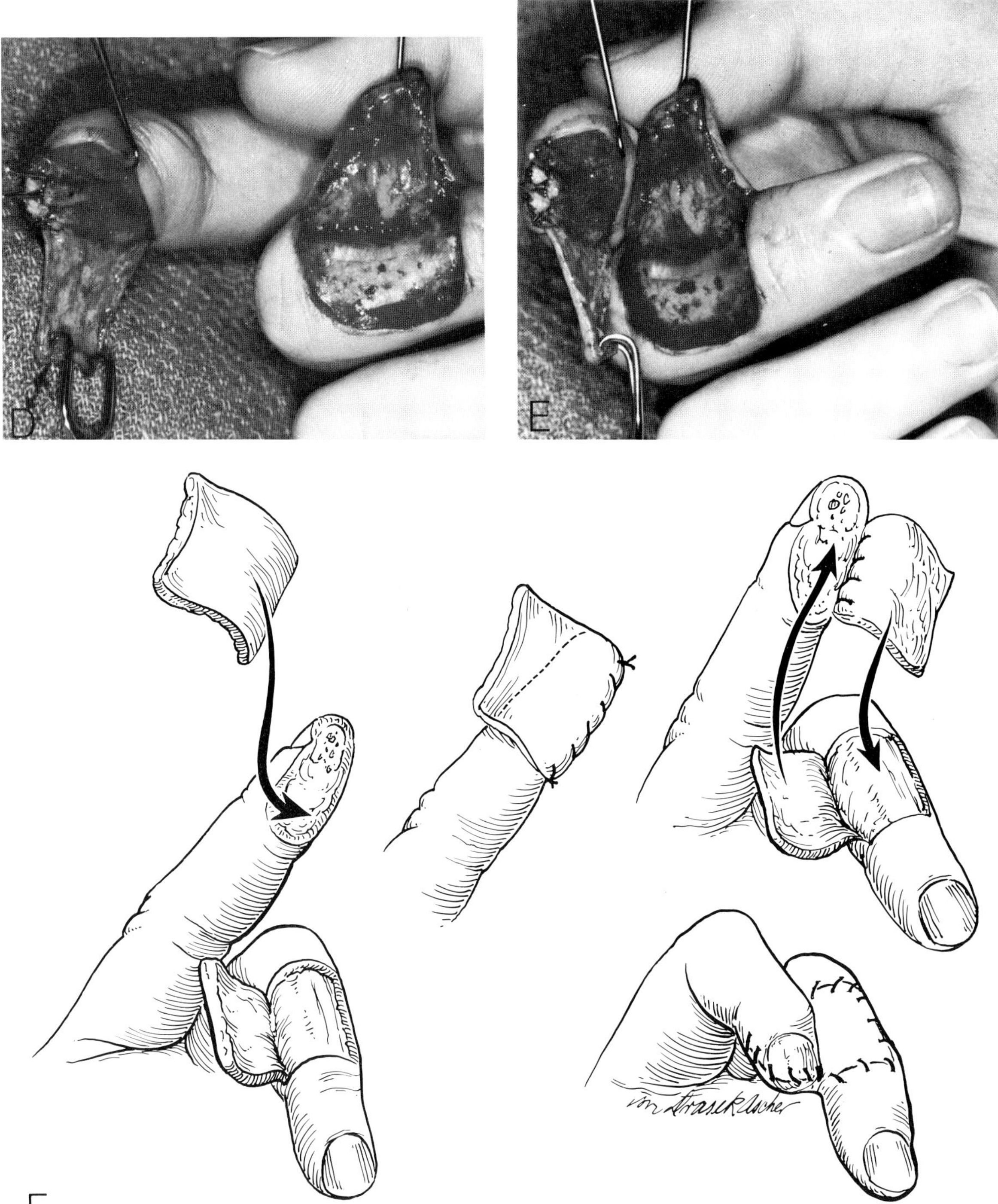

Fig. 49-25 *(Continued).* **(D&E)** The two "flaps" are now swung outward. It can be seen that this approximates the flaps to the defects with full closure of the bridge segment. **(F)** This is shown diagrammatically.

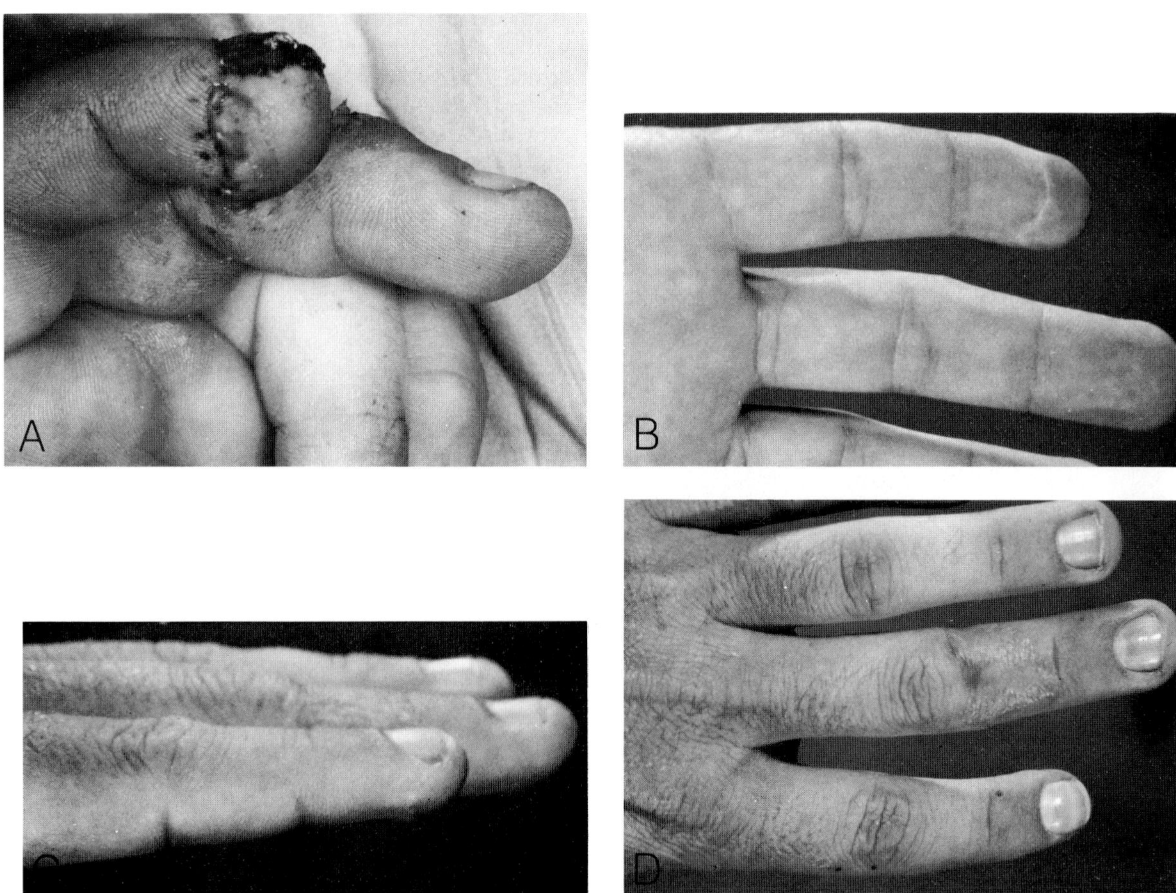

Fig. 49-26. Cross-finger flap to an amputation. **(A)** The orientation of the flap on the tip of an amputation has been achieved by making the proximal cut in the donor finger significantly longer than the distal cut, thus causing the flap to face proximally (see Fig. 49-41B). **(B–D)** The result.

flap. The vessels to the flap penetrate the more superficial part of the ligament and may be damaged unless care is taken to incise it at its depth, against the skeleton.

Once the flap has been raised satisfactorily, a pattern of the full-thickness graft required for the secondary defect should be taken. The tourniquet should be released at this juncture and hemostasis achieved. During this process, the full-thickness graft to cover the secondary defect is obtained. This is commonly taken from the same limb, at the wrist, the elbow, or the inner aspect of the upper forearm or arm. This practice is unacceptable in all except perhaps the older working man in whom scars will be good and possibly of little consequence. In the young and especially the female, the infliction of a wound in any of these sites is to be condemned. Rather, the grafts should be taken from the inguinal region. Before puberty, the skin that has the potential of bearing pubic hair can be avoided by staying at least one centimeter lateral to the femoral pulse.

As in all flaps, it is desirable to close all raw surfaces. When one considers the hinge of the cross-finger design, the only free edge to which the skin graft can be sutured is the hinge margin of the primary defect, which is very inaccessible after the flap has been sutured in place, lying as it does between the fingers. To overcome this difficulty, the skin grafts should be first laid on the *primary* defect as if it were intended to use it to cover the primary wound rather than the flap already raised. The graft is then sutured to the hinge margin of the primary defect (Fig. 49-25C). It will be appreciated that there are now two "flaps," the cross-finger and the graft, with contiguous hinges. If both are swung 180 degrees around their hinges, the flap will come to lie on the primary and the graft on the secondary defect (Fig. 49-25D and E). For one last time the positioning of the flap is checked. If the flap has been well chosen, any kinks can be eliminated by lengthening the extension cut. The flap can now be inset and sutured into position, trimming as necessary since the flap was not designed to fit the primary defect. The skin graft is sutured to the secondary defect. The circulation to the flap should be good, although a little blanching around the margins is common and acceptable. If the flap appears very pale and has been designed and raised correctly, it may be that the recipient finger is extending, thereby exerting undue pressure on the flap and its pedicle. This can be overcome by flexing the recipient finger until circulation returns and then maintaining the position by inserting a K-wire between the fingers, usually transfixing the middle phalanx of the injured finger and the proximal phalanx of the donor.[168] This is rarely necessary.

Variants of the Cross-Finger Flap

Reversed Cross-Finger Flap. Primary defects on the dorsum of the finger cannot be covered by a standard dorsal cross-finger flap as described above. They can be treated with a flap taken from the palmar surface, but the skin is rather unsuitable and the secondary defect would be in a more significant area functionally than the primary, never a satisfactory solution. In such circumstances a reversed cross-finger flap should be used.[11] This is designed on the dorsal aspect of the middle phalanx of the adjacent finger as with the standard flap, the hinge being adjacent to the primary defect (Fig. 49-27A). The first step, however, is to raise a full-thickness skin graft from the donor site, commencing the elevation at the hinge and leaving it attached on the opposite margin of the design. This should be done at the level of the deep dermis, below the hair follicles, and requires a scalpel (Fig. 49-27B). The underlying subcutaneous tissue is then raised in the same manner as the standard cross-finger flap, with its hinge adjacent to the defect (Fig. 49-27C). When this flap is swung through 180 degrees around the hinge, its superficial surface lies on the primary defect and the deep surface becomes superficial. A full-thickness skin graft is harvested, laid on the flap, and both are sutured to the margins of the primary defect. The full-thickness graft previously raised from the donor finger is sutured in place to cover the secondary defect (Fig. 49-27D).

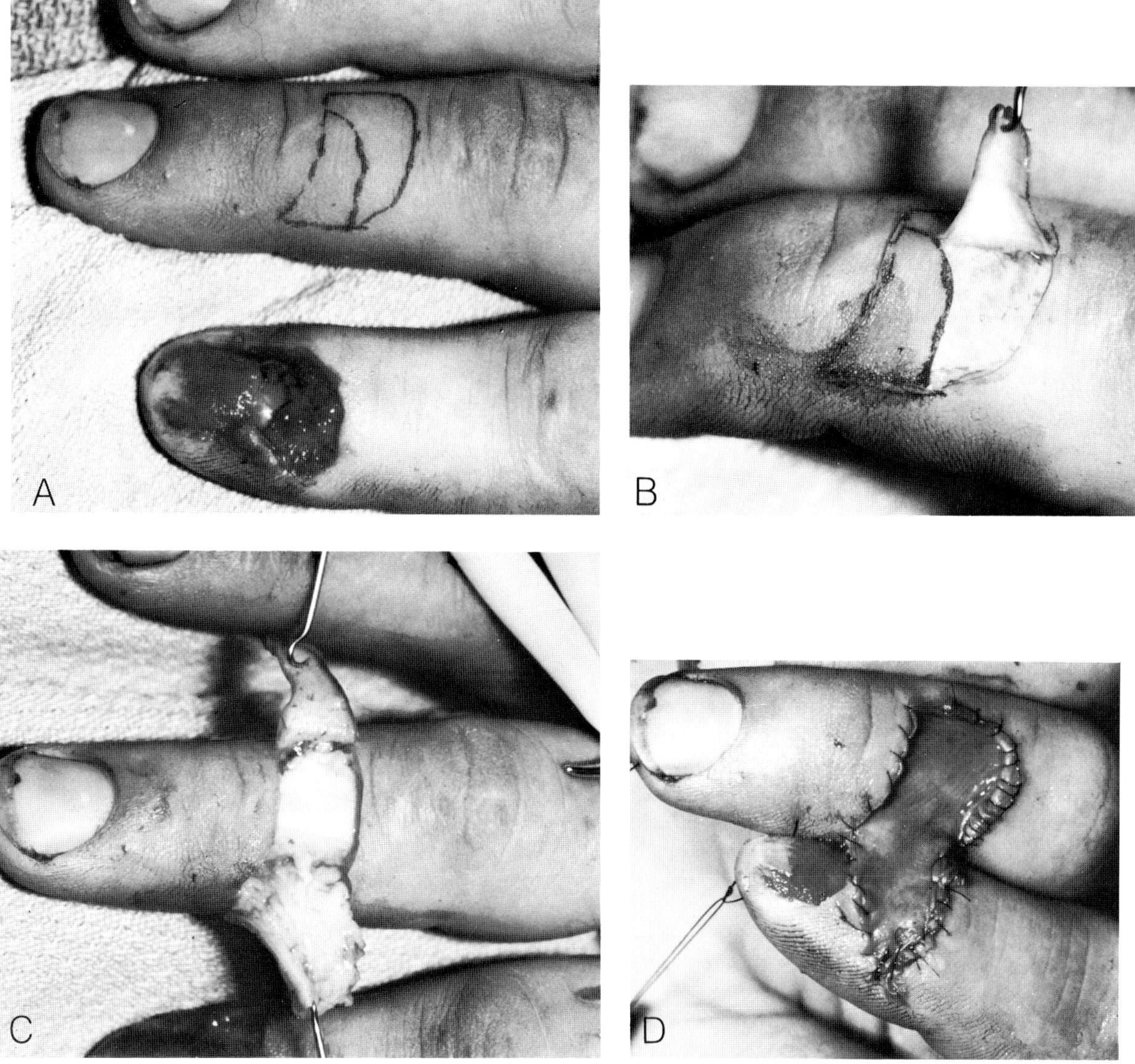

Fig. 49-27. Reversed cross-finger flap. **(A)** A dorsal defect, including the proximal nailfold, was inflicted on the index finger by a router. A flap has been drawn out that includes a segment of skin to replace the superficial surface of the nail cul-de-sac. **(B)** The reversed cross-finger flap is commenced by raising a layer of skin at the subdermal level based on the aspect of the design opposite to the injured finger, leaving skin on the portion that will form the cul-de-sac when the flap is turned over. **(C)** The remainder of the flap is raised as for a cross-finger flap, the hinge being adjacent to the primary defect. **(D)** Both the primary and secondary defects are covered together with a thin full-thickness skin graft.

Variations in the position of the hinge are necessary in certain situations. The standard position along the lateral margin of the donor finger that is adjacent to the injured digit brings the flap to the palmar surface of the injured finger. Where the defect is more complex, various hinge positions should be tested by making a pattern of the primary defect, laying it on the donor finger, bringing the injured finger to meet it and adjusting the location and hinge of the pattern until the most comfortable posture is achieved. Thus, for example, an amputation that extends on to the dorsal aspect on the distal phalanx may be best covered by a distally based flap with the hinge almost transversely across the finger.

Innervated Cross-Finger Flap. Cohen[56] has described a technique for innervation of the standard cross-finger flap. The dorsal branch of the proper digital nerve of the donor finger, on the side away from the injured finger, which supplies the dorsum of the middle phalanx, is divided proximally in the course of raising the free margin of the flap. It is then joined to the proper digital nerve of the injured finger on the side opposite the donor digit. Thus the ulnar dorsal digital branch of the middle would be joined to the radial digital nerve of the index. While attractive theoretically, one is deterred from incorporating this additional complexity by the excellent sensory results of the standard cross-finger flap. Kleinert and others[169] reported 70 percent of patients as having two-point discrimination less than 8 mm in standard cross-finger flaps. Johnson and Iverson[146] noted that all their patients had better sensation than that present in an area equivalent to the donor site in the opposite hand, and Nicolai and Hentenaar[242] reported that 53 percent had two-point discrimination within 2 mm of that of the same pulp in the opposite hand.

For resurfacing the thumb, a cross-finger flap from the dorsum of the proximal phalanx of the index finger can be innervated by transposition of the radial nerve supplying that skin[4,107,226] (see also Chapter 57). Before this flap is used, the radial nerve should be blocked at the wrist to delineate its dermatome. The flap is raised with either a proximal or radial base, care being taken to preserve the branches of the radial nerve. At the time of division, the nerve is isolated and dissected back through an incision extending proximally to a point close to the snuffbox sufficiently so that the nerve can be transposed to a further incision made on the dorsum of the thumb to the proximal edge of the previously transposed flap. This technique is not of value in providing coverage where almost all of the thumb length has been maintained, as sensation in such circumstances often deteriorates with use. This is presumably due to the tension exerted on the transposed nerve with extension and abduction of the thumb. As with the innervated cross-finger flap, results must be compared with those reported for standard flaps. With the radial nerve innervated flap, Bralliar[30] reported 64 percent of patients with two-point discrimination less than 15 mm, results that are poorer than those reported above for standard cross-finger flaps.

Cross-Thumb Flap. Cross-thumb flaps[10] (see also Chapter 57) are indicated where the primary defect is on the radial aspect of the index finger, or in pulp injuries of that digit where the normal donor finger for a routine cross-finger flap, the middle, is injured or absent (Fig. 49-28). The cross-thumb flap is invariably taken from the dorsal aspect of the proximal phalanx of the thumb with a proximal pedicle. The flap is raised and applied in the same manner as a standard cross-finger flap, except that it is necessary to apply the full-thickness graft to the secondary defect before suturing the flap in place (Fig. 49-28).

Thenar Flap

The thenar flap was first described by Gatewood,[106] who was distinguished in several ways, not least of which by his lack of first names.[219] The procedure has been much criticized because of joint contracture and tenderness of the donor site, but has received strong support from Beasley.[23] His description places the thenar flap high on the thenar eminence in a position almost identical to that illustrated by Gatewood. In a series of 150 cases, Melone[222] showed only 4 percent persistent PIP joint contracture and 3 percent hypersensitivity of the palmar scar. With respect to the likelihood of joint contracture, simple observation shows that the PIP joint of the injured finger is flexed almost equally when either a cross-finger or a properly designed thenar flap are applied.

The injured finger is flexed to meet the thenar eminence with the thumb abducted so that the point of contact is adjacent to the metacarpophalangeal crease of the thumb. The *palmar,* proximal margin of the primary defect is marked on the thenar eminence and serves as the marking for the hinge of the intended thenar flap, which is customarily based on the radial (proximal) aspect of the thumb. The flap is marked out distal to that base (Fig. 49-29B). The flap should be a little longer than the length of the defect from palmar to dorsal margins. It should also be wider than the primary defect by 50 percent. This is because the contour of the lost pulp is semicircular and the shape can be restored by making the width of the flap equal to 1.5d, where d is the width of the primary defect measured as a straight line. The flap is raised at the level of the underlying thenar muscle so as to include as much subcutaneous tissue as possible (Fig. 49-29C). The only potential hazard is damage to the radial digital nerve of the thumb, which should be sought and protected. A full-thickness graft is applied to the secondary defect (Fig. 49-29D) and the flap sutured to the primary defect. In so doing, the distal end of the flap should not be sutured to the nailbed, but should be left a little long (Fig. 49-29E). This excess can be trimmed after division of the flap, recreating the hyponychium of the finger. The pedicle of the flap as described is proximal, but it may be ulnar for predominantly ulnar defects[20] and radial for radial. Dellon[65] suggested a distal pedicle, which he termed a "proximal inset thenar flap," believing that this design offered the potential to cover a larger defect and to close the secondary defect primarily. He reported six cases and his claims were refuted by Beasley in discussion.

Division of Random Regional Flaps

Flatt[88] has recommended that thenar flaps be divided at 2 weeks, and this is the standard practice for all random regional flaps. To divide them earlier invites necrosis, although some surgeons test and divide these flaps as early as 7 days.[168] To do so later than 2 weeks might be expected to increase the incidence of joint stiffness. Division is usually performed under

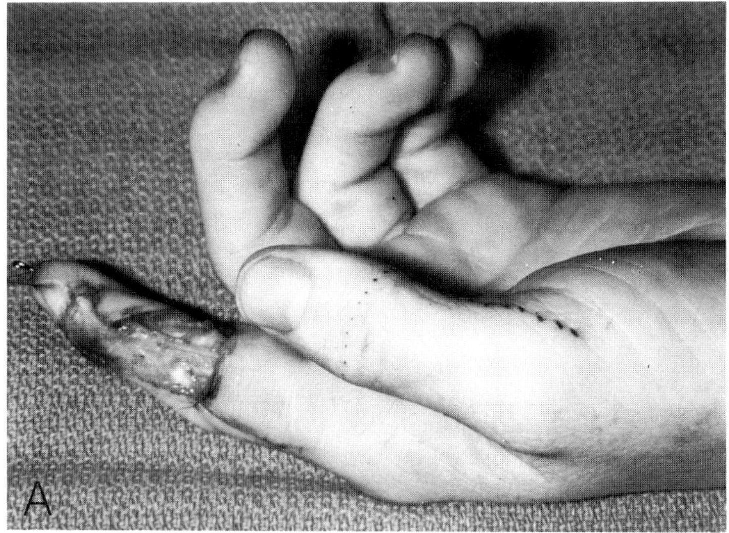

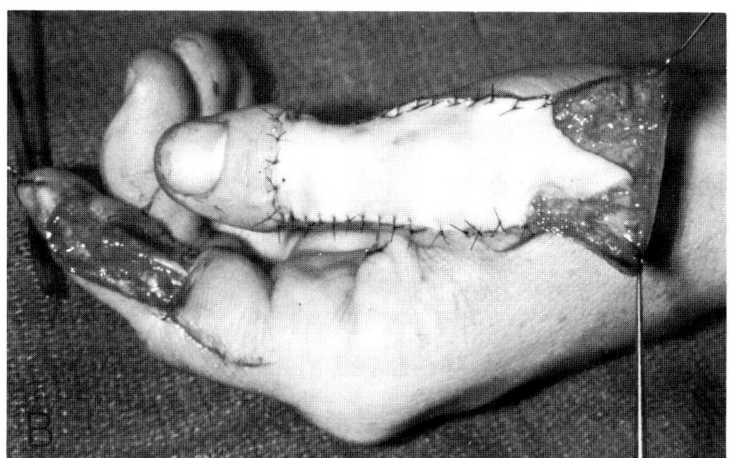

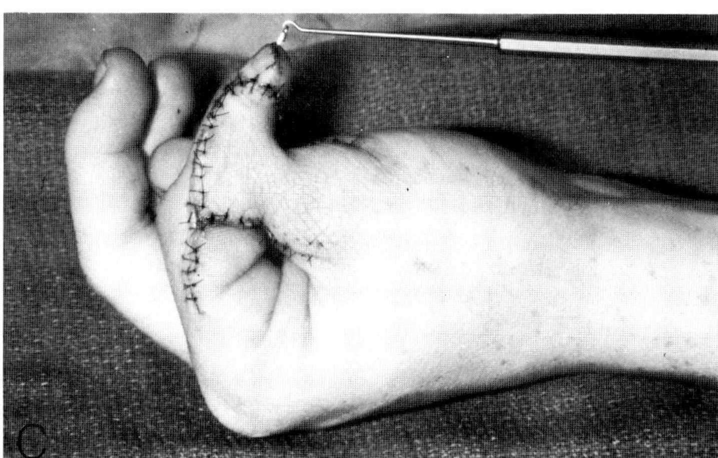

Fig. 49-28. Cross-thumb flap. **(A)** A defect on the radial aspect of the index finger is to be covered by a proximally based cross-thumb flap. **(B)** The secondary defect is covered with a split-thickness skin graft that also covers the bridge segment. This must be done before **(C)** suturing the flap into position.

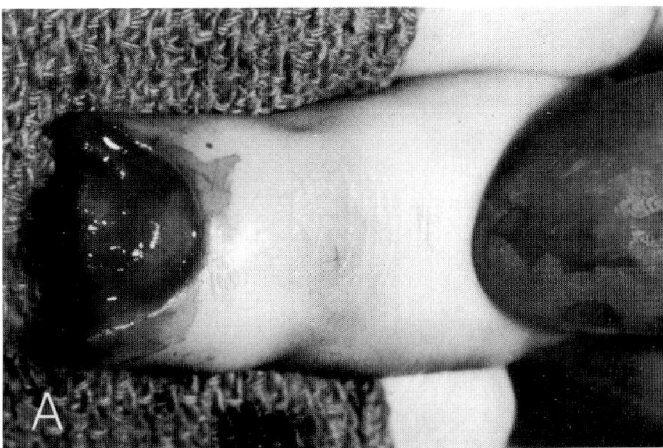

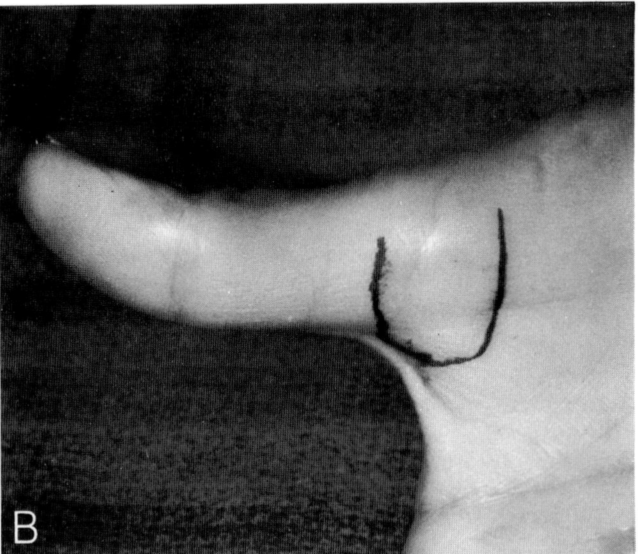

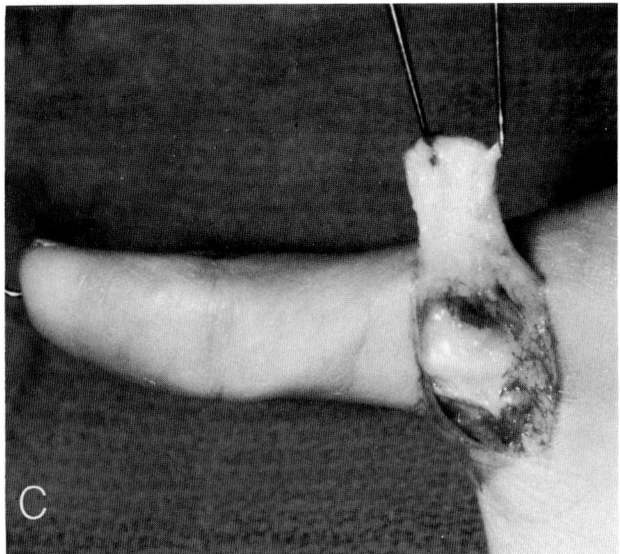

Fig. 49-29. Thenar flap. **(A)** An amputation in a girl of the tip of the index finger in which approximately one-half of the nailbed remains with good bony support is an appropriate indication for a thenar flap. **(B)** The finger has been carried to the thumb and the proximal margin of the primary defect has been used as the proximal marking of a proximally (radially) based thenar flap. This is designed in the region of the metacarpophalangeal crease of the thumb. **(C)** The flap is raised taking care to avoid damage to the digital nerves but carrying as much subcutaneous tissue as possible. *(Figure continues.)*

local infiltration anesthesia. The pedicle may be inset or not, but Beasley[23] and Dellon[65] emphasized the possibility of necrosis if too vigorous dissection is done at this stage. Immediate mobilization is mandatory, and the one benefit of regional over local anesthesia is that the joints can be taken gently through a full range of motion under its protection.

Axial-Pattern Regional Flaps

Regional flaps applicable to the upper extremity that have a known pedicle are the neurovascular island flap, the fillet flap, and those axial cutaneous, fasciocutaneous, and musculocutaneous flaps that may be used in the upper extremity.

Neurovascular Island Flap[201]

Hailed by Hueston in 1965 as "the most important development in hand surgery in the past decade," [139] the neurovascular island flap was first described in the English literature by Littler[191,192] (see also Chapter 57). The technique was initially popular since it had the potential of transferring sensibility to the functionally significant pulp of the thumb from a less important part of the hand, such as the middle or ring finger. However, after Hueston's comment and Tubiana's 1961 report of 10 cases with almost normal two-point discrimination,[335] there were four adverse reports in the decade commencing in 1966,[171,214,236,267] expressing dissatisfaction on the grounds of high or absent two-point discrimination, cold intol-

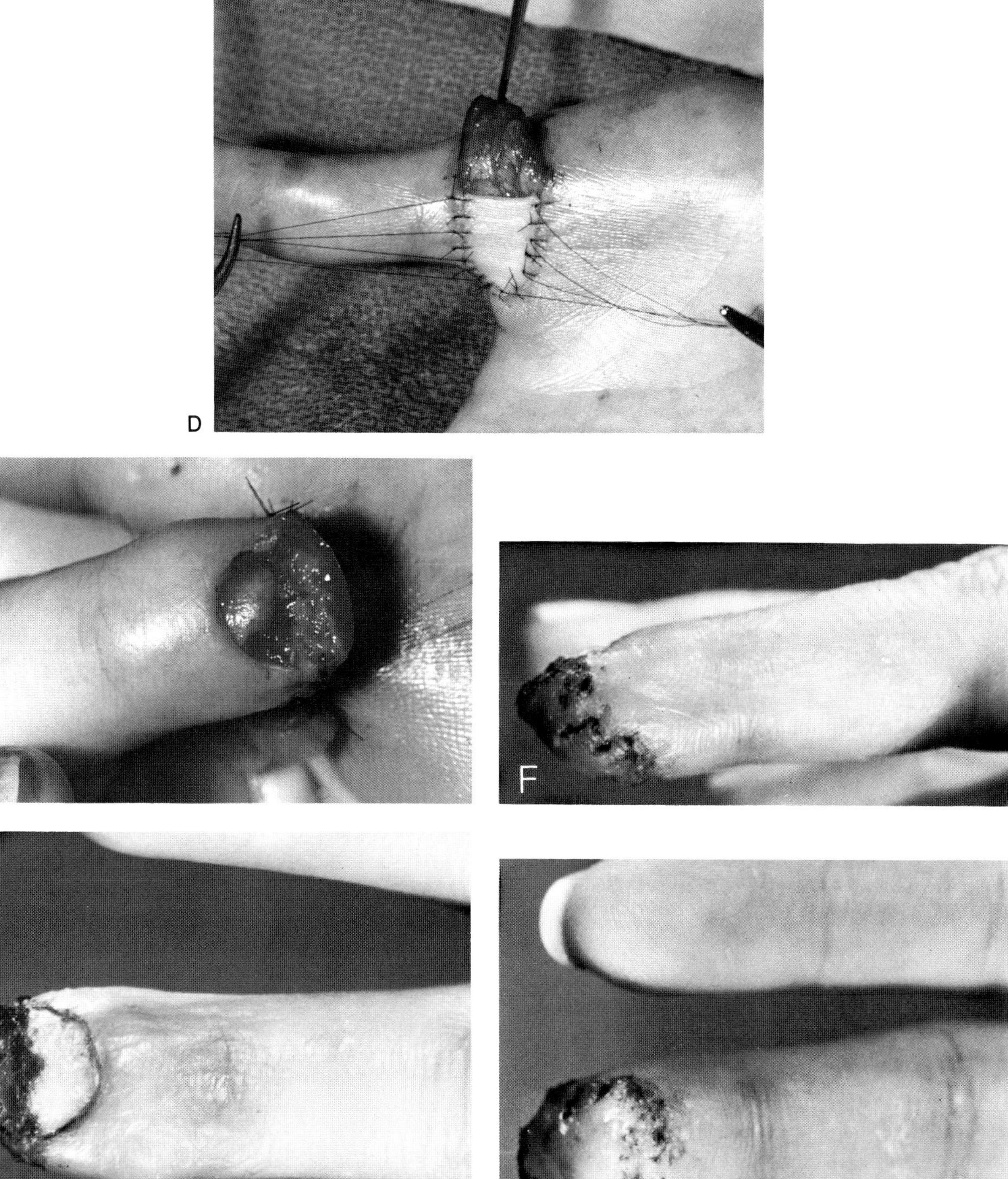

Fig. 49-29 *(Continued).* **(D)** The secondary defect is covered with a full-thickness graft. **(E)** The flap is sutured in position but the free margin is left a little long in order to support the advancing nail. **(F–H)** The early result shows good contour of the tip with satisfactory support for later nail growth.

erance, hyperesthesia and failure of reorientation. There has been much debate on this latter score, both on the grounds of whether it can happen and if so, how often. That it *can* has been demonstrated by elegant cortical mapping studies in primates.[52] That it *does* occur in 25 percent of patients was shown by both Murray, Ord, and Gavelin[236] and Henderson and Reid.[129] To overcome this problem, European surgeons[344] have divided the nerve of the flap at the time of transfer and sutured it to that of the thumb. This seemingly attractive solution has two potential hazards. First, dissecting in the pedicle may impair the venous return of the flap (see below). Second, a painful neuroma may remain on the unsatisfied nerve of the pedicle, as it may, of course, on that of the thumb if this division and resuture is *not* done. Both possible neuromas can be eliminated from the thumb by dissecting the nerve in question in the palm, dividing it and turning it back into the carpal tunnel where it will be protected from contact. The tide of adverse comment was turned in 1977 with a paper from Markley,[200] who pointed out several important technical reasons for the previous poor results, reporting no loss of two-point discrimination in his cases. Henderson and Reid[129] reported an average of 9 mm in 20 cases, and in 12 cases done by the author over 3 years ending in 1980, two-point discrimination ranged from 3 to 10 mm with an average of 6.4.

The major indication for neurovascular island transfer is damage to the thumb, sufficient to produce a scarred tender pulp, anesthesia, or relative ischemia. Stated conversely, a neurovascular island pedicle can provide robust padding, good sensation or increased blood flow, or any combination of the three. The flap may be taken from any digit, preference being given to one that is in other respects unsatisfactory but that contains an intact neurovascular pedicle. For example, a digit that is being considered for ray amputation due to lack of motion or previous partial amputation may be an excellent donor. Otherwise, either neurovascular island from the third web space is selected. My preference is for the ulnar aspect of the middle finger, as it is longer and makes less contact in normal handling than does the radial aspect of the ring finger. Before surgery the flow to the hand must be assessed by Doppler. Not only is good flow necesssary in both vessels of the proposed donor digit to supply both the flap and that finger, but it is also essential in the contralateral vessel of the digit adjacent to the flap pedicle, since the other vessel to that digit will be divided in the course of raising the pedicle. Thus, in taking an island flap from the ulnar aspect of the middle finger, flow must be present in the ulnar proper digital artery of the ring finger, as well as in the radial proper digital artery of the middle finger (Fig. 49-30).

The operation is commenced by creating the primary defect on the thumb (Fig. 49-31A). The margins of the defect should be undermined quite generously to accommodate the pedicle of the intended flap. In particular the proximal margin should be elevated, and there the distal end of the tunnel from the palm through which the pedicle will pass should be made of as large a caliber as possible by scar excision and blunt scissor dissection toward the palm. The digital nerves should be dealt with appropriately. If one is to be joined to the nerve of the flap, as in the European technique, the ulnar digital nerve should be selected and prepared if in good condition. If the nerves are not

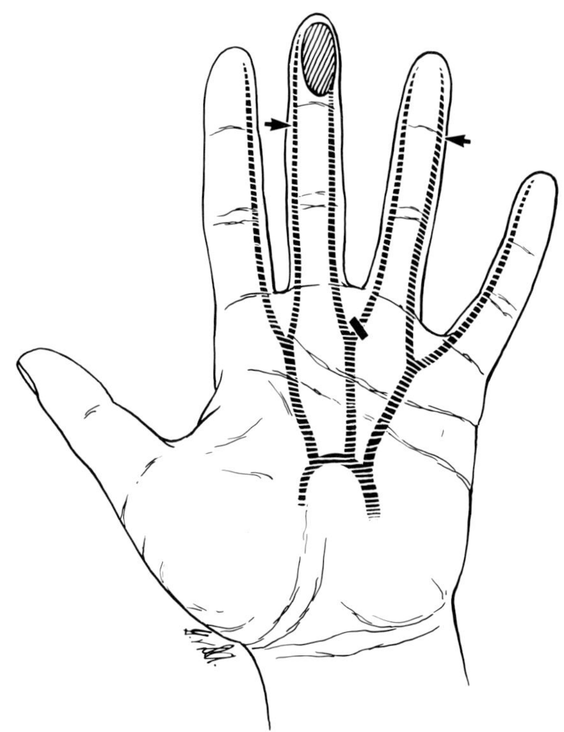

Fig. 49-30. Neurovascular island flap—preliminary evaluation. It is necessary to ensure by Doppler studies that flow exists not only in the vessel that will supply the flap and in the vessel that will maintain the donor digit after the flap has been raised *(left arrow),* but also in the contralateral digital artery of the adjacent finger *(right arrow)* because the ipsilateral vessel will be divided *(bar)* in mobilizing the pedicle.

to be used and have been the source of discomfort, they should be dissected proximally to the muscle bellies of the flexor pollicis brevis and there transected. A pattern of the defect is then taken, making it sufficiently generous to accommodate the unusual bulk of the pedicle and pulp tissue that will be transferred. The pattern is then applied to the ulnar aspect of the middle finger, carrying the distal point out to or even beyond the tip of the digit on to the radial aspect. Where necessary, the flap can extend as far proximally as the web.[139] The proximal incision is then marked out in the midlateral line as far as the web and into the palm as a zigzag as far proximal as the distal margin of the flexor retinaculum (Fig. 49-31B). The initial dissection is performed in the palm to ensure that there are no anomalies of the vascular tree. If any are found that preclude transfer, the procedure should be abandoned in most instances for some better alternative, although the transfer can be done on the metacarpal artery arising from the deep palmar arch.[283] Where the anatomy is normal, the dissection can proceed into the finger. A most important point should be made with respect to the dissection in the finger. The veins that accompany the nerve and artery are not the main drainage of the pulp and as such are small, irregular, and unpredictable. To ensure their survival and therefore that of the flap, the pedicle in the finger as far proximal as the bifurcation of the common digital artery must be raised as a monobloc of fatty tissue containing all the unidentified elements of the pedicle (Fig. 49-31C). Thus, once

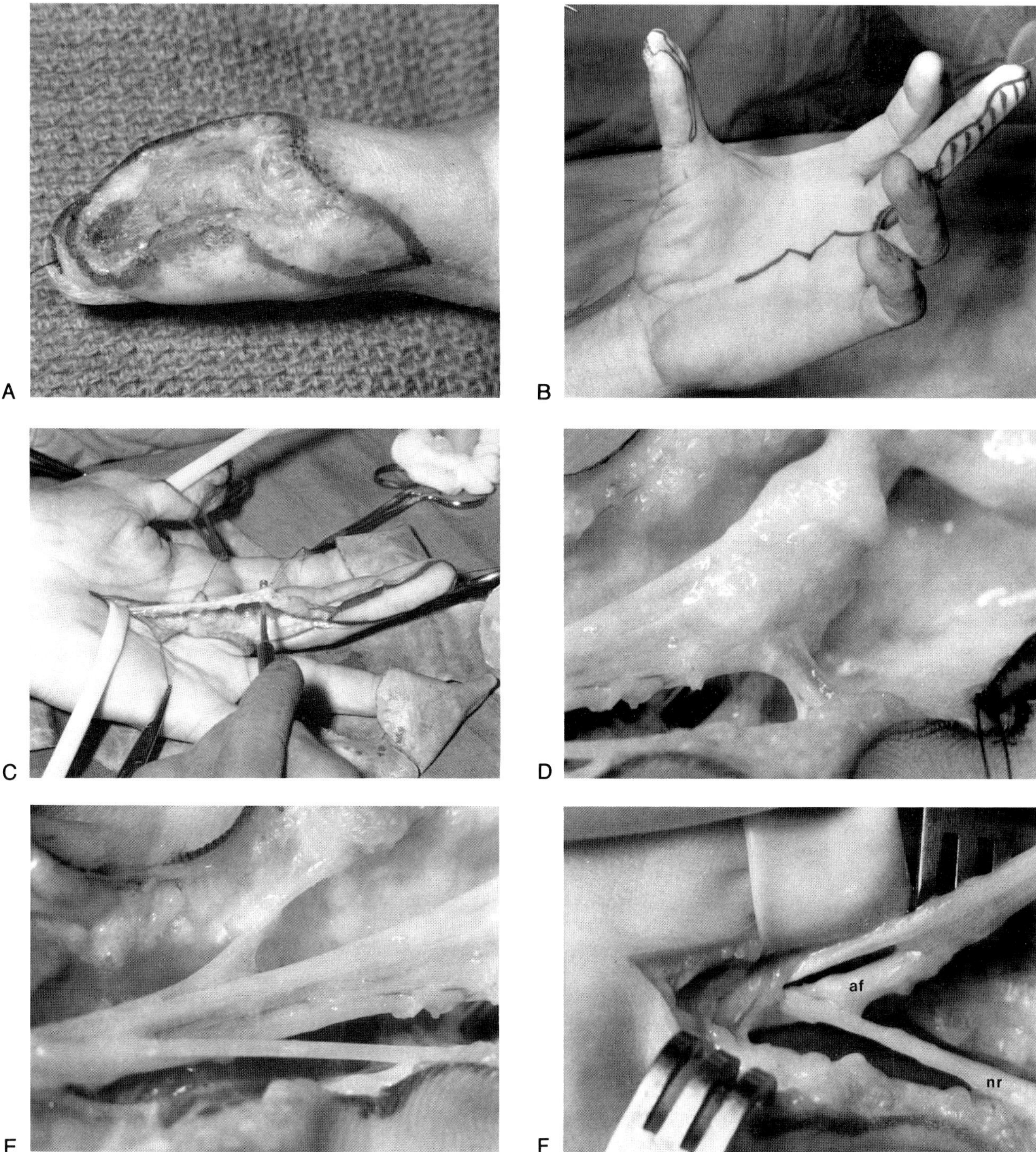

Fig. 49-31. Neurovascular island flap. **(A)** A defect of the thumb caused by a paint injection injury is anesthetic, adherent, and painful. The pattern of the neurovascular island replacement has been marked out. **(B)** Here in another patient, again with an adherent and painful scar of the thumb, a long neurovascular island has been marked out not only to replace soft tissue, but also to increase the blood supply to this relatively avascular thumb. A long flap has been marked out on the ulnar border of the middle finger and the proximal incision marked on the palm of the hand. **(C)** The neurovascular island is shown here at a later stage in dissection to emphasize the manner in which the pedicle should be dissected in the substance of the finger, that is, with a significant surrounding fatty cover that contains the small veins important for drainage. **(D)** The proper digital artery to the adjacent ring finger is displayed for division. **(E)** The common digital nerve is split as far proximally as the superficial palmar arch. **(F)** When the flap is carried over toward the thumb, it can be seen that the artery *(af)* passes around the proper digital nerve to the ring finger *(nr)* and may be kinked by it. *(Figure continues.)*

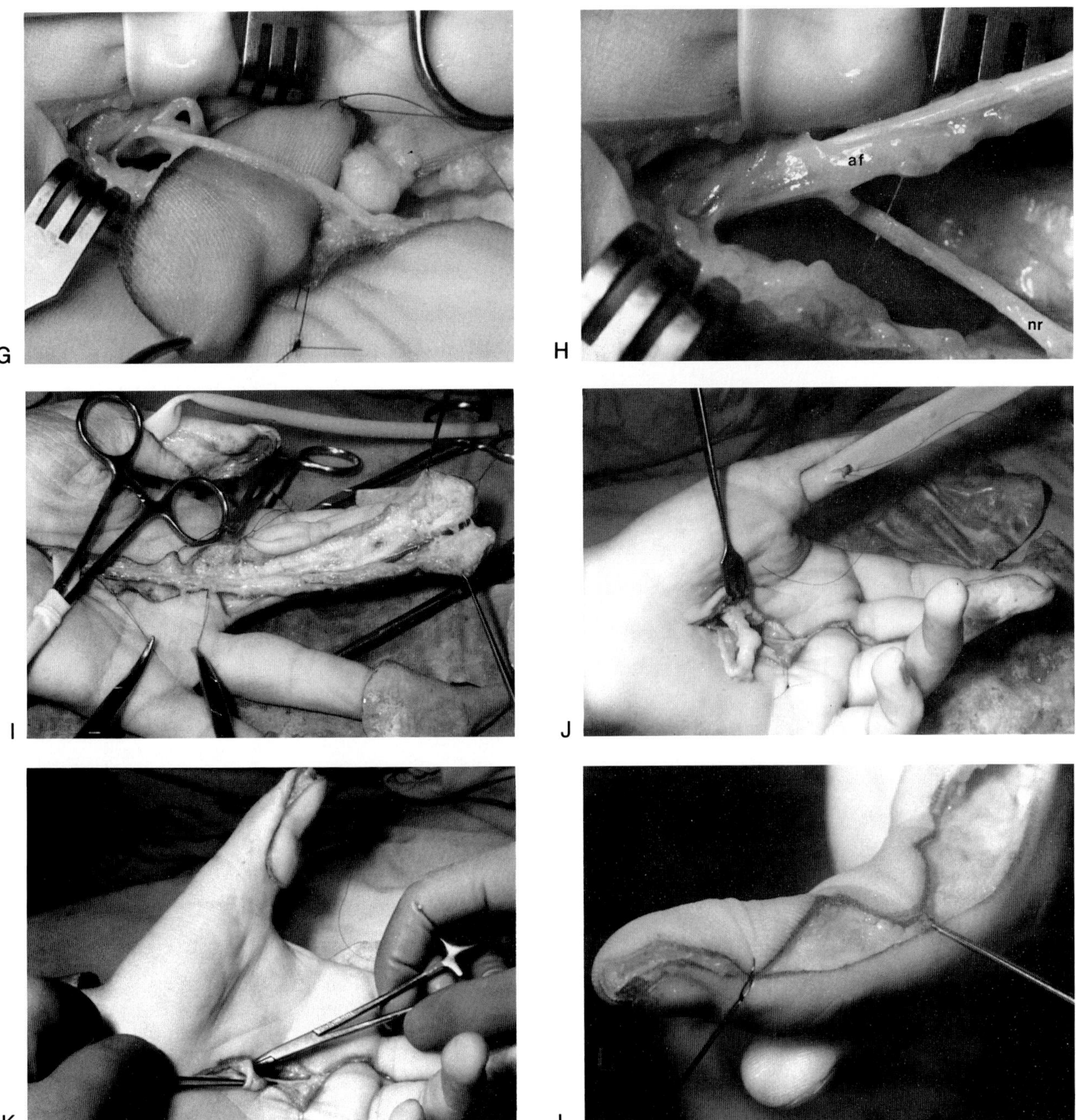

Fig. 49-31 *(Continued).* **(G)** The flap is therefore passed beneath that proper digital nerve to the ring finger and **(H)** the vessel *(af)* released from this kinking *nr*, digital nerve to ring finger. **(I)** A Penrose drain is placed in the tunnel prepared out to the thumb. A small incision is made in the Penrose and a hemostat is advanced through that incision to the ulnar end of the drain. The flap is now released from the tip of the middle finger and placed immediately into the Penrose drain by drawing the stay suture out with the hemostat. **(J)** The flap can now be drawn through the tunnel in the Penrose without torsion on the pedicle. **(K)** With the flap in place and the thumb fully extended and abducted, the pedicle is checked in the palm to ensure that it is under no tension and is not kinked. **(L)** In narrow neurovascular flaps, the donor defect can be closed directly at the pulp, with skin grafts being required more proximally. *(Figure continues.)*

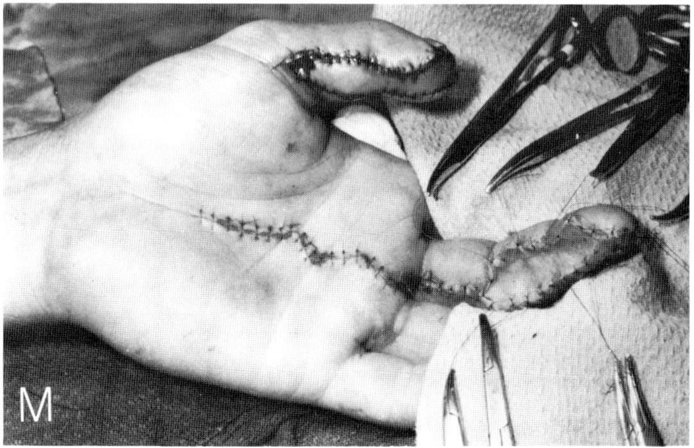

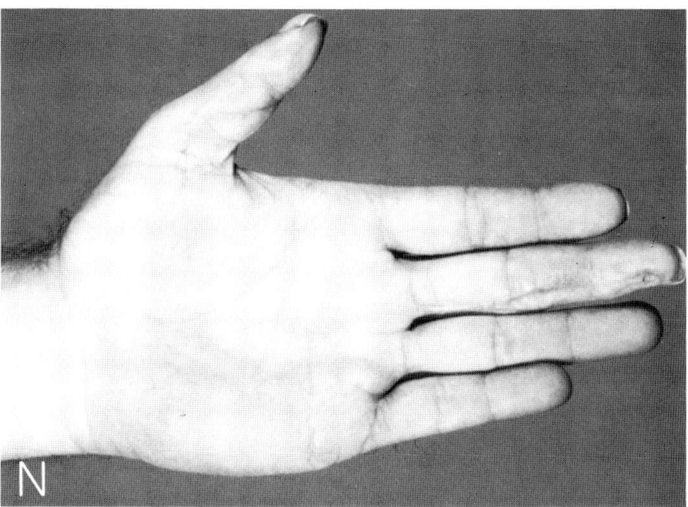

Fig. 49-31 *(Continued).* **(M)** In larger defects, a full-thickness or split-thickness graft is applied to the secondary defect. **(N)** The result.

the incision is made in the side of the finger, the palmar skin is raised off the subcutaneous tissue to almost the midline of the finger. At that point the subcutaneous tissue is incised down to the tendon sheath and then lifted off the sheath, proceeding dorsally until the skeleton of the finger is reached. There it meets the plane of dissection of the dorsal edge of the incision. Blunt scissor dissection will now separate the bloc of pedicle tissue from the skeleton and a vessel loop of soft rubber can be passed around it. Gentle traction away from the skeleton will display the branches of the vessels and nerve to the flexor tendons and interphalangeal joints, which can be divided. The dissection in the finger completed, further progress is made proximally by isolating (Fig. 49-31D) and ligating the branch of the common digital artery to the ring finger. There is commonly a communication from the metacarpal artery to the bifurcation of the common digital, and this also must be sought and ligated.

The proper digital nerves of the third web space should be split from each other in the substance of the common digital nerve (Fig. 49-31E). It is possible also in this way to preserve the dorsal digital branches of these nerves. The vessel loop previously passed around the pedicle is moved proximally as dissection proceeds, lifting the pedicle from its bed and preventing unnecessary dissection within the pedicle itself, which could harm the veins. The proximal advance should only be halted at the superficial palmar arch. Mobilization proceeds this far for two reasons. First, it gives the maximum pedicle length, of importance for reasons discussed below. Second, it allows the surgeon to study the relationship of the pedicle to the intact digital nerve to the ring finger. In some instances if the pedicle is passed directly to the thumb it would be kinked by that nerve to a degree that may impair the circulation (Fig. 49-31F). This potential problem can be eliminated simply by passing the entire neurovascular island beneath that digital nerve before its transfer to the thumb (Fig. 49-31G and H).

The tunnel to the primary defect should now be prepared by blunt scissor dissection in the subcutaneous plane superficial to the palmar fascia. It should be made sufficiently wide to permit the withdrawal of the scissors from primary defect to palm with the tips open by 2 cm. Should the margin of the palmar fascia offer a potential hazard to the pedicle, it should be divided transversely. A 1-inch Penrose drain is passed from the palmar wound to the primary defect, leaving a generous length lying across the ulnar border of the hand. A partial cut is made in the drain close to the palmar wound and a hemostat is passed through it and along the drain, to emerge at its ulnar end (Fig. 49-31I). A stay suture of 4–0 nylon is placed through the tip of the island flap, which can now finally be raised from its bed. By leaving it in place throughout the dissection thus far, the risk of torsion or traction on the pedicle has been minimized. Such risks would damage not only the vascular supply, but might also contribute to reduced digital nerve function with the loss of fine sensibility referred to above. Where the flap is being taken mainly to provide better sensibility or blood supply and little skin is required or has been taken, the palmar aspect of the incision should be undermined to the midline, both to ensure inclusion of all branches of nerve and artery and to facilitate direct closure of the donor pulp. The flap is raised with a scalpel kept close to the skeleton, coagulating the many branches of the digital artery in so doing. Once freed from the finger, the flap is immediately put inside the Penrose drain by placing the stay suture of the flap in the hemostat previously inserted into the drain, and withdrawing the hemostat from the drain. The flap is thereby carefully introduced into the Penrose. This can now be pulled out of the tunnel into the primary defect, maintaining traction on the stay suture to prevent the flap from being extruded from the ulnar end of the drain (Fig. 49-31J). Once the flap is in place, the drain can be discarded.

An important test should now be performed (Fig. 49-31K). With one stitch securing the flap in position in the primary defect, the thumb should be fully abducted and extended. With the thumb in this position, the pedicle should be checked at the proximal end of the palmar wound for any evidence of tension or kinking. Providing the steps outlined above have been followed this should not exist. If it does, it should be eliminated, for traction on the nerve with increasingly vigorous use after full healing is the only likely explanation of the phenomenon of decreasing two-point discrimination reported by some authors.[171,248] The flap should now be sutured into position, prior to release of the tourniquet. All hemostasis should have been achieved in raising the flap and further attempts after release of the tourniquet may damage the pedicle. The tourniquet can now be released and flow to the flap should be immediate. If it is not, the pedicle should be inspected in the palm for any obvious kinks and hot packs should be applied for 10 minutes. If flow is still unsatisfactory, release of a few marginal sutures may improve it. This should not be necessary, however, where the technique described above has been followed. During the waiting period a full-thickness graft is harvested for the secondary defect (Fig. 49-31L–N). Postoperative care should include early institution of sensory rehabilitation[63,66] of the island transfer.

Rose[275] has described a modification of the Littler flap in which the skin island is taken from some juncture along the course of the neurovascular pedicle, not necessarily the pulp. Dissection is similar, except that the nerve is left in place. This method is useful for small, difficult defects which do not require innervation, only cover. Rose described six cases with a maximum flap dimension of 5.5 × 2.5 cm. The secondary defect is covered with a full-thickness graft.

Fillet Flap

Fillet flaps are developed from a well-vascularized digit that is otherwise worthless due to extensive injury to skeleton, nerves, or tendons and commonly to all three.[43,44,250] The technique of filleting a finger requires that the skeleton and tendons be removed, preserving all other soft tissues on one or both vascular pedicles. As the circumference of a finger at the free edge of the web is equal to the distance from the web to a point just proximal to the nail fold, a fillet flap as described below will be roughly a square, the sides of which are equal to that measure. The difficulties in planning to use such a flap are first that of determining whether or not it can reach the presenting primary defect, and second incising it to ensure that it does. Measuring the distance from the web of the digit to be sacrificed to the nearest point of defect will provide only a rough guide, particularly in the secondary situation where scar in the soft tissues of the digit reduces their elasticity significantly.

In preparing to fillet a finger, the patency or otherwise of the two proper digital vessels should be determined. With this knowledge, the surgeon should then plan the longitudinal incision in the digit by visualizing how the flap will first open in a lateral direction and then fold over proximally into the defect. For example, if the middle finger is to be filleted for a defect on the dorsum of the hand, the incision in the finger should be on its radial aspect if that defect is predominantly to the ulnar side of the third metacarpal, on the ulnar if the defect is radial. A further consideration where middle or ring fingers are to be sacrificed is whether or not the adjacent ray—index or small, respectively—is to be transposed into the defect left by the ray ablation (Fig. 49-32). If it is, then the fillet flap is best reduced to an island flap by appropriate excision of palmar skin. While technically more demanding, this gives a more mobile flap and a more pleasing final result. Once these decisions have been made the appropriate longitudinal incision is made down to the skeleton. At its distal end a circumferential incision is made around the finger at a point 5 mm proximal to the nail fold. This means discarding the pulp tissue as its bulk makes it rather unsatisfactory cover for its new location. At the proximal end of the longitudinal incision, its continuation depends upon whether or not the metacarpal of the digit is to be resected and an adjacent digit transposed. If the metacarpal is not to be resected, then a transverse incision is made over the dorsum of the finger so as to create a hinge along the side of the finger opposite the incision. All dorsal veins should be ligated with the exception of that end of the proximal venous arcade that corresponds to the hinge. This single vein alone will give excellent venous drainage. If it is intended to transpose a digit, thereby making the fillet an island flap, the incision should again be circumferential at the level of the proximal digital crease; that is, at the free margin of the web. A further incision should be made in zigzag manner proximally into the palm, through which the necessary neurovascular bundle should be dissected exactly in the manner described in the section on Neurovascular Island Flap. This should always be done before the skeleton is removed as dissection of supported tissues is

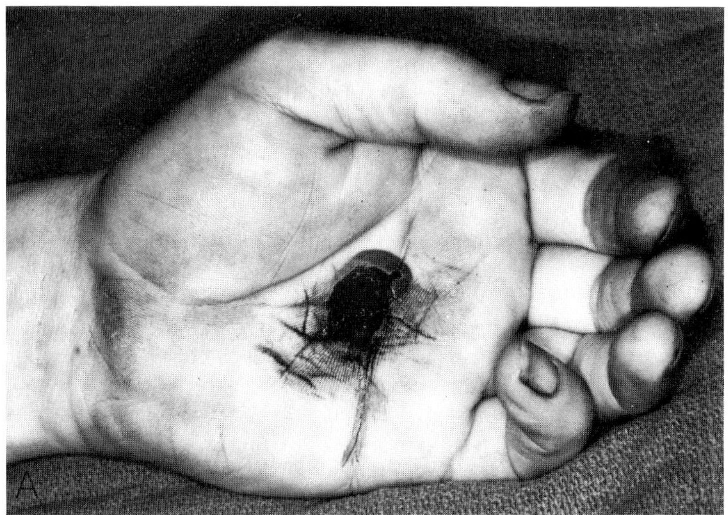

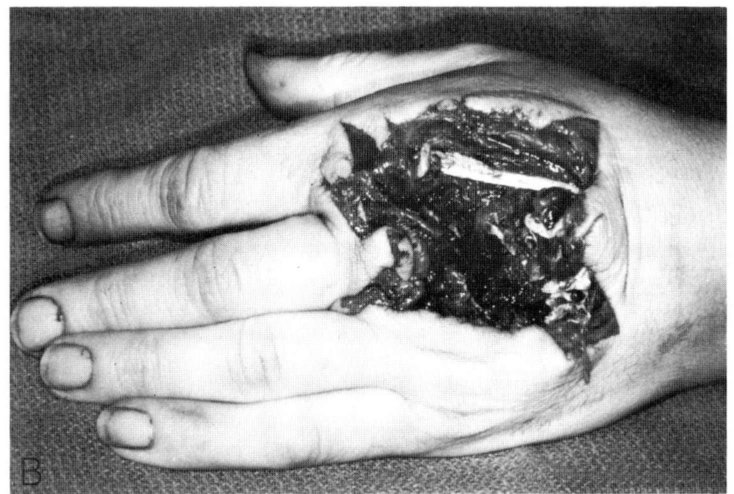

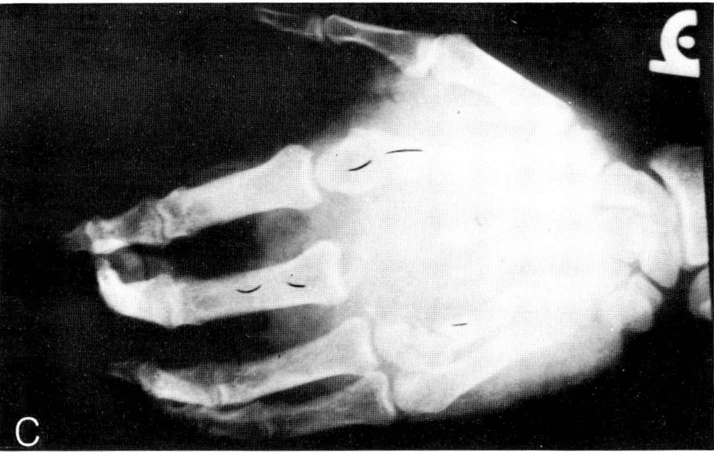

Fig. 49-32. Fillet flap. This patient sustained a gunshot wound of the palm of the nondominant hand **(A)** at close range, producing a large dorsal exit wound **(B)** and destroying the metacarpal of the middle finger **(C)**. As the extensor tendons were also disrupted and the flexor tendons heavily contaminated, it was deemed appropriate to sacrifice the middle finger, which was well-vascularized. *(Figure continues.)*

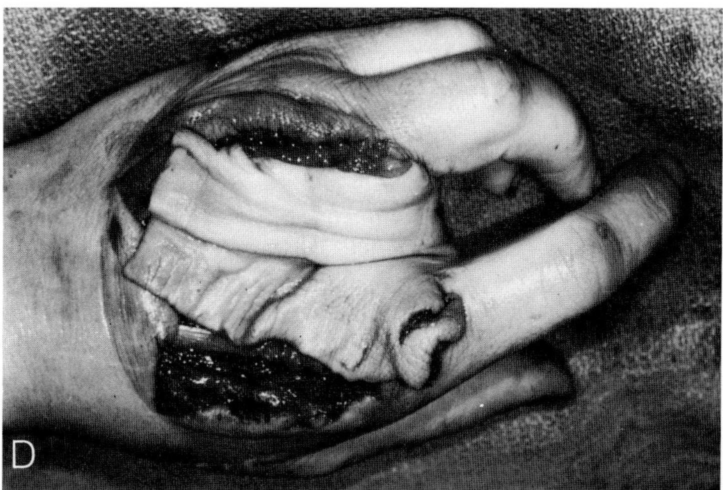

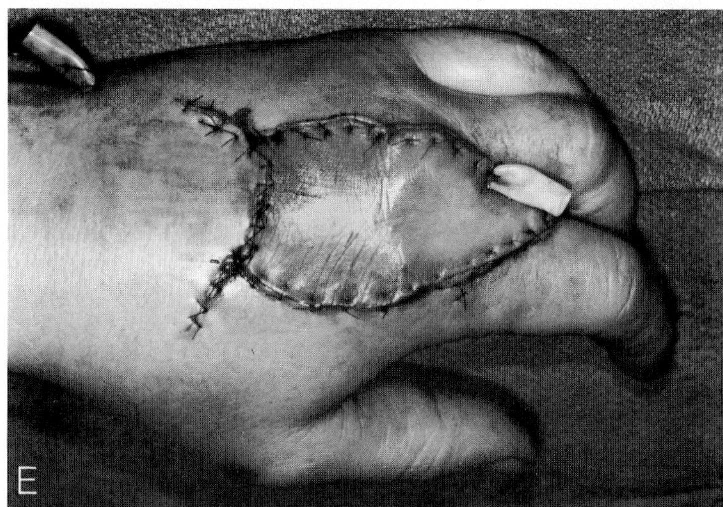

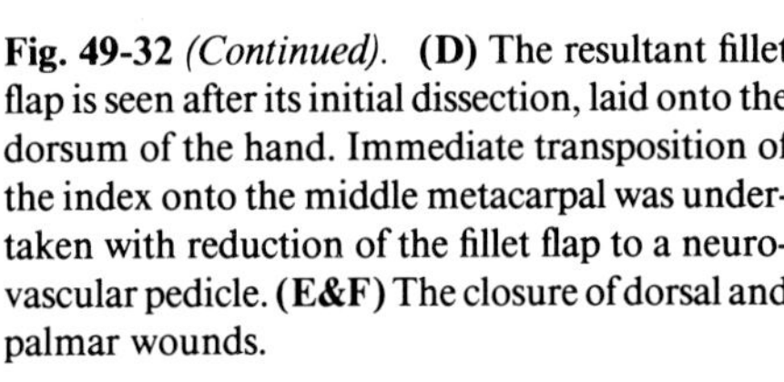

Fig. 49-32 *(Continued).* **(D)** The resultant fillet flap is seen after its initial dissection, laid onto the dorsum of the hand. Immediate transposition of the index onto the middle metacarpal was undertaken with reduction of the fillet flap to a neurovascular pedicle. **(E&F)** The closure of dorsal and palmar wounds.

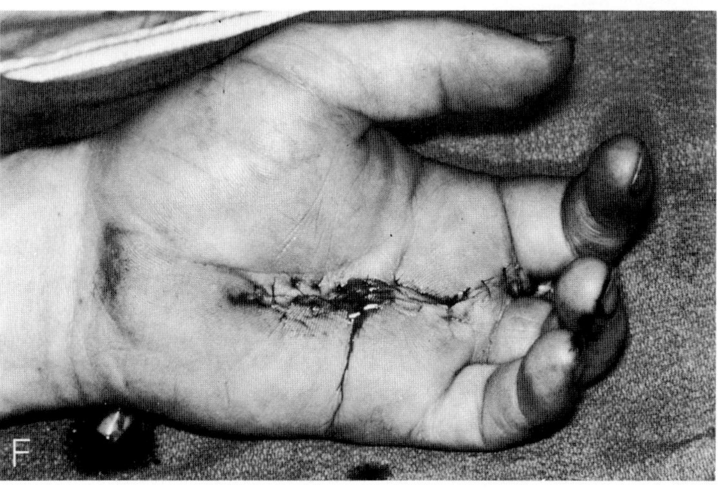

easier. To remove the digital skeleton, skin hooks are applied to the margins of the longitudinal incision distally, and the soft tissues are peeled off the underlying extensor tendon, bone, and flexor tendon sheath. The deep branches and tributaries of the vessels should be ligated as this is done. The flap can now be opened and folded onto the primary defect. The necessary movement of the flap is more readily obtained if the injury to the donor digit is fresh and if the fillet has been raised as an island. Now, for the first time, the surgeon can really judge whether or not the flap will fit the primary defect. If it is too small, other solutions must be added. If it is too large, but the defect is deep, the excess should not be discarded; rather it should be de-epithelialized and turned in to fill the depths of the wound. If the hole in the depths of the wound is due to a segmental bony defect, a portion of phalanx can be taken as a vascularized bone graft with the fillet flap.[105]

Axial Cutaneous Flap

The scapular flap,[75] commonly used as a free flap, can reach the upper extremity as an island and has been described for use after the release of burn contractures of the axilla.[70] Its disadvantage as an island is that its pedicle is rather short and likely to kink unless the surgeon divides the considerable bulk of the teres major and latissimus dorsi muscles. If those muscles are not cut—and I can see no justification for so doing—the flap cannot reach beyond the axilla. If the axilla is sufficiently impaired as to require a flap, it is probable that the subscapular artery, from which the pedicle of the scapular flap originates, may have also been damaged.

Fasciocutaneous Flap

Regional fasciocutaneous flaps have been described from the forearm to the periolecranon region[38] and from the medial arm for release of axillary and elbow burn contractures.[37] However, the major fasciocutaneous flaps of the upper extremity are the lateral arm flap, the radial artery, forearm, or "Chinese" flap, the ulnar artery flap, and the posterior interosseous artery flap.[234,304,348] While the lateral arm flap, based on the posterior radial collateral artery, is an invaluable adjunct to hand surgery as a free flap, its location and rather limited pedicle length make its use as an axial regional flap rarely feasible. By contrast, the reversed radial artery flap, with its potential area of much of the forearm skin and a pedicle located at the anatomic snuffbox, is capable of covering almost any defect in the hand.[22,305]

Radial Artery, Forearm Flap. The reversed forearm flap is not more widely used for three reasons. First, it depends upon the presence of good flow through the ulnar artery and the palmar arches into the radial artery, which must be divided proximally. The radial artery may be the only patent vessel to the hand. When it is not, it is the dominant vessel in 12 percent of hands.[233] While not necessarily placing the hand in jeopardy, acute ischemia[148] and[138] cold intolerance may be a consequence of its use.[31] This potential problem can be overcome by reconstructing the radial artery with a reversed vein graft at the time of preparing the flap. In 3.6 percent of 220 dissections the palmar arch was incomplete.[142] Rarely, the radial artery may be anomalous, pursuing a dorsal course.[128] The second drawback is the secondary defect[120,319] which is unsightly. The third reason why the reversed radial artery flap is used relatively rarely is that the surgeon who is familiar with its preparation is also likely to be familiar with other axial flaps that can be imported as free tissue transfers, such as the groin or lateral arm flap. In those relatively uncommon cases in which a vascularized segment of radius is harvested in addition,[204] fracture may occur.[16,319] If it is decided to disregard these considerations, the flap certainly offers unrivalled quality of skin, for it is thin and mobile, similar in its characteristics to the skin of the dorsum of the hand.[48,116,220,265,271]

The radial artery (Fig. 49-33) pursues a relatively superficial course in the forearm from its source at the division of the brachial artery to the point where it passes deep to the tendon of the abductor pollicis longus to reach the anatomic snuffbox. In the proximal forearm it lies on the superficial surface of the pronator teres, just beneath the anterior margin of the muscle belly of the brachioradialis. Leaving the pronator teres, it comes to lie in turn on the radial head of the flexor digitorum superficialis and the flexor pollicis longus, here being palpable through the skin. Throughout its course the artery gives branches to a plexus of vessels in the overlying deep fascia, and this plexus supplies the skin of the anterior and radiodorsal surfaces of the forearm. By similar fascial branches it also supplies the periosteum of the distal half of the radius between the insertions of pronator teres and brachioradialis. This allows construction of osteocutaneous flaps where desired.[26,93] The artery is accompanied by two or more venae comitantes. The multiple anastomoses between these veins permit reversal of flow in the venae comitantes without valvular obstruction.[182] Thus the artery and veins can be divided proximally and no venous engorgement will result (valvulotomy has been described to enhance flow[254]).

The minimum precaution that should be taken before raising a forearm flap is a timed Allen test[108] to ensure that flow is present and adequate through both vessels. Preferably full noninvasive vascular studies should be performed to determine vessel dominance. The course of the radial artery should be mapped out with a Doppler and marked on the skin, as should the course of the major veins in the region of the flap. Using a soft inelastic material, the distance from the radial styloid to the closest margin of the primary defect should be measured and transposed to the forearm to determine the location of the distal edge of the flap outline. The pattern of the primary defect is drawn out proximal to this point, remembering to place proximal pattern to distal flap, since the flap will be reversed on its pedicle. The margins of the flap are then incised. A zigzag incision is extended distally from the flap margin over the course of the radial artery. The skin margins adjacent to the flap are elevated from the underlying deep fascia. In elevating the radial edge, the cephalic vein should be identified and preserved, for it will be used to reconstruct the radial artery. Once the skin has been elevated for 1 cm or so from the flap margin, the deep fascia should be incised all around the flap, thereby gaining the plane of dissection. At this point, the deep fascia and the skin can with benefit be sutured one to the other at several points around the margin. This serves to prevent shearing between the two during subsequent mobilization. If the

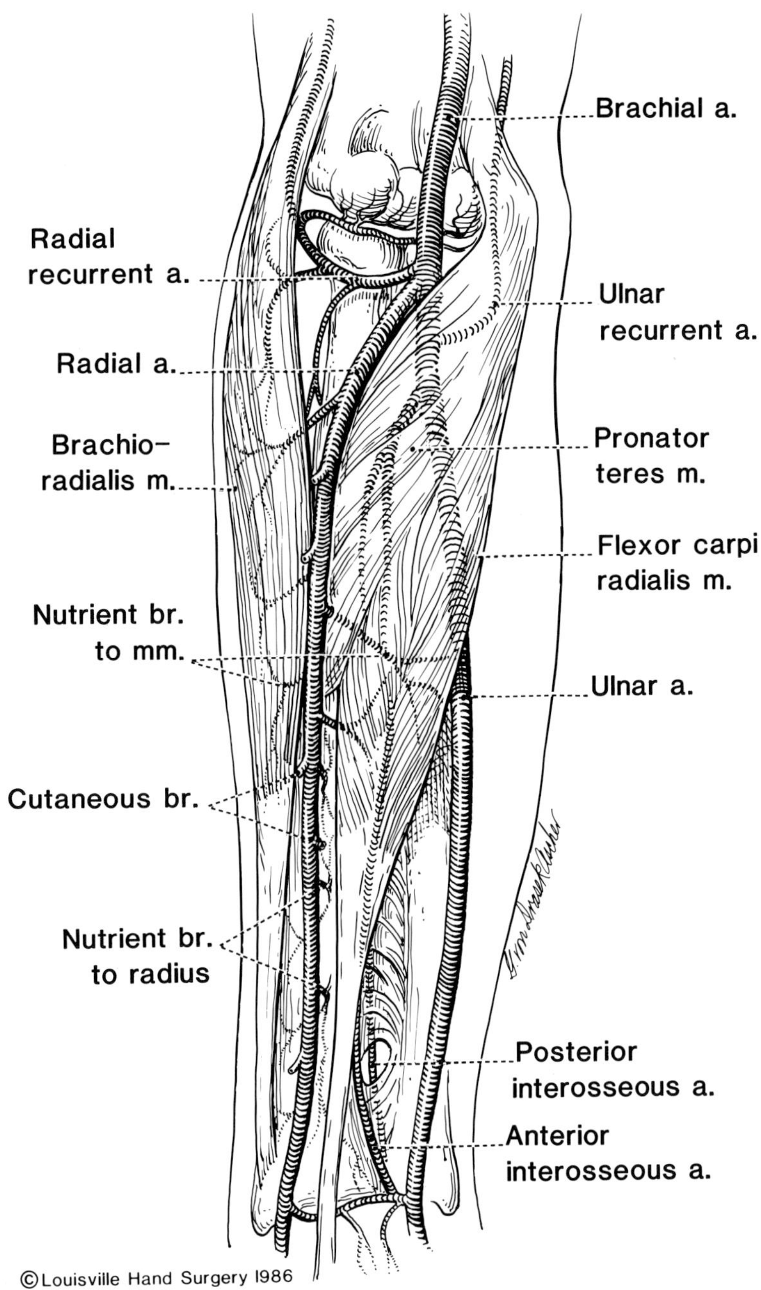

Fig. 49-33. The course of the radial artery is superficial throughout much of the forearm, lying just beneath the margin of the brachioradialis on the pronator teres and the flexor digitorum superficialis. The cutaneous branches supply the overlying skin and nutrient branches of the radius.

ends of these sutures are left a little long, they can be grasped in turn with hemostats and elevated to give the necessary tension during dissection. The flap is now raised by dissecting in the loose areolar tissue beneath the deep fascia. In larger flaps, some intermuscular deep extensions may be encountered, which should be incised. In the pedicle forearm flap here described it is less likely that the secondary defect will lie distally over the wrist tendons as when it is used as a free flap. Nonetheless, wherever tendon is encountered in elevating the flap, care must be taken to preserve the overlying epitenon. Once the flap has been raised across the flexor carpi radialis from the ulnar margin, traction will reveal the radial artery and its venae comitantes (Fig. 49-34). The vessels will be similarly revealed as the fascia is lifted from the brachioradialis radially. Retracting

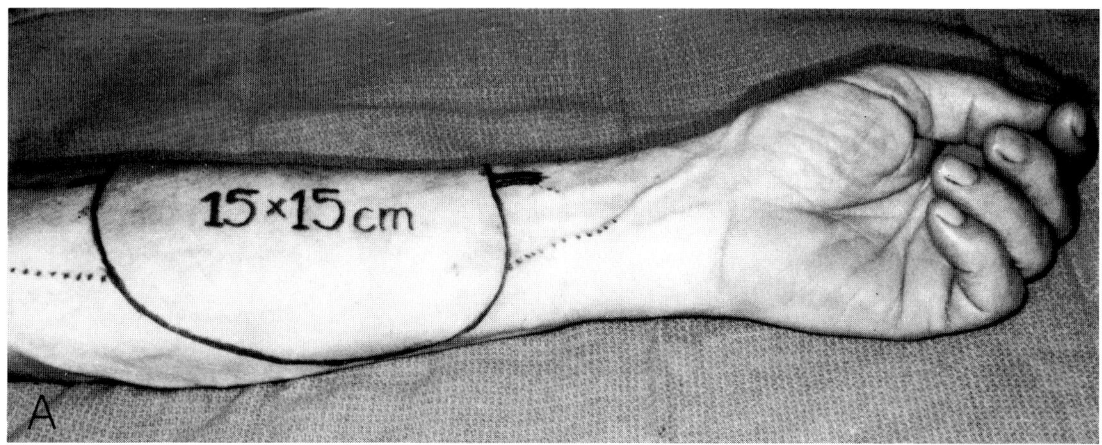

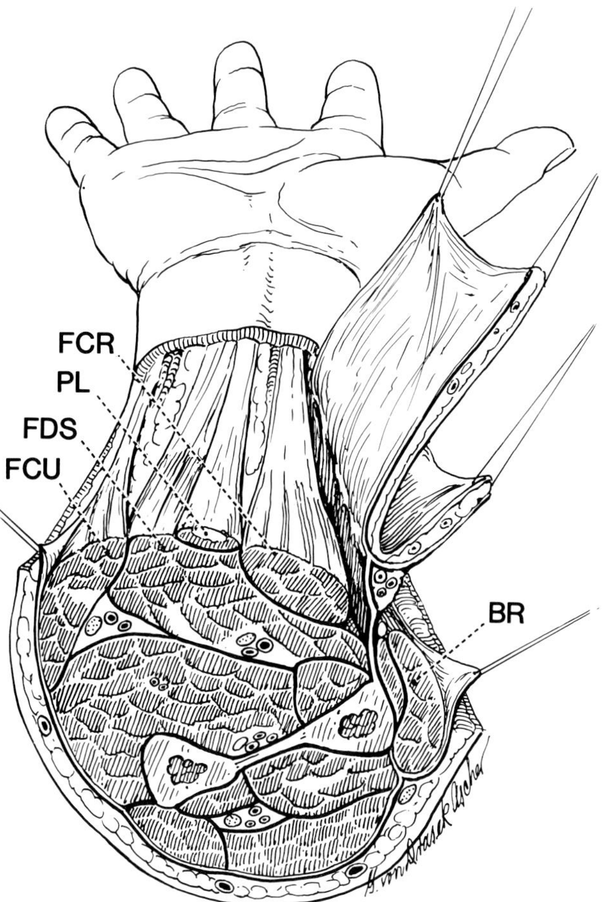

Fig. 49-34. Radial forearm flap. **(A)** The marking for a radial forearm flap is shown (to be used here as a free flap). **(B)** Incision of the fascia lifts the entire flap off the underlying muscles of the forearm. *(Figure continues.)*

both the aforementioned muscles away from one another, the lateral intermuscular septum in which the artery runs should be incised parallel and deep to the radial artery. The pedicle is now dissected distally, elevating it from the underlying tissues as far as the radial styloid. The radial artery can now be ligated proximally and the flap transposed to the primary defect (Fig. 49-35A–E), passing it through a tunnel beneath intervening intact skin where it is present, using the technique described in the section on Neurovascular Island Flaps.

Once in place, the previously proximal radial artery in the

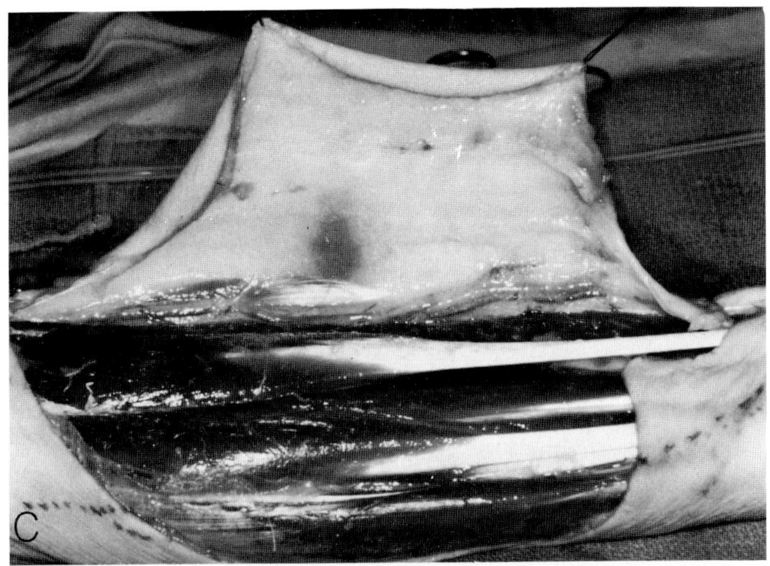

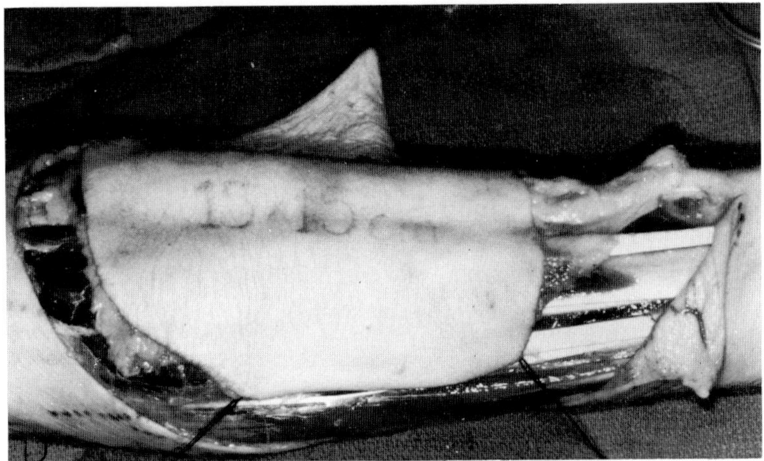

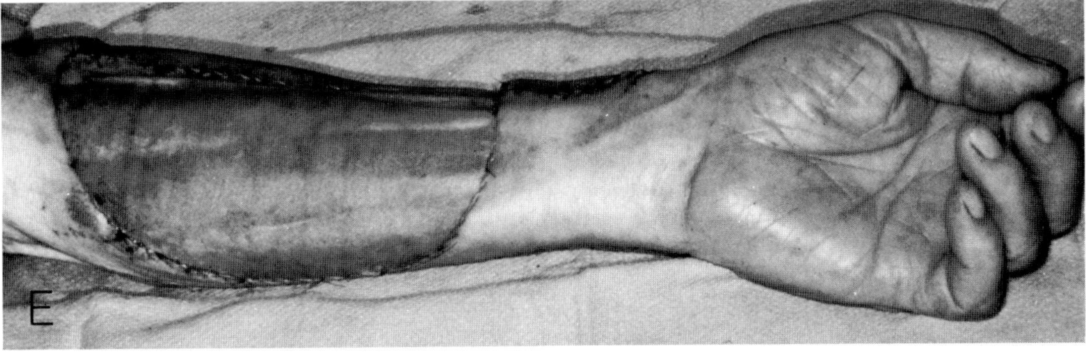

Fig. 49-34 *(Continued).* **(C)** Clinical photograph of **(B)**. These are seen from the ulnar aspect. The radial artery and its venae comitantes run at the lower margin of the flap **(D)**. The flap and **(E)** the secondary defect covered with a split-thickness skin graft.

A
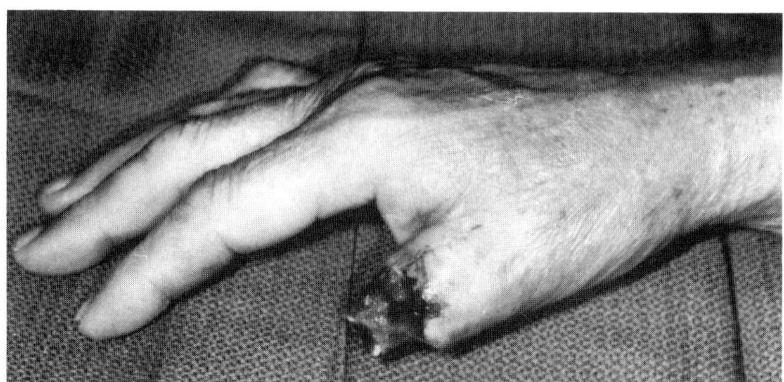

B
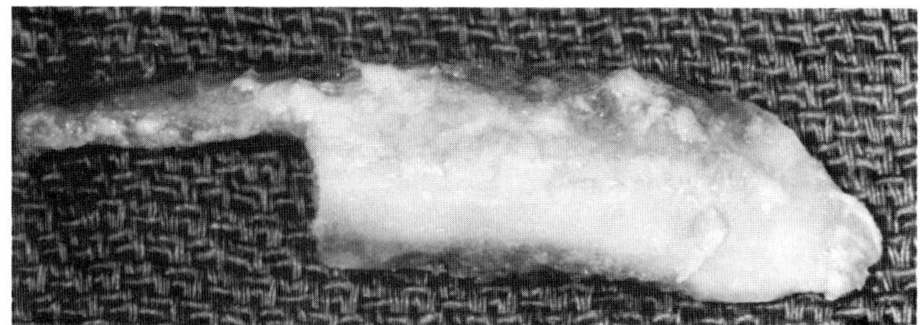

C
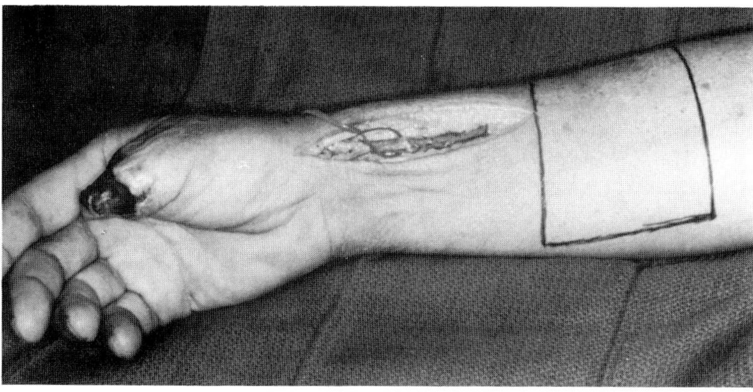

Fig. 49-35. **(A)** This patient suffered an amputation of the thumb in a roping injury. **(B)** The thumb is lengthened using a cortico-cancellous iliac crest bone graft. **(C)** A radial forearm flap has been marked out and the radial artery dissected. *(Figure continues.)*

flap, now distal, can be anastomosed either immediately or at a later procedure to supply more distal tissues, such as a devascularized finger or a toe transfer.[92,199] The forearm flap can be used for forearm defects provided only that their location is appropriate (Fig. 49-36A–D). In such cases one or more superficial veins can be rejoined proximally to make venous drainage more efficient.[111] In the secondary defect, the gap between the end of the radial artery proximally and the radial artery at the pivot point adjacent to the snuffbox is measured. A vein graft of that length is harvested from the cephalic vein and interposed end-to-end proximally and end-to-side distally, using the microsurgical techniques described in Chapter 26. The secondary skin defect is closed with a split-thickness skin graft. This will be cosmetically unsightly, but rarely if ever causes the problems of distal edema that were feared when this flap was first used. The poor appearance of the secondary defect can be eliminated by raising the flap as fascia alone. This in turn has the disadvantage that split skin grafts over fascial flaps do not always show perfect "take."

Ulnar Artery, Forearm Flap. Like the radial artery flap, the ulnar artery flap can be based proximally to cover defects around the elbow,[110,144] or distally for hand cover.[119,180,279] First described in 1984,[194] it has gained less popularity than the radial artery, forearm flap, despite offering the advantages of less hairy skin and a less obvious secondary defect which, having more muscle and less tendon, should take skin grafts more readily. Dissection is similar to the radial artery, forearm flap save only that the vascular septum from artery to skin lies between the flexor carpi ulnaris and flexor digitorum muscles and that care must be taken not to harm the ulnar nerve lying immediately deep to the vessel.

Reversed Posterior Interosseous Artery Flap. In 1986 the anatomic basis[256] and clinical application[352] of a flap based on the posterior interosseous artery was first reported. Initially used as a proximally based flap to cover the elbow,[239] its popularity has increased since description of more detailed anatomy and also because of its use as a reversed flap.[21,59,71,125,353]

The posterior interosseous artery (PIA) arises in the anterior compartment from the common interosseous artery, which also gives rise to the anterior vessel. The PIA immediately passes dorsally through the interosseous membrane some six centimeters distal to the lateral epicondyle emerging just below

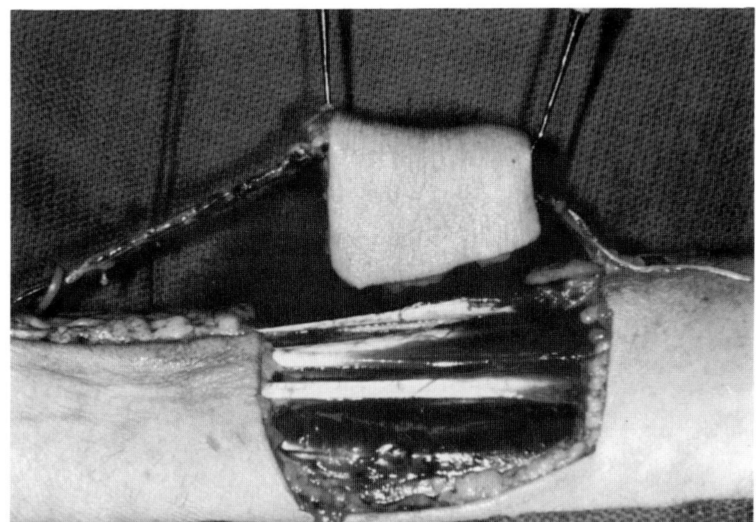

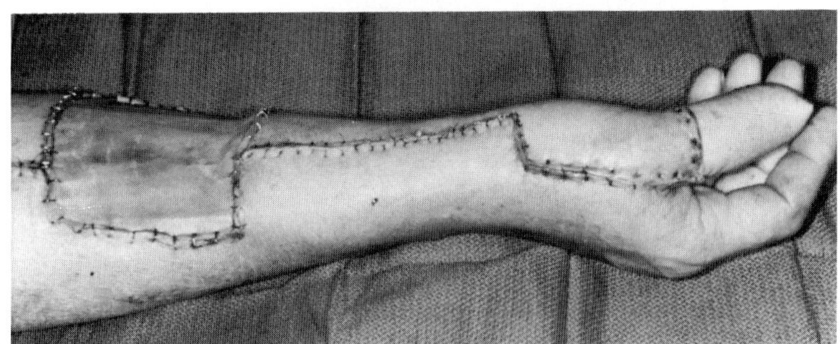

Fig. 49-35 *(Continued).* **(D)** The flap is raised on its pedicle. **(E)** The flap has been transposed and sutured in position and the secondary defect closed with a split-thickness skin graft.

the distal edge of the supinator. Throughout its course it lies between the extensor carpi ulnaris and the extensor digiti minimi, initially lying on the abductor pollicis longus muscle belly in close approximation to the posterior interosseous nerve. Some 2 cm proximal to the ulnar styloid it has an anastomosis with the anterior interosseous artery, passing then on to the dorsum of the carpus where it anastomoses with branches of the radial artery. Throughout its course the PIA gives septocutaneous perforators which supply the skin over the dorsum of the forearm.

To raise the flap, a line is first drawn from the lateral epicondyle to the distal radio-ulnar joint. A point on this line 2 cm proximal to the ulnar styloid is marked, which represents the pivot point of the distally based flap. Measurements are taken from the point to the proximal and distal edges of the primary defect. These represent the distances from the pivot point along the line initially drawn at which are marked the distal and proximal margins of the flap outline, respectively. The radial margin of the flap and a distal extension to the distal radio-ulnar joint are incised. The distal extension can with merit be made 1 cm radial to the previously marked surface marking of the PIA.[36] The flap is raised and the fascia over the extensor digiti minimi is incised 5 mm radial to the thick fascial septum. Retracting the muscle radially, the posterior interosseous artery, its branches, and the anastomosis to the anterior interosseous artery distally are dissected, taking care to preserve the perforating vessels to the skin. Provided no anomalies are encountered, a similar skin and fascial incision is now made on the ulnar aspect over the extensor carpi ulnaris, which is again mobilized by division of the muscular branches of the PIA. The relationship of the motor branch of the extensor carpi ulnaris to the PIA and its most proximal relevant perforator (MPRP)[36] must now be inspected, for if it passes superficial to the PIA and the MPRP is the major septocutaneous perforator, which it may be,[59] then the surgeon may decide to divide and repair the nerve, as recommended by Büchler and Frey[36] in that circumstance. Once the pedicle and flap have been fully mobilized so that they are attached only by the proximal and distal vascular connections, there is merit in placing a microvascular clamp on the PIA proximal to the MPRP and releasing the tourniquet. If flow is good, ligation can replace the clamp and the flap can be turned into place on the hand. The reach of the flap has not been clearly defined. It can certainly reach the first web space and the metacarpophalangeal joints. Büchler and Frey[36] have taken the flap to the proximal interphalangeal joint, but they did report a 21 percent incidence of partial necrosis. While statistical analysis of their results indicated that this necrosis was not related to pedicle length, this incidence of partial flap loss is higher than that encountered in other series with only one case of remediable venous congestion out of 32 flaps performed.

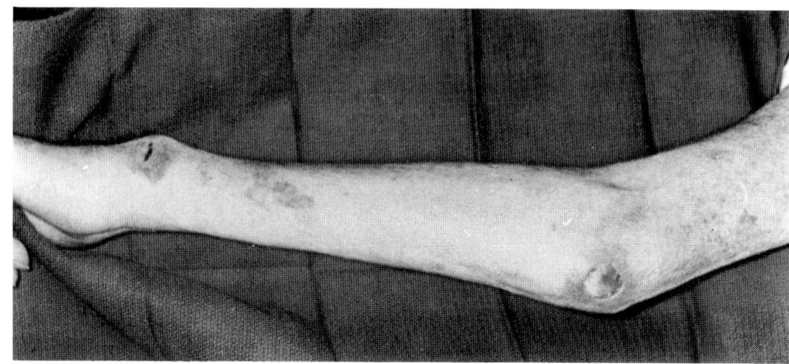

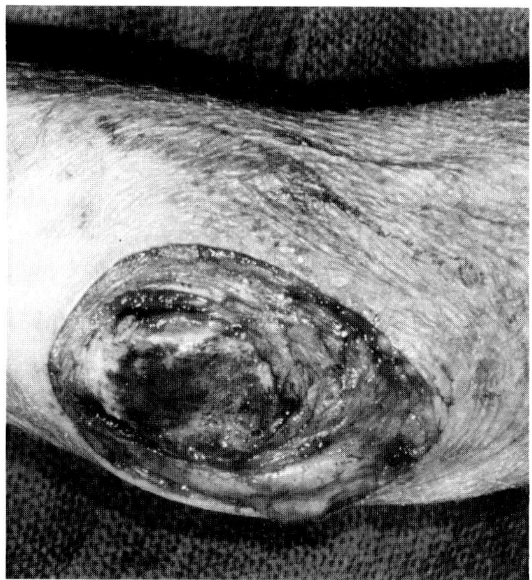

Fig. 49-36. This patient with scleroderma has undergone over 20 operations in an attempt to close the ulcerating olecranon bursa **(A)**. Pseudo-tumor resection of the olecranon bursa together with underlying bone yields a clean defect **(B)**. *(Figure continues.)*

Musculocutaneous Flap

The blood supply of muscles has been classified into five types,[206] which are listed here.

I One vascular pedicle	Example—Tensor fascia lata
II One dominant plus other minor	Example—Gracilis
III Two dominant	Example—Gluteus maximus
IV Several, equal, segmental	Example—Sartorius
V One dominant plus peripheral	Example—Latissimus dorsi

In Types I, II, and V one so-called "dominant" pedicle[211] is capable of supporting the entire muscle if the others are ligated. Theoretically therefore, any muscle in the upper extremity that belongs to one of these three types can be transposed on its pedicle. Several have been described: coracobrachialis to the axilla[134]; deltoid to the shoulder[121]; brachioradialis,[174] extensor carpi radialis longus,[245] and flexor carpi ulnaris[163] (Fig. 49-37A,B) all to the elbow; flexor digitorum superficialis to the antecubital fossa[135]; extensor carpi ulnaris and flexor digitorum profundus to the proximal ulna[54]; pronator quadratus[67] and abductor digit minimi[225,270] to the wrist; the first dorsal interosseous to the first metacarpal[207] and to the third metacarpal.[195] As the majority of these lie beneath a well-vascularized deep fascia, most have been used as muscle flaps to which have been applied split-thickness skin grafts. These flaps have limited value for they all eliminate a functioning motor. Furthermore, their contour is only good when the defect has a volume similar to that of the muscle belly. Where defects are smaller, muscle can be tailored to fit, but where they are significantly larger, stretching it unphysiologically will impair its blood supply. The function of the transposed muscle can be preserved where necessary,[45,205] provided the correct tension is maintained.[99] The fascia overlying a muscle, if it is thick, will have a rich plexus supplied through vessels of the intermuscular septa. In the absence of a direct axial cutaneous vessel, that plexus will supply the overlying skin, which will therefore be best raised as a fasciocutaneous flap, leaving the muscle in place. Where the fascia is thin or absent, the supply to the skin comes more from small branches that perforate the muscle; Olivari[247] described 27 such vessels in the latissimus dorsi. In this case, the muscle and the skin overlying it can be moved efficiently as a block to provide skin cover and, where needed, function. Whether the cover achieved is better when the muscle alone is moved and then skin-grafted, or when a musculocutaneous flap is used is still a matter of debate.[238] Two muscles of Type V

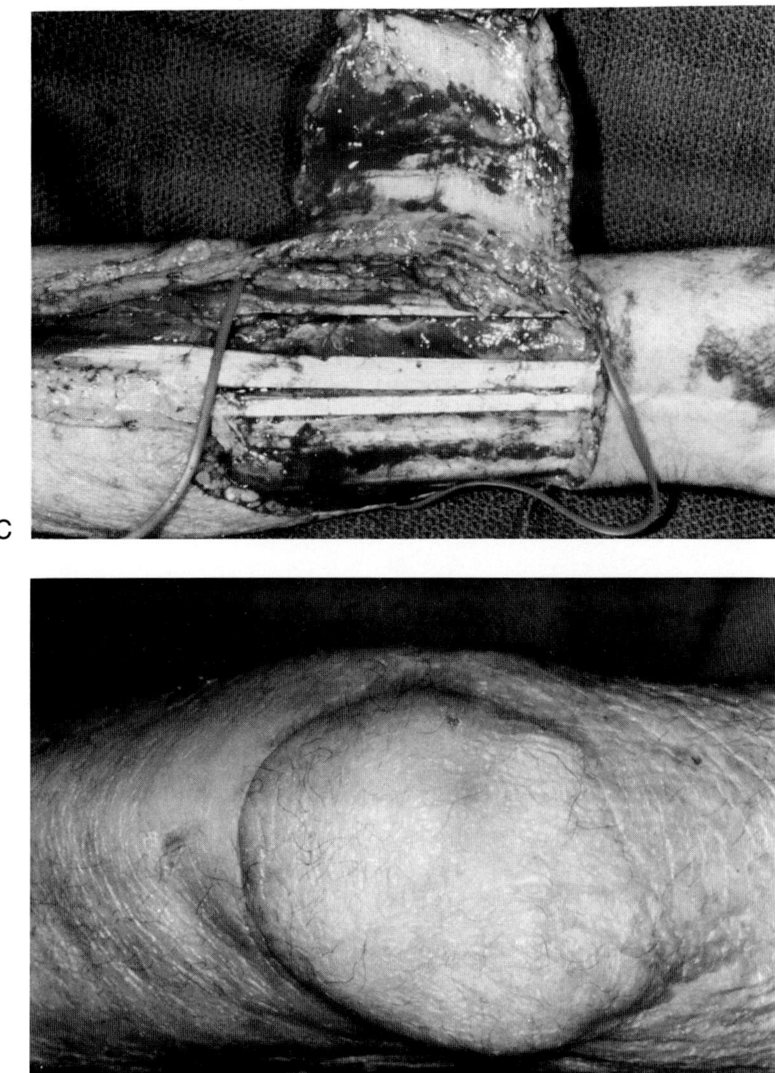

Fig. 49-36 *(Continued).* A radial forearm flap is raised and transposed on its proximal pedicle **(C)**, producing a flap that healed satisfactorily and has remained so **(D)**.

in the classification above have been used in this manner to the upper extremity—pectoralis major and latissimus dorsi. As an axial flap, the pectoralis major was first described for head and neck reconstruction.[8,35] As with other Type V muscles, the main vascular pedicle of the pectoralis major—the pectoral branch of the acromiothoracic axis supplemented by the lateral thoracic artery[97,266]—enters close to its insertion. There are numerous small vessels entering the periphery or origin of the muscle, notably from the internal mammary artery. Unlike all of the regional axial muscle flaps listed above, the pectoralis is left attached at its insertion and released from its origin. It can be split longitudinally to cover two adjacent defects.[230] The pectoralis muscle without skin—in one series, with the addition of pectoralis minor[331]—has long been used for restoration of elbow flexion lost as a result of nerve injury[33,51] or arthrogryposis.[13,77] With an island of overlying skin it has been used as an axial regional flap for reconstruction of the axilla[95] and shoulder.[76] However, the secondary defect, even when it can be closed directly is entirely unacceptable to the female and largely so to the male. Since all primary defects in the upper extremity that could be reached by the pectoralis can be covered with ease and with a much more acceptable donor site by the latissimus dorsi flap, the latter is preferred in virtually all cases.

Latissimus Dorsi Flap. The latissimus dorsi as an axial pattern regional flap was first described in 1906 by Tansini[322] for breast reconstruction.[208] It was used only sporadically until Olivari[246] reintroduced it for coverage of radiation defects of the anterior chest wall in 1976. Its wide arc of rotation around its pedicle makes it currently popular for reconstruction of the breast, the abdominal wall, the head and neck[28] and the shoul-

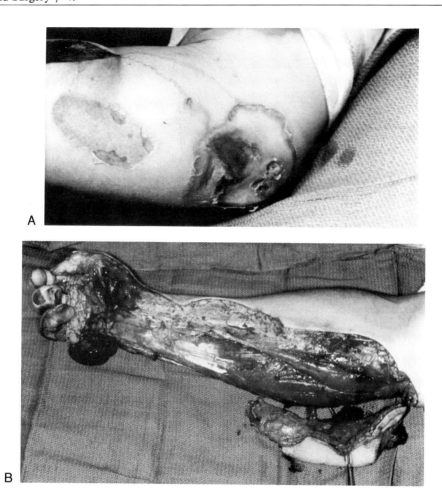

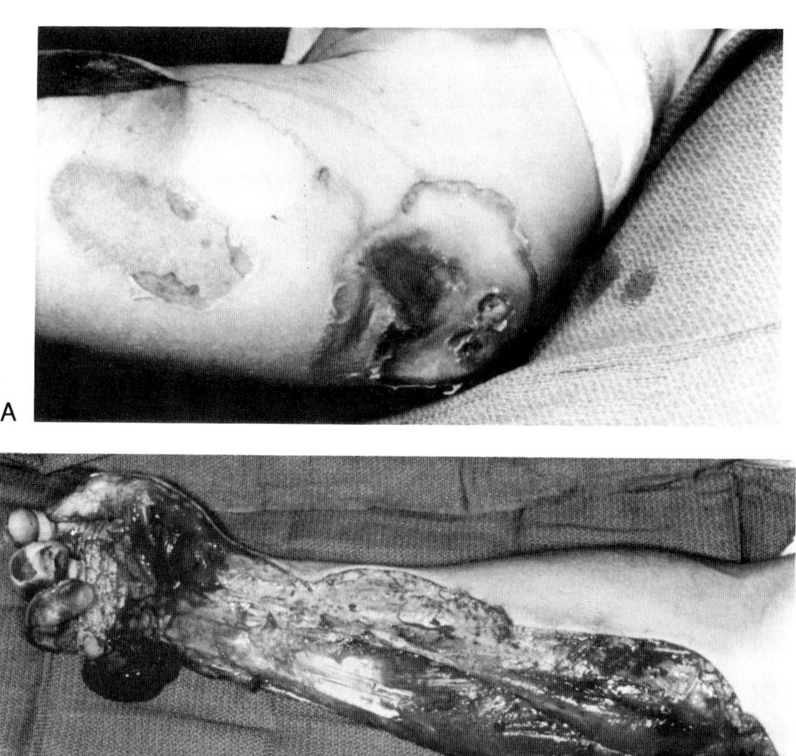

Fig. 49-37. **(A)** A full-thickness thermal burn is located over the cubital tunnel. **(B)** The flexor carpi ulnaris has been destroyed in its distal portion by the same thermal injury. It is possible therefore to transpose it on the proximal ulnar artery, which was thrombosed distally, to cover the defect in the region of the olecranon and medial epicondyle after primary excision of the burn (This is the same patient seen in Fig. 28-22 in Chapter 28 on free skin and composite flaps).

der.[55,76,223] The diameter of the artery (1 to 2.5 mm) and the length of the pedicle (11 cm[19]) has made it the most robust and therefore popular tissue for free transfer, especially to the extremities.[112] Functional transposition of the latissimus dorsi to restore lost biceps function has been known to the orthopaedic surgeon for over thirty years.[286,320,354] Its use to restore both function and skin cover[32,177,311] and to restore cover alone[1,294] is a more recent development.

The latissimus dorsi arises from the lower six thoracic vertebrae, from the thoracolumbar fascia and from the posterior part of the iliac crest. From this extensive origin the muscle fibers converge to wrap around the lower border of the teres major and end in a quadrilateral tendon that inserts into the intertubercular sulcus of the humerus. Together with the teres major it forms the posterior axillary fold. Furnas[103] has reported one patient in whom the lower part of the muscle was absent, but its anterior border felt quite normal preoperatively. Its main blood supply derives from the vessel popularly known as the thoracodorsal artery, which is the continuation of the subscapular artery after it gives off its circumflex scapular branch some 2 cm distal to its origin from the axillary artery (Fig. 49-38). The thoracodorsal artery gives a variable number of branches to the chest wall, notably one to the serratus anterior, before reaching its hilum on the latissimus dorsi some 11 cm from the axillary artery.[19] Immediately distal to the hilum the artery divides into two branches in 94 percent of specimens.[329] The upper branch runs parallel to, and 3.5 cm from, the upper margin of the muscle; the lateral parallel to, and 2.1 cm from, the lateral margin of the muscle. This arrangement permits the surgeon to split the muscle longitudinally when a narrow flap is required.[329] One might suppose that absence of the artery would preclude use of the latissimus dorsi flap, and routine angiography to ensure its presence has been suggested.[277] However, this need was disputed[72] in the belief that previous injury to the vessel served as a delay. Certainly, if the serratus branch remains intact, it has been shown that collateral circulation is established and the flap can be safely transposed.[85] This would, however, severely limit the reach of the flap when it is taken to the arm, and carries the risk of kinking the pedicle. The muscle can also be used in "reverse"[313] based on the vessels of T9, 10, and 11 intercostal spaces, but rarely to the upper extremity. Any significant defect of the upper arm

Fig. 49-38. The vascular pedicle of the latissimus dorsi flap is displayed here in the course of its dissection. The subscapular artery arises from the axillary artery and soon gives off the circumflex scapular, which passes between the teres major and the latissimus dorsi. **(A)** The next branch to arise is that to the serratus. The thoracodorsal artery passes beneath the epimysium of the latissimus dorsi and there divides into two branches. The upper branch runs parallel to and 3.5 cm from the upper margin of the muscle, the lateral parallel to and 2.1 cm from the lateral margin of the muscle. **(B)** The first, distal cut of the flap has been made through skin and muscle. *(Figure continues.)*

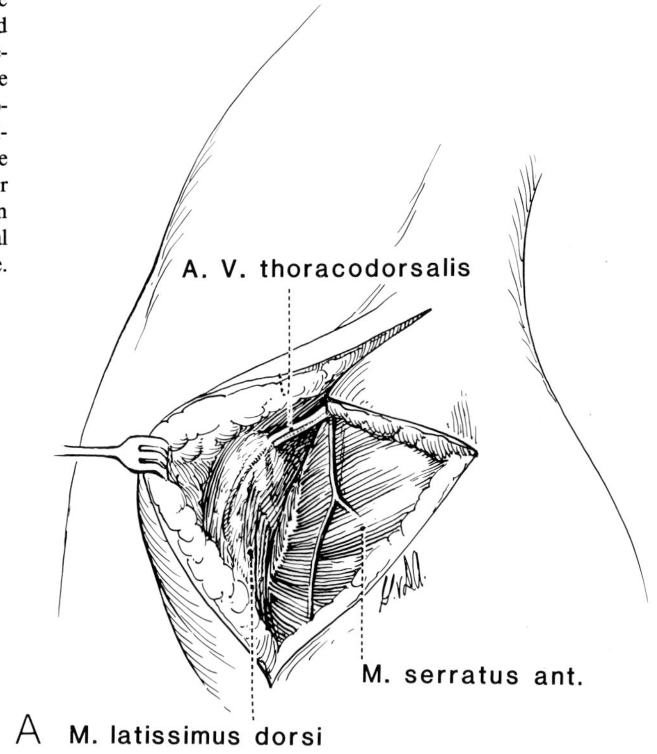

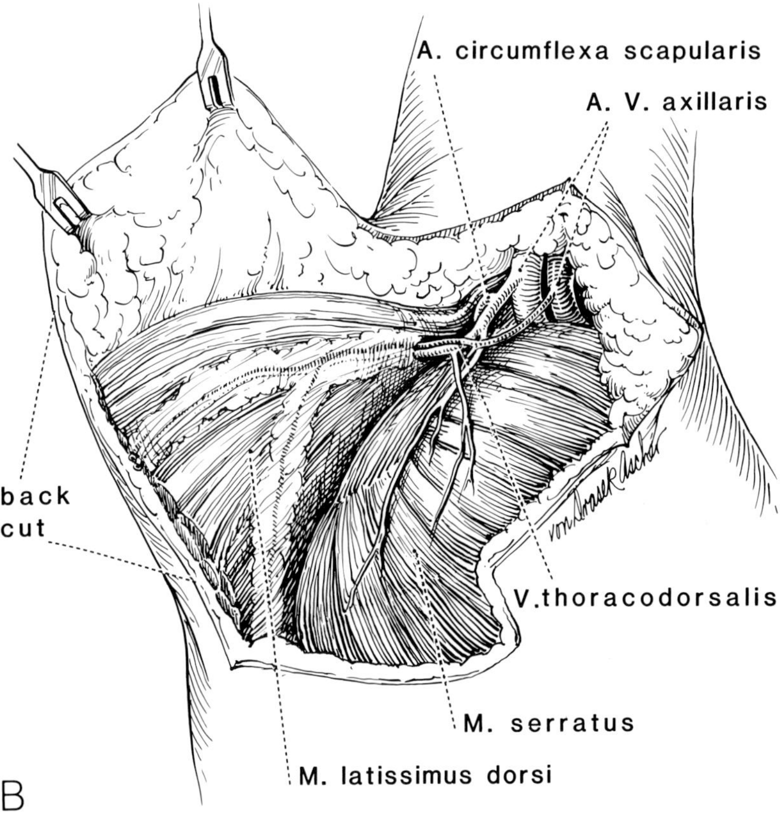

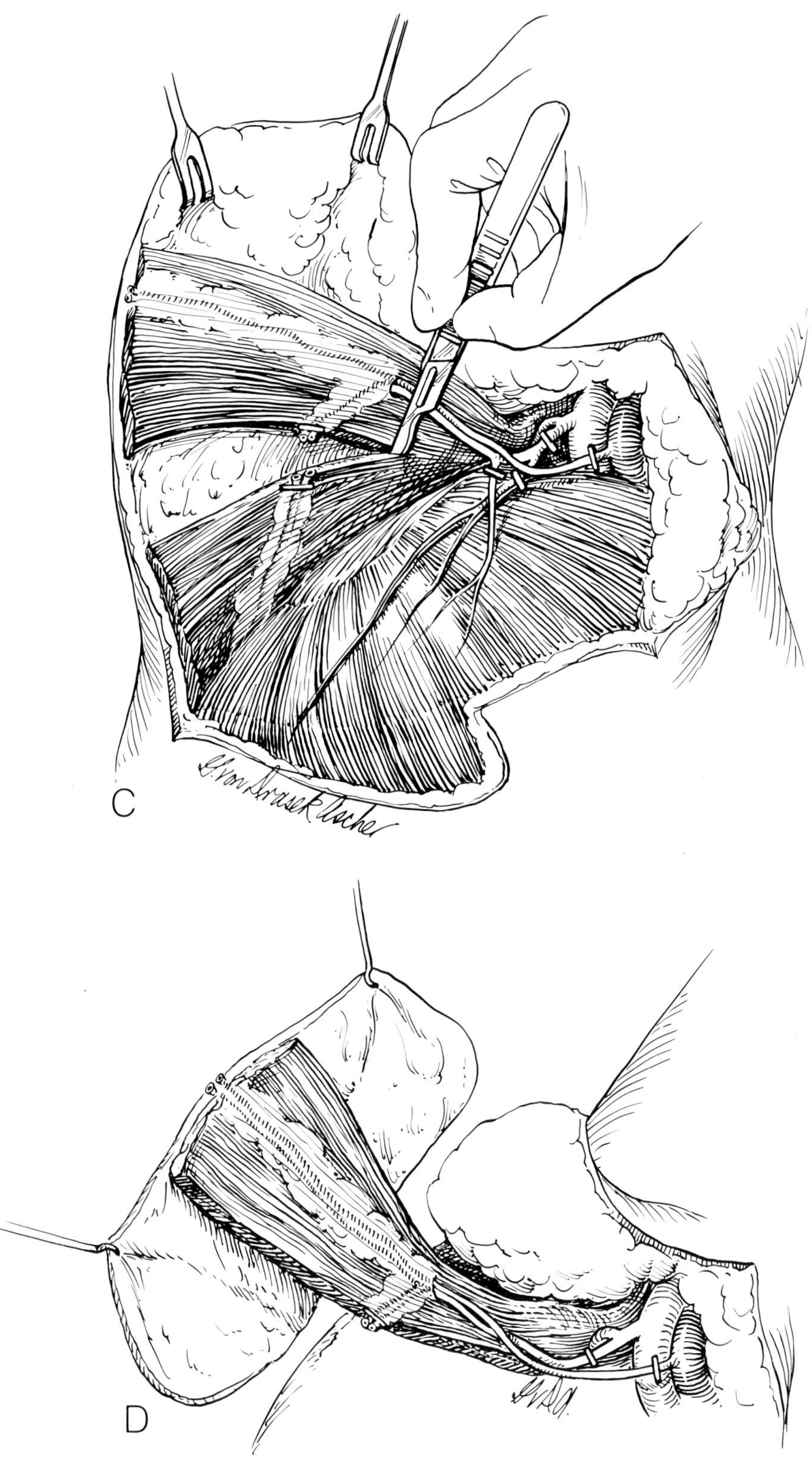

Fig. 49-38 *(Continued).* **(C)** The lateral or anterior portion of the muscle is being used alone in designing this small flap. The posterior or upper branch of the thoracodorsal has therefore been divided and the muscle is split either with a knife, as shown here, or better with cutting diathermy through both muscle and skin as required. **(D)** The proximal margin of the flap has been divided here through skin and will then be divided through muscle just proximal to the point at which the thoracodorsal artery passes beneath the epimysium of the latissimus dorsi. In this way a thin, well-tailored latissimus dorsi is created. (The clips shown here on the artery and vein of the pedicle would not, of course, be applied in using the latissimus as a regional flap.) (Modified from Godina,[113] with permission.)

and elbow can be covered with a pedicle latissimus dorsi flap (Fig. 49-39), and it has been transferred successfully to the forearm.[198]

Preoperatively, it may be of some benefit to have the patient abduct the arm against resistance and tattoo four or five points along the posterior axillary fold with methylene blue and a hypodermic needle. The patient should be placed in the lateral position with padding beneath the torso sufficient to protect circulation to the arm on the operating table.[104] Where the latissimus dorsi is to be transposed to a defect in the upper extremity, the involved limb, together with the entire ipsilateral hemithorax and distally to the iliac crest, should be prepared and draped. The axilla is displayed by wrapping the forearm with soft padding and then applying upward traction to a ceiling fixture so as to achieve 100 degrees of abduction. A similar position can be less satisfactorily achieved by taping the forearm to a sterile Mayo stand. In either case, there is considerable danger of brachial plexus neurapraxia with consequent paresis.[193] Checking the radial pulse regularly is no guarantee that all is well. This complication can only be avoided by a

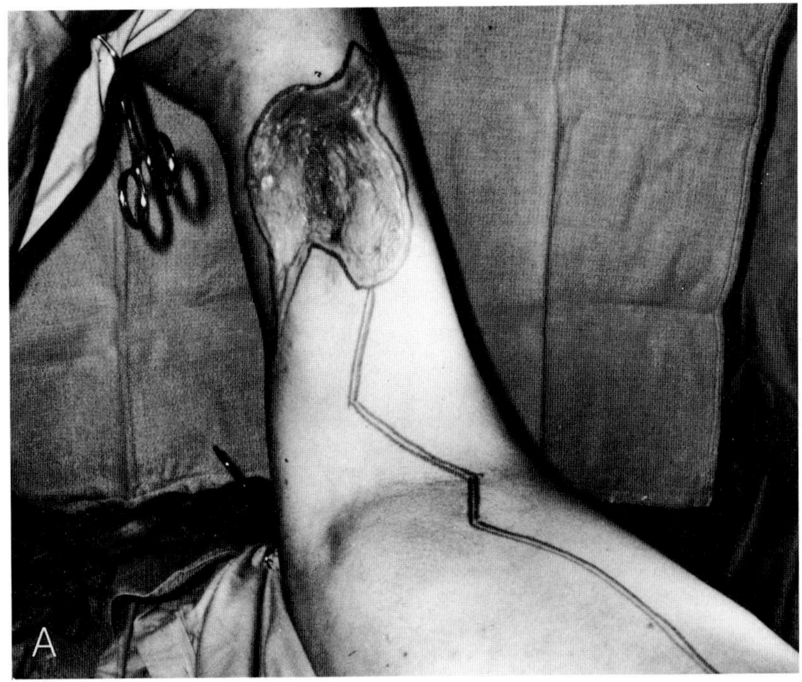

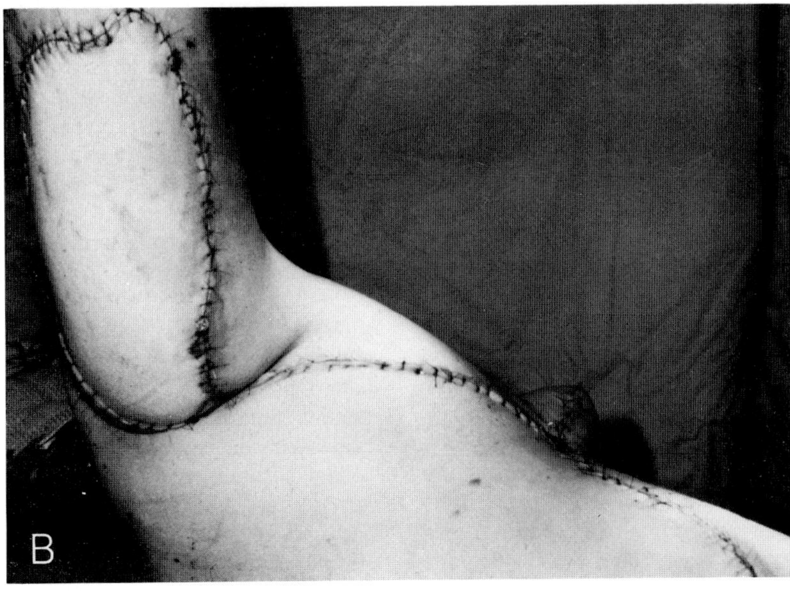

Fig. 49-39. Latissimus dorsi pedicle flap. **(A)** A forearm defect resulting from a gunshot wound is covered with a large latissimus dorsi pedicle flap **(B)**.

strict practice of returning the limb to the patient's side for 5 minutes out of every hour, monitored by the anesthesiologist.

A zigzag incision is made in the axilla, avoiding the hair-bearing area, extending down toward the previous tattoo points marking the posterior axillary fold.[113] Through this incision, the anterior border of the latissimus is located and everted using heavy stay sutures placed in the muscle margin. The thoracodorsal vessel can best be found where it approaches the muscular hilum. This is approximately at the nipple line in the male or a child. With good retraction and light, the vessel can be traced proximally, identifying first the serratus branch and then the circumflex scapular artery. These should be ligated and divided. If they are not, they tether and kink the pedicle after transposition. The most proximal extent of the dissection constitutes the pivot point or axis of the flap.

At this juncture the distance from this pivot point to the proximal margin of the defect in the limb should be measured and transposed to the anterior border of the latissimus dorsi previously marked. This second point represents the proximal edge of the proposed flap. Using a pattern of the primary defect the flap can now be marked out over the posterolateral thorax. The anterior margin should be incised and the anterior border of the latissimus elevated with the overlying skin. The inferior border of the flap can now be raised with benefit by incising through skin, subcutaneous tissue, and muscle, using cutting diathermy for all but the skin. The benefit accrued is that the latissimus dorsi can now be swung away and posterior from the trunk, permitting a clear view of the vascular tree of the thoracodorsal artery. Where a narrow flap is all that is needed, the lateral branch should be located and the posterior border of the flap incised as was the inferior border, while carefully avoiding that lateral branch. The upper (situated also medial and posterior) branch should be ligated and divided. The thoracodorsal artery is now dissected off the latissimus dorsi, working from the axilla distally as far as possible without injury to it or its muscular branches. The proximal margin of the flap can now be incised in a similar manner to the inferior (or distal) and posterior, while retracting the pedicle anteriorly and so protecting it from harm. Raising the flap in this manner rather than taking the whole muscle as in the past yields a flap tailored exactly to the primary defect.[113] In particular it avoids both a bulky proximal portion to the flap and the difficult task of separating latissimus dorsi from teres major. The bulk proximally was not only unsightly but was also difficult to fit into the upper arm. This was particularly so in the common circumstance where the flap was to be passed beneath an intact skin bridge. The flap can now be passed to the primary defect and sutured in place. The secondary defect should always be closed directly, for a skin graft in this location presents a very difficult nursing problem. Seroma formation is common[264] and prolonged suction drainage is indicated. More tissue is available for superior to inferior closure than in the line of the trunk. Small defects are therefore best closed transversely. Larger defects may require transposition of loose tissue from the waistline anteriorly, using a rhomboid design (Type II transposition flap, described on page 1747). No significant loss of function has been shown following use of the latissimus dorsi.[175]

DISTANT FLAPS

Distant flaps come from body parts outside of the upper extremity. Both random and axial pattern varieties exist. All distant flaps require a period of attachment between the operated limb and the donor part. They therefore all require at least two stages, attachment and division. Where the blood supply to a random-pattern flap is doubtful, preliminary delay and later inset operations may be necessary, making four operations in total. While distant random-pattern flaps were formerly the routine method of providing skin cover to the hand where free grafts would not suffice,[34,41] the necessary hospitalization time was long and the outcome unpredictable.[314] When these factors—attachment, multiple stages, prolonged hospital stay, and doubtful result—are considered together, it is readily understood why the random-pattern distant flap has been largely superseded by the axial-pattern distant flap and it in turn by free microvascular transfer of skin. There are, however, still indications for the use of both types of conventional distant flaps. The axial flaps all have defined territories based on pedicles that run in the vascular strata previously defined. The need to ensure that the vessel is included in the flap restricts the surgeon's ability to invade its vascular territory too boldly in trying to harvest a flap for a small defect. Even more, the license to thin an axial flap is strictly controlled by the need to preserve the nutrient vascular plane. It follows that for small defects or for ones requiring thin skin, distant axial flaps, either conventional or by free transfer, are unsuitable. Normally, local or regional flaps will satisfy the need, but where they are not suitable or available, distant random-pattern flaps are still required. Such a circumstance may arise in loss of palmar skin, circumferential avulsion of soft tissue from the thumb, and small but significant defects—as, for example, where bone is exposed on the dorsum of the thumb—in a hand already extensively injured.

Conventional distant axial flaps are indicated in quite different circumstances. They are the most reliable form of coverage when microsurgical expertise is not available. Where it is, free flap transfer will become the method of choice, not only because it eliminates the problems of attachment and multiple procedures detailed above, but also because it ensures a permanent, vigorous blood supply to the injured area. It is difficult, however, to transfer much "spare" soft tissue with a free flap. Thus, if it is intended at a later stage to transfer the index finger by pollicization[310] or toes from the foot to restore an amputated thumb or fingers, then a conventional axial-pattern flap should be used for skin cover. Its tube pedicle can provide the additional skin necessary to clothe the proximal portion of the later digital transfer. In our series, 77 percent of toe transfers required preliminary groin flaps.[188] The presence of such additional skin allows a minimum of skin to be taken from the foot so that closure there can be achieved entirely with local skin, a very desirable objective. In the case of toe transfer, the use of a conventional flap has the additional benefit over free flap transfer of preserving the vessels of the hand untouched for the later anastomosis to those of the toe. As experience in microvascular surgery increases, this consideration becomes less valid.

Random-Pattern Distant Flaps

As the blood supply of the random-pattern flap derives from the subdermal or subcutaneous plexus, it can be raised at any site on the body. This apparent freedom is severely restricted by considerations of suitability, availability, positioning, and appearance. To give extreme examples, scalp skin is not suitable, penile skin is not available, leg skin would not be comfortable, and neck skin is not cosmetically acceptable. Indeed, when all factors are weighed, few donor sites remain. In the male patient, any site on the torso or the other uninjured arm may be used if no better alternative is available. In the female, only the inguinal region where the defect can be closed directly and concealed beneath a two-piece swimsuit is universally acceptable. In practice this means that random-pattern flaps are rarely used in females, primarily to transfer thin skin from the region of the iliac crest. In males the opposite infraclavicular region is used for selected thumb defects and the opposite arm for palmar defects.

As they have no axial vessel, random-pattern flaps should be designed with considerable attention to the 1 : 1 rule. This inevitably means that the bridge segment between the donor and recipient sites will be of very limited length. This further means that it cannot be tubed and thereby protected from torsional impairment of its blood flow. Both these limitations dictate that the positioning of the limb and the planning of the flap must be meticulous. The general location of the flap should be selected preoperatively in consultation with the patient. Once the patient is anesthetized and the areas are prepared and draped, the primary defect should be created and a pattern taken as previously described (Fig. 49-40A). The limb should now be brought to the prospective donor site. The margin of the primary defect that most comfortably meets the donor skin is noted and its endpoints marked, on the edge of the primary defect, on the donor site, and on the pattern. The limb is lifted and the pattern is laid on the donor site, with the marked endpoints corresponding. It can, with benefit, be secured in place with two sutures at the endpoints, forming a hinge. The

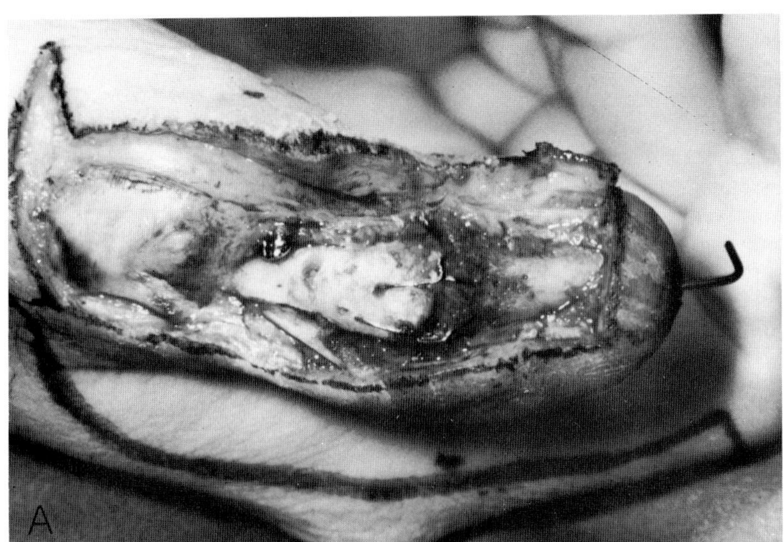

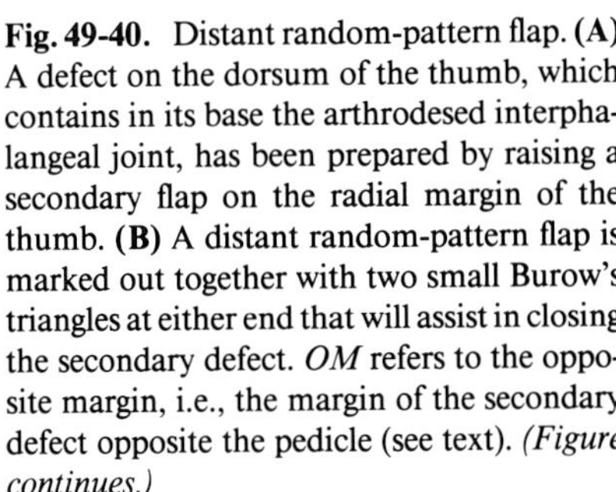

Fig. 49-40. Distant random-pattern flap. **(A)** A defect on the dorsum of the thumb, which contains in its base the arthrodesed interphalangeal joint, has been prepared by raising a secondary flap on the radial margin of the thumb. **(B)** A distant random-pattern flap is marked out together with two small Burow's triangles at either end that will assist in closing the secondary defect. *OM* refers to the opposite margin, i.e., the margin of the secondary defect opposite the pedicle (see text). *(Figure continues.)*

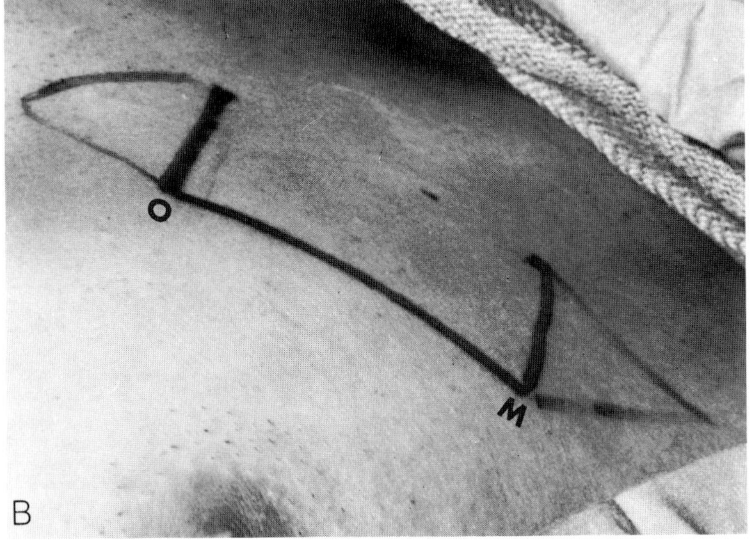

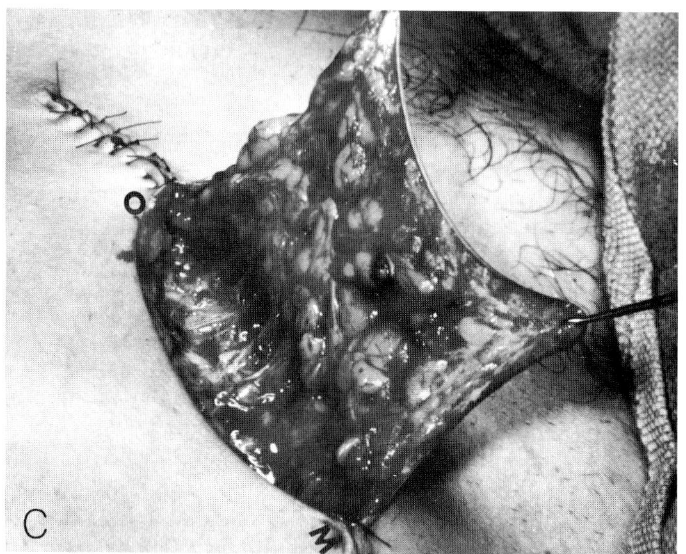

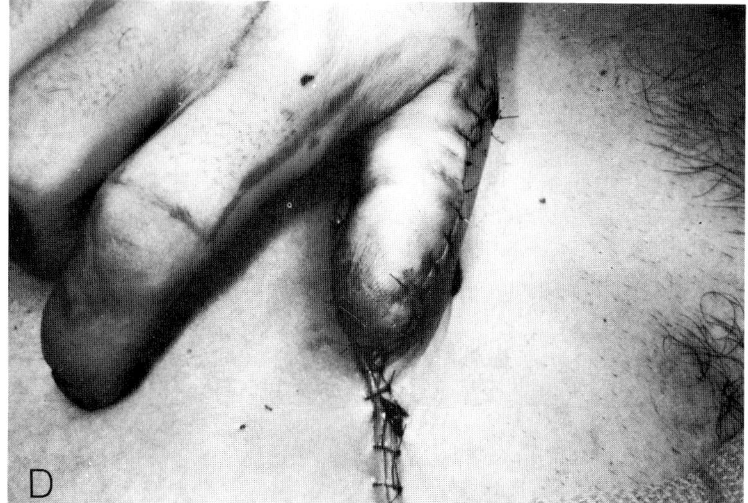

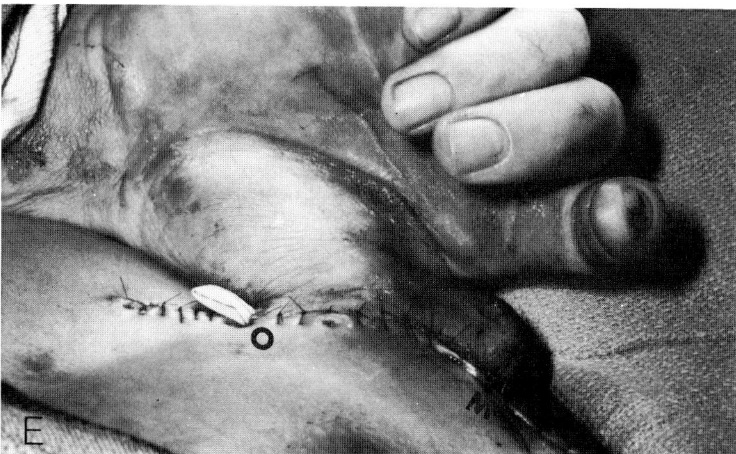

Fig. 49-40 *(Continued).* **(C)** The two Burow's triangles have been excised and the flap raised. This brings a free margin up to the bridge segment of the flap. This free margin will be sutured to the secondary flap on the thumb. **(D&E)** The flap sutured into position. The suture of the secondary flap to the free margin has ensured that avulsion of this flap will be much less likely.

skin of the donor site at the margins of the pattern is inspected to ensure that it is acceptable. For example, an infraclavicular flap must not encroach on the areola, nor an inguinal flap on the pubic hair. The limb is returned to the donor area and the pattern raised on the hinge to ensure that it fits the primary defect. If it is intended to cover the secondary defect with a skin graft, the proposed flap can now be marked around the pattern, the pattern can be removed, and the flap raised. This is necessary in very large random-pattern flaps, now rarely performed; in cross-arm flaps where direct closure may cause edema in the donor limb; and in construction of a tube pedicle for thumb reconstruction. However, if the preferable procedure of direct closure of the primary defect is to be done, then further planning is necessary.

The secondary defect may be closed in several ways. On rare occasions, it may be closed simply by approximating the two sides of the defect, leaving the pedicle at one end and excising a dog-ear at the other to facilitate closure. This is done even less often than could be, for the closure brings together the two endpoints of the pedicle, making the flap too small for the primary defect. While the flap can be made longer to accommodate this closure of the pedicle where there is an axial vessel, this is done in the random pattern only at considerable risk of losing the end of the flap. Where the necessary flap is wider than it is long, the margin of the secondary defect opposite the pedicle (here called OM) can be brought adjacent to the pedicle by excising two triangles of normal skin from the two lateral margins of the secondary defect (Fig. 49-40B). Once the flap is sutured in place and the secondary defect closed, the free margin OM lies closely approximated to that edge of the primary defect on which the endpoints of the hinge were marked (Fig. 49-40C). By raising a "secondary flap" on this edge of the primary defect (Fig. 49-40A), complete closure can be achieved by suturing that secondary flap to the free margin OM of the secondary defect (Fig. 49-40D and E). The secondary flap is raised by making incisions at the two previously marked endpoints, 5 to 10 mm long, perpendicular to the margin of the primary defect. The flap is then elevated at the subcutaneous level. This device serves not only to close all wounds directly with all the attendant benefits of so doing, but also adds security to the fixation of the flap. If it is not done, and the margin of the primary defect that corresponds to the pedicle is left free, the security of attachment of the flap to the hand depends on the strength of two sutures, those at either end of the free margin that attach the pedicle to the hand. If one pulls free, the next in line then takes the strain, and so on. The sutures may give way like a zipper, with all the embarrassment that commonly attends such an unwanted event.

A third method of closing the primary defect requires that one lateral margin of the flap, and therefore also of the secondary defect, be made longer than the other by a distance that approximates the width of the flap (Fig. 49-41). If the secondary defect is now closed directly, commencing at the margin OM opposite the pedicle, excising the dogear that results, a free margin adjacent to the underside of the pedicle will again result (Fig. 49-41C). This free margin will be the incision that extended one lateral margin. Once again this can be sutured to a secondary flap raised on the margin of the primary defect. Closure in this fashion has an important effect on the flap that must be borne in mind during planning. It rotates the flap around its long axis through 90 degrees toward the lateral margin of the secondary defect that was made longer. Returning to the planning stage, where such a closure is intended the pattern should be so positioned on the donor area that when it rotates with closure of the secondary defect it comes to lie comfortably on the primary defect (Fig. 49-42C and D). If the pattern is sutured in place as suggested above, this movement can be practiced by pulling the margins of the proposed flap together with skin hooks or stay sutures. A further consequence of this closure will be apparent. If the pattern of the primary defect is marked out on the donor area and then one side is extended as

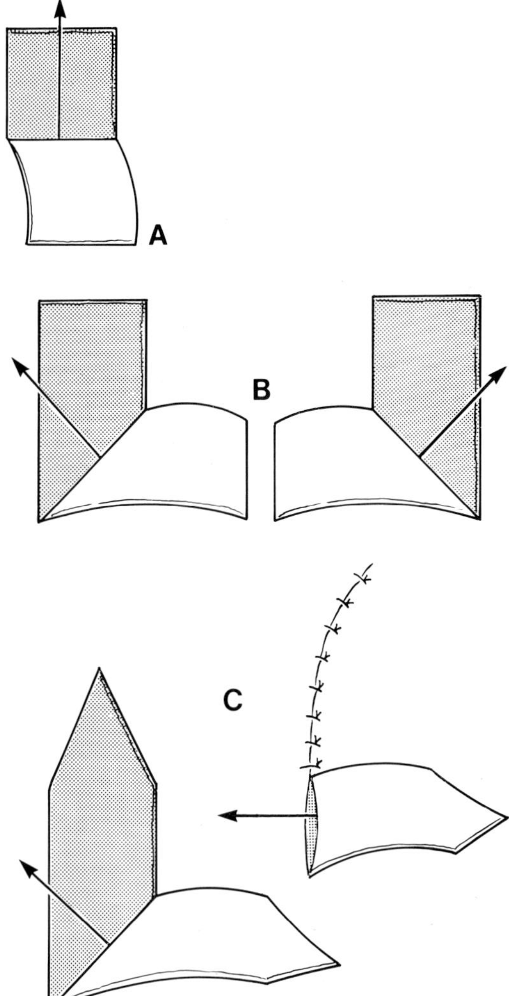

Fig. 49-41. Secondary defect closure and orientation of random flaps. **(A)** If a random flap is lifted from the secondary defect and that defect is then skin grafted, the flap will face in the same direction as when it was first raised. (This can be represented as north in this diagram, indicated as the tip of the arrow.) **(B)** If one or the other lateral margins is made longer than its counterpart, then the flap can be made to face either northeast or northwest. **(C)** By excising a Burow's triangle in the upper part of the secondary defect and suturing the defect margin-to-margin, the flap can be made to face either due east or due west depending on the location of the extension cut.

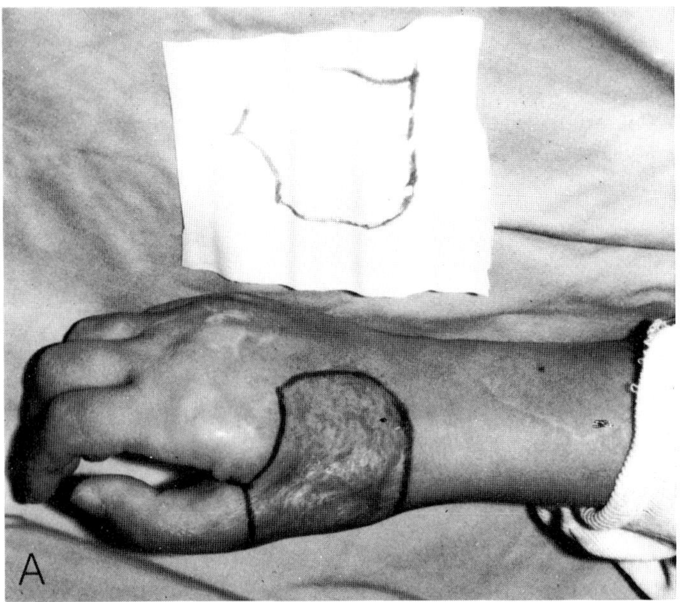

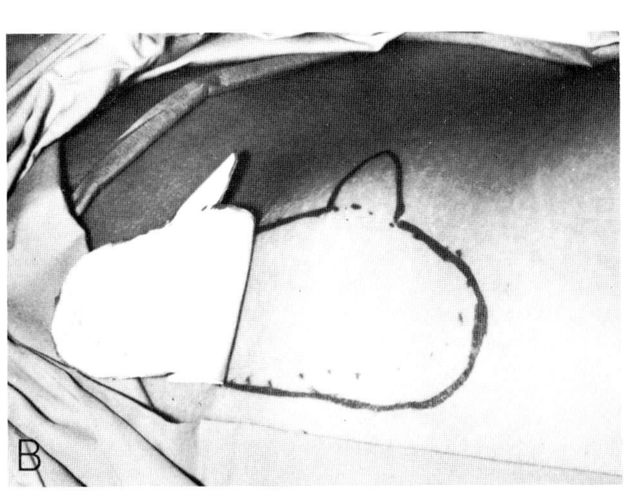

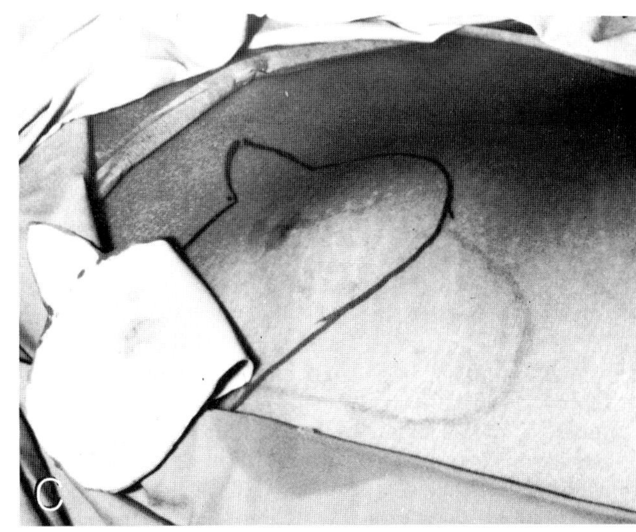

Fig. 49-42. Random-pattern flap. **(A)** The proposed primary defect has been marked out with ink and a pattern taken by moistening a portion of Esmarch bandage with alcohol. **(B)** The pattern cut out of the Esmarch bandage has been applied to the region of the iliac crest and sutured in position. If the secondary defect were to be covered with a skin graft, this would be the flap appropriate to this primary defect giving comfortable positioning of the limb. **(C)** Since, however, the intention is to close the secondary defect directly, the location of the flap donor site has to be adjusted. In this photograph, the initial design is seen faintly and the new design well marked. This has been tested by practicing closure of the defect using skin hooks, ensuring that the flap will finally face in the correct direction. *(Figure continues.)*

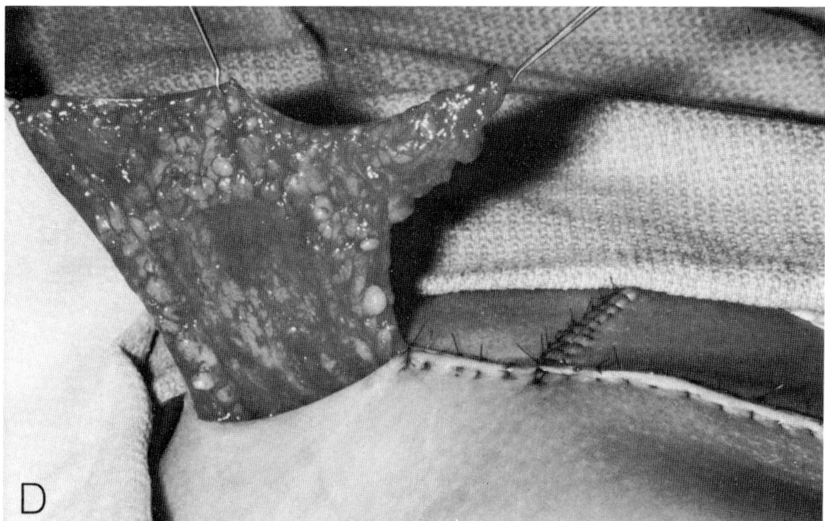

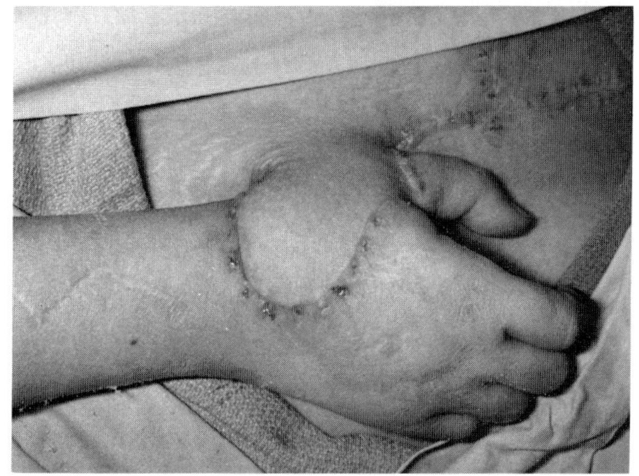

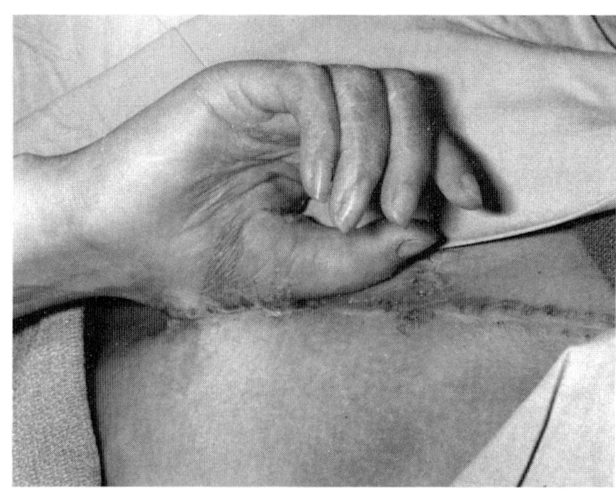

Fig. 49-42 *(Continued).* **(D)** The secondary defect has been closed directly and it can be seen that the flap now faces in a direction quite different from that seen in **(C)**. The free margin shown at the bridge segment of the flap will be sutured to the secondary flap raised on the primary defect. **(E&F)** The flap sits comfortably in position and all wounds are closed. *(Figure continues.)*

required, the flap will clearly be larger by the area encompassed by this extension cut. If it were a rectangular flap and the design were rigidly geometric, the fact that one lateral margin is longer than the other would angle the flap away from that side. Closure would cause the flap to rotate to the left and lean to the right, or vice versa! In practice, the elasticity of the skin is very forgiving. Because of it, the extension cut need not be made so long as to equal the breadth. By differential suturing, closure can be effected without distorting the flap. However, the extension cut must be made and the altered shape of the flap must be fitted to the pattern and topography of the primary defect. It will be appreciated from all these considerations that the planning and positioning of the random-pattern flap requires time and thought. Once drawn out on the donor site, the flap is, by contrast, simple to raise. The incision is carried down through the subdermal plexus to the subcutaneous tissue. The plane of dissection can be at any level in the subcutaneous tissue, which is of a thickness that varies with the patient's fat content. However, fat is a poor bed for a skin graft so if it is intended to graft the secondary defect, the flap should be raised on the superficial surface of the deep fascia and then defatted to the required thickness. Where the defect is to be closed directly, the subcutaneous layer should be incised at the necessary depth. Once the flap is elevated, the secondary defect is closed and, if a skin graft has been used, a bolus applied. The limb is then returned to the donor site and the flap sutured into place (Fig. 49-42E and F).

As the pedicle can be easily kinked, considerable care should be taken to apply strapping to the limb and torso in such a way as to immobilize the limb in the position that assures best

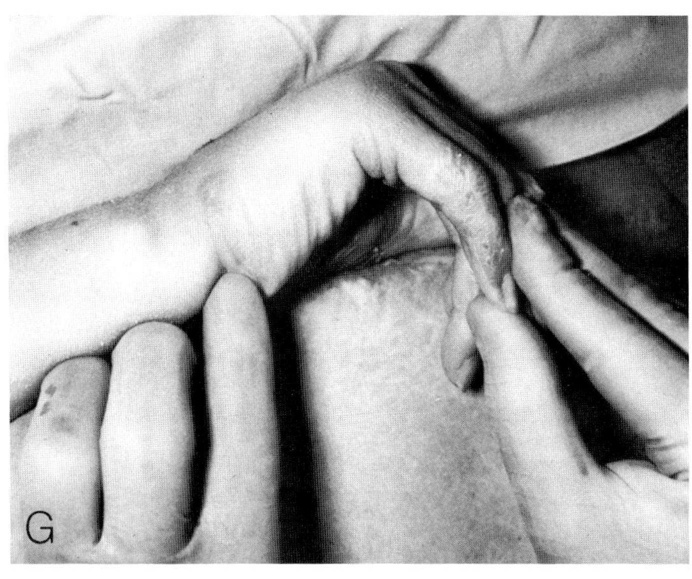

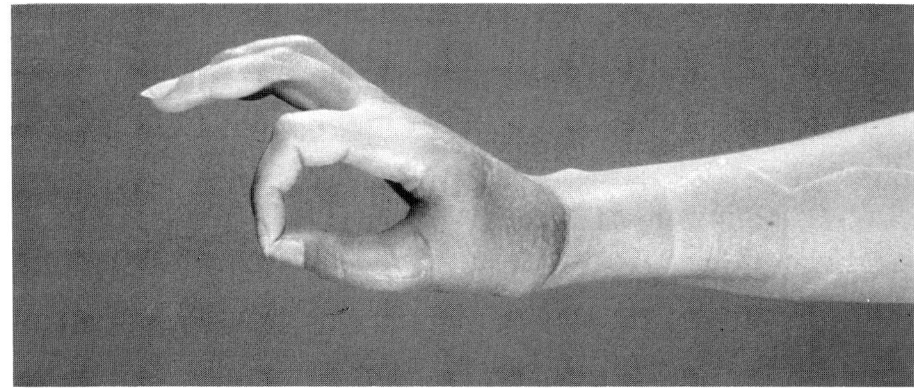

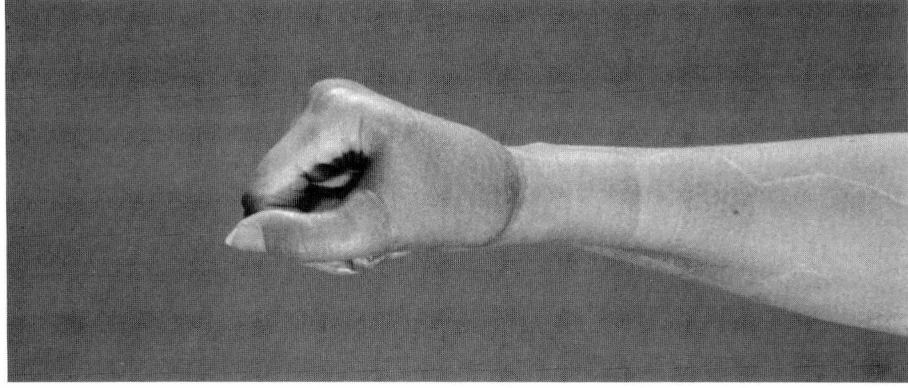

Fig. 49-42 *(Continued).* **(G)** The small joints of the hand can be mobilized. **(H&I)** The result. The similarity of the primary defect here to that in Figure 49-50 is apparent. A random-pattern flap was selected in this case because the patient was a rather obese female. A random flap could be thinned more radically than the axial groin flap used in the relatively thin male patient shown in Figure 49-50.

perfusion of the flap, yet permits exercise of the joints of the hand (Fig. 49-42G–I). This should be done while the patient is still anesthetized. The surgeon should remain as the patient awakens to add any additional restraints that prove necessary.

As emphasized, random-pattern flaps are limited in size by their blood supply. Their size can be increased by a prior delay procedure performed 10 days previously. A similar effect recently has been reported experimentally using preliminary tissue expansion: the mean increase in surviving length after expansion was on average 117 percent compared with a control. A flap delayed by traditional methods showed a mean increase of 73 percent.[47] The size can also be increased by creating a bipedicle flap; that is, one raised with only two lateral incisions. Such bipedicle flaps are deemed to be safe with a length-breadth ratio of 2.5 : 1. Bipedicle flaps constructed on the opposite arm have been used successfully to resurface both palmar and dorsal defects.[210] Colson[58] has stressed the merits of radical thinning of such flaps in producing good contour and function.

Other modifications of the random distant flap include suture of cutaneous nerves in the flap to branches of the radial nerve in the defect to reinnervate a thumb reconstruction[73]; the use of double flaps to cover both dorsal and palmar wounds[228] and to create a new first web[227,338]; and the use of several interdigitating flaps to resurface multiple finger injuries.[140]

Where osteoplastic reconstruction[192,337] (see also Chapter 57) is deemed to be the best method of restoring an amputated thumb,[184] the necessary random-pattern flap is best fashioned in the contralateral infraclavicular fossa (Fig. 49-43). That choice virtually limits the procedure to the male patient. The circumference of the adult male thumb at the MP joint is a surprising 9 cm. The flap is therefore planned as a square with 9-cm sides, the base being directed toward the shoulder joint. The resultant defect cannot be closed directly. As the envelope required should be as thin as possible, and as it is a random-pattern flap, it can be thinned radically. This is best done by having an assistant hold the flap under tension with skin hooks. The subcutaneous fat is then grasped with toothed forceps and

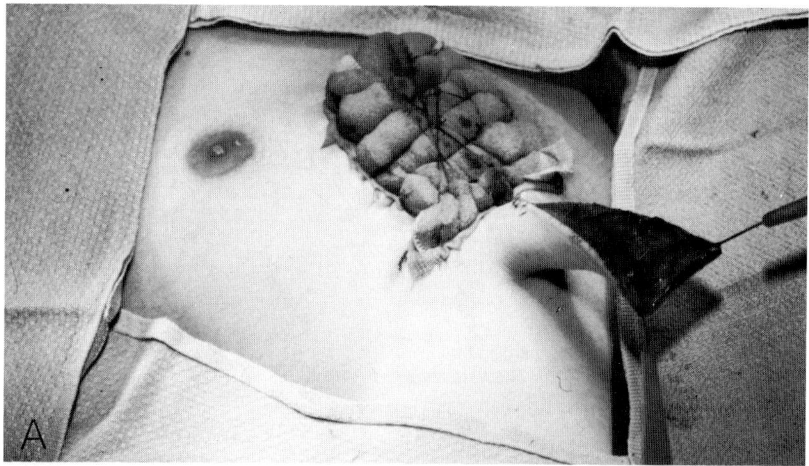

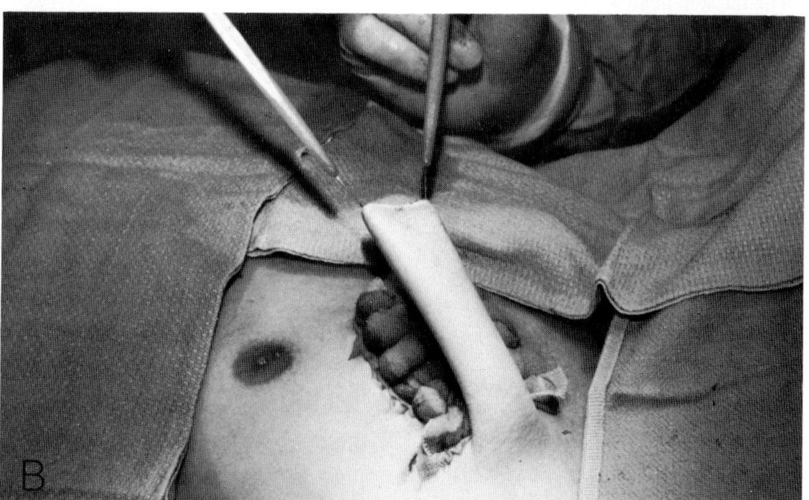

Fig. 49-43. Tube pedicle for thumb coverage. **(A)** A random-pattern flap has been raised in the infraclavicular region, thinned, tubed, and the secondary defect covered with a split-thickness skin graft held firmly in place by a bolus. **(B)** The length of the flap. *(Figure continues.)*

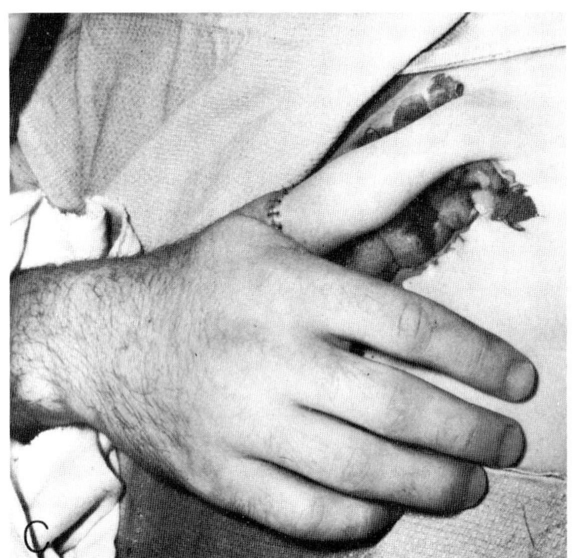

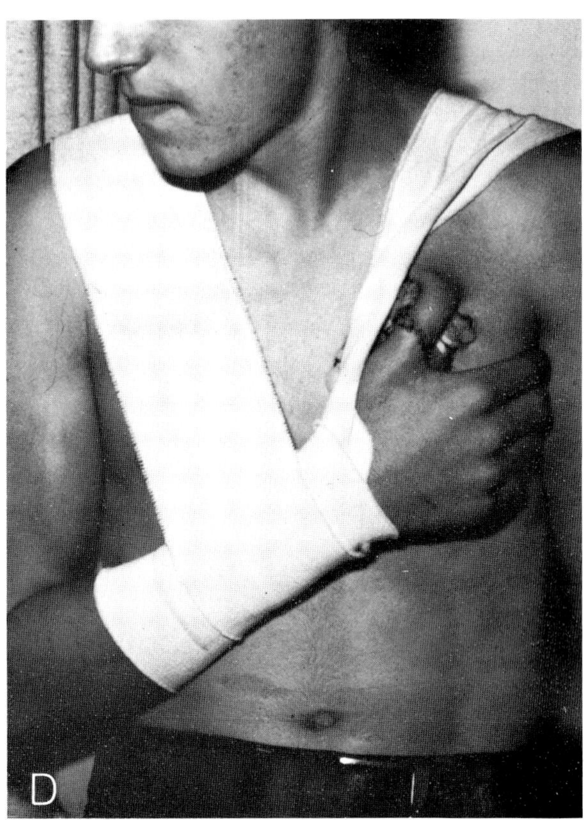

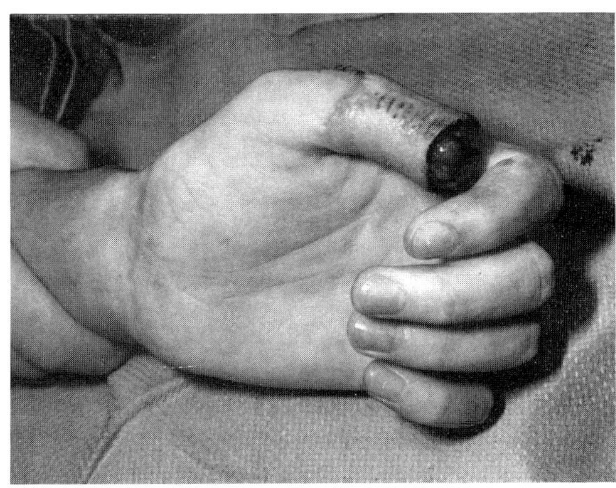

Fig. 49-43 *(Continued).* **(C)** The flap is placed in position and **(D)** the hand is maintained in position with strapping. **(E)** At the time of division, it can be seen that the seam of this flap was placed incorrectly on the dorsoradial aspect. Fortunately, it was well healed and it was possible to proceed with a pedicle neurovascular island through an incision in an appropriate position on the tube.

trimmed away with curved tenotomy scissors held with the convexity to the underside of the flap. This can continue until the subdermal vessels can be clearly seen. The flap is tubed throughout its length, starting by approximating the two distal corners of the flap, proceeding toward the base. It should be possible to do this for some 6 cm, producing an adequate tube to cover the iliac crest bone graft (or the original skeleton in the case of an acute avulsion). The remaining 3 cm of each lateral side will now be in line with one another, creating a straight border to the secondary defect at the base of the pedicle. The split-thickness skin graft that is then applied to the secondary defect can be sutured to skin on all four margins, creating a closed wound. A bolus dressing is applied (Fig. 49-43A and B). The thumb is now introduced into the tube, flexing the wrist so that the fingers lie in the axilla. In this way the seam of the tube can be brought to the midline of the palmar surface of the thumb (Fig. 49-43C and D). At the next definitive stage, this seam can be opened to introduce a neurovascular island flap. This should be done at the time of division of the tube pedicle (Fig. 49-43E), not only because it brings needed sensation to the thumb, but also because of its beneficial influence on the circulation of the reconstruction. The additional skin it provides eliminates any need to close the newly divided tube under tension. Also, its axial vessel revascularizes the tip much more satisfactorily than those of the tube pedicle, which derive their flow from the new vessels that have grown across the wound of attachment during the preceding weeks. So marginal is this flow and so important the reconstruction, that it is wise to stimulate that flow by a delay incision halfway across the base of the tube pedicle at 3 weeks, leaving final division for a further week.

Axial-Pattern Distant Flaps

The concept that a large vessel supplying a block of tissue will assure good perfusion is simple. That concept was recognized in 1863 by Wood[345] who emphasized the importance of including the superficial inferior epigastric artery in a flap to release a burn contracture in a child. This vessel was the basis of the flap used in the first modern description of an axial-pattern flap in 1946 by Shaw and Payne.[290] The same flap has since been described by various authors under different names, including the Shaw flap,[17] the abdominohypogastric flap,[284] and the superficial inferior epigastric artery flap.[130,312] The use of a large abdominal flap based on both superficial inferior epigastric arteries and both superficial circumflex iliac arteries for large upper extremity defects has been reported by Kelleher and others.[162] Despite the successes reported by all of these authors, neither this hypogastric flap nor other axial flaps from the torso, such as the transverse rectus[39] and thoracoumbilical flaps,[29] have achieved the popularity enjoyed by the groin flap.[94,217]

Groin Flap

The groin flap is an axial-pattern flap of the cutaneous variety (Fig. 49-44). Its axial vessel is the superficial circumflex iliac artery,[301] which is a relatively constant vessel, being present in 96 percent of a series of angiograms.[158] The vessel arises from the femoral artery in the femoral triangle, which forms a vascular "hub"[323] for the axes of several flaps converge here. The superficial circumflex iliac artery emerges from the triangle by passing over the medial border of the sartorius immediately after giving a deep muscular branch. Initially below the deep fascia, the vessel emerges through that fascia as it crosses the sartorius. It passes laterally, parallel to, and some 2 cm below, the inguinal ligament. At a point below the anterior superior iliac spine, the vessel divides and supplies the skin immediately below the iliac crest. The vascular territory of the superficial circumflex iliac artery therefore ends at some point lateral to the anterior superior iliac spine. Common wisdom and practical experience dictate that the flap can safely be extended beyond the spine by a distance at least equal to the width of the flap. The venous drainage[255]—which is of importance equal to the arterial supply[298]—and lymphatic outflow[53] of the flap have both been studied in detail. The former report

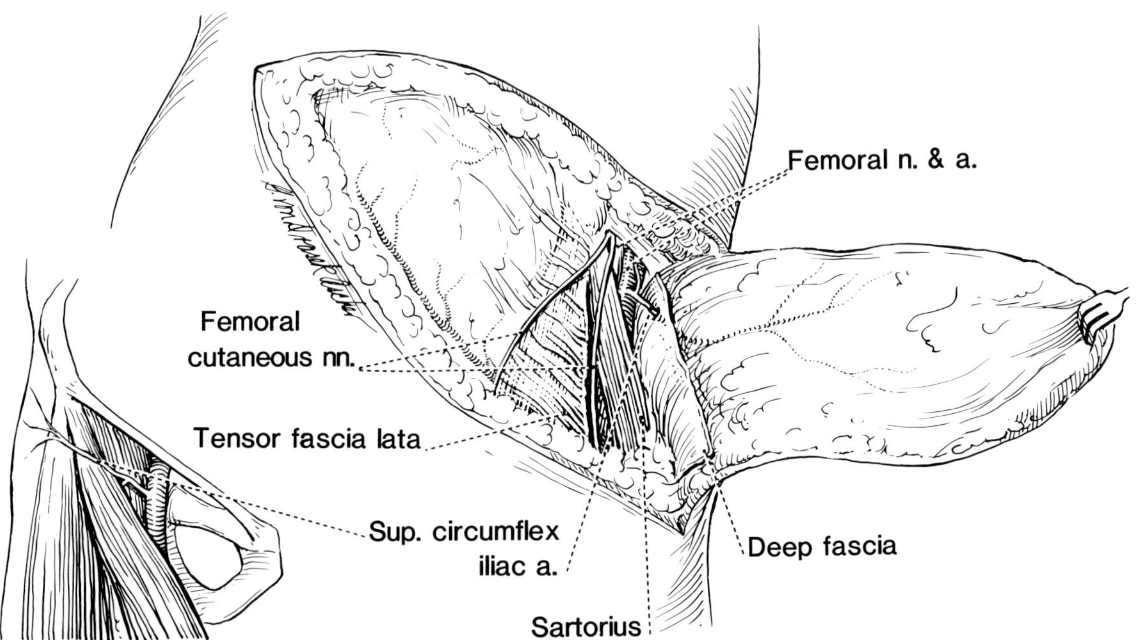

Fig. 49-44. Groin flap. The groin flap is based on the superficial circumflex iliac artery, which runs parallel to and approximately one inch inferior to the inguinal ligament. It emerges through the deep fascia as it crosses the sartorius and breaks up into branches at the level of the anterior superior iliac spine. When the flap is raised the lateral femoral cutaneous nerve should be preserved or, in certain instances (see text), divided and repaired. The fascia that is divided at the lateral margin of the sartorius can be seen.

by Penteado gives details of venous variations in the femoral triangle important to the microsurgeon; the surgeon intent upon using the flap as an axial pedicle need only know that all drainage of this region is to the femoral triangle and therefore will lie within the pedicle. Commonly, no reinnervation of the flap is attempted, but Joshi[155] has pointed out that the lateral cutaneous branch of the subcostal or twelfth thoracic nerve consistently crosses the iliac crest 5 cm posterior to the anterior superior iliac spine. This can be dissected, divided and sutured to any available cutaneous nerve ending in the hand. The groin flap can provide skin cover for any defect on any aspect of the hand or of the forearm in its distal two-thirds.[50] It can safely be made wide enough to replace massive loss, with the only drawback being that the widest secondary defect that can be readily closed directly is 12 cm. For defects on both aspects of the hand, the flap can be split longitudinally or used in conjunction with a hypogastric flap,[300] a tensor fascia lata musculocutaneous flap,[340] or with a contralateral groin flap.[127] Where a relatively large block of bone is required in the hand in the depths of a soft tissue defect, the iliac crest (Fig. 49-45) immediately beneath the flap can be taken as a vascularized composite extension.[40,83,269]

In planning the groin flap less attention is paid to the primary defect than in planning a random-pattern flap. However, preparation of a pattern of the primary defect is still helpful. It should next be decided from which direction the flap should approach the defect. For example, for defects primarily on the dorsal aspect of the wrist, the flap pedicle could lie to either the radial or ulnar side. Time should be taken with this decision, for the obvious choice is not always the correct one. Factors to be considered are the precise location of the defect, the resulting configuration of the tube pedicle, the freedom of pronation and supination of the forearm, and the patient's comfort and exercise postoperatively. The major fact to be appreciated with respect to the configuration of the pedicle is that it will do well if stretched gently, and poorly if kinked; flaps always perfuse more satisfactorily on a convex surface than on a concave. To take another example, a defect on the dorsal aspect of the hand extending on to the radial border might be best approached by a pedicle around the ulnar border, for full pronation and supination would place little stress on the suture line and would not kink the pedicle. The previously prepared pattern can well be extended with a portion to represent the pedicle so that various approaches and positions can be tested. Once the approach and eventual position has been chosen, that edge of the primary defect that will be closest to the pedicle will be known. The original pattern should be laid on the skin immediately below and behind the anterior superior iliac spine, for the more medial, inguinal portion of the flap will be largely used to construct the tube.

A few words about constructing the tube are appropriate at this juncture. Two extreme possibilities should be considered. If a flap is not tubed at all, then its distal and lateral margins can be made to fit precisely to the primary defect. The other margin of the defect, adjacent to the pedicle, has to be left unsutured, but the eventual contour of the flap to the hand is excellent, without revision. At the other extreme, if the flap is raised as a rectangle and tubed throughout its length, it could cover a circular defect, but it would approach the defect perpendicularly and would be most difficult to inset after division. Since the first (untubed) flap is unacceptable because of the open wound, poor flap fixation to the defect margins, and difficulties with postoperative exercise, and the latter because of contour, a compromise must be sought. The distal margin of the flap is cut to conform to the edge of the distal half of the defect. When this design is tubed the distal few centimeters of the *lateral* edges of the flap come to meet the edge of the proximal half of the defect. After division of the flap there will be too much skin at the proximal margin, which will require excision as dog-ears at division or at a later stage. The surgeon's ability to tube the groin flap depends on the width of the flap, but also on its thickness. Since its axial vessel emerges through the deep fascia, the flap cannot be thinned appreciably in the part to be tubed. Thus, in choosing the width of the flap, the surgeon must pay heed not only to the width of the primary defect but also to the weight/height ratio of the patient. If this is high, the flap will be thick and must therefore be wide. Skin grafts may be necessary to close the secondary defect. Therefore, if the flap is being planned on an elective basis the overweight patient should be encouraged to reduce.

Once all these factors have been considered, and the patient prepared and draped, the midline of the flap should be drawn out 2 cm inferior and parallel to the inguinal ligament. In children this vessel can be located by measuring below the inguinal ligament by a distance equal to the breadth of the child's index and middle fingers. The elected width of pedicle to be tubed should be measured out as far as the anterior superior iliac spine, and the distal, lateral margin of the flap should be made to conform to the distal half of the pattern of the primary defect. The part of the flap to cover the primary defect can be wider than the pedicle. There must be a limit to the extent by which it can be wider, but this is never challenged in normal practice. The entire margin of the flap is incised down to the superficial surface of the deep fascia. The distal edge of the flap is placed under tension and the subcutaneous plane is developed with a knife as far as the anterior superior iliac spine, making sure not to create a cave beneath the midportion of the flap (see page 1743). At this point the flap should be laid in a cephalad direction and retraction applied to the inferior incision. The deep fascia should be incised at the level of this inferior incision and retracted toward the abdomen to reveal the sartorius, the tensor fascia lata lateral to it, and the intervening intermuscular septum. Maintaining traction on the flap cephalad and away from the thigh, the deep fascia should be divided in the line of the fibers of the sartorius from inferior to superior, and at its lateral border, just medial to the septum between tensor and sartorius. As this incision in the deep fascia proceeds, the subcutaneous plane previously developed laterally is advanced to meet it. The superficial circumflex iliac artery will be seen in the deep fascia as it is lifted from the sartorius. Incision of the fascia proceeds cephalad beyond the artery as far as the origin of the sartorius from the anterior superior iliac spine. Here the flap should be drawn in the opposite direction, caudally, to facilitate dissection of the upper margin. The upper incision, if carried down to the external oblique aponeurosis, will, in the majority of cases, divide a significant artery. This may cause alarm, but should not, for this is the superficial inferior epigastric artery, which must be

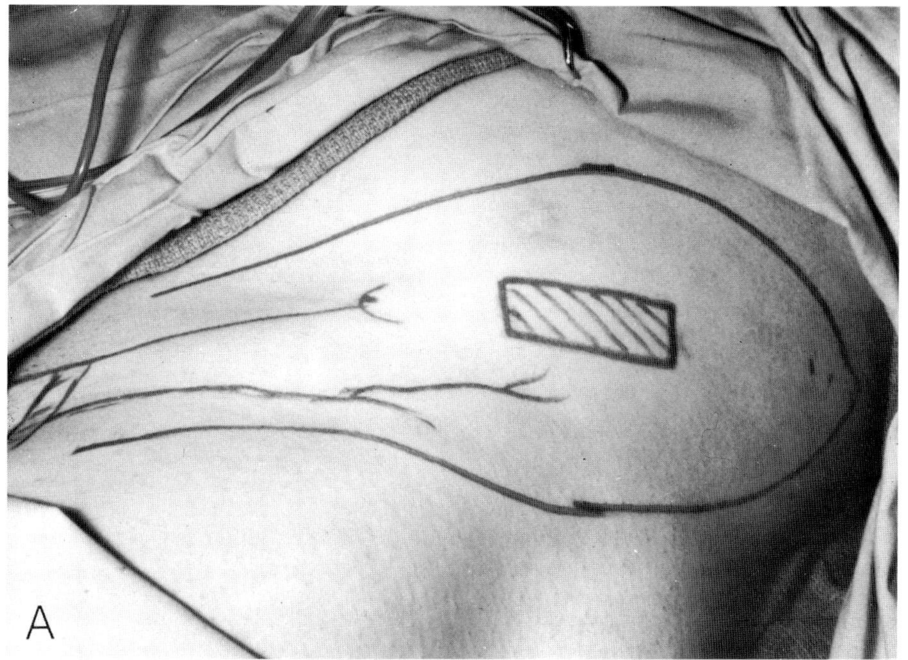

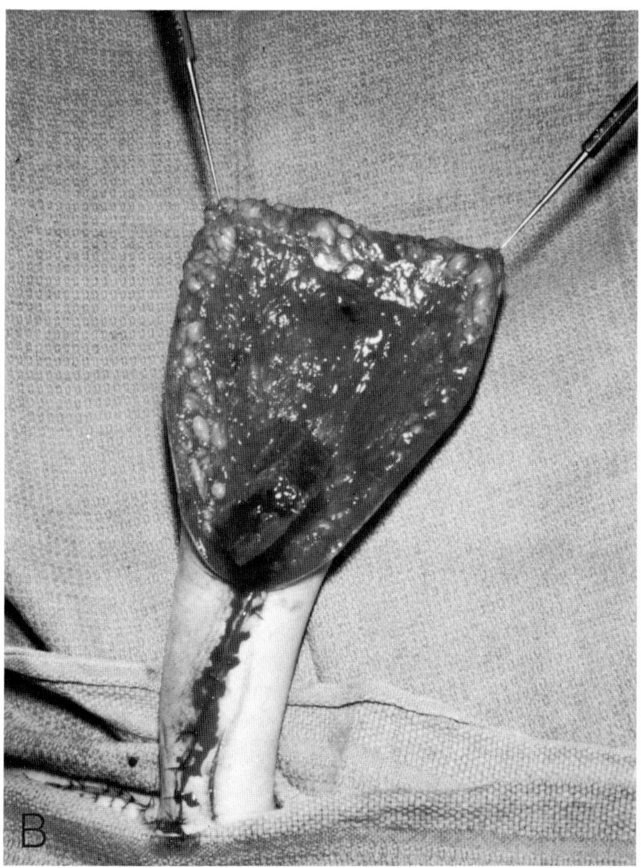

Fig. 49-45. Groin flap with iliac crest. **(A)** The groin flap has been marked out with the inguinal ligament and the expected course of the superficial circumflex iliac artery. A monobloc of iliac crest has been taken with the groin flap and it can be seen to be bleeding well in the distal portion of the tube **(B)**. (This is the same patient as shown in Fig. 49-51.)

cut. Furthermore, its division indicates that the relevant vascular stratum has been cut and the level of dissection is now in the correct plane. The flap is retracted caudally off the aponeurosis until the level of the anterior superior iliac spine is reached. The incision previously made in the sartorius fascia is located and turned medially to free the deep fascia of the thigh from the inguinal ligament. In the course of this incision the lateral cutaneous nerve of the thigh will be encountered. Care must be taken not to injure this, for meralgia paresthetica may result.[231] While this nerve usually passes deep to the vessel of the flap, in which case it can be freed by dissection, on occasion it or one of its usual two branches may be superficial and, therefore, more likely to be injured and also more likely to kink the vessel of the flap. Any such branches superficial to the artery should be divided, placed deep to the vessel, and repaired. All fascial incisions are now completed.

It should be noted that it is possible to raise a groin flap without ever dividing either the fascia or the vessel. However, the consequences may be dire, for the superficial circumflex iliac artery is tethered by the intact fascia. The relaxed and redirected flap will pull on the vessel and may kink it severely (Fig. 49-46). Herein lies the explanation for necrotic edges on otherwise well-designed and executed groin flaps. The fascia must *always* be incised!

Applying upward traction to the flap, the fascia is dissected from the underlying fibers of the sartorius, paying due heed to the vessels, which can usually be seen through the elevated fascia. In preparing a pedicle groin flap, dissection can cease at the medial border of the sartorius. In dissecting for free tissue transfer, or where the flap is to be taken to the opposite hand, the pedicle should be dissected further, using scissors and forceps. The main hazard is the muscular branch of the superficial circumflex iliac artery. This should be isolated by retracting the sartorius laterally with instruments on either side of the pedicle, caudad and cephalad. Once dissected free under loupe magnification, the muscular branch should be divided. The vessel can then be freed as far as its origin.

The flap can now be thinned. This is done by having an assistant hold the flap vertically with hooks or stay sutures and proceeding with curved tenotomy scissors and forceps. Using the scissors with concave surface uppermost, the surgeon can thin the flap quite radically *at the margins* by trimming away fat. In the midline of the flap, he must be more cautious or the pedicle may be damaged. Lobules of fat can be lifted with forceps and trimmed away, between periphery and midline, but the deep fascia that has been lifted *must not be transgressed.* Therefore any fat that lies between it and the skin must be left alone. If there is a significant amount, it makes the tube necessarily bulky.

Closure should commence at the lateral end of the secondary defect. It may be difficult, but the surgeon should *not* undermine the margins in an attempt to facilitate closure. Such action only increases the area of the potential dead space and does little to relax the skin. Instead, the surgeon should flex the thigh, take up a heavy suture, and go to it with the knowledge that closure is always possible if the defect was 12 cm or less *when first outlined* (Fig. 49-47). (The tension created will inevitably result in postoperative inflammation along the closure. *Do not remove sutures!* To do so would open the entire cavity

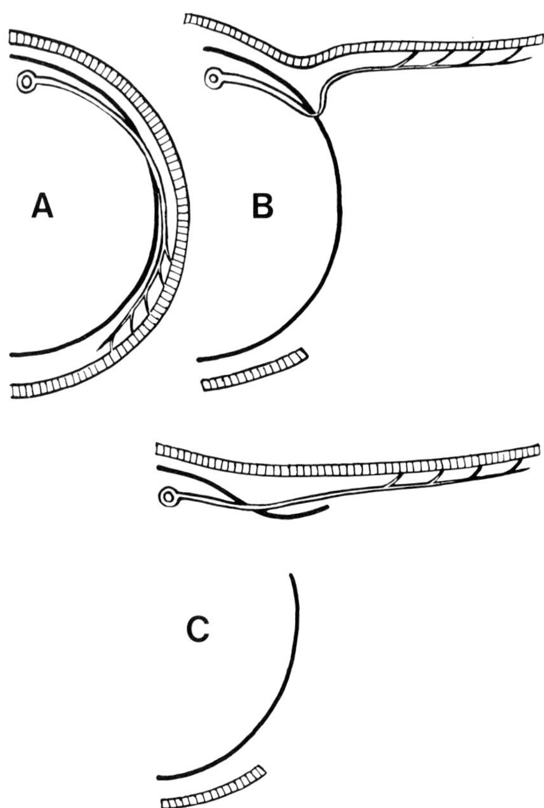

Fig. 49-46. In cross-sectional diagram, the course of the superficial circumflex iliac artery is shown in **(A)**. The black line represents the deep fascia, and it can be seen that the superficial circumflex iliac artery pierces that fascia. **(B)** If the flap is raised without dividing the fascia, the vessel is restrained and kinked by that deep fascia, reducing significantly the blood flow to the flap. **(C)** If the fascia is divided, as recommended, at the lateral margin of the sartorius, this kink in the vessel is eliminated.

created by the closure. If this then becomes infected, as is almost inevitable, one has created a disaster akin to a bedsore.) Closure of the secondary defect could continue medially all the way to the pedicle. However, a more comfortable closure is achieved if, in the last few centimeters, the flap is resutured from whence it came (Fig. 49-48). Where these three suture lines meet, the tubing of the flap commences. This should be easily achieved provided the width has been well tailored to the thickness. If it has not, further marginal thinning should be done. The tube is closed with interrupted sutures. The closure should continue until the portion of flap remaining open for the defect is clearly too small. That is, the tube should be closed too far. The reason for this is that once the flap is sutured to the hand it is simple to release sutures from the tube, but very awkward to insert them. The limb is now brought to the flap, the planned posture adopted, any minor adjustments made, and the flap sutured in place. It is good to commence this at the center point of the distal margin of the flap and then proceed progressively around both margins alternately toward the pedicle. In this way, little or no distortion is applied to the flap. With each stitch, the skin of the flap should be stretched slightly

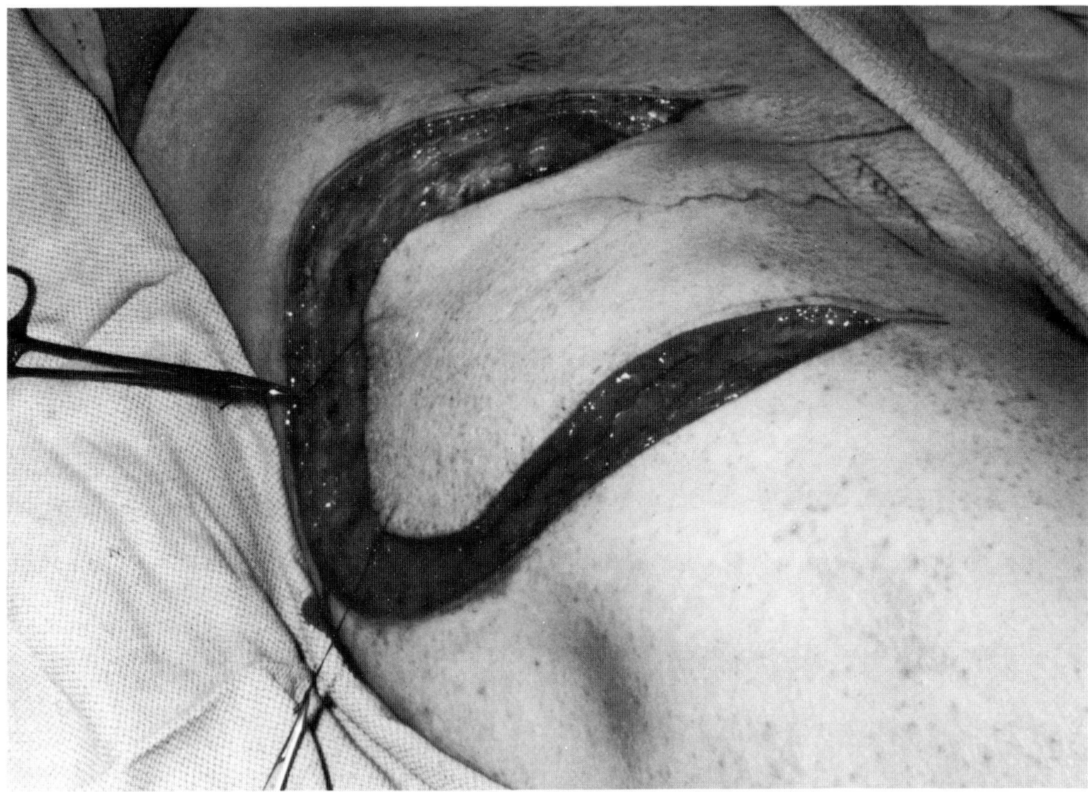

Fig. 49-47. A groin flap here has been raised and the size of the resultant secondary defect can be seen. The stay sutures have been kept in place to support the flap during the thinning progress (see text). This is the same patient shown in Figure 49-50.

to reproduce tension similar to that present in the margin of the defect. Whether or not this has been done correctly can be determined by looking at the wound edges between each stitch: neither should sit above the other.

On completion of application of the flap, the involved limb should be immobilized. It has been suggested that this be done with external fixation between the iliac crest and the radius[78,240] but this is not necessary and is positively disadvantageous if it limits motion of the hand throughout the period of flap attachment. Temporary control can be achieved by placing rolled bandages between the limb and the torso and then strapping the arm in place with tape from the abdomen, around the arm to the back. The intent of this strapping is to control the arm in such a way that the flap is not kinked; indeed, it is held under gentle traction. Once the patient is fully recovered from anesthesia, on the first or second postoperative day, all restraints should be removed and the patient placed in charge of his own flap. Clear instructions should be given to him to maintain a little traction and avoid kinking the flap. He should be shown how to exercise all joints. By depressing the shoulder and carrying the hand toward the umbilicus, the elbow can be flexed to 90 degrees. By elevating the shoulder and carrying the hand toward the knee, it can be fully extended. Full pronation and supination, flexion and extension of the wrist and motion of all the digital joints can be attained, and should be, every waking hour. It is in this respect that the axial flap with its tube pedicle is incontestably superior to even the best-designed random-pattern flap. Patients can be dressed soon after surgery by wearing either dungarees, or trousers with a pocket removed and a fastening incorporated in the waistband above the pocket.

The groin flap can be used in young children[209] with no increased incidence of flap avulsion during the postoperative period. Unless unforeseen circumstances are encountered, the complete survival of the groin flap can be predicted[189] with sufficient confidence that the practiced exponent should not hesitate to undertake extensive reconstruction in the bed of the primary defect, including joint replacement and tendon graft.[309]

Problems with circulation are more likely to arise after division of the pedicle,[346] understandably, for the flap, previously nourished by an axial vessel, is now dependent on flow across the wounds of attachment. The optimum time at which to perform the division varies considerably, as shown by fluorescin studies.[213] The first requirement for safe division is perfect healing of the wound of attachment. The second requirement is that the wound of attachment be long when compared to the area of flap skin required on the hand. This is not so, for example, where much or all of the tube pedicle is required for later use. Division of such a flap should be preceded by a delay procedure. The third requirement is that the surrounding skin of the limb should be supple and unscarred. If all these are met, then the flap an be safely divided at 3 weeks and inset. If one or more are not met, then one or more of the

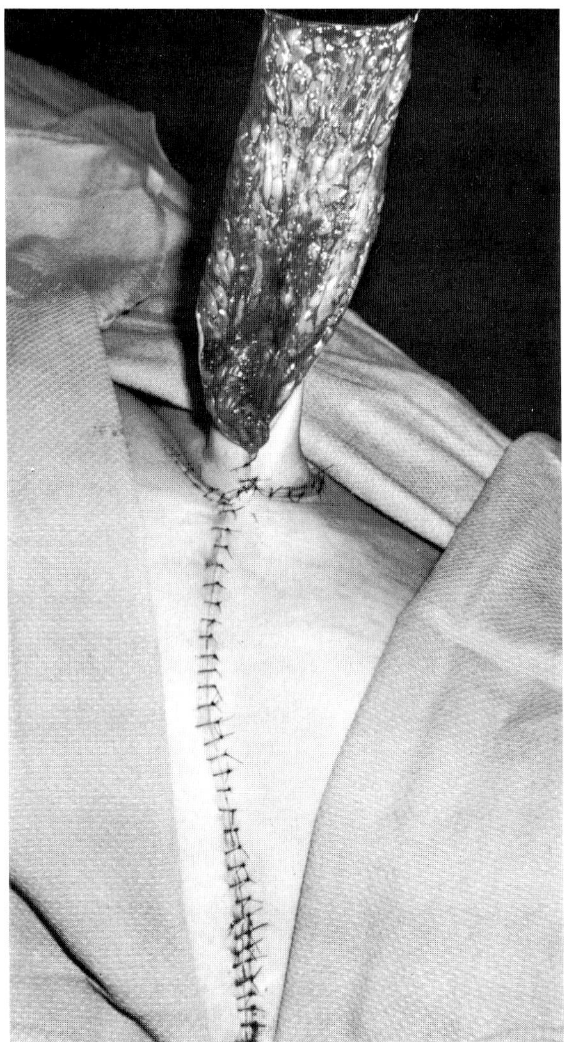

Fig. 49-48. Closure of the secondary defect. Direct closure of the secondary defect should in all instances be attempted. The junction of the secondary defect and the tube is shown. It is important not to close the secondary defect too far medially, or kinking in the base of the tube may result.

following steps should be taken. First, wait. No harm comes from a longer attachment. Second, test the flow. This is done by placing a rubber tourniquet around the tube pedicle and testing whether flow to the flap remains good. Flow can be assessed by the use of systemic fluorescin or by injecting atropine into the flap and measuring the time until the onset of visual disturbance. It may also be assessed by the simple clinical tests of sticking a needle into the flap or observing whether or not reactive hyperemia develops in the flap after 20 minutes of occlusion. Third, if the flap is divided, and bleeding from the flap on the hand is poor, do not inset it, but simply wrap the hand and return 1 week later. Fourth, and this is my routine practice where I need the tube pedicle to cover a later digital transfer, perform a delay procedure. This is done under local anesthetic and consists of making an incision half-way around the tube pedicle, through which all deep soft tissue in the tube is divided. The wound is then closed and the flap divided completely and with confidence 1 week later.

AUTHOR'S PREFERRED METHODS

Contrary to other opinion, I am firmly committed to the belief that definitive skin cover at the time of injury is preferable to delayed closure, provided only that debridement is adequate.[112,114] It will have become evident from the above account of local, regional, and distant flaps, all with both random and axial designs, that I have a rich storehouse from which to select that skin cover. Since I have microsurgical training, to that store must be added all of the free tissue transfers described elsewhere in this book. Much of this bounty has been harvested in my lifetime,[46,215] and by keeping abreast of these developments, I have been able to incorporate each new addition into the process by which I make my selection. However, for the younger surgeon these very riches may be a source of confusion, causing him to make less than the best choice, or worse, to disregard or remain ignorant of the older techniques in favor of the more complex and more expensive, but more exciting, free skin transfers.[24] In an attempt to offer guidance, I will approach the matter of skin cover not from the viewpoint used throughout this chapter, namely, which flaps are available, but rather by the nature of the presenting skin defect (Table 49-2). I have assumed in all that follows that the possibility of a free skin graft has been weighed and rejected. I will look at defects on the fingers separately from those of the thumb, and palmar defects apart from dorsal. Dorsal defects can be subdivided further into small and large. *All* small dorsal defects I manage by transposition or rotation flaps (see page 1746) taken from either the adjacent dorsal skin or from the lateral aspect of the fingers.

Palmar defects distal to the PIP joint are most commonly fingertip injuries.[117,141] In such injuries where more skin is in fact lost dorsally, or the amputation is transverse, V-Y advancement flaps (see page 1760) are indicated. Where more is lost from the palmar surface, a regional flap is required. In patients under 40 years of age—and, of course, this can be adjusted to circumstance and "physiological condition," which I judge by whether or not the proximal interphalangeal joints can be hyperextended—the digit can safely be immobilized in flexion for the necessary 14 days. In the female, who may be dismayed by the secondary defect of a cross-finger flap, I would use a thenar flap (see page 1771); in the male, who tends to be less supple, the cross-finger flap (see page 1776). In those over 40, if the digit is of considerable functional importance, for example the thumb or a finger where others have been lost, a neurovascular island flap (see page 1773) is justified, taken either from the toe or from the ulnar aspect of the middle fingers. Where the digit is of less importance, I explain the thoughts outlined above to the patient and recommend revision of the amputation. If he balks, I then proceed as if he were under 40, knowing that he understands the potential problems. On the *dorsal* aspect of the finger distally, if the defect is sufficiently large that I cannot use a local flap, a reversed cross-finger flap is indicated (see page 1770). Defects around the *PIP joint* I cover with cross-finger flaps; conventional for the palmar surface, reversed for the dorsal.

Table 49-2. Author's Preferred Methods for Specific Situations

	Palmar	Dorsal–Larger Defects
Distal to PIP Joint	Loss more dorsal—*V-Y Advancement* (p. 1760) Loss more palmar—<40—female—*Thenar* (p. 1771) —male—*cross-finger* (p. 1766) —>40—important—*Neurovascular island* (p. 1773) —not important—revise amputation	*Reversed cross-finger* (p. 1770)
PIP Joint	*Cross-finger* (p. 1766)	*Reversed cross-finger* (p. 1770)
Proximal phalanx	Small defect—*Transposition from lateral aspect* (p. 1752) Large defect —Palmar alone—*Cross-finger* (p. 1766) —+Lateral—Index/middle—*Axial flag* (p. 1757) —Ring/small—*Vascular island* (p. 1773)	*Reversed cross-finger* (p. 1770)
MP Joint	Index/middle—*Axial flag* (p. 1757) Ring/small—*Vascular island* (p. 1773)	Index/middle—*Axial flag* (p. 1757) Ring/small—*Vascular island* (p. 1773)
Metacarpus or several fingers syndactylized	Worthless digit—*Fillet* (p. 1779) Small defect—*Vascular island* (p. 1773) —*SDMA* (p. 1778) Large defect—*(Free lateral arm)* —*Forearm fascia* (p. 1782) + skin graft	Worthless digit—*Fillet* (p. 1779) *(Free lateral arm)*
Thumb	Loss more dorsal—*V-Y Advancement* (p. 1760) More palmar—<2/3 pulp—*Moberg* (p. 1760) —>2/3 pulp—(*Neurovascular island* from toe) —*Neurovascular island* (p. 1773) —No donor digit, no micro skills —*FDMA or SDMA* (p. 1778)	*FDMA* from index (p. 1778) *Forearm* (preferably PIA) No donor digit, no vessel —Male—*Infraclavicular* (p. 1795) —Female—*Iliac*

Small defects on the *palmar aspect of the proximal phalanx,* such as are produced in releasing burn contractures, require transposition flaps from the lateral or dorsal aspect of the finger, as described by Green and Dominquez[118] and by Harrison and Morris,[123] respectively. Larger defects that are confined strictly to the palmar surface can be covered with an extended cross-finger flap. For defects that extend onto the lateral aspect to any great extent, I find it difficult to use a conventional cross-finger flap for cover, and I fear problems with kinking of the pedicle. In such circumstances, the axial flag flap (see page 1757) is ideal for defects on the index and middle fingers. However, the vessel of the flag flap is not always reliable in the third and fourth web spaces. I listen for it there with a Doppler. If I cannot hear the vessel, I take a vascular island from the adjacent digit, as described by Rose[275] (see page 1779). For *dorsal defects over the proximal phalanx* I use an axial flag flap in those digits with a demonstrable vessel, for the quality of the skin is identical to that lost. In others, the reversed cross-finger flap is adequate.

Palmar defects around the MP joint, as with palmar-lateral defects of the proximal phalanx, do well with an axial flag flap, taking care to ensure that the injury did not damage the pedicle. Where the vessel cannot be heard, I employ a vascular island. *Dorsal defects* should be treated similarly. Thus, for example, for full-thickness loss over the middle MP joint I might use an axial flag from the proximal phalanx of the index finger; over that of the ring finger a second dorsal metacarpal arterial flap (SDMA) or a vascular island from the small finger might be used.

Injuries over the metacarpus are of course to the palm or dorsum of the hand. Although skin loss from several adjacent digits over the proximal phalanx can usually be covered by multiple local and regional flaps (Fig. 49-49), on occasion this is not possible and they should be considered as one large defect and managed as if at the metacarpus. The defects on the digits are temporarily made one by suturing their adjacent margins, thereby creating a syndactyly, which is later divided. Small *defects in the palm* can be covered with an SDMA or a vascular island. This may be in the form of a fillet flap where a vascularized digit is deemed of no functional value. This solution is also applicable to *dorsal defects,* a situation most commonly encountered in gunshot wounds. For larger defects on either aspect of the metacarpus I use a free lateral arm flap: fasciocutaneous where its subcutaneous layer is not too thick; fascial where it is so. Where microsurgical expertise is not available and the patient is compliant, a cross-arm flap can be used for *palmar defects.* If the defect is more ulnar, the flap can be from the dorsum of the forearm, the lateral aspect of the arm, proximally based, or the medial aspect of the arm, distally based. If it is more radial, the flap can be from the lateral aspect of the arm, distally based, or the medial aspect, proximally based. However, I would rarely use these flaps, for the defect is unsightly and therefore unacceptable to the female, while in the male the flap is often hair-bearing and therefore unsuitable for resurfacing the palm. I would rather adopt a reversed forearm flap (see page 1786), using the fascia alone or an ulnar artery flap in those where the cosmetic defect of a fasciocutaneous flap would be distressing. For *dorsal defects* of the

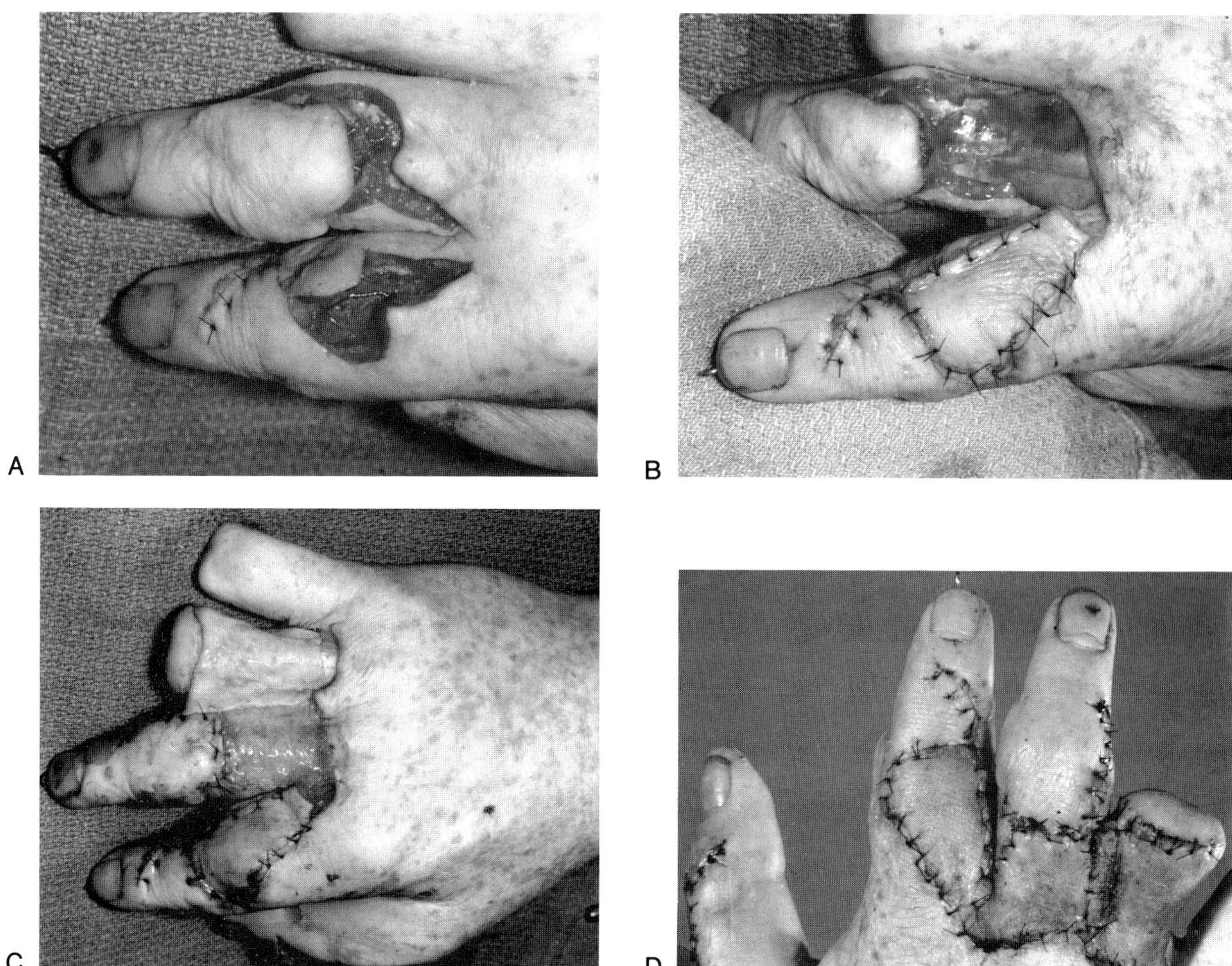

Fig. 49-49. Multiple flaps. **(A)** Defects on the index and middle fingers resulting from the management of multiple nonunions following a fan injury. **(B)** The defect on the index finger has been closed by use of an axial flag flap from the middle finger. **(C)** The resultant defect in the middle finger has been closed using a reversed cross-finger flap from the ring finger. **(D)** The viability of all flaps 1 week later.

metacarpus a forearm flap is similarly appropriate, the reversed posterior interosseous artery flap being preferred to the radial artery flap, provided only that the vessel is present. In the compliant, young patient had I no microsurgical skills the groin flap (page 1803) offers good skin cover (Fig. 49-50), with none of the potential for cosmetic and vascular problems that exist with the forearm flap. In my practice, however, the groin flap is now reserved for those circumstances where I know that I will need the skin of the tube to give additional cover; for example, to a later toe transfer (Fig. 49-51).

For *dorsal defects on the thumb* I would raise a first dorsal metatarsal artery flap (see page 1778) from the dorsal aspect of the proximal phalanx of the index finger. Where that is not available due to the extent of injury, I would use a reversed PIA flap; if no vessel is to be found, a random flap, from the infraclavicular region in the male, and from the iliac crest in the female. Tip amputations in the thumb with more loss dorsally require a V-Y advancement (see page 1760). Those with loss that is more *palmar,* but which is less than two-thirds of the pulp, are ideal for a Moberg advancement or some variant thereof (see page 1760). Where the entire pulp is lost, I replace it with a neurovascular island flap, preferably from the toe, but acceptable from a suitable finger (see page 1773. If no donor digit is available—usually where an island transfer is judged unsuitable for a particular patient—an FDMA or SDMA flap (see page 1778) must be employed.

Circumferential degloving injuries of the thumb require immediate cover with a random-pattern tube pedicle, from the

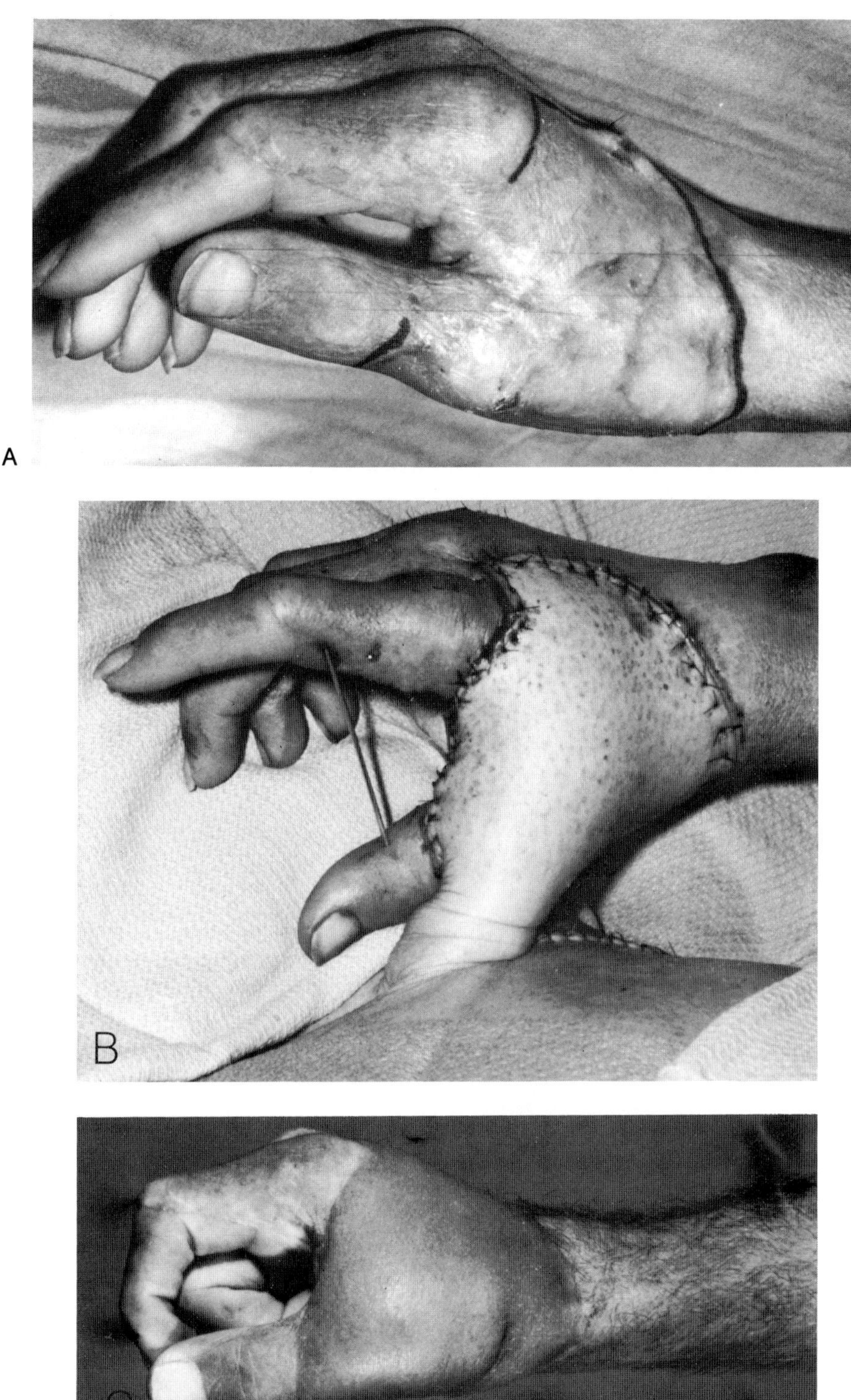

Fig. 49-50. Groin flap. **(A)** A defect on the dorsoradial aspect of the hand. **(B)** A pedicle groin flap in position. Note the kinks in accordion-like fashion at the base of the tube. These kinks are dangerous and must be eliminated in later positioning. **(C)** The result.

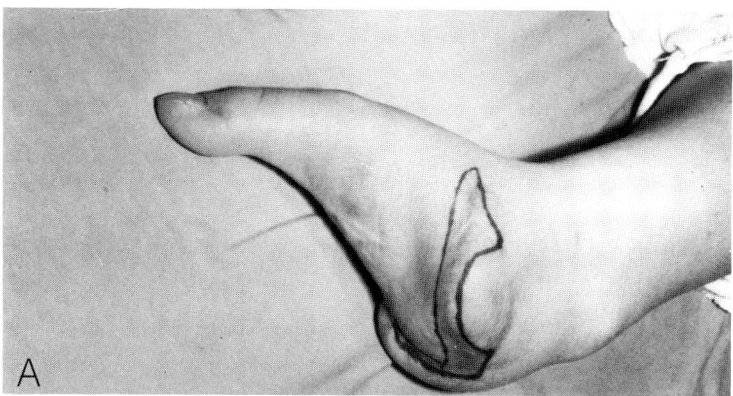

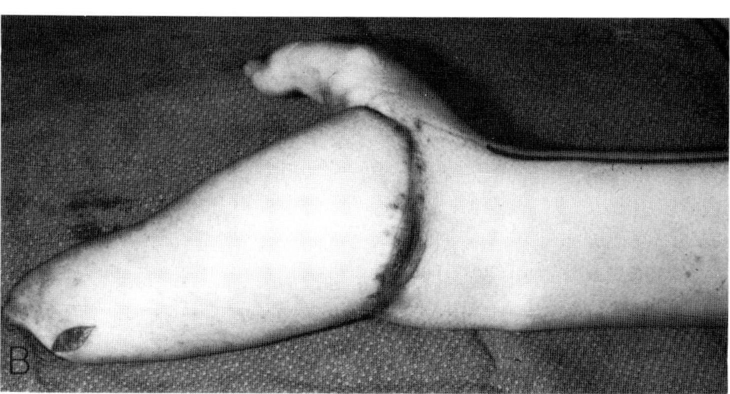

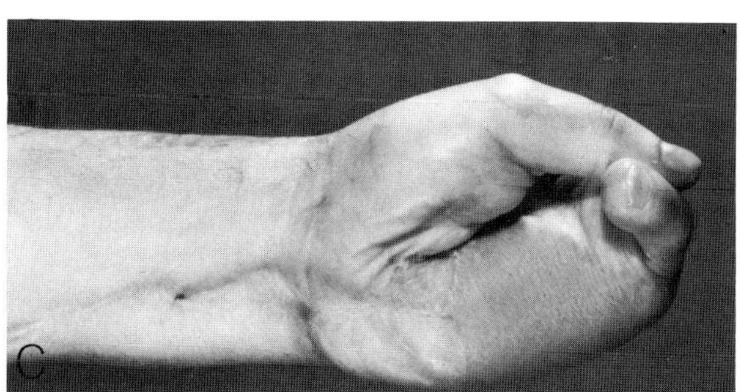

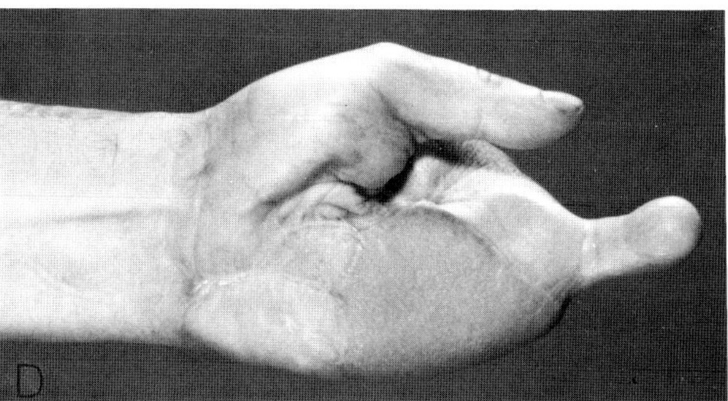

Fig. 49-51. **(A)** Following a bomb explosion, this patient lost all digits from his dominant left hand, together with the metacarpus. **(B)** The metacarpus was replaced with a vascularized iliac crest bone graft in conjunction with a groin flap (see Fig. 48-45). **(C&D)** A long tube pedicle was retained in order to provide all cover necessary for transfer of a toe to the finger position **(C&D)**.

infraclavicular region in the male or from the iliac in the female. The axial portion of the groin flap should not be used, for the resulting tube is invariably too thick to create a good thumb. The exception is where a significant portion of the skeleton of the thumb has been lost also and osteoplastic reconstruction is deemed unsatisfactory. In such circumstances, toe-to-hand transfer or pollicization will both require skin additional to that required simply to cover the primary defect on the thumb. In such circumstances, the pedicle groin flap (see page 1803) is ideal. Degloving of a single finger, in the presence of other normal digits, requires amputation. Where several digits have been degloved, I cover them all with a tube pedicle groin flap. Thereafter, for short stumps I remove the skin of the flap and skin graft the soft tissue over the stumps. In longer fingers, I leave the flap in place and the digits are used as a mitten. These can only be separated if the blood supply is improved. I have done this by transferring a neurovascular island, either from the foot or from the thumb, if an arteriogram shows the presence of two sufficiently long digital vessels in that digit.

For *defects of the wrist, forearm, and elbow,* I prefer free tissue transfers because the patient is not immobilized and because a permanent pedicle is provided to the skin cover. I use the lateral arm flap for small defects, the scapular flap for medium, and the tailored latissimus flap for large. Where these are not indicated or available, the groin flap (page 1803) can reach defects of both dorsal and palmar aspects as far proximally as the midpoint of the forearm. The pedicle latissimus dorsi flap (page 1789) can reach the elbow with ease and the forearm with difficulty. Defects of the proximal one-half of the forearm, where no local flaps suffice, can be covered with a random-pattern abdominal flap (page 1795), or better, with an axial fasciocutaneous flap of the external oblique aponeurosis.[86]

The *first web space* is the remaining specialized region worthy of mention. Contracture here is common, both of congenital and traumatic origin, and the solutions are numerous.[190] I release relatively long yet tight first web contractures, which are composed of normal skin, with a simple 60 degree Z-plasty or by some variant thereof (page 1751). Where the web is shorter and the tight web margin produces a very acute ridge angle, a four-flap Z-plasty (page 1751) works well. In other circumstances, where the skin is scarred or the adduction contracture is severe, skin must be brought in to the web space, by transposition from the dorsum of the thumb (page 1752) or index finger (page 1754), or by rotation from the dorsum of the hand (page 1759). Where these do not suffice or the donor sites are themselves scarred, other skin must be used. It is important that this skin be as thin as possible, for it is pointless to dig a hole that you need—the web space—and promptly fill it with a fat flap. Therefore I favor a reversed forearm flap, preferably the PIA. If distant flaps are used, they must be random so that they can be vigorously thinned; the cross-arm and the iliac are suitable.

The injury that created the primary defect is of significance mainly where its nature makes it difficult or impossible to define the extent of eventual skin loss. One instance of clinical significance is the chemical injury resulting from extravasation of chemotherapeutic agents,[287] of which the most common is doxorubicin hydrochloride (Adriamycin). Identification of the agent in the tissues has been the subject of some debate.[57,61] However, all are agreed that wide excision of all potentially damaged tissues should be undertaken. A period of observation before applying definitive skin cover has been recommended.[183] The cover eventually chosen should be robust and for this reason, free skin transfer is appropriate where available.

POSTOPERATIVE CARE

Postoperative care should be directed at the comfort of both patient and flap, and should be the responsibility of a team of trained, trusted nurses. The comfort of the patient is pursued through the usual channels and should not be neglected due to concern for the flap. It is important that the patient be up and about as soon as possible, preferably starting on the first postoperative day. All joints should be mobilized (see page 1807). Comfort of the flap is achieved mainly by avoiding kinks in its pedicle. This should be ensured by correct positioning of the involved upper limb and of the patient. Once attained, other patient positions that similarly avoid kinking should also be sought. If conscious, the patient should be shown that part of the flap to inspect for kinking and the positions that are acceptable. The earlier he takes charge of his flap, the better. If he is not conscious, the position must be maintained by strapping. Skin-to-skin contact produces maceration and the chance of consequent infection. Therefore, padding should be used to ensure that all skin surfaces are exposed to air. A routine of wound cleansing should be established, using hydrogen peroxide followed by a thin smear of antibiotic ointment. This routine has many benefits. It eliminates a nutritious medium for bacteria. It ensures that color assessment is neither obscured by blood-staining nor impaired by vivid contrast within the observer's visual field. It permits assessment of the rate of bleeding from the wound, in itself a valuable index of venous insufficiency. Finally, it has an inestimable effect on the morale of the patient who can see his wound.

Flap Failure

Flaps fail for a number of reasons, some of which are still debated.[164,295] Therefore, having made the patient and the flap comfortable, the nurse should observe the flap regularly to ensure its continued good health. There are several steps in this process.

1. *Observe the color of the flap.* Difficult to learn and impossible to convey adequately, color assessment yet remains a mainstay of care. The lighting must always be good. The observer can well start by neutralizing his color perception by looking for some 10 seconds at an area of normal skin, similar to the flap. He should then assess the flap. The random and axial pattern flaps differ in their color. A healthy random-pattern flap is pink. If arterial supply is inadequate it will become pale with a faint blue-grey tinge. If venous drainage is occluded, it will be first an angry red and then progressively purple-red and purple-blue. The

axial-pattern flap, especially the groin flap, is pale to a degree that makes the novice nervous. It is not a pure white, as can be detected by comparing it with a sheet of white paper, but rather a very pale pink. Changes in a failing flap are much more rapid and dramatic in the random than in the axial. Within 48 hours the failed portion of a random-pattern flap becomes cyanosed and then blistered, and the margin between the part that will fail and that which will survive is represented by a clear line. The sick axial flap at first assumes a waxy pallor—that is, white tinged with yellow or brown—that differs from its healthy pink pallor by a margin so subtle that only the experienced are pessimistic. The failed margin then becomes indurated and may blister, but doubts concerning the extent of loss persist for as long as a week.

2. *Observe the refill after blanching by fingertip pressure or by running a blunt point across the flap.* If refill after blanching is slow and the flap is pale, arterial insufficiency is the likely cause. Very slow refill may be seen in a flap with no flow whatsoever, being due to the movement of stagnant blood by surrounding tissue pressures. If it is too swift and the flap has a bluish hue, then venous outflow is impaired. This may be due to kinking and should be corrected. Kinking of a flap pedicle is similar to strangulation of bowel. In both cases, the pressure is not high enough initially to occlude the arterial flow, but it impedes the venous drainage. The occluded area therefore becomes engorged and tissue tension rises to a point at which arterial inflow is finally also arrested and the tissue dies in engorgement.[334]
3. *Measure the temperature of the flap.* This may be done with the dorsum of the middle phalanx of the observer, comparing the flap with tissue adjacent both to the pedicle and to the primary defect. A marked difference is a significant index of impaired flow. Where there is little or no difference, it cannot be concluded that the flap is undoubtedly well, for the warmth may be largely or entirely transmitted from the underlying bed.
4. *Stick the flap and adjacent tissue with an 18-gauge needle or a #11 scalpel blade, taking care to go to the same depth, and observe the bleeding.* While this cannot be done repeatedly, it is permissible where the three clinical tests above leave serious doubt. A healthy flap should yield blood of the same color as the control and should bleed just a little longer. If no bleeding occurs or does so only briefly, arterial inflow is inadequate. If the blood is darker and bleeding persists much longer, there is venous congestion. For the same reason, persistent bleeding from the marginal wounds of a flap indicates venous inadequacy.

Many more complex tests of flap viability have been introduced. They fall into three broad categories: *detection of an alteration in local tissue constituents; observation of the presence in the flap of systemically administered agents; monitoring of pulsatile flow within the flap.* In the first category tissue gases have been assessed: Achauer[2,3] showed that if any oxygen was detected transcutaneously a flap would survive; Raskin[263] showed that PO_2[298] was less reliable than pH. Kerrigan and Daniel[165] tested the pH[69] and hematocrit of blood from a stab wound in the flap and found that the former fell by 0.4 and the latter rose by 19 percent in the presence of inadequate circulation and when compared to normal blood. In the second category, injection of fluorescin and evaluation of its presence in the flap with ultraviolet light has been used by many authors[212,237,259,293,295,327] and all report that bright fluorescence indicates eventual survival.[68] Clearance studies of radioactive isotopes have been performed, notably with technetium,[351] xenon, and chromium.[259] In the third category, pulse detection has long been practiced with the Doppler[334] photoplethysmography[150,282] and more recently with the laser Doppler,[84,131,317] the duplex scanner[74] and, for subcutaneous flaps, impedance monitoring.[122] Outside of these three categories, Jones assessed quantitative measurement of the two most popular clinical parameters, color and temperature: he showed that color spectrophotometry was swift and reliable,[149] and that differential thermometry was slow to reveal flap problems.[147] An exhaustive list would be exhausting; it would also be sterile, for very few of the techniques developed experimentally, and of which the above are only a sampling, have become useful clinically. In monitoring axial flaps I routinely use a photoplethysmograph. In assessing replantations, toe transfers, and neurovascular island flaps I use a thermocouple. With the former, I seek to maintain a regular pulse, observed first in the operating room.[282] With the latter, I consider any sudden fall and any temperature below 30°C an indication for action.

Salvage of a Failing Flap

What actions can be taken to salvage a failing flap? A checklist can be given.

1. *Seek out and eliminate any kinks in the pedicle.* Multiple small kinks produce an accordion-like appearance and are equally as harmful as one large obstruction. Flaps do best if they lie on a convex surface and are gently stretched, thereby eliminating all possible occlusion and reducing edema to a minimum. This should be explained to the patient at an early stage so that he may take care of his own flap.
2. *Check the patient's general condition.* Hypotension, cardiopulmonary impairment, or a low circulating volume as revealed by urinary output may all affect oxygenation of the flap. Cold extremities may be due to circumstances as grave as advanced shock or as simple as a low room temperature. Both should be evaluated and corrected.
3. *Look for signs of hematoma and evacuate if found.* Wherever the possibility of hematoma exists, the

surgeon should have inserted a suction drain. Ensure that it is functioning. If none is present, the flap is swollen and discolored, there is persistent serosanguinous oozing from the flap wounds, and edema is revealed by pitting on pressure, then a hematoma is likely. This has been shown to cause loss of a flap, which can be saved by its evacuation.[235] This should be done in the operating room as a formal procedure as soon as the hematoma is detected.
4. *Look for any unduly tight stitches and release.* This should be done only by the operating surgeon for only he knows fully their significance.
5. *Reposition the patient.* Determine in particular if elevation or dependency of the limb improves the flow. If it does, make the patient comfortable in this new position.

There are as many publications in the literature concerning methods of enhancing flap survival as there are of monitoring it—possibly more. They appear to be equally fruitless. Once again they fall into three main categories: *alteration of the environment; physical applications; administration of drugs.* In the first, flap survival has been shown to increase in a moist environment[281] and with the use of local or systemic oxygen.[159] Blood flow has been shown to have a linear relationship to the ambient temperature.[15] Hyperbaric oxygen[352] at both 21 percent and 100 percent concentration has been shown to double the area of flap survival.[321] In the second category, ultrasound and local heat have been shown to be of no benefit.[288] In the third category, many drugs have been tried: streptokinase,[100,115,260] allopurinol and prednisolone,[224,285] chlorpromazine,[6] calcium antagonists,[133,308] free radical scavengers,[5,124,167,221,249,278,317] prostaglandins,[292] antiadrenergics,[156] Ancrod to lower the blood viscosity,[14] topical nitroglycerin,[274,339] ketamine,[160] and isoxuprine[82,356] represent but a small sample. While all have been reported to be beneficial at one time or another, usually in experimental animals, there are also a lesser number of negative reports: nitroglycerin does not work[160]; pentoxifylline does not work[49,96]; chlorpromazine does not work[136] Phenoxybenzamine, isoxuprine and reserpine do not work[166]; isoxuprine, propanolol and heparin do not work.[347] In the end, the surgeon is left with the knowledge that the only way to ensure that a flap will survive is to follow simple rules: assess the primary defect carefully; select the correct flap for that defect and execute it properly; and train nurses who can be trusted to protect and care for the work.

ACKNOWLEDGMENT

I thank Danny Smith, formerly of Louisville and now of Salt Lake City, and Grace von Drasek Ascher, Medical Illustrator of Louisville Hand Surgery, for the hours of work to which the figures in this chapter bear testimony. The copyright to much of the artwork is held by Louisville Hand Surgery, which I thank for permission to publish it here.

REFERENCES

1. Abu Jamra FN, Akel SR, Shamma AR: Repair of major defect of the upper extremity with a latissimus dorsi myocutaneous flap: A case report. Br J Plast Surg 34:121–123, 1981
2. Achauer BM, Black KS: Transcutaneous oxygen and flaps. Plast Reconstr Surg 74:721–722, 1984
3. Achauer BM, Black KS, Litke DK: Transcutaneous PO_2 in flaps: A new method of survival prediction. Plast Reconstr Surg 65:738–745, 1980
4. Adamson JE, Horton CE, Crawford HH: Sensory rehabilitation of the injured thumb. Plast Reconstr Surg 40:53–57, 1967
5. Angel MF, Mellow CG, Knight KR, O'Brien BMcC: The effect of deferoxamine on tolerance to secondary ischaemia caused by venous obstruction. Br J Plast Surg 42:422–424, 1989
6. Angel MF, Schieren G, Jorysz M, Knight KR, O'Brien BMcC: The beneficial effect of chlorpromazine on dorsal skin flap survival. Ann Plast Surg 23:492–497, 1989
7. Argamaso RV: Rotation transposition method for soft tissue replacement on the distal segment of the thumb. Plast Reconstr Surg 54:366–368, 1974
8. Ariyan S: The pectoralis major myocutaneous flap. A versatile flap for reconstruction in the head and neck. Plast Reconstr Surg 63:73–82, 1979
9. Arons MS: Fingertip reconstruction with a palmar advancement flap and free dermal graft: A report of six cases. J Hand Surg 10A:230–232, 1985
10. Atasoy E: The cross thumb to index finger pedicle. J Hand Surg 5:572–574, 1980
11. Atasoy E: Reversed cross-finger subcutaneous flap. J Hand Surg 7:481–483, 1982
12. Atasoy E, Ioakimidis E, Kasdan ML, Kutz JE, Kleinert HE: Reconstruction of the amputated finger tip with a triangular volar flap. A new surgical procedure. J Bone Joint Surg 52A:921–926, 1970
13. Atkins RM, Bell MJ, Sharrard WJW: Pectoralis major transfer for paralysis of elbow flexion in children. J Bone Joint Surg 67B:640–644, 1985
14. Awwad AM, White RJ, Lowe GDO, Forbes CD: The effect of blood viscosity on blood flow in the experimental saphenous flap model. Br J Plast Surg 36:383–386, 1983
15. Awwad AM, White RJ, Webster MHC, Vance JP: The effect of temperature on blood flow in island and free skin flaps: An experimental study. Br J Plast Surg 36:373–382, 1983
16. Bardsley AF, Soutar DS, Elliot D, Batchelor AG: Reducing morbidity in the radial forearm flap donor site. Plast Reconstr Surg 86:287–292; discussion 293–294, 1990
17. Barfred T: The Shaw abdominal flap. Scand J Plast Reconstr Surg 10:56–58, 1976
18. Barron JN: Cock another hat at the thumb. Hand 9:39–41, 1977
19. Bartlett SP, May JW Jr, Yaremchuk MJ: The latissimus dorsi muscle: A fresh cadaver study of the primary neurovascular pedicle. Plast Reconstr Surg 67:631–636, 1981
20. Barton NJ: A modified thenar flap. Hand 7:150–151, 1975
21. Bayon P, Pho RWH: Anatomical basis of dorsal forearm flap. Based on posterior interosseous vessels. J Hand Surg 13B:435–439, 1988
22. Beasley RW: Hand Injuries. WB Saunders, Philadelphia, 1981
23. Beasley RW: Principles of soft tissue replacement for the hand. J Hand Surg 8:781–784, 1983
24. Bennett JE: Grafts and flaps (letter). Plast Reconstr Surg 83:194, 1989
25. Biddulph SL: The neurovascular flap in fingertip injuries. Hand 11:59–63, 1979
26. Biemer E, Stock W: Total thumb reconstruction: A one-stage

reconstruction using an osteo-cutaneous forearm flap. Br J Plast Surg 36:52–55, 1983
27. Bonnel F: New concepts of the arterial vascularization of skin and muscle. Plast Reconstr Surg 75:552–559, 1985
28. Bostwick J III: Latissimus dorsi flap: Current applications. Ann Plast Surg 9:377–380, 1982
29. Boyd JB, Mackinnon SE: An evaluation of the pedicled thoracoumbilical flap in upper extremity reconstruction. Ann Plast Surg 22:236–242, 1989
30. Bralliar F, Horner RL: Sensory cross-finger pedicle graft. J Bone Joint Surg 51:1264–1268, 1969
31. Braun FM, Hoang Ph, Merle M, Van Genechten F, Foucher G: Technique and indications of the forearm flap in hand surgery. A report of thirty-three cases. Ann Chir Main 4:85–97, 1985
32. Brones MF, Wheeler ES, Lesavoy MA: Restoration of elbow flexion and arm contour with the latissimus dorsi myocutaneous flap. Plast Reconstr Surg 69:329–332, 1982
33. Brooks DM, Seddon HJ: Pectoral transplantation for paralysis of the flexors of the elbow. A new technique. J Bone Joint Surg 41B:36–43, 1959
34. Brown JB, Cannon B, Graham WC, Lischer CE, Scarborough CP, Davis WB, Moore AM: Direct flap repair of defects of the arm and hand. Preparation of gunshot wounds for repair of nerves, bones and tendons. Ann Surg 122:706–715, 1945
35. Brown RG, Fleming WH, Jurkiewicz MJ: An island flap of the pectoralis major muscle. Br J Plast Surg 30:161–165, 1977
36. Büchler U, Frey H-P: Retrograde posterior interosseous flap. J Hand Surg 16A:283–292, 1991
37. Budo J, Finucan T, Clarke J: The inner arm fasciocutaneous flap. Plast Reconstr Surg 73:629–632, 1984
38. Bunkis J, Ryu RK, Walton RL, Epstein LI, Vasconez LO: Fasciocutaneous flap coverage for periolecranon defects. Ann Plast Surg 14:361–370, 1985
39. Burstein FD, Salomon JC, Stahl RS: Elbow joint salvage with the transverse rectus island flap: A new application. Plast Reconstr Surg 84:492–497; discussion 498, 1989. Comment in: Plast Reconstr Surg 85:830–831, 1990
40. Button M, Stone EJ: Segmental bony reconstruction of the thumb by composite groin flap: A case report. J Hand Surg 5:488–491, 1980
41. Cannon B, Trott AW: Expeditious use of direct flaps in extremity repairs. Plast Reconstr Surg 4:415–419, 1949
42. Carriquiry CE: Versatile fasciocutaneous flaps based on the medial septocutaneous vessels of the arm. Plast Reconstr Surg 86:103–109, 1990
43. Chase RA: The damaged index digit: A source of components to restore the crippled hand. J Bone Joint Surg 50A:1152–1160, 1968
44. Chase RA: Belaboring a principle. Ann Plast Surg 11:255–260, 1983
45. Chase RA, Hentz VR, Apfelberg D: A dynamic myocutaneous flap for hand reconstruction. J Hand Surg 5:594–599, 1980
46. Chase RA: Historical review of skin and soft tissue coverage of the upper extremity. Hand Clinics 1:599–608, 1985
47. Cherry GW, Austad E, Pasyk K, McClatchey K, Rohrich RJ: Increased survival and vascularity of random-pattern skin flaps elevated in controlled, expanded skin. Plast Reconstr Surg 72:680–685, 1983
48. Cherup LL, Zachary LS, Gottlieb LJ, Petti CA: The radial forearm skin graft-fascial flap. Plast Reconstr Surg 85:898–902, 1990
49. Chu BC, Deshmukh N: The lack of effect of pentoxifylline on random skin flap survival. Plast Reconstr Surg 83:315–318, 1989. Comment in: Plast Reconstr Surg 85:641–643, 1990
50. Chuang DC, Colony LH, Chen HC, Wei FC: Groin flap design and versatility. Plast Reconstr Surg 84:100–107, 1989
51. Clark JM: Reconstruction of biceps brachii by pectoral muscle transplantation. Br J Surg 34:180–182, 1946
52. Clark S, Chase R, Allard T, Jenkins W, Merzenich M: Changes in the somatosensory cortex following peripheral tissue transfers in the hand (abstract). J Hand Surg 11A:768–769, 1986
53. Clodius L, Smith PJ, Bruna J, Serafin D: The lymphatics of the groin flap. Ann Plast Surg 9:447–458, 1982
54. Cohen BE: Local muscle flap coverage of the proximal ulna without functional loss. Plast Reconstr Surg 70:745–748, 1982
55. Cohen BE: Shoulder defect correction with island latissimus dorsi flap. Plast Reconstr Surg 74:650–656, 1984
56. Cohen BE, Cronin ED: An innervated cross-finger flap for fingertip reconstruction. Plast Reconstr Surg 72:688–697, 1983
57. Cohen FJ, Manganaro J, Bezozo RC: Identification of involved tissue during surgical treatment of doxorubicin-induced extravasation necrosis. J Hand Surg 8:43–45, 1983
58. Colson P, Hovot R, Cangolphe M et al: Utilisation des lambeaux degraisses (lambeaux-greffes) en chirurgie reparatrice de la main. Ann Chir Plast 12:298, 1967
59. Costa H, Soutar DS: The distally based island posterior interosseous flap. Br J Plast Surg 41:221–227, 1988
60. Cuono CB: Double Z-plasty repair of large and small rhombic defects: The double-Z rhomboid. Plast Reconstr Surg 71:658–666, 1983
61. Cuono CB: Doxorubicin-induced extravasation necrosis. J Hand Surg 8:497–498, 1983
62. Cuono CB: Double Z-rhombic repair of both large and small defects of the upper extremity. J Hand Surg 9A:197–202, 1984
63. Dellon AL: Evaluation of Sensibility and Re-education of Sensation in the Hand. Williams & Wilkins, Baltimore, 1981
64. Dellon AL: The extended palmar advancement flap. J Hand Surg 8:190–194, 1983
65. Dellon AL: The proximal inset thenar flap for fingertip reconstruction. Plast Reconstr Surg 72:698–702, 1983
66. Dellon AL, Curtis RM, Edgerton MT: Re-education of sensation in the hand after nerve injury and repair. Plast Reconstr Surg 53:297–305, 1974
67. Dellon AL, Mackinnon SE: The pronator quadratus muscle flap. J Hand Surg 9A:423–427, 1984
68. Dibbell DC, Hedberg JR, McGraw JB, Rankin JHC, Souther SG: A quantitative examination of the use of fluorescein in predicting viability of skin flaps. Ann Plast Surg 3:101–105, 1979
69. Dickson MG, Sharpe DT: Continuous subcutaneous tissue pH measurement as a monitor of blood flow in skin flaps: An experimental study. Br J Plast Surg 38:39–42, 1985
70. Dimond M, Barwick W: Treatment of axillary burn scar contracture using an arterialized scapular island flap. Plast Reconstr Surg 72:388–390, 1983
71. Ding Y, Sun G, Lu Y, Ly S: The vascular microanatomy of skin territory of posterior forearm and its clinical application. Ann Plast Surg 22:126–134, 1989
72. Dinner M: Value of angiography prior to use of the latissimus dorsi myocutaneous flap. Plast Reconstr Surg 64:553, 1979
73. Dolich BH, Olshansky KJ, Babar AH: Use of cross-forearm neurocutaneous flap to provide sensation and coverage in hand reconstruction. Plast Reconstr Surg 62:550–558, 1978
74. Dooley TW, Welsh CF, Puckett CL: Noninvasive assessment of microvessels with the duplex scanner. J Hand Surg 14A:670–673, 1989
75. Dos Santos LF: The vascular anatomy and dissection of the free scapular flap. Plast Reconstr Surg 73:599–603, 1984
76. Dowden RV, McCraw JB: Muscle flap reconstruction of shoulder defects. J Hand Surg 5:382–390, 1980
77. Doyle JR, James PM, Larsen LJ, Ashley RK: Restoration of

elbow flexion in arthrogryposis multiplex congenita. J Hand Surg 5:149–152, 1980
78. Drabyn GA, Porterfield HW, Mohler LR, Nappi JF: Ideas and innovations: Wrist-iliac crest fixation for groin flap-thumb immobilization. Plast Reconstr Surg 70:98–99, 1982
79. Earley MJ: The second dorsal metacarpal artery neurovascular island flap. J Hand Surg 14B:434–440, 1989
80. Earley MJ, Milner RH: Dorsal metacarpal flaps. Br J Plast Surg 40:333–341, 1987
81. Esser JSF: Island flaps. NY State Med J 106:264–265, 1917
82. Finseth F: Clinical salvage of three failing skin flaps by treatment with a vasodilator drug. Plast Reconstr Surg 63:304–309, 1979
83. Finseth F, May JW, Smith RJ: Composite groin flap with iliac-bone for primary thumb reconstruction. Case report. J Bone Joint Surg 58A: 130–132, 1976
84. Fischer JC, Parker PM, Shaw WW: Comparison of two laser Doppler flowmeters for the monitoring of dermal blood flow. Microsurgery 4:164–170, 1983
85. Fisher J, Bostwick J, Powell RW: Latissimus dorsi blood supply after thoracodorsal vessel division: The serratus collateral. Plast Reconstr Surg 72:502–509, 1983
86. Fisher J: External oblique fasciocutaneous flap for elbow coverage. Plast Reconstr Surg 75:51–59, 1985
87. Fisher JC, Hurn I, Rudolph R, Utley J, Arganese T: The effect of delay on flap survival in an irradiated field. Plast Reconstr Surg 73:99–102, 1984
88. Flatt AE: The thenar flap. J Bone Joint Surg 39B:80–85, 1957
89. Flatt AE, Wood VE: Multiple dorsal rotation flaps from the hand for thumb web contractures. Plast Reconstr Surg 45:258–262, 1970
90. Flint MH, Harrison SH: A local neurovascular flap to repair loss of the digital pulp. Br J Plast Surg 18:156–163, 1965
91. Foucher G, Braun JB: A new island flap transfer from the dorsum of the index to the thumb. Plast Reconstr Surg 63:344–349, 1979
92. Foucher G, Van Genechten F, Merle N, Michon J: A compound radial artery forearm flap in hand surgery: An original modification of the Chinese forearm flap. Br J Plast Surg 37:139–148, 1984
93. Foucher G, Van Genechten F, Merle M, Michon J: Single stage thumb reconstruction by a composite forearm island flap. J Hand Surg 9B:245–248, 1984
94. Freedlander E, Dickson WA, McGrouther DA: The present role of the groin flap in hand trauma in the light of a long-term review. J Hand Surg 11B:187–190, 1986
95. Freedlander E, Lee K, Vandervord JC: Reconstruction of the axilla with a pectoralis major myocutaneous island flap. Br J Plast Surg 35:144–146, 1982
96. Freedman AM, Hyde GL, Luce EA: Failure of pentoxifylline to enhance skin flap survival in the rat. Ann Plast Surg 23:31–34, 1989
97. Freeman JL, Walker EP, Wilson JSP, Shaw HJ: The vascular anatomy of the pectoralis major myocutaneous flap. Br J Plast Surg 34:3–10, 1981
98. Freiburg A, Manktelow R: The Kutler repair for fingertip amputations. Plast Reconstr Surg 50:371–375, 1972
99. Frey M, Gruber H, Freilinger G: The importance of the correct tension in muscle transplantation: Experimental and clinical aspects. Plast Reconstr Surg 71:510–518, 1983
100. Fudem GM, Walton RL: Microvascular thrombolysis to salvage a free flap using human recombinant tissue plasminogen activator. J Reconstr Microsurg 5:231–234, 1989
101. Furlow LT Jr: V-Y "cup" flap for volar oblique amputation of fingers. J Hand Surg 9B:253–256, 1984
102. Furnas DW: Z-plasties and related procedures for the hand and upper limb. Hand Clinics 1:649–665, 1985
103. Furnas DW, Furnas H: Absence of the lower part of the latissimus dorsi muscle: An important anatomical variation. Ann Plast Surg 10:70–71, 1983
104. Furnas H, Canales F, Buncke GM, Rosen JM: Complications with the use of an axillary roll. Ann Plast Surg 25:208–209, 1990
105. Gainor BJ: Osteocutaneous digital fillet flap: A technical modification. J Hand Surg 10B:79–82, 1985
106. Gatewood: A plastic repair of finger defects without hospitalization. JAMA 87:1479, 1926
107. Gaul JS: Radial innervated cross-finger flap from index to provide sensory pulp to injured thumb. J Bone Joint Surg 51A:1257–1263, 1969
108. Gelberman RH, Blasingame JP: The timed Allen test. J Trauma 21:477–479, 1981
109. Gibraiel EA: A local finger flap to treat post-traumatic flexion contractures of the fingers. Br J Plast Surg 30:134–137, 1977
110. Glasson DW, Lovie MJ: The ulnar island flap in hand and forearm reconstruction. Br J Plast Surg 41:349–353, 1988
111. Godfrey AM, Poole MD, Rowsell AR, Rohrich RJ: Local transposition of a distally-based island forearm flap to close a complicated excisional wrist defect in a nonagenarian: Some anatomical and clinical considerations. Br J Plast Surg 37:493–495, 1984
112. Godina M: Early microsurgical reconstruction of complex trauma of the extremities. Plast Reconstr Surg 78:285–292, 1986
113. Godina M: The tailored latissimus dorsi free flap. Plast Reconstr Surg 80:304–306, 1987
114. Godina M, Bajec J, Baraga A: Salvage of the mutilated upper extremity with temporary ectopic implantation of the undamaged part. Plast Reconstr Surg 78:295–299, 1986
115. Goldberg JA, Pederson WC, Barwick WJ: Salvage of free tissue transfers using thrombolytic agents. J Reconstr Microsurg 5:351–356, 1989
116. Govila A, Sharma D: The radial forearm flap for reconstruction of the upper extremity. Plast Reconstr Surg 86:920–927, 1990
117. Grad JB, Beasley RW: Fingertip reconstruction. Hand Clin 1:667–676, 1985
118. Green DP, Dominguez OJ: A transpositional skin flap for release of volar contractures of a finger at the MP joint. Plast Reconstr Surg 64:516–520, 1979
119. Guimberteau JC, Goin JL, Panconi B, Schuhmacher B: The reverse ulnar artery forearm island flap in hand surgery: 54 cases. Plast Reconstr Surg 81:925–932, 1988
120. Hallock GG: The radial forearm donor site: a locus minoris resistentiae (letter). Plast Reconstr Surg 83:579, 1989
121. Handle N, Winspur I, Hoehn R: Coverage of a shoulder wound with a deltoid muscle flap. Ann Plast Surg 3:277–279, 1979
122. Harrison DH, Mott G: Impedance monitoring for subcutaneous free flap transfers. Br J Plast Surg 42:318–323, 1989
123. Harrison SH, Morris A: Dupuytren's contracture: The dorsal transposition flap. Hand 7:145–149, 1975
124. Hawkes JS, Young CMA, Cleland LG: Ischaemia reperfusion injury in pedicle skin flaps in the pig: lack of protective effect of SOD and allopurinol. Br J Plast Surg 42:668–674, 1989
125. Hayashi A, Maruyama Y: Anatomical study of the recurrent flaps of the upper arm. Br J Plast Surg 43:300–306, 1990
126. Healy C, Mercer NSG, Earley MJ, Woodcock J: Focusable Doppler ultrasound in mapping dorsal hand flaps. Br J Plast Surg 43:296–299, 1990
127. Heath PM, Jackson IT, Cooney WP, Morgan RG: Simultaneous bilateral staged groin flaps for coverage of mutilating injuries of the hand. Ann Plast Surg 11:462–468, 1983
128. Hedén P, Gylbert L: Anomaly of the radial artery encountered during elevation of the radial forearm flap. J Reconstr Microsurg 6:139–141, 1990

129. Henderson HP, Reid DAC: Long term follow-up of neurovascular island flaps. Hand 12:113-122, 1980
130. Hester TR, Nahai F, Beegle PE, Bostwick J: Blood supply of the abdomen revisited, with emphasis on the superficial inferior epigastric artery. Plast Reconstr Surg 74:657-666, 1984
131. Hickerson WL, Colgin SL, Proctor KG: Regional variations of laser Doppler blood flow in ischemic skin flaps. Plast Reconstr Surg 86:319-326; discussion 327-328, 1990
132. Him FP, Casanova R, Vasconez LO: Myocutaneous and fasciocutaneous flaps in the upper limb. Hand Clinics 1:759-768, 1985
133. Hira M, Tajima S, Sano S: Increased survival length of experimental flap by calcium antagonist nifedipine. Ann Plast Surg 24:45-48, 1990
134. Hobar PC, Rohrich RJ, Mickel TJ: The coracobrachialis muscle flap for coverage of exposed axillary vessels: A salvage procedure. Plast Reconstr Surg 85:801-804, 1990
135. Hodgkinson DJ, Shepard GH: Muscle musculocutaneous and fasciocutaneous flaps in forearm reconstruction. Ann Plast Surg 10:400-407, 1983
136. Höft H-D, Oswald P, Tilgner A, Schumann D: Can chlorpromazine prevent flap necrosis? Br J Plast Surg 43:587-589, 1990
137. Holevich J: A new method of restoring sensibility to the thumb. J Bone Joint Surg 45B:496-502, 1963
138. Hosokawa K, Hata Y, Yano K, Matsuka K, Ito O, Ogli K: Results of the Allen test on 2,940 arms. Ann Plast Surg 24:149-151, 1990
139. Hueston J: The extended neurovascular island flap. Br J Plast Surg 18:304-305, 1965
140. Hurwitz PJ: The many-tailed flap for multiple finger injuries. Br J Plast Surg 33:230-232, 1980
141. Idler R, Strickland JW: Management of soft tissue injuries to the fingertip. Orthop Rev 11:25-39, 1982
142. Ikeda A, Ugawa A, Kazihara Y, Hamada N: Arterial patterns in the hand based on a three-dimensional analysis of 220 cadaver hands. J Hand Surg 13A:501-509, 1988
143. Iselin F: The flag flap. Plast Reconstr Surg 52:374-377, 1973
144. Jawad AS, Harrison DH: The island sensate ulnar artery flap for reconstruction around the elbow. Br J Plast Surg 43:695-698, 1990
145. Johnson MK, Cohen MJ: The Hand Atlas. Charles C Thomas, Springfield, IL, 1975
146. Johnson RK, Iverson RE: Cross-finger pedicle flaps in the hand. J Bone Joint Surg 53A:913-919, 1971
147. Jones BM, Dunscombe PB, Greenhalgh RM: Differential thermometry as a monitor of blood flow in skin flaps. Br J Plast Surg 36:83-87, 1983
148. Jones BM, O'Brien CJ: Acute ischaemia of the hand resulting from elevation of a radial forearm flap. Br J Plast Surg 38:396-397, 1985
149. Jones BM, Sanders R, Greenhalgh RM: Monitoring skin flaps by colour measurement. Br J Plast Surg 36:88-94, 1983
150. Jones JW, Glassford EJ, Hillman WCJ: Remote monitoring of free flaps with telephonic transmission of photoplethysmograph waveforms. J Reconstr Microsurg 5:141-144, 1989
151. Joshi BB: One-stage repair for distal amputation of the thumb. Plast Reconstr Surg 45:613-614, 1970
152. Joshi BB: Problem of sensory loss in fingertip injuries in the blind. Br J Plast Surg 23:283, 1970
153. Joshi BB: Dorsolateral flap from the same finger to relieve flexion contracture. Plast Reconstr Surg 49:186-189, 1972
154. Joshi BB: A local dorso lateral island flap for restoration of sensation after avulsion injury of fingertip pulp. Plast Reconstr Surg 54:175-182, 1974
155. Joshi BB: Neural repair for sensory restoration in a groin flap. Hand 9:221-225, 1977
156. Jurell G, Hjemdahl P, Fredholm BB: On the mechanism by which antiadrenergic drugs increase survival of critical skin flap. Plast Reconstr Surg 72:518-523, 1983
157. Kappel DA, Burech JG: The cross-finger flap: An established reconstructive procedure. Hand Clinics 1:677-684, 1985
158. Katai K, Kido M, Numaguchi Y: Angiography of the iliofemoral arteriovenous system supplying free groin flaps and free hypogastric flaps. Plast Reconstr Surg 63:671-679, 1979
159. Kaufman T, Hurwitz DJ: Systemic and local oxygen effects on rat axial pattern flap survival. Chir Plast 7:201-209, 1983
160. Kaufman Th, Angel MF, Levin M, Eichenlaub EH, Futerell JW: The effect of I.M. ketamine HCl and 2% topical nitroglycerine cream on the survival of experimental flaps. Chir Plast 8:45-49, 1984
161. Kawabata H, Kawai H, Masada K, Ono K: Computer-aided analysis of Z-plasties. Plast Reconstr Surg 83:319-325, 1989
162. Kelleher JC, Sullivan JG, Baibak GJ, Robinson JH, Yanik MA: Large combined axial vessel pattern abdominal pedicle flap: Indications for its use in surgery of the hand. Orthop Rev 11:33-48, 1982
163. Kenney JG, Morgan RF, McLaughlin R, Edgerton MT: The "fold-back" flexor ulnaris muscle flap for repair of soft tissue losses about the elbow. Contemp Orthop 7:63-66, 1983
164. Kerrigan CL: Skin flap failure: Pathophysiology. Plast Reconstr Surg 72:766-774, 1983
165. Kerrigan CL, Daniel RK: Monitoring acute skin flap failure. Plast Reconstr Surg 71:519-524, 1983
166. Kerrigan CL, Daniel RK: Pharmacologic treatment of the failing skin flap. Plast Reconstr Surg 70:541-548, 1982
167. Kim YS, Im MJ, Hoopes JE: The effect of a free-radical scavenger, N-2-mercaptopropionylglycine, on the survival of skin flaps. Ann Plast Surg 25:18-20, 1990
168. Kislov R, Kelly AP: Cross-finger flaps in digital injuries, with notes on Kirschner wire fixation. Plast Reconstr Surg 25:312-322, 1960
169. Kleinert HE, McAlister CG, MacDonald CJ, Kutz JE: A critical evaluation of cross-finger flaps. J Trauma 14:756-763, 1974
170. Kojima T, Tsuchida Y, Hirase Y, Endo T: Reverse vascular pedicle digital island flap. Br J Plast Surg 43:290-295, 1990
171. Krag C, Rasmussen B: The neurovascular island flap for defective sensibility of the thumb. J Bone Joint Surg 57B:495-499, 1975
172. Kutler WA: A new method for finger tip amputation. JAMA 133:129, 1947
173. Lai C-S, Lin S-D, Yang C-C: The reverse digital artery flap for fingertip reconstruction. Ann Plast Surg 22:495-500, 1989
174. Lai MF, Krishna BV, Pelly AD: The brachioradialis myocutaneous flap. Br J Plast Surg 34:431-434, 1981
175. Laitung JKG, Peck F: Shoulder function following the loss of the latissimus dorsi muscle. Br J Plast Surg 38:375-379, 1985
176. Lamberty BGH, Cormack GC: The forearm angiotomes. Br J Plast Surg 35:420-429, 1982
177. Landra AP: The latissimus dorsi musculocutaneous flap used to resurface a defect on the upper arm and restore extension to the elbow. Br J Plast Surg 32:275-277, 1979
178. Langer K: On the anatomy and physiology of the skin. III. The elasticity of the cutis. Br J Plast Surg 31:185-199, 1978
179. Lesavoy MA: The dorsal index finger neurovascular island flap. Orthop Rev 9:91-95, 1980
180. Li Z, Liu K, Cao Y: The reverse flow ulnar artery island flap: 42 clinical cases. Br J Plast Surg 42:256-259, 1989
181. Limberg AA: Design of local flaps. In Gibson T (ed): Modern Trends in Plastic Surgery, 2nd Ed. Butterworths, London, 1966

182. Lin SD, Lai CS, Chiu CC: Venous drainage in the reverse forearm flap. Plast Reconstr Surg 74:508–512, 1984
183. Linder RM, Upton J, Osteen R: Management of extensive doxorubicin hydrochloride extravasation injuries. J Hand Surg 8:32–38, 1983
184. Lister G: The choice of procedure following thumb amputation. Clin Orthop 195:45–51, 1985
185. Lister G: Local flaps to the hand. Hand Clin 1:621–640, 1985
186. Lister GD: The theory of the transposition flap and its practical application in the hand. Clin Plast Surg 8:115–128, 1981
187. Lister GD, Gibson T: Closure of rhomboid skin defects: The flaps of Limberg and Dufourmentel. Br J Plast Surg 25:300–314, 1972
188. Lister GD, Kalisman M, Tsai TM: Reconstruction of the hand with free microneurovascular toe-to-hand transfer: Experience with 54 toe transfers. Plast Reconstr Surg 71:372–386, 1983
189. Lister GD, McGregor IA, Jackson IT: Groin flap in hand injuries. Injury (Br J Accident Surg) 4:229–239, 1973
190. Lister GD, Milward TM: Skin contracture of the first web space. Trans Sixth Intl Congress Plast Reconstr Surg 594–604, Paris, 1976
191. Littler JW: Neurovascular skin island transfer in reconstructive hand surgery. Trans Second Intl Congress Soc Plast Surgeons 175–179, 1960
192. Littler JW: On making a thumb: One hundred years of surgical effort. J Hand Surg 1:35–51, 1976
193. Logan AM, Black MJM: Injury to the brachial plexus resulting from shoulder positioning during latissimus dorsi flap pedicle dissection. Br J Plast Surg 38:380–382, 1985
194. Lovie MJ, Duncan GM, Glasson DW: The ulnar artery forearm free flap. Br J Plast Surg 37:486–492, 1984
195. Lubahn JD, Carlier A, Lister GD: The denervated first dorsal interosseous muscle flap. A case report. J Hand Surg 10A:684–686, 1985
196. Lueders HW, Shapiro RL: Rotation finger flaps in reconstruction of burned hands. Plast Reconstr Surg 47:176, 1971
197. Macht SD, Watson HK: The Moberg volar advancement flap for digital reconstruction. J Hand Surg 5:372–376, 1980
198. MacKinnon SE, Weiland AJ, Godina M: Immediate forearm reconstruction with a functional latissimus dorsi island pedicle myocutaneous flap. Plast Reconstr Surg 71:706–710, 1983
199. Mahoney J, Naiberg J: Toe transfer to the vessels of the reversed forearm flap. J Hand Surg 12A:62–65, 1987
200. Markley JM: The preservation of close two-point discrimination in the interdigital transfer of neurovascular island flaps. Plast Reconstr Surg 59:812–816, 1977
201. Markley JM: Island flaps of the hand. Hand Clinics 1:689–700, 1985
202. Marty FM, Montandon D, Gumener R, Zbrodowski A: The use of subcutaneous tissue flaps in the repair of soft tissue defects of the forearm and hand: An experimental and clinical study of a new technique. Br J Plast Surg 37:95–102, 1984
203. Maruyama Y: The reverse dorsal metacarpal flap. Br J Plast Surg 43:24–27, 1990
204. Matev I: The osteocutaneous pedicle forearm flap. J Hand Surg 10B:179–182, 1985
205. Mathes SJ, Nahai F: Muscle flap transposition with function preservation: Technical and clinical considerations. Plast Reconstr Surg 66:242–249, 1980
206. Mathes SJ, Nahai F: Classification of the vascular anatomy of muscles: Experimental and clinical correlation. Plast Reconstr Surg 67:177–187, 1981
207. Mathes SJ, Vasconez LO, Jurkiewicz MJ: Extension and further applications of the muscle flap transposition. Plast Reconstr Surg 60:6–13, 1977
208. Maxwell GP: Iginio Tansini and the origin of the latissimus dorsi musculocutaneous flap. Plast Reconstr Surg 65:686–692, 1980
209. May JW, Bartlett SP: Staged groin flap in reconstruction of the pediatric hand. J Hand Surg 6:163–171, 1981
210. McCash CR: Cross-arm bridge flaps in the repair of flexion contractures of the fingers. Br J Plast Surg 9:25–33, 1956
211. McCraw JB, Dibbell DG, Carraway JH: Clinical definition of independent myocutaneous vascular territories. Plast Reconstr Surg 60:341–352, 1977
212. McCraw JB, Myers B, Shanklin KD: The value of fluorescein in predicting the viability of arterialized flaps. Plast Reconstr Surg 60:710–719, 1977
213. McGrath MH, Adelberg D, Finseth F: The intravenous fluorescein test: Use in timing of groin flap division. J Hand Surg 4:19–22, 1979
214. McGregor IA: Less satisfactory experiences with neurovascular island flaps. Hand 1:21–22, 1969
215. McGregor IA: Flap reconstruction in hand surgery: The evolution of presently used methods. J Hand Surg 4:1–10, 1979
216. McGregor IA: Fundamental Techniques of Plastic Surgery. 7th Ed. Churchill Livingstone, Edinburgh, 1980
217. McGregor IA, Jackson IT: The groin flap. Br J Plast Surg 25:3, 1972
218. McGregor IA, Morgan G: Axial and random pattern flaps. Br J Plast Surg 26:202–213, 1973
219. Meals RA, Brody GS: Gatewood and the first thenar pedicle. Plast Reconstr Surg 73:315–319, 1984
220. Meland NB, Lincenberg SM, Cooney WP III, Wood MB, Hentz VR: Experience with the island radial forearm flap in local hand coverage. J Trauma 29:489–493, 1989
221. Mellow CG, Knight KR, Angel MF, O'Brien BMcC: The effect of thromboxane synthetase inhibition on tolerance of skin flaps to secondary ischemia caused by venous obstruction. Plast Reconstr Surg 86:329–334, 1990
222. Melone CP, Beasley RW, Carstens JH: The thenar flap: An analysis of its use in 150 cases. J Hand Surg 7:291–297, 1982
223. Mendelson BC, Masson JK: Treatment of chronic radiation injury over the shoulder with a latissimus dorsi myocutaneous flap. Plast Reconstr Surg 60:681–691, 1977
224. Mes LGB: Improving flap survival by sustaining cell metabolism within ischemic cells: A study using rabbits. Plast Reconstr Surg 65:56–65, 1980
225. Milward TM, Stott WG, Kleinert HE: The abductor digiti minimi muscle flap. Hand 9:82–85, 1977
226. Miura T: Thumb reconstruction using radial-innervated cross-finger pedicle graft. J Bone Joint Surg 55A:563–569, 1973
227. Miura T: Use of paired abdominal flaps for release of adduction contractures of the thumb. Plast Reconstr Surg 63:242–245, 1979
228. Miura T, Nakamura R: Use of paired flaps to simultaneously cover the dorsal and volar surfaces of a new hand. Plast Reconstr Surg 54:286–289, 1974
229. Moberg E: Aspects of sensation in reconstructive surgery of the upper extremity. J Bone Joint Surg 46A:817–825, 1964
230. Morain WD, Geurkink NA: Split pectoralis major myocutaneous flap. Ann Plast Surg 5:358–361, 1980
231. Moscona AR, Hirshowitz B: Meralgia paresthetica as a complication of the groin flap. Ann Plast Surg 4:161–163, 1980
232. Moss SH, Schwartz KS, Von Drasek-Ascher G, Ogden LL, Wheeler CS, Lister GD: Digital venous anatomy. J Hand Surg 10A:473–482, 1985
233. Mozersky DJ, Buckley CJ, Hagood CO, Capps WF Jr, Dannemiller FJ Jr: Ultrasonic evaluation of the palmar circulation — A useful adjunct to radial artery cannulation. Am J Surg 126:810–812, 1973

234. Muhlbauer W, Herndl E, Stock W: The forearm flap. Plast Reconstr Surg 70:336–342, 1982
235. Mulliken JB, Healey NA: Pathogenesis of skin flap necrosis from an underlying hematoma. Plast Reconstr Surg 63:540–546, 1979
236. Murray JF, Ord JVR, Gavelin GE: The neurovascular island pedicle flap. An assessment of late results in sixteen cases. J Bone Joint Surg 49A:1285–1297, 1967
237. Myers B, Donovan W: An evaluation of eight methods of using fluorescein to predict the viability of skin flaps in the pig. Plast Reconstr Surg 75:245–250, 1985
238. Nahai F, Mathes SJ: Musculocutaneous flap or muscle flap and skin graft? Ann Plast Surg 12:199–203, 1984
239. Nakajima H, Fujino T, Adachi S: A new concept of vascular supply to the skin and classification of skin flaps according to their vascularization. Ann Plast Surg 16:1–17, 1986
240. Nappi JF, Drabyn GA: External fixation for pedicle-flap immobilization: A new method providing limited motion. Plast Reconstr Surg 72:243–245, 1983
241. Nathan PA: Double V-Y flap for correction of proximal interphalangeal joint flexion contractures. J Hand Surg 9A:48–53, 1984
242. Nicolai JPA, Hentenaar G: Sensation in cross-finger flaps. Hand 13:12–16, 1981
243. O'Brien B: Neurovascular island pedicle flaps for terminal amputations and digital scars. Br J Plast Surg 21:258–261, 1968
244. Ogunro O: Dorsal transposition flap for reconstruction of lateral or medial oblique amputations of the thumb with exposure of bone. J Hand Surg 8:894–898, 1983
245. Ohtsuka H, Imagawa S: Reconstruction of a posterior defect of the elbow joint using an extensor carpi radialis longus myocutaneous flap: Case report. Br J Plast Surg 38:238–240, 1985
246. Olivari N: The latissimus flap. Br J Plast Surg 29:126–128, 1976
247. Olivari N: Use of thirty latissimus dorsi flaps. Plast Reconstr Surg 64:654–661, 1979
248. Omer GE, Day DJ, Ratliff H, Lambert P: Neurovascular cutaneous island pedicles for deficient median nerve sensibility. J Bone Joint Surg 52A:1181–1192, 1970
249. Ono I, Ohura T, Murazumi M, Sakamura R, Chiba S: A study on the effectiveness of a thromboxane synthetase inhibitor (OKY-046) in increasing the survival length of skin flaps. Plast Reconstr Surg 86:1164–1173, 1990
250. Peacock EE: Reconstruction of the hand by the local transfer of composite tissue island flaps. Plast Reconstr Surg 25:298–311, 1960
251. Pearl RM, Johnson D: The vascular supply to the skin: An anatomical and physiological reappraisal—Part I. Ann Plast Surg 11:99–105, 1983
252. Pearl RM, Johnson D: The vascular supply to the skin: Anatomical and physiological reappraisal—Part II. Ann Plast Surg 11:196–205, 1983
253. Pearl RM, Arnstein D: A vascular approach to the prevention of infection. Ann Plast Surg 14:443–450, 1985
254. Pederson WC, Eades E, Occhialini A, Schuster J, Demas C: The distally-based radial forearm free flap with valvulotomy of the cephalic vein; a preliminary report. Br J Plast Surg 43:140–144, 1990
255. Penteado CV: Venous drainage of the groin flap. Plast Reconstr Surg 71:678–682, 1983
256. Penteado CV, Masquelat AC, Chevrel JP: The anatomic basis of the fascio-cutaneous flap of the posterior interosseous artery. Surg Radio Anat 8:209–215, 1986
257. Pho RWH: Local composite neurovascular island flap for skin cover in pulp loss of the thumb. J Hand Surg 4:11–15, 1979
258. Posner MA, Smith RJ: Advancement pedicle flap for thumb injuries. J Bone Joint Surg 53A:1618–1621, 1971
259. Prather A, Blackburn JP, Williams TR, Lynn JA: Evaluation of tests for predicting the viability of axial pattern skin flaps in the pig. Plast Reconstr Surg 63:250–258, 1979
260. Puckett CL, Misholy H, Reinisch JF: The effects of streptokinase on ischemic flaps. J Hand Surg 8:101–104, 1983
261. Quaba AA, Davison PM: The distally-based dorsal hand flap. Br J Plast Surg 43:28–39, 1990
262. Rae PS, Pho RWH: The radial transposition flap: A useful composite flap. Hand 15:96–102, 1983
263. Raskin DJ, Nathan R, Erk Y, Spira M: Critical comparison of transcutaneous PO_2 and tissue pH as indices of perfusion. Microsurgery 4:29–33, 1983
264. Reddick LP: Seroma after latissimus dorsi myocutaneous flap for breast reconstruction (letter). Plast Reconstr Surg 85:826, 1990. Commenting upon Slavin SA: Drainage of seromas after latissimus dorsi myocutaneous flap breast reconstruction (letter). Plast Reconstr Surg 83:925–926, 1989
265. Reid CD, Moss ALH: One-stage flap repair with vascularised tendon grafts in a dorsal hand injury using the "Chinese" forearm flap. Br J Plast Surg 36:473–479, 1983
266. Reid DAC, Taylor GI: The vascular territory of the acromiothoracic axis. Br J Plast Surg 37:194–212, 1984
267. Reid DAC: The neurovascular island flap for thumb reconstruction. Br J Plast Surg 19: 234–244, 1966
268. Reid DAC: The Gillies thumb lengthening operation. Hand 12:123–129, 1980
269. Reinisch JF, Winters R, Puckett CL: The use of the osteocutaneous groin flap in gunshot wounds of the hand. J Hand Surg 9A:12–17, 1984
270. Reisman NR, Dellon AL: The abductor digiti minimi muscle flap: A salvage technique for palmar wrist pain. Plast Reconstr Surg 72:859–863, 1983
271. Reyes FA, Burkhalter WE: The fascial radial flap. J Hand Surg 13A:432–437, 1988
272. Rivet D, Boileau R, Saiveau M, Baudet J: Restoration of elbow flexion using the latissimus dorsi musculocutaneous flap. Ann Chir Main 8:110–123, 1989
273. Roggendorf E: The planimetric z-plasty. Plast Reconstr Surg 71:834–842, 1983
274. Rohrich RJ, Cherry GW, Spira M: Enhancement of skin-flap survival using nitroglycerin ointment. Plast Reconstr Surg 73:943–948, 1984
275. Rose EH: Local arterialized island flap coverage of difficult hand defects preserving donor digit sensibility. Plast Reconstr Surg 72:848–857, 1983
276. Roth JH, Urbaniak JR, Boswick JM: Comparison of suture ligation, bipolar cauterization, and hemoclip ligation in the management of small branching vessels in a rat model. J Reconstr Microsurg 1:7–9, 1984
277. Rubinstein ZJ, Shafir R, Tsur H: The value of angiography prior to the use of the latissimus dorsi myocutaneous flap. Plast Reconstr Surg 63:374–377, 1979
278. Sagi A, Ferder M, Yu H-L, Gordon MJV, Strauch B: pH balanced solutions with superoxide dismutase (SOD): An attempt to increase island groin flap survival in rats. Ann Plast Surg 24:521–523, 1990
279. Sakai S, Soeda S, Endo T, Shojima M: Distally based ulnar artery island forearm flap for the large defect of the ulnar side of the hand. Ann Plast Surg 23:266–268, 1989
280. Sandzen SC: Dorsal pedicle flap for resurfacing a moderate thumb-index web contracture release. J Hand Surg 7:21–24, 1982

281. Sasaki A, Fukuda O, Soeda S: Attempts to increase the surviving length in skin flaps by a moist environment. Plast Reconstr Surg 64:526–531, 1979
282. Scheker LR, Slattery PG, Firrell JC, Lister GD: The value of the photoplethysmograph in monitoring skin closure in microsurgery. J Reconstr Microsurgery, 2:1–4, 1985
283. Schlenker JD: Transfer of a neurovascular island pedicle flap based upon the metacarpal artery: A case report. J Hand Surg 4:16–19, 1979
284. Schlenker JD, Atasoy E, Lyon JW: The abdominohypogastric flap—An axial pattern flap for forearm coverage. Hand 12:248–252, 1980
285. Schmidt JH, Caffee HH: The efficacy of methylprednisolone in reducing flap edema. Plast Reconstr Surg 86:1148–1151, 1990
286. Schottstaedt ER, Larsen LJ, Bost FC: Complete muscle transposition. J Bone Joint Surg 37A:897–919, 1955
287. Seyfer AE, Solimando DA: Toxic lesions of the hand associated with chemotherapy. J Hand Surg 8:39–42, 1983
288. Shamberger RC, Talbot TL, Tipton HW, Thibault LE, Brennan MF: The effect of ultrasonic and thermal treatment on wounds. Plast Reconstr Surg 68:860–870, 1981
289. Shaw DT, Li CS, Richey DG, Nahigian SH: Interdigital butterfly flap in the hand (the double-opposing Z-plasty). J Bone Joint Surg 55A:1677–1679, 1973
290. Shaw DT, Payne RL: One-stage tubed abdominal flaps. Surg Gynecol Obstet 83:205, 1946
291. Shepard GH: The use of lateral V-Y advancement flaps for fingertip reconstruction. J Hand Surg 8:254–259, 1983
292. Silverman DG, Brousseau DA, Norton KJ, Clark N, Weinberg H: The effects of a topical PGE_2 analogue on global flap ischemia in rats. Plast Reconstr Surg 84:794–799, 1989
293. Silverman DG, LaRossa D: Fluorescein and flap viability (letter). Plast Reconstr Surg 73:326, 1984
294. Silverton JS, Nahai F, Jurkiewicz MJ: The latissimus dorsi myocutaneous flap to replace a defect of the upper arm. Br J Plast Surg 31:29–31, 1978
295. Sloan GM, Reinisch JF: Flap physiology and the prediction of flap viability. Hand Clinics 1:609–620, 1985
296. Small JO, Brennen MD: The second dorsal metacarpal artery neurovascular island flap. Br J Plast Surg 43:17–23, 1990
297. Smith AR, Sonneveld GJ, Kort WJ, van der Meulen JC: Clinical application of transcutaneous oxygen measurements in replantation surgery and free tissue transfer. J Hand Surg 8:139–145, 1983
298. Smith PJ: The importance of venous drainage in axial pattern flaps. Br J Plast Surg 31:233–237, 1978
299. Smith PJ: A sliding flap to cover dorsal skin defects over the proximal interphalangeal joint. Hand 14:271–278, 1982
300. Smith PJ: The Y-shaped hypogastric-groin flap. Hand 14:263–270, 1982
301. Smith PJ, Foley B, McGregor IA, Jackson IT: The anatomical basis of the groin flap. Plast Reconstr Surg 49:41–47, 1972
302. Smith PJ, Harrison SH: The "seagull" flap for syndactyly. Br J Plast Surg 35:390–393, 1982
303. Snow JW: Use of a volar flap for repair of fingertip amputations. A primary report. Plast Reconstr Surg 40:163–168, 1967
304. Song R, Gao Y, Song Y, Yu Y, Song Y: The forearm flap. Clin Plast Surg 9:21, 1982
305. Soutar DS, Tanner NSB: The radial forearm flap in the management of soft tissue injuries of the hand. Br J Plast Surg 37:18–26, 1984
306. Spinner M: Fashioned transpositional flap for soft tissue adduction contracture of the thumb. Plast Reconstr Surg 44:345–348, 1969
307. Stark GB, Dorer A, Jaeger K, Narayanan K: The influence of the calcium channel blocker nimodipine on flap survival. Ann Plast Surg 23:306–309, 1989
308. Stell PM: The effects of varying degrees of tension on the viability of skin flaps in pigs. Br J Plast Surg 33:371–376, 1980
309. Stern PJ, Amin AK, Neale HW: Early joint and tendon reconstruction for a degloving injury to the dorsum of the hand. Plast Reconstr Surg 72:391–394, 1983
310. Stern PJ, Lister GD: Pollicization after traumatic amputation of the thumb. Clin Orthop 155:85–94, 1981
311. Stern PJ, Neale HW, Gregory RO, Kreilein JG: Latissimus dorsi musculocutaneous flap for elbow flexion. J Hand Surg 7:25–30, 1982
312. Stevenson TR, Hester TR, Duus EC, Dingman RO: The superficial inferior epigastric artery flap for coverage of hand and forearm defects. Ann Plast Surg 12:333–339, 1984
313. Stevenson TR, Rohrich RJ, Pollock RA, Dingman RO, Bostwick J: More experience with the "reverse" latissimus dorsi musculocutaneous flap: Precise location of blood supply. Plast Reconstr Surg 74:237–243, 1984
314. Stranc MF, Labandter H, Roy A: Review of 196 tube pedicles. Br J Plast Surg 28:54–58, 1975
315. Strauch B: Dorsal thumb flap for release of adduction contracture of the first web space. Bull Hosp Joint Dis 36:34–39, 1975
316. Suzuki S, Miyachi Y, Niwa Y, Isshiki N: Significance of reactive oxygen species in distal flap necrosis and its salvage with liposomal SOD. Br J Plast Surg 42:559–564, 1989
317. Svensson H, Svedman P, Holmberg J, Jacobsson S: Detecting arterial and venous obstruction in flaps. Ann Plast Surg 14:20–23, 1985
318. Swanson E, Boyd JB, Manktelow RT: The radial forearm flap: Reconstructive applications and donor-site defects in 35 consecutive patients. Plast Reconstr Surg 85:258–266, 1990
319. Swanson E, Boyd JB, Mulholland RS: The radial forearm flap: A biomechanical study of the osteotomized radius. Plast Reconstr Surg 85:267–272, 1990
320. Takami H, Takahashi S, Ando M: Latissimus dorsi transplantation to restore elbow flexion to the paralysed limb. J Hand Surg 9B:61–63, 1984
321. Tan CM, Im MJ, Myers RAM, Hoopes JE: Effects of hyperbaric oxygen and hyperbaric air on the survival of island skin flaps. Plast Reconstr Surg 73:27–28, 1984
322. Tansini I: Sopra il mio nuovo processo di amputazione della mamella. Riforma Medica 12:757, 1906; Gas Med Ital 57:141, 1906
323. Taylor GI: Blood supply of the abdomen revisited, with emphasis on the superficial inferior epigastric artery: Discussion. Plast Reconstr Surg 74:667–670, 1984
324. Taylor GI, Caddy CM, Watterson PA, Crock JG: The venous territories (venosomes) of the human body: Experimental study and clinical implications. Plast Reconstr Surg 86:185–213, 1990
325. Taylor GI, Doyle M, McCarten G: The Doppler probe for planning flaps: Anatomical study and clinical applications. Br J Plast Surg 43:1–16, 1990
326. Thomson JG, Kerrigan CL: Dermofluorometry: Thresholds for predicting flap survival. Plast Reconstr Surg 83:859–864; discussion 865, 1989
327. Timmons MJ: Landmarks in the anatomical study of the blood supply of the skin. Br J Plast Surg 38:197–207, 1985
328. Tobin GR, Moberg AW, DuBou RH, Weiner LJ, Bland KI: The split latissimus dorsi myocutaneous flap. Ann Plast Surg 7:272–280, 1981
329. Tobin GR, Schusterman M, Peterson GH, Nichols G, Bland KI: The intramuscular neurovascular anatomy of the latissimus

dorsi muscle: The basis for splitting the flap. Plast Reconstr Surg 67:637–641, 1981
330. Tranquilli-Leali E: Ricostruzione dell'apice delle falangi ungueali mediante autoplastica volare peduncolata per scorrimento. Infort Traum Lavoro 1:186–193, 1935
331. Tsai T, Kalisman M, Burns J, Kleinert HE: Restoration of elbow flexion by pectoralis major and pectoralis minor transfer. J Hand Surg 8:186–190, 1983
332. Tsuchida Y, Tsuya A, Uchida M, Kamata S: The delay phenomenon in types of deltopectoral flap studied by xenon-133. Plast Reconstr Surg 67:34–41, 1981
333. Tsuzuki K, Yanai A, Bandoh Y: A contrivance for monitoring skin flaps with a Doppler flowmeter. J Reconstr Microsurg 6:363–366, 1990
334. Tsuzuki K, Yanai A, Tange I, Bandoh Y: The influence of congestion and ischemia on survival of an experimental vascular pedicle island flap. Plast Reconstr Surg 84:789–793, 1989
335. Tubiana R, DuParc J: Restoration of sensibility in the hand by neurovascular skin island transfer. J Bone Joint Surg 43B:474–480, 1961
336. Venkatasawami R, Subramanian N: Oblique triangular flap: A new method of repair for oblique amputations of the fingertip and thumb. Plast Reconstr Surg 66:296–300, 1980
337. Verdan C: The reconstruction of the thumb. Surg Clin North Am 48:1033–1061, 1968
338. Vilain R, Dupuis JF: Use of the flag flap for coverage of a small area on a finger or the palm. 20 years experience. Plast Reconstr Surg 51:397–401, 1973
339. Waters LM, Pearl RM, Macaulay RM: A comparative analysis of the ability of five classes of pharmacological agents to augment skin flap survival in various models and species: An attempt to standardize skin flap research. Ann Plast Surg 23:117–122, 1989
340. Watson ACH, McGregor JC: The simultaneous use of a groin flap and a tensor fasciae latae myocutaneous flap to provide tissue cover for a completely degloved hand. Br J Plast Surg 34:349–352, 1981
341. Weston PAM, Wallace WA: The use of locally based triangular skin flaps for the repair of finger tip injuries. Hand 8:54–58, 1976
342. Winspur I: Distant flaps. Hand Clinics 1:729–740, 1985
343. Winspur I: Single-stage reconstruction of the subtotally amputated thumb: A synchronous neurovascular flap and Z-plasty. J Hand Surg 6:70–72, 1981
344. Wintsch K: Transport von fingerteilen mittels. Bauchhautlappen zur finger—und danmenanfbauplastik. Handchirurgie 13:56–61, 1981
345. Wood J: Extreme deformity of the neck and forearm. Med Chir Trans 46:151, 1863
346. Wray RC, Wise DM, Young VL, Weeks PM: The groin flap in severe hand injuries. Ann Plast Surg 9:459–462, 1982
347. Wray RC, Young VL: Drug treatment and flap survival. Plast Reconstr Surg 73:939–942, 1984
348. Yang G et al: Forearm free skin flap transplantation. Natl Med J China 61:139, 1981
349. Yeschua R, Wexler MR, Neuman Z: Cross-arm triangular flaps for correction of adduction contracture of the first web space in the hand. Case report. Plast Reconstr Surg 59:859–861, 1977
350. Young CMA, Hopewell JW: The isotope clearance technique for measuring skin blood flow. Br J Plast Surg 36:222–230, 1983
351. Zamboni WA, Roth AC, Russell RC, Nemiroff PM, Casas L, Smoot EC: The effect of acute hyperbaric oxygen therapy on axial pattern skin flap survival when administered during and after total ischemia. J Reconstr Microsurg 5:343–347; discussion 349–350, 1989
352. Zancolli EA, Angrigianni C: Colgajo dorsal de antebrazo (en "isla" con pedianco de vasos interoseos postemomes). Rev Asoc Arg Ortop Traumatos 51:161–168, 1986
353. Zancolli EA, Angrigiani C: Posterior interosseous island forearm flap. J Hand Surg 13B:130–135, 1988
354. Zancolli E, Mitre H: Latissimus dorsi transfer to restore elbow flexion. J Bone Joint Surg 55A: 1265–1275, 1973
355. Zide B, Buncke HJ, Finseth F: A study of the treatment time necessary for the vasodilator drug isoxuprine to prevent necrosis in a skin flap. Br J Plast Surg 33:383–387, 1980

50

Flexor Tendons—Acute Injuries

Joseph P. Leddy

Flexor tendon injuries are common. The exact incidence is unknown. Prolonged disability following such an injury can cause physical and emotional suffering and socioeconomic disaster for the patient. The initial treatment is of the utmost importance, because it often determines the final outcome. Flexor tendon injuries present difficult problems, even for the experienced hand surgeon who, unfortunately, is not always involved in the primary care. Surgical repair of flexor tendon injuries requires an exact knowledge of the pertinent anatomy, careful adherence to some basic surgical principles, sound clinical judgment, strict atraumatic surgical technique, and a well-planned postoperative program.

There is now general agreement among hand surgeons regarding the treatment of most flexor tendon injuries. Tendon lacerations in Bunnell's "no-man's land," or Zone II, at one time caused a major controversy. Should primary or delayed primary repair be done, or should the wound be debrided and closed and the patient referred for a flexor tendon graft at a later date? Virtually all would now agree that primary or delayed primary repair is the treatment of choice when possible. Should both tendons be repaired or just the flexor digitorum profundus? Should the sheath be excised or repaired? What types of sutures should be utilized? Is early controlled postoperative motion beneficial and if so, which type is the best? The list of questions and controversies goes on and on. Prominent surgeons in the field seem to have diametrically opposite views, making it difficult for the practitioner or resident in hand surgery to form an opinion by reading the literature. Many of these questions cannot yet be answered on a statistical basis, and more information is necessary. As Boyes advised, we should follow the example of the clinical surgeons at the turn of the century by "making accurate observations, recording our findings and our results carefully and in detail, and arriving at our conclusions honestly and logically."[36] We need to know more about the exact nature of tendon healing. We must find a way to control the inevitable scar formation that interferes with the beautiful gliding mechanism within the flexor tendon system. Much basic research is being directed to these problems, and the knowledge derived from this work will, in the future, help us to restore function to the damaged hand.

There is yet no internationally accepted system of assessing results after flexor tendon repair. The most commonly used systems in this country are those devised by the American Society for Surgery of the Hand[143] and by Strickland.[268] So and associates studied five different methods and concluded that the Buck-Gramcko system was the most comprehensive but had many drawbacks.[258] It is critically important to establish a universal system to assess these results so that meaningful progress can be made.

ANATOMY

For ease in the classification and discussion of flexor tendon injuries, a modification of Verdan's zone system[284,285] is used in this chapter (Fig. 50-1).

The flexor tendons begin in the distal third of the forearm at the musculotendinous junctions. The independent superficialis tendons lie palmar to the conjoined profundus tendon group[282] in this location, covered by loose subcutaneous tissue and skin. This is Zone V. Just proximal to the deep transverse carpal ligament, the flexor pollicis longus tendon enters its continuous sheath, which becomes the radial bursa. The superficialis and profundus tendons also enter a large sheath that terminates just distal to the deep transverse carpal ligament for the index, middle, and ring finger flexor tendons but is continuous for the flexor tendons of the little finger. This portion of

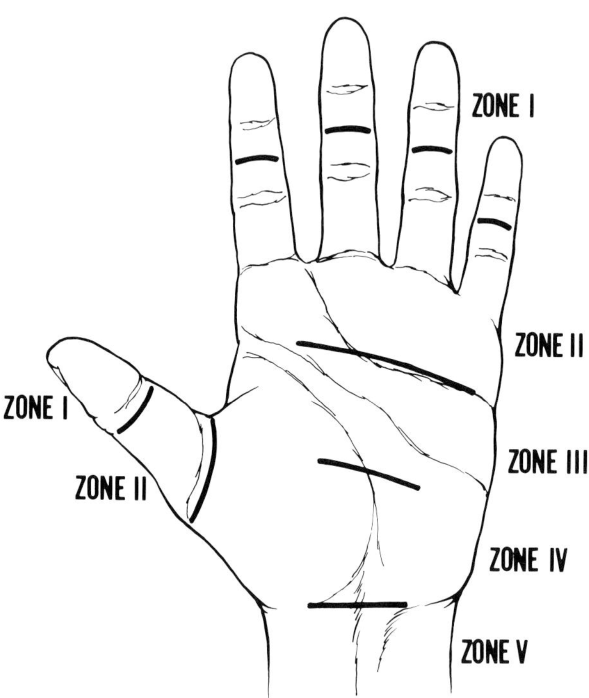

Fig. 50-1. Zone classification of flexor tendon injuries.

the sheath becomes the ulnar bursa (Fig. 50-2). There are multiple anatomic variations of this norm.[101,128,239,287]

Proceeding distally, nine flexor tendons and the median nerve then pass through the tight carpal canal, surrounded on three sides by bone and on top by the tough, unyielding, deep transverse carpal ligament. The superficialis tendons again lie palmar to the deep flexors. This is Zone IV.

The lumbrical muscles originate from the flexor digitorum profundus tendons in the palm distal to the carpal canal[214]; this area up to the level of the fibroosseous tunnel is known as Zone III.

The flexor synovial sheath for the index, middle, and ring fingers begins at the level of the neck of the metacarpal or, according to Kaplan,[128] 10 mm proximal to the proximal border of the deep transverse metacarpal ligament. The sheath for each finger is a double-walled hollow tube sealed at both ends,[70,121] and consisting of a visceral and a parietal layer, which provide low friction gliding and bathe the tendons with synovial fluid for nutritional purposes.[67,68,185] The retinacular portion of the flexor tendon sheath overlies these synovial layers and consists of five annular (A) pulleys and three cruciform (C) pulleys. There is also a palmar aponeurosis pulley.[67-69,187] The annular and cruciform pulleys are thickened areas within the flexor sheath (Fig. 50-3). The very thick annular pulleys prevent tendon bowstringing during finger flexion while the thinner cruciate pulleys give the sheath the ability to conform to the position of flexion by allowing the annular pulleys to approximate each other.[67,68,70,116,117,122,154] The A2

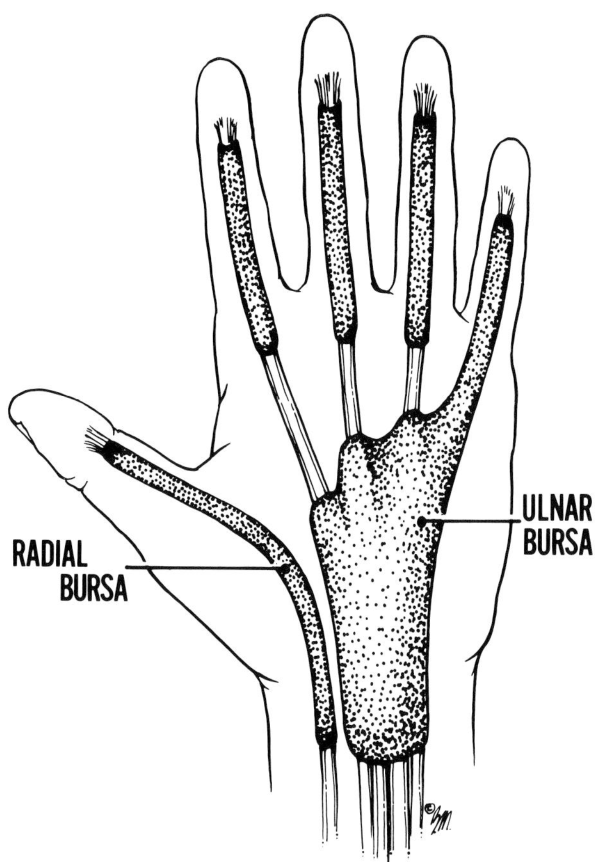

Fig. 50-2. Normal anatomic configuration of synovial sheaths.

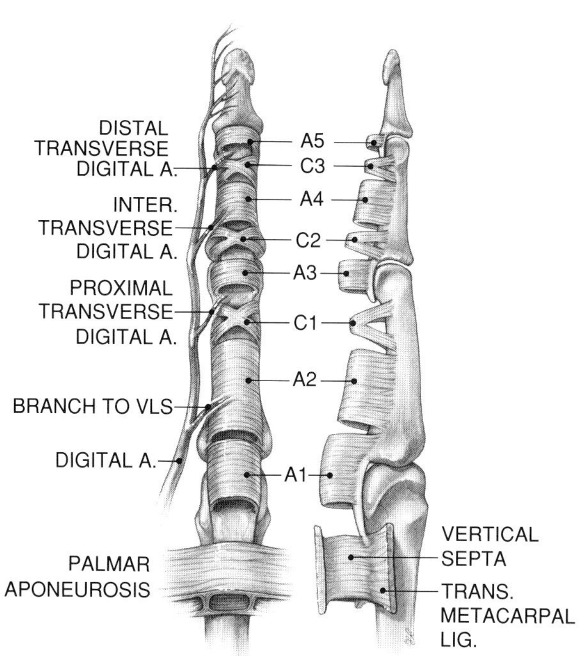

Fig. 50-3. The fibrous retinacular sheath starts at the neck of the metacarpal and ends at the distal phalanx. It can be divided into five heavier annular bands and three filmy cruciform ligaments. Note the palmar aponeurosis pulley proximal to A1.

and A4 pulleys are the most important, both clinically and experimentally, and should be preserved or reconstructed for optimal digital function.[35,45,62,70,137,154,162] The palmar aponeurosis pulley is composed of the transverse fibers of the palmar fascia, which are attached by vertical septa to the deep transverse metacarpal ligament.[67-69] These transverse fibers lie directly over the flexor tendons and thus form a pulley that definitely improves finger flexion in the absence of an A1 and/or A2 pulley.[187] This palmar aponeurosis pulley should be preserved if at all possible during flexor tendon surgery.

The flexor synovial sheath of the thumb starts proximal to the carpal canal and is also a double-walled hollow tube sealed at both ends.[71] There is a visceral and a parietal layer. The retinacular portion of the sheath consists of three constant pulleys on top of the sheath and closely applied to it (Fig. 50-4). In the thumb, the A1 and oblique pulleys are the most important. The reader is referred to excellent works in the literature for the length, width, thickness, and other details of the pulley system in the fingers and thumb.[15,16,70,71,116-118,121,122,154,262]

The flexor tendons enter the synovial sheaths starting at the level of the distal palmar crease. From this point to the insertion of the superficialis tendon into the midportion of the middle phalanx is Bunnell's "no-man's land," or Zone II. Both flexor tendons pass through a tight fibroosseous tunnel in this region, lubricated by a thin layer of synovial fluid. The floor of the tunnel is formed by the periosteum of the underlying bones and by the palmar plates of the MP and PIP joints. Distal to the MP joint, overlying the proximal phalanx, Camper's chiasma tendinum digitorum manus is formed,[128] which allows the profundus tendon to pass through the superficialis on the way to its insertion in the distal phalanx. The superficialis tendon, palmar to the profundus, splits into two slips that roll around the sides of the profundus and join dorsal to this tendon, separating it from the proximal phalanx and palmar plate of the PIP joint. Proceeding distally, the superficialis tendon bifurcates again and reaches its insertion along the midportion of the middle phalanx.[101,128,287] Distal to this level is Zone I. Here, the profundus tendon lies in its synovial sheath beneath the A4, C3, and A5 pulleys as it proceeds to its broad, fan-shaped insertion into the distal phalanx.

There is no general agreement regarding the zones of the thumb. There is a tight fibroosseous tunnel here, but only one tendon, the flexor pollicis longus, passes through it, making comparison with the fingers difficult. For this chapter, I will designate the area between the proximal end of the A1 pulley and the distal portion of the oblique pulley as Zone II (see Fig. 50-4). Distal to this is Zone I, and the proximal zones will correspond to the zones of the finger flexor tendons, although it is recognized that the flexor pollicis longus has its own continuous sheath in Zones III and IV, and there is no lumbrical muscle arising from it.

Tendon Nutrition

Many elaborate studies have outlined the vascular anatomy of the flexor tendons,[9,10,15,41,52,56,63,73,74,109,116,152,171,174,203,213,215,253,257,300] and not all authors are in agreement. From their origin in the distal forearm all the way into the palm, the flexor tendons receive their blood supply from segmental vessels arising from the paratenon. These vessels enter the tendons and travel longitudinally, located between the fascicles. It is now generally agreed that these blood vessels supply the nutritional needs of the flexor tendons in this area.

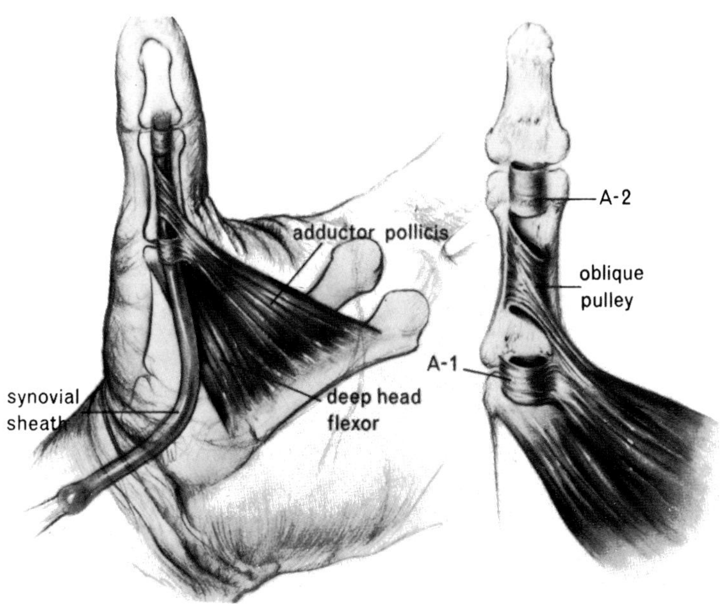

Fig. 50-4. The thumb flexor synovial sheath is a double-walled, hollow tube sealed at both ends. The sheath begins 2.0 cm proximal to the radial styloid and ends just distal to the interphalangeal joint. On top of the sheath and closely applied to it are three constant pulleys—two annular and one oblique. The first annular, located at the MP joint, is 7 to 9 mm wide and 0.5 mm thick. The oblique pulley courses from ulnar-proximal to radial-distal and is 9 to 11 mm wide at its middle aspect. The second annular pulley is near the site of insertion of the flexor pollicis longus and is 8 to 10 mm wide but quite thin. (From Doyle and Blythe,[71] with permission.)

Although the existence of a blood supply to the flexor tendons within the sheath is certain, its relative importance in the nutritional supply and healing process of these tendons is still being investigated. According to Ochiai and co-workers,[213] the crossover zone between the longitudinally arranged intrinsic system and the vincular system in the digital sheath occurs at the level of the midproximal phalanx. The vincula are folds of mesotenon carrying blood supply to both tendons. Although there are many variations, normally there is a short and a long vinculum for each of the superficialis and profundus tendons. This vincular system exists on the dorsal surface of the tendons and is supplied by transverse communicating branches of the common digital artery (Fig. 50-5). Since most of the intratendinous vessels in the digital sheath are in the dorsal portion of the tendons, some authors[52] recommend placing sutures in the palmar half of the tendons during repair so as not to disturb these vessels.

Some investigators, noting the tenuous blood supply to the tendons within the sheath, postulated that the tendons were nourished not only by vascular perfusion, but also by diffusion from the synovial fluid. According to Manske,[181,190] this controversy began at the turn of the century and still remains unsettled. Potenza,[227] in 1963, postulated that flexor tendons in their sheath could get "all or most of their nutritional requirements" by diffusion from the synovial fluid. McDowell and Snyder[206] suggested that synovial fluid is formed by a vascular loop system and diffused through canaliculi in the tendon by repetitive loading and unloading forces. Manske and co-workers[181-183,185,186,188-192,221,222] have done much to help our understanding of the relative importance of diffusion from the synovial fluid to the flexor tendons. They used tracer materials to compare the role of vascular perfusion and synovial diffusion in supplying the nutritional needs of the flexor tendons within the sheath. They concluded, through their experiments, that there is a dual source of nutrients, but that diffusion is a more effective pathway than perfusion. Other authors have confirmed this.[172,173] They also found that diffusion could adequately nourish a tendon that had been stripped of its vascular connections. Their perfusion studies showed that the dorsal half of the tendon was better perfused than the palmar half. They confirmed the findings of previous investigators, showing that the longitudinal vessels from the palm supplied the proximal portion of the tendon in the sheath, while the vincular system supplied the remainder.

In summary then, the flexor tendons in the distal forearm and palm receive their nutritional supply via vascular perfusion from longitudinally oriented vessels from the surrounding paratenon. Flexor tendons within the digital sheath have a dual source of nutritional supply, which is vascular perfusion via the vincular system and diffusion of nutrients from the synovial fluid. Most studies indicate that diffusion is more important than perfusion within the digital sheath.

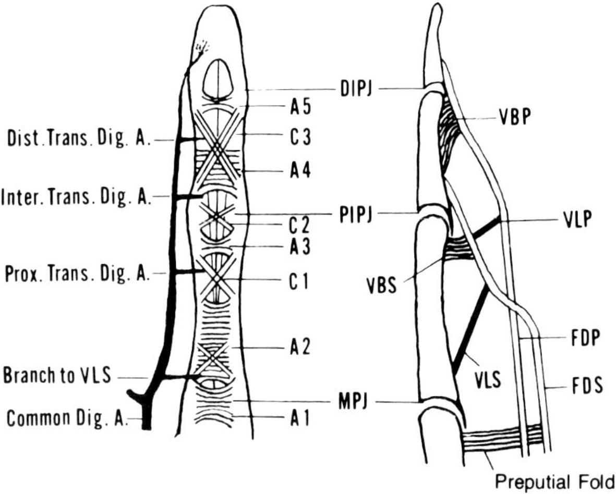

Fig. 50-5. A diagrammatic representation of the fibrous pulley system, the vincular system, and the four transverse communicating branches of the common digital artery. (*Dist. Trans. Dig. A.*, distal transverse digital artery; *Inter Trans. Dig. A.*, interphalangeal transverse digital artery; *Prox. Trans. Dig. A.*, proximal transverse digital artery, *Common Dig. A.*, common digital artery; *DIPJ*, distal interphalangeal joint; *PIPJ*, proximal interphalangeal joint; *VBS*, vinculum breve superficialis; *MPJ*, metacarpophalangeal joint; *VBP*, vinculum breve profundus; *VLP*, vinculum longum profundus; *VLS*, vinculum longum superficialis, *FDP*, flexor digitorum profundus; *FDS*, flexor digitorum superficialis.) (From Ochiai et al,[213] with permission.)

TENDON HEALING

The exact nature of tendon healing is still not completely understood.[181,182] The controversy regarding tendon healing really applies to the flexor tendons within the digital sheath. Lindsay,[156-161,211,278] Matthews,[200-202] Potenza,[226-228] Peacock,[216] Furlow,[81] and others[63,195] have studied the mechanism of tendon healing here extensively. More recently, the studies of Manske,[181-183,185,186,188-192] Gelberman,[83-95] Mass[197,198] and others[59,78,82,102,127,157,170,172,175,219-222,250] have greatly increased our understanding of this process. At one time, it was believed that tendons within the sheath healed by the fibroblastic response of the sheath and surrounding tissues following injury. It is now generally agreed that flexor tendons possess an intrinsic capacity to heal themselves with diffusion without depending on extratendinous cells or surrounding adhesions. Lundborg[170,175] showed in rabbits that flexor tendons deprived of their blood supply can heal without adhesion formation. He removed flexor profundus tendons from the sheaths of rabbit toes, cut them in half, sutured them together, and placed them in a rabbit's knee in the suprapatellar pouch. The tendons were analyzed macroscopically and microscopically at periods ranging from 1 to 6 weeks. Healing without adhesion formation took place, and Lundborg concluded that flexor tendons did possess an intrinsic capacity for healing with nutrients supplied by diffusion from the synovial fluid. Potenza and Herte,[229] and others,[59] however, disagreed with this conclusion, believing that cells from the synovium actually seeded onto the surface of the tendons to "heal" them. Manske,[183,188,189] Gelberman,[88,92] Mass[197,198] and others[82,250] have recently shown, in various animal models, that flexor tendons do have an intrinsic capacity for healing. They placed cut segments of flexor tendons in tissue culture media and demonstrated the presence of a healing process by light and electron microscopy. However, it has also been shown recently that there is neovascularization present within the sheath of healing flexor tendons, which suggests that vascular perfusion does play a role in the healing of intrasynovial tendinous connective tissue.[85] The presence of an intact vincular system does improve the results of flexor tendon repair in Zone II.[5]

Even though the exact process of tendon healing is not completely understood, it is now known that flexor tendons do possess an intrinsic capacity to heal themselves. Whether or not adhesion formation from the surrounding soft tissues is an integral part of the repair process is questionable, although recent evidence suggests that it is not necessary.

During the past several years, Gelberman and his associates[83–95,273] have carefully evaluated the healing processes of flexor tendons with in vivo and in vitro studies. They compared repaired flexor tendons that were totally immobilized to tendons treated with varying degrees of protected passive mobilization. The tensile strength and gliding function were consistently greater in the mobilized tendons. In the immobilized tendons, there were adhesions surrounding the repair site attaching it to the sheath. In contrast, there was a smooth gliding surface and good healing in the mobilized tendons, showing that adhesions are not necessary for healing at the repair site. They also studied the cellular mechanism of repair extensively with their in vitro studies, demonstrating phagocytosis of debris by epitenon cells and collagen synthesis by endotenon cells. These studies provided us with the first true experimental evidence that early, controlled, passive mobilization of repaired flexor tendons within the digital sheath could be beneficial. Their recent studies indicate that increasing the duration and frequency of protected passive mobilization following flexor tendon repair can have a beneficial effect on the tensile strength of the healing flexor tendon and ultimately improve tendon function. Current studies are underway with the use of a continuous passive motion machine.

Much attention has been paid recently to the utilization of early active motion following flexor tendon repair.[42,65,106,176,249,255] There is no clinical study to date showing that this is superior to early protected passive mobilization of the flexor tendons, although many experimental and clinical studies are investigating this possibility.

Some investigators[8,12–14,49,99,203,215,228,296] have tried to wrap the tendon juncture with various substances to prevent the ingrowth of adhesions; others[6,27,64,66,110,133,146–148,218,271] have tried to modify adhesion formation with different biochemical agents. Neither of these approaches has any clinical application at this time, although advances may be made in this field in the future.

What then is the nutritional pathway for the flexor tendon within the digital sheath? How does the severed tendon heal in the sheath? If diffusion from the synovial fluid is a more effective nutritional pathway than perfusion, should the digital flexor sheath be repaired or reconstructed at the time of tendon repair? How should early protected passive mobilization be carried out following tendon repair? Should one use elastic band traction with a palmar pulley or a continuous passive motion machine on an intermittent basis? Is early active flexion motion beneficial? Unfortunately, the answers to some of these questions and others remain unknown, and more basic research must be done. In formulating a treatment plan for flexor tendon injuries, therefore, considerable reliance should be placed on clinical results and experience until some of these basic questions are definitively answered.

GENERAL CONSIDERATIONS

Diagnosis

The diagnosis of flexor tendon injuries is not always easy. A careful examination of superficialis and profundus function is essential (Fig. 50-6). It has been shown that an intact vinculum can flex the PIP joint when both flexor tendons are cut and, therefore, the strength of flexion should also be carefully examined.[247] Avulsion of the profundus tendon insertion is frequently missed because of an incomplete examination.[149,150] Tendon and nerve damage may be difficult to assess in an uncooperative, frightened child, although some information can be obtained by observing the position of the finger at rest. In this instance, the only way to be absolutely sure about flexor tendon injury may be to explore the wound. Partial flexor tendon lacerations can also pose a diagnostic and therapeutic problem. There may be a full range of motion of the finger, but the patient will usually have weakness or pain when the examiner tests for function against resistance in the individual superficialis and profundus tendons. In this case, particularly in Zones I and II, when the sheath has been violated, consideration should be given to exploration of the wound and repair or debridement of the partially divided tendon, depending on the extent of injury.[284] This can prevent a subsequent rupture of the involved tendon and may also prevent triggering, which can occur[22] even after a small partial laceration. If the wound is not explored, the extremity should be splinted for 2 to 3 weeks to prevent rupture of the damaged tendon. In general, if there is any question in the examiner's mind that a tendon is damaged, exploration is warranted.

Not all tendon lacerations have to be repaired. For instance, laceration of the superficialis tendon only in the ring finger of an elderly or sick patient may not cause enough functional disability to warrant the risks of surgical repair. The general condition and functional needs of the patient must always be considered.

Basic Principles

All flexor tendon repairs should be done in the operating theater. Proper assistance, lighting, instrumentation, and magnification are essential. I prefer either general or axillary block anesthesia to intravenous regional anesthesia (Bier block) and I believe that the tourniquet should be deflated prior to wound closure to obtain good hemostasis. A culture is taken of each wound preoperatively, and I give most patients intravenous antibiotics just before, during, and for 4 to 6 hours after surgery. A pneumatic tourniquet is used unless contraindicated. The wound should be carefully cleansed and debrided and the extent of injury determined. If the original laceration has to be

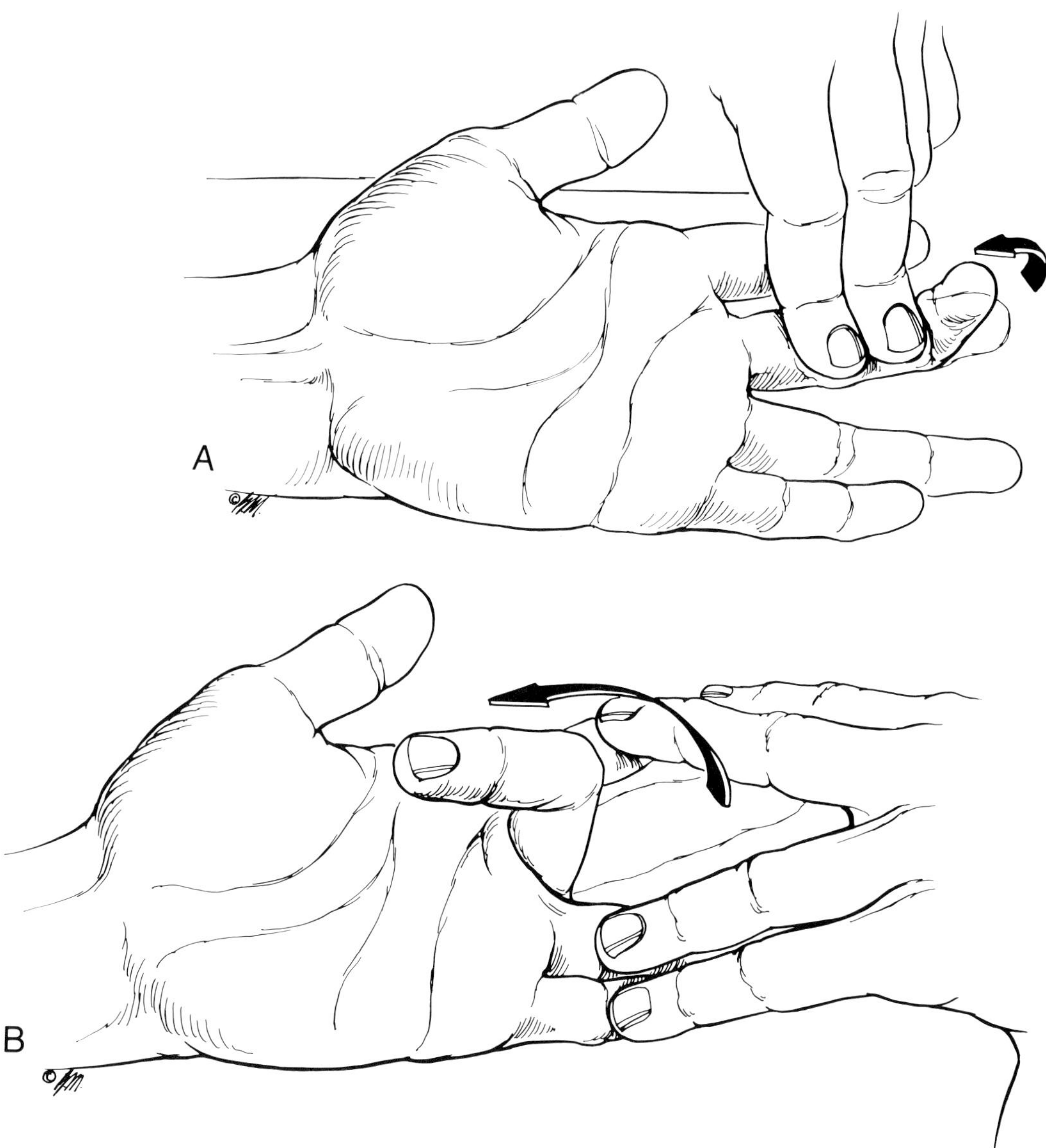

Fig. 50-6. **(A)** The correct method of testing the flexor digitorium profundus. The intact profundus tendon actively flexes the DIP joint. **(B)** The correct method of testing for flexor digitorum superficialis. The intact superficialis tendon actively flexes the PIP joint, while the profundus unit is inactivated by passive extension of the other fingers.

extended for better exposure and repair, proper incisions must be used[34,43,44,140,169] (Fig. 50-7). Careful consideration should be given to the viability of any skin flap created by extending the wound. Straight and midline palmar incisions that cross flexor creases and damage the pulley system will eventually contract and make secondary reconstruction difficult or impossible. Poor placement of incisions is an almost certain invitation to disaster.

Bunnell's "atraumatic" technique[45] should be used. Minimal debridement of tendons is necessary, and only the cut ends should be handled. In a clean, sharply incised, fresh wound, it is usually not necessary to debride the tendon ends at all. If necessary, the cut ends can be squared off using a sharp blade. A technique to debride and prepare the tendon ends utilizing a nerve cutting instrument has recently been described[254] and may prove helpful to some surgeons.

Suture Technique

The ideal suture material should be nonreactive, pliable, of small caliber, strong, easy to handle, and able to hold a good knot. Some of the more commonly used materials are Ethibond, Prolene, nylon, Supramid, Mersilene, Tevdek, monofilament stainless steel wire, and silk. Numerous reports[1,2,46,135,136,180,234,260,274,280] have detailed the properties of these and other materials. Several suture techniques[18–20,35,42,105,131,132,140,141,144,151,165,176,234,248,252,265,266,272,275,

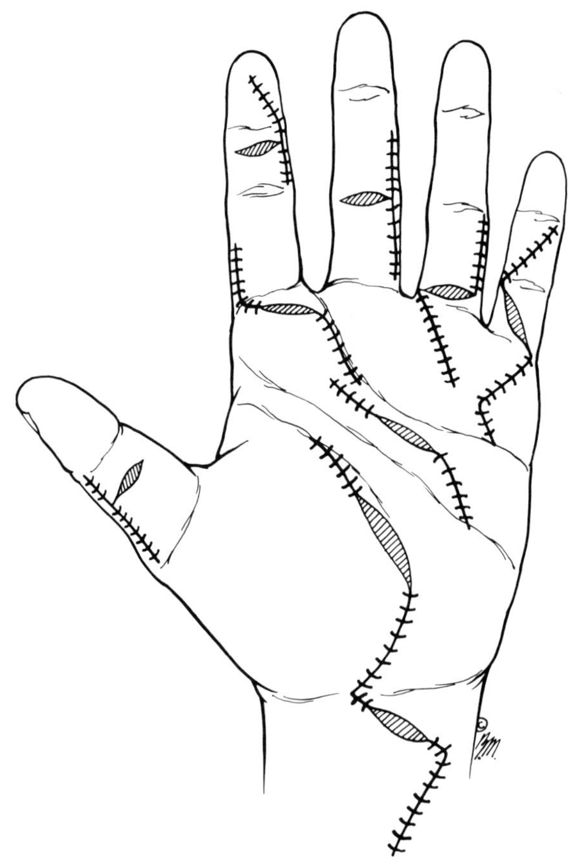

Fig. 50-7. The original wound should be extended only as far as necessary, using proper incisions.

[281,284,289,290,299] have been devised for tendon repair, and some of the more common methods used for primary repair are depicted in Figure 50-8. Urbaniak, Cahill, and Mortenson[280] tested the tensile strengths of eight different tendon suture techniques, not all of which are applicable in primary repair. The Bunnell and Kessler sutures provided nearly equal strength initially, but the Kessler suture was three times stronger on the fifth day postrepair. From the tenth day onward, there was no significant difference between the strengths of the two methods. Urbaniak and co-workers reasoned that the Bunnell double figure-of-eight technique appeared to have more of a "strangling" effect on the intact tendon than the "grasping" suture of Kessler. For the core stitch, I prefer to use the modified Kessler technique[131,132] with two sutures or the technique of Strickland.[265,266] Both are easy to use, are strong, and give good tendon approximation with little accordion effect and minimal strangulation of tissue. The true Kessler stitch leaves knots of suture material exposed, which is a theoretical disadvantage, particularly in the fibroosseous flexor tendon sheath.

I currently use 4-0 Ethibond (a synthetic, braided material) for the core suture. There is some concern that use of the smoother monofilament sutures may result in stretching or gapping at the repair site.[76] This can result in increased adhesion formation and/or the possibility of rupture. A running 6-0 epitendinous suture is added to the repair whenever possible. It has been demonstrated, that besides "tidying up" the repair, the running epitendinous suture adds significantly to its strength.[155,230] A running locking suture has proven to be stronger than a simple running suture.[155] The Halsted horizontal mattress suture utilized for the peripheral stitch has been shown to markedly increase the load where gap formation will occur and also to greatly increase the maximum strength of the repair.[290]

The standard repair should include a core stitch followed by a running type of epitendinous suture. Many new suture techniques[42,151,176,248,290] are being investigated in an effort to increase the strength of repair so that early active motion may be possible. To date, none of these new techniques have been universally accepted, and protected passive mobilization of the flexor tendon is still the treatment of choice.

Postoperative Splinting

The pneumatic tourniquet should be deflated and good hemostasis obtained prior to wound closure. Hematoma formation can lead to wound healing problems, tendon adherence, rupture, and infection. Wounds are closed with fine, interrupted, nonabsorbable sutures. A sterile dressing is applied, followed by a dorsal plaster splint, extending from beyond the fingertips to the proximal forearm in adults and to above the elbow in children. The wrist is held in approximately 20 to 30 degrees palmar flexion, and the MP joints are flexed approximately 60 degrees. The splint should allow full extension of the PIP and DIP joints so that troublesome flexion contractures of these joints can be avoided. The palmar surfaces of the fingers should not be blocked by a constrictive bandage but should be relatively free (Fig. 50-9). Voluntary and involuntary contractions of the fingers against a constrictive dressing can cause tension with resultant gapping or rupture at the repair site.

Postoperative Mobilization

The desire for early motion after tendon repair is certainly not new.[18-20,42,57,58,60,61,65,72,78,80,83,84,86,89,90,93-95,106,132,139,151,153,165,176,208,249,255,269,270,273,290,301] Due to the disastrous effects that adhesion formation has on the gliding mechanism of the flexor tendons, many techniques have been devised to permit early motion and to prevent adhesion formation. Both clinically and experimentally, it has been shown that early mobilization techniques following flexor tendon repair within the digital sheath have improved tendon healing and the final end result.

In 1967, Kleinert and colleagues[139] popularized the use of elastic band traction originally described by Young and Harmon.[301] They placed a double loop of 5-0 nylon suture through the nail and knotted it. A rubber band was attached to the nylon loop and then to a safety pin fastened proximal to the wrist, slightly on the radial side. Under the appropriate tension, the rubber band held the finger in flexion but allowed it to be actively extended against the dorsal plaster splint. The patients were instructed to attach the rubber band for several half-hour periods daily and to leave it unattached for the rest of the day

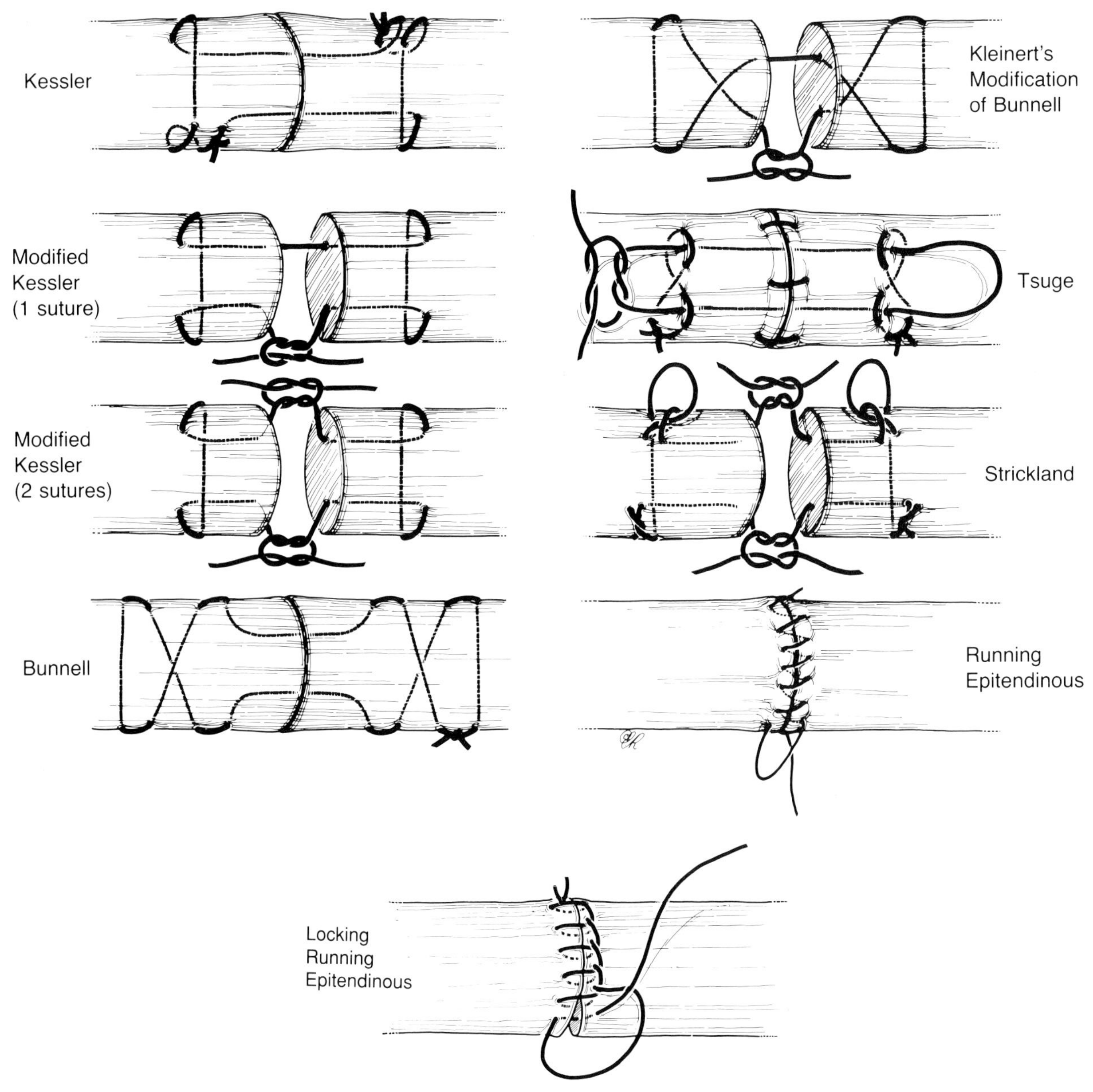

Fig. 50-8. Some suture techniques used in flexor tendon repair.

and at night in order to lessen the tendency for the development of flexion contractures. A new version of this splint that incorporates a "palmar pulley" (see below) has been developed, and excellent results have been reported with its use.[295]

Duran and Houser[72] were among the first to recommend a method of controlled passive mobilization following repair of both superficialis and profundus tendons in tidy Zone II injuries. They determined both clinically and experimentally that 3 to 5 mm of extension motion at the repair site is sufficient to prevent firm adhesion formation. Following flexor tendon repair, the wrist is placed in 20 to 30 degrees flexion and the MP joint is stabilized in its normal balanced position. Then, under direct vision in the operating room, the distal phalanx is extended enough to see the repair site of the flexor digitorum profundus move 3 to 5 mm. Next, the middle phalanx is extended until both repair sites move 3 to 5 mm. These motions are recorded and used later as a guide for the passive motion exercises, which are begun immediately. The exercises are done in the morning and evening with six to eight motions for each tendon per session. The patients (or parents) are trained to do the exercises themselves. Controlled passive motion is used alone for 4½ weeks, at which time, the dorsal splint is removed and rubber band traction is attached to a wrist band. The passive exercises, along with gentle active exercises, are done for 1 more week. The rubber band traction is then removed, and active flexion and extension exercises are increased. The repair is protected for another 2 weeks because the authors fear an increased risk of rupture due to the early mobilization. This technique of Duran and Houser has been further modified by Strickland[51,264,266,269] (see Author's Preferred Method below).

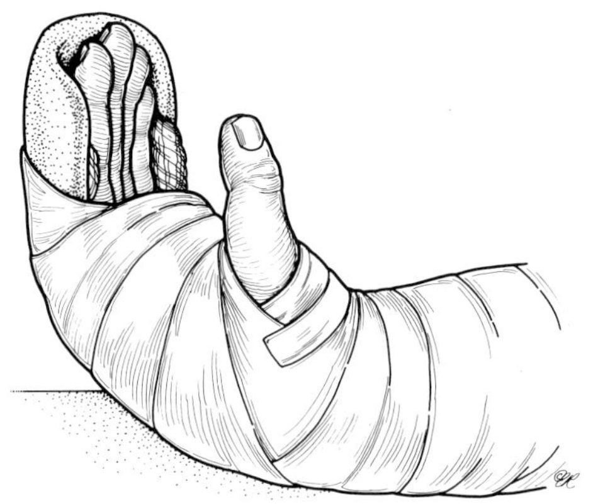

Fig. 50-9. A dorsal splint holding the wrist and MP joints in flexion and allowing full extension of the PIP and DIP joints.

Recent studies have shown that increasing the duration and frequency of passive flexion exercises can increase the tensile strength of the repair and have a beneficial effect on the end result.[90,273] The exact duration and frequency for these exercises has not yet been established. Some investigators are using continuous passive motion machines in their postoperative regimen and we will await the results of these studies.

Recently, Chow and colleagues[57,58] reported excellent results in the treatment of flexor tendon lacerations in Zone II using a combination of the "palmar pulley" and passive exercises. Their tendon repair was a standard technique consisting of a core suture with a running epitendinous suture, with no attempt to close the flexor tendon sheath. In their postoperative rehabilitation program, they modified the use of the rubber band passive flexion orthosis by incorporating a palmar pulley utilizing a safety pin to redirect the line of pull. This modification increased the passive flexion of the interphalangeal joints by pulling the tip of the finger towards the distal palmar crease (Fig. 50-10). They reasoned that by increasing interphalangeal flexion, the tendon excursion in the sheath was maximized. This could also increase the differential gliding between the superficialis and profundus tendons, which has been shown to be important.[293] During the first 2 weeks after tenorrhaphy, full passive extension and flexion exercises of the PIP and DIP joints were performed daily under supervision of the physician or hand therapist to prevent contracture at the interphalangeal joints. This passive motion was carried out in addition to the hourly program of active extension against the rubber band traction. The passive extension exercises were discontinued by the fourteenth day. At 4 weeks, the rubber band traction was completely discontinued, and during the fifth and sixth weeks, the patient performed hourly finger motion exercises of active flexion followed by passive flexion and active extension. These patients were cared for in a military setting and often were seen daily by the physician and/or hand therapist. Nevertheless, the results achieved utilizing this regimen in 44 digits are superior to other comparable series. The use of the "palmar pulley" for those who utilize postoperative rubber band traction is now almost universal.

Other investigators are attempting to use early *active* flexion exercises following flexor tendon repair in Zone II.[42,65,106,151,176,248,255,290] New suture techniques are being devised in order to strengthen the repair so that active flexion exercises will be possible without fear of gapping or rupture at the repair site. The concept is intriguing, but more work needs to be done to define the role of early active motion after tendon repair.

Author's Preferred Method

I use a modification of the controlled passive mobilization technique of Duran and Houser that has been basically described by Strickland.[51,264,266,269] A dorsal block splint is applied holding the wrist in 20 to 30 degrees flexion and the MP joints in 50 degrees flexion while the PIP and DIP joints are allowed to extend fully. For the flexor pollicis longus, the MP and interphalangeal joints of the thumb are held in 15 to 20 degrees of flexion. I do not use Velcro straps across the volar surface of the fingers because a voluntary or involuntary contraction

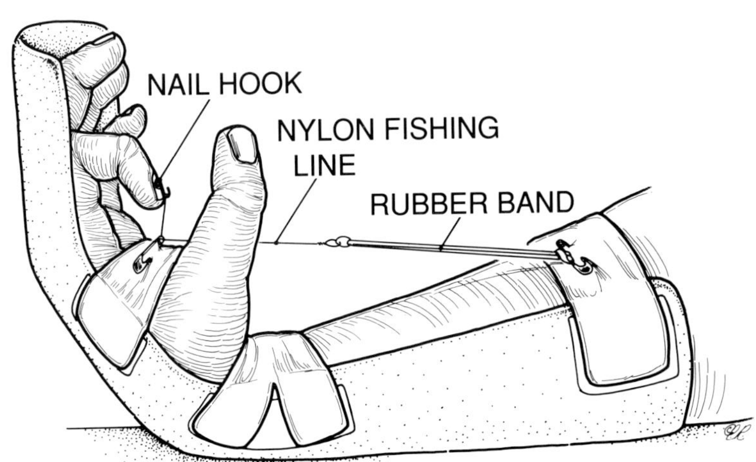

Fig. 50-10. Chow's modification of rubber band traction incorporating a "palmar pulley," which increases passive flexion at the PIP and DIP joints.

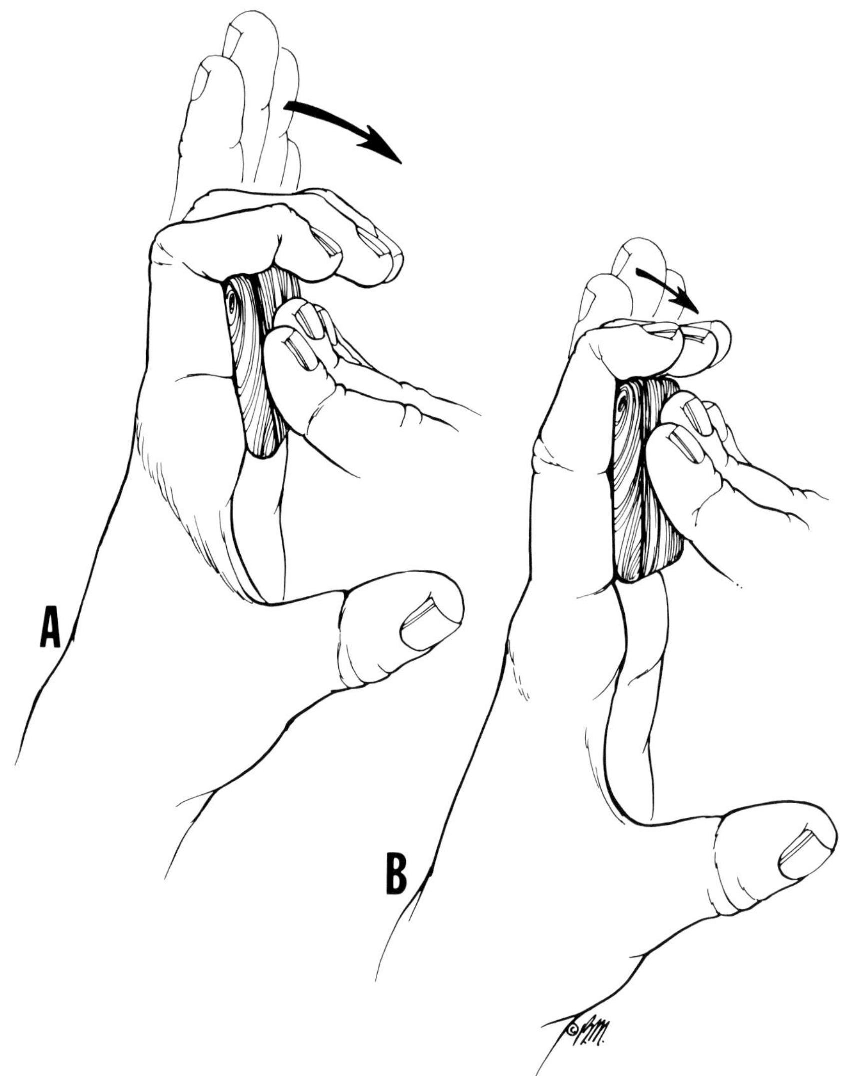

Fig. 50-11. The use of the Bunnell block to improve active flexion of the PIP and DIP joints by blocking motion at the next most proximal joint.

against them could cause tension at the repair site. I have been increasing the frequency and duration of the exercises so that the patient spends at least a total of an hour a day performing them. If both tendons have been repaired, the PIP and DIP joints are taken separately through several repetitions of full passive flexion and extension. Complete passive flexion of MP, PIP, and DIP joints is then performed several times. This regimen begins within 72 hours of surgery and continues for 4 weeks, at which time, gentle, active flexion and extension exercises of the wrist and fingers are instituted. Splinting is discontinued after 5 weeks. (Children wear above-elbow splints for 4 weeks, but the passive exercises can be carried out by their parents if the surgeon so desires.) Close supervision by the operating surgeon is essential during this period of time. If hand therapy is contemplated, it should be carried out only by a specially trained therapist working closely with the surgeon.

The Bunnell block can be used as an aid to improve active flexion after 5 weeks (Fig. 50-11). The patient can also be instructed to block the MP joint of the affected finger in extension and in varying degrees of flexion with the opposite hand while actively flexing the PIP joint. Similarly, the PIP joint can be held in extension and varying degrees of flexion while the DIP joint is actively flexed. These maneuvers are referred to as "blocking" exercises; they will help the repaired tendon glide actively in the finger instead of using up its restricted amplitude to flex the more proximal joints.[35]

If there is restriction of extension beyond 6 weeks, dynamic splinting may be necessary. Different splints are used depending on the zone of injury. At this time also, for Zone I and Zone II injuries, if passive extension is limited, the surgeon can hold the wrist in neutral and the MP joint in the acutely flexed position, while gently passively extending the PIP joint. This maneuver can free some adhesions and increase motion, but must be used with great care to prevent rupture. No heavy lifting is allowed for 16 weeks or more. Emphasis is placed on improving the range of motion. Grip strengthening exercises are not initiated for 3 to 4 months and not until satisfactory motion has been achieved. Improvement in motion can continue for 6 months or longer following tenorrhaphy, particularly in children. Therefore, the surgeon may sometimes await this period of time before considering tenolysis, although it may be advisable to proceed earlier in some selected cases.[267]

If postoperative rubber band traction is utilized, Chow's method and regimen[57,58] are carefully followed so that troublesome flexion contractures can be avoided.

Flexor Tendon Sheath

In the past, for Zone I and II injuries, most surgeons removed a portion of the sheath around the repair site in the fingers and thumb after a flexor tendon repair.[134,194] Theoretically, this would prevent the development of adhesions between the tendons and the sheath and would allow some motion of the tendon repair without interference by the sheath and pulley system. As previously mentioned, our concepts of tendon nutrition and healing have changed. Recently, emphasis has been placed on the role of diffusion of nutrients from the synovial fluid in the nourishment of flexor tendons. We have learned that flexor tendons within the digital sheath do have an intrinsic capacity for healing and, therefore, it may not be necessary for adhesions to form for the healing process to take place. With these concepts in mind, some surgeons recommend closure of the sheath when possible with fine suture material after flexor tendon repairs in Zones I and II.[75,163,164] Theoretically and experimentally, since the synovial sheath and fluid are maintained, nutrition of the tendons is improved and there will be less tendency for adhesion formation.[7,130,219–222,242,250,263] The tendon repair is less likely to "catch" on or adhere to the resected ends of the synovial sheath when motion is begun. One carefully done study in dogs showed that reconstruction of the sheath did not significantly improve various characteristics of repaired tendons treated with early motion rehabilitation.[94]

Lister has developed a technique for preserving the digital flexor sheath during primary and delayed primary repair of flexor tendons.[163,164] He calls the areas between the annular pulleys "retinacular windows" (Fig. 50-12). To expose the ten-

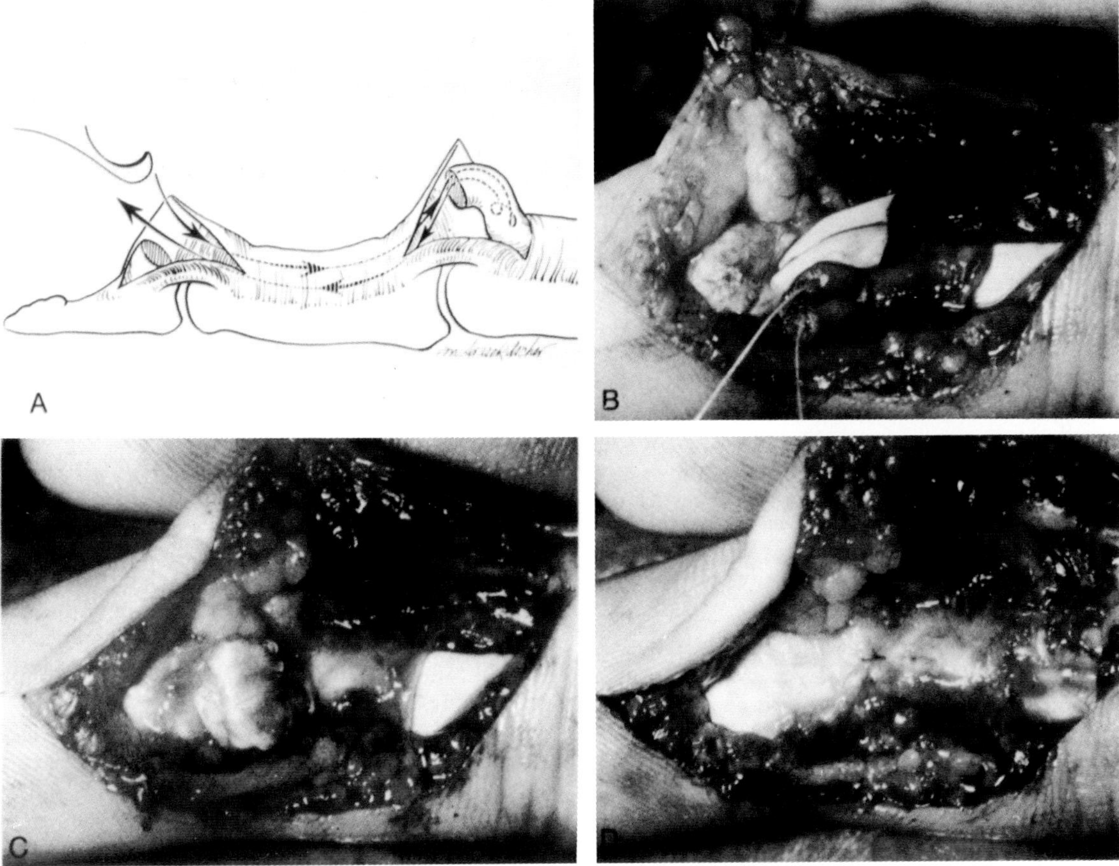

Fig. 50-12. Lister's technique for preserving the flexor sheath. **(A)** This diagram illustrates the L-shaped cuts that facilitate passage of the tendon from one window to another. The technique for a "distal combined" repair is illustrated; it is simply the reverse of the technique for proximal combined repair. Since the core suture is placed in the tendon ends in two windows, it is a combined repair, and because the peripheral running suture is placed in the distal window, it is called a "distal combined" repair. **(B)** In this patient, the proximal tendon end has been drawn beneath the intervening pulley after the proximal core suture was placed. An L-shaped cut has been employed in the proximal window to facilitate passage of the tendon end. Note the relatively undamaged epitenon on the end that has been passed beneath the pulley. **(C)** The repair has been completed in the distal window, and the two windows have been closed. **(D)** Close inspection of the photograph reveals the peripheral running suture in the tendon lying beneath the pulley intervening between the two windows. (From Lister,[164] with permission.)

don for repair, a longitudinal incision should be made only in these "retinacular windows" and not in the annular pulleys. The finger is opened and the distal cut end of the tendon is located. The site of repair will be determined and an L-shaped incision is made in the retinacular window in this level. The finger may be flexed to bring the distal cut end into a more proximal window or extended to bring it into a more distal window. The proximal cut end of the tendon can always be brought to the level of the appropriate window. If 10 mm or more of the distal cut end can be brought to a retinacular window by flexion of the digit, then "a proximal single window" repair can be done. A central core suture is placed in both ends of the tendon using separate sutures. Following tendon repair, the L-shaped opening in the sheath is closed with interrupted sutures of 6-0 monofilament nylon suture. If only 5 to 10 mm of the distal end can be brought into the proximal window, then the core suture must be placed in the distal end of the tendon in the next most distal window by making a L-shaped incision in the sheath distal to that annular pulley. The suture is placed, the tendon is brought back proximally beneath the annular pulley, and the distal window is closed with a 6-0 monofilament suture. The tendon repair is then accomplished through the proximal window and the sheath is closed with 6-0 monofilament nylon suture. Lister calls this a "proximal combined repair." If less than 5 mm of the distal cut end is available, the core suture must be placed in the proximal cut end of the tendon and in the distal cut end in the distal window. This is a "distal combined" repair. It is a combined repair if the core sutures are placed in the tendon ends in two different windows. The technique of closure of the sheath is the same in both with a suture of 6-0 monofilament suture. Closure of the sheath is possible in most cases of primary and delayed primary repair.

In clinical series reported to date, there is still no clear statistical evidence to support the contention that closure of the sheath will improve the final end result.[166,244] However, in light of the research regarding nutrition and healing of flexor tendons, closure of the sheath theoretically may be the proper thing to do. Further clinical studies are being undertaken. During primary and delayed primary repairs, when possible, I repair the sheath in the manner described by Lister.

Primary and Delayed Primary Repair

In this chapter, primary repair is defined as repair done within 18 to 24 hours of injury. Direct end-to-end repair of the tendon ends after this period of time is termed delayed primary repair regardless of the length of time that has passed. Some use an arbitrary time to differentiate between a delayed primary repair and a secondary repair. In general, primary repair of flexor tendon lacerations is preferable, but if the facilities and personnel are not available or if the patient is not seen until a few days postinjury, delayed primary repair can be done without adversely effecting the end result.[11,54,103,124,177,178,199,245,251] In such cases, tetanus prophylaxis is administered, and the wound should be cultured, cleansed, debrided, and closed, if possible. Oral antibiotics are administered. In my opinion, delayed primary repair should be done as soon as there is evidence of wound healing without any sign of infection.

A word of caution is appropriate here regarding delayed primary repair. In some instances, it is possible to do this 6 weeks or more following the injury, and in other cases, it may be impossible to achieve end-to-end repair as early as 2 weeks after the injury. Factors influencing this include the level of tendon laceration, the extent of loss of the nutritional supply to the tendon, and the amount of retraction that has taken place proximally. The surgeon should have an alternative plan in case delayed primary repair is not feasible (see Chapter 51).

If the injury is a clean, incised wound, or can be converted to one by proper debridement, and if there is good skin coverage, direct end-to-end repair should be carried out, either primarily or delayed. Tendon repair, however, is not the first priority in a massive, crush injury, or in a dirty, contaminated wound that cannot be converted to a clean wound by debridement, such as a human bite. The surgeon's primary objective in these cases is to cleanse and debride the damaged part, stabilize fractures if necessary, and achieve good wound healing without infection.[32,33,47] Similarly, if there is a large skin loss over the flexor tendon mechanism, good coverage must be obtained prior to any repair or reconstruction.[145] Last, but certainly not least, the surgeon must possess the knowledge, training, and experience to perform this surgery. Attempts at repair by an unqualified person can lead to disaster, making later reconstruction more difficult or impossible.

TREATMENT

The treatment of flexor tendon lacerations in each specific zone is discussed separately in this section.

Zone I

Tendon lacerations in Zone I involve only the flexor digitorum profundus tendon. There is loss of flexion at the DIP joint, instability in pinch, and loss of grip strength. If conditions permit, these should be treated with primary or delayed primary repair. The tendon can be repaired directly or advanced and reinserted into the distal phalanx,[138,237] but it should not be advanced more than 1 cm.[179] In the thumb, there is loss of flexion at the interphalangeal joint and instability and weakness of pinch. The treatment options are the same.

Author's Preferred Method

The laceration is debrided and extended as previously described, if necessary. The proximal end of the tendon is normally not hard to find because it is prevented from retracting by the intact vinculum. If the palmar plate has been damaged, it should be repaired with a fine, nonreactive suture, such as 6-0 Mersilene. The A4, C3, and A5 pulleys are found in the finger in Zone I. The A4 pulley is the most important functionally, and every attempt should be made to preserve it. If this is excised completely at the time of repair, only about 20 to 30 degrees useful flexion in the DIP joint will be obtained, and although there is minimal bowstringing, usually there will be a 30-degree flexion contracture of the DIP joint. If the tendon laceration is more than 1 cm proximal to the insertion, end-to-end repair is done, followed by a running epitendinous 6–0 suture. The sheath may be repaired as previously described. If not, a small portion should be excised surrounding the repair. It may be necessary to narrow the A4 pulley, but it will still retain its function if it is not completely excised.

If the tendon laceration is 1 cm or less from the insertion, advancement and reinsertion into the distal phalanx may be preferable, particularly if the distal portion of the tendon is too small to accept a core suture or if it had been severely damaged at the time of the injury. The A4 pulley can usually be preserved. Various methods of reinsertion have been advocated, and I prefer to use a modification of the standard Bunnell pull-out wire and button technique[35] (Fig. 50-13). An osteoperiosteal flap of bone is raised in the distal phalanx just distal to the insertion of the palmar plate. A 4–0 Prolene suture is used in the tendon instead of the 4–0 monofilament stainless steel wire, and therefore no proximal pull-out wire is necessary. The suture is passed through a drill hole starting in the bone at the level of the osteoperiosteal flap and exiting dorsally at the midnail level. The 4–0 Prolene is tied over a button on the nail in the usual fashion, and when healing has taken place, the entire suture can be removed by cutting one end and pulling the remainder of the suture out through the tendon and distal phalanx. This provides a strong attachment and is a relatively simple technique, leaving no foreign material in the finger when the suture is removed 3 to 4 weeks later. When reinserting the tendon, damage to the volar plate should be avoided, and the insertion should not be placed too far distally in the phalanx; either of these can result in a flexion contracture of the DIP joint. I have not seen a late problem with the nail or nail bed utilizing this technique. Some authors prefer to place the suture around the distal phalanx rather than through it, and this method is perfectly acceptable.

Delayed primary repair in this zone can often be performed up to 6 weeks or longer, provided the profundus tendon is held in place by an intact vinculum and does not become too contracted.

Thumb

In the thumb, the oblique and A2 pulleys are located in Zone I. The oblique pulley is the most important, but it can be excised if necessary without great functional loss, provided the A1 pulley is intact. The same treatment principles apply here. However, if more than 1 cm of advancement is necessary, the flexor pollicis longus tendon can be Z-lengthened proximal to the wrist[279] or a fractional lengthening at the musculotendinous junction may be performed. I prefer the latter technique. It is possible to gain 2 to 3 cm in length in this fashion. The sheath may also be repaired in Zone I injuries of the thumb.

Postoperative Management

For Zone I injuries of the fingers and thumb, I use the passive mobilization program outlined previously. However, Gerbino and associates[96] reported a 35 percent complication rate following repair of Zone I injuries treated with dynamic traction splinting. If extension splinting is necessary at 5 to 6 weeks following tendon repair, a clock-spring type of splint may be utilized.

Complications

If the tendon is advanced too far distally, flexion contracture at the DIP and PIP joints can result. This is especially true in the index finger, where these contractures produce the largest functional deficit.

If the tendon has been repaired in Zone I and fails to glide, a tenodesis effect may be produced at the DIP joint. This often requires no further treatment, provided the joint is in acceptable position.

Rupture of the tendon repair or detachment of the reinserted tendon, if recognized immediately, should be treated with prompt reexploration and repair.

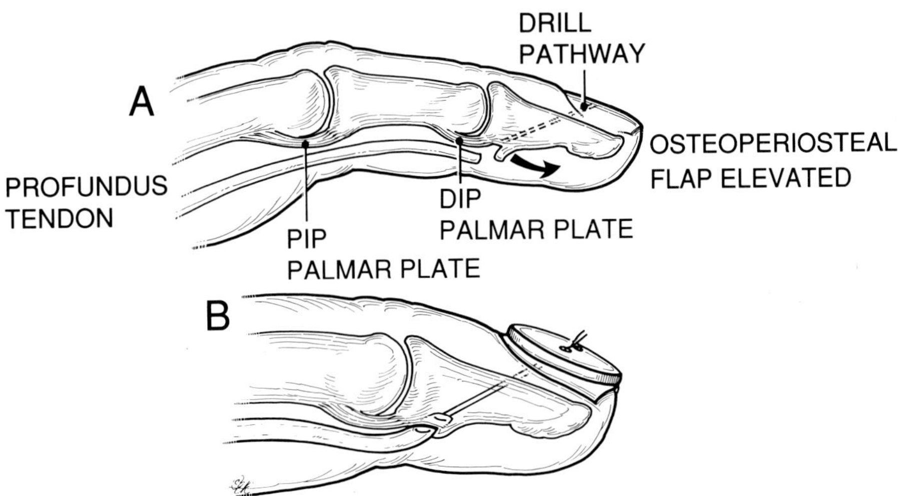

Fig. 50-13. Pull-out suture and button technique for reinsertion of the profundus tendon.

Zone II

There is almost universal agreement that primary or delayed primary repair of flexor tendon lacerations in Zone II is now the treatment of choice. Bunnell coined the term "no-man's land" to describe that area where the superficialis and profundus tendons are held closely together in a common sheath and fibroosseous tunnel, which is the area now designated as Zone II. Bunnell felt that the results of primary repair in this area were usually so poor that no one should attempt it.[48] He and others[28,29,32,33,35,37,217,231,233] advised debridement and wound closure followed by tendon grafting at a later date. Results of this type of treatment have been well documented, particularly in 1971 by Boyes and Stark[37] in their study on the factors influencing results in 1,000 cases. They showed that flexor tendon grafting was not as successful following failed primary repair as it was when the original wound was closed primarily followed by a flexor tendon graft done as a secondary procedure. In a later report, Boyes and Stark[38] suggested that primary repair might be justified in patients under 6 and over 40 years of age because these people did not fare as well following their tendon grafts. Bunnell,[48] Boyes,[29-31,37,38] Pulvertaft,[231-233] Mason and Shearon,[196] Koch,[145] Littler,[167-169] and others[3,40,50,77,107,111,224,235,236,276,277,292,297] have also contributed significantly to our knowledge of flexor tendon reconstructions. Hunter[115,119,120] and others[17,114,243,292,298] have pioneered the development of staged flexor tendon reconstruction.

Some surgeons, apparently including Bunnell[46] himself, performed primary repair of tendon lacerations in Zone II, while continuing to advise against it in their teachings. Perhaps this reflected their concern that these cases might be done by unqualified surgeons, causing many more problems.

Verdan,[281-285] Kleinert and colleagues,[139-144] and others,[21,24,25,103,108,112,126,129,132,158,193,194,200,204,207,210,223,238,291] must be given credit for promoting the cause of primary repair of flexor tendon lacerations in Zone II. There are several advantages: (1) the problem is taken care of immediately and the period of disability is lessened, (2) there is often no need for a second operation, (3) there is no stiffness or joint contracture to overcome preoperatively because it has no time to develop, and (4) most authors now agree that the results of primary repair are equal or superior to the results of flexor tendon grafts.[57,58,123,139-144,255,281,284,285,295] The great disadvantage is that failure of primary repair in Zone II can leave a finger contracted with scar that may be difficult or impossible to correct with reconstructive surgery. I agree with Kleinert et al's statement that "the likelihood of the inexperienced or unqualified surgeon attempting primary tenorrhaphy is the greatest disadvantage in encouraging the use of this technique.[140]

In a clean, incised wound, or in an injury that can be converted to one by proper debridement, primary or delayed primary repair should be done in Zone II. Primary repair, however, is contraindicated in massive crush injuries, in a dirty or contaminated wound, and when there is significant skin loss over the flexor tendon mechanism. Injury to the neurovascular bundles, the palmar plate, periosteum, or even the bone, is not a contraindication to primary repair. These structures may be repaired along with the flexor tendons. In these instances, the surgeon must make an important decision. Using all of his knowledge and experience, he must decide whether, in his hands, primary repair offers the patient a good chance for a successful result. If not, primary tenorrhaphy should not be attempted, and tendon grafting in one or two stages may be done at a later date. As their experience in primary repairs grows, most surgeons are becoming more aggressive in its use. However, in general, the more severe the injury and associated trauma, the less successful is the result (see Chapter 45 for more discussion about the management of these complex injuries).

Delayed primary repair in Zone II is done usually from 2 to 14 days postinjury. As soon as the wound shows sign of healing without infection, surgery should be considered. If the proximal end of the tendon has not retracted far and is held in place by an intact vinculum or by the lumbrical origin in a proximal Zone II injury, delayed primary repair can be done up to 6 weeks or more postinjury, especially in children.

Author's Preferred Method

After careful wound debridement, the extent of injury can be evaluated. Usually, the level of tendon damage and the skin laceration do not correspond. Most lacerations occur with the finger in flexion, which places the level of tendon damage distal to the skin laceration. The opposite is true if the laceration occurs with the finger in extension. The wound should be extended only as far as necessary to complete the repair. Sharp angles in the skin flaps should be avoided to prevent tip necrosis. In general, if the laceration over the palmar aspect of the finger is oblique, I prefer to extend the wound using the palmar zigzag approach that has been popularized by Bruner.[43,44] If the skin laceration is transverse, I tend to extend the wound via the midlateral approach. The midlateral incision can, in theory, damage the vincular blood supply to the tendons,[152] but it leaves no further skin scar over the flexor mechanism. The palmar zigzag approach affords excellent exposure, but does extend the scar over the flexor tendon mechanism.

The sheath is opened between the annular pulleys with an L-shaped incision. The distal ends of the tendons can be located by flexing the finger. The location of the distal cut ends determines the site of repair. If the sheath can be repaired, the appropriate "window" between the annular pulleys must be selected, as described on page 1833. If damage to the sheath has been extensive and repair is not possible, I excise a portion of the sheath around the repair site. There must be sufficient annular pulley remaining to prevent bowstringing, and enough of the sheath should be excised to prevent the repair site from catching on it during flexion and extension movements. The proximal ends of the tendons are found by milking the finger distally with the wrist and MP joint in flexion. If this is unsuccessful, a tendon retriever can be used carefully without damaging the sheath. If this does not work, the tendon is not held by its vinculum and has probably slipped into the palm beneath the A1 pulley. It can then be located through a transverse incision in the palmar crease by pulling it proximally from under the A1 pulley. I use a small red rubber catheter or #8 infant-feeding gastrostomy tube to pull the tendon distally to the appropriate "window." A Hunter prosthesis can also be used as a tendon passer. For example, if the profundus has retracted into the palm, the tube is passed retrograde through the rent in the sheath, through the superficialis chiasm, and beneath the pulleys and sheath. The tendon is attached to the tube using a 4–0 Ethibond core suture. Then, with the wrist and MP joints flexed, pulling the tube distally will deliver the tendon to the desired level (Fig. 50-14). It can then be held in place during repair by transfixing it with a Keith needle proximally through the skin and sheath (Fig. 50-15). Lister[164] places the core suture in the proximal end of the tendon and then passes a piece of intravenous connecting tubing of sufficient caliber proximally through the rent in the sheath. He then passes the suture through the intravenous connecting tube, pulls the end of the tendon into the tube, and pulls the tube distally, delivering the tendon to the desired level. Sourmelis and McGrouther[259] suggested an ingenious method to retrieve the retracted flexor tendon in the palm. They make an incision in the palm and locate the tendon without retrieving the proximal cut end. They then pass a catheter from proximal to distal through the distal opening in the sheath. They then connect the tendon and catheter side-to-side proximal to the A1 metacarpal pulley and pull the catheter distally, delivering the proximal cut end of the tendon or tendons into the distal opening in the sheath.

Minimal debridement of the tendon is recommended, but both cut ends may be squared off, if necessary, using a sharp knife, razor blade, or a nerve cutting instrument.[254] In a clean, sharp wound, it is not necessary to debride the tendon at all. Only the cut ends should be handled since injury to the epitenon layer can provoke adhesion formation. A firm, grasping, fine-tooth forceps is sufficient here because the proximal end of the tendon is held in position by a Keith needle, and the distal end can be brought into the wound by simply flexing the finger. The forceps should be used only to control the tendon during placement of the suture. For the core stitch, I use a modified Kessler type of stitch (see Fig. 50-8) with 4–0 Ethibond and a separate suture in each tendon end (also known as the Tajima stitch). With loupe magnification, the edges of the tendon are carefully repaired with a running, locking 6–0 epitendinous suture. Sanders[246] has described a clever technique of bringing the tendon ends together first with the epitendinous suture, followed by the core suture. It is not always possible to use this technique, but when the situation allows its use, the method offers the advantage of ending up with less "bunching" of the tendon at the suture line.

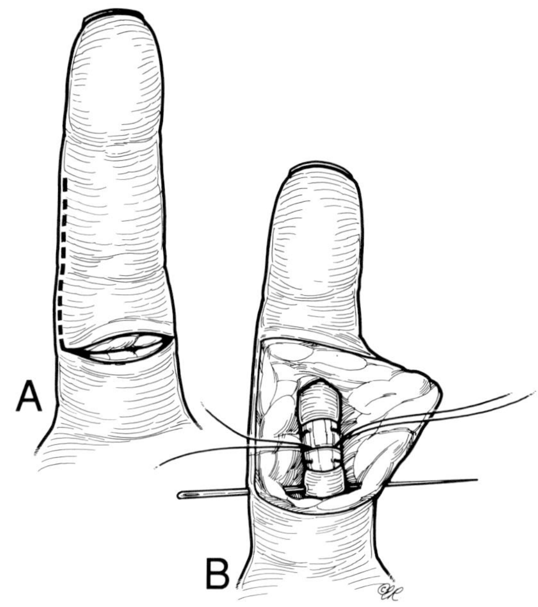

Fig. 50-15. Temporary fixation of the proximal tendon stump with a Keith needle facilitates repair.

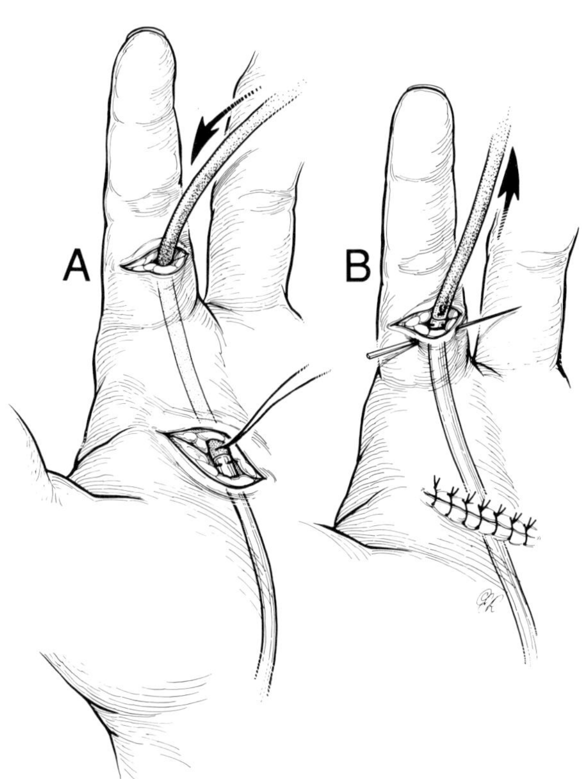

Fig. 50-14. Technique for retrieving a tendon that has retracted into the palm. (A) The tube is passed retrograde into the palm and the tendon is sutured to it. (B) The tube is pulled distally, bringing the tendon to the desired level.

When both superficialis and profundus tendons have been divided, both should be repaired if feasible. To repair a slip of the superficialis tendon, interrupted sutures of 5–0 Ethibond are used in a vertical mattress fashion. If for some reason the superficialis is not repaired, the distal stump should be left intact distal to the vinculum to preserve the blood supply to the profundus tendon and to prevent the development of a hyperextension deformity at the PIP joint. Through a separate incision in the palm, the proximal end of the superficialis tendon is pulled distally, cut, and allowed to retract.

At this point, the sheath is repaired, if possible, with a 6–0 suture. If the sheath is not repaired, approximately 1.5 cm of it is removed during the tendon repair. The A1, A2, A3, C1, and C2 pulleys are found in Zone II. The A1 and A2 pulleys are the most important and are spared, if possible, although they may be trimmed. At least one of these two pulleys must be intact to prevent bowstringing, loss of motion, and/or flexion contracture. Every attempt should also be made to preserve the palmar aponeurosis pulley during the repair.

Repair of both superficialis and profundus tendons has several advantages: (1) the blood supply of the profundus tendon is better preserved through the vincular system; (2) if successful, there is more independent motion of the finger and flexion power is stronger; (3) the smooth bed for the profundus tendon is retained; (4) there is no tendency for hyperextension at the PIP joint; (5) the incidence of rupture is probably less; and (6) according to some authors,[140,141,144,285] the results are better when both tendons are repaired. The disadvantages are (1) the surgery is more difficult; and (2) there is a possibility that adhesions at the repair sites will bind the tendons together, thus preventing motion, although this does not seem to be the case clinically.

Good hemostasis must be obtained prior to wound closure to prevent hematoma formation. A dorsal splint is applied and the postoperative regimen of early passive mobilization as outlined earlier is followed. If extension splinting is necessary at 5 to 6 weeks postoperative, a clock-spring type of splint may be utilized.

Thumb

Zone II in the thumb is different because there is only one tendon in the fibroosseous tunnel. The A1 and oblique pulleys are both here, and one of them must be preserved or motion will be compromised and bowstringing will result. A portion of the sheath is usually excised. The sheath in the thumb in Zone II is different than it is in the fingers and I do not attempt to repair it normally. The proximal portion of the tendon is easily found if it is held by an intact vinculum. If not, it slips into the palm, making retrieval difficult. Through the rent in the sheath, a tube can be passed retrograde to the level of the distal forearm where it is easily palpable. Through a small transverse incision proximal to the wrist crease, the tendon is located and attached to the tube, taking care not to damage the palmar cutaneous branch of the median nerve. With the wrist flexed, the tendon is pulled distally through the carpal canal to the desired level and transfixed proximally with a Keith needle. Alternatively, the technique of Sourmelis and McGrouther[259] may be utilized to retrieve the tendon (see page 1837). Repair then proceeds as just described for Zone II injuries in the finger. Acute flexion of MP and IP joints is avoided in the splint. I use early passive mobilization for Zone II injuries in the thumb as previously outlined.

I prefer not to explore the thenar eminence or to open the carpal tunnel when looking for the proximal end of the flexor pollicis longus tendon. Postoperatively, with the wrist held in flexion, the contents of the carpal canal can tend to bowstring, causing further problems. With the simple technique described above, it is not necessary to expose the thenar eminence or the carpal tunnel area.

In a retrospective study of 94 flexor pollicis longus repairs involving all five zones, Noonan and Blair found that the zone of injury had very little effect on the postoperative range of motion.[212]

Zone III

Primary or delayed primary repair is the treatment of choice in Zone III injuries. Frequently, there is accompanying damage to the neurovascular structures that must be repaired. Both superficialis and profundus tendons should be repaired. I use the same suture technique here with 4-0 Ethibond as in Zone I and Zone II injuries. A running, locking 6-0 epitendinous suture is also utilized. Good hemostasis must be secured prior to wound closure. The same postoperative regimen is followed. Early passive mobilization is used.

Delayed primary repair can be done up to 3 weeks or more postinjury in this area because the proximal end of the profundus tendon is held by the lumbrical origin. If extension splinting is necessary 6 weeks postoperatively, I prefer to use a splint with outriggers. This should hold the wrist in approximately 10 degrees extension and should provide a stop at the MP joints, preventing hyperextension here. Rubber band traction can then be employed through the outrigger to gain extension at the PIP and DIP joints (Fig. 50-16).

Zone IV

Injuries in Zone IV (within the carpal tunnel) are uncommon because of the protection the normal anatomic configuration provides. Here nine flexor tendons and the median nerve lie in close proximity in the carpal canal. Flexor tendon injuries in this area are usually associated with such things as injuries to the median nerve, palmar arch, or motor branch of the ulnar nerve. Again, if possible, primary repair of all tendons, except perhaps the superficialis of the small finger, is recommended. A modified Kessler suture of 4-0 Ethibond is used. In order to prevent bowstringing of the flexor tendons and median nerve postoperatively, the MP joints can be more acutely flexed and the wrist should be immobilized in nearly neutral position. The same postoperative regimen is followed. Usually multiple tendons are involved and early passive mobilization can be used unless contraindicated by nerve or vessel repair.

Delayed primary repair should be done within 3 weeks of injury, if possible. If the delay is much longer than this, myostatic contraction of the muscle may take place making end-to-end repair difficult or impossible. If extension splinting is necessary after 5 or 6 weeks, I prefer a splint holding the wrist in 10 degrees dorsiflexion with an MP stop and outriggers to gain extension at the PIP and DIP joints (see Fig. 50-16).

Zone V

Tendon lacerations in this area are usually multiple, and the injury often involves the median and ulnar nerves and the radial and ulnar vessels. Primary repair of all the tendons is the recommended treatment. This can be done with 4-0 Ethibond, using the same suture techniques. A running, locking, epitendinous, 6-0 suture is utilized if time permits. Delay of more than 3 or 4 weeks may result in myostatic contracture of the forearm flexor musculature, making end-to-end repair im-

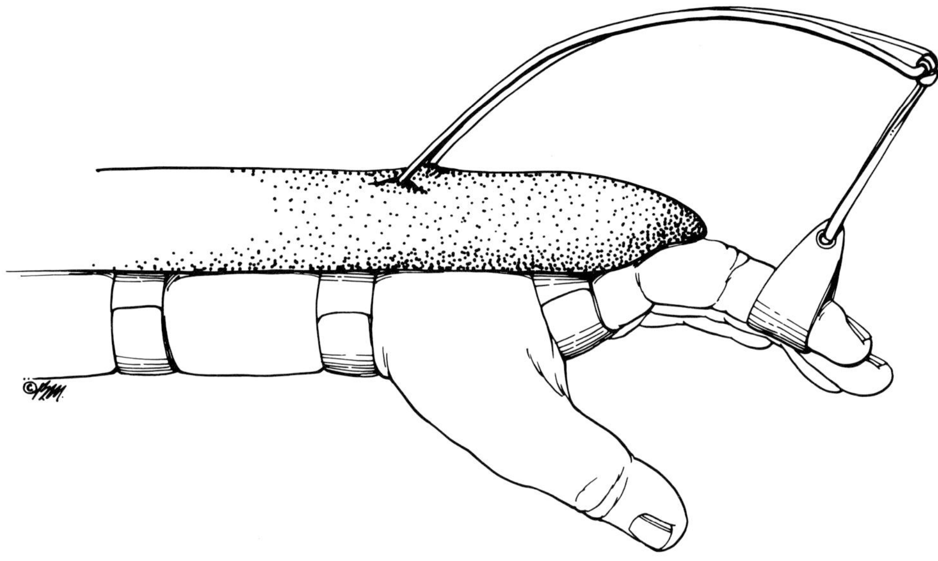

Fig. 50-16. A dynamic splint with an MP hyperextension stop and outrigger for elastic band traction to gain extension at the PIP and DIP joints.

possible. If this occurs, bridge grafts may be necessary to restore tendon continuity. The early postoperative regimen is the same. Early passive mobilization is utilized unless contraindicated by nerve and/or vessel repair. If extension splinting is necessary, the same procedure is used here as was recommended for injuries in Zones III and IV.

Following extensive injuries in Zone V, return of satisfactory active motion is the rule,[241] but it may take several months. With the utilization of proper exercise and splinting programs, the prognosis is good and tenolysis is not often necessary. The patient should be continually encouraged during this long, difficult period.

Complications in Zones II to V

Tendon rupture following primary repair is uncommon. It most commonly occurs around the tenth postoperative day, but can occur as late as 6 to 7 weeks. The preferred treatment is prompt reexploration and repair even in Zone II.[4] A useful digit can be salvaged, although tenolysis may be necessary at a later date.

Infection is rare and its treatment is discussed elsewhere. Failure of primary repair may necessitate secondary reconstruction, which is discussed in Chapter 51.

AVULSION OF PROFUNDUS TENDON INSERTION

Avulsion of the insertion of a profundus tendon is a relatively common injury, particularly in athletes. Several reports of flexor tendon ruptures[23,39,53,55,79,97,100,104,113,149,150,225,240,256,294] have been published since an early report by Von Zander[288] in 1891. Each has emphasized the necessity for prompt diagnosis and treatment, but some controversy remains regarding the management of late, untreated cases. In 1933, McMaster[209] stated that the tendon was the strongest link in the musculotendinous chain and that rupture rarely occurred in the substance of a normal tendon. He showed experimentally that a normal tendon usually ruptures at its bony insertion and less often at the musculotendinous junction. This injury occurs most frequently in young adult males participating in football, flag football, and rugby. However, it can occur at any age in either sex. The vast majority of cases occur in the ring finger (Fig. 50-17), but any digit can be involved. Often there is a delay in treatment because the nature and extent of the injury are not immediately recognized.

Gunter[104] postulated that the presence of a common flexor muscle belly of the profundus to the middle, ring, and little fingers makes the ring finger more susceptible to this injury. Manske and Lesker[184] have shown that the insertion of the profundus tendon is anatomically weaker in the ring finger than in the middle finger. I believe that the anatomic arrangement of the extensor tendons may also be a factor. When the MP joints of the middle and little fingers are flexed 90 degrees, the ring finger cannot be extended fully. The ring finger extensor tendon is pulled distally by the intertendinous connections between the extensor tendons. These act as check-reins to prevent passive extension of the ring finger, making it more susceptible to injury by hyperextension or to rupture of the tendon when the finger flexes against an unyielding object.

Many of these injuries occur in football, when, in an attempt to make a tackle, the fingers grasp the pants or jersey of the opposing player. As the little finger continues to flex and the opposing player pulls away, the ring finger, still caught in the pants or jersey, is extended forcibly while the profundus is maximally contracting. This can result in avulsion of the tendon insertion.[149,150] Often, the diagnosis is not made initially.

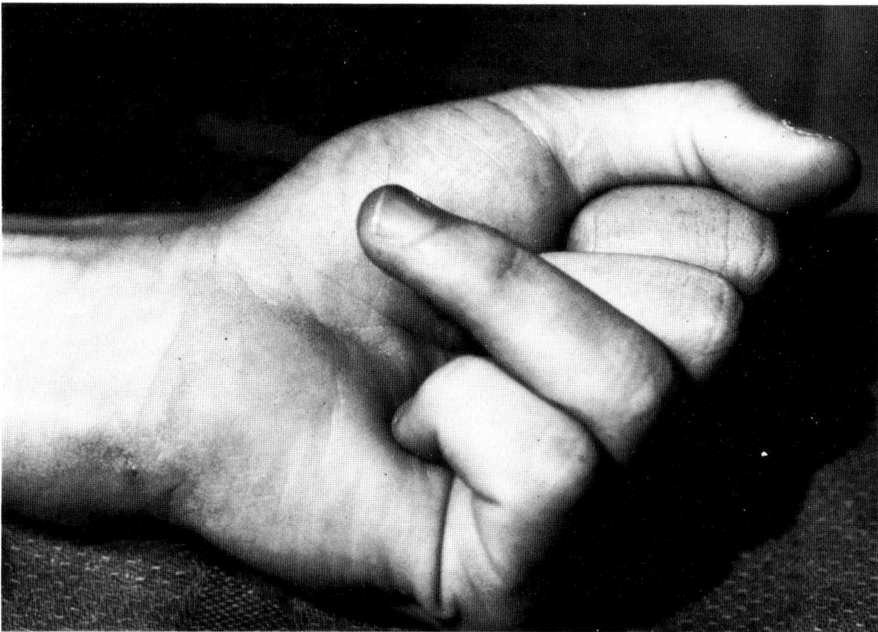

Fig. 50-17. Incomplete flexion of the ring finger seen in a patient with avulsion of the flexor digitorum profundus.

The player may continue in the game and not report his injury immediately. Unless the trainer, coach, or physician is aware of the entity, takes an accurate history, and tests specifically for active flexion at the DIP joint, the injury will not be recognized. Radiographs are usually normal, and the patient is told he has a "jammed finger." Unfortunately, delay in diagnosis and treatment can severely compromise the function of the finger. Acute vascular compromise of the finger has been reported after bony avulsion of the flexor digitorum profundus tendon.[100] Gibson and Manske recorded a case of isolated avulsion of the flexor digitorum superficialis tendon, and this is a rare injury indeed.[97]

The nutritional supply of the flexor tendons has been discussed elsewhere in this chapter. The main factors influencing prognosis and treatment of this injury include (1) the level to which the tendon retracts; (2) the remaining nutritional supply (vascular perfusion and synovial fluid diffusion) of the avulsed tendon; (3) the length of time between injury and treatment; and (4) the presence, size and location of a bony fragment seen radiographically.

Classification

Leddy and Packer[150] described three main types of avulsion of the profundus tendon insertion.

Type I

In Type I, the tendon retracts into the palm beneath the A1 pulley, the vincula rupture, and therefore, a substantial portion of the blood supply is lost. The diffusion of nutrients from the synovial fluid is also interrupted. There is no active flexion at the DIP joint level, and there is a tender mass in the palm. There is excellent flexion at the PIP joint. This tendon should be reinserted within 7 to 10 days before it becomes contracted (Fig. 50-18). This is the most rare type.

Type II

Type II is the most common type. The tendon retracts to the level of the PIP joint, leaving the vinculum at this level intact, thereby retaining more of its blood supply. Since the tendon remains in the sheath, presumably diffusion of nutrients from the synovial fluid continues. Occasionally, a small fleck of bone is avulsed with the tendon and can be seen on lateral radiographs at the PIP joint level (Fig. 50-19). There is no active flexion at the DIP joint, and there is pain, swelling, tenderness, and some loss of flexion at the PIP joint. This type is best treated by early reinsertion of the tendon into the distal phalanx. However, in contrast to Type I injuries, the tendon can be reinserted at a later date because it has retained a better nutritional supply and does not become too contracted. These can be repaired up to 3 or more months postinjury with a satisfactory result. It is not unusual for the tendon to first retract to the PIP joint level and later when the vinculum gives way, to slip into the palm, thus becoming a Type I injury.

Type III

In Type III, there is a large bony fragment. The A4 pulley catches the fragment and prevents proximal retraction. Both vincula are usually intact, and tendon length and nutrition are preserved. There is swelling, ecchymosis, and tenderness over the middle and distal phalanges, and inability to flex the DIP

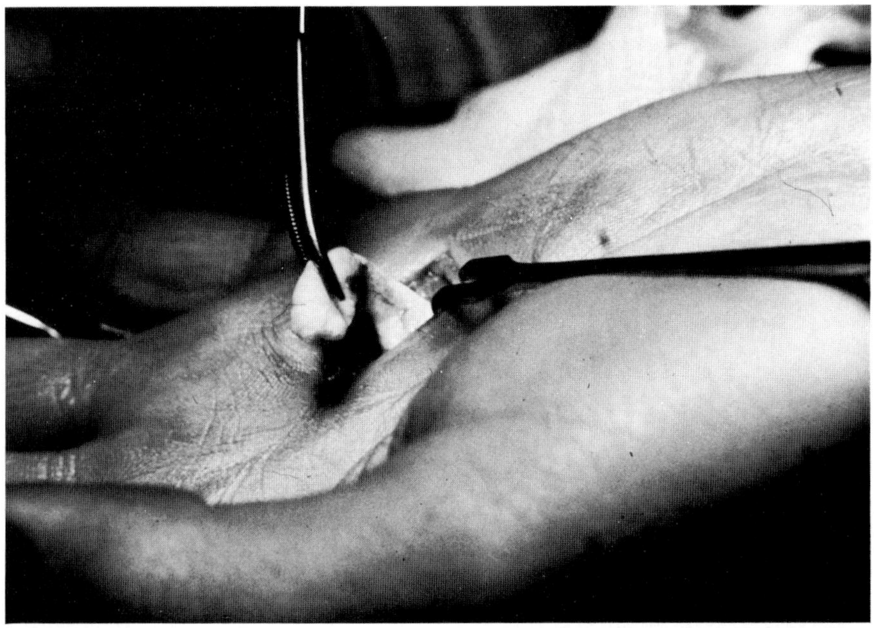

Fig. 50-18. A necrotic contracted avulsed tendon in the palm that cannot be reinserted. (From Leddy and Packer,[150] with permission.)

joint. A large bony fragment can be seen just proximal to the DIP joint on the lateral radiograph (Fig. 50-20) and may sometimes be palpated just proximal to the DIP joint crease. Early reinsertion of the fragment with internal fixation will give a satisfactory result. Robins and Dobyns[240] in 1975 and Smith[256] in 1981 each described a Type IIIA injury with simultaneous avulsion of the profundus tendon from the fracture fragment. This is an unusual injury (Fig. 50-21). In this instance, bony continuity should be restored by open reduction and internal fixation if possible. The avulsed flexor profundus tendon should then be treated as a Type I or Type II injury, depending on the level of retraction. Postoperative care is the same. Occasionally, there is a comminuted intraarticular fracture dislocation of the DIP joint with large bony avulsions of both the extensor and flexor tendon mechanisms. Open reduction and internal fixation with multiple small K-wires, some crossing the joint, is usually the treatment of choice but may be a very difficult procedure (Fig. 50-22).

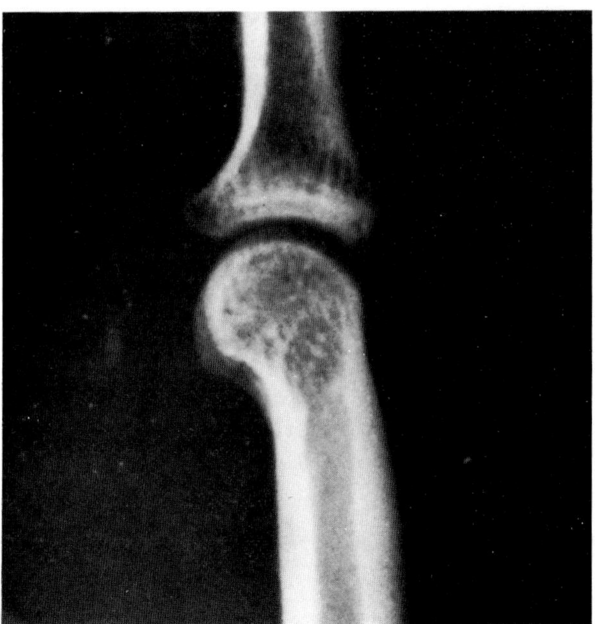

Fig. 50-19. The small bony fleck opposite the condyles of the proximal phalanx indicates the level to which the profundus tendon has retracted. (From Leddy and Packer,[150] with permission.)

Treatment

Most authors agree that early diagnosis and prompt reinsertion of the tendon is the treatment of choice.

Author's Preferred Method

Type I

A midlateral or palmar zigzag incision is made on the affected finger, exposing the flexor sheath from just proximal to the PIP joint to the area of insertion of the profundus tendon. A transverse incision is made in the sheath just distal to the A2 pulley. If the tendon is not at this level, it has retracted into the palm beneath the A1 pulley, and an incision is made in the palm at the base of the finger, paralleling the distal palmar crease. There is usually some hemorrhage within the sheath, and an incision is made here proximal to the A1 metacarpal pulley, exposing the distal end of the profundus tendon. A small pliable catheter, such as an infant feeding gastrostomy tube, is then passed retrograde beneath the sheath and pulleys and through the superficialis decussation to exit proximal to

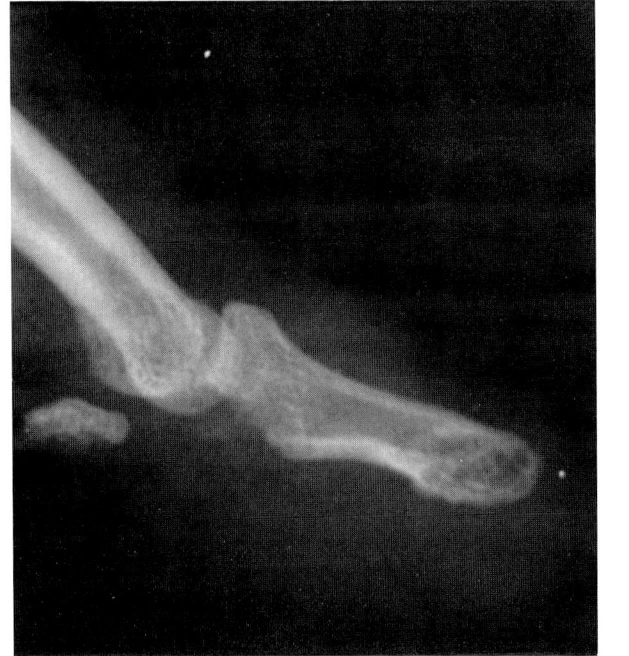

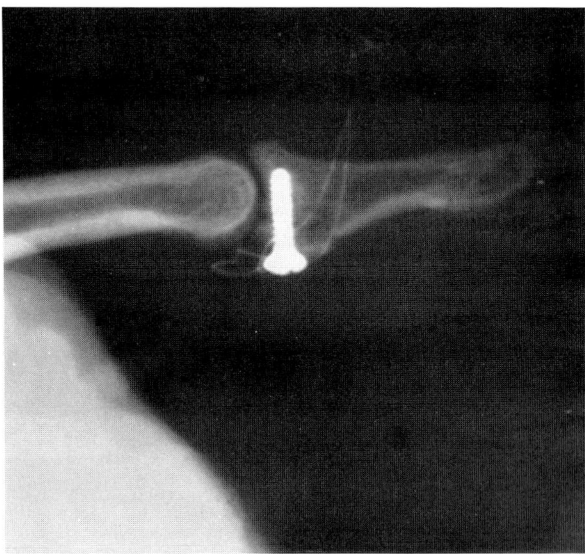

Fig. 50-20. Type III profundus tendon avulsion. **(A)** A large bony fragment held up at the A4 pulley. **(B)** After open reduction and internal fixation.

the A1 pulley through the incision previously made in the sheath. The distal end of the flexor tendon is then attached to the catheter with nonabsorbable sutures. The phalangeal portion of the tendon is handled as little as possible. When the catheter is pulled distally, the profundus tendon is threaded back beneath the pulleys and through the superficialis chiasm to the level of the previously made incision in the sheath distal to the A2 pulley. Alternatively, the technique of Sourmelis and McGrouther[259] may be utilized here (see page 1837). The distal phalanx is then exposed and an osteoperiosteal flap is elevated

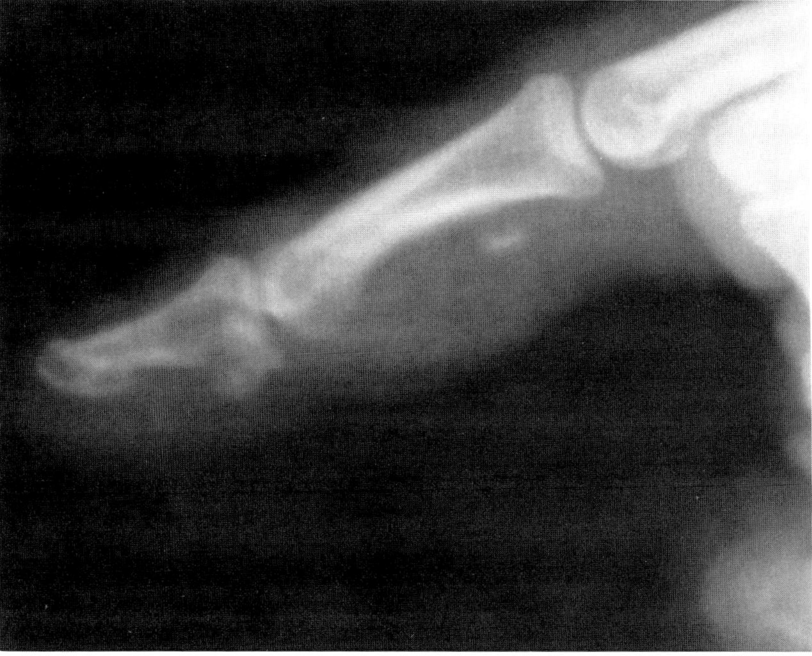

Fig. 50-21. Type IV profundus tendon avulsion. A large bony fragment at the base of distal phalanx and a small bony fragment just distal to the PIP joint. The profundus tendon is attached to the small fragment.

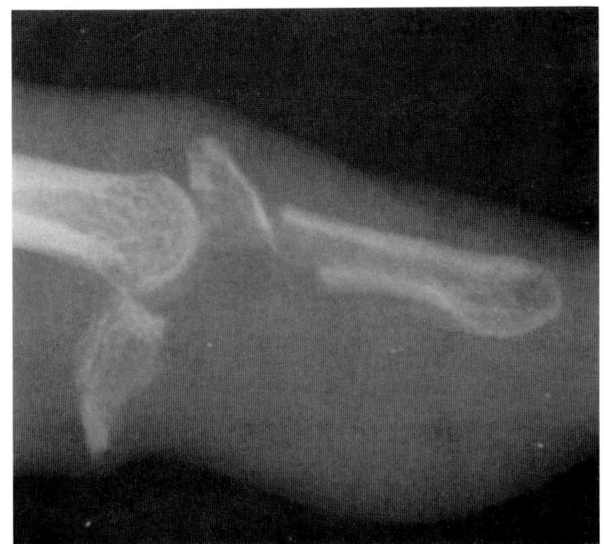

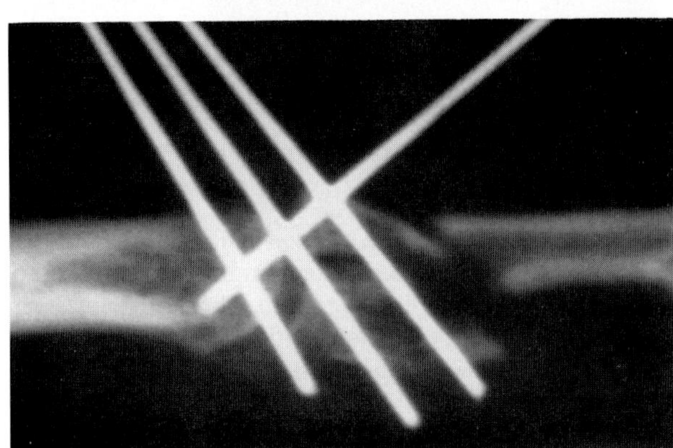

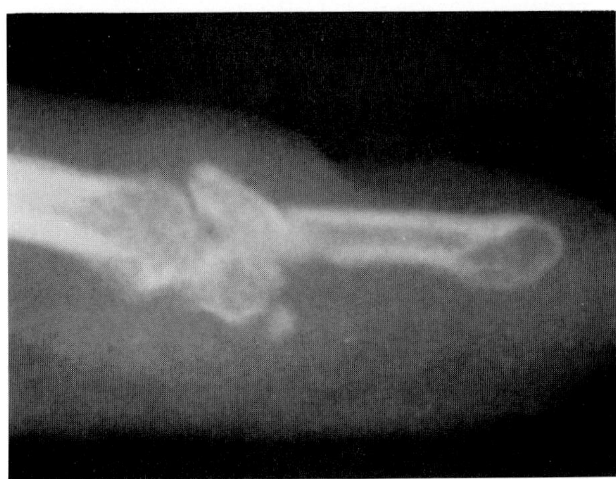

Fig. 50-22. **(A)** A comminuted intraarticular fracture—dislocation of the DIP joint. **(B)** After open reduction and internal fixation. **(C)** End result with 40 degrees active motion in the DIP joint.

for reinsertion of the tendon as described earlier in this chapter. The tendon is then passed distally through the remainder of the sheath and pulleys to the level of the distal phalanx. It is imperative to preserve the A4 pulley even though it may be difficult to pass the distal end of the avulsed tendon beneath this pulley. In order to accomplish this, the fan-shaped distal portion of the tendon may be sutured to itself to narrow its diameter. The tendon is then reinserted into the base of the distal phalanx through the raised osteoperiosteal flap with a 4–0 Prolene suture tied over a button (Fig. 50-23). In my experience, suturing the tendon to the surrounding periosteum and soft tissues following avulsion of the insertion is an unsatisfactory way of anchoring the tendon into the distal phalanx. Care must be taken not to damage the palmar plate of the DIP joint, which can cause a late flexion contracture.

A dorsal plaster splint is applied, holding the wrist in slight flexion, the MP joints in 60 to 70 degrees flexion, and the PIP and DIP joints in extension. Passive flexion exercises may be instituted early. The splint is removed at 3 weeks and active exercises are begun. The tendon suture and button may be removed at 3 to 4 weeks postoperatively. The remaining care is similar to that for other flexor tendon injuries.

Type II

In Type II injuries, a midlateral or zigzag incision is made on the affected finger, exposing the flexor tendon mechanism. A transverse incision is made in the sheath just distal to the A2 pulley. The tendon is usually found at this level, held in place by the long vinculum. If the injury is more than a few weeks old, any granulation tissue at the level of the PIP joint should be excised and a full passive range of motion restored prior to reinsertion. The tendon should be passed beneath the sheath and pulleys to the level of the distal phalanx and reinserted as described above. Postoperative care is the same. It is sometimes possible to repair these a few months postinjury with a satisfactory result. A Type II injury often converts to a Type I injury when the tendon slips away from the level of the PIP joint into the palm, thus rupturing the long vinculum. It is then treated as a Type I injury.

Type III

In Type III injuries, there is usually a large bony fragment. There may be some comminution of the fragment, a comminuted intraarticular fracture of the DIP joint, or both. The A4 pulley prevents retraction of the bony fragment beyond the distal portion of the middle phalanx. Open reduction and internal fixation of the fragment will usually give a satisfactory result (see Fig. 50-20). Postoperative care is the same. Active motion is instituted when bony healing permits.

Type IIIA

In Type IIIA injuries, there is a large bony fragment held up at the A4 pulley, but, in addition, the tendon has pulled away from this bony fragment and will be found either at the level of the PIP joint or in the palm (see Fig. 50-21). The treatment is open reduction and internal fixation of the large bony fragment and then reinsertion of the tendon into the base of the distal phalanx. Postoperative care is the same as in Type III injuries.

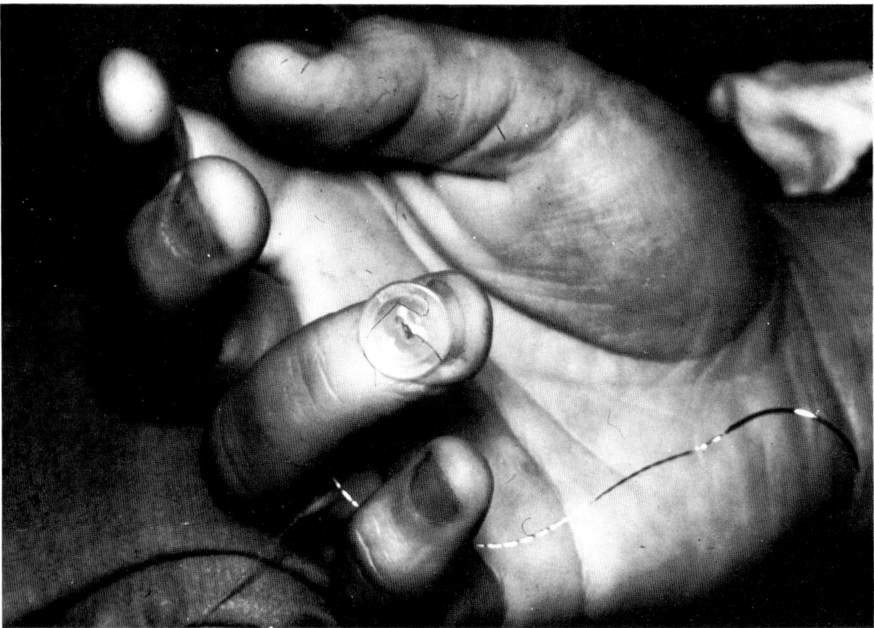

Fig. 50-23. Normal tension restored to the ring finger after reinsertion of an avulsed profundus tendon.

Late Treatment

There is still some disagreement regarding the management of old, untreated cases that are too late for reinsertion. Those that are relatively asymptomatic are best left alone, in my opinion. It is rare to see limitation of motion at the PIP joint 6 months or more postinjury. If there is no instability at the DIP joint and no special requirement for active flexion at this joint, no surgical treatment is indicated. If there is instability of the DIP joint with weakness of pinch or recurrent dorsal dislocation, fusion or tenodesis of this joint should be considered. Following this injury, tenodesis can be a difficult procedure. A portion of the retracted tendon may be utilized, but it has to be inserted into both the distal and middle phalanges, since there is no tendon remaining on the distal phalanx. It can also stretch out with the passage of time. In my opinion, fusion is preferable, since it provides a stable joint and it will not interfere with the function of the superficialis tendon (Fig. 50-24). If there is a tender lump in the palm, the retracted tendon can be excised at the time of fusion.

The use of a free flexor tendon graft in the presence of an intact, functioning superficialis tendon has been reported by several authors.[26,53,55,98,104,125,205,232,261] Pulvertaft recommended it only for the index and middle fingers in children.[232] Goldner and Coonrad believed that it was justifiable in the growing child or young adult.[98] Stark et al recommended this procedure only in carefully selected patients.[261] They suggested that the ideal age is between 10 and 21 years and that it is worthwhile for the index and middle fingers, but rarely for the little finger. The procedure was recommended for the ring finger only when there was a specific need. McClinton, Curtis and Wilgis,[205] in a series of 100 cases, believed that age was not a contraindication to this operation in properly motivated patients. Unless the profundus tendon remained in the superficialis decussation, they placed their tendon graft *around* rather than through the superficialis tendon. Other authors have reported good to excellent results with two-stage flexor tendon grafting following avulsion of the profundus tendon insertion.[113,286,298] Whether it is performed in one or two stages, a flexor tendon graft in the presence of an intact, functioning superficialis tendon is an exacting procedure that should not be undertaken by the occasional hand surgeon. Most authors agree that it can be worthwhile in the index and middle fingers of a young person. As stated earlier, 75 percent or more of the

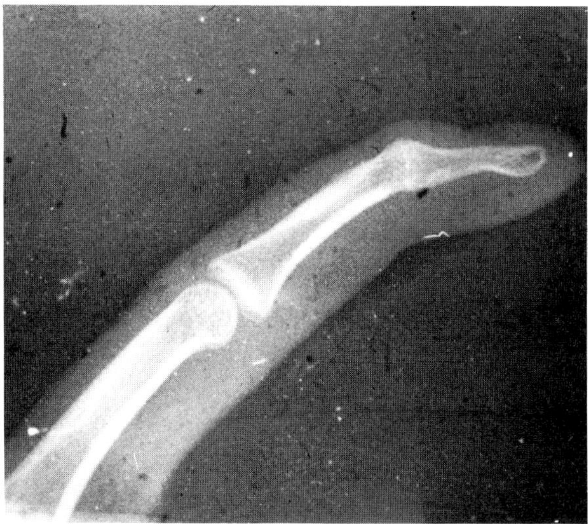

Fig. 50-24. In some cases, fusion of the DIP joint may be the preferred treatment for late flexor profundus avulsion (see text).

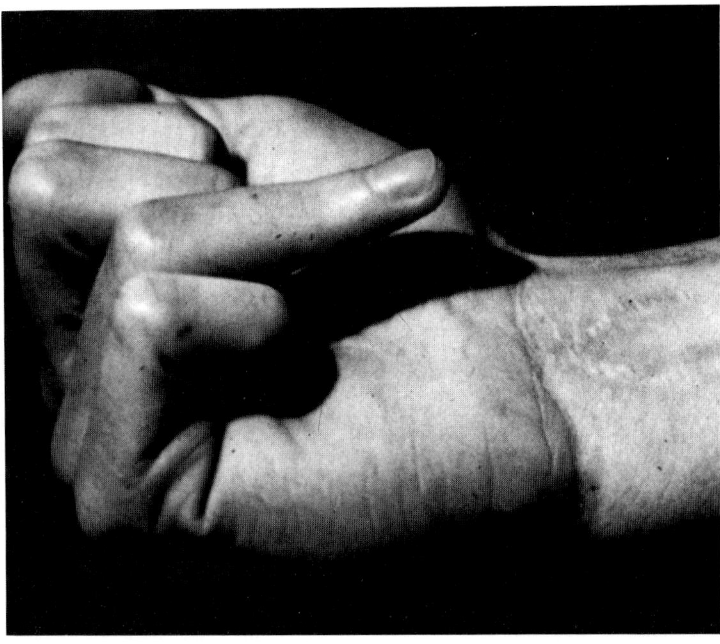

Fig. 50-25. Following avulsion of the flexor digitorum profundus tendon of the ring finger, this patient had six separate surgical procedures, including two attempts at tendon grafting. He has now lost his pulley mechanism, and has hyperextension at the DIP joint and some loss of flexion at the PIP joint. (From Leddy,[149] with permission.)

flexor tendon avulsion injuries occur in the ring finger. Some people, such as musicians or skilled technicians, may require active flexion at the DIP joint of the ring finger and in these instances, the procedure may be indicated. However, in addition to all of the possible complications associated with tendon grafting, this operation may interfere with the previously normal function of the superficialis tendon, and both active and passive motion may be lost at the PIP joint, making the finger worse than it was before (Fig. 50-25). The possible complications should be carefully understood by the patient before the physician embarks on any such reconstruction.

In those patients who are seen and treated early with reinsertion of the tendon, a satisfactory result can generally be anticipated. There may be a 10- to 15-degree loss of extension at the DIP joint, but grip strength approaches normal. Grip strength in those patients with fusion or tenodesis will be no different than in the late, untreated group. A fusion or tenodesis, although improving stability of the DIP joint, cannot be expected to improve strength. A successful tendon graft will stabilize the DIP joint and increase grip strength.

REFERENCES

1. Adamson JE: Suture materials and tissue replacements. p. 279. In Symposium on Reconstructive Hand Surgery. CV Mosby, St. Louis, 1974
2. Adamson JE, Srouji S, Mladick R, Horton C: Tissue reaction to contemporary tendon suture. J Bone Joint Surg 53A:815, 1971
3. Adamson JE, Wilson JN: The history of flexor tendon grafting. J Bone Joint Surg 43A:709, 1961
4. Allen BN, Frykman GK, Unsell RS, Wood VE: Ruptured flexor tendon tenorrhaphies in Zone II: Repair and rehabilitation. J Hand Surg 12A:18-21, 1987
5. Amadio PC, Hunter JM, Jaeger SH, Wehbe MA, Schneider LH: The effect of vincular injury on the results of flexor tendon surgery in Zone 2. J Hand Surg 10A:626-632, 1985
6. Amiel D, Ishizue K, Billings E Jr, Wiig M, Vande Berg J, Akeson WH, Gelberman R: Hyaluronan in flexor tendon repair. J Hand Surg 14A:837-843, 1989
7. An-Min L, Shi-Bi L: Reconstruction of sheath with fascial graft in flexor tendon repair. An experimental study. J Hand Surg 16B:179-184, 1991
8. Anzel SH, Lipscomb PR, Grindlay JH: Construction of artificial tendon sheaths in dogs. Am J Surg 101:355, 1961
9. Armenta E, Fisher J: Anatomy of flexor pollicis longus vinculum system. J Hand Surg 9A:210-212, 1984
10. Armenta E, Lehrman A: The vincula to the flexor tendons of the hand. J Hand Surg 5:127-134, 1980
11. Arons MS: Purposeful delay of the primary repair of cut flexor tendons in "some man's land" in children. Plast Reconstr Surg 53:638-642, 1974
12. Ashley FL, Polak T, Stone RS, Marmor L: An evaluation of the healing process in avian and mammalian digital-flexor tendons following the application of an artificial tendon sheath (silastic) (abstract). J Bone Joint Surg 44A:1038, 1962
13. Ashley FL, Stone RS, Alonso-Artieda M, Syverud JM, Edwards JW, Sloan RF, Mooney SA: Experimental and clinical studies on the application of monomolecular cellulose filter tubes to create artificial tendon sheath in digits. Plast Reconstr Surg 23:526-534, 1959
14. Ashley FL, Stone RS, Edwards JW, Sloan RF: Further studies on the application of monomolecular cellulose filter tubes to create artificial tendon sheaths in the hand and wrist. West J Surg 68:156, 1960
15. Azar CA, Culver JE, Fleegler EJ: Blood supply of the flexor pollicis longus tendon. J Hand Surg 8:471-475, 1983

16. Azar CA, Fleegler TL, Culver JE: Dynamic anatomy of the flexor pulley system of the fingers and thumb (abstract). J Hand Surg 9A:595, 1984
17. Bassett AL, Carroll RE: Formation of tendon sheath by silicone rod implants (abstract). J Bone Joint Surg 45A:884, 1963
18. Becker H: Primary repair of flexor tendons in the hand without immobilization—preliminary report. Hand 10:37-47, 1978
19. Becker H, Davidoff M: Eliminating the gap in flexor tendon surgery. A new method of suture. Hand 9:306, 1977
20. Becker H, Orak F, Duponselle E: Early active motion following a beveled technique of flexor tendon repair. Report on fifty cases. J Hand Surg 4:454-460, 1979
21. Bell JL, Mason ML, Koch SL, Stromberg WB: Injuries to flexor tendons of the hand in children. J Bone Joint Surg 40A:1220-1230, 1958
22. Bilos ZJ, Hui PWT, Stamelos S: Trigger finger following partial flexor tendon laceration. Hand 9:232, 1977
23. Blazina ME, Lane C: Rupture of the insertion of the flexor digitorum profundus tendon in student athletes. J Am Coll Health Assoc 14:248, 1966
24. Bolton H: Primary repair of the severed flexor tendon. Hand 1:102, 1969
25. Bolton H: Primary tendon repair. Hand 2:56, 1970
26. Bora FW Jr: Profundus tendon grafting with unimpaired sublimus function in children. Clin Orthop 71:118-123, 1970
27. Bora FW Jr, Lane JM, Prockop DJ: Inhibitors of collagen biosynthesis as a means of controlling scar formation in tendon injury. J Bone Joint Surg 54A:1501-1508, 1972
28. Boyes JH: Immediate vs. delayed repair of the digital flexor tendons. Ann West Med Surg 1:145, 1947
29. Boyes JH: Flexor tendon grafts in the fingers and thumb. J Bone Joint Surg 32A:489-499, 1950
30. Boyes JH: Operative technique of digital flexor tendon grafts, p. 263. AAOS Instr Course Lectures. Vol 10. CV Mosby, St. Louis, 1953
31. Boyes JH: Evaluation of results of digital flexor tendon grafts. Am J Surg 89:1116, 1955
32. Boyes JH: Why tendon repair? J Bone Joint Surg 41A:577, 1959
33. Boyes JH: The primary treatment of the injured hand. Kansas City Med J 35:14, 1959
34. Boyes JH: Incisions in the hand. Am J Orthop 4:308, 1962
35. Boyes JH: Bunnell's Surgery of the Hand. 5th Ed. JB Lippincott, Philadelphia, 1970
36. Boyes JH: The philosophy of tendon surgery. pp. 1-5. In AAOS Symposium of Tendon Surgery in the Hand. CV Mosby, St. Louis, 1975
37. Boyes JH, Stark HH: Flexor tendon grafts in the fingers and thumb. A study of factors influencing results in 1000 cases. J Bone Joint Surg 53A:1332-1342, 1971
38. Boyes JH, Stark HH: Flexor tendon grafts in the fingers and thumb. p. 85. In Verdan C (ed): Tendon Surgery of the Hand. Churchill Livingstone, Edinburgh, 1979
39. Boyes JH, Wilson JN, Smith JW: Flexor tendon ruptures in the forearm and hand. J Bone Joint Surg 42A:637-646, 1960
40. Brand PW: Tendon grafting. J Bone Joint Surg 43B:444-453, 1961
41. Brockis JG: The blood supply of the flexor and extensor tendons of the fingers in man. J Bone Joint Surg 35B:131-138, 1953
42. Brunelli G, Vigasio A, Brunelli F: Slip knot flexor tendon suture in Zone II allowing immediate mobilization. Hand 15:352-358, 1983
43. Bruner JM: The zig-zag volar-digital incision for flexor tendon surgery. Plast Reconstr Surg 40:571-574, 1967
44. Bruner JM: Surgical exposure of flexor tendons in the hand. Ann R Coll Surg Engl 53:84, 1973
45. Bunnell S: Repair of tendons in the fingers and description of two new instruments. Surg Gynecol Obstet 26:103-110, 1918
46. Bunnell S: Primary repair of severed tendons. The use of stainless steel wire. Am J Surg 47:502, 1940
47. Bunnell S: The early treatment of hand injuries. J Bone Joint Surg 33A:807-811, 1951
48. Bunnell S: Surgery of the Hand. 3rd Ed. JB Lippincott, Philadelphia, 1956
49. Burman MS: The use of a nylon sheath in the secondary repairs of torn finger flexor tendons. Bull Hosp Joint Dis 5:122, 1944
50. Burton RI: Severed tendons and nerves distal to the metacarpophalangeal joint. p. 117. In Symposium on Reconstructive Hand Surgery. CV Mosby, St. Louis, 1974
51. Cannon NM, Strickland JW: Therapy following flexor tendon surgery. Hand Clin 1(1):147-165, 1985
52. Caplan HS, Hunter JM, Merklin RJ: Intrinsic vascularization of flexor tendons. pp. 48-58. In AAOS Symposium on Tendon Surgery in the Hand. CV Mosby, St. Louis, 1975
53. Carroll RE, Match RM: Avulsion of the profundus tendon insertion. J Trauma 10:1109, 1970
54. Carter SJ, Mersheimer WL: Deferred primary tendon repair. Results in 27 cases. Ann Surg 164:913, 1966
55. Chang WH, Thoms OJ, White WL: Avulsion injury of the long flexor tendons. Plast Reconstr Surg 50:260, 1972
56. Chaplin DM: The vascular anatomy within normal tendons, divided tendons, free tendon grafts and pedicle tendon grafts in rabbits. A microradioangiographic study. J Bone Joint Surg 55B:369-389, 1973
57. Chow JA, Thomes LJ, Dovelle S, Milnor WH, Seyfer AE, Smith AC: A combined regimen of controlled motion following flexor tendon repair in "no man's land." Plast Reconstr Surg 79:447-453, 1987
58. Chow JA, Thomes LJ, Dovelle S, Monsivais J, Milnor WH, Jackson JP: Controlled motion rehabilitation after flexor tendon repair and grafting. A multi-centre study. J Bone Joint Surg 70B:591-595, 1988
59. Chow SP, Hooper G, Chan CW: The healing of freeze-dried rabbit flexor tendon in a synovial fluid environment. Hand 15:136-142, 1983
60. Chow SP, Stephens MM, Ngai WK, So YC, Pun WK, Chu M, Crosby C: A splint for controlled active motion after flexor tendon repair. Design, mechanical testing, and preliminary clinical results. J Hand Surg 15A:645-651, 1990
61. Citron ND, Forster A: Dynamic splinting following flexor tendon repair. J Hand Surg 12B:96-100, 1987
62. Cleveland M: Restoration of the digital portion of a flexor tendon and sheath in the hand. J Bone Joint Surg 15:762, 1933
63. Colville J, Callison JR, White WL: Role of mesotendon in tendon blood supply. Plast Reconstr Surg 43:53-60, 1969
64. Craver JM, Madden JW, Peacock EE Jr: Biological control of physical properties of tendon adhesions: Effect of Beta-Aminopropionitrile in chickens. Ann Surg 167:697, 1968
65. Cullen KW, Tolhurst P, Lang D, Page RE: Flexor tendon repair in Zone 2 followed by controlled active mobilisation. J Hand Surg 14B:392-395, 1989
66. Douglas LG, Jackson SH, Lindsay WK: The effects of Dexamethasone, Norethandrolone, Promethazine and tension relieving procedure on collagen synthesis in healing flexor tendons as estimated by tritiated proline uptake studies. Can J Surg 10:36, 1967
67. Doyle JR: Anatomy of the finger flexor tendon sheath and pulley system. J Hand Surg 13A:473-484, 1988
68. Doyle JR: Anatomy of the flexor tendon sheath and pulley system: A current review. J Hand Surg 14A:349-351, 1989

69. Doyle JR: Anatomy and function of the palmar aponeurosis pulley. J Hand Surg 15A:78-82, 1990
70. Doyle JR, Blythe W: The finger flexor tendon sheath and pulleys: anatomy and reconstruction. pp. 81-87. In AAOS Symposium on Tendon Surgery in the Hand. CV Mosby, St. Louis, 1975
71. Doyle JR, Blythe WF: Anatomy of the flexor tendon sheath and pulleys of the thumb. J Hand Surg 2:149-151, 1977
72. Duran RJ, Houser RG: Controlled passive motion following flexor tendon repair in zones 2 and 3. pp. 105-114. In AAOS Symposium on Tendon Surgery in the Hand. CV Mosby, St. Louis, 1975
73. Edwards DAW: The blood supply and lymphatic drainage of tendons. J Anat 80:147, 1946
74. Edwards EA: Organization of the small arteries of the hand and digits. Am J Surg 99:837, 1960
75. Eiken O, Hagberg L, Rank P: The healing process of transplanted digital tendon sheath synovium. Scand J Plast Reconstr Surg 12:225-229, 1978
76. Ejeskar A, Irstram V: Elongation in profundus tendon repair. Scand J Plast Reconstr Surg 15:61, 1981
77. Entin MA: Philosophy of tendon repair. Orthop Clin North Am 4:859, 1973
78. Feehan LM, Beauchene JG: Early tensile properties of healing chicken flexor tendons: Early controlled passive motion versus postoperative immobilization. J Hand Surg 15A:63-68, 1990
79. Folmar RC, Nelson CL, Phalen GS: Ruptures of the flexor tendons in hands of non rheumatoid patients. J Bone Joint Surg 54A:579, 1972
80. Furlow LT Jr: Early active motion in flexor tendon healing. J Bone Joint Surg 54A:911, 1972
81. Furlow LT: Role of tendon tissues in tendon healing. Plast Reconstr Surg 57:39, 1976
82. Garner WL, McDonald JA, Kuhn C III, Weeks PM: Autonomous healing of chicken flexor tendons in vitro. J Hand Surg 13A:697-700, 1988
83. Gelberman RH, Amiel D, Gonsalves M, Woo S, Akeson WH: The influence of protected passive mobilization on the healing of flexor tendons: A biochemical and microangiographic study. Hand 13:120-128, 1981
84. Gelberman RH, Botte MJ, Spiegelman JJ, Akeson WH: The excursion and deformation of repaired flexor tendon treated with protected early motion. J Hand Surg 11A:106-110, 1986
85. Gelberman RH, Khabie V, Cahill CJ: The revascularization of healing flexor tendons in the digital sheath. A vascular injection study in dogs. J Bone Joint Surg 73A:868-881, 1991
86. Gelberman RH, Manske PR: Factors influencing flexor tendon adhesions. Hand Clin 1(1):35-42, 1985
87. Gelberman RH, Manske PR, Akeson WH, Woo SL-Y, Lundborg G, Amiel D: Flexor tendon repair. J Orthop Res 4:119-128, 1986
88. Gelberman RH, Manske PR, Vande Berg JS, Lesker PA, Akeson WH: Flexor tendon repair *in vitro:* Comparative histologic study of the rabbit, chicken, dog, and monkey. J Orthop Res 2:39-48, 1984
89. Gelberman RH, Menon J, Gonsalves M, Akeson WH: The effects of mobilization on vascularization of healing flexor tendons in dogs. Clin Orthop 153:283-289, 1980
90. Gelberman RH, Nunley JA II, Osterman AL, Breen TF, Dimick MP, Woo SL-Y: Influences of the protected passive mobilization interval on flexor tendon healing. A prospective randomized clinical study. Clin Orthop 264:189-196, 1991
91. Gelberman RH, Siegel DB, Woo SL-Y, Amiel D, Takai S, Lee D: Healing of digital flexor tendons: Importance of the interval from injury to repair. A biomechanical, biochemical, and morphological study in dogs. J Bone Joint Surg 73A:66-75, 1991
92. Gelberman RH, Steinberg D, Amiel D, Akeson W: Fibroblast chemotaxis after tendon repair. J Hand Surg 16A:686-693, 1991
93. Gelberman RH, Vande Berg JS, Lundborg GN, Akeson WH: Flexor tendon healing and restoration of the gliding surface. An ultrastructural study in dogs. J Bone Joint Surg 65A:70-80, 1983
94. Gelberman RH, Woo SL-Y, Amiel D, Horibe S, Lee D: Influences of flexor sheath continuity and early motion on tendon healing in dogs. J Hand Surg 15A:69-77, 1990
95. Gelberman RH, Woo SL-Y, Lothringer K, Akeson WH, Amiel D: Effects of early intermittent passive mobilization on healing canine flexor tendons. J Hand Surg 7:170-175, 1982
96. Gerbino PG II, Saldana MJ, Westerbeck P, Schacherer TG: Complications experienced in the rehabilitation of Zone I flexor tendon injuries with dynamic traction splinting. J Hand Surg 16A:680-686, 1991
97. Gibson CT, Manske PR: Isolated avulsion of a flexor digitorum superficialis tendon insertion. J Hand Surg 12A:601-602, 1987
98. Goldner JL, Coonrad RW: Tendon grafting of the flexor profundus in the presence of a completely or partially intact flexor sublimis. J Bone Joint Surg 51A:527-532, 1969
99. Gonzales RI: Experimental tendon repair within the flexor tunnels: Use of polyethylene tubes for improvement of function results in the dog. Surgery 26:181, 1949
100. Gordon L, Monsanto EH: Acute vascular compromise after avulsion of the distal phalanx with the flexor digitorum profundus tendon. J Hand Surg 12A:259-261, 1987
101. Goss CM: Gray's Anatomy. 27th Ed. Lea & Febiger, Philadelphia, 1959
102. Graham MF, Becker H, Cohen IK, Merritt W, Diegelmann RF: Intrinsic tendon fibroplasia; Documentation by *in vitro* studies. J Orthop Res 1:251-256, 1984
103. Green WL, Niebauer JJ: Results of primary and secondary flexor tendon repairs in no man's land. J Bone Joint Surg 56A:1216, 1974
104. Gunter GS: Traumatic avulsion of the insertion of flexor digitorum profundus. Aust NZ J Surg 30:1, 1960
105. Haddad RJ Jr, Kester MA, McCluskey GM, Brunet ME, Cook SD: Comparative mechanical analysis of a looped-suture tendon repair. J Hand Surg 13A:709-713, 1988
106. Hagberg L, Selvik G: Tendon excursion and dehiscence during early controlled mobilization after flexor tendon repair in Zone II: An x-ray stereophotogrammetric analysis. J Hand Surg 16A:669-680, 1991
107. Harrison SH: Repair of digital flexor tendon injuries in the hand. Br J Plast Surg 14:211, 1961
108. Hauge MF: The results of tendon suture of the hand. A review of 500 patients. Acta Orthop Scand 24:258, 1955
109. Hergenroeder PT, Gelberman RH, Akeson WH: The vascularity of the flexor pollicis longus tendon. Clin Orthop 162:298-303, 1982
110. Herzog M, Lindsay WK, McCain WG: Effect of beta-aminoproprionitrile on adhesions following digital flexor tendon repair in chickens. Surg Forum 21:509-511, 1970
111. Holm CL, Embick RP: Anatomical considerations in the primary treatment of tendon injuries of the hand. J Bone Joint Surg 41A:599-608, 1959
112. Holms W: Primary suture of flexor tendons in the danger zone. Hand 6:17, 1974
113. Honner R: The late management of the isolated lesion of the flexor digitorum profundus tendon. Hand 7:171-174, 1975
114. Honner R, Meares A: A review of 100 flexor tendon reconstructions with prosthesis. Hand 9:226-231, 1977
115. Hunter JM: Artificial tendons—early development and application. Am J Surg 109:325, 1965
116. Hunter JM: Anatomy of flexor tendons—pulley, vincular, syno-

via, and vascular structures. pp. 65-92. In Spinner M (ed): Kaplan's Functional and Surgical Anatomy of the Hand. 3rd Ed. JB Lippincott, Philadelphia, 1984
117. Hunter JM, Cook JF Jr: The pulley system: rationale for reconstruction. pp. 94-102. In Strickland JW, Steichen JB (eds): Difficult Problems in Hand Surgery. CV Mosby, St. Louis, 1982
118. Hunter JM, Cook JF, Ochai N, Konikoff JJ, Merklin RJ, Mackin GA: The pulley system. J Hand Surg 5:283, 1980
119. Hunter JM, Salisbury RE: Use of gliding artificial implants to produce tendon sheaths. Techniques and results in children. Plast Reconstr Surg 45:564-572, 1970
120. Hunter JM, Salisbury RE: Flexor tendon reconstruction in severely damaged hands. J Bone Joint Surg 53A:829-858, 1971
121. Idler RS: Anatomy and biomechanics of the digital flexor tendons. Hand Clin 1(1):3-11, 1985
122. Idler RS, Strickland JW: The effects of pulley resection on the biomechanics of the proximal interphalangeal joint (abstract). J Hand Surg 9A:595, 1984
123. Ikuta Y, Tsuge K: Postoperative results of looped nylon suture used in injuries of the digital flexor tendons. J Hand Surg 10B:67-72, 1985
124. Iselin M: "Delayed emergency" in fresh wounds of the hand. Proc R Soc Med 51:713, 1958
125. Jaffe S, Weckesser E: Profundus tendon grafting with the sublimis intact. J Bone Joint Surg 49A:1298-1308, 1967
126. Jensen EG, Weilby A: Primary tendon suture in the thumb and fingers. Hand 6:297, 1974
127. Kain CC, Russell JE, Burri R, Dunlap J, McCarthy J, Manske PR: The effect of vascularization on avian flexor tendon repair. A biochemical study. Clin Orthop 233:295-303, 1988
128. Kaplan EB: Functional and Surgical Anatomy of the Hand. 2nd Ed. JB Lippincott, Philadelphia, 1965
129. Kelly AP: Primary tendon repairs. A study of 789 consecutive tendon severances. J Bone Joint Surg 41A:581-598, 1959
130. Kessler FB, Epstein MJ, Lannick D, Maher D, Pappu S: Fascia patch graft for a digital flexor sheath defect over primary tendon repair in the chicken. J Hand Surg 11A:241-245, 1986
131. Kessler I: The "grasping" technique for tendon repair. Hand 5:253-255, 1973
132. Kessler I, Nissimi F: Primary repair without immobilization of flexor tendon division within the digital sheath. Acta Orthop Scand 40:587, 1969
133. Ketchum LD: Effects of triamcinolone on tendon healing and function. A laboratory study. Plast Reconstr Surg 47:471-484, 1971
134. Ketchum LD: Primary tendon healing: A review. J Hand Surg 2:428-435, 1977
135. Ketchum LD: Suture materials and suture techniques used in tendon repair. Hand Clin 1(1):43-53, 1985
136. Ketchum LD, Martin NL, Kappel DA: Experimental evaluation of factors affecting the strength of tendon repairs. Plast Reconstr Surg 59:708, 1977
137. Kleinert HE, Bennett JB: Digital pulley reconstruction employing the always present rim of the previous pulley. J Hand Surg 3:297, 1978
138. Kleinert HE, Forshew FC, Cohen MJ: Repair of zone 1 flexor tendon injuries. pp. 115-122. In AAOS Symposium on Tendon Surgery in the Hand. CV Mosby, St. Louis, 1975
139. Kleinert HE, Kutz JE, Ashbell TS, Martinez E: Primary repair of lacerated flexor tendon in no man's land (abstract). J Bone Joint Surg 49A:577, 1967
140. Kleinert HE, Kutz JE, Atasoy E, Stormo A: Primary repair of flexor tendons. Orthop Clin North Am 4:865, 1973
141. Kleinert HE, Kutz JE, Cohen MJ: Primary repair of zone 2 flexor tendon lacerations. pp. 91-104. In AAOS Symposium on Tendon Surgery in the Hand. CV Mosby, St. Louis, 1975
142. Kleinert HE, Smith DJ: Primary and secondary repairs of flexor and extensor tendon injuries. In Flynn JE (ed): Hand Surgery. 3rd Ed. Williams & Wilkins, Baltimore, 1982
143. Kleinert HE, Verdan C: Report of the Committee on Tendon Injuries. J Hand Surg 8:794-798, 1983
144. Kleinert HE, Weiland AJ: Primary repair of flexor tendon lacerations in Zone II. pp. 71-75. In Verdan C (ed): Tendon Surgery of the Hand. Churchill Livingstone, Edinburgh, 1979
145. Koch SL: Division of the flexor tendons within the digital sheath. Surg Gynecol Obstet 78:9-22, 1944
146. Kulick MI, Smith S, Hadler K: Oral ibuprofen: Evaluation of its effect on peritendinous adhesions and the breaking strength of tenorrhaphy. J Hand Surg 11A:110-120, 1986
147. Lane JM, Black J, Bora FW Jr: Gliding function following flexor-tendon injury. A biomechanical study of rat tendon function. J Bone Joint Surg 58A:985-990, 1976
148. Lane JM, Bora FW Jr, Black J: Cis-hydroxyproline limits work necessary to flex a digit after tendon injury. Clin Orthop 109:193, 1975
149. Leddy JP: Avulsions of the flexor digitorum profundus. Hand Clin 1(1):77-83, 1985
150. Leddy JP, Packer JW: Avulsion of the profundus tendon insertion in athletes. J Hand Surg 2:66, 1977
151. Lee H: Double loop locking suture: A technique of tendon repair for early active mobilization. Part I: Evaluation of technique and experimental study and Part II: Clinical experience. J Hand Surg 15A:945-958, 1990
152. Leffert RD, Weiss C, Athanasoulis C: The vincula. J Bone Joint Surg 56A:1191, 1974
153. Lexer E: Verwethung des freien Sehnetransplantation. Arch Klin Chir 98:818, 1912
154. Lin G-T, Amadio PC, An K-N, Cooney WP: Functional anatomy of the human digital flexor pulley system. J Hand Surg 14A:949-956, 1989
155. Lin G-T, An K-N, Amadio PC, Cooney WP III: Biomechanical studies of running suture for flexor tendon repair in dogs. J Hand Surg 13A:553-558, 1988
156. Lindsay WK: Tendon healing: A continuing experimental approach. pp. 35-39. In Verdan C (ed): Tendon Surgery of the Hand. Churchill Livingstone, Edinburgh, 1979
157. Lindsay WK, Birch JR: The fibroblast in flexor tendon healing. Plast Reconstr Surg 34:223-232, 1964
158. Lindsay WK, McDougall EP: Direct digital flexor tendon repair. Plast Reconstr Surg 26:613-621, 1960
159. Lindsay WK, Thomson HG: Digital flexor tendons: An experimental study. Part I. The significance of each component of the flexor mechanism in tendon healing. Br J Plast Surg 12:289-316, 1959
160. Lindsay WK, Thomson HG, Walker FG: Digital flexor tendons: An experimental study. Part II. The significance of a gap occurring at the line of suture. Br J Plast Surg 13:1-9, 1960
161. Lindsay WK, Tustanoff ER, Birdsell DC: The uptake of tritiated proline in regenerating tendon. Surg Forum 15:459, 1964
162. Lister GD: Reconstruction of pulleys employing extensor retinaculum. J Hand Surg 4:461-464, 1979
163. Lister GD: Incision and closure of the flexor tendon sheath during tendon repair. Hand 15:123-135, 1983
164. Lister G: Indications and techniques for repair of the flexor tendon sheath. Hand Clin 1(1):85-95, 1985
165. Lister GD, Kleinert HE, Kutz JE, Atasoy E: Primary flexor tendon repair followed by immediate controlled mobilization. J Hand Surg 2:441-451, 1977

166. Lister GD, Tonkin M: The results of primary flexor tendon repair with closure of the tendon sheath (abstract). J Hand Surg 11A:767, 1986
167. Littler JW: Free tendon grafts in secondary flexor tendon repair. Am J Surg 74:315, 1947
168. Littler JW: The severed flexor tendon. Surg Clin North Am 39:435, 1959
169. Littler JW: Hand, wrist, and forearm incisions. p. 87. In Symposium on Reconstructive Hand Surgery. CV Mosby, St. Louis, 1974
170. Lundborg G: Experimental flexor tendon healing without adhesion formation—a new concept of tendon nutrition and intrinsic healing mechanisms. A preliminary report. Hand 8:235, 1976
171. Lundborg G: The vascularization of the human flexor pollicis longus tendon. Hand 11:28, 1979
172. Lundborg G, Hansson HA, Rank F, Rydevik B: Superficial repair of severed flexor tendons in synovial environment—an experimental study on cellular mechanisms. J Hand Surg 5:451–461, 1980
173. Lundborg G, Holm S, Myrhage R: The role of the synovial fluid and tendon sheath for flexor tendon nutrition. Scand J Plast Reconstr Surg 14:99–107, 1980
174. Lundborg G, Myrhage R, Rydevik B: The vascularization of human flexor tendons within the digital synovial sheath region—structural and functional aspects. J Hand Surg 2:417–427, 1977
175. Lundborg G, Rank F: Experimental intrinsic healing of flexor tendons based upon synovial fluid nutrition. J Hand Surg 3:21–31, 1978
176. MacMillan M, Sheppard JE, Dell PC: An experimental flexor tendon repair in Zone II that allows immediate postoperative mobilization. J Hand Surg 12A:582–589, 1987
177. Madsen E: Delayed primary tendon suture. J Bone Joint Surg 46B:357, 1964
178. Madsen E: Delayed primary suture of flexor tendons cut in the digital sheath. J Bone Joint Surg 52B:264–267, 1970
179. Malerich MM, Baird RA, McMaster W, Erickson JM: Permissible limits of flexor digitorum profundus tendon advancement—An anatomic study. J Hand Surg 12A:30–33, 1987
180. Mangus D, Brown F, Byrnes W, Habal A: Tendon repairs with nylon and a modified pull-out technique. Plast Reconstr Surg 48:32, 1971
181. Manske PR: Flexor tendon healing. J Hand Surg 13B:237–245, 1988
182. Manske PR, Gelberman RH, Lesker PA: Flexor tendon healing. Hand Clin 1(1):25–34, 1985
183. Manske PR, Gelberman RH, Vande Berg JS, Lesker PA: Intrinsic flexor tendon repair: A morphological study in vitro. J Bone Joint Surg 66A:385–396, 1984
184. Manske PR, Lesker PA: Avulsion of the ring finger flexor digitorum profundus tendon: An experimental study. Hand 10:52–55, 1978
185. Manske PR, Lesker PA: Nutrient pathways of flexor tendons in primates. J Hand Surg 7:436–444, 1982
186. Manske PR, Lesker PA: Comparative nutrient pathways to the flexor profundus tendons in zone II of various experimental animals. J Surg Res 34:83–93, 1983
187. Manske PR, Lesker PA: Palmar aponeurosis pulley. J Hand Surg 8:259–263, 1983
188. Manske PR, Lesker PA: Biochemical evidence of flexor tendon participation in the repair process. An in vitro study. J Hand Surg 9B:117–120, 1984
189. Manske PR, Lesker PA: Histological evidence of flexor tendon repair in various experimental animals. An in vitro study. Clin Orthop 182:297–304, 1984
190. Manske PR, Lesker PA: Flexor tendon nutrition. Hand Clin 1(1):13–24, 1985
191. Manske PR, Lesker PA: Diffusion as a nutrient pathway to the flexor tendon. pp. 86–90. In Hunter JM, Schneider LH, Mackin EJ (eds): Tendon Surgery in the Hand. CV Mosby, St. Louis, 1987
192. Manske PR, Whiteside LA, Lesker PA: Nutrient pathways to flexor tendons using hydrogen washout technique. J Hand Surg 3:32–36, 1978
193. Mason ML: Primary and secondary tendon suture. A discussion of the significance of technique in tendon surgery. Surg Gynecol Obstet 70:392, 1940
194. Mason ML: Primary tendon repair. J Bone Joint Surg 41A:575, 1959
195. Mason ML, Allen HS: The rate of healing of tendons. An experimental study of tensile strength. Ann Surg 113:424, 1941
196. Mason ML, Shearon CG: The process of tendon repair—an experimental study of tendon suture and tendon graft. Arch Surg 25:615, 1932
197. Mass DP, Tuel R: Human flexor tendon participation in the in vitro repair process. J Hand Surg 14A:64–71, 1989
198. Mass DP, Tuel RJ: Intrinsic healing of the laceration site in human superficialis flexor tendons in vitro. J Hand Surg 16A:24–30, 1991
199. Matev I, Karagancheva S, Trichkova P, Tsekov P: Delayed primary suture of flexor tendons cut in the digital theca. Hand 12:158–162, 1980
200. Matthews P: The pathology of flexor tendon repair. Hand 11:233, 1979
201. Matthews P, Richards H: The repair potential of digital flexor tendons. An experimental study. J Bone Joint Surg 56B:618–625, 1974
202. Matthews P, Richards H: Factors in the adherence of flexor tendon after repair. An experimental study in the rabbit. J Bone Joint Surg 58B:230–236, 1976
203. Mayer L: The physiological method of tendon transplantation. I. Historical: Anatomy and physiology of tendons. Surg Gynecol Obstet 22:182, 1916
204. McCash CR: The immediate repair of flexor tendons. Br J Plast Surg 14:53, 1961
205. McClinton MA, Curtis RM, Wilgis EFS: One hundred tendon grafts for isolated flexor digitorum profundus injuries. J Hand Surg 7:224–229, 1982
206. McDowell CL, Snyder DM: Tendon healing: An experimental model in the dog. J Hand Surg 2:122, 1977
207. McFarlane RM, Lamon R, Jarvis G: Flexor tendon injuries within the finger. A study of the results of tendon suture and tendon graft. J Trauma 8:987, 1968
208. McLean NR: Some observations on controlled mobilisation following flexor tendon injury. J Hand Surg 12B:101–104, 1987
209. McMaster PE: Tendon and muscle ruptures. Clinical and experimental studies on the causes and location of subcutaneous ruptures. J Bone Joint Surg 15:705, 1933
210. Miller RC: Flexor tendon repair over the proximal phalanx. Am J Surg 122:319, 1971
211. Munro IR, Lindsay WK, Jackson SH: A synchronous study of collagen & mucopolysaccharide in healing flexor tendons of chickens. Plast Reconstr Surg 45:493, 1970
212. Noonan KJ, Blair WF: Long-term follow-up of primary flexor pollicis longus tenorrhaphies. J Hand Surg 16A:653–662, 1991
213. Ochiai N, Matsui T, Miyaji N, Merklin RJ, Hunter JM: Vascular anatomy of flexor tendons. I. Vincular system and blood supply

of the profundus tendon in the digital sheath. J Hand Surg 4:321, 1979
214. Parkes A: The lumbrical plus finger. Hand 2:164, 1970
215. Peacock EE Jr: A study of the circulation in normal tendons and healing grafts. Ann Surg 149:415, 1959
216. Peacock EE Jr: Biological principles in the healing of long tendons. Surg Clin North Am 45:461, 1965
217. Peacock EE Jr: Some technical aspects and results of flexor tendon repair. Surgery 58:330, 1965
218. Peacock EE Jr, Madden JW: Some studies on the effects of β-aminopropionitrile in patients with injured flexor tendons. Surgery 66:215-223, 1969
219. Peterson WW, Manske PR, Dunlap J, Horwitz DS, Kahn B: Effect of various methods of restoring flexor sheath integrity on the formation of adhesions after tendon injury. J Hand Surg 15A:48-56, 1990
220. Peterson WW, Manske PR, Kain CC, Lesker PA: Effect of flexor sheath integrity on tendon gliding: A biomechanical and histologic study. J Orthop Res 4:458-465, 1986
221. Peterson WW, Manske PR, Lesker PA: The effect of flexor sheath integrity on nutrient uptake by chicken flexor tendons. Clin Orthop 201:259-263, 1985
222. Peterson WW, Manske PR, Lesker PA: The effect of flexor sheath integrity on nutrient uptake by primate flexor tendons. J Hand Surg 11A:413-416, 1986
223. Pho RWH, Sanguin R, Chacha PB: Primary repair of flexor tendons within the digital theca of the hand. Hand 10:154, 1978
224. Posch JL: Primary tenorrhaphies and tendon grafting procedures in hand injuries. Arch Surg 73:609, 1956
225. Posch JL, Walker PJ, Miller H: Treatment of ruptured tendons of the hand and wrist. Am J Surg 91:669, 1956
226. Potenza AD: Tendon healing within the flexor digital sheath in the dog. J Bone Joint Surg 44A:49, 1962
227. Potenza AD: Critical evaluation of flexor tendon healing and adhesion formation without artificial digital sheaths. An experimental study. J Bone Joint Surg 45A:1217-1233, 1963
228. Potenza AD: The healing process in wounds of the digital flexor tendons and tendon grafts. An experimental study. pp. 40-54. In Verdan C (ed): Tendon Surgery of the Hand. Churchill Livingstone, Edinburgh, 1979
229. Potenza AD, Herte MC: The synovial cavity as a "tissue culture in situ"—science or nonsense. J Hand Surg 7:196-199, 1982
230. Pruitt DL, Manske PR, Fink B: Cyclic stress analysis of flexor tendon repair. J Hand Surg 16A:701-707, 1991
231. Pulvertaft RG: Tendon grafts for flexor tendon injuries in the fingers and thumb. J Bone Joint Surg 38B:175, 1956
232. Pulvertaft RG: The treatment of profundus division by free tendon graft. J Bone Joint Surg 42A:1363, 1960
233. Pulvertaft RG: Problems of flexor tendon surgery of the hand. J Bone Joint Surg 47A:123, 1965
234. Pulvertaft RG: Suture materials and tendon junctures. Am J Surg 109:346, 1965
235. Rank BK, Wakefield AR: The repair of flexor tendons in the hand. Br J Plast Surg 4:244, 1952
236. Rank BK, Wakefield AR, Hueston JT: Surgery of Repair as Applied to Hand Injuries. 4th Ed. Williams & Wilkins, Baltimore, 1973
237. Reid DAC: The isolated flexor digitorum profundus lesion. Hand 1:115, 1969
238. Richards HJ: Digital flexor tendon repair and return of function. Ann R Coll Surg Engl 59:25, 1977
239. Robb JE: The termination of flexor tendon sheaths. Hand 11:17, 1979
240. Robins PR, Dobyns JH: Avulsion of the insertion of the flexor digitorum profundus tendon associated with fracture of the distal phalanx. A brief review. pp. 151-156. In AAOS Symposium on Tendon Surgery in the Hand. CV Mosby, St. Louis, 1975
241. Rogers GD, Henshall AL, Sach RP, Wallis KA: Simultaneous laceration of the median and ulnar nerves with flexor tendons at the wrist. J Hand Surg 15A:990-995, 1990
242. Rothkopf DM, Webb S, Szabo RM, Gelberman RH, May JW Jr: An experimental model for the study of canine flexor tendon adhesions. J Hand Surg 16A:694-700, 1991
243. Sakellarides HT: Severe injuries of the flexor tendons in no man's land with excess scarring and flexion contracture treated with silicone rod and tendon grafting. Orthop Rev 6(6):51, 1977
244. Saldana MJ, Ho PK, Lichtman DM, Chow JA, Dovelle S, Thomes LJ: Flexor tendon repair and rehabilitation in Zone II open sheath technique versus closed sheath technique. J Hand Surg 12A:1110-1114, 1987
245. Salvi V: Delayed primary suture in flexor tendon division. Hand 3:181, 1971
246. Sanders WE: Advantages of "epitenon first" suture placement technique in flexor tendon repair. Clin Orthop 280:198-199, 1992
247. Sasaki Y, Nomura S: An unusual role of the vinculum after complete laceration of the flexor tendons. J Hand Surg 12B:105-108, 1987
248. Savage R: In vitro studies of a new method of flexor tendon repair. J Hand Surg 10B:135-141, 1985
249. Savage R: The influence of wrist position on the minimum force required for active movement of the interphalangeal joints. J Hand Surg 13B:262-268, 1988
250. Schepel SJ: Intrinsic healing of flexor tendons in primates. pp. 61-66. In Hunter JM, Schneider LH, Mackin EJ (eds): Tendon Surgery in the Hand. CV Mosby, St. Louis, 1987
251. Schneider LH, Hunter JM, Norris TR, Nadeau PO: Delayed flexor tendon repair in no man's land. J Hand Surg 2:452-455, 1977
252. Seradge H: Elongation of the repair configuration following flexor tendon repair. J Hand Surg 8:182-185, 1983
253. Setti GC, Verdan C: Lymphatic circulation in tendons and sheaths. pp. 13-15. In Verdan C (ed): Tendon Surgery of the Hand. Churchill Livingstone, Edinburgh, 1979
254. Shaw JA: Flexor tendon surgery: Technical note. J Hand Surg 14A:150-152, 1989
255. Small JO, Brennen MD, Colville J: Early active mobilisation following flexor tendon repair in Zone 2. J Hand Surg 14B:383-391, 1989
256. Smith JH: Avulsion of the profundus tendon with simultaneous intraarticular fracture of the distal phalanx. Case report. J Hand Surg 6:600-601, 1981
257. Smith JW: Blood supply of tendons. Am J Surg 109:272, 1965
258. So YC, Chow SP, Pun WK, Luk KDK, Crosby C, Ng C: Evaluation of results in flexor tendon repair: A critical analysis of five methods in ninety-five digits. J Hand Surg 15A:258-264, 1990
259. Sourmelis SG, McGrouther DA: Retrieval of the retracted flexor tendon. J Hand Surg 12B:109-111, 1987
260. Srugi S, Adamson JE: A comparative study of tendon suture material in dogs. Plast Reconstr Surg 50:31, 1972
261. Stark HH, Zemel NP, Boyes JH, Ashworth CR: Flexor tendon graft through intact superficialis tendon. J Hand Surg 2:456, 1977
262. Strauch B, de Moura W: Digital flexor tendon sheath: An anatomic study. J Hand Surg 10A:785-789, 1985
263. Strauch B, de Moura W, Ferder M, Hall C, Sagi A, Greenstein B: The fate of tendon healing after restoration of the integrity of the tendon sheath with autogenous vein grafts. J Hand Surg 10A:790-795, 1985
264. Strickland JW: Functional recovery after flexor tendon sever-

ance in the finger: The state of the art. In Strickland JW, Steichen JB (eds): Difficult Problems in Hand Surgery. CV Mosby, St. Louis, 1982

265. Strickland JW: The management of acute flexor tendon injuries. Orthop Clin North Am 14:827-849, 1983
266. Strickland JW: Flexor tendon repair. Hand Clin 1(1):55-68, 1985
267. Strickland JW: Flexor tenolysis. Hand Clin 1(1):121-132, 1985
268. Strickland JW: Results of flexor tendon surgery in Zone II. Hand Clin 1(1):167-179, 1985
269. Strickland JW: Biologic rationale, clinical application, and results of early motion following flexor tendon repair. J Hand Ther 2:71-83, 1989
270. Strickland JW, Glogovac SV: Digital function following flexor tendon repair in Zone II: A comparison of immobilization and controlled passive motion techniques. J Hand Surg 5:537-543, 1980
271. Szabo RM, Younger E: Effects of indomethacin on adhesion formation after repair of Zone II tendon lacerations in the rabbit. J Hand Surg 15A:480-483, 1990
272. Tajima T: History, current status, and aspects of hand surgery in Japan. Clin Orthop 184:41-49, 1984
273. Takai S, Woo S, Tung D, Gelberman R: The effects of frequency and duration of controlled passive mobilization on tendon healing. J Orthop Res 9:705-713, 1991
274. Trail IA, Powell ES, Noble J: An evaluation of suture materials used in tendon surgery. J Hand Surg 14B:422-427, 1989
275. Tsuge K, Ikuta Y, Matsuishi Y: Repair of flexor tendons by intratendinous suture. J Hand Surg 2:436, 1977
276. Tubiana R: Incisions and techniques in tendon grafting. Am J Surg 109:339, 1965
277. Tubiana R: Technique of flexor tendon grafts. Hand 1:108-114, 1969
278. Tustanoff ER, Birdsell DC, Lindsay WK: In vivo incorporation of Proline-H3 and its subsequent hydroxylation during collagen synthesis in regenerating tendon. Proc Can Fed Biol Soc 8:54, 1965
279. Urbaniak JR: Repair of the flexor pollicis longus. Hand Clin 1(1):69-76, 1985
280. Urbaniak JR, Cahill JD Jr, Mortenson RA: Tendon suturing methods: analysis of tensile strengths. pp. 70-80. In AAOS Symposium on Tendon Surgery in the Hand. CV Mosby, St. Louis, 1975
281. Verdan CE: Primary repair of flexor tendons. J Bone Joint Surg 42A:647-657, 1960
282. Verdan CE: Syndrome of the quadriga. Surg Clin North Am 40:425, 1960
283. Verdan CE: Half a century of flexor-tendon surgery. Current status and changing philosophies. J Bone Joint Surg 54A:472-491, 1972
284. Verdan C: Reparative surgery of flexor tendons in the digits. pp. 57-66. In Verdan C (ed): Tendon Surgery of the Hand. Churchill Livingstone, Edinburgh, 1979
285. Verdan CE, Michon J: Le traitement des plaies des tendons fléchisseurs des dogits. Rev Chir Orthop 47:285, 1961
286. Versaci AD: Secondary tendon grafting in isolated flexor digitorum profundus surgery. Plast Reconstr Surg 46:57, 1970
287. Von Lanz T, Wachsmuth W: Praktische Anatomie. 2nd Ed. Springer-Verlag, Berlin, 1959
288. Von Zander: Trommlerlahmung. Inaug. Dissertation. Berlin, 1891
289. Wade PJF, Muir IFK, Hutcheon LL: Primary flexor tendon repair: The mechanical limitations of the modified Kessler technique. J Hand Surg 11B:71-76, 1986
290. Wade PJF, Wetherell RG, Amis AA: Flexor tendon repair: Significant gain in strength from the Halsted peripheral suture technique. J Hand Surg 14B:232-235, 1989
291. Wakefield AR: Hand injuries in children. J Bone Joint Surg 46A:1226, 1964
292. Weeks PM, Wray RC: Rate and extent of functional recovery after flexor tendon grafting with and without silicone rod preparation. J Hand Surg 1:174-180, 1976
293. Wehbe MA, Hunter JM: Flexor tendon gliding in the hand. Part I. In vivo excursions. Part II. Differential gliding. J Hand Surg 10A:570-579, 1985
294. Wenger DR: Avulsion of the profundus tendon insertion in football players. Arch Surg 106:145, 1973
295. Werntz JR, Chesher SP, Briedenbach WC, Kleinert HE, Bissonnette MA: A new dynamic splint for postoperative treatment of flexor tendon injury. J Hand Surg 14A:559-566, 1989
296. Wheeldon T: The use of cellophane as a permanent tendon sheath. J Bone Joint Surg 21:393, 1939
297. White WL: Secondary restoration of finger flexion by digital tendon graft. An evaluation of seventy-six cases. Am J Surg 91:662, 1956
298. Wilson RL, Carter MS, Holdeman VA, Lovett WL: Flexor profundus injuries treated with delayed two-staged tendon grafting. J Hand Surg 5:74-78, 1980
299. Wray RC, Weeks PM: Experimental comparison of technics of tendon repair. J Hand Surg 5:144-148, 1980
300. Young L, Weeks PM: Profundus tendon blood supply within the digital sheath. Surg Forum 21:504-506, 1970
301. Young RES, Harmon JM: Repair of tendon injuries of the hand. Ann Surg 151:562-566, 1960

51

Flexor Tendons—Late Reconstruction

Lawrence H. Schneider
James M. Hunter

The progress made in reconstruction of flexor tendon injuries is based on the work of leaders who pioneered the development of techniques widely used today. We surgeons who perform reconstructive procedures on the flexor tendon system are greatly in debt to our predecessors. The technical and philosophic works of Mayer,[263,265,269] Bunnell,[51,53,54] Mason et al,[257] Boyes,[38,39] Verdan,[431,432,435] and Pulvertaft[328,330] set a background for all of our efforts and should be appreciated and understood. The articles by Mason et al,[254] Peacock and Hartrampf,[307] Ketchum,[194] Meals,[280] and Strickland[401-403] provide an excellent background for a review of this topic.

TENDON HEALING

To achieve successful repair of divided flexor tendons, as measured by return of gliding function, is a great challenge to the surgeon, chiefly because of the nature of tendon healing. The very process by which an injured and repaired tendon heals may also cause it to adhere indiscriminately to its surrounding bed, thereby preventing the smooth gliding necessary for movement of the fingers. The presence of local tissue injury secondary to the original traumatizing force, or that injury added to the wound by the treating surgeon, further complicates healing and increases the incidence and density of the tendon adhesions. The surgeon's objective, therefore, is to create an environment in which the repaired tendon can heal with a minimal amount of tissue reaction and then, after an initial period of protection, to institute physical measures to mobilize the repaired tendon, thereby stretching adhesions associated with the healing process without endangering the continuity of the repair. The difficulty in achieving this goal is underlined by the great variability and unpredictability in the end results of tendon repair.

While the surgical literature is replete with articles by various authors expressing preference for their own particular techniques, it is apparent that there is no substitute for thorough anatomic knowledge combined with gentle technique so as not to inflict additional damage to the delicate tissues. This, however, is not a simple proposition. Experiments have shown that even the passage of a wire suture through an intact tendon will cause significant adhesion formation.[224] Every site where the tissue forceps punctures the tendon surface is a site of potential tendon adhesion.[314,316]

It was formerly believed that tendon union could only occur through the process in which paratendinous tissues invaded the healing area, and that the tendon itself was completely passive in the healing process.[28,85,307,315,319,424] However, more recent research has shown that the tendon itself can play an active role in the repair phenomenon in experimentally controlled injury conditions.[26,112,194,202,259-261,276,380] Nutrition can also reach the tendon through the synovial fluid as well as by adhesions carrying capillaries.[240,251,252,260]

It is likely that both extrinsic and intrinsic healing mechanisms play active roles in tendon healing. Other papers of interest have expounded viewpoints on this topic.[114,220,221,250,305,320,380]

Unfortunately, in actual clinical situations the tissue response to injury is such that the formation of adhesions, which limits tendon gliding, is difficult, if not impossible, to avoid.[261,314-318] Many of the factors important in determining the end result attained cannot be controlled. These include:

1. Age of the patient. In general, younger patients do better than the aged, although there are technical and management problems in the very young.
2. Mechanism and extent of the injury. Wounds complicated by crushing of soft tissue, fractures, joint injuries, nerve and artery damage, skin loss, or infection have a much poorer prognosis than the cleanly incised tendon injury with minimal tissue damage.
3. Level of the tendon laceration. As a rule, tendons injured outside of the flexor sheath yield much better results after repair than do those injured within the sheath (Zone II).
4. Healing response of the individual patient. This factor cannot be overestimated. There are undoubtedly patients whose healing collagen is of a different quality than others. These patients form adhesions that are more subtle, filmy, and pliable than others and, given equal conditions, will attain better gliding after tendon repair. When we are fortunate enough to encounter one of these "soft scar formers," we attain outstanding results but are probably being presumptuous in our self-laudatory claims.

Assuming the repair is done by a well-trained and experienced surgeon, the above factors are more likely to determine the end result of a tendon repair than the actual technique of suture, the type of suture material chosen, or the timing of the procedure.

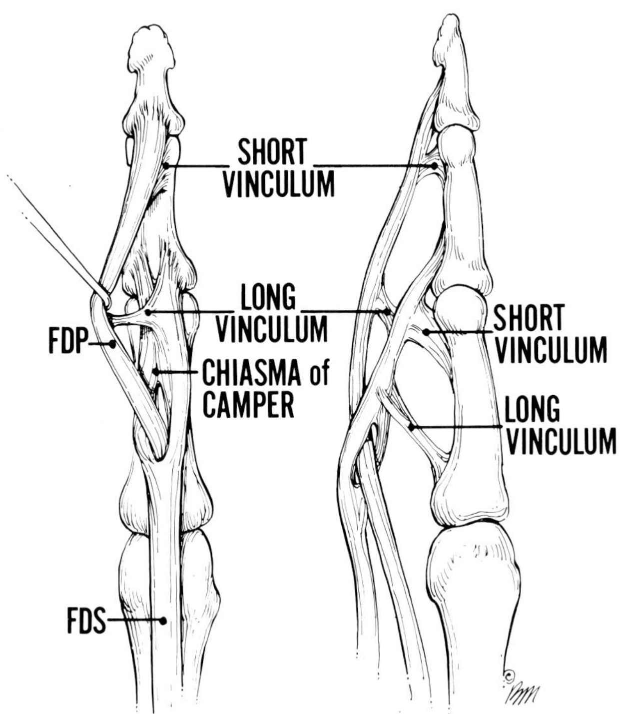

Fig. 51-1. The flexor digitorum profundus *(FDP)* passes through the tails of the flexor digitorum superficialis *(FDS)* on the way to its insertion into the distal phalanx.

ANATOMY

Much interest has been focused on the vascular anatomy of the flexor tendons, both on gross and microscopic levels. The blood supply that enters the tendon via the mesotenon vincular systems has been implicated in the healing reaction of the tendon and the subsequent formation of limiting adhesions.[5,10,26,42,46,60,67,76,92,214,236–238,290,294,303,323,324,351,382,407,474]

The flexor system of the fingers consists of two tendons for each finger and one for the thumb.[98,103,137,172,186,209,210,469,470] These tendons, whose muscles originate from the distal humerus and forearm, pass through the carpal canal and proceed to their respective fingers. The flexor digitorum superficialis inserts on the middle phalanx and the flexor digitorum profundi and flexor pollicis longus insert at the bases of the distal phalanges (Fig. 51-1).

The actual level of tendon injury in relation to its surrounding tissues is of significance when discussing treatment techniques and particularly in arriving at a prognosis. The skin wound level is not as significant as the level of the tendon injury itself, the latter being dependent on the position of the fingers at the time of wounding. Tendons lacerated in flexion are injured at a level distal to the skin wound. When the hand is examined in the emergency room with the finger in extension, the exact level of the tendon severance is sometimes difficult to delineate. When reporting injuries by level, evaluation should be standardized; it is now our opinion that this is most accurate if done in the operating room with the repaired finger lying in full extension. The level of the repair is then noted as it relates to the landmarks of the various zones.[358] Ochiai and colleagues[294] and Amadio and colleagues[5] recently advised relating tendon injury levels to the vincular blood supply, which is thought to be important to the healing process.

Flexor Tendon Zones in the Fingers

Many authors have divided (and subdivided) the flexor system into horizontal zones.[90,138,202,403] As far as treatment method is concerned, these are not as important now if one subscribes to the concept of direct early repair of flexor tendon injuries.[11,63,176,201,252,255,347,370,379,428,431,433] At an earlier time, when most authorities advocated delayed care of injuries within the flexor retinaculum by free tendon grafts,[37,111,121,122,230,323–325,440] these zone levels assumed a more prominent position in determination of treatment. The controversy between those advocating early direct repair and those who do delayed tendon grafts is barely active now, with the great majority of hand surgeons using direct repair as the procedure of choice.[32,138,181,253,277,312,426] It is our belief that the advantages of a direct repair, expertly done at an early period, outweigh the advantages of a free tendon graft.[370]

In a previous edition of this chapter[367] we had divided the flexor system into four zones, but reconsideration has made it apparent that the use of five zones or levels is more appropriate (Fig. 51-2).

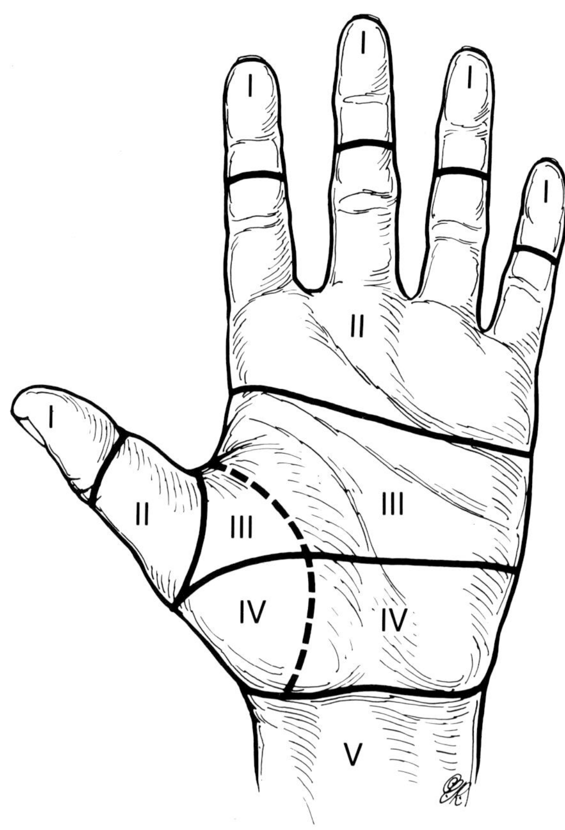

Fig. 51-2. The flexor system has been divided into five zones or levels for purposes of discussion.

Zone I. Distal to the insertion of the flexor digitorum superficialis on the middle phalanx. Only the flexor digitorum profundus will be injured.

Zone II. Within the flexor retinaculum, from the midportion of the middle phalanx to the neck of the metacarpal. This area, where two tendons glide in an unyielding fibrous retinaculum, has been further divided into three parts by Duran and Houser.[90] Depending on the position of the finger and the nature of the wounding force, lacerations here can sever either one or both of the flexor tendons.

Zone III. Proximal to the metacarpal neck to the distal edge of the transverse carpal ligament. This zone has also been subdivided in relation to the lumbrical origin. Both tendons or the superficialis alone will be injured here. Additional injury to the common digital nerves or the main trunk of the major nerves is not infrequent.

Zone IV. Under the carpal ligament. Here nerve division accompanying the tendon laceration is very frequent. This level, the carpal canal, is very crowded, and the tendons are covered with a double layered synovial membrane.

Zone V. The forearm extending from the proximal edge of the carpal ligament to the musculotendinous juncture. Injury in this area is frequently accompanied by major nerve injury, which greatly complicates the rehabilitation of the patient.

Flexor Tendon Zones in the Thumb

The flexor system of the thumb presents a simpler anatomic arrangement. Only one flexor tendon—the flexor pollicis longus—is present here, and the system has one less phalanx. Restoration of function here is greatly simplified by these anatomic factors.

For our discussion purposes there are five zones in the thumb (Fig. 51-2):

Zone I. Distal, at the insertion of the flexor tendon

Zone II. From the neck of the proximal phalanx to the neck of the metacarpal; coincides with the flexor retinaculum of the thumb

Zone III. The area of the thenar muscles

Zone IV. The carpal canal—also with thenar muscles overlying

Zone V. Proximal to the proximal edge of the carpal ligament

Influence of Anatomy on Prognosis

The anatomy peculiar to the flexor system is highly significant as far as prognosis is concerned in the difficult Zone II. Called "no man's land" by Bunnell and the "critical zone" by Boyes, this area presents the greatest challenge to the surgeon.[32] Results have always been significantly better in Zones I, III, IV, and V, and all authorities on tendon surgery will concur that direct repair, either primarily or deferred, is reasonable in these areas. Controversy at one time existed about the timing and type of procedure to be done in Zone II (see Chapter 50). This controversy has now waned, and all hand surgeons agree that early direct repair is the technique of choice when wound conditions allow.

The Retinacular Pulley System

The flexor retinaculum is a firm, fibrous sheath that functions to keep the flexor tendons approximated to the underlying bony structure and thereby provides the mechanical leverage for full finger motion. Anatomic dissections reveal that, encircling the synovial sheath in the fingers, there is a series of annular bands and cruciform fibers often referred to as the flexor pulleys. It should be noted that the word *pulley,* which describes a wheel and implies a moving structure, is not an accurate description of these stationary fibrous rings, which are better described by the term *fairlead.* However, the literature is imbued with the term pulley, so this semantic point will not be further belabored.

The Flexor Retinaculum in the Fingers

With the proximal pull of the long flexor tendons, the fingers are drawn into a functional flexion arc.[309] This smoothly integrated motion requires gliding of the flexor tendons through the tissues they traverse. Gliding is aided by a double-layered synovial sheath that envelops the tendons. The two layers consist of a visceral layer closely applied to the tendon itself and an outer parietal layer.[74] By virtue of being joined at each end, a potential space is created between these layers, and the tendons move on a plane of synovial fluid in this space between the membranes. This arrangement is found in the finger and thumb flexor tendon systems in the region of Zone II, where the tendons must glide under the fixed retinaculum, and in the wrist area where a similar retinaculum is present—the transverse carpal ligament. Within the synovial sheath the mesotenon connects the two synovial layers.[53] As it is analogous to a mesentery, it conveys blood vessels to the tendon. In the fingers, this mesotenon is condensed and represented as the vincula brevia and longa.[74,146,151,152,172,214]

A fibrous retinacular sheath encloses the synovial sheath and its tendons. This sheath, which is of utmost importance to the surgeon, starts at the neck of the metacarpal and ends at the distal phalanx. Doyle and Blythe[86,87] performed careful dissections of cadaver fingers and defined this flexor sheath, showing it to be divided into four heavy annular bands and three more filmy cruciform components. Hunter and colleagues[152] identified a distal fifth annular pulley at the DIP joint. Others have recently studied the pulley system.[397] Details of the anatomy of the pulleys are described on page 1892.

INCISIONS USED IN FLEXOR TENDON SURGERY

The zigzag volar incision advocated by Bruner[49,50] has many advantages over the midlateral finger incision, which was more generally used by tendon surgeons before 1967[416] (Fig. 51-3A and B). The incision crisscrosses the course of the flexor tendon and can have extensions that can carry it proximally into the palm and wrist. It can be combined with a transverse palmar incision in the case of palm-to-fingertip tendon grafting.

This direct approach to the flexor system has provided excellent exposure of the flexor sheath as well as the digital nerves, and all surgery on the volar aspect of the hand and finger can be performed through this approach.

The midlateral finger incision[35,38,55,120,233,306,329,416] is used by many surgeons doing flexor tendon work (Fig. 51-3C). It has the advantage of leaving scar on the nontactile area of the finger, but it does increase risk of injury to the dorsal branch of the digital nerve when the neurovascular bundle is carried with the volar flap. It is our feeling that it provides an inferior exposure when compared to the volar zigzag incision, which we use to the exclusion of all others in reconstructive flexor tendon surgery.

FLEXOR TENDON GRAFTING (ZONE II INJURIES)

For flexor tendon injury in the area of poorest prognosis for function (i.e., Zone II) application of the tendon graft allows the surgeon to place the tendon junctures outside the confines of the flexor sheath, [i.e., distally at the base of the distal phalanx, with the proximal juncture generally in the palm (in Zone III) (Fig. 51-4A and B)]. This bypass of no man's land was offered as a solution to the problems of tendon severance in this difficult area. Interest in the free tendon graft grew out of animal experimentation carried out in the nineteenth century. A review of the early literature is confusing, as the term *graft* was used interchangeably with the technique of tendon transfer, which is obviously quite a different procedure. Although Missa is given credit[443] for the first "tendon graft" in 1770, when he sutured the irreparable distal end of the middle finger extensor tendon to the intact extensor of the ring finger, this, of course, was a tendon transfer. The first free autogenous tendon graft removed and used at a different site was reported in 1889 when Robeson[342] transplanted 4½ inches of a flexor tendon from a damaged finger to restore extensor function in the index finger. Robeson himself stated that he could find no earlier report of a whole autogenous tendon graft being used, although Adamson and Wilson[1] reported that in 1882 Heuch used a free tendon graft of the long thumb extensor to repair itself in an accidental division of the tendon during surgery.

The first series of free flexor tendon grafts in the hand was reported by Lexer[216] of Jena in 1912. For tendon material he used the palmaris longus or a long toe extensor as well as adjacent flexor tendons. This study was followed by the work of Mayer,[263-268,270] Biesalski,[101] Lange,[211] and Bunnell.[51-54]

A few stalwarts held out for primary (direct) repair[253,255,256,379] of flexor tendons in Zone II, if conditions were optimal and the time elapsed from injury was short. However, the generally poor results from direct repair witnessed by hand surgeons led to the recommendation that it would be better to close the skin only and then prepare the patient for a secondary tendon graft 3 or more weeks later when soft tissues began to heal.[231] Many series of free tendon grafts were presented with reasonable results obtained.[2,33,36,40,41,108,111,121,122,129,199,206,208,230,279,312,323,325,333,396,411,423,440,460] It is noted that there is a great deal of difficulty in comparing these various series due to many variables in the injuries and techniques used, and also in the methods and standards of measuring results.[363]

In the 1950s and 1960s[201,222,255,428-430] it became apparent that some surgeons were disenchanted with the demanding procedure of tendon grafting and particularly with their inability to achieve functional results that gratified either themselves or their patients. Thus, interest in direct repair in Zone II was renewed. Because of better techniques, improved suture material, and availability of trained people interested in hand surgery, direct repair is by far more commonly done now than in the past few decades. The time interval allowed for direct repair has now increased from less than 2 hours to as long as 3 weeks or longer under some conditions.[11,63,176,245,347,370] Wakefield[440] and Harrison[130] have even made a case for primary and delayed primary tendon grafting, if wound conditions permit.

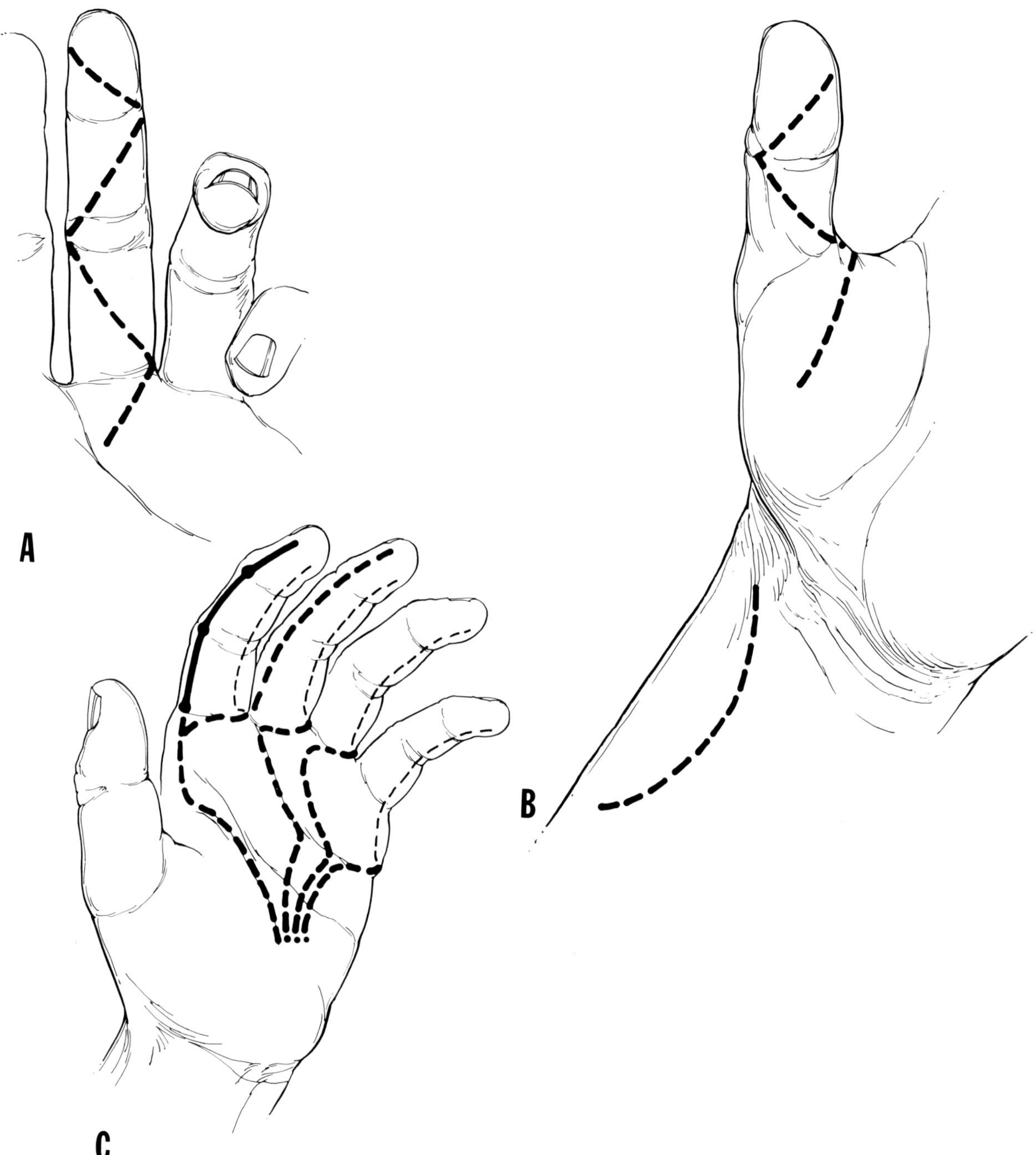

Fig. 51-3. Incisions. **(A)** The volar zigzag incision advocated by Bruner provides an approach adequate for all surgery on the volar aspect of the finger. It can be carried proximally across the palm or be combined with a transverse palmar incision. **(B)** The volar zigzag incision in the thumb. **(C)** The midlateral incision connects the tips of the flexor creases along the midlateral aspect of the fingers. It can be continued proximally in a variety of ways as shown, but care must be taken not to cross the flexion crease at the base of the finger at a right angle.

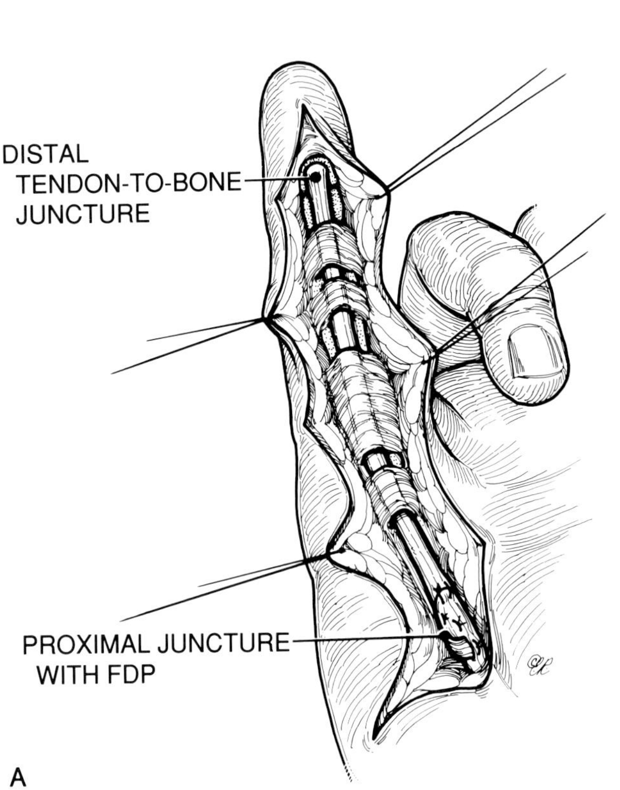

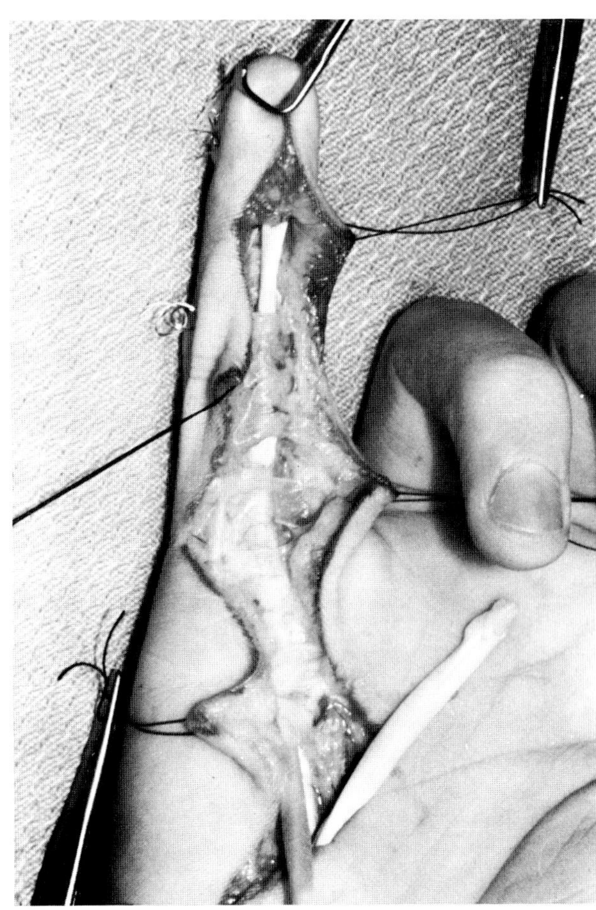

Fig. 51-4. **(A)** A flexor tendon graft. The tendon junctures are placed outside the confines of the flexor sheath (Zone II). **(B)** In this clinical case the graft has been fixed into the distal phalanx, and the proximal juncture will be completed in the palm using the flexor digitorum profundus as the motor.

Despite the rightful popularity of direct early repair, there still exists a group of patients in whom a free tendon graft is indicated.[75,328,331,332,362,467] These are patients in whom there is a delay in their definitive repair, which makes it impossible to do an end-to-end repair. Here the injured tendons are removed and replaced with a palm-to-distal phalanx free graft. This situation arises in patients in whom the wound or general conditions did not allow direct repair or whose treating surgeon felt that delayed grafting was the better treatment alternative for their Zone II injuries. The delay can also be caused by late referral for definitive treatment or in cases where the flexor tendon injury was missed at the time of injury. The closed rupture of the flexor digitorum profundus is an example of an injury whose significance is often underestimated by the initial examiner, leading to considerable delay before definitive treatment and consequently a need for the use of a tendon graft if distal joint motion is to be restored.

Indications for Tendon Graft

The palm-to-fingertip free tendon graft is usually performed in those fingers that have had both flexor tendons severed in Zone II. The wound should be well healed, and the joints should be supple with as much passive motion as possible (Boyes' Grade 1[33,34] (Table 51-1). Certainly the surgeon's judgment must prevail. The surgeon must decide whether a surgically acceptable situation can be created based on gross examination, knowing that all the factors that govern the end result cannot be fully controlled. Some of the patients will have had failed primary surgery and may do better with the staged

Table 51-1. Boyes' Preoperative Classification

Grade	Preoperative Condition
1	Good. Minimal scar with mobile joints and no trophic changes.
2	Cicatrix. Heavy skin scarring due to injury or prior surgery. Deep scarring due to failed primary repair or infection.
3	Joint damage. Injury to the joint with restricted range of motion.
4	Nerve damage. Injury to the digital nerves resulting in trophic changes in the finger.
5	Multiple damage. Involvement of multiple fingers with a combination of the above problems.

(From Boyes,[33] with permission.)

reconstruction discussed later in this chapter. The patient should be prepared preoperatively for any of the operative alternatives, which will be presented later in this chapter, that might prove necessary, so that the surgeon can keep options open during the operation.

Timing for Flexor Tendon Grafts

In patients with relatively benign wounds, 3 or 4 weeks usually suffice to prepare the hand. This allows time for skin healing and softening and for recovery or maintenance of full passive range of motion. The importance of passive range of motion cannot be overstressed. It is disconcerting to see that tendon grafting is at times still proposed in a finger that is markedly restricted in range of motion.

Technique

All flexor tendon surgery should be carried out under tourniquet control. A Bruner-type incision is used and the tendon system exposed (Fig. 51-5). The neurovascular bundles are protected, and if nerve repair is indicated, the nerve ends are prepared at this time. The area of injury in the sheath is noted, and the damaged sheath is minimally resected with the scalpel. As much of the uninjured flexor sheath is preserved as possible.[444] This is in contradistinction to the older teachings of many leading tendon surgeons[34,35,54,208,319,327,334,335] who believed that all the sheath, except for critical narrow bands (pulleys), should be removed. No careless handling, pinching, or probing is allowed because of the risk of increasing the number and density of adhesions. Approximately 1 cm of profundus stump is preserved distally. The remainder of the injured profundus is sharply excised proximally to the lumbrical origin in the palm. The more resilient tendon, either the flexor digitorum superficialis or flexor digitorum profundus (usually the latter), is selected for the motor. The proximal stump of the flexor digitorum superficialis is pulled distally, transected, and allowed to retract proximally. The distal flexor digitorum superficialis is excised sharply, leaving only about 1 or 2 cm of its insertion undisturbed. It is not excised completely, as an undisturbed insertion provides a more favorable posterior bed for the graft than a ripped-out, freshly granulating area. The superficialis tail may, be virtue of adhesion to the floor of the flexor canal, provide stability at the PIP joint, thereby helping to prevent hyperextension deformity at this joint, a problem oc-

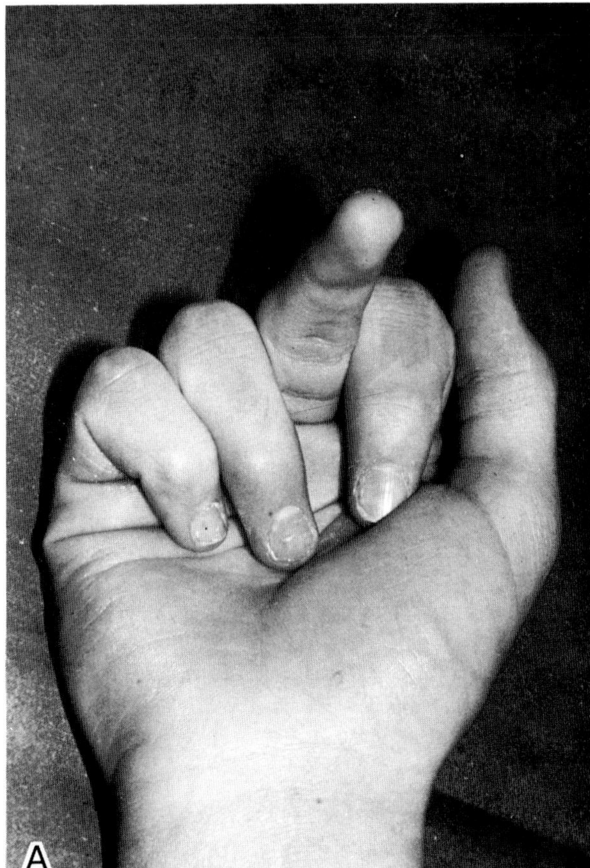

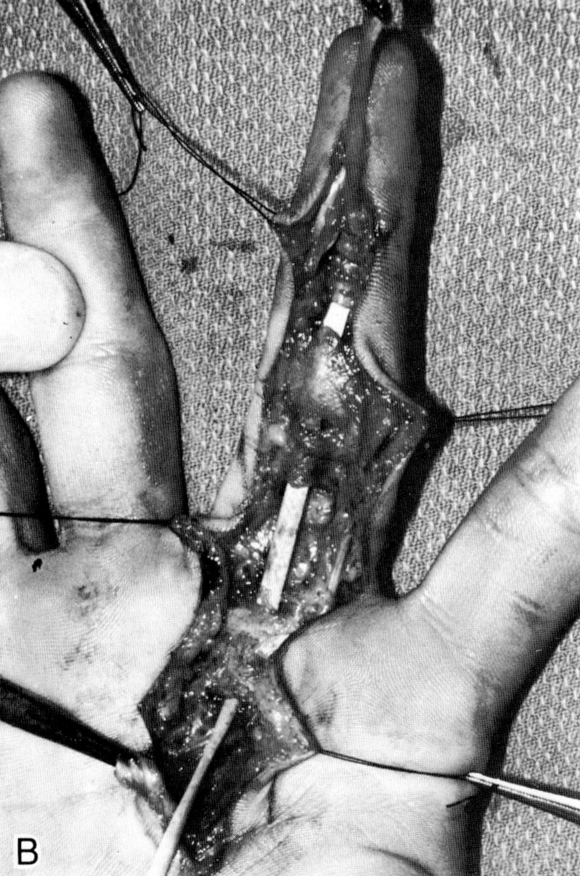

Fig. 51-5. Example of a flexor tendon graft. **(A)** A 16-year-old boy with a 3-month-old laceration in Zone II in which both flexor tendons had been severed. The patient maintained supple joints and had minimal scarring. **(B)** As much uninjured flexor sheath was preserved as possible. The tendon graft (palmaris longus) has been threaded into the retinacular system in preparation for distal and proximal junctures. (Note preservation of pulleys.) *(Figure continues.)*

casionally seen in fingers without a superficialis tendon.[463] Since this problem is more frequent in hands with loose hyperextensible PIP joints, in such cases one tail of the superficialis can be left long and sutured with nonabsorbable material to the flexor sheath proximal to the joint, providing a tenodesis of this joint in 10 to 20 degrees flexion.

At this point the wound can be covered with a moist temporary dressing while attention is directed to obtaining graft material. If it is necessary to go to the lower extremity for the tendon graft, the tourniquet is released at this time (see section on procedure for obtaining tendon graft on page 1864).

After the finger wound bleeding has been controlled, the extremity is exsanguinated and the tourniquet reinflated. The graft is threaded under the pulleys using a silk-holding suture. Various techniques can be used to facilitate the passing of the graft, but our preferred method is to use a commercially available disposable suture passer or a length of 0 monofilament wire twisted into a loop that can be passed beneath the pulleys and the suture passed through the loop. The graft can then be fed into the pulley system. A flexible silicone rod to which the graft can be sutured can also be used as a tendon passer. Leddy[213] and Sourmelis and McGrouther[388] have used a flexible rubber catheter as a passer but, regardless of which method is used, care must be taken to minimize trauma to the intact sheath. A clamp is placed at each end of the graft to prevent inadvertent withdrawal while work on the junctures progresses.

Distal Juncture

We prefer to perform the distal juncture first, as in this way the finger can be closed more easily in the extended position and graft length determination can be carried out in the palm when the proximal juncture is accomplished. Some surgeons prefer to do the proximal juncture first, making their length adjustment out at the fingertip. Pulvertaft[329] and others[386,393,453,465] reported that they perform the distal juncture after the proximal is completed.

The distal juncture must be strong.[249] Motion does not occur at this point, so its only requirement is a firm union between the tendon and the stump of profundus or preferably to bone, as the latter is felt to be a stronger form of bonding.[109,188,427,458] A study of the tendon/bone interface in rabbits by Jones et al,[182] published in 1987, showed that the normal bone tendon interface was not restored by this surgical technique. In their study the union occurred only between the tendon and the periosteum, and although adequate mechanical strength may occur in time, it was not equivalent to the normal juncture. Despite these findings, in our clinical experience this juncture is quite adequate.

Methods of Distal Juncture

Transverse Tunnel (Pulvertaft,[325,329] Koch[204]) (Fig. 51-6). A transverse drill hole is made across the base of the distal phalanx and the graft is threaded through and sutured to itself. It is

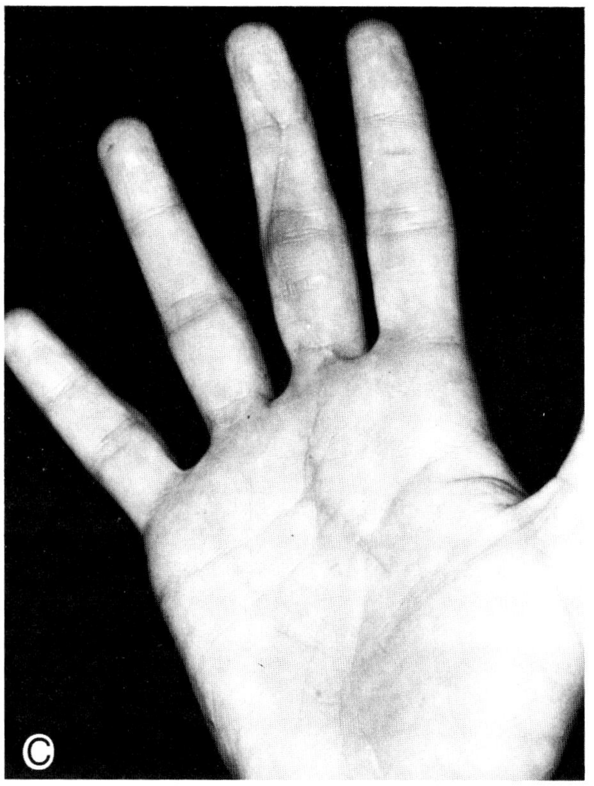

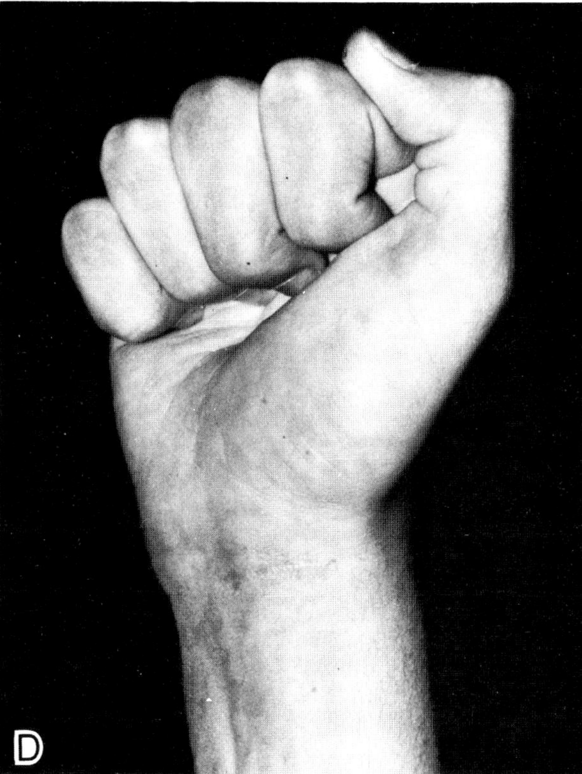

Fig. 51-5 *(Continued).* **(C&D)** Extension and flexion 6 months postoperatively.

relatively simple to judge tension on the graft, when tension is to be set at the distal juncture by this technique, but Pulvertaft warns that the graft must be thin. This technique is not recommended in children because of risk of damage to the open epiphyseal plate.

Through the Finger Pulp (Pulvertaft[329] (Fig. 51-7). The graft itself is drawn through the pulp using a large needle and the projecting end is temporarily clipped at the tip of the pulp. This allows adjustment for tension with precision, and then additional sutures are placed between the graft and the profundus stump through which it has been passed. Similar techniques had been described by others.[386,393,453,465] There has been a case report of infection when using[352] this technique.

Tendon-to-Tendon Juncture (Fig. 51-8). The distal stump of profundus is split longitudinally and the graft laid within the split. An interweave suture using 4–0 nonabsorbable material is then carried out. This is a preferred technique in children.

Authors' Preferred Method

We prefer the classic Bunnell tendon-to-bone pull-out technique[35,233,329,396,417,444] (Fig. 42-9). The stump of profundus is elevated to clear an area for a hole to be created in the volar cortex. This is started with a bone awl and enlarged with a small curette, providing access to the medullary canal of the distal phalanx. A Keith needle is then driven through this hole with a hand drill, emerging dorsally through the middle third of the nail.

The previously used wire pull-out technique of Bunnell as described in the earlier editions of this chapter[367] (Fig. 51-9A) has given way to a modification of that technique. While the wire pull-out technique gave satisfactory service for many years, the need to extract this suture in a proximal direction, against the newly healing distal juncture, gave some discomfort to the surgeon (as well as the patient). The modified technique allows distal withdrawal of the suture (Fig. 51-9B).

A 3–0 Prolene double armed suture is placed in the Bunnell configuration in the distal end of the graft. The suture is crisscrossed two times, taking care not to impale the suture with the crisscross. The suture is pulled tight to snug up the Prolene within the graft. The needles are cut off and the Prolene is threaded onto a previously placed Keith needle, which is withdrawn, bringing the suture out through the nail. The end of the graft is fed into the medullary canal and pulled tightly into the bone. The suture is tied over a button on the nail. A strip of fine mesh gauze is then wrapped beneath the button to take up any slack in the system. For extra security, the juncture is reinforced with two 4–0 nonabsorbable sutures that catch the graft, tendon stump, and, if possible, some periosteum. Care is taken not to interfere with the pull-out system. The pull-out suture is removed at 4 weeks by cutting the button off and pulling one end of the Prolene out distally at the nail. This technique has an advantage in that the direction of removal is more favorable; it also does away with the need for the separate pullout loop used in the original technique. Moreover, Prolene suture slides out much more easily than wire and is therefore much less painful for the patient.

For completeness the older wire technique is described. A Bunnell-type suture is placed in the distal end of the tendon graft using 4–0 monofilament wire on straight needles, taking care not to put a kink in the wires. The pull-out loop must be placed prior to the first crisscross. The ends of the wires are now placed in the previously placed Keith needles and pulled through into the bone. The wires are tied over a button on the nail with gauze wrapped between the button and the nail to snug up the system. The pull-out loop needle is passed proximally, dorsal to the neurovascular bundle and out through the skin.

After completion of the distal juncture, nerve repair, if necessary, is carried out at this time. The finger wound is then closed, and the proximal juncture is carried out.

Proximal Juncture

All of the end-to-end suture techniques to join tendons of similar sizes together have been used in tendon grafting by various authors. As these techniques leave little margin for error as far as tension adjustment is concerned, and because the graft is often a different size than the motor tendon, interweave techniques are usually better utilized at the proximal juncture of a free tendon graft. An additional advantage is the inherent strength of this type of repair.[79,421] It is desirable to create a juncture that can withstand muscle pull in the early healing period and prevent gapping of the repair. A gap will lengthen the repair, making the graft too long, and also creates an area of potential rupture.[195,197,225,421]

The proximal juncture is made into the profundus tendon just distal to the lumbrical origin. The lumbrical muscle itself is left undisturbed unless it is involved in scarring, in which case this scar tissue is excised. Severe scarring may be an indication for staged tendon reconstruction.

Methods of Proximal Juncture

The Bunnell Crisscross Suture (Fig. 51-10). Using 4–0 monofilament wire on straight needles, a double crisscross is placed in the motor tendon and carried over into the graft. This can also be done using a Dacron suture, but the needles must be passed simultaneously to prevent snagging by the needle and weakening of the suture material within the tendon. A modification in which two sutures are used, one in each end of the tendons to be joined, and then tied at each side of the juncture, simplified this suture and is preferred when using this technique.

Despite a long history of successful application of this technique by many, including the authors, work by Bergljung[26] suggests that gapping of this repair is not uncommon and that this technique may cause undue impingement on the microcirculation of the tendon. However, a study by Wray and Weeks[472] concluded that this repair used by a hand surgeon would give satisfactory results.

Grasping Suture (Kessler,[191,192] Mason,[253–257] Allen,[2] Koch[204–207]) (Fig. 51-11). The authors' modification, which has been described by Tajima,[406] makes use of two polyester sutures, whereas Kessler described using only one. The 4–0 suture enters the cut surface and exits about 0.5 cm above, grasping

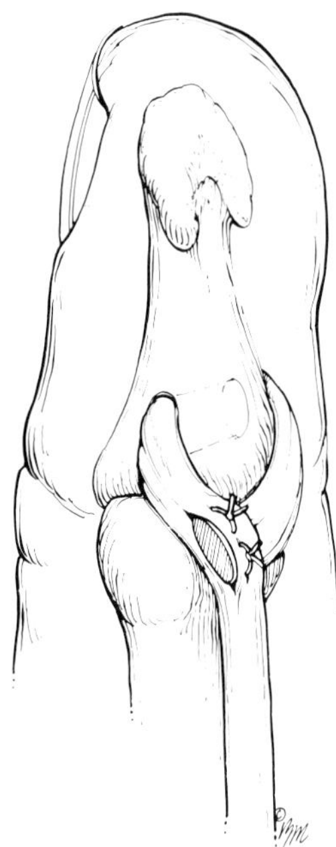

Fig. 51-6. Distal juncture technique. The tendon graft, which must be thin, is passed through a transverse drill hole in the distal phalanx.

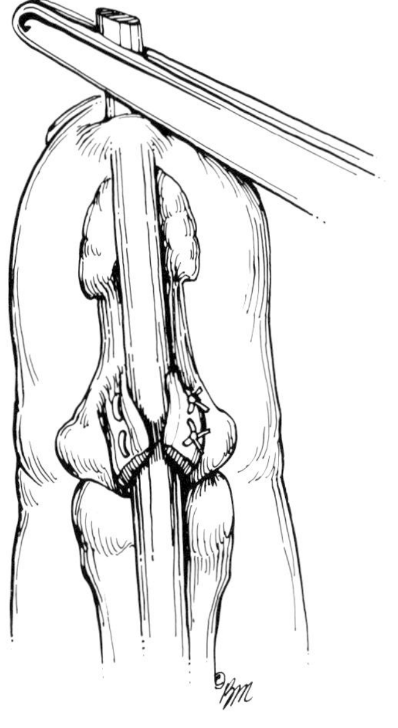

Fig. 51-7. Distal juncture technique. The graft itself is drawn through the pulp and, after tension adjustments are made, is sutured to the profundus stump.

some fibers. The needle is then reintroduced transversely, exiting 180 degrees on the other side of the tendon. Here fibers are grasped, and the needle reenters the tendon longitudinally to emerge at the cut surface. A similarly placed suture is applied through the other stump, and two knots are tied simultaneously, burying the knots within the juncture. While some surgeons have used a 6–0 circumferential running suture to oversew the repair, this suture has little tensile strength, as shown in a recent in vitro study done in dogs.[218] This same study, however, showed that a rather complex locking peripheral suture added considerable strength to the repair and would suggest further study in an in vivo model.

Another recent study reported that a properly applied peripheral suture added to the core stitch helped prevent early gap formation in direct repair.[439] The oversew suture is not recommended outside of Zone II. We make frequent use of the Kessler suture in our tendon work.

Authors' Preferred Method

Our preferred method is interlace suture (Pulvertaft[325–329]) (Fig. 51-12). This technique is especially useful for tendon grafts or in any area outside the flexor sheath, within which it would be too bulky. The motor tendon is slit with a fine blade at its end or a tendon braider instrument is used, and the graft is threaded into the slit. A tendon braider is a fine clamp which has been sharpened for use in penetrating the recipient tendon. The graft is then threaded transversely in a different plane. Buried 4–0 polyester sutures are used to join the tendons, and the fish mouth created is closed to embrace the graft. This type of juncture appears to be stronger than the end-to-end suture techniques.[79,84,421]

There are many other end-to-end techniques[22,23,84,197,253,341,349,414–417,421,429,447] that may be suitable for tendon grafting, each with its advantages and disadvantages. The reader is referred to the literature for details.

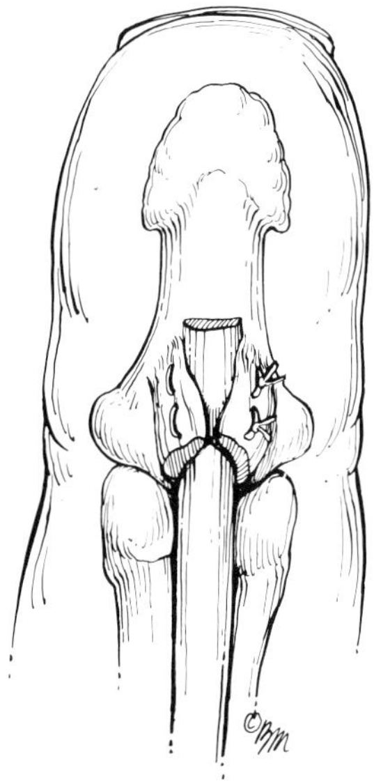

Fig. 51-8. Distal juncture technique. In this tendon-to-tendon technique an interweave suture is used to fix the graft to the stump of flexor digitorum profundus.

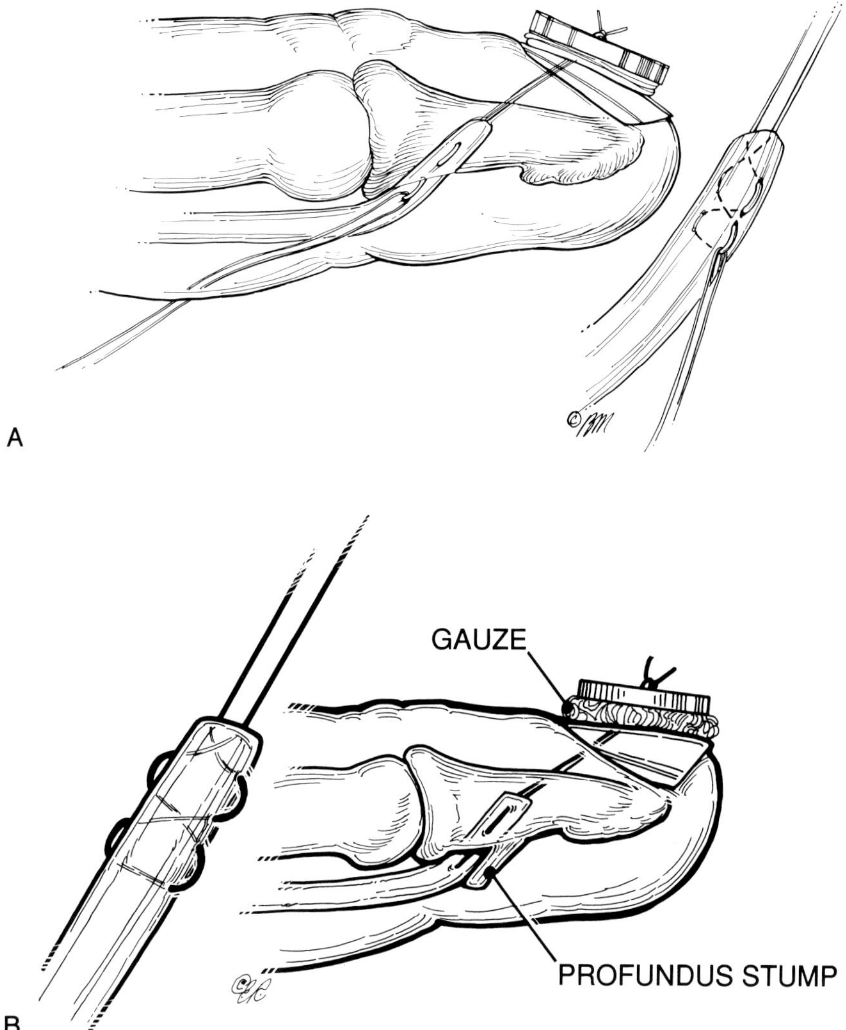

Fig. 51-9. Distal juncture technique. **(A)** The classic Bunnell technique provides a strong distal juncture. The suture is done using #32 wire. **(B)** It can be used without the proximal pull-out wire, removing the suture distally by pulling on one of the ends of the Prolene suture at the time of button removal.

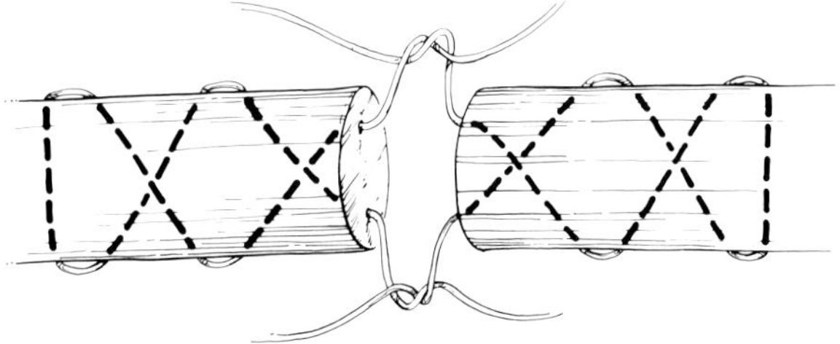

Fig. 51-10. Proximal juncture technique. The Bunnell crisscross suture modified by using two separate sutures tied within the tendon juncture.

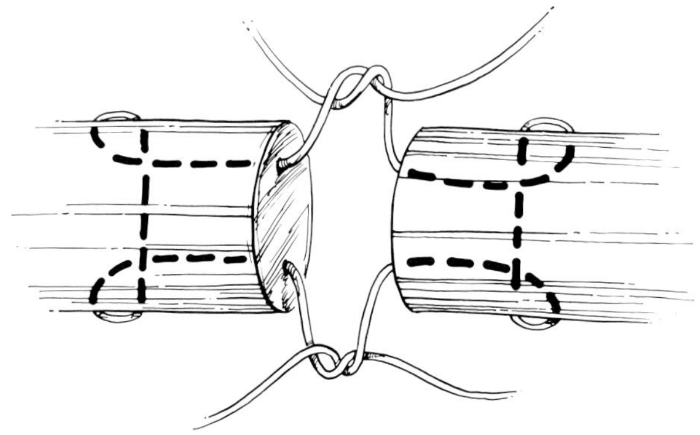

Fig. 51-11. Proximal juncture technique. The grasping suture using two separate sutures tied within the juncture.

Obtaining Free Tendon Grafts

The tendons of the palmaris longus, plantaris, and long extensors of the three middle toes are available for use as free tendon grafts.[366,461,462] The flexor superficialis tendon can also be utilized under certain conditions, and the proprius extensors [extensor indicis proprius (EIP) and extensor digiti minimi (EDM)] have their advocates.[385] The selection of a graft in any particular instance is determined by its presence and then by the particular demands of the surgical procedure. The tendon graft, once obtained, is handled with the utmost care. It should be placed in a sponge moistened with saline or Ringer's solution to protect it from drying. There should be no careless handling of the graft, and it must be protected from injury to its surface. Clamps or suture on each end can be used to facilitate handling of the graft.

Considerable controversy surrounds the role of paratenon in free tendon grafts. Bunnell[54] defined paratenon as the specialized loose fatty tissue that fills the space between tendons and the immovable fascial compartments through which they run. He believed that it serves to assist gliding, and in the intact, uninjured situation this sounds reasonable. However, is paratenon likely to be helpful on the surface of a tendon graft by participating in establishing a new gliding system? This is the question that reconstructive surgeons must consider. Transfer of paratenon with the graft was believed to be necessary by Bunnell[54] and others.[41,108,204,230,237,262,354,453,461,462] Strandell,[396] Peacock,[306] and others[35,315,417,440,444,454] have questioned the desirability of paratenon on grafts, believing that it may contribute to adhesion formation. The question comes down to whether this material should be regarded as "slippery stuff" or "sticky stuff." We tend to support the latter concept, and our policy is to carefully remove the paratenon from our tendon grafts, with every effort being made not to injure the delicate surface of the graft. We may leave a small margin of the fatty material on the graft rather than risk injury to the surface of the graft[306] (Fig. 51-13).

Palmaris Longus

As a general rule, we prefer the palmaris longus for use in the palm-to-fingertip graft, as it is in the same field of surgery and is easily accessible. The presence of the palmaris longus is easily determined by examination preoperatively. The patient is asked to oppose the thumb to the little finger while flexing the wrist against resistance. The palmaris longus tendon should be readily visible, superficial, and palpable in the midline of the wrist. This tendon is present in 85 percent of people,[338] but due

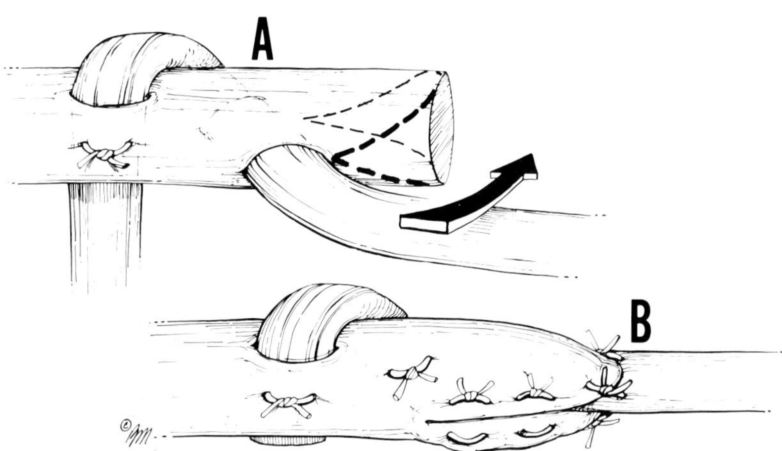

Fig. 51-12. Proximal juncture technique. The Pulvertaft interlace suture. This can be used in the palm or distal forearm; it greatly simplifies the establishment of proper tension in the reconstructed flexor system.

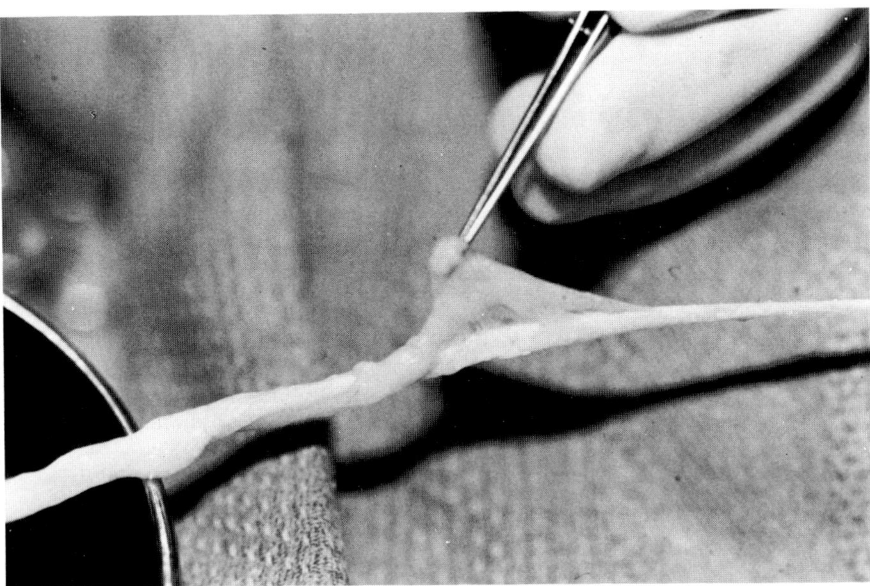

Fig. 51-13. Paratenon. This fatty tissue on the surface of the plantaris tendon is carefully removed so that the surface of the graft is not injured.

to variations its presence does not guarantee its usefulness, as it may be very fine or have a long muscle belly, which makes it an inadequate graft. In its usual form, however, it provides sufficient length for one palm-to-fingertip graft and is of satisfactory diameter to serve as an excellent tendon graft.

Technique. A transverse incision is made at the wrist. The tendon is identified by blunt dissection along the long axis of the tendon. Positive identification is made. The skin is elevated and retracted, and the tendon mobilized subcutaneously under direct vision. A transverse incision is then made 6 to 8 cm above the first incision, and the tendon is pulled into this second wound after transection at the wrist crease. A third and occasionally fourth wound may be necessary to obtain the entire length of tendon.

Authors' Preferred Method (Fig. 51-14). A transverse incision is made at the wrist, and the palmaris longus is positively identified. After transection at the wrist crease, a holding suture of 4–0 silk is placed in the distal end of the graft. The tendon is then mobilized proximally, under direct vision, for 6 to 8 cm and threaded through a circular tendon stripper. Holding tension on the graft at its distal end with a clamp, the stripper is firmly advanced with a slight twisting motion. As the stripper advances into the proximal forearm, the muscle belly will fill the circular cutting blade and be divided, allowing the tendon to be withdrawn through one incision. At times a second proximal incision is made over the stripper in the proximal forearm if the surgeon feels undue resistance to the stripper.

Plantaris Tendon

When multiple grafts are needed or one long distal forearm-to-fingertip graft is required, it is necessary to go to the lower extremity and seek out tendons longer than the palmaris. The presence of the plantaris tendon cannot be predicted preoperatively, and although it is said to be absent in only 7 percent of cadavers,[83] our experience suggests that it is absent far more frequently. This has been verified by Harvey and colleagues,[131] who found that the tendon was present in about 80 percent of limbs. They also reported that if absent in one limb the chance of finding it in the other was only one in three. It is also unusable at times because of variations in its girth or by virtue of attachments to the triceps surae, which make its removal in one length impossible. However, at its best, the plantaris is an excellent graft and can supply two, and occasionally three, palm-to-fingertip grafts or one long distal forearm-to-fingertip graft.

Technique[43,461] (Fig. 51-15). A 5-cm vertical incision is made just anterior to the medial aspect of the Achilles tendon starting at the insertion and proceeding proximally. The tendon is identified, using blunt dissection, anterior to the Achilles tendon and divided near its insertion. With a holding suture securely fixed in its cut end, the tendon is mobilized bluntly as far as possible under direct vision. This gives the tubular stripper through which tendon is threaded a nonangled start up the leg. The stripper should be held parallel to the leg and advanced with a wiggling motion while the tendon graft is held under tension. The knee should be extended. When the belly of the plantaris muscle fills the stripper it divides the muscle, allowing the entire plantaris tendon to be withdrawn from the wound. Care must be taken to keep the stripper parallel to the long axis of the tendon or else the tendon may be severed prematurely.

Long Toe Extensors

The long toe extensors can serve as excellent grafts. Their presence is assured and their diameter is appropriate to most needs. As many as three long tendon grafts are provided when the tendons to the second, third, and fourth toes are harvested.

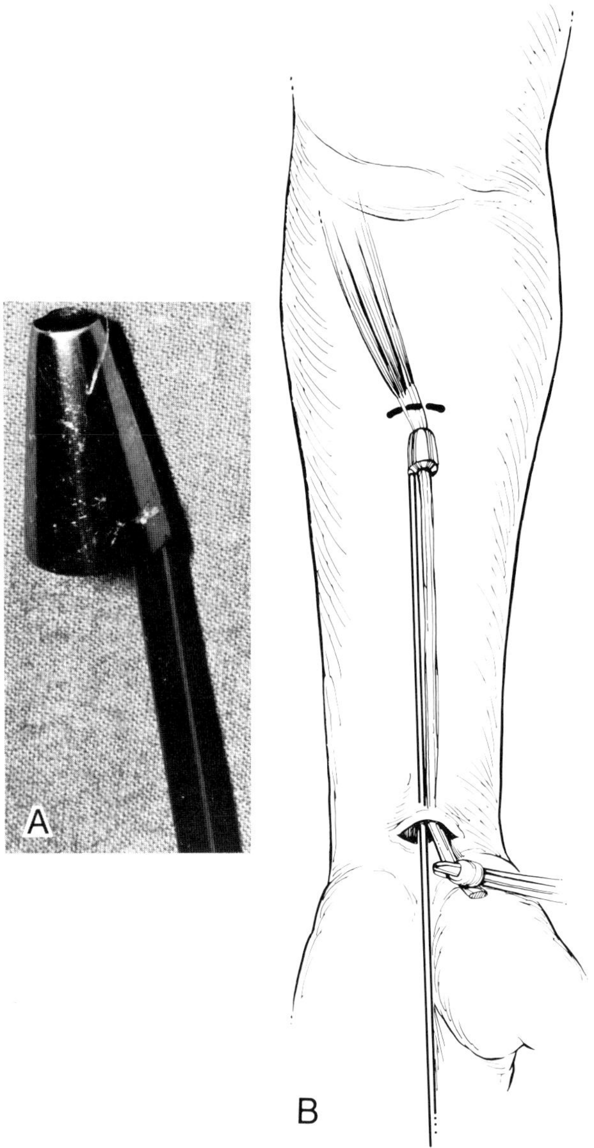

Fig. 51-14. Palmaris longus. Our preferred technique for obtaining the graft uses a tendon stripper, which is a circular knife passed along the surface of the tendon. **(A)** The stripper. **(B)** Technique. The stripper is advanced until it cuts off the graft at the muscle belly, or a second proximal incision can be used to obtain the proximal end of the tendon graft.

The problem frequently arising is that the individual tendons may fuse distal to the ankle, and three long grafts may be unobtainable. Although we formerly removed these through a large longitudinal incision,[462] we believe that wound morbidity is reduced by using multiple transverse incisions and a tendon stripper.

Technique (Fig. 51-16). A generous transverse incision is made on the dorsum of the foot at the level of the metatarsophalangeal joint. The long toe extensor is isolated proximal to the hood and prepared for the stripper by placing a holding suture in the tendon and transecting it. After mobilization, a small stripper is advanced proximally but stopped when resistance is encountered. A second transverse incision is made at this level, and the cause of obstruction is checked under direct vision. Further direct dissection can be carried out, the tendon withdrawn into this second wound, and the stripper again utilized. Distal to the ankle level, the cruciate crural ligament encloses the tendons and this must be opened. From this point proximally, the tendon can be stripped up into the leg. In some cases all the long extensors will have merged, making it impossible to obtain a high-quality long graft. When this problem is encountered, more and larger incisions are used and the tendons are actually dissected out individually. This, of course, compromises the graft because it will have some raw surfaces created by the dissection.

Flexor Digitorum Superficialis

The superficialis is rarely used as a free tendon graft but can occasionally be useful. A segment of injured superficialis tendon can serve as a free graft to the profundus within the same finger, provided the level of injury allows for sufficient length of the graft. The use of a normal superficialis tendon would be an unlikely free graft source, although the entire intact muscle-tendon unit is useful as a tendon transfer under certain conditions.[313,376] An example would be reconstruction of the flexor system of the little finger or thumb using the entire flexor digitorum superficialis muscle-tendon unit of the long or ring finger. This technique has been particularly useful in reconstruction of the flexor pollicis longus system.

Short segments of the flexor digitorum superficialis are also useful as interposition grafts in the reconstruction of Zone III injuries in which end-to-end repair is not possible.

Extensor Proprius Tendons

The two proprius tendons (EIP and EDM) are available for grafting material. Each can provide sufficient length for one palm-to-fingertip graft. We rarely use this source.

Technique. The tendon is exposed through a transverse incision over the MP joint of either the index or little finger. The proprius tendon lies ulnar to the corresponding extensor digitorum communis tendon and is transected about 1 cm proximal to the hood after a holding suture is placed in the tendon end. The tendon is then mobilized subcutaneously, and a second incision is made over the musculotendinous junction proximal to the wrist. The tendon can usually be pulled into the second wound and transected. If the tendon does not withdraw easily, a third incision halfway between the first and second may be necessary. Synovial connections can be freed under direct vision through this incision. In the case of the proprius extensor to the little finger, usually represented by two tendon slips, Snow recommends taking only the ulnar half as a graft.[385]

Tendon Allografts

Tendons taken from fresh cadavers or from amputated limbs have been preserved in a mercurial solution; these have been used extensively by Iselin[174,175] for free tendon grafts. The

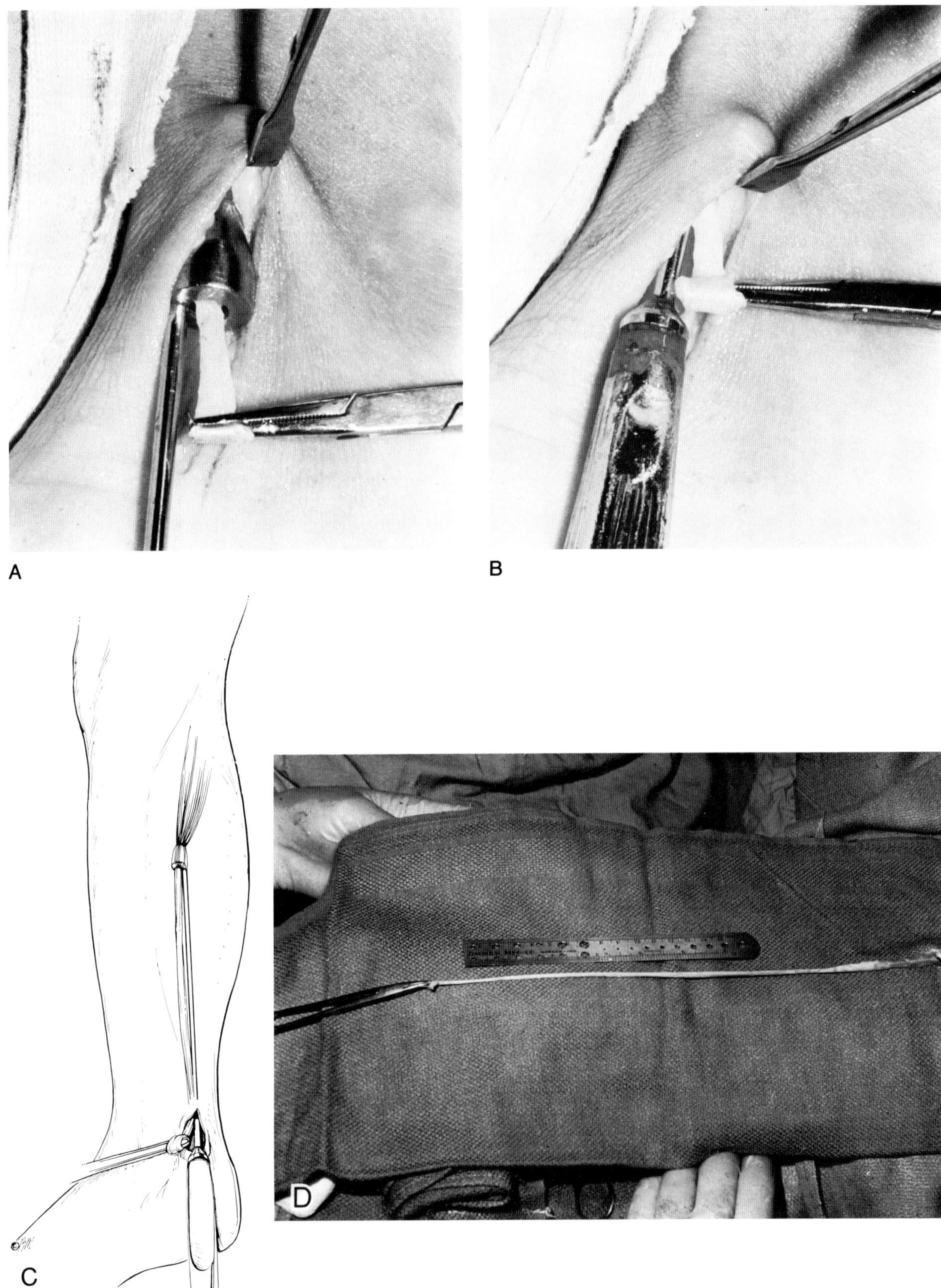

Fig. 51-15. Plantaris. **(A)** The tendon is located anterior and medial to the Achilles tendon. After division distally, it is passed through the circular stripper. **(B)** The stripper is advanced up the leg. **(C)** When the stripper engages the muscle belly, it divides it, enabling the surgeon to withdraw the tendon. **(D)** The plantaris graft can supply two fingertip-to-palm grafts.

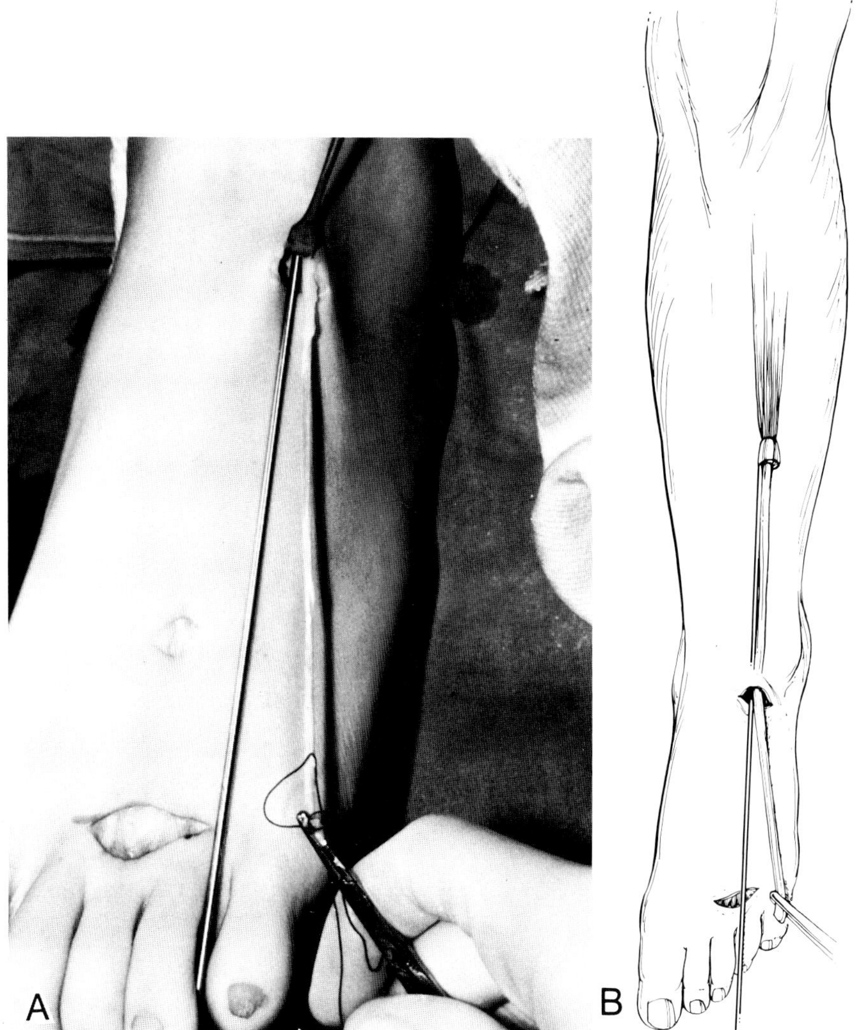

Fig. 51-16. Long toe extensors. These tendons are best obtained through multiple transverse incisions on the foot. **(A)** Graft obtainable when the long toe extensor is used. **(B)** Once proximal to the ankle, the stripper can be advanced up the leg until the muscle is severed.

advantages of using this material are obvious, but the concept has not had widespread acceptance.[321] Other authors have written of the use of tendon allografts.[234,235,284,381,446] We have no clinical experience with the use of tendon allografts or heterografts.

Tendon Graft Length: Adjusting Tension in the Flexor System

Bunnell[54] believed that grafts tend to shrink with time; therefore, he recommended a graft in excess of normal length. Pulvertaft[325] noted that grafts did better if they were put in slightly more tension than is normally present, believing that with exercise the muscle stretches out somewhat. Others have studied methods to determine more exactly the length of the graft needed to restore the ideal tension in the flexor system.[394] Williams[465] used electrical stimulation of the motor nerves at surgery to cause profundus contraction, enabling him to exactly determine the length of the graft. Electrical stimulation was also used by Omer and Vogel.[296] Mayou and Harrison[271] measured the length of tendon removed at primary and delayed primary tendon grafting and developed a chart that gave estimates of tendon graft lengths needed in each finger. Kaplan[185] and Colville and Dickie[77] developed techniques for estimating graft lengths.

Another approach to estimating length of the graft uses the patient's active cooperation, and on occasion we have performed tendon grafts under local anesthesia[163] in which we were able to determine critical graft length by active flexion and extension of the finger by the patient (see Neuroleptanalgesia in Chapter 2).

In general, most surgeons agree that length is estimated in the anesthetized patient by the relaxed positioning of the fingers with the wrist in neutral position.[35,230,444] Each finger should fall into semiflexion, slightly less flexed than its ulnar neighbor or more flexed than its adjacent radial finger (Fig.

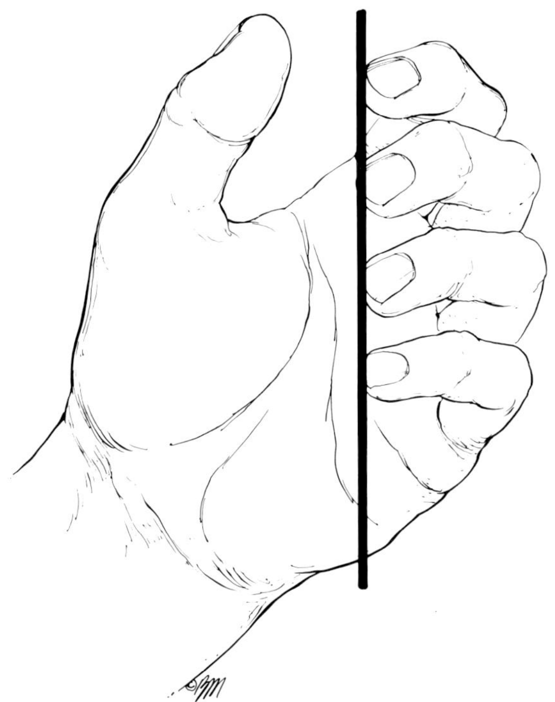

Fig. 51-17. Determining tension in a reconstructed flexor system at the time of suturing the proximal juncture. With the wrist in neutral position, each finger falls into slightly less flexion than its ulnar neighbor.

51-17). Using the interweave technique,[325,444] this can be studied with one suture in place and, if the posture of the hand is satisfactory, the juncture is completed.

Postoperative Management of Tendon Grafts

Traditional treatment called for a period of 3 weeks immobilization in which a posterior molded plaster splint is applied from fingertips to below the elbow, with the wrist flexed approximately 35 degrees, the MP joints at 60 to 70 degrees, and the interphalangeal joints at rest in extension. The dressings are changed at 10 days when the skin sutures are removed. The splint is replaced and worn full time for a total of 21 days, at which time an active exercise program is instituted.[418] The patient wears the splint in between exercise periods for 1 or 2 additional weeks. The pull-out suture is removed at 28 days, at which time more vigorous exercises can be started.

Since the earliest edition of this chapter we have expanded our use of "controlled mobilization"[229] used in primary and secondary tendon repairs to our tendon grafts. The use of this technique, adopted from the aftercare used in primary repair, has been supported by other clinicians.[70,173,258,412] This is set up at surgery by placing a nylon suture through the nail, to which an elastic band is attached allowing for active extension and passive flexion in the postoperative period. Details for this procedure are presented in the section on secondary tendon repairs (page 1880).

Regardless of the postoperative technique selected, patients whose tendon grafts glide well, as demonstrated by an early recovery of range of motion, are protected by splinting for a longer period of time, as these "soft-healers" are more likely to rupture their junctures if overstressed in the early postoperative period. Therefore, when full excursion recovers rapidly postoperatively, resistive exercises are deferred for 6 to 8 weeks from surgery.

Resistive exercises, such as blocking, in which the patient blocks flexion at the MP joint while attempting active flexion at the distal joints, will put stress on the junctures as well as on limiting adhesions. This, however, is the most valuable method used to obtain gliding and is used, blocking the MP and PIP joints, gently at 4 weeks and more vigorously at 5 weeks. Judgment must be used in guiding the more active patient and prodding the reluctant. Blocking is best done using the other hand (Fig. 51-18A), but wood blocks ("Bunnell blocks") cut to fit in the hand also have been useful (Fig. 51-18B and C). Flexion deformities are treated by gentle passive stretching as well as by elastic traction splints, interval finger casting, and static splints.

Tendon repairs strengthen[255,256] and fingers improve functionally over the next 6 months.

A program in which immediate active motion was allowed has been advocated,[19] but this required hospitalization for direct supervision.

The Fate of a Tendon Graft

If a grafted tendon is reexplored after a period of 6 or more months, it is often seen to be of normal appearance, and is, indeed, histologically a replica of the original tendon. Whether the tendon is in reality the original graft or a new creation brought about by fibroblasts from the host building on a scaffold provided by the graft is a question pondered by many writers. The answer, according to Lindsay and McDougall,[223] is that the graft as a whole survives and is reconstructed by a repair process manifested by an increase in number of mature fibroblasts, a revascularization of the graft, and a gradual reconstruction of the original collagen. This concept was confirmed in a later study by the same group.[28] It is likely that the graft is nourished by local synovial fluids prior to revascularization of its tissue. Blood supply is then carried in by local granulation tissue in the form of adhesions. Others have written about the fate of tendon grafts.[125,221,308]

Complications[227,360]

The most common problem after flexor tendon grafting, as in all flexor tendon surgery, is adhesion formation along the surface of the graft and at the level of the proximal juncture, which by immobilizing or tethering the free passage of the graft through the tissues, prevents gliding necessary for finger motion.[360] To help reduce this problem the surgeon must practice gentle handling of the tissues, use fine instruments, and adhere to proven surgical indications. Each injury to the surface of the tendon will result in an adhesion at that level. The assistance of a good hand therapy program will often help mobilize adhesions and guide the patient through the critical 8-week period

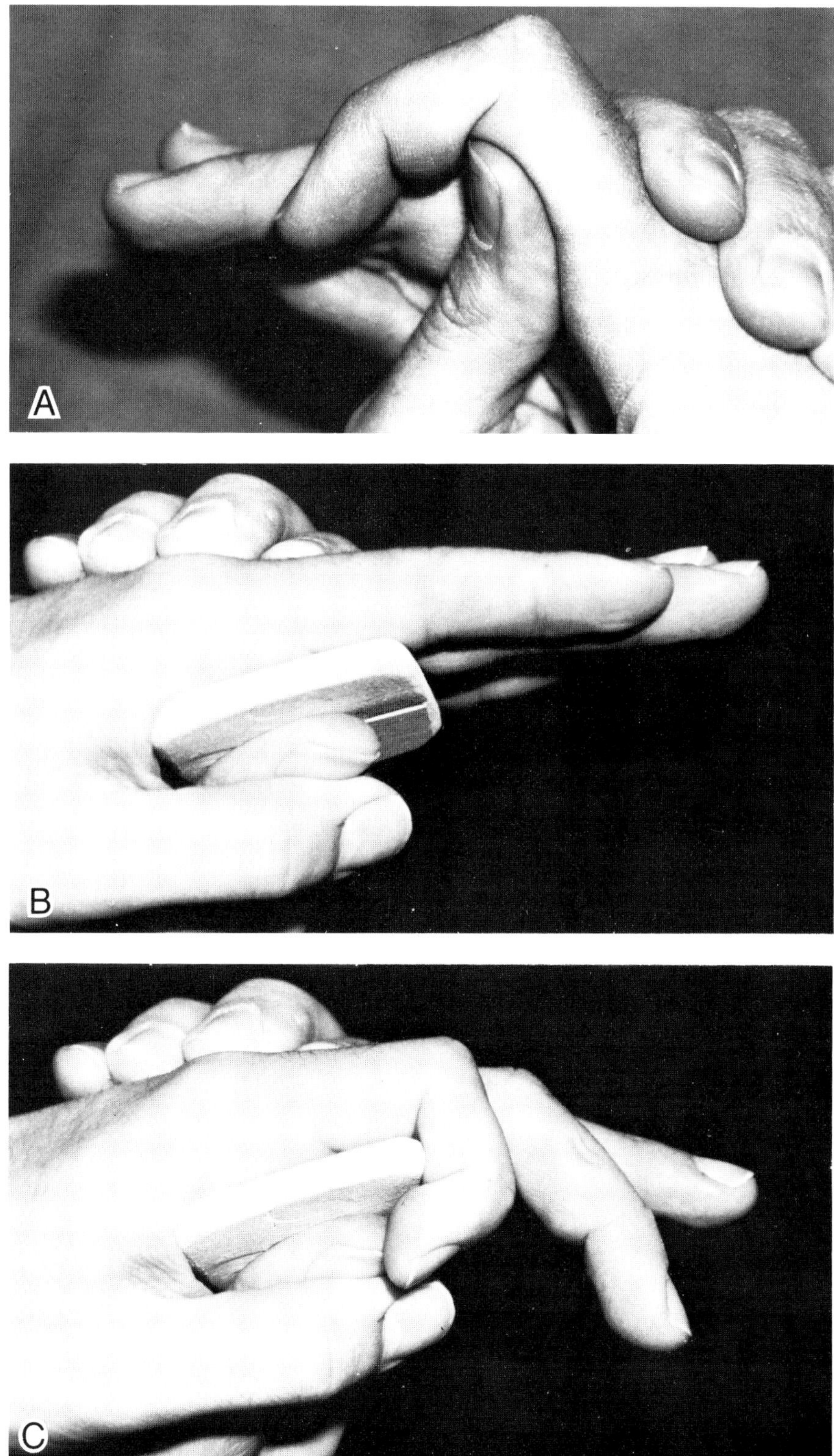

Fig. 51-18. Blocking used at the PIP or DIP joint is accomplished by stabilizing the more proximal joint and forcing the tendon to actively pull through distally. This can be done by using the fingers of the other hand **(A)** or a pre-cut wood block **(B&C).**

after surgery. Tenolysis (see page 1881) is effective in salvaging some tendon grafts with adhesion problems, provided the patient has reached a plateau and at least 3 to 6 months have elapsed since the grafting procedure.

Rupture of the junctures, either proximal or distal, can occur, but should be minimized to a large degree by careful attention to the technical details of the procedure. Close supervision postoperatively will help control the patient who overuses his hand too early in the program.

When a separation of a graft juncture is recognized early, rapid reexploration and reattachment can occasionally salvage the situation. Exploration is done under local-sedative anesthesia, and if distal reattachment is not possible a "superficialis finger" [164,368] can be created by reattachment into the middle phalanx (see page 1898). If the bed is still satisfactory and reattachment is not possible, regrafting can be considered. When the bed is known to be poor, the finger should be passively mobilized and prepared for staged tendon reconstruction.

Absence of the superficialis tendon in a grafted finger may, by interfering with the delicate finger balance,[293,383,384,463] result in a hyperextension deformity at the PIP joint, and create a problem in initiating flexion at that joint. The surgeon who anticipates this problem in hyperextensile, loose-jointed patients should tenodese one tail of the superficialis across the PIP joint as part of the grafting procedure. Also notable if the graft is too long is the lumbrical-plus finger described by Parkes.[300,301] This occurs when, with proximal movement of the graft, the lumbrical origin is also normally pulled proximally. If the graft is too long, excessive traction is exerted on the lumbrical muscle, which will "paradoxically" cause extension at the interphalangeal joints. This problem can be avoided by ensuring proper length at the time of placement of the graft. This problem is not seen frequently, partly because our grafts are not perfect enough in their gliding to allow this situation to occur.[417] Those who advocate wrapping the lumbrical muscle around the proximal juncture in the palm incur increased risk of creating this problem, and, therefore, this technique is not advocated at this time.

TENDON GRAFTING IN THE FINGER WITH AN INTACT SUPERFICIALIS (ZONE I INJURIES)

In patients with an injury to the flexor profundus but an intact flexor superficialis, a careful early direct repair is indicated, provided the lesion is recognized and referred in time.[213] It is unusual that direct repair can be performed after 3 to 4 weeks have elapsed unless the short vinculum to the flexor digitorum profundus has remained intact and has kept the tendon well out in the finger. This may not be determinable until exploration. At times in the closed injury the tendon is avulsed with a piece of the bony insertion; a radiograph may thus be of value in determining the location of the proximal tendon end.

When more than 4 weeks have elapsed and the flexor digitorum superficialis is fully functional, careful consideration and much caution should be exercised before offering the patient a free tendon graft to restore distal joint function.[362] Much of the useful arc of motion of the finger has been maintained if the flexor digitorum superficialis is fully functional[232] (Fig. 51-19), and there is considerable risk to this function if, while passing the tendon graft through or around the superficialis one does injury to this delicate system and adhesions intervene, resulting in an overall loss of function. In short, the patient can be made worse if this procedure fails. Many surgeons have voiced conservatism here.[139,286,289,337,341,440]

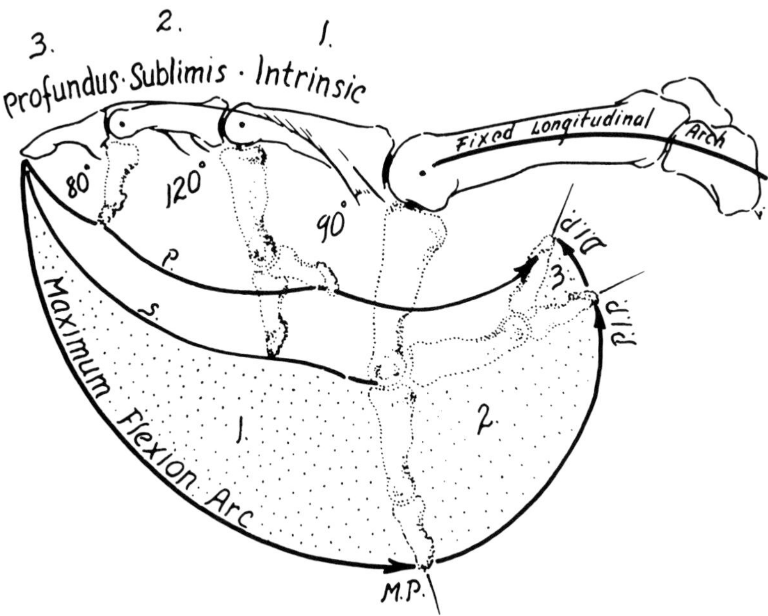

Fig. 51-19. The flexion arc. In isolated injuries to the flexor profundus where the flexor superficialis is fully functional, the greatest part of the flexion arc is maintained (denoted by stippled areas *1* and *2*). Restoration of active profundus function provides only that portion of the arc denoted by the small stippled area *3*. (From Littler,[232] with permission.)

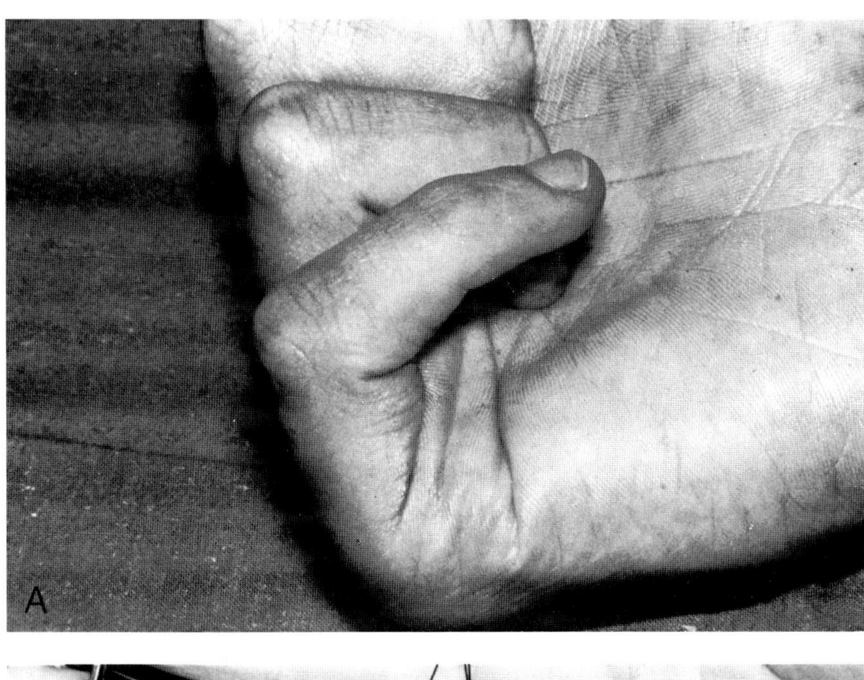

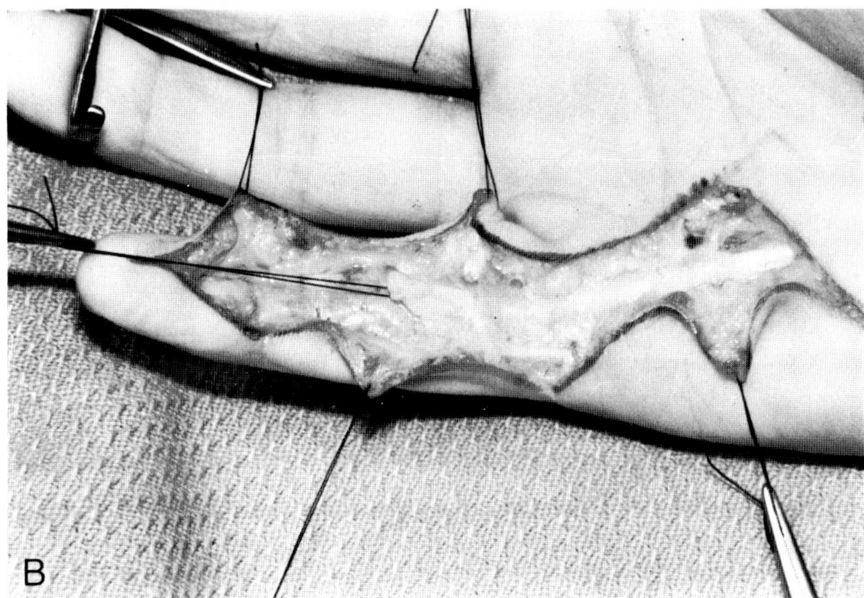

Fig. 51-20. Tendon graft through an intact superficialis. **(A)** This 17-year-old boy had ruptured the flexor digitorum profundus and demonstrated incomplete superficialis function 3 months after injury. **(B)** The flexor digitorum profundus was retrieved and mobilized, but it was not possible to advance it to the insertion. A tendon graft was then placed. *(Figure continues.)*

Despite the difficulties and not inconsiderable risks, others[30,117,177,273,326,392] have presented outstanding results with this lesion in carefully selected patients. Frankly, it is our opinion that much of the variability in results here could be attributed to different techniques used by the authors in the evaluation of their patients.[292,357,362]

The procedure should be restricted to young people with supple joints and a reasonable need for active DIP joint function. The graft is probably more frequently justified on the ulnar side of the hand (i.e., in the ring and little fingers for power grip) than on the radial side of the hand (Fig. 51-20). A thinner graft is easier to pass, and the plantaris should be useful here. The technique is similar to free tendon grafting discussed earlier. We usually pass the graft through the superficialis decussation but, if this area appears tight, we may elect to pass the graft around the superficialis. Under *no* conditions is it ever justifiable to remove an intact, fully functioning flexor superficialis tendon. Harrison did suggest removal of one tail of the tendon for passage of the graft.[129] The grafting of the isolated flexor profundus lesion is even better indicated when the superficialis is not pulling through completely. On occasion the procedure has been done in two stages,[139,438,468] placing a tendon implant as the first stage, particularly if there has been some element of injury to the superficialis or the flexor tendon bed or pulley system. The use of the staged tendon graft has been gratifying here but should be restricted to those fingers

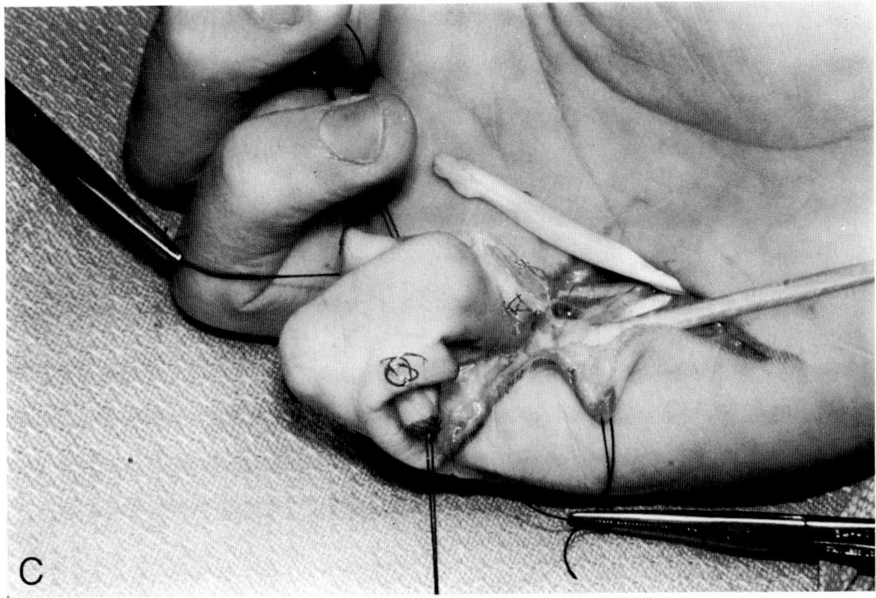

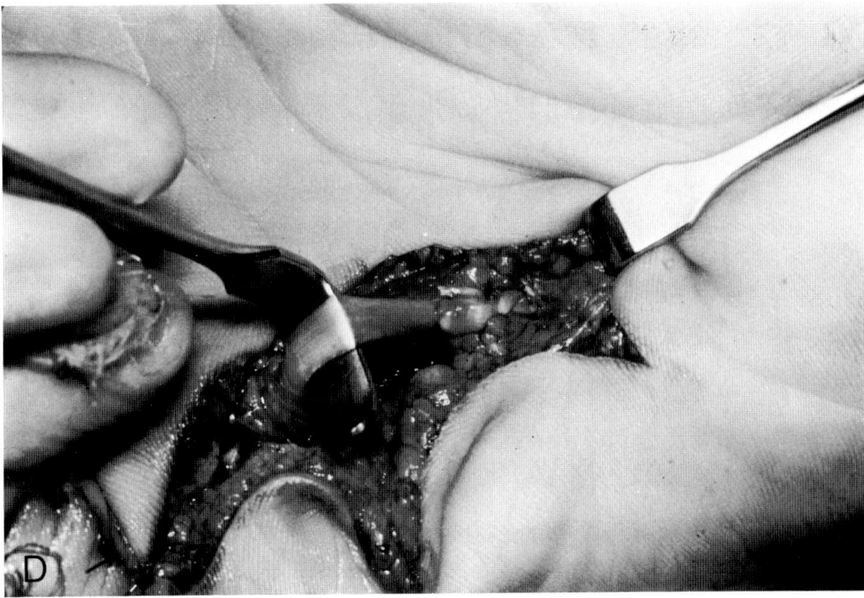

Fig. 51-20 *(Continued).* **(C)** The graft in place. The finger will be closed prior to completing the proximal juncture. **(D)** An interlace juncture in the palm using the flexor digitorum profundus as the motor. *(Figure continues.)*

with a poor bed.[404] In the one-stage procedure a thin graft passed through the superficialis decussation is preferred. It was noted that a considerable number of patients who underwent this one-stage graft procedure required tenolysis as a second stage.[362]

Other Methods of Treatment in the Finger with a Severed Profundus and an Intact Superficialis

Some patients who have this lesion may adapt to it quite well and will need no treatment. This is especially likely in those people with tight joints in whom the distal joint does not go into hyperextension. In view of the risks, it is not unreasonable to accept this condition in many patients, especially the aged and the heavy laborer. In those patients troubled by instability at the tip or by the lack of involvement of the distal portion of the finger in grip, stabilization of the DIP joint by tenodesis[183] or arthrodesis can be recommended.

RECONSTRUCTION OF THE FLEXOR POLLICIS LONGUS

There are only a few articles written on the repair of this tendon,[8,274,285] and, as pointed out by Urbaniak[419] and Urbaniak and Goldner,[422] the long flexor tendon of the thumb is different from the other digital flexor tendons. Despite this, many studies of flexor tendon repairs include repairs of this

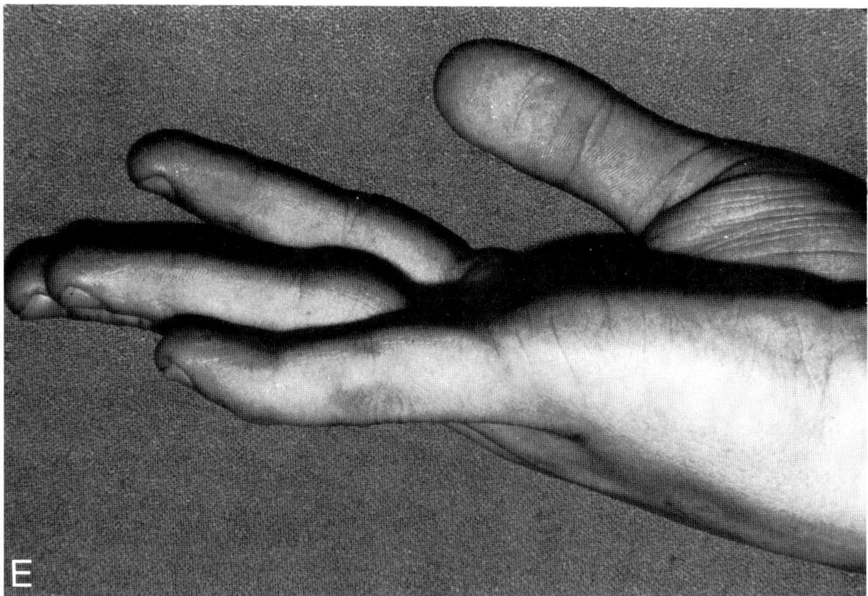

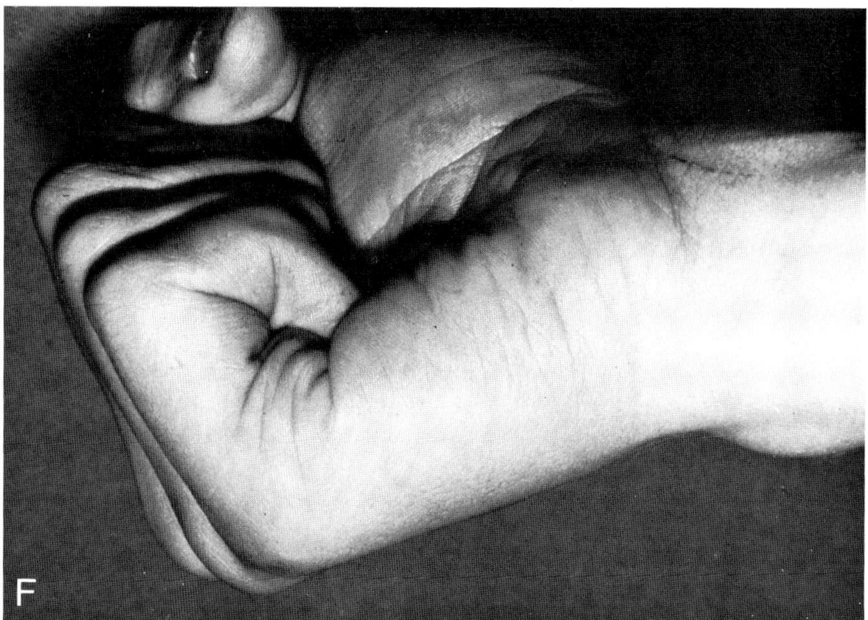

Fig. 51-20 *(Continued).* **(E&F)** End result at 1 year. There is a flexion deformity at the tip but a total of 50 degrees strong flexion has been gained at the DIP joint.

tendon when evaluating overall results. The flexor system of the thumb is considerably less complicated than that of the fingers, because there is one joint less in the system and only one long flexor tendon is involved. It should also be noted that the modest recovery of 30 to 40 degrees active flexion at the interphalangeal joint can provide an excellently functioning thumb. While some surgeons have questioned the advisability of reconstructing lesions in this area,[198] we believe that the attempt at restoration of active motion at the interphalangeal joint is generally justified.

Reconstructive procedures in flexor pollicis longus injuries are indicated when a satisfactory range of passive motion exists at the interphalangeal joint after expiration of the time when direct repair can be satisfactorily carried out. This would be seen in those situations in which the wound was deemed unfavorable at the time of injury, the significance of the injury was underestimated, or no trained surgeon was available at the time of injury.

Direct repair at all levels of injury may be possible as late as 3 to 4 weeks after wounding and even later in those cases where the tendon ends have not widely separated, as when the wound is distal and the proximal segment is prevented from retracting proximally by an intact vinculum. When doing delayed direct repair, preservation of as much pulley system as possible is recommended, provided it does not restrict proximal or distal movement of the repaired tendon as needed to accomplish active motion at the interphalangeal joint.

In those instances where the tendon ends cannot be rejoined

secondarily, the surgeon has several options if active motion is to be restored to the thumb tip.

Free Tendon Graft in the Thumb

Basically the same technique is utilized as that previously described for free tendon grafting in the fingers. The flexor system is approached through the volar zigzag incision[50] from the distal phalanx proximal to the MP joint (see Fig. 51-3B). Pulleys are preserved with care and the injured tendon is excised. A second incision is made, curvilinear, at the volar-radial aspect of the distal forearm starting distally at the wrist crease and proceeding about 6 cm proximally. The musculotendinous junction of the flexor pollicis longus is identified and the tendon pulled into this incision. The palmaris longus or plantaris is obtained and threaded through the system using a tendon passer. The distal juncture is carried out with the distal pull-out suture technique (or any of the distal juncture techniques) and the thumb wound closed. The proximal juncture is made by interweaving the graft into the tendon of the flexor pollicis longus. Tension in this system is critical. This is estimated by placing the wrist in 0 degrees (neutral) position, the thumb abducted in front of the index finger metacarpal, and the interphalangeal joint of the thumb in 30 degrees flexion. With tension set at the proximal juncture, the thumb should adopt this position. After wound closure and dressing, a dorsal splint is applied with the wrist in 30 degrees flexion and the thumb protected in about 30 degrees abduction at the carpometacarpal joint. The metacarpolphalangeal and interphalangeal joints are allowed full flexion by the dorsal splint, and an elastic band is attached via a suture through the nail. This band is then pinned to the dressing at the level of the pisiform with sufficient tension to keep the IP joint flexed about 30 degrees but allow full active extension against the splint. The patient is followed closely in this device for 3 to 4 weeks. Generally the patient is allowed to actively mobilize the joints at 3 weeks with the protective splint reapplied in between exercise sessions. At 4 weeks the button and pull-out suture is removed, and more strenuous activities, including blocking techniques, are allowed.

Flexor Digitorum Superficialis Transfer[313,376]

An alternative method to tendon grafting, especially useful when the flexor pollicis longus muscle is not functional, is the utilization of the superficialis flexor of the ring finger as both motor and tendon.

Technique

The zigzag volar approach to the flexor system of the thumb is used along with the second, curved, vertical incision in the distal forearm (Fig. 51-21). The injured tendon is removed with preservation of as much uninjured pulley system as possible. A transverse incision is made at the base of the ring finger, and the superficialis is identified and transected about 2 cm proximal to the PIP joint after a suture has been placed in one of the tails. The tendon is then located in the forearm wound and withdrawn into the wound. At times this may be difficult because of synovial interconnections, in which case a transverse wound in the palm is needed to free these connections. The tagging of distal end of the tendon with a silk suture facilitates the manipulations necessary to mobilize the donor tendon. With the tendon now in the forearm wound, it can be redirected into the thumb flexor system and a distal juncture carried out as in the free tendon graft. It must be noted, however, that the critical tension is more difficult to establish at the distal juncture, especially if the Bunnell tendon-to-bone technique is planned. For this reason one of the other techniques, which more easily allows readjustments to be made, is preferable (page 1860). In this situation, we prefer the split tendon-to-tendon technique described earlier. The repair is fixed with one suture, and tension is evaluated prior to completion of the juncture. The follow-up splint period for 3 to 4 weeks postoperatively is similar to that used in grafting. Mobilization of the transfer by combining active ring finger flexion with thumb flexion is helpful in learning to use the transfer.

Staged Tendon Reconstruction in the Thumb

In those patients in whom it is imperative to restore active thumb flexion and in whom prior surgery has failed or there is a severely scarred tendon bed, staged flexor tendon reconstruction offers an opportunity for salvage. This approach becomes even more pertinent where the retinacular pulley system has been destroyed. Pulley reconstruction over the implant at the level of the proximal half of the proximal phalanx will usually suffice if the oblique pulley has been destroyed. The details of the technique are similar to that in the fingers and are covered in that section (see page 1895). It is noted that in the thumb the surgeon can use a free graft or a superficialis transfer at Stage II.[376]

Other Options in Flexor Pollicis Longus Disruption

In patients who have lost flexor pollicis longus function but have a stable distal joint, it may be acceptable to do nothing if the time period for direct repair has passed, especially if the carpometacarpal and the MP joints are functioning normally. This is certainly reasonable in the aged.

When strong pinch is required, especially in the presence of intraarticular damage at the interphalangeal joint, or in those patients with a hyperextensile interphalangeal joint, arthrodesis of the joint in 10 to 20 degrees flexion is a predictable method to improve function.

For distal lacerations, advancement of the end of the cut tendon to the insertion can be performed, provided the advancement is limited to approximately 1 cm. As in the fingers, advancement must be used with caution, as making up a gap more then this amount will create a flexion deformity at the interphalangeal joint. If a greater advancement is needed, lengthening of the tendon at the musculocutaneous juncture has been advocated by Urbaniak and Goldner.[422] They used a Z-type lengthening, interweaving the ends and reinforcing the repair with a free tendon graft obtained from one-half of the flexor carpi radialis taken in the same wound. We have had little experience with this technique and would prefer to use a tendon graft if advancement is not practical.

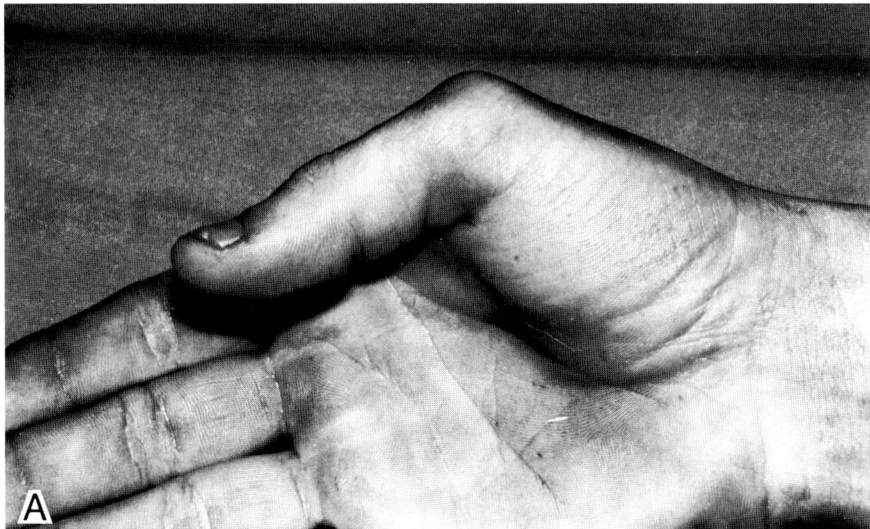

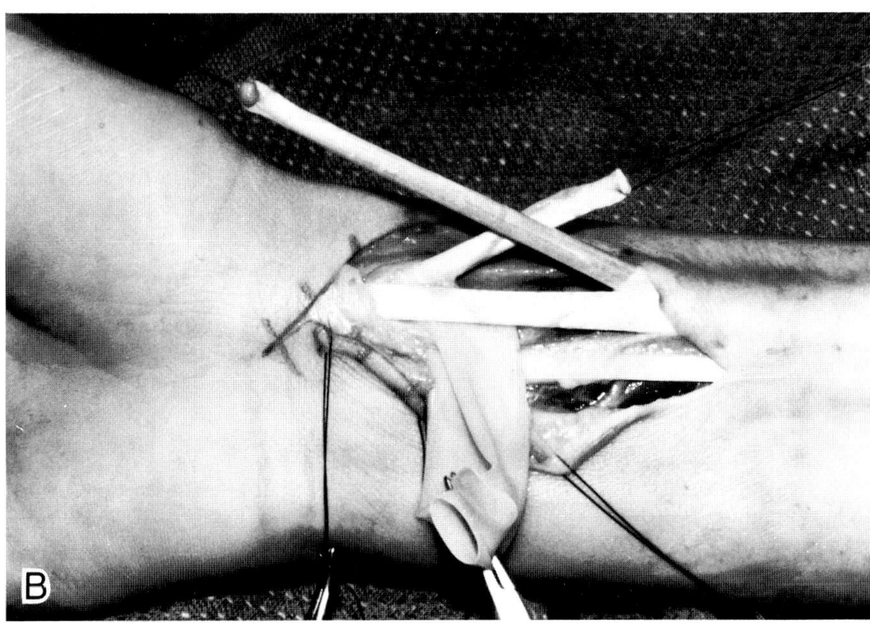

Fig. 51-21. Flexor pollicis longus reconstruction using the flexor digitorum superficialis from the ring finger. **(A)** Loss of active flexion at the interphalangeal joint of the right thumb in a 28-year-old machinist with an old Zone V laceration. **(B)** The distal flexor pollicis longus stump is obtained and the flexor superficialis is brought over into the same wound. An interlace juncture is utilized. *(Figure continues.)*

SECONDARY RECONSTRUCTION OF TENDON INJURIES IN ZONES III, IV, AND V

When flexor tendons are injured in the palm, wrist, carpal tunnel, or distal forearm, all authorities agree that direct repair at an early date is desirable. In those patients in whom direct repair was not carried out, secondary reconstruction usually carries a more favorable prognosis than reconstruction in Zone II injuries.[436] In fact, tendon injuries do relatively well when repaired at these levels. Impairment problems usually are more directly related to concomitant nerve injury in Zones IV and V.

Prior to secondary tendon surgery, the wounds should be well healed and the hand soft and fully mobile, if optimal results are to be obtained. A generous longitudinal, curvilinear exposure is needed to correctly identify and repair the injured structures. Surgery is technically easier to do through ample incisions, and the likelihood of additional damage is lessened if all structures are first identified proximally and distally in unscarred areas of normal anatomy and then followed into the

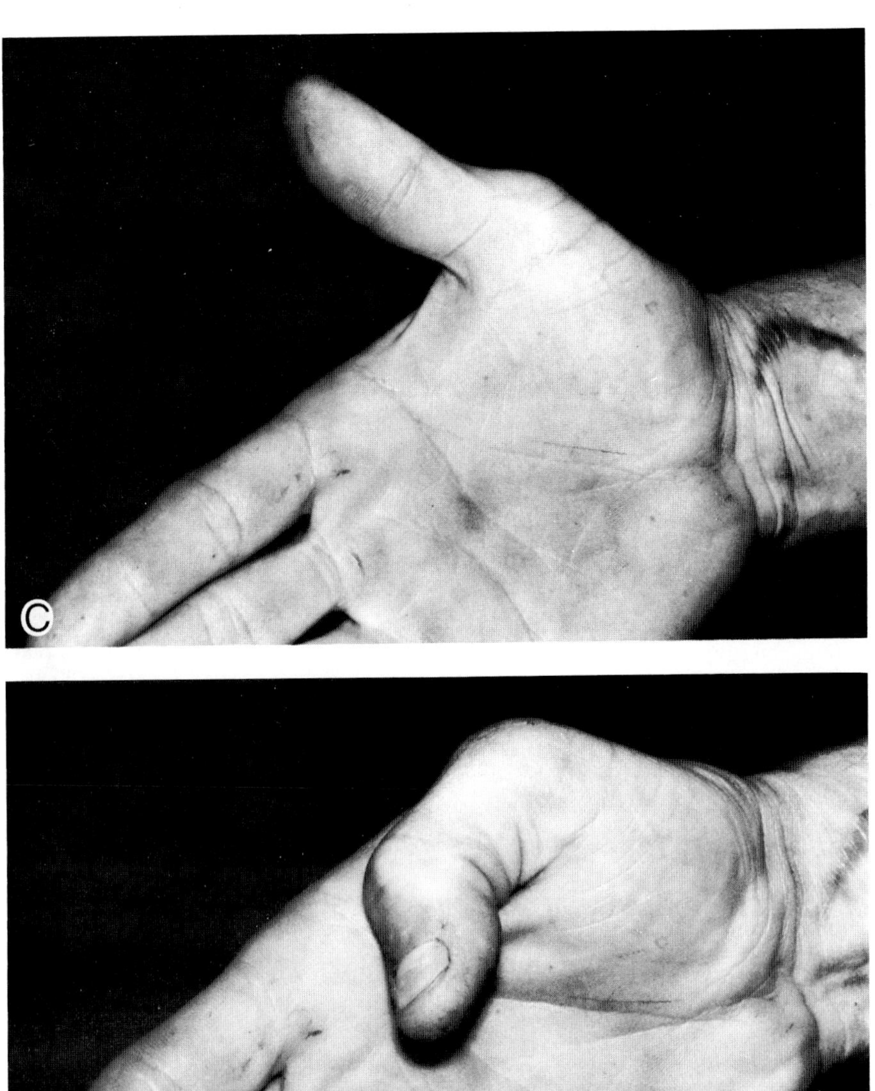

Fig. 51-21 *(Continued).* **(C&D)** Range of extension and flexion after 6 months. It should be noted that the flexor superficialis is long enough to use for any level of laceration of the flexor pollicis longus, even out at the insertion.

area of injury. If synovial connections and adhesions have prevented proximal migration of the tendons, direct end-to-end repairs using any of the techniques mentioned earlier can be utilized. The question of whether to repair both the superficialis and profundus or just the profundus often arises. This is a judgment decision. While it is advantageous to have independent superficialis and profundus function for any finger, this situation is not always attainable after injury, and excessive operative trauma can sometimes yield a lesser result. If the tendon injury had a crushing element or if tendon damage has been severe, discretion may indicate repair of the profundus only at these secondary procedures. A gliding profundus is more valuable than an adherent flexor superficialis-to-profundus repair!

Methods of Reconstruction

When the tendons cannot be brought together without undue tension, three techniques have proven useful at these levels (Zones III, IV, V).

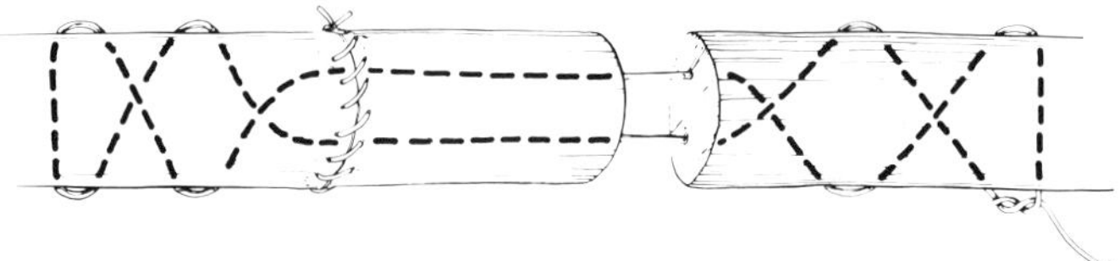

Fig. 51-22. Interposition graft. By using short segments of available graft material, a gap can be closed in the late repair of Zone III, IV, or V injuries.

Interposition Graft (Fig. 51-22)

When trying to reunite the profundus tendon ends in the palm or wrist after delay, the surgeon often finds a gap of 2 to 5 cm needed to bring the tendons to normal functional length. A short tendon graft is carried out by estimating the length needed and obtaining this from a segment of the injured superficialis or palmaris longus.[390] A Bunnell crisscross suture is placed in the proximal motor end of the tendon using #32 monofilament wire. The graft is threaded on the straight needles, and the distal juncture is completed by another crisscross suture in the distal portion, snugging up the suture until the appropriate resting posture of the finger is obtained. If the graft is found to slide along the suture, it may be tacked at each juncture with a fine nonabsorbable encircling stitch. Proper tension is critical here, and in the palm this procedure is often carried out under local anesthesia with active cooperation of the patient utilized to determine the appropriate tension in the system.

Superficialis Transfer[267,374,375] (Fig. 51-23)

The gap in the palm or wrist level can be overcome by an end-to-end transfer of an adjacent intact superficialis tendon, passed deep to the neurovascular bundle or median nerve, into the distal segment of the injured tendon. This is sutured using any of the techniques described for end-to-end repair. Again, tension is critical and the use of local-sedative anesthesia, if possible, is advocated.

In both of the above techniques, if a juncture is found to be under the proximal pulley when the finger is extended, thereby

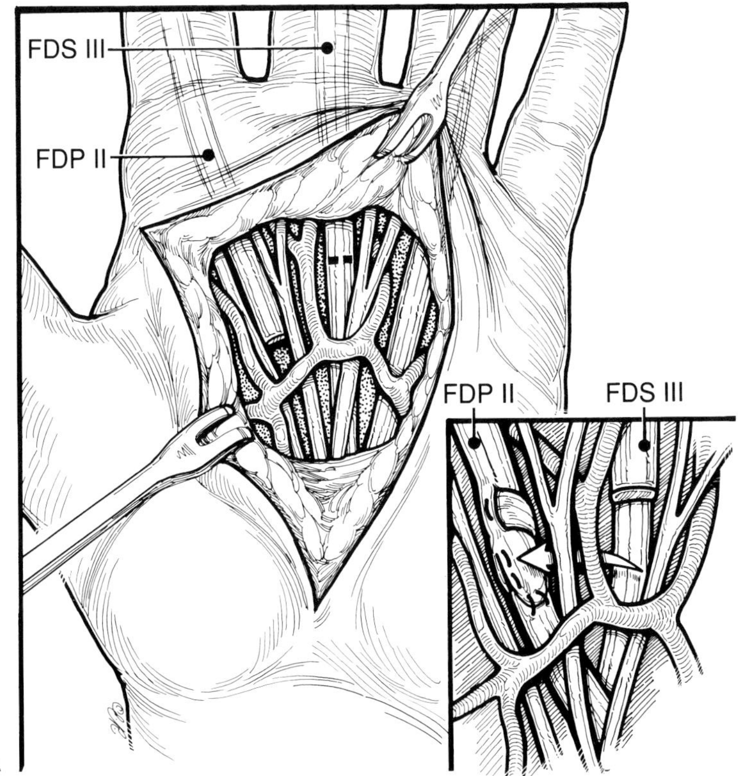

Fig. 51-23. Superficialis transfer for flexor digitorum profundus injuries in another finger. **(A)** Illustration of the technique. *(Figure continues.)*

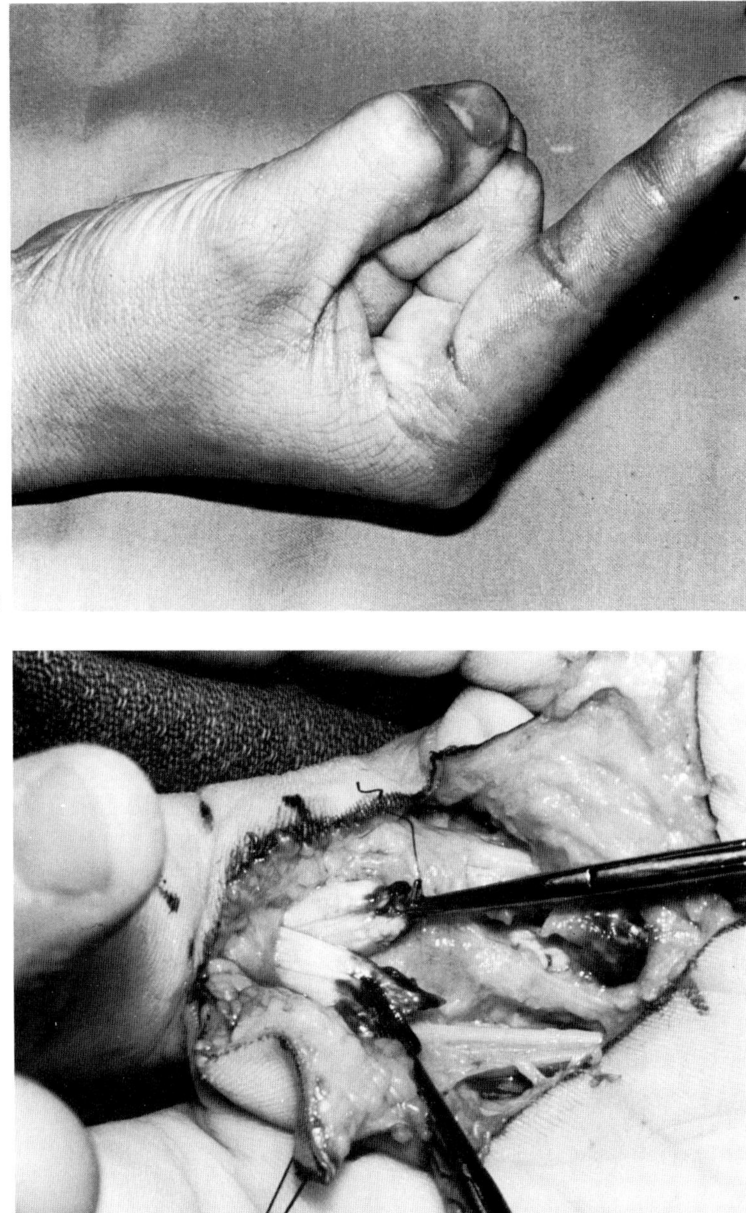

Fig. 51-23 *(Continued).* **(B)** Long-standing injury to flexor tendons in Zone III in a 20-year-old man. There is no active motion at the interphalangeal joints. **(C)** The distal tendon stumps have been recovered at the A1 pulley level. There is good distal pull-through of the tendons within the retinacular system. *(Figure continues.)*

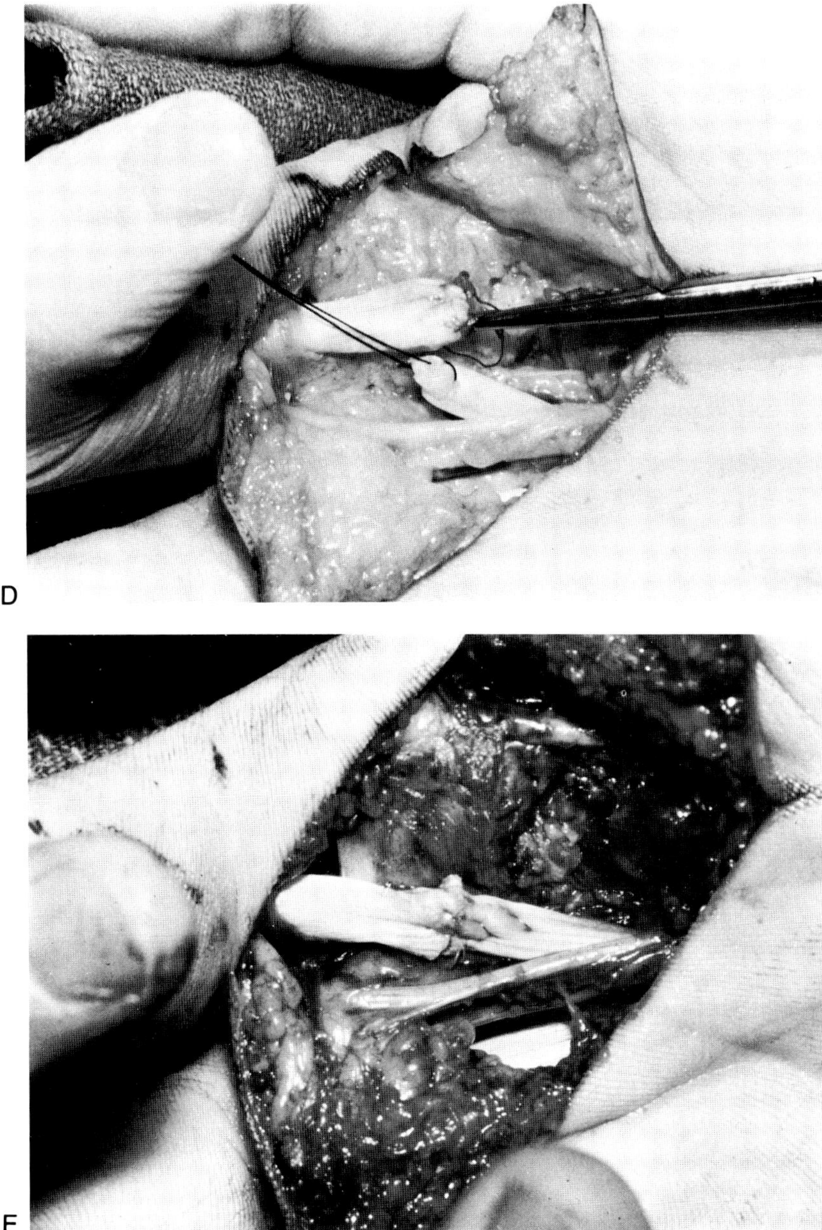

Fig. 51-23 *(Continued).* **(D)** The superficialis tendon of the long finger is transected and brought over to the profundus of the index finger. **(E)** An end-to-end juncture has been created. *(Figure continues.)*

placing the repair in Zone II, the proximal pulley (A1) can be sacrificed. This converts a Zone II injury into a more favorable Zone III problem. If this is possible, it is recommended over removing an essentially normal finger flexor system from the Zone II level to do a palm-to-fingertip tendon graft.

End-to-Side Profundus Juncture

Occasionally it is possible to attach the distal end of a severed profundus tendon to the side of an intact adjacent profundus (Fig. 51-24). This can be done best with an interweave technique. More useful in the Zone V area (forearm), this technique should be used with care in the distal portion of Zone III (palm), as the juncture could hang up on the A1 pulley in extension.

Postoperative Management

A short arm posterior molded plaster splint is applied from fingertips to below the elbow over the dressing, with the wrist in 35 degrees flexion and the MP joints in 60 to 70 degrees flexion. The fingers are in the extended position at the interphalangeal joints. Generally, in repairs at these levels, controlled mobilization is carried out by attaching a weak elastic band to a 2–0 nylon suture that has been placed through the distal nail. The

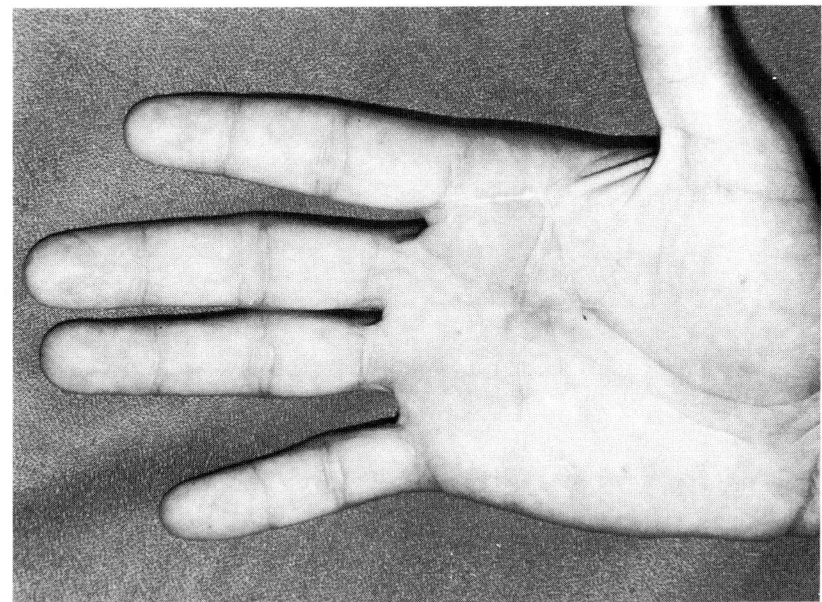

F

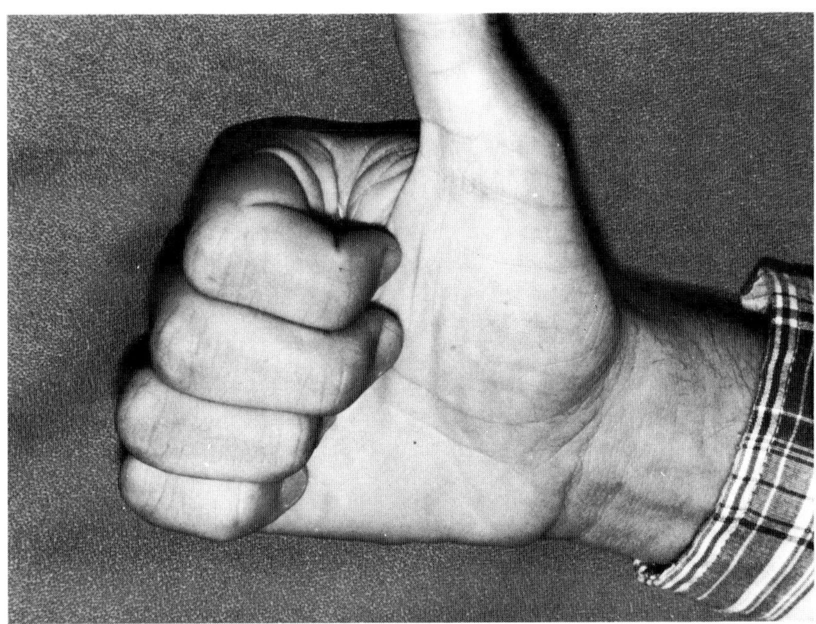

G

Fig. 51-23 *(Continued).* **(F&G)** Extension and flexion 6 months postoperatively.

proximal end of the band is fixed to the dressing at the distal forearm level with sufficient tension to hold the fingers in flexion (Fig. 51-25). The patient is taught to extend the finger actively until the dorsum of the finger touches the splint, and the rubber band then passively pulls the finger into flexion. The patient should be seen preferably twice a week to check and adjust the splint. Flexion contractures develop rapidly if the splint does not allow full extension at the proximal interphalangeal joint. The patient should be taught correct usage of the splint and report for care if any slippage or loosening occurs. Splint protection is continued for 4 weeks, at which time it is removed and the elastic band attached to a wrist band for an additional 2 to 3 weeks. Blocking techniques at each of the interphalangeal joints are allowed at 4 to 5 weeks after the repair.[59,73] The reader is referred to the literature for other modifications of early mobilization.[56,456]

FLEXOR TENOLYSIS

Indications

Surgical release of nongliding adhesions that form along the surface of a tendon after injury and repair is a useful procedure in the salvage of tendon function.[107,115,171,180,371,372,399,400,403,434,437,459] Tendon adhesions occur whenever the surface

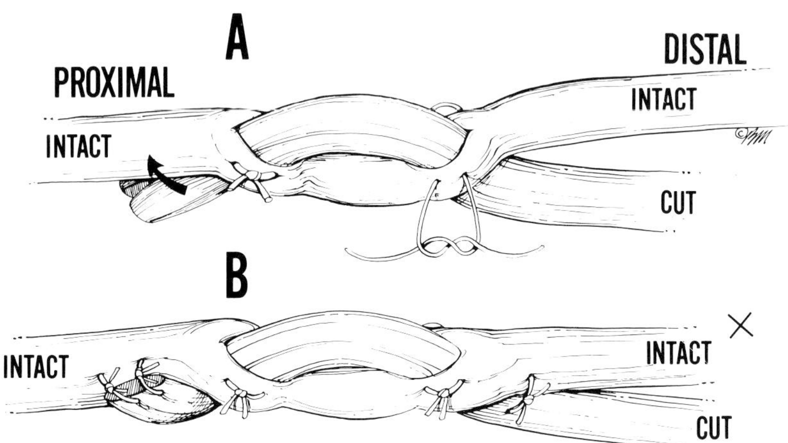

Fig. 51-24. End-to-side interweave suture technique useful in Zone V injuries.

of a tendon is violated, either through the injury itself or during surgical manipulation.[128,224,261,305,314,445] Because active motion is based on the ability of the flexor tendon to glide smoothly in its bed, the formation of nonpliable adhesions causes a number of patients to be unable to achieve full gliding even with the most conscientious postoperative program. These patients present with a varying degree of deficiency in range of active motion. After they have reached a plateau in their progress through exercise and splinting, they become candidates for tenolysis, assuming that the flexor tendon is intact and the involved joints are not irreparably damaged. Another preoperative criterion to be considered is the importance of the limitation of active motion in relation to the age, occupational needs, and desires of the individual patient. For example, 50 percent of a normal range of motion may be reasonable to accept, especially in an aged person or in someone who has concurrent arthritis or joint surface injury. The sensory status of the involved finger, as well as the degree of circulatory sufficiency, is of prime importance. An atrophic, cold finger is a poor digit, even if a satisfactory range of motion could be attained. The risk of further decreasing the vascular supply and innervation to a borderline finger by tenolysis is considerable.

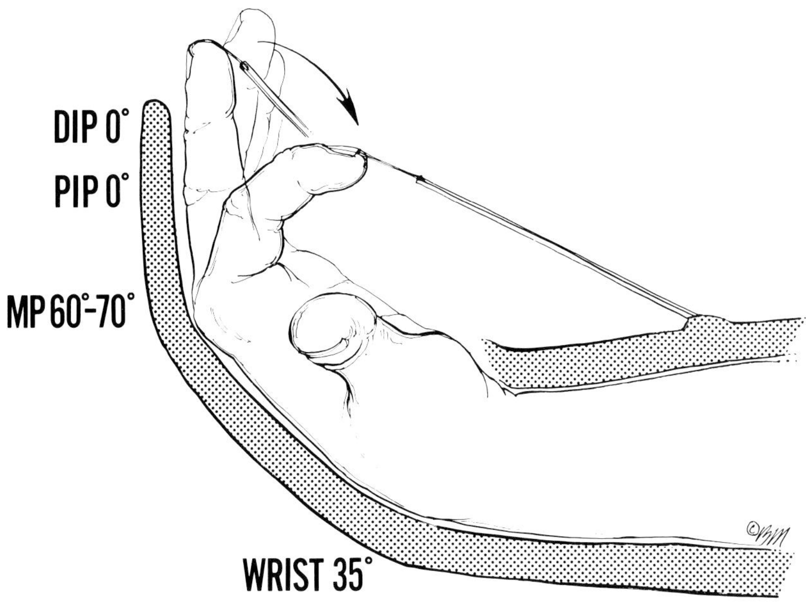

Fig. 51-25. Postoperative care after secondary repair in Zones III, IV, and V injuries. A rubber band has been fixed to the nail of the involved finger and the opposite end fastened to the dressing with a safety pin. Full active extension at the interphalangeal joints is encouraged with the MP joint blocked at 60 to 70 degrees flexion. With relaxation of the extensor system, the rubber band passively flexes the finger. It is important that the splint not restrict full extension of the PIP joint.

Flexor tenolysis is as technically difficult and demanding as tendon repair itself, and its undertaking cannot be treated lightly. It represents another surgical onslaught in an area of previous trauma and/or surgery. If unsuccessful, the patient's hand may show no improvement or may even be worse.[47] A finger that has undergone multiple insults may be better treated at times by arthrodesis or amputation.

Ideally, the best candidate for tenolysis is the patient whose repaired tendon has a localized adhesion that limits gliding. Following surgical release of such an adhesion, full range of motion is regained. More frequently, however, the adhesions involve a long segment of the involved tendon and require extensive exposure for release. Joint contracture, which can occur secondary to the tendon fixation, may also require correction, and this further complicates both the surgical procedure and the patient's recovery.

Timing of Flexor Tenolysis

There is some disagreement about the exact timing of tenolysis. Certainly all surgeons would agree that a reasonable period of time should be allowed for healing; i.e., for softening of the wound and spontaneous remodeling of adhesions and scar tissue while the patient is trying to regain gliding movement through hand therapy measures. Improvement through these techniques should reach a standstill before tenolysis is considered. Fetrow,[107] after reviewing Pulvertaft's cases, stated that 6 months should be allowed after a free tendon graft to lessen the risk of graft rupture. He also suggested that a minimum of 3 months be allowed to elapse after tendon repair to prepare the tissues for lysis. Rank and Wakefield[334] originally waited 3 months but later advocated a delay of 6 to 9 months before considering tenolysis.[335] Weeks and Wray[449] showed that most of the active function obtained after a tendon graft was achieved by 22 weeks postoperatively, which suggests that this point is a good time to perform lysis when indicated.

The judgment of the surgeon should prevail, and we do not perform tenolysis earlier than 3 months in cases of direct repair or graft. The necessity of stripping the tendon of soft tissue connections greatly endangers the circulation of the tendon and increases the liability of rupture. Delay is believed, although not guaranteed, to reduce the incidence of this disastrous complication.

Prognosis

Certainly a soft finger with good skin, supple joints, and an adherent flexor system in a cooperative and well-motivated patient would present the best prognosis for successful lysis. Unfortunately, such is rarely the case. Successful tenolysis demands immediate mobilization and any concomitant surgery preventing this will detract from the attainable result. Verdan stated[434] that this would include tendon lengthening or shortening, as well as free skin grafts or osteotomies. Verdan also included the necessity for capsulotomy as a poor prognostic factor and we concur, although we are not infrequently forced to perform capsulotomy at the time of tenolysis. He also concluded that patients over 40 years of age, nerve suture, late tenolysis (more than 1 year postoperatively), and tenolysis requiring a prolonged operative time were poor prognostic factors.[434,437] Others[226,399] have even built pulleys in association with flexor tenolysis but, in general, we find the need for major pulley reconstruction a strong indication to go on to staged tendon reconstruction. As a rule, additional procedures that require immobilization or protection in the post-tenolysis period will tend to compromise the results of the primary procedure.

In our cases of flexor tenolysis,[365] most of the patients had adherent flexor repairs or grafts performed by ourselves or other surgeons. In an additional group of patients who were subjected to lysis, the tendon injury was only partial where the adhesions formed in response to incomplete laceration or in association with crush injuries, fractures, or healed infections. A review of our cases reveals that there are no absolute indications for the advisability of tenolysis in any one case because of the great variability in patient factors.[364,365,373] All aspects of the problem have to be considered, including the prognosticators discussed above. Each of these must be evaluated, along with the patient's motivation, before the procedure is decided upon. Because the exact nature of the tendon problem may not be discovered until the surgical exploration is underway (i.e., juncture rupture or gap may accompany the adhesion problem), all patients are prepared preoperatively for the possibility that staged tendon reconstruction may be needed.

Technique

Active participation of the patient in the operative procedure, we believe, is the key to improved results in flexor tenolysis. This is achieved by using local anesthesia supplemented by an intravenous sedative drug.[163] The addition of the systemic medication provides sedation for the patient and will increase tourniquet tolerance to over 1 hour. Easily awakened, the patient cooperates dynamically in the surgery. The surgeon can be certain that the tendon has been completely freed and that the tendon motor can actively pull the finger fully into flexion. It should be noted that others do perform this procedure under general anesthesia. Whitaker, Strickland, and Ellis[459] recommend a "traction flexor check" by pulling on the involved tendon through a separate incision at the wrist. This gives an estimate of the potential range of motion and has the additional benefit of breaking up any adhesions that may have been missed. The active capability of the muscle to pull through is not tested, however, if the operation is done under general anesthesia. Strickland more recently reported that he now makes use of the local anesthesia-sedation technique wherever possible.[399]

Most of our patients have been prepared for the possibility of two-stage flexor tendon reconstruction, and, if direct evaluation shows that successful lysis is unfeasible, we proceed immediately with staged flexor reconstruction, putting in a silicone rubber implant as the first stage.[364]

The involved flexor system is approached through an ample zigzag incision[49,50] sufficiently long to uncover the entire length of the flexor tendon, if necessary (Fig. 51-26). All limiting

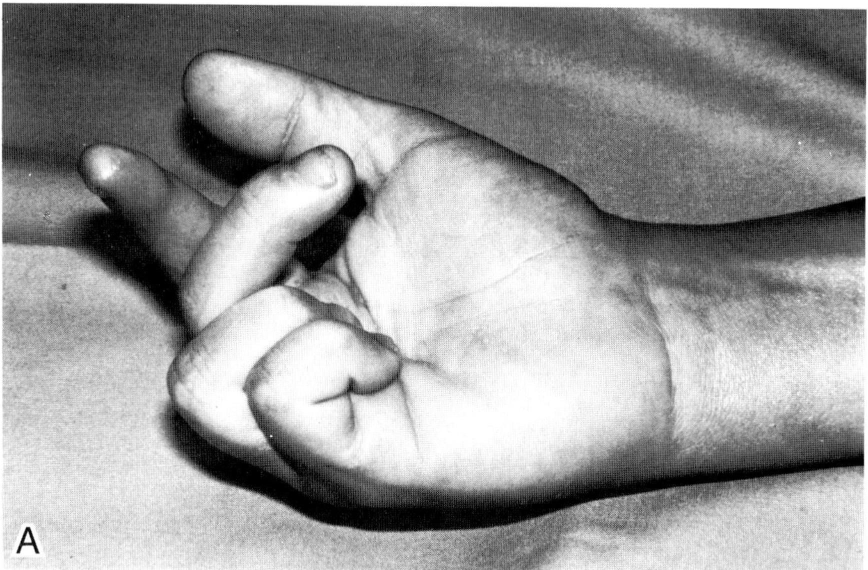

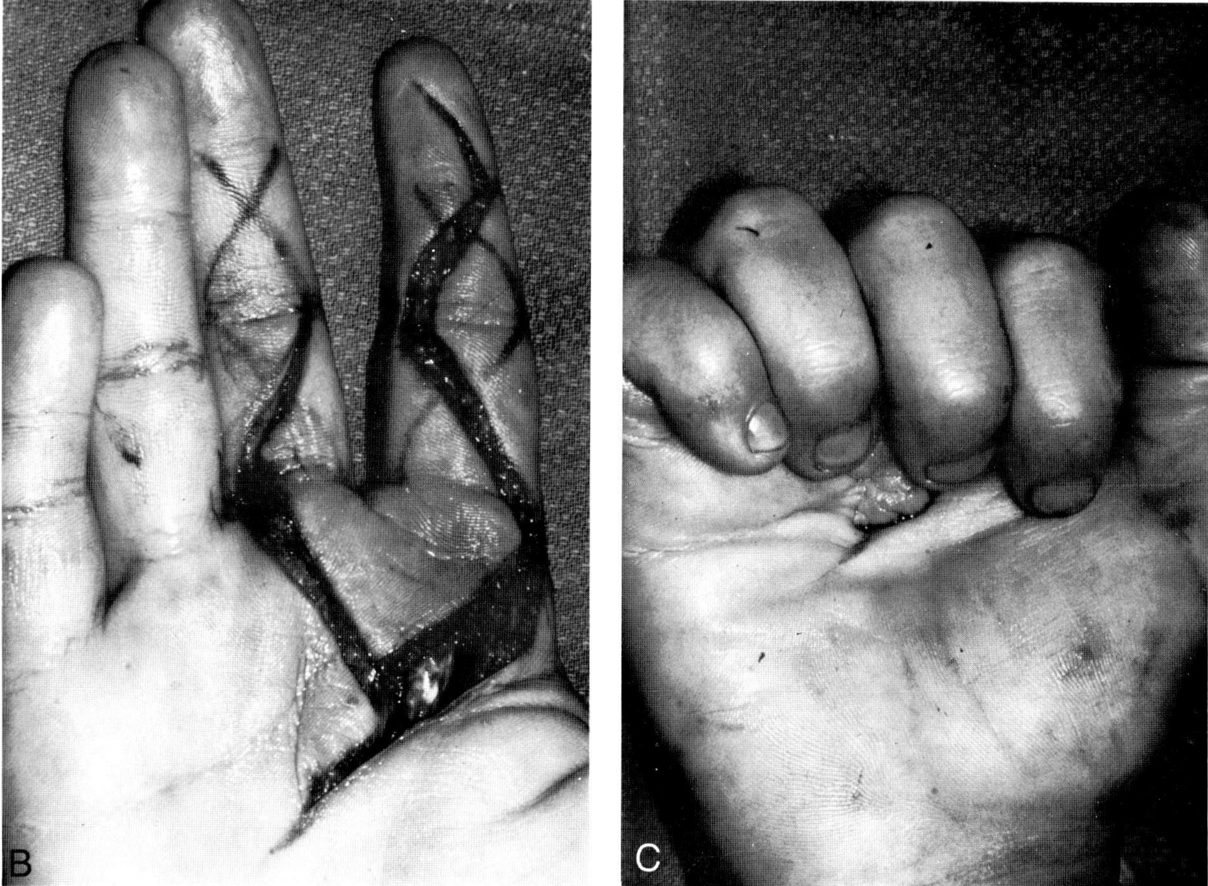

Fig. 51-26. Flexor tenolysis. A 25-year-old man 4 months following flexor digitorum profundus repairs in Zone II in both index and long fingers. **(A)** Active flexion attempted. There is essentially no pull-through in the index finger and incomplete range of motion in the long finger. **(B&C)** Under local sedative anesthesia the tenolysis has been performed as described in the text. The tourniquet has been deflated, and active range of motion is demonstrated by the patient. *(Figure continues.)*

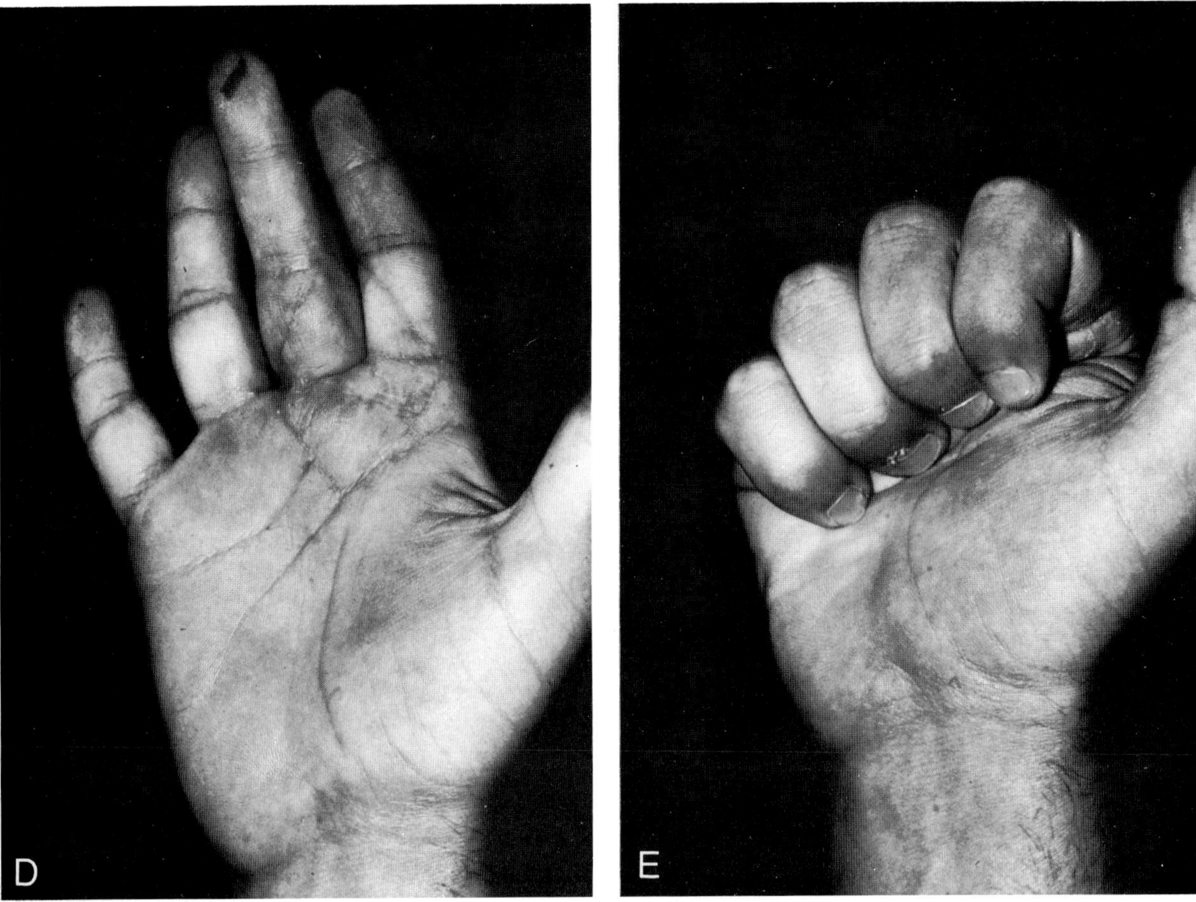

Fig. 51-26 *(Continued).* **(D&E)** Active range of motion demonstrated at 4 months.

adhesions are methodically excised and care is taken to define the border of the tendon, a task that is not simple in a heavily scarred area. Filmy, nonlimiting adhesions are, if possible, left intact. The retinacular pulley system is preserved with great care. If this is not possible, new pulleys can be constructed at the time of lysis,[226,399] but this greatly reduces the probability for success. A staged tendon implant should be considered when an adequate retinacular pulley system cannot be preserved at the time of lysis. During the procedure, the patient's active motion is reevaluated frequently as each area of blockage is attacked. Tourniquet paralysis intervenes between 20 and 30 minutes in most patients, and, if the procedure is prolonged, it can be continued without the patient's activity for over 1 hour. The tourniquet is then released, bleeding controlled by pressure and cautery, and in a few minutes the patient is actively reevaluated. If necessary, the tourniquet can be reinflated, but this is rarely needed.

After closure, a dorsal plaster splint is provided and the dressing placed so that immediate (continued) flexion can be performed within the bandage to maintain the gliding obtained through lysis.[115,116] Most authors find that, if the patient shows improving motion in the first week and maintains this gain through the first 3 to 4 weeks, a good improvement will be maintained. To help the patient get through the difficult and often painful first week after lysis, an indwelling polyethylene catheter can be left in the area of tenolysis at the time of surgery in selected patients.[154,345] Small amounts of local anesthetic are instilled into the area during exercise periods. This catheter is left in place for 5 days, after which time it is hoped that satisfactory active range has been established. Because of the risks of wound complications, we are currently using this technique infrequently.

Continuous motion devices may have a part to play in maintaining motion after tenolysis,[196,272] but it is clear that they will not substitute for the immediate active pull through of the lysed tendon system. *Active* range of motion exercises must be the primary therapeutic modality after tenolysis.

Anesthesia (Neuroleptanalgesia) Technique[163]

We use 1 or 2 percent lidocaine (without epinephrine) infiltrated locally in the skin or as digital nerve blocks at the metacarpal level. Nerve blocks at the wrist can also be useful, but with resultant paralysis of the intrinsic muscles some of the benefits of this technique will be sacrificed.

The administration of intravenous medication relieves anxiety and alleviates tourniquet pain. The anesthesia technique has been modified since our first report[163] in that the anesthesiologists now use a wide variety of newer sedative and analgesic medications. The patient's response is titrated throughout the procedure, and medication is then added as required for the patient's comfort and allowed by the vital signs. Obviously too much sedation will interfere with the patient's ability to cooperate, thereby nullifying the main advantage of this technique.

It is said that tourniquet time can also be prolonged by a subcutaneous ring of local anesthetic to block the superficial nerves in the arm, but we do not use this technique (see Chapter 2).

Monitoring of the patient's vital signs by experienced anesthesia personnel in an operating room environment is mandatory. Careful titration of the medication is also necessary. Too much medication depresses the patient's function and his ability to cooperate.

Adjuncts to Tenolysis

Steroids

In addition to the surgical lysis of tendon adhesions, some authors[61,62,119,180,197,473] have used steroid preparations injected into the tendon bed upon completion of the surgical procedure. Steroids have been shown experimentally to modify the production of fibrous tissue, thereby reducing the density and strength of the adhesions about the injured tendon surface. As this drug also alters the strength of the healing tendon, it has not been strongly advocated for use after tendon repair but, according to Whitaker, Strickland, and Ellis,[459] it is useful in tenolysis. We do not use steroids in association with tenolysis.

Interpositional Materials

Interpositional materials have been used after tenolysis in an effort to prevent the reinvasion of the lysed tendon by the unfavorable healing process that tends to fix the tendon in its bed. Many of these materials have also been used as blocking devices in tendon repair in unfavorable areas. In general, those materials used to completely encircle the repair or lysis have failed because restricting adhesions, which formed at the ends of the tube, prevented gliding. Use of artificial membranes inserted as an interpositional material, however, has many advocates, and many materials[81,343] have been tried, among them cellophane,[457] silicone rubber sheeting,[18,391,464] polyethylene film,[391] gelatin sponge,[288] amnionic membrane,[311] fascia,[406] partenon,[391] and tunica vaginalis,[466] Cutwright and Reid[81] reported on experiments with a biodegradable overlay that was absorbed in about 8 weeks and showed some promise. Stark and colleagues[391] presented a large series of tenolyses in which the procedure was supplemented by the use of paratenon, polyethylene film, or silicone rubber sheeting. They believed that this adjunct improved results over tenolysis alone in selected instances. While we have made limited use of silicone rubber sheet underlays in tenolysis in the past, our current technique, which stresses immediate and continued active range of motion in an intense postoperative hand therapy program, has obviated the need for these materials.

FLEXOR TENDON GRAFTING IN LESS THAN OPTIMAL SITUATIONS (STAGED TENDON RECONSTRUCTION)

Indications

There are patients with flexor tendon injury in whom reconstruction by conventional tendon grafting techniques is likely to yield a very low probability of success. The reasons for this are numerous and include the severity of the original trauma, i.e., crushing injuries associated with underlying fracture or overlying skin damage and failure of a previous operation or excessive scarring of the tendon bed, secondary to the patient's particular healing response or due to complications of healed infection. At times, the retinacular pulley system may have been lost either at the time of injury or prior to surgery. Joints that are restricted by contractures that are not responsive to therapy measures are also poor prognostic factors in flexion tendon surgery. The presence of double digital nerve injury also should be mentioned as a negative factor.[359]

Patients with all or some of the problems described above, in whom conventional tendon grafting is not likely to offer a reasonable chance of success, may undergo staged tendon reconstruction as an alternative method in the attempt to salvage finger function.

Historical Review

Prior to the relatively recent development of interest in this staged procedure, it was believed justifiable to perform the one-stage flexor graft even with the expectation of only modest improvement, as a better procedure was not available. Articles advocating this approach were published by Wakefield[441] in 1960 and McCormack, Demuth, and Kindling[275] in 1962. In experimental conditions, Butler, Burkhalter, and Cranston[58] tested the possibility of scar excision in dogs as a preliminary procedure prior to a later tendon graft operation. They were sufficiently pleased with the results to consider offering this procedure to their patients. In 1960 Pulvertaft[327] published a series of late flexor tendon grafts performed 10 years or more after injury. He attained improved function in most of his patients, as did Millar, Dickie, and Colville.[283]

Another interesting approach to the problem of the severe tendon injury was published by Paneva-Holevich in 1969.[302] In this staged technique, the proximal cut end of the superficialis is sutured to the proximal cut end of the profundus tendon in the palm. This will become the proximal juncture. At the second stage the superficialis is used as a pedicle graft by severing it more proximally and bringing this proximal end out distally to be inserted at the distal phalanx. This technique has been combined with the silicone rod technique by several authors.[4,48,69,71,189]

In retrospect, we believe that most of the patients presented in the above studies would have been candidates for the two-stage tendon reconstruction as presented here.

In 1965 Hunter[143] first published his personal experience with a tendon implant and in 1971, with Salisbury,[160] presented more than 10 years experience with this technique, in which severely damaged flexor tendons were excised and the system rebuilt around a silicone-Dacron reinforced implant. A Dacron woven tape was added within the rubber to give body to the implant, to enhance its gliding in the passive motion program, and to supply better hold for the distal sutures. The implant, attached only at its distal end, was left free at its proximal end in the distal part of the forearm. During wound healing, a passive exercise program was utilized to mobilize the finger prior to the second stage. In response to the implant, a smooth, well-organized pseudosheath was formed, ideally creating order in a previously chaotic tendon bed. The proximal end of the implant was placed in the distal forearm as many of the patients had severe scarring that involved the palm as well as Zone II. This also gave the surgeon the option to create the proximal juncture above the wrist, bypassing the scarred palm and using an area relatively favorable for tendon juncture.

At the second stage, performed 3 months postoperatively, the implant was replaced with a long tendon graft, an operation carried out with as little disturbance as possible to the newly formed sheath. The second stage was therefore a tendon graft carried out in a manner greatly simplified by the tendon implant. This work was based on earlier studies of artificial tendon and tendon implants by Bassett and Carroll.[21]

Many investigators have applied various approaches in an effort to combat the effects of proliferating adhesions that inevitably follow injury to a flexor tendon and its supportive gliding mechanism. In reviewing the literature, it can be seen that attempts to alter the effects of adhesions have fallen into four general categories:

1. The first approach involved the use of artificial tendon materials in which a gap in the tendon was bridged by some foreign material. Lange,[211] in 1900, worked with silk,[133] which was very reactive. Other materials used by the pioneers in this work included wire,[9] polyethylene and nylon,[348] and polyethylene and silk.[123] Silk threaded through a vein was also used.[447] These materials were far from inert, and excessive tissue reaction and adhesions prevented successful gliding. Experiments in which a graft of artery was used to complete a gap in tendon found the material too elastic to be effective.[395]
2. A second approach was the use of blocking devices that interposed a barrier between the tendon and the surrounding tissue in an effort to prevent scar invasion. Many materials were tried, including cellophane,[106,343,457] artery,[207] vein,[7,16,25,110,124] polyethylene,[118,315] fascia,[406,448] milipore,[15] nylon,[57] Ivalon tubes,[136] tygon,[127] Teflon,[120] gelatin sponge,[247] Silastic sheeting,[13,14,340] tunica vaginalis,[37] amnion,[82,311] metal tubes,[278] and fibrin film.[343]

   These materials promoted additional scarring, which further immobilized the healing tendon. If blocking was effective, then healing was greatly delayed.

   Probably the most elegant of techniques devised that might be classified under the blocking approach was the use of homograft of the entire flexor system, tendon, and supportive structures transplanted into a damaged finger. This procedure, published by Peacock,[304] showed that such grafts were well tolerated. Hueston, Hubble, and Rigg[142] also presented an encouraging series of cases using homografts, but, because of difficulty in obtaining these grafts, widespread use of this technique did not ensue. More recently, Chacha[64] used autologus composite grafts from the toe to the flexor system of the hand with overall modest results.
3. A different approach to this problem is the use of drug therapy for control of adhesion formation. Beta-amino proprionitrile was tried and was found to be toxic.[308] Several additional agents, including CIS-hydroxy-proline, were tried experimentally by Bora, Lane, and Prockop,[31] and inhibition of scar formation was shown. However, it was felt that further studies were needed before considering clinical usage. Cortisone preparations have been shown to reduce fixation of healing tendons by adhesions.[61] Although Ketchum[193] showed increased tendon function in dogs after the administration of triamcinolone, Carstam[62] showed that there was an increased risk of tendon juncture breakdown due to a significant reduction in the tensile strength of the tendon repair in the early weeks, and the agent has not been advocated as a clinical tool after tendon repair.
4. A fourth group of investigators tried to build a "pseudosheath" through which a tendon could glide. The classic work published by Mayer and Ransohoff in 1936[270] explained this concept. Nonflexible materials, such as glass, metal,[282,409] or celloidin[268,269] were well tolerated by the tissues, but their use led to joint stiffness since their rigidity did not allow for passive motion of the finger joints while the sheath was being formed. Unfortunately, a flexible, inert material was not available at that time, and this method was largely abandoned.

In the 1950s, Bassett and Carroll[21] began working with flexible silicone rubber rods to build pseudosheaths. The rod served as a template on which a new sheath would be created with minimal reaction. This would thereby organize a severely scarred area, one in which standard one-stage tendon grafting would certainly fail, and grade such a finger up to the point at which tendon grafting would have a reasonable chance for success.

Hunter, under the influence of Carroll, used this method and began to perfect a silicone rubber tendon that would be reinforced for strength and have appropriate end devices for fixation both proximally and distally. It could then be used as a one-stage, true artificial tendon graft.

Over the next few years, many prototypes were developed.[143] They varied in size, shape, and material used for reinforcement, as well as in the type of end devices incorporated for distal and proximal fixation. It became apparent that firm, permanent fixation (i.e., bonding of the tendon distally and proximally to living tissue) could not be developed under the then current technology, and Hunter temporarily abandoned the active tendon implant in favor of the two-stage passive motion program. The search for a permanent active tendon implant goes on, and is discussed on page 1900. The one-stage artificial tendon has been undergoing clinical trial in our center[143,144,150,166–168] as well as by other authors.[17,80,153,154,161,190,348]

Many authors have written of their experience in tendon salvage using the staged technique in which the silicone rubber implant is placed at the first stage.[3,6,66,113,132,140,212,215,291,345,346,353,355,356,358,359,425,449,452,455]

Patient Selection for Staged Tendon Reconstruction

Many factors must be taken into account, both general and local, when this procedure is considered. The patient should be helped to understand the complexity of the problem and be willing to undertake a difficult postoperative therapy program. The surgeon should ask himself whether it is justifiable to subject a severely damaged finger to two more surgical procedures; in some instances, arthrodesis or amputation may be a better reconstructive alternative. A helpful approach is to start the patient on a range of motion and softening therapy program[242–244] to allow further healing and attain maximum preoperative passive range of motion. This gives the surgeon an opportunity to better evaluate the patient's willingness to work actively in the program. It is probable that those patients with severe neurovascular impairment will at best make very limited gains and should be rejected as candidates for staged reconstruction.

Technique of Staged Tendon Reconstruction

Preoperative Plan

There are various options open, which have to be presented to the patient preoperatively. In some instances at exploration conditions may be deemed favorable for a one-stage free tendon graft. If the case is one of a previous repair bound down by adhesions, it may be possible to salvage the finger through tenolysis. Accordingly, the patient is informed preoperatively and the exploration is started under local anesthesia, supplemented by intravenous sedation to define the situation better (see Tenolysis on page 1881). If the repair is found to be intact and, in the judgment of the surgeon, active motion obtained through the lysis is adequate, the procedure can be terminated at this point. If the repair is found to have gapped or ruptured, if the bed is very poor, or if the retinacular pulley system is inadequate, formal staged reconstruction is carried out. It is usually necessary to change over to general anesthesia if the first stage of reconstruction is going to be carried out.

Stage I[144,145,147,150,161]

The flexor system of the involved finger is exposed through the volar zigzag approach and continued to the lumbrical origin level in the palm. Incisions healed earlier can be partially utilized, when feasible, combining them with the modified Bruner[49] incision. If a midlateral incision was previously used, it should be ignored and the volar approach used. All potential pulley material, injured or uninjured, is preserved. The flexor tendons are then excised, leaving a stump of the profundus approximately 1 cm long attached to the distal phalanx. If a superficialis tail is preservable, it is left attached to the middle phalanx and saved for pulley reconstruction if needed. The excised tendon material is also set aside in moist sponges for possible use in pulley reconstruction. The proximal profundus is transected at the lumbrical origin level, and, if the lumbrical is scarred, it is also excised. As much of the original flexor retinaculum is preserved as possible. If joint flexion deformities are not corrected with excision of the injured tendons, volar plate and accessory collateral ligament release are performed at this time.

A second curvilinear incision is made above the wrist in the ulnar one-half of the volar aspect of the forearm. The involved superficialis tendon is identified, drawn into the wound, and transected near the musculotendinous junction.

A trial set of Hunter tendon implants is useful here to determine the appropriate size needed. The adult male generally can take a 5- or 6-mm tendon implant. We now prefer smaller (4 mm) implants, which are closer in size to the expected tendon graft, thereby creating a snugger tendon sheath. The implant is threaded into the pulley system and should be movable with only minimal resistance. A minimal requirement is the presence of the A2 and A4 pulleys at the proximal and middle phalangeal levels, respectively. However, there is evidence that a four-pulley system is superior, and this is discussed under the section on pulley reconstruction. The pulleys must be strong and snug but nonbinding, so as to allow passive gliding of the implant.

If nerves have been injured, the ends are identified and prepared for suture. The tourniquet is released and bleeding controlled. After an appropriate delay, the tourniquet is reinflated and the actual implant is removed from its sterile package and placed in the retinacular system. This is done in a distal to proximal direction with the slight stiffness of the reinforced implant of assistance here. The implant is passed from the proximal palm to the distal forearm in the plane between the profundus and superficialis, using a tendon passer.[213,378,388] A finger placed in the distal forearm wound, proximally in the muscle plane, ensures a space for migration of the proximal end of the implant during passive exercise after Stage I.

The distal juncture is now carried out. The technique used depends on which of the two Hunter tendons is selected.[144]

Technique #1—Wire Suture Technique (Fig. 51-27).[160] First, the distal end of the implant is trimmed by pulling the proximally pointed end up to a point 3 to 5 cm proximal to the wrist crease and removing the excess distally. A #32 monofilament stainless steel wire suture is used in a figure-of-eight stitch, fixing the implant beneath the profundus stump. This is

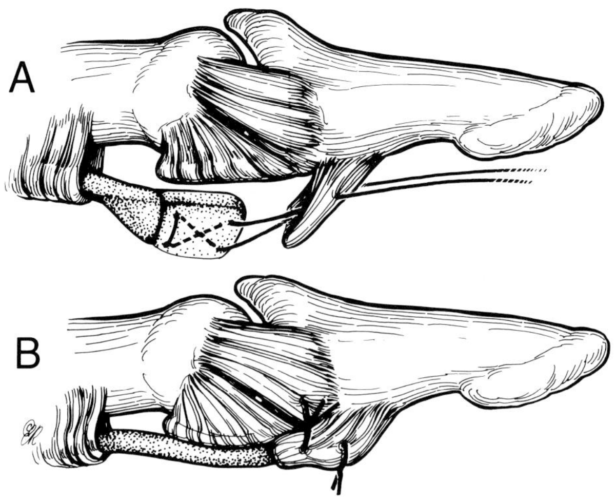

Fig. 51-27. Stage I flexor reconstruction. The distal juncture wire suture technique. A figure-of-eight suture of #32 monofilament wire is placed in the implant and sutured to the profundus stump. Additional sutures are placed on each side of the implant. (From Hunter and Salisbury,[160] with permission.)

reinforced by two nonabsorbable 4–0 sutures that go through the stump, local periosteum and the implant. The surgeon must be certain that these added sutures catch the Dacron tape within the silicone rubber, as the sutures will have little holding power in the rubber alone.

Technique #2—Screw-Plate Technique (Fig. 51-28). (See also the section on the active tendon implant.) A metal endpiece for the implant has been provided (Phoenix Bioengineering design), which is fixed beneath the profundus stump directly to bone with a screw (a 2-mm Woodruff self-tapping screw, available in various lengths). The screw hole is prepared using the appropriate bit or a 0.035-inch K-wire. (A preoperative radiograph will help estimate the length.) The screw should engage, but not penetrate, the dorsal cortex of the phalanx or it will create a painful area on the dorsum. Care is exercised to place the screw in the proximal one-third of the phalanx to avoid damage to the germinal matrix of the nail. After fixation, the profundus tendon stump is placed over the end piece.

Traction is now exerted on the proximal end of the implant to ensure its free passage under the pulleys and to observe potential range of motion. If the tendon bowstrings anteriorly to the joints such that loss of range of motion is observable, tighter or additional pulleys must be constructed. The surgeon should not hesitate to reconstruct the needed pulleys at this time. If there is any question of bowstringing of the implant or ineffective passive gliding or buckling, pulleys should be built. If any portion of the salvaged retinacular system is tight, it is stretched with a curved hemostat or removed, and this area reconstructed.

Prior to skin closure, records are made of the passive potential achieved by pulling on the proximal end of the implant. This test also verifies the competence of the pulley system. Digital nerve repairs are done prior to wound closure.

A bulky dressing is applied with a posterior plaster splint used to keep the wrist in about 35 degrees flexion. This ensures

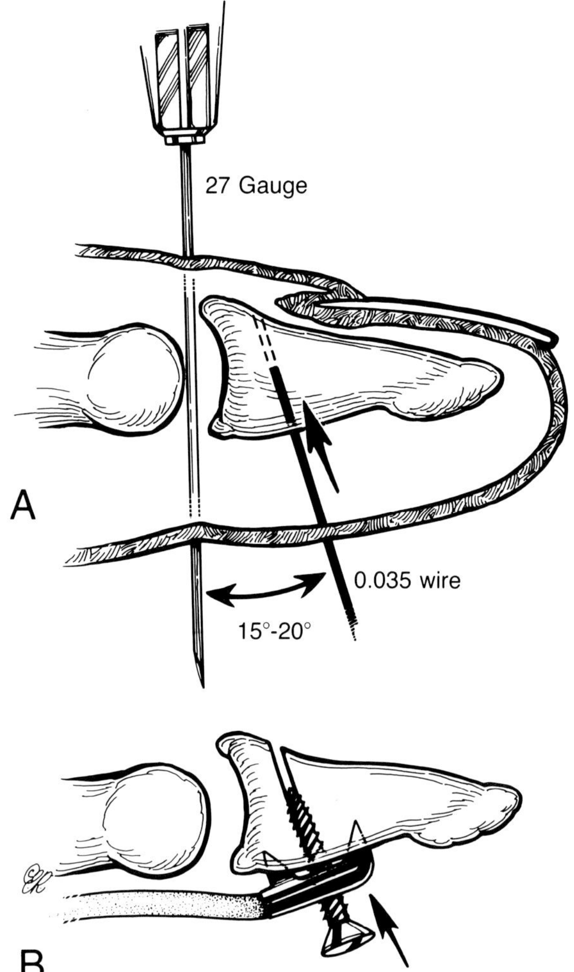

Fig. 51-28. Technique of fixation using screw-plate. A self-tapping 2-mm Woodruff screw is used in a hole drilled using a 0.035-inch K-wire. (see text for details).

more proximal placement of the implant, which creates a longer proximal extension of the sheath in the forearm and gives the implant more room in the forearm to move without buckling during the passive motion program between Stages I and II. The splint should extend past the fingertips, keeping the MP joints in 60 to 70 degrees flexion and the interphalangeal joints relaxed in the extended position.

Passive motion is usually started 7 days after Stage I. In fingers with significant joint contractures requiring release, range of motion exercises may be started earlier in the Hand Therapy department.[242–244] In these situations, the application of elastic traction splinting is helpful. Patients are taught passive motion exercises, including the use of trapping with adjacent normal fingers to regain mobilization in the operated finger. Of course, the combination of nerve repair with Stage I may delay the onset of some of these activities until approximately 3 weeks after performing Stage I.

The appropriate interval between Stages I and II is the time needed for development of the gliding sheath to form in response to the implant and also to allow for wound healing and softening. The joints are mobilized in an effort to regain full passive mobility. Lateral radiographs in flexion and extension, after Stage I and when range of passive motion is restored, will demonstrate the excursion of the implant and reveal whether buckling is interfering with the smooth movement of the implant, a phenomenon associated with synovitis. The time interval generally allowed is 3 months; clinically this seems to be adequate. Occasionally, conditions allow or demand an earlier Stage II, and treatment of each patient is individualized. The decision to do the second stage is made by the surgeon based on the condition of the hand. Generally, at 3 months, the hand is soft, the joints are well mobilized, and the patient is ready for Stage II.

Stage II (Fig. 51-29)

The distal portion of the finger incision is opened to about the middle of the middle phalanx. The implant is located at its attachment to the profundus stump. Care is taken not to injure the most distal pulley over the middle phalanx. The proximal incision is then reopened in the distal forearm. The forearm fascia is excised and the sheath is located. Ideally, the sheath should be soft, thin, and translucent. This is opened with exposure of the proximal end of the implant. The motor is selected — most commonly the profundus mass to the long, ring, and little fingers. For index finger reconstruction, the profundus to index is chosen. The superficialis muscle can also be used.[356] In the case of flexor reconstruction of the thumb, the flexor pollicis longus or one of the superficialis muscles is used as a motor. The full length of the superficialis of the ring finger is occasionally used as the motor (as a tendon transfer), thereby obviating the need for a graft.[313,376]

The wounds are then packed and the tourniquet is released while a tendon graft is obtained (see discussion on obtaining tendon graft on page 1864).

As an alternative technique, Stage II can be performed under local-sedative anesthesia,[160,163] thereby allowing active participation of the patient in the procedure. In this situation, the tendon graft is obtained prior to opening the finger in order to conserve tourniquet time. The graft is then placed before releasing the tourniquet.

After bleeding is controlled, the tourniquet is reinflated and the graft is pulled into the flexor system by suturing it to the proximal end of the implant and pulling it through the sheath (Fig. 51-29A). The implant is then discarded. The distal juncture is secured with the distal pullout technique (see page 1860) and the finger wound is closed. Attention is now directed to the proximal juncture. The graft is woven into the motor tendon or tendons (Fig. 51-29B). When only one motor is used, the technique of Pulvertaft is advised (see page 1862). In the instances where the profundus of the long, ring, and little fingers is chosen as a common motor, an interweave juncture is created. Excess sheath is resected, and at times it will be necessary to remove the proximal sheath to allow the juncture to pass distally when the fingers are extended. The need for this will be recognized if passive extension is carried out at the table.

In almost all of our cases, the proximal juncture is placed in the forearm, a favorable level for tendon gliding. In the rare

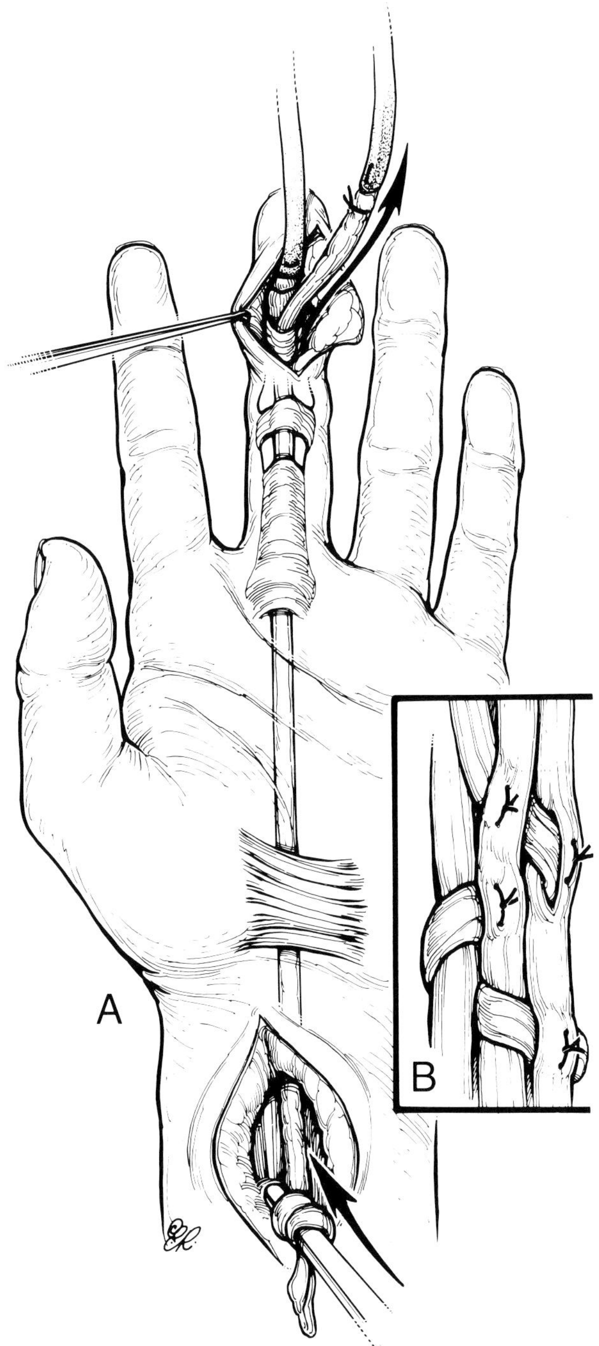

Fig. 51-29. Stage II flexor reconstruction. **(A)** The distal portion of the finger wound and the distal forearm wound are opened, and both ends of the implant are located. The tendon graft is now sutured to the proximal end of the implant and drawn into the newly created sheath. **(B)** The proximal juncture is either an interweave of the graft into the adjacent flexor profundus motor in the case of the long, ring, and little fingers or an interlace into the flexor profundus of the index finger. (See Fig. 51-12 for the Pulvertaft interlace technique.) (From Hunter and Salisbury,[160] with permission.)

instance in which the palm is not involved in the trauma or in prior surgery, a shorter graft can be used, motoring it with the profundus tendon at the lumbrical origin.[344] The option of using an adjacent superficialis as motor is also open in the palm if the profundus is not deemed adequate. Proper tension in the graft is essential for success (see page 1868).

With completion of the proximal juncture, wound closure is accomplished and a bulky dressing applied. A short arm posterior splint is applied, keeping the wrist in 30 degrees flexion and the MP joints in 70 degrees flexion. The fingers themselves are protected in almost full extension. At the present time, these patients are managed with an early controlled motion program.[242,389] This program requires close supervision by the therapy department. An elastic band is attached to the distal portion of the finger by a suture in the nail at 1 to 3 days postsurgery, and a protected mobilization program[229] is used, similar to that described for Zones III, IV, and V injuries earlier in the chapter (page 1880) (see Fig. 51-25). Gentle active motion is allowed at 3 weeks.[450,451] At 4 weeks, the pull-out suture is removed, and the rubber band then used with a wrist cuff, giving further protection for an additional 1 to 2 weeks. Blocking is used at 4 to 5 weeks. If there is a history of flexion contracture prior to Stage I or a tendency to develop a flexion deformity after Stage II, a resting static extension splint is worn at night for up to a year. Dynamic and static splints are added to the program as needed. This may be as early as 4 to 5 weeks in the patient with poor pull-through of the graft and significant contracture, or later (6 to 8 weeks) in those with satisfactory gliding. The latter patients with good pull-through of their grafts are more likely to separate their junctures if heavy resistance is added too early in the program.

If the patient demonstrates less than full ability to cooperate, the hand may be splinted without traction for 3 postoperative weeks and started on the mobilization program after that time. This would include active and passive range exercise at 3 weeks with blocking added at 4 weeks. The program is then continued as in the early mobilization program described above (Fig. 51-30).

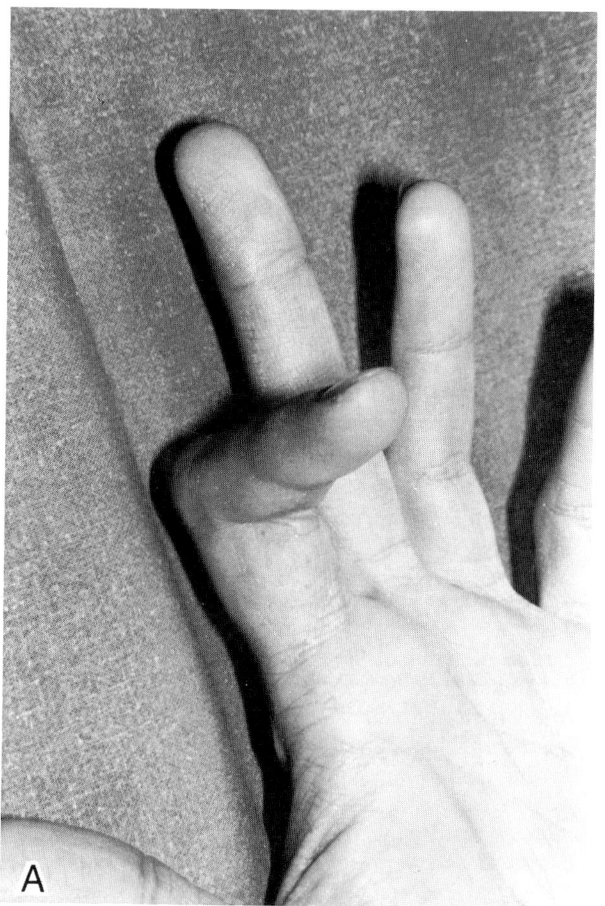

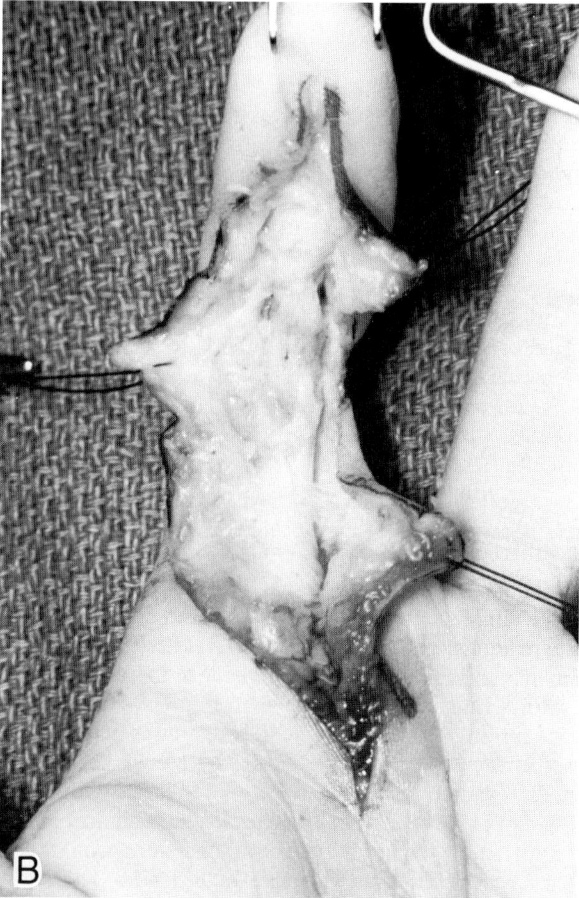

Fig. 51-30. Staged tendon reconstruction. A 31-year-old school teacher had had primary repair of both flexor tendons followed by tenolysis 2 years prior to treatment by this technique. **(A)** Demonstrating maximal possible extension. A 75-degree fixed flexion contracture of the PIP joint was present. **(B)** Stage I. On exploration, massive scarring was found. *(Figure continues.)*

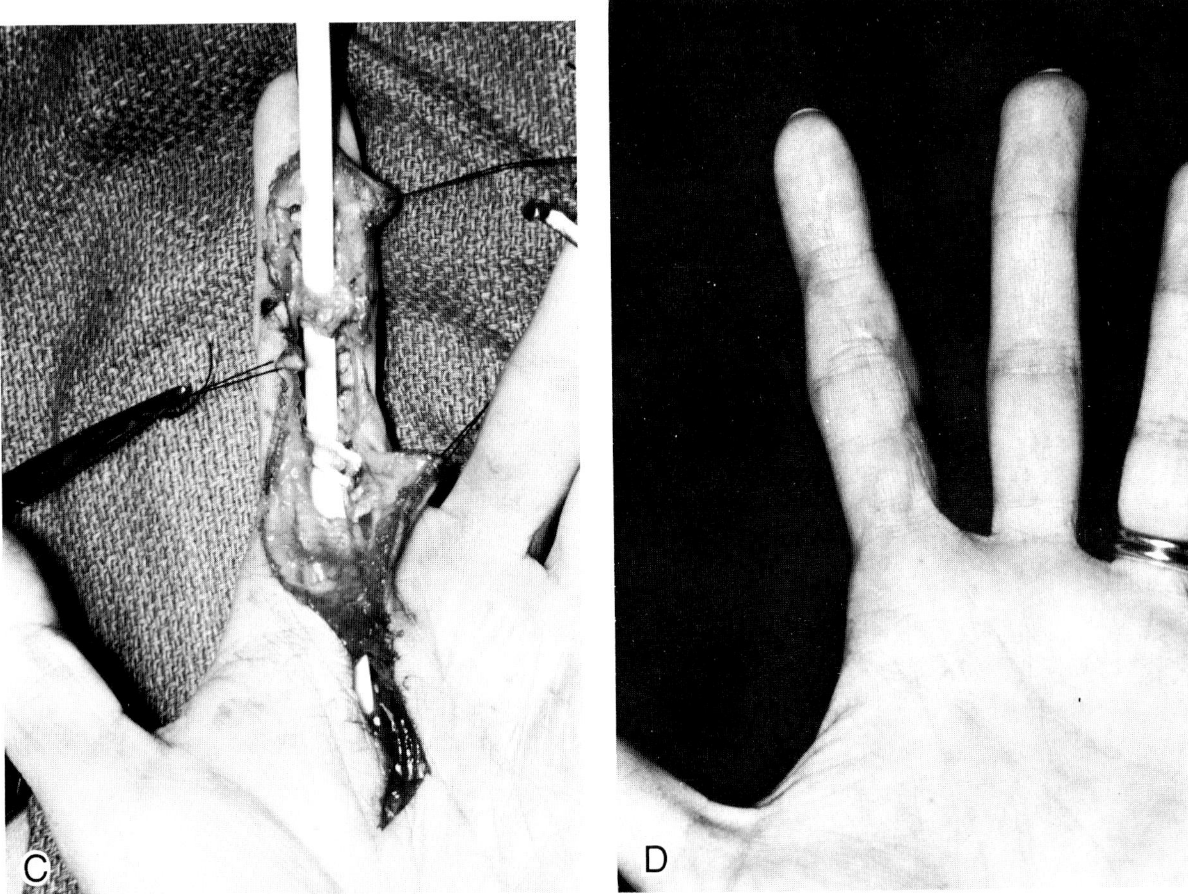

Fig. 51-30 *(Continued).* **(C)** Stage I. The flexion contracture has been released by scar tissue excision and PIP joint capsulotomy. The A1, part of the A2, and the A4 pulleys were preservable. A tendon graft pulley was constructed over the implant at the distal A2 level. **(D)** End result. *(Figure continues.)*

Response of Tissues to the Silicone Rubber Implant

The exact nature and the activity of the pseudosheath formed in response to a flexible rubber implant has been debated.[158,315,336] Before an inert, yet flexible material was available, Milgram[282] implanted rigid bands of stainless steel, tantalum, and Vitallium in an effort to attain a smooth-gliding bed prior to tendon graft or transplantation. He described the formation of a smooth bursa-like sac clinging to the implant contour with a liquid that was similar to synovial fluid on the implant surface. Microscopically, the sheath was lined by flat "mesothelial cells," surrounded by a fibrovascular supportive layer. This wall became thicker and more fibrous with time. The rigid implant would not allow passive motion during the important sheath-building stage and, therefore, could not create a favorable situation when used in the fingers. The availability of medical grade silicone rubber improved the possibilities for this reconstructive approach.

The nature of the silicone-induced sheath has been studied in many laboratories.[65,102,134,156,246,287] Hunter's group, working in the late 1960s, published studies on the sheath formed when silicone implants were placed in the paravertebral soft tissues of dogs[169] and found an orderly pattern of cellular organization of the surface of the implant. He did not believe that this was a foreign body reaction. A parallel study was designed to evaluate the response to an actively gliding implant in the extensor system of the dog.[170] Evidence was obtained that the system could function as a physiologic sheath that would support a long tendon graft by fluid nutrition and with time by the formation of vascular, yet mobile, adhesions. Conway, Smith, and Elliott[78] and Urbaniak and colleagues[420] confirmed these observations. Urbaniak's experiments were carried out in the flexor system and actually demonstrated revascularization of the dog tendon by infratendinous vessels in the sheath. At 1 year, he believed that these vessels appeared to be normal. In chicken experiments, Farkas and colleagues[105] showed a response which by ultrastructional examination could resemble the normal tendon sheath. This study suggested that, with time the sheath became rigid and that the implant should be replaced at about 1 month. Farkas agreed with Hunter that motion was most important for the remodeling of adhesions formed within the sheath when tendon grafts were performed.

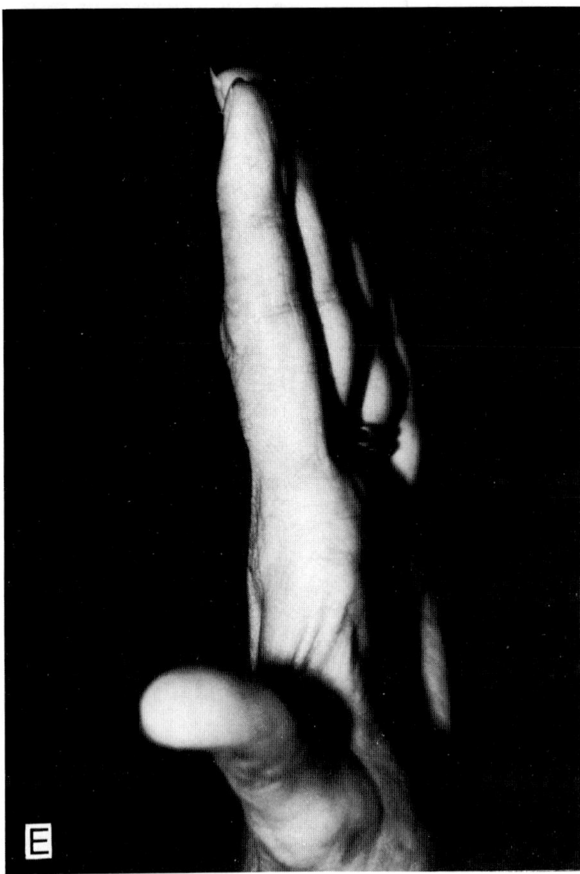

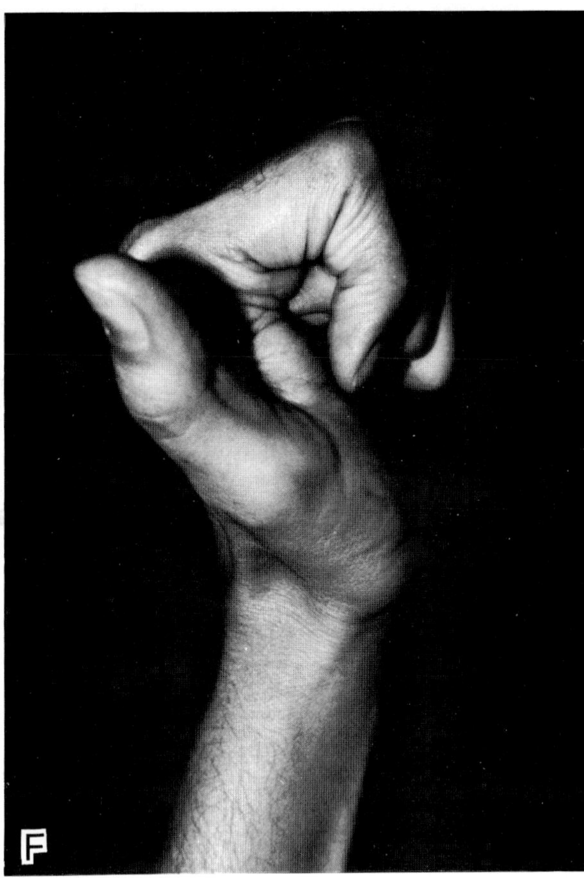

Fig. 51-30 *(Continued).* **(E&F)** Range of motion maintained at 1 year after Stage II.

Electron microscopic studies of the silicone-rubber-induced sheath in chickens by Salisbury and colleagues[346] and Takasugi, Inoue, and Akahori[408] showed that the pseudosheath closely resembled normal synovium in reference to architecture and biologic properties.

In 1976 Rayner[336] pointed out that histologic appearances are deceiving and that the lining of the induced sheath did not fulfill the criteria of the normal synovium. He believed that the cell lining is not mesothelial but fibroblastic, although it could secrete a synovial-like fluid. He conceded that this fluid may be helpful in the nutrition of the second stage tendon graft, particularly in the first 4 to 5 weeks prior to blood vessel invasion and adhesion formation. Rayner's studies suggested that grafts should not be done too early when the fibroblastic potential and vascularity of the sheath are at their highest level of activity. He recommended a delay of 3 to 4 months to wait for the most favorable conditions for grafting.

Eiken and his group concurred with Rayner that the pseudosheath produced in response to the silicone rod implantation consisted mainly of connective tissue, which they expected would contract like scar tissue.[95,96] They believed that the rubber induced a foreign body-type reaction in the healing flexor system.[93,97] This would question the findings of earlier investigators,[78,160,287,420] but they also agreed that implantation of the material in the muscle,[134,336] rather than in synovial systems, was not a fair test of the implant's sheath-inducing potential. Placing grafts of synovium about the tendon implant in chickens may improve the sheath quality,[93] they reasoned, and success here has prompted them to study this technique in 40 patients.[94] Their conclusions were that while silicone rubber is not perfect, it is the best material available for creating a tendon sheath at this time, and we concur. Farkas and Lindsay[104] showed that in experimental conditions, in chickens, the placing of the newly formed sheath over the graft junctures at Stage II led to significantly greater flexion recovery.

In summary, the final work on the exact nature of the sheath created in response to a low reactive flexible implant used in a passive gliding program, in humans, is still debated. Some of the varying observations may be a result of species differences and conditions of the experiments. The presence of a soft, pliable, translucent sheath, seen with frequency in clinical cases and associated with an uncomplicated Stage I, encourages us in using this technique in the salvage of severely damaged flexor systems.

RECONSTRUCTION OF THE PULLEY SYSTEM

Successful reconstruction of the flexor tendon system within the finger is not only dependent on the treatment of the tendon itself, but also must involve the important structural aspects of the pulley system and the vincular blood supply. The long flexor muscles have a maximum ability to shorten or contract, pulling the fingers into flexion. Because their amplitude of excursion is constant, the pulley system plays an important role in controlling the effect of range of motion at the joints in the system.[87,141,203,233] In the ideal, uninjured situation the pulley system serves to prevent bowstringing of the tendon across the volar aspect of the joint in flexion. This provides for the most efficient use of the flexor tendon excursion, thereby allowing maximum range of motion of the digital joints. As the pulleys are resected, the efficiency of the flexor system is reduced. With increasing volar displacement of the tendon, the effective range of motion decreases. Bunnell[51] suggested that pulley loss results in the tendon taking the shortest distance between the next two adjacent pulleys, i.e., bowstringing. If significant, bowstringing will result in a decreased range of joint motion as well as a flexion deformity at the involved joint. Tendon adhesions and increased risk of rupture of the remaining pulleys, due to stress, also become a possibility.

A reconstructed pulley, therefore, should be not only optimally located but also of the proper diameter and strong enough to resist breakdown or attenuation. It must hold the tendon as close to the underlying bone as possible without restricting gliding. The relative importance of the individual pulleys has been studied by Doyle and Blythe,[86-88] Hunter and colleagues,[151,152] and others[45,89,217,219,350,387] who confirmed the work of Barton,[20] who stated in 1969 that at least two pulleys (A2 and A4) need to be retained or reconstructed, including one over the middle phalanx. We agree with this, but recently a paper by Savage[350] suggested that the A2 and A4 pulleys did not seem to be more important mechanically than the other pulleys, provided that the majority of the sheath was intact. We also believe that two pulleys may not be enough; in general, a three- or even four- or five-pulley system should be reconstructed for optimal efficiency. Practically speaking, because reconstruction may interfere with volar plate or collateral ligament function, pulleys should be reconstructed just distal to the MP and PIP joints at the bases of the proximal and middle phalanges as a minimum requirement. In the clinical situation, it is often necessary to settle for less than optimal conditions when reconstructing the pulley system.

When considering the literature on flexor tendon grafting, it is interesting to find that some authors concerned themselves with the problems related to pulley disruption[16,51,54,205,444,449] while others completely ignored this aspect of flexor tendon reconstruction. Cleveland[72] reported the reconstruction of what he called "vircula" using fascia lata in a case report published in 1933. These were pulleys built over a tendon graft and located at each joint in the finger. It is interesting that he also used some kind of elastic traction for postoperative exercise in this case, although the details of the technique were not amplified.

Anatomy of the Pulley System in the Fingers (Fig. 51-31)

The fibrous retinacular sheath, which encloses the synovial sheath, starts at the neck of the metacarpal and ends at the distal phalanx. Dissections demonstrate that different areas of the sheath vary in width and can be divided into five heavier annular bands and three filmy cruciform ligaments. It is noted that A2 and A4 arise exclusively from bone, while A1, A3, and A5 originate from bone as well as volar plate.[86,136,141,397] The mechanical properties of human pulleys have been studied by

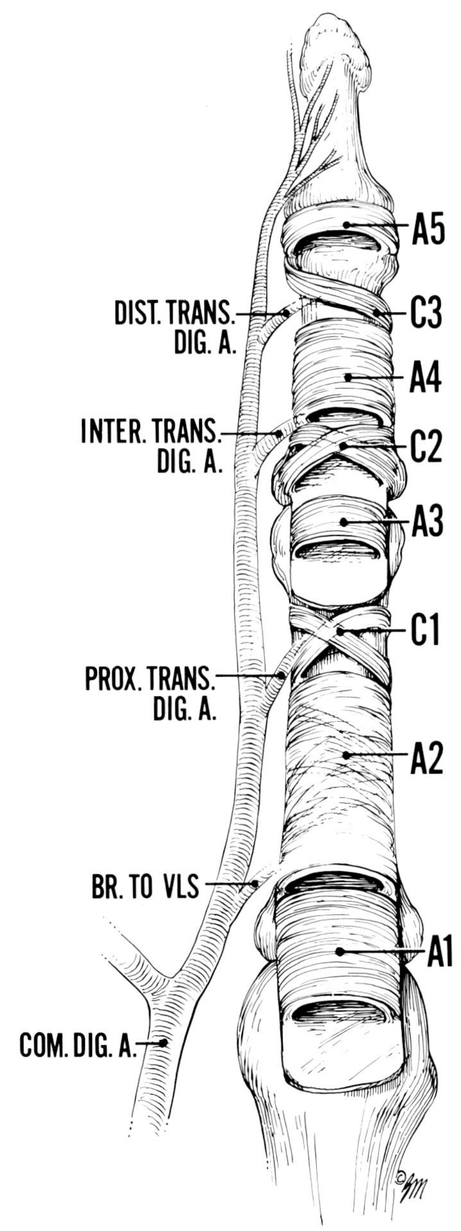

Fig. 51-31. The fibrous retinacular sheath starts at the neck of the metacarpal and ends at the distal phalanx. It can be divided into five heavier annular bands and three filmy cruciform ligaments (see text).

Lin et al and they found that the A2 and A4 pulleys were mechanically stronger than the other pulleys.[219]

Annulus 1. The A1 pulley is about 10 mm long, extending from 5 mm proximal to the MP joint to the distal end of the base of the proximal phalanx. It arises in part from the volar plate of the MP joint.

Annulus 2. The A2 pulley begins about 2 mm distal to A1, with a small 2-mm gap between them, and runs about 20 mm, arising entirely from the proximal phalanx. This long pulley has been divided into a proximal A2a and distal A2b by Hunter.

Cruciform 1. The C1 pulley consists of thin oblique fibers that crisscross over the flexor tendons. It originates from bone at the distal end of A2 and is about 4 mm long, overlying the distal portion of the proximal phalanx.

Annulus 3. The A3 pulley is a narrow band, 3 mm wide, arising from the volar plate of the PIP joint. The existence of this pulley has been recently questioned.[281]

Cruciform 2. The C2 pulley arises at the level of the base of the middle phalanx. It is usually very filmy and only 3 mm wide.

Annulus 4. The A4 pulley is a thick structure, 12 mm in length, in the middle of the middle phalanx, from which it arises.

Cruciate 3. The C3 pulley begins at the distal end of A4 and may be represented by only one oblique band.

Annulus 5. The A5 pulley, described by Hunter and colleagues,[152] is located at the DIP joint.

Anatomy of the Pulley System In the Thumb

Dissections of the retinacular system in the thumb carried out by Doyle and Blythe[88] revealed a synovial sheath similar to the one in the fingers that began at the wrist proximal to the radial styloid and ended at the interphalangeal joint.

These authors were able to identify three constant overlying pulleys as follows (Fig. 51-32):

Annulus 1. At the level of the MP joint, the A1 pulley is 9 mm wide and arises from the volar plate and base of the proximal phalanx.

Oblique pulley. Centered on the proximal phalanx, this pulley is 11 mm wide; its fibers take an oblique direction, proximal-ulnar to distal-radial. Fibers of the adductor pollicis insertion blend into this pulley at its proximal end.

Annulus 2. This thin pulley, 10 mm wide, is attached to the volar plate of the interphalangeal joint.

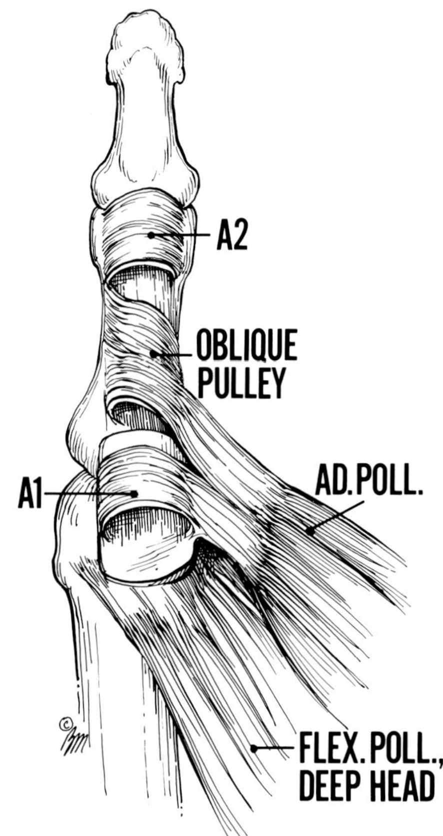

Fig. 51-32. The retinacular system in the thumb. (Modified from Doyle and Blythe,[88] with permission.)

Technique of Flexor Pulley Reconstruction

When exploring a relatively intact system, it appears preferable to surgically enter the tendon sheath at the cruciate pulley areas,[152] bearing in mind that the blood supply to the vincula enters the sheath in these areas also.[294] Removal of the cruciates and the A5 pulley when other annular ligaments are intact results in no obvious loss in potential range of motion.

When preparing a finger for a standard one-stage tendon graft, all uninjured pulley material is retained.[93,96,160,350] Supporting this technique are the multiple studies showing favorable healing potential of flexor tendons within the uninjured sheath.[96,112,237,239,251,259,260,276] This is in contradistinction to the earlier teachings of Boyes,[33] Brand,[43] Littler,[230] Pulvertaft,[325] Rank and Wakefield,[333] and Tubiana[417] who believed that only narrow critical bands should be left to keep the tendon from prolapsing. If pulley material is absent because of injury or prior surgery, reconstruction must be carried out. We have done the greatest number of our pulley reconstructions in association with staged tendon reconstruction, not being satisfied with pulley reconstruction over a standard one-stage graft. In our opinion, the staged tendon procedure is indicated if extensive pulley reconstruction is necessary.

In a staged reconstruction, even an injured pulley may be acceptable over the implant if the pulley is reparable by suture. Damaged pulleys, if strong, are also useful, as they will not adhere to the implant as they would to a tendon graft. For this reason, all pulley material is saved at Stage I if possible. If a pulley is constricted, an attempt is made to dilate the tissue available to accept the implant. If the material is unsalvageable or absent, reconstruction must be carried out.

Methods of Pulley Reconstruction

The tail of the superficialis can be used as a pulley if it is long enough (Fig. 51-33A). It can be left attached at its insertion and the free end sutured over the implant to the contralateral side to either periostium or the rim of the original pulley, or sutured via small drill holes to bone. This is done with 4–0 nonabsorbable Dacron used in all of our pulley reconstructions. This makes an excellent pulley in the A3 area.

When doing staged tendon reconstruction, there is generally sufficient tendon material available to construct free tendon graft pulleys. Various techniques have been advocated for the fixation of this material. As pointed out by Kleinert and Bennett,[200] there is often a remnant of the destroyed pulley left to which one can suture this free graft material. They[200] interwove the pulley material in the rim itself; if the rim is adequate, we utilize this technique (Fig. 51-33B). The material should be thin and the remnant strong enough to hold the pulley graft (Fig. 51-33C).

Another technique uses tendon graft encircling the phalanx[12,54,203] superficial to the extensor apparatus in the middle phalanx and deep to the extensor mechanism in the area of the proximal phalanx (Fig. 51-33D). It is desirable to support the flexor system with a long pulley at the important A2 area; thus, if possible, the phalanx is encircled two times in the proximal phalangeal area, creating a pulley 10 mm long. Approximately 6 to 8 cm of graft is required to encircle the phalanx one time, so adequate material must be available. We have been building stronger pulleys with this encircling technique, and it is now a

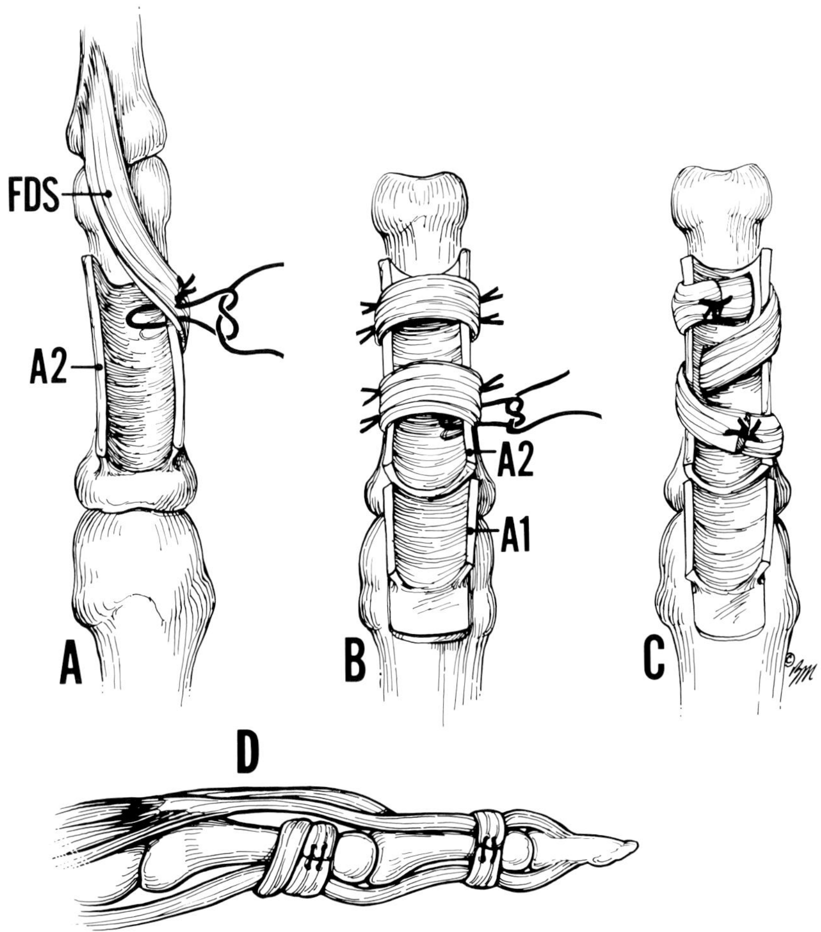

Fig. 51-33. Methods of reconstruction of the pulley system. **(A)** The tail of the superficialis, when left attached to its insertion, can be sutured over the implant to the periosteum or to the rim of the original A2 pulley. **(B)** A free tendon graft pulley can be constructed by suturing graft material to the rim of the destroyed pulley. This can take the form of an interweave **(C)** into the rim, or if the rim is inadequate, the graft can be sutured through drill holes in the bone (not shown). **(D)** Free tendon graft pulleys encircling the phalanx, deep to the extensor mechanism at the proximal phalanx and superficial to the extensor mechanism at the middle phalanx.

preferred method when critical pulleys are built at the A2 level. In a study by Lin and colleagues,[217] it was reported that this type of reconstruction used in a triple loop around the proximal phalanx was very strong and approached in vitro the normal annulus.[295] Care must be taken not to include the neurovascular bundle. Although this type of pulley may be bulky, it does not seem to have an adverse effect on the extensor system.

Doyle and Blythe[88] quoted Riordan as using a technique in which a hole is drilled completely through the bone, through which tendon material is passed and sutured to itself as a pulley. This weakens the phalanx, and, although we occasionally use this technique, the possibility of phalangeal fracture during the procedure and afterward is of concern.

Lister[226,228] has described good results with a technique in which a segment of the extensor retinaculum from the dorsum of the wrist is passed around the phalanx for pulley reconstruction. The advantages of this technique are (1) the undersurface of the retinaculum is an ideal gliding surface (the broad fourth dorsal compartment segment of the retinaculum is rotated into position overlying the flexor tendon or silicone implant), and (2) the new pulley is strong enough to allow early motion (e.g., following tenolysis). The major disadvantage is that harvesting the 6- to 8-cm length of retinaculum is technically somewhat difficult and time-consuming and also requires a separate incision.

A technique that uses the volar plate in reconstruction of the pulleys has been published.[187] Recent articles have suggested that this "belt-loop" technique is nearly as strong as a normal annular band[219] but did not provide as normal joint motion as reconstruction of the A2 and A4 pulleys.[217] We have no experience with this technique.

The reconstructed pulley must be strong[248] and should be vigorously tested under direct visualization at the operating table. The forces generated against the pulley in flexion are considerable.

Artificial materials have been utilized in the reconstruction of pulleys. These materials include knitted Dacron arterial graft,[471] silicone rubber sheeting,[18] Xenograft materials,[68] polytetrafluoroethylene (PTFE),[184] woven nylon and fascia lata[89,310] The plentiful availability at operation of tendon remnants to be used as pulley grafts is such that we are not tempted to try these artificial materials.

Complications of Staged Tendon Reconstruction

Synovitis in the sheath forming in response to the implant was formerly recognized in about 15 to 20 percent of post-Stage I patients.[331,335] It is noted now that this complication has been reduced to 8 percent in the most recent evaluation of our cases.[452] This problem is characterized by increased heat, crepitus, and obvious swelling with fluid in the sheath, and will be associated with a thickened, less pliable sheath at Stage II (Fig. 51-34). This serious complication is often, but not necessarily always, followed by a less successful end result after Stage II. Cultures for bacteria in the fluid found within these sheaths have consistently shown no growth.[360]

While the inciting cause for this inflammatory reaction is not always apparent, there are certain occurrences that seem to be associated with the development of synovitis. Breakdown of the distal juncture after Stage I will usually be followed by the clinical picture of synovitis. Careful attention to the details of Stage I and use of the Dacron reinforced implant have all but eliminated this cause of mechanical irritation within the sheath.

Buckling or binding of the implant because of tight or inadequate pulleys is another situation that is seen with synovial reaction in the sheath, and may be an inciting cause. Appropriate pulley reconstruction should eliminate this problem. Passive movement of the finger at Stage I will usually demonstrate potential problem areas where further dilation or reconstruction of a pulley will be of value. Postoperative lateral radiographs in flexion and extension will identify the amount of excursion present and will often demonstrate buckling, particularly in patients with synovitis.

The problem of foreign materials, such as talc, on the implant surface is reduced by minimizing handling of the implant and careful cleansing of the surgeon's gloves. Sterile packaging of the implant has reduced this potential source of problems, and breaking the actual implant out of the package as late as possible in the procedure has further shortened the exposure time.

When synovitis is recognized, the patient's exercise program should be decreased, with return to resting splints except for limited periods of passive range of motion exercises. An earlier Stage II may be advisable if the problem is not controllable.

Postoperative infection following Stage I is a disastrous complication, as in any implant procedure. When confronted with infection in the sheath, we have tried antibiotic irrigations using small bore catheters and, on at least one occasion, have salvaged the sheath. In general, however, established infection calls for removal of the implant, with a healing period of 3 to 6 months, and, if feasible, later replacement with a new implant.

One other source of problems that we hear about after Stage I is in the patient in whom the surgeon had ill-advisably sutured the proximal end of the implant, designed for the passive motion program, to a flexor motor. This juncture will usually disrupt and create additional irritation and scarring in the region of the future proximal tendon graft juncture. If this unnecessary proximal juncture is stronger than the distal juncture, the distal end will most certainly break free and thereby reduce the benefit of the operation. Tendon implants designed with both proximal and distal end devices for active function are discussed on page 1900.

Complications after Stage II

Breakdown at the proximal or distal juncture of the graft has been seen in staged tendon reconstruction as with any tendon graft.[360] Good surgical technique should make this a rare complication, and the application of a closely supervised postoperative hand therapy program is also advisable. When rupture of a graft juncture is recognized early, the procedure can often be salvaged by early reoperation. The patient usually can localize the juncture that has pulled free, and exploration may allow reattachment. This complication occurs more frequently at the

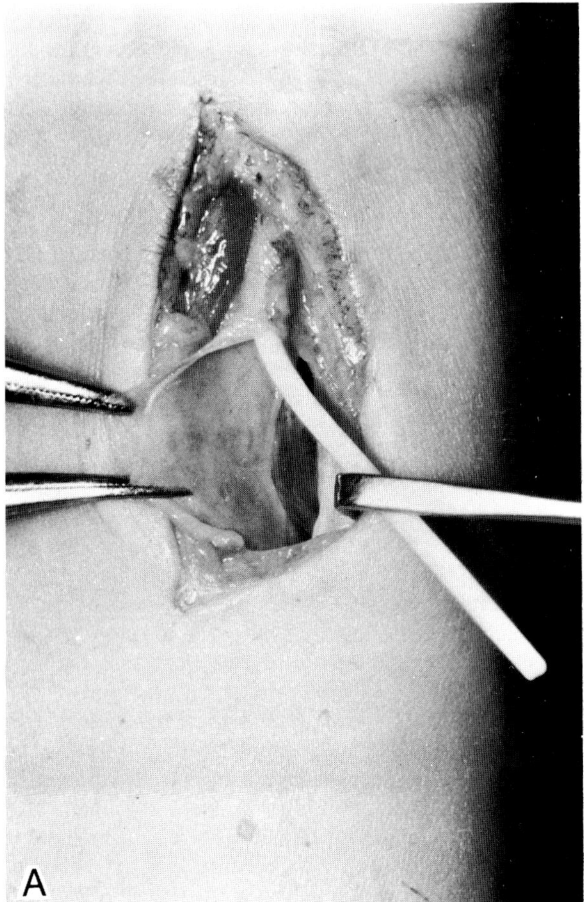

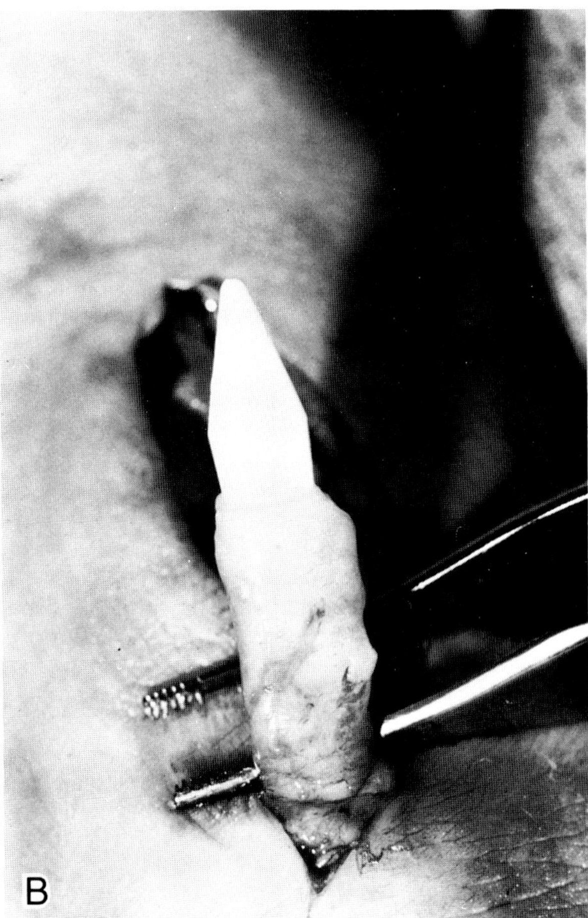

Fig. 51-34. The sheath formed in response to the implant as seen at Stage II. **(A)** A soft, translucent sheath seen at 3 months in a patient with a benign postoperative course. **(B)** A thickened sheath seen in a patient with synovitis after Stage I.

distal juncture, and if the tendon cannot be advanced to the original insertion, the end of the graft can be inserted into the middle phalanx, creating a superficialis finger[164] (see below).

A proximal level juncture disruption is usually represented by a distal slippage of the graft interweave. Exploration of the distal forearm wound will often allow reattachment and salvage.

Pulley breakdown is another failure point seen and is confirmed by reduction in regained range of motion, with bowstringing of the tendon graft. Blocking support of the flexor tendon using the patient's other hand, a wood block, or an external ring will help maintain tendon gliding while consideration for secondary pulley reconstruction is undertaken. Use of the encircling method for A2 pulley reconstruction has virtually eliminated this problem.

Late flexion deformity is seen mostly in less than ideal cases and may be related to a poor nutritional status in the finger or by a particular patient's collagen formation. This deformity is rarely seen in a patient with a good range of movement early after Stage II.[356,360] This problem is aggravated by inadequate pulley structure and bowstringing. In addition to complete release of joints at Stage I and the construction of stronger pulleys, we advocate a prolonged retentive splinting program (up to 1 year), along with gentle stretching in the postoperative period.

THE FLEXOR DIGITORUM SUPERFICIALIS FINGER: A SALVAGE PROCEDURE

In flexor tendon reconstruction, an effort is usually made to restore active motion in both the PIP and DIP joints. Occasionally, under specific conditions, efforts are directed at regaining motion only in the PIP joint in a more modest attempt to salvage function. This procedure has been called the superficialis finger,[71,164,297,298,368,417] although most of these reconstructions, in our experience, have been motored by the profundus tendon inserted into the middle phalanx. Perhaps the term proximal interphalangeal joint finger would be more appropriate.

In the following three clinical types, where there is flexor system disruption and distal joint motion is likely to be unattainable, consideration for salvage via restoration of motion at the PIP joint might be undertaken:

Type I. Digits in which the DIP joint is inadequate because of intraarticular damage or through destruction of the extensor mechanism.

Type II. Digits with a gliding flexor system that functions poorly due to bowstringing of the tendon caused by pulley failure or inadequate pulleys.

Type III. Digits in which the distal insertion ruptured following tendon grafting.

Technique (Fig. 51-35)

In Type I, a standard tendon graft is carried out as described earlier, but the graft is inserted into the middle phalanx by the pull-out technique as used in the standard tendon graft. Particular attention is directed to padding placed between the button and the skin to distribute skin pressure over as wide an area as possible. Alternately, the graft can be sutured by various techniques to the middle phalanx via the use of the pulley remnants, the superficialis tail, or local periosteum.

In the anesthetized patient, tension must be adjusted so that, with the wrist in neutral, the finger adopts a flexion posture at the PIP joint similar to that of the adjacent fingers. We prefer, whenever possible, to do this procedure under local-sedative anesthesia so the patient can directly cooperate in the setting of tension at the distal juncture at the middle phalangeal level.

In situations where the distal joint is not stable, arthrodesis or tenodesis in 20 to 30 degrees flexion is also carried out.

In Types II and III, the motor tendon end is identified through a volar approach to the finger and reattached preferably to bone. The technique is the same as in Type I cases, except that pulley reconstruction is needed in Type II. Again, the use of local anesthesia technique to allow active participation of the patient is extremely useful.

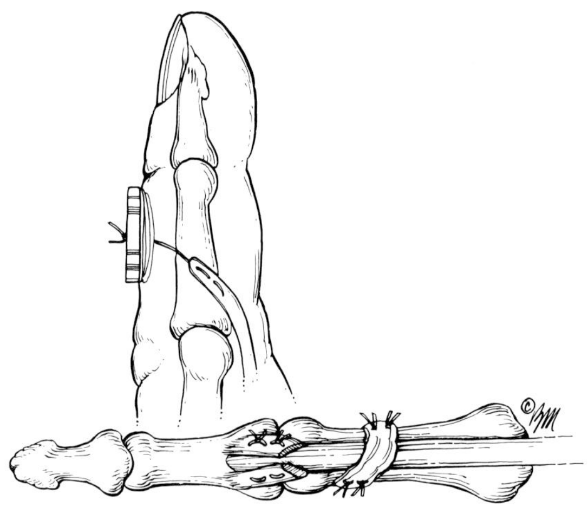

Fig. 51-35. The flexor digitorum superficialis finger. The graft is inserted into the middle phalanx by one of several techniques. If the distal joint is not stable, tenodesis or arthrodesis of the DIP joint can be carried out at the same operation.

Postoperative Management

The tendon grafts (Type I) are treated exactly as we treat the standard graft. In Types II and III, early nonresistive motion is allowed in a splint, combined with gentle rubber band traction on the fingernail. The MP joints are placed in 70 degrees, with the posterior splint allowing the PIP joints to be fully extended. The wrist is flexed approximately 30 degrees. When a pulley is reconstructed, an orthoplast ring is fabricated, measuring about 2 cm in width, and is worn to protect the pulley. At 3 to 4 weeks, the splint is removed but the rubber band, attached to a wrist cuff, is continued for a total of 6 weeks. The ring is worn for at least 8 weeks postoperatively.

FLEXOR TENDON RECONSTRUCTION IN CHILDREN

Children present a somewhat different problem after flexor tendon injury. The very young, especially, present difficulties with diagnosis, but, with careful observation and the use of various tricks geared to stimulate withdrawal of the fingers into flexion, a diagnosis can usually be made. A positive consideration is that children heal rapidly and rarely develop contractures, provided the joint has not been directly injured. They also do not have the economic problems that can hinder progress in the adult.[91]

As a general rule, direct early repair, at all levels of injuries, is agreed upon,[99,100,135,222,335,361,442] provided wound conditions permit. This is even more pertinent in the youngest age group, those under 4 to 6 years of age, in whom flexor tendon grafting is particularly difficult.[24]

The appropriate time to perform a flexor tendon graft in children has been debated. Hage and Dupius[125] studied this question and concluded that age was no contraindication to grafting, although others[122,325] have hesitated doing flexor grafts in children. The latter cited technical difficulties, due to the small size of the tendons and the inability of children to cooperate in postoperative care and rehabilitation.

We do occasionally perform tendon grafts in young children in selected cases,[159] but generally plan to wait until the patient is over 7 years of age for the reasons mentioned above. While magnification helps eliminate some of the technical objections to tendon surgery in the young, the small size of the injured tendon and material used for grafting will not always hold sutures well and separation of the juncture in the postoperative period can easily occur.

Technique

The technique in children is essentially the same as that in adults, except that the distal juncture is not placed in the distal phalangeal bone. Our preferred method in children is a juncture to the distal profundus stump as shown in Fig. 51-8. If there is no distal stump, we would be forced to suture the graft directly into bone with nonabsorbable sutures through drill holes placed distal to the epiphysis.

The graft material preferred is the palmaris longus or superficialis of the injured finger. The plantaris in children is often too thin to hold sutures, although not all surgeons have found this to be an objection.[154]

Another minor modification in the young is the closure of the skin with absorbable suture material, thereby avoiding an unpleasant confrontation in the office postoperatively. We strongly oppose the use of general anesthesia for suture removal as advocated by some surgeons.

The flexor tendon graft, if successful, will probably grow along with the child's hand. This is a clinical observation that could not be proven by Hage and Dupius.[125] They did report that, despite good function, the involved finger did lag slightly in growth, remaining minimally smaller than the uninjured fingers.

In general, flexor tendon injuries present difficult problems both for the young patient and for the surgeon. Careful attention to surgical principles and details will reward both surgeon and patient. Direct repair of injured flexor tendons is, in general, a better procedure than late reconstruction. This fact is even more pertinent in children because of the aforementioned difficulties with grafting.[361] When injury of the flexors is diagnosed, surgical repair of both tendons, if possible, is carried out at all levels (with the possible exception of the Zone IV carpal tunnel level, where it may be better to repair only the flexor profundus). At this time we would defer surgical reconstruction by graft in one or two stages until after the age of 7 or 8 years.

FLEXOR TENDON RECONSTRUCTION AND REHABILITATION USING ACTIVE TENDON IMPLANTS

James M. Hunter
Scott Jaeger

The advantages of an active tendon implant are apparent. There would be a need for only one operative procedure. The gliding motion felt to be necessary for pseudosheath formation would be provided by the patient's own muscular activity rather than by passive movement of the finger. Muscle function and strength as well as joint motion would be more easily maintained. When and if a tendon graft is to be necessary at a second stage it would be simplified, as the gliding sheath would have been formed and the gliding tissue planes at the proximal level had already been established. The motor muscle would be actively kept "in tune." The problems with an active tendon are related mainly to those of creation of a permanent attachment of the implant both proximally to the motor tendon and distally to the distal phalanx. It is in this area that efforts are being directed both in the laboratory and in the operating room.[148,167]

Considerations for tendon reconstruction in the 1990s should include, in addition to the passive tendon sheath formation alternative to tendon grafting, active power-driven tendon sheath formation, with the goal of earlier return of function in the hand.

During the past two decades, hand therapists called our attention to softer, more pliable fingers following reconstruction using passive implants.[168] The reinforced Silastic rod, attached to bone at the distal end, glides during flexion and extension. This induces a new sheath that must produce synovial lubrication fluid to support implant gliding,[156] which satisfies not only the implant rheology, but also scar bed surface remodeling. The sheath is a closed system that forces fluid diffusion, resulting in "softening" of the ligamentous connective tissues in the fingers. Softening of the connective tissue, therefore, helps to improve joint motion and enhances neurovascular recovery of the finger and hand.

Since 1980, our experience with active tendon implants has added power-induced flexion to the new sheath system.[166,168] This has been made possible by attaching the motor muscle tendon to the tendon implant in the forearm. The new sheath cul-de-sac at the tendon-implant juncture becomes elongated in extension and folds in flexion. The adjacent tissues "learn" these same patterns by developing soft adhesions to support muscle contraction and tendon gliding. The quest that started in the 1960s with Merseline sutures and homemade loop attachment is nearly complete.[143] Two helical formed polyester fiber twill cords are molded into the silicone body of the implant. This design has resulted in a strong tendon replacement with improved reliability. The surgeon has two options for the proximal tendon juncture:

1. On the single unit tendon, the loop (proximal end) enables the tendon loop interweave juncture to be completed immediately. Function is dependable for 2 years or longer.
2. On the adjustable length implant, the two free porous cords (proximal end) require a woven juncture by motion-induced geotaxis. This juncture becomes stronger with time, resulting in a connection that is actually stronger than the implant itself.

The active tendon implant with the new sheath and power-induced proximal interface has now reached the fourth decade of study and development. Permanent patient benefits have become a positive force in flexor tendon reconstruction. In our opinion, this program should be considered early after failed flexor tendon repair and later in flexor tendon reconstruction.

The first positive benefit of power-induced gliding following Stage I is the flexibility in delaying Stage II. The Stage II benefit is tendon grafting with an adhesion-free juncture, overcoming one of the problems reported after use of the two-stage passive tendon. These positive advances can be achieved with reasonable assurance with active tendon reconstruction when certain *key factors* are addressed.

Extensor Tendon System

When the proximal and distal joints are passively positioned into flexion, the patient should be able to actively extend the finger. Extensor tenolysis is often necessary in the early steps of

Stage I surgery before and after release of IP joint flexion contractures.

Flexor Retinaculum (Pulley) Reconstruction

The flexor retinaculum must be efficiently reconstructed and of sufficient strength to support the powerful vector forces of "adhesion-free" flexor tendon function.

The authors' experience suggests that the best method of pulley reconstruction is a free tendon graft wrapped around bone. The tendon is passed under the extensor tendon hood for A2 and A4 reconstruction. A minimum of two wraps (if possible, four wraps) is recommended for sufficient strength to allow early active motion. A separate small dorsal incision in the skin and extensor tendon will facilitate passing the free graft under the extensor tendon hood Bunnell-style.

For A1 deficiency, the tendon graft is wrapped two or three times around the metacarpal neck. For superficialis finger constructions, the A2 reconstruction should not only be wide, but also should be close to the radius of the proximal interphalangeal joint. The A1 pulley fair-leads (see page 1855) and protects the A2 pulley by reducing the angular power drive at the proximal edge of the construct. Firm manual pressure on the A1 pulley during rehabilitation training is important.

Construction of a Superficialis Finger

This concept is based on the principle of a one-tendon/two-joint finger; the distal fixation of the implant is placed on the proximal one-third of the middle phalanx with the proximal tendon implant juncture in the forearm.[29,156,367] (see page 1898). We recommended that the superficialis finger construction be done when the following problems in reconstruction are encountered: (1) reconstruction of more than two flexor pulleys is necessary; (2) poor extensor tendon control of the distal interphalangeal joint; (3) arthritis of the distal interphalangeal joint; (4) multiple finger injuries in one hand and partial or complete amputations of adjacent fingers, either ulnarly or radially; and (5) vascular deficiencies of the finger characteristic of Boyes Grade V or Salvage VI.

Active Tendon Implant Technique

Flexor tendon reconstruction using active tendon implants[29,147–150,155,166–168] takes advantage of the muscle tendon dynamics during Stage I. The new sheath that develops on the implant surface also develops a functioning interface with the motor tendon at the proximal juncture in the forearm. In selected patients, excellent function may be expected, and Stage I may be extended for indefinite periods. The prerequisites for an active rather than a passive tendon are (1) a patient of appropriate age with social motivation for predicted compliance; (2) a functioning extensor tendon system sufficient to balance the known or projected passive range of joint motion of the finger or thumb; (3) patient understanding that a superficialis finger reconstruction with DIP joint arthrodesis may be elected by the surgeon if the extensor tendon function is not fully recovered or if more than two pulleys will require reconstruction.

The surgeon considering active tendon reconstruction should understand the details of the passive two-stage tendon reconstruction method and the significance of placing the proximal tendon juncture in the forearm, bypassing the palm tissues compromised by the previous injury or operations. There are fixed-length implants of four sizes and adjustable length implants in which the silicone cover can be removed from porous Dacron cords (Fig. 51-36).

Stage I

Active tendon implants follow the same general guidelines for insertion as described for passive tendon implants, and the same incisions are used (see page 1888). The motor tendon in the forearm is exposed and tested for excursion. The profundus of the injured digit or digits is the preferred choice, but if excursion is insufficient, another available motor tendon unit is chosen. A superficialis motor unit can be chosen if necessary, but its excursion potential is less than that of an intact profundus tendon. However, superficialis muscle power may be used to advantage to motor the finger when the surgeon elects to use only the PIP joint while performing an arthrodesis on the distal joint—the superficialis finger (Fig. 51-37). The length of the implant is estimated by measuring the distance from the distal phalanx or middle phalanx to the motor tendon unit in the forearm.

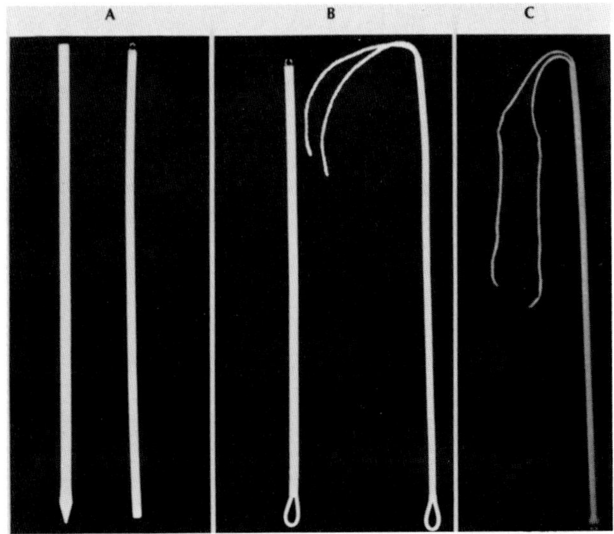

Fig. 51-36. **(A)** Passive, gliding tendon implants. **(B)** Active, gliding tendon implants. Left, metal end-screw fixation and fixed-length loop system. Right, porous Dacron fiber replaces the loop system. **(C)** Active, gliding tendon implant. Metal end-screw fixation with two free, porous Dacron cords with adjustable-length design.

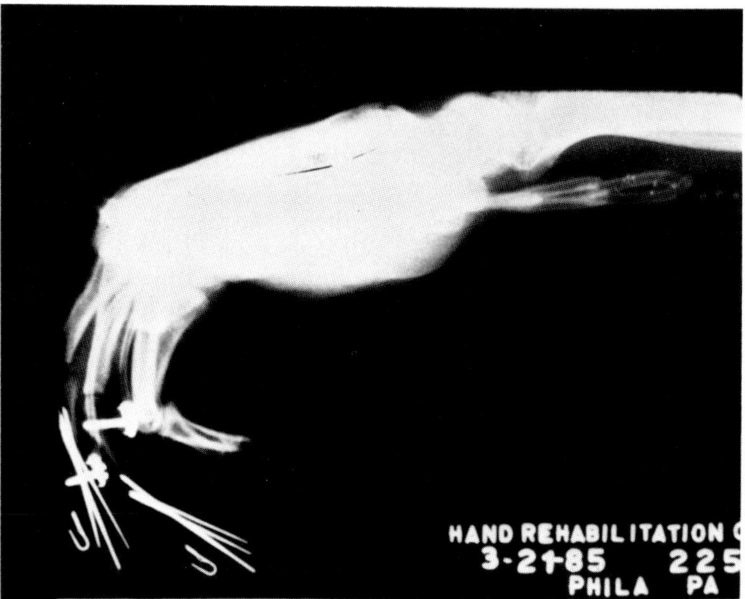

Fig. 51-37. Superficialis finger active tendon reconstruction. Note: *(1)* arthrodesis of distal joints; *(2)* metal ends fixed with screws to the middle phalanx; *(3)* proximal implant loops in the forearm; *(4)* hooks on nails distally for rubber band training.

Types of Active Tendon Implants

Two types of active tendon are available for use in flexor tendon reconstruction.

Fixed Length Active Tendon Implant (Fig. 51-36B)

This implant is designed as a single unit (metal plate distally, Dacron silicone flexible shaft, and a preformed Dacron silicone loop proximally).

It is available in four lengths—16, 18, 20, and 22 cm. All are 4 mm in overall diameter.

Adjustable Length Active Tendon Implant (Fig. 51-36C)

This implant permits length adjustment by pulling the silicone away from the two porous woven Dacron cords. It is available in three designs:

1. Distal—a metal plate, a 27-cm shaft, and two free porous cords proximally
2. Distal—two free porous cords, a 27-cm shaft, and a Dacron silicone loop proximally
3. Distal—two porous Dacron cords, a 27-cm shaft, and two porous Dacron cords proximally

The stainless steel distal component is passed from the palm through the pulleys in the finger using a no-touch technique. Moistening the device with Ringer's solution will facilitate this process. The distal component should pass through the normal A1 and A2 pulleys with gentle manipulation. A generous length of wet umbilical tape or heavy nonabsorbable, nonmetallic suture is threaded through the distal component screw hole. Both ends of the tape or suture are grasped and used to guide the distal component through the A1 and A2 pulleys. In some cases the normal A2 retinaculum should be opened for implant placement. The A2 retinaculum is cut along the periosteal rim on the middle phalanx. The A2 pulley is repaired exactly with multiple Dacron sutures using small drill holes if necessary. The adjustable active tendon with two porous Dacron cords at the proximal end is passed through the pulley system distal to proximal with ease.

If good *retinaculum* cannot be salvaged, (Fig. 51-38) free tendon graft material is preferred, either a portion of an excised flexor tendon or the palmaris longus. The preferred technique is to pass the tendon graft around the bone extraperiosteally under the extensor apparatus (Fig. 51-39). A small dorsal, extensor-tendon splitting skin incision will assist passage of the tendon around bone. It is wrapped at least twice around the phalanx and sutured to itself and to the periosteal rim of the fibroosseous canal. [Note: Three tendon turns (four if possible) are preferred for A2 pulley construction.]

To pass the implant loop to the proximal wrist, the loop is manually compressed and passed from palm to forearm through the carpal canal. If necessary, a tendon passer having a diameter slightly larger than that of the device can be used to carry the implant into the carpal canal. Again, the use of wet umbilical tape looped through the implant proximal loop and carried into the forearm on a tendon passer will facilitate passage of the implant. It is imperative to protect the silicone coating on the loop against tear damage.

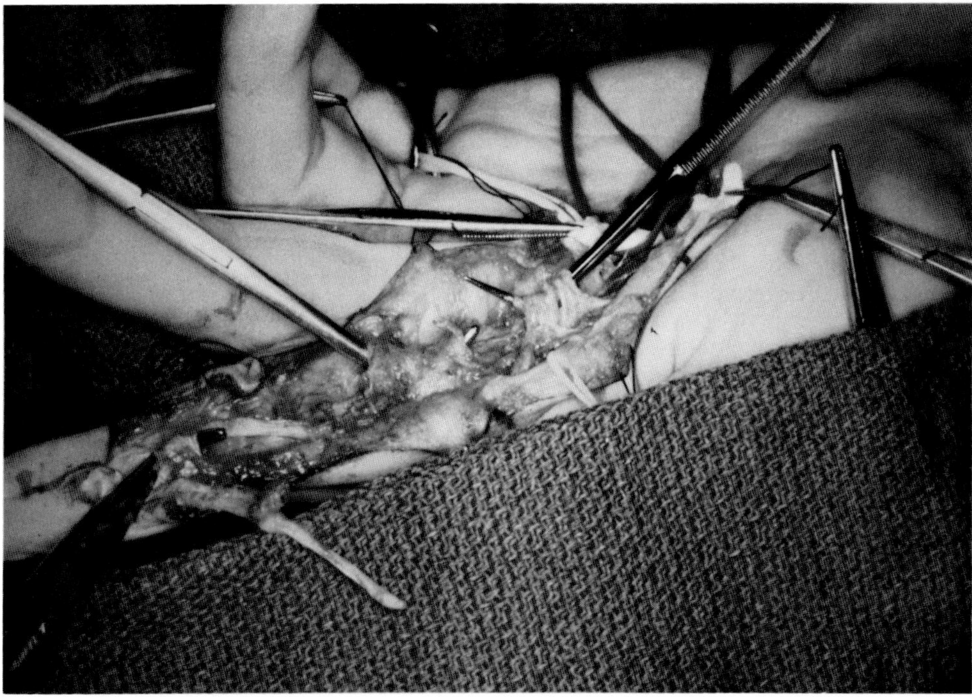

Fig. 51-38. In this patient, retinaculum could be salvaged for the A1, A2, and A4 pulleys.

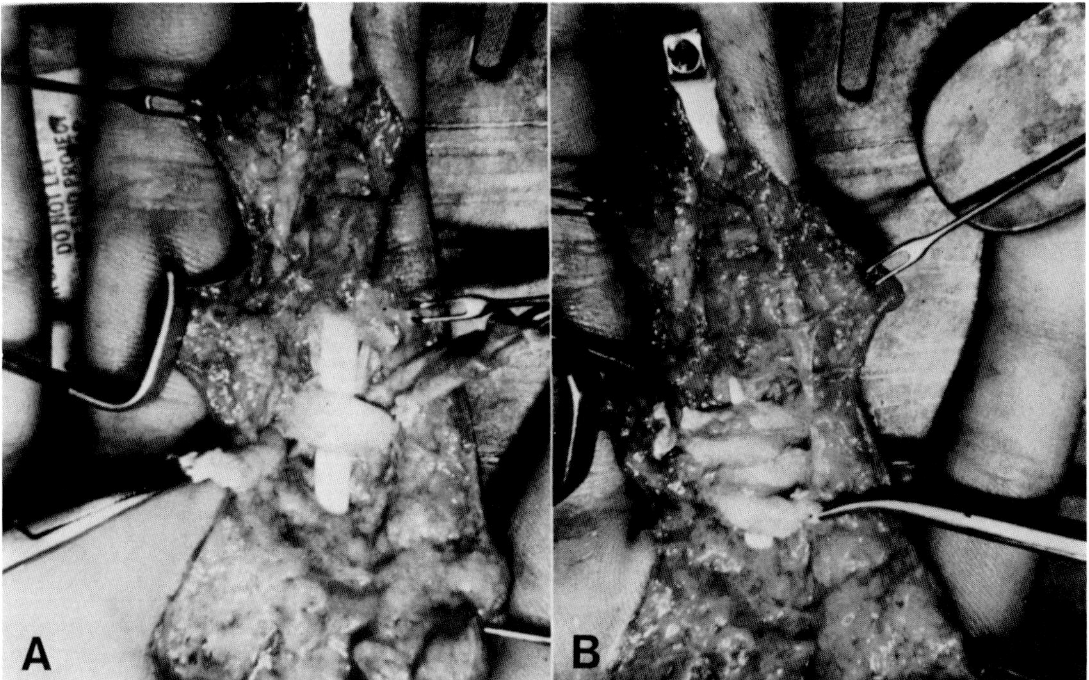

Fig. 51-39. Pulley reconstruction. **(A)** A remnant of superficialis tendon is wrapped under the extensor apparatus and over the implant to reconstruct the A2 pulley. **(B)** After the tendon is wrapped around the finger twice, it is sewn to itself and the rim of the fibroosseous canal. The reconstructed pulley should be as wide as possible without blocking motion.

Distal Fixation

The distal component must be secured to bone in a way that will achieve a strong, durable, immediate juncture. A 27-gauge needle is passed through the lateral space of the distal IP joint and out of the dorsum. With the joint identified, the base of the distal phalanx is stripped of volar periosteum. The needle point is used as a reference point in the following steps:

1. Bear in mind that the ideal position of the distal metal (fixation plate) is with its proximal edge at least 3 mm distal to the joint. With the joint identified, the point where the screw should enter bone is visualized or measured. The 2-mm AO screw system is preferred. One end of a K-wire is placed on the determined point, holding it parallel to the needle. The uppermost tip of the K-wire is tilted distally approximately 15 degrees and the bone of the phalanx is marked.
2. The tendon implant bone plate is centered over the marked bone. All negotiable parts, (i.e., gloved finger) are removed from the plate. The dorsum of the patient's finger is placed on a firm part of the operative table. A bone impacter is positioned against the plate and "struck firmly," driving the four sharp spikes into the bone so that the plate is secure and evenly aligned on the bone.
3. The 1.5-mm drill bit is passed through both cortices of bone. The finger is turned for a lateral x-ray view. The K-wire should have missed the joint and base of nail and be in cortical bone. Drill location should be central.
4. The recommended bone screw is the 2-mm AO screw. Holding the joint securely, the drill is carefully removed, the threads are tapped, and the proper screw length is chosen. The distal end of the device is secured by carefully turning the screw through both cortices of bone to thumb tightness. The screw should appear dorsally. A minimum amount (less than 1 mm) is acceptable, but if there is more than 1 mm protruding, it is trimmed through a small dorsal transverse incision. The screw fit should feel firm all the way, and final fixation should be secure (Fig. 51-40). If the final screw turns are loose, the system may not stand cyclic force. If the screw fixation is not firm, it should either be reinserted more distally in bone or the alternate technique (fixing the endpiece to bone with twisted wire) should be used.
5. The profundus tendon stump may be drawn over the distal component and sutured laterally to provide a soft tissue buffer, minimizing irritation of the overlying skin (Fig. 51-41).
6. A strip of superficialis tendon may be drawn over the distal component and sutured laterally at the middle phalanx level in the superficialis finger procedure.
7. The tourniquet is released, the wounds are irrigated, and the distal incision is closed.

The distal component is also designed to permit fixation by two twisted wires through bone, as well as by screw. If the bone has been fractured or shows osteoporosis, wiring is preferred. The four sharp metal spikes, if driven securely into bone, do the real work, as distal plate security is set by the fifth bone contact, the screw through two cortices.

The active tendon may be fixed to the distal phalanx for a one-tendon, three-joint finger or to the middle phalanx for a one-tendon, two-joint finger (the superficialis finger).

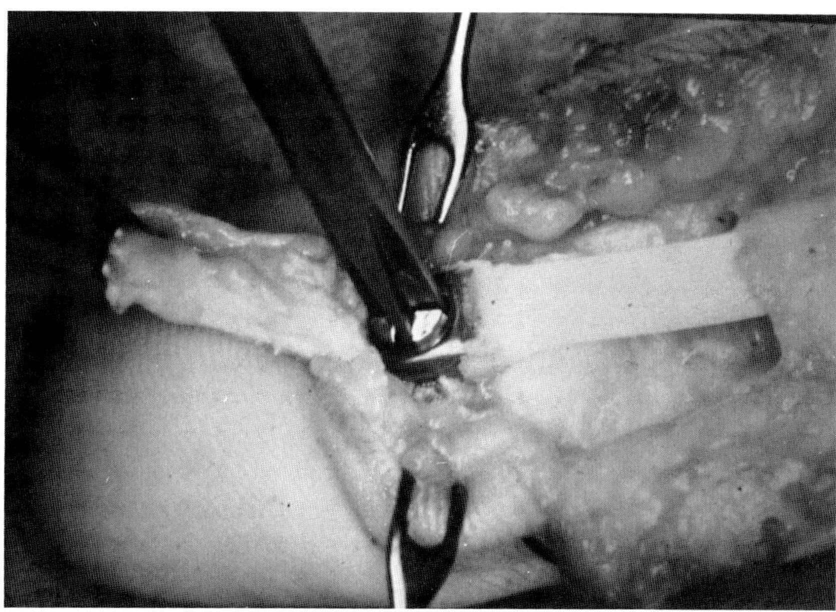

Fig. 51-40. Setting the tension in the distal screw.

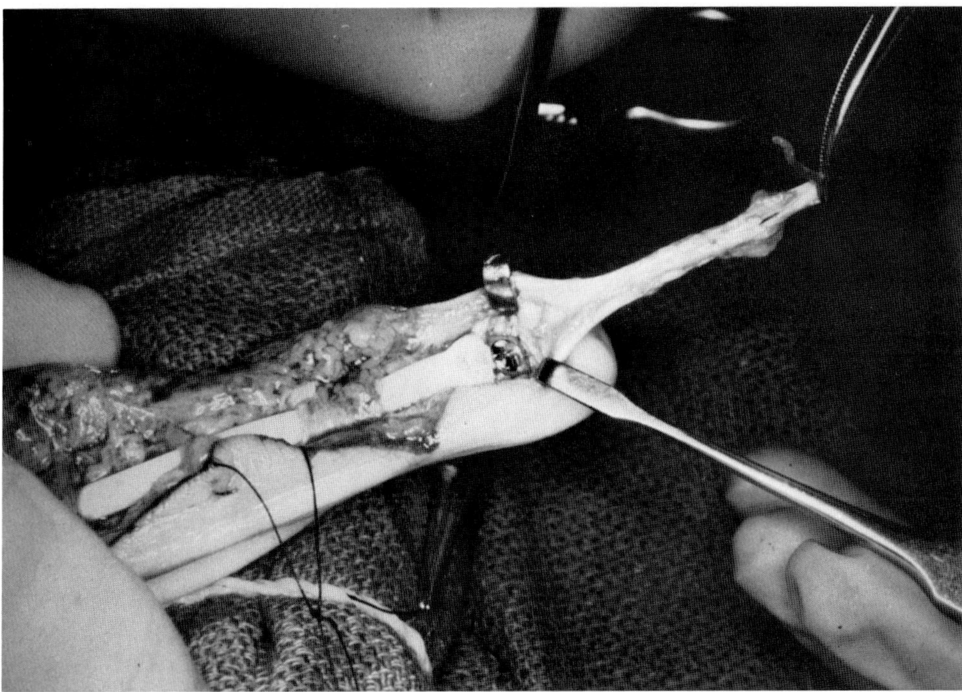

Fig. 51-41. The distal profundus stump may be drawn over the distal component to minimize skin irritation.

Proximal Juncture: Loop Method

The length of the motor tendon must be sufficient to pass through the proximal loop and return proximally for at least two 90-degree passes through the tendon. Desired excursion of the motor tendon is 4 cm for the flexor digitorum profundus and 3 cm for the flexor digitorum superficialis. If the patient can be aroused from anesthesia during this last phase of tendon surgery, an accurate assessment of the muscle amplitude is possible. Otherwise, the traditional technique of passively flexing and extending the wrist to secure a cascade in the fingers is effective.

The selected tendon is passed through the implant loop and then through a small longitudinal split in the tendon. (Fig. 51-42) One suture is placed through the tendon and the tension is tested. Tension is tested by moistening the implant surface, followed by flexion and extension of the wrist. The finger should lie in extension during wrist flexion and show a position of balance with the adjacent fingers on wrist extension. If balance is acceptable, a second suture is placed and the tendon is turned 90 degrees through one or two additional longitudinal splits in the tendon. Tendon balance is retested to be sure there has been no loss of tendon tension.

Adjustable Length Active Tendon Implants

One of the three types has the same metal four-prong distal plate for screw fixation as the fixed length implant, with the free two-cord proximal end. This is a good multipurpose implant, passing easily through the pulleys to the forearm for tendon juncture (see Fig. 51-36C).

Design Characteristics of Porous Dacron Cords

A helical weave of thousands of fine high-density Dacron fibers forms the two-cord center of the Hunter Flexible Silicone Dacron Tendon Implant. The two cords, measuring $\frac{1}{32}$-inch in diameter, have a compliance that favors a secure fixation in tendon or bone for connective tissue or bone ingrowth. The combined stimulus of tension and delicate movement gives the helical weave a geometric memory. Energy transmission and heat retention favor a plan of "geotaxis" that integrates the new fibrous cell system and encourages collagen formation. Providing the system does not loosen, fixation is assured, and proximal juncture strength can be expected to approach or surpass a standard tendon-to-tendon juncture.

Indication and Technique

The porous Dacron and tendon weave technique is useful when very short or very long tendon defects are encountered. With care, the silicone rubber can be peeled away from the Dacron and the silicone part of the tendon can therefore be shortened. Using magnification, care is taken not to damage the fine Dacron weave during this technique.

Distal Juncture to Bone Using Two Porous Dacron Cords. This technique is an alternative to the metal plate and screw fixation to bone. Long-term results are not available for this specific type of distal fixation; however, considerable data are available using this porous cord material in bone for small joint collateral ligament reconstruction with and without Swanson implants. Good bone acceptability and strength is the rule. This type of bone juncture is uniquely useful for digital salvage

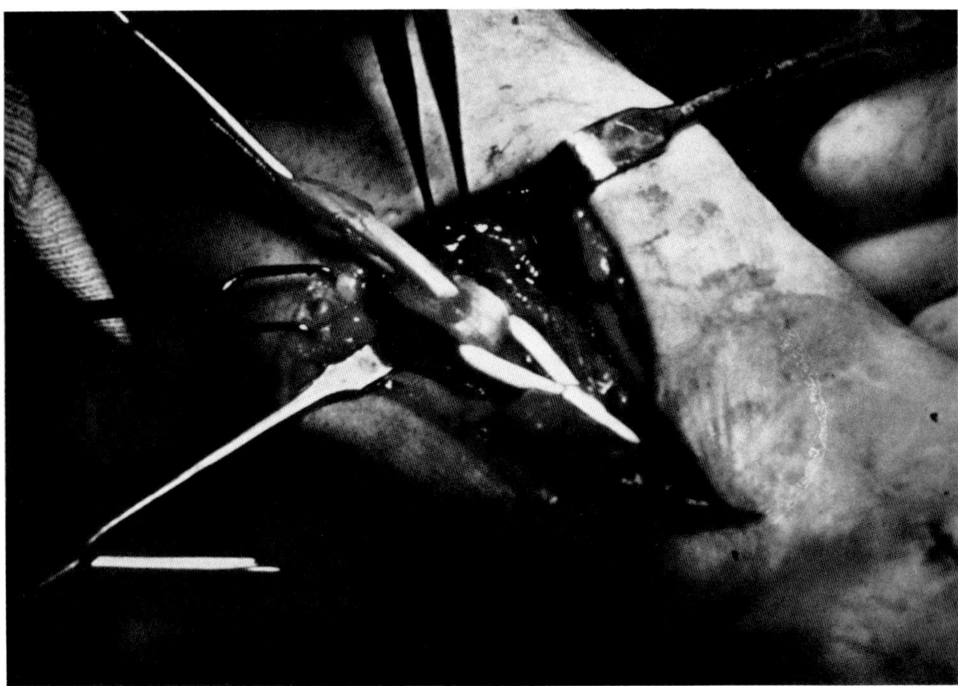

Fig. 51-42. Proximal juncture with the loop method.

when a PIP joint arthroplasty with intramedullary stems is necessary in superficialis finger reconstruction.

Proximal Juncture of Adjustable Length Active Tendons. The Dacron is woven into the lateral borders of the tendon and fixed with nonabsorbable sutures at points of exit. Tendon balance is tested after the first two sutures, and readjusted if necessary. After three or four passes, the Dacron can be tied securely with a square knot, reinforced with 3–0 Dacron sutures, and the ends cut with electric cautery. (Fig. 51-43) *Tapercut needles only* are used during all reinforcement procedures; cutting needles will seriously damage the delicate Dacron weave. The final resting balance of the fingers is reestablished by repeated flexion and extension of the wrist. When satisfied with tendon tension, and pulley integrity (Fig. 51-44), the proximal juncture is tucked beneath the muscle folds and the muscle is gently closed with 5-0 chromic sutures. The tourniquet is released, and the wound is closed when hemostatis is achieved. X-rays at 12 weeks postoperative should show full excursion of the gliding tendon implant (Fig. 51-45). This is measured by drawing a line between the distal ulna and the proximal excursion of the implant.

Stage II

The interval between stage I and stage II can be quite variable when the functioning active tendon implant is used. The active tendon implant should be retained for at least 4 months, so that the patient can derive the full benefit of the implant, especially the maturing of the proximal juncture and the biologic softening of connective tissues. In the event of a proximal juncture failure, if there is full passive gliding on radiographic reexamination, stage II surgery can be delayed, providing no signs of synovitis are noted. Patients who have returned to work and a normal life-style can benefit beyond 1 year before stage II tendon grafting.

At operation, the limits of extension and flexion of the finger are measured and recorded. A short Bruner zigzag incision is made to locate the distal end of the device where it is attached to the phalanx. This attachment is left intact and a second ulnarly curved incision is made through the previous stage I incision in the distal volar forearm to expose the proximal end of the device.

Either the palmaris longus, plantaris, or long toe extensor tendon is obtained for use as the graft. The palmaris longus tendon or segments of a superficialis tendon will suffice for short tendon grafts; for example, thumb, fifth finger, and superficialis finger reconstruction. The proximal end of the device is extricated from the motor tendon by cutting the Dacron and silicone loop. (If the proximal weave technique has been used, the Dacron cord is cut through at the sheath juncture.) When the device and tendon have been sufficiently separated, the proximal end of the device is trimmed to a straight edge. One end of the tendon graft is sutured to the proximal end of the implant with a suture. Leaving the distal end of the device attached to the distal phalanx, the rest of the device with the attached tendon graft is pulled distally. The distal end is now removed and the graft is freed for distal juncture to bone. The Stage II procedure is completed by following established techniques for tendon grafting with one important exception—the connective tissue around the proximal juncture should be carefully preserved and closed around the new tendon graft juncture with fine sutures. When the biologic proximal end of the sheath is undisturbed, the formation of regional adhesions is minimized.

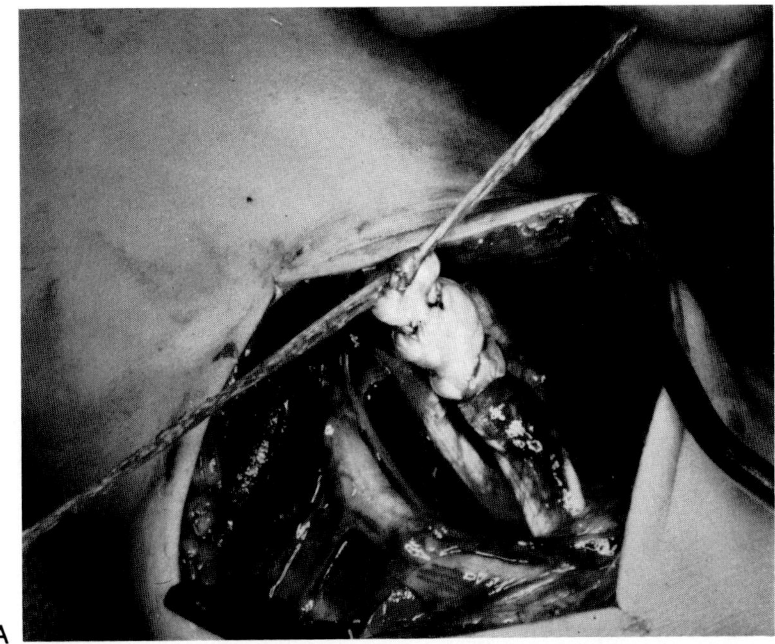

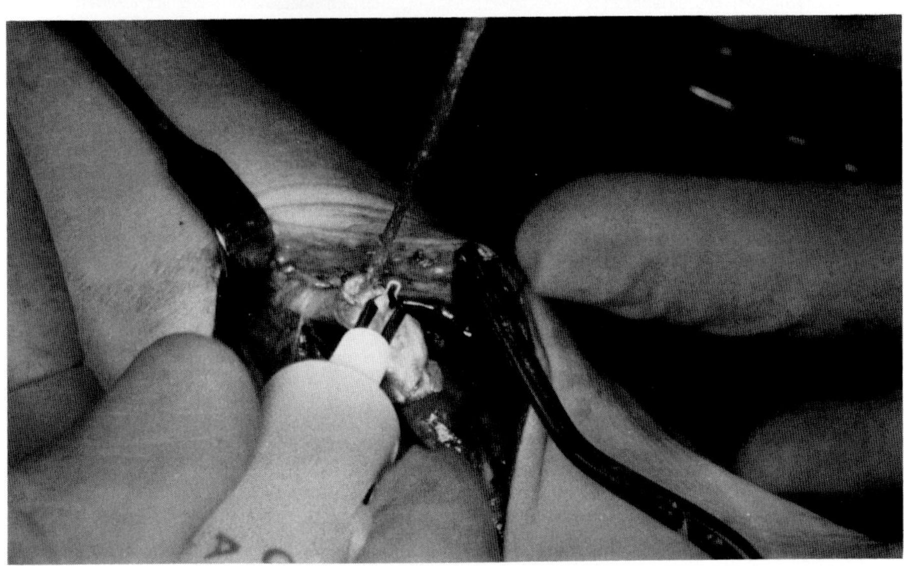

Fig. 51-43. Proximal juncture with the Dacron cord method. **(A)** The Dacron is tied securely with a square knot, and **(B)** the ends are cut with an electric cautery.

Postoperative Management*

Rehabilitation Following Stage I

Stage I reconstruction requires careful, structured postoperative care to facilitate orderly pseudosheath development around the tendon implant and to prepare the patient's hand for a return to work. Therapy begins the first postoperative day and is the same as for a tendon graft; that is, Stage II without rubber band, although slightly more rigorous. It begins with the passive hold exercise described earlier. Hand dressings must permit full passive flexion of the digits into the palm. At 2 weeks, when the patient demonstrates good tendon gliding, elastic band traction is added. The passive hold exercise is continued, however; the elastic band adds protection.

Pulley reconstruction at Stage I surgery using a passive tendon implant attached only distally does not require protection, since the patient will be performing passive motion. Reconstructed pulleys in the presence of an active tendon implant must be protected from rupture. Protection during the early postoperative days may be with a Velcro-and-felt pulley ring

* Consultant: Evelyn Mackin, R.P.T., Hand Rehabilitation Foundation, Philadelphia, Pennsylvania.

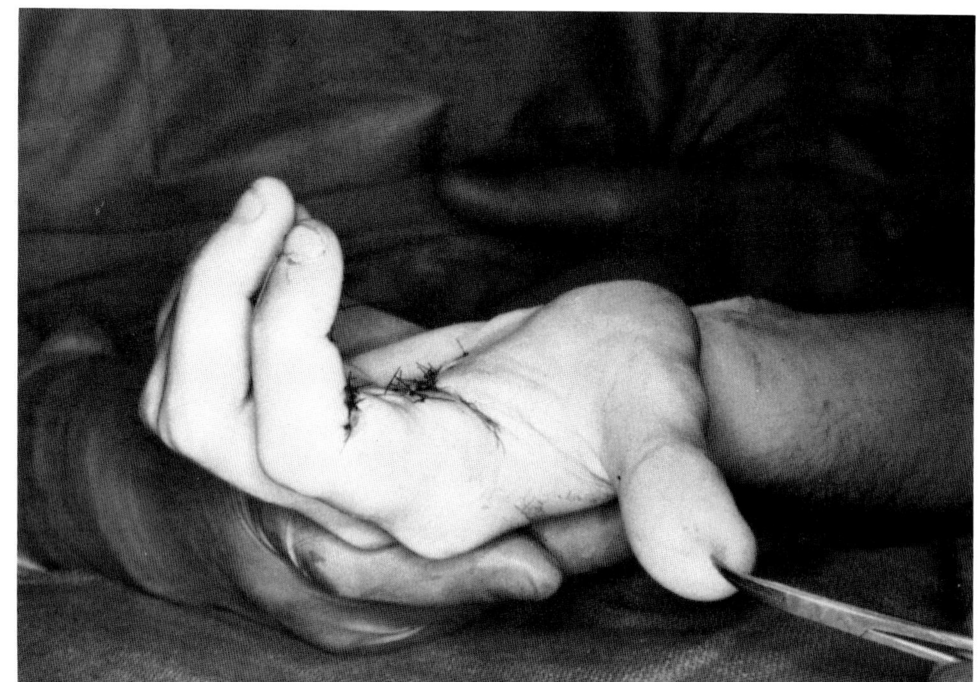

A

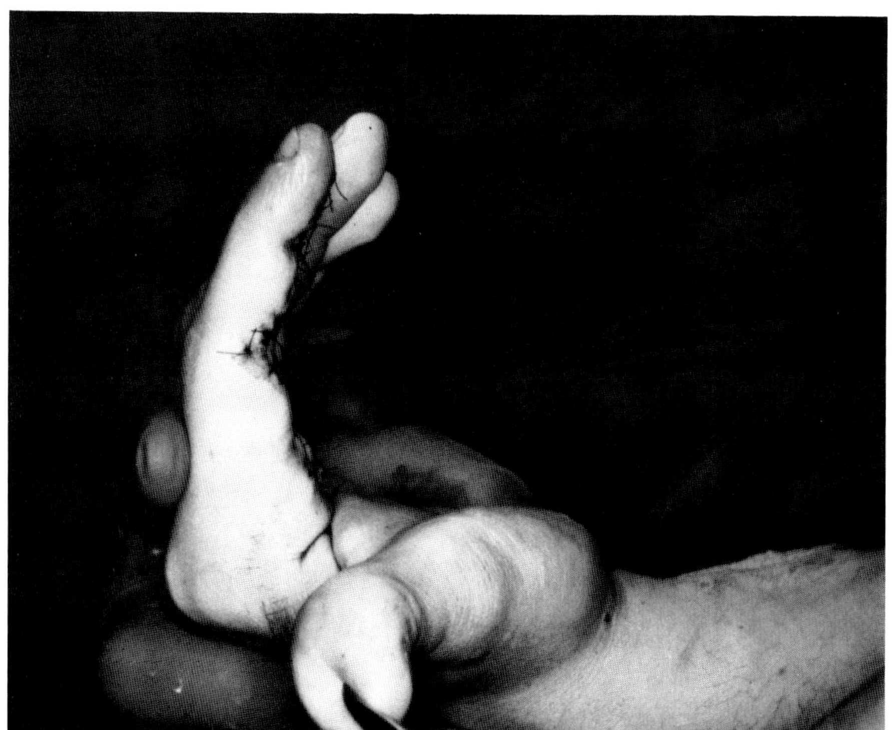

B

Fig. 51-44. **(A&B)** Setting the balance of an active tendon in the superficialis finger.

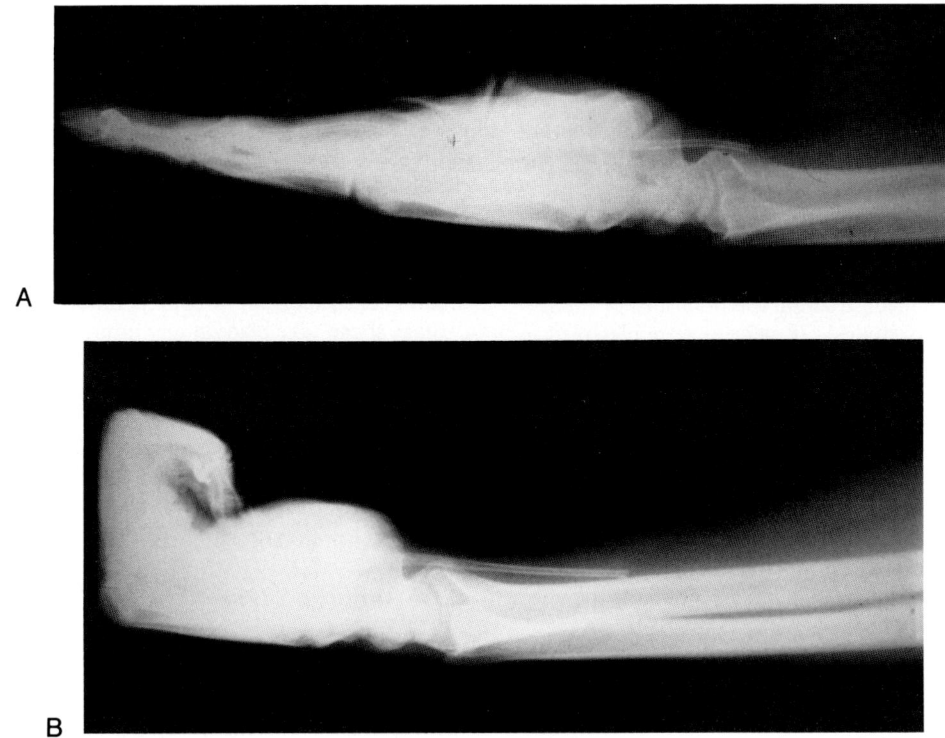

Fig. 51-45. Lateral x-rays in extension **(A)** and flexion **(B)** show full excursion of the implant with no buckling.

and/or support with pressure from a finger on the opposite hand. When postoperative edema decreases, the soft pulley ring can be replaced with a thermoplastic pulley ring, and eventually a metal ring in some cases. Pulley reconstruction is as sensitive as tendon repair, and protection should be considered for up to 6 months.

If the patient does not have full active IP joint extension, a contracture control program as discussed earlier must be initiated during the first week. The IP joint passive extension splint is fitted within the dorsal splint. As the contracted joint is pulley gently into extension, a counterforce is applied over the reconstructed pulley to prevent attenuation of the pulley.

Squeezing a piece of foam is allowed after 3 weeks and light putty squeezing after 4 weeks, 10 repetitions a day. The passive hold exercise is continued. Overzealous use of the digit soon after surgery is to be avoided, as this may result in a synovitis that generally responds to rest and splinting.

At 6 weeks, the protective dorsal splint may be removed and a wristlet and elastic band traction applied permitting wrist extension to neutral and full extension of the MP and IP joints. An active implant patient may necessitate the use of the dorsal splint for more than 6 weeks, with freedom from the splint for exercising under supervision.

Usually by 8 weeks patients are permitted full activities, with restrictions on full power grip until 12 weeks after surgery.

The immature mesothelial sheath is formed around the tendon implant by 72 hours postoperative, becoming a functioning organ by 4 weeks. Sheath maturity is stabilized by 4 months. Four to 5 months between Stage I and Stage II are required to facilitate hand reconditioning. When tendon and joint function is satisfactory, and patient compliance and morale are good, Stage II is often delayed for up to 1 year or longer. In principle, as time passes with the tendon implant actively gliding in the digit, the motor unit becomes stronger, range of motion is maximized, and soft tissue becomes more pliable. The digit is better prepared for Stage II.

Rehabilitation Following Stage II

Stage II surgery consists of removal of the active tendon implant and insertion of a tendon graft through the new pseudosheath, followed by postoperative therapy to facilitate gliding of the tendon graft and achieve maximum digital motion.

Postoperatively the patient's hand is kept in a protective dorsal splint; the wrist in 30 degrees flexion, the MP joints at 70 degrees and the IP joints in full extension. Early mobilization with elastic band traction begins the first postoperative day. The patient actively extends the finger, then reciprocally releases, permitting the elastic band to flex the finger. This is repeated with 10 repetitions several times a day, with care being given to extensor tendon attenuation and attention to contracture control. Postoperative therapy is similar to the Stage I period. However, because very early pain-free gliding generally occurs, protective splinting may be extended beyond the usual 6-week period if necessary to protect against excessive force on the tendon junctures. Initiation of the wristlet at 6 weeks may be extended to 8 weeks and active exercise at 8 to 10 weeks. Timetables should always be adjusted to the patient's progress.

Results

A group of patients with 73 active tendon, two-stage procedures, done over the past decade, were compared with a larger number of passive two-stage procedures. These were complicated cases to assess, but a pattern of improvement with the active tendon over the average passive two-stage tendon grafting was observed, and recent results suggest even further improvements since the 1988 report.[168]

A 5-year study of the results of the active tendon implants used in flexor tendon reconstruction was published in 1988.[143] Of 45 active implants studied, 78 percent were classified as Boyes grade 5. The improvement in total active motion (TAM) averaged 72 degrees *during* Stage I implant function.

Twenty-seven digits evaluated after implant replacement by tendon autograft (Stage II) showed average improvement of 62 degrees for active implants and 74 degrees for the passive implant in a comparative study from our Hand Center.[153] These results, however, are skewed in favor of passive tendon implants because active tendon implants included 70 percent salvage digits, whereas the passive tendon implants included only 45 percent salvage digits.

In studying the results, it becomes clear that the increase in TAM is directly dependent on the preoperative condition of the digit.[160,168] The authors concluded that the results are comparable between active and passive tendon implants. Active tendon implant surgery, however, is more demanding than passive implant surgery: "It is our impression that gliding after Stage II is far easier to obtain and occurs earlier when the active tendon implant is used."[153] The following case studies illustrate this concept.

Illustrative Cases

Case Report #1 (Fig. 51-46)

A 22-year-old male college student and bartender sustained a glass laceration of the flexor tendons of the left index finger. Immediate tendon repair at a University Center resulted in tendon rupture at 6 weeks. There was no infection. The patient was seen 1 month after failed repair. At Stage I, 3 months after injury, the flexor tendons were removed, along with portions of the new scarred tendon bed (Boyes Grade II). A 16-cm long single unit implant, 4 mm wide, was introduced. The distal metal end was secured to the distal phalanx with a 2-mm Woodruff bone screw after the four points were impacted into bone cortex.

The flexor tendons were divided distal to the lumbricals in the palm. The four main pulleys were preserved, and the superficialis bed proximal to and at the PIP joint was left intact. The flexor profundus tendon in the forearm was passed through the loop of the implant and interwoven three times, Pulvertaft-style. Tension was adjusted to a one-tendon, three-joint balance.

This patient had 80 percent TAM by 3 weeks and returned to work at 8 weeks post-operative. Stage II autografting was carried out 4 months after Stage I.

Active tendon Stage I has the advantage of permitting the surgeon to judge the adequacy of the reconstructed pulleys before Stage II. Thus, the surgeon has *a second chance* to reconstruct a failed flexor pulley system around the new sheath and tendon graft.

Certain situations that had been considered failures in the past are now considered acceptable occurrences in Grade V and VI salvage. One such problem is loosening or separation of the distal plate from bone. Appropriate management is earlier Stage II reconstruction.[156] If basic bone stock is good, the same distal plate of the active implant can be reset to bone with a new screw. If the technique recommended in this chapter for active tendon construct is followed, separation distally is unlikely.

Stage II can take place at any future date after Stage I, providing the surgeon and patient are in agreement. The longest functioning Stage I in this series of 73 patients was 8 years prior to completing the Stage II tendon grafting. (See case report #2).

Patients selected for the active tendon benefited by power induced gliding and early hand function. The patients that were able to return to work improved the results of the overall reconstructive program.

Case Report #2 (Fig. 51-47)

This 22-year-old college woman had an infection of the right middle finger at 3 years of age. Motion was lost, and the PIP joint had a 40-degree contracture at age 13. Other motion in the finger was good; the finger was considered to be a Boyes Grade V or VI.

At age 13, the scarred flexor tendons were removed, joint contractures released, and a power-driven active single unit (plate and loop) tendon implant was inserted. The A2 pulley was reconstructed, and the A4 pulley was salvaged and repaired.

Conclusions

The potential advantages of the active tendon implant in flexor tendon reconstruction are:

1. Reorganization of the proximal juncture adhesion problem by a "biologic tune up" of the motor tendon sheath unit
2. Physiologic maturity of the tendon sheath and retinaculum plus softening of the finger connective tissues and joints
3. Opportunity to critically assess the status of the A1 and A2 pulleys prior to Stage II
4. Improved patient morale and motivation with early observable functional programs
5. Opportunities to augment sound rehabilitation programming by returning to work before Stage II tendon implant surgery

The active tendon implant is now in its fourth decade of study and development. The dividends from early and continued muscle-powered implant gliding are substantial enough to recommend the active tendon over the passive tendon in many instances. In very complex or multiple reconstructions, however, and in children, the passive tendon implant two-stage program is usually preferred.

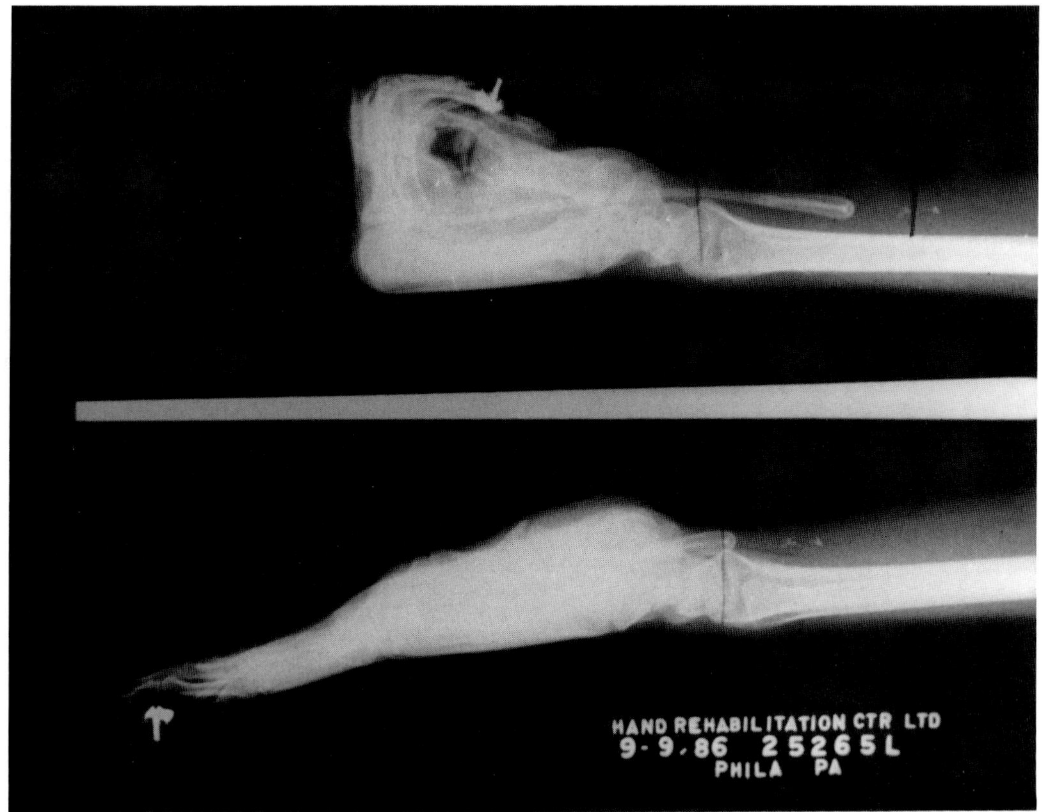

A

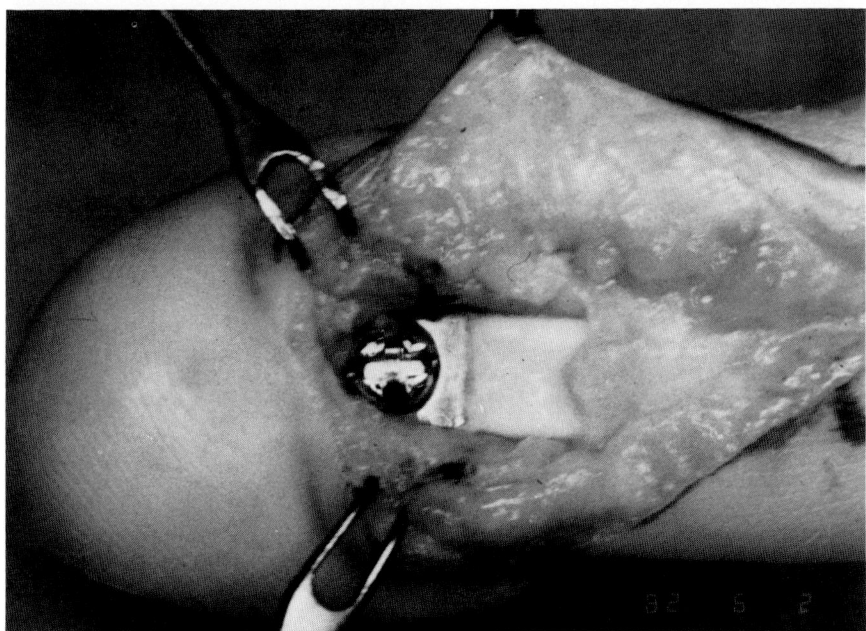

B

Fig. 51-46. Case #1. **(A)** Four months post-Stage I, showing active power-induced profundus motion. The upper view shows 80 percent flexion (5 cm proximal excursion is seen on 95 percent flexion). The lower view is extension of the hand; note the proximal edge of the implant at the wrist level. **(B)** Stage II. Four months following Stage I, the distal end screw is secure. (Metal stain is from Stage I screw driver technique.) *(Figure continues.)*

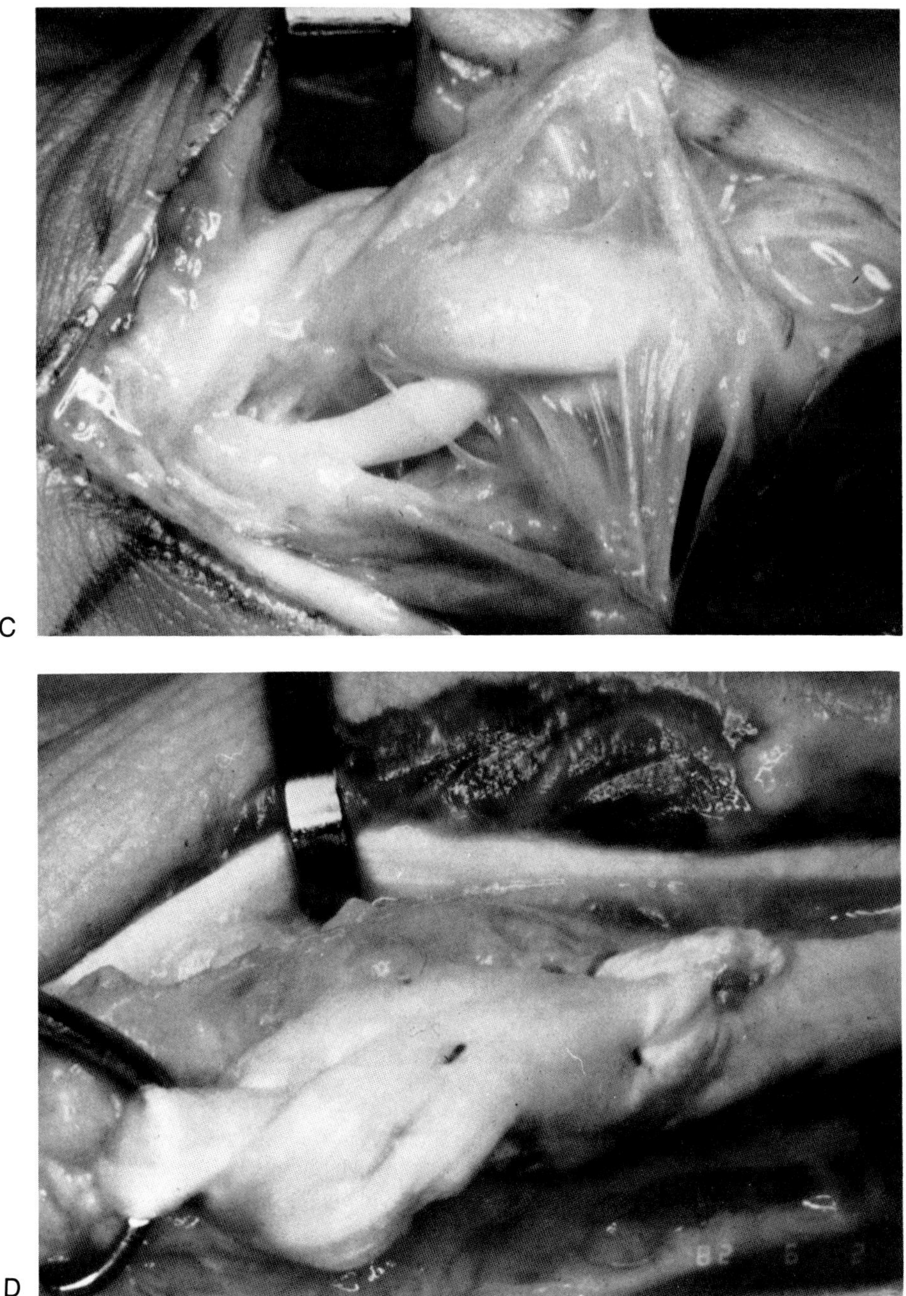

Fig. 51-46 *(Continued).* **(C)** Proximal tendon juncture at Stage II showing the sheath formed by profundus-powered excursion. The loop of the implant is on the left; the tendon loop is on the right. *The soft tissue around the connection must be preserved to protect the tendon graft juncture.* Excursion was 5 cm. **(D)** Stage II autograft showing preservation of the proximal sheath tendon juncture interface. A palmaris longus graft (left) has been woven into the tendon of the index flexor digitorum profundus. It is important to close the sheath around the tendon juncture with fine sutures. *(Figure continues.)*

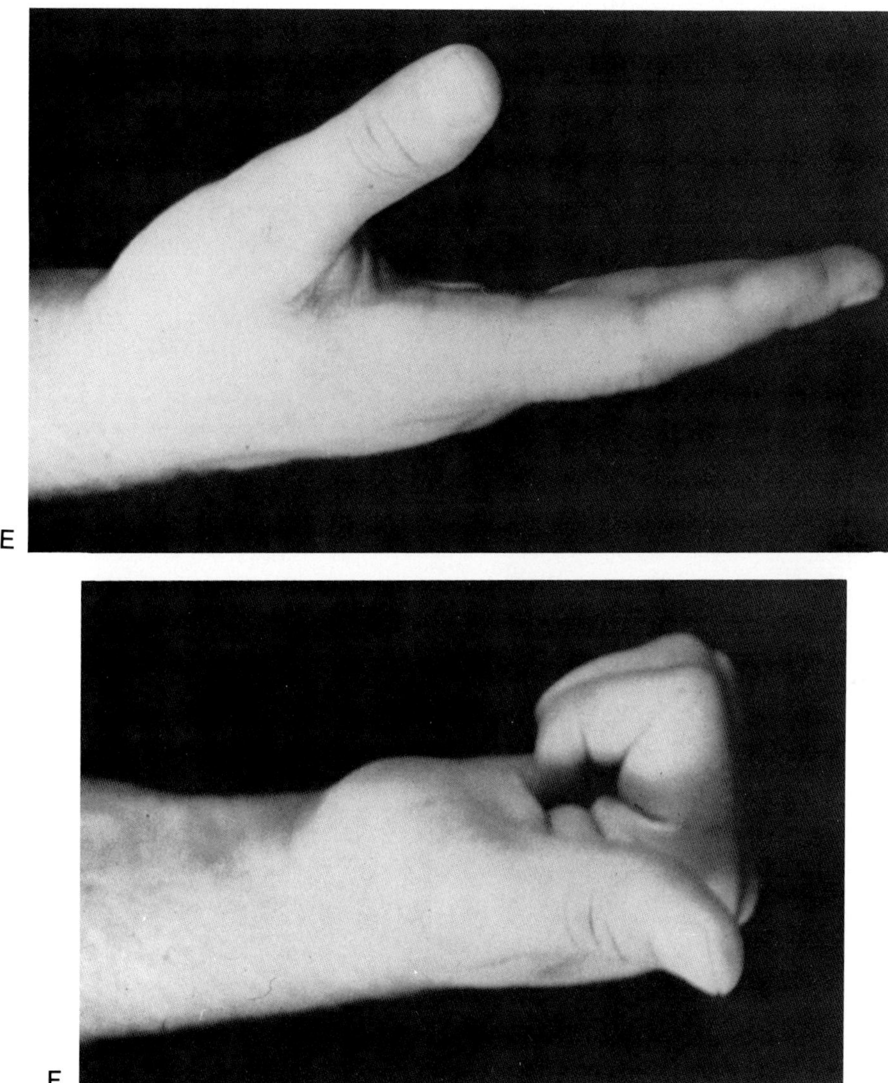

Fig. 51-46 *(Continued).* **(E&F)** Final function of the left index finger 9 months after Stage II autograft. This result was maintained at 5 years.

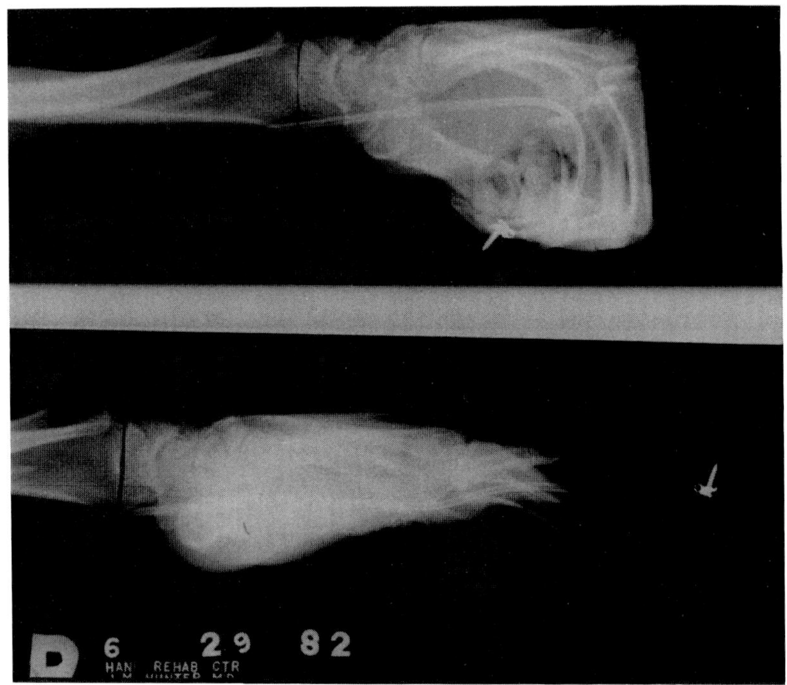

A

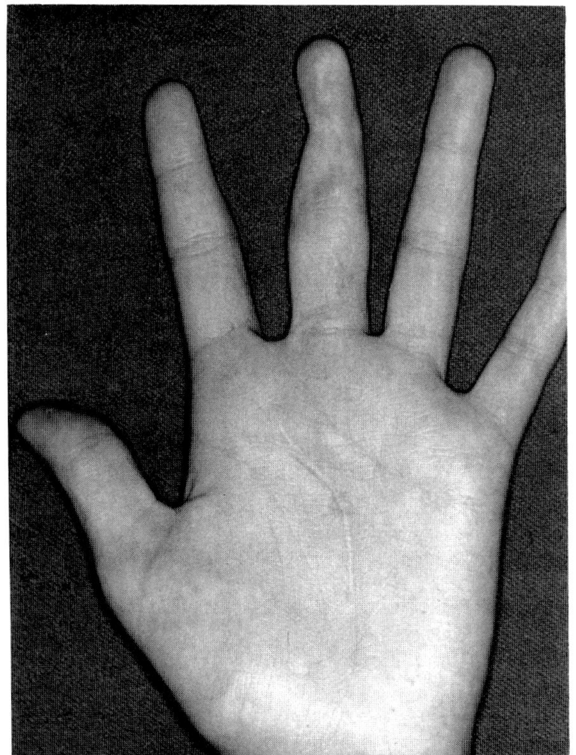

B

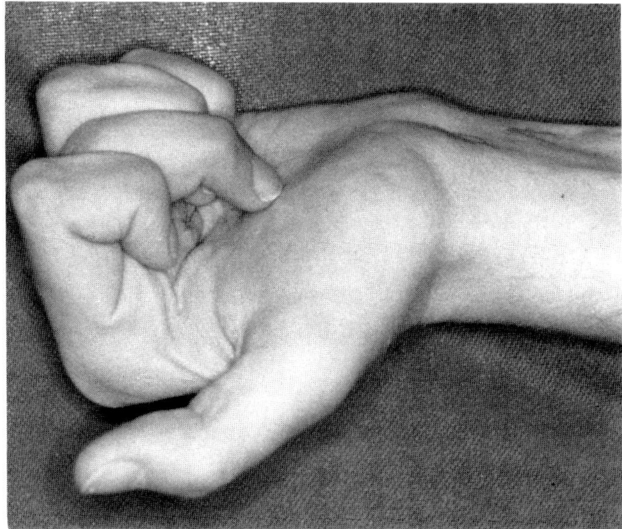

C

Fig. 51-47. Case #2. **(A)** X-ray of gliding after Stage I. Function was recovered early and the patient, through her teens, retained 90 percent of finger function, with implant excursion of 4 cm. Seven years following Stage I, the DIP joint was arthrodesed in 30 degrees leaving the screw plate and implant in place. The conversion to a superficialis finger followed an injury and gradual loss of DIP joint extension. The patient finally pulled the distal plate loose in a hockey game 8 years later. Stage II autografting was then done with no loss of pre-Stage II motion. **(B&C)** Active range of motion of the right index finger 7 years following Stage I. Stage I was converted to Stage II at 8 years with no loss of active MP or PIP joint function.

REFERENCES

1. Adamson JE, Wilson JN: The history of flexor tendon grafting. J Bone Joint Surg 43A:709–716, 1961
2. Allen HS: Flexor tendon grafting to the hand. Arch Surg 63:362, 1951
3. Allieu Y, Asencio G, Bahri H, Pascal M, Gomis R, Louchahi N: Two-step reconstruction of the flexor tendons (Hunter's technique) in the treatment of fingers "en crochet." Ann Chir Main 2:341–344, 1983
4. Alms A: Pedicle tendon graft for flexor tendon injuries of the fingers. J Bone Joint Surg 55B:881, 1973
5. Amadio PC, Hunter JM, Jaeger SH, Wehbe MA, Schneider LH: The effect of vincular injury on the results of flexor tendon surgery in zone 2. J Hand Surg 10A:626–632, 1985
6. Amadio PC, Wood MB, Cooney WP III, Bogard SD: Staged flexor tendon reconstruction in the fingers and hand. J Hand Surg 13A:559–562, 1988
7. Anzel SH, Lipscomb PR, Grindby JH: Construction of artificial tendon sheaths in dogs. Am J Surg 101:355–356, 1961
8. Apfelberg DB, Maser MR, Lash H, Keoshian L: "I-P flexor lag" after thumb flexor reconstruction—causes and solution. Hand 12:167–172, 1980
9. Arkin AM, Siffert RS: Use of wire in tenoplasty and tenorrhaphy. Am J Surg 85:795, 1953
10. Armenta E, Lehrman A: The vincula to the flexor tendons of the hand. J Hand Surg 5:127–133, 1980
11. Arons MS: Purposeful delay of the primary repair of cut tendons in "some man's land" in children. Plast Reconstr Surg 53:638–642, 1974
12. Arons MS: A new tendon pulley passer. J Hand Surg 10A:758–759, 1985
13. Ashley FL, McConnell DV, Polak T, Stone RS, Marmor L: An evaluation of the healing process in avian digital flexor tendons and grafts following the application of an artificial tendon sheath. Plast Reconstr Surg 33:411–421, 1964
14. Ashley FL, McConnell DV, Polak T, Stone RS, Marmor L: Further studies on the use of irradiated homografts and artificial sheaths in avian and mammalian tendon injuries. Plast Reconstr Surg 33:522–531, 1964
15. Ashley FL, Stone RS, Alonso Artieda M, Syverud JM, Edwards JW, Sloan RF, Mooney SA: Experimental and clinical studies on the application of monomolecular cellulose filter tubes to create artificial tendon sheaths in digits. Plast Reconstr Surg 23:526–534, 1959
16. Auchincloss H: Tendon transplantation. Ann Surg 89:145–148, 1929
17. Bader KF, Curtin JW: A successful silicone tendon prosthesis. Arch Surg 97:406–411, 1968
18. Bader KF, Sethi G, Curtin JW: Silicone pulleys and underlays in tendon surgery. Plast Reconstr Surg 41:157–164, 1968
19. Bakalim G: Primary mobilization after secondary flexor tendon surgery. Scand J Plast Reconstr Surg 9:240–244, 1975
20. Barton NJ: Experimental study of optimal location of flexor tendon pulleys. Plast Reconstr Surg 43:125–129, 1969
21. Bassett AL, Carroll RE: Formation of tendon sheaths by silicone rod implants. In proceedings of the American Society for Surgery of the Hand. J Bone Joint Surg 45A:884, 1963
22. Becker H: Primary repair of flexor tendons in the hand without immobilization. Preliminary report. Hand 10:37–47, 1978
23. Becker H, Orak F, Duponselle E: Early active motion following a beveled technique of flexor tendon repair: Report on fifty cases. J Hand Surg 4:454–460, 1979
24. Bell JL, Mason ML, Koch SL, Stromberg WB: Injuries to flexor tendons of the hand in children. J Bone Joint Surg 40A:1220–1230, 1958
25. Benjamin HB, Wagner U, Zeit W, Ausman RK: The use of endothelial cuff in tendon repair. Med Times 83:697–699, 1955
26. Bergljung L: Vascular reactions after the tendon suture and tendon transplantation. A stereo-micro-angiographic study on the calcaneal tendon of the rabbit. Scand J Plast Reconstr Surg suppl 4: 1968
27. Birch JR, Lindsay WK: Histochemical studies of the fate of autologous digital flexor tendon grafts in the chicken. Can J Surg 7:454–461, 1964
28. Birdsell DC, Tustanoff ER, Lindsay WK: Collagen production in regenerating tendon. Plast Reconstr Surg 37:504–511, 1966
29. Blackmore SM, Hunter JM, Kobus RJ: Superficialis finger reconstruction: A new look at a last-resort procedure. Hand Clin 7(3):461–469, 1991
30. Bora FW: Profundus tendon grafting with unimpaired sublimus function in children. Clin Orthop 71:118–123, 1970
31. Bora FW, Lane JM, Prockop DJ: Inhibitors of collagen biosynthesis as a means of controlling scar formation in tendon injury. J Bone Joint Surg 54A:1501–1508, 1972
32. Boyes JH: Immediate vs delayed repair of the digital flexor tendons. Ann West Med Surg 1:145, 1947
33. Boyes JH: Flexor tendon grafts in the fingers and thumb. An evaluation of end results. J Bone Joint Surg 32A:489–499, 1950
34. Boyes JH: Operative technique in surgery of the hand. p. 181. AAOS Instructional Course Lectures. Vol 9. JW Edwards, Ann Arbor, 1952
35. Boyes JH: Operative technique of digital flexor tendon grafts. AAOS Instructional Course Lectures. Vol 10. JW Edwards, Ann Arbor, 1953
36. Boyes JH: Evaluation of results of digital flexor tendon graft. Am J Surg 89:1116–1119, 1955
37. Boyes JH: Why tendon repair? J Bone Joint Surg 41A:577–579, 1959
38. Boyes JH: Bunnell's Surgery of the Hand. 4th Ed. JB Lippincott, Philadelphia, 1964
39. Boyes JH: The philosophy of tendon surgery. pp. 1–5 AAOS Symposium on Tendon Surgery in the Hand. CV Mosby, St. Louis, 1975
40. Boyes JH, Stark HH: Flexor tendon grafts in the fingers and thumb. A study of factors influencing results in 1000 cases. J Bone Joint Surg 53A:1332–1342, 1971
41. Boyes JH, Stark HH: Flexor tendon grafts in the fingers and thumb. p. 85. In Verdan C (ed): Tendon Surgery of the Hand, Churchill Livingstone, Edinburgh, 1979
42. Braithwaite F, Brockis JG: The vascularization of the tendon graft. Br J Plast Surg 4:130–138, 1951
43. Brand PW: Tendon grafting. J Bone Joint Surg 43B:444–453, 1961
44. Brand PW: Clinical Mechanics of the Hand. CV Mosby, St. Louis, 1985
45. Brand PW, Cranor KC, Ellis JC: Tendon and pulleys at the metacarpophalangeal joint of a finger. J Bone Joint Surg 57A:779–784, 1975
46. Brockis JG: The blood supply of the flexor and extensor tendons of the fingers in man. J Bone Joint Surg 35B:131–138, 1953
47. Brooks DM: Problems of restoration of tendon movements after repair and grafts. Proc R Soc Med 63:67, 1970
48. Brug E, Stedtfeld HW: Experience with a two stage pedicled flexor tendon graft. Hand 11:198–205, 1979
49. Bruner JM: The zig-zag volar-digital incision for flexor tendon surgery. Plast Reconstr Surg 40:571–574, 1967
50. Bruner JM: Surgical exposure of the flexor pollicis longus tendon. Hand 7:241–245, 1975

51. Bunnell S: Repair of tendons in the fingers and description of two new instruments. Surg Gynecol Obstet 26:103–110, 1918
52. Bunnell S: An essential in reconstructive surgery, "atraumatic technique". Calif State J Med 19:204, 1921
53. Bunnell S: Repair of tendons in the fingers. Surg Gynecol Obstet 35:88–97, 1922
54. Bunnell S: Surgery of the Hand. JB Lippincott, Philadelphia, 1944
55. Bunnell S: Surgery of the Hand. 3rd Ed. JB Lippincott, Philadelphia, 1956
56. Burge PD, Brown M: Elastic band mobilisation after flexor tendon repair; splint design and risk of flexion contracture. J Hand Surg 15B:443–448, 1990
57. Burman MS: The use of nylon sheaths in the secondary repair of torn finger tendons. Bull Hosp Joint Dis 3:122, 1944
58. Butler B, Burkhalter WE, Cranston JP: Flexor tendon grafts in the severely scarred digit. J Bone Joint Surg 50A:452–457, 1968
59. Cannon NM, Strickland JW: Therapy following flexor tendon surgery. Hand Clin 1:147–165, 1985
60. Caplan HS, Hunter JM, Merklin RJ: Intrinsic vascularization of flexor tendons, pp. 48–58. AAOS Symposium on Tendon Surgery in the Hand, CV Mosby, St. Louis, 1975
61. Carstram N: Prevention of experimental tendon adhesions by cortisone. Acta Orthop Scand 22:15–24, 1953
62. Carstam N: The efforts of cortisone on the formation of tendon adhesions and on tendon healing. Acta Chir Scand suppl 182: 1953
63. Carter SJ, Mersheimer WL: Deferred primary tendon repair. Ann Surg 164:913–916, 1966
64. Chacha P: Free autologous composite tendon grafts for division of both flexor tendons within the digital theca of the hand. J Bone Joint Surg 56A:960–978, 1974
65. Chamay A, Gabbiani G: Digital contracture deformity after implantation of a silicone prosthesis: Light and electron microscopic study. J Hand Surg 3:266–270, 1978
66. Chamay A, Verdan C, Simonetta C: The two-stage graft: A salvage operation for the flexor apparatus (A clinical study of 28 cases). pp. 109–112. In Verdan C (ed): Tendon Surgery of the Hand. Churchill Livingstone, Edinburgh, 1979
67. Chaplin DM: The vascular anatomy within normal tendons, divided tendons, free tendon grafts and pedicle tendon grafts in rabbits. A microangiographic study. J Bone Joint Surg 55B:369–389, 1973
68. Cheng JCY, Hsu SYC, Chong YW, Leung PC: Use of bioprosthetic tendon in digital pulley reconstruction—An experimental study. J Hand Surg 11B:225–230, 1986
69. Chong JK, Cramer LM, Culf NK: Combined two-stage tenoplasty with silicone rods for multiple flexor tendon injuries in "no-man's-land." J Trauma 12:104–121, 1972
70. Chow JA, Thomes LJ, Dovelle S, Monsivais J, Milnor WH, Jackson JP: Controlled motion rehabilitation after flexor tendon repair and grafting. A multi-centre study. J Bone Joint Surg 70B:591–595, 1988
71. Chuinard RG, Dabezies EJ, Mathews RE: Two stage superficialis reconstruction in severely damaged fingers. J Hand Surg 5:135–143, 1980
72. Cleveland M: Restoration of the digital portion of a flexor tendon and sheath in the hand. J Bone Joint Surg 15:762–765, 1933
73. Cohen J: Occupational therapy following hand tendon surgery. pp. 292–300. AAOS Symposium on Tendon Surgery in the Hand. CV Mosby, St. Louis, 1975
74. Cohen MJ, Kaplan L: Histology and ultrastructure of the human flexor tendon sheath. J Hand Surg 12A:25–29, 1987
75. Colville J: Tendon graft function. Hand 5:152–154, 1973
76. Colville J, Callison JR, White WL: Role of mesotenon in tendon blood supply. Plast Reconstr Surg 43:53–60, 1969
77. Colville J, Dickie WR: Tendon graft length. Br J Plast Surg 22:37–40, 1969
78. Conway H, Smith JW, Elliott MP: Studies on the revascularization of tendons grafted by the silicone rod technique. Plast Reconstr Surg 46:582–587, 1970
79. Cowan RJ, Courtemanche AD: An experimental study of tendon suturing techniques. Can J Surg 2:373–380, 1959
80. Crabbe WA: Some experiences with artificial tendons. pp. 247–248. In Stack HG, Bolton H (eds): The Proceedings of the Second Hand Club. The British Society for Surgery of the Hand, London, 1975
81. Cutright DE, Reid RL: A biodegradable tendon gliding device. Hand 7:228–237, 1975
82. Davis L, Aries LJ: An experimental study upon the prevention of adhesions about repaired nerves and tendons. Surgery 2:877–888, 1937
83. Daseler EH, Anson BJ: The plantaris muscle. An anatomical study of 750 specimens. J Bone Joint Surg 25:822–827, 1943
84. Defino HLA, Barbieri CH, Gonçalves RP, Paulin JBP: Studies on tendon healing. A comparison between suturing techniques. J Hand Surg 11B:444–450, 1986
85. Dodd RM, Sigel B, Dunn MR: Localization of new cell formation in tendon healing by tritiated thymidine autoradiography. Surg Gynecol Obstet 122:805–806, 1966
86. Doyle JR: Anatomy of the finger flexor tendon sheath and pulley system. J Hand Surg 13A:473–484, 1988
87. Doyle JR, Blythe W: The finger flexor tendon sheath and pulleys: anatomy and reconstruction. pp. 81–87. AAOS Symposium on Tendon Surgery in the Hand. CV Mosby, St. Louis, 1975
88. Doyle JR, Blythe WF: Anatomy of the flexor tendon sheath and pulleys of the tendon sheath and pulleys of the thumb. J Hand Surg 2:149–151, 1977
89. Dunlap J, McCarthy JA, Manske PR: Flexor tendon pulley reconstructions—A histological and ultrastructural study in nonhuman primates. J Hand Surg 14B:273–277, 1989
90. Duran RJ, Houser RG: Controlled passive motion following flexor tendon repair in Zones 2 and 3. pp. 105–114. AAOS Symposium on Tendon Surgery in the Hand. CV Mosby, St. Louis, 1975
91. Eaton RG: Hand problems in children. Pediatr Clin North Am 14:643–658, 1967
92. Edwards DAW: The blood supply and lymphatic supply of tendons. J Anat 80:147, 1946
93. Eiken O, Hagberg L, Rank F: The healing process of transplanted digital tendon sheath synovium. Scand J Plast Reconstr Surg 12:225–229, 1978
94. Eiken O, Holmberg J, Ekerot L, Salgeback S: Restoration of the digital tendon sheath. Scand J Plast Reconstr Surg 14:89–97, 1980
95. Eiken O, Lundborg G: Experimental tendon grafting within intact tendon sheath. Scand J Plast Reconstr Surg 17:127–131, 1983
96. Eiken O, Lundborg G, Rank F: The role of the digital synovial sheath in tendon grafting. Scand J Plast Reconstr Surg 9:182–189, 1975
97. Eiken O, Rank F: Experimental restoration of the digital synovial sheath. Scand J Plast Reconstr Surg 11:213–218, 1977
98. Enna CD, Dyer RE: Tendon plasticity: A property applicable to reconstructive surgery of the hand. Hand 8:118–124, 1976
99. Entin MA: Flexor tendon repair and grafting in children. Am J Surg 109:287–290, 1965
100. Entin MA: Flexor tendon surgery in children. pp. 132–144.

AAOS Symposium on Tendon Surgery in the Hand. CV Mosby, St. Louis, 1975
101. Erlacher P: The development of tendon surgery in Germany. AAOS Instruc Course Lec XIII:110-117, 1956
102. Eskeland G, Eskeland T, Hovig T, Teigland J: The ultrastructure of normal digital flexor tendon sheath and of the tissue formed around silicone and polyethylene implants in man. J Bone Joint Surg 59B:206-212, 1977
103. Fahrer M: The anatomy of the deep flexor and lumbrical muscles. pp. 16-24. In Verdan C (ed): Tendon Surgery of the Hand. Churchill Livingstone, Edinburgh, 1979
104. Farkas LG, Lindsay WK: Functional return of tendon graft protected entirely by pseudosheath—experimental study. Plast Reconstr Surg 65:188-193, 1980
105. Farkas LG, McCain WG, Sweeney P, Wilson W, Hurst LN, Lindsay WK: An experimental study of the changes following Silastic rod preparation of a new tendon sheath and subsequent tendon grafting. J Bone Joint Surg 55A:1149-1158, 1973
106. Farmer AW: Experiments in the use of cellophane as an aid in tendon surgery. Plast Reconstr Surg 2:207-213, 1947
107. Fetrow KO: Tenolysis in the hand and wrist. A clinical evaluation of two hundred and twenty flexor and extensor tenolyses. J Bone Joint Surg 49A:667-685, 1967
108. Flynn JE: Flexor tendon grafts in the hand. N Engl J Med 241:807-812, 1949
109. Foreward AD, Cowan RJ: Experimental suture of tendon to bone. Clinical Congress XI: Surg Forum:458-460, 1960
110. Forgon M, Biro V: Reconstruction of the digital sheath in "no man's land" with autologous transplanted vein graft. Hand 10:28-36, 1978
111. Frackelton WH: Salvaging the injured hand. Conn State Med J 19:554-557, 1955
112. Furlow LT: The role of tendon tissues in tendon healing. Plast Reconstr Surg 57:39-48, 1976
113. Gaisford JC, Hanna DC, Richardson GS: Tendon grafting. A suggested technique. Plast Reconstr Surg 38:302-308, 1966
114. Garlock JM: The repair process in wounds of tendon and in tendon grafts. Ann Surg 85:92, 1927
115. Gelberman RH, Manske PR: Factors influencing flexor tendon adhesions. Hand Clin 1:35-42, 1985
116. Gelberman RH, Woo SL-Y, Lothringer K, Akeson WH, Amiel D: Effects of early intermittent passive mobilization on healing canine flexor tendons. J Hand Surg 7:170-175, 1982
117. Goldner JL, Coonrad RW: Tendon grafting of the flexor profundus in the presence of a completely or partially intact flexor sublimis. J Bone Joint Surg 51A:527-532, 1969
118. Gonzalez RI: Experimental tendon repair within the flexor tunnels: Use of polyethylene tubes for improvement of functional results in the dog. Surgery 26:181-198, 1949
119. Gonzalez RI: Experimental tendon repair within the flexor tunnels. The use of hydrocortisone without improvement of function of the dog. J Bone Joint Surg 35A:991-993, 1953
120. Gonzalez RI: Experimental use of Teflon in tendon surgery. Plast Reconstr Surg 22:562, 1958
121. Graham WC: Flexor tendon grafts to the finger and thumb. J Bone Joint Surg 29:553-559, 1947
122. Graham WC: Delayed tendon repairs. Am J Surg 80:776-779, 1950
123. Grau HR: The artificial tendon. An experimental study. Plast Reconstr Surg 22:562-566, 1958
124. Gueukdjian SA: A new method of canalizing tendon sutures with vein grafts. Arch Surg 73:1018-1022, 1956
125. Hage J, Dupius CC: The intriguing fate of tendon grafts in small children's hands and their results. Br J Plast Surg 18:341-349, 1965
126. Hall RF Jr, Vliegenthart DH: A modified midlateral incision for volar approach to the digit. J Hand Surg 11B:195-197, 1986
127. Hanisch CM, Kleiger B: Experimental production of tendon sheaths. A preliminary report of a flexible plastic in the tissues of rabbits and guinea pigs. Bull Hosp Joint Dis 9:22, 1948
128. Hansson HA, Lundborg G, Rydevik B: Restoration of superficially damaged flexor tendons in synovial environment. Scand J Plast Reconstr Surg 14:109, 1980
129. Harrison SH: Repair of digital flexor tendon injuries in the hand. Br J Plast Surg 14:211, 1961
130. Harrison SH: Delayed primary flexor tendon grafts. Hand 1:106-107, 1969
131. Harvey JF, Chu G, Harvey PM: Surgical availability of the plantaris tendon. J Hand Surg 8:243-247, 1983
132. Helal B: The use of silicone rubber spacers in flexor tendon surgery. Hand 5:85-90, 1973
133. Henze CW, Mayer L: An experimental study of silk-tendon plastics with particular reference to the prevention of post operative adhesions. Surg Gynecol Obstet 19:10-24, 1914
134. Hernandez-Jauregui P, Esperanza GC, Gonzalez-Angulo A: Morphology of the connective tissue grown in response to implanted silicone rubber: A light and electron microscopic study. Surgery 75:631-637, 1974
135. Herndon JH: Treatment of tendon injuries in children. Orthop Clin North Am 7:717-731, 1976
136. Hochstrausser AE, Broadbent TR, Woolf R: Sheath replacement in tendon repair. Rocky Mt Med J 57:30-33, 1960
137. Hollinshead WH: Anatomy for Surgeons. Hoeber-Harper, New York, 1958
138. Holm C, Embick R: Anatomical considerations in the primary treatment of tendon injuries of the hand. J Bone Joint Surg 41A:599-608, 1959
139. Honnor R: The late management of the isolated lesion of the flexor digitorum profundus tendon. Hand 7:171-174, 1975
140. Honnor R, Meares A: A review of 100 flexor tendon reconstructions with prosthesis. Hand 9:226-231, 1977
141. Hoving EW, Hillen B: Functional anatomy of the vagina fibrosa of the flexors of the fingers. J Hand Surg 14B:99-101, 1989
142. Hueston JJ, Hubble B, Rigg BR: Homografts of the digital flexor tendon system. Aust NZ J Surg 36:269-274, 1967
143. Hunter JM: Artificial tendons. Early development and application. Am J Surg 109:325-338, 1965
144. Hunter JM: Two-stage tendon reconstruction using gliding tendon implants. p. 601. In Pulvertaft RG (ed): Operative Surgery. 3rd Ed. Butterworths, London, 1977
145. Hunter JM: Staged flexor tendon reconstruction. J Hand Surg 8:789-793, 1983
146. Hunter JM: Anatomy of flexor tendons-pulley, vincular, synovia, and vascular structures. pp. 65-92. In Spinner M (ed): Kaplan's Functional and Surgical Anatomy of the Hand. 3rd Ed. JB Lippincott, Philadelphia, 1984
147. Hunter JM: Staged flexor tendon reconstruction. pp. 288-313. In Hunter JM, Schneider LH, Mackin EJ, Callahan AD (eds): Rehabilitation of the Hand. 2nd Ed. CV Mosby, St. Louis, 1984
148. Hunter JM: Tendon salvage and the active tendon implant: A perspective. Hand Clin 1:181-186, 1985
149. Hunter JM: Active tendon prosthesis: Technique and clinical experience. pp. 282-292. In Hunter JM, Schneider LH, Mackin EJ: Tendon Surgery in the Hand. CV Mosby, St. Louis, 1987
150. Hunter JM, Aulicino PL: Salvage of the scarred tendon system using the Hunter tendon implant. In Flynn JE (ed): Hand Surgery. 3rd Ed. Williams & Wilkins, Baltimore, 1981
151. Hunter JM, Cook JF Jr: The pulley system: rationale for reconstruction. pp. 94-102. In Strickland JW, Steichen JB (eds): Difficult Problems in Hand Surgery. CV Mosby, St. Louis, 1982

152. Hunter JM, Cook JF, Ochiai N, Konikoff JJ, Merklin RJ, Mackin GA: The pulley system. Orthop Trans 4:4, 1980
153. Hunter JM, Jaeger SH: The active gliding tendon prosthesis: progress. pp. 275-282. AAOS Symposium on Tendon Surgery in the Hand. CV Mosby, St. Louis, 1975
154. Hunter JM, Jaeger SH: Tendon implants: Primary and secondary usage. Orthop Clin North Am 8:473-489, 1977
155. Hunter JM, Jaeger SH: Flexor tendon implants and prostheses. pp. 624-643. In Rubin LR (ed): Biomaterials in Reconstructive Surgery. CV Mosby, St. Louis, 1983
156. Hunter JM, Jaeger SH, Matsui T, Miyaji N: The pseudosynovial sheath—Its characteristics in a primate model. J Hand Surg 8:461-470, 1983
157. Hunter JM, Kobus RJ, Kirkpatrick WH: The superficialis finger: Results and indications in flexor tendon surgery. Presented at the ASSH 46th Annual Mtg., Orlando, October 1991
158. Hunter JM, Matsui T, Miyaji N, Jaeger SH: The characteristics and long term fate of the pseudosynovial sheath formed in response to gliding tendon implants in primates. Orthop Trans 1:9, 1977
159. Hunter JM, Salisbury RE: Use of gliding artificial implants to produce tendon sheaths. Techniques and results in children. Plast Reconstr Surg 45:564-572, 1970
160. Hunter JM, Salisbury RE: Flexor tendon reconstruction in severely damaged hands. A two stage procedure using a silicone Dacron reinforced gliding prosthesis prior to tendon grafting. J Bone Joint Surg 53A:829-858, 1971
161. Hunter JM, Schneider LH: Staged flexor tendon reconstruction: current status. pp. 271-274. AAOS Symposium on Tendon Surgery in the Hand. CV Mosby, St. Louis, 1975
162. Hunter JM, Schneider LH: Staged tendon reconstruction. p. 134. AAOS Instructional Course Lectures. Vol 26. CV Mosby, St. Louis, 1977
163. Hunter JM, Schneider LH, Dumont J, Erickson JC: A dynamic approach to problems of hand function using local anesthesia supplemented by intravenous fentanyl-droperidol. Clin Orthop 104:112-115, 1974
164. Hunter JM, Schneider L, Fietti VG: Reconstruction of the sublimis finger. Orthop Trans 3:321-322, 1979
165. Hunter JM, Seinsheimer F, Mackin EJ: Tenolysis: Pain control and rehabilitation. pp. 312-318. In Strickland JW, Steichen JB (eds): Difficult Problems in Hand Surgery. CV Mosby, St. Louis, 1982
166. Hunter JM, Singer DI, Jaeger SH, Mackin EJ: Active tendon implants in flexor tendon reconstruction. Presented at the American Society for Surgery of the Hand Annual Mtg., New Orleans, Feb 1986
167. Hunter JM, Singer DI, Jaeger SH, Mackin EJ: Active tendon implants in flexor tendon reconstruction. J Hand Surg 13A:849-859, 1988
168. Hunter JM, Singer DI, Mackin EJ: Staged flexor tendon reconstruction using passive and active tendon implants. pp. 427-457. In Hunter JM, Schneider LH, Mackin EJ, Callahan AD (eds): Rehabilitation of the Hand: Surgery and Therapy. 3rd Ed. CV Mosby, St. Louis, 1990
169. Hunter JM, Steindel C, Salisbury R, Hughes D: Study of early sheath development using static non-gliding implants. J Biomed Mater Res 5:155, 1974
170. Hunter JM, Subin D, Minkow F, Konikoff J: Sheath formation in response to limited active gliding implants (animals). J Biomed Mater Res 5:155, 1974
171. Hurst LN, McCain WG, Lindsay WK: Results of tenolysis. A controlled evaluation in chickens. Plast Reconstr Surg 52:171-173, 1973
172. Idler RS: Anatomy and biomechanics of the digital flexor tendons. Hand Clin 1:3-11, 1985
173. Ipsen T, Barfield T: Early mobilization after flexor tendon grafting for isolated profundus tendon lesions. Scand J Plast Reconstr Surg 22:163, 1988
174. Iselin F: Preliminary observations on the use of chemically stored tendinous allografts in hand surgery. pp. 66-69. AAOS Symposium on Tendon Surgery in the Hand. St. Louis, CV Mosby, 1975
175. Iselin F, Peze W: Use of chemically preserved tendon allografts in hand surgery. Hand 8:167-172, 1976
176. Iselin M: Delayed emergencies in fresh wounds of the hand. Proc R Soc Med 51:713-714, 1958
177. Jaffe S, Weckesser E: Profundus tendon grafting with the sublimis intact. The end result of thirty patients. J Bone Joint Surg 49A:1298-1308, 1967
178. Jaeger SH, Schneider PJ, Clemow AJT, Chen EH, Hunter JM: Development of a long-term flexor tendon prosthesis. pp. 491-500. In Hunter JM, Schneider LH, Mackin EJ (eds): Flexor Tendon Surgery in the Hand. CV Mosby, St. Louis, 1986
179. James JIP: The use of cortisone in tenolysis. J Bone Joint Surg 41B:209-210, 1959
180. James JIP: The value of tenolysis. Hand 1:118-119, 1969
181. James JIP: Suture or tendon graft? (editorial). J Bone Joint Surg 52B:203-204, 1970
182. Jones JR, Smibert JG, McCullough CJ, Price AB, Hutton WC: Tendon implantation into bone: An experimental study. J Hand Surg 12B:306-312, 1987
183. Kahn S: A dynamic tenodesis of the distal interphalangeal joint for use after severance of the profundus alone. Plast Reconstr Surg 51:536-540, 1973
184. Kain CC, Manske PR, Reinsel TE, Rouse A, Peterson WW: Reconstruction of the digital pulley in the monkey using biologic and nonbiologic materials. J Orthop Res 6:871-877, 1988
185. Kaplan EB: Device for measuring length of tendon graft in flexor tendon surgery of the hand. Bull Hosp Joint Dis 3:97, 1942
186. Kaplan EB: Functional and Surgical Anatomy of the Hand. JB Lippincott, Philadelphia, 1965
187. Karev A: The "belt loop" technique for the reconstruction of pulleys in the first stage of flexor tendon grafting. J Hand Surg 9A:923-924, 1984
188. Kerwein GA: A study of tendon implantations into bone. Surg Gynecol Obstet 75:794-796, 1942
189. Kessler FB: Use of a pedicled tendon transfer with a silicone rod in complicated secondary flexor tendon repairs. Plast Reconstr Surg 49:439-443, 1972
190. Kessler FB, Homsy CA, Prewitt JM III, Anderson MS: An active tendon prosthesis: Development and present status. Orthop Trans 1:8-9, 1977
191. Kessler I: The "grasping" technique for tendon repair. Hand 5:253-255, 1973
192. Kessler I, Nissim F: Primary repair without immobilization of flexor tendon division within the digital sheath. Acta Orthop Scand 40:587-601, 1969
193. Ketchum LD: Effects of triamcinolone on tendon healing and function. A laboratory study. Plast Reconstr Surg 47:471-484, 1971
194. Ketchum LD: Primary tendon healing: A review. J Hand Surg 2:428-435, 1977
195. Ketchum LD: Suture materials and suture techniques used in tendon repair. Hand Clin 1:43-53, 1985
196. Ketchum LD, Hubbard A, Hassanein K: Follow-up report on the electrically driven hand splint. J Hand Surg 4:474-481, 1979
197. Ketchum LD, Martin NL, Kappel DA: Experimental evaluation of factors affecting the strength of tendon repairs. Plast Reconstr Surg 59:708-719, 1977
198. Kilgore ES, Newmeyer WL, Graham WP, Brown G: The

dubiousness of grafting the dispensable flexor pollicis longus. Am J Surg 132:292–296, 1976

199. Kinmonth JB: The cut flexor tendon. Experiences with free grafts and steel wire fixation. Br J Surg 35:29–36, 1947
200. Kleinert HE, Bennett JB: Digital pulley reconstruction employing the always present rim of the previous pulley. J Hand Surg 3:297–298, 1978
201. Kleinert HE, Kutz JE, Ashbell T, Martinez E: Primary repair of flexor tendons in no man's land. J Bone Joint Surg 49A:577, 1967
202. Kleinert HE, Kutz JE, Cohen MJ: Primary repair of zone 2 flexor tendon lacerations. p. 91. AAOS Symposium on Tendon Surgery in the Hand. CV Mosby, St. Louis, 1975
203. Kleinert H, Schepel S, Gill T: Flexor tendon injuries. Surg Clin North Am 61:267–286, 1981
204. Koch SL: Complicated contractures of the hand; their treatment by freeing fibrosed tendons and replacing destroyed tendons with grafts. Ann Surg 98:546–580, 1933
205. Koch SL: Division of the flexor tendons within the digital sheath. Surg Gynecol Obstet 78:9–22, 1944
206. Koch SL: The use of tendon grafts in injuries of the flexor tendons of the hand. South Surg 13:449, 1947
207. Koth DR, Sewell WH: Freeze-dried arteries used as tendon sheaths. Surg Gynecol Obstet 101:615–620, 1955
208. Kyle JB, Eyre-Brook AL: The surgical treatment of flexor tendon injuries in the hand. Br J Surg 41:502–511, 1954
209. Landsmeer JMF: Atlas of Anatomy of the Hand. Churchill Livingstone, Edinburgh, 1976
210. Landsmeer JMF: An introduction to the functional analysis of the fingers of the hand. p. 25. In Verdan C (ed): Tendon Surgery of the Hand. Churchill Livingstone, Edinburgh, 1979
211. Lange F: Ueber periostale Sehnenver-Pflanzungen bei Lahmungen. Munchener Med Wochenschr 47:486, 1900
212. LaSalle WB, Strickland JW: An evaluation of the two-stage flexor tendon reconstruction technique. J Hand Surg 8:263–267, 1983
213. Leddy JP: Flexor tendons-Acute injuries. pp. 1347–1373. In Green DP: Operative Hand Surgery. Churchill Livingstone, New York, 1982
214. Leffert RD, Weiss C, Athanasoulis CA: The vincula with reference to their vessels and nerves. J Bone Joint Surg 56A:1191–1198, 1974
215. Leonard AG, Dickie WR: Observations on the use of silicone rubber spacers in tendon graft surgery. Hand 8:66–68, 1976
216. Lexer E: Die Verwehtung der freien Schnens-transplantation. Arch Klin Chir 98:918, 1912
217. Lin G-T, Amadio PC, An K-N, Cooney WP, Chao EYS: Biomechanical analysis of finger flexor pulley reconstruction. J Hand Surg 14B:278–282, 1989
218. Lin G-T, An K-N, Amadio PC, Cooney WP III: Biomechanical studies of running suture for flexor tendon repair in dogs. J Hand Surg 13A:553–558, 1988
219. Lin G-T, Cooney WP, Amadio PC, An K-N: Mechanical properties of human pulleys. J Hand Surg 15B:429–434, 1990
220. Lindsay WK: Tendon healing: A continuing experimental approach. p 35. In Verdan C (ed): Tendon Surgery of the Hand. Churchill Livingstone, Edinburgh, 1979
221. Lindsay WK, Birch JR: The fibroblast in flexor tendon healing. Plast Reconstr Surg 34:223–232, 1964
222. Lindsay WK, McDougall EP: Direct digital flexor repair. Plast Reconstr Surg 26:613–621, 1960
223. Lindsay WK, McDougall EP: Digital flexor tendons: An experimental study. Part III. The fate of autogenous digital flexor tendon grafts. Br J Plast Surg 13:293–304, 1961
224. Lindsay WK, Thomson HG: Digital flexor tendons: An experimental study. Part I. The significance of each component of the flexor mechanism in tendon healing. Br J Plast Surg 12:289–316, 1959
225. Lindsay WK, Thomson HG, Walker FG: Digital flexor tendons: An experimental study. Part II. The significance of a gap occurring at the line of suture. Br J Plast Surg 13:1–9, 1960
226. Lister GD: Reconstruction of pulleys employing extensor retinaculum. J Hand Surg 4:461–464, 1979
227. Lister G: Pitfalls and complications of flexor tendon surgery. Hand Clin 1:133–146, 1985
228. Lister G: Indications and techniques for repair of the flexor tendon sheath. Hand Clin 1:85–95, 1985
229. Lister GD, Kleinert HE, Kutz JE, Atasoy E: Primary flexor tendon repair followed by immediate controlled immobilization. J Hand Surg 2:441–451, 1977
230. Littler JW: Free tendon grafts in secondary flexor tendon repair. Am J Surg 74:315–321, 1947
231. Littler JW: The severed flexor tendon. Surg Clin North Am 39:435, 1959
232. Littler JW: The physiology and dynamic function of the hand. Surg Clin North Am 40:259, 1960
233. Littler JW: The digital flexor-extensor system. p. 366. In Converse JM (ed): Reconstructive Plastic Surgery. 2nd Ed. WB Saunders, Philadelphia, 1977
234. Liu TK: Transplantation of preserved composite tendon allografts. An experimental study in chickens. J Bone Joint Surg 57A:65–70, 1975
235. Liu TK: Clinical use of refrigerated flexor tendon allografts to replace a silicone rubber rod. J Hand Surg 8:881–887, 1983
236. Lundborg G: The microcirculation in rabbit tendon. In vivo studies after mobilization and transection. Hand 7:1–10, 1975
237. Lundborg G: Experimental flexor tendon healing without adhesion formation—a new concept of tendon nutrition and intrinsic healing mechanisms. A preliminary report. Hand 8:235–238, 1976
238. Lundborg G: The vascularization of the human flexor pollicis longus tendon. Hand 11:28–33, 1979
239. Lundborg G, Myrhage R, Rydevik B: The vascularization of human flexor tendons within the digital sheath region—structural and functional aspects. J Hand Surg 2:417–427, 1977
240. Lundborg G, Rank F: Experimental intrinsic healing of flexor tendons based upon synovial fluid nutrition. J Hand Surg 3:21–31, 1978
241. Lundborg G, Rank F: Experimental studies of cellular mechanisms involved in healing of animal and human flexor tendon in synovial environment. Hand 12:3–11, 1980
242. Mackin EJ: Physical therapy and the staged tendon graft: preoperative and postoperative management. pp. 283–291. AAOS Symposium on Tendon Surgery in the Hand. CV Mosby, St. Louis, 1975
243. Mackin EJ: Therapist's management of staged flexor tendon reconstruction. pp. 314–323. In Hunter JM, Schneider LH, Mackin EJ, Callahan A (eds): Rehabilitation of the Hand. 2nd Ed. CV Mosby, St. Louis, 1984
244. Mackin EJ, Maiorano L: Postoperative therapy following staged flexor tendon reconstruction. pp. 247–261. In Hunter JM, Schneider LH, Mackin EJ, Bell JA (eds): Rehabilitation of the Hand. CV Mosby, St. Louis, 1978
245. Madsen E: Delayed primary suture of flexor tendons cut in the digital sheath. J Bone Joint Surg 52B:264–267, 1970
246. Mahoney J, Farkas LG, Lindsay WK: Silastic rod pseudosheaths and tendon graft healing. Plast Reconstr Surg 66:746–750, 1980
247. Mangus DJ, Brown F, Byrnes W, Habal A: Tendon repairs with nylon and a modified pull-out technique. Plast Reconstr Surg 48:32–35, 1971
248. Manske PR, Lesker PA: Strength of human pulleys. Hand 9:147–152, 1977

249. Manske PR, Lesker PA: Avulsion of the ring finger flexor digitorum profundus tendon. An experimental study. Hand 10:52–55, 1978
250. Manske PR, Lesker PA: Palmar aponeurosis pulley. J Hand Surg 8:259–263, 1983
251. Manske PR, Lesker PA, Birdwell K: Experimental studies in chickens on the initial nutrition of tendon grafts. J Hand Surg 4:565–575, 1979
252. Manske PR, Whiteside LA, Lesker PA: Nutrient pathways to flexor tendons using hydrogen washout technique. J Hand Surg 3:32–36, 1978
253. Mason ML: Primary and secondary tendon suture. Surg Gynecol Obstet 70:392–402, 1940
254. Mason ML: Fifty years progress in surgery of the hand. Inter Abs Surg (In Surg Gynecol Obstet) 101:541, 1955
255. Mason ML: Primary tendon repair. J Bone Joint Surg 41A:575, 1959
256. Mason ML, Allen HS: The rate of healing of tendons. Ann Surg 113:424–459, 1941
257. Mason ML, Shearon CG: The process of tendon repair, and experimental study of tendon suture and tendon graft. Arch Surg 25:615–692, 1932
258. Matthews JP: Early mobilisation after flexor tendon repair. (editorial) J Hand Surg 14B:363–367, 1989
259. Matthews P: The fate of isolated segments of flexor tendons within the digital sheath—a study in synovial nutrition. Br J Plast Surg 29:216–224, 1976
260. Matthews P, Richards H: The repair potential of digital flexor tendons. J Bone Joint Surg 56B:618–625, 1974
261. Matthews P, Richards H: Factors in the adherence of flexor tendons after repair. J Bone Joint Surg 58B:230–236, 1976
262. May H: Tendon transplantation in the hand. Surg Gynecol Obstet 83:631–638, 1946
263. Mayer L: The physiologic method of tendon transplantation. Surg Gynecol Obstet 22:182–197, 1916
264. Mayer L: Free transplantation of tendons. Am J Surg 35:571, 1921
265. Mayer L: Physiologic method of tendon transplantation. Surg Gynecol Obstet 33:528–543, 1921
266. Mayer L: Repair of damaged finger tendons. Am J Surg 31:56, 1936
267. Mayer L: Repair of severed tendons. Am J Surg 42:714–722, 1938
268. Mayer L: Celloidin tube reconstruction of extensor communis sheath. Bull Hosp Joint Dis 1:39, 1940
269. Mayer L: The physiological method of tendon transplantation reviewed after forty years. p. 116. AAOS Instruc Course Lectures. Vol 12. JW Edwards, Ann Arbor, 1955
270. Mayer L, Ransohoff N: Reconstruction of the digital tendon sheath. A contribution to the physiological method of repair of damaged finger tendons. J Bone Joint Surg 18:607–616, 1936
271. Mayou BJ, Harrison SH: The length of flexor tendon grafts. Hand 10:48–51, 1978
272. McCarthy JA, Lesker PA, Peterson WW, Manske PR: Continuous passive motion as an adjunct therapy for tenolysis. J Hand Surg 11B:88–90, 1986
273. McClinton MA, Curtis RM, Wilgis EFS: 100 tendon grafts for isolated flexor digitorum profundus injuries. J Hand Surg 7:224–229, 1982
274. McCollough FH: Repair of the flexor pollicis longus tendon. US Armed Forces Med J 2:1579, 1951
275. McCormack RM, Demuth RJ, Kindling PH: Flexor tendon grafts in the less-than-optimal situation. J Bone Joint Surg 44A:1360–1364, 1962
276. McDowell CL, Snyder DM: Tendon healing: An experimental model in the dog. J Hand Surg 2:122–126, 1977
277. McFarlane RM, Lamon R, Jarvis G: Flexor tendon injuries within the finger. A study of the results of tendon suture and tendon graft. J Trauma 8:987–1003, 1968
278. McKee GK: Metal anastomosis tubes in tendon suture. Lancet 1:659–660, 1945
279. McKenzie AR: Function after reconstruction of severed long flexor tendons of the hand. A review of 297 tendons. J Bone Joint Surg 49B:424–439, 1967
280. Meals RA: Flexor tendon injuries—Current concepts review. J Bone Joint Surg 67A:817–821, 1985
281. Micks JE, Hager DL: The A-3 pulley—fact or fiction? Orthop Trans 7:44–45, 1983
282. Milgram JE: Transplantation of tendons through performed gliding channels. Bull Hosp Joint Dis 21:250–295, 1960
283. Millar R, Dickie WR, Colville J: The results of long delayed flexor tendon grafting. Hand 4:261–262, 1972
284. Minami A, Usui M, Ishii S, Kobayashi H: The in vivo effects of various immunoreactive treatments on allogeneic tendon grafts. J Hand Surg 8:888–893, 1983
285. Murphy FG: Repair of laceration of flexor pollicis longus tendon. J Bone Joint Surg 19:1121–1123, 1937
286. Nalebuff EA: The intact sublimis. p. 76. In Verdan C (ed): Tendon Surgery of the Hand. Churchill Livingstone, Edinburgh, 1979
287. Neuman Z, Ben-Hur N, Tritsch IE: Induction of tendon sheath formation by the implantation of silicone tubes in rabbits. Br J Plast Surg 19:313–316, 1966
288. Nichols HM: Discussion of tendon repair with clinical and experimental data on the use of gelatin sponge. Ann Surg 129:223–234, 1949
289. Nichols HM: The dilemma of the intact superficialis tendon. Hand 7:85–86, 1975
290. Nichols HM, Lehman WL, Meek EC: Alteration of the blood supply of flexor tendons following injury. Am J Surg 87:379–383, 1954
291. Nicolle FV: A silastic tendon prosthesis as an adjunct to flexor tendon grafting: An experimental and clinical evaluation. Br J Plast Surg 22:224–236, 1969
292. Nielsen AB, Jensen PØ: Methods of evaluation of the functional results of flexor tendon repair of the fingers. J Hand Surg 10B:60–61, 1985
293. North ER, Littler JW: Transferring the flexor superficialis tendon: technical considerations in the prevention of proximal interphalangeal joint disability. J Hand Surg 5:498–501, 1980
294. Ochiai N, Matsui T, Miyaji N, Merklin RJ, Hunter JM: Vascular anatomy of flexor tendons. I. Vincular system and blood supply of the profundus tendon in the digital sheath. J Hand Surg 4:321–330, 1979
295. Okutsu I, Ninomiya S, Hiraki S, Inanami H, Kuroshima N: Three-loop technique for A2 pulley reconstruction. J Hand Surg 12A:790–794, 1987
296. Omer GE, Vogel JA: Determination of physiological length of a reconstructed muscle-tendon unit through muscle stimulation. J Bone Joint Surg 47A:304–312, 1965
297. Osborne GV: The sublimis tendon replacement technique in tendon injuries. J Bone Joint Surg 42B:647, 1960
298. Osborne GV: Redemption operations for flexor tendon injuries. p. 248. In Stack HG, Bolton H (eds): Proceedings of the Second Hand Club. The British Society for Surgery of the Hand. London, 1975
299. O'Shea MC: The treatment and results of 870 severed tendons and 57 severed nerves of the hand. Am J Surg 43:346–366, 1939

300. Parkes A: "Lumbrical plus" finger. Hand 2:164-165, 1970
301. Parkes A: The "lumbrical plus" finger. J Bone Joint Surg 53B:236-239, 1971
302. Paneva-Holevich E: Two-stage tenoplasty in injury of the flexor tendons of the hand. J Bone Joint Surg 51A:21-32, 1969
303. Peacock EE: A study of the circulation in normal tendons and healing grafts. Ann Surg 149:415, 1959
304. Peacock EE: Homologous composite tissue grafts of the digital flexor mechanism in human beings. Plast Reconstr Surg 25:418-421, 1960
305. Peacock EE: Biological principles in the healing of long tendons. Surg Clin North Am 45:461-476, 1965
306. Peacock EE: Some technical aspects and results of flexor tendon repair. Surgery 58:330-342, 1965
307. Peacock EE, Hartrampf CR: The repair of flexor tendons in the hand. Int Abstr Surg (In Surg Gynecol Obstet) 113:411-424, 1961
308. Peacock EE, Madden JW: Some studies on the effects of B-aminopropriontrile in patients with injured flexor tendons. Surgery 66:215-223, 1969
309. Peterson WW, Manske PR, Bollinger BA, Lesker PA, McCarthy JA: Effect of pulley excision on flexor tendon biomechanics. J Orthop Res 4:96-101, 1986
310. Peterson WW, Manske PR, Lesker PA, Kain CC, Schaefer RK: Development of a synthetic replacement for the flexor tendon pulleys—An experimental study. J Hand Surg 11A:403-409, 1986
311. Pinkerton MC: Amnionplastin for adherent digital flexor tendons. Lancet 1:70-72, 1942
312. Posch JL: Primary tenorrhaphies and tendon grafting in hand injuries. Arch Surg 73:609-624, 1956
313. Posner MA: Flexor superficialis tendon transfers to the thumb—an alternative to the free tendon graft for treatment of chronic injuries within the digital sheath. J Hand Surg 8:876-881, 1983
314. Potenza AD: Tendon healing within the flexor digital sheath in the dog. J Bone Joint Surg 44A:49-64, 1962
315. Potenza AD: Critical evaluation of flexor tendon healing and adhesion formation within artificial digital sheaths. J Bone Joint Surg 45A:1217-1233, 1963
316. Potenza AD: Prevention of adhesions to healing digital flexor tendons. JAMA 187:187-191, 1964
317. Potenza AD: The healing of autogenous tendon grafts within the flexor digital sheaths in dogs. J Bone Joint Surg 46A:1462-1484, 1964
318. Potenza AD: Mechanisms of healing digital flexor tendons. Hand 1:40, 1969
319. Potenza AD: Flexor tendon injuries. Orthop Clin North Am 1:355-373, 1970
320. Potenza AD: The healing process in wounds of the digital flexor tendons and tendon grafts. p. 40. In Verdan C (ed): Tendon Surgery of the Hand. Churchill Livingstone, Edinburgh, 1979
321. Potenza AD, Melone CP: Functional evaluation of freeze-dried flexor tendon grafts in the dog. Orthop Trans 1:8, 1977
322. Pring DJ, Amis AA, Coombs RRH: The mechanical properties of human flexor tendons in relation to artificial tendons. J Hand Surg 10B:331-336, 1985
323. Pulvertaft RG: Repair of tendon injuries in the hand. Ann R Coll Surg Engl 3:3, 1948
324. Pulvertaft RG: Reparative surgery of flexor tendon injuries in the hand. J Bone Joint Surg 36B:689, 1954
325. Pulvertaft RG: Tendon grafts for flexor tendon injuries in the fingers and thumb. A study of technique and results. J Bone Joint Surg 38B:175-194, 1956
326. Pulvertaft RG: The treatment of profundus division by the free tendon graft. J Bone Joint Surg 42A:1363-1371, 1960
327. Pulvertaft RG: The results of tendon grafting for flexor injuries in fingers and thumb after long delay. Bull Hosp Joint Dis 21:317-321, 1960
328. Pulvertaft RG: Problems of flexor tendon surgery of the hand. J Bone Joint Surg 47A:123-132, 1965
329. Pulvertaft RG: Suture materials and tendon junctures. Am J Surg 109:346-352, 1965
330. Pulvertaft RG: Twenty-five years of hand surgery. Personal reflections. J Bone Joint Surg 55B:32-55, 1973
331. Pulvertaft RG: Indications for tendon grafting. p. 123. AAOS Symposium on Tendon Surgery in the Hand. CV Mosby, St. Louis, 1975
332. Pulvertaft RG: Indications for tendon grafting. pp. 277-279. In Hunter JM, Schneider LH, Mackin EJ, Callahan AD: Rehabilitation of the Hand. CV Mosby, St. Louis, 1984
333. Rank BK, Wakefield AR: The repair of flexor tendons in the hand. Br J Plast Surg 4:244-253, 1952
334. Rank BK, Wakefield AR: Surgery of Repair as Applied to Hand Injuries. 2nd Ed. E & S Livingstone, Edinburgh, 1960
335. Rank BK, Wakefield AR, Hueston JJ: Surgery of Repair as Applied to Hand Injuries. 4th Ed. Williams & Wilkins, Baltimore, 1973
336. Rayner CRW: The origin and nature of pseudosynovium appearing around implanted Silastic rods, an experimental study. Hand 8:101-109, 1976
337. Reid DAC: The isolated flexor digitorum profundus lesion. Hand 1:115-117, 1960
338. Reimann AF: The palmaris longus muscle. Anat Rec 89:495, 1944
339. Reis ND: Experimental tendon repair. Modification of natural healing by silicone rubber sheath. Br J Plast Surg 22:134-142, 1969
340. Rigg BM: A simple tendon transfer for the isolated division of the flexor digitorum profundus. Hand 7:246-249, 1975
341. Robertson DC: The place of flexor tendon grafts in the repair of flexor tendon injuries to the hand. Clin Orthop 15:16-21, 1959
342. Robson AWM: A case of tendon-grafting. Trans Clin Soc London 22:289, 1889
343. Rogers NB: A review of the use of prosthetic materials in tendon surgery. Med Ann DC 39:411, 1970
344. Rowland SA: Palmar fingertip use of silicone rubber followed by free tendon graft. p. 145. AAOS Symposium on Tendon Surgery in the Hand. CV Mosby, St. Louis, 1975
345. Sakellarides HT: Severe injuries of the flexor tendons in no man's land and with excess scarring and flexion contracture. Orthop Rev 6:51, 1977
346. Salisbury RE, Levine NS, McKeel DW, Pruitt BA, Wade CWR: Tendon sheath reconstruction with artificial implants: A study of ultrastructure. pp. 59-65. AAOS Symposium on Flexor Tendon Surgery in the Hand. CV Mosby, St. Louis, 1975
347. Salvi V: Delayed primary suture in flexor tendon division. Hand 3:181-183, 1971
348. Sarkin TL: The plastic replacement of severed flexor tendons of the fingers. Br J Surg 44:232, 1956
349. Savage R: In vitro studies of a new method of flexor tendon repair. J Hand Surg 10B:135-141, 1985
350. Savage R: The mechanical effect of partial resection of the digital fibrous flexor sheath. J Hand Surg 15B:435-442, 1990
351. Schatzker J, Branemark P: Intravital observations on the microvascular anatomy and microcirculation of the tendon. Acta Orthop Scand suppl. 126, 1969
352. Schlenker JD: Infection following pulp pull-through technique of flexor tendon grafting. J Hand Surg 6:550-552, 1981
353. Schmitz PW, Stromberg WB: Two-stage flexor tendon reconstruction in the hand. Clin Orthop 131:185-190, 1978

354. Schneewind J, Kline IK, Monsour CW: The role of paratenon in healing of experimental tendon transplants. J Occup Med 6:429-436, 1964
355. Schneider LH: Staged flexor tendon reconstruction using the method of Hunter. Orthop Trans 2:1, 1978
356. Schneider LH: Staged flexor tendon reconstruction using the method of Hunter. Clin Orthop 171:164-171, 1983
357. Schneider LH: Letter to the editor re: One hundred tendon grafts for isolated flexor digitorum profundus injuries. J Hand Surg 8:225, 1985
358. Schneider LH: Flexor Tendon Injuries. Boston, Little, Brown and Company, 1985
359. Schneider LH: Staged tendon reconstruction. Hand Clin 1:109-120, 1985
360. Schneider LH: Complications in tendon injury and surgery. Hand Clin 2:361-371, 1986
361. Schneider LH: Injuries to tendons in children. pp. 91-119. In Bora FW: The Pediatric Upper Extremity. WB Saunders, Philadelphia, 1986
362. Schneider LH: Treatment of isolated flexor digitorum profundus injuries by tendon grafting. pp. 518-525. In Hunter JM, Schneider LH, Mackin EJ: Flexor Tendon Surgery in the Hand. CV Mosby, St. Louis, 1986
363. Schneider LH: Evaluation in flexor tendon surgery. pp. 321-345. In Hunter JM, Schneider LH, Mackin EJ: Flexor Tendon Surgery in the Hand. CV Mosby, St. Louis, 1986
364. Schneider LH: Flexor tenolysis. pp. 348-361. In Hunter JM, Schneider LH, Mackin EJ: Flexor Tendon Surgery in the Hand. CV Mosby, St. Louis, 1986
365. Schneider LH, Hunter JM: Flexor tenolysis. pp. 157-162. AAOS Symposium on Tendon Surgery in the Hand. CV Mosby, St. Louis, 1975
366. Schneider LH, Hunter JM: Tendon injuries in the hand. p. 723. In Cotler J (ed): Cyclopedia of Medicine, Surgery and Specialties. FA Davis, Philadelphia, 1975
367. Schneider LH, Hunter JM: Flexor tendons—Late reconstruction. pp. 1375-1440. In Green DP (ed): Operative Hand Surgery. Churchill Livingstone, New York, 1982
368. Schneider LH, Hunter JM, Fietti VG: The flexor superficialis finger: A salvage procedure. pp. 528-532. In Hunter JM, Schneider LH, Mackin EJ: Flexor Tendon Surgery in the Hand. CV Mosby, St. Louis, 1986
369. Schneider LH, Hunter JM, Fietti VC: The flexor superficialis finger: A salvage procedure. pp. 312-316. In Hunter JM, Schneider LH, Mackin EJ (eds): Tendon Surgery in the Hand. CV Mosby, St. Louis, 1987
370. Schneider LH, Hunter JM, Norris TR, Nadeau PO: Delayed flexor tendon repair in no-man's land. J Hand Surg 2:452-455, 1977
371. Schneider LH, Mackin EJ: Tenolysis. pp. 229-234. In Hunter JM, Schneider LH, Mackin EJ, Bell JA (eds): Rehabilitation of the Hand. CV Mosby, St. Louis, 1978
372. Schneider LH, Mackin EJ: Tenolysis: dynamic approach to surgery and therapy. pp. 280-287. In Hunter JM, Schneider LH, Mackin EJ, Callahan AD (eds): Rehabilitation of the Hand, 2nd Ed. CV Mosby, St. Louis, 1984
373. Schneider LH, Mackin EJ: Tenolysis: dynamic approach to surgery and therapy. pp. 417-426. In Hunter JM, Schneider LH, Mackin EJ, Callahan AD (eds.): Rehabilitation of the Mackin EJ, Callahan AD (eds.): Rehabilitation of the Hand: Surgery and Therapy, 3rd Ed. CV Mosby, St. Louis, 1990
374. Schneider LH, Wehbe MA: Reconstruction of the flexor profundus tendon injury by superficialis transfer. Abstracts of the 2nd International Congress, International Federation of Societies for Surgery of the Hand, Boston, October 1983
375. Schneider LH, Wehbe MA: Delayed repair of flexor profundus tendon in the palm (zone 3) with superficialis transfer. J Hand Surg 13A:227-230, 1988
376. Schneider LH, Wiltshire D: Restoration of flexor pollicus longus function by flexor digitorum superficialis transfer. J Hand Surg 8:98-101, 1983
377. Schreiber DR: Arthroscopic blades in flexor tenolysis of the hand. J Hand Surg 11A:144-145, 1986
378. Seradge H, Homan ES, Spiegel PG: Tendon passer. Clin Orthop 155:307-308, 1981
379. Siler VE: Primary tenorrhaphy of the flexor tendons in the hand. J Bone Joint Surg 32A:218-225, 1950
380. Skoog T, Persson BH: An experimental study of the early healing of tendons. Plast Reconstr Surg 13:384-399, 1954
381. Smith DJ Jr, Jones CS, Hull M, Kleinert HE: Evaluation of glutaraldehyde-treated tendon xenograft. J Hand Surg 11A:97-106, 1986
382. Smith JW: Blood supply of tendons. Am J Surg 109:272, 1965
383. Smith RJ: Non-ischemic contracture of the intrinsic muscles of the hand. J Bone Joint Surg 53A:1313-1331, 1971
384. Smith RJ: Balance and kinetics of the fingers under normal and pathological conditions. Clin Orthop 104:92-111, 1974
385. Snow JW: Ulnar half of extensor digiti-quinti proprius tendon for flexor grafts. Plast Reconstr Surg 42:603-604, 1968
386. Snow JW, Littler JW: A non-suture distal fixation technique for tendon grafts. Plast Reconstr Surg 47:91-92, 1971
387. Solonen KA, Hoyer P: Positioning of the pulley mechanism when reconstructing deep flexor tendons of the fingers. Acta Orthop Scand 38:321-328, 1967
388. Sourmelis SG, McGrouther DA: Retrieval of the retracted flexor tendon. J Hand Surg 12B:109-111, 1987
389. Stanley BG: Flexor tendon injuries: Late solution. Therapist's management. Hand Clin 2:139-147, 1986
390. Stark HH, Anderson DR, Boyes JH, Zemel NP, Rickard TA, Ashworth CR: Bridge grafts of flexor tendons. Orthop Trans 7:44, 1983
391. Stark HH, Boyes JH, Johnson L, Ashworth CR: The use of paratenon, polyethylene film or Silastic sheeting to prevent restricting adhesions to tendons in the hand. J Bone Joint Surg 59A:908, 1977
392. Stark HH, Zemel NP, Boyes JH, Ashworth CR: Flexor tendon graft through intact superficialis tendon. J Hand Surg 2:456-461, 1977
393. Stenstrom S: A new method for distal anastomosis in flexor tendon grafting. Scand J Plast Reconstr Surg 1:64-67, 1967
394. Stenstrom SJ: Functional determination of the flexor tendon graft length. Plast Reconstr Surg 43:633-634, 1969
395. Stenstrom S, Bergman F: Homologous vessel graft as substitute for flexor tendon graft. Scand J Plast Reconstr Surg 9:177-181, 1975
396. Strandell G: Tendon grafts in injuries of the flexor tendons in the fingers and thumb. End results in a consecutive series of 74 cases. Acta Chir Scand 111:124-141, 1956
397. Strauch B, de Moura W: Digital flexor tendon sheath: an anatomic study. J Hand Surg 10A:785-789, 1985
398. Strauch B, de Moura W, Ferder M, Hall C, Sagi A, Greenstein B: The fate of tendon healing after restoration of the integrity of the tendon sheath with autogenous vein grafts. J Hand Surg 10A:790-795, 1985
399. Strickland JW: Flexor tenolysis. Hand Clin 1:121-132, 1985
400. Strickland JW: Flexor tenolysis: A personal experience. pp. 216-233. In Hunter JM, Schneider LH, Mackin EJ: Tendon Surgery in the Hand. CV Mosby, St. Louis, 1987
401. Strickland JW: Flexor tendon injuries—Part 3: Free tendon grafts. Orthop Rev 16(1):56-64, 1987

402. Strickland JW: Flexor tendon injuries—Part 4: Staged flexor tendon reconstruction and restoration of the flexor pulley. Orthop Rev 16(2):39–51, 1987
403. Strickland JW: Flexor tendon surgery. Part 2: Free tendon grafts and tenolysis. J Hand Surg 14B:368–382, 1989
404. Sullivan DJ: Disappointing outcomes in staged flexor tendon grafting for isolated profundus loss. J Hand Surg 11B:231–233, 1986
405. Suzuki K: Delayed flexor tendon repair in the digital sheath with end to end suture and fascial graft. Hand 8:141–144, 1976
406. Tajima T: History, current status, and aspects of hand surgery in Japan. Clin Orthop 184:41–49, 1984
407. Takasugi H, Akahori O, Nishihara K, Tada K: Three dimensional architecture of blood vessels of tendons demonstrated by corrosion casts. Hand 10:9–15, 1978
408. Takasugi H, Inoue H, Akahori O: Scanning electron microscopy of repaired tendon and pseudo-sheath. Hand 8:228–234, 1976
409. Thatcher HV: The use of stainless steel rods to canalize flexor tendon sheaths. South Med J 32:13–18, 1939
410. Thomas SC, Jones LC, Hungerford DS: Hyaluronic acid and its effect on postoperative adhesions in the rabbit flexor tendon. A preliminary look. Clin Orthop 206:281–289, 1986
411. Thompson RV: An evaluation of flexor tendon grafting. Br J Plast Surg 20:21–44, 1967
412. Tonkin M, Hagberg L, Lister G, Kutz J: Post-operative management of flexor tendon grafting. J Hand Surg 13B:277–281, 1988
413. Trail IA, Powell ES, Noble J: An evaluation of suture materials used in tendon surgery. J Hand Surg 14B:422–427, 1989
414. Tsuge K, Ikuta Y, Matsuishi Y: Intra-tendinous tendon suture in the hand. A new technique. Hand 7:250–255, 1975
415. Tsuge K, Ikuta Y, Matsuishi Y: Repair of flexor tendons by intratendinous tendon suture. J Hand Surg 2:436–440, 1977
416. Tubiana R: Incisions and techniques in tendon grafting. Am J Surg 109:339–345, 1965
417. Tubiana R: Technique of flexor tendon grafts. Hand 1:108–114, 1969
418. Tubiana R: Post-operative care following flexor tendon grafts. Hand 6:152–154, 1974
419. Urbaniak JR: Repair of the flexor pollicis longus. Hand Clin 1:69–76, 1985
420. Urbaniak JR, Bright DS, Gill LH, Goldner JL: Vascularization and the gliding mechanism of free flexor tendon grafts inserted by the silicone rod method. J Bone Joint Surg 56A:473–482, 1974
421. Urbaniak JR, Cahill JD, Mortenson RA: Tendon suturing methods: Analysis of muscle strengths. p. 70. AAOS Symposium on Tendon Surgery in the Hand. CV Mosby, St. Louis, 1975
422. Urbaniak JR, Goldner JL: Laceration of the flexor pollicis longus tendon: Delayed repair by advancement, free graft or direct suture. J Bone Joint Surg 55A:1123–1148, 1973
423. Van Demark RE: Tendon graft replacement of the finger flexors. J Lancet 68:259, 1948
424. Van Der Meulen JC: Healing and repair of tendons. Hand 1:79–82, 1969
425. Van Der Meulen JC: Silastic spacers in tendon grafting. Br J Plast Surg 24:166–173, 1971
426. Van't Hof A, Heiple KG: Flexor tendon injuries in the fingers and thumb, a comparative study. J Bone Joint Surg 40A:256–262, 1958
427. Vercimak MP, Hendel PM: A permanent tendon-to-bone suture technique in the distal phalanx. J Hand Surg 9A:146–147, 1984
428. Verdan CE: Primary repair of flexor tendons. J Bone Joint Surg 42A:647–657, 1960
429. Verdan C: Primary repair of flexor tendons—A summary. Surg Clin North Am 40:426, 1960
430. Verdan C: Practical considerations for primary and secondary repair in flexor tendon injuries. Surg Clin North Am 44:951, 1964
431. Verdan CE: Half a century of flexor tendon surgery: Current status and changing philosophies. J Bone Joint Surg 54A:472–491, 1972
432. Verdan C: The decades of tendon surgery. p. 6. AAOS Symposium on Tendon Surgery in the Hand. CV Mosby, St. Louis, 1975
433. Verdan C: Primary and secondary repair of flexor and extensor tendon injuries. p. 144. In Flynn JE (ed): Hand Surgery. 2nd Ed. Williams & Wilkins, Baltimore, 1975
434. Verdan C: Tenolysis. pp. 137–142. In Verdan C (ed): Tendon Surgery of the Hand. Churchill Livingstone, Edinburgh, 1979
435. Verdan C: An introduction to tendon surgery. pp. 1–3. In Verdan C (ed): Tendon Surgery of the Hand. Churchill Livingstone, Edinburgh, 1979
436. Verdan C: Repair of flexor tendon division outside the digital canal. pp. 113–115. In Verdan C (ed): Tendon Surgery of the Hand. Churchill Livingstone, Edinburgh, 1979
437. Verdan C, Crawford G, Martini-Ben Keddach Y: The valuable role of tenolysis in the digits. p. 192. In Cramer LM, Chase RA (eds): Symposium on the Hand. Vol 3. CV Mosby, St. Louis, 1971
438. Versaci AD: Secondary tendon grafting for isolated flexor digitorum profundus injury. Plast Reconstr Surg 46:57–60, 1970
439. Wade PJF, Muir IFK, Hutcheon LL: Primary flexor tendon repair: The mechanical limitations of the modified Kessler technique. J Hand Surg 11B:71–76, 1986
440. Wakefield AR: The management of flexor tendon injuries. Surg Clin North Am 40:267, 1960
441. Wakefield AR: Late flexor endongrafts. Surg Clin North Am 40:399, 1960
442. Wakefield AR: Hand injuries in children. J Bone Joint Surg 46A:1226–1234, 1964
443. Waterman, JH: Tendon transplantation: Its history, indications and techniques. Med News 81:54–61, 1902
444. Watson AB: Some remarks on the repair of flexor tendons in the hand, with particular reference to the technique of free grafting. Br J Surg 43:35–42, 1955
445. Watson M: The determinants of flexor tendon fibrosis following trauma: An experimental study in rabbits. Hand 10:150–153, 1978
446. Webster DA, Werner FW: Mechanical and functional properties of implanted freeze-dried flexor tendons. Clin Orthop 180:301–309, 1983
447. Weckesser EC: Technique of tendon repair. p. 116. In Flynn JE (ed): Hand Surgery. 2nd Ed. Williams & Wilkins, Baltimore, 1975
448. Weckesser EC, Shaw BW, Spears GN, Shea PC: A comparative study of various substances for the prevention of adhesions about tendons. Surgery 25:361–369, 1949
449. Weeks PM, Wray RC: Rate and extent of functional recovery after flexor tendon grafting with and without silicone rod preparation. J Hand Surg 1:174–180, 1976
450. Wehbe MA, Hunter JM: Flexor tendon gliding in the hand. Part I. In vivo excursions. J Hand Surg 10A:570–574, 1985
451. Wehbe MA, Hunter JM: Flexor tendon gliding in the hand. Part II. Differential gliding. J Hand Surg 10A:575–579, 1985
452. Wehbé MA, Hunter JM, Schneider LH, Goodwyn BL: Two-stage flexor-tendon reconstruction. Ten-year experience. J Bone Joint Surg 68A:752–763, 1986
453. Weiner DL, Hoffman S, Barsky AJ: Improved method for distal attachment of flexor tendon grafts. Modification of Stenstrom technique. Plast Reconstr Surg 41:71–74, 1968
454. Weiner LJ, Peacock EE: Biologic principles affecting repair of flexor tendons. Adv Surg 5:145–188, 1971

455. Weinstein SL, Sprague BL, Flatt AE: Evaluation of the two-staged flexor tendon reconstruction in severely damaged digits. J Bone Joint Surg 58A:786-791, 1976
456. Werntz JR, Chesher SP, Breidenbach WC, Kleinert HE, Bissonnette MA: A new dynamic splint for postoperative treatment of flexor tendon injury. J Hand Surg 14A:559-566, 1989
457. Wheeldon T: The use of cellophane as a permanent tendon sheath. J Bone Joint Surg 21:393-396, 1939
458. Whiston TB, Walmsley R: Some observations on the reaction of bone and tendon after tunnelling of bone and insertion of tendon. J Bone Joint Surg 42B:377-386, 1960
459. Whitaker JH, Strickland JW, Ellis KK: The role of flexor tenolysis in the palm and digits. J Hand Surg 2:462-470, 1977
460. White WL: Secondary restoration of finger flexion by digital tendon grafts. Am J Surg 91:662-668, 1956
461. White WL: The unique, accessible and useful plantaris tendon. Plast Reconstr Surg 25:133-144, 1960
462. White WL: Tendon grafts: A consideration of their source, procurement and suitability. Surg Clin North Am 40:402, 1960
463. White WL: Restoration of function and balance of the wrist and hand by tendon transfer. Surg Clin North Am 40:427, 1960
464. Williams CW, Dickie WR, Colville J: Silastic sheeting in hand surgery. Hand 4:273-276, 1972
465. Williams SB: New dynamic concepts in the grafting of flexor tendons. Plast Reconstr Surg 36:377-419, 1965
466. Wilmouth CL: Tendoplasty of flexor tendons of the hand: Use of tunica vaginalis in reconstructing tendon sheaths. J Bone Joint Surg 19:152-156, 1937
467. Wilson RL: Flexor tendon grafting. Hand Clin 1:97-107, 1985
468. Wilson RL, Carter MS, Holdeman VA, Lovett WL: Flexor profundus injuries treated with delayed two-staged tendon grafting. J Hand Surg 5:74-78, 1980
469. Wilson WF, Hueston JT: The intra-tendinous architecture of the tendons of the flexor digitorum profundus and flexor pollicis longus. Hand 5:33-38, 1973
470. Winckler G: Normal anatomy of the flexor and extensor tendons of the hand. p. 7. In Verdan C (ed): Tendon Surgery of the Hand. Churchill Livingstone, Edinburgh, 1979
471. Wray RC, Weeks PM: Reconstruction of digital pulley. Plast Reconstr Surg 53:534-536, 1974
472. Wray RC, Weeks PM: Experimental comparison of technics of tendon repair. J Hand Surg 5:144-148, 1980
473. Wrenn RN, Goldner JL, Markee JL: An experimental study of the effect of cortisone on the healing process and tensile strength of tendons. J Bone Joint Surg 36A:588-601, 1954
474. Young L, Weeks PM: Profundus tendon blood supply within the digital sheath. Surg Forum 21:504, 1970

52

Extensor Tendons—Acute Injuries

James R. Doyle

Surgeons who treat hand injuries have developed a great respect for injuries of the flexor tendons.[31] There is widespread knowledge about the pitfalls and complications encountered in the management of these injuries. Injuries of the extensor mechanism, by contrast, may seem relatively simple to treat, but this is not so.[40] Extensor injuries have not been given the same degree of attention, despite the advice of many authors.[31,36,40,61,74,134] Repair of the complex extensor mechanism is often performed by the youngest or least skilled surgeon, with anticipation of success by simple approximation of the tendon ends.[1,61] The management of injuries to the extensor mechanism demands the same amount of skill and knowledge required for the care of flexor tendon injuries. The extensor mechanism in the finger, in comparison to that of the flexors, is thinner, less substantial, and less likely to hold sutures well.[46,63] At the wrist and forearm, however, the extensors' substance and cross-sectional area are much more like the flexor tendons.[63] Injuries to the extensor tendons are common due to their relatively exposed and superficial location. The dorsal aspect of the hand and wrist is covered with a thin layer of supple skin with minimal subcutaneous tissue. In many areas, such as the distal finger joint, the tendon is very thin and subject to rupture with sufficient force. Injury may be secondary to laceration, deep abrasion, crush, or avulsion, and the majority of extensor tendon injuries are at joint levels. Penetrating wounds that disrupt the tendon are also prone to enter the joint; this is true not only at the interphalangeal joints but also at the MP joint.[40] The degree of joint contamination must be evaluated and considered in the treatment plan.

Simple loss of continuity due to laceration or avulsion of the extensor mechanism in the hand and fingers is usually not associated with immediate retraction of the tendon ends because of the multiple soft tissue attachments and interconnections at various levels.[59,85] Furthermore, the extensor mechanism in the hand is extrasynovial, except at the wrist where the tendons are covered with a synovial sheath.[59,60] Paratenon surrounds the extensor tendons over the dorsum of the hand, and tendons covered with paratenon do not separate widely when lacerated.[85] Therefore, divided extensor tendons are usually free to retract only on the dorsum of the wrist. Because of this, many tendon injuries, especially in the fingers, may be treated successfully by splinting alone. In the hand and fingers, any gap in the tendon following laceration or avulsion is usually due to unopposed flexion of the joints rather than to retraction of the tendon.[85]

Traditional wisdom had suggested that extensor tendon injuries seen and treated early and properly usually responded well to treatment.[61,89] However, a recent retrospective analysis by Newport, Blair, and Steyers[93] of long-term results of extensor tendon repair has suggested that this is not always true. Their study reported the results of extensor tendon repair in 62 patients with 101 digits and revealed that (1) 60 percent of all fingers sustained an associated injury such as fracture, dislocation, joint capsule, or flexor tendon damage, (2) patients with an associated injury achieved 45 percent good to excellent results with total active motion (TAM) of 212 degrees, (3) patients without associated injuries achieved 64 percent good to excellent results with total active motion of 230 degrees, (4) distal zone injuries (Zones I to IV) had a less favorable result than proximal injuries (Zones V to VIII), (5) the percentage of fingers that lost flexion was greater than the percentage that lost extension, and (6) the average degree of loss of flexion was greater than the average loss of extension. Ninety-five percent of patients were satisfied with their functional result. Total active motion for all patients was 83 percent of normal; for those without associated injuries, TAM was 89 percent of normal. For those fingers with associated injuries TAM was 82 percent of normal. Grip strength for all patients averaged 95 percent of the unaffected hand. The authors noted, however, that TAM and grip strength, although useful in evaluating results in flexor tendon injuries, may not adequately reflect the loss of function at the PIP joint or the ability to use tools effectively. These authors concluded that loss of flexion might be a more significant complication in extensor tendon injuries than previously thought.[93] Most patients in this study were treated by static splinting with the affected joints held in extension. The authors observed that splinting in extension may result in loss of flexion but noted that it was not clear to what degree splinting might be implicated in loss of flexion. Recent published reports on the concept of dynamic splinting for extensor tendon injuries was acknowledged by the authors.[9,21,38] Newport and colleagues[93] noted that Evans[38] reported TAM averaging 212 degrees for finger and wrist injuries with periosteal or soft-tissue injury. Browne and Ribik,[9] and Chow et al[21] were noted to have 98 and 100 percent good to excellent results, respectively, with dynamic splinting in patients without associated injuries. Newport and colleagues[93] suggested that a well-controlled prospective study comparing static versus dynamic splinting in patients with simple tendon lacerations as well as those with associated injuries would be the most valid confirmation of the apparent efficacy of dynamic splinting. Because of the complex and delicate balance of the extensor mechanism in the finger, delayed or late treatment of injuries does not carry the same prognosis since, it is often impossible to restore the delicate balance of the various components of the extensor mechanism.[49,59,85,134] This is especially true in injuries over the PIP joint.[42]

ANATOMY

Extension of the finger is a complex act and is considered to be more intricate than finger flexion. This mechanism is composed of two separate and neurologically independent systems —namely, the radial nerve-innervated extrinsic extensors and the intrinsic systems supplied by the ulnar and median nerves.[28] Considerable differences of opinion exist regarding the mechanics of finger extension.[49] There have been many contributions to the understanding of this complex mechanism, and the reader is referred to these reports for a detailed review of the subject.[28,36,49,59,60,69,70,74,86–88,122,135,136] However, a brief description of the anatomy of the extensor mechanism is important in understanding the proper treatment, and the following discussion is useful in this regard.

The extensor mechanism arises from multiple muscle bellies in the forearm. The extensor pollicis longus (EPL), extensor pollicis brevis (EPB), extensor indicis proprius (EIP), and extensor digiti quinti proprius (EDQP) have a comparatively independent origin and action.[59] The proprius tendons at the MP joint level are almost always to the ulnar side of the communis tendons. The little finger proprius tendon over the metacarpal and wrist level is usually represented by two distinct tendinous structures. Kaplan and others, however, noted that the variations in the disposition and the number of tendons are numerous.[23,59] Kaplan believed that the extensor digitorum communis (EDC) usually had four distinct tendons and was characterized by limited independent action in contrast to the proprius tendons.[59] My own operative experience parallels the cadaver observations of Schenck[113] and von Schroeder, Botte, and Gellman[139] that the EDC tendon to the little finger is present less than 50 percent of the time. When it is absent it is almost always replaced by juncturae tendinum from the ring finger to the extensor aponeurosis of the little finger.[139] Traditional knowledge has suggested that independent extension of the index and little fingers was due solely to the proprius tendons to these digits (Fig. 52-1). Loss of independent extension, especially of the index finger, was said to be highly probable if the index proprius was injured and not repaired, or was transferred. This concept as it applies to the index finger was not confirmed by Moore, Weiland, and Valdata,[91] who noted independent index extension in all of their of 27 patients after extensor indicis transfer. They suggested that the reasons for the presence of independent action after extensor indicis transfer were (1) the EDC in all cases had four distinct muscle bellies with separate and distinct innervation from the posterior interosseous nerve and (2) the junctura tendinum between the index and long fingers was filamentous and poorly developed in comparison to the more ulnar digits, which had well developed and thick juncturae that limited independent extension. They noted also that despite complete release of the juncturae tendinum, full independent excursion of the long or ring finger MP joint was not obtained, which suggested that extracapsular constraints limited independent extension of the long and ring fingers when adjacent fingers were held in flexion. Anatomic variations in the EIP have been described by Caudwell and colleagues,[19] including double tendon slips, an accessory slip to the long finger, and slips to the index finger and thumb.

The wrist, thumb, and finger extensors gain entrance to the hand beneath the extensor retinaculum through a series of six tunnels, five fibroosseous and one fibrous (the fifth dorsal compartment, which contains the EDQP).[97] The extensor retinaculum is a wide fibrous band that prevents bowstringing of the tendons across the wrist joint. Its average width is 4.9 cm (range 2.9 to 8.4 cm) as measured over the fourth compartment[97] (Fig. 52-1). At this level the extensor tendons are covered with a synovial sheath. The extensor retinaculum consists of two layers: the supratendinous and the infratendinous. The infratendinous layer is limited to an area deep to the ulnar three compartments. The six dorsal compartments are separated by septa that arise from the supratendinous retinaculum and insert onto the radius.[133] Just proximal to the MP joint level, the communis tendons are joined together by oblique interconnections called juncturae tendinum (Fig. 52-1). These connecting bands usually run in a distal direction from the ring finger communis to the little and middle fingers and from the middle to the index finger.[59,113,127] An anomalous junctura tendinum has been observed between the EPL and EDC.[127] In a recent description of the juncturae tendinum, von Schroeder, Botte, and Gellman[139] noted that the EDQP received a junctura from the ring finger extensor if the little finger EDC was absent. They described three distinct morphologic types of junctura tendinum. Because of these interconnections, laceration of the middle finger communis tendon just proximal to this junctura may result in only partial extension loss of the middle finger.[94]

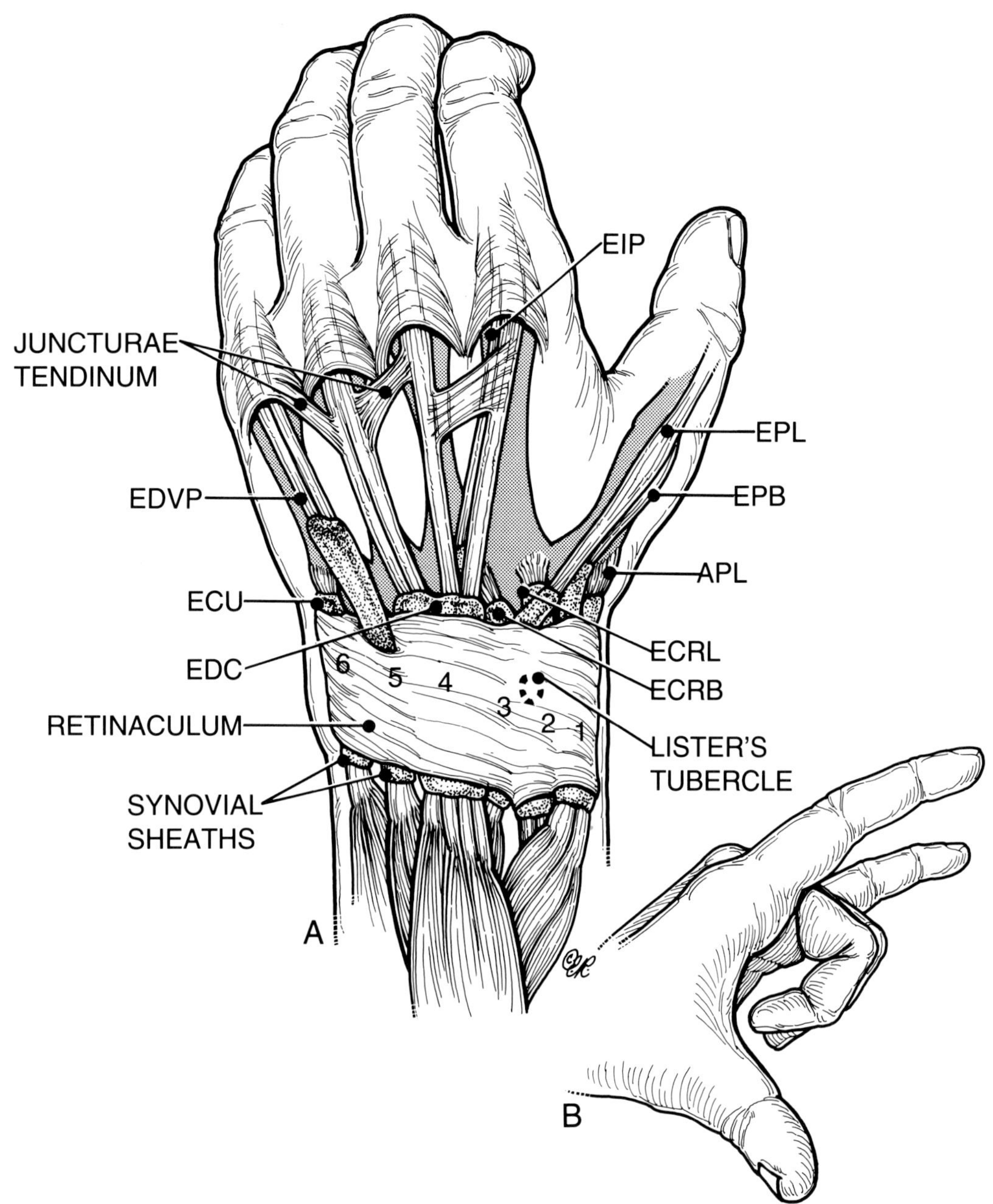

Fig. 52-1. **(A)** The extensor tendons gain entrance to the hand from the forearm through a series of six canals, five fibroosseous and one fibrous (the fifth dorsal compartment, which contains the extensor digiti quinti proprius [*EDQP*]).[97] The first compartment contains the abductor pollicis longus (*APL*) and extensor pollicis brevis (*EPB*); the second the radial wrist extensors; the third the extensor pollicis longus (*EPL*), which angles around Lister's tubercle; the fourth the extensor digitorum communis (*EDC*) to the fingers, as well as the extensor indicis proprius (*EIP*); the fifth the *EDQP*; and the sixth the extensor carpi ulnaris (*ECU*). The communis tendons are joined distally near the MP joints by fibrous interconnections called *juncturae tendinum.* These juncturae are usually found only between the communis tendons and may aid in surgical recognition of the proprius tendon of the index. The proprius tendons are always positioned to the ulnar side of the adjacent communis tendons. Beneath the retinaculum, the extensor tendons are covered with a synovial sheath. **(B)** The proprius tendons to the index and little fingers are capable of independent extension, and their function may be evaluated as depicted. With the middle and ring fingers flexed into the palm, the proprius tendons can extend the ring and little fingers. Independent extension of the index, however, is not lost following transfer of the indicis proprius.[91] *ECRB,* extensor carpi radialis brevis; *ECRL,* extensor carpi radialis longus.

The extensor tendon at the MP joint level is held in place over the dorsum of the joint by the conjoined tendons of the intrinsic muscles and the transverse lamina or sagittal band, which together tether and keep the extensor tendons centralized over the joint.[59] The sagittal band arises from the volar plate and the intermetacarpal ligaments at the neck of the metacarpals.[28,59] Any injury to this extensor hood or expansion may result in subluxation or dislocation of the extensor tendon.[16,28,59,86,107] The extensor mechanism at the level of the proximal aspect of the finger is composed of a layered criss-crossed fiber pattern, which changes its geometric arrangement as the finger flexes and extends. This arrangement allows the lateral bands to be displaced volarly in flexion and to return to the dorsum of the finger in extension.[114] The intrinsic tendons from the lumbricals and interosseous muscles join the extensor mechanism at about the level of the proximal and midportion of the proximal phalanx and continue distally to the DIP joint of the finger.[59,114]

At the MP joint level, the intrinsic muscles and tendons are volar to the joint axis of rotation. At the PIP joint, however, they are dorsal to the joint axis. The extensor mechanism at the PIP joint is best described as a trifurcation of the extensor tendon into the central slip, which attaches to the dorsal base of the middle phalanx and the two lateral bands[49] (Fig. 52-2). The lateral bands pass on either side of the PIP joint and continue distally to insert at the dorsal base of the distal phalanx. The extensor mechanism is maintained in place over the PIP joint by the transverse retinacular ligaments. The extensor tendon achieves simultaneous extension of the two finger joints by a mechanism in which the central slip extends the middle phalanx and the lateral bands bypass the PIP joint to extend the distal phalanx. The fibers overlying the PIP joint are differen-

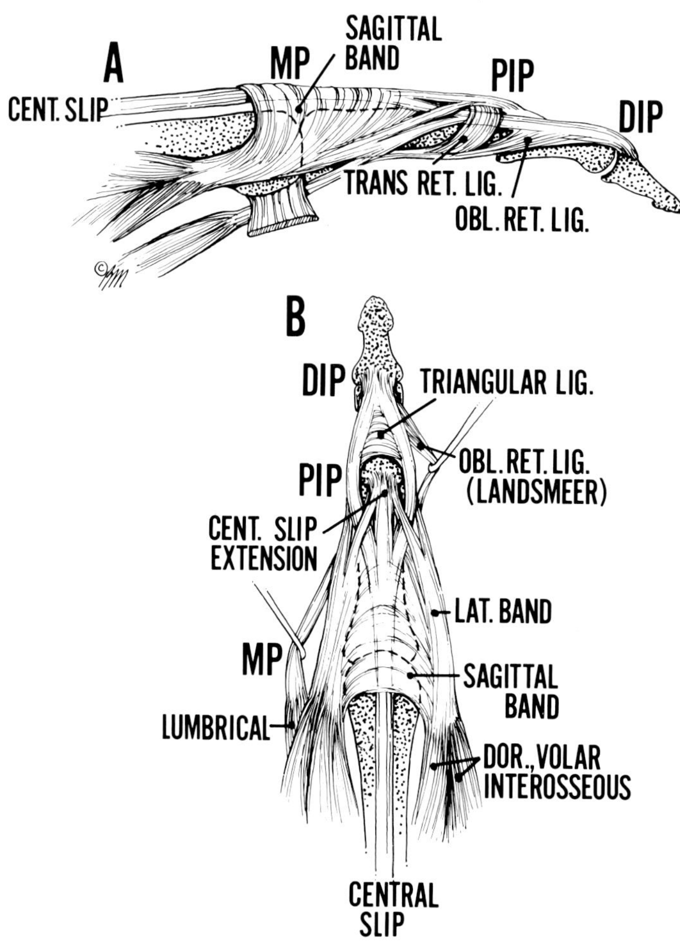

Fig. 52-2. The extensor tendon at the MP joint level is held in place by the transverse lamina or sagittal band, which tethers and centers the extensor tendons over the joint. This sagittal band arises from the volar plate and the intermetacarpal ligaments at the neck of the metacarpals. Any injury to this extensor hood or expansion may result in subluxation or dislocation of the extensor tendon. The intrinsic tendons from the lumbrical and interosseous muscles joint the extensor mechanism at about the level of the proximal and midportion of the proximal phalanx and continue distally to the DIP joint of the finger. The extensor mechanism at the PIP joint is best described as a trifurcation of the extensor tendon into the central slip, which attaches to the dorsal base of the middle phalanx, and the two lateral bands. These lateral bands continue distally to insert at the dorsal base of the distal phalanx. The extensor mechanism is maintained in place over the PIP joint by the transverse retinacular ligaments.

tially loaded as the finger moves. In the flexed position, the most central fibers are tensed, whereas in extension the lateral fibers are tensed.[69,87] The most important feature of this mechanism is that the three elements are in balance.[49,134] Specifically, the lengths of the central slip and two lateral bands must be such that extension of the PIP and DIP joints takes place together, so that when the middle phalanx is brought up into alignment with the proximal phalanx, the distal phalanx reaches alignment at the same time.[49] This mechanism depends on the relative length of the central slip and two lateral bands. This precise and consistent length relationship is what is so difficult to restore when the mechanism has been damaged.[49,85,134] Loss of this critical relationship at the PIP joint level with relative lengthening of the central slip results in the characteristic boutonnière deformity.[49]

DYNAMIC SPLINTING FOR EXTENSOR TENDON INJURIES

Extensor tendon injuries traditionally have been immobilized in extension for 3 to 4 weeks after surgical repair.[40,61,77,83,89] The sutured tendons are protected by maintaining the wrist in 40 to 45 degrees extension and the fingers in slight flexion. However, in some instances this resulted in adhesions between the extensor tendon and the surrounding tissues. This is especially true when the tendon injury is associated with a crush injury, surrounding soft tissue loss, infection, underlying fracture, joint capsule, or flexor tendon injury.[93] Significant and extensive research (both basic and clinical) has focused on the best methods of postoperative management of *flexor* tendon injuries.[27,43,45,67,73,79,81,95,99,131,138,143,144] Controlled and early passive motion of the tendon suture site provided by dynamic splinting has proved to be a very useful method to promote a well-healed smooth, nonadherent gliding flexor tendon surface with improved tensile strength. This body of evidence regarding the rehabilitation of flexor tendon injuries with dynamic splinting may be applicable to extensor tendon injuries, and several clinical studies have supported this statement[9,21,38,39,54] (Fig. 52-3). However, as noted by Newport and colleagues,[93] valid confirmation of the value of dynamic splinting awaits a well-controlled prospective study comparing static versus dynamic splinting in patients with simple extensor tendon lacerations as well as in patients with associated injuries. These principles may be especially applicable when multiple extensor tendons are injured beneath the extensor retinaculum and when there are associated injuries. The extensor tendons at the wrist level are surrounded by a synovial sheath and constrained by fibroosseous and fibrous tunnels. Indiscriminate sacrifice of the extensor retinaculum results in altered biomechanics and poor function. The use of controlled passive motion has been clearly shown to improve results in flexor tendon injuries, and these principles are now being applied to extensor tendon injuries. Following this principle, extensor tendon injuries can be placed in an outrigger splint that maintains passive extension using elastic traction but allows limited active flexion.

Zones of extensor tendon injury have been described[68] and are depicted in Figure 52-4. These zones are useful in understanding the following discussion of dynamic splinting.

Evans and Burkhalter,[39] in a pilot study of 66 digits in 36 patients, reported their 6-year experience with controlled passive motion in untidy extensor tendon injuries. They noted, based on their review of the literature, biomechanic and anatomic considerations, and intraoperative studies, that depending on the involved finger, 27.3 to 40.9 degrees of MP joint flexion would create 5 mm of EDC tendon glide in Zones V, VI, and VII (index 28.3 degrees, long 27.5 degrees; ring 40.9 degrees; little 38.3 degrees). They also noted that the EPL would glide 5 mm at Lister's tubercle with 60 degrees of IP joint flexion. Five millimeters of passive tendon glide was found to be safe as well as effective in limiting adhesions after an untidy extensor tendon injury.

Their method of postoperative management for extensor tendon injuries in finger Zones V, VI, and VII and thumb Zones IV and V began with dynamic splinting at 3 days postoperative. The wrist was positioned in an appropriate amount of extension to relieve tension at the repair site, usually 40 to 45 degrees. The MP and IP joints were supported at 0 degrees in elastic traction slings attached to an outrigger device (Fig. 52-3). A palmar block limited MP flexion to that arc of motion previously noted to result in 5 mm of extensor tendon excursion. The patient was instructed to actively flex the MP joints but to allow the elastic traction on the outrigger device to passively return the digital joints to 0 degrees. This exercise was done 10 times per hour. In thumb injuries involving Zones IV and V the EPL was splinted with the wrist extended, CMC joint at neutral, and MP joint at 0 degrees. Dynamic traction maintained the IP joint at 0 degrees but allowed 60 degrees active flexion.

In their study, Evans and Burkhalter[39] discontinued dynamic splinting between the third and fourth week; active motion was then started using the usual protocol for extensor tendon rehabilitation. Evans[38] in a companion publication, explained that this treatment included gentle active and active assistive exercises that emphasized extension at the MP joint with the wrist supported in extension. Between 4 and 5 weeks, individual finger extension and the claw position were emphasized to direct controlled stress to the adhesions.[38] At 5 to 6 weeks finger flexion was emphasized. At 7 weeks, resistance, functional electrical stimulation, and dynamic flexion splinting were considered to be safe modalities to encourage full finger flexion. During the phase of dynamic splinting, resting the digital joints at 0 degrees prevented extensor lag; controlled MP motion prevented extension contractures, maintained the integrity of the collateral ligaments, and lessened the effects of adhesions at the repair site. With the wrist and MP joints fully extended the therapist could passively move the IP joints without effecting tendon excursion in Zones V, VI, and VII, and thus avoid stiffness in these joints.

In a review of 70 patients who sustained 119 complete extensor injuries, Browne and Ribik[9] verified the efficacy of early dynamic splinting for extensor tendon injuries. In order to minimize the chance of tendon rupture, only those patients who were considered to be well motivated and reliable were treated with dynamic splinting. Fifty-two patients were selected for this treatment plan based on these criteria. An outrigger device using elastic traction was fitted that provided for passive extension and allowed active flexion. A similar splint

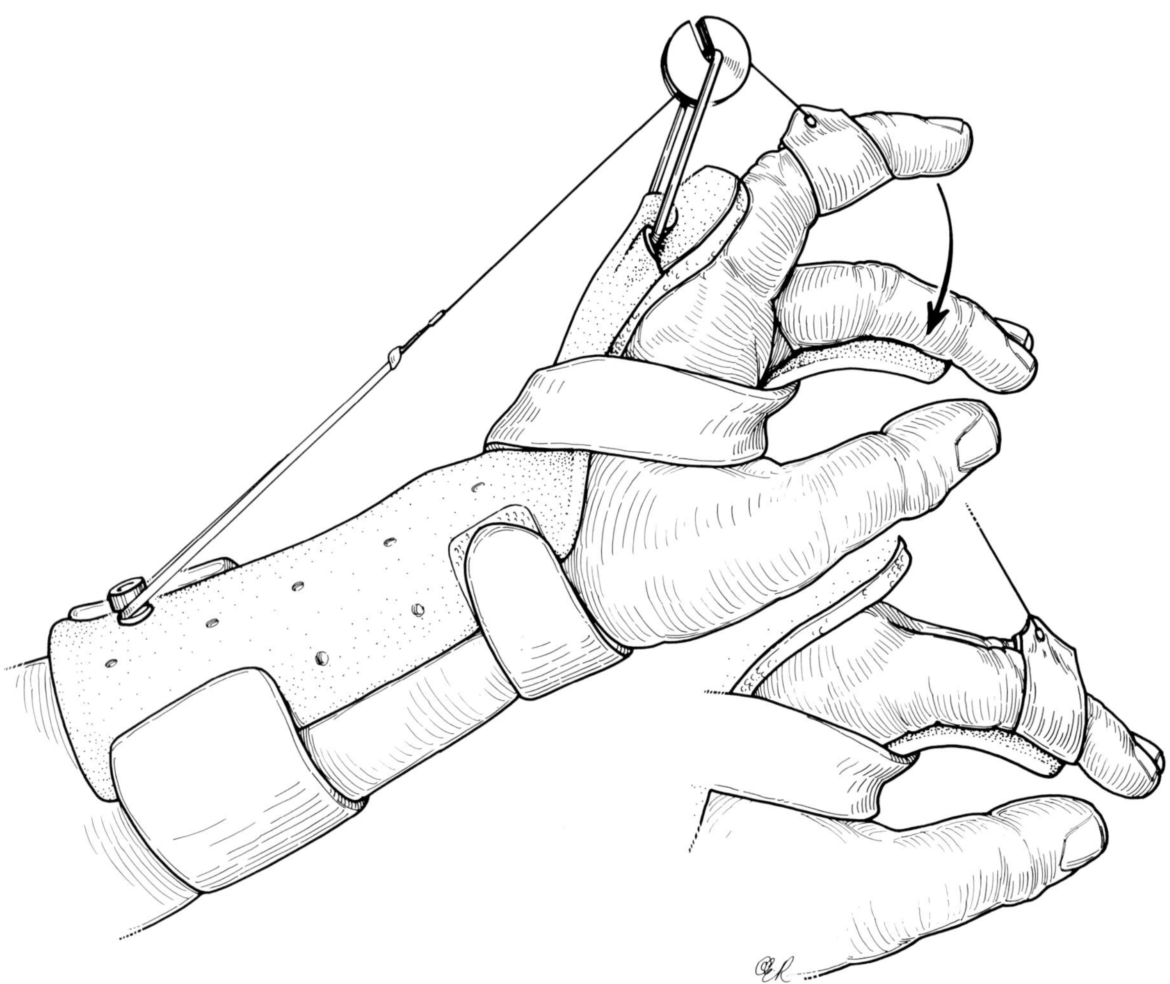

Fig. 52-3. Dynamic splint for early motion of extensor tendon injuries. Elastic traction maintains the fingers in extension. Excursion of the repaired extensor tendon is achieved by active flexion. Splinting is started 3 to 5 days after surgery and is maintained for 5 weeks. Active flexion is performed 10 times an hour. See text for details.

was used for the thumb extensor that maintained the thumb in extension and abduction to allow flexion motion across the palm. Splinting was started 3 to 5 days after repair and was maintained for 5 weeks. Patients were evaluated by the therapist 2 to 3 times per week for splint adjustment and verification of proper activity. The goal of therapy was to flex 10 times per hour and to achieve a minimum range of 70 degrees MP flexion, 90 degrees PIP flexion and 50 degrees DIP flexion. Patients slept with the fingers in extension; some used a static rather than a dynamic splint. Dynamic splinting was discontinued after 5 weeks but an extension night splint was used for another month. During the sixth week active motion with light resistance was performed, followed by 2 weeks of active motion with moderate resistance, followed by 2 additional weeks of motion with maximum resistance. Therapy was stopped after 10 weeks in all cases. No tendon ruptures were noted in any of the 52 patients. Full extension was achieved in 77 of 82 digits. All patients were able to make a complete fist. The earliest return to work was 8 weeks and the longest, 11 weeks. Although the patients treated by this method were preselected based on motivation and reliability, it was observed that the patients treated by static splinting were also vigorously treated by the same treatment team and the results in this group, although not nearly as good as in the dynamic splinting group, probably compared favorably with the results of extensor tendon repair reported in other series. The authors concluded that this intensive therapy protocol is justified in circumstances in which one might expect a poor result such as multiple tendon lacerations, especially under the extensor retinaculum, lacerations involving the metacarpal periosteum or MP joint, or patients with a history of excessive scarring. The authors observed that for this treatment plan to be carried out appropriately the patient must be reliable and well motivated, and an experienced and capable hand therapist must be available.[9]

Hung and colleagues, in a prospective study on early controlled active mobilization with dynamic splinting, reviewed 38 patients with 48 digit injuries.[54] Dynamic splinting was started on the third postoperative day and continued for 5 to 6 weeks. Injuries involving the fingers showed an average total active motion of 229 degrees whereas injuries involving the thumb averaged 118 degrees. Injuries in Zones II, III, and IV showed the worst results with an average total active motion of 188 degrees. No tendon ruptures were noted in this series. Only patients with predominant extensor tendon injuries were in-

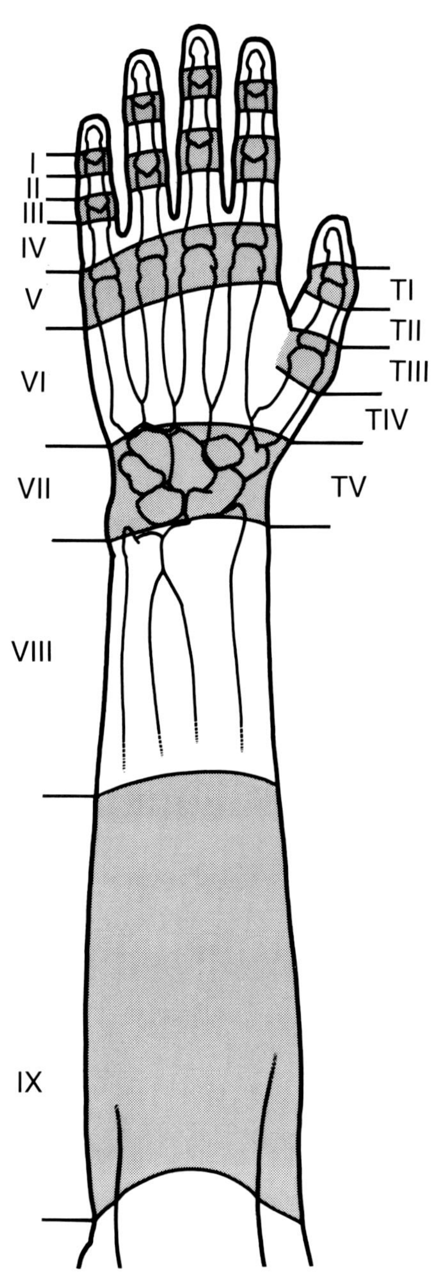

Fig. 52-4. Zones of extensor tendon injury. The extensor mechanism can be injured from the finger tip to the mid- and proximal forearm. Nine zones (I to IX) have been identified to aid in ease of classification and discussion of treatment as follows:

Zone	Finger	Thumb
I	DIP joint	IP joint
II	Middle phalanx	Proximal phalanx
III	PIP joint	MP joint
IV	Proximal phalanx	Metacarpal
V	MP joint	CMC joint/radial styloid
VI	Metacarpal	
VII	Dorsal retinaculum	
VIII	Distal forearm	
IX	Mid- and proximal forearm	

cluded in the study. A variable amount of skin and bony injuries were noted. Patients with unstable fractures, severe joint dislocations, and flexor tendon or neurovascular injuries were excluded as were mallet deformities. Four groups of patients were identified:

Group I: Zones II, III, IV

Group II: Zone V

Group III: Zones VI, VII

Group IV: Division of EPL at all levels

Injuries distal to the MP joints were splinted in 70 to 90 degrees of MP flexion for 3 weeks, then gradually extended. Injuries at the MP joints and proximal were held with the MP joint in extension. The details of the postoperative programs are given in Table 52-1.

The authors noted that their Groups I and II (Zones II to V) were injuries of the extensor mechanism overlying the phalanges and MP joint and as such were different than Zone VII injuries. They noted that controlled mobilization in Zone VII extensor injuries was analogous to controlled mobilization of flexor tendon injuries. However, when controlled mobilization is applied to other zones that are extrasynovial, the major effect is more on mobilization of the joints, although there may also be beneficial side effects on tendon healing. The authors concluded that controlled active mobilization is a reliable and effective means of rehabilitation of extensor tendon injuries. No immediate complications were noted and most patients regained a good range of motion. Although the use of dynamic splinting was noted to be expensive and labor-intensive when compared to static splinting, the good results obtained and the average return to work in 8.5 weeks were considered to be money and effort well spent.[54]

Author's Comment

Dynamic splinting has been demonstrated to be a very useful method for the postoperative management of both complex and simple extensor tendon injuries in Zones V to VIII. Its usefulness in Zones II to IV is less apparent at this time. It is most likely to yield a good result in a cooperative patient. The technique is most advantageous to the surgeon and patient when a skilled hand therapist is available to fabricate the splint and to monitor the patient. Standard forms of immobilization may prove to be most useful in children and uncooperative adults.

EVALUATION OF RESULTS IN EXTENSOR TENDON INJURIES

The results following extensor tendon injury and treatment may be evaluated by:

1. TAM[9,38,39,54]
2. Extension lag[54,132]
3. Extension lag and flexion loss[89,93]
4. Grip strength[54,93]

Table 52-1. Position of Splinting and Programs for Mobilization for Extensor Tendon Injuries[a]

	Group I Dorsum of Finger (Zones II, III, IV)	Group II Knuckle (Zone V)	Group III Dorsum of Hand (Zones VI, VII)	Group IV Thumb (All EPL)
Initial position	Wrist 40° extension MP 70° flexion Adjustable palmar Block at PIP	Wrist 40° extension Adjustable palmar Block at MP	Wrist 40° extension	Wrist 40° extension Thumb in midabduction and midextension Adjustable palmar block at IP joint
1st week	DIP 0–90° PIP 0–30° Active flexion Assisted extension MP 70–90° Wrist not moving	DIP 0–90° PIP 0–90° MP 0–30° Active flexion Wrist not moving	Free mobilization of IP joints MP 0–90° Active flexion Wrist not moving	IP 0–45° Active flexion Assisted extension Wrist and MP joint not moving
2nd week	PIP 0–60° Other joints same	MP 0–60° Other joints same	Same as 1st week	IP full flexion Other joint same
3rd week	PIP 0–90° Other joints same	MP 0–90° Other joints same	Dynamic component removed Wrist extension Splint only Free mobilization of all finger joints	Dynamic pulley moved to proximal phalanx IP 0–90° MP 0–45° Active flexion Assisted extension Wrist not moving
4th week	Dynamic component removed Wrist extension Splint only Free mobilization of all finger joints	Dynamic component removed Wrist extension Splint only Free mobilization of all finger joints	Same as 3rd week	MP joint full flexion Other joint same
5th week	Splint removed	Splint removed	Splint removed	Dynamic component removed Wrist extension splint 1st metacarpal in midabduction and extension Free mobilization of MP and IP joints
6th week	—	—	—	Splint removed

[a] This treatment protocol was developed by Hung and colleagues and used in a prospective study involving 38 patients and 48 digits (see text). (From Hung et al,[54] with permission.)

Newport and colleagues[93] found that relatively little had been published concerning the quality of result after extensor tendon repair. They noted that loss of extension was addressed as a potential problem but that overall range of motion or loss of flexion was not. They endorsed a rating system that they ascribed to Miller.[89] This system was considered to be the most accurate and discriminating in reflecting the quality of outcome. This system or classification of extensor repair results is as follows:

Excellent: Full flexion and full extension.

Good: 10 degrees or less of extension lost, 20 degrees or less of flexion lost.

Fair: 11 to 45 degrees of extension lost, 21 to 45 degrees of flexion lost.

Poor: 45 degrees or more of both extension and flexion lost.

These authors also noted that it was not clear what significance should be placed on TAM and grip strength in outcome evaluation of extensor tendon injuries. Although these 2 measurements are accepted indicators of hand function after flexor tendon repair, they may not adequately reflect the loss of function at the PIP joint or the ability to use tools effectively. They also observed that many patients with extensor tendon injuries were heavy laborers in whom the ability to make a tight fist is paramount.[93]

ZONES OF INJURY

The extensor mechanism may be injured at any level from the distal joint of the finger to the proximal forearm. The physical characteristics of the extensor tendon varies at each level, and a zone system is utilized to aid in ease of classification and discussion of treatment. The zones of injury are depicted in Fig. 52-4. Although the original classification by Kleinert and Verdan[68] ended at Zone VIII (the distal forearm), an additional zone is required to include the muscular area of the extensor mechanism at the middle and proximal forearm, which is considered to be Zone IX.

EXTENSOR MECHANISM INJURIES AT SPECIFIC ZONES

Zone I Finger

DIP Joint

Mallet Finger

Loss of continuity of the conjoined lateral bands at the distal joint of the finger results in a characteristic flexion deformity of the distal joint called *mallet, baseball,* or *drop finger.* Although the term mallet finger is a misnomer, it is, by common usage, defined as a loss of continuity of the extensor tendon over the distal finger joint.[1,102,126] The distal joint assumes varying degrees of flexion and the patient cannot actively extend the distal segment, although full passive extension is usually present. Hyperextension of the middle joint may also be observed and is due to unopposed central slip tension at the PIP joint and joint laxity.[37] In recent injuries, there is swelling and tenderness over the dorsum of the distal joint.

Mechanism of Injury

The mallet finger deformity may be an open or closed injury. The injury may be due to a variety of sports or occupational activities.[1] Open injuries may be due to sharp or crushing-type lacerations. Closed injuries are more common, and by far the most common cause is sudden, acute forceful flexion of the extended digit, which results in rupture of the extensor tendon or avulsion of the tendon with or without a small fragment of bone from the insertion. A torsion injury with associated rupture of one of the lateral bands has been reported and is a very rare cause of mallet finger.[1] Forced hyperextension of the distal joint may result in a fracture of the dorsal base of the distal phalanx involving one-third or more of the phalanx.[1] Although a mallet finger deformity may be associated with this injury, the lesion should be considered primarily a fracture with a secondary mallet finger deformity. This fracture should not be confused with a small avulsion fracture, which occurs in some mallet finger cases, since the mechanism of the injury and treatment are different. The same comments apply to transepiphyseal plate fracture in a growing child. In Stark, Boyes, and Wilson's series,[126] although many patients noted the lesion following significant trauma associated with some sports or occupational activity, in 42 percent of cases the lesion was associated with such a minor degree of trauma that the patients were surprised at the resultant deformity.

Incidence

The sex and age incidence of mallet finger deformity, as well as the finger involved, may vary with the population studied. In Hallberg and Lindholm's 127 cases in Sweden[47] 91 were men (one with two ruptures) and 35 were women. The mean age in males was 35.5 years and in females 47.8 years. Injuries in males were most common in the young (13- to 25-year age group), in contrast to females, whose injuries were evenly distributed in all age groups. In men, the fourth and fifth digits were most commonly involved. In women, the lesion was most common in the middle finger. In Stark, Boyes, and Wilson's series in the United States,[126] the highest incidence of injury in males was in the 36- to 49-year range and in females, in patients over 50. In this series, no gender distinction was made as to the finger involved. The middle finger was the most commonly involved, followed by the little finger. In a review of 75 patients, Robb (Scotland)[108] noted a peak incidence in the 50- to 60-year age group, with the ring and little fingers most commonly involved. The males with injuries outnumbered the females. In 148 cases, Abouna and Brown (England)[1] noted more injuries in males than in females. The highest age incidence in males was in the adolescent and young adult group (11 to 40 years), while in females the incidence was higher in middle-aged women (41 to 60 years). In both sexes, there was a progressive increase in incidence from the radial to ulnar side of the hand. An epidemiologic survey of 24 members of a three-generation family by Jones and Peterson[58] found 20 mallet fingers in seven family members, suggesting a familial predisposition. Multiple mallet fingers (range: 2 to 6) occurred in four individuals. Eighty-five percent of the cases resulted from minimal trauma or occurred spontaneously.

Anatomy of Mallet Finger

The lateral bands from each side of the digit merge and conjoin to form one tendon just distal to the dorsal tubercle on the proximal portion of the middle phalanx. This tendon continues distally to form a wide unit for insertion into the dorsal base of the distal phalanx. The tendon attaches to the dorsal part of the capsule and inserts into a ridge distal to the articular cartilage from one collateral ligament to the other.[60] Warren and colleagues, in a study of the microvascular anatomy of distal digital extensor tendon, noted an area of deficient blood supply in this area and suggested that this zone of avascularity might have implications in the cause and treatment of mallet finger.[140]

Classification of Mallet Finger

Mallet finger deformities may result from several causes, and the following classification is given as an aid in establishing a proper treatment plan:

Type I: Closed or blunt trauma with loss of tendon continuity with or without a small avulsion fracture

Type II: Laceration at or proximal to the DIP joint with loss of tendon continuity

Type III: Deep abrasion with loss of skin, subcutaneous cover, and tendon substance

Type IV: (A) Transepiphyseal plate fracture in children; (B) Hyperflexion injury with fracture of articular surface of 20 to 50 percent; (C) Hyperextension injury with fracture of the articular surface usually greater than 50 percent and with early or late volar subluxation of distal phalanx

The most common type of mallet finger is Type I, which is due to loss of continuity either from tearing of the substance of the tendon just proximal to the joint or avulsion of the tendon from its insertion, with or without a small piece of bone. One-fourth of Stark, Boyes, and Wilson's cases were associated with a small bone fragment. In their series, the presence of a small bone fragment did not alter the end result of treatment in any way.[121] McFarlane and Hampole,[85] however, noted that in their series of 50 cases of mallet finger, injuries with fracture did not obtain results as good as those injuries without fracture, but they included all fractures of varying sizes in this nine-patient group. Abouna and Brown[1] noted no significant difference in the results with the presence of a small fragment of bone on x-ray examination.

The degree of deformity in this injury may vary from a few degrees of extension loss to a 75 to 80 degree drop finger deformity. Although the finger deformity is usually immediate in its onset, in some cases it may be delayed by a few hours or days.[1] This is especially true of those closed injuries with a crushing element to the dorsum of the distal joint. In partial or incomplete tears of the tendon, the lesion may be represented by a small amount of extension loss that becomes progressively worse following additional trauma or repeated active flexion of the joint.

A laceration over or near the DIP joint that transects the tendon also produces a characteristic mallet deformity. Lacerations directly over the joint more often than not enter the joint, and this must be considered in treatment because of the potential for joint contamination. Deep abrasion-type injuries over the distal joint may result in significant loss of soft tissue cover and a portion or all of the underlying tendon mechanism. The joint is almost always exposed. The management of this injury is far different than that for a simple closed mallet deformity, and staged surgical reconstruction is required.

A blow on the end of a finger with a hyperextension force may be associated with a fracture of the dorsal base of the distal phalanx. There is often a resultant mallet deformity and early or late volar subluxation of the distal phalanx.[71,145] This injury must be distinguished from the usual closed mallet finger, since its treatment is based on the management of the lesion as a fracture and not as a tendon injury as such. The same applies to a fracture of the basal epiphysis of the distal phalanx in a child. Management of these fractures is discussed on page 1939. These comments do serve to establish the need for radiographic evaluation in all patients with mallet finger deformity. A true lateral x-ray of the individual finger is mandatory.

Methods of Treatment of Closed (Type I) Mallet Finger Injuries

The primary goal in all methods of treatment is restoration of the continuity of the injured tendon with maximum recovery of function. Both non-operative and operative (invasive) treatments have been advocated to achieve this goal.[14,52] Non-operative treatment includes the use of plaster cast immobilization and various types of finger splints. Surgical treatment includes K-wire fixation, external tendon suture, and direct repair of the tendon with or without K-wire fixation. The following comprehensive review of many of the published methods of treatment of mallet finger may seem redundant and of historical interest only. However, their inclusion seems appropriate since some of these techniques may be useful in certain circumstances. Also, older methods of treatment are often "discovered" and presented as a new concept. Finally, their chronological presentation may offer guidance to the surgeon about their respective hazards and relative usefulness.

Plaster Cast

In 1937 Smillie[116] described his plaster technique for correction and immobilization of the mallet finger deformity. Others have used this method with certain modifications, including Watson-Jones (1940),[142] Howie (1947),[53] Williams (1947),[148] and more recently, Stark, Boyes, and Wilson (1962),[126] and Green and Rowland (1975).[46] These plaster casts are applied so that the DIP joint is in slight hyperextension and the PIP joint is at approximately 60 degrees flexion. Bunnell[11] explained the rationale for this position by stating that flexion of the PIP joint resulted in advancement of the lateral bands for a distance of 3 mm, which, along with hyperextension of the DIP joint, promoted approximation of the torn extensor tendon at the DIP joint. In 1959, however, Kaplan[59] noted that this position should not be used for treatment of mallet finger. Specifically, he observed that the extensor mechanism was moderately relaxed over all three finger joints when the finger was held in moderate extension. In recent years, Kaplan's viewpoint has been affirmed by clinical experience. That is, most authors have not found it necessary to immobilize the PIP joint in the treatment of mallet finger except in those cases with a swan-neck tendency or deformity.[1] Smillie's method (Fig. 52-5), however, is useful in patients who are unreliable or who are unable to understand or consistently apply a splint correctly.[46] If there is doubt about a patient's reliability or ability to follow instructions, a plaster cast may be advantageous. Stark, Boyes, and Wilson noted that a plaster cast properly applied gives satisfactory results; this technique includes a precut plaster splint that avoids pressure over the PIP and DIP joints. It

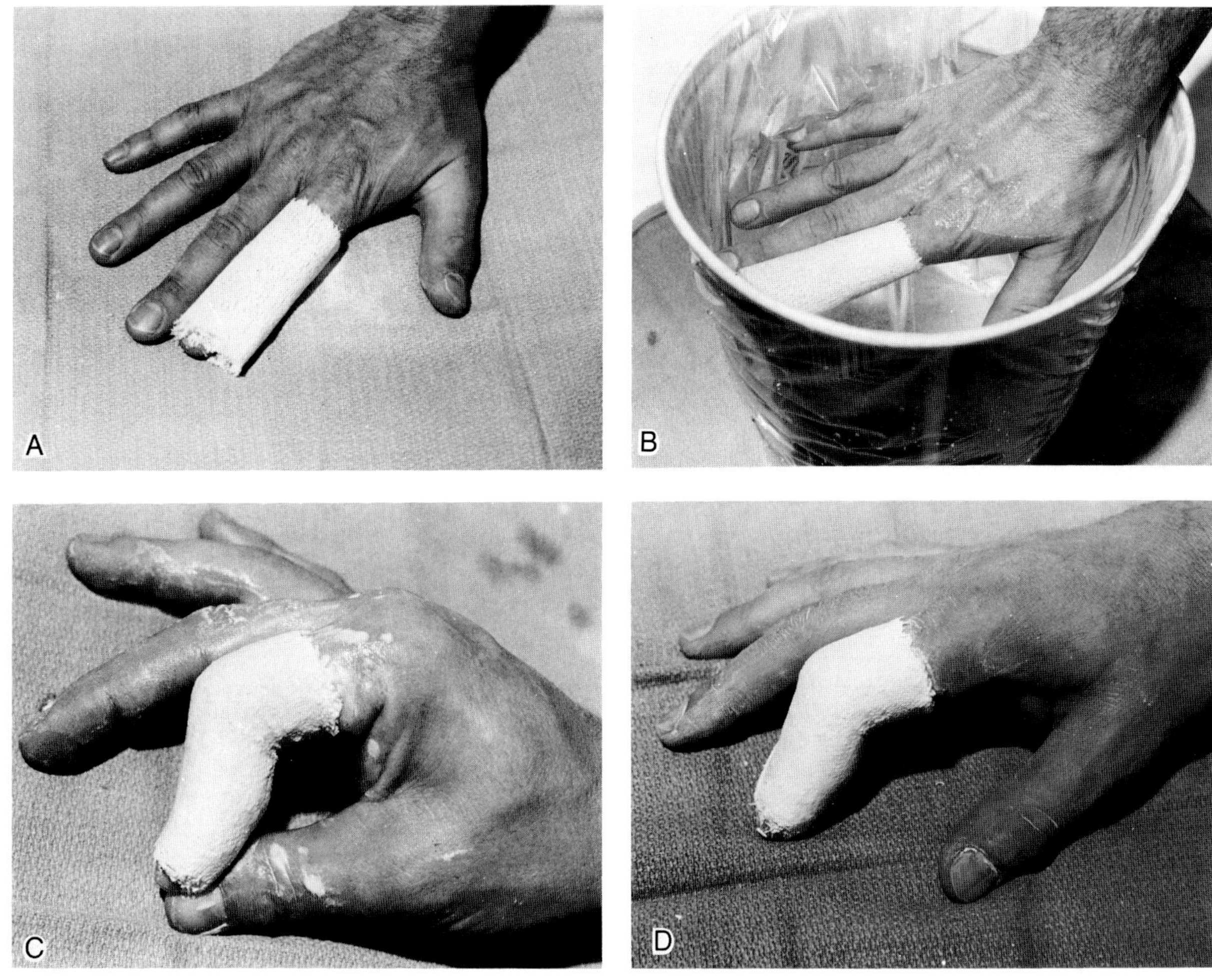

Fig. 52-5. Plaster cast immobilization for mallet finger is sometimes a useful procedure in patients who are unreliable or unable to understand or consistently apply a splint. This technique has been described by Smillie[116] and Green.[46] **(A)** An 18-inch strip of 3- or 4-inch dry plaster is rolled into a tube and slipped over the end of the injured finger. No padding is used. **(B)** The patient dips his hand into a bucket of water, holding the tube of plaster in place over the finger. **(C)** The patient holds the finger in the correct position of immobilization while the physician smooths out the plaster. **(D)** The completed cast. Removal is facilitated by soaking the plaster in water. (From Green and Rowland,[46] with permission.)

avoids hyperextension at the distal joint and does not exceed 60 degrees flexion at the PIP joint.[126] Although it may be argued that PIP joint immobilization is not required in the management of this lesion, from a practical viewpoint it is highly unlikely that a finger cast applied without flexion at the PIP joint would remain in place for a significant period of time. Flexion of the PIP joint, and its subsequent incorporation in plaster, seems to be a practical solution to keeping a finger cast in place. Hallberg and Lindholm[47] in 1960 reported on 76 patients with mallet finger treated by plaster immobilization and noted a 5 degree extension loss in 28 patients, a 5 to 20 degree loss in 11, and a greater than 20 degree loss in 37.

Splints

Lewin[72] in 1925 described a tubular metal splint that maintained the DIP and PIP joints in full extension. Numerous splints of metal, wood, and plastic have been described and used since that time.[32,46,55,66,120,124,137,141] Most authors agree that splinting should be continuous for a 6-week period. Night splinting for an additional 2 weeks has been advocated by some authors. The majority of splints are placed on the volar side of the digit, although Newmeyer[92] has applied his padded aluminum splint dorsally. These splints are shaped to fit the individual finger and are usually held in place by tape; they are designed to hold the terminal joint in full extension or slight hyperextension. A great variety of splints have been designed and used. McFarlane and Hampole[85] in 1973 reviewed 50 cases of mallet finger personally treated by them with splinting of the distal joint for 6 weeks. The series included closed injuries, open injuries, and avulsions, whether seen at the time of injury or some months later. Eighty percent of their cases obtained an excellent to good result with splinting alone. The results were satisfactory even when the patient was seen late. Kaplan[59] also noted that even cases that are several months old may yield a good result. In his series, both early and late cases were treated with 6 weeks of continuous splinting, followed by 2 weeks of night splinting. McFarlane and Hampole noted that even 3 months after injury, splinting alone will probably yield a satisfactory result.[85] They noted that fair and poor results were not due to treatment but to poor patient cooperation or inadequate immobilization. Even mallet fingers due to laceration of the extensor mechanism at or near the distal joint that were treated by splint alone demonstrated results comparable to closed injuries treated by splinting. McFarlane and Hampole further noted that when some component of the extensor mechanism within the digit was torn or divided, the tendon ends did not retract very far, and, even in untreated injuries, scar tissue would bridge the gap. If this scar tissue reaction is minimized by splinting the joint in extension, normal relationships can be restored.[85] Engelbrecht[34] expressed a similar opinion when he observed that in placing the distal joint in full extension, a perfect opposition of the tendon ends was obtained, and that after careful suturing there was often a small gap between the tendon ends, causing unsatisfactory postoperative results. Abouna and Brown[1] in 1968, in a series of 110 cases followed for 6 months to 3 years and treated by continuous splinting of the distal joint for 6 weeks, noted that 72 percent of the cases had an extension defect of less than 5 degrees, 13.4 percent had an extension loss of 5 to 15 degrees, and 14.6 percent had an extension loss greater than 15 degrees.

Warren and colleagues compared the efficacy of the Stack and Abouna splints in a series of mallet finger injuries in which the majority were Type I.[141] The criteria used to assess the effect of treatment was developed by Abouna and Brown[1] as follows:

Success: Extension loss 0 to 5 degrees, no stiffness, normal flexion/extension;

Improved: Extension loss 6 to 15 degrees, no stiffness, normal flexion;

Failure: Extension loss more than 15 degrees, stiffness or impaired flexion.

Based on these criteria, success or improved status was achieved in 52 percent of patients using the Stack splint and 53 percent with the Abouna splint.

These results are compared to the series reported by Crawford,[22] who used only the Stack splint in 62 patients with Type I injuries without fracture. Splinting was maintained for 8 weeks followed by 2 weeks of night splinting. His slightly less rigid criteria for evaluation of results were as follows:

Excellent: Full extension, full flexion, no pain

Good: 0–10 degrees extension loss, full flexion, no pain

Fair: 10–25 degrees extension loss, any flexion loss, no pain

Poor: > 25 degrees extension loss, any patient with persistent pain

Excellent to good results were achieved in 49 of 62 patients (79 percent). The fair and poor results were noted in patients who were treated on a delayed basis or who wore or changed the splint improperly.

K-wire Fixation

Pratt[100] in 1952 described a technique for internal immobilization of the mallet finger deformity in which a longitudinal K-wire was placed across the DIP joint and into the neck of the proximal phalanx with the PIP joint flexed. This method was designed to provide constant and rigid fixation of the mallet finger deformity and at the same time provide flexion of the PIP joint. Watson-Jones (1956)[142] spoke against this method, as did others who noted technical difficulties with proper insertion of the K-wire, as well as residual joint stiffness at the PIP joint level. Pratt's method has been abandoned because of these problems.

Casscells and Strange[17] in 1957 advised immobilization of only the DIP joint with a K-wire. They reaffirmed their recommendation for this method in 1969.[18] Longitudinal K-wire immobilization has also been recommended by Flinchum (1959),[41] Engelbrecht (1966),[34] and Elliott (1970).[31] Tubiana (1968)[134] abandoned use of the longitudinal K-wire in favor of an oblique transarticular wire after he observed a few cases of fibrous scarring of the pulp. Weinberg, Stein, and Wexler[146] in 1976 described another method of fixation of the distal joint by means of two K-wires placed from dorsal to volar into the distal and middle phalanges respectively, with the two wires diverging at a 15 to 20 degree angle. A rubber band is then wrapped around the protruding wires on the dorsum of the finger to bring the joint into extension. A light plaster dressing is then applied. Some of their patients developed loss of flexion of the terminal joint. This method was discussed by Littler,[75] who expressed concern that only 6 of 15 cases in the author's series regained full DIP joint flexion. Littler believed this was due to damage within the flexor sheath or fixation of the extensor mechanism over the middle phalanx caused by insertion of the K-wires. I agree with Littler's opinion and advise that other simpler and safer methods are available and should be used.

External Tendon Suture

Hillman[51] in 1956 described a technique for treatment of the mallet finger and associated fractures of the distal phalanx by insertion of a #2 silk suture beginning at the pulp and continuing distally along the dorsal aspect of the distal joint. The silk suture was tied over small vinyl tubes applied to the pulp of the finger and to the dorsum of the PIP joint. Hillman described nine cases with satisfactory results following this method. I do not recommend Hillman's method because of potential problems with scar formation in the soft tissues.

Direct Repair

Mason[82] in 1930 recommended immediate operative repair of closed mallet finger injuries. However, Rosenzweig[109] subsequently noted that the results of operative repair are not always satisfactory, since the extensor tendon at the distal joint is extremely thin and sutures almost always tear out. Robb,[108] as well as Stark, Boyes, and Wilson,[126] found that operative repair was not necessary in closed mallet finger deformity. Nichols,[94] Stark, Boyes, and Wilson,[126] and Elliott[31] did, however, recommend suture of acute lacerations of the extensor mechanism over the DIP joint with mallet finger deformity, followed by internal or external splinting. Nichols[94] advised interrupted mattress sutures of 6–0 silk or a fine pull-out wire anchored to the nail. Elliott[31] advised repair of this lesion with a continuous 4–0 monofilament wire suture, the ends of which were left protruding from the skin on either side of the phalanx for ease of removal after the tendon had healed.

Complications

Stern and Kastrup[128] reviewed the short- and long-term complications encountered in the treatment of 123 mallet fingers treated operatively and nonoperatively. Eighty-four digits were splinted with a complication rate of 45 percent, represented mostly by transient skin problems including dorsal maceration, dorsal ulceration, and tape allergy. Fifty percent of the skin ulcerations and 67 percent of the macerations appeared during the second week. Other complications, including transverse nail grooves and pain from the splint, were noted less commonly. Residual scarring from skin ulcers, however, did not cause any limitation of flexion.

Stern and Kastrup noted that these complications were often dependent upon the type of splint used. Compared to other splints, the dorsal DIP aluminum foam splint had a higher rate of dorsal ulceration and maceration and incidence of nail grooves. The only long-term splint-related complication was a nail groove in one patient. Most splint-related nail grooves were noted to disappear at about 6 months. Based on the large number of complications with the dorsal DIP aluminum foam splint, the authors discouraged its use. If used, they emphasized the importance of placing tubular gauze or moleskin beneath the splint as advised by Evans[38] to prevent maceration and ischemia.[128] Careful observation of the skin at weekly intervals for at least 3 weeks was advised regardless of the type of splint used.

Rayan and Mullins reported two patients with full-thickness skin necrosis over the DIP joint after dorsal splint immobilization in hyperextension to treat acute mallet finger.[103] They noted in a series of 66 fingers that the average total passive hyperextension of the DIP joint was 28.3 degrees and that skin blanching occurred at approximately 50 percent of the total passive hyperextension. Based on their observations they recommended that (1) when the distal joint was splinted the degree of hyperextension at which the dorsal skin blanches be determined and that this amount of hyperextension not be exceeded, and (2) the angle of the dorsal splint should not exceed that of the DIP joint in order to prevent localized pressure over the dorsal skin.[103]

In Stern and Kastrup's[128] study, 53 percent of the 45 surgically treated patients developed complications, and of these complications 76 percent were long-term. Surgical complications included permanent nail deformities, joint incongruities, infection, pin or pull-out wire failure, and radial or ulnar prominence or deviation of the DIP joint. Loss of surgical reduction occurred in seven digits necessitating additional surgery. The outcome for these seven digits was: four had an arthrodesis; one had an amputation; one had a fixed flexion contracture and a mallet deformity more severe than before surgery; and in one, the final result was unknown.

Author's Preferred Method of Treatment(Type I)

My personal preferences for treatment of the mallet finger (Type I) are a commercially available volar splint made of plastic (Stack finger splint) or an aluminum foam splint (Fig. 52-6). The Stack splint is available in eight sizes, can be used to fit almost all fingers with mallet finger deformity using appropriate selection and padding, and has a high level of patient satisfaction.[124,141] The splint is taped in place and used continuously for a minimum of 6 weeks. The patient is advised to remove the splint only for cleansing of the finger and is cautioned to maintain the distal joint in extension at all times during removal of the splint. The splint is then reapplied by the patient and carefully retaped to maintain the distal joint in extension. This method is found to be quite satisfactory in a cooperative patient who understands the nature of the injury and the recommended treatment. The method has been found to be quite successful in the majority of patients with early as well as late mallet finger deformity—even in patients seen as late as 6 months following injury.

At the end of 6 weeks, the splint is removed and the finger inspected. The patient is allowed to begin guarded flexion exercises at that time but the splint is used at night for another 2 weeks. The patient should carry the splint with him, and if an extension loss is noted at any time following removal of the splint, the splint is immediately reapplied and left in place for another 2 weeks. The same process is then repeated. In spite of the high incidence of transient skin complications reported by Stern and Kastrup[128] with the aluminum foam splint, I have used it successfully both on the dorsal and volar aspects of the DIP joint (Fig. 52-6). This splinting material is inexpensive and readily available in most emergency rooms. The splint is carefully shaped and applied to avoid hyperextension of the DIP joint and the associated potential for skin ischemia and possible necrosis. (This skin ischemia can be demonstrated by hyperextending your own finger at the DIP joint.) Most patients require two visits during the first week of treatment and weekly visits thereafter to monitor their progress. It is not always possible to achieve full extension at the DIP joint on the initial splinting, especially if treatment has been delayed. At the second visit, 3 to 4 days later, the DIP joint can usually be fully extended. Skin maceration may be prevented by placing a small piece of circular gauze bandage around the middle and distal phalanx. In patients who are uncooperative or who, for one reason or another, are unable to wear a splint as just described, the Smillie[116] plaster cast is applied as described by Green[46] (see Fig. 52-5).

In rare circumstances, such as in a health professional (dentist, surgeon, etc.), an external splint may be difficult if not impossible to wear. In these unusual circumstances, a 0.045-inch K-wire is placed obliquely across the distal joint to main-

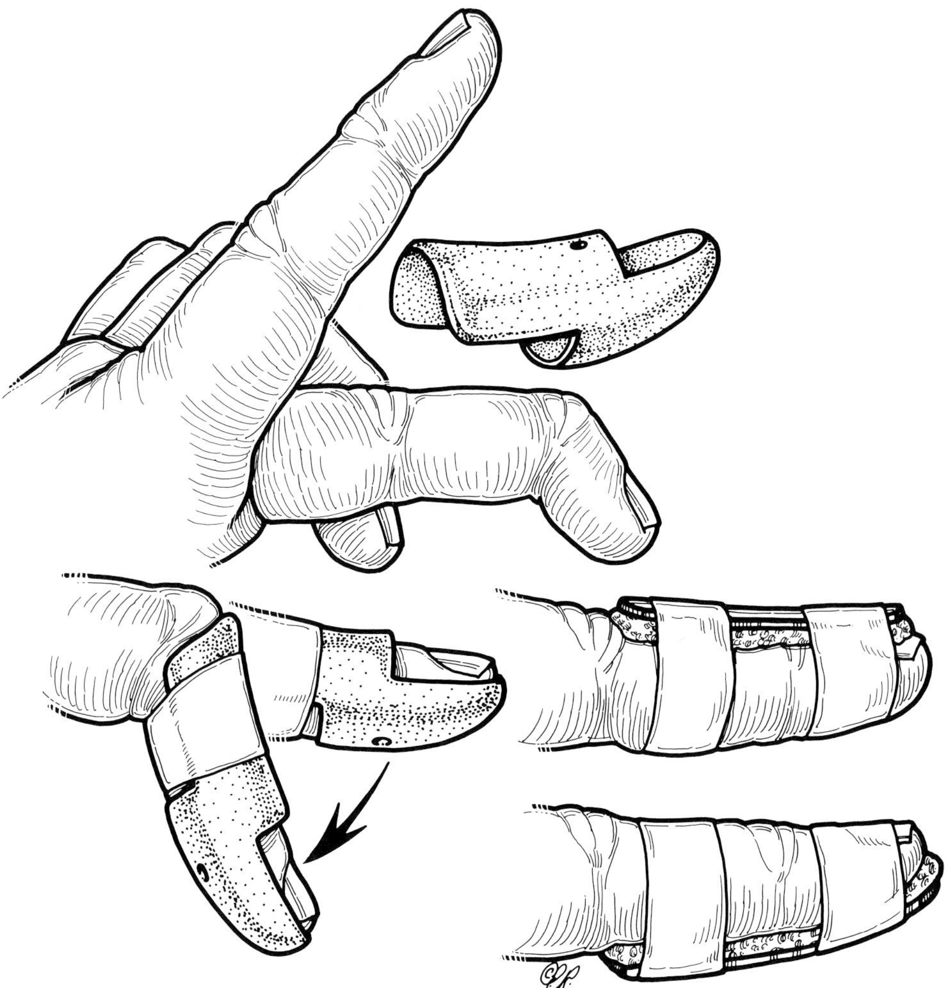

Fig. 52-6. The author's personal preferences for treatment of Type I mallet finger injuries are a commercially available volar plastic splint (Stack mallet finger splint) or an aluminum foam splint, which is taped either to the dorsal or volar aspect of the finger to immobilize the DIP joint in extension. The Stack splint is available in eight sizes and, with appropriate selection and padding, can be used to fit almost all fingers with the mallet finger deformity. The splint is taped in place and is used continuously for a minimum of 6 weeks. The patient is advised to remove the splint only for cleansing of the finger and is cautioned to maintain the distal joint in full extension at all times during removal of the splint. The aluminum foam splint is cut to the appropriate length, bent to the proper shape and taped in place either dorsally or volarly depending on the patient's preference and needs. Skin maceration may be avoided by placing a circular gauze bandage between the foam pad and the finger. Both splints (Stack and padded aluminum) have been found to be equally effective in treating Type I mallet injuries.

tain it in full extension.[46,134] The wire is cut off beneath the skin, and the patient is warned to protect the joint against strenuous flexion since the wire can be bent or broken. The K-wire is left in place for 6 weeks, followed by 2 weeks of night splinting.

Methods of Treatment of Open Mallet Finger Injuries (Types II and III)

Fresh lacerations of the extensor mechanism over the distal joint with mallet finger deformity are repaired by a simple figure-of-eight or roll-type suture, which reapproximates the skin and tendon simultaneously (Figure 52-7). A small dressing is applied incorporating a splint, which maintains the distal joint in full extension. The suture is removed at about 10 to 12 days, and the distal joint is maintained in the extended position by the previously described Stack or aluminum foam splint. The splint is maintained in position continuously for a minimum of 6 weeks, followed by protected range of motion. The splint is reapplied if any extension loss is noted following removal of the splint. Type III mallet deformities with loss of tendon substance and soft tissue coverage require reconstructive surgery to provide skin coverage, with late reconstruction by free tendon graft to restore tendon continuity or arthrodesis of the joint (see Chapter 53).

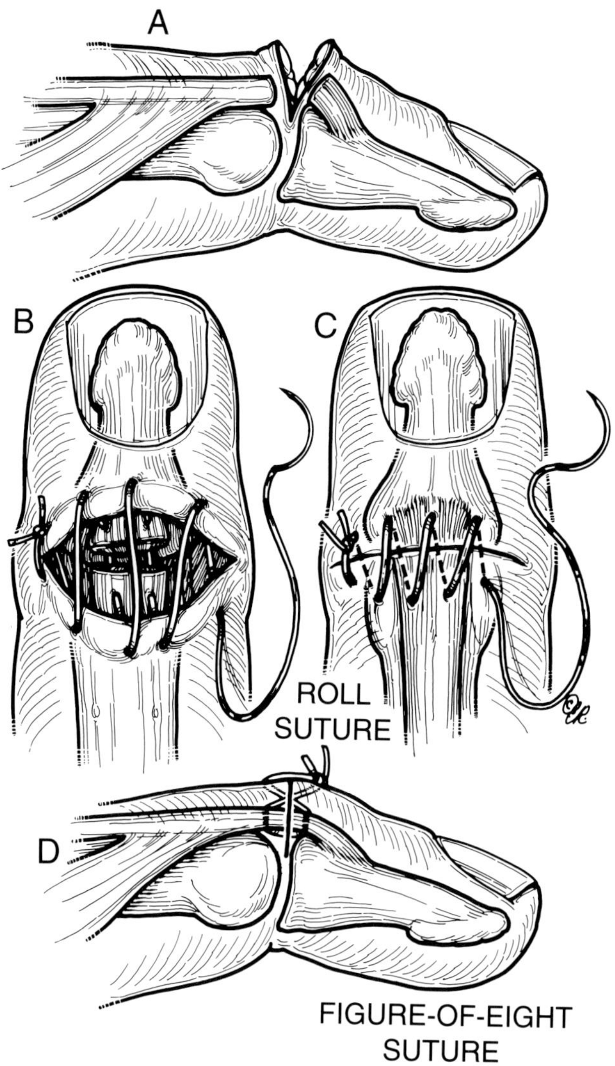

Fig. 52-7. Fresh lacerations of the extensor mechanism over the distal joint with mallet finger deformity **(A)** are repaired by a roll-type suture, which simultaneously approximates the skin and tendon **(B&C)**. A small dressing is applied along with a splint, which maintains the joint in full extension. The sutures are removed at 10 to 12 days but the splint is continued for a total of 6 weeks. One or two figure-of-eight vertical sutures **(D)** may be used, which also simultaneously close the defect in the tendon and skin. Splinting is mandatory for 6 weeks.

Methods of Treatment of Mallet Finger with Fracture (Type IV)

Mallet finger deformity resulting from a fracture of the distal phalanx in a child is usually a transepiphyseal fracture of the phalanx.[30] The extensor mechanism is attached to the basal epiphysis, and closed reduction of the fracture results in correction of the deformity. Continuous external splinting of the distal joint in full extension for 3 to 4 weeks results in union of the fracture and correction of the deformity.

In an adult, Type IV mallet finger injuries are associated with significant fracture fragments. Type IV-B is a hyperflexion injury and the fracture fragment is usually 20 to 50 percent of the dorsal articular surface of the distal phalanx.[71] Type IV-C mallet fracture is a hyperextension injury and is generally associated with a fracture fragment that is greater than 50 percent of the articular surface of the distal phalanx and is accompanied by volar subluxation of the distal phalanx.[71] Loss of the normal balance of forces between the extensor and flexor mechanisms and significant disruption of the dorsal joint capsule results in volar subluxation of the distal phalanx on the middle phalanx. This type of fracture with an associated mallet finger deformity is said to be a relatively uncommon injury. Stark, Boyes, and Wilson[126] described only five such cases in a series of 168 mallet finger deformities treated over a 13-year period. Abouna and Brown[1] noted only eight Type IV lesions in 148 mallet injuries. Wehbe and Schneider,[145] however, reported 44 mallet fractures in 160 mallet injuries, 13 of which demonstrated volar subluxation of the distal phalanx. *This fracture is not to be confused with the more common small bone fragment associated with a tendon avulsion and mallet finger deformity.* The mallet finger with a small avulsion fracture should be managed the same as a Type I closed mallet finger injury (see page 1934).

Operative treatment has been recommended for fracture fragments involving greater than one-third of the articular surface. An accurate reduction is advocated to prevent joint deformity with secondary arthritis and stiffness.[46,48,125] Stark[125] advised a dorsal approach with division of the ulnar collateral ligament as an aid in reduction. One or two small (0.028- or 0.035-inch) K-wires or a pull-out suture is used for fixation of the fracture. The collateral ligament is repaired prior to closure. Postoperative management includes a metal splint that holds the PIP joint in moderate flexion and the distal joint in extension (but not hyperextension). PIP joint splinting is discontinued after 3 weeks, but continuous splinting of the distal joint is done until the fracture has healed radiographically, at which time the K-wires are removed. Stark noted that, in his experience, this technique prevented painful and limited motion in the distal joint.[125]

Hamas, Horrell, and Pierret[48] described an alternative surgical technique in which a midlateral incision is extended to the corner of the nail. The dorsal skin flap of cuticle and subcutaneous tissue is raised from the nail and paratenon. The extensor tendon is divided 5 mm proximal to its insertion. The distal phalanx is flexed and the joint distracted to expose the articular surface. An 0.035-inch K-wire is drilled into the articular surface of the distal phalanx volar to the fracture line and withdrawn distally. The fracture is then reduced under direct vision and held with an Allis clamp while one or two 0.028-inch K-wires are drilled across the fracture site in a volar-lateral direction. The distal phalanx is then brought up into neutral and any volar subluxation corrected, after which the longitudinal K-wire is driven across the joint into the middle phalanx. Radiographs are used to confirm the reduction, and the extensor tendon is repaired with fine interrupted nylon. Care is taken to align the cuticle during skin closure. The K-wires are left in place for 6 to 8 weeks until union is demonstrated by radiograph. This time coincides with the duration required for tendon healing. Hamas, Horrell, and Pierret described consistently good results with this method.

In contrast to these recommendations for open reduction, Wehbe and Schneider[145] recommended nonoperative treatment by extension splinting of all mallet fractures, including the hyperextension type with subluxation of the distal phalanx. They believe that restoration of joint congruity does not influence the end result, since remodeling of the articular surface is reported to lead to a near-normal painless joint in spite of persistent joint subluxation. Lange and Engber[71] suggested that hyperextension mallet fractures with volar subluxation require accurate reduction. They observed that application of standard extension splint management to hyperextension injuries results in unacceptable volar subluxation and has been associated with quite unsatisfactory results. Crawford[22] has obtained encouraging results with nonoperative treatment of these fractures by the use of the molded polythene (Stack) splint even with relatively large fracture fragments. He has abandoned open reduction and internal fixation except for those occasional cases where volar subluxation of the distal phalanx is present. Eighty-nine of his 151 cases had fracture fragments comprising 20 to 50 percent of the joint surface. Eleven of these 89 mallet fracture cases had volar subluxation. Seven of these 11 cases required surgery due to inability to reduce or maintain the reduction of the volar subluxation in a splint. Surgery was in the form of open reduction and K-wire fixation of the distal joint in extension. Crawford further advised that in some cases with large fracture fragments (35 to 50 percent of the joint surface) the distal joint should not be hyperextended in the splint, since this may encourage palmar subluxation of the distal phalanx.[22]

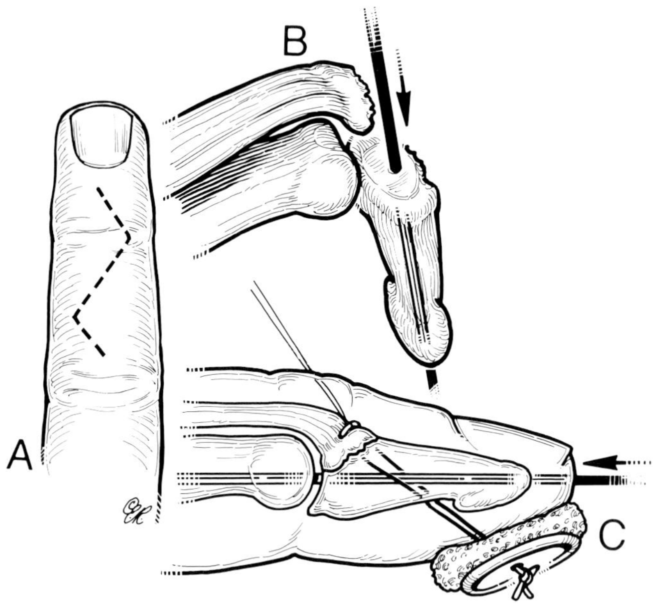

Fig. 52-8. Author's recommended technique for reduction and fixation of the mallet fracture with volar subluxation of the distal phalanx. **(A)** The joint is exposed through a dorsal zigzag incision. **(B)** A 0.035-inch double-ended K-wire is drilled longitudinally through the distal phalanx. **(C)** The joint is reduced, the K-wire is driven proximally across the joint, and the fracture fragment is reduced. If the fracture fragment cannot be maintained in position, a loop of 4–0 wire is passed through the fragment and distal phalanx and tied over a padded button. Intraoperative radiographs are made to determine anatomic reduction. The transarticular K-wire is protected with a splint for 6 weeks. The pull-out wire may be removed in 3 or 4 weeks.

Author's Comment and Preferred Method for Treatment of Type IV (B–C) Mallet Fractures

Operative repair of a mallet fracture is a technically difficult and potentially hazardous operation. Attempted fixation of the fracture fragment by K-wire or wire loop may result in comminution of the fragment and loss of attachment of the extensor mechanism. I agree with Crawford[22] that open reduction of mallet fractures should be reserved for those fractures with associated volar subluxation of the distal phalanx. Excellent remodeling of the articular surface occurs in most mallet fractures. In those cases of mallet fracture with volar subluxation of the distal phalanx, the joint is exposed through a zigzag dorsal incision, a 0.035-inch K-wire is passed longitudinally through the distal phalanx, the joint reduced, the fracture fragment manipulated into place and the K-wire passed across the joint, holding it in full extension (Fig. 52-8). X-rays in two planes are taken in the operating room to verify reduction. If the fracture fragment cannot be maintained in close apposition to the major fragment, a pull-out suture is used to hold it in position. The transarticular K-wire is protected by a splint for 6 weeks, after which the K-wire is removed and motion started.

Zone I Thumb

IP Joint

Mallet Thumb

Stark and colleagues[126] reported that mallet thumb is rare and did not include these cases in their study. Hallberg and Lindholm[47] noted that 3 cases out of 127 involved the thumb. Robb had only one case in the 75 patients he studied. Abouna and Brown[1] noted two thumbs involved in 148 cases of mallet finger. Din and Meggitt[24] in 1983 reported 4 cases of mallet thumb; 3 were closed and one was due to a laceration over the IP joint. They advised operative treatment for 3 reasons: (1) no reports of successful conservative treatment of the deformity, (2) the EPL tendon is thicker than the finger extensor at the DIP joint and holds sutures well, and (3) the finding of a fairly large gap due to retraction of the proximal tendon end. They noted excellent results in their series. In contrast, Patel, Lipson, and Desai[98] noted excellent results in 4 mallet thumbs treated by 8 weeks of continuous splinting. Two of their cases were due to laceration of the extensor tendon at the

IP joint and 2 were closed avulsion injuries. Miura, Nakamura, and Torii[90] reported their experience in 25 patients with mallet thumb treated by continuous splinting for 4 to 6 weeks followed by splinting for 8 to 12 hours per day for 3 to 6 months. Only 5 of the patients had closed ruptures; 20 (80 percent) were caused by open injuries. The patients who were splinted within 2 weeks after injury attained significantly better results than those treated 2 weeks or later after injury. Satisfactory extension was obtained in 21 of the 25 patients (84 percent). This series of 25 patients was compared to 9 patients who were treated by tendon suture. In these 9 patients favorable results were achieved in 5 treated by the authors in their clinic, but 4 patients sutured elsewhere did not obtain satisfactory extension or flexion in spite of splint treatment. They concluded that primary suture of a clean tendon laceration was best, but that splinting was preferred if the skin was closed. Primiano[101] noted excellent results in 2 cases of mallet thumb treated by a dorsal splint that immobilized the IP joint in extension for 6 weeks. He concluded that splinting was the treatment of choice for closed mallet thumb injuries.

Author's Preferred Method of Treatment for Mallet Thumb

Closed mallet thumb deformity is treated with a Stack-type or aluminum foam dorsal splint for 6 to 8 weeks. Mallet thumb injuries due to laceration require wound care and it seems appropriate to suture the tendon and skin with a roll or figure-of-eight suture followed by splinting as for a closed mallet thumb (see Fig. 52-7).

Zone II: Finger Middle Phalanx and Thumb Proximal Phalanx

In contrast to Zone I, Zone II extensor tendon injuries both in the fingers and thumb are usually secondary to a laceration or crush injury rather than an avulsion. Most lacerations to the extensor tendon in this zone can be treated as described for Zone I lacerations. Both crush and laceration injuries in Zone II may result in incomplete or partial division of the tendon because of its increased width and curved shape over the middle phalanx in the finger and proximal phalanx in the thumb. A partial laceration in Zone II involving less than 50 percent of the tendon substance can be treated by skin wound care followed by active motion in 7 to 10 days. Complete lacerations without associated injuries in Zone II in the fingers are treated by buried core or interrupted sutures followed by static splinting of the DIP joint in full extension for 6 weeks. Active flexion of the PIP is performed during this time. If associated injuries are present which might compromise the end result, consideration should be given to dynamic splinting as described by Hung and colleagues[54] for Zone II injuries (see Table 52-1). Complete laceration of the EPL in Zone II without associated injuries is treated by static splinting of the IP joint in full extension. The MP joint is left free for active exercises. If associated injuries are present consideration should be given to dynamic splinting as noted above.

Zone III Finger

PIP Joint Level

Boutonnière Lesion

Disruption of the central slip of the extensor tendon at the PIP joint level along with volar migration of the lateral bands will result in the so-called boutonnière deformity, with subsequent loss of extension at the middle joint and compensatory hyperextension at the distal joint. This lesion may be secondary to closed blunt trauma with acute forceful flexion of the PIP joint, producing avulsion of the central slip from its insertion on the dorsal base of the middle phalanx with or without fracture and laceration of the extensor tendon at or near its insertion.[119] Volar dislocation of the PIP joint may also result in avulsion of the central slip and subsequent boutonnière deformity.[119,121,129]

In closed injuries, the characteristic boutonnière deformity may not be present at the time of injury and usually develops over a 10- to 21-day period following injury. This condition is often missed even in an open wound. A painful, tender, and swollen PIP joint that has been recently injured should arouse suspicion. Active motion is decreased and the finger is held semiflexed. Carducci[15] reviewed 43 of 71 patients treated in an emergency room with the diagnosis of jammed or sprained finger over a 14-month period and noted that 2 of the 43 patients developed a boutonnière deformity. He described two diagnostic tests that are useful in early recognition of this lesion: (1) a 15 to 20 degree or greater loss of active extension of the PIP joint when the wrist and MP joint are fully flexed, and (2) extravasation of intraarticular radio-opaque dye dorsal and distal to the PIP joint. Lovett and McCalla[77] also noted that weak extension against resistance is an excellent diagnostic finding and is suggestive if not diagnostic of central slip injury. Boyes[6] noted that early diagnosis may be facilitated by holding the PIP joint in full extension and testing the amount of passive flexion of the distal joint. With disruption of the central slip and volar migration of the lateral bands, flexion of the distal joint is markedly decreased.[6] In fresh cadavers, Harris and Rutledge[49] and Micks and Hager[86] observed that section of the central slip alone did not result in the boutonnière deformity. However, the boutonnière deformity did develop if the PIP joint was repetitively flexed while tension was applied to the extrinsic extensor. The lateral bands tore away from the other fibers, producing a boutonnière deformity.

The boutonnière deformity illustrates the problem of imbalance in the finger, which is a chain of joints with multiple tendon attachments. This chain collapses into an abnormal posture or deformity when there is an imbalance of the critical forces maintaining equilibrium.[119,123] Zancolli has divided this sequence into three stages. At first, there is flexion of the PIP joint due to loss of the central slip and the unopposed force of the flexor digitorum superficialis. Later, with stretching of the expansion (transverse retinacular ligament and triangular ligament) between the central and lateral slips, the lateral bands migrate volarward to a position volar to the axis of joint rotation. Finally, in this position of the lateral bands, the pull of the intrinsic muscles is directed exclusively to the distal joint, which progressively hyperextends. The MP joint is also hyperextended by action of the long extensor tendon.[149] In the discussions that follow, treatment of the early acute boutonnière deformity is arbitrarily divided into closed or avulsion injuries, and open injuries with laceration of the extensor tendons at or near the PIP joint.

Methods of Treatment of Closed Acute Boutonnière Deformity

Correction of this deformity is dependent on restoration of the normal tendon balance and the precise length relationship of the central slip and lateral bands. In acute cases, before fixed contractures have occurred, this may be achieved by two basic means: (1) splinting of the PIP joint into progressively full extension, or (2) insertion of a transarticular K-wire to maintain the PIP joint in full extension. At the same time, active and passive flexion exercises of the distal joint are performed as recommended by Boyes.[6] Splinting of the PIP joint and active flexion of the DIP joint have been said to draw the lateral bands distally and dorsally and to reduce the separation of the torn ends of the central slip of the extensor tendon. This allows repair by contracture of the disrupted tendon ends at their anatomic length and migration of the lateral bands to their normal anatomic position above the joint axis of rotation at the PIP joint.[8,20]

Stewart[129,130] has achieved the same good results by a plaster cylinder finger cast with the distal joint flexed (the mallet finger posture) and the PIP joint in extension. The plaster is maintained for 6 weeks, and the MP joint is free to move during that time. After removal of the plaster, the DIP joint is mobilized first before unrestricted motion of the PIP joint is allowed, since, according to Stewart, the lateral bands made tight by DIP joint flexion would otherwise exert more than normal traction on the healed central slip during PIP joint flexion.[129] King[65] and Stewart[130] have emphasized the importance of early recognition and closed treatment of the boutonnière deformity, because of the fact that surgical correction of this late or established deformity is unpredictable.

Metal, plastic, plaster, and dynamic splints have been used for the maintenance of the PIP joint in extension. Most authors agree that only the PIP joint needs to be splinted, although McFarlane and Hampole[85] advised immobilization of the wrist and MP joint because of difficulties encountered in maintaining the PIP joint in full extension. They also noted that a K-wire placed obliquely across the joint affords firm immobilization and is a more reliable way of holding the PIP joint in extension. A shorter splint that immobilizes only the MP and PIP joints can then be used. McFarlane and Hampole continued the splint for 4 weeks and removed the K-wire in 3 weeks. In older patients, they reduced the time of absolute immobility to 2 weeks.[85] Tubiana also advised splinting the wrist in extension, along with immobilization of the MP joint in 10 degrees flexion, the PIP joint in extension, and the DIP joint in 45 degrees flexion for 4 weeks. At the end of that time, only the PIP joint is kept immobilized in extension for another week.[134] Both Boyes[6] and King[65] have used the Bunnell-type safety-pin splint with good success. Boyes[5] has used this method since 1957 and has noted satisfaction with the method in early boutonnière cases. The splint is worn for 5 weeks. If the middle joint cannot be fully extended passively, it is brought into extension by dynamic splinting with the safety-pin splint and strap. The distal joint must be left free. The patient is advised to use the splint constantly and to perform strong active flexion of the distal joint. If the distal joint can be fully flexed with the PIP joint extended, all components of the extensor mechanism have been restored to their normal relationships and balance, and the splint may be discontinued[5,6] (Fig. 52-9).

In closed boutonnière deformity, Boyes[6] advocated operative treatment under two circumstances: (1) when the central slip has been avulsed with a bone fragment and is lying free over the PIP joint, it should be replaced or excised and the tendon reattached with a pull-out suture; and (2) a long-

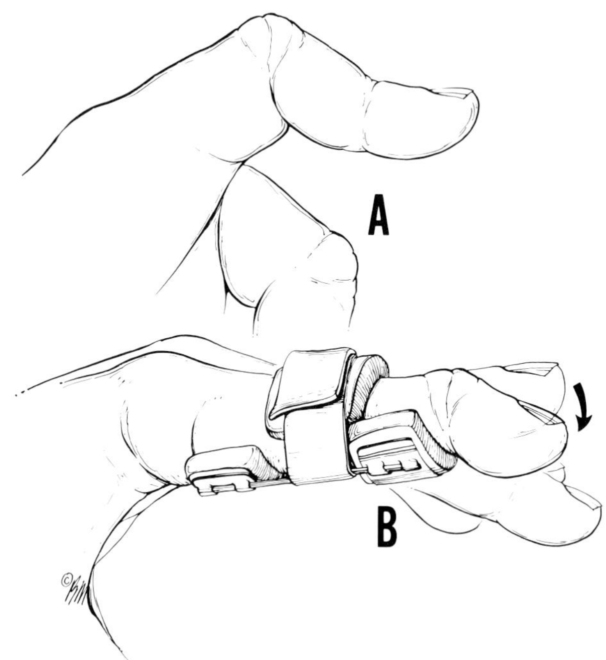

Fig. 52-9. The Bunnell-type safety-pin splint is the author's preferred method for the management of a closed boutonnière deformity **(A).** The splint is worn constantly, and the strap on the splint is tightened on a daily basis until full extension of the PIP joint is achieved. The terminal crossbar does not go beyond the distal joint flexion crease **(B),** and the patient is instructed to actively and passively flex the distal joint while the proximal joint is held in maximum extension. The splint is used on a continuous basis for several weeks until full passive extension of the PIP joint can be achieved along with full or nearly full flexion of the DIP joint. When this occurs, the length relationships and balance between the central slip and the lateral bands have been achieved, and the splint can be discontinued.

standing boutonnière deformity in a young person. Tubiana[134] also favors surgery in recent closed ruptures with avulsion of a bone fragment. Depending on its size, the fragment is excised or reattached. If the fragment is excised, the central slip should be reattached to the base of the middle phalanx. The joint is transfixed with a K-wire for 10 days followed by a splint.

Spinner and Choi have noted that closed anterior or volar dislocations of the PIP joint usually result in rupture of the central slip along with rupture of a collateral ligament and volar plate and subsequent boutonnière deformity.[121] They have observed that these potentially disabling soft tissue injuries must be recognized and repaired. Spinner and Choi recommend prompt reduction and primary repair of all ruptured structures (central slip, collateral ligament, and volar plate), combined with stabilization of the PIP joint in extension with a K-wire for 3 weeks, followed by gradual mobilization over the next 3 to 4 weeks while the PIP joint is protected. Motion of the distal joint is encouraged in the early postoperative period. It can be anticipated that this method will produce satisfactory results, although joint stiffness can be a problem because of the extensive soft tissue injury.[121] Transarticular K-wire fixation of the PIP joint in full extension is preferred by Elliott[31] and Sakellarides.[112] Elliott used a light volar splint as additional protection, leaving the distal joint free for active flexion exercises.[31] The K-wire is left in place for 5 weeks, and an external splint is worn for another week, followed by a night splint for a second week. After removal of the splint, active extension exercises are encouraged and distal joint flexion is continued with manual support of the middle phalanx in extension. Maximum recovery may take 9 months.[31] Sakellarides noted that external splinting of the PIP joint is often not satisfactory in maintaining full PIP joint extension, and it is his practice to insert an oblique transarticular 0.035-inch K-wire to maintain this joint in extension. The wire is removed after 6 weeks and active exercises are begun.[112]

A difference of opinion exists concerning the definition of early and late boutonnière deformity. The definition is important in terms of splinting versus surgical repair of the boutonnière deformity. Boyes[8] noted that splinting is effective as late as 30 days after injury. King[65] stated that if the joints are loose, particularly in a young patient, a trial of splinting was worthwhile after 6 weeks and even up to 12 weeks. Sakellarides[112] categorizes the lesion as a late case if the rupture is several weeks old and advocates excision of scar tissue and repair or tendon ends in late cases. According to McFarlane and Hampole[85] and Chase,[20] the time interval between date of injury and treatment seems to be less important than the presence or absence of a fixed flexion contracture at the PIP joint. McFarlane and Hampole noted that if the PIP joint can be extended passively, the lateral bands are probably not fixed volar to the axis of movement and splinting alone is likely to yield a good result. They noted that the finger should be splinted for 6 weeks continuously and then for another 3 weeks at night to allow the scar tissue that has reestablished the continuity of the extensor mechanism to shorten enough to correct the deformity.[85] Chase expressed a similar viewpoint that scar tissue in the boutonnière deformity will contract when given the opportunity. In his opinion, splinting is useful except in a fixed deformity.[20]

Author's Preferred Method of Treatment for Closed Boutonnière Injuries

My personal preference for management of the acute closed finger boutonnière is the safety-pin splint, which is used to achieve extension in the PIP joint. The terminal crossbar does not go beyond the distal joint flexion crease, and the patient is instructed to actively flex the distal joint while the PIP joint is held in maximum extension (see Fig. 52-9). The web strap on the splint is tightened on a daily basis until full extension of the PIP joint is achieved. This may require several days or even weeks. The splint is used in this manner on a continuous basis for several weeks until full passive extension of the PIP joint can be achieved, along with full or nearly full flexion of the DIP joint. When this occurs, the normal length relationships and balance between the central slip and the lateral bands have been achieved and the splint can be discontinued. Some temporary loss of flexion at the PIP joint may be noted, but this will resolve with additional exercise of the finger. If partial recurrence of the deformity is noted, the splint is reapplied and the same exercise plan carried out. This method has been used with success in closed boutonnière deformity of greater than 6 months duration, as well as the recent closed acute boutonnière deformity. One advantage of this method over a transarticular K-wire is that any passive motion lost at the PIP joint (fixed flexion contracture) can be gradually corrected by the splint. Although this technique can correct passive loss of joint motion at the PIP joint in an established boutonnière deformity, it of course cannot restore tendon substance lost as a result of a deep abrasion or burn to the dorsum of the PIP joint. Reconstructive procedures are required in these instances; these are discussed in Chapter 53.

Methods of Treatment of Lacerations Over the PIP Joint (Open Boutonnière)

Lacerations over the PIP joint are likely to enter the joint space. The first aim of treatment should be to prevent infection.[134] This requires cleansing, debridement, and appropriate antibiotics as indicated. Most authors agree that a laceration of the central slip and/or lateral bands at the PIP joint levels should be primarily repaired.[3,31,85,112] In an acute laceration over the PIP joint with laceration of the central slip and lateral bands, McFarlane and Hampole first pass a K-wire across the joint with the joint in full extension. The various components of the extensor mechanism need not be identified, in their opinion, but are simply clustered together with figure-of-eight sutures; the hand and wrist are immobilized as done for a closed boutonnière deformity. The K-wire is removed in 3 weeks, and only the PIP joint is immobilized for another week.[85] Elliott also noted that acute lacerations at this level require K-wire fixation of the PIP joint in extension along with repair of the tendon with a pull-out suture or with interrupted buried sutures. The K-wire is removed after 5 weeks, and then a continuous external splint is worn for another week.[31] Sakellarides[112] treats open lacerations over the PIP joint by capsular and tendon repair with 4–0 Mersilene and a transarticular K-wire for 5 to 6 weeks. In my experience the skin and tendon may be brought together with a figure-of-eight or roll-type stitch, or the lacerated tendon ends may be reapproximated with buried interrupted sutures. After repair, the PIP joint must be maintained in extension; this may be done with a splint or K-wire.[85] I agree with Evans[38] that the PIP joint must be maintained in full extension for 6 weeks. The DIP joint is left free and active joint exercise performed. If insufficient distal stump of the central slip is available for repair, the central slip must be reattached to bone.[59,94] This may be done with a pull-out suture technique or by anchoring the tendon to the dorsal base of the middle phalanx by a nonabsorbable suture passed through a small transverse drill hole over the base of the phalanx. If the lateral bands are also injured along with the central slip, they should also be repaired with interrupted buried sutures.

Although simple laceration of the extensor mechanism at this level can be treated by relatively simple sutures, Snow[118] and Aiche, Barsky, and Weiner[2] noted difficulties in repair of primary acute boutonnière deformities associated with loss of substance of the extensor mechanism at this level. In an attempt to resolve this problem, Snow[118] described a retrograde (distal-based) flap taken from the central slip and applied as a reinforcing batten over the central slip repair (Fig. 52-10). After the lacerated extensor has been sutured in the routine end-to-end manner, this retrograde flap is brought over the entire area proximal and distal to the repair. The donor site of the tendon flap is closed primarily. The hand is dressed in the position of function for 3 weeks, and then guarded motion is started. The method is also found to be useful in cases where a gap is present in the extensor mechanism, as in grinding wheel injuries. Aiche, Barsky, and Weiner[2] similarly have noted cases of acute disruption of the extensor mechanism over the PIP joint with badly shredded tendon and loss of tendon substance. Primary reconstruction of the central slip is performed by identifying and dissecting free the two lateral bands from the oblique and transverse retinacular ligaments. These bands are then split longitudinally for about 2 cm, and their middle segments are reapproximated in the midline over the base of the middle phalanx with 5-0 silk (Fig. 52-11). The lateral segments are left in position and represent the lumbrical insertions and retinacular ligaments. The wrist is splinted in extension, the MP joint in 20 degrees flexion, and the PIP joint in extension for 3 weeks after which range of motion is started. The authors state that this procedure will aid in prevention of the boutonnière deformity.

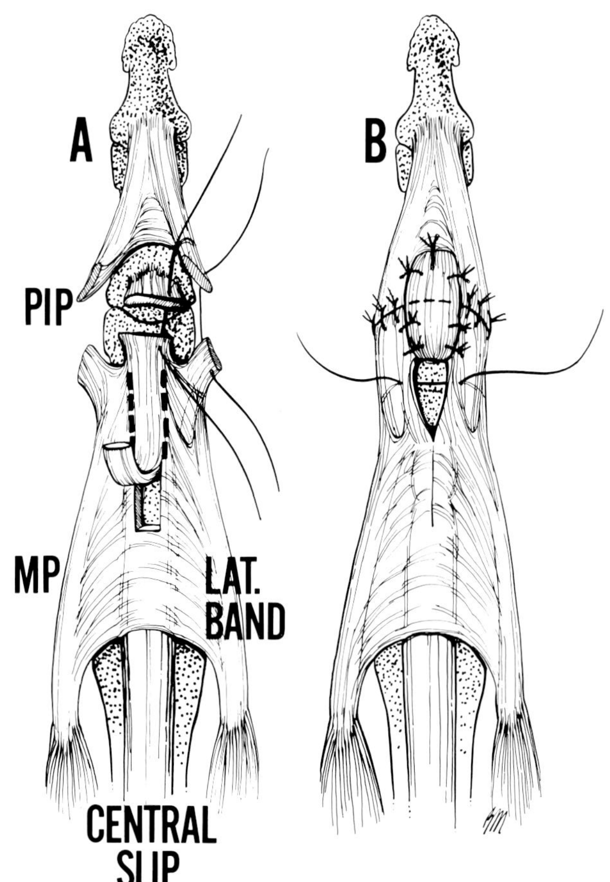

Fig. 52-10. Acute boutonnière deformities associated with loss of substance of the extensor mechanism at the PIP joint are difficult to treat. In an attempt to solve this problem, Snow[118] described a retrograde flap taken from the central slip of the extensor **(A)** and applied it as a reinforcing batten over the central slip repair. The retrograde flap is carefully sutured into place over the repair site to act as a reinforcement in the area of repair. The defect in the central slip is then closed with interrupted sutures **(B).**

Author's Preferred Method of Treatment for Open Boutonnière Injuries

A fresh or acute laceration of the extensor mechanism over the PIP joint will result in a drop finger at the PIP joint level, which soon develops into a boutonnière deformity if not properly treated. The acute laceration is repaired with nonabsorbable suture such as 4-0 or 5-0 nylon, or a figure-of-eight suture is used to coapt the tendon ends and skin margins simultaneously. Any method that joins the tendon ends is satisfactory. The PIP joint is splinted in full extension. After soft tissue healing has occurred and the sutures have been removed, a safety-pin splint is applied, as described under treatment of the closed boutonnière deformity, and active flexion exercises of the distal joint are started. The safety-pin splint is maintained on a continuous basis for 5 to 6 weeks with the PIP joint in full extension, and active flexion exercises of the distal joint are performed. As recommended by Evans, when active exercises are started at 5 to 6 weeks the patient is advised to support the proximal phalanx in flexion as the PIP joint is extended.[38] This directs the force of the extensor tendon more distally and the finger is in a more effective position for extension.[130] The PIP joint is splinted in extension between these exercise sessions for another 2 to 4 weeks. At 8 to 10 weeks active flexion and extension exercises are increased. Dynamic flexion splinting of the PIP joint can be used to augment recovery of flexion if there is no extensor lag at the PIP joint.[38] Repairs of the extensor mechanism over the PIP joint result in a condition quite analogous to a closed boutonnière deformity. Specifically, the PIP joint must be maintained in full extension for at

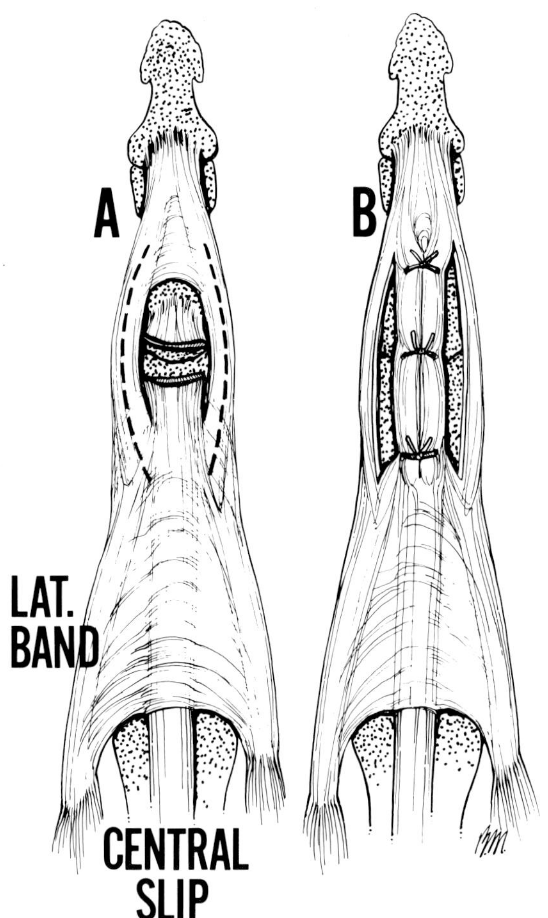

Fig. 52-11. Aiche, Barsky, and Weiner[2] have described cases of acute disruption of the extensor tendon over the PIP joint with shredded tendon and loss of tendon substance. In their technique, primary reconstruction of the central slip is performed by identifying and dissecting free the two lateral bands from the oblique and transverse retinacular ligaments. These bands are then split longitudinally for about 2 cm **(A)** and their middle segments reapproximated in the midline over the base of the middle phalanx using 5–0 nonabsorbable suture **(B).** The lateral segments are left in position and represent the lumbrical insertions and retinacular ligaments. The authors state that this procedure will aid in prevention of the boutonnière deformity.

least 5 to 6 weeks, and, at the same time, active flexion of the distal joint must be performed. In my experience, this method has proved to be satisfactory for correction of the drop finger following laceration of the central slip and for prevention of the boutonnière deformity. In lacerations at or near the insertion, a pull-out wire technique is used, which firmly reattaches the tendon to bone. Careful attention must be given to restoration of the normal length relationships of the central slip and the adjacent lateral bands. The recovery of flexion in the DIP joint can be augmented by gentle and intermittent rubber band traction between a dress hook attached to the fingernail distally and a small proximal hook attached to a plaster finger cylinder cast as recommended by Evans.[38] I have not found it necessary to immobilize the DIP joint for 4 weeks in acute lacerations over the PIP joint that include the central slip and lateral bands as advised by Lovett and McCalla.[77] Acute injuries that result in loss of significant substance in the extensor mechanism at this level may be treated by the methods previously described by Snow[118] and by Aiche, Barsky, and Weiner.[2] If these methods fail, a secondary reconstructive procedure is required as discussed in Chapter 53.

Zone III Thumb

MP Joint Level

Injuries at this level over the MP joint of the thumb may involve one or both of the extensor tendons (EPL and EPB). Isolated injury of the EPB usually results in some loss of extension of the MP joint that may be immediate or late. Acute lacerations of these tendons may be repaired by suturing the tendons with a buried core-type suture and the capsule, if involved, with interrupted sutures. Closed injuries at this level are rare in the nonrheumatoid patient, although I have seen boutonnière-like deformities in the thumb with flexion of the MP joint and hyperextension of the IP joint in older males who perform heavy labor.

Postoperative management includes maintaining the wrist in 40 degrees extension and slight radial deviation with the thumb MP joint in full extension for 3 to 4 weeks. If the EPL is injured, the thumb should be held in extension and slight abduction with a dynamic traction sling over the IP joint that allows controlled active flexion of the MP and IP joints, following the principles and methods of Evans.[38] Hung and colleagues[54] do not begin MP joint flexion until the third week (see Table 52-1). If only the EPB is injured, the IP joint may be left free and the dynamic traction sling placed beneath the MP joint to maintain it in full extension. Additional splint protection is used for 2 weeks.

Zone IV Finger

Proximal Phalanx

Injuries at this level are usually partial lacerations of the extensor mechanism because of the broad configuration of the tendon over the curved shape of the underlying phalanx and consequent protection of the lateral bands.[94,138] These partial injuries can be diagnosed only by direct inspection.[92,94] Laceration of an isolated lateral band may be repaired with fine nonabsorbable suture and early protected motion started. Complete lacerations of the central tendon should be repaired with fine nonabsorbable suture since relative lengthening of the central tendon may occur with resultant imbalance between the central slip and the lateral bands. The PIP joint should be maintained in full extension for 6 weeks as in the boutonnière injury over the PIP joint. The DIP joint is left free for flexion exercises.

Zone IV Thumb

Metacarpal Level

At this level the EPB and EPL are easily distinguished and can be repaired with a buried core type suture. Postoperative management is the same as in Zone III thumb injuries.

Zone V Finger

MP Joint Level

Human Bite Wounds

Injuries at this level are most often associated with open wounds. A small penetrating wound over the MP joint may be due to striking someone in the mouth with a clenched fist, and a careful history must be taken. Most, if not all, patients will deny this mechanism of injury. This is a contaminated wound, and the organisms involved are capable of producing a significant wound infection. Gram-positive bacteria (usually streptococci and staphylococci) are most frequently cultured. The incidence of gram-negative organisms is lower; they are usually found in association with gram-positive organisms. The incidence of complications is directly related to the time span from injury to treatment.[26] A radiograph should be obtained to note the presence or absence of fracture or foreign body. The wound must be extended proximally and distally to permit inspection of the joint, and a culture should be taken. The wound is debrided, irrigated, and *left open.* Appropriate antibiotics should be started immediately (preferably preoperatively).[104] Under no circumstances should a human bite wound be closed.[6,80] Most tendon injuries associated with this type of wound are partial and need not be repaired immediately. The hand is splinted with the wrist in 40 to 45 degrees extension and the MP joints in 15 to 20 degrees flexion. The soft tissues, including the capsule and extensor hood, are allowed to seek their own position over the joint. Partial or even complete lacerations are seldom if ever associated with significant retraction at this level. The tendon laceration may be repaired secondarily as needed in 5 to 7 days or even later, depending on the nature of the wound at the time of inspection. When the infection is under control, dynamic splinting should be started.

Simple Lacerations

Simple lacerations of the extensor tendon or hood at the MP joint level should be repaired using simple sutures of nonabsorbable material. Injuries of the extensor tendon at this level are not associated with retraction of the ends, and tendon suture followed by dynamic splinting is appropriate treatment using the method described by Browne and Ribik[9] or Evans.[38] Lacerations of the hood or sagittal bands at this level must be repaired so that the extensor tendon will remain centralized over the dorsum of the joint. Failure to repair this type of injury may result in subluxation of the extensor tendon and associated loss of extension. Buried interrupted sutures of 4–0 or 5–0 nylon are usually sufficient to repair these lacerations. Gentle flexion and extension exercises are started in 3 to 5 days. Abduction and adduction motions are avoided and these forces are minimized by "buddy strapping" the injured and an adjacent finger together.

Traumatic Dislocation of Extensor Tendon (Rupture of Extensor Hood)

Subluxation or dislocation of the extensor tendon may occur at the MP joint following laceration of the hood, or may occur following forceful flexion or extension injury of the finger.[33,56,62] In traumatic dislocation without laceration, the middle finger is most commonly involved. The lesion is secondary to a tear of the sagittal band and oblique fibers of the hood, usually on the radial side, although rupture of the ulnar sagittal band and radial dislocation has been reported.[62,107] Ulnar dislocation is the usual finding and is associated with incomplete finger extension and ulnar deviation of the involved digit[62,147] (Fig. 52-12). The middle finger is most commonly involved. This may be due to an inherent anatomic weakness, since the extensor tendon of the long finger is situated on top of the transverse fibers and has a comparatively loose attachment at this level.[62] Ishizuki, in a series of 16 cases all involving the middle finger, classified 5 as traumatic and 11 as spontaneous according to the provoking cause. Those classified as spontaneous had no history of trauma and occurred during a common daily activity such as flicking the finger or crumpling paper. Traumatic dislocations were caused by a direct blow or forced flexion of the MP joint as a result of a contusion or fall.[56] Ishizuki identified a superficial and deep layer of the sagittal band and noted disruption of only the superficial layer in spontaneous cases and *both layers* in traumatic cases. Thirteen of 16 cases were treated by local repair and three cases by a junctura tendinum reinforcement as described by Wheeldon.[56,147] Postoperative management included a splint with the MP joint in neutral or slight flexion for 4 weeks. Although acute tears can be satisfactorily treated by primary suture of the defect,[50,62] Ritts, Wood, and Engber reported two cases of acute traumatic dislocation of the middle finger extensor, one with ulnar subluxation and one with radial subluxation that were successfully treated by plaster cast immobilization with the MP joints in full extension for 4 weeks. These two cases were unique in that diagnosis and treatment was made within hours of the injury.[107] Carroll, Moore, and Weiland similarly reported four cases of ulnar subluxation treated successfully by 6 weeks of splinting of the MP joint in 0 degrees extension. The four successful cases were compared to five fingers that were either diagnosed long after the injury or had failed initial splinting who required reconstructive surgery.[16] These authors agreed with Bunnell that initial treatment should be nonoperative.[12,16] The authors described the successful use of a portion of the extensor tendon as a sling around the radial collateral ligament and noted its similarity to a procedure described by Kilgore et al.[64] If primary suture is not possible, the transverse fibers of the hood are anchored to the MP joint capsule.[62] Reefing of the radial fibers over the hood, along with release of the ulnar side of the hood, also

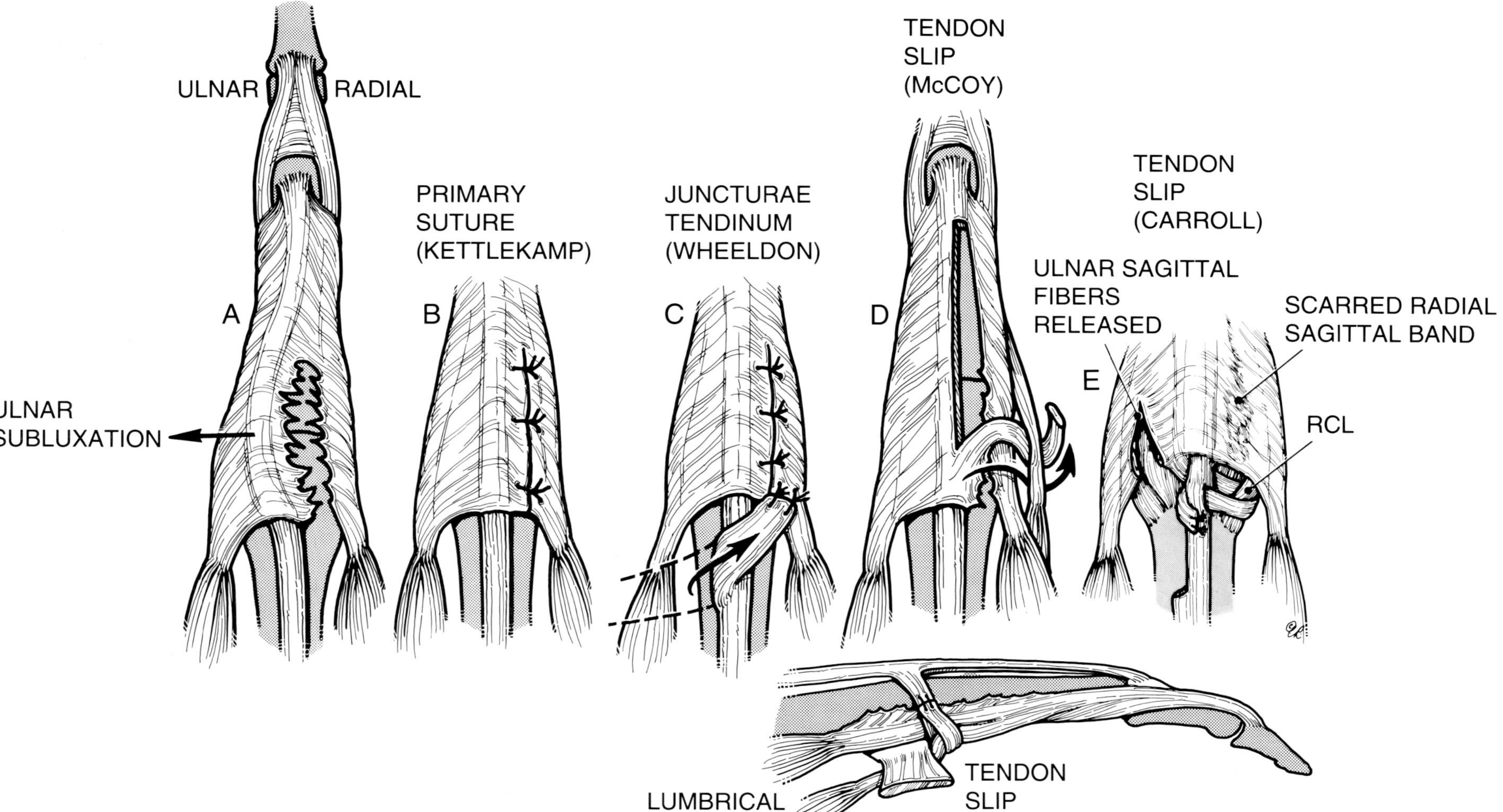

Fig. 52-12. Subluxation or dislocation of the extensor tendon at the MP joint may occur following laceration of the hood or following forceful flexion or extension of the finger. The lesion is secondary to a tear of the radial portion of the sagittal band **(A),** which allows ulnar subluxation of the extensor tendon. Acute or fresh injuries are satisfactorily treated by primary suture of the defect in the hood and sagittal band **(B).** Late cases may require additional reconstruction. Wheeldon[147] has described a method using a portion of the junctura tendinum to stabilize the tendon over the dorsum of the joint **(C).** The junctura is lapped over the extensor tendon and sutured to the joint capsule on the radial side. McCoy and Winsky[84] have also devised a technique **(D)** for stabilizing the extensor by removing a portion of the extensor tendon on the radial side of the finger, passing it around the lumbrical tendon, and suturing it back to itself. **(E)** Carroll and colleagues[16] modified a technique originally described by Kilgore et al[64] for stabilizing the extensor by forming a distally based slip of tendon from the ulnar side of the extensor digitorum communis (*EDC*), wrapping it around the radial collateral ligament (*RCL*) and then suturing it back to itself under proper tension. *(Figure continues.)*

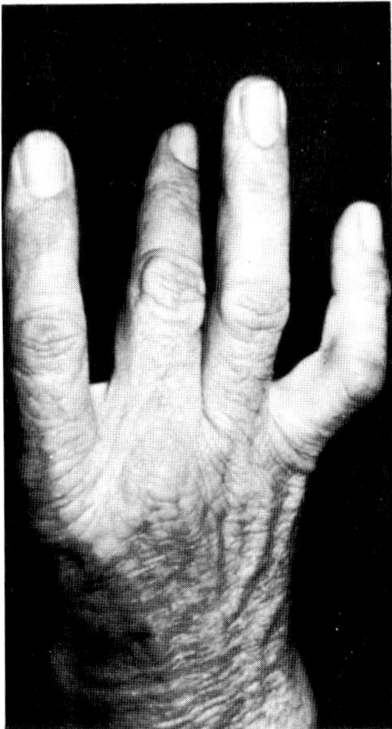

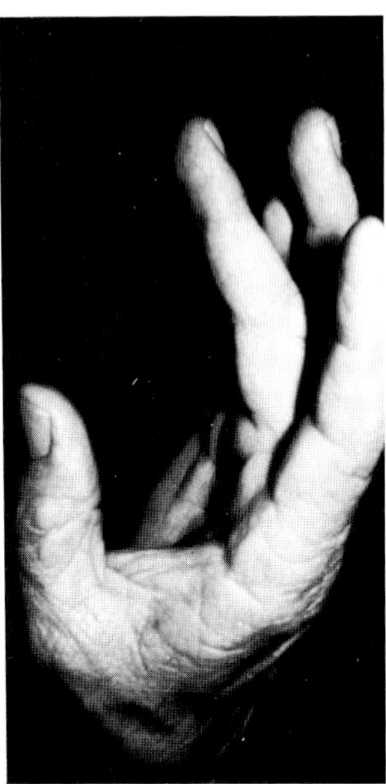

Fig. 52-12 *(Continued).* **(F&G)** The clinical picture of ulnar subluxation of the extensor tendon in the long finger.

provides an acceptable repair.[62] The tendon must be accurately centered over the MP joint, and the repair must be strong enough to resist recurrence of the subluxation during flexion of the finger. If the radial portion of the hood is absent or not suitable for repair, some type of tether must be made to centralize the tendon. A portion of junctura tendinum may be used for this purpose; it is lapped over the extensor and sutured to the joint capsule on the radial side.[147] A retrograde slip of extensor may also be used and is anchored to the deep transverse intermetacarpal ligament[33] or passed around the lumbrical tendon and sutured back to itself[84] (see Fig. 52-12).

Author's Preferred Method for Treatment of Extensor Tendon Dislocation

Although early splinting has been reported to be successful in the management of traumatic dislocation of the extensor tendon, my personal preference is to repair the acute tears in the sagittal band followed by splinting for four weeks of the involved MP joint in 15 to 20 degrees flexion. The PIP joint is left free for exercises.

Chronic cases are treated by recentralization of the EDC by first releasing the ulnar sagittal band as needed. The tendon is then stabilized by either a tether made from a portion of an adjacent junctura tendinum[147] or a slip of the EDC passed around the radial collateral ligament[16] (see Fig. 52-12). Tension on the repair is adjusted to allow normal flexion of the MP joint while maintaining centralization of the tendon throughout flexion and extension. Active ROM and stability can be checked easily if the patient is under local anesthesia. Postoperatively, only the involved digit is splinted. Both the MP and PIP joints are held in 15 to 20 degrees flexion. The MP joint is splinted for a total of 4 weeks but active PIP joint motion is started at 2 weeks.

Zone V Thumb

CMC Joint Area

Injuries in this area involve lacerations of the EPB and APL, the latter having two to four tendon slips. Associated structures that may also be injured are the sensory branches of the radial nerve and the radial artery in the anatomic snuff box. The tendons are repaired with a buried core suture. If the APL is lacerated near its insertion into the thumb metacarpal it should be firmly reattached to the bone without undue shortening of the tendon. Postoperative management includes immobilization of the wrist in 40 to 45 degrees extension and slight radial deviation for 5 weeks followed by 2 weeks of splint protection. Dynamic splinting is applied to the thumb to maintain it in extension and moderate abduction using a traction sling just distal to the MP joint. Active flexion of the MP joint as described by Browne and Ribik is performed.[9]

Zone VI Finger

Metacarpal Level

Zone VI injuries have been noted to have a better prognosis than more distal lesions (Zones II to V).[54,93] This may be due to the fact that (1) Zone VI injuries are unlikely to have associated joint injuries, (2) decreased tendon surface area in Zone VI lessens the potential for adhesion formation,[93] (3) increased subcutaneous tissue lessens the potential for adhesions, (4) there is greater tendon excursion in Zone VI, and (5) complex tendon imbalances are less likely to occur.

The extensor tendons in this zone have sufficient substance to accept substantial buried core type sutures, and dynamic splinting can be performed with the assurance that disruption of the suture site is unlikely.

Postoperative management includes dynamic splinting beginning at 3 to 5 days with the wrist in 40 to 45 degrees of extension and the MP joints in 0 to 15 degrees flexion for 5 weeks. The treatment protocol of Evans and Burkhalter is followed[38,39] (see page 1929).

Secretan's Disease (Peritendinous Fibrosis)

In 1901, Henri Secretan[115] described 11 cases of persistent hard edema on the dorsum of the hand associated with work-related injuries. All patients were covered by worker's compensation insurance, sustained trauma not sufficient to produce fracture, and had prolonged symptoms and findings. This condition has been called dorsal hard edema of the hand, peritendinous fibrosis of the dorsum of the hand, and factitious lymphedema of the hand.[105,106,117] Typically, a worker, usually male, describes a blow to the dorsum of the hand without fracture or laceration and then develops firm, persistent swelling over the back of the hand with subsequent loss of finger flexion and prolonged time out of work. Since Secretan's 1901 report, controversy has developed regarding the etiology and treatment of this condition.

Etiology

A number of factors have been reported in association with this condition including (1) proven or suspected self-inflicted trauma such as repeated blows to the back of the hand or application of tourniquets, (2) compensable work-related injuries, and (3) neurosis, psychosis, or suicidal tendency.[76,117] Boyes surmised that this condition is an example of reflex dystrophy in which edema is the major sign, just as pain is the principal finding in causalgia.[7] Bureau et al[13] stated that this condition is a form of reflex vasomotor edema. In 1969, Omer et al[96] reported their experimental efforts to produce this condition in monkeys by blunt trauma, injection of autologous blood, and tight wrist to elbow cast to cause venous and lymphatic obstruction. No one single modality produced the condition but any two in combination did produce the lesion.

Treatment

Most authors advise nonoperative management of this condition. Boyes[7] advised studious neglect, avoiding all passive manipulation, heat, and massage but encouraging patient exercise by voluntary means. Saferin and Posch[111] noted poor results in three patients operated on to excise this lesion. They observed prolonged disability of 2 to 5 years and advised splinting and active exercise as treatment. Bureau et al[13] reported 2 patients who had excision of the mass and failed to improve; they advocated gentle therapy and relaxation techniques. They also noted encouraging results with steroid injections in two cases. Reading[105] described four cases of hard edema of the dorsum of the hand who had resection of the lesions by other surgeons. Each demonstrated prolonged difficulties in healing and none was improved by surgery. All hands improved when protected by a plaster dressing. Redfern et al[106] described their experience with this condition in 15 patients in which 13 had excision of a dorsal fibroma (dense fibrous tissue with vascular proliferation, thickened vessel walls, an occasional organized intravascular thrombus and perivascular lymphocytic infiltration) and extensor tenolysis when necessary. Eleven of 15 patients were able to return to work. The average time from injury to return to work was 14 months. Almost all authors have noted a prolonged recovery time and a high recurrence rate with or without surgery. Louis[76] and Smith[117] agree that confrontation of the patient with factitious disease is dangerous for the patient and the doctor.

Author's Preferred Method of Treatment

This condition must be recognized as a factitious illness. Patients with factitious illnesses are not feigning illness, they are causing it.[76,117] Confrontation in the form of accusation can be potentially harmful to both the patient and doctor and should be avoided.[76,117] The physical problem or lesion may resolve when compensation is terminated. In spite of the report by Redfern et al,[106] this is *not* a surgical lesion. Best results have been achieved by psychotherapy.[105] Protective casting, although it may result in immediate improvement and confirm a diagnostic impression, may not be effective as definitive treatment. However, this technique may demonstrate to the therapist or patient on some level (conscious or unconscious) the self-inflicted nature of the problem.[105] Active physical therapy may be useful in many cases in conjunction with psychotherapy.

Zone VII

Wrist Level

Injuries of the extensor mechanism at the wrist level are associated with damage to the retinaculum.[3,5,31,112] The retinaculum prevents bowstringing of the extensor tendons, and lacerations of the extensors at this level are said to be associated with subsequent adhesions to the overlying retinaculum.[5,31,38,39] For this reason, many authors in the past have advised that *portions* of the extensor retinaculum located over the site of tendon repair should be excised to prevent adhesions.[3,31,77,112] However, Newport, Blair, and Steyers[93] noted no statistical differences in their results when comparing Zones VI, VII, and VIII. They repaired each retinacular rent primarily and used traditional postoperative immobilization. The excellent results with early dynamic splinting noted by Browne and Ribik,[9] Evans,[38] Evans and Burkhalter,[39] and Hung and colleagues[54] suggest that excision of portions of the retinaculum over the tendon repair site may not be as important as previously believed. However, it is my opinion that limited excision of portions of the retinaculum does no harm and may facilitate tendon exposure and gliding, especially in those repairs in which there might be some impingement between the suture site and the adjacent retinaculum. If the surgeon is concerned about maintaining the anatomic integrity of the retinaculum, the traumatic openings in the retinaculum may be extended distally and proximally at each end of the retinacular laceration to facilitate tendon repair and then reapproximated. The tendon (tendons) is repaired using a standard core-type suture of appropriate nonabsorbable material. The adequacy of retinacular restraint is verified by passive flexion and extension of the fingers and wrist. Multiple tendon injuries at this level may be dealt with by appropriate excision of the retinaculum as needed. Portions of the retinaculum should be preserved either proximal or distal to the suture line to prevent bowstringing; this is usually technically feasible to do. Although it has been recommended that complete excision of the extensor retinaculum be performed in lacerations at multiple levels,[31] it is my opinion that complete excision of the retinaculum is seldom if ever necessary even in this type of injury. Some portion of the retinaculum can usually be preserved, and adhesions that limit function are unlikely, especially if early dynamic splinting is utilized.[9,38,39] The anatomy of the area must be well understood; Figure 52-1 demonstrates the appropriate anatomic relationships in this area. Tendons lacerated at this level retract, and traumatic wounds must be extended proximally and distally to find the tendon ends. In addition to injury by laceration, the extensor tendons may rupture following a closed fracture or dislocate following injury to the retinaculum. The EPL and EDC tendons may rupture following a Colles' fracture, and the extensor carpi ulnaris (ECU) tendon may dislocate ulnarward with forceful supination, palmar flexion and ulnar deviation.[29,35,78,82,110] Itoh et al[57] noted extensor tendon entrapment and rupture in Smith's and Galeazzi's fractures. In one case of Smith's fracture the EIP tendon was entrapped and ruptured and in another case the EDC of the index was lacerated by a fracture fragment. In a third case of Smith's fracture the long extensor tendons of the thumb and index were trapped beneath a dorsally displaced fracture fragment, making closed reduction impossible.

In Galeazzi's fracture the ECU was trapped between the dorsally displaced ulnar head and avulsed ulnar styloid in one case and in the other the extensor digiti minimi tendon was caught beneath the radial border of the dorsally dislocated ulnar head.[57] Impending rupture of the EPL has been treated by subcutaneous transposition from its canal.[10] Treatment of acute ruptures of the EPL tendon is by transfer of the EIP tendon (or intercalary graft) and the ruptured communis tendons by intercalary graft or suturing of the distal tendon stump to adjacent extensor tendons (see Chapter 53). Dislocation of the ECU tendon is treated by repair of the fibroosseous sheath with a free tendon graft or a portion of the extensor retinaculum[29] (see Chapter 24).

Author's Recommended Postoperative Treatment for Zone VII Injuries

Postoperative management of lacerations of the digital extensors is the same as for Zone VI. Postoperative management of lacerations of the extensor carpi radialis longus (ECRL) and brevis (ECRB) and ECU includes immobilization of the wrist at 40 to 45 degrees extension for 4 to 5 weeks with the fingers free.

Progressive active and gentle passive range of motion is started after 4 to 5 weeks and a night splint with the wrist in 40 to 45 degrees extension is used for an additional 2 weeks.

Injuries of the EPL in Zone VII are treated by postoperative dynamic splinting as described for Zone V thumb injuries.

Zone VIII

Distal Forearm Level

Injuries at the muscle tendon junction require careful reapproximation of the separated parts. Although the distal tendon accepts and holds sutures well, the proximal muscle belly does not, and reapproximation of the separated parts is facilitated by multiple nonabsorbable sutures that coapt the tendon and muscle together. Tendons characteristically originate from a fibrous tissue raphe in the substance of the muscle belly several centimeters proximal to the area where the tendon is grossly identifiable as a distinct structure. To obtain a significant purchase on the muscle belly with the sutures, these septa should be identified and the sutures placed in this fibrous tissue area as much as possible in order to keep the sutures from pulling out. The knots are buried between the tendon and the muscle. Care is taken to avoid strangulation of the muscle with the sutures, which may cause necrosis of the muscle. Small absorbable sutures may be used to repair the fascial margins of the muscle. Postoperative management includes static immobilization of the wrist in 40 to 45 degrees of extension, and the MPs in 15 to 20 degrees of flexion for 4 to 5 weeks. Flexion of the MP joints may be started at 2 weeks against elastic traction resistance. A static night splint that maintains the wrist in extension is used for an additional 2 weeks. The thumb is splinted in extension and moderate abduction if the EPL, EPB, or APB are involved. Thumb MP joint flexion may be started against elastic traction at 2 weeks.

Zone IX

Proximal Forearm Level

The wrist and common finger extensors, as well as the little finger proprius, arise from the region of the lateral epicondyle at the elbow. The thumb extensors and abductors, along with the proprius tendon of the index finger, arise from the forearm below the elbow. Injuries at this level are usually due to a penetrating wound with a knife or piece of broken glass. The size of the skin wound may give little indication of the magnitude of the injury. Single or multiple functional units may be injured. The demonstrated loss of function may be due to muscle transection, nerve injury, or both. Such loss of function in a penetrating injury in the proximal forearm may defy accurate preoperative diagnosis. The radial nerve at the level of the distal arm gives off branches to the brachialis, brachioradialis, and extensor carpi radialis longus. A major division of this nerve then occurs into the sensory branch and posterior interosseous nerve (motor branch). The superficial (sensory) branch continues distally under cover of the brachioradialis into the forearm, wrist, and hand areas. The posterior interosseous nerve gives branches to the ECRB and supinator, which it penetrates and supplies, and then innervates the remainder of the extensor muscle group.

A penetrating wound in the proximal one-third of the forearm with functional loss must be carefully explored to determine the exact etiology of the loss. Under tourniquet control and appropriate anesthesia, the wound margins are debrided and then extended proximally and distally and the extent of damage is noted. If it can be determined that the wounds extend only into the muscle belly, a careful repair of the muscle belly is performed with multiple figure-of-eight sutures of polyglactin (Vicryl-Ethicon). Experimental data on repaired muscle lacerations in laboratory animals (rabbits) imply that useful but not complete function can be restored with adequate repair of skeletal muscle.[44] A muscle segment totally isolated from its motor point may not contribute to the contractile function of the innervated muscle.[44] Botte et al,[4] in a series of patients with forearm flexor muscle lacerations, noted that tendon grafting was an effective method of repair to overcome extensive defects. Their indications for the technique were laceration of two or more muscle bellies with at least 50 percent of the muscle substance lacerated. The palmaris longus or long toe extensor were utilized and passed through the superficial epimysium, muscle belly, and deep epimysium proximally and distally and sutured to themselves with a Pulvertaft side-weave technique. One to three grafts were used as required. The limb was immobilized for 3 weeks with the elbow at 90 degrees. Protected motion was started at 3 weeks and progressive motion at 6 weeks. If there is evidence of nerve involvement, the appropriate branches are identified and traced out to their insertions. Penetrating wounds may often injure the nerve at or near its entrance into the muscle belly. Retraction of the distal nerve stump into the muscle belly may occur and defy location and subsequent repair. Many times it is impossible to determine nerve damage at the time of surgery in the immediate postinjury period. However, after 7 to 10 days a denervated muscle will spontaneously contract for several minutes under the influence of succinylcholine used during induction of general anesthesia.[25] Additional information may be gained by electrodiagnostic studies 3 to 4 weeks following injury. The decision for secondary nerve repair or reconstruction versus tendon transfer will depend on the judgment and experience of the surgeon.

If the lesion is confined to the muscle belly, definitive repair is carried out using sutures or tendon graft and sutures as previously described.[4,44] The muscle is usually quite hemorrhagic and muscle planes are difficult to identify. Identification is aided by evacuation of the hematoma, irrigation, and gentle sponging of the cut muscle ends. The identification of intramuscular fibrous septa and fascia for placement of sutures will aid in preventing the sutures from pulling out of the muscle. Coaptation of the cut ends of those muscles that arise at or distal to the elbow is facilitated by wrist extension.

Postoperative Management

Postoperatively, the extremity is supported in a plaster splint or cast that maintains the wrist in 45 degrees extension (dorsiflexion) and the MP joints in 15 to 20 degrees flexion. The elbow joint is immobilized in 90 degrees flexion if the muscles involved arise at or above the lateral epicondyle. Immobilization is continued for 4 weeks postinjury, and then protected range of motion is permitted but a night splint is used to maintain the wrist in extension for another 2 weeks.

REFERENCES

1. Abouna JM, Brown H: The treatment of mallet finger, the results in a series of 148 consecutive cases and a review of the literature. Br J Surg 55:653–667, 1968
2. Aiche A, Barsky AJ, Weiner DL: Prevention of boutonnière deformity. Plast Reconstr Surg 46:164–167, 1979
3. Blue AI, Spira M, Hardy SB: Repair of extensor tendon injuries of the hand. Am J Surg 132:128–132, 1976
4. Botte MJ, Gelberman RH, Smith DG, Silver MA, Gellman H: Repair of severe muscle belly lacerations using a tendon graft. J Hand Surg 12A:406–412, 1987
5. Boyes JH: Bunnell's Surgery of the Hand, 4th Ed. pp. 469–470. JB Lippincott, Philadelphia, 1964
6. Boyes JH: Bunnell's Surgery of the Hand, 5th Ed. pp. 439–442, 616–618. JB Lippincott, Philadelphia, 1970
7. Boyes JH: Bunnell's Surgery of the Hand, 5th Ed. p. 653. JB Lippincott, Philadelphia, 1970
8. Boyes JH: Boutonniere deformity (discussion). p. 56. In Cramer LM, Chase RA (eds): Symposium on the Hand. Vol 3. CV Mosby, St. Louis, 1971
9. Browne EZ Jr, Ribik CA: Early dynamic splinting for extensor tendon injuries. J Hand Surg 14A:72–76, 1989
10. Bunata RE: Impending rupture of the extensor pollicis longus tendon after a minimally displaced Colles fracture. A case report. J Bone Joint Surg 65A:401–402, 1983
11. Bunnell SB: Surgery of the Hand. 1st Ed. pp. 490–493. JB Lippincott, Philadelphia, 1944
12. Bunnell SB: Surgery of the Hand, 3rd Ed. pp. 470–471. JB Lippincott, Philadelphia, 1964
13. Bureau H, Decaillet J, Magalon G: Le syndrome de Secretan existe-t-il. Sem Hop Paris 55:449, 1979
14. Burke F: Mallet finger (editorial). J Hand Surg 13B:115–117, 1988
15. Carducci AT: Potential boutonnière deformity. Its recognition and treatment. Orthop Rev 10:121–123, 1981
16. Carroll C IV, Moore JR, Weiland AJ: Posttraumatic ulnar subluxation of the extensor tendons: A reconstructive technique. J Hand Surg 12A:227–231, 1987
17. Casscells SW, Strange TB: Intramedullary wire fixation of mallet finger. J Bone Joint Surg 39A:521–526, 1957
18. Casscells SW, Strange TB: Intramedullary wire fixation of mallet finger. J Bone Joint Surg 51A:1018–1019, 1969
19. Caudwell EW, Anson BJ, Wright RR: The extensor indicis proprius muscle. A study of 263 consecutive specimens. Quart Bull Northwestern Univ M School 17:267–279, 1963
20. Chase RA: Boutonniere deformity (discussion). p. 56. In Cramer LM, Chase RA (eds): Symposium on the Hand. Vol 3. CV Mosby, St. Louis, 1971
21. Chow JA, Dovelle S, Thomas LJ, Callahan D: Postoperative management of repair of extensor tendons of the hand—dynamic splinting versus static splinting. Orthop Trans 11(2):258–259, 1987
22. Crawford GP: The molded polythene splint for mallet finger deformities. J Hand Surg 9A:231–237, 1984
23. Cusenz BJ, Hallock GG: Multiple anomalous tendons of the fourth dorsal compartment. J Hand Surg 11A:263–264, 1986
24. Din KM, Meggitt BF: Mallet thumb. J Bone Joint Surg 65B:606–607, 1983
25. Doyle JR, Semenza J, Gilling B: The effect of succinylcholine on denervated skeletal muscle. J Hand Surg 6:40–42, 1981
26. Dreyfuss UY, Singer M: Human bites of the hand: A study of one hundred six patients. J Hand Surg 10A:884–889, 1985
27. Duran RJ, Houser RG, Stover MG: Management of flexor tendon lacerations in zone 2 using controlled passive motion postoperatively. pp. 217–224. In Hunter JM, Schneider LH, Mackin EJ, Bell JA (eds): Rehabilitation of the Hand. CV Mosby, St. Louis, 1978
28. Eaton RG: The extensor mechanism of the fingers. Bull Hosp Joint Dis 30:39–47, 1969
29. Eckhardt WA, Palmer AK: Recurrent dislocation of the extensor carpi ulnaris tendon. J Hand Surg 6:629–631, 1981
30. Edmonson AS, Crenshaw AH: Campbell's Operative Orthopedics. 6th Ed. pp. 162–163. CV Mosby, St. Louis, 1980
31. Elliott RA: Injuries to the extensor mechanism of the hand. Orthop Clin North Am 1:335–354, 1970
32. Elliott RA: Splints for mallet and boutonniere deformities. Plast Reconstr Surg 52:282–285, 1973
33. Elson RA: Dislocation of the extensor tendons of the hand. Report of a case. J Bone Joint Surg 49B:324–326, 1967
34. Engelbrecht JA: A method for repair of extensor tendons. S Afr Med J 40:623, 1966
35. Engkvist O, Lundborg G: Rupture of the extensor pollicis longus tendon after fracture of the lower end of the radius—a clinical and microangiographic study. Hand 11:76–86, 1979

36. Entin MA: Repair of the extensor mechanism of the hand. Surg Clin North Am 40:275–285, 1960
37. Evans D, Weightman B: The pipflex splint for treatment of mallet finger. J Hand Surg 13B:156–158, 1988
38. Evans RB: Therapeutic management of extensor tendon injuries. Hand Clin 2:157–169, 1986
39. Evans RB, Burkhalter WE: A study of the dynamic anatomy of extensor tendons and implications for treatment. J Hand Surg 11A:774–779, 1986
40. Flatt AE: The Care of Minor Hand Injuries 4th Ed. CV Mosby, St. Louis, 1979
41. Flinchum D: Mallet finger. J Med Assoc Ga 48:601–603, 1959
42. Froehlich JA, Akelman E, Herndon JH: Extensor tendon injuries at the proximal interphalangeal joint. Hand Clin 4:25–37, 1988
43. Furlow LT Jr: Early active motion in flexor tendon healing (abstract). J Bone Joint Surg 54A:911, 1972
44. Garrett WE Jr, Seaber AV, Boswick J, Urbaniak JR, Goldner JL: Recovery of skeletal muscle after laceration and repair. J Hand Surg 9A:683–692, 1984
45. Gelberman RH, Woo SL-Y, Lothringer K, Akeson WH, Amiel D: Effects of early intermittent passive mobilization on healing canine flexor tendons. J Hand Surg 7:170–175, 1982
46. Green DP, Rowland SA: Fractures and dislocations in the hand. pp. 446–453. In Rockwood CA, Green DP (eds): Fractures. 3rd. Ed. JB Lippincott, Philadelphia, 1991
47. Hallberg D, Lindholm A: Subcutaneous rupture of the extensor tendon of the distal phalanx of the finger: "Mallet finger." Brief review of the literature and report on 127 cases treated conservatively. Acta Chir Scand 119:260–267, 1960
48. Hamas RS, Horrell ED, Pierret GP: Treatment of mallet finger due to intra-articular fracture of the distal phalanx. J Hand Surg 3:361–363, 1978
49. Harris C, Rutledge GL Jr: The functional anatomy of the extensor mechanism of the finger. J Bone Joint Surg 54A:713–726, 1972
50. Harvey FJ, Hume KF: Spontaneous recurrent ulnar dislocation of the long extensor tendons of the fingers. J Hand Surg 5:492–494, 1980
51. Hillman FE: New technique for treatment of mallet fingers and fractures of the distal phalanx. JAMA 161:1135–1138, 1956
52. Hovgaard C, Klareskov B: Alternative conservative treatment of mallet-finger injuries by elastic double-finger bandage. J Hand Surg 13B:154–155, 1988
53. Howie H: The treatment of mallet finger: A modified plaster technique. NZ Med J 46:513, 1947
54. Hung LK, Chan A, Chang J, Tsang A, Leung PC: Early controlled active mobilization with dynamic splintage for treatment of extensor tendon injuries. J Hand Surg 15A:251–257, 1990
55. Hunter JM, Schneider LH, Mackin EJ, Bell JA: Rehabilitation of the Hand. CV Mosby, St. Louis, 1978
56. Ishizuki M: Traumatic and spontaneous dislocation of extensor tendon of the long finger. J Hand Surg 15A:967–972, 1990
57. Itoh Y, Horiuchi Y, Takahashi M, Uchinishi K, Yabe Y: Extensor tendon involvement in Smith's and Galeazzi's fractures. J Hand Surg 12A:535–540, 1987
58. Jones NF, Peterson J: Epidemiologic study of the mallet finger deformity. J Hand Surg 13A:334–338, 1988
59. Kaplan EB: Anatomy, injuries and treatment of the extensor apparatus of the hand and fingers. Clin Orthop 13:24–41, 1959
60. Kaplan EB: Functional and Surgical Anatomy of the Hand. 2nd Ed. JB Lippincott, Philadelphia, 1965
61. Kelly AP: Primary tendon repairs. A study of 789 consecutive tendon severances. J Bone Joint Surg 41A:581–598, 1959
62. Kettelkamp DB, Flatt AE, Moulds R: Traumatic dislocation of the long finger extensor tendon. A clinical, anatomical, and biomechanical study. J Bone Joint Surg 53A:229–240, 1971
63. Kilgore ES, Graham WP: The Hand. Surgical and Nonsurgical Management. Lea & Febiger, Philadelphia, 1977
64. Kilgore ES, Graham WP, Newmeyer WL, Brown LG: Correction of ulnar subluxation of the extensor communis. Hand 7:272–284, 1975
65. King T: Injuries of the dorsal extensor mechanism of the fingers. Med J Aust 2:213–217, 1970
66. Kinninmonth AWG, Holburn F: A comparative controlled trial of a new perforated splint and a traditional splint in the treatment of mallet finger. J Hand Surg 11B:261–262, 1986
67. Kleinert HE, Kutz JE, Cohen MJ: Primary repair of zone II flexor tendon lacerations. pp. 91–104. In AAOS Symposium on Tendon Injury. CV Mosby, St. Louis, 1975
68. Kleinert HE, Verdan C: Report of the committee on tendon injuries. J Hand Surg 8:794–798, 1983
69. Landsmeer JMF: Anatomy of the dorsal aponeurosis of the human finger and its functional significance. Anat Rec 104:31–44, 1949
70. Landsmeer JMF: The coordination of finger joint motions. J Bone Joint Surg 45A:1654–1662, 1963
71. Lange RH, Engber WD: Hyperextension mallet finger. Orthopedics 6:1426–1431, 1983
72. Lewin P: A simple splint for baseball finger. JAMA 85:1059, 1925
73. Lister GD, Kleinert HE, Kutz JE, Atasoy E: Primary flexor tendon repair followed by immediate controlled mobilization. J Hand Surg 2:441–451, 1977
74. Littler JW: The finger extensor mechanism. Surg Clin North Am 47:415–423, 1967
75. Littler JW: A new method of treatment for mallet finger (commentary). Plast Reconstr Surg 58:499–500, 1976
76. Louis DS, Lamp MK, Greene TL: The upper extremity and psychiatric illness. J Hand Surg 10A:687–693, 1985
77. Lovett WL, McCalla MA: Management and rehabilitation of extensor tendon injuries. Orthop Clin North Am 14:811–826, 1983
78. Mackay I, Simpson RG: Closed rupture of extensor digitorum communis tendon following fracture of the radius. Hand 12:214–216, 1980
79. Madden JW: Wound healing: the biological basis of hand surgery. pp. 105–112. In Hunter JM, Schneider LH, Mackin EJ, Bell JA (eds): Rehabilitation of the Hand. CV Mosby, St. Louis, 1978
80. Mann RJ, Hoffeld TA, Farmer CB: Human bites of the hand: Twenty years experience. J Hand Surg 2:97–104, 1977
81. Manske PR, Lesker PA, Gelberman RH, Rucinsky TE: Intrinsic restoration of the flexor tendon surface in the nonhuman primate. J Hand Surg 10A:632–637, 1985
82. Mason ML: Rupture of the tendons of the hand. Surg Gynecol Obstet 50:611–624, 1930
83. Mason ML, Allen HS: The rate of healing of tendons: An experimental study of tensile strength. Ann Surg 113:424–459, 1941
84. McCoy FJ, Winsky AJ: Lumbrical loop operation for luxation of the extensor tendons of the hand. Plast Reconstr Surg 44:142–146, 1969
85. McFarlane RM, Hampole MK: Treatment of extensor tendon injuries of the hand. Can J Surg 16:366–375, 1973
86. Micks JE, Hager D: Role of the controversial parts of the extensor of the finger. J Bone Joint Surg 55A:884, 1973
87. Micks JE, Reswick JB: Confirmation of differential loading of lateral and central fibers of the extensor tendon. J Hand Surg 6:462–467, 1981
88. Milford LW: Retaining Ligaments of the Digits of the Hand. WB Saunders, Philadelphia, 1968
89. Miller H: Repair of severed tendons of the hand and wrist. Surg Gynecol Obstet 75:693–698, 1942

90. Miura T, Nakamura R, Torii S: Conservative treatment for a ruptured extensor tendon on the dorsum of the proximal phalanges of the thumb (mallet thumb). J Hand Surg 11A:229–233, 1986
91. Moore JR, Weiland AJ, Valdata L: Independent index extension after extensor indicis proprius transfer. J Hand Surg 12A:232–236, 1987
92. Newmeyer WL: Primary Care of Hand Injuries. Lea & Febiger, Philadelphia, 1979
93. Newport ML, Blair WF, Steyers CM Jr: Long-term results of extensor tendon repair. J Hand Surg 15A:961–966, 1990
94. Nichols HM: Manual of Hand Injuries. 2nd Ed. pp. 180–181, 191. Year Book Medical Publishers, Chicago, 1960
95. Nissenbaum M: Early care of flexor tendon injuries: application of principles of tendon healing and early motion. pp. 187–196. In Hunter JM, Schneider LH, Mackin EJ, Bell JA (eds): Rehabilitation of the Hand. CV Mosby, St. Louis, 1978
96. Omer GE Jr, Riordan DC, Conran PB, Winter R: Peritendinous fibrosis of the dorsum of the hand in monkeys. An experimental approach. Clin Orthop 62:251–259, 1969
97. Palmer AK, Skahen JR, Werner FW, Glisson RR: The extensor retinaculum of the wrist: An anatomical and biomechanical study. J Hand Surg 10B:11–16, 1985
98. Patel MR, Lipson L-B, Desai SS: Conservative treatment of mallet thumb. J Hand Surg 11A:45–47, 1986
99. Peacock EE: Repair of tendons and restoration of gliding function. pp. 263–331. In: Wound Repair. 3rd Ed. WB Saunders, Philadelphia, 1984
100. Pratt DR: Internal splint for closed and open treatment of injuries of the extensor tendon at the distal joint of the finger. J Bone Joint Surg 34A:785–788, 1952
101. Primiano GA: Conservative treatment of two cases of mallet thumb. J Hand Surg 11A:233–235, 1986
102. Ramsay RA: Mallet finger (letter). Lancet 2:1244, 1968
103. Rayan GM, Mullins PT: Skin necrosis complicating mallet finger splinting and vascularity of the distal interphalangeal joint overlying skin. J Hand Surg 12A:548–552, 1987
104. Rayan GM, Putnam JL, Cahill SL, Flournoy DJ: *Eikenella corrodens* in human mouth flora. J Hand Surg 13A:953–956, 1988
105. Reading G: Secretan's syndrome: hard edema of the dorsum of the hand. Plast Reconstr Surg 65:182–187, 1980
106. Redfern AB, Curtis RM, Wilgis EFS: Experience with peritendinous fibrosis of the dorsum of the hand. J Hand Surg 7:380–383, 1982
107. Ritts GD, Wood MB, Engber WD: Nonoperative treatment of traumatic dislocations of the extensor digitorum tendons in patients without rheumatoid disorders. J Hand Surg 10A:714–716, 1985
108. Robb WAT: The results of treatment of mallet finger. J Bone Joint Surg 41B:546–549, 1959
109. Rosenzweig N: Management of the mallet finger. S Afr Med J 24:831–832, 1950
110. Sadr B: Sequential rupture of extensor tendons after a Colles fracture. J Hand Surg 9A:144–145, 1984
111. Saferin EH, Posch JL: Secretan's disease, post-traumatic hard edema of the dorsum of the hand. Plast Reconstr Surg 58:703–707, 1976
112. Sakellarides HT: The extensor tendon injuries and the treatment. RI Med J 61:307–313, 1978
113. Schenck RR: Variations of the extensor tendons of the fingers. Surgical significance. J Bone Joint Surg 46A:103–110, 1964
114. Schultz RJ, Furlong J, Storace A: Detailed anatomy of the extensor mechanism at the proximal aspect of the finger. J Hand Surg 6:493–498, 1981
115. Secretan H: Oedeme dur et hyperplasie traumatique du metacarpe dorsal. Rev Med Suisse Romande 21:409, 1901
116. Smillie IS: Mallet finger. Br J Surg 24:439–445, 1937
117. Smith RJ: Factitious lymphedema of the hand. J Bone Joint Surg 57A:89–94, 1975
118. Snow JW: Use of a retrograde tendon flap in repairing a severed extensor tendon in the PIP joint area. Plast Reconstr Surg 51:555–558, 1973
119. Souter WA: The bountonniere deformity. A review of 101 patients with division of the central slip of the extensor expansion of the fingers. J Bone Joint Surg 49B:710–721, 1967
120. Spigelman L: New splint management of mallet finger. JAMA 153:1362, 1953
121. Spinner M, Choi BY: Anterior dislocation of the proximal interphalangeal joint, a cause of rupture of the central slip of the extensor mechanism. J Bone Joint Surg 52A:1329–1336, 1970
122. Stack HG: Muscle function in the fingers. J Bone Joint Surg 44B:899–909, 1962
123. Stack HG: Buttonhole deformity. Hand 3:152–154, 1971
124. Stack HG: A modified splint for mallet finger. J Hand Surg 11B:263, 1986
125. Stark HH: Troublesome fractures and dislocations of the hand. pp. 130–149. AAOS Instructional Course Lectures, Vol. 19. CV Mosby, St. Louis, 1970
126. Stark HH, Boyes JH, Wilson JN: Mallet finger. J Bone Joint Surg 44A:1061–1068, 1962
127. Steichen JB, Petersen DP: Junctura tendinum between extensor digitorum communis and extensor pollicis longus. J Hand Surg 9A:674–676, 1984
128. Stern PJ, Kastrup JJ: Complications and prognosis of treatment of mallet finger. J Hand Surg 13A:329–334, 1988
129. Stewart IM: Boutonniere finger. The Proceedings of the Second Hand Club. p. 87. 10th meeting, Nov. 1960
130. Stewart IM: Boutonniere finger. Clin Orthop 23:220–226, 1962
131. Strickland JW, Glogovac SV: Digital function following flexor tendon repair in zone II: A comparison of immobilization and controlled passive motion techniques. J Hand Surg 5:537–543, 1980
132. Stuart D: Duration of splinting after repair of extensor tendons in the hand: A clinical study. J Bone Joint Surg 47B:72–79, 1965
133. Taleisnik J, Gelberman RH, Miller BW, Szabo RM: The extensor retinaculum at the wrist. J Hand Surg 9A:495–501, 1984
134. Tubiana R: Surgical repair of the extensor apparatus of the fingers. Surg Clin North Am 48:1015–1031, 1968
135. Tubiana R, Valentin P: Anatomy of the extensor apparatus and the physiology of the finger extension. Surg Clin North Am 44:897–918, 1964
136. Valentin P: Physiology of extension of the fingers. In Tubiana R (ed): The Hand. WB Saunders, Philadelphia, 1981
137. Van Denmark RE: A simple method of treatment for recent mallet finger. Milit Surg 106:385–386, 1950
138. Verdan CE: Primary and secondary repair of flexor and extensor tendon injuries. p. 149. In Flynn, JE (ed): Hand Surgery. 2nd Ed. Williams & Wilkins, Baltimore, 1975
139. von Schroeder HP, Botte MJ, Gellman H: Anatomy of the juncturae tendinum of the hand. J Hand Surg 15A:595–602, 1990
140. Warren RA, Kay NRM, Norris SH: The microvascular anatomy of the distal digital extensor tendon. J Hand Surg 13B:161–163, 1988
141. Warren RA, Norris SH, Ferguson DG: Mallet finger: A trial of two splints. J Hand Surg 13B:151–153, 1988
142. Watson-Jones R: Fractures and Joint Injuries. 4th Ed. Vol. 2. p. 645. E & S Livingstone, Edinburgh, 1956
143. Weeks PM, Wray RC: Management of Acute Hand Injuries. A Biologic Approach. 2nd Ed. pp. 292–325. CV Mosby, St. Louis, 1978

144. Weeks PM, Wray RC: Tendon gliding and repair. pp. 76–108. In Management of Acute Hand Injuries: A Biological Approach. 2nd Ed. CV Mosby, St. Louis, 1978
145. Wehbe MA, Schneider LH: Mallet fractures. J Bone Joint Surg 66A:658–669, 1984
146. Weinberg H, Stein HC, Wexler M-R: A new method of treatment for mallet finger. A preliminary report. Plast Reconstr Surg 58:347–349, 1976
147. Wheeldon FT: Recurrent dislocation of extensor tendons. J Bone Joint Surg 36B:612–617, 1954
148. Williams EG: Treatment of mallet finger. Can Med Assoc J 57:582, 1947
149. Zancolli E: Structural and Dynamic Bases of Hand Surgery. pp. 105–106. JB Lippincott, Philadelphia, 1968

53

Extensor Tendons—Late Reconstruction

Richard I. Burton

ANATOMY AND FUNCTION

The function of the extensor tendon assembly has been described by Littler[76] as a "fugue of movement." The extensor mechanism is a system of subtlety, complex in its interrelationships, yet simple in that this tendon system extends three joints and flexes one joint.[62–67,76,78,80]

Simply cataloged, the finger *extrinsic* extensor system originates in the forearm, is radially innervated, and has four insertions (into the MP joint volar plate and into the dorsal base of each phalanx) (Fig. 53-1). The finger *intrinsic* system is composed of the seven interosseous and four lumbrical muscles, all passing volar to the axis of movement at the MP joints and then dorsal to the interphalangeal joints (Fig. 53-2), arborizing and interrelating with the components of the extrinsic extensor tendons (Fig. 53-3). The extrinsic extensors extend the finger MP joints, and the intrinsics flex the MP joints and extend the interphalangeal joints (Fig. 53-4).

The thumb, with its prerequisite for mobility with stability, has an independent extensor motor for each joint—extensor pollicis longus for the interphalangeal joint, extensor pollicis brevis for the MP joint, and abductor pollicis longus for the carpometacarpal joint. The thumb intrinsic musculotendinous units primarily provide rotational control of the thumb axis, although these muscles do also flex the MP joint and extend the interphalangeal joint. Because of this relatively independent control of each thumb joint, functional deficits are more straightforward to correct than most of the late disorders of the finger extensor system.

Certain general concepts about the function of the finger extensor tendon system merit emphasis. An understanding of these concepts will clarify the altered dynamics of established extensor mechanism disorders and permit rational treatment selection from the several options available.

1. *The movement of finger extension is synergistic with wrist flexion,* and the effective excursion of the extrinsic extensor tendons is increased by wrist flexion[22,76,78,80] (Fig. 53-5A and B). Thus, (1) active wrist control is important for normal finger extensor mechanics, (2) wrist flexors are excellent donor musculotendinous units for transfer to replace absent extrinsic extensors of the MP joints, and (3) such transfers will be more functional in the presence of active wrist motion with greater effective transfer excursion.
2. *Distal to the MP joint the extensor mechanism* (including extrinsic and intrinsic components) *is a single fascial-tendon expansion* with four firm attachments to fixed points—one insertion at the dorsal base of each phalanx (the distal and middle being stout and the proximal more tenuous) and the fourth into the MP joint volar plate via the sagittal (shroud) fibers.[76,80] Thus, this single aponeurotic tendon expansion, which must extend three joints, is secured to bone at all three joints with fixed tendon lengths between these points of fixation without any interposed muscular units (Fig. 53-6). This is very different from the flexor system, which has an independent flexor for each joint, each with a different excursion.
3. *This extensor tendon complex is based on a series of overlapping linkage systems*[22,76,80] (Fig. 53-5B). The components normally pass volar to the axis of rotation at one joint and dorsal to the next most distal joint—the intrinsic musculotendinous units at the MP and PIP joints and the oblique retinacular ligament at the PIP and DIP joints.[63–67,76,80]

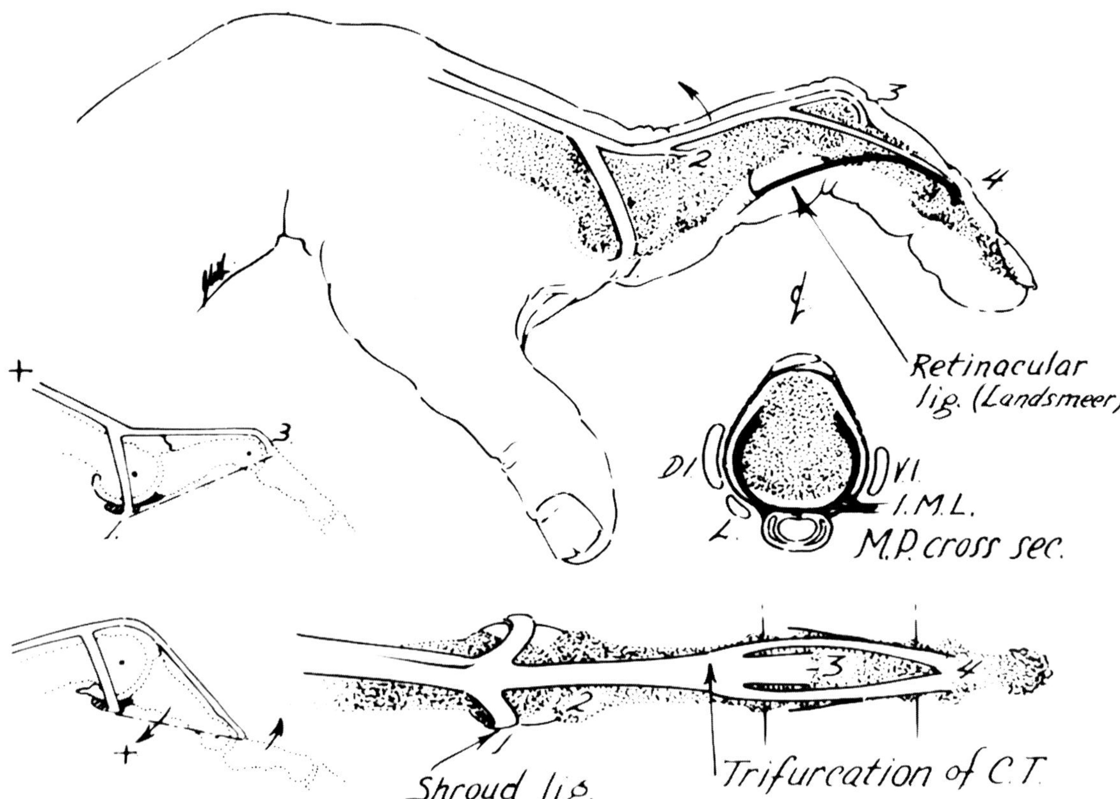

Fig. 53-1. The extrinsic extensor tendon system passes dorsal to the axis of motion at all three finger joints and has four insertions. Those into the dorsal base of the middle and distal phalanges are functionally the most important in a normal digit, although the insertion through the shroud fibers at the MP joint assumes prime importance in the pathomechanics of the claw hand. The prime functional insertion is into the dorsal base of the middle phalanx (see text and Fig. 53-11). (From Eaton,[22] with permission.)

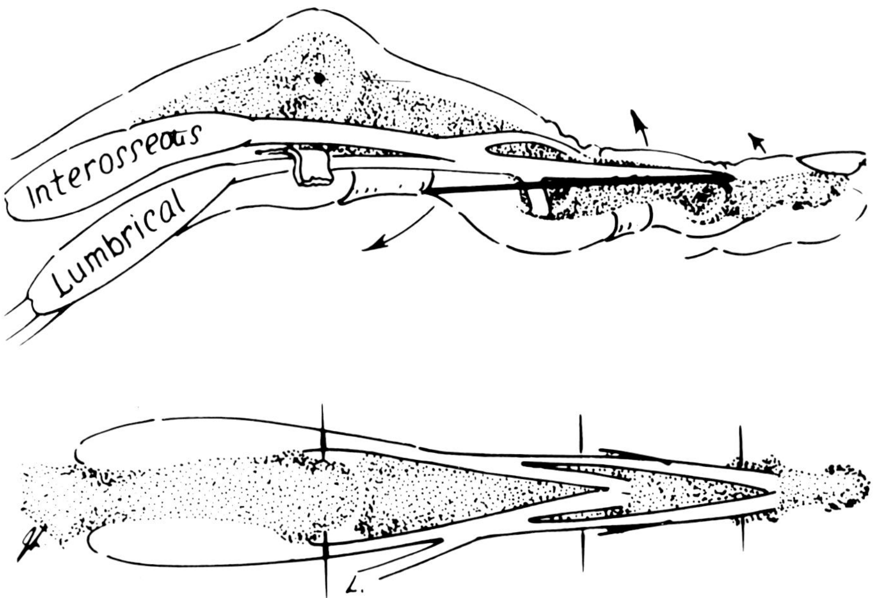

Fig. 53-2. The intrinsic musculotendinous systems are comprised of the interossei and lumbricals. The interossei abduct and adduct the fingers, as well as flex the MP joints and extend the interphalangeal joints. The lumbricals function as extensors of the interphalangeal joints. They pass volar to the axis of the MP joint and are thus flexors, as is attested to by the absence of the claw posture for the index and long fingers in the ulnar nerve deficient hand. (From Littler et al,[80] with permission.)

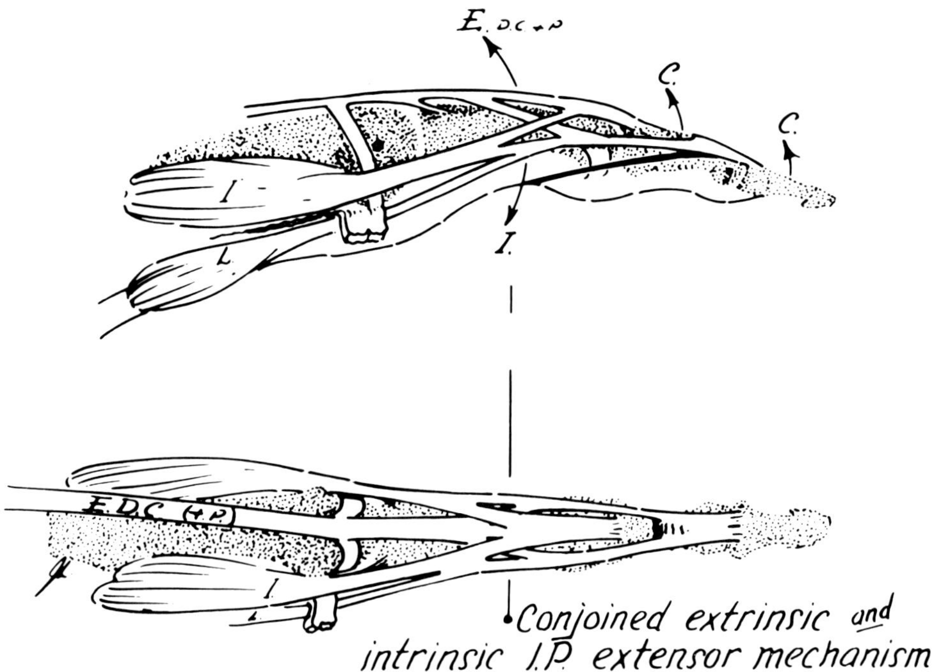

Fig. 53-3. The intrinsic and extrinsic extensor tendon systems arborize and interdigitate to form a complex of interconnected tendons spanning the three finger joints. As there is no longitudinal elasticity or motor unit distal to the MP joint, synchronous joint movements are contingent upon the shifting of this tendon complex relative to the axis of joint motion (see text). (From Eaton,[22] with permission.)

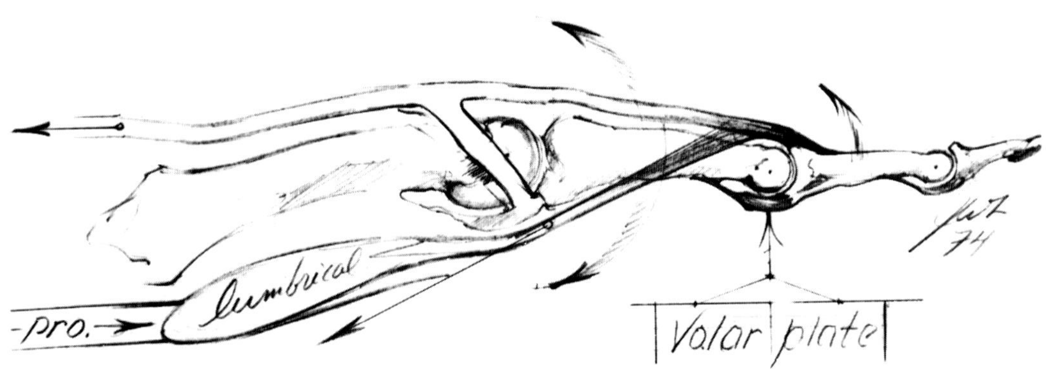

Fig. 53-4. The extrinsic system and intrinsic extensor system (represented here by the lumbrical) serve as antagonists at the MP joint, thereby "balancing" the joint. They combine to act as an extensor of the PIP joint. Their site of insertion into the dorsal base of the middle phalanx is the prime functional insertion of the extensor mechanism, and the integrity of its normal function depends on the intact PIP volar plate mechanism. Deficiency of this volar plate mechanism will alter the extensor mechanics at this joint and secondarily at the distal joint (see text). (From Littler et al,[80] with permission.)

4. *Tension in the normal extensor tendon mechanism at any given joint is dependent on the position of that joint and the adjacent joints.* The dorsovolar location of the extensor system changes with joint flexion and extension. For example, the dorsal to volar displacement of the lateral bands with PIP joint flexion relaxes distal extensor system tension enough to allow simultaneous DIP joint flexion[47,76,80] (Fig. 53-7). Alternation of this in the pathologic state imposes a restraint to distal joint motion.
5. *The deformities of late extensor mechanism disorders are reciprocal at adjacent joints* because of the factors described above in points 2, 3, and 4.[22,63-67,76,80] There are many examples: (1) in the mallet finger, secondary PIP joint hyperextension may occur in maximum attempted digital extension (see Fig. 53-27); (2) in the boutonnière deformity,

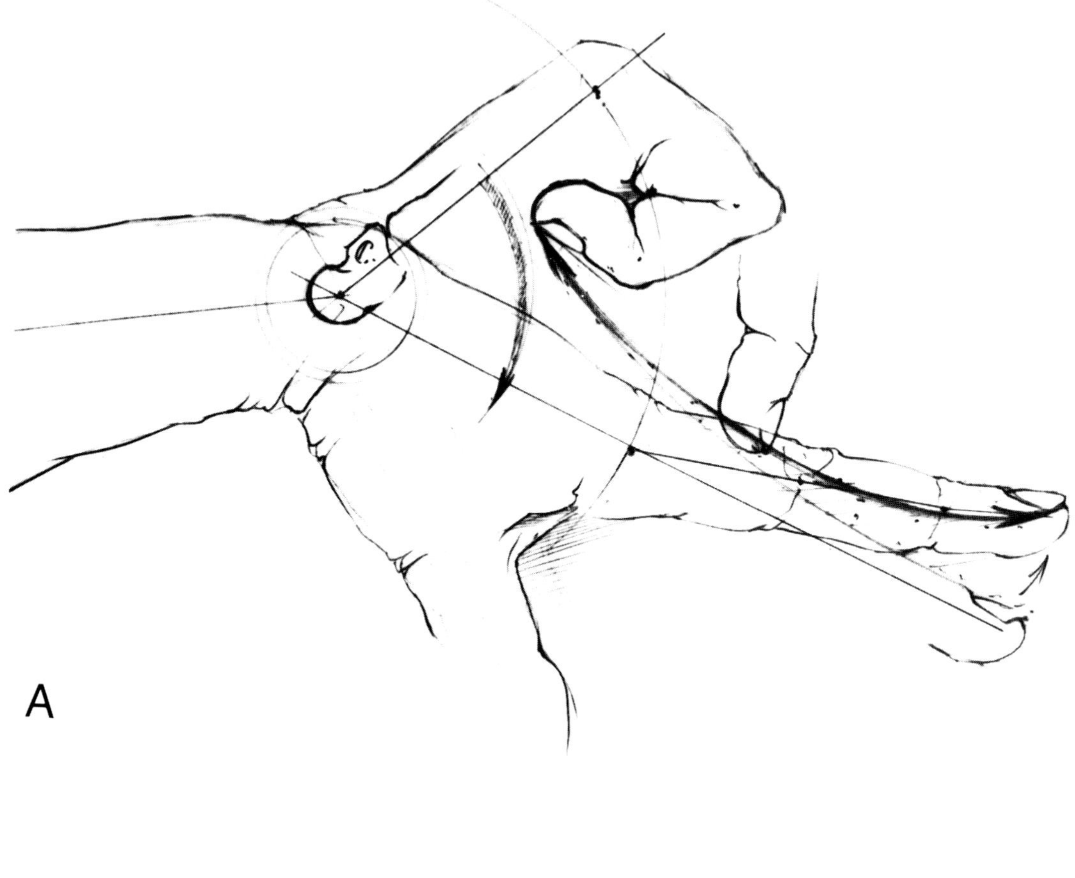

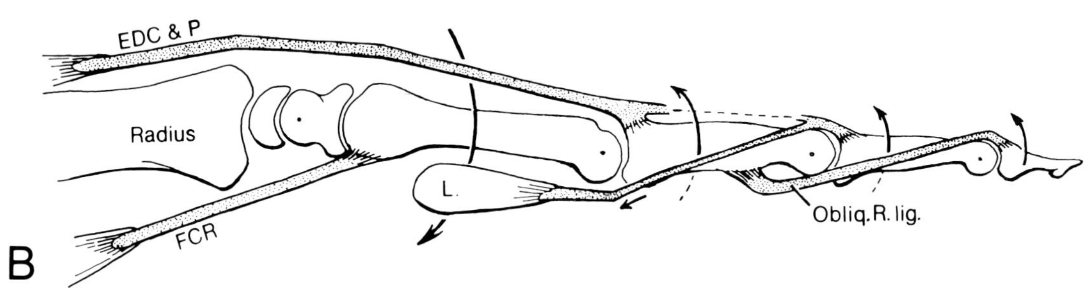

Fig. 53-5. **(A)** The motion of digital extension is potentiated by and synergistic with wrist flexion. **(B)** As the wrist is flexed by the flexor carpi radialis *(FCR)* and the flexor carpi ulnaris, tone is increased in the extensor digitorum communis and proprius systems *(EDC & P)*, thus passively bringing the MP joint into extension. Extension of this joint increases the tone in the intrinsic system (represented here by the lumbrical *[L]*) by tenodesis action, thereby extending the PIP joint. The oblique retinacular ligament *(Obliq.R.lig.)* by a similar mechanism will tenodese the distal joint into extension. (Fig. A from Littler et al,[80] with permission; Fig. B adapted from Littler,[76] with permission.)

PIP joint flexion is associated with DIP joint hyperextension (see Figs. 53-19, 53-20, and 53-21); (3) in the swan-neck finger, PIP joint hyperextension causes DIP joint droop (see Figs. 53-15, 53-16, and 53-17); (4) in intrinsic tightness, MP extension limits PIP joint flexion (see Fig. 53-13); and (5) in the rheumatoid hand, the deformity of MP joint extensor lag and ulnar drift is commonly associated with PIP joint hyperextension, i.e., swan-neck deformity.

6. *The extensor mechanism has far less tolerance than the flexor system to changes in tendinous lengths.*[70,76,80,82] The efficiency and power of the extensor system can be lost and deformity imposed by only a few millimeters of tendon displacement in relation to joint axes, or by only a few millimeters of shortening or lengthening of the critical tendon lengths, which pass between the fixed points of the extensor mechanism at each of the three finger joints (see Fig. 53-1).

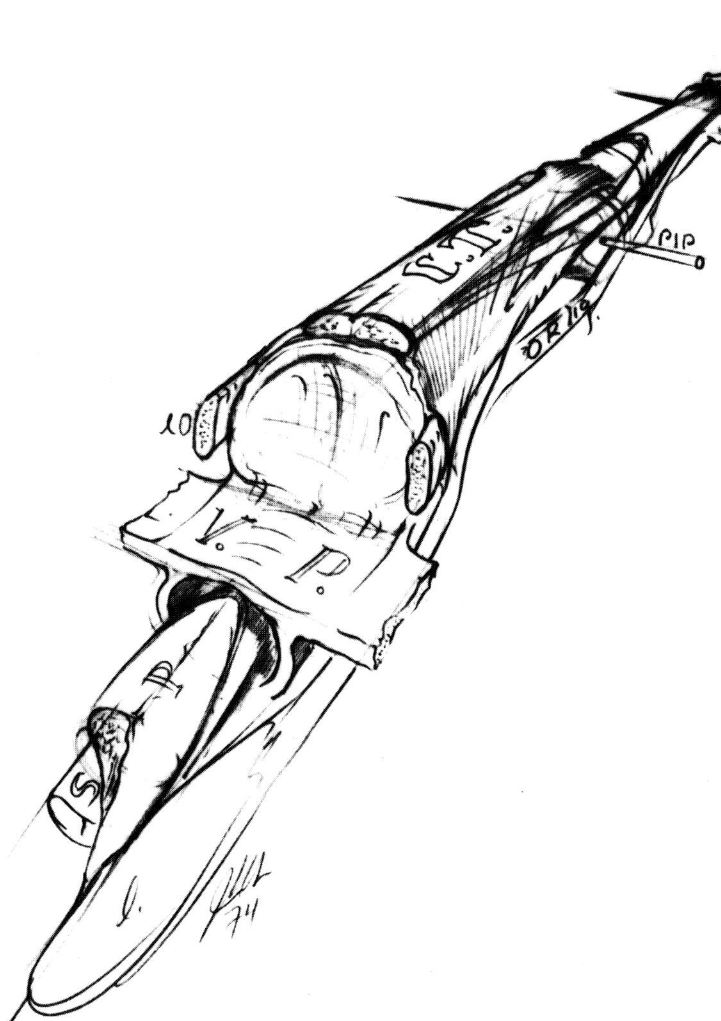

Fig. 53-6. The extensor mechanism distal to the MP joint is a truncated cone of a single tendon system controlling three joints. Note the relationship of the various components to the axis of joint motion. (Flexor digitorum profundus, *P*; flexor digitorum superficialis, *S*; lumbrical, *L*; volar plate, *V.P.*; interosseous, *io*; central tendon, *C.T.*; oblique retinacular ligament, *O.R.lig.*) (From Littler,[80] with permission.)

7. The linkage system and critical tolerances result in four dynamic concepts that should be emphasized if established extensor mechanism deformities are to be understood and proper treatment selected.[80] (1) *The component parts of this dynamic system of tenodeses are interrelated.* This system is a series of fixed tendinous and retinacular lengths, whose distal function is normally determined by the more proximal joint position. In established pathologic states, joint deformity may be imposed by the dynamic imbalance at the adjacent more proximal joint. *Thus, any evaluation of a late established extensor mechanism disorder must include a very careful assessment of extensor mechanism function at all three joints.* (2) *An imbalance at one joint will cause a predictable deformity in the next adjacent joint.* The fixed lengths of these tendinous structures dictate that the position of any one joint in this triarticular system will exert a particular effect on the others. This accounts for the complicated nature of normal active finger extension and causes the predictable reciprocal joint deformities. For example, if the MP joint goes into hyperextension in the hand devoid of median and ulnar nerve function, the PIP joint flexes, producing the so-called claw hand. In the boutonnière deformity with extensor lag of the PIP joint, hyperextension deformity is induced in the distal joint. Thus, to correct the PIP joint extensor lag of the claw hand, the treatment is *not* directed to the tendon at the PIP joint, but is meant to rebalance the MP joint. Similarly, to correct the DIP joint hyperextension of boutonnière, primary treatment must be directed *not* to the DIP joint, but instead to the PIP joint (Fig. 53-7 and see Fig. 53-19). (3) *The importance of tendon pathway in relation to the flexion-extension axis must be emphasized.* As mentioned, the intrinsic system originates volar to the axis of motion at the MP joint and passes dorsal to it at the PIP joint (Figs. 53-2, 53-4, and 53-5). Thus, in the normal state, active MP joint extension will potentiate PIP joint extension. The oblique retinacular ligament has an analogous course (one joint distally) volar to the

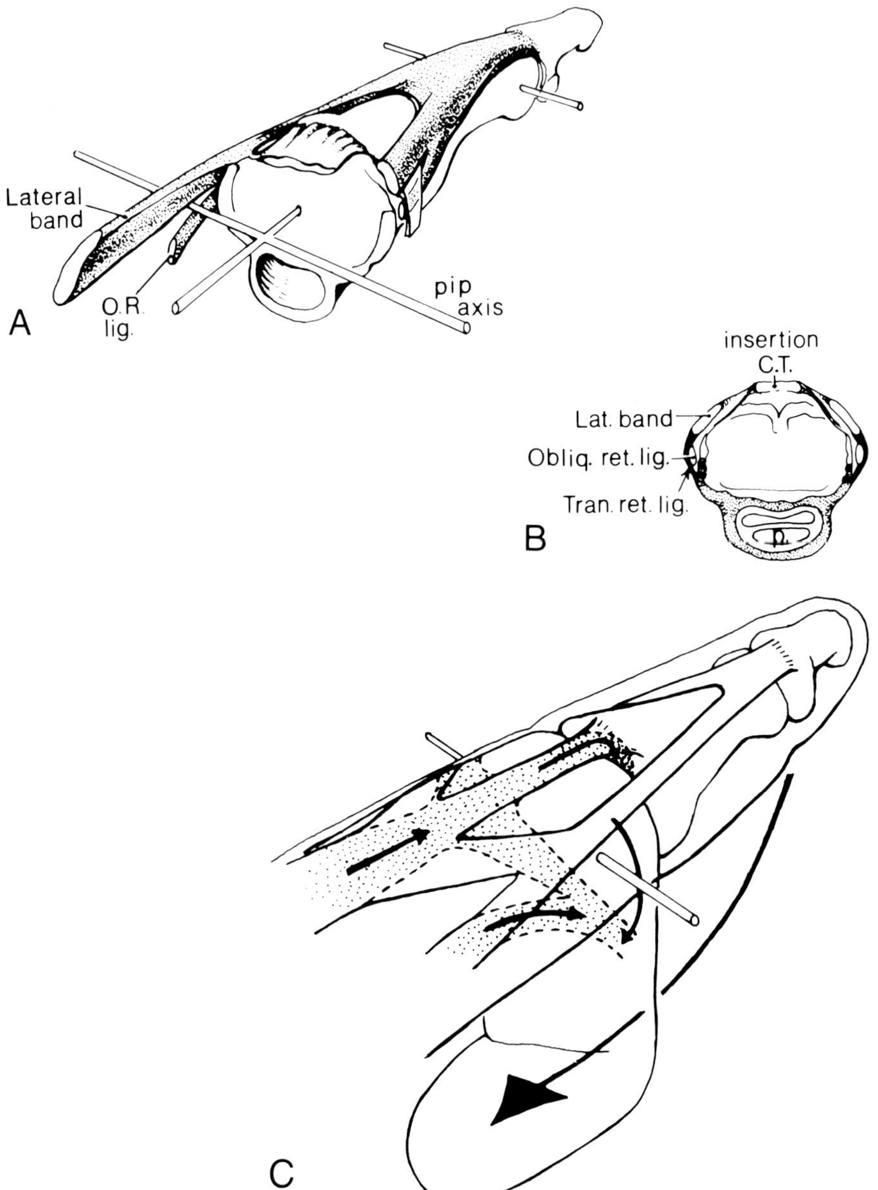

Fig. 53-7. (A&B) An understanding of the relationship of the lateral band and oblique retinacular ligament *(O.R.lig.)* to the axis of motion at the PIP joint is essential. Note that the lateral band is dorsal to the joint axis when the finger is extended. **(C)** With PIP joint flexion, the lateral bands move distally and volar to the axis of motion at the PIP joint, thus relaxing tension on the lateral bands and allowing simultaneous flexion of the distal joint. Loss of this normal lateral band mobility at the PIP joint will impose restraint to distal joint flexion. When the lateral bands are adherent dorsally, PIP joint flexion is limited; if combined with PIP joint hyperextension, distal joint droop occurs and the swan-neck deformity is present. When the lateral bands at the PIP joint adhere and foreshorten volarly, distal joint hyperextension results, with a boutonnière deformity (see text). (Figs. A and B adapted from Littler et al,[80] with permission.)

PIP joint and dorsal to the DIP joint.[63,76,80] Thus, deformity at one joint invariably induces a reciprocal deformity at the next joint—a collapse of the linkage system. In planning the correction of any established extensor mechanism imbalance, tendon pathways must be precisely evaluated. This assessment must consider not only the accepted traditional concepts of direction of pull to the point of insertion, but also the relationship of the transfer line of pull to the axis of motion for each joint position of each joint it passes, and whether it will properly shift its position to the axes of each of the joints as they flex and extend. (4) *As mentioned, the extensor system has a critical amplitude in three dimensions.* Any increase or decrease in length of these tendons may induce major disability, whether from the original pathology or from a well-intentioned surgeon.

TREATMENT OPTIONS

This functional complexity of the extensor mechanism, when altered in certain pathologic states, can result in late tendon imbalance with or without fixed joint contractures. The physician must be accurate in the assessment of the deformity, and treatment must be precise. Before making final decisions regarding treatment, the surgeon must consider the following four factors.

1. *Patient education is essential.* The patient should be informed of the complexity of the established deformity and the details and chronicity of treatment. The patient may initially be incredulous when learning what is involved to treat these problems, such as an established boutonnière, which is the late result of "just a jammed finger." There must be a commitment of time and effort by physician, therapist, *and* patient. If the patient is unwilling or unable to follow very specific long-range exercise and splinting instructions, surgical reconstruction of the extensor mechanism is best avoided.
2. *The potential functional gain or risk must be realistically assessed.* Many of these patients will present with a concern about the appearance of a "crooked finger," rather than with a functional deficit. For example, most patients with a boutonnière deformity have normal grasp. To lose full PIP joint flexion in order to regain full extension may be very helpful in certain situations, but very detrimental in others. This will depend on the digit involved, the patient's occupation, and the amount of discomfort present.
3. *A surgical rebalancing or reconstruction of the extensor mechanism should never be attempted if fixed joint deformity is present.* This is true at the MP, PIP, and DIP joint levels (an example of each is given below). A tendon transfer (e.g., the extensor indicis propius to extensor digiti quinti) to reestablish active MP joint extension of the little finger following rupture will fail if a fixed flexion deformity of that joint exists. Littler's boutonnière reconstruction will not be successful unless full passive PIP joint extension-flexion is first present. Tendon reconstruction for mallet deformity cannot be done without full passive DIP joint extension. This prerequisite of passive joint mobility can often be obtained with a careful, conscientious splinting and exercise program. Occasionally, passive mobility will not be regained with the exercise and splinting program and a two-stage surgical program will be needed. First the joint release is done. This must be followed by the maintenance of full passive motion of all three joints with a compulsive exercise and splinting program. Then, the extensor tendon reconstruction is performed as a second stage. After appropriate immobilization for tendon healing, the patient again must follow a compulsive long-term splinting and exercise program to sustain the gains from the surgery and to prevent both stiffness and/or recurrence of deformity.
4. *Many established extensor mechanism imbalances will respond to nonoperative treatment.* Very few chronic extensor mechanism disorders distal to the metacarpals should have surgery done as the initial treatment. Those patients without fixed deformity often respond to a conscientious exercise and splinting program. In those with fixed contractures, as these joints respond to the exercise and splinting program, the dynamic extensor mechanism imbalance may also correct. With or without joint contractures, the extensor assembly pathology involves only a few millimeters of abnormal length or aberrant pathway. The extensor system may "self-adjust" with the discipline of hand therapy. The foreshortened structures are actively stretched out to normal length by the patient, and the attenuated components contract the necessary 1 or 2 mm in response to control of joint position by splinting.

Specific Operative Procedures

The operative procedures pertinent to extensor mechanism reconstruction are presented sequentially in this chapter, starting with the reestablishment of more proximal joint extension and considering, in turn, the next most distal joint. Because of the above-described concept of collapse reciprocal deformities with the more proximal joint influencing the adjacent distal joint, the surgeon must start proximally and work distally.

The established chronic extensor mechanism disorders to be discussed in this chapter are: (1) loss of extrinsic extensor function secondary to old musculotendinous injury proximal to the MP joint; (2) subluxation of extrinsic extensor at the MP joint level; (3) extrinsic extensor tendon tightness; (4) intrinsic tightness; (5) swan-neck deformity; (6) boutonnière deformity; (7) late extensor hood problems; and (8) mallet finger, with and without fracture.

Many of the surgical procedures essential for the adequate treatment of established extensor mechanism disorders are described in detail in other chapters in this book. For these specific entities, the reader is referred as follows:

1. Extrinsic extensor musculotendinous deficit secondary to radial nerve injury (Chapter 38) or rheumatoid arthritis (Chapter 46)
2. Claw hand with loss of intrinsic extensor musculotendinous PIP joint extension secondary to median and/or ulnar nerve dysfunction (Chapters 39, 40, and 41)
3. Swan-neck deformity secondary to the spasticity

of cerebral palsy or stroke (Chapters 9 and 10) or rheumatoid arthritis (Chapter 46)
4. Boutonnière deformity secondary to Dupuytren's contracture (Chapter 13), burns (Chapter 55), or rheumatoid arthritis (Chapter 46)
5. Congenital extensor mechanism deficits at the wrist, as in arthrogryposis, or in the digits, as in camptodactyly (Chapter 11)
6. Details of intrinsic tightness (Chapter 15)
7. Extensor mechanism disruptions secondary to infection, such as in septic boutonnière at the PIP joint in the drug addict or in the human bite at the MP joint (Chapter 25)
8. Techniques for the essential adjunctive procedures of small joint fusion (Chapter 4), arthroplasty (Chapter 7), and surgical release of stiff or contracted joints (Chapter 12)

Late Extrinsic Extensor Tendon Reconstruction in the Forearm, Wrist, and Dorsum of the Hand

The extrinsic extensor tendon system powers extension in the wrist and the finger MP joints, abduction in the thumb metacarpal, and extension in the thumb MP and interphalangeal joints.

If the patient is unable to extend actively the finger MP joint or radially abduct the thumb metacarpal in the presence of intact radial nerve function, the tendon deficit may be anywhere proximal to the MP joint. These injuries are the most straightforward of the extensor mechanism problems to reconstruct. Unless the injury is distal to the juncturae tendinum, the motor unit contracts with tendon retraction. The myostatic muscle contracture that develops imposes a gap between the disrupted tendon ends. This precludes the secondary tendon repair in all but the most unusual cases. It is rare that repair by direct suture is either possible or advisable. To try direct repair of the irreversibly contracted motor unit to the distal tendon will commit the patient to severe extrinsic extensor tightness and limit active flexion secondary to the dorsal tenodesis (see page 1966).

The reasonable alternatives for surgical treatment are tendon transfers or intercalated tendon "minigrafts."[44]

Tendon transfer is the most reliable treatment. The reader is referred to Chapters 38, 39, 40, 41, and 46 for the principles of tendon transfers in regard to synergism, excursion, motor power, direction of pull, and choice of insertion; to Chapters 38 and 46 for operative technique; and to Chapter 50 for technique of tendon repair. In late reconstruction of the extrinsic extensor after trauma, there are certain specific considerations that should be emphasized.

1. If the tendon repair site will pass beneath the extensor retinaculum at the wrist with active digital flexion and extension, the path of the transfer should be placed in the subcutaneous fat rather than beneath the retinaculum. This ensures a straight line of pull and minimizes the risk of adherence and scarring of the transfer into its bed. The amount of bowstring at the wrist is not a functional problem, because wrist flexion is synergistic with finger and thumb extension and thus the carpus itself will function as a pulley with the wrist in the flexed position. The insertions of the wrist extensors and thumb abductor are close to the center of rotation for the wrist, and thus the amount of tendon prolapse imposes much less functional limitation than would scarring and adherence to the retinaculum if the tendon repair were to pass beneath it.
2. If the transfer is that of a flexor into an extensor (e.g., flexor carpi ulnaris or, less commonly, flexor digitorum superficialis), the path around the subcutaneous border of the forearm is better than through the interosseous membrane. There is less chance of scarring of the transfer to the bed in the path of the transfer.
3. A *normal* wrist joint should rarely be fused in order to provide wrist extensor motors as transfers for finger and/or thumb function.
4. In some patients, the original injury may have involved loss of overlying skin and subcutaneous tissue such that the path of the proposed transfer is through an area of heavy scar or beneath a skin graft adherent to scar and/or bone. In these situations the area may have to be resurfaced with a flap first. At the time of flap attachment, the proposed path of the transfer can be prepared with a silicone tendon rod placed beneath the flap and flap margins to facilitate the subsequent transfers.

Author's Preferred Methods for Chronic Extensor Tendon Deficit Proximal to the MP Joint

Later reconstruction by tendon transfer, if it involves loss of all extrinsic extensor musculotendinous function, presents an almost identical situation to that of a radial palsy distal to the triceps innervation. The ideal transfers for this deficit are pronator teres to extensor carpi radialis brevis to regain wrist extension, flexor carpi ulnaris to extensor digitorum communis for finger extension, and palmaris longus to reestablish the thumb abduction-extension arc (see Chapter 38 for alternative transfers). Obviously, if the active motor units are not sufficiently long to reach the distal recipient tendon, the proximal unit can be prolonged by the use of an intercalated tendon graft.

In less severe injuries involving loss of only one or two extensor units, some commonly used transfers not requiring graft prolongation are outlined in Table 53-1.

The technique of minigrafts has been used as an alternative to tendon transfers.[44] The gap between the retracted tendon ends is bridged with a segment of tendon graft. The author prefers the use of tendon transfers unless the unusual situation outlined below is found at surgery. Success of the minigraft technique is predicated on two assumptions: (1) the myostatic muscle contracture has not become irreversible, and (2) the muscle belly or contractility can still impart adequate excur-

Table 53-1. Commonly Used Transfers in Less Severe Injuries

Function Lost	Transfer Possibilities
Extensor pollicis longus	Extensor indicis proprius or palmaris longus
Abductor pollicis longus	Brachioradialis
Extensor digitorum communis	Extensor indicis proprius or side-to-side to adjacent extensor digitorum communis (Fig. 53-8); flexor carpi ulnaris
Extensor carpi radialis longus, brevis	Pronator teres

sion to the distal tendon for full range of motion. There is one situation in which these assumptions are often valid. If the original injury is distal to the wrist and the proximal tendon retraction is limited by adherence, the distal end of the proximal tendon has some effective attachment distal to the wrist. Thus, (1) some motor unit length is retained; and (2) active wrist motion will impart some passive excursion to the muscle. These preclude a myostatic contracture.

Operative Techniques

Except as discussed above, the operative technique for tendon transfer is the same as that for tendon transfer to reestablish active extension of the thumb, fingers, and/or wrist in radial nerve palsy (Chapter 38), and in rheumatoid arthritis (Chapter 46) (Fig. 53-8).

In the transfer repair for wrist extension, the tension should be snug with the wrist in 30 to 40 degrees extension. In transfer or minigraft for MP extension, the tension should be as tight as reasonable tendon traction will allow while the wrist is in maximum extension and the digits in a fist. In the operating room after these latter repairs are completed, passive wrist extension should allow full passive fist formation and passive wrist flexion should tenodese the involved digits into extension.

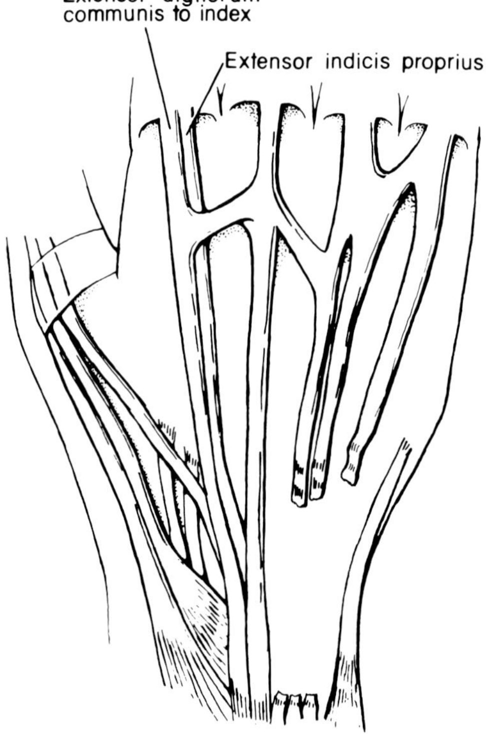

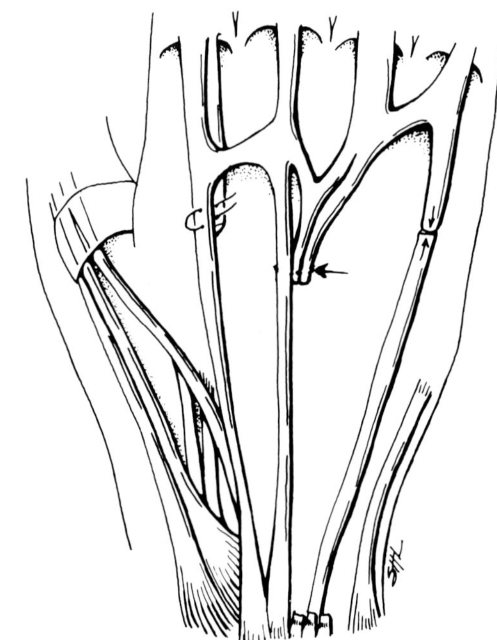

Fig. 53-8. The technique of tendon transfer for long-standing disruption of the extrinsic extensor tendons varies with the situation encountered at surgery. Principles and techniques are similar to those for transfers in radial nerve palsy. The choice of motor units and the type of repair used must be adapted to the individual situation. A typical finding is loss of the extensor digitorum communis to the ring and little fingers and loss of the extensor digiti quinti. An example of the type of transfers that can be used is shown here. The distal stump of the extensor indicis proprius is sutured side to side to the extensor digitorum communis. The proprius is then divided just proximal to this repair site and transferred to the extensor digiti quinti. The repair site, if possible, should be well distal to the retinaculum and should be away from areas of previous scar, as these are points of potential tendon adherence. The extensor digitorum communis tendon to the ring finger can be repaired side to side to that of the long finger. The tendon repair done may be one of several types, depending on the size of the tendons involved. The repair of the ring communis to that of the long is frequently of an interweaving type, secured by multiple horizontal mattress sutures. The proprius transfer may be sutured with a modified Kessler or interweaving technique. (See Chapter 50 for techniques of specific types of tendon junctures.)

Postoperative Care

The immobilization is specific. The small joints of the hand should be in the "safe position" with the MP joints flexed 60 to 70 degrees, interphalangeal joints extended, and thumb in the fist projection. The wrist is held in 10 degrees less than maximum extension. If the transfers involve units that originate proximal to the elbow, the elbow should be immobilized in 90-degree flexion with the forearm rotation positioned according to that which will minimize static tension on the repairs; for example, in supination for flexor carpi ulnaris around the ulnar border of forearm into extensor digitorum communis, in pronation for pronator teres into extensor carpi radialis brevis, and in neutral if both transfers have been done.

Duration of continuous immobilization is 4 to 6 weeks. Exercises are started after that interval. If begun at 4 weeks, the exercises must be done very carefully with active assisted extension and limited active flexion to avoid rupture. Splinting is continued, except during therapy exercises, for a total of 2 months after surgery, and then the patient is gradually weaned from the splint during the third month.

Complications

Four potential complications are noteworthy.

1. Scarring of the tendons, especially at the repair sites, is the most common complication. This risk can be minimized by careful attention to the preoperative assessment and the postoperative hand therapy as detailed above. This complication may present as (1) simple failure of the transfer to function or (2) extrinsic extensor tendon tightness (see page 1966). The treatment of this complication should start with a specific therapy program of exercises and splinting in an attempt to improve muscle control and amplitude of the musculotendinous unit. Should this fail after several months, consideration should be given to tenolysis. If the soft tissue coverage is poor (i.e., secondary to previous injury), a local or distant flap may be indicated as well.
2. Rupture and/or attenuation does occur, even under favorable conditions. This problem can be best avoided by precise secure tendon repairs, by proper (not excessive) tension in the musculotendinous unit at the initial repair, by continuing the immobilization for an adequate interval after surgery, and by compulsive following of the subsequent exercise program and gradual weaning from a splint with the graduated resumption of hand activities.

   If the musculotendinous unit is in continuity but attenuated, it is occasionally possible to salvage the situation nonoperatively with a dynamic assist splint accompanied by static splinting at night. Otherwise, it is necessary to redo the tendon repair.

   If the musculotendinous repair has ruptured, it should be repaired immediately before the motor unit contracts. If not, another transfer may be needed.
3. Donor deficits may complicate the result. Deficits may be secondary to either a too-weak muscle used for transfer, or weak or absent function originally performed by the muscle used for the transfer. The former is usually the result of failure to appreciate weakness in the donor prior to transfer, the latter the result of failure to recognize weakness in muscles that will be needed to substitute for the transfer donor function. An example of this latter situation is use of an extensor indicis proprius transfer for extensor pollicis longus deficit, not recognizing coexistent absent extensor digitorum communis index function.
4. Joint stiffness can be a problem, especially in the finger MP or PIP joints. Contributing factors may be the sequelae of old injury, immobilization in other than "safe position," or failure to follow the specific exercise and splinting program. Treatment must be prompt (see Chapter 12).

Subluxation of Extrinsic Extensor at the MP Joint Level

As the extensor tendons (the communi and proprii) pass over the metacarpal head, a modification of the retinacular system, in the form of sagittal (or shroud) fibers, stabilizes the extensor tendons.[22,76,79] These fibers arise from the extrinsic extensor, embrace the metacarpal head, and insert into the volar plate (Fig. 53-9). With MP joint motion, these sagittal (coronal) fibers pass to and fro in a sagittal plane, not unlike a bucket handle or helmet visor, as the central tendon moves distal to proximal with MP joint flexion and extension[76,79] (Fig. 53-10).

One essential function of these shroud fibers is the maintenance of the central position of the extensor tendon over the apex of the metacarpal head during MP joint flexion and extension. This is absolutely necessary for the mechanics of MP joint flexion and extension because, to extend actively the flexed MP joint, the functional pulley of the extrinsic extensor is the metacarpal head[80] (Fig. 53-9). The sagittal fibers have several other functions, the most important being related to the pathomechanics of the claw hand and not pertinent to this chapter.

With rupture or attenuation of these sagittal fibers (more common on the radial aspect) the extrinsic extensor tendon slips off the apex of the metacarpal head. The power dissipated by abnormal lateral-volar or downward displacement of the central extensor tendon is diverted excessively to the PIP joint level.[80] With time (especially if PIP joint disease is present as in rheumatoid arthritis), the structures restraining PIP joint hyperextension are overwhelmed. A secondary and disabling PIP joint recurvatum deformity can then develop. The abnormal path of the central tendon is then acting to cause not only PIP joint recurvature but also ulnar deviation, as well as the obvious extensor deficit at the MP joint.[80]

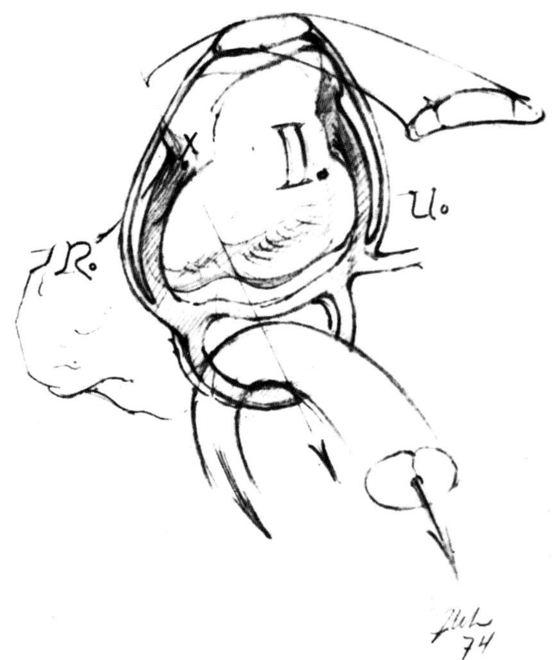

Fig. 53-9. The metacarpal head *(II)* serves as a pulley for the extrinsic extensor tendon, which passes over the apex of the metacarpal head. The extrinsic extensor is stabilized in this position by the sagittal bands (shroud fibers), which embrace the metacarpal head and attach to the volar plate mechanism. Suspended from this volar plate mechanism is the A1 pulley of the flexor mechanism. Rupture of a sagittal band from trauma or attenuation from arthritis will cause the extrinsic extensor tendon to subluxate from the apex of the metacarpal head pulley, thus losing its mechanical advantage for extension (see text). (From Littler et al,[80] with permission.)

Diagnosis

This condition is simple to diagnose in the nonrheumatoid patient. Usually there is a history of blunt trauma to the metacarpal head. The patient will have excellent active MP joint flexion, but will be unable to extend the MP joint from the flexed position. If the joint is passively extended to 0 degrees, the tendon reduces to the apex of the metacarpal head and the patient will then be able to hold the MP joint in full extension against resistance. This is the critical point in differentiating extensor tendon subluxation at the MP joint from a more proximal extrinsic extensor tendon rupture or laceration.

Nonoperative Treatment

If the diagnosis is made early, the shroud fibers on the side toward which the tendon subluxates will not have contracted. These patients often do very well with splint treatment. The splint must hold the involved MP joint at 0 degrees to allow healing of the ruptured or attenuated shroud fibers without tension while the extrinsic extensor rests over the apex of the metacarpal head. Active PIP joint motion is encouraged. At 3 to 4 weeks the splint is removed three times a day for gentle active MP joint flexion with *passive* MP joint extension. Except for these exercises, splinting is continuous for 2 months.

Operative Techniques

There are three types of surgical repair for this clinical problem. All are best exposed as would be done for MP joint arthroplasty (see Chapter 7). These procedures are for isolated digital imbalance secondary to trauma and are *not* adequate for the rheumatoid patient unless combined with multiple other procedures, such as intrinsic releases, collateral ligament releases, and, frequently, joint arthroplasties (see Chapter 46).

Delayed Primary Repair. If the disruption is diagnosed and referred for treatment in the subacute situation (usually after laceration or closed crush injury), delayed primary repair of the ruptured sagittal fibers is possible. This may be technically difficult for two reasons: (1) the shroud fibers are normally quite thin, and the fiber orientation is such that sutures do not hold well. Small horizontal mattress sutures are the most effective; and (2) because the metacarpal head is rounded and there is considerable tension on the extrinsic extensor with the joint flexed, the tendon will snap off the apex of the metacarpal head into the "valley" unless the sagittal fiber repair is stout and of the perfect length. If the sagittal fibers are too friable or if the surgery is done late after the fibers have contracted, either of the following two procedures is effective. Of these two operations, I prefer the dorsal tenodesis to the sling procedure because it is technically easier.

Dorsal Tenodesis. A dorsal tenodesis is created as a carefully adjusted new distal juncturae tendinum (Littler JW: personal

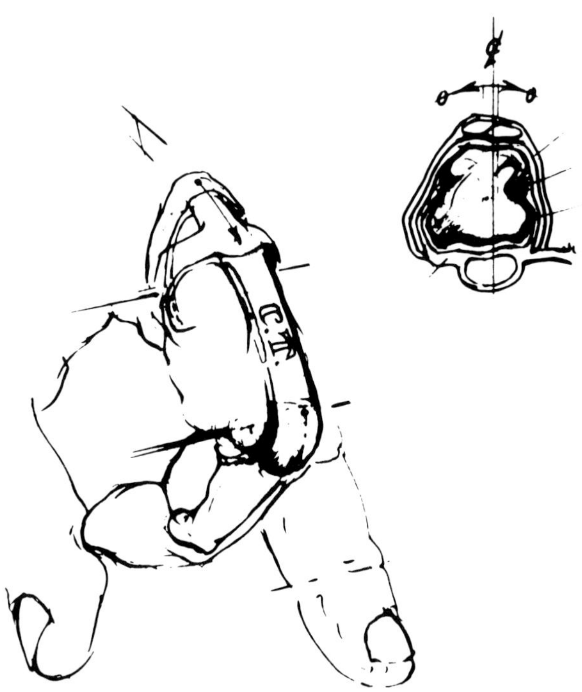

Fig. 53-10. The sagittal fibers move to and fro with extrinsic extensor tendon excursion, thus maintaining the extrinsic extensor over the apex of the metacarpal head throughout the arc of active MP joint motion. (From Littler et al,[80] with permission.)

communication, 1970). The exposure is the same as that used for arthroplasty of the MP joint of the involved ray and the adjacent finger to the side of the ruptured sagittal fibers. I prefer a gently curved longitudinal incision. The extensor digitorum communis tendon of this *adjacent* digit is split longitudinally for its distal 3 cm over the metacarpal, and one limb is transected at the proximal extent of the split. A horizontal mattress suture is placed at the distal margin to prevent propagation of this split distally. This distally based tendon slip is then passed through or around the extensor digitorum communis of the involved digit and sutured back to itself. The tension is carefully adjusted before the tenodesis is sutured, to ensure that the recipient extensor digitorum communis remains centralized with MP flexion and extension. The procedure can be done under wrist block anesthesia to permit active motion when the tenodesis repair is being adjusted.

Sling Procedure. A sling is constructed to the intrinsic tendon of the involved digit. In a fashion similar to the dorsal tenodesis, a distally based strip of extensor digitorum communis is raised, with one critical difference. In the dorsal tenodesis, the tendon strip is raised from the tendon of the *adjacent* finger. In the sling procedure, the tendon strip is raised from the *subluxating* tendon itself.[76,78] This strip is then sutured to the intervolar plate (deep transverse metacarpal) ligament. As an alternative, this strip is passed volarly around the leading margin of the intrinsic wing tendon on the side of the digit with the deficient shroud fibers. The tension is similarly adjusted and the tenodesis sutured back to itself.

Postoperative Care

The hand is immobilized with the MP joint in 0 degrees and the PIP joints free. At 5 to 7 days the patient is started on active PIP joint exercises (similar to the acute nonoperative treatment, these active PIP flexion-extension exercises must be done with the MP joint passively supported either at neutral or slight hyperextension). The purpose of these exercises is to gain some excursion of the involved reconstruction. At 2 weeks, gentle active MP joint flexion is started with a dorsal extension assist splint. Unprotected use of the hand is not permitted for 10 weeks.

Extrinsic Extensor Tendon Tightness (Dorsal Tenodesis)

The extrinsic extensor tendon passes dorsal to both the MP and PIP joints on the way to its prime functional insertion into the tubercle at the dorsal base of the middle phalanx (Fig. 53-11). In some situations the muscle belly is contracted in the forearm. More commonly, the tendon is scarred to the bone or

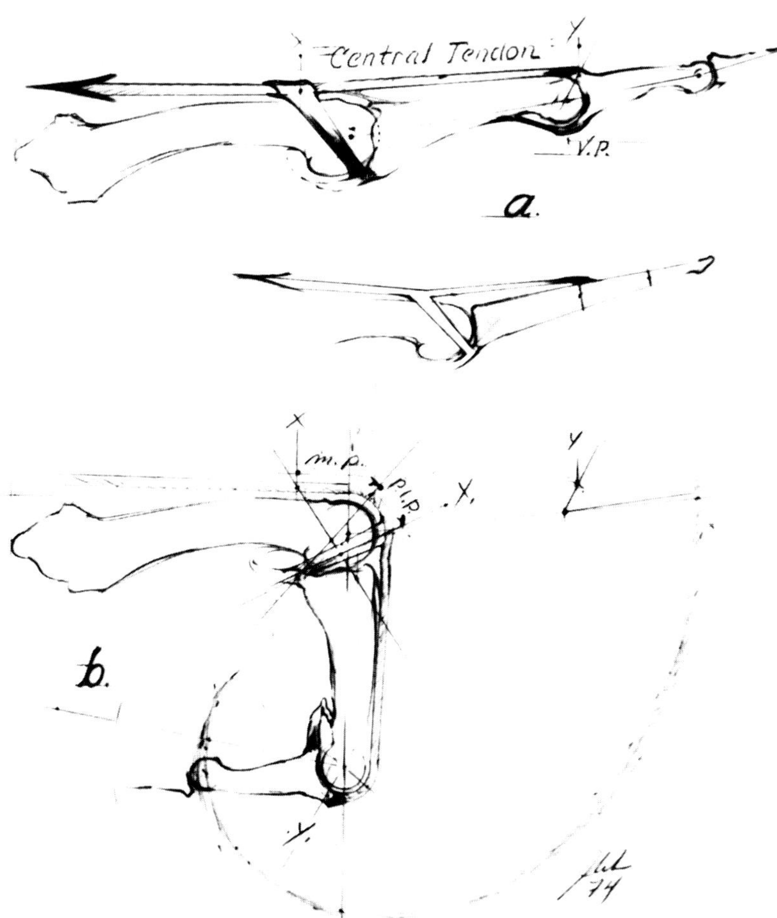

Fig. 53-11. In the normal digit, the prime functional insertion of the extrinsic extensor tendon is through the central tendon into the dorsal base of the middle phalanx. Traction on the extrinsic extensor will lift the finger as a beam if the volar plate at this PIP joint is competent. Thus, normal extrinsic extensor tone may impose PIP joint recurvature if the volar plate *(V.P.)* is lax. However, once the MP joint starts to hyperextend, the prime insertion of the extrinsic extensor shifts to the sagittal fibers into the volar plate at the MP joint, and extrinsic extensor tone is lost at the PIP joint. In the absence of normal intrinsic MP joint flexor power, the extrinsic extensor tendon is unable to extend the PIP joint as the MP joint comes into the hyperextended position (claw hand). (From Littler et al,[80] with permission.)

retinaculum at the wrist or adherent to a metacarpal on the dorsum of the hand. When this occurs, the tendon lacks the necessary excursion to permit simultaneous flexion of the MP and PIP joints.[73,78,80]

Thus, if the extrinsic extensor becomes adherent over the metacarpal or foreshortened, active or passive MP joint flexion imposes, by dorsal tenodesis restraint, an unyielding extension force at the PIP joint (Fig. 53-12). As seen clinically, PIP joint flexion imposes MP joint hyperextension and MP joint flexion imposes PIP joint extension.[22] This condition is known as "extrinsic extensor tendon tightness." These patients complain of inability to flex fully the involved finger(s).

On examination, the patient can actively flex the PIP joint with the MP joint extended or flex the MP joint with the PIP joint extended. Simultaneous full flexion of both joints, however, is not possible either actively or passively. When the MP joint is passively brought into full flexion by the examiner, the PIP joint is tenodesed into extension; both passive and active flexion of the PIP joint are limited. If the MP joint is placed in neutral or extension by the examiner, the PIP joint can be flexed (Fig. 53-12).

This condition is seen in a variety of clinical situations: (1) after metacarpal fractures, particularly open injuries or those requiring open reduction and internal fixation; (2) following extensive soft tissue injuries over the dorsum of the hand or wrist, especially if grafts are required for closure; (3) subsequent to any extrinsic extensor tendon repair after laceration, transfer, or graft if there is scarring of the tendon to adjacent fascia or bone; (4) consequent to crush injuries of the dorsum of the hand; and (5) after extensor tendon repairs or transfers that are sutured under excessive tension.

Nonoperative Treatment

In a high percentage of patients, the condition responds well to a program of exercises and static or dynamic splinting. This is particularly true if the diagnosis is made early and the therapy program is instituted before the dorsal scarring becomes mature and/or joint contractures develop. In this context, it should be noted that the problem can often be prevented if it is anticipated and exercises started 2 to 8 weeks after injury or surgery. The specific exercises commence as soon as they can be done safely (very carefully under close supervision and in combination with protective splinting) without jeopardizing soft tissue, tendon, or osseous healing. These exercises are designed to emphasize active extrinsic extensor tendon excursion.

If tendon and bony unions are secure by 8 weeks, the exercises can include active assisted flexion of the MP and PIP joints simultaneously and active assisted extension. Frequently the use of a flexion glove or flexion assist splint is helpful, especially at night. Care must be taken to ensure that the increasing flexion is from improved tendon excursion and not from stretching or attenuation of the tendon. For this rea-

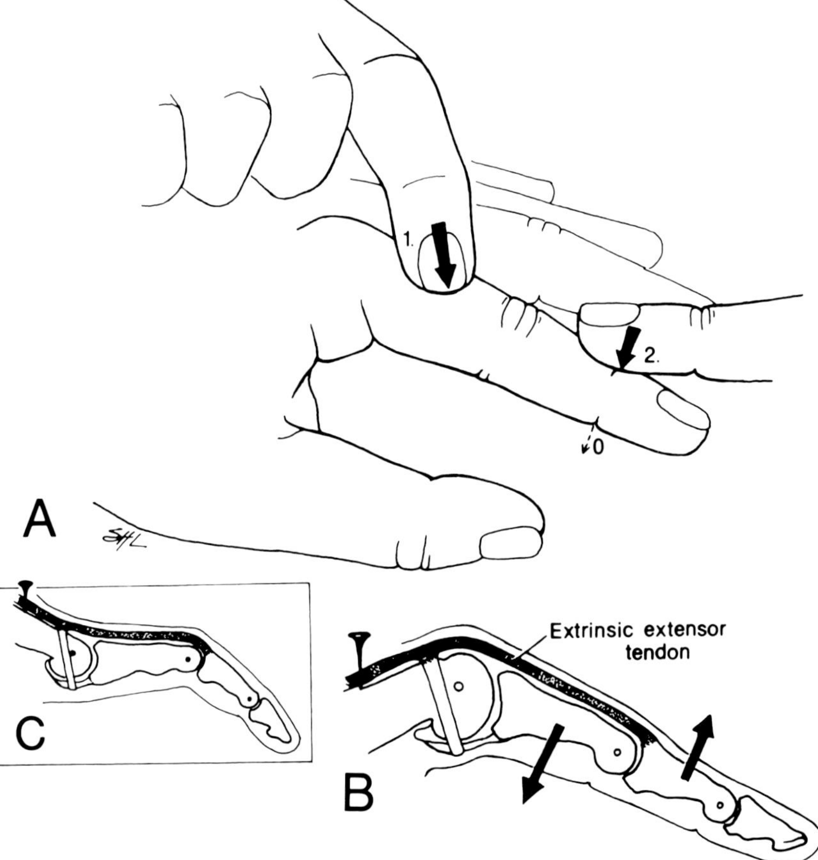

Fig. 53-12. The test for *extrinsic* tightness. If the extrinsic extensor tendon is adherent to the metacarpal, the limitation of excursion distal to that point will limit or preclude simultaneous flexion of the MP and PIP joints. **(A&B)** As the MP joint is flexed, the PIP joint is pulled into extension. **(C)** Conversely, as the PIP joint flexes, the MP joint is tenodesed into hyperextension. The clinical test for this condition is demonstrated in A. With passive MP joint flexion *(1),* the PIP joint is felt to tenodese into extension *(2).*

son the splinting program may also need to include extension assist splints and exercises.

Operative Techniques

Two types of procedures, each entirely different in concept, may be helpful: tenolysis or extrinsic extensor release. Neither should be considered until 6 months of hand therapy have failed to achieve the desired mobility. If MP and/or PIP joint fixed contractures are present, simultaneous joint release is essential (see Chapter 12 for technique).

Author's Preferred Method for Extrinsic Extensor Tendon Tightness

The author prefers tenolysis if the condition and length of the tendon are reasonable, and the problem is one of adherence and scarring of the tendon. Obviously the shorter the length of tendon involvement the easier the procedure and the more favorable the result. If the problem is one of inadequate tendon length (i.e., the tendon is too short), or scarring for a long length of tendon proximal to the junctura tendinum (to retain active MP extension from adjacent normal digits), I prefer the Littler extrinsic tendon release.

Extensor Tendon Tenolysis. Tenolysis is discussed in detail in Chapter 51 as it is applied to the flexor system. The principles and techniques are the same for the extrinsic extensors, except there is no critical annular restraint (pulley) system that has to be preserved, although the sagittal bands at the MP joint must be protected. The extensor retinaculum at the wrist is expendable, for digital extension normally occurs simultaneously with wrist flexion. Thus, extensor tendon bowstring at the wrist does not occur significantly with normal hand use.

Extrinsic Extensor Tendon Release. Extrinsic extensor tendon release is a concept developed by Littler.[22,73,76] It is predicated on a separation of the intrinsic and extrinsic extensor tendon systems and a separation of the dual extrinsic-intrinsic extensor control of the PIP joint (see Fig. 53-14). The extrinsic extensor tendon release is contraindicated in the hand with weak or absent intrinsic musculotendinous function.

The central portion of the extensor assembly is excised over the proximal phalangeal shaft.[73] Both the sagittal bands at the MP joint and the central tendon insertion at the dorsal base of the middle phalanx must be carefully protected and preserved. This leaves the extrinsic extensor to extend the MP joint only and relies on the intrinsic system to extend the PIP joint. Thus, the distal extent of tendon resection must be 5 to 8 mm proximal to the PIP joint so as not to disturb the confluence of the lateral bands and the extensor mechanism insertion into the dorsal base of the middle phalanx. If the tendon excision is carried too far distally, a boutonnière may result.

This procedure is best done with digital block anesthesia. The patient can thus actively flex and extend the fingers after the release, permitting the surgeon to be certain as to the adequacy of tendon resection. A wrist block should not be used as this will also block intrinsic muscle innervation.

Postoperative Care

The postoperative program is very similar for the two procedures and is identical to that outlined under the section on nonoperative treatment. Gentle active assisted range of motion, both flexion and extension, within the limits of discomfort, is begun on the first day. These exercises are done several times daily. Sutures are removed at 2 weeks, but exercises and splinting may be necessary for many months.

If the extrinsic extensor tendon release has been done, the window in the tendon aponeurosis over the proximal phalanx fills with a "pseudotendon" scar within 8 weeks. During this time the patient must be carefully checked to be certain that no PIP joint extensor lag is developing. Should this start to occur, the PIP joint should be splinted in 0 degrees between the exercise periods.

Intrinsic Extensor Tendon Tightness

The topic of intrinsic extensor tendon tightness is covered in detail in Chapter 15. To avoid confusion with extrinsic tendon tightness, one must contrast and emphasize the differences on physical examination, because both entities can follow crush injury with or without metacarpal fracture and both are associated with limitation of PIP joint flexion. In intrinsic tightness, when the MP joint is passively brought into full extension by the examiner, active or passive PIP joint flexion is limited[22] (Fig. 53-13). The finger with intrinsic tightness frequently responds to an appropriate exercise program.

If the exercises provide incomplete correction, this condition is similarly treated with a procedure that eliminates the dual control of PIP joint extension by excision of the wing tendons[30,31,33,71,76,80] (Fig. 53-14). This procedure eliminates intrinsic PIP joint extension, leaving the extrinsic tendon to extend the PIP joint (this latter is possible because interosseous muscle MP joint flexion remains intact). Note that this is *not* an operation for correction of the swan-neck deformity, because it does not address the major problem of PIP joint volar plate laxity.[75,80]

Swan-neck Deformity

Swan-neck deformity describes a posture of the finger in which the PIP joint is hyperextended and the DIP joint is flexed. Initially this is a dynamic imbalance that occurs when the patient attempts maximal active digital extension. This dynamic finger imbalance can progress to a fixed deformity with joint changes.

There are many etiologies for this pathologic state. Swan-neck deformity is seen consequent to (1) injuries resulting in volar plate laxity at the PIP joint, (2) spastic conditions—both stroke and cerebral palsy (Chapters 9 and 10), (3) rheumatoid arthritis (Chapter 46), (4) fractures of the middle phalanx healed in hyperextension, (5) mallet deformity at the distal joint when there is coexistent volar plate laxity at the PIP joint (see page 1983), and (6) generalized systemic ligamentous laxity.

An understanding of the altered functional dynamics is essential. The prime functional insertion of the conjoined exten-

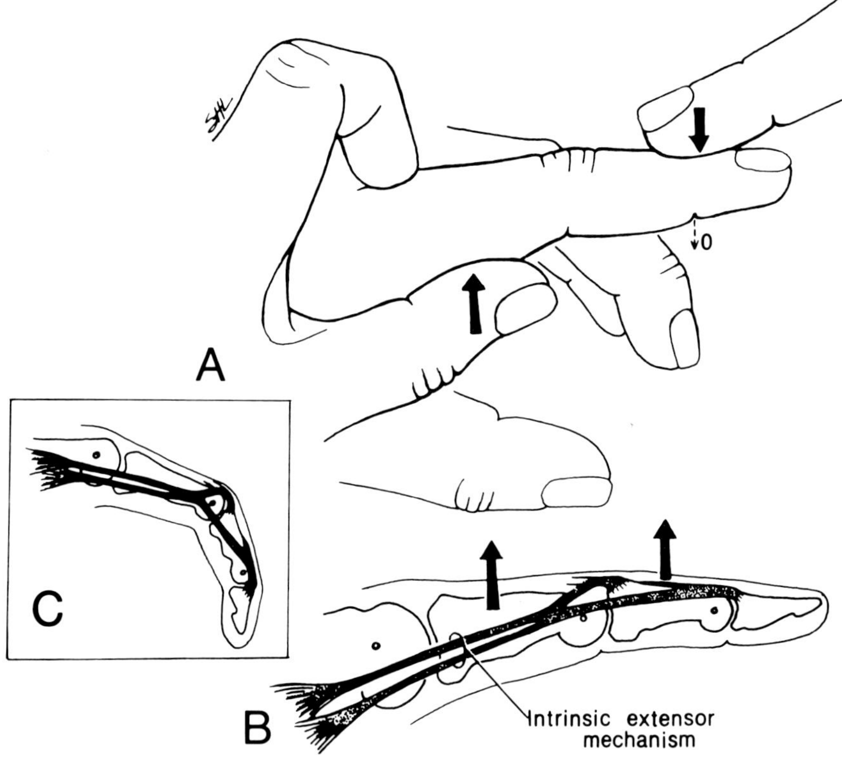

Fig. 53-13. The test for *intrinsic* tightness. If the intrinsic musculotendinous system is foreshortened, extension of the MP joint either actively or passively will increase the tone in this system and thus impose a restraint to flexion of the PIP joint. **(A&B)** This is tested by the examiner: (1) by passively extending the MP joint and (2) by testing for passive flexion of the proximal joint. If flexion of the PIP joint is greater when the MP joint is flexed than when it is extended, an element of intrinsic tightness is present. **(C)** As the MP joint is allowed to flex, tone decreases in the intrinsic system and the PIP joint is able to flex further.

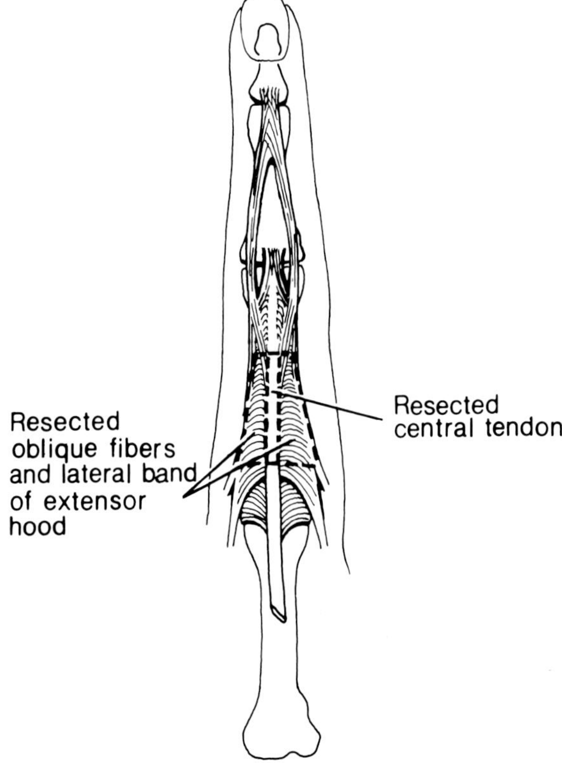

Fig. 53-14. Extrinsic or intrinsic extensor tendon release. Partial resection of the appropriate portion of the extensor mechanism in carefully selected cases is very helpful in the treatment of intrinsic tightness or extrinsic extensor tendon tightness. In patients with *extrinsic* extensor tendon tightness, the central tendon portion is resected. In those with *intrinsic* tightness, only the lateral bands are resected as indicated. (See text for details.)

sor mechanism is into the tubercle at the dorsal base of the middle phalanx.[76,79,80] Thus, normal digital extension is predicated upon a competent PIP joint volar plate mechanism that will not permit PIP joint hyperextension as the exensor mechanism lifts the finger into full extension (see Figs. 53-4 and 53-11). In the abnormal state of PIP joint hyperextension, there is a dorsal displacement of the lateral bands at the PIP joint. This dorsal prolapse of the lateral bands slackens the distal tension because of the fixed attachment of the central tendon at the PIP joint level (Fig. 53-15A and B). Thus, a droop of the distal joint is imposed as the flexor digitorum profundus becomes an unopposed, deforming force.[76,79,80]

There are definite similarities in the pathomechanics and surgical treatment of the claw and swan-neck deformities.[80] Both have the important pathology of a hyperextended proximal joint and flexed distal joint. Both have fixed points for the extensor tendon assembly at the proximal joint that limit active extension at the distal joint. These fixed points are the sagittal fibers at the MP joint for the claw and the central tendon insertion at the PIP joint for the swan-neck. Both have a flexor tendon acting as a deforming force at the distally involved joint—the flexor digitorum superficialis at the PIP joint in the claw and the flexor digitorum profundus at the DIP joint for the swan-neck. Both have a yoke tendon restraint at the proximally involved hyperextended joint—the sagittal fibers at the PIP joint in the claw and the transverse retinacular fibers at the PIP joint in the swan-neck. With these similar pathomechanics, it is not surprising that both deformities are rebalanced by the reestablishment of flexion (or limitation of hyperextension) at the proximal joint imbalance (Table 53-2).

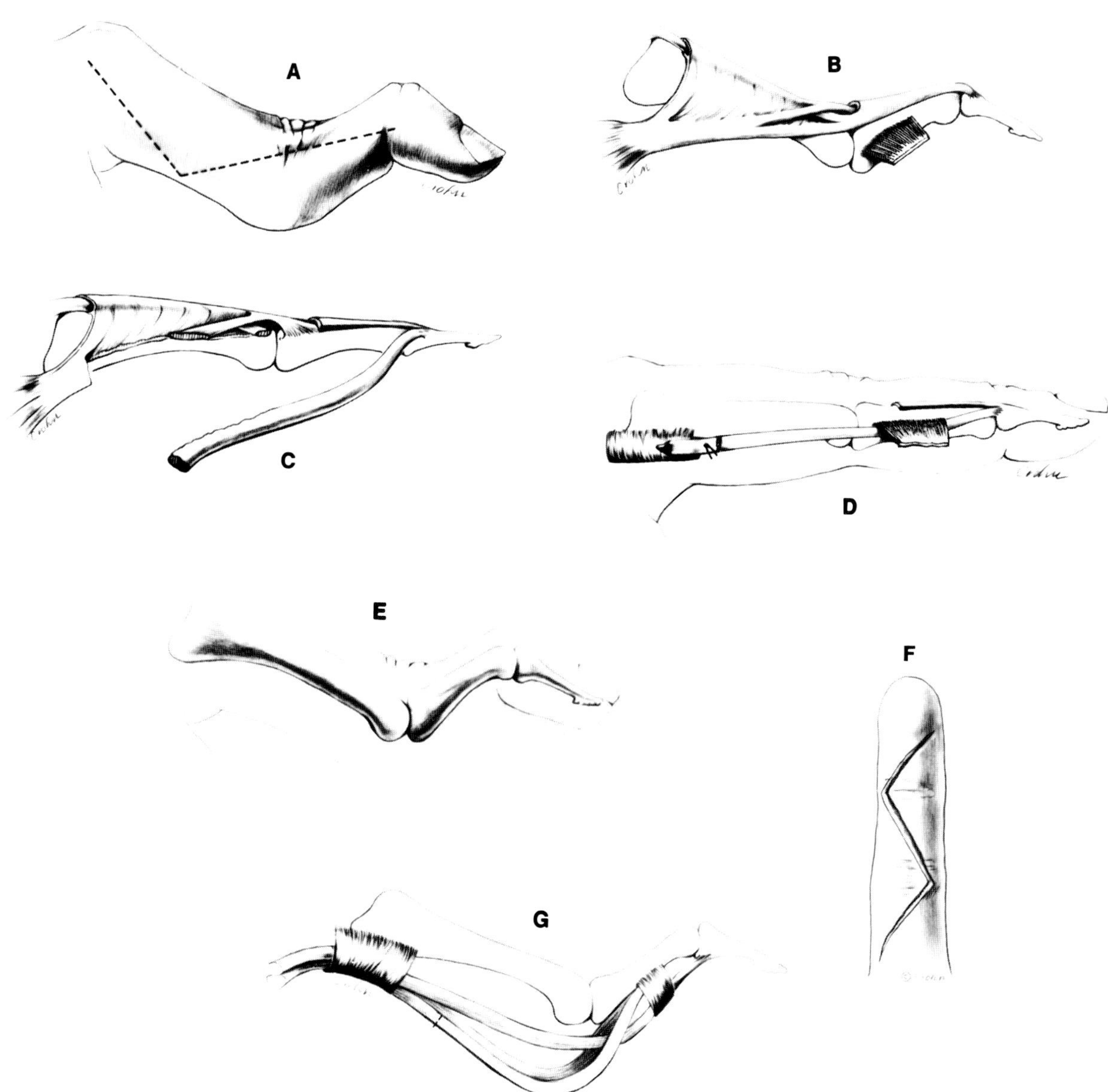

Fig. 53-15. (A–D) Littler oblique retinacular ligament reconstruction (see text). **(E–K)** Littler superficialis tenodesis (see text). *(Figure continues.)* (Figs. A–D adapted from Littler,[76] with permission; Figs. E–K from Burton,[10] with permission.)

Patients with swan-neck deformity can be subdivided into those with full active PIP joint flexion who simply have a dynamic imbalance of the finger with attempted active maximum extension, and those who have developed fixed deformity with secondary contractures and joint changes. As already mentioned, no swan-neck dynamic rebalancing is possible in the presence of joint deformity (see Chapter 12 for treatment of stiff joints).

Nonoperative Treatment

Swan-neck deformity is one of the few extensor mechanism imbalances that does not respond to a conservative splinting and exercise program. Such a program may relieve fixed contractures and/or intrinsic tightness, but the volar plate laxity will persist, as will the dynamic imbalance at the interphalangeal joints.

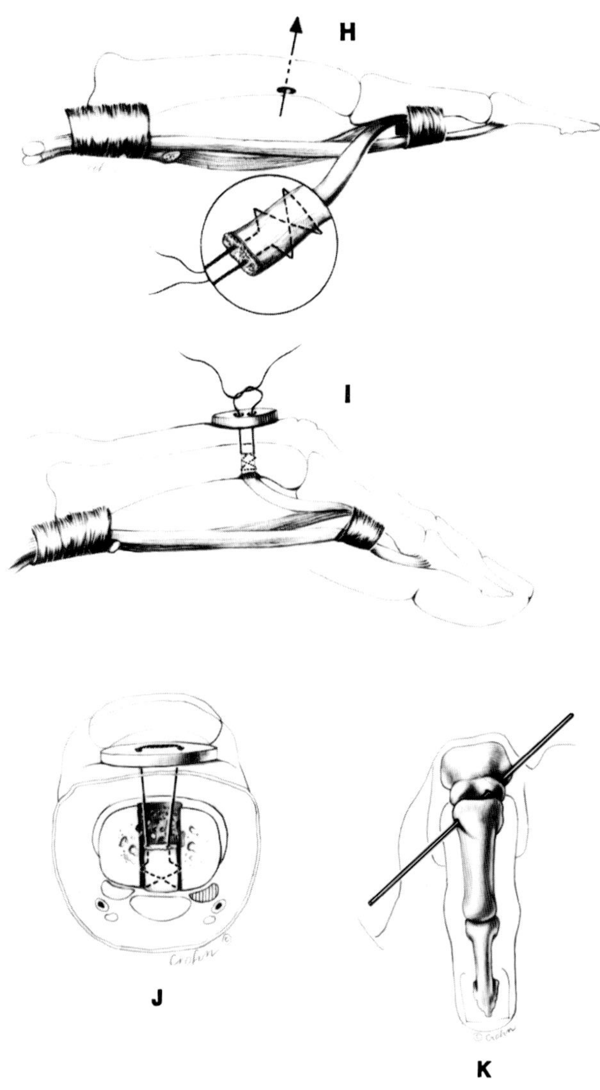

Fig. 53-15 *(Continued).*

Operative Techniques

In deciding the most appropriate surgical procedure for swan-neck deformity, the entire hand must be considered. Four examples are given: (1) if the imbalance is secondary to a mallet deformity, only the mallet need be corrected because restoration of proper distal joint balance will correct the excess PIP joint extensor tone; (2) if the condition is from a fracture of the middle phalanx healed in hyperextension, correction of this bony malalignment is the best treatment for the deformity (see Chapter 18) since reestablishing the alignment and length of the skeleton will rebalance the extensor system; (3) in swan-neck associated with severe spasticity or in a patient whose postoperative adherence to splinting and exercises is doubtful, arthrodesis of the PIP joint is an excellent choice of procedure (see Chapter 4 for technique); (4) in the patient with rheumatoid arthritis, it is absolutely essential to correct any tendon imbalance or flexion contracture at the MP joint before treating a swan-neck deformity. Failure to correct this more proximal MP flexion deformity or imbalance will predetermine failure of the attempt at swan-neck reconstruction in the rheumatoid hand.

Furthermore, it must be repeatedly emphasized that correction of intrinsic tightness will *not* correct swan-neck deformity unless the PIP joint volar plate laxity is also corrected.

If the swan-neck deformity is associated with severe joint changes, such as those seen with advanced rheumatoid arthritis, old fracture dislocations, etc., the PIP joint itself may require arthroplasty (see Chapters 7 and 46) or arthrodesis (see Chapter 4).

In the supple swan-neck deformity, the altered extensor mechanism dynamics at the PIP joint disrupt the linkage of the extensor mechanism. The posture of the DIP joint is totally dependent on the extensor balance and joint position at the PIP joint (and secondarily, and in turn, at the MP joint).

If the swan-neck deformity is a matter of extensor mechanism rebalancing with correction of PIP joint volar plate incompetence, there are two commonly used methods of reconstruction: the oblique retinacular ligament reconstruction and the superficialis tenodesis at the PIP joint.

Oblique Retinacular Ligament Reconstruction (Littler). There are two techniques for this procedure—the original one as described by Littler[75,76,79,81] and the improved modification as more recently reported by Thompson, Littler, and Upton as the "spiral oblique" ligament reconstruction.[139] Both techniques must be done in the digit without fixed deformity and without joint destruction. The principle is the same in each technique, i.e., a tenodesis that (1) passively tightens as the PIP joint actively extends, thus serving as a checkrein to prevent PIP hyperextension; (2) is held volar to the PIP joint axis; and (3) passively tenodeses the DIP joint into extension as the PIP actively extends. Thus, the oblique and spiral retinacular ligament reconstruction directly corrects both interphalangeal joints. The original procedure uses the lateral band, and the modification uses a free tendon graft (palmaris longus or other suitable donor).

Lateral Band Technique (Littler). The exposure is through a long hockey stick incision on the ulnar dorsolateral aspect (Fig.

Table 53-2. Dynamic Similarities of Two Common Collapse Deformities

Dynamic Factor	Claw Deformity	Swan-neck Deformity
Hyperextension proximal joint	MP	PIP
Loss of proximal joint restraint	Intrinsics	Volar plate
Fixed point at proximal joint	Sagittal fibers at MP	Central tendon insertion at PIP
Flexor tendon as deforming force at distal joint	Flexor digitorum superficialis at PIP	Flexor digitorum profundus at DIP
Surgical correction	MP capsulodesis (Zancolli); or tendon transfer for MP flexion	PIP tenodesis (Swanson or Littler)

53-15A–D). The ulnar lateral band is left attached distally and is divided at the musculotendinous junction proximally near the level of the MP joint. The lateral band should be handled minimally, with only skin hooks or fine forceps, as it is sharply incised from the transverse retinacular fibers of the extensor assembly. This freed and distally based lateral band is rerouted volar to Cleland's ligaments. Thus, the new path of the lateral band is dorsal to the DIP joint and volar to the PIP joint. Proximally, at the base of the proximal phalanx, the rerouted lateral band is secured with sufficient tension to restrain the PIP joint in a position 20 degrees short of full extension, at which point the tenodesis tension should be such to lift the DIP joint to 0 degrees. The proximal attachment may be done by passing the lateral band through a window in the proximal flexor tendon sheath (A2 level) and then suturing it back to itself. As a more secure alternative, the proximal lateral band is placed through a hole in the bone of the proximal phalangeal base with a pull-out suture over a button at the opposite side of the digit. For an even more secure repair, the lateral band may be routed volarly across the digit and then through the bone of the proximal phalanx (Fig. 53-16).

Tendon Graft Technique (SORL* Reconstruction) (Thompson and Littler).[139] The exposure of the digit is similar to that of the lateral band technique. Two through-and-through holes are made with gouges (Fig. 53-17)—the first being in the anteroposterior direction at the base of the distal phalanx, with care taken to protect the germinal nail matrix and flexor digitorum profundus insertion, and the second going transversely through the base of the proximal phalanx. The path of the graft (palmaris longus, if available) starts distally at the dorsum of the distal phalanx and passes volarly and proximally along the side of the middle phalanx and anteriorly and obliquely across the front of the PIP joint to the opposite side of the digit at the proximal metaphysis of the proximal phalanx. Thus, the free tendon graft is spiraled around the digit in a subcutaneous plane, but deep to the neurovascular bundles. The path of this tendon graft tenodesis is identical to that of the oblique retinacular ligament reconstruction as illustrated in Figure 53-16, the essential difference being that the former utilizes a free tendon graft and the latter a lateral band from that digit. The proximal end of the tenodesis graft is passed through the hole in the proximal phalanx and secured either to the periosteum or over a button with a pull-out suture. The distal end of the graft is slid through its distal insertion in a dorsal to volar direction. The tenodesis tension is adjusted by slowly pulling more of the graft through the terminal phalanx until the proximal joint rests in 20 degrees flexion with the distal joint at 0 degrees.

* SORL = Spiral Oblique Retinacular Ligament.

Superficialis Tenodesis (Littler). This tenodesis utilizes one slip of the flexor digitorum superficialis as described by Littler[70] (Fig. 53-15E–K). This forms a very stout tenodesis at the PIP joint, reconstituting a check-rein restraint to prevent hyperextension that is secure enough even for the spastic hand. However, it does not rebalance the extensor mechanism at the distal joint and may or may not correct the distal joint extensor lag completely, depending upon the severity of the distal joint droop and the condition of the tendon at that location.

Exposure is via the volar zigzag incision as described by Littler[74] and later by Bruner,[7] and usually requires only the limbs of the incision over the proximal and middle phalanges. The flexor tendon sheath is resected between the A2 and A4 pulleys. One slip of the flexor digitorum superficialis is transected as far proximally as can be safely and gently reached and is left attached distally. The proximally divided and distally based slip is then passed through a drill hole in a volar to dorsal direction through the proximal phalanx and sutured to a button over the dorsum. The PIP joint is then stabilized in 20 degrees flexion with a percutaneous K-wire.

Other operations have been described to provide a passive volar restraint to excessive PIP joint extension. These include suturing the superficial flexor into the neck of the proximal phalanx without tendon transection (Swanson)[136]; fascial or tendon graft, bridging the joint anteriorly (Adams)[1]; tightening of the volar capsule (Bate)[3]; and reattachment of the ruptured volar plate (Portis).[107]

Author's Preferred Method for Swan-neck Deformity

There is no single preferred method for all situations. The author favors the spiral oblique reconstruction with the pathway illustrated in Figures 53-16 and 53-17 to that of the procedure as first described by Littler (Fig. 53-15A–D). The spiral pathway is more secure, as it does preclude the chance of the tenodesis migrating dorsal to the axis of motion at the PIP joint.

The spiral technique using the lateral band is preferable if intrinsic tendon tightness is present, as the harvesting of the lateral band will simultaneously effect an intrinsic release on

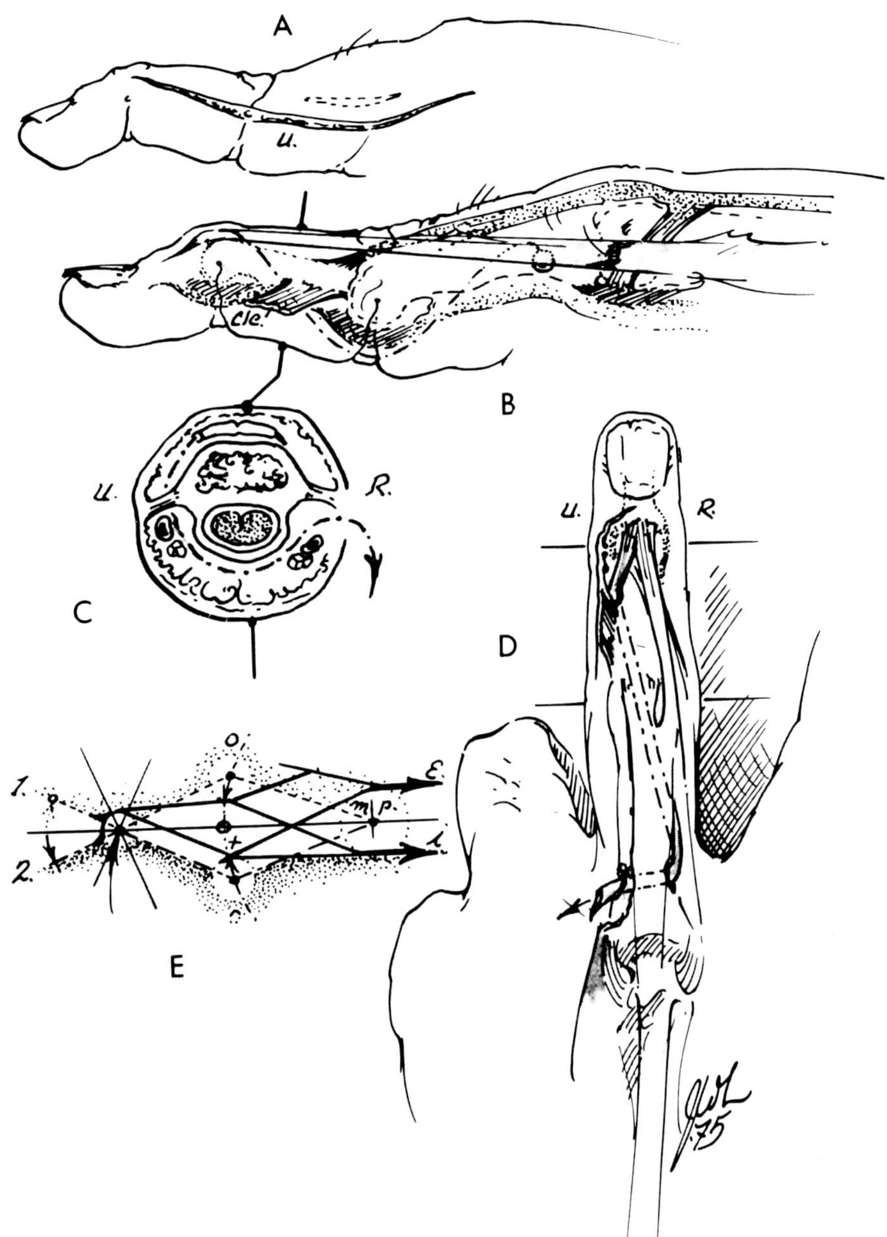

Fig. 53-16. Oblique retinacular ligament reconstruction for swan-neck deformity as modified by Littler from his original procedure to provide more secure repair. The oblique retinacular ligament is routed obliquely across the volar aspect of the digit volar to the flexor sheath but deep to the neurovascular bundles. This precludes any chance of the tenodesis migrating dorsal to the axis of motion at the PIP joint. In addition, the proximal end of the oblique retinacular ligament is passed through the bone and secured to a button, thus providing a far more secure proximal fixation than that originally described by Littler, in which the tenodesis is secured by sutures into the flexor sheath as illustrated in Figure 53-15A–D. (From Littler,[78] with permission.)

one side of the digit. If the opposite lateral band is also tight, it should be released as shown in Figure 53-14.

If the droop of the terminal joint is severe, or if the quality of the extensor tendon complex is poor distal to the PIP joint, the tendon graft technique is definitely preferred by the author.

There are two circumstances in which the author favors the superficialis tenodesis. The first is that where a particularly stout repair is advisable—for example, the spastic hand of cerebral palsy. The second is the situation of correcting three or four fingers at the same operative procedure, as this tenodesis is somewhat easier and can be done more quickly.

If the PIP joint itself is involved with collateral ligament adherence, volar plate scarring, fibrous ankylosis, or joint arthritic changes, the surgeon will need to consider arthrodesis or arthroplasty (see Chapters 4, 7, and 46), as the soft tissue procedures described in this section alone will not suffice.

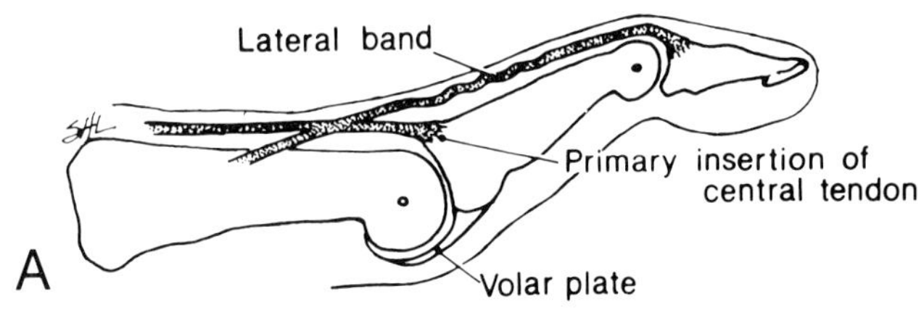

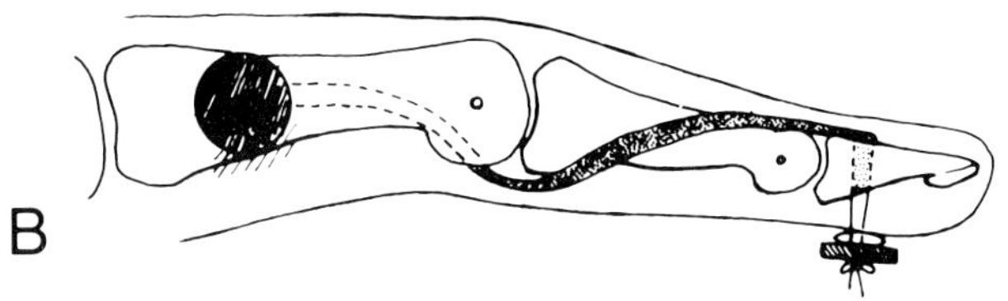

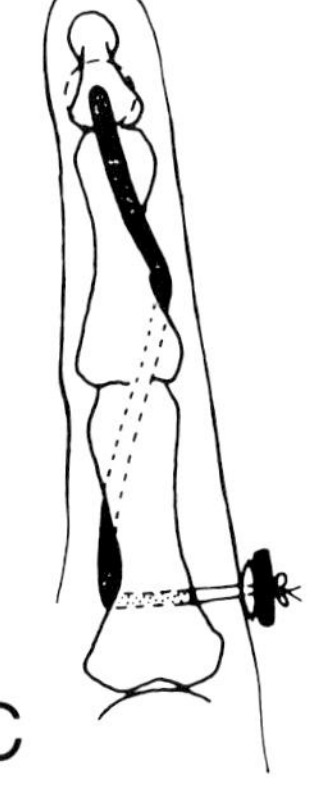

Fig. 53-17. Palmaris longus tenodesis for oblique retinacular ligament reconstruction for swan-neck deformity, called the spiral oblique retinacular ligament (SORL). The pathology of the swan-neck deformity involves hyperextension of the PIP joint with extensor lag at the distal joint, combined with a laxity of the volar plate **(A)**. The palmaris longus can be used to provide a tenodesis to correct the imbalance at both joints in a fashion analogous to that illustrated in Figure 53-16. The essential differences are (1) the use of the palmaris longus tendon as a graft rather than the oblique retinacular ligament, thus making a simpler dissection; and (2) it is easier to adjust the tension of this tenodesis. (See text for operative details.) (Adapted from Thompson et al,[139] with permission.)

Postoperative Care

For all of the above techniques, the protective dressing and K-wire are removed at 4 weeks. Thereafter, the involved digit is protected with a dorsal splint that holds the PIP joint in 20 degrees flexion and the DIP joint in 0 degrees. The patient is started on active assisted PIP flexion exercises with active extension, using the splint as a "back stop" to block active PIP extension at a position of 20 degrees flexion. This protective splint is gradually straightened to 5 to 10 degrees from 6 to 10 weeks after surgery.

It should be noted that the intended goal of these surgical procedures for swan-neck deformity is to prevent hyperextension of the PIP joint. Ideally, the joint should be limited at 0 degrees, but, practically and realistically speaking, the best long-term results without recurrence will be obtained when the proximal joint is check reined at 5 to 10 degrees flexion. This is the desirable goal, and attempts should not be made to stretch out the contracture with dynamic splinting and exercises to 0 degrees extension.

Complications

The major postoperative difficulties are (1) stretching out or rupture of these tenodeses with recurrence of deformity, (2) placing the tenodesis too tight, resulting in excessive PIP joint flexion deformity and potentially a boutonnière (especially with the oblique retinacular ligament procedure), and (3) loss of joint flexion mobility from flexon tendon scarring (especially after superficialis tenodesis).

The attenuation or rupture of the tenodesis is best prevented by careful adherence to the postoperative program. Should such complications occur from overenthusiastic and premature use of the unprotected digit by the patient, the situation can often be salvaged by resumption of extension block splinting for several months to allow rehealing and/or contracture of the tenodesis.

Excessive fixed flexion contracture of the PIP joint, with or without the distal joint recurvature of boutonnière, is a very difficult problem to correct. Fortunately, it does not occur often, especially with careful attention to surgical technique and postoperative care.

If the repair is done with excess tension or if the exercise program is not carefully followed, an unacceptable amount of flexion deformity of the PIP joint may result. This is best treated with a very closely supervised exercise and splinting hand therapy program, as would be used for a boutonnière deformity (see page 1977).

Scarring of the flexor tendons will not happen often, but when it does occur, the digital function is seriously compromised. It may respond well to a hand therapy program or may require tenolysis (see Chapter 51).

Late Extensor Hood Adherence

Following lacerations of the extensor mechanism over the proximal phalanx, especially if fractures are present, the extensor hood may adhere to the bone or periosteum of the proximal phalanx. There are two anatomic reasons for this: (1) the tendon normally is in direct proximity to the periosteum, separated only by a very thin layer of areolar tissue; and (2) this extensor tendon assembly surrounds the proximal phalanx on three sides (Fig. 53-18).

Should this pathologic state exist, it may be of two types: (1) following tangential lacerations, the scar is limited in its extent, involving only a portion of the extensor mechanism, such as only the central tendon or only a lateral band; and (2) following a comminuted fracture, crush injury, or old shredding-type extensor tendon injuries, the scarring is extensive with broad areas of tendon adherence to two or three sides of the proximal phalanx.

Regardless of which of the two types of adherence is present, on examination, these patients have an obvious limitation of active PIP joint extension. More importantly, they have a loss of active and passive PIP joint flexion because of the extensor tenodesis tethering restraint.

Treatment

Usually these injuries present as a limitation of PIP joint motion and are best treated by an exercise and splinting program that emphasizes active assisted PIP joint flexion and extension.

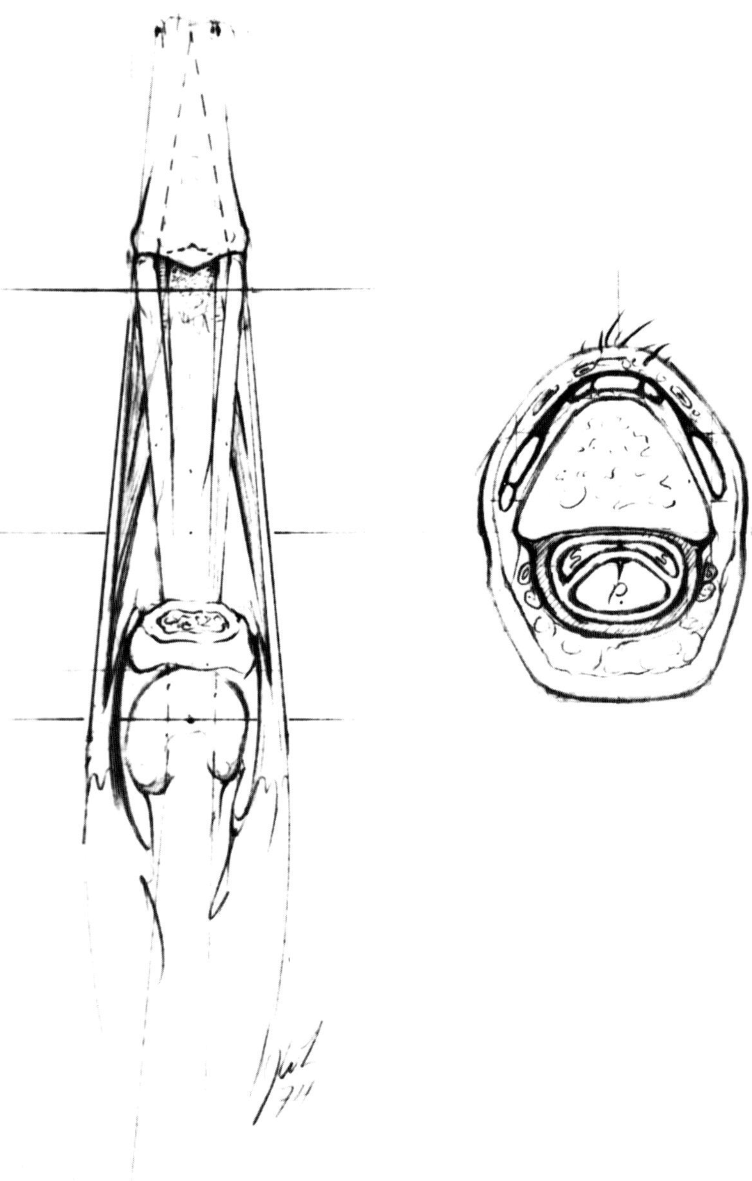

Fig. 53-18. The proximity of the extrinsic extensor mechanism to the bone of the proximal phalanx combined with its anatomic distribution on three sides of the proximal phalanx imposes a high risk of extensor mechanism scarring to the proximal phalanx after tendon injuries at this level and in fractures of the proximal phalanx (see text). (From Littler et al,[80] with permission.)

Occasionally a patient will not respond to this conservative program. In the patient with scarring of just the central tendon or one lateral band, the offending portion of the extensor assembly is best resected, as would be done for extrinsic or intrinsic release as described on page 1968 (Fig. 53-14).

Should the area of adherence be of the broad, latter type, conservative treatment is difficult and results are limited. The effort is well justified, however, for the results from extensive surgical extensor tenolysis over the proximal phalanx are poor.

Boutonnière Deformity

If the extensor mechanism linkage system dynamics is primarily disrupted at the PIP joint, a boutonnière deformity develops. A boutonnière is *not* synonymous with a PIP joint flexion deformity.[80,82] Simply stated, a boutonnière deformity refers to a finger posture with the PIP joint flexed and the DIP joint hyperextended. It occurs secondary to dorsal disruption of the extensor assembly at the PIP joint and initially is a dynamic imbalance of the extensor linkage system (Fig. 53-19). When left untreated, the condition will progress to a fixed deformity, in which case there are fixed contractures in this posture that will not passively correct (Fig. 53-20).

The basic initial pathomechanics are attenuation, attrition, or rupture of the central tendon over the PIP joint or off the dorsal base of the middle phalanx, and prolapse of the lateral bands volar to the PIP joint axis[10,11,80,82] (Fig. 53-19). This central tendon change may be secondary to laceration, closed avulsion, crush injury, or the synovitis of rheumatoid arthritis or osteoarthritis. By whatever etiology, there is damage to the central tendon and the dorsal transverse retinacular fibers. It is critical to realize that the boutonnière does not merely involve damage to the central tendon, but also alterations of the transverse retinacular fibers, which permit the volar subluxation of the lateral bands. In the acute situation, the patient will have full active flexion and full passive extension of both interphalangeal joints. In fact, some patients with the PIP joint placed at 0 degrees are able to maintain *full* active PIP extension. Once the joint flexes enough for volar lateral band displacement, however, active extension arc is lost, as the lateral bands do not pass dorsal to the axis of PIP motion.

If the condition is left untreated, the dorsal central tendon and dorsal transverse retinacular fibers continue to lengthen, the volar transverse retinacular fibers tighten, and the lateral bands are restrained anterior to the PIP joint axis. The fixed or rigid boutonnière is thus established as the lateral bands shorten, the oblique retinacular ligaments thicken and shorten, and secondary joint changes occur[80,82] (Fig. 53-20).

In this imbalance of the late boutonnière deformity, all flexor and extensor power is concentrated for PIP joint flexion. Not only the flexor digitorum profundus and superficialis, but all of the extensor mechanism via the dislocated lateral bands, act as PIP joint flexors (Fig. 53-20). Therefore, the deformity is "self-accelerating" from this unopposed PIP joint flexion force.[80]

Thus, there are three types (or stages) of the boutonnière deformity:

Stage 1. The dynamic imbalance, passively supple,

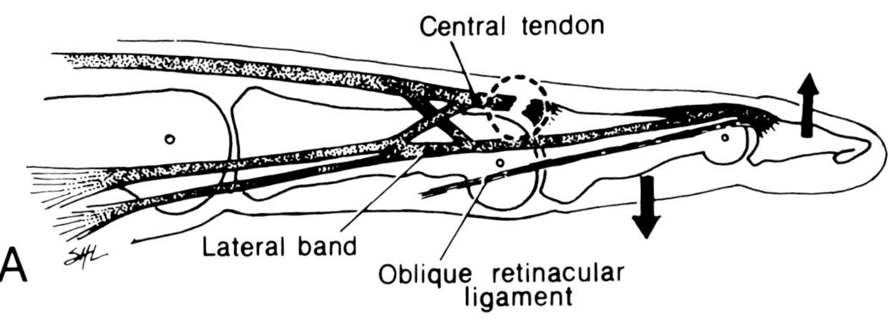

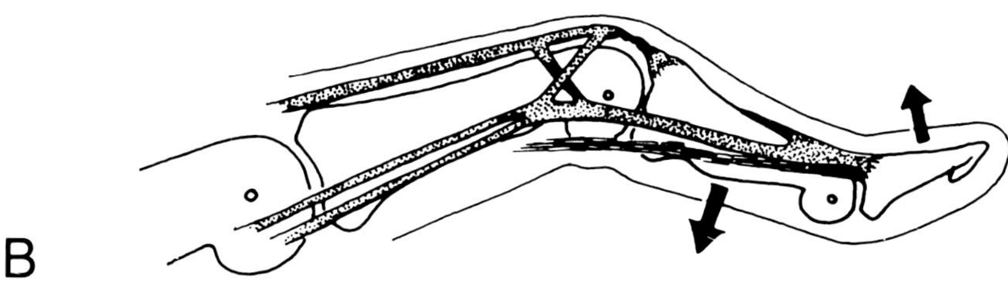

Fig. 53-19. Pathomechanics of the boutonnière deformity. **(A)** As the central tendon either ruptures or attenuates, extensor tone is decreased at the dorsal base of the middle phalanx, allowing the PIP joint to drop into flexion. **(B)** As the joint flexes, the lateral bands move volar to the axis of motion. They will adhere in that position, and the central tendon heals in the attenuated position. The pathomechanics of the established boutonnière involve not only the attenuation of the central tendon, but the displaced, adherent, and foreshortened lateral bands resting volar to the axis of motion at the PIP joint. Excess extensor pull thus secondarily bypasses the PIP joint and is imposed dorsally at the DIP joint, causing a recurvature at this distal joint (see text and Fig. 53-20). (Adapted from Burton and Eaton,[11] with permission.)

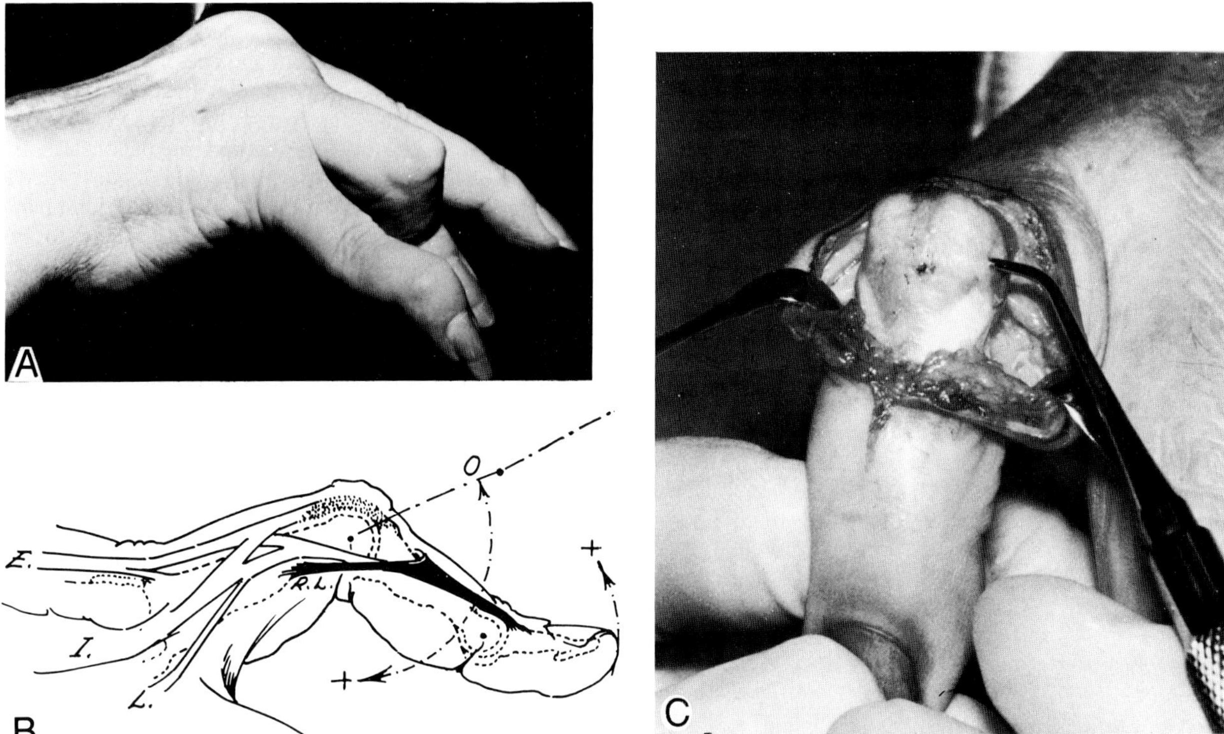

Fig. 53-20. **(A)** Established boutonnière deformity (see text). **(B)** In the late established boutonnière, all power at the PIP joint serves to flex the joint. The extrinsic and intrinsic extensor tone at the PIP joint is absent due to the attenuation. All of the extrinsic and intrinsic extensor tone passes through the lateral bands volar to the axis of motion at the PIP joint. Obviously, the flexor tendons impart only flexor tone at this joint. Thus, there is no extensor power, only flexor power at the proximal joint. All of the extensor tone is diverted to the distal joint imposing hyperextension. At this stage, the contracted lateral bands limit even passive extension of the PIP joint. **(C)** Operative findings in the patient with late established boutonnière deformity. The dental probe is at the axis of joint motion. The lateral bands are seen well volar to this axis of motion. The attenuation of the central tendon is impressive. (Fig. B adapted from Littler and Eaton,[82] with permission.)

in which the lateral bands are subluxated but not adherent anteriorly

Stage 2. Established extensor tendon contracture in which the deformity *cannot* be passively corrected as the lateral bands are shortened and thickened, but the joint itself is not involved

Stage 3. Secondary joint changes, such as volar plate scarring and contracture, collateral ligament scarring, and intraarticular fibrosis

Nonoperative Treatment

The best treatment is to recognize the potential problem before it occurs and by doing so prevent the problem (Chapter 52). Surgical correction of the established boutonnière deformity is fraught with difficulties and pitfalls, although it is technically possible. Fortunately, many of these deformities will respond to a specific and conscientious splinting and exercise program. Certain generalities merit emphasis: (1) the earlier the splints and exercises are begun the better, for the dynamic imbalance of Stage 1 will almost always respond extremely well to conservative management; (2) attention must be paid to regaining DIP joint flexion as well as PIP joint extension; (3) almost all those fingers in Stage 1 and many of those in Stage 2 are best treated without surgery; (4) unless bone or joint changes have occurred, surgery should not be considered without first trying the therapy program for several weeks and, if early objective measureable improvement is noted, continuing the conservative program; and (5) surgery cannot take the place of any exercise and splinting program, but is used in *addition* to such a program. Thus surgery is *not* a shortcut in either time or patient effort. Finally, in those fingers that respond conservatively, the result equals or exceeds that possible from surgery.

The critical exercise involves two sequential maneuvers (Fig. 53-21). The *first* is active assisted PIP joint extension. This will stretch the tight volar structures, such as the volar plate, flexor sheath, and volar transverse retinacular fibers. This initial part of the exercise will cause the lateral bands to ride dorsal to the PIP joint axis and will put longitudinal tension on the lateral bands and oblique retinacular ligaments. This in turn will *increase* the tenodesis of the DIP joint into hyperextension. In other words, passive correction of the proximal deformity will increase the distal deformity.

The *second* maneuver is maximal active forced flexion of the DIP joint *while the PIP joint is held at 0 degrees* (or as close to that position as the PIP joint will allow). This will gradually

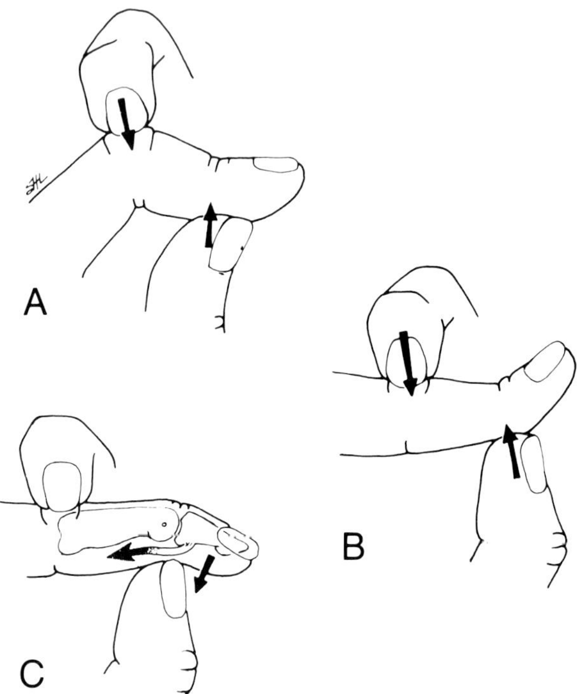

Fig. 53-21. Exercise program for boutonnière deformity. Many patients with boutonnière deformity respond very well to a carefully structured exercise and splinting program. The exercise is done in three steps. **(A)** The patient is instructed to place the index finger of the opposite hand on the dorsum of the PIP joint of the involved finger. The thumb of the uninvolved hand is placed on the flexor aspect of the DIP joint. **(B)** The PIP joint is then passively extended by the patient as far as can be tolerated. This will passively correct the deformity at the proximal joint, but will increase the tone in the lateral bands and oblique retinacular ligament, increasing the hyperextension at the DIP joint. As a third step to the exercise **(C)**, the patient then actively flexes the DIP joint over the thumb of the opposite hand, thus stretching the oblique retinacular ligaments and lateral bands (see text).

stretch the lateral bands and oblique retinacular ligaments to their physiologic length.

The splinting program involves a combination of active and static splints worn during the day and static splints worn at night (Fig. 53-22A–D). The splint supports only the PIP joint and the proximal two phalanges, leaving the MP and DIP joints free.

This exercise and splinting program must be maintained for a minimum of 2 to 3 months and often much longer, to gain the maximum possible correction and prevent recurrence.

Operative Techniques

There are many surgical procedures for boutonnière deformity. Seven considerations must be strongly emphasized.

1. These operations must be precisely done. They are deceptively difficult and should not be attempted by the surgeon who only occasionally operates on the hand.
2. Operative treatment should rarely be necessary in the supple boutonnière, as this condition usually responds to conservative management.
3. The procedure should be done within the context of a pre- and postoperative exercise and splinting program. The exercises and splints are needed for several months after surgery.
4. The tendon procedure is best done after the joint has full passive mobility. In some difficult problems with a very stiff joint, the surgical correction must be done in two stages. The first stage is the release of the joint (see Chapter 12), and the second is the tendon reconstruction. In many patients, after the joint release is completed and the exercise program resumed, the extensor mechanism rebalances with the conscientious performance of the two-stage exercise program and the splinting/cast support of the PIP joint. In these patients the second surgical stage is not required.
5. If the radiograph shows significant arthritic changes, extensor mechanism rebalancing must be combined with implant arthroplasty (see Chapter 7) or with PIP joint fusion (see Chapter 4).
6. Most patients with a boutonnière deformity retain full flexion and, therefore, full grip function; thus, most patients, even with this deformity, have good function. As surgery is planned, the surgeon must be constantly aware of the need not to jeopardize flexor function in an attempt to gain extension.
7. All procedures involve a rebalancing of the extensor system, decreasing the tone at the distal joint and diverting it to the proximal joint.

Extensor Tendon Division. Many different types of operations have been described for treatment of the established boutonnière deformity. In my opinion, the most reliable procedure is that advocated by Eaton and Littler.[23] This is similar in principle to the essential first part of their initial procedure[82] and not unlike that described by Dolphin,[21] Fowler,[31-33] and Nalebuff[98] (Fig. 53-23). A favorable surgical result is much more predictable in the patient who has full passive extension *preoperatively*. This operation is best done via a dorsal bayonet incision centered over the PIP joint. The extensor mechanism is divided transversely over the junction of the mid and proximal thirds of the middle phalanx, distal to the dorsal transverse retinacular fibers. This thus separates the fixed point of the extensor mechanism at the dorsal base of the middle phalanx from the fixed point at the distal phalanx. This allows the mechanism to slide proximally at the proximal metaphyseal level of the middle phalanx. The lateral band tendon heals in this lengthened position. This release is identical to the critical first step of the procedure described in 1967,[82] except that any redundancy of lateral band is allowed to slide proximally (rather than be sutured dorsally). The results are increased tone of the central tendon insertion at the base of the proximal phalanx, decrease of the excessive tone of the extensor tendon at the DIP joint level, and dorsal shift of the lateral bands relative to the PIP joint axis as the converging bands slide proximally. Note that the oblique retinacular ligament is not divided; its preservation is necessary or the distal joint will droop.

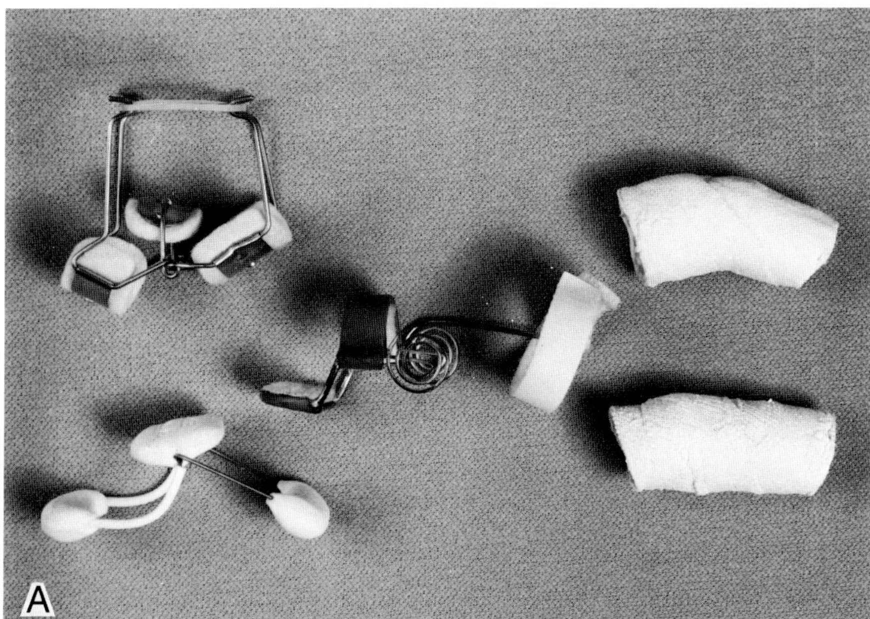

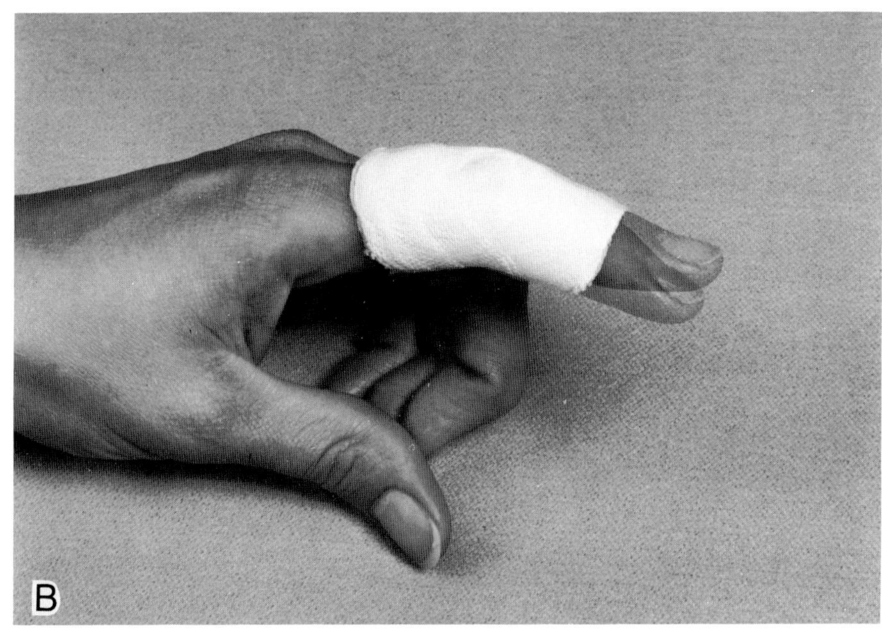

Fig. 53-22. Many types of splints are helpful in the nonoperative treatment of boutonnière deformity. **(A)** These splints may be one of a number of types of dynamic splints, or may involve the use of static splinting, such as small cylinder casts, etc. **(B)** In the patient with some fixed flexion contracture of the PIP joint, a cylinder cast can be made that the patient can remove for skin care and bathing, but wear at all other times. This splint holds the proximal joint in its maximally corrected position. The distal joint is left free to flex. Thus, throughout the day the patient is flexing the distal joint and gradually stretching the contracted oblique retinacular ligaments and lateral bands. *(Figure continues.)*

Postoperative Care. The digit is covered with a small sterile dressing, and active assisted range of motion exercises are resumed. Between exercises the PIP joint is splinted in full extension. Usually the DIP joint is left free, but if a slight droop is noted, the distal joint is splinted in full extension between exercises. This splinting is continued for 6 to 8 weeks, and then the patient is weaned from the splint.

Littler's Boutonnière Reconstruction.[79,82] The traditional Littler procedure is recommended if the lateral bands are so foreshortened and heavily scarred that they contribute significantly to the fixed flexion deformity at the PIP joint (Fig. 53-20). In this procedure, the lateral bands (except for the lumbrical and the oblique retinacular ligaments) are divided at the middle phalanx, identical to the operation described above. The lateral bands are then rolled dorsally and sutured to the central tendon insertion (Fig. 53-24). Thus, the extensor mechanism is simplified, and the component parts of the extensor mechanism to the PIP and DIP joints are separated. Note the similarity in principle to the more recent operation.[23] The lateral bands and central tendon act only to extend the PIP joint and have no effect on the DIP joint. A very important concept is that the previously displaced lateral bands no longer restrain PIP joint extension, the volar restraint having been transferred to an active extensor. The oblique retinacular ligament and lumbrical (on the radial side) are left to control the extensor tone at the DIP joint. As the PIP joint is actively extended, the tone increases in the oblique retinacular ligament, passively lifting the DIP joint into extension.

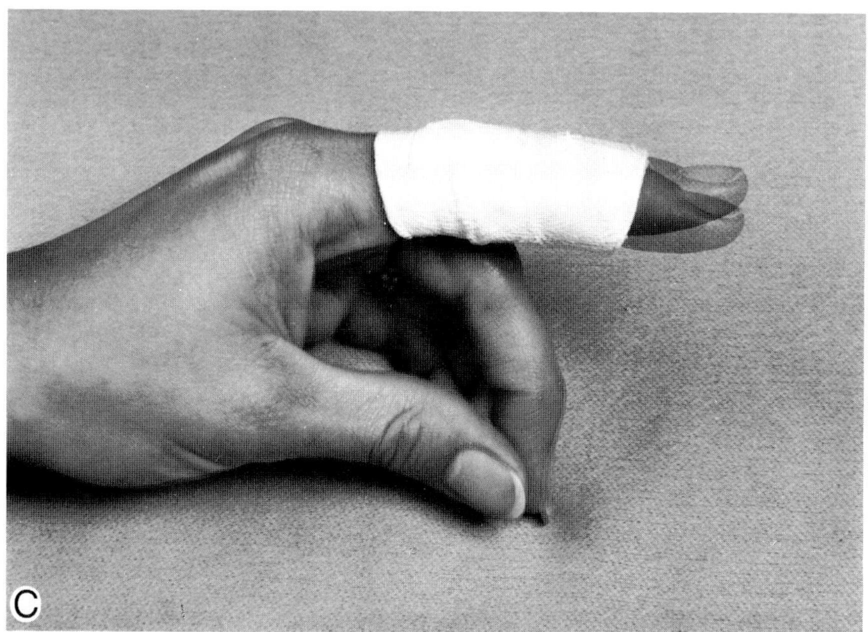

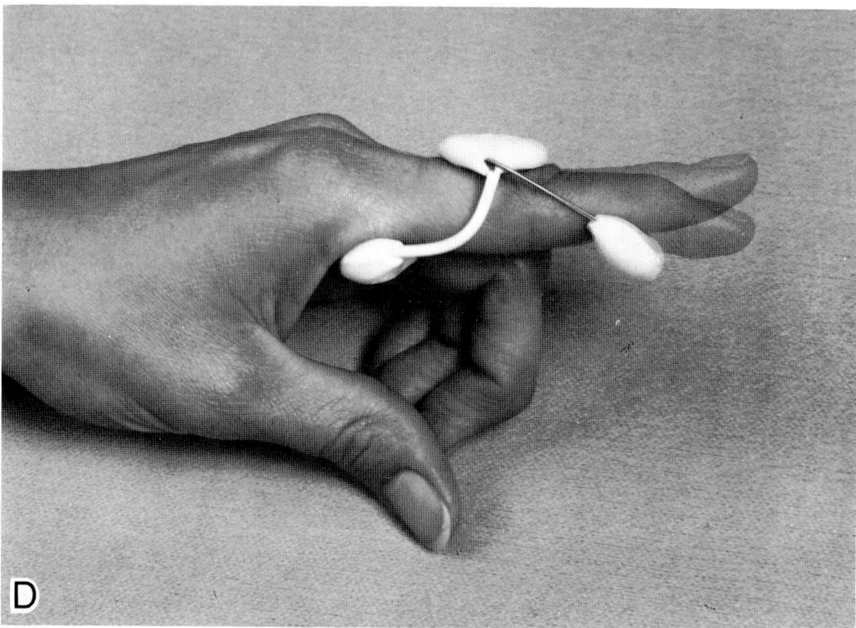

Fig. 53-22 *(Continued).* **(C)** As passive correction of the proximal joint is obtained with the exercise program illustrated in Figure 53-21, increasingly straighter cylinder casts are made for the patient. By continuing the exercise program and the serial cylinder cast, the boutonnière deformity can frequently be gradually corrected. **(D)** The correction of the joint contracture at the proximal level is frequently aided by the use of dynamic splints (see text).

The PIP joint is stabilized in full extension with an oblique K-wire (0.045 inch).

Note that this reconstruction cannot be done if the boutonnière is acute or if the chronic state is such that the central tendon is too thinned to accept the sutures from the lateral bands.

Postoperative Care. The finger and hand are supported in a hand dressing with an external plaster shell or splint for 3 weeks. At 3 weeks the K-wire and sutures are removed, and the PIP joint is splinted dorsally in full extension, with the MP and DIP joints left free. If the distal joint tends to droop, it is also included in the splint in full extension. At 4 weeks gentle active range of motion exercises for both interphalangeal joints are begun but the dorsal splint is continued between exercises for a total of 2 to 4 months after surgery, depending on the clinical progress.

Tendon Graft Procedure. On occasion, the central tendon deficit will be so large or attenuated as to preclude the use of these procedures, and a tendon graft will be required, as described by Fowler,[33] Nichols,[99] and, more recently, Littler[79] (Fig. 53-25). This procedure should be done only if full passive extension of the joint is present preoperatively. A long slender strip of the palmaris longus or extensor digiti quinti is passed through two adjacent holes in the dorsal base of the middle

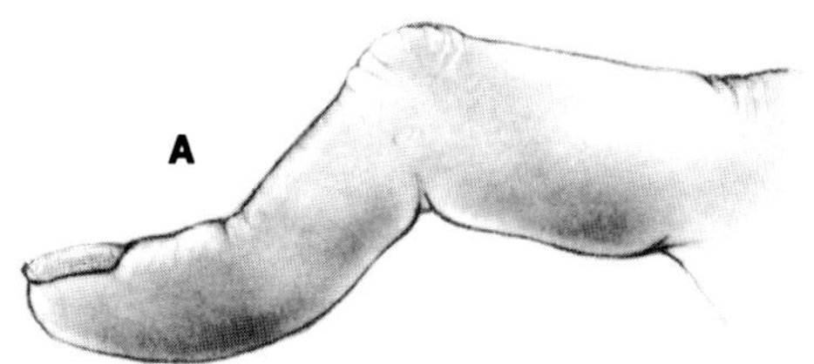

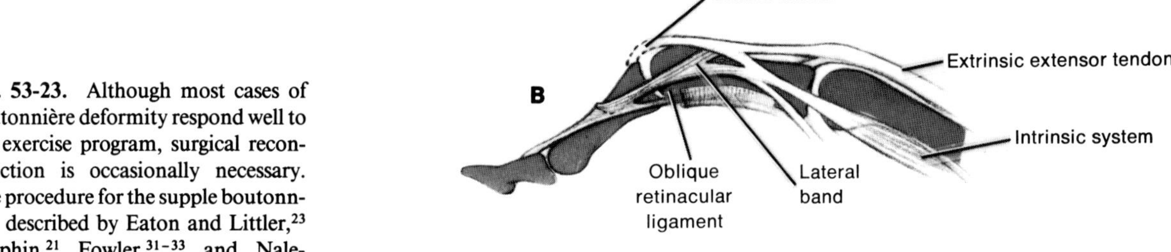

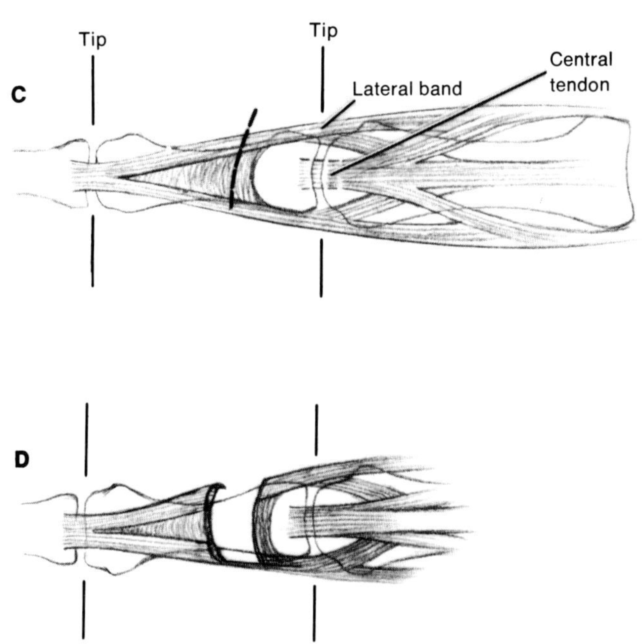

Fig. 53-23. Although most cases of boutonnière deformity respond well to the exercise program, surgical reconstruction is occasionally necessary. The procedure for the supple boutonnière described by Eaton and Littler,[23] Dolphin,[21] Fowler,[31-33] and Nalebuff[98] uses the surgical principle of decreasing the extensor tone at the distal joint by incomplete transection of the extensor mechanism (leaving the oblique retinacular ligament intact), allowing the lateral bands of the extensor mechanism to slide proximally and increase the tone at the PIP joint (see text). (From Burton,[10] with permission.)

phalanx. Each end of the tendon slip is passed through and sutured to the contralateral lateral band. The holes in the middle phalanx must be carefully placed: they must be as dorsal as possible to obtain mechanical advantage for the graft insertion, and great care must be exercised not to fracture the bone bridge between the holes. The joint is stabilized in full extension with an oblique 0.045-inch K-wire. The postoperative care is identical to that described above for the traditional Littler procedure.

Lateral Band Tendon Transfer Procedures. A lateral band transfer,[73] as an alternative to this type of tendon graft, has also been described by Littler. This procedure utilizes the ulnar lateral band as a tendon transfer. The lateral band is transected over the distal end of the middle phalanx and left attached to its proximal muscles. Both radial and ulnar lateral bands are released from the volar transverse retinacular fibers. The ulnar lateral band is then passed (as a tendon transfer) through the radial lateral band at the PIP joint level and then through two holes in the dorsal base of the middle phalanx (placed as for the tendon graft described above). The postoperative care is similar to that for the graft.

Another lateral band transfer procedure has been described by Matev.[88,89] The ulnar lateral band is transected at the level of the DIP joint, the radial band at the midshaft level of the middle phalanx. Both lateral bands are transferred, the longer proximal ulnar one across the dorsum of the middle phalanx to

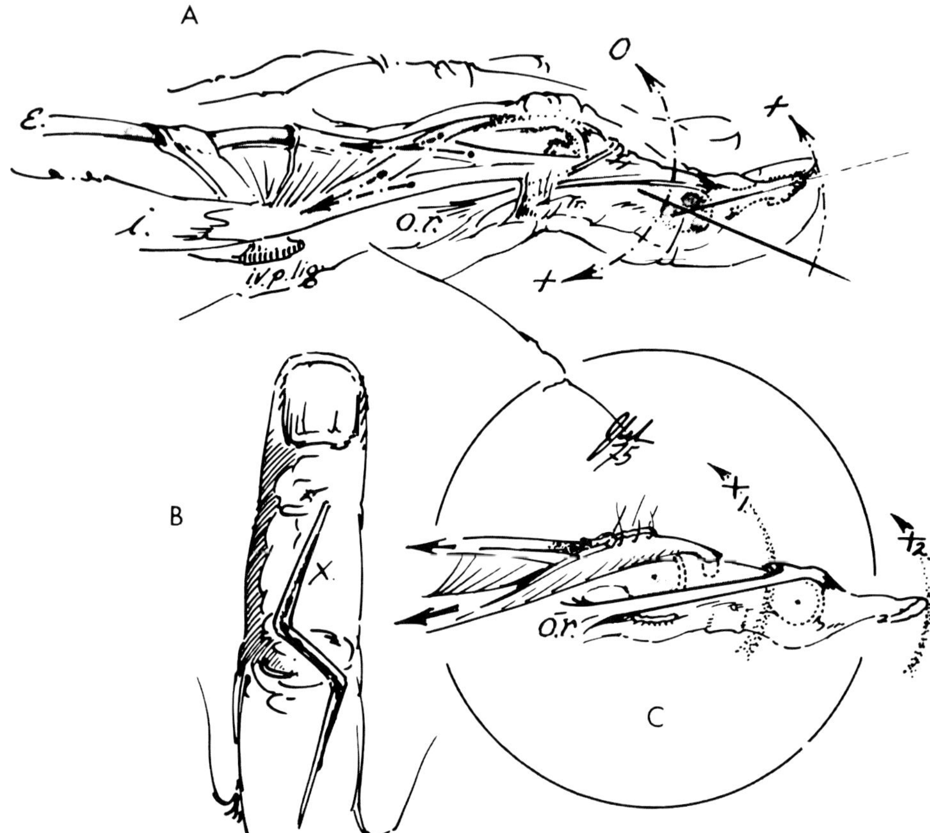

Fig. 53-24. In patients with the severely contracted boutonnière deformity, it may be necessary to transect the lateral bands and divert all of their power to the dorsal base of the middle phalanx, relying upon the oblique retinacular ligament to control the distal joint. This is known as the Littler procedure (see text). (From Littler,[78] with permission.)

the distal radial stump, and the shorter proximal radial one through the central tendon and into the periosteum at the dorsal base of the middle phalanx. Matev recommends 3 weeks of immobilization with the MP joint flexed 45 degrees and the interphalangeal joints in full extension, followed by a graduated active exercise and splinting program.

Secondary Direct Central Tendon Repair. Mason[86] described primary surgical repair of the central tendon in the acute injury. This concept has been applied to the chronic state by Kilgore and Graham[56] and later by Elliott.[24] Kilgore and Graham do a Y-V type advancement, whereas Elliott simply resects the redundant attenuated central tendon and then performs a direct repair. Note that both these procedures are successful only if there is no restraint to full passive PIP joint extension. As these are the patients with supple deformities, many will respond very well to the exercise and splinting program without surgery. This conservative program should be attempted first.

Author's Preferred Method

The difficulty of surgical reconstruction for late boutonnière deformity is indicated by the number of these and many other procedures described in the past. The results from some are less predictable than from those described above. Other procedures for the less severe boutonnière deformity have been replaced by the much more reliable results obtained from the careful exercise and splinting program described on page 1977.

For the boutonnière deformity, the enthusiastic surgeon must be ever mindful that (1) even the most careful operative techniques may not overcome the fibroblastic response of the extensor mechanism paratenon with its destruction of gliding surfaces and loss of a few millimeters of excursion; (2) the most encouraging early surgical result may be destroyed by a few millimeters of attenuation as a repair site stretches out from poor attention to the exercise and splinting program; and (3) if a good joint is present, as seen on radiograph, the result from a carefully designed and closely followed exercise and splinting program may equal or exceed that obtained with surgery.

Should surgery be necessary as a final resort in those patients not responding to the conscientious splinting and exercise program the summary of the author's preferences is as follows.

1. Initially all established boutonnière fingers should be treated with the splinting and exercise program as outlined in the text and in Figures 53-21 and 53-22.
2. In the occasional Stage 1 and Stage 2 (see page 1976) boutonnière that does not respond, the

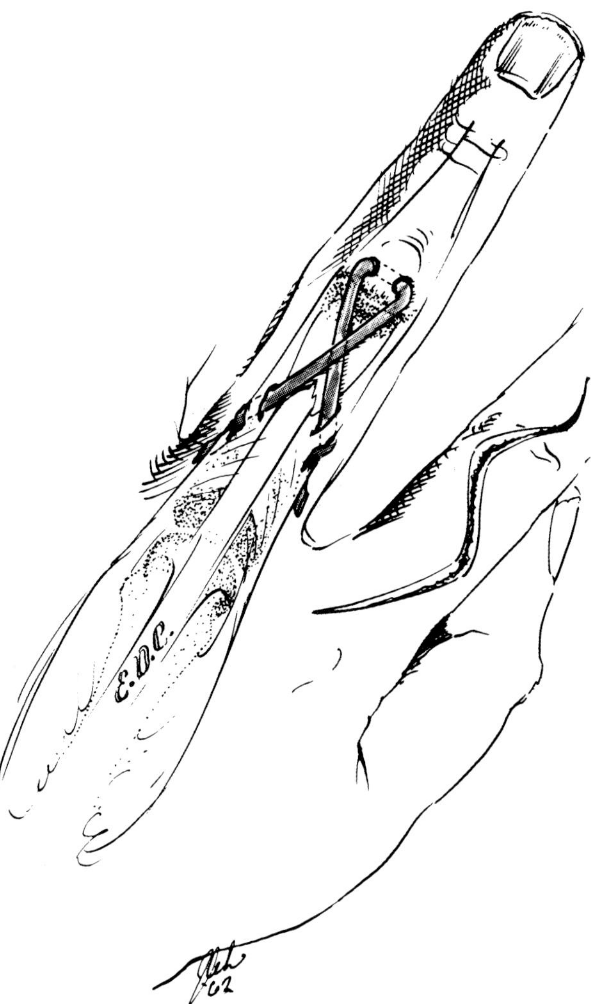

Fig. 53-25. In those patients with marked extensor lag at the PIP joint with absence of the central tendon insertion and deficient lateral bands, tendon graft may be necessary. The procedure, as described by Fowler and illustrated by Littler, involves a tendon graft using the palmaris longus, as shown here. (From Littler,[78] with permission.)

Eaton-Littler procedure (Fig. 53-23), the Littler-Eaton procedure (Fig. 53-24), or the Matev procedure are recommended. The Eaton-Littler is the simplest to do technically, but does require some competence of the extensor insertion into the dorsal base of the middle phalanx. If I find this extensor insertion inadequate once the Eaton-Littler release is completed, I then prefer to add the repair of the Littler-Eaton.

3. If at surgery it is obvious that the central tendon insertion is deficient and the lateral bands inadequate, the Littler-Fowler tendon graft (Fig. 53-25) can be used.
4. If the joint is involved with fibrous ankylosis or arthritis, then fusion (Chapter 4) or arthroplasty (Chapters 7 and 46) is recommended.

DIP Joint Extensor Disorders (Mallet Finger Deformity)

The terminal joint of the finger has no extensor function independent of the position of the more proximal joint[79,80] (Fig. 53-26). The range of active extension of the DIP joint from a flexed position is predicated on active extension of the PIP joint. Because of the fixed tendon and retinacular lengths already described on page 1958, active extension of these two interphalangeal joints is interrelated.

With either DIP joint hyperextension or flexion deformity, the PIP joint mechanics must always be examined, for the prime pathology may be at that more proximal level in the boutonnière or swan-neck deformity. Absence of normal lateral band mobility at the PIP joint, if associated with anterior displacement and shortening, will impose DIP joint hyperextension. If the lateral bands bowstring dorsally at the PIP joint, DIP joint extensor lag may occur (see previous discussions on boutonnière and swan-neck deformities).

The most common extensor mechanism disorder at the DIP joint is an extensor lag, the so-called mallet deformity, secondary to loss of extensor power to the terminal segment. This causes the extensor mechanism to shift proximally, increasing the extensor tone at the PIP joint relative to the DIP joint. If the patient has a lax PIP joint volar plate, this joint will hyperex-

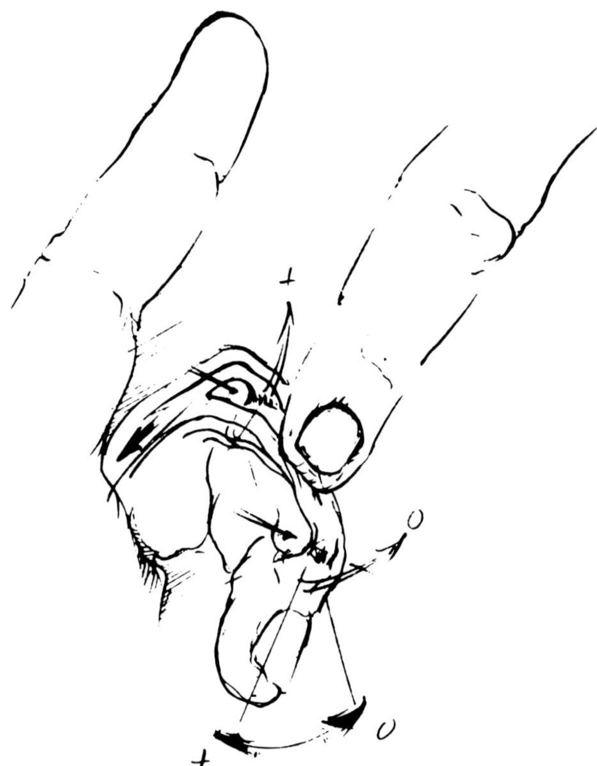

Fig. 53-26. The DIP joint has little independent active extension. When the PIP joint is in maximum flexion, the tone in the lateral bands is maximally relaxed to permit simultaneous active flexion of the distal joint. This laxity, however, precludes active extension of the distal joint in this position. (From Littler,[80] with permission.)

tend as a secondary deformity.[79,80] A secondary swan-neck will thus develop (Fig. 53-27). Parenthetically, it should be noted that this increase in PIP joint extensor tendon tension by distal disruption is the principle of the Littler-Eaton, Fowler, Dolphin, and Nalebuff release procedures for early boutonnière.

Initially, the acute mallet deformity can be one of three types: tendon disruption, tendon avulsion with small fleck of bone, and tendon avulsion with an intraarticular bone fragment comprising a significant portion of the joint surface and with volar joint subluxation[11] (Fig. 53-28). The initial treatment of these is detailed in Chapter 52. These can be treated as fresh injuries up to 4 weeks.[92]

Should the patient be seen later with a chronic mallet deformity, one of several situations may exist, each condition with or without a secondary swan-neck deformity: (1) *supple* or *fixed* following old injury of the type seen in Figure 53-28A or B (no fracture); these joints usually have congruous surfaces. (2) *supple* or *fixed* following old injury of the type seen in Figure 53-28C or D (with fracture); these joints usually have incongruity, and (3) established secondary osteoarthritis.

There are several situations that may justify the patient's seeking late treatment for mallet deformity: pain in the joint, concern about appearance, secondary swan-neck deformity, or the complaint, "the finger is hooked and gets in my way."

Operative Techniques

If the deformity is fixed and does not respond to exercises and splinting, if the joint surfaces are incongruous, or if significant degenerative arthritis is present, the distal joint is best treated with arthrodesis (see Chapter 4).

If the droop is passively correctable with joint congruity, the extensor insertion is exposed dorsally as for an acute injury. Three types of tendon reconstruction by shortening are feasible because of the pseudotendon (scar tissue), which fills the gap from the old rupture.

First, a tuck may be taken in the tendon. Second, a segment of tendon is resected and an end-to-end repair done under appropriate tension.[24] Third, the insertion of the pseudotendon is divided, and the tendon is advanced into the bone of the dorsal base of distal phalanx. All three techniques simply involve a shortening of the tendon length between the fixed points at the dorsal bases of the distal and middle phalanges.

It must be emphasized that only 2 to 3 mm of tendon usually needs to be resected, so critical and small is the amplitude of the extensor at this level. Excess shortening will impose distal joint hyperextension deformity.

Regardless of the technique used for the tendon shortening, a K-wire is used to stabilize the terminal joint at 0 degrees for 4 to 6 weeks, and the DIP joint is immobilized with a dorsal splint at all times for 6 to 8 weeks. When the DIP flexion exercises are commenced, they must be carefully regulated and the splint gradually weaned so that the repaired tendon will "slide and glide" and not stretch out.

If the deformity is supple following an old injury of the type seen in Figure 53-28C, surgical correction is possible but may be very difficult because of the foreshortened and contracted collateral ligaments and volar plate, if the anterior joint subluxation is such that some proximal migration of the terminal phalanx has occurred as well. The joint is exposed dorsally. The germinal nail matrix must be carefully protected. The fracture is freed from adhesions. Part of the collateral ligaments may require section in order to gain sufficient length to correct the volar subluxation. The fracture is then reduced, stabilized, and followed postoperatively as for an acute injury (see Chapter 52). The secondary late open reduction of these chronic fractures can be difficult, and the results disappointing. Accurate reduction may be elusive, bony union slow, and final joint motion limited.

A

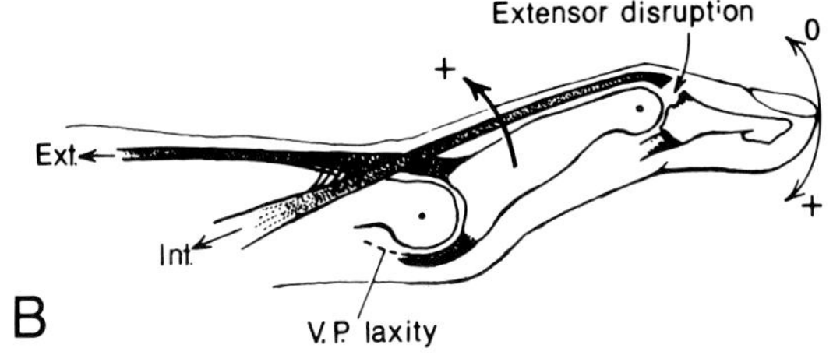

Fig. 53-27. **(A)** With disruption of the extensor mechanism at the distal joint, an extensor lag occurs. In this situation tone of the extensor mechanism at the proximal joint is increased. This patient with a lax volar plate at the PIP joint then developed a swan-neck deformity secondary to the old extensor tendon laceration at the distal joint. **(B)** The altered extensor mechanism imposes the swan-neck deformity as the tendon assembly slides proximally in the presence of a lax PIP volar plate *(V.P.)*. Both the intrinsic *(Int.)* and extrinsic *(Ext.)* extensors contribute to this proximal imbalance. (Fig. A from Littler et al,[80] with permission; Fig B adapted from Littler et al,[80] with permission.)

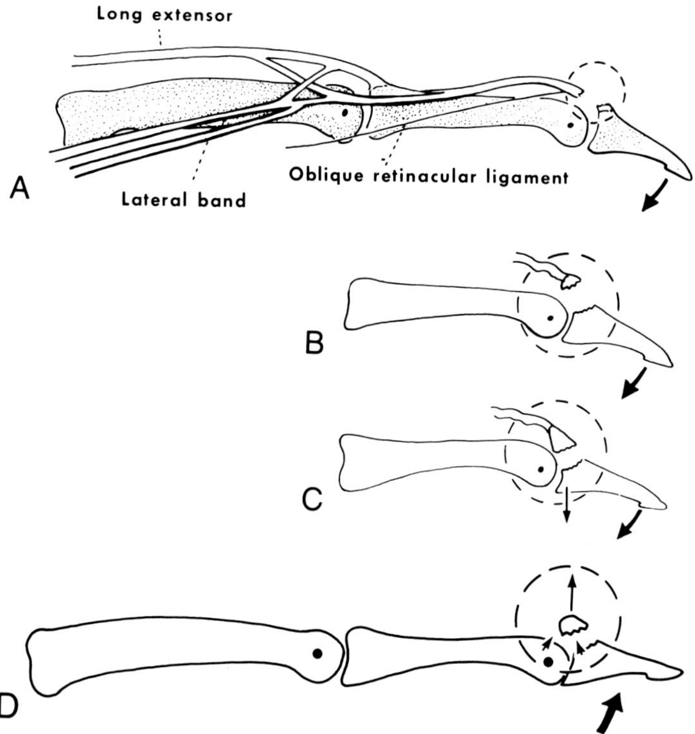

Fig. 53-28. Mallet deformity can occur secondary to tendon rupture **(A)**, tendon avulsion with a small fleck of attached bone **(B)**, or a significant intraarticular fracture with joint incongruity and anterior subluxation **(C)**. This latter type usually cannot be reduced closed because of fracture displacement. **(D)** With attempted closed reduction of a large fracture fragment, the realignment of the distal phalanx on the middle may extrude the fragment dorsally. When seen late, Type A, B, or C may be a supple or fixed deformity, with or without swan-neck. Types A and B usually result in congruous joint surfaces, but Type C in joint incongruity (see text). (From Burton and Eaton,[11] with permission.)

Fowler's central slip release is another technique that can yield good results in carefully selected patients with chronic mallet finger injuries. However, the operation and the postoperative management must be meticulously performed according to the precise guidelines described by Bowers and Hurst.[6]

Postoperative Care

Following late repair, the treatment is similar to that for acute injury. The joint must be protected in 0 degrees for 8 weeks and is then gradually weaned from the immobilization.

Author's Preferred Method for Late Mallet Deformity

If only the tendon at the terminal joint is involved (i.e., no fracture, no degenerative arthritis, and no secondary PIP hyperextension), a well secured tuck in the tendon is effective if carefully rehabilitated as outlined above.

If both the PIP and DIP joints are without old fracture and without arthritic changes, but the mallet has resulted in a secondary swan-neck posture (Fig. 53-27), the spiral oblique ligament reconstruction with a tendon graft (see Fig. 53-17) is recommended. This has the great advantage of directly addressing the problem at both of the joints.

If there is an old displaced fracture present (the type illustrated in Fig. 53-28C) that is symptomatic, or if there are traumatic arthritic changes present, arthrodesis of this DIP joint is recommended if the patient's symptoms are sufficient to warrant the surgical intervention.

Summary

The extensor mechanism is complex, yet elegant—a single tendon system of interrelated components controlling three joints. The concepts of fixed points and lengths and reciprocal deformities are critical for understanding the pathomechanics and treatment of established deformities of the extensor mechanism. Deformities are common secondary to disruption by trauma or arthritis. Diagnosis and treatment must be precise and based on an intimate knowledge of functional dynamics of the normal and of the disordered extensor tendon mechanism.

REFERENCES

1. Adams JP: Correction of chronic dorsal subluxation of the proximal interphalangeal joint by means of a criss-cross volar graft. J Bone Joint Surg 41A:111–115, 1959
2. Ambrose J, Goldstone R: Anomalous extensor digiti minimi proprius causing tunnel syndrome in the dorsal compartment. Report of a case. J Bone Joint Surg 57A:706–707, 1975
3. Bate JT: An operation for the correction of locking of the proximal interphalangeal joint of the finger in hyperextension. J Bone Joint Surg 27:142–144, 1945
4. Bevin AG, Hothem AL: The use of silicone rods under split-thickness skin grafts for reconstruction of extensor tendon injuries. Hand 10:254–258, 1978
5. Bingham DLC, Jack EQ: Buttonholed extensor expansion. Br Med J 2:701–702, 1937
6. Bowers WH, Hurst LC: Chronic mallet finger: The use of Fowler's central slip release. J Hand Surg 3:373–376, 1978
7. Bruner JM: The zigzag volar digital incision for flexor tendon surgery. Plast Reconstr Surg 40:571–574, 1967

8. Bunnell S, Doherty EW, Curtis RM: Ischemic contracture, local, in the hand. Plast Reconstr Surg 3:424-433, 1948
9. Burkhalter WE, Carneiro RS: Correction of the attritional boutonnière deformity in high ulnar nerve paralysis. J Bone Joint Surg 61A:131-134, 1979
10. Burton RI: The hand. pp. 137-170. In Goldstein LA, Dickerson RC (eds): Atlas of Orthopaedic Surgery. 2nd Ed. CV Mosby, St Louis, 1981
11. Burton RI, Eaton RG: Common hand injuries in the athlete. Orthop Clin North Am 4:809-838, 1973
12. Cleland J: On the cutaneous ligament of the phalanges. J Anat Physiol 12:526-527, 1878
13. Crawford GP: The molded polythene splint for mallet finger deformities. J Hand Surg 9A:231-237, 1984
14. Curtis RM: Capsulotomy of the interphalangeal joints of the fingers. J Bone Joint Surg 36A:1219-1232, 1954
15. Curtis RM: Treatment of injuries of proximal interphalangeal joints of fingers. p. 1410. In Adams JP (ed): Current Practice in Orthopaedic Surgery. CV Mosby, St Louis, 1964
16. Curtis RM: Management of the stiff proximal interphalangeal joint. Hand 1:32-37, 1969
17. Curtis RM, Reid RL, Provost JM: A staged technique for the repair of the traumatic boutonnière deformity. J Hand Surg 8:167-171, 1983
18. Dargan EL: Management of extensor tendon injuries of the hand. Surg Gynecol Obstet 128:1269-1273, 1969
19. Dawson RLG: Anatomy of the joints of the finger. p. 24. Proceedings of the Second Hand Club. British Society for Surgery of the Hand, London, 1958
20. Devos R: Conservative treatment of mallet finger. Acta Orthop Belg 43:203-205, 1977
21. Dolphin JA: Extensor tenotomy for chronic boutonnière deformity of the finger. Report of two cases. J Bone Joint Surg 47A:161-164, 1965
22. Eaton RG: The extensor mechanism of the fingers. Bull Hosp Joint Dis 30:39-47, 1969
23. Eaton RG, Littler JW: Personal communication, 1979
24. Elliott RA Jr: Injuries to the extensor mechanisms of the hand. Orthop Clin North Am 1:335-354, 1970
25. Elliot D, McGrouther DA: The excursions of the long extensor tendons of the hand. J Hand Surg 11B:77-80, 1986
26. Elson RA: Dislocation of the extensor tendons of the hand. Report of a case. J Bone Joint Surg 49B:324-326, 1967
27. Entin MA: Repair of extensor mechanism of the hand. Surg Clin North Am 40:275-285, 1960
28. Eyler DL, Markee JE: The anatomy and function of the intrinsic muscles of the fingers. J Bone Joint Surg 36A:1-9, 1954
29. Fetrow KO: Tenolysis in the hand and wrist. A clinical evaluation of 220 flexor and extensor tenolyses. J Bone Joint Surg 49A:667-685, 1967
30. Finochietto R: Retraction de Volkman de los musculos intrinsecos de la mans. De la Sociedad de Cirugia de Buenos Aires, Tomo IV, 1920
31. Fowler SB: Extensor apparatus of the digits. Proceedings of the British Orthopaedic Association. J Bone Joint Surg 31B:477, 1949
32. Fowler SB: The management of tendon injuries. J Bone Joint Surg 41A:579-580, 1959
33. Fowler SB: As quoted by Littler in principles of reconstructive surgery of the hand. pp. 1630-1631. In Converse JM (ed): Reconstructive Plastic Surgery. WB Saunders, Philadelphia, 1964
34. Furnas DW, Spinner M: The sign of "horns" in the diagnosis of injury or disease of the extensor digitorum communis of the hand. J Plast Surg 31:263-265, 1978
35. Gainor BJ, Hummel GL: Correction of rheumatoid swan neck deformity by lateral band mobilization. J Hand Surg 10A:370-375, 1985
36. Gama C: Results of the Matev operation for correction of boutonnière deformity. Plast Reconstr Surg 64:319-324, 1979
37. Gardner RC: Hypertrophic infiltrative tendinitis (hit syndrome) of the long extensor. The abused karate hand. JAMA 211:1009-1010, 1970
38. Georgitis J: Extensor tenosynovitis of the hand from cold exposure. J Maine Med Assoc 69:129-131, 1978
39. Goldner JA: Deformities of the hand incidental to pathological changes of the extensor and intrinsic muscle mechanisms. J Bone Joint Surg 35A:115-131, 1953
40. Haines RQ: The extensor apparatus of the fingers. J Anat 85:251-259, 1951
41. Hakstian RW, Tubiana R: Ulnar deviation of the fingers. The role of joint structure and function. J Bone Joint Surg 49A:299-316, 1967
42. Hallberg D, Lindholm A: Subcutaneous rupture of the extensor tendon of the distal phalanx of the finger; "mallet finger." Acta Chir Scand 119:260-267, 1960
43. Hamas RS, Horrell ED, Pierret GP: Treatment of mallet finger due to intra-articular fracture of the distal phalanx. J Hand Surg 3:361-363, 1978
44. Hamlin C, Littler JW: Restoration of the extensor pollicis longus tendon by an intercalated graft. J Bone Joint Surg 59A:412-414, 1977
45. Harris C Jr, Riordan DC: Intrinsic contracture in the hand and its surgical treatment. J Bone Joint Surg 36A:10-20, 1954
46. Harris C Jr, Rutlege GL: The functional anatomy of the extensor mechanism of the finger. J Bone Joint Surg 54A:713-726, 1972
47. Hauck G: Die Ruptur der Dorsal Aponeurose am ersten Interphalangeal Gelenk, zugleich eim Beitrag zur Anatomic and Physiologic der Dorsal Aponeurose. Arch Klin Chir 123:197-232, 1923
48. Herschel M: "Swan neck" deformity in rheumatoid arthritis. Ned Tijdschr Geneeskd 106:2017-2018, 1962
49. Heywood AWB: Correction of the rheumatoid boutonnière deformity. J Bone Joint Surg 51A:1309-1314, 1969
50. Hueston JT: The extensor apparatus in Dupuytren's disease. Ann Chir Main 4:7-10, 1985
51. Kaplan EB: Extension deformities of the proximal interphalangeal joint of the fingers. An anatomical study. J Bone Joint Surg 18:781-783, 1936
52. Kaplan EB: Anatomy, injuries and treatment of the extensor apparatus of the hand and the digits. Clin Orthop 13:24-41, 1959
53. Ketchum LD, Thompson D, Pocock G, Wallingford D: A clinical study of forces generated by the intrinsic muscles of the index finger and the extrinsic flexor and extensor muscles of the hand. J Hand Surg 3:571-578, 1978
54. Kettlekamp DB, Flatt AE, Moulds R: Traumatic dislocation of the long finger extensor tendon. A clinical, anatomical, and biomechanical study. J Bone Joint Surg 53A:229-240, 1971
55. Kilgore ES Jr, Graham WP: Operative treatment of swan-neck deformity. Plast Reconstr Surg 39:468-471, 1967
56. Kilgore ES, Graham WP: Operative treatment of boutonnière deformity. Surgery 64:999-1000, 1968
57. Kilgore ES Jr, Graham WP, Newmeyer WL, Brown LG: Correction of ulnar subluxation of the extensor communis. Hand 7:272-274, 1975
58. Kilgore ES Jr, Graham WP, Newmeyer WL, Brown LG: The extensor plus finger. Hand 7:159-165, 1975
59. King T: Injuries of the dorsal extensor mechanism of the fingers. Med J Aust 2:213-217, 1970
60. Kleinert HE, Kasdan ML: Reconstruction of chronically sublux-

ated proximal interphalangeal finger joint. J Bone Joint Surg 47A:958-964, 1965
61. Kleinman WB, Petersen DP: Oblique retinacular ligament reconstruction for chronic mallet finger deformity. J Hand Surg 9A:399-404, 1984
62. Laine VAI, Sairanen E, Vainio K: Finger deformities caused by rheumatoid arthritis. J Bone Joint Surg 39A:527-533, 1957
63. Landsmeer JMF: Anatomy of the dorsal aponeurosis of the human finger and its functional significance. Anat Rec 104:31-44, 1949
64. Landsmeer JMF: A report on the coordination of the interphalangeal joints of the human finger and its disturbances. Acta Morph Neerl Scand 2:59-84, 1953
65. Landsmeer JMF: Anatomical and functional investigation on the articulation of the human fingers. Acta Anat suppl. 24, 25:1-69, 1955
66. Landsmeer JMF: Report on the coordination of the interphalangeal joints of the human finger and its disturbances. Acta Morphol Neerl Scand 2:59-84, 1958
67. Landsmeer JMF: Atlas of Anatomy of the Hand. Churchill Livingstone, New York, 1976
68. Larson DL, Wofford BH, Evans EB, Lewis SR: Repair of the boutonnière deformity of the burned hand. J Trauma 10:481-487, 1970
69. Littler JW: Tendon transfers and arthrodesis in combined median and ulnar nerve paralysis. J Bone Joint Surg 31A:225-234, 1949
70. Littler JW: The hand and wrist. p. 284. In Howorth MB (ed): A Textbook of Orthopedics. WB Saunders, Philadelphia, 1952
71. Littler JW: Quoted by Harris C, and Riordan DC, in Intrinsic contracture in the hand and its surgical treatment. J Bone Joint Surg 36A:10-20, 1954
72. Littler JW: Principles of reconstructive surgery of the hand. Am J Surg 92:88-93, 1956
73. Littler JW: Principles of reconstructive surgery of the hand. pp. 1612-1632. In Converse JM (ed): Reconstructive Plastic Surgery. WB Saunders, Philadelphia, 1964
74. Littler JW: The hand. pp. 1287-1313. In Cooper P (ed): The Craft of Surgery. Little, Brown, Boston, 1964
75. Littler JW: Restoration of the oblique retinacular ligament for correction of hyperextension-deformity of the proximal interphalangeal joint. In Fourniee A (ed): La Main Theumatismale. Expansion Scientifique Francaise, Paris, 1966
76. Littler JW: The finger extensor mechanism. Surg Clin North Am 47:415-432, 1967
77. Littler JW: On the adaptability of man's hand. With reference to the equiangular curve. Hand 5:187-191, 1973
78. Littler JW: The digital extensor-flexor system. pp. 3166-3183. In Converse JM (ed): Reconstructive Plastic Surgery. Vol. 6. WB Saunders, Philadelphia, 1977
79. Littler JW: The digital extensor-flexor system. pp. 3166-3214. In Converse JM (ed): Reconstructive Plastic Surgery. Vol. 6. WB Saunders, Philadelphia, 1977
80. Littler JW, Burton RI, Eaton RG: The dynamics of digital extension. AAOS Sound Slide Program: #467, #468, 1976
81. Littler JW, Colley SGE: Restoration of the retinacular system in hyperextension deformity of the interphalangeal joint. Proceedings of the American Society for Surgery of the Hand. J Bone Joint Surg 47A:637, 1965
82. Littler JW, Eaton RG: Redistribution of forces in correction of boutonnière deformity. J Bone Joint Surg 49A:1267-1274, 1967
83. Long C, Brown ME: Electromyographic kinesiology of the hand. Muscles moving the long finger. J Bone Joint Surg 46A:1683-1706, 1964
84. Maisals DO: The middle slip or boutonnière deformity in burned hands. Br J Plast Surg 18:117-129, 1965
85. Manske PR: Redirection of the extensor pollicis longus in the treatment of spastic thumb-in-palm deformity. J Hand Surg 10A:553-560, 1985
86. Mason ML: Ruptures of tendons of the hand. Surg Gynecol Obstet 50:611-624, 1930
87. Mason MD, Allen HS: The rate of healing of tendons—An experimental study of tensile strength. Ann Surg 113:424-459, 1941
88. Matev I: Transposition of the lateral slips of the aponeurosis in treatment of long-standing "boutonnière deformity" of the fingers. Br J Plast Surg 17:281-286, 1964
89. Matev I: The boutonnière deformity. Hand 1:90-95, 1969
90. McCoy FJ, Winsky AJ: Lumbrical loop operation for luxation of the extensor tendons of the hand. Plast Reconstr Surg 44:142-146, 1969
91. McFarlane RM: Observations on the functional anatomy of the intrinsic muscles of the thumb. J Bone Joint Surg 44A:1073-1088, 1962
92. McFarlane RM, Hampole MD: Treatment of extensor tendon injuries of the hand. Can J Surg 16:366-375, 1973
93. McMurtry RY, Jochims JL: Congenital deficiency of the extrinsic extensor mechanism of the hand. Clin Orthop 125:36-39, 1977
94. Micks JE, Reswick JB: Confirmation of differential loading of lateral and central fibers of the extensor tendon. J Hand Surg 6:462-467, 1981
95. Milford LW Jr: Retaining Ligaments of the Digits of the Hand. Gross and Microscopic Anatomic Study. WB Saunders, Philadelphia, 1968
96. Miura T, Nakamura R, Torii S: Conservative treatment for a ruptured extensor tendon on the dorsum of the proximal phalanges of the thumb (mallet thumb). J Hand Surg 11A:229-233, 1986
97. Nalebuff EA, Millender LH: Surgical treatment of the swan-neck deformity in rheumatoid arthritis. Orthop Clin North Am 6:733-752, 1975
98. Nalebuff EA, Millender LH: Surgical treatment of the boutonnière deformity in rheumatoid arthritis. Orthop Clin North Am 6:753-763, 1975
99. Nichols HM: Repair of extensor tendon insertions in the fingers. J Bone Joint Surg 33A:836-841, 1951
100. Palmer AK, Skahen JR, Werner FW, Glisson RR: The extensor retinaculum of the wrist: An anatomical and biomechanical study. J Hand Surg 10B:11-16, 1985
101. Pardini AG, Costa RD, Morais MS: Surgical repair of the boutonnière deformity of the fingers. Hand 11:87-92, 1979
102. Parkes AR: Traumatic ischaemia of peripheral nerves, with some observations on Volkmann's ischaemic contracture. Br J Surg 32:403-414, 1945
103. Parkes A: The lumbrical plus finger. Hand 2:164-165, 1970
104. Patel MR, Lipson LB, Desai SS: Conservative treatment of mallet thumb. J Hand Surg 11A:45-47, 1986
105. Peacock EE Jr: The dynamic splinting for the prevention and correction of hand deformities. A simple and inexpensive method. J Bone Joint Surg 34A:789-796, 1952
106. Planas J: Buttonhole deformity of the fingers. J Bone Joint Surg 45B:424, 1963
107. Portis RB: Hyperextensibility of the proximal interphalangeal joint of the finger following trauma. J Bone Joint Surg 36A:1141-1146, 1954
108. Pratt DR, Bunnell S, Howard LD Jr: Mallet finger classification and methods of treatment. Am J Surg 93:573-579, 1957

109. Primiano GA: Conservative treatment of two cases of mallet thumb. J Hand Surg 11A:233–235, 1986
110. Rabischong P: L'innervation proprioceptive des muscles lombricaus de la mainchez l'homme. Rev Chir Orthop 48:234–245, 1962
111. Reef TC, Brestin SG: The extensor digitorum manus and its clinical significance. J Bone Joint Surg 57A:704–706, 1975
112. Riddell DM: Spontaneous rupture of the extensor pollicis longus; the results of tendon transfers. J Bone Joint Surg 45B:506–510, 1963
113. Riordan DC, Stokes HM: Synovitis of the extensors of the fingers associated with extensor digitorum brevis manus muscle. A case report. Clin Orthop 95:278–280, 1973
114. Rothwell AG: Repair of the established post traumatic boutonnière deformity. Hand 10:241–245, 1978
115. Saldana MJ, McGuire RA: Chronic painful subluxation of the metacarpal phalangeal joint extensor tendons. J Hand Surg 11A:420–423, 1986
116. Salisbury RE, Bervin AG: Boutonnière deformity. pp. 164–167. Atlas of Reconstructive Surgery. 1981
117. Salvi V: Tcchnique for the buttonhole deformity. Hand 1:96–97, 1969
118. Sarrafian SK, Kazarian LE, Topouzian LK, Sarrafian VK, Siegelman A: Strain variation in the components of the extensor apparatus of the finger during flexion and extension. A biomechanical study. J Bone Joint Surg 52A:980–990, 1970
119. Schenck RR: Variations of the extensor tendons of the fingers—surgical significance. J Bone Joint Surg 46A:103–110, 1964
120. Schultz RJ: Traumatic entrapment of the extensor digiti minimi proprius resulting in progressive restriction of motion of the metacarpophalangeal joint of the little finger. J Bone Joint Surg 56A:428–429, 1974
121. Schultz RJ, Furlong JP: Observations on the fiber pattern of the extensor mechanism of the finger at the level of the proximal interphalangeal joint. Bull Hosp Joint Dis 39:100–101, 1978
122. Schultz RJ, Furlong J, Storace A: Detailed anatomy of the extensor mechanism at the proximal aspect of the finger. J Hand Surg 6:493–498, 1981
123. Shrewsbury MM, Johnson RK: A systematic study of the oblique retinacular ligament of the human finger: Its structure and function. J Hand Surg 2:194–199, 1977
124. Smith RJ: Non-ischemic contractures of the intrinsic muscles of the hand. J Bone Joint Surg 53A:1313–1331, 1971
125. Smith RJ: Balance and kinetics of the finger under normal and pathological conditions. Clin Orthop 104:92–111, 1974
126. Snow JW: Use of a retrograde tendon flap in repairing a severed extensor at the PIP joint area. Plast Reconstr Surg 51:555–558, 1973
127. Snow JW: A method for reconstruction of the central slip of the extensor tendon of a finger. Plast Reconstr Surg 57:455–459, 1976
128. Snow JW, Switzer H: Method of studying the relationships between the finger joints and the flexor and extensor mechanism. Plast Reconstr Surg 55:242–243, 1975
129. Souter WA: The boutonnière deformity. A review of 101 patients with division of the central slip of the extensor expansion of the fingers. J Bone Joint Surg 49B:710–721, 1967
130. Souter WA: The problem of boutonnière deformity. Clin Orthop 104:116–133, 1974
131. Spoor CW, Landsmeer JM: Analysis of the zigzag movement of the human finger under influence of the extensor digitorum tendon and the deep flexor tendon. J Biomech 9:561–566, 1976
132. Stack HG: Muscle function in the fingers. J Bone Joint Surg 44B:899–910, 1962
133. Stack HG: Mallet finger. Hand 1:83–89, 1969
134. Stack HG: Buttonhole deformity. Hand 3:152–154, 1971
135. Stack HG: The anatomy of the muscles and tendons of the hand. p. 95. Proceedings of the Second Hand Club, Copenhagen, 1961. British Society for Surgery of the Hand, London, 1975
136. Swanson AB: Surgery of the hand in cerebral palsy and the swan-neck deformity. J Bone Joint Surg 42A:951–964, 1960
137. Suzuki K: Reconstruction of post-traumatic boutonnière deformity. Hand 5:145–148, 1973
138. Taleisnik J, Gelberman RH, Miller BW, Szabo RM: The extensor retinaculum of the wrist. J Hand Surg 9A:495–501, 1984
139. Thompson JS, Littler JW, Upton J: The spiral oblique retinacular ligament. SORL. J Hand Surg 3:482–487, 1978
140. Tubiana R: Surgical repair of the extensor apparatus of the fingers. Surg Clin North Am 48:1015–1031, 1968
141. Tubiana R, Valentin P: Anatomy of the extensor apparatus and the physiology of finger extension. Surg Clin North Am 44:897–906, 1964
142. Tubiana R, Valentin P: The physiology of the extension of the fingers. Surg Clin North Am 44:907–918, 1964
143. Urbaniak JR, Hayes MG: Chronic boutonnière deformity—An anatomic reconstruction. J Hand Surg 6:379–383, 1981
144. Vainio K, Oka M: Ulnar deviation of the fingers. Ann Rheum Dis 12:122–124, 1953
145. van der Meulen JC: Causes of prolapse and collapse of the proximal interphalangeal joint. Hand 4:147–153, 1972
146. van der Meulen JC: The treatment of prolapse and collapse of the proximal interphalangeal joint. Hand 4:154–162, 1972
147. Varian JW, Pennington DG: Extensor digitorum brevis manus used to restore function to a ruptured extensor pollicis longus. Br J Plast Surg 30:313–315, 1977
148. Weeks PM: The chronic boutonnière deformity: A method of repair. Plast Reconstr Surg 40:248–251, 1967
149. Wehbé MA, Schneider LH: Mallet fractures. J Bone Joint Surg 66A:658–669, 1984

54

Tenosynovitis and Tennis Elbow

Avrum I. Froimson

DE QUERVAIN'S DISEASE

Stenosing tenosynovitis of the first dorsal compartment of the wrist is a common cause of wrist and hand pain and disability. De Quervain has been credited with the first description, in 1895, of a specific entity involving the abductor pollicis longus and extensor pollicis brevis sheaths at the radial styloid process.[21,28,33,36,48,50] The diagnosis is made without difficulty after eliciting the complaint of several weeks or months of pain localized to the radial side of the wrist aggravated by movement of the thumb, with a history of chronic overuse of the wrist and hand. Most patients are middle-aged women, although men and women of all ages can develop the condition with sufficient provocation at work or other activity requiring repetitive thumb abduction and extension, combined with radial and ulnar wrist movements.

The findings of local tenderness and swelling of the extensor retinaculum of the wrist over its first compartment and a positive Finkelstein's[13,17,49] test confirm the diagnosis of de Quervain's disease. Crepitus or squeaking with movement of the involved tendons ("wet leather sign") may be palpable. Triggering occurs rarely.[9,61,63] A small ganglion may occasionally arise from the roof of the first dorsal compartment.

De Quervain's disease must be differentiated by radiographic and physical examination from arthritis of the thumb carpometacarpal joint, although the two lesions may coexist as both are most frequently seen in middle-aged women.[43] Radiographic study also excludes scaphoid fracture and arthrosis involving radiocarpal or intercarpal joints. Radionucleotide bone scanning with technitium polyphosphonate may show increased uptake in the distal radius deep to the de Quervain's tenosynovitis. Occasionally plain radiographs show osteoporosis localized to the radial styloid area.[45]

First compartment tenosynovitis must also be differentiated from a less commonly recognized painful condition, the intersection syndrome,[20] in which pain, swelling, and in severe cases crepitus is found 4 cm proximal to the wrist (see page 1992).

Rheumatoid arthritis can be another cause of stenosing tenosynovitis of the wrist, in which case management includes specific antirheumatic medication as well as localized treatment of the first compartment.

Nonoperative treatment with local steroid injections, thumb and wrist immobilization, heat, hydrotherapy, and systemic antiinflammatory medication may give temporary relief of pain and swelling. However, upon resumption of activity, the problem frequently recurs. Although some authors have had remarkable success with injection therapy,[22,47] most authors have made appeals for early surgical release to shorten the period of morbidity and prevent recurrence.[3,10,32,65] Only when tenosynovitis is associated with pregnancy or a medically correctable condition, such as an endocrinopathy, should nonoperative treatment be prolonged. Tenography has been advocated as a method of identifying those patients more likely to respond favorably to injection therapy.[14]

Anatomy

There are six separate compartments under the dorsal carpal ligament, each lined with a synovial sheath membrane. The first of these over the styloid process of the radius contains the abductor pollicis longus and extensor pollicis brevis tendons. These tendons pass through an unyielding osteoligamentous tunnel formed by a shallow groove in the radial styloid process and a tough overlying roof composed of the transverse fibers of the dorsal ligament attached by vertical septa to bone. This fibrous tunnel is about 1 cm long, while the synovial sheath extends from each musculotendinous junction proximally to the tendon insertions well beyond the tunnel itself.

Although early anatomic textbooks showed one long thumb abductor tendon accompanying one extensor brevis tendon through a unified first dorsal compartment as the normal anatomy, numerous modern anatomic and surgical studies have shown this is not usually the case.[2,4,30,33,37,44,58] In most reports, fewer than 20 percent of cases showed the so-called normal anatomy.[27,58,61]

In fact, the first dorsal compartment of the wrist is probably the site of the most numerous variations in tendon structure and organization in the upper limb. Failure to recognize these variations can cause persistence or recurrence of pain due to incomplete surgical release of the tendon sheaths.[2,3,39]

In 20 to 30 percent of reported cases, the first compartment is subdivided by a longitudinal ridge and septum into two tunnels, the ulnar one for the extensor pollicis brevis and the other containing one or more slips of the abductor pollicis longus. A third deep tunnel containing an anomalous tendon has also been reported.

The extensor pollicis brevis is a phylogenetically young structure found only in humans and gorillas as a separate muscle distinct from the thumb abductor. The muscle is always narrower than the abductor and is absent in 5 to 7 percent of people. The larger abductor pollicis longus often has two and sometimes three or more tendinous slips inserting variously into the base of the first metacarpal, trapezium, volar carpal ligament, opponens pollicis, or abductor pollicis brevis.[58] As noted in various published reports of operative findings, as well as in my own experience, either one or both subdivisions of the first dorsal compartment may be stenotic.

The relationship of the radial artery and nerve to this compartment must be understood to prevent complicating injury to these structures during surgical release of the tendons (Fig. 54-1). The radial artery passes diagonally across the anatomic snuffbox from the volar aspect of the wrist to the dorsum of the first web space deep to the thumb abductor and both extensors. It is separated from the first compartment sheath by enough areolar tissue that it need not be exposed during the dissection if the surgeon does not perforate the floor of the sheath distal to the radial styloid. However, two or three terminal divisions of the radial sensory nerve lie immediately superficial to the first dorsal compartment and must be identified and protected during the operation described below.[1,53]

Operative Technique

I prefer to perform the operation using only local infiltration anesthesia. The pneumatic tourniquet routinely employed is well tolerated for the short duration of this procedure. A bloodless surgical field is essential for the identification of radial sensory nerve branches, as well as the anatomical variations discussed above.

A 2-cm transverse skin incision is made over the first dorsal compartment about 0.5 cm proximal to the tip of the radial styloid process (Fig. 54-2A). Care is taken to identify and

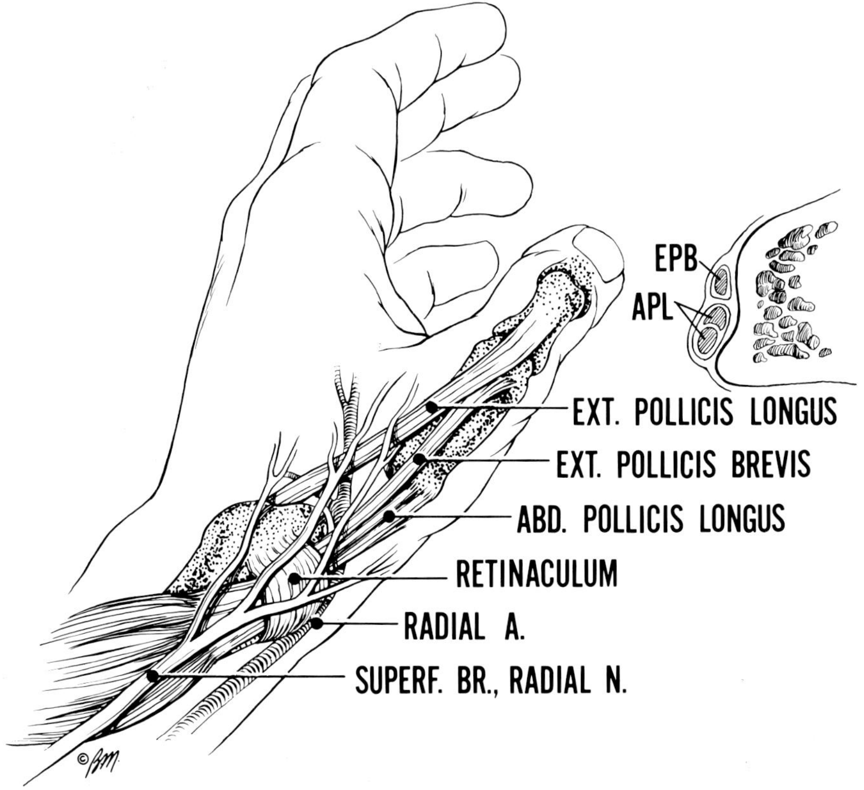

Fig. 54-1. Anatomic relations of the first dorsal compartment.

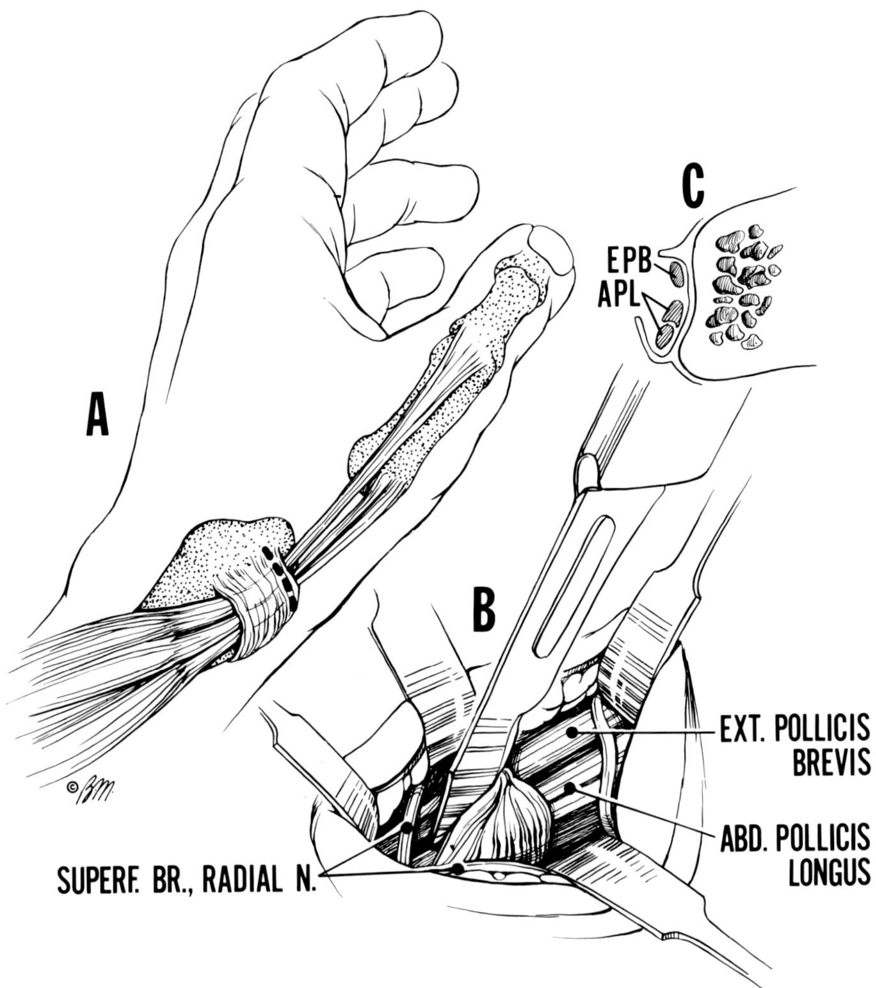

Fig. 54-2. Tenovaginotomy for de Quervain's disease. **(A)** The first dorsal compartment is approached by a short transverse skin incision. **(B)** The annular ligament is incised with a scalpel from the snuffbox to the musculotendinous junctions. **(C)** Separate compartments are sought and completely opened, excising the septa between tunnels.

gently retract the one to three radial sensory branches that cross the compartment obliquely, using gentle, blunt longitudinal dissection as soon as the deepest dermal layer of skin has been incised. A common technical error is to transversely incise the subcutaneous fat with the skin knife, severing a nerve branch before it has been dissected and protected. The exposed annular ligament covering the compartment is sharply incised longitudinally with a scalpel, which in my experience is less painful than scissors (Fig. 54-2B).

If they are markedly thickened, the entire sheath and ligament covering the compartment are excised. Separate compartments are sought and each is completely opened, excising the septa between separate tunnels (Fig. 54-2C). If the synovial tissue covering the tendons is thick and opaque, tenosynovectomy is performed. (This is especially necessary in rheumatoid arthritis.) The tendons are lifted by hook or blunt retractors out of the tunnel to assure complete decompression from their musculotendinous junctions to a point at least 1 cm distal to the tunnel. The tendons are replaced and the patient moves the thumb to demonstrate free and independent movement of the long abductor and short extensor. If the operation is done under general or regional anesthesia gentle retraction on each of the tendons will identify them correctly. It is imperative that the separate tendon of the extensor pollicis brevis be specifically identified by demonstrating passive extension of the thumb MP joint. Although others have advocated leaving a radiovolar-based flap of retinaculum to prevent volar prolapse of the abductor with wrist flexion,[1,3,7] I have not found this to be necessary.

Hemostasis is established using cautery after tourniquet release and the skin is closed with absorbable subcuticular sutures and sterile tape strips. The postsurgical compression dressing should immobilize the thumb to minimize discomfort. Two or three days later, at the first postoperative office visit, only a small wrist bandage is applied, permitting use of the hand as tolerated. One week later, after a second office examination to confirm wound healing, the patient can be discharged from active care.

Complications

The most serious complication of this operation follows iatrogenic injury of a superficial sensory branch of the radial nerve with subsequent formation of a painful neuroma.[1,2,34] Overly vigorous retraction of a radial nerve branch without apparent injury may cause a painful neuroma-in-continuity. Management of an inadvertently lacerated radial sensory nerve is a controversial subject. Some authors advise resection of the lacerated nerve to put the resultant neuroma well above the operative scar, where it will be less exposed to repeated contusion. However, I agree with those[34] who advocate immediate nerve reapproximation using appropriate microsurgical techniques to reduce the likelihood of neuroma formation and minimize hypoesthesia in the thumb and index finger. (For more detailed discussion on the management of this problem the reader is referred to Chapter 37.)

Volar subluxation of the tendons of the first dorsal compartment after de Quervain's release may rarely cause a painful tenosynovitis, requiring pulley reconstruction.[41,62]

INTERSECTION SYNDROME

Pain and swelling of the muscle bellies of the abductor pollicis longus (APL) and the extensor pollicis brevis (EPB) are characteristic of the intersection syndrome. This area about 4 cm proximal to the wrist joint may show increased swelling of a normally prominent area (Fig. 54-3), and in severe cases, redness and crepitus. Although previously thought to be the result of friction between the APL and EPB muscle bellies and the radial wrist extensor tendons,[5,11,25,64] Grundberg has demonstrated the basic pathology to be a tenosynovitis of the second dorsal compartment.

This syndrome is frequently associated with repetitive use of the wrist in the work place.[5] Initial nonoperative treatment consists of modification of work activities to reduce stress, a thermoplastic molded wrist splint in 15 degrees of extension, and in some patients steroid injected into the second dorsal compartment. The majority of patients so treated improve and remain permanently asymptomatic.

For those with persistent pain, Grundberg[20] suggests a longitudinal incision to approach the radial wrist extensors beginning at the wrist and extending proximal to the swollen area. After incising the deep fascia, release of the second dorsal compartment demonstrates synovitis (Fig. 54-4). Pathological examination of the removed synovium reveals acute and chronic synovitis. Postoperative management with a plaster splint holding the wrist in slight extension for 10 days is recommended. Thereafter the patients are advised to use the hand and wrist as tolerated. Although bowstringing of the tendons is a theoretical problem after incising the dorsal retinaculum, Grundberg did not report this in his cases.

My experience with this syndrome has been limited to seven cases, treated as recommended above, all with successful outcome. This condition is probably more common than generally recognized.

TRIGGER THUMB AND FINGERS

Stenosing tenovaginitis or tenosynovitis of the thumb or finger flexors is another common cause of hand pain and disability. As the patient flexes and extends the involved digit, painful triggering or snapping occurs. Although the flexor tendon sheath is constricted at the MP joint, the patient or examining physician often localizes the phenomenon incorrectly to the PIP joint and misinterprets the problem as a dislocation. This erroneous diagnosis is especially likely to be made by the physician who "reduces" the locked finger by manipulation of the digit into extension. Less common is locking in extension when the finger or thumb flexors are trapped distal to the stenotic annulus.

Except for the rare instances of locking caused by a tumor of tendon or sheath,[31,46,52] a loose body in the MP joint or entrapment of intrinsic tendon on an irregularity on the metacarpal head,[51] the phenomenon of triggering is due to disproportion between a flexor tendon and its tendon sheath[29] and should not

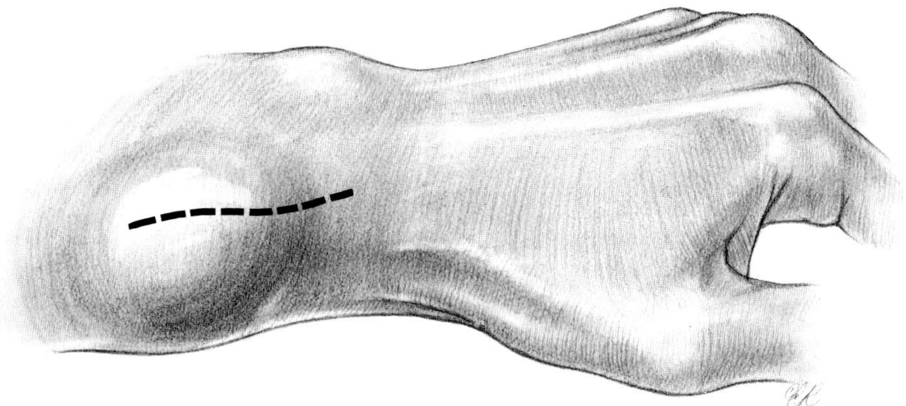

Fig. 54-3. A patient with intersection syndrome manifests swelling in the area where the APL and EPB cross the common radial wrist extensors. The dotted line indicates the location of the surgical incision. (Adapted from Grundberg and Reagan,[20] with permission.)

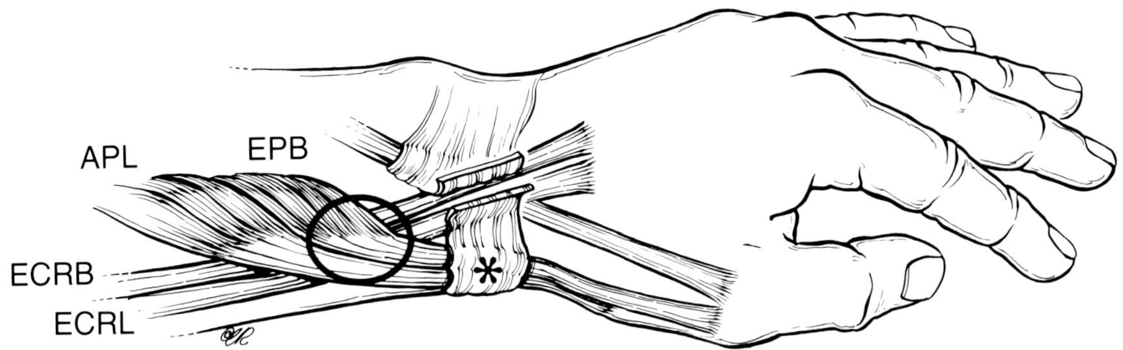

Fig. 54-4. The circled area shows where the extensor pollicus brevis *(EPB)* and abductor pollicus longus *(APL)* cross the common radial wrist extensors. The location of the first dorsal compartment where de Quervain's disease occurs is indicated with a star. The second dorsal compartment has been released in the manner recommended for treatment of intersection syndrome.

present a problem in diagnosis. The most common form of trigger finger is the primary type, most often found in otherwise healthy middle-aged women with a much lower incidence in men. Trigger thumbs are especially more frequent in women, up to four times as common as in men.[40]

Secondary trigger finger can be seen in rheumatoid arthritis, gout, and other metabolic disorders, such as diabetes, that cause connective tissue changes.[10] Trigger finger and thumb not infrequently coexist with de Quervain's disease and carpal tunnel syndrome, which are other manifestations of stenosing tenosynovitis in the hand.[36] Trigger thumb and finger occur with approximately the same frequency as de Quervain's disease,[32] and involvement of several fingers at the same time is not unusual. A congenital or developmental form of trigger thumb or finger presenting in an infant is much less common (see Chapter 11). As in the adult, the ring and middle digits are the most frequently affected of the four fingers. Index finger triggering is uncommon.[4]

Nonoperative treatment (i.e., local steroid injection) is not used in infants or children. In adults, splinting and steroid injection into the flexor sheath has been reported by a few authors[18,40] to yield a high percentage of cures, while others have found that only trigger fingers of a few weeks' duration respond favorably to injection.[7,10,29,32] In my experience recurrence of medically treated triggering is frequent. Few patients are content to spend many weeks being treated with so-called conservative measures when a simple and reliable surgical operation can quickly and permanently relieve triggering. The irreducibly locked trigger finger, often with flexion contracture of the proximal interphalangeal joint, should certainly not be treated by injections.

Anatomy

Thumb

The long thumb flexor tendon passes through a narrow tunnel formed by the grooved palmar surface of the first metacarpal neck and the transverse fibers of the annular ligament of the flexor sheath. On each side in the capsule of the MP joint is a sesamoid bone, into which a tendon of one head of the flexor pollicis brevis is inserted. It is at this narrowest point in the sheath of the flexor pollicis that constriction develops.

Fingers

Sesamoid bones in the fingers are inconsistent. Flexor digitorum profundus and superficialis tendons enter a narrow fibroosseous tunnel formed by a groove in the palmar surface of the metacarpal neck and the annular ligament.[10,32] Doyle and Blythe[12,13] have demonstrated that the flexor sheath in the finger is a double-walled, hollow, synovial-lined, connective tissue tube that encloses the flexor tendons. These authors have identified four annular and three cruciform pulleys (Fig. 54-5). The annular pulleys are thick and rigid. The second pulley (A2) attached to the proximal phalanx and the fourth pulley (A4) are the most important functionally. It was shown experimentally that section of only the first annular pulley (A1), as is done in surgical release of trigger finger or thumb, produces no loss of flexor function. However, division of both the A1 and A2 pulleys causes significant postoperative bowstringing and limitation of active flexion.

Topographical Anatomy and Skin Incisions

A study of the relationship of surface anatomy to deep structures in the palm shows that the proximal edge of the first annular pulley almost exactly coincides with the distal palmar crease in the fourth and fifth rays, the proximal palmar crease in the index, and halfway between the two creases in the middle finger (Fig. 54-6). The proximal edge of the flexor pollicis longus sheath annulus is directly deep to the MP flexion crease of the thumb.[38] Short transverse incisions placed within the appropriate crease, or for the middle finger release halfway between the two creases, thus provide excellent exposure of the A1 pulley to be divided. This site also locates the healed incision away from the underlying bone prominence of metacarpal head, lessening direct pressure on a tender scar in grasping spherical or cylindrical objects.[33] Digital nerves and arteries

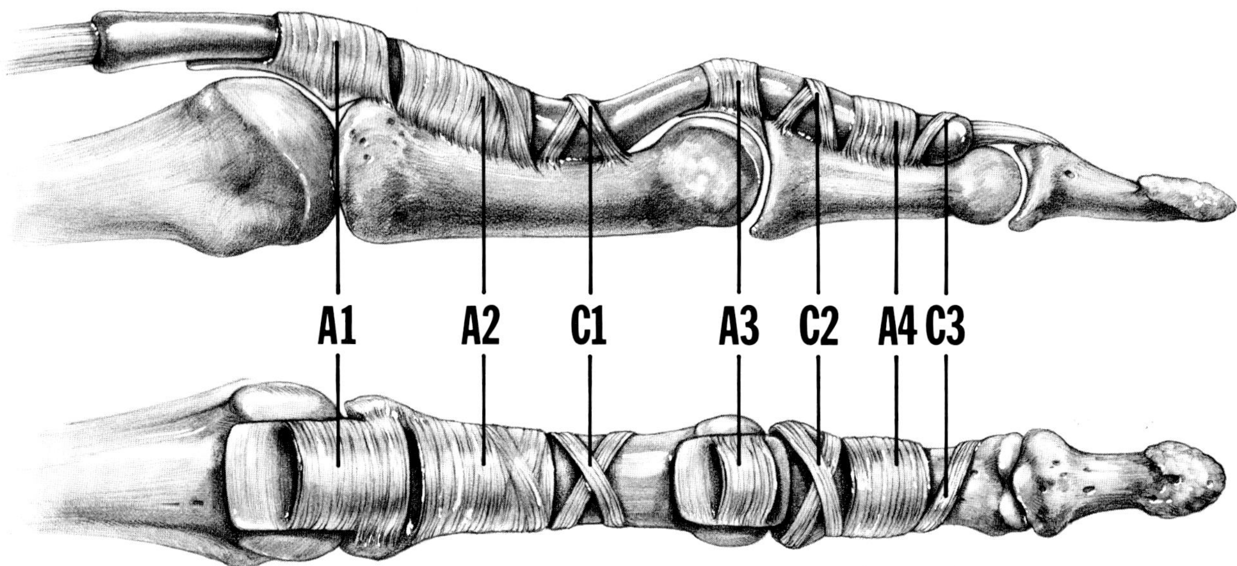

Fig. 54-5. Doyle and Blythe have identified four annular and three cruciform pulleys in the fingers. A slight modification of this configuration is shown in Chapter 50. (Adapted from Doyle and Blythe,[12] with permission.)

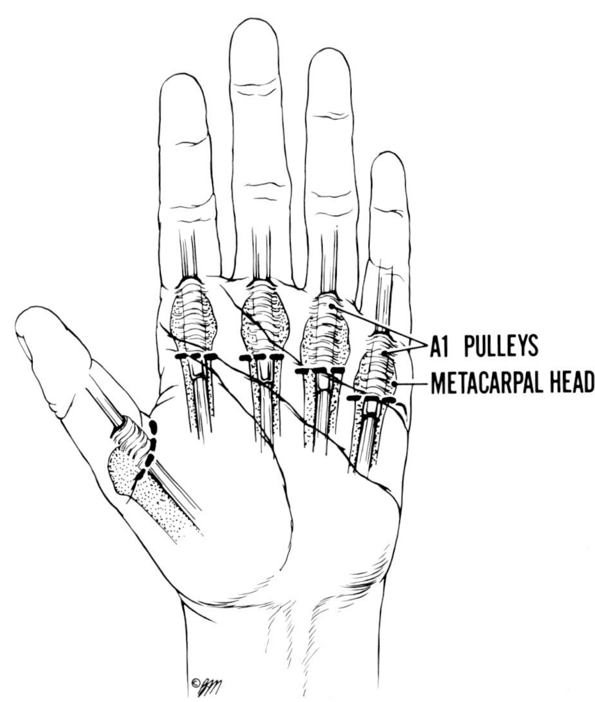

Fig. 54-6. Incisions for release of trigger fingers and thumb. The index is released through an incision in the proximal palmar crease, ring and little in the distal crease, and the middle midway between the two palmar creases. The thumb flexor is approached through its MP crease. In each instance the resultant scar will lie proximal to the metacarpal head prominence.

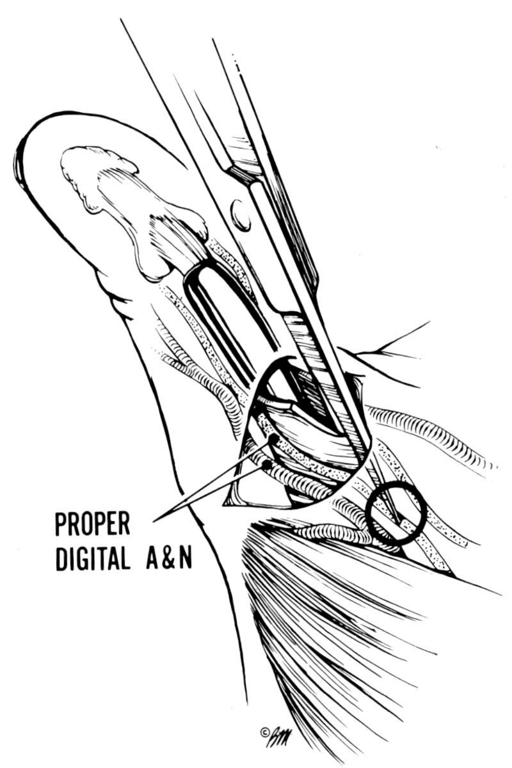

Fig. 54-7. The thumb digital nerves are vulnerable to injury if the skin incision is deepened too quickly or if scissors are inserted too far proximally without visualizing the nerves *(circle).*

that closely parallel each flexor sheath in the fingers must be identified and protected. The two digital nerves of the thumb are more vulnerable, especially the radial one lying quite close to the deep layer of dermis at the flexion crease where it will be lacerated if the initial incision is carried too deeply.[8,60] The same nerve can also be injured by blind scissors dissection more proximally where it diagonally crosses the thumb flexor sheath (Fig. 54-7).

Operative Technique

Pneumatic arm tourniquet and local anesthesia are used. Although the use of a longitudinal incision is advocated by some surgeons,[4,56] I recommend a transverse skin incision 1.0 to 1.5 cm long made in or next to the appropriate crease as discussed above. As soon as the skin has been incised, longitudinal blunt dissection is used to spread the subcutaneous tissues and the palmar fascia to expose the flexor strength. Digital nerves and vessels are protected by right-angle retractors, but they are not subjected to extensive dissection. The thick proximal edge of the tough flexor tunnel is identified. A #11 scalpel blade is inserted beneath the annulus and pushed distally to divide the A1 pulley longitudinally in the tendon's midline (Fig. 54-8). (I have found the knife to cause less pain than scissors.) Only the first annular pulley (A1) is sectioned, a distance of about 1.5 cm in the adult but only 0.5 cm in the infant. The patient actively moves the involved finger or thumb to confirm that triggering and locking have been abolished. The tourniquet is released to permit hemostasis to be achieved with cautery, and the wound is approximated with a few interrupted fine monofilament nonabsorbable sutures. The compression dressing applied in the operating room permits finger motion. In 2 to 3 days a small patch dressing is applied and full hand function is encouraged.

Percutaneous Trigger Finger Release

As more hand surgery is being performed in ambulatory settings, surgical techniques have evolved to further simplify the release of trigger fingers and trigger thumbs, to reduce morbidity and economic cost and to permit the performance of surgery in out-patient clinics and offices. Several authors have reported their techniques and favorable results with subcutaneous or percutaneous trigger finger release, stipulating that this procedure is reserved for the experienced and careful hand surgeon.[38,59] I have performed more than 100 of those procedures in an office treatment room, releasing trigger fingers and trigger thumbs under local infiltration anesthesia without use of tourniquet, reserving the more formal procedure described above for selected cases. A thickened annulus must be palpable and locking of the finger definitely present to provide a reliable endpoint to confirm cessation of the triggering after the A1 pulley has been cut. Patients with diabetes, rheumatoid arthritis, or excessive subcutaneous tissue are not treated with the percutaneous technique.

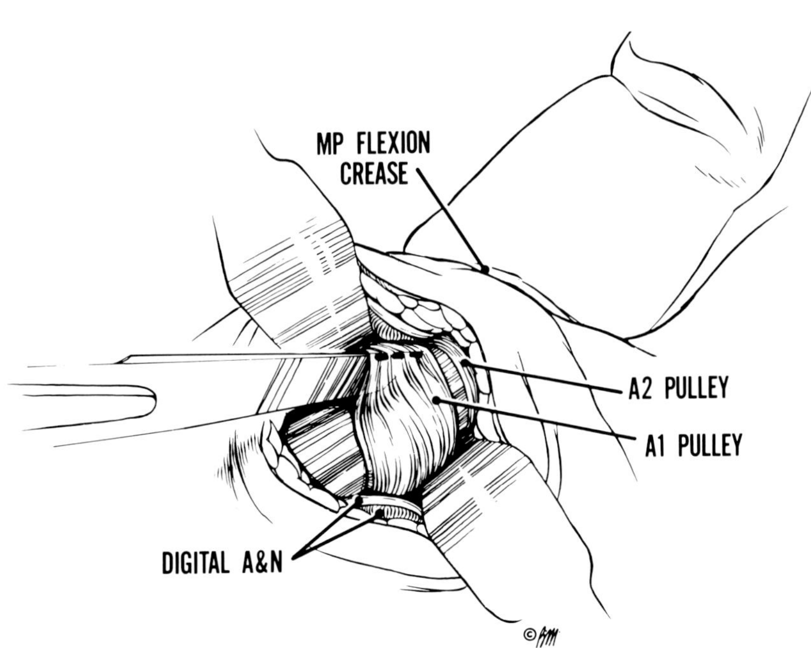

Fig. 54-8. A #11 knife blade is used to divide the first annular pulley to relieve triggering in the finger.

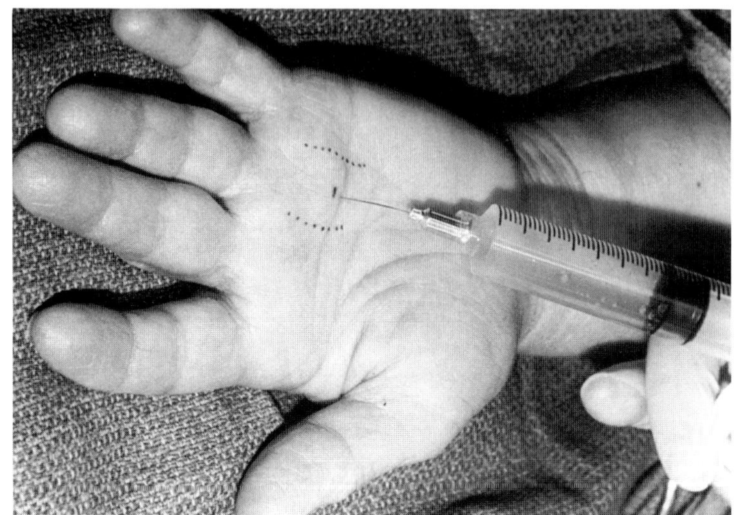
A

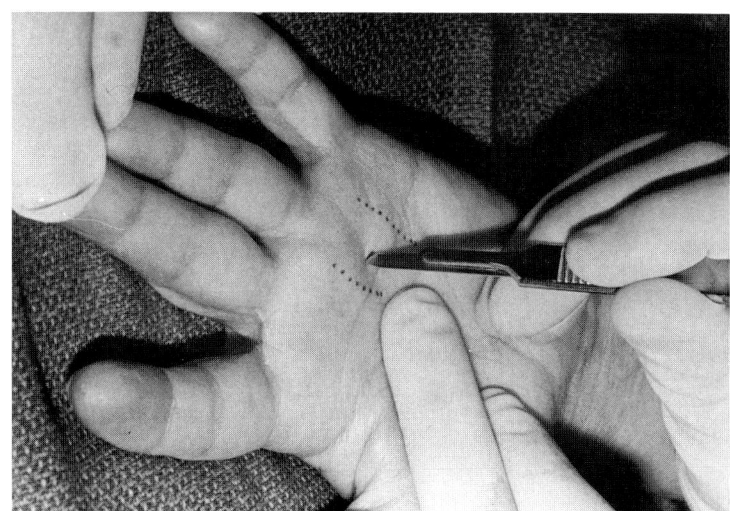
B

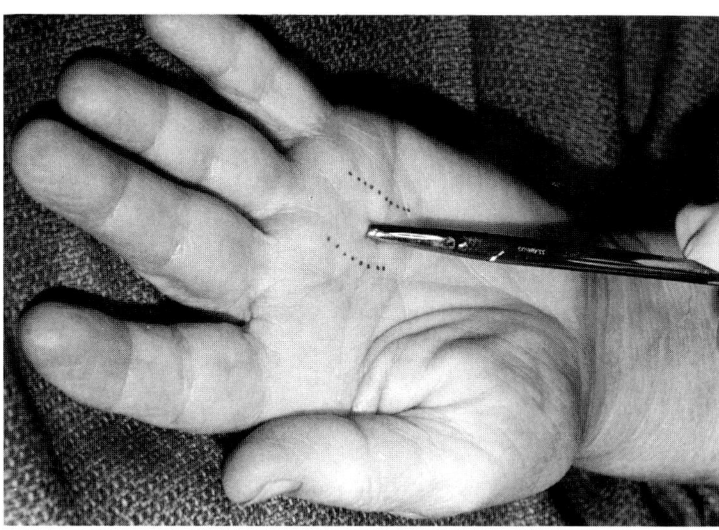
C

Fig. 54-9. Percutaneous trigger finger release. **(A)** The operation is done under local anesthetic. **(B)** A #11 blade is used to make a skin incision no longer than 3 mm in length. **(C)** Scissors are introduced into the wound to spread the fat and feel the proximal end of the A1 pulley. *(Figure continues.)*

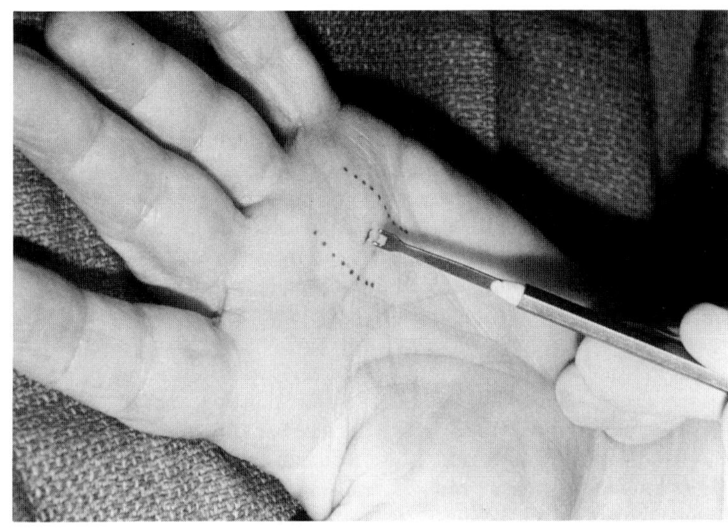

D

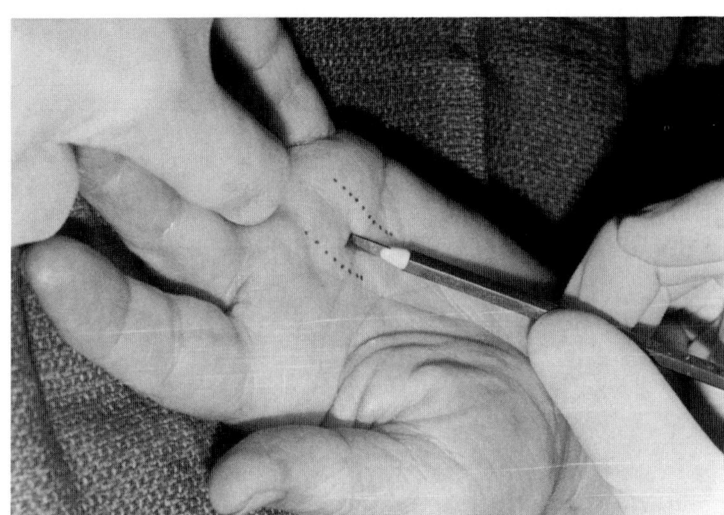

E

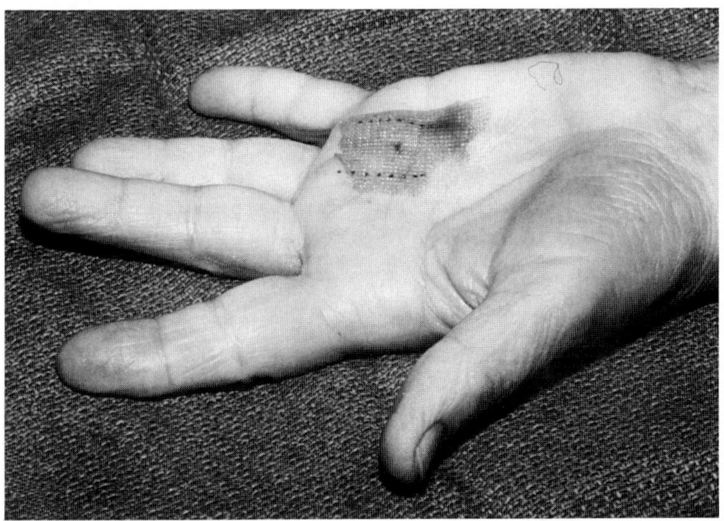

F

Fig. 54-9 *(Continued).* **(D&E)** A small meniscotome blade is inserted to divide the A1 pulley; the surgeon's finger stops the knife from cutting the A2 pulley **(F)**. The wound is not sutured **(F)**. See text for more details.

Technique

After appropriate skin preparation with a soap or antiseptic solution that does not leave residual sticky material on the skin (as this causes the fingers to stick together and makes it difficult to detect correction of the triggering), the skin and underlying annulus are anesthesized using a small caliber needle (Fig. 54-9). A #11 blade is introduced vertically through skin and subcutaneous tissue, creating an opening no longer than 3 mm in length. The tip of the #11 scalpel blade or alternatively a small meniscotome blade is inserted through this opening to divide the first annular pulley distally as far as the metacarpophalangeal flexor crease and proximally to the proximal end of the pulley. In release of trigger fingers dissection proceeds from proximal to distal. For trigger thumbs the entry point of incision is just distal to the nodule over the proximal phalanx, and division of the annulus proceeds carefully proximally. The wound is not sutured. A dressing is immediately applied and the patient instructed in early motion, removal of the bandage and application of a small bandage dressing on the second day, and the use of the hand as tolerated thereafter. *It is emphasized that this procedure is reserved for the experienced hand surgeon.*

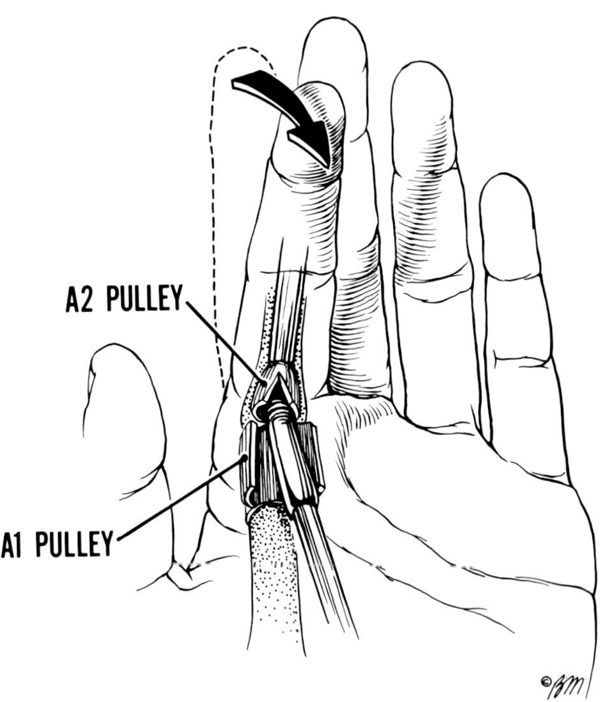

Fig. 54-10. Incising the second annular pulley can cause bowstringing or ulnar deviation of the finger.

Complications

If the trigger finger has been locked in flexion for awhile before operation, the patient may require hand therapy and dynamic splinting to overcome a flexion contracture of the PIP joint.

Digital nerve injury is the most frequently reported complication of trigger finger release by the open method.[60] Prompt nerve suture is indicated with this injury.

Section of the second annular pulley (A2) can cause bowstringing with resultant loss of full finger flexion[23] and, in the case of the index finger, an ulnar deviation deformity[7] (Fig. 54-10). If these problems do not resolve, pulley reconstruction may be required (see Chapter 51).

Reduction Tenoplasty

Triggering and loss of full finger flexion occasionally persists after release of the first annular pulley. This may be due to bulbous enlargement of the flexor tendon distally to the second annular pulley.[55] Since it is imperative to preserve the second annular pulley, reduction flexor tenoplasty[55] is used to narrow the bulbous tendon at the level of the proximal phalangeal joint to correct the stenotic triggering. Release of the third annular pulley has also been reported in the management of this unusual problem.[54]

Operative Technique

The flexor tendon sheath is exposed at the level of the proximal interphalangeal (PIP) joint through a midaxial incision. The bulbous thickening of the flexor tendon is palpated while the interphalangeal joints are passively flexed and extended. The flexor sheath is opened by excising the second *cruciform* pulley, and the distal flexor tendons are brought into the wound by traction and position of the wrist and digit. The A3 pulley may also have to be incised.[54] A lateral incision is made in the bulbous enlargement of tendon through peritenon. Superficial tendon fibers along the edges of the tendon are retracted by fine skin hooks, and a central core of tendon material is excised sufficient to restore the contour of the tendon to normal diameters (Fig. 54-11A–C).

The tenotomy is closed with fine absorbable suture (Fig. 54-11D) material and restoration of passive motion confirms that the reduced tendon is able to easily slide through the second annular pulley. Postoperatively, active range of motion exercise is begun immediately but avoidance of heavy power grip for 1 month is advised.

EXTENSOR POLLICIS LONGUS TENOSYNOVITIS

Tenosynovitis of the extensor pollicis longus occurs rarely but requires early diagnosis and urgent operative treatment to prevent tendon rupture, a complication that is seldom seen in de Quervain's disease, trigger finger, or trigger thumb. The condition is recognized by pain, swelling, tenderness, and often crepitus on the dorsum of the distal radius at Lister's tubercle, around which the long thumb extensor tendon veers towards its insertion in the thumb. Its separate synovial sheath-lined tunnel beneath the extensor retinaculum may be compromised by Colles' fracture, even though it is anatomically reduced or initially undisplaced. Tenosynovitis may be caused by rheumatoid disease or very rarely by overuse, the classical "drummer boy palsy."

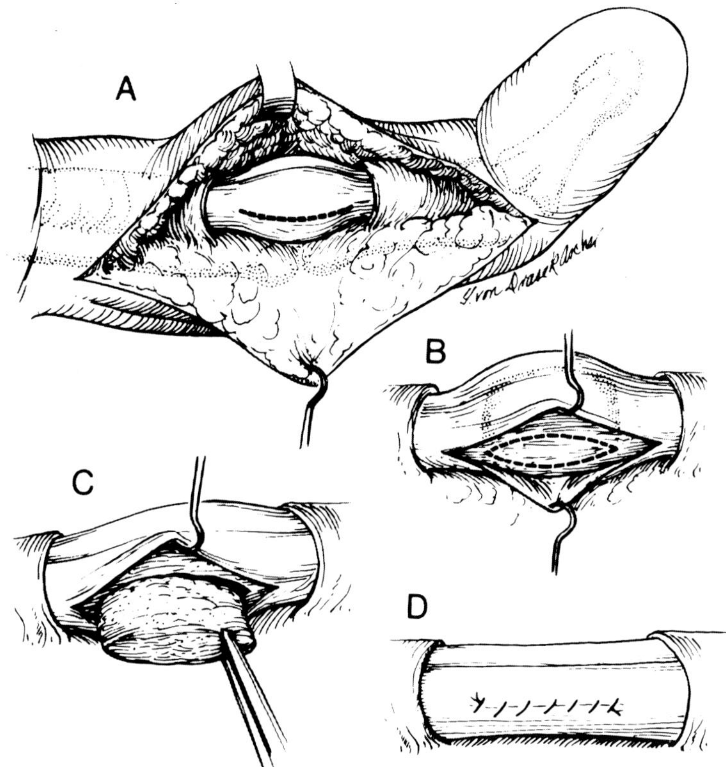

Fig. 54-11. **(A)** Fusiform enlargement of the flexor tendon approached through a Bruner incision. The dotted line shows the location of a lateral incision along the tendon. **(B)** The epitenon is retracted and an elliptical core incison is carried out. Care must be exercised to avoid further penetration of the epitenon. **(C)** Enough central matrix is removed to leave no abnormal convexity on the tendon. **(D)** The tenotomy site is closed and free gliding of the tendon through the second annular pulley is verified. (From Seradge and Kleinert,[55] with permission.)

Operative Technique

Using tourniquet and local anesthesia, a transverse incision 2 cm long is made centered over Lister's tubercle. After the extensor pollicis longus tendon is identified proximal to the tunnel, scissors are used to incise the roof of its tunnel along the course of the tendon, far enough distally to allow the tendon to be completely lifted out of its groove. The tendon is displaced to the radial side of the tubercle into a subcutaneous path opened by blunt dissection, taking care not to injure the distal sensory branches of the radial nerve. To prevent later spontaneous relocation of the tendon into its original groove the tunnel is closed with several sutures (Fig. 54-12).

After subcuticular skin closure, a light dressing is applied permitting full use of the hand. Splinting is not required.

OTHER TENOSYNOVITIS

Other examples of stenosing tenosynovitis that are seen less commonly involve the flexor carpi radialis, the extensor carpi ulnaris, extensor indicis proprius, and even the extensor digit minimi. These conditions are also treated by the injection of water soluble steroid, nonsteroidal antiinflammatory agents, and rest. Failure of response to nonoperative measures can be managed by surgical division of the offending annulus.[24,57]

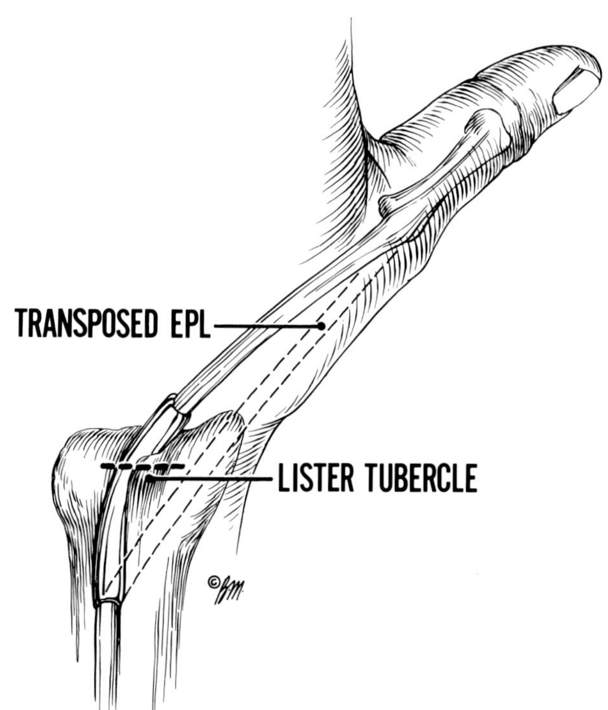

Fig. 54-12. The extensor pollicis longus *(EPL)* tendon is rerouted superficially radial to Lister's tubercle to relieve tenosynovitis.

Flexor Carpi Radialis Tendinitis

Flexor carpi radialis tendinitis is being diagnosed more frequently in recent years as a cause of pain over the flexor aspect of the wrist, especially in laborers and others who do repetitive wrist motions. The diagnosis is made by palpating tenderness over the osteofibrous flexor carpi radialis tunnel. There is usually increased pain with resisted wrist flexion and resisted radial deviation of the wrist. This tendinitis frequently co-exists with other conditions about the wrist, such as arthritis of the scaphotrapezial joint and carpal tunnel syndrome, and may occur after direct contusion trauma to the area. Injection of local anesthetic and water soluble steroid into the painful area frequently resolves the problem without resort to surgery, or serves as a useful confirmatory diagnostic test if pain is completely relieved by the injection of local anesthetic into the FCR tunnel.

The tunnel begins about 3 cm proximal to the wrist and extends to the insertion of the flexor carpi radialis. The tendon crosses close to the scaphoid tubercle, the scaphoid-trapezial-trapezoid (STT) joint and the trapezoid-trapezial joint. The tendon itself frequently has three insertions, the most significant into the base of the second metacarpal, but other smaller insertions into the crest of the trapezium and frequently a slip to the base of the third metacarpal. The tunnel is formed by the covering of the transverse carpal ligament, and along the ulnar border a fairly thick fibrous septum is present.

In patients requiring surgical decompression the roof of the tunnel is incised from proximal to distal through a 1 cm transverse incision over the flexor carpi radialis at the wrist. Care is taken to avoid trauma to the palmar cutaneous branch of the median nerve. The tendon has often been found frayed and on one occasion completely ruptured.

Postoperative results have been satisfactory with no bowstringing or tendon subluxation. Early postoperative management includes a volar splint that holds the wrist in slight extension for approximately 2 weeks, followed by restoration of motion and strengthening.[57]

TENNIS ELBOW

Because of the common use of the expression for over a century, the term tennis elbow has generally become accepted as the standard diagnosis of a syndrome characterized by epicondylar pain and tenderness and related disability,[88,89] even though the condition is much more common in nonathletes than in tennis players. Also known as epicondylitis or epicondylalgia, the condition is seen seven to ten times more often on the lateral than on the medial side of the elbow. Tennis elbow usually affects patients in the fourth and fifth decades of life[70] and is clinically characterized by tenderness and pain at the involved humeral epicondyle, aggravated by wrist extension if lateral and by wrist flexion if the medial side is affected. Occasionally both are painful.

Differentiation of tennis elbow from the much less common problem of radial tunnel syndrome (see Chapter 36) is not always easy, and sometimes the two lesions coexist.[82,85,97] However, certain characteristics of each can be identified. In tennis elbow the point of maximal tenderness is at the lateral epicondyle, while in radial tunnel syndrome tenderness is most severe where the radial nerve is palpated through the mobile muscle mass just distal to the radial head. In radial tunnel syndrome, pain is produced by resisting middle finger extension or forearm supination with the elbow extended.[85] The typical pain of tennis elbow or lateral epicondylitis is reproduced by passively flexing the fingers and wrist with the elbow fully extended. Electromyographic confirmation of radial nerve involvement is diagnostic of tunnel syndrome, but a negative examination does not rule out the problem.

Heyse-Moore[79] has shown by anatomic dissection studies that the origins of extensor carpi radialis brevis and the superficial part of the supinator are blended and inseparable, both originating from the lateral epicondyle, elbow joint capsule, and articular ligament. He therefore theorized that the relief of tennis elbow symptoms that followed surgical division of the fibrous arch of supinator was due to lessening of tension at the lateral epicondyle rather than to radial nerve decompression. He advocated abandonment of the concept that resistant tennis elbow is a radial tunnel syndrome.

Several different pathologic lesions at the elbow have been described in the literature to explain the signs and symptoms of tennis elbow, and each hypothesis has generated an operative technique to be used in cases resistent to conservative management. Synovial fringes have been excised,[67,88,91,93,95] the orbital ligament sectioned,[67,69,74,84,93] the radial nerve decompressed,[79,81,82,96,98] diseased articular cartilage excised,[86] tendon lengthened or released,[66,67,74,76,78,83,86,93,94,99] tendon excised,[87,90] tendon origin repaired,[69,72,77,87–90] or combinations of these.

The studies of Coonrad and Hooper[72] and of Nirschl,[87–90] however, have confirmed earlier works by Goldie[78] and Cyriax,[73] which demonstrated that the lesion in tennis elbow is a tear in the common extensor or flexor origin at or near the respective epicondyle. These tears are produced by mechanical overload in sports or at work in degenerating or aging tendon fibers. The tears range in magnitude from microscopic to gross rupture or avulsion.

My preferred method of surgical management, described later in this chapter, is derived from this understanding of the true nature of the problem in tennis elbow.

Nonoperative Treatment

Tennis elbow usually responds to nonsurgical treatment with an initial period of rest followed by a program of exercises to strengthen the forearm and hand muscles. Various modalities of heat therapy, including an electric heating pad, ultrasound, or diathermy supplement antiinflammatory medication, such as the salicylates or nonsteroidal drugs, to quell acute pain and swelling. Manipulation therapy has been proposed.[97] Local injections of a water-soluble steroid preparation and local anesthetic into the tender tear are administered at intervals up to three times in severe cases. As recovery is noted, a forearm support band[75] is prescribed for use during the sport or occupational activity that provokes pain. For tennis players, changes in racquet size, weight, or composition and a course of professional instruction may be recommended.[89]

Indications for Operative Treatment

Surgical management is indicated in the 5 to 10 percent of cases in which nonoperative treatment fails to provide lasting relief in a reasonable length of time. Assessment of the individual patient's functional requirements provides the critical factor in timing. Some may be willing and able to endure a year or more of pain and disability, while others, particularly professional athletes and manual workers, are given the option of earlier surgical repair to shorten the period of disability.

Anatomy

The tendon of the common extensor originates from the lateral humeral epicondyle. This conjoined tendon consists of fibers of the extensor carpi radialis brevis, extensor digitorum communis, extensor digiti minimi, and extensor carpi ulnaris, as well as part of the origin of the supinator. In considering the pathology and treatment of tennis elbow, one is interested primarily in that portion of the common tendon belonging to the extensor carpi radialis brevis, since the tears associated with tennis elbow are found in these fibers. The long radial wrist extensor arising more proximally along the supracondylar ridge of the humerus is spared (Fig. 54-13).

The extensor carpi radialis brevis also arises in small part from the radial collateral ligament of the elbow joint, and this ligament in turn attaches to the annular or orbicular ligament containing the radial head. This interrelationship of parts has been used by some authors[67–70,88–90] as the rationale to explore the elbow joint surgically for this lesion. In my experience, this is both unnecessary and undesirable.

On the inner side of the elbow, the common flexor origin arises from the medial epicondyle. The tendinous fibers of the flexor carpi radialis and less frequently, of the flexor digitorum superficialis, are those torn or avulsed in this less common variety of tennis elbow producing medial pain. The proximity of the ulnar nerve[90] within the adjacent cubital tunnel must be remembered in dissections in this region (Fig. 54-14).

Types of Operations

The various operations for tennis elbow may be classified into four types: (1) those that repair the extensor or flexor origin after excision of torn tendon, granulation tissue, and part of the epicondyle[69,72,75,77,87–89]; (2) those that relieve tension on the common extensor or flexor origin by fasciotomy or by direct release by dissection of the extensor (or flexor) origin from the respective epicondyle[66,78,80,83,94,99] or by lengthening the extensor carpi radialis brevis tendon distally[76]; (3) those directed at the radial nerve, either by denervating the outside of the elbow by severing sensory fibers[81] or by decompressing the posterior interosseous nerve[82,85,92,98]; and (4) those that involve intraarticular procedures such as partial or complete division of the orbicular ligament,[67,68,70,74,84,93] reshaping of the radial head or synovectomy,[86,91,95] separately or in combination with fasciotomy, or release of the extensor origin.

Since the lesion in tennis elbow is extraarticular, in my opinion the procedures in Category 4 are not warranted. The synovitis with effusion that may be present will resolve after extensor origin repair.[72] The procedure of denervation was published with only three cases,[81] so it cannot be recommended. The uncommon problem of posterior interosseous nerve compression (radial tunnel syndrome) is a condition other than tennis elbow; thus, those operative procedures devised to relieve it will not be described here (see Chapter 36).

While fasciotomy and extensor (or flexor) release have been

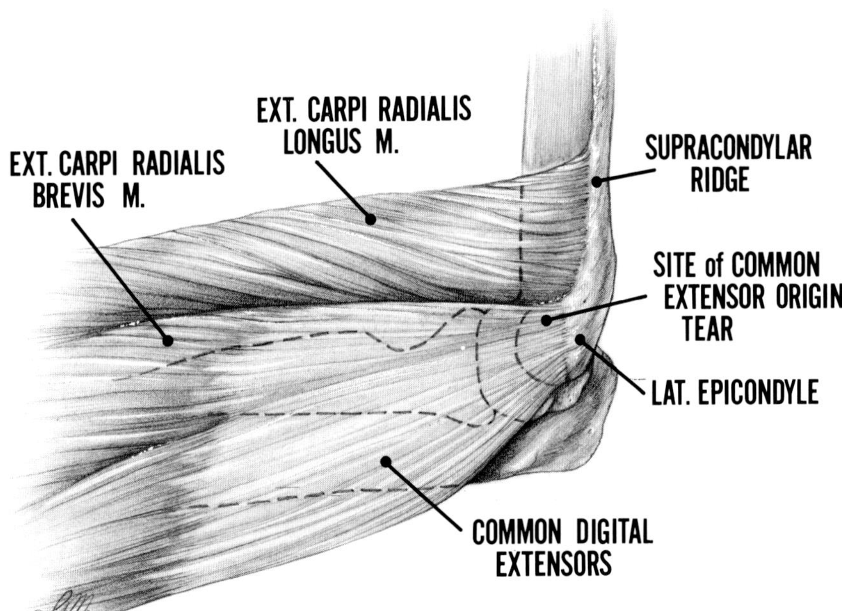

Fig. 54-13. Anatomic features of the lateral side of the elbow showing the site of the common extensor origin tear found in cases of tennis elbow.

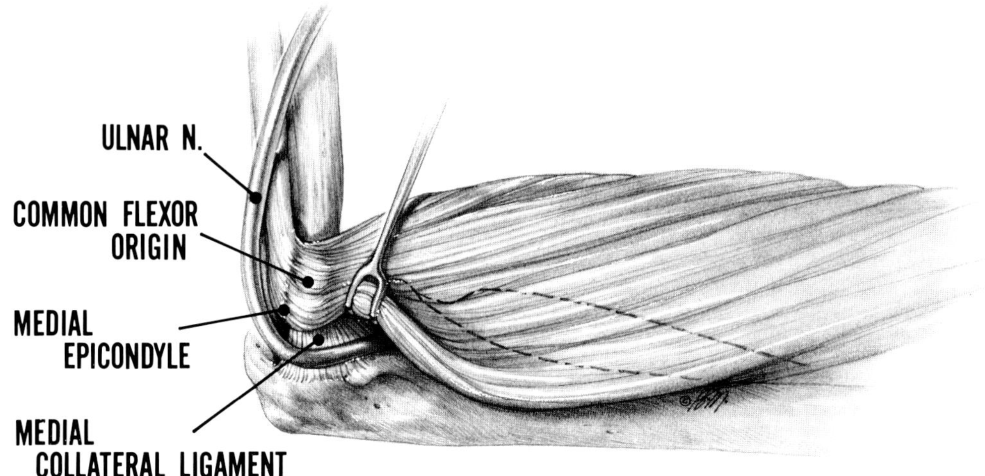

Fig. 54-14. The proximity of the ulnar nerve must be remembered in repairing tears of the flexor origin in medial tennis elbow.

lauded by their proponents as simple operative methods, I stopped doing these procedures after finding that loss of strength often resulted, hampering effectiveness in tennis and other activities, especially in the more advanced player. I also found it difficult to determine the necessary extent of the fasciotomy since the transection has to be done across normal tendon fibers. The idea of relieving the pain resulting from a partly torn tendon by creating a larger defect in tendon and fascia seems illogical.

In my experience, wrist extensor tendon lengthening at the wrist[71,79] relieved pain in only about one-half of the cases.

The operative method that I practice has proved reliable in over 200 cases during the past 30 years and is, therefore, the recommended procedure. It consists of direct exposure of the lesion in the extensor or flexor origin, excision of damaged tendon fibers and granulation tissue, partial excision of the epicondyle, and then reattachment of healthy tendon to adja-

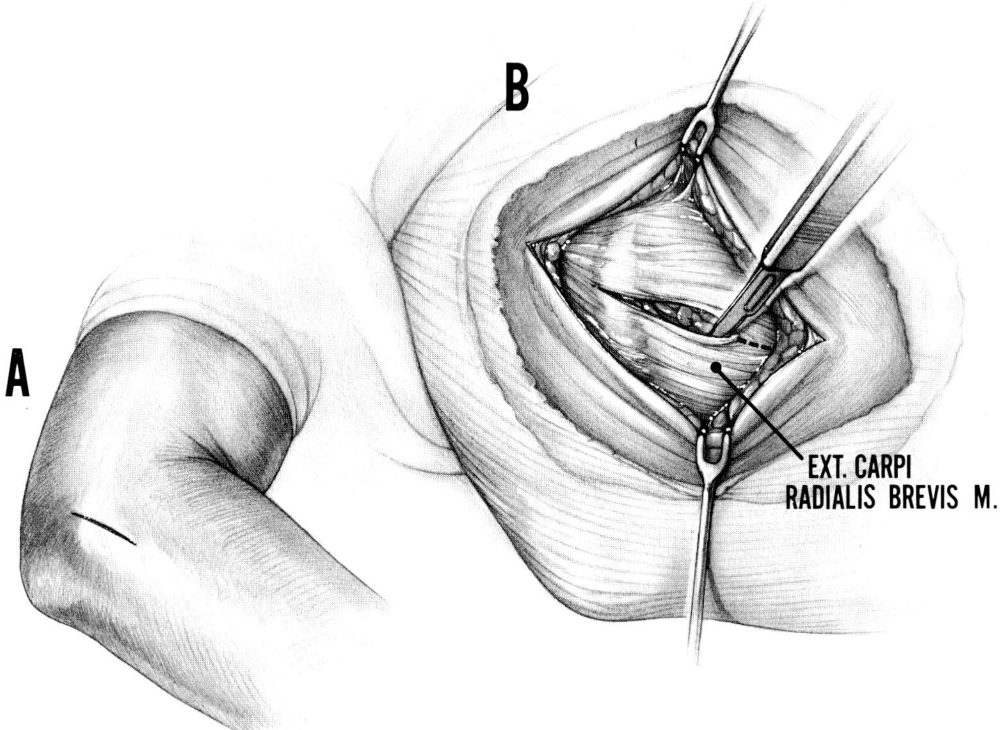

Fig. 54-15. Operative steps in the repair of lateral tennis elbow. **(A)** Longitudinal skin incision across the lateral epicondyle. **(B)** The common extensor tendon is longitudinally split and dissected off the lateral epicondyle. *(Figure continues.)*

cent soft tissue over exposed bone. The elbow joint is not entered intentionally unless another problem, such as a loose body, requires treatment.

Author's Preferred Operative Technique

This operation should be performed under general anesthesia or axillary block since a pneumatic tourniquet must be used to obtain the bloodless field essential to precise recognition and excision of damaged and inflamed tissue.

Lateral (Extensor) Side

In the operation for repair of the extensor origin, the patient is supine, although turned slightly toward the opposite side by a large pillow or blanket roll placed beneath the ipsilateral shoulder, elbow, and buttock. The arm then lies across the chest.

A longitudinal skin incision is made extending from 1 cm above the lateral humeral epicondyle to 4 cm distal to it to expose the common extensor origin (Fig. 54-15A). The deep antebrachial fascia is also incised longitudinally and retracted. The superficial fibers of origin of the extensor carpi radialis brevis may be intact and appear normal, they may be edematous and hyperemic, or they may be grossly disrupted or actually avulsed. In any case, the common extensor tendon is split by longitudinal incision and then sharply dissected off of the lateral epicondyle approximately 0.8 cm both anteriorly and posteriorly (Fig. 54-15B). The tear in the substance of the tendon or subaponeurotic space is identified. (The use of magnifying operating loupes is advised). Necrotic and torn tendon fibers are excised along with any granulation tissue in the tendon or subaponeurotic space (Fig. 54-15C).

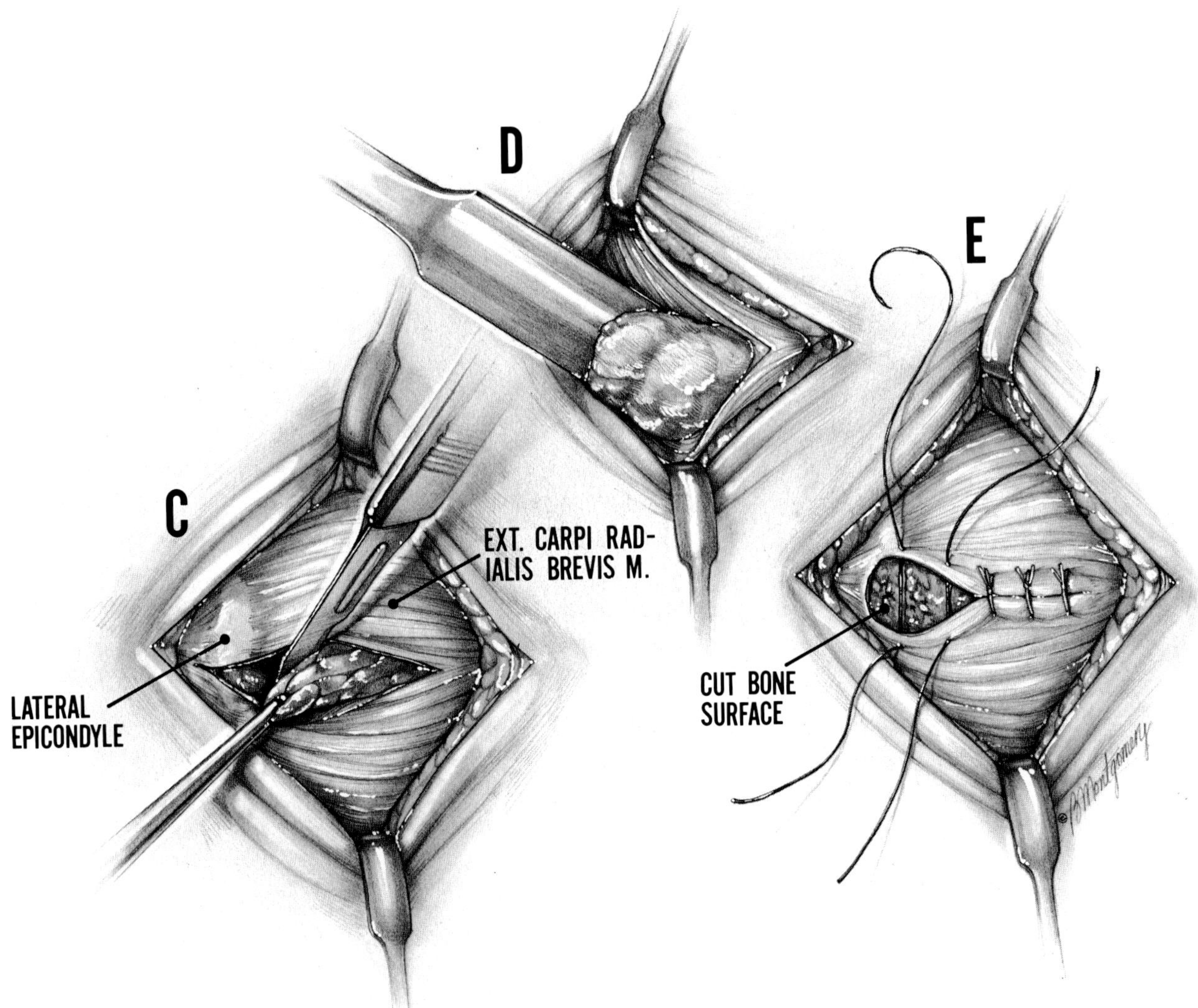

Fig. 54-15 *(Continued).* **(C)** Necrotic and torn tendon fibers and granulation tissue are excised. **(D)** The tip of the lateral epicondyle is removed. **(E)** The cut edges of the common extensor tendon are approximated over the cut bone surface to complete the repair.

With a narrow osteotome, enough of the tip of the lateral epicondyle is excised to produce a raw cancellous bone surface and to permit approximation of the edges of the debrided extensor tendon over bone without tension (Fig. 54-15D). The excised piece of epicondyle is usually 0.5 cm thick. The elbow joint is not entered. Care is taken to avoid injury to the radial collateral ligament. The operation is completed by closing the defect by approximating the edges of the common extensor tendon over the cut bone surface and suturing this tendon to adjacent soft tissue, such as the periosteum and triceps fascia margin (Fig. 54-15E) if necessary to ensure complete closure.

Medial (Flexor) Side

To repair the flexor origin on the medial side of the elbow, the patient lies supine with the arm abducted and resting on an arm board or hand table. The operation is conducted as for lateral repair, taking precautions to avoid injury to the ulnar nerve in the cubital tunnel.[90] Ulnar neurolysis and transposition are done only if ulnar nerve dysfunction is proven.[87,88]

Postoperative Treatment

After subcuticular skin closure a laterally reinforced posterior plaster splint is applied extending from the axilla to the palmar crease with the elbow at a right angle, the forearm in midposition, and the wrist in slight extension. After 2 weeks the splint is removed to allow active elbow exercises without resistance. At the end of the first month, the patient is encouraged to regain grip strength by using a handheld spring exerciser, an elastic or rubber device, or exercise putty. At 6 weeks resistive elbow and wrist flexion and extension exercises are done using dumbbell weights or other gym apparatus. By the end of 2 months, the patient should have regained adequate strength to resume sports or hard work with little or no discomfort. A forearm support band[75] should be worn while working or playing for several months to prevent recurrence of injury.

Complications

Transient ulnar paresthesias, which occurred after medial repairs in two cases, completely resolved without specific therapy. Failure to relieve the patient's pain after lateral side repair has been uncommon in my experience, and only two patients have required re-operation.

REFERENCES

Tenosynovitis

1. Alegado RB, Meals RA: An unusual complication following surgical treatment of de Quervain's disease. J Hand Surg 4:185-186, 1979
2. Arons MS: De Quervain's release in working women: A report of failures, complications, and associated diagnoses. J Hand Surg 12A:540-544, 1987
3. Belsole RJ: De Quervain's tenosynovitis: Diagnostic and operative complications. Orthopedics 4:899-903, 1981
4. Bonnici AV, Spencer JD: A survey of 'trigger finger' in adults. J Hand Surg 13B:202-203, 1988
5. Brooker AF Jr: Extensor carpi radialis tenosynovitis. An occupational affliction. Orthop Rev 6(5):99-100, 1977
6. Burman M: Stenosing tendovaginitis of the dorsal and volar compartments of the wrist. Arch Surg 65:752-762, 1952
7. Burton RI, Littler JW: Tendon entrapment syndrome of first extensor compartment (de Quervain's disorder). Curr Probl Surg 12:32-34, 1975
8. Carrozzella J, Stern PJ, Von Kuster LC: Transection of radial digital nerve of the thumb during trigger release. J Hand Surg 14A:198-200, 1989
9. Chow SP: Triggering due to de Quervain's disease. Hand 11:93-94, 1979
10. Conklin JE, White WL: Stenosing tenosynovitis and its possible relation to the carpal tunnel syndrome. Surg Clin North Am 40:531-540, 1960
11. Dobyns JH, Sim FH, Linscheid RL: Sports stress syndromes of the hand and wrist. Am J Sports Med 6:236-254, 1978
12. Doyle JR, Blythe W: The finger flexor tendon sheath and pulleys: Anatomy and reconstruction. p. 81. AAOS Symposium on Tendon Surgery in the Hand. CV Mosby, St. Louis, 1975
13. Doyle JR, Blythe WF: Anatomy of the flexor tendon sheath and pulleys of the thumb. J Hand Surg 2:149-151, 1977
14. Engel J, Luboshitz S, Israeli A, Ganel A: Tenography in de Quervain's disease. Hand 13:142-146, 1981
15. Fahey JJ, Bollinger JA: Trigger-finger in adults and children. J Bone Joint Surg 36A:1200-1218, 1954
16. Fenton R: Stenosing tenosynovitis at the radial styloid process involving an accessory tendon sheath. Bull Hosp Joint Dis 11:90-95, 1950
17. Finkelstein H: Stenosing tendovaginitis at the radial styloid process. J Bone Joint Surg 12:509-540, 1930
18. Freiberg A, Mulholland RS, Levine R: Nonoperative treatment of trigger fingers and thumbs. J Hand Surg 14A:533-558, 1989
19. Freund EI, Weigl K: Foreign body granuloma. A cause of trigger thumb. J Hand Surg 9B:210, 1984
20. Grundberg AB, Reagan DS: Pathologic anatomy of the forearm: Intersection syndrome. J Hand Surg 10A:299-302, 1985
21. Hall CL, Berg C: Chronic stenosing tenovaginitis of the wrist. J Int Coll Surg 14:48-51, 1950
22. Harvey FJ, Harvey PM, Horsley MW: De Quervain's disease: Surgical or nonsurgical treatment. J Hand Surg 15A:83-87, 1990
23. Heithoff SJ, Millender LH, Helman J: Bowstringing as a complication of trigger finger release. J Hand Surg 13A:567-570, 1988
24. Hooper G, McMaster MJ: Stenosing tenovaginitis affecting the tendon of extensor digiti minimi at the wrist. Hand 11:299-301, 1979
25. Howard NJ: Peritendinitis crepitans. J Bone Joint Surg 19:447-459, 1937
26. Hueston JT, Wilson WF, Soin K: Trigger thumb. Med J Aust 2:1044-1045, 1973
27. Jackson WT, Viegas SF, Coon TM, Stimpson KD, Frogameni AD, Simpson JM: Anatomical variations in the first extensor compartment of the wrist. A clinical and anatomical study. J Bone Joint Surg 68A: 923-926, 1986
28. Janssen JT, Teasley JL: De Quervain's disease: Stenosing tenosynovitis of the first dorsal compartment. Wis Med J 69:95-97, 1970
29. Kolind-Sorensen V: Treatment of trigger fingers. Acta Orthop Scand 41:428-432, 1970
30. Lacey T II, Goldstein LA, Tobin CE: Anatomical and clinical study of the variations in the insertions of the abductor pollicis longus tendon, associated with stenosing tendovaginitis. J Bone Joint Surg 33A:347-350, 1951
31. Laing PW: A tendon tumour presenting as a trigger finger. J Hand Surg 11B:275, 1986

32. Lapidus PW: Stenosing tenovaginitis. Surg Clin North Am 33:1317–1347, 1953
33. Leão L: De Quervain's disease; A clinical and anatomical study. J Bone Joint Surg 40A:1063–1070, 1958
34. Linscheid RL: Injuries to radial nerve at wrist. Arch Surg 91:942–946, 1965
35. Lipscomb PR: Stenosing tenosynovitis at the radial styloid process (de Quervain's disease). Ann Surg 134:110–115, 1951
36. Lipscomb PR: Tenosynovitis of the hand and the wrist: Carpal tunnel syndrome, de Quervain's disease, trigger digit. Clin Orthop 13:164–180, 1959
37. Loomis LK: Variations of stenosing tenosynovitis at the radial styloid process. J Bone Joint Surg 33A:340–346, 1951
38. Lorthier J: Surgical treatment of trigger-finger by a subcutaneous method. J Bone Joint Surg 40A:793–795, 1958
39. Louis DS: Incomplete release of the first dorsal compartment—A diagnostic test. J Hand Surg 12A:87–88, 1987
40. Marks MR, Gunther SF: Efficacy of cortisone injection in treatment of trigger fingers and thumbs. J Hand Surg 14A:722–727, 1989
41. McMahon M, Craig SM, Posner MA: Tendon subluxation after de Quervain's release: Treatment by brachioradialis tendon flap. J Hand Surg 16A:30–32, 1991
42. Medl WT: Tendonitis, tenosynovitis, "trigger finger," and Quervain's disease. Orthop Clin North Am 1:375–382, 1970
43. Melone CP Jr, Beavers B, Isani A: The basal joint pain syndrome. Clin Orthop 220:58–67, 1987
44. Miller LF: Stenosing tendovaginitis, a survey of findings and treatment in 49 cases. Indust Med Surg 19:465–467, 1950
45. Nyska M, Floman Y, Fast A: Osseous involvement in de Quervain's disease. Clin Orthop 186:159–161, 1984
46. Oni OOA: A tendon sheath tumour presenting as trigger finger. J Hand Surg 9B:340, 1984
47. Otto N, Wehbé MA: Steroid injections for tenosynovitis in the Hand. Orthop Rev 15(5):45–48, 1986
48. Patterson DC: De Quervain's disease; Stenosing tendovaginitis at the radial styloid. N Engl J Med 214:101–103, 1936
49. Pick RY: De Quervain's disease: A clinical triad. Clin Orthop 143:165–166, 1979
50. Piver JD, Raney RB: De Quervain's tendovaginitis. Am J Surg 83:691–694, 1952
51. Posner MA, Langa V, Green SM: The locked metacarpophalangeal joint: Diagnosis and treatment. J Hand Surg 11A:249–253, 1986
52. Rankin EA, Reid B: An unusual etiology of trigger finger: A case report. J Hand Surg 10A:904–905, 1985
53. Rask MR: Superficial radial neuritis and de Quervain's disease, report of three cases. Clin Orthop 131:176–178, 1978
54. Rayan GM: Distal stenosing tenosynovitis. J Hand Surg 15A:973–975, 1990
55. Seradge H, Kleinert HE: Reduction flexor tenoplasty. Treatment of stenosing flexor tenosynovitis distal to the first pulley. J Hand Surg 6:543–544, 1981
56. Stefanich RJ, Peimer CA: Longitudinal incision for trigger finger release. J Hand Surg 14A:316–317, 1989
57. Stern PJ: Tendinitis, overuse syndromes, and tendon injuries. Hand Clinics 6(3):467–476, 1990
58. Strandell G: Variations of the anatomy in stenosing tenosynovitis at the radial styloid process. Acta Chir Scand 113:234–240, 1957
59. Tanaka J, Muraji M, Negoro H, Yamashita H, Nakano T, Nakano K: Subcutaneous release of trigger thumb and fingers in 210 fingers. J Hand Surg 15B:463–465, 1990
60. Thorpe AP: Results of surgery for trigger finger. J Hand Surg 13B:199–201, 1988
61. Viegas SF: Trigger thumb of de Quervain's disease. J Hand Surg 11A:235–237, 1986
62. White GM, Weiland AJ: Symptomatic palmar tendon subluxation after surgical release for de Quervain's disease: A case report. J Hand Surg 9A:704–706, 1984
63. Witczak JW, Masear VR, Meyer RD: Triggering of the thumb with de Quervain's stenosing tendovaginitis. J Hand Surg 15A:265–268, 1990
64. Wood MB, Linscheid RL: Abductor pollicis longus bursitis. Clin Orthop 93:293–296, 1973
65. Woods THE: De Quervain's disease: A plea for early operation: A report on 40 cases. Br J Surg 51:358–359, 1954

Tennis Elbow

66. Baumgard SH, Schwartz DR: Percutaneous release of the epicondylar muscles for humeral epicondylitis. Am J Sports Med 10:233–236, 1982
67. Bosworth DM: The role of the orbicular ligament in tennis elbow. J Bone Joint Surg 37A:527–533, 1955
68. Bosworth DM: Surgical treatment of tennis elbow: A follow-up study. J Bone Joint Surg 47A:1533–1536, 1965
69. Boyd HB, McLeod AC: Tennis elbow. J Bone Joint Surg 55A:1183–1187, 1973
70. Cabot A: Tennis elbow, A curable affliction. Orthop Rev 16(5):69–73, 1987
71. Carroll RE, Jorgensen EC: Evaluation of the Garden procedure for lateral epicondylitis. Clin Orthop 60:201–204, 1968
72. Coonrad RW, Hooper WR: Tennis elbow: Its course, natural history, conservative and surgical management. J Bone Joint Surg 55A:1177–1182, 1973
73. Cyriax JH: The pathology and treatment of tennis elbow. J Bone Joint Surg 18:921–940, 1936
74. Friedlander HL, Reid RL, Cape RF: Tennis elbow. Clin Orthop 51:109–116, 1967
75. Froimson AI: Treatment of tennis elbow with forearm support band. J Bone Joint Surg 53A:183–184, 1971
76. Garden RS: Tennis elbow. J Bone Joint Surg 43B:100–106, 1961
77. Gardner RC: Tennis elbow: Diagnosis, pathology and treatment. Nine severe cases treated by a new reconstructive operation. Clin Orthop 72:248–253, 1970
78. Goldie I: Epicondylitis lateralis humeri (epicondylitis or tennis elbow). Acta Chir Scand (suppl) 339:1–119, 1964
79. Heyse-Moore GH: Resistant tennis elbow. J Hand Surg 9B:64–66, 1984
80. Hohl M: Epicondylitis—Tennis elbow. Clin Orthop 19:232–238, 1961
81. Kaplan EB: Treatment of tennis elbow (epicondylitis) by denervation. J Bone Joint Surg 41A:147–151, 1959
82. Lister GD, Belsole RB, Kleinert HE: The radial tunnel syndrome. J Hand Surg 4:52–59, 1979
83. Michele AA, Krueger FJ: Lateral epicondylitis of the elbow treated by fasciotomy. Surgery 39:277–284, 1956
84. Mills GP: The treatment of "tennis elbow." Br Med J 1:12–13, 1928
85. Moss SH, Switzer HE: Radial tunnel syndrome: A spectrum of clinical presentations. J Hand Surg 8:414–420, 1983
86. Newman JH, Goodfellow JW: Fibrillation of head of radius as one cause of tennis elbow. Br Med J 2:328–330, 1975
87. Nirschl RP: Soft-tissue injuries about the elbow. Clin Sports Med 5:637–652, 1986
88. Nirschl RP: Tennis elbow. Orthop Clin North Am 3:787–800, 1973
89. Nirschl RP: The etiology and treatment of tennis elbow. J Sports Med 2:308–323, 1974

90. Nirschl RP, Pettrone FA: Tennis elbow: The surgical treatment of lateral epicondylitis. J Bone Joint Surg 61A:832–839, 1979
91. Osgood RB: Radiohumeral bursitis, epicondylitis, epicondylalgia (tennis elbow): A personal experience. Arch Surg 4:420–433, 1922
92. Roles NC, Maudsley RH: Radial tunnel syndrome: Resistant tennis elbow as a nerve entrapment. J Bone Joint Surg 54B:499–508, 1972
93. Savastano AA, Kamioneck S, Knowles K, Gibson T: Treatment of resistant tennis elbow a combined surgical procedure. Int Surg 57:470–474, 1972
94. Spencer GE, Herndon CH: Surgical treatment of epicondylitis. J Bone Joint Surg 35A:421–424, 1953
95. Trethowan WH: Tennis elbow. Br Med J 2:1218–1219, 1929
96. Van Rossum J, Buruma OJS, Kamphuisen HAC, Onvlee GJ: Tennis elbow—A radial tunnel syndrome? J Bone Joint Surg 60B:197–198, 1978
97. Wadsworth TG: Tennis elbow: Conservative, surgical, and manipulative treatment. Br Med J 294:621–624, 1987
98. Werner CO: Lateral elbow pain and posterior interosseous nerve entrapment. Acta Orthop Scand (suppl) 174:1–62, 1979
99. Yerger B, Turner T: Percutaneous extensor tenotomy for chronic tennis elbow: An office procedure. Orthopedics 8:1261–1263, 1985

55

The Burned Hand and Upper Extremity

Roger E. Salisbury
George Peter Dingeldein

As the hand is used in manipulatory and exploratory functions, it is not surprising to learn that the upper extremity is the most frequently injured part of the human anatomy. In a study of product-related injuries, it has been estimated that 35.8 percent involved the hand or upper extremity, and 39 percent of burn wounds involved some portion of the hand or arm.[12] The hand and arm are frequently involved as a part of a much larger burn complex, illustrated by a 2-year study at the US Army Institute of Surgical Research in which 89 percent of 568 burn patients had thermal injury of the arm or hand on either or both sides.[62]

Although some burns will be minor, creating an inconvenience rather than a therapeutic challenge, others will have great potential for causing chronic disability and expense for the patient, employers, and insurance carriers. Thus, it is important that severe burns of the hands and upper extremities be managed by physicians with specific knowledge of burn therapy and reconstruction/rehabilitation in order to maximize the ultimate functional results.

ACUTE THERMAL BURNS OF THE UPPER EXTREMITY

Management of Superficial Burns

First degree burns of the hand and arm require only symptomatic treatment, consisting of analgesia and early active range of motion exercises. In small areas of superficial second degree injury, debris is removed and the wound lavaged with saline before a dressing is applied. Intact blisters should not be opened unless rupture seems imminent. The blister is a form of biologic dressing and may even mitigate against infection, as it has been shown that antibiotics will diffuse into the fluid.[25] Small areas of intermediate second degree burn can be treated in an open fashion, allowing a crust to form, or may be covered for comfort with a non-adherent impregnated gauze. The latter treatment is preferable because in the case of outpatient treatment the wound is better protected. Larger areas of intermediate second degree injury or small areas of third degree burn may be managed with topical antibiotics (silver sulfadiazine, mafenide acetate) and dressing changes, twice daily. Such injuries frequently can be cared for in the outpatient clinic after assessing the patient's reliability for follow-up visits. Commercial wound care dressings proliferate each year, touting superior efficacy. Clinical studies, often anecdotal, are offered as evidence of the worthiness of product X. In actuality, the small injury will heal regardless of the treatment if it is protected from further trauma and infection. Oral antibiotics (penicillin or cephalosporin) are prescribed for 5 days and appropriate analgesia is given. The patient is informed of the significance of increasing edema or erythema and is instructed to return if cellulitis occurs. The principle and methods of elevation of the hand and arm are also explained.

For all burns, even minor ones, the patient's tetanus immunization status must be ascertained, as fatal cases have resulted from relatively small burns[38,42] (even those that are only partial thickness). A tetanus booster should be given when necessary. If the patient has not been previously immunized or if the immunization history is in doubt, tetanus immune globulin (250 units, adult dose) is given by injection, and the patient is scheduled to complete a full immunization program (see Chapter 44).

Management of Deep Burns

Larger areas of deep second degree or third degree burns involving the hands and arms will usually require hospitalization of the patient. The size of the wound, however, should not be the only criterion for deciding on inpatient treatment. Age, coexisting medical problems, and the patient's reliability should all be considered. It is better to admit the patient to the hospital in marginal clinical situations than to risk the possible conversion of a partial-thickness wound to a full-thickness one by neglect and subsequent infection.

Since many thermal injuries of the hand are part of a larger total body burn, it is imperative that a complete physical examination of the patient be done and that initial first aid and resuscitation take precedence over the management of the upper extremity. Inadequate early examination and management of the burned hand and arm, however, may have subsequent limb-threatening results.

The most important principle in the initial management of the burned upper extremity is maintenance of perfusion, which is assured by adequate fluid resuscitation to maintain circulating volume and removal of any mechanical obstruction of flow to the extremity. Marked edema formation is characteristic of severe burns, due to both increased capillary permeability and the massive fluid loads often required to maintain the intravascular volume. The situation may be worsened by the tourniquet effect of an unyielding circumferential burn eschar, and the potential for vascular insufficiency is great. It is useful to consider the arm and each individual digit as vascular pedicles and to direct the initial therapy toward maintaining the arterial and venous flow in the pedicles.

Vascular insufficiency due to edema must be differentiated from hypovolemia secondary to inadequate resuscitation. For instance, decreased capillary filling of the nail beds and cool skin may be secondary to the shunting of blood away from the extremity to the viscera and to decreased cardiac output. The presence of adequate urine output (30 to 50 cc/hour in an adult and 1 cc/kg/hour in an infant) is a good indication of internal organ perfusion, and thus an absent pulse would reflect obstruction to local flow.

Palpable radial and ulnar pulses are a reassuring indication of limb perfusion, but their presence does not always guarantee adequate flow into the hand. If the equipment is available, a Doppler ultrasound examination should be done to determine flow in the palmar arch. If the pulse is present, the limb should be elevated, exercised, and checked hourly for continued evidence of perfusion. The presence of sensation is helpful, but its subsequent loss does not necessarily mean worsening of perfusion, as increasing edema in deeper second degree wounds may reduce sensibility. The Wick catheter technique has been found to be very accurate in measuring intramuscular pressure in the circumferentially burned upper extremity and as a warning of ischemia. Warden[73] discovered a dangerously high level in 42 percent of the extremities he studied. Furthermore, there was a very poor correlation between increased pressures and Doppler pulse recordings. Specifically, pressures as high as 64 mmHg were noted in the presence of intact Doppler pulses.

Many therapists and surgeons will not permit unlimited exercise of fingers that are circumferentially burned because of the danger of ischemic necrosis and rupture of the extensor mechanism. If one is concerned about blood supply to the fingers, then small individual volar splints may be applied to prevent proximal interphalangeal joint flexion. Wrist and MP joint flexion can be performed as often as possible without jeopardizing the extensor surface of the fingers.

Escharotomies should be done immediately for evidence of vascular insufficiency, especially if the patient is to be transported to another facility for definitive treatment.[56] Decompression is performed if the flow in the palmar arch is lost on ultrasonic examination, or, lacking this instrumentation, if palpable radial and ulnar pulsations cease. In electrical injuries, sensory deficit in the distribution of the median or ulnar nerve is an indication for fasciotomy and decompression of the involved nerve.

Technique of Escharotomy

If escharotomy is necessary, it can be done effectively at the bedside. Bleeding may be brisk, and blood should be available for transfusion if necessary (replacement usually is not required). Good lighting, an adequate supply of surgical instruments (particularly hemostats), and an electrocautery with a cutting current are prerequisites. The use of electrocautery will facilitate the procedure by minimizing bleeding while cutting the constricting burn wound.

The eschar is insensitive, but pain may be significant in some deep second degree burns. Intravenous sedation and analgesia are obtained with small doses of narcotics (usually morphine), which can be titrated to the clinical requirements. If necessary, additional anesthesia can be obtained by injecting the prospective incision with a dilute (0.5 percent) solution of lidocaine. The lateral (radial) incision to decompress the hand and arm is performed first, because there is no chance of injury to an important peripheral nerve except the superficial branch of radial nerve. The incision extends the entire length of the constricting burn (Fig. 55-1) on the axis from the tip of the acromion along the lateral edge of the antecubital flexion crease to the radial aspect of the distal flexion crease of the wrist. If blood flow is not restored (evidenced by the return of either palpable or Doppler-audible pulses), a medial incision is added.[62] The medial escharotomy is on a line from the axilla to the medial aspect of the antecubital flexion crease. If this landmark is obscured by edema or the burn wound, the medial epicondyle must be palpated and the incision made anterior to the epicondyle to avoid injury to the ulnar nerve at the elbow. From this point, the incision is extended to the ulnar aspect of the distal flexion crease of the wrist. Either escharotomy (medial or lateral) should be continued onto the hand, whether used singly or in combination. The tendons of the abductor pollicis longus and extensor pollicis brevis should be avoided in making the lateral (radial) incision across the wrist. Whenever there are circumferential burns of the fingers, digital escharotomies should be done as well. The lateral escharotomy is extended along the radial aspect of the thenar eminence and the midlateral aspect of the thumb. If a medial escharotomy has been necessary, it may be extended in a similar fashion along the hypothenar eminence to the midlateral line of the ulnar border of the little finger. The index, long, and ring fingers are decom-

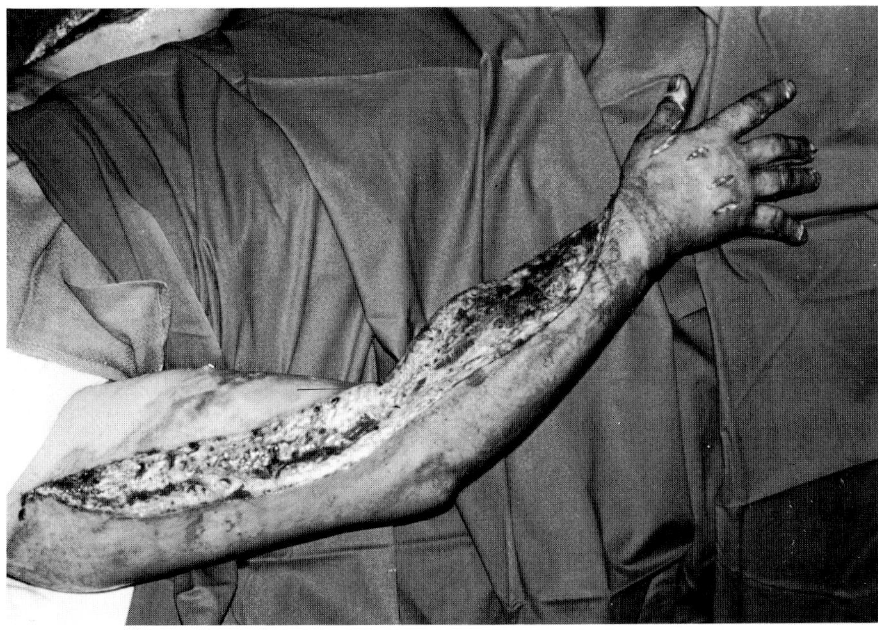

Fig. 55-1. A lateral (radial) escharotomy demonstrating wide separation of wound edges with decompression.

pressed with similar midlateral incisions on the ulnar aspect of each finger (Fig. 55-2). The ulnar sides of the fingers are preferred for escharotomy to minimize the possibility of a painful scar where the thumb opposes the fingers. It has been shown that there is a statistically significant improvement in the survival of digits with escharotomy over those that are not decompressed.[66] Lastly, decompression of the dorsal interossei should be performed if there is significant edema of the hand and diminished flexion. Small vertical incisions (Fig. 55-3) are made on the dorsum of the hand between the metacarpals, a hemostat is used to spread the edematous tissue, and the investing fascia is cut with a scalpel. Intrinsic muscle ischemia may be more prevalent than is clinically obvious on admission and may account for significant postburn disability of the hand.

Frequently, the increased range of motion provided by escharotomy is impressive (Fig. 55-4), and patients may have near-normal flexion and extension of the fingers within a few

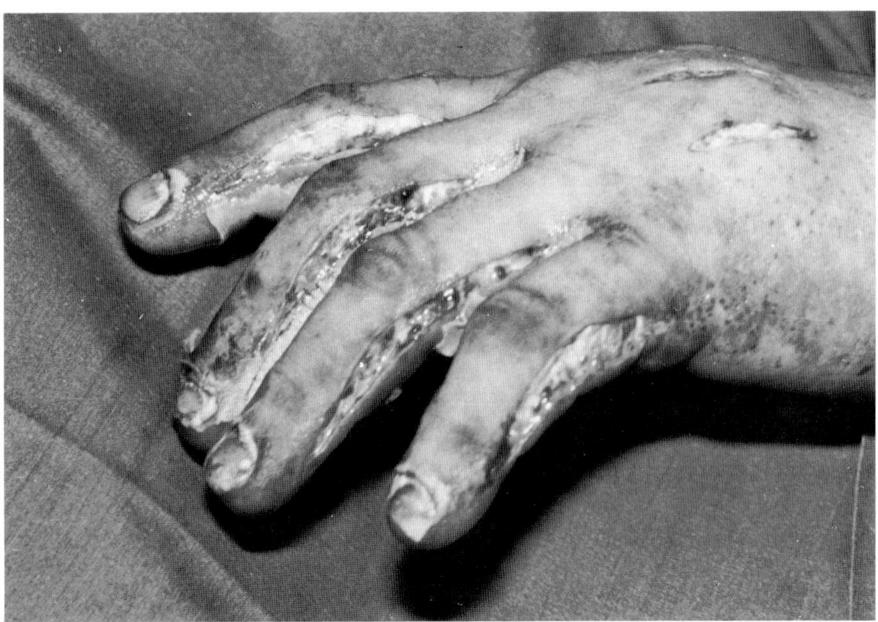

Fig. 55-2. Midlateral incisions used for digital escharotomy in circumferential burns.

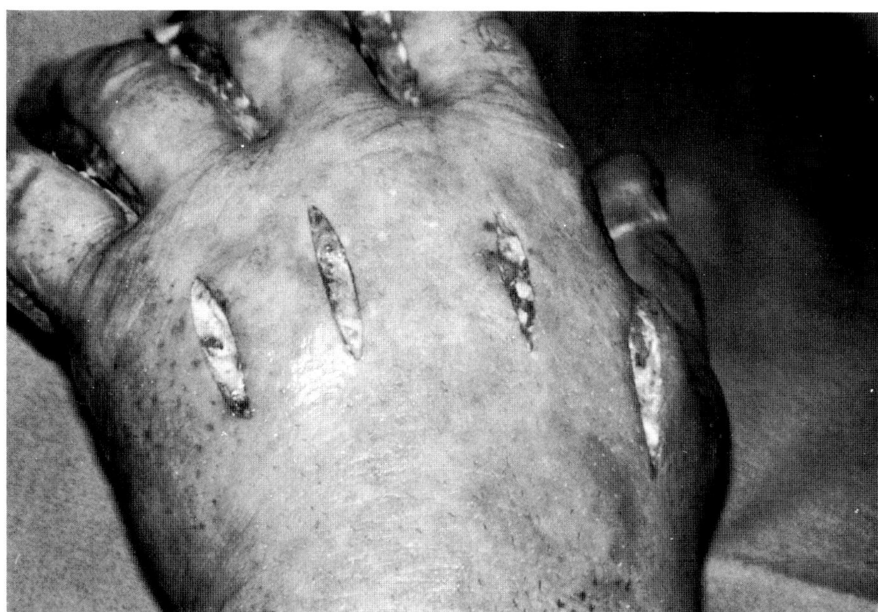

Fig. 55-3. Incisions for decompression of dorsal interossei musculature.

hours of decompression. It has been suggested that escharotomy incisions should not extend through the fascia,[56] but in very deep burns the subfascial edema may be significant. In electrical burns, where the primary injury is usually in the muscle, fasciotomy is mandatory. The fascia can be opened with electrocautery with minimal bleeding if the muscle is not cut. Hemostasis should be achieved with cautery or suture and should be complete, because pressure dressings to control escharotomy site bleeding clearly are contraindicated. If hemostasis is adequate, the wounds can be treated open with a topical chemotherapeutic agent like the rest of the burn wounds. Elevation of the hand and arm is immediately instituted. Subsequent grafting of escharotomy sites of the arm may be necessary (Fig. 55-5) but the digital incisions always close by secondary intention and, if properly placed, are compatible with satisfactory function of the fingers.

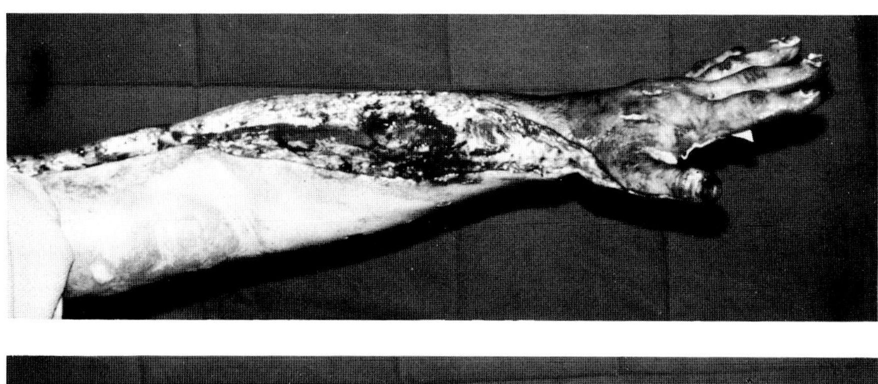

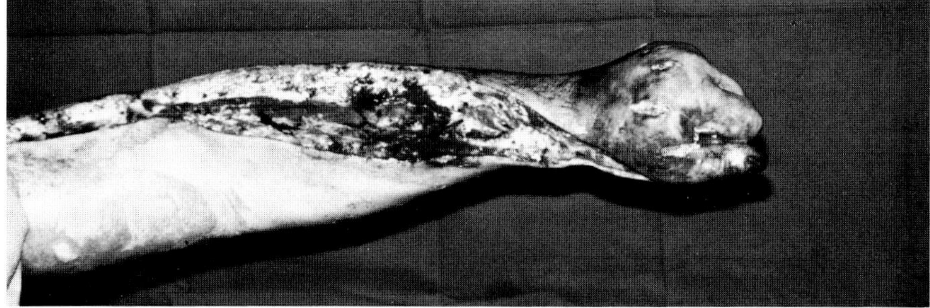

Fig. 55-4. Good motion is restored to a circumferentially burned hand and arm 24 hours after decompression of arms, digits, and dorsal interosseous muscles.

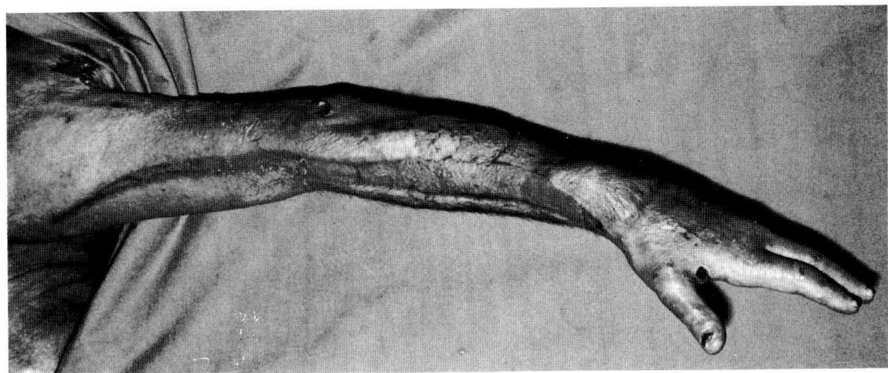

Fig. 55-5. Healed lateral (radial) escharotomy site after grafting.

Edema and Splinting

The effects of pain and edema combine to position the burned hand in a characteristic attitude: the wrist flexed, the MP joints extended, and the interphalangeal joints flexed. If the arm is involved, typically the elbow is flexed and the shoulder adducted. If maintained, this position of greatest comfort results in a position of greatest functional disadvantage in the healed burned extremity.

The edema is treated by a combination of early elevation and active exercise. The hands and arms are elevated on pillows or suspended in troughs (Fig. 55-6) elevated to intravenous poles. The troughs, made from thermoplastic materials, provide elevation while also extending the elbow and abducting the shoulder. Occlusive pressure dressings have not proved to be more effective in reducing edema than elevation,[67] and since they would interfere with clinical evaluation of perfusion, such dressings are not used. Physical therapy is begun early by therapists and nurses to maintain range of motion. Care is taken not to flex the fingers forcefully (either passively or actively), to avoid rupture of the extensor tendons in the hand with a deep dorsal burn. Exercises of daily living activities are begun as early as possible, employing adaptive tools as necessary.

After the edema has begun to subside (48 to 72 hours), night splinting is instituted to combat the deformity of comfort described above. It has been noted that the hand is not placed in the "position of function," but more in a "position of advantage" to combat the deforming action of the healing burn scar. A thermoplastic splint is constructed to maintain the wrist in dorsiflexion (15 to 20 degrees), the MP joints in flexion (75 to 80 degrees), and the interphalangeal joints in slight flexion (10 degrees). The thumb is abducted. Because the splint is made of thermoplastic material, it can be individualized to the specific needs of each patient and is compatible with open wound care with topical antibiotics. Splints should be worn at night by all patients with significant hand burns. Comatose or uncooperative individuals may require constant splinting except during periods of supervised exercise.

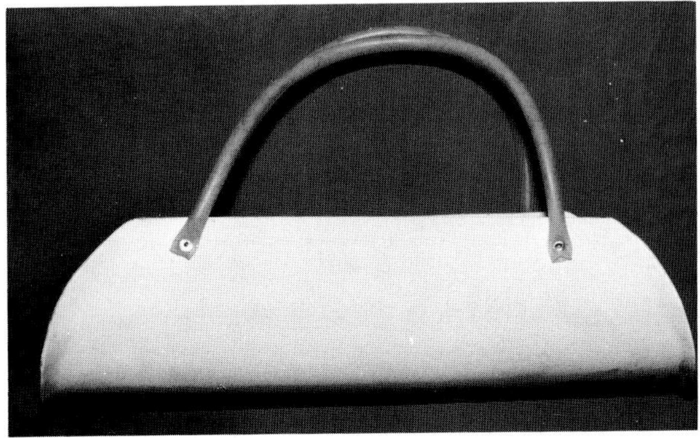

Fig. 55-6. Trough splint used to provide elevation of the extremity, shoulder abduction, and elbow extension.

Wound Closure

The proper technique for achieving closure of the burned hand is an unsettled issue in the minds of most surgeons. In the past, the weight of the literature favored early excision of deep dermal and third degree wounds with immediate grafting.[5,9,30,37,50] The recommendations for the timing of such procedures varied widely, from a few days to 2 weeks,[35] but unfortunately, no prospective controlled studies were done. With the advent of reliable topical chemotherapeutic agents that penetrated the eschar, surgery could be delayed more safely. It became clear that many wounds that were previously judged to be full thickness were instead partial-thickness injuries with regenerative capabilities and healed spontaneously with excellent functional results. Critics of a nonexcisional approach claimed that spontaneous healing resulted in thick hypertrophic scar and diminishing function with time.[21] Three prospective studies, however, do not seem to bear out this argument. In one study,[17] deep partial-thickness burns excised at 14 days and grafted were compared to deep partial-thickness burns that were allowed to heal spontaneously. Equal attention in each group was given to physical therapy, splinting, and scar compression. Follow-up at 6 to 12 months failed to show any difference in the total degrees of flexion between the two groups, nor was the number of reconstructive procedures subsequently required different. In another prospective study of deep second and third degree injuries, three treatment techniques were studied:[76] (1) early primary excision with grafting, (2) spontaneous healing with topical chemotherapy, and (3)

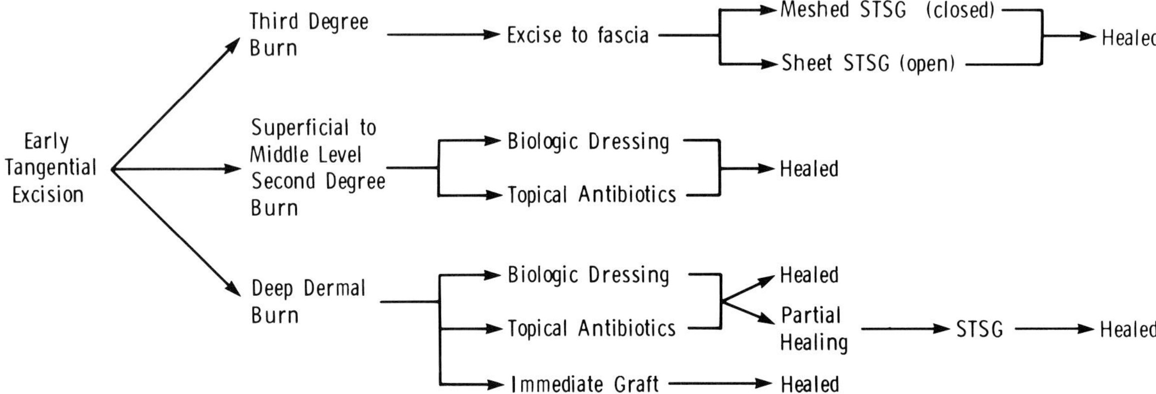

Fig. 55-7. Suggested schema for the management of the burned hand by sequential ("tangential") excision.

grafting following separation of eschar. At 1 year, no significant difference in results of clinically measured parameters could be detected among the three groups.

Tangential excision with grafting has also been reported to give good results and has the advantage of preserving viable dermal elements.[31,41,72,74] However, other investigators have compared tangential excision with grafting to spontaneous healing with intensive physiotherapy and have achieved comparable results. These investigators[23] object to grafting a partial-thickness injury that would heal spontaneously.

Good results with deep second degree burns have been achieved with enzymatic debridement and grafting.[20] The advantages obviously include reduced operative time and blood loss, and early healing. One must question, however, the advisability of using valuable donor skin to graft a wound that would heal anyway.

Faced with such conflicting opinions, the surgical regimen for management of the burned hand outlined in Figure 55-7 seems reasonable and will give good results, assuming the availability of a knowledgeable and active therapist, a cooperative nursing team, and good patient follow-up. This outline of treatment has the advantages of rapidly removing eschar, diagnosing the depth of the burn, and preserving dermal elements, where present. No clinical protocol will always fit each patient's needs, and adjustment for age, other medical problems, and availability of donor sites will need to be made.

Technique of Early Excision and Grafting

If full-thickness excision is decided upon, specific surgical details are to be observed. Prospective finger excisions (Fig. 55-8) extend to the midlateral plane; if they are made more volar, linear contractures will result. The dissection is done

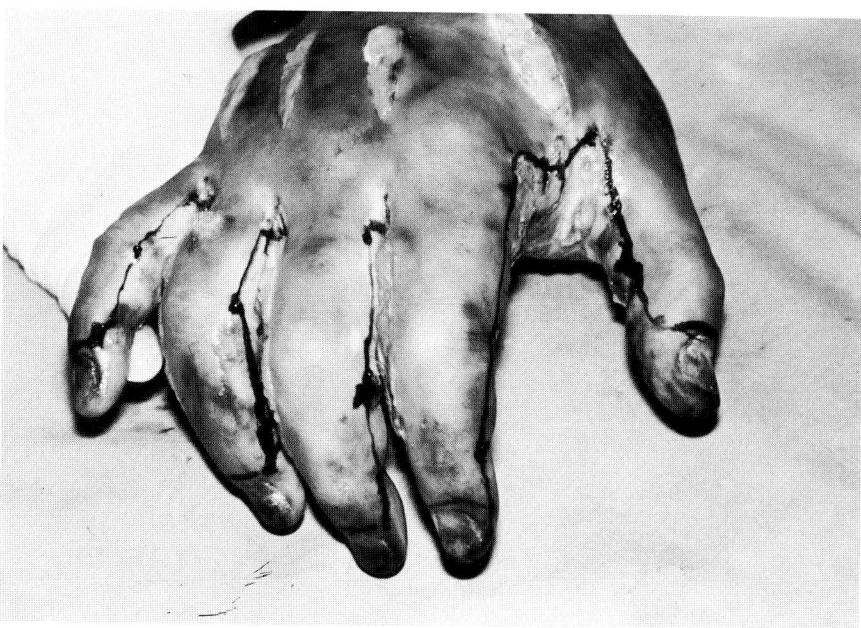

Fig. 55-8. Planned lines of excision in full-thickness dorsal hand burn. Note the "dart" carried into the first web space.

under the control of a pneumatic tourniquet to facilitate the identification and preservation of the veins, paratenon, and tendons. A plane of dissection is developed (Fig. 55-9) just above the level of the dorsal veins, which must be preserved to avoid postsurgical edema. Excision of eschar is taken onto the thenar and hypothenar eminences if necessary. The MP joints are pinned in 80 degrees flexion for immobilization and to increase the amount of skin required for coverage of the dorsum of the hand. Some surgeons prefer to use a hayrake splint with K-wires, or fingertip traction with silk sutures inserted through the fingernails and connected to a resting splint. Both techniques will permit open treatment of the grafted hand. In all three techniques mentioned, the emphasis is on maintaining the proper position of the fingers. Merely placing the hand in a static splint often leads to loss of positioning and hyperextension of the MP joints with subsequent graft shortening. The tourniquet is then deflated and hemostasis achieved. Occasionally, persistent bleeding from a number of small vessels may preclude immediate grafting. If so, a pressure dressing, placed over cadaver allograft or meshed pigskin, is applied and delayed autografting done 24 to 48 hours later. Sheet grafts may be used to achieve coverage, but good results also have been obtained with the use of unexpanded meshed (1.5:1) autograft (Fig. 55-10). Grafts may be held in place with sutures,

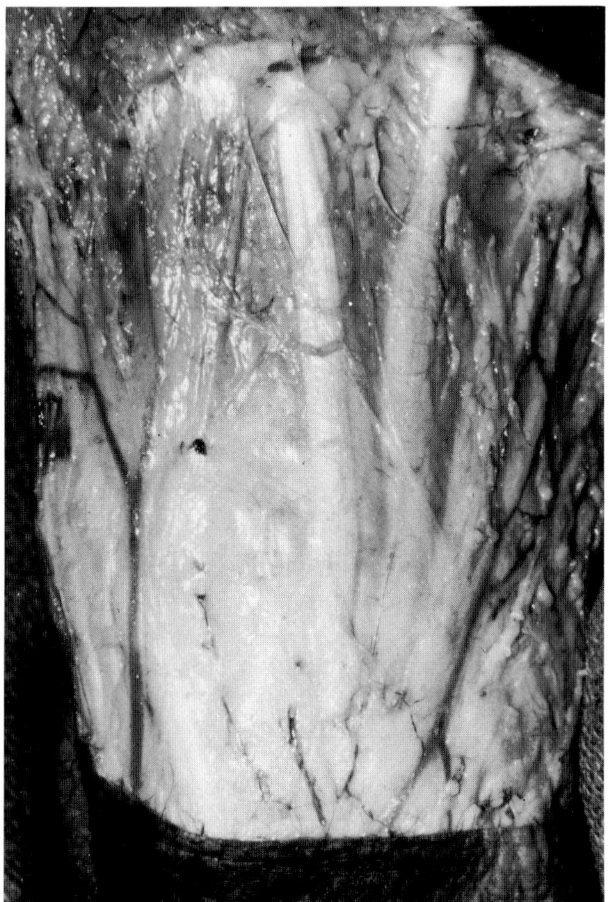

Fig. 55-9. Full-thickness excision in the proper plane retains dorsal veins and paratenon.

staples, or Steristrips. The grafts must be darted into the web spaces to prevent dorsal hooding. Meshed split-thickness grafts are treated closed and kept moist with 0.5 percent silver nitrate or GU (antibiotic) irrigant. The dressings are changed first at 48 hours, and then daily until graft take is assured. The dressing is designed to maintain the wrist in flexion to avoid shortening of the dorsal graft. The pins are extracted on the seventh to tenth day, and the hand is mobilized. Dynamic splinting with fingernail traction is effective in cases where dorsal pressure on newly vascularized grafts is not desirable.[68]

Although tangential excision can be used in third degree burns (see below), full-thickness excision to fascia has certain advantages. If done in the first 3 to 5 days (after resuscitation is complete), there is an edema plane that lies between the subcutaneous fat and the dorsal veins. This plane is relatively avascular and facilitates the dissection.

Technique of Tangential Excision

For partial-thickness injury, tangential excision may be performed with a guarded knife, the air-driven Brown dermatome, or dermabrader. With the knife or dermatome, sequential thin excisions (0.008 to 0.010 inch) are done until the level of injury to the dermis is determined[39] (Fig. 55-11). Since the depth of the injury may vary, the wound is excised in sections. The procedure can be done under tourniquet, but this deprives the surgeon of one of his major guides to the depth of excision, namely punctate dermal bleeding (Figs. 55-12 and 55-13).

Following excision, the wound can be treated with topical antibiotics or biologic dressings (cadaver homograft or porcine heterograft). The biologic dressing is preferable in that it assists with hemostasis, often needs to be applied only once, and better prevents drying of the freshly exposed dermis. If the dermis is allowed to dry, a new eschar will form, and the depth of the wound will increase.

Very deep dermal injury requires grafting, as the dermal elements remaining will not heal quickly or provide adequate stable epidermis. The skin may be applied as unexpanded meshed grafts (meshed 1.5:1) or as sheets. Both have given satisfactory results, although the open technique of managing sheet grafts of the hand and arm may call for "creative splinting" to provide adequate immobilization. Alternatively, skeletal suspension by radial or metacarpal pins[19] or a "hayrake" will provide immobilization as well as access to the wounds. Serum is initially rolled from beneath the graft to the edge with cotton-tipped applicators, but as the skin begins to adhere to the wound, individual collections of fluid are opened with a scalpel and flattened. Continued rolling of the fluid collection to the edge of the graft after adherence of the skin to the wound serves to disrupt any neovascularization.

Concomitant Bone Injury

The most serious bone problem accompanying acute injury may be a fracture under the burn wound. Lack of stabilization and an infected hematoma can lead to systemic sepsis and death. Once the patient is resuscitated (48 to 72 hours), the burn should be excised from the extremity and open reduction

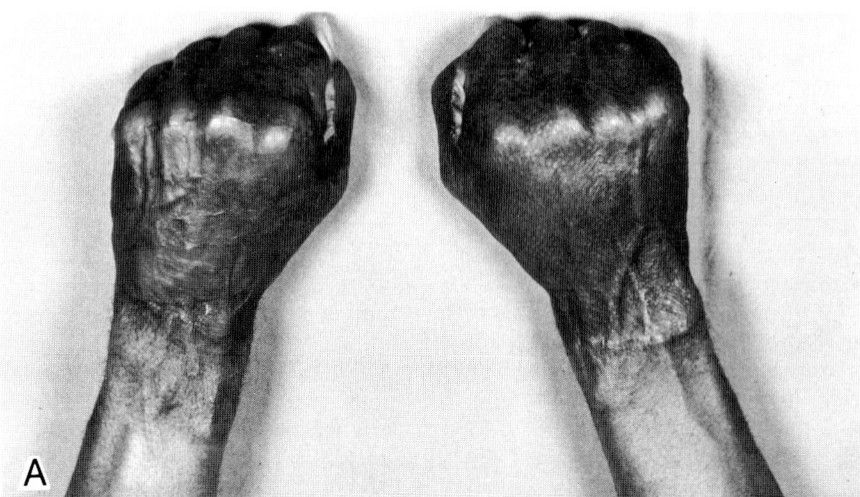

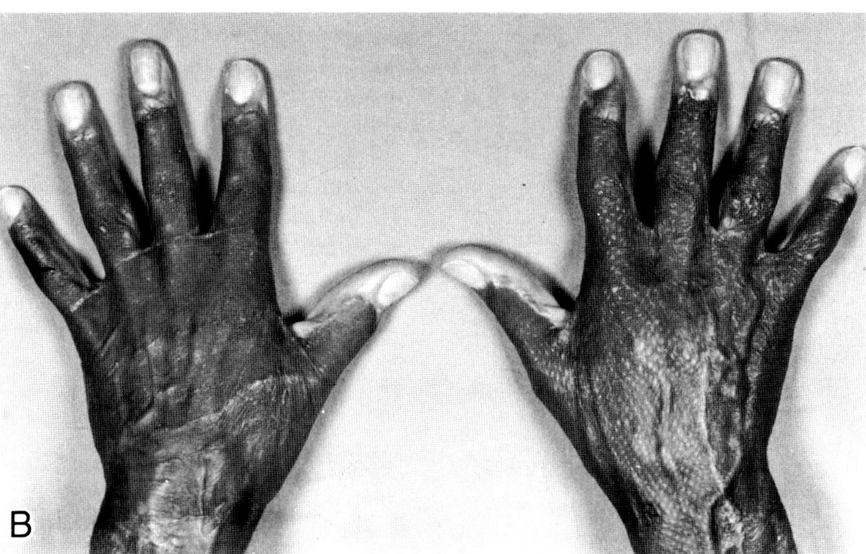

Fig. 55-10. Full flexion **(A)** and extension **(B)** of fingers bilaterally, following excision of shortened hypertrophic dorsal scar.

and fixation done, followed by skin grafting. Thus, infection is minimized. Attempting open reduction after 5 days through a heavily seeded burn wound without excision invites osteomyelitis.

Deep burns of the fingers may destroy not only the overlying soft tissue but the bone itself. While the radiograph may be compatible with osteomyelitis, clinically the bone is obviously necrotic. Debridement reveals nonviable marrow, and disarticulation is necessary.

Full-thickness burns of the dorsum may involve all tissue down to but not including the bone. When debridement exposes bone and an unstable joint, it should be rongeured to bleeding marrow and the joint pinned in a functional position. Once granulations have formed, the finger is skin grafted.

Evans[19] has described the management of concomitant orthopaedic problems in the severely burned patient.

Choice of Treatment for Acute Burns

It is clear that the surgeon treating the burned hand and arm has a number of options for acute treatment open to him. Evidence is accumulating that full-thickness excision of deep partial-thickness burns with immediate grafting does not produce uniformly better results than spontaneously healing wounds in long-term follow-up, when meticulous attention to pre- and postoperative (inpatient and outpatient) physical and occupational therapy is maintained.[23,37] Appropriate therapy, massage, compression, and splinting are absolute requirements for excellent results, as they are in so many other types of surgery.

It is also necessary for the hand surgeon to be flexible in his choice of treatment modalities for the acutely burned hand and arm. The patient's age, general health, size of burn, and coex-

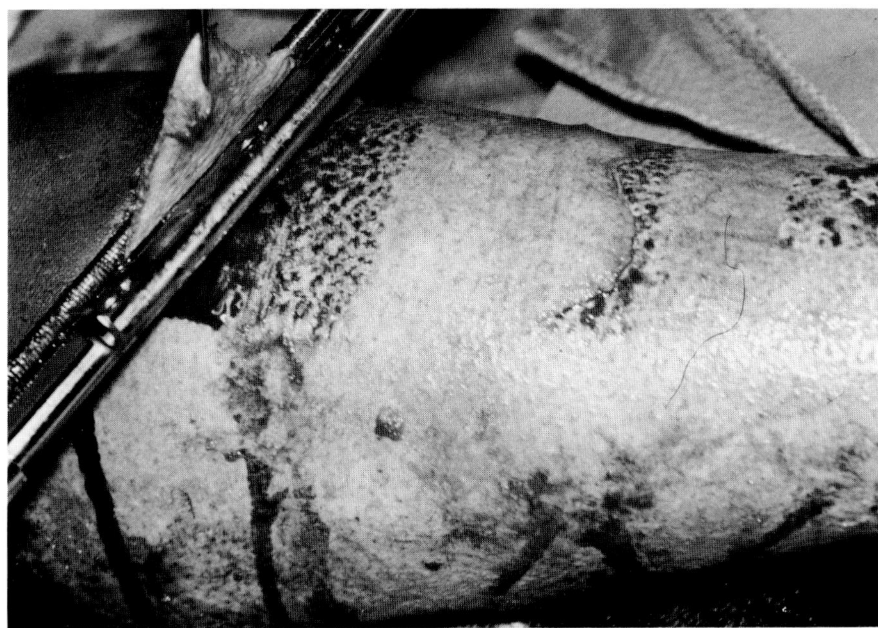

Fig. 55-11. Sequential ("tangential") excision with a guarded knife. Punctate dermal bleeding demonstrates adequate depth of excision.

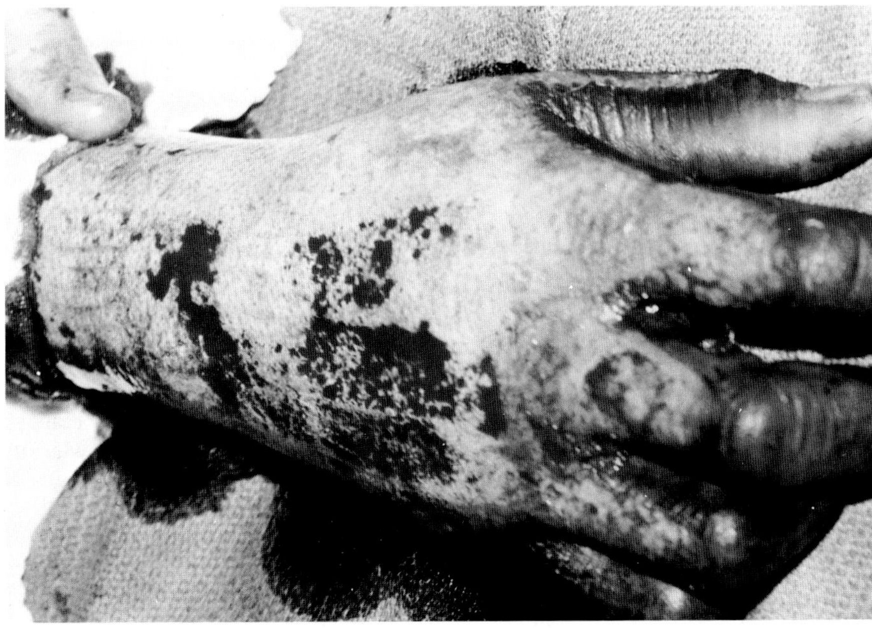

Fig. 55-12. Punctate dermal bleeding indicates viable tissue.

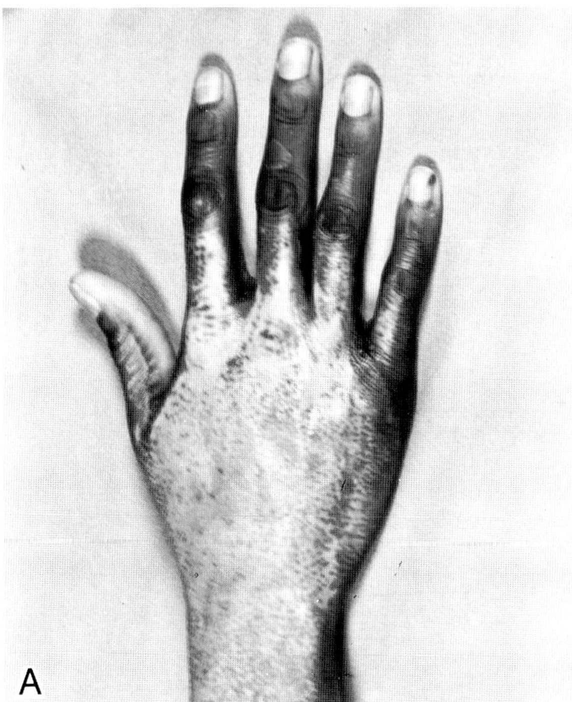

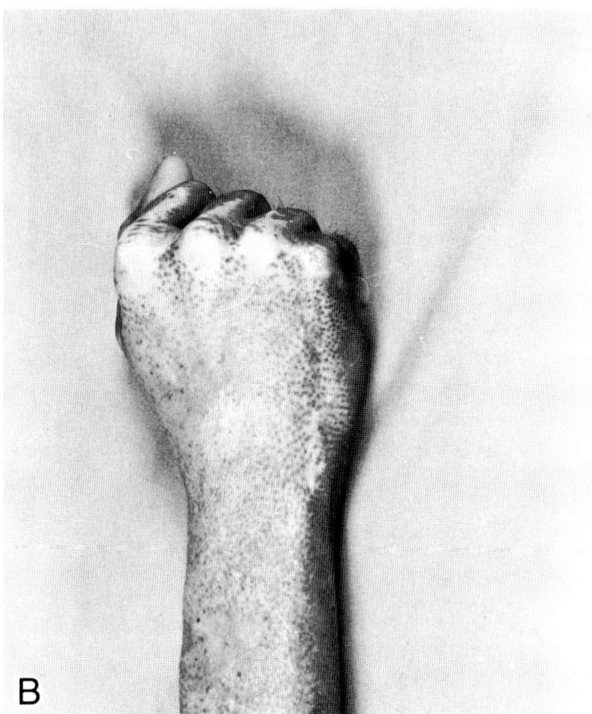

Fig. 55-13. Healed functional result 6 weeks after sequential ("tangential") excision and application of heterograft.

isting injuries must be considered. What is the patient's occupation? If the total body burn size is small and mostly confined to the upper extremity, then early excision and grafting may lead to a more rapid return to work. In the same way that "a splint that fits everyone fits no one," the acute treatment regimen for the thermally injured upper extremity must be individualized.

ELECTRICAL INJURY OF THE UPPER EXTREMITY[53,65]

The underlying pathology of the high-voltage electrical injury is completely different from a gasoline or scald burn and requires different evaluation and treatment. The amount of tissue damage is the result of the complex interplay[71] of a number of factors, including amperage, voltage, tissue resistance, type and duration of current, and the surface area over which the current makes contact. Associated injuries may include thermal burns from secondary clothing fire, fractures and internal injuries associated with falling from heights (power poles, roofs), and fractures associated with tetanic contraction of muscles. The hand and upper extremity are the most frequent sites of entry in electrical wounds, and in the case of high-voltage injury, males are almost exclusively the victims (i.e., job-related accidents).

The key to assessing any electrical wound, including that in the hands and arms, is to realize that the degree of injury is frequently more extensive than indicated by cutaneous examination. Often extensive muscle necrosis is present under viable skin, even in the presence of palpable peripheral pulses, which may lead to a serious underestimation of the total injury and the volume of fluid necessary to prevent shock. The presence of hemochromogens in the urine is indicative of muscle injury, and high urine flows must be maintained to prevent acute tubular necrosis. Ringer's lactate must be given in sufficient quantity to maintain urine flow in the range of 75 to 100 cc/hour, employing a mannitol diuresis if necessary, until the urine clears of pigment.

Additional initial management includes attention to tetanus immunization, as discussed earlier under thermal burns. Coexisting injuries (fractures, thermal and internal injuries) must be sought and managed. Internal tissue damage may occur anywhere along the course of the current, and the patient should be monitored acutely for electrically induced arrhythmias.

The initial local management of the electrically injured hand and upper extremity is similar to the management of the thermally wounded limb, including early elevation and splinting and careful monitoring of peripheral pulses. Because electrical injuries often involve deep structures, subfascial edema is more common than in thermal burns, and therefore when pulses are lost, fasciotomy in association with escharotomy is more likely to be required. Even though cutaneous wounds may be small in an electrical injury, the physician must monitor peripheral pulses diligently, as underlying muscle damage may make decompression necessary.

Although peripheral nerves have very low resistance to electrical current, they also seem to have a high potential for recovery, particularly if not associated with cutaneous injury. For this reason, absent median nerve function in the hand following an electrical injury to the hand and forearm may be due to the direct effect of current or to local edema in the carpal tunnel, suggesting the need for decompression by division of the transverse carpal ligament.

Evaluation of the extent of deep tissue damage in electrical injury is difficult even for the experienced clinician. Preoperative evaluation of the degree of muscle injury has involved arteriography, xenon washout, and ^{99m}Tc stannous pyrophosphate scintigraphy, all particularly useful in patients with palpable distal pulses in the face of obvious proximal clinical injury. Arteriography should be done only after the patient is adequately resuscitated, as the contrast dye induces an osmotic diuresis that can result in hypovolemia.

In addition to the initial difficulty in determining the magnitude of deep tissue injury, definitive debridement of nonviable tissue is further hampered by the apparent clinical progression of tissue necrosis over several days. The mechanism of this phenomenon is not clear and may be more apparent than real, in that the full extent of the injury may be underestimated at the time of the original insult, and hence not truly "progressive."

Whatever the mechanism, this apparent gradual loss of tissue must be taken into account in the management of the extremity. Two schools of thought have emerged as to the management of this clinical problem. The first advocates waiting a week or more to allow full demarcation of nonviable structures, and then proceeding with amputations, grafting, or flaps. The second philosophy advocates early debridement to avoid septic complications, but potentially risking the removal of viable tissue. A compromise position is to proceed with early debridement of clearly nonvital structures, grossly guided by the previously mentioned radiographic techniques. Any tissue showing clinical evidence of viability (contraction on electrical stimulation, bleeding on cut surface, normal color) is spared. Fluorescein staining is also useful intraoperatively to determine vital muscle. The wounds are then dressed with biologic dressing and reexamined 72 to 96 hours later. Additional necrotic tissue is excised employing clinical diagnostic parameters as well as fluorescein injection. Wound closure by grafting or flap coverage is then usually possible. Any protocol must be tailored to the patient's individual problems, as well as his general condition and associated injuries. Functional deficiencies due to initial extirpation of necrotic nerves and tendons, as well as late functional loss secondary to intraneural fibrosis, require exploration for possible neurolysis, nerve grafting, or tendon transfer.

The clinical research by Wang Xue Wei[72] and colleagues in revascularizing the electrically injured upper extremity is very provocative and deserves more study before being recommended in a textbook. Essentially, these authors have been doing vigorous early debridement and extirpation of necrotic muscle. When there is obvious injury to the radial and ulnar arteries resulting in limb jeopardy, saphenous vein bypass grafts are inserted with microsurgical technique from proximal viable to distal uninjured vessels. Free flaps from the foot have been also used in some cases, with subsequent limb survival. Because of the poor results obtained with severe high voltage injuries using conventional techniques, this work deserves close study. The effect of interposition grafts on the partially injured nutrient arterioles or veins remains to be elucidated.

CHEMICAL INJURY OF THE UPPER EXTREMITY

Chemical "burns" of the upper extremity do not present any special long-term management problems that have not already been discussed under thermal and electric injuries. The same careful attention must be given to tetanus immunization status, elevation, immobilization, and the monitoring of pulses as in the other burns. The acute management of chemical injuries of the hand and arm is unique perhaps only in the question of specific neutralization of individual agents. Extensive lists of exact neutralizing agents are available,[32] but unless extreme foresight has made such solutions readily accessible, water lavage should be begun at once without losing time to seek out specific agents.

There are several specific exceptions,[58,64] however, to the rule of copious water dilution for chemical injuries that deserve mention. Phenol should be removed from the skin with glycerol, propylene, or polyethylene glycol because of the limited solubility of phenol in water. Lime is removed by first brushing the powder from the skin and then beginning water lavage. Hydrofluoric acid is a common industrial chemical and is absorbed into the exposed tissues. Continued burning after lavage indicates persistant chemical action and is an indication for the injection of calcium gluconate into the affected area to bind the active fluoride ion. Alternatively, the affected area may be excised and grafted.

Particulate white phosphorus in the skin is treated first with water lavage and then is covered with a copper sulfate rinse in concentrations no greater than 1 percent to avoid hemolysis and renal damage. This rinse retards further oxidation of the phosphorus by forming a film of cupric phosphide on the phosphorous particles. The dark color of the cupric phosphide aids in locating the embedded chemical and in the subsequent debridement.

RECONSTRUCTION OF THE BURNED HAND

The problems of "what to do" and "when to do" burn reconstruction following healing of the acute injury are best understood by studying the pathologic involvement of the individual tissues of the hand, i.e., skin and soft tissue, tendons, nerves, and bones and joints.

Once the complex injury has been dissected into its components, the physician, patient, vocational rehabilitation worker, and employer can meet as a team and decide what procedures have priority in returning the injured patient to work. The hand surgeon must be aware of the other parts of the body with burn deformities that might necessitate surgery. A time-related plan with specific recovery goals is imperative because it has been shown that if the patient is not back to work within 18 months following injury, his changes of employment fall off geometrically. Thus, the logical approach is to carefully record all the anatomic abnormalities secondary to burn injury. The surgeon must then listen to what the patient desires corrected. The expectations of thermally injured patients are notoriously unrealistic, and the operations must be carefully explained to them in a simple, honest fashion.

The presence of an abnormality is obviously not an automatic indication for reconstructive surgery. So often in the patient recovering from a large thermal injury, the number of physical problems seems overwhelming to all. Fortunately, it is possible to group the procedures to decrease the number of admissions and general anesthetics. For example, part of the team may operate on the hand while others simultaneously reconstruct the face, creating eyebrows, relieving microstomia with flaps, or replacing an aesthetic unit of the face. Many of our patients have had bilateral upper extremity injuries, and the issue of whether to correct both hands at the same time is often addressed. It is unwise to reconstruct both hands simultaneously in an outpatient or someone who is going home in 24 hours to convalesce because of their helplessness and inability to perform the activities of daily living. Occasionally the patient who will convalesce for a week in the hospital (where nursing staff can support him) is a good candidate. In the last 15 years of grouping procedures in this fashion, we have not experienced any increased incidence of complications (infection, wound breakdown, etc.).

Skin and Soft Tissue Contractures

The most common skin and soft tissue problem of the burned hand is contracture formation, which may be due to (1) skin grafts of inadequate dimension and thickness, (2) hypertrophic scar or keloid formation, or (3) an inadequate exercise program and failure to splint in the antideformity position.

On the extensor surface, inadequate skin coverage results in a feeling of "tightness" or even MP joint hyperextension and limitation of flexion of the fingers. Inability to fully flex the fingers or recurrent ulceration from thin, unstable skin is an indication for excision and grafting the dorsum of the hand. The technique is not different from early excision (previously described) except that it is more difficult. There is no edema plane separating injured from intact tissue. Therefore dissection must begin proximal to the injury to identify normal tissue. Once the normal intact dorsal veins and paratenon are identified, all distal tissue is dissected off them and discarded. Seeing the thickness of the hypertrophic scar in the hand shown in Figure 55-14 makes one appreciate why there was limitation of flexion. If there has been severe dorsal shortening (a large wound healed by contraction, not by skin grafting), the MP joints will be hyperextended (Fig. 55-15) or even dislocated, and the PIP joints hyperflexed. The extensor tendons are markedly shortened, fixed in scar, and not amenable to tenolysis or step cut lengthening. Thus, dissection of the scar off the tendons will not result in release of the contracture. The tendons must be transected, and perhaps excised, to allow MP joint flexion. If release is still not complete, MP joint capsulectomies will often be helpful.[15] Once there is good passive range of motion of the MP joints, one must create a soft tissue base through which tendons will glide. Abdominal (Fig. 55-16), groin, myocutaneous (tensor fascia lata), and free flaps have all given excellent results, and the choice partly depends on the distribution of the patient's burn and the surgeon's experience. (Discussion of these individual flaps is presented in Chapter 28). Regardless of the flap chosen, the most common error is to make the flap too small, which compromises future surgery.

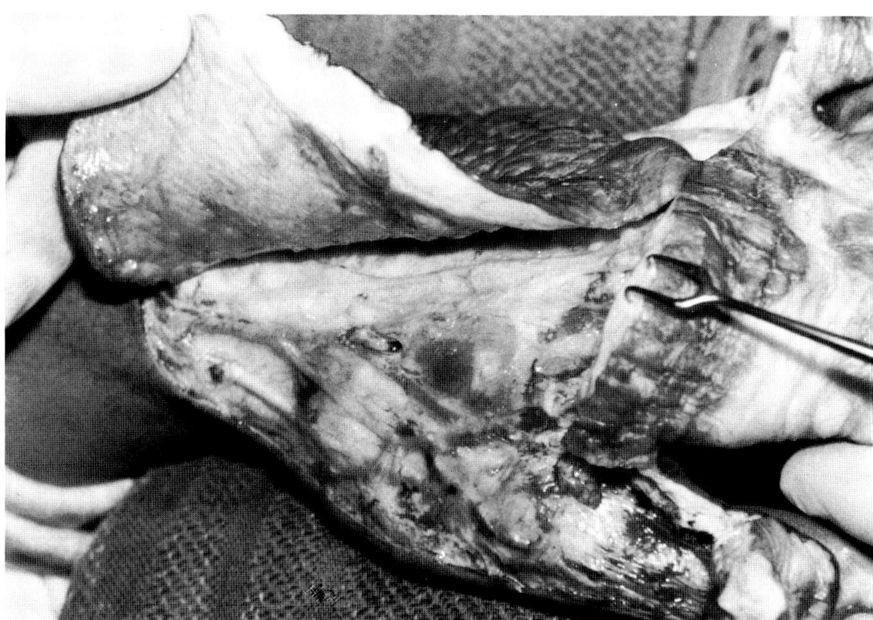

Fig. 55-14. Excision of hypertrophic scar from the dorsum of the hand after primary healing. The plane of dissection preserves the dorsal veins. Note the thickness of the scar.

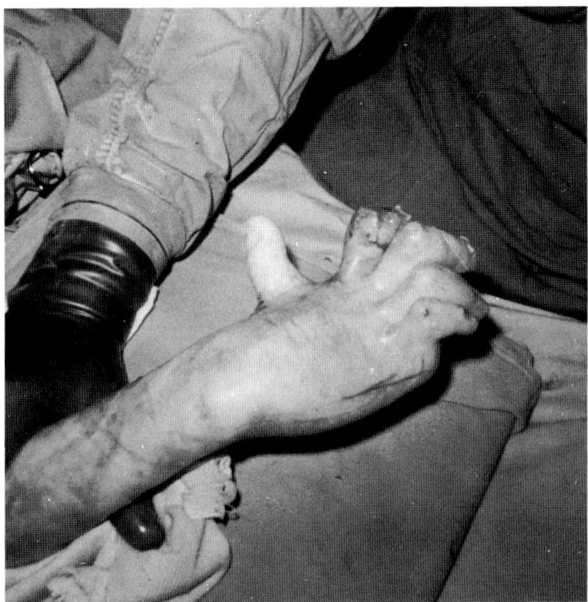

Fig. 55-15. Severe shortening of the dorsal skin in a neglected burned hand, resulting in dorsal dislocation of the MP joints.

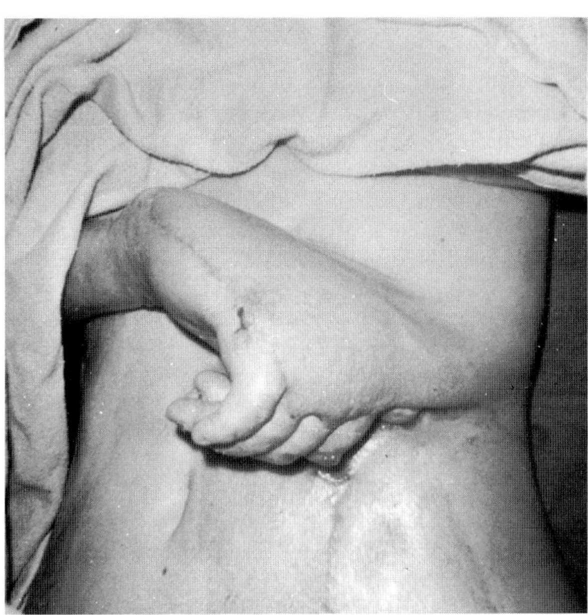

Fig. 55-16. Exposed bone and joint structures necessitates flap coverage of the hand. Note that the wrist and MP joints were flexed to fully open the defect, ensuring that a sufficiently large flap would be applied.

The wrist and MP joints must be placed in flexion (Fig. 55-16) to fully appreciate the magnitude of tissue deficit. The abdominal flap extends from the wrist over the MP joints. Reconstruction of the PIP joint is not usually attempted at this operation because of prolonged tourniquet time. In this type of hand injury with compromised vascularity, it is unwise to subject the limb to more than 2 hours of ischemia, even by deflating and reinflating the tourniquet.

Volar contractures of the hand and upper extremity may be managed by many different techniques, depending on the severity of the injury and the condition of the surrounding tissues. Deep second or third degree burns of the palm (Fig. 55-17) may result in extensive shortening of all structures of the fingers, as well as loss of width of the palm. Obviously, aggressive early splinting will prevent or minimize these contractures in most cases and may even be successful in reversing an early deformity. *Excision* of palmar skin is only rarely performed because the sensory qualities are usually superior to a skin

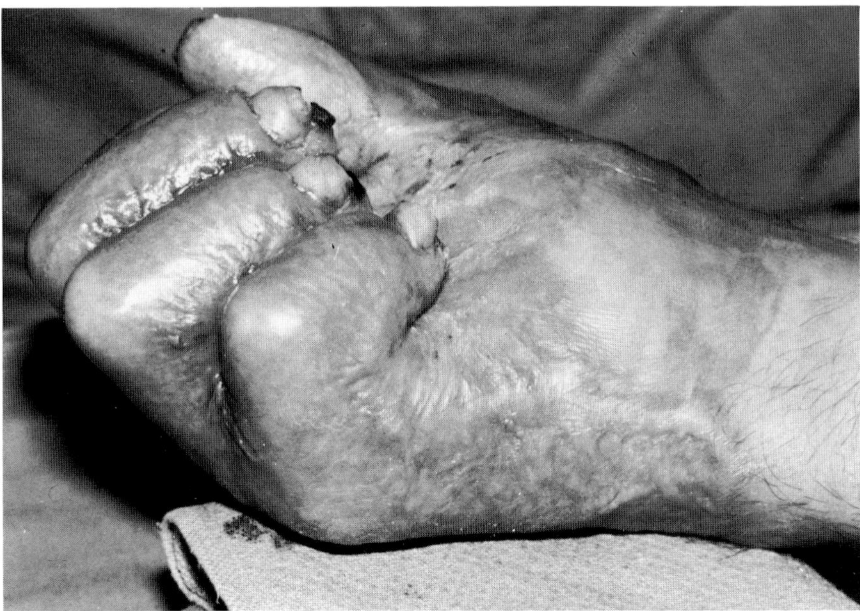

Fig. 55-17. Neglected palmar burn resulted in severe flexion contracture from shortened volar skin.

graft. Thus, *incision* and grafting are preferable in most cases.

Transverse incisions are planned to straighten the fingers. The location depends on the severity of the contracture, either at the MP or PIP level or both. In the case shown in Figure 55-18, incision was made at the MP joint. The fingers are extended enough to allow identification of the neurovascular bundles. No attempt to straighten the fingers with the tourniquet elevated is done, or vascular spasm and irreversible ischemia may result. The tourniquet is lowered and the fingers are slowly straightened. The contracted PIP volar plate may have to be incised and released to permit finger extension. If the fingers blanch before they are straightened, they should be released slightly into flexion until normal color returns and then pinned in that position with a single longitudinal K-wire (Fig. 55-18). The remaining range of motion will have to be gained through postoperative therapy (Fig. 55-19). Incisions parallel to the distal palmar and thenar creases will aid in opening the width and breadth of the palm. Skin grafts are sutured in place and maintained with a hand dressing. For fingers that have been contracted a long time, it is wise to leave the K-wires in place for 2 weeks to allow healing of all structures in a lengthened position (Fig. 55-19). Night splinting for 1 year, in the antideformity position with wrist and fingers fully extended, and the early use of pressure garments and supplemental silicone inserts, are all necessary to maintain operative gains.

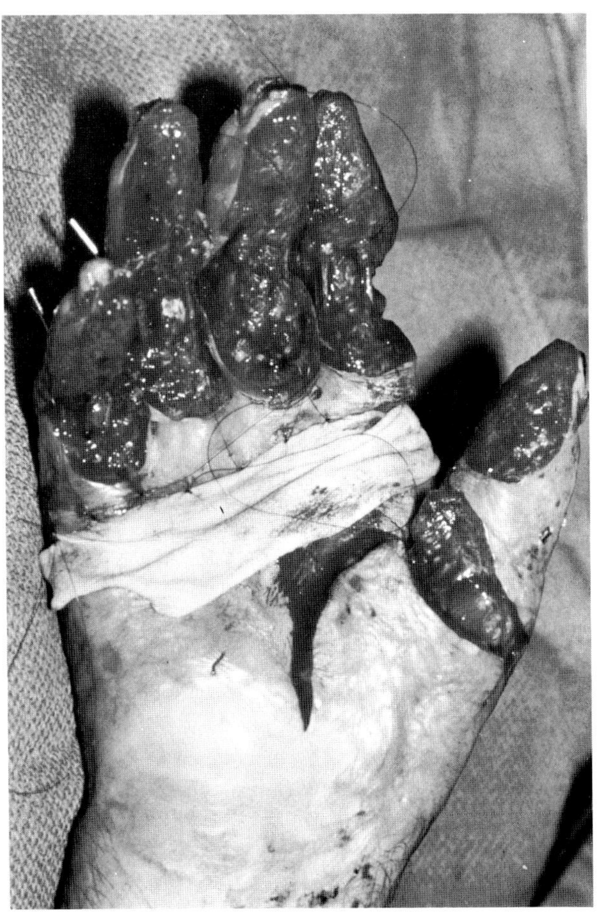

Fig. 55-18. Sheet grafting of the digits and palm after release of the flexion contractures of the fingers and palm, and release of the adduction contraction of the first web space. K-wires hold the fingers extended.

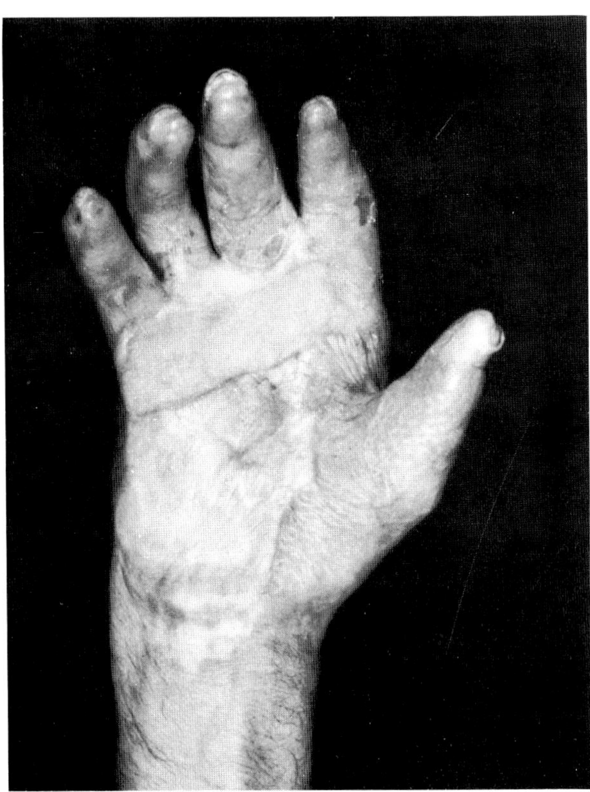

Fig. 55-19. Skin grafting results in an improved volar surface for an "assist" hand.

Reconstruction of the web spaces deals with three common problems: dorsal hooding, syndactyly, and adduction contracture of the first web space.

Dorsal Hooding

Dorsal hooding results from a scar or graft contracture across the dorsal leading edge of the web. Because the fingers at rest are in a shortened, adducted position, the burned web often heals in a contracture. It is seldom of functional significance, but usually a cosmetic problem that can be corrected by Z-plasty. If the bands, however, are thick scar, blood supply to the small flaps would be tenuous with a high incidence of necrosis. Thus, incision and grafting of the defect are done.

Syndactyly (Fig. 55-20), actual union of two fingers in scar due to the burn, necessitates resurfacing of the sides of the fingers to reestablish their integrity as well as web space reconstruction.[2,36] The technique described (Bevin)[3] utilizes a dorsal pedicle flap (Fig. 55-21) and relies on the constant normal contour anatomy of an interdigital web. The key points to mark with methylene blue or brilliant green dye are (the num-

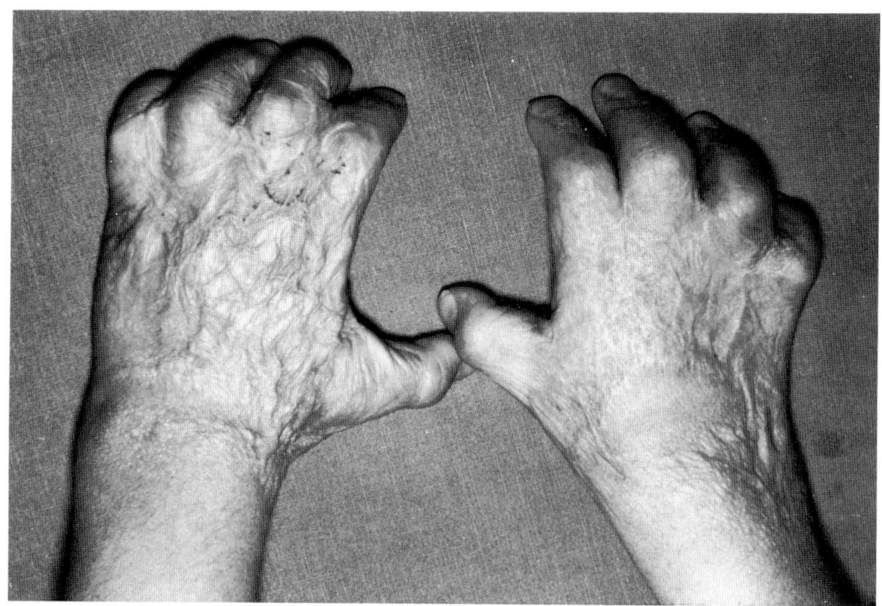

Fig. 55-20. Burn syndactyly involving multiple web spaces of both hands.

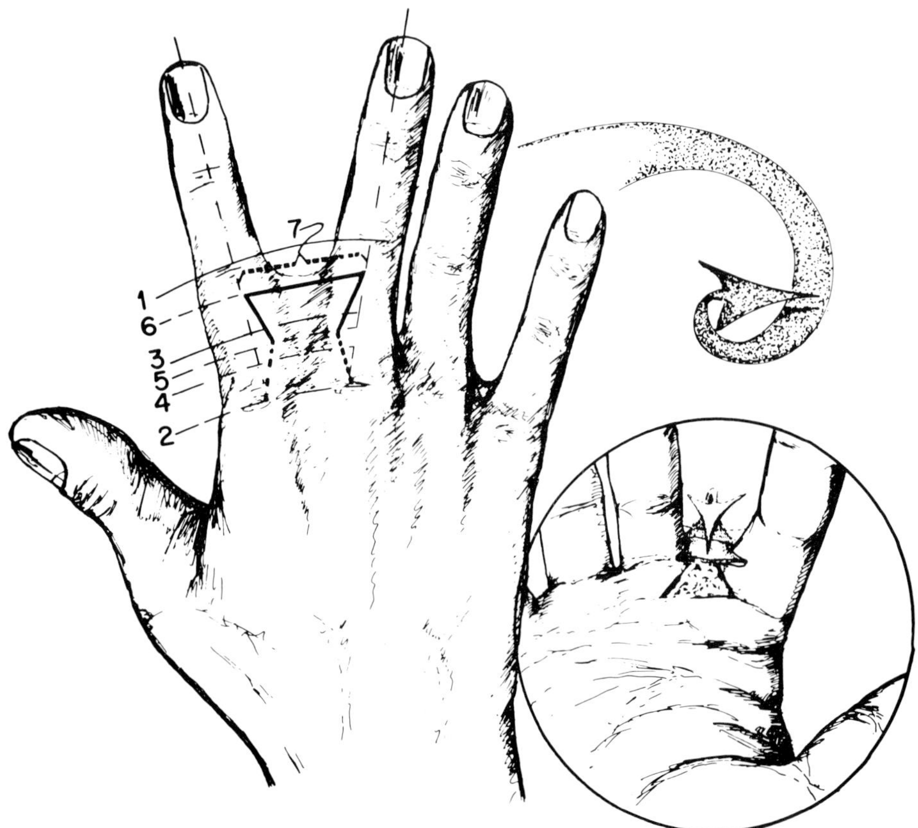

Fig. 55-21. Bevin's "hourglass" technique for treatment of burn syndactyly. The key points for flap reconstruction are represented by numbers *1* to *7*. (See text for description of landmarks.) (From Salisbury and Bevin,[63] with permission.)

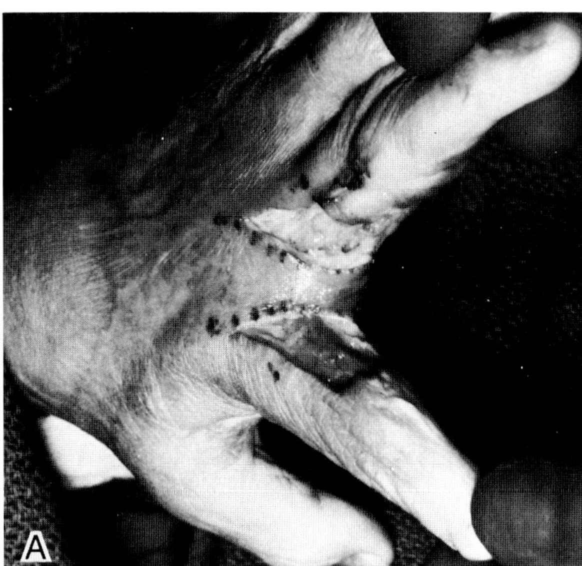

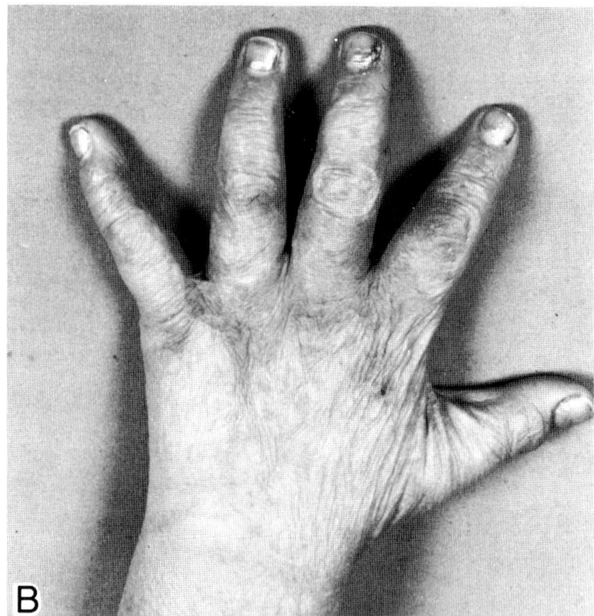

Fig. 55-22. **(A)** The flap is advanced volarly. The sides of the fingers are skin grafted. **(B)** Postoperative result shows a well-defined web space.

bers refer to the anatomic landmarks noted in Fig. 55-21):

1. The level of the PIP joint
2. The level of the MP joint
3. The distal edge of the interdigital web (one-half the distance between 1 and 2)
4. The distal lumbrical canal (one-half the distance between 2 and 3)
5. The narrow portion of the dorsal pedicle flap (one-half the distance between 3 and 4)
6. The distal point of the dorsal pedicle flap (one-half the distance between 1 and 3)
7. The width of the distal flap

An "hourglass"-shaped dorsal pedicle flap, proximally based, is drawn that will be sufficiently long to create both the dorsal surface, new web, and volar surface of the web. On the dorsal surface, the flap is dissected from distally to Point 4. The palmar skin is cut in the midline back to Point 4. The flap is then folded volarly (Fig. 55-22), and a small trapezoid of nor-

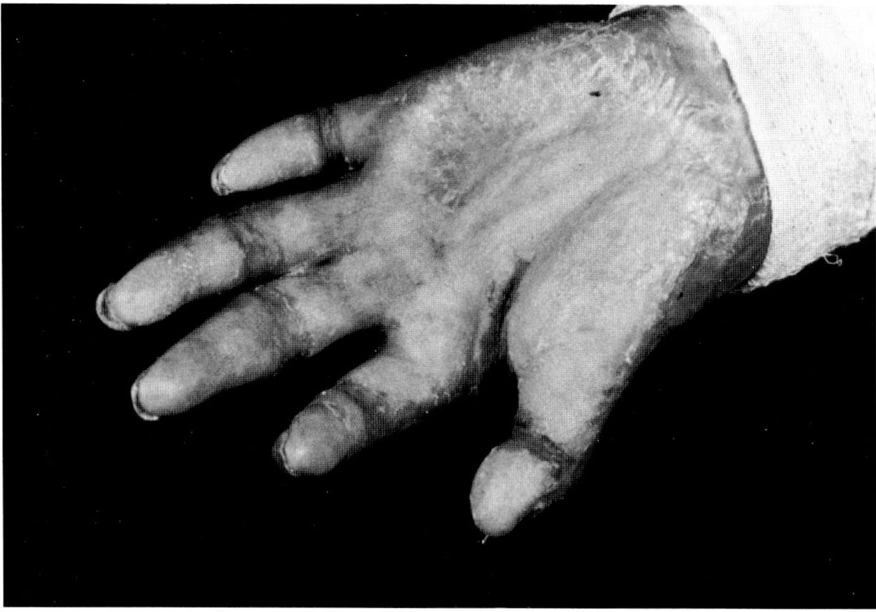

Fig. 55-23. First web space adduction contracture.

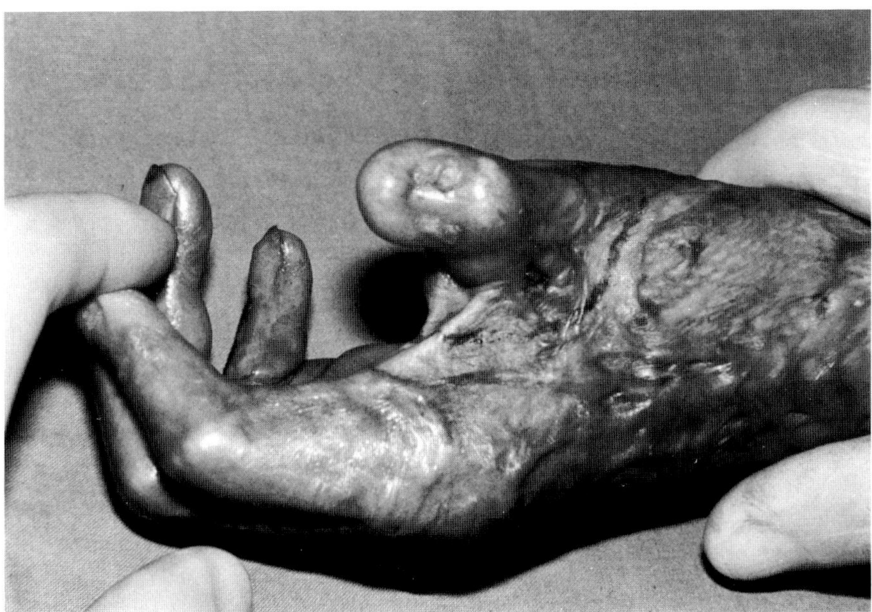

Fig. 55-24. Adduction contracture of the first web space with hyperextended MP joint of the thumb.

mal distal palmar skin or healed burn scar in that area is excised to receive the flap. The rectangular wounds on the sides of the fingers are covered with split-thickness or full-thickness skin grafts. The hand is dressed with the digits in slight abduction and the MP joints in 30 to 45 degrees flexion. Severe scarring, especially when associated with adduction contractures at the MP level, limits the use of this technique. However, supple scar tissue or skin grafts may be successfully incorporated into the "hourglass" format.

Adduction Contracture of the Thumb Web

A first web space adduction contracture (Fig. 55-23) may be due to shortening of scarred skin or, in the chronic severe case, fibrosis of the adductor muscle. Unless the scar is a discrete band (which is very unusual), Z-plasty will not yield the desired release. Although incision and release of the first web space are technically not difficult, the potential for significant complications is great.

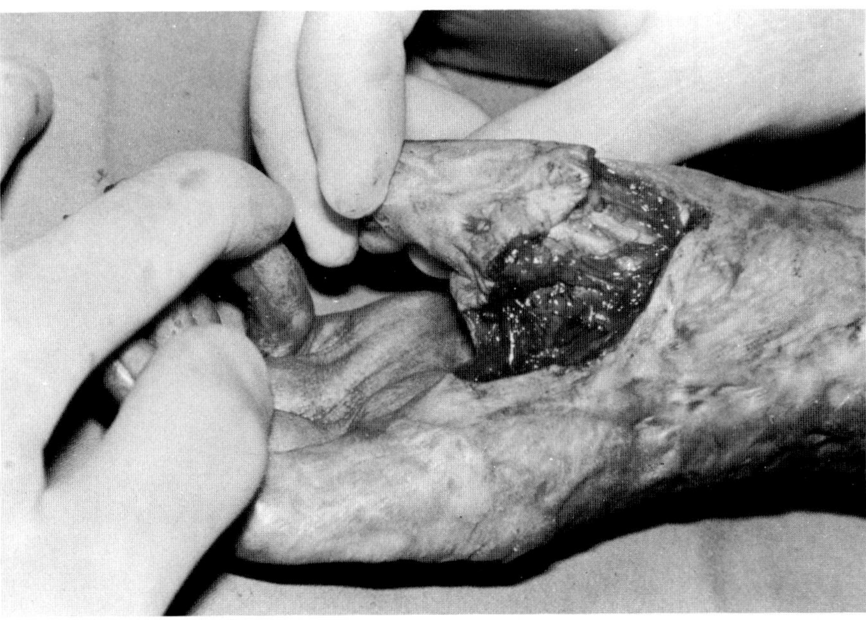

Fig. 55-25. Release of adduction contracture of the thumb with incision of the first web space. Note that the incision begins over the dorsum of the contracted MP joint.

With the thumb in a fixed adducted position, the MP joint is often hyperextended (Fig. 55-24) by dorsal scar. Thus, the releasing incision should extend from dorsally (Fig. 55-25) over the MP joint through the web and volarly along the thenar crease. The potential exists for cutting the sensory branch of the radial nerve, neurovascular bundles to the ulnar side of the thumb (Fig. 55-26) and radial side of the index finger, and even the motor branch of the median nerve. Thus, once the incision is made through the skin, the tissue is spread with blunt-tipped scissors in a longitudinal dissection to avoid cutting the nerves. Full expansion of the first web space may be limited by the scarred adductor muscle, and its insertion is incised subperiosteally. It is stripped only far enough to bring the thumb into opposition. If the MP joint of the thumb is in hyperextension, the dorsal capsule is incised to allow full joint flexion. Before grafting, the first and second metacarpals are abducted and pinned apart. The MP joint is then pinned in maximum flexion. The graft is inserted into the convolutions and confines of the wound and stented in place (Fig. 55-27).

Contractures of the Elbow and Axilla

Volar contractures of the wrist, elbow, and axilla require surgery if they are functionally disabling and splinting has been unproductive. Treatment rarely involves excision and grafting because the extremity can be covered easily with a shirt, and donor skin is usually at a premium. Incision and grafting or flap reconstruction is the most common form of treatment. Several large joints may be released at the same operation, saving extra hospitalization time and surgery, the only limiting factor being enough donor skin.

For example, in the elbow contracture shown in Figure 55-28, note the narrow restrictive band and the normal medial skin and soft tissue. The band is incised and the contracture released. A broad-based flap is raised at the fascial level. The tip of the flap is round to help avoid ischemic necrosis. Occasionally, the superficial veins, fascia, or even part of the biceps must be cut to achieve full extension. The flap is inset with half-buried mattress sutures tied over cotton bolsters and a running subcuticular suture. Early postoperative splinting is in mild flexion to avoid any tension on the flap. The splint is removed in 2 weeks and motion begun (Fig. 55-29). Even though extension is complete, splinting with the elbow in extension should be maintained at least at night for 1 year.

Often the extent of contracture (and tissue defect) is deceptively larger than it appears. In the axilla shown in Figure 55-30, the appearance of bands suggests that flap release is possible, but the surrounding tissue was heavily scarred and previously mesh grafted, and nutritional support of a flap was highly doubtful. Incision and release (Fig. 55-31) revealed a large defect requiring several drums of skin for closure.

The use of free flaps is rarely appropriate for correction of these contractures for several reasons. First, the procedures just described yield functional and cosmetic results that are as good. Secondly, virgin donor tissue is usually at a premium. Potential free flaps should be saved for more worthy problems involving the face or hand. Lastly, the burned patient is usually very sensitive about further disfigurement and may view free flap donor sites as another significant loss.

Tendon Injury

Tendon involvement most commonly consists of adhesions secondary to prolonged disuse or deep tissue injury and scarring. On the flexor surface, a conventional tenolysis may be

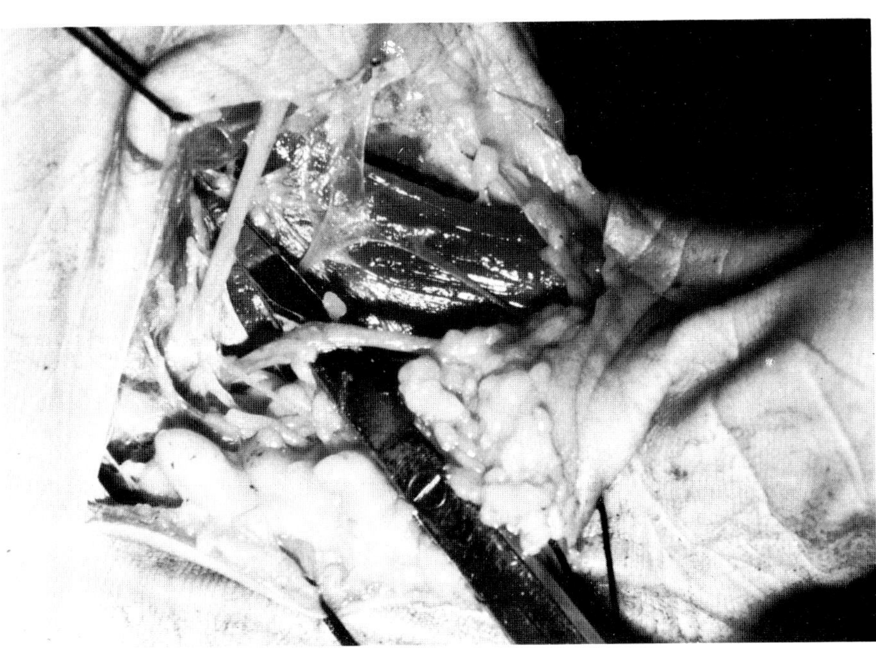

Fig. 55-26. Release of the first web space contracture can easily cause inadvertent injury to digital nerves of the thumb and index finger.

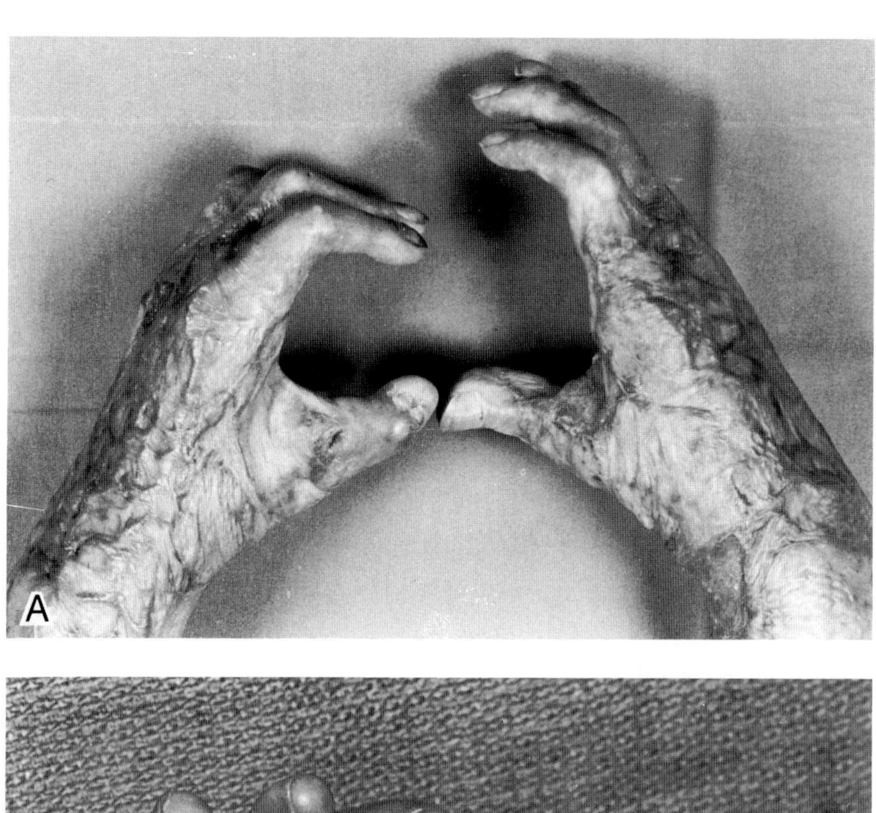

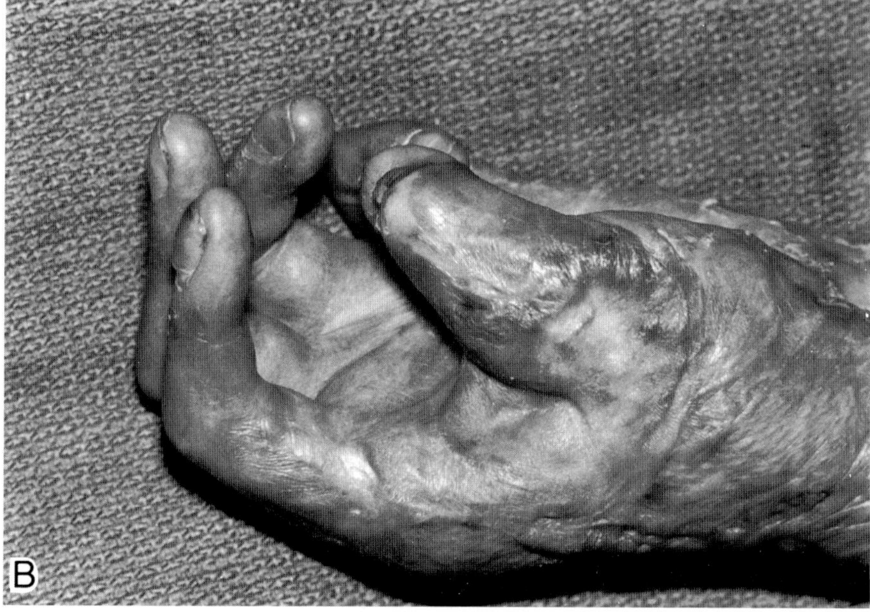

Fig. 55-27. **(A)** Improved abduction of the thumb following release of first web space. **(B)** Improved opposition of the thumb after release of contracted first web space and MP joint, and sheet grafting of the defect.

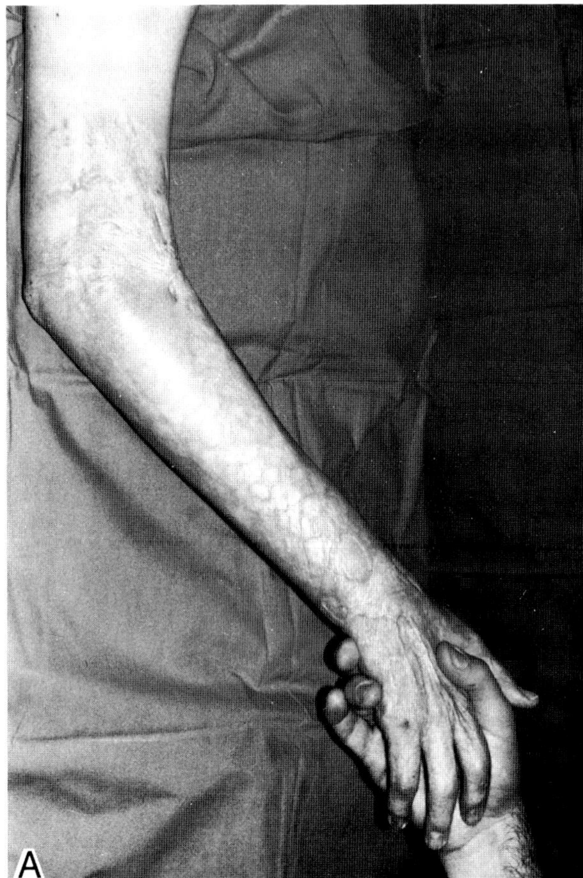

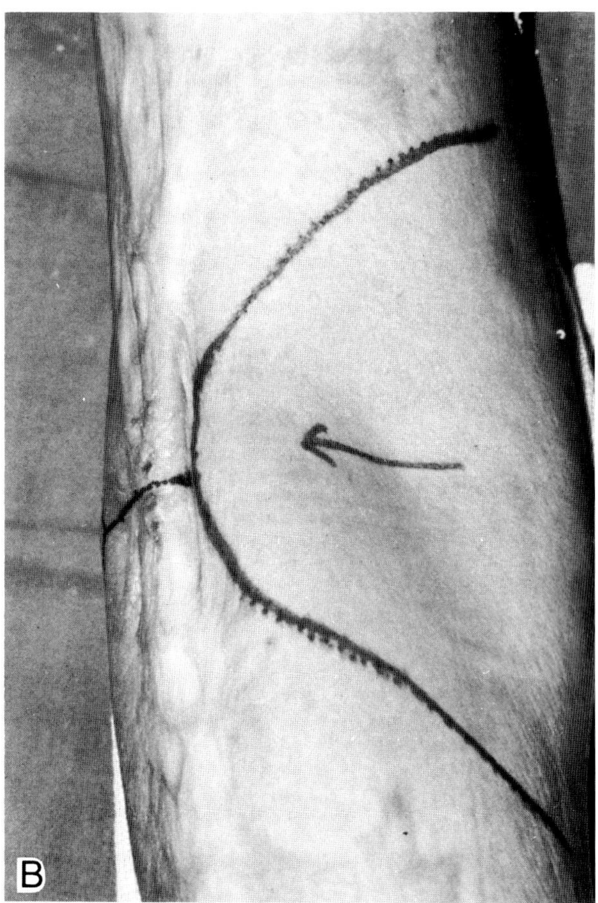

Fig. 55-28. **(A)** Elbow extension limited by contracted scar band. **(B)** Design of advancement flap from adjacent unburned skin from the medial antecubital fossa to fill defect created by incising the contracted scar band.

done. On the dorsum, the scar bed may be so extensive that tenolysis is not feasible. If shortening is severe in a long neglected case with soft tissue replacement by scar, the tendons must be cut and excised and a flap applied before tendon grafts are done.

Burn Boutonnière Deformity

Tendon reconstruction of the boutonnière deformity is appropriate only in a few cases. Some early cases may be splinted successfully and surgery thus avoided. Often, the dorsal skin is too fragile and ulcerates due to dorsal pressure with attempts at splinting. This patient, if neglected, develops a severe fixed PIP flexion deformity that can only be corrected by arthrodesis. If seen early, this type of patient may be amenable to tendon reconstruction.

Elliot's technique[18] of reconstruction is anatomical and the results have been satisfying. The scar bridge-central tendon is dissected to normal central slip (Fig. 55-32), and the attenuated scar is excised. The shortened transverse retinacular ligaments are incised (Fig. 55-33), allowing the extensor tendon to slide dorsally to its normal position. The central slip is reinserted to the middle phalanx with a 3–0 monofilament suture. With two 5–0 monofilament sutures (Fig. 55-34), the lateral bands are approximated distally to "recreate" the triangular ligament. At this point it is imperative to test if passive flexion is possible. If not, these sutures should be removed. If the lateral bands are sutured too far dorsally or too many sutures are inserted proximally, a tenodesis will be created that prevents flexion. The PIP joint is pinned in 10 degrees flexion. The pin is left in place for 6 weeks and active exercise begun at that time (Fig. 55-35).

Nerve Injury

Nerve destruction is rarely seen with thermal injury, unless the extremity has been cooked or a compressive phenomenon secondary to heterotopic ossification has occurred. Electrical injuries commonly result in nerve defects, and reconstruction depends on the extent of injury. Because of its low resistance to current, damage may be extensive. If there is a persistent deficit, after allowing adequate time for clinical return, exploration may reveal intact nerve but longitudinal fibrosis and some fiber destruction. Neurolysis is indicated. Sometimes the pathology is only fully appreciated at exploration, and the surgeon must be ready to perform neurolysis or nerve graft. That

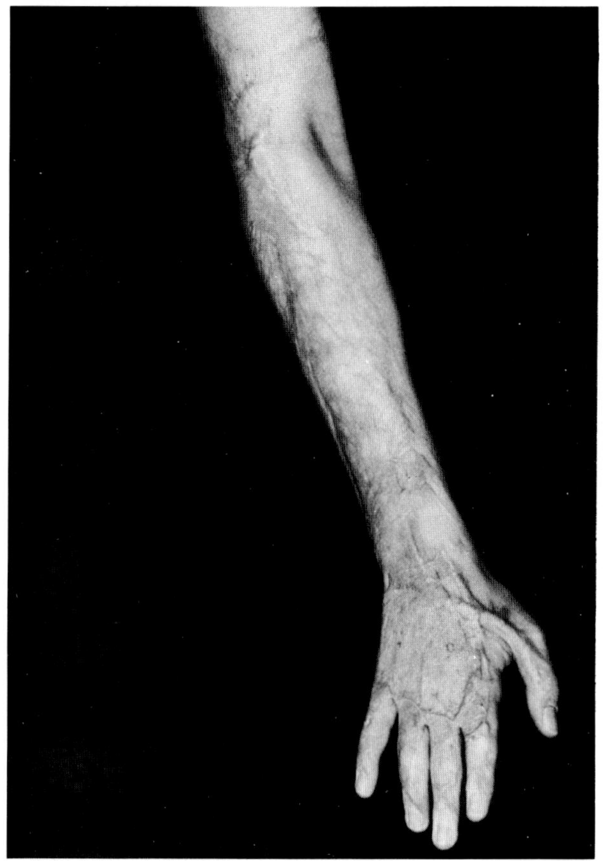

Fig. 55-29. Full extension of the elbow after release of contracture and advancement of the medial flap.

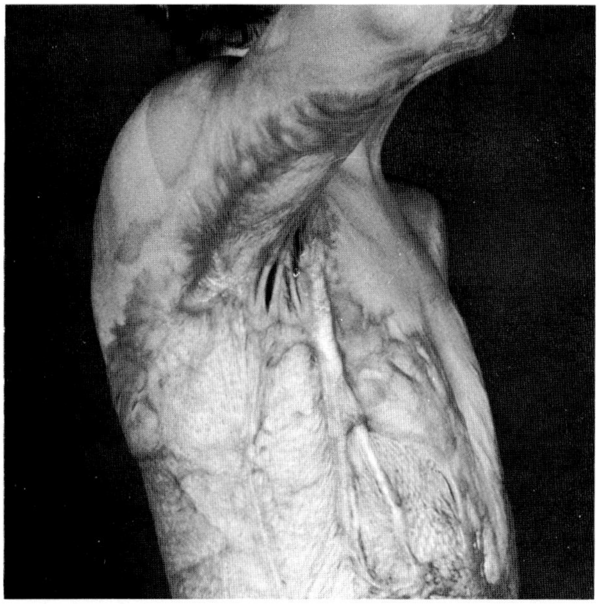

Fig. 55-30. Axillary contracture not amenable to flap reconstruction because of scarred adjacent tissue.

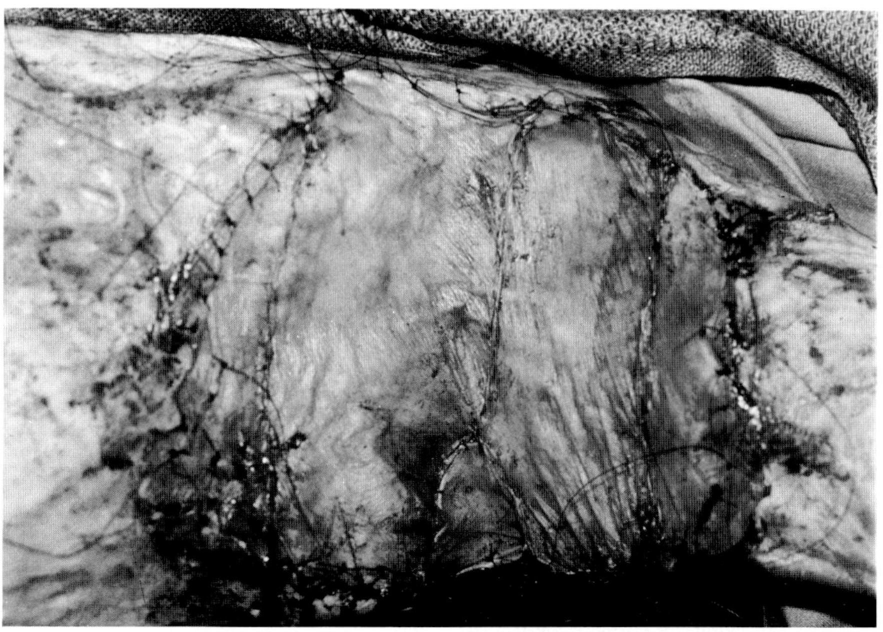

Fig. 55-31. Sheet grafting of axillary contracture after incision of scar. No tissue was excised. Note the large dimensions of the graft needed.

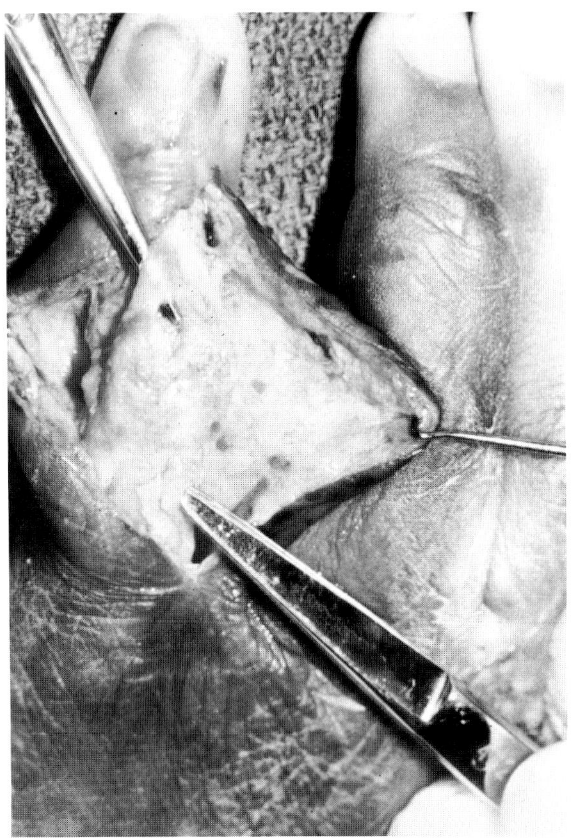

Fig. 55-32. Burn boutonnière deformity. The dissected central slip is identified by forceps. Scissors are inserted under one lateral band.

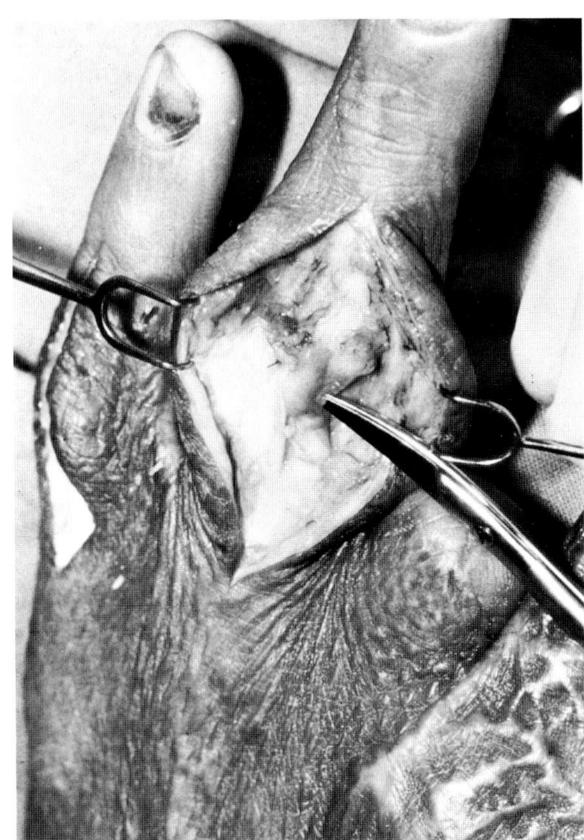

Fig. 55-33. Scissors demonstrate that the transverse retinacular ligament has been cut and the tendon has been mobilized dorsally.

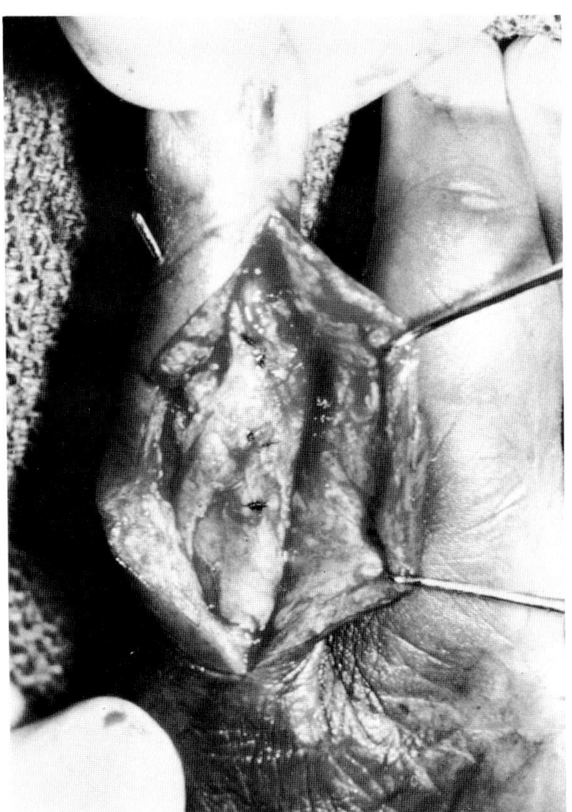

Fig. 55-34. The lateral bands are apposed dorsally distal to the PIP joint to recreate the triangular ligament, and the PIP joint is pinned in full extension.

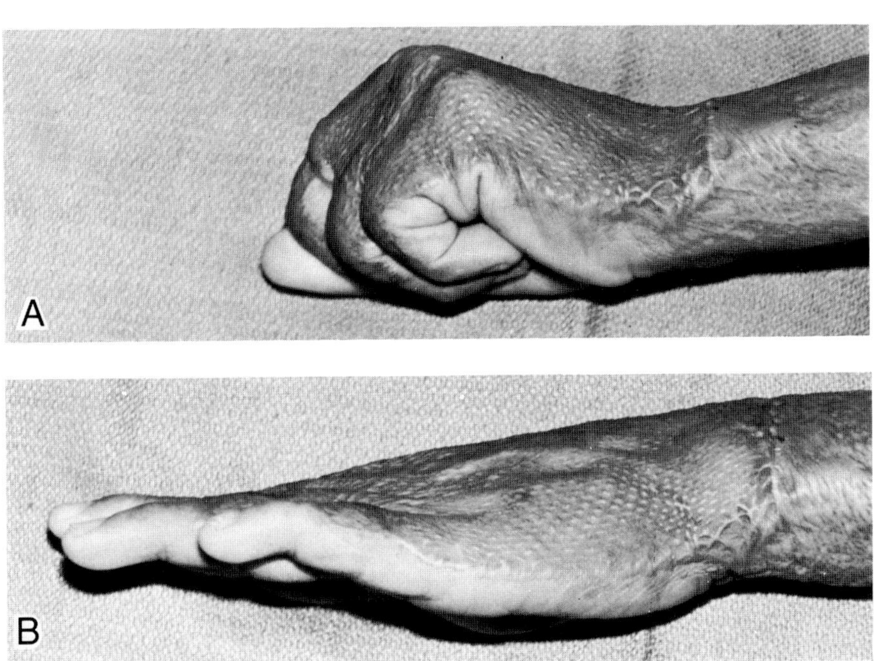

Fig. 55-35. Postoperative result following repair of boutonnière deformity showing full flexion **(A)** and extension **(B)** of the operated digit.

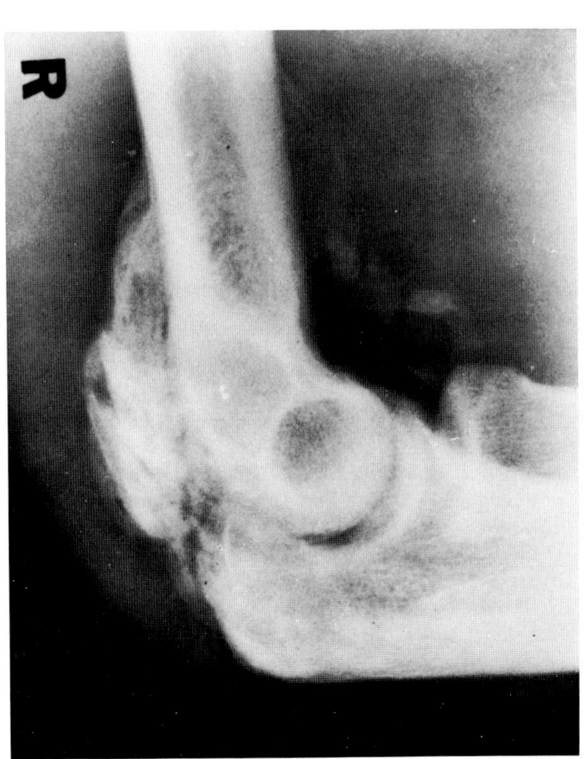

Fig. 55-36. Radiographic appearance of heterotopic calcification of the elbow following a burn of the arm.

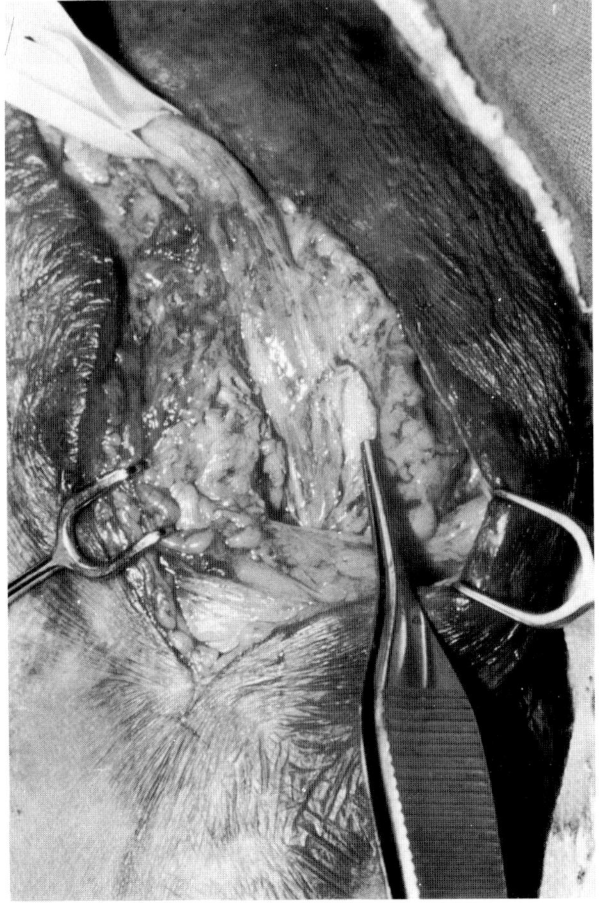

Fig. 55-37. Encasement of the ulnar nerve (Penrose drain) in bone at the elbow. Note the shelf of calcified tissue reflected by the forceps.

long segments are destroyed is the rule. Therefore resection and end-to-end suture are rarely feasible.

Heterotopic ossification[6,28] and nerve entrapment most often occur at the elbow and involve the ulnar nerve with symptoms of weakness or diminished sensation along the nerve distribution. Diagnosis may be confirmed by radiograph, showing abnormal bone formation (Fig. 55-36), and electrical conduction studies.

Exploration is through an incision posterior to the medial epicondyle and should begin proximal to the area of involvement. A tape is placed around normal nerve and dissection carried distally (Fig. 55-37). Once nerve disappears into calcified bone, dissection is begun distal to the involved area and normal nerve once again identified and taped. Bone is carefully rongeured from over the nerve to avoid injury. Once dissection is complete, the nerve is transposed into normal soft tissue anterior to the medial epicondyle and maintained in this position by several sutures in the overlying soft tissue. The extremity is splinted for 2 weeks in mild elbow flexion. Unlimited activity after neurolysis can precipitate a neuritis.

The possible permutations and combinations of burn injury requiring reconstruction would fill a textbook. Many of the techniques have been merely glanced at in this chapter as they are described in detail elsewhere in the text (arthrodesis, neurolysis, flaps, etc.). For instance, microvascular surgery and free flaps for reconstruction, as described in length elsewhere, are applicable in many instances, depending on the deformity. Reconstruction of the partially amputated thumb has been improved by May's[43] technique of advancement pollicization of the second ray remnant. This technique and others[33,40,47,70] described in the chapters on microvascular surgery have produced marked increase in function for many patients who previously were not surgical candidates.

The critical key to rehabilitation of this type of patient is the physician's appreciation that many surgical procedures may be required over a number of years with full recovery still not always possible. Therefore, each patient's career and personal goals must be analyzed carefully with other members of the burn team to reduce the patient's disability time.

REFERENCES

1. Achauer BM, Bartlett RH, Furnas DW, Allyn PA, Wingerson E'L: Internal fixation in the management of the burned hand. Arch Surg 108:814–820, 1974
2. Alexander JW, MacMillan BG, Martel L: Correction of Postburn Syndactyly: An analysis of children with introduction of the VM-Plasty and postoperative pressure inserts. Plast Reconstr Surg 70:345–352, 1982
3. Bevin AG: A different approach to the repair of syndactylism of the fingers—the "hourglass" operation. J Bone Joint Surg 55A:880, 1973
4. Bondoc CC, Quinby WC, Burke JF: Primary surgical management of the deeply burned hand in children. J Pediatr Surg 11:355–362, 1976
5. Boswick JA Jr: The management of fresh burns of the hand and deformities resulting from burn injuries. Clin Plast Surg 1:621–631, 1974
6. Boyd BM, Roberts WM, Miller GR: Periarticular ossification following burns. South Med J 52:1048–1051, 1959
7. Braithwaite F, Watson J: Some observations on the treatment of the dorsal burn of the hand. Br J Plast Surg 2:21–31, 1949
8. Burke JF, Bondoc CC, Quinby WC: Primary burn excision and immediate grafting: A method shortening illness. J Trauma 14:389–395, 1974
9. Burke JF, Bondoc CC, Quinby WC, Remensynder JP: Primary surgical management of the deeply burned hand. J Trauma 16:593–598, 1976
10. Cannon B, Murray JE: Reflections on skin grafting in hand repairs. JAMA 200:663–668, 1967
11. Cannon B, Zuidema GD: The care and treatment of the burned hand. Clin Orthop 15:111–117, 1959
12. Consumer Product-Related Injuries Treated in Hospital Emergency Rooms, Jan 1–Dec 31, 1976. US Consumer Product Safety Commission, Washington, DC, April 1978
13. Cope O, Langohr JL, Moore FD, Webster RC: Expeditious care of full thickness burn wounds by surgical excision and grafting. Ann Surg 125:1–22, 1947
14. Covey MH, Dutcher K, Heimbach DM, Marvin JA, Engrav CH: Return of hand function following major burns. J Burn Care Rehabil 8:224–226, 1987
15. Curtis RM: Capsulectomy of the interphalangeal joints of the fingers. J Bone Joint Surg 36A:1219–1232, 1954
16. Earle AS, Fratianne RB: Delayed definitive reconstruction of the burned hand: Evolution of a program of care. J Trauma 19:149–152, 1979
17. Edstrom L, Robson MC, Macchiaverna JR, Scala AD: Management of deep partial thickness dorsal hand burns. Orthop Rev 8:27–33, 1979
18. Elliott RA Jr: Boutonnière deformity. pp. 42–54. In Cramer LM, Chase RA (eds): Symposium on the Hand. CV Mosby, St Louis, 1971
19. Evans EB: Orthopaedic measures in the treatment of severe burns. J Bone Joint Surg 48A:643–669, 1966
20. Gant TD: The early enzymatic debridement and grafting of deep dermal burns of the hand. Plast Reconstr Surg 66:185–190, 1980
21. Goodwin CW, Maguire MS, McManus WF, Pruitt BA: Prospective study of burn wound excision of the hands. J Trauma 23:510–517, 1983
22. Grant GH: The "intact" hand after crush and burn (editorial). JAMA 227:1305, 1974
23. Habal MB: The burned hand: A planned treatment program. J Trauma 18:587–595, 1978
24. Hartrampf CR: Management of the burned hand. South Med J 57:1342–1345, 1964
25. Heggers JP, Robson MC: Evaluation of burn blister fluid. Presented at the Proceedings of the 48th Annual Convention of the American Society of Plastic and Reconstructive Surgeons, its Educational Foundation, and the American Society of Maxillofacial Surgeons, Toronto, Ontario, Oct 1979
26. Helm PA, Head MD, Pullium G, O'Brien M, Cromes GF Jr: Burn rehabilitation—A team approach. Surg Clinics NA 58:1263–1278, 1978
27. Helm PA, Walker SC, Peyton SA: Return to work following hand burns. Arch Phys Med Rehabil 67:297–298, 1986
28. Hoffer MM, Brody G, Ferlic F: Excision of heterotopic ossification about elbows in patients with thermal injury. J Trauma 18:667–670, 1978
29. Huang TT, Larson DL, Lewis SR: Burned hands. Plast Reconstr Surg 56:21–28, 1975
30. Hunt JL, Sato RM: Early excision of full thickness hand and digit burns: Factors affecting morbidity. J Trauma 22:414–419, 1982

31. Jackson DM, Stone PA: Tangential excision and grafting of burns: The method, and report of 50 consecutive cases. Br J Plast Surg 25:416–426, 1972
32. Jelenko C: Chemicals that "burn." J Trauma 14:65–72, 1974
33. Kartchinov K: Reconstruction and sensitization of the amputated thumb. J Hand Surg 9A:478–484, 1984
34. Kiehn CL, DesPrez JD: The burnt hand. Am J Surg 97:421–427, 1959
35. Krizek TJ, Flagg SV, Wolfort FG, Jabaley ME: Delayed primary excision and skin grafting of the burned hand. Plast Reconstr Surg 51:524–529, 1973
36. Krizek TJ, Robson MC, Flagg SV: Management of burn syndactyly. J Trauma 14:587–593, 1974
37. Labandter H, Kaplan I, Shavitt C: Burns of the dorsum of the hand: Conservative treatment with intensive physiotherapy vs. tangential excision and grafting. Br J Plast Surg 29:352–354, 1976
38. Larkin JM, Moylan JA: Tetanus following a minor burn. J Trauma 15:546–548, 1975
39. Leonard LG, Munster AM, Su CT: Adjunctive use of intravenous fluorescein in the tangential excision of burns of the hands. Presented at the Proceedings of the 48th Annual Convention of the American Society of Plastic and Reconstructive Surgeons, its Educational Foundation, and the American Society of Maxillofacial Surgeons, Toronto, Ontario, Oct 1979
40. Leung PC: Thumb reconstruction using second-toe transfer. Hand 15:15–21, 1983
41. Mahler D, Hirshowitz B: Tangential excision and grafting for burns of the hand. Br J Plast Surg 28:189–192, 1975
42. Marshall JH, Bromberg BE, Adrizzo JR, Heurich AE, Samet CM: Fatal tetanus complicating a small partial-thickness burn. J Trauma 12:91–93, 1972
43. May JW, Donelan MB, Toth BA, Wall J: Thumb reconstruction in the burned hand by advancement pollicization of the second ray remnant. J Hand Surg 9A:484–489, 1984
44. Moncrief JA: Third degree burns of the dorsum of the hand. Am J Surg 96:535–544, 1958
45. Moncrief JA, Switzer WE, Rose L: Primary excision and grafting in the treatment of third-degree burns of the dorsum of the hand. Plast Reconstr Surg 33:305–316, 1964
46. Munster AM, Bruck HM, Johns LA, Von Prince K, Kirkman EM, Remig RL: Heterotopic calcification following burns: A prospective study. J Trauma 12:1071–1074, 1972
47. Ohmori S: Correction of burn deformities using free flap transfer. J Trauma 22:103–111, 1982
48. Peacock EE Jr: Management of the burned hand. South Med J 56:1094–1099, 1963
49. Peacock EE Jr, Madden JW, Trier WC: Some studies on the treatment of burned hands. Ann Surg 171:903–914, 1970
50. Pegg SP, Cavaye D, Fowler D, Jones M: Results of early excision and grafting in hand burns. Burns 11:99–103, 1984
51. Peterson HD: Tangential excision. pp. 235–249. In Artz CP, Moncrief JA, Pruitt BA Jr (eds): Burns: A Team Approach. WB Saunders, Philadelphia, 1979
52. Peterson HD, Elton R: Reconstruction of the thermally injured upper extremity. In Salisbury RE, Pruitt BA Jr (eds): Management of Burns of the Upper Extremity. WB Saunders, Philadelphia, 1976
53. Peterson RA: Electrical burns of the hand; treatment by early excision. J Bone Joint Surg 48A:407–424, 1966
54. Poticha SM, Bell JL, Mehn WH: Electrical injuries with special reference to the hand. Arch Surg 85:852–861, 1962
55. Pruitt BA: Epidemiology and general considerations. p. 3. In Salisbury RE, Pruitt BA Jr (eds): Management of Burns of the Upper Extremity. WB Saunders, Philadelphia, 1976
56. Pruitt BA Jr, Dowling JA, Moncrief JA: Escharotomy in early burn care. Arch Surg 96:502–507, 1968
57. Pruitt BA Jr: Complications of thermal injury. Clin Plast Surg 1:667–691, 1974
58. Pruitt BA Jr: The burn patient: I. Initial care. Curr Probl Surg 16(4): April 1979
59. Pruitt BA Jr: The burn patient: II. Later care and complications of thermal injury. Curr Probl Surg 16(5): May 1979
60. Robertson DC: The management of the burned hand. J Bone Joint Surg 40A:625–632, 1958
61. Ross WPD: The treatment of recent burns of the hand. Br J Plast Surg 2:233–253, 1950
62. Salisbury RE: Burns of the upper extremity. pp. 320–329. In Artz CP, Moncrief JA, Pruitt BA (eds): Burns: A Team Approach. WB Saunders, Philadelphia, 1979
63. Salisbury RE, Bevin AG: Atlas of Reconstructive Burn Surgery. WB Saunders, Philadelphia, 1981
64. Salisbury RE, Bevin AG: Burn induced peripheral nerve injury. In Omer GE, Spinner M (eds): Management of Peripheral Nerve Problems. WB Saunders, Philadelphia, 1980
65. Salisbury RE, Hunt JL, Warden GD, Pruitt BA: Management of electrical injuries of the upper extremity. Plast Reconstr Surg 51:648–652, 1973
66. Salisbury RE, Levine NS: The early management of upper extremity thermal injury. pp. 36–46. In Salisbury RE, Pruitt BA Jr (eds): Management of Burns of the Upper Extremity. WB Saunders, Philadelphia, 1976
67. Salisbury RE, Loveless S, Silverstein P, Wilmore DW, Moylan JA, Pruitt BA: Postburn edema of the upper extremity; evaluation of present treatment. J Trauma 13:857–869, 1973
68. Salisbury RE, Palm L: Dynamic splinting for dorsal burns of the hand. Plast Reconstr Surg 51:226–228, 1973
69. Salzberg CA, Salisbury RE: Thermal injury of peripheral nerve. pp. 671–678. In Gelberman RH (ed): Operative Nerve Repair and Reconstruction. JB Lippincott, Philadelphia, 1991
70. Seljavaara S, Pitkanen J, Sundell B: Microvascular free flaps in early reconstruction of burns of the hand and forearm. Case reports. Scand J Plast Reconstr Surg 18:139–144, 1984
71. Sturim HS: The treatment of electrical burns. Surg Gynecol Obstet 128:129–133, 1969
72. Wang XW, Sun YH, Zhang GZ, Zhang ZM, Davies JW: Tangential excision of eschar for deep burns of the hand: Analysis of 156 patients collected over 10 years. Burns 11:92–98, 1984
73. Warden GD, Zeluff GR, Saffle JR: Intramuscular pressure in the burned arm: measurement and response to escharotomy. Amer J Surg 140:825–831, 1980
74. Wexler MR, Yeschua R, Neuman Z: Early treatment of burns of the dorsum of the hand by tangential excision and skin grafting. Plast Reconstr Surg 54:268–273, 1974
75. Whitson TC, Allen BD: Management of the burned hand. J Trauma 11:606–614, 1971
76. Wright PC, Salisbury RE: Early excision and grafting versus nonoperative treatment in deep 2° and 3° burns of the hand. Presented at the Rehabilitation of the Burned Patient: A Symposium sponsored by the American Burn Association and the University of North Carolina Jaycee Burn Center, Chapel Hill, Sept 1979

56

Frostbite of the Hand

James H. House
Michael O. Fidler

Frostbite is one of the two major groups of cold injuries. Trench foot, immersion foot, and chilblains are cold injuries resulting from prolonged exposure at temperatures above freezing, often associated with some degree of wetness and frequently resulting in irreversible neurovascular changes.[39] *Frostbite* may be defined as damage to tissue as a result of exposure to low environmental temperatures,[8] and most experts agree that the injury involves the actual formation of ice crystals within living tissues.[15,38,45,57]

Historically, interest in frostbite has coincided with major military campaigns in which cold exposure has played a significant role—including the American Revolution, the retreat from Moscow of Napoleon's Grand Army, the European theater of World War II, and the Korean Conflict. American soldiers suffered over 55,000 cases of cold injury in World War II,[59] and 8,000 cases were reported in the Korean operation.[17] The problem in civilian medical practice is small by comparison,[24,26] but frostbite represents a recurring injury that merits careful analysis and an adequate knowledge of the proper modes of management.

Considerable work has been done with experimentally induced frostbite in an effort to elucidate the precise mechanism of injury.[2,29,58] Two distinct events seem to take place within living tissues upon contact with extreme cold. The first is a *direct injury to the cells* through the formation of ice crystals in the extracellular fluid, with the establishment of an osmotic gradient producing pronounced dehydration, electrolyte imbalance, and metabolic disruption.[36] The second event is one of *vascular impairment.* This results both from *direct endothelial injury,* causing thrombus formation, hemoconcentration, and increased viscosity, and from *increased sympathetic tone,* producing intense vasoconstriction, shunting, and stasis.[45,57,58] Marzalla and co-workers[32] have shown that the endothelial cell is the target of injury by freezing. It is likely that this acute injury ultimately compromises blood flow and leads to skin necrosis.

It has been customary in the past to try to describe the injury as first, second, third, or fourth degree frostbite.[60] However, this system is subjective at best and may have little clinical usefulness with regard to treatment, as it is difficult, if not impossible, to determine the depth of the initial injury clinically. Mills, Whaley, and Fish[38] have proposed a simpler classification wherein *superficial frostbite* signifies injury only to skin, while *deep frostbite* implies damage to deeper structures within the extremity. This classification has prognostic significance and recognizes the difficulty of judging the true extent of injury on initial examination.

Multiple factors that may influence the severity of injury and the eventual prognosis have been identified. Paramount among these is the degree of cold penetrating the tissues and the duration of exposure.[29] Also of major importance are factors that promote heat loss, such as immobility, hyperventilation, loss of or inadequate protective clothing, contact with moisture or bare metal, and high wind velocity.[29,57] The exposure of bare skin to high wind velocities has been given particular attention due to its contribution to significantly increased heat dissipation and therefore to frostbite. According to the windchill factor calculations, flesh exposed to 0°F in a 10-mile-an-hour wind would freeze in 1 hour. However, under identical conditions but with a wind velocity of 40 miles per hour (not uncommon in many parts of this country), frostbite would occur in only *10 minutes.*[55] Thawing and subsequent refreezing of an extremity will produce uniformly disastrous results,[37] a phenomenon that may be related to evidence that thawing causes tissue injury even greater than that from the original freezing.[36]

Variations in peripheral circulation, due to preexisting occlusive arterial disease,[29] smoking,[12,51] or previous frostbite,[19] may enhance the development of cold injury. There is evidence that suggests that differences in thermoregulatory responses may predispose blacks to a higher incidence of cold injury than whites or native Alaskans.[34] Conversely, according to Rasmusen, Shikata, and others, natives of colder climates may develop an increased resistance to the effects of extreme cold.[45,50] Mills, Whaley, and Fish's Alaskan series failed to corroborate this conclusion.[38] Finally, such factors as diet, physical conditioning, coexisting injuries, and alcohol intoxication may influence the development of frostbite.[57] The typical frostbite victim has been profiled as an alcohol-abusing male, dressed inappropriately for the conditions, and often suffering related psychiatric illness. Lower extremity involvement, infection, and delay in seeking medical attention are associated with increased risk of poor outcome and amputation.[61]

MANAGEMENT OF ACUTE FROSTBITE

Most cases of cold injury occur in situations of prolonged exposure, inadequate nutrition, fatigue, and some degree of panic. Associated serious injury may have precipitated the exposure resulting in frostbite. It becomes obvious, therefore, that the initial management of an acute frostbite injury should include attention to the condition of the entire patient as well as the frozen extremity. Important steps in early treatment are (1) restoration of normal core body temperature by the application of external warming devices or blankets and by oral administration of warm fluids, and (2) management of shock, fractures, and malnutrition. Protection of the frostbitten hand through careful handling and bulky dressings will help prevent further tissue damage through abrasion of the anesthetic tissues. Specific treatment of deep frostbite should only be undertaken when the patient can be provided with adequate and ongoing care to the frostbitten part. Otherwise, the patient will become further disabled with the onset of severe pain, and the likelihood of increased tissue loss will be greatly magnified should the hand become refrozen.[37,39] Reports of patients who were able to travel on frozen feet for 3 to 4 days with relatively minor eventual tissue loss attest to the durability of the frozen extremity,[57] but once thawed, the epithelium and blisters can be easily abraded and thereby become secondarily infected.

General agreement among the experts now supports the concept of *rapid rewarming* of the frozen extremity at 40°C to 44°C as the single most important step in salvage of tissue and limb function.[24,37,53,57] The details of this important technique are discussed below. It seems almost incredible that only a few years ago physicians were teaching first-aid groups to rub the frostbitten area with snow. Manipulating the injured part, plunging it into cold water baths, or allowing it to thaw at room temperature were also suggested, in the belief that rewarming should be done slowly.[24] A wealth of experimental and clinical evidence now exists to thoroughly condemn this concept.[28,30,53]

On the other hand, considerable controversy has persisted regarding the value of other techniques in the treatment of acute frostbite. Recommendations for the local care of the extremity have ranged from compressive bandaging and plaster casts[10] to completely open exposure.[37] As long as meticulous care is taken to avoid secondary infection, the results of each method appear to be similar.[24,29] Early excision of large blisters and mobilization in flamazine bags were found to be beneficial by Page and Robertson,[42] but they agreed that surgical debridement of necrotic tissue should typically be delayed, often for several weeks, in order to preserve digital length. Rutin (a vitamin) and certain antihistamine drugs have been used in an effort to reduce capillary membrane permeability and, thus, local edema, but these have met with little clinical success.[47] Systemic antibiotic therapy, initially advocated routinely,[14,41] is now usually withheld until wound infection becomes evident and culture and sensitivity are obtained.[37] Tetanus has been reported following frostbite injuries, and adherence to appropriate tetanus prophylaxis protocols is recommended[19,44] (see Chapter 44). Ultrasound treatments may actually do more harm than good by increasing pain and tissue necrosis.[39] Lange, Boyd, and Loewe reported dramatic reduction in the incidence of gangrene with systemic anticoagulation in experimental animal studies,[27] but others have been unable to reproduce these results or show similar efficacy in man.[53] In an effort to reverse intracapillary sludging and red cell aggregation, antisludging agents, such as low molecular weight Dextran, have been studied extensively, with inconclusive results.[26,40,43,59] Experimental work in animals with the antifibrinolytic agents urokinase and streptokinase suggests a decrease in tissue necrosis if infusion is done within 12 to 48 hours of injury.[32,35] Clinical confirmation of the efficacy of these techniques is still lacking.

Robson and Heggers[50] have demonstrated the presence of vasoconstricting metabolites of arachidonic acid in blister fluid of frostbite wounds. Further experimental work has defined the role of the metabolite thromboxane TxA2 as a mediator of progressive dermal ischemia.[13] Morbidity from progressive dermal ischemia has been reduced by the therapeutic use of inhibitors of the arachidonic acid cascade, specifically topical aloe vera (dermaide aloe) and systemic ibuprofen. The potential benefit and low risk of these agents justified inclusion in the treatment protocol.

It is suggested that use of systemic steroid therapy may inhibit the pathogenic role of these metabolites in frostbite. McCauley et al[33] treated 38 consecutive frostbite patients with a protocol using aspirin as an antiprostaglandin agent and aloe vera as a topical thromboxane inhibitor. All patients recovered without significant tissue loss.

There is evidence that regional sympathectomy provides significant diminution of the late sequelae of frostbite: circulation is improved; hyperhidrosis and pallor disappear; vasospastic symptoms and pain on cold exposure are reduced; and the extremity may actually perceive cold more readily than a previously frozen extremity without sympathectomy.[21,51,52] The benefits in the treatment of acute frostbite are not as certain. Several investigators have suggested that surgical sympathectomy within 36 to 72 hours following the injury probably results in less eventual tissue edema, more rapid resolution of the edema, and earlier cessation of pain.[14,21,51] However, disagreement persists regarding assertions of faster healing and diminished ultimate tissue loss.[24,37] Bouwman and coworkers[4] found in a comparative study that early regional sympathectomy—either surgical or via intraarterial reserpine

Table 56-1. Management of Acute Frostbite—Summary

1. Restore core body heat
2. Rapid rewarming of frozen extremity
   40°C to 44°C water bath
   Sedation and/or analgesics
   Continue rewarming until digital flush appears
3. Tetanus prophylaxis
4. Open dressing technique
   Keep blebs intact
   Topical aloe vera (Dermaide Aloe) q6h
   Silvadene cream to ruptured blebs, mummified skin
5. Oral ibuprofen 12 mg/kg/day (200 mg QID)
6. Antibiotics only for confirmed infection
7. BID physical therapy
   Whirlpool debridement
   Gentle active range of motion
8. Await clear demarcation before amputation or surgical debridement

injection—was not effective therapy for acute frostbite. Coyle and Leddy[5] also reported that sympathectomy was not effective therapy for acute frostbite, even when achieved early and in conjunction with immediate intraarterial reserpine. Engkvist[23] found no benefit with regional intravenous guanethidine in the treatment of acute frostbite. Surgical sympathectomy for multiple extremities has significant morbidity, and therefore this technique has been employed infrequently in the early management of frostbite since most patients with frostbite of the hands also have frostbitten feet. A summary of acute frostbite management is given in Table 56-1.

Authors' Preferred Method

Management of the frostbitten part is carried out in accordance with the guidelines popularized by Mills.[37] Emergency management must also include a thorough assessment of the patient's general condition and stabilization of other disorders in a routine system of priorities. Of major importance is the restoration of normal body temperature through provision of a warm environment and oral administration of warm liquids. Rapid rewarming of the frozen part is undertaken by complete immersion in a water bath at a temperature carefully maintained between 40°C and 44°C. A whirlpool bath is ideal for this purpose. There is evidence that higher temperatures will cause further tissue damage, while lower temperatures may be injurious due to prolongation of the frozen state.[16] Rewarming is continued until flushing of the digital pads is observed, usually within 30 minutes. This process is associated with considerable pain and usually requires administration of parenteral sedatives or analgesics. An open technique is then employed for skin care, avoiding the use of occlusive bandages. Surface blebs will appear within the first several hours after rewarming, and great care is exercised to maintain these intact. Nevertheless, inevitable ruptures require meticulous aseptic handling to prevent secondary infection and its potentially disastrous consequences. Our current recommendation is to apply topical aloe vera (dermaide aloe) to intact blisters every 6 hours. Ruptured blebs or mummified tissue is treated with 1 percent silver sulfadiazine cream (silvadene) in an effort to control surface bacterial growth. Systemic antibiotics are used only in the presence of frank infection and are selected according to culture and sensitivity reports. Whirlpool treatments are administered

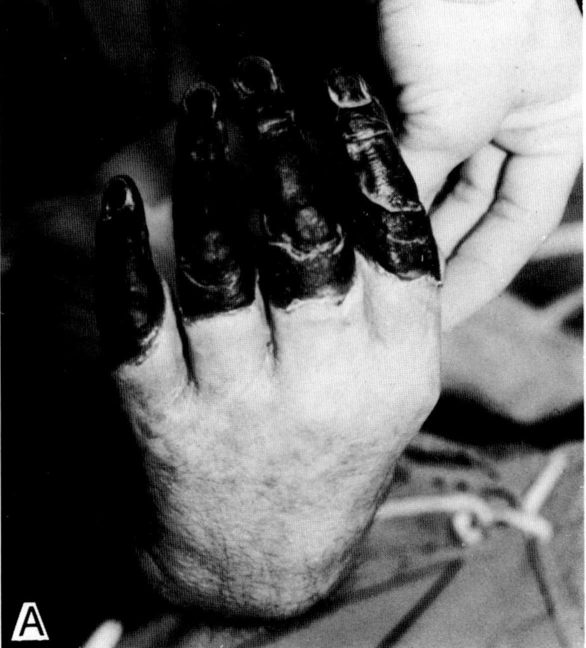

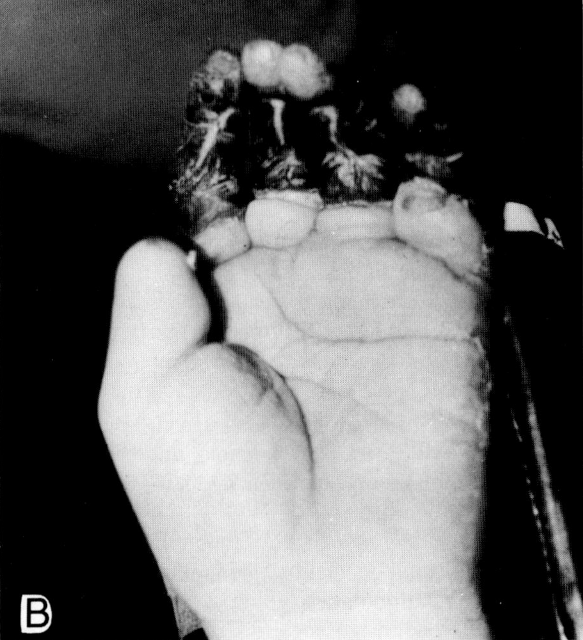

Fig. 56-1. **(A)** Clear demarcation and mummification of the fingers are seen in this 53-year-old man, 40 days following frostbite. **(B)** The margins of the viable tissue are distinct and remain free of infection. The thumb had been lost in a previous accident.

twice daily and provide atraumatic debridement of bacterial accumulation and necrotic tissue, as well as facilitating gentle, active range of motion exercise of the injured hand. Topical enzymatic debridement compounds have had little effect on frostbite eschars.[56] Prolonged dependency of the hand must be avoided to prevent increased edema. Of equal importance is that the exercises provide the patient with a break in his monotonous hospital routine and a sense of active participation in his treatment program. Functional splinting, with custom-made thermoplastic orthoses, may be helpful in the occasional patient who shows evidence of progressive deformity due to contracture.

Early surgical intervention in frostbite is to be condemned. Surgical debridement or early amputation prior to clear demarcation and mummification greatly increases the risk in infection and will routinely result in increased tissue loss. Demarcation of nonviable tissue may take as long as 2 to 3 months and should be patiently awaited[29] (Fig. 56-1). A possible exception to this rule involves the technique of escharotomy, which may be indicated in situations where the dry, contracting eschar is believed to be producing necrosis of healthy underlying tissues by circumferential constriction, thereby impeding blood flow to distal viable tissues.[39] When escharotomy of a digit is necessary because of circumferential constriction, midlateral incisions made down to the level of healthy tissues are preferred. This may provide improved mobility of the digit and enhance early shedding of the eschar.

Systemic anticoagulation or antisludging agents, such as low molecular weight Dextran, have not been used. Our experience with regional sympathetic blockade is encouraging, but has been too limited to draw useful conclusions, and surgical sympathectomy has not been used.

MANAGEMENT OF THE SEQUELAE OF FROSTBITE (LATE TREATMENT)

Mummified Digits

Avoidance of premature amputation is essential and cannot be overemphasized. Radionuclide imaging techniques can help predict the extent of soft tissue ultimately requiring surgical resection.[42] Triple-phase bone scans, with delayed imaging, enhance the clinical usefulness of this technique. Even small amounts of tracer in the frostbitten region indicate deep tissue viability. This information can encourage the physician to continue aggressive conservative therapies and provide more reliable data for counseling the patient about the probability of amputation.[48]

However, when clear demarcation and mummification of a digit occurs, collateral circulation in adjacent viable tissue is better, and amputation can be more safely performed and maximum functional length preserved. It is usually desirable to resect sufficient bone to permit loose skin closure, as in routine terminal amputations. If skin is insufficient to preserve functional length and allow for primary closure, split-thickness skin grafts are applied secondarily when the bed of granulation tissue is adequate. Occasionally, local or remote flaps may be indicated to preserve length.

In the presence of uncontrolled local infection in the digit, open guillotine amputation becomes necessary. The stump is then either revised secondarily to simply allowed to granulate and epithelialize.

Necrosis of Critical Skin

In our experience, certain patients have suffered patchy full-thickness skin necrosis with resultant exposure of vital underlying tissues. This has occurred over the extensor mechanism at the PIP joints of the fingers. In these instances, local skin flap rotation or construction of full-thickness pedicle flaps may become necessary to preserve useful function. Considerable ingenuity is required in order to construct flaps that do not further jeopardize function of the hand.

Vasopastic Syndromes

Reference has already been made to the frequent appearance of sympathetic overactivity and cold sensitivity complaints following frostbite. This is evidenced by heightened pain and vasoconstriction on exposure to cold, and often by hyperhidrosis and development of trophic skin changes.[51] Regional sympathectomy may offer relief from these sequelae. The proper timing of such procedures is uncertain, since it is not possible to predict which patients will show long-lasting, chronic symptoms. Edwards and Leeper have suggested that the surgeon wait no longer than 2 years for spontaneous disappearance of symptoms before performing sympathectomy.[12] In addition, Flatt has suggested late distal sympathectomy at the level of the digital arteries for relief of debilitating vasopastic states.[19,20] He considers the operation experimental but reported that two patients demonstrated increased skin temperature during the subsequent winter.[20] The procedure involves segmental stripping of the adventitia from the digital vessels in the distal palm to remove the sympathetic nerve fibers.

Intrinsic Muscle Atrophy

The intrinsic muscles of the hand may be particularly sensitive to the ravages of severe frostbite injury. Flatt observed varying degrees of fibrosis of the muscle bellies and attributed this to local ischemia.[19] Rigorous attention to a program of early, active physiotherapy and functional splinting may obviate the need for surgical intervention, although in extreme cases release of fibrosed muscles and joint contractures may be required. The extent of the surgical release becomes individualized according to the severity of the deformity. In the authors' experience, surgery has not been necessary for the correction of intrinsic deformities due to frostbite.

FROSTBITE IN THE JUVENILE HAND

Since an initial report by Lohr in 1930, the literature has carried numerous descriptions of a complex of unique skeletal abnormalities following cold injury to the hands of growing children.[3,11,22,49] The major lesion is premature closure of phalangeal epiphyses and is believed to result from a direct injury to vulnerable chondrocytes in the cartilaginous growth plate. Children in an intermediate age-group appear to be most susceptible, probably due to a combination of carelessness and decreased adult supervision. A review of 20 such patients in Minnesota by Dowdle and coworkers[10] showed that radiographic evidence of epiphyseal closure did not become apparent until about 6 to 12 months after the cold exposure, and followed a pattern of decreasing frequency from distal to prox-

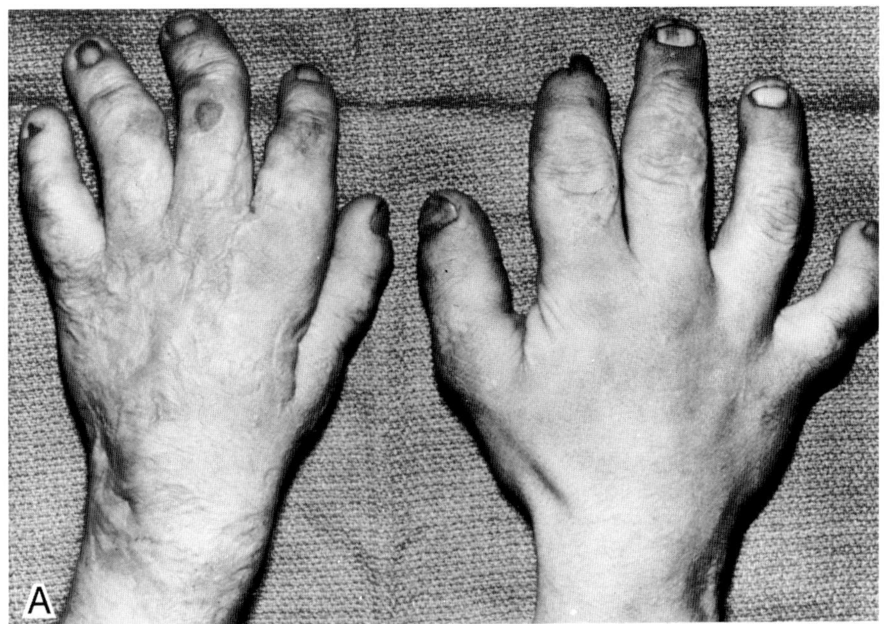

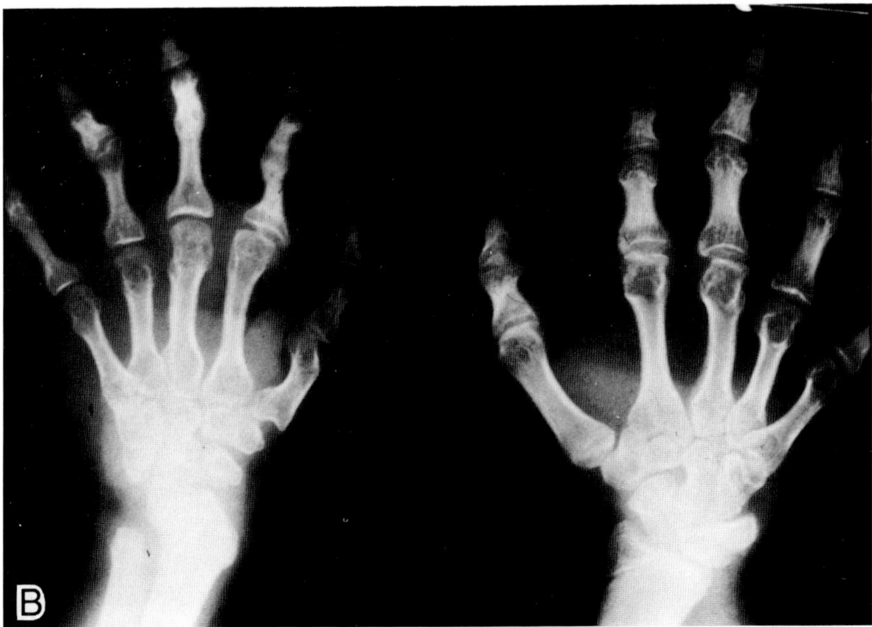

Fig. 56-2. (**A**) The hands of a 16-year-old boy who sustained deep frostbite of both hands 8 years previously. His fingers are shortened and show angular deformities and hypertrophic cutaneous scarring, particularly of the left hand. (**B**) A radiograph of this patient's hands reveals closure of the physes of both hands, including the thumb metacarpal on the left. This is the first case reported with involvement of the epiphyseal plate of the thumb metacarpal. There is significant distortion of the carpal anatomy of the left wrist, as well as premature closure of the distal physis of the radius and ulna.

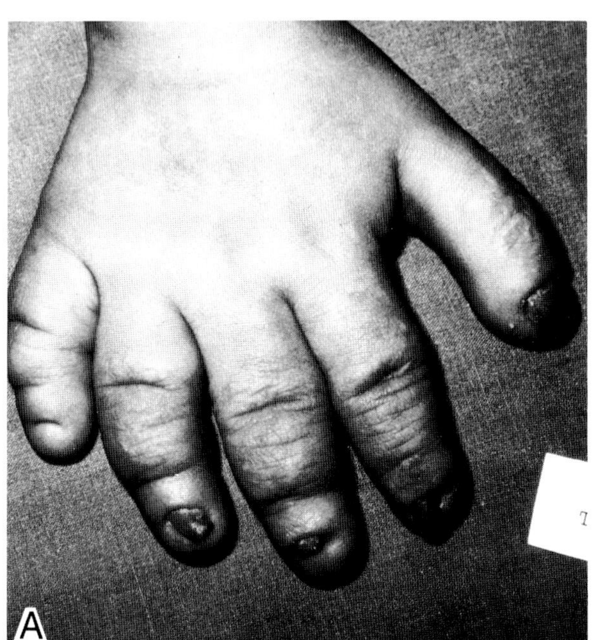

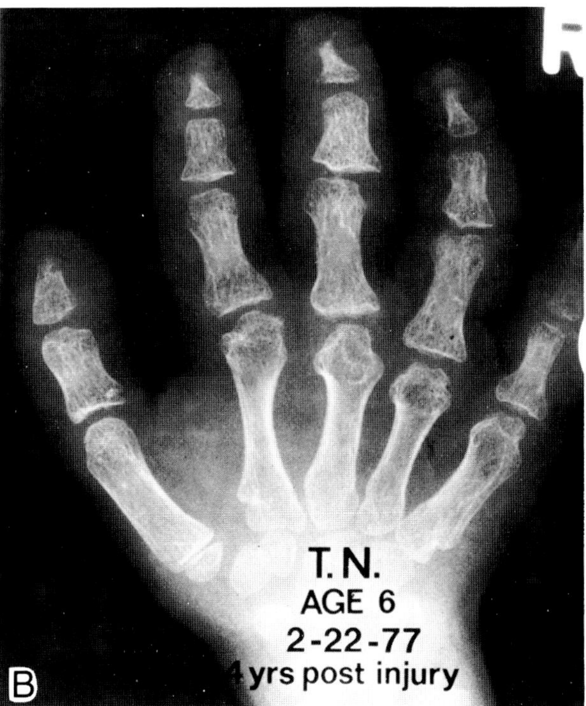

Fig. 56-3. (**A**) The hand of a 6-year-old child who suffered frostbite at age 2. Growth retardation, skin redundancy, abnormal nails, and joint laxity are present. (**B**) A radiograph of this child's hand shows closure of all physes except the physis of the thumb metacarpal. There is considerable bony irregularity with preservation of the joint spaces.

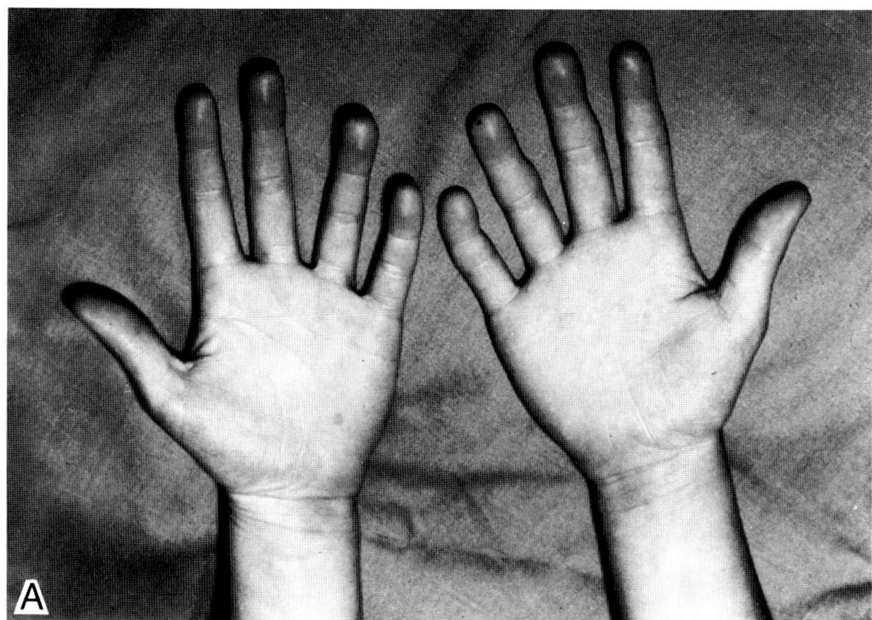

Fig. 56-4. (**A**) The hands of a 19-year-old man who suffered frostbite at age 3. He shows distal segment shortening and angular deformities of the little fingers. *(Figure continues.)*

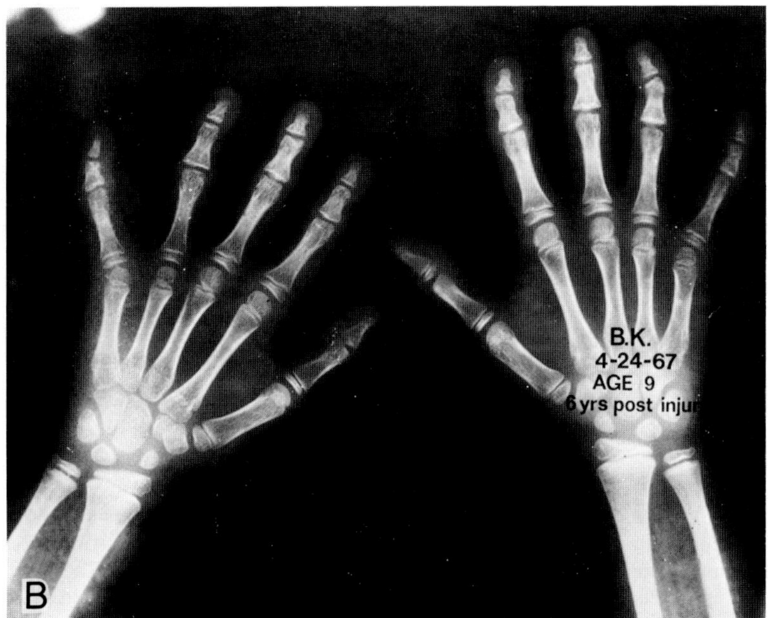

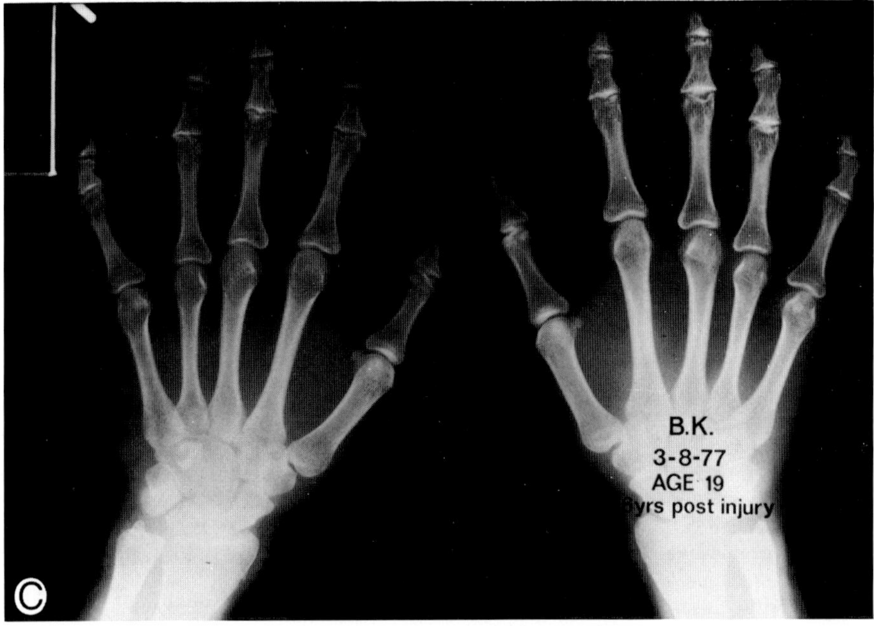

Fig. 56-4 *(Continued).* **(B)** A radiograph of this patient at 9 years of age shows closure of the middle and distal phalangeal physes with angular deformities apparent in the left little and right ring fingers. **(C)** At age 19, there are relatively small middle and distal phalanges with irregularity and angulation at several of the interphalangeal joints.

imal epiphyses. This series included the only report in the literature of closure of the thumb metacarpal epiphysis, a structure usually protected by the surrounding envelope of the thenar muscles and the proximity of the radial artery (Fig. 56-2). Presenting complaints were usually joint pain, stiffness, and weakness of the fingers. Patients followed longer than 10 years invariably developed typical degenerative joint changes, and shortening of the digits, skin redundance, and joint laxity were frequent sequelae (Fig. 56-3). Radial deviation of the DIP joint of the little finger was the most common angular deformity (Fig. 56-4).

In children there is a striking lack of correlation between the extent of initial soft tissue injury to the hand and the eventual skeletal changes. Twenty-five percent of the children in the Minnesota series had not even sought medical attention for the initial injury. The relative absence of significant soft tissue ischemic changes combined with late evidence of epiphyseal damage supports the hypothesis that direct cellular injury to the epiphyseal chondrocyte is the likely etiologic mechanism.

Very few children require surgical treatment.[10,22] When deformities do require treatment, epiphyseal arrest, arthrodesis, or angular osteotomy may be performed as indicated. Function of the hand, however, generally remains satisfactory without surgery.

REFERENCES

1. Ahle NW, Hamlet MP: Enzymatic frostbite eschar debridement by bromelain. Annals Emergency Med 16:1063-1065, 1987
2. Baxter H, Entin MA: Experimental and clinical studies of reduced temperatures in injury and repair in man. Plast Reconstr Surg 5:193, 1950
3. Bigelow DR, Ritchie GW: The effects of frostbite in childhood. J Bone Joint Surg 45B:122-131, 1963
4. Bouwman DL, Morrison S, Lucas CE, Ledgerwood AM: Early sympathetic blockade for frostbite—Is it of value? J Trauma 20:744-749, September 1980
5. Coyle MP Jr, Leddy JP: Injuries of the distal finger. Primary Care 7:245-258, June 1980
6. Crimson JM, Fuhrman FA: Studies on gangrene following cold injury. VIII. The use of casts and pressure dressings in the treatment of severe frostbite. J Clin Invest 26:486-496, 1947
7. Dejong P, Golding MR, Sawyer PN, Wesolowski SA: The role of regional sympathectomy in the early management of cold injury. Surg Gynecol Obstet 115:45-48, 1962
8. Didlake RH, Kukora JS: Tetanus following frostbite injury. Contemporary Orthopaedics 10:69-72, April 1985
9. Dorland's Illustrated Medical Dictionary. 24th Ed. WB Saunders, Philadelphia, 1965
10. Dowdle JA, Kleven LH, House JH, Thompson WW: Frostbite—effect on the juvenile hand (Abstract). Orthop Trans 2:13, 1978
11. Dreyfuss JR, Glimcher MJ: Epiphyseal injury following frostbite. N Engl J Med 253:1065-1068, 1955
12. Edwards EA, Leeper RW: Frostbite—an analysis of 71 cases. JAMA 149:1199-1205, 1952
13. Engkvist O: The effect of regional intravenous guanethidine block in acute frostbite. Case report. Scand J Plast Reconstr Surg 20:243-245, 1986
14. Ervasti E: Frostbite of the extremities and their sequelae—a clinical study. Acta Chir Scand suppl: 299, 1-69, 1962
15. Ferrer MI: Cold injury. Transactions of the First Conference. Bristol. Josiah Macy, Jr., Foundation, 1952
16. Ferrer MI: Cold injury. Transactions of the Second Conference. New York, Josiah Macy, Jr, Foundation, 1954
17. Ferrer MI: Cold injury; Transactions of the Fourth Conference. New York, Josiah Macy, Jr, Foundation, 1955
18. Finneran JC, Shumacker HB Jr: Studies in experimental frostbite. V. Further evaluation of early treatment. Surg Gynecol Obstet 90:430-438, 1950
19. Flatt AE: Frostbite of the extremities: A review of current therapy. J Iowa Med Soc 52:53-55, 1962
20. Flatt AE: Digital artery sympathectomy. J Hand Surg 5:550-556, 1980
21. Golding MR, deJong P, Sawyer PN, Hennigar GR, Wesolowski SA: Protection from early and late sequelae of frostbite by regional sympathectomy: Mechanism of "cold sensitivity" frostbite. Surgery 53:303-308, 1963
22. Hakstian RW: Cold-induced digital epiphyseal necrosis in childhood. Can J Surg 15:168-178, 1972
23. Heggers JP, Robson MC, Manavalen K, Weingarten MD, Carethers JM, Boertman JA, Smith DJ Jr, Sachs RJ: Experimental and clinical observations on frostbite. Annals Emergency Med 16:1056-1062, 1987
24. Hermann G, Schechter DC, Owens JC, Starzl TE: The problem of frostbite in civilian medical practice. Surg Clin North Am, 43:519-536, 1963
25. Irving L, Nelms JB, Ellsner R: Frostbite. Experience with rapid rewarming and ultrasonic therapy. Alaska Med 3:28-36, 1961
26. Knize DM, Weatherley-White RCA, Paton BC: Use of anti-sludging agents in experimental cold injuries. Surg Gynecol Obstet 129:1019-1026, 1969
27. Lange K, Boyd LJ, Loewe L: Functional pathology of frostbite and prevention of gangrene in experimental animals and humans. Science 102:151-152, 1945
28. Lange K, Weiner D, Boyd LJ: Frostbite—physiology, pathology, and therapy. N Engl J Med 237:383-389, 1947
29. Lapp NL, Juergens JL: Frostbite. Mayo Clin Proc 40:932-948, 1965
30. Lempke RE, Shumacker HB Jr: Studies in experimental frostbite. III. An evaluation of several methods for early treatment. Yale J Biol Med 21:321-334, 1949
31. Littell ET: Frostbite. Sci Am 186:52-56, 1952
32. Marzella L, Jesudass RR, Manson PN, Myers RAM, Bulkley GB: Morphologic characterization of acute injury to vascular endothelium of skin after frostbite. Plast Reconstr Surg 83:67-75, 1989
33. McCauley RL, Hing DN, Robson MC, Hegger JP: Frostbite injuries: A rational approach based on the pathophysiology. J Trauma 23:143-147, 1983
34. Meehan JP Jr: Individual and racial variations in a vascular response to a cold stimulus. Milit Med 116:330-334, 1955
35. Mehta RC, Wilson MA: Frostbite injury: Prediction of tissue viability with triple-phase bone scanning. Radiology 170:511-514, 1989
36. Meryman HT: Mechanics of freezing in living cells and tissues. Science 124:515-521, 1956
37. Mills WJ Jr: Frostbite: A method of management including rapid thawing. Northwest Med 65:119-125, 1966
38. Mills WJ Jr, Whaley R, Fish W: Frostbite: Experience with rapid rewarming and ultrasonic therapy. Alaska Med 2:1-3, 114-122, 1960
39. Mills WJ Jr, Whaley R, Fish W: Frostbite: Experience with rapid rewarming and ultrasonic therapy. Alaska Med 3:28-36, 1961
40. Mundth ED, Long DM, Brown RB: Treatment of experimental frostbite with low molecular weight dextran. J Trauma 4:246-257, 1964
41. Orr KD, Fainer DC: Cold injuries in Korea during winter of 1950-51. Medicine 31:177-220, 1952
42. Page RE, Robertson GA: Management of the frostbitten hand. Hand 15:185-191, 1983
43. Penn I, Schwartz SI: Evaluation of low molecular weight dextran in the treatment of frostbite. J Trauma 4:784-790, 1964
44. Perry CR, Lowry WE, Pankovich AM, Kallick CA: Tetanus in a patient with frostbite: A case report. Orthopaedics 4:907-908, 1981
45. Rasmusen DL, Zook EG: Frostbite: A review of pathophysiology and newest treatments. J Indiana State Med Assoc 65:1237-1241, 1972
46. Robson MC, Heggers JP: Evaluation of hand frostbite blister fluid as a clue to pathogenesis. J Hand Surg 6:43-46, 1981
47. Salimi Z, Vas W, Tang-Barton P, Eachempati RG, Morris L, Carron M: Assessment of tissue viability in frostbite by ^{99m}Tc pertechnetate scintigraphy. Am J Radiology 142:415-419, 1984
48. Salimi Z, Wolverson MK, Herbold DR, Vas W, Salimi A: Treatment of frostbite with IV streptokinase: An experimental study in rabbits. AJR 149:773-776, 1987
49. Selke AC Jr: Destruction of phalangeal epiphyses by frostbite. Radiology 93:859-860, 1969
50. Shikata J, Shumacker HB Jr, Nash FD: Studies in experimental frostbite. Arch Surg 81:817-823, 1960

51. Shumacker HB Jr: Frostbite in Hand Surgery. pp. 405–412. 2nd Ed. Williams and Wilkins, Baltimore, 1975
52. Shumacker HB Jr, Kilman JW: Sympathectomy in the treatment of frostbite. Arch Surg 89:575–584, 1964
53. Shumacker HB Jr, Lempke RE: Recent advances in frostbite. Surgery 30:873–904, 1951
54. Shumacker HB Jr, Lempke RE: Vascular surgery. Cold injuries. National Research Council 64–126, 1951
55. Siple PA, Passel CF: Measurements of dry atmosphere cooling in subfreezing temperatures. Proc Am Philos Soc 89:177–199, 1945
56. Urschel JD: Frostbite: Predisposing factors and predictors of poor outcome. J Trauma 30:340–342, 1990
57. Washburn B: Frostbite. What it is. How to prevent it. Emergency treatment. N Engl J Med 266:974–989, 1962
58. Weatherley-White RCA, Knize DM, Geisterfer DJ, Paton BC: Experimental studies in cold injury. V Circulatory hemodynamics. Surgery 66:208–214, 1969
59. Weatherley-White RCA, Paton BC, Sjostrom B: Experimental studies in cold injury. III Observations on the treatment of frostbite. Plast Reconstr Surg 36:10–18, 1965
60. Whayne TF, Debakey ME: Cold injury, ground type. U.S. Printing Office, Washington, D.C., 1958
61. Zdeblick TA, Field GA, Shaffer JW: Treatment of experimental frostbite with urokinase. J Hand Surg 13A:948–953, 1988

57

Thumb Reconstruction

James W. Strickland
William B. Kleinman

The long-standing respect of hand surgeons for the functional value of the thumb, their fertile imaginations, and steady advances in surgical technology have combined to produce a profusion of procedures for the restoration, reconstruction, and replacement of this important part of the hand, in cases both of traumatic loss and congenital failure of formation. Fortunately, the development and subsequent refinement of microvascular techniques has made it possible to replant complete or revascularize partial thumb amputations under ideal circumstances. Microvascular transplantation of whole or partial toes to the hand can now be performed with excellent success rates. There is universal agreement that reconstruction of an opposable thumb should be attempted whenever possible, using whatever technical pathways are available to the surgeon.

Thumb reconstruction by means of free-tissue transfer has become well accepted after an initial period of skepticism. Great and second toe transplants, wrap-around flaps, and other resourceful methods have proven their value, and have rendered some of the more traditional techniques of thumb reconstruction nearly obsolete.[79] Many patients adjust quite well to a loss of all or a portion of their thumb and do not seek or require any reconstructive efforts; others will opt not to sacrifice either a toe or other uninjured tissue in order to regain thumb use. These patients are best served by more conservative measures using techniques of bone, joint, and soft tissue rearrangement and transfer. The more traditional, nonmicrovascular procedures have evolved over a considerable period of time and have undergone numerous revisions, as we will elucidate in this chapter. Results using these techniques are predictable, and satisfactory restoration of thumb function can usually be assured. Whether used for congenital reconstruction, or for thumb salvage following trauma, many of these procedures are technically difficult; they require skills that are no less demanding than those required for employing methods of microvascular surgery and the operating microscope. In this chapter, we will delineate selected time-honored, nonmicrovascular techniques of reconstruction for either congenital absence or traumatic partial or complete thumb loss. Surgical indications, operative techniques, postoperative management, and potential complications for each method will be described, and pertinent bibliographic information provided. In particular, the many excellent articles and chapters authored by Littler,[59–69] Reid,[102–112] and Buck-Gramcko,[13] establish these clinicians as some of the most prolific contributors to this area of hand reconstruction. Excellent monographs have also been published that review and describe the many methods of thumb reconstruction.[41,77] In addition, many of the operations described in this chapter, as they specifically apply to the thumb, are discussed in more general terms in other chapters of this book.

GENERAL CONSIDERATIONS FOR THUMB RECONSTRUCTION

Functional requirements of the thumb include (1) adequate sensibility to perceive its environment; (2) sufficient length and mobility to oppose any of the medial digits; and (3) freedom from pain.[4,14,16,17,21,28,40,54,57,58,67,68,77,80,82,83,88,90,98,99,101,102,103,109,110,112,121–123,133,136,137] Careful consideration of each of these factors is important when planning a reconstructive procedure either to rebuild a congenital deficiency, or following thumb injury. There is considerable controversy regarding the amount of thumb shortening that can exist before significant functional impairment occurs.[23,27,98,99,109,110] Amputations (those both trauma-induced and those secondary to congenital failure of formation), that retain most of the proximal phalanx will provide adequate function without the need for surgical lengthening or first web space-deepening procedures.[98,101,108-110,121,122,124,137] However, thumb loss at the base of the proximal phalanx, through the metacarpophalangeal joint, or more proximal, may result in a residual stump inadequate for pinch and grasp functions.[100,120]

The importance of restoring at least an acceptable level of sensory cognition following thumb salvage or reconstruction cannot be overstated.[16,17,37,41,43,58,84,85,108,121,127,137] Procedures should be selected to provide a predictably satisfactory level of tactile perception and stereognosis. Failure to achieve this quality was the most consistent reason for patient thumb disuse following many early reconstructive techniques (despite the fact that other functional requirements may have been met by the procedures). Before a patient will consistently use a reconstructed thumb, it must have painless skin coverage, be durable enough for normal use, and have at least protective—if not normal—sensation.[137] The use of neurovascular island pedicle techniques, sensory-innervated cross-finger flaps, and other methods of transferring innervated skin have greatly enhanced the ability to restore sensation when carrying out thumb salvage following either trauma, or after congenital insult.

To function correctly, the thumb must be positioned so that it can oppose the adjacent medial border fingers and grasp objects securely from an antiposed (abducted, slightly extended and pronated) position.[86,108,127] Although normal motion is usually not required at the metacarpophalangeal (MP) or interphalangeal (IP) joints, thumb function is greatly dependent on preserving a full arc of circumduction at the carpometacarpal (CMC) joint.[17,37,86,108] If a substantial range of CMC motion cannot be attained, the thumb should be positioned in nearly full abduction-opposition (40 degrees abduction, 15 degrees extension, 120 degrees metacarpal pronation),[54] so that other mobile digits can be flexed to meet it. In addition, all three thumb joints must be sufficiently stable to provide resistance during grasp and pinch.

In recent years, the development and refinement of microvascular techniques have produced a high level of predictability for digital replantation under ideal circumstances. The rationale for attempting replantation following thumb amputation is undeniable, and hand function has benefitted more from the successful replantation of a severed thumb than it has from other digital replantation efforts. Excellent restoration of thumb function has been reported by numerous authors describing techniques, complications, and results of thumb replantation.[3,6,11,12,26,32,36,41,46,47,52,53,55,72,73,80,87,94,96,112-114,116,119,121,123,126,128,129-131,135,138,139] Although replantation is not discussed in this chapter, it is clear that when successful, the technique provides more functional benefit than any other type of thumb reconstruction, even in the face of obligatory skeletal shortening and possible loss of motion of either the MP joint, the IP joint, or both.

Factors to be taken into consideration when selecting a reasonable surgical option for thumb reconstruction following either trauma, or for congenital deficiency, include age, sex, occupational demands, hand dominance, and the subjective needs of the patient. Once the patient or family (in cases of congenital reconstruction) has expressed interest in a restorative or reconstructive effort, an open and honest dialogue between patient and surgeon is necessary before any final decision can be made.

The procedures we describe in this chapter are reserved for those patients who have experienced a significant functional loss to the hand because of their thumb deficiency. Almost without exception these operative efforts require a skillful surgeon, well-experienced in the wide spectrum of hand surgical techniques.

PART I. THUMB RECONSTRUCTION FOR CONGENITAL ABSENCE

FAILURE OF THUMB FORMATION

Throughout the last century of thumb reconstructive surgery, an appreciation has existed for the importance of an opposable unit to the prehensile human hand.[67] Since 1874, when Huguier[45] reported deepening a remaining cleft between a partial traumatic thumb and index finger amputation in an adult, exhaustive surgical efforts have been directed towards salvage and reconstruction of an opposable thumb unit. The issue of thumb reconstruction has been controversial throughout the last century. Established doctrines have been frequently challenged; thoughtful new principles and techniques have been regularly introduced into the literature. Only a few of these innovations have endured to become contemporary hallmarks of reconstruction of the *congenitally* absent thumb.

The differences between congenital failure of thumb formation and traumatic thumb loss cannot be overstated, and must be appreciated by the reconstructive hand surgeon during his assessment of the functionally compromised patient.[54] The child with congenital thumb deficiency has either a markedly reduced or absent cerebrocortical representation for thumb function, normally a rather large portion of the sensory cortex (Fig. 57-1A & B). The child afflicted by complete or partial thumb aplasia may insidiously develop a progressive pronatory curve of the index ray, enlargement of the interdigital cleft between index and long fingers, and gradually increased breadth of the index pulp to compensate for inadequacies of prehensile thumb function (Fig. 57-2). Even in the absence of thumb cortical representation, a primitive but functional level of prehensile grasp and pinch can be achieved between the index and long fingers.

Historical Review

Contemporary principles of thumb reconstruction for the congenitally compromised hand are based on surgical experience following traumatic thumb loss. In the latter part of the nineteenth and early twentieth centuries, two distinct surgical philosophies evolved: (1) local thumb phalangealization following partial amputation, essentially a deepening of the first

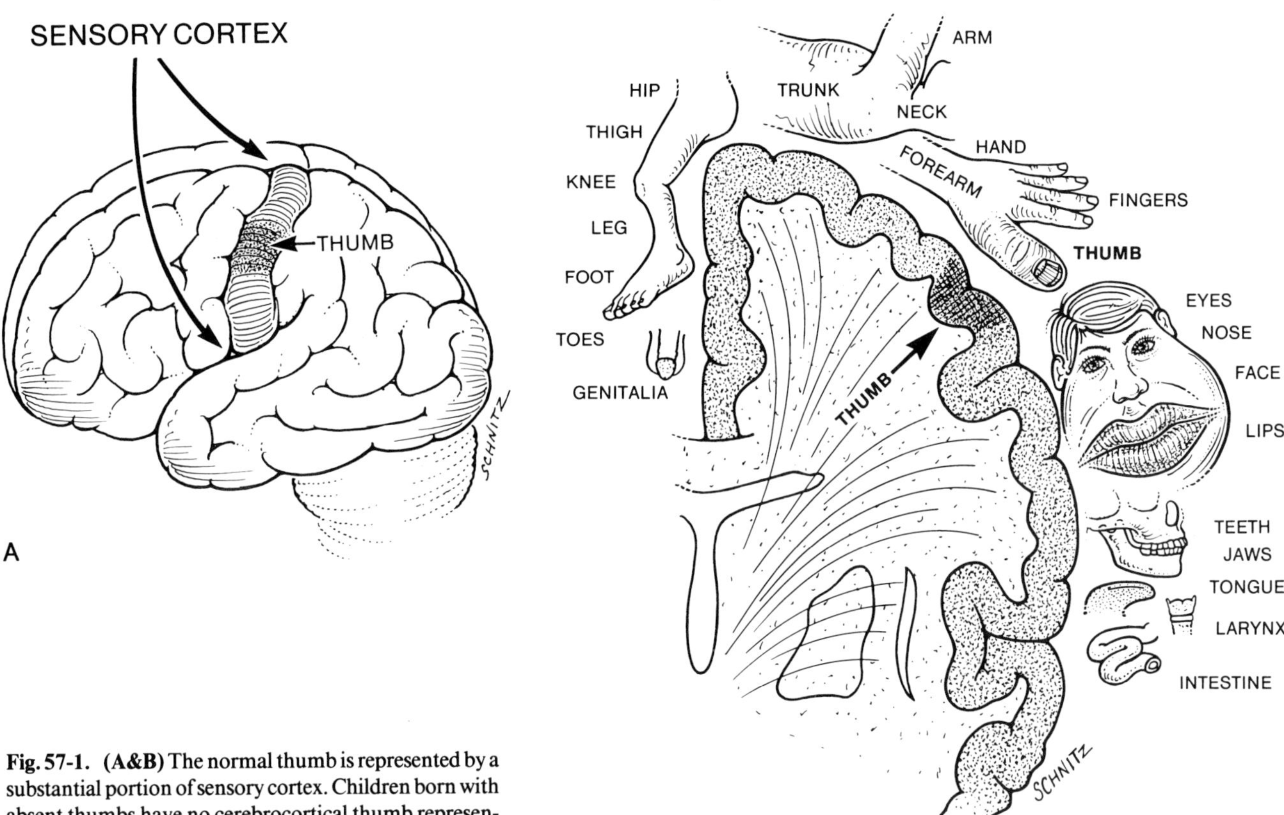

Fig. 57-1. (A&B) The normal thumb is represented by a substantial portion of sensory cortex. Children born with absent thumbs have no cerebrocortical thumb representation.

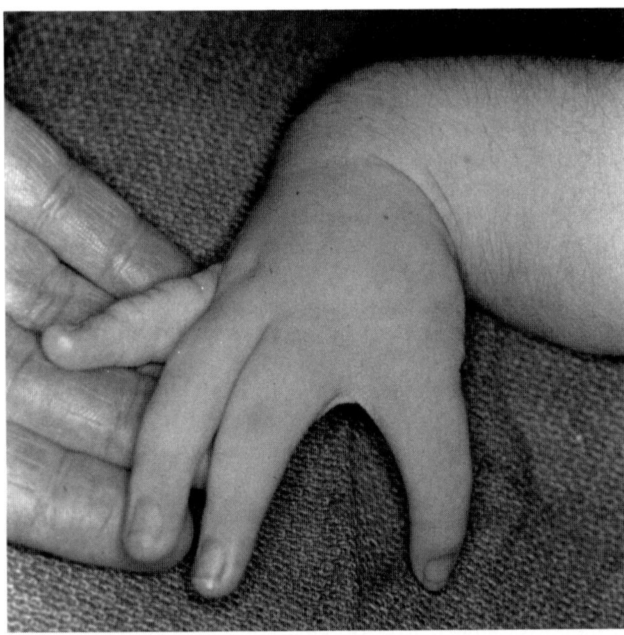

Fig. 57-2. Children with congenital thumb absence develop progressive widening of the index-long interdigital cleft, pronation of the index ray, and broadening of its pulp. These adaptive changes facilitate elementary grasp and pinch between the index and long fingers.

webspace as first described by Huguier[45]; and (2) distant pedicle flap attachment with delayed secondary detachment, described in 1897 by Nicoladoni.[91] Nicoladoni approached the tedious task of rebuilding the thumb following traumatic amputation by a staged, attached great toe-to-thumb transfer, which was a reconstructive effort of substantial technical magnitude for its time, requiring an enormous degree of patient motivation and cooperation. In 1966, Tubiana and coauthors[1,134] reported that on long-term follow-up of Nicoladoni's three patients in whom this technique was used, each was found to have refused subsequent bone grafting procedures and remained with unstable, floppy "thumbs" following detachment from the foot. Clarkson,[23] as recently as 1955, however, reported the largest known series using Nicoladoni's principles of two-staged distant pedicle toe transfer in 15 digits transferred in six patients, one of whom underwent a five-toe transfer for the treatment of complete congenital transverse failure of formation at the midpalmar level. Results of this case were reported as completely successful, the patient requiring only a later web space deepening between the great and second toes.

The idea of using distant pedicle flaps in rebuilding amputated thumbs was also proposed by Luksch[70] in 1903, first describing the use of the contralateral index finger as a staged pedicle transfer. His work was based on an earlier reconstructive experience by Guermonprez,[33-35] which unfortunately went essentially unnoticed and unappreciated for more than a half-century. Joyce,[49] in 1918, reported reconstruction of an amputated thumb with the ring finger of the opposite hand in a manner similar to Guermonprez's work, relying on the principles of a distant pedicle flap with delayed detachment.

"Osteoplastic" reconstruction,[2,92–95,118] used extensively prior to World War II, was performed in either one or two stages. Reconstruction involved attaching the injured thumb stump to a random tubed pedicle of vascularized skin and subcutaneous tissue from the abdomen or groin, with iliac crest corticocancellous bone grafting for skeletal reconstruction (see page 2116).

The historical principles that slowly evolved during the early decades of this century continued in 1931 when Sterling Bunnell[15] reported the first use of an index finger remnant (distal metacarpal and proximal phalanx) to reconstruct the lost basilar joint of a thumb. But it was not until 1949, following an extensive experience with post-World War II traumatic reconstructions, that Gosset,[31] in Paris, reported the first transfer of an index finger isolated on its neurovascular pedicle to a remote position on the hand. In introducing this technique, Gosset not only revolutionized contemporary traumatic thumb reconstruction, but pioneered the seminal principles of congenital reconstruction for the absent thumb.

An international exchange of medical information and creative new ideas in surgery occurred after World War II; Gosset's techniques, for example, attained worldwide use in centers for hand reconstruction. Over the past four decades, his initial recommendations have been significantly modified from those involving simple lateral displacement of the index ray without bony shortening, to metacarpal recession and rotation, intrinsic muscle transfers, and skin flaps especially designed to produce a wide first web space, free of scar and the potential for contracture.

Before these principles gained wide acceptance, Barsky[4–6] and others[50,132] sought to improve prehensile grasp in the congenitally deficient hand by surgical enhancement of the natural tendency of the index finger to progressively pronate in those children with complete thumb absence. Barsky advocated simple surgical deepening of the index-long finger web space, with rotational osteotomy of the index metacarpal. The pulps of the "repositioned" index finger could be opposed for pinch and primitive grasp (Fig. 57-3A–D). Although at the time these principles were quite sound and widely practiced, following World War II the technique was quickly replaced by the principles of neurovascular pedicle transfer with index recession and repositioning, adapted from techniques utilized for traumatic thumb loss by Bunnell, Littler, and others.

For historic accuracy, Gersuny,[30] in Vienna in 1887, was actually the first to describe the principle of the neurovascular island pedicle flap; however, his reports identified no named artery. Not until 1893, when Dunham,[24] of New York, described a permanently vascularized island pedicle flap with identifiable blood vessels, were clear principles established for this technique. These principles were widely applied throughout the first half of this century in the field of plastic surgery and craniofacial reconstruction,[21] and became the basis for Gosset's later historic work in post-World War II France.

A plethora of respectable contributions to the field of digital neurovascular pedicle transfer followed Gosset's original description.[31] Success with index ray transfer led to the use of the long,[10,29,39,48,71,78] ring,[9,18,19,89,95,117] and little[51,56] fingers for reconstruction of thumb position, length, and sensibility (Fig. 57-4). As recently as 1955, even the traditional osteoplastic staged pedicle-and-graft reconstruction received a boost by Moberg's[83] introduction of the "island pedicle" transfer of vascularized, sensible, cornified skin from an uninjured portion of the hand, used to restore stereognosis to the tactile portion of the osteoplastic thumb. Thus, this type of staged reconstruction combined principles of tubed abdominal pedicle, iliac crest corticocancellous bone graft, and neurovascular island pedicle transfer from another digit (usually the ulnar border of the long finger), with subsequent cosmetic debulking. This technique has been widely practiced, and remains a fundamental approach in complex thumb reconstruction following trauma.[21]

The thalidomide tragedy in Europe resulted in a devastating number of drug-induced congenital deformities of the upper and lower extremities between 1959 and 1962. Over a 10-year period Buck-Gramcko, of Hamburg, then West Germany, performed an unprecedented series of 100 index finger pollicizations for congenital failure of thumb formation, mostly drug-induced. After careful study and revision of both principles and technique, Buck-Gramcko presented the results of his work at the 1971 meeting of the American Society for Surgery of the Hand in a landmark paper on congenital thumb reconstruction.[13] He emphasized in his report that digital transposition should be performed during infancy, as Riordan had advocated.[80,97,115] Using contributions from Gosset,[31] Hilgenfeldt,[42] Littler,[59–61,64] Harrison,[37–39] and Riordan,[80,81,115] Buck-Gramcko designed a surgical approach for the thumbless child, using the index finger. His technique resulted in stability, mobility, and optimum position and strength for prehensile grasp and pinch. His theoretical and practical contributions, including intrinsic muscle transfers, carpometacarpal reconstruction, and the geometry of skin flaps to avoid first web space contracture, have become hallmarks of contemporary congenital thumb reconstruction[54] (see page 2058).

Pollicization for Congenital Failure of Formation: The Aplastic Thumb and the *Pouce Flottant*

There are wide variations in the phenotypic expressivity of congenital deformity of the thumb, including failure of formation of the entire osteoarticular column (including trapezium and scaphoid) (Fig. 57-5A & B), and the so-called floating thumb *(pouce flottant)* (Fig. 57-6A & B).

A useful classification of the spectrum of congenital thumb involvement was suggested by Muller[89] in 1937 as a "teratologic sequence," and later by Blauth[8] in 1967. Buck-Gramcko (D. Buck-Gramcko, MD: personal communication, 1989) has refined and detailed these earlier contributions, and classified thumb hypoplasia into five reasonably distinct categories (Fig. 57-7A–E).[54] Severe thumb involvement with absence of the entire osteoarticular column and all soft tissue is classified as

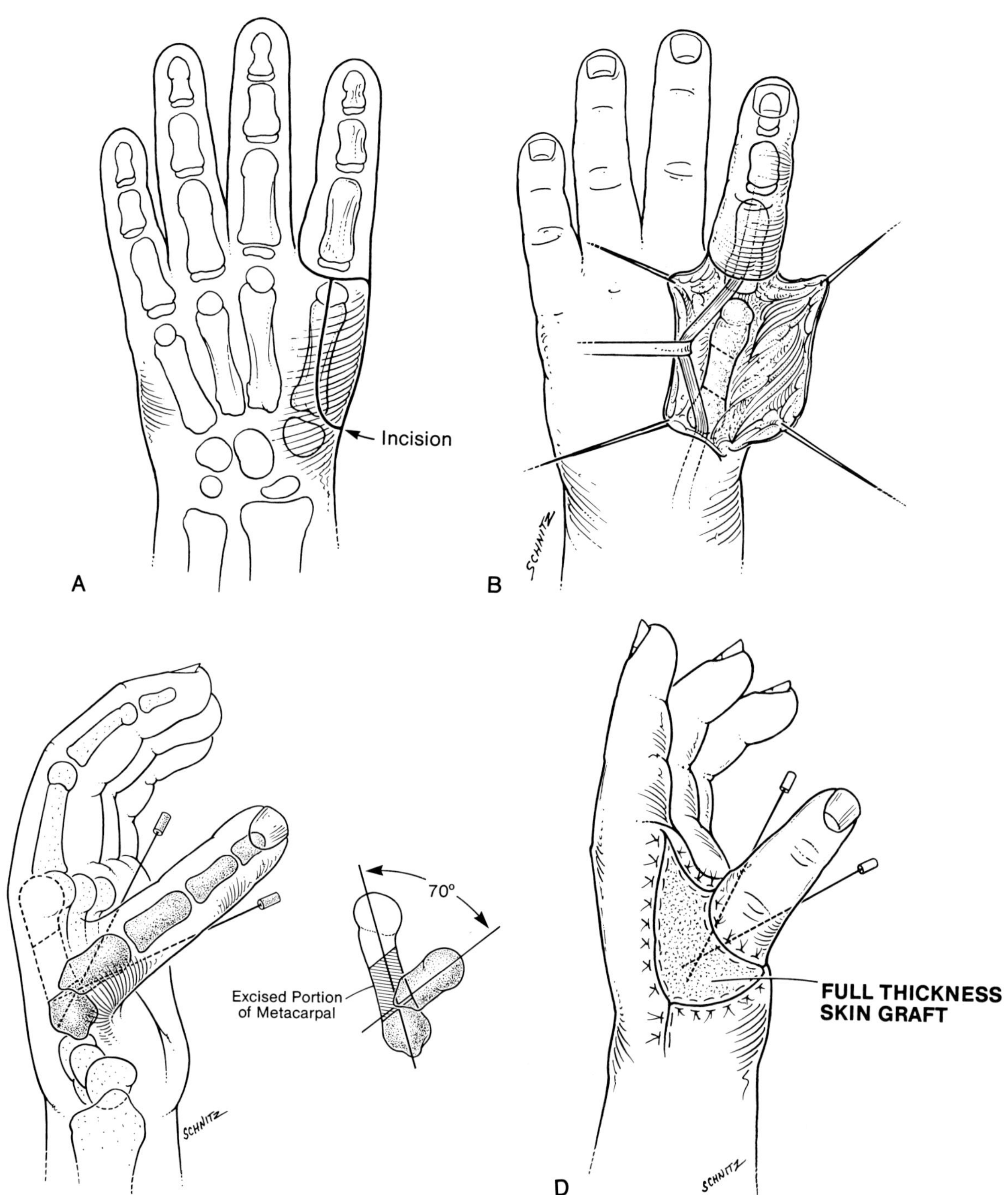

Fig. 57-3. (A–D) Barsky's technique for surgical improvement of grasp and pinch in the hand afflicted by congenital absence of the thumb. The index-long finger web space is deepened, and an abduction/rotation osteotomy used to "reposition" the index ray. Except for applying a full thickness skin graft directly to the first web space, the principles of reconstruction were sound. Historically, however, the long-term results were disappointing.[4–6]

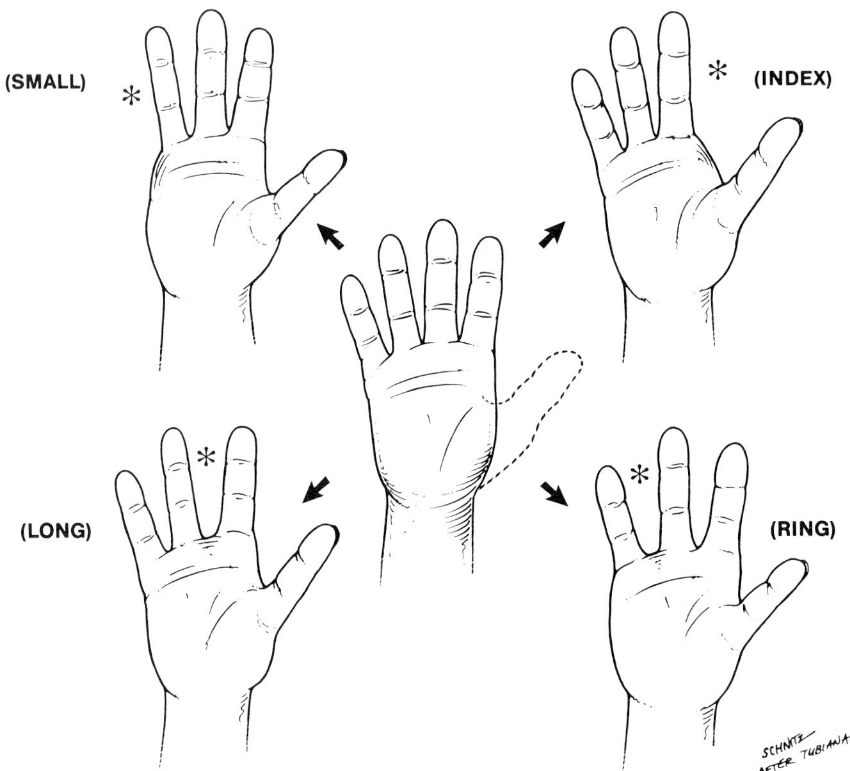

Fig. 57-4. Pollicization has been described using each ray for reconstruction of traumatic loss of thumb; in each approach Gosset's original principles of the neurovascular pedicle technique, described in 1949, are followed. (Adapted from Tubiana,[134a] with permission.)

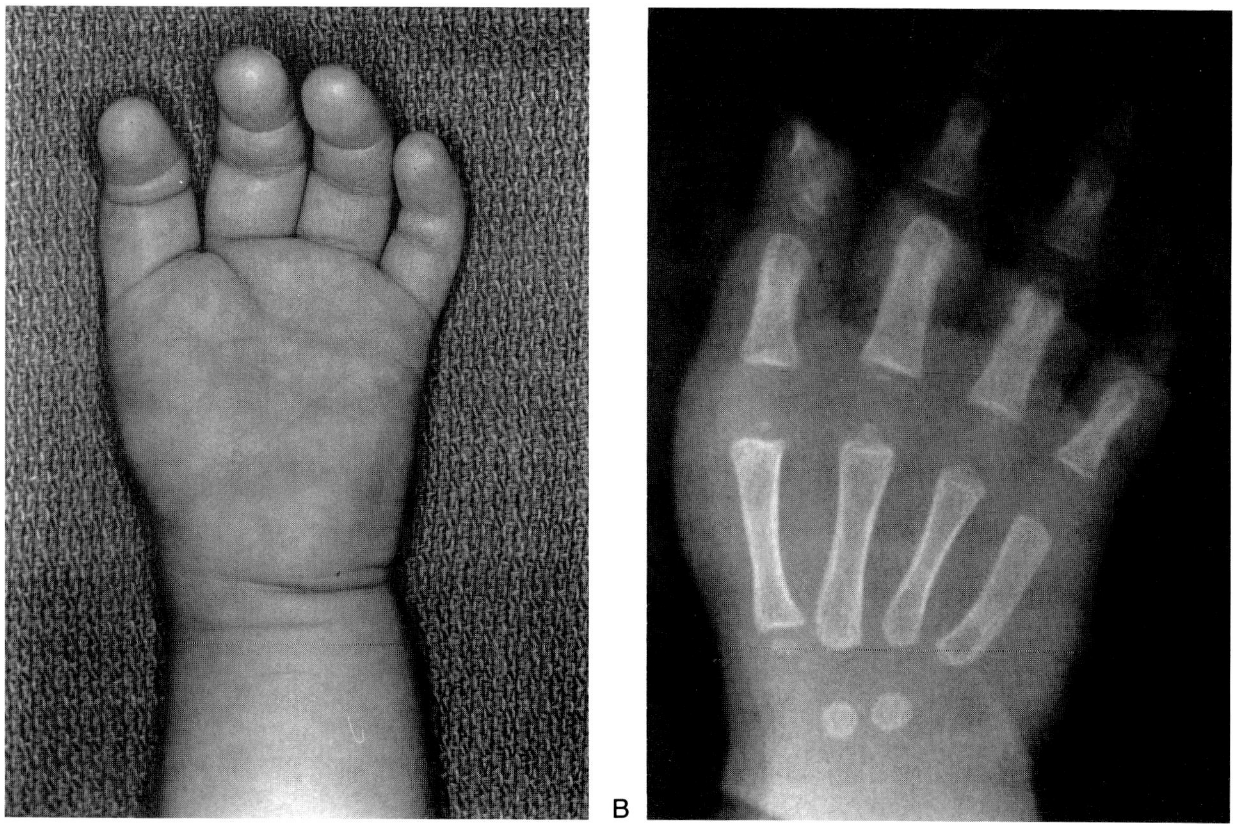

Fig. 57-5. (A&B) Complete failure of formation of the thumb consists of neither soft tissue nor bony thumb remnants. The entire osteoarticular column, including trapezium and scaphoid, is absent (Buck-Gramcko grade V thumb hypoplasia; see Fig. 57-7).

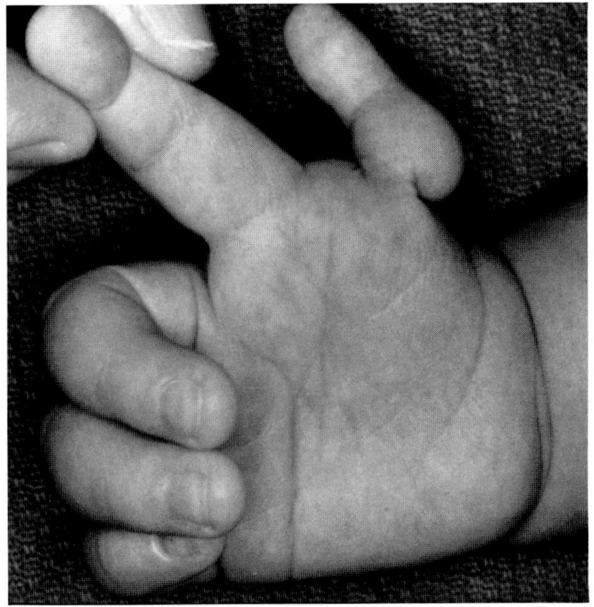

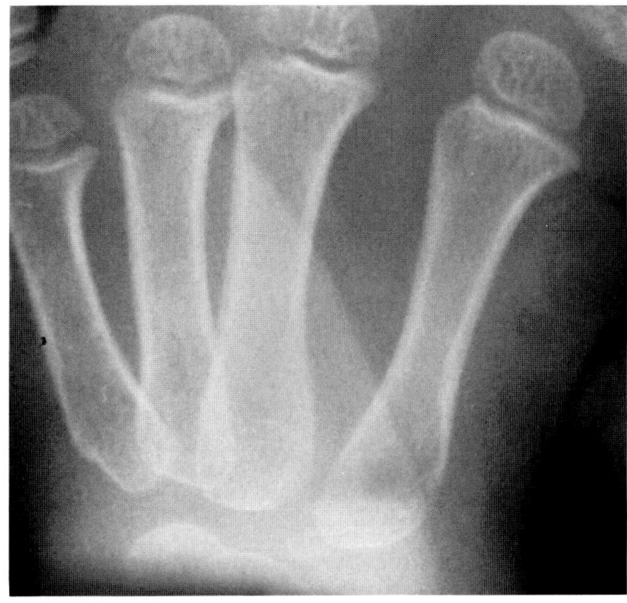

Fig. 57-6. (A&B) The origin of the base of the *pouce flottant* (Buck-Gramcko grade IV thumb hypoplasia; see Fig. 57-7) is distal and dorsal along the radial midaxial border of the hand. The part is nonfunctional, and devoid of metacarpal or bony base. The neurovascular status of the floating thumb, however, is normal.

grade V hypoplasia, or aplasia (the final, most severe stage of thumb reduction in Muller's "teratologic sequence"). Grade IV hypoplasia describes the *pouce flottant,* or *floating thumb,* a rudimentary appendage connected to the hand by a small skin tag, and usually containing two hypoplastic phalanges and a single well-developed neurovascular bundle; the remainder of the thumb osteoarticular column is absent. The origin of this severely deficient appendage is consistently along the radial midaxial line of the hand, and lies quite distal (Fig. 57-8A & B); the appendages vary in size.

Assuming fundamental understanding and cooperation of both patient and family, complete absence of the thumb (grade V hypoplasia) should be treated early in life by pollicization of the index finger using the principles of Gosset, Littler, Riordan, and Buck-Gramcko. Progressive moderate pronation of the index ray, widening of the index-long interdigital space, and broadening of the index pulp, all predispose the untreated patient to permanent functional scissoring between index and long fingers unless treated (Fig. 57-9).[54]

Index ray development in patients afflicted by either complete thumb absence or *pouce flottant* (grade V or IV thumb hypoplasia) demands pollicization. Attempts to mobilize poorly developed and contracted joints, and to reestablish a functional orientation to the base of a grade IV floating thumb, are unjustified, even without considering the problems inherent in performing the multiple tendon transfers required to motor the reconstructed digit.

In spite of the skin constriction at the base of the *pouce flottant,* digital survival during the postnatal period is assured. Proximal to the constriction the thumb unit is severely hypoplastic, usually devoid of metacarpal, trapezium, and scaphoid, and has neither intrinsic nor extrinsic tendons; the proximal and distal phalanges may be only cartilage remnants (see Fig. 57-7D). A thumb nail is usually present and developed to an extent similar to the general development of the entire distal thumb unit. It is important to emphasize that within the narrowed base of the grade IV hypoplastic thumb there is always a distinct neurovascular pedicle (Fig. 57-10A & B).

The *pouce flottant* should be amputated, either as an independent procedure or in conjunction with pollicization. In the newborn nursery, the base of the thumb can be anesthetized locally and a sterile silk tie applied tightly at the base to induce ischemic necrosis. A small amount of local long-acting anesthetic prevents the pain associated with crushing a well-developed digital nerve with the tie.[54]

Whether the part is ablated as an independent procedure or removed at the time of pollicization, no efforts should be made to reconstruct a grade IV hypoplastic thumb with a functional five-finger hand as a surgical goal. The results of such efforts are functionally and cosmetically poor. The child will invariably —after many surgical procedures—bypass the reconstructed unit, preferring the more natural index-long finger scissoring action. Dexterity of the medial four fingers and the paucity of cerebrocortical representation outweigh any effort to create a functional thumb unit from the *pouce flottant.*

There are exceptions, however, to any rule. Particularly in Oriental cultures in which a five-fingered hand has extreme importance, select cases may justify efforts to reconstruct a grade IV hypoplastic thumb. In these rare instances, the site of origin of the thumb base should be shifted to a more palmar

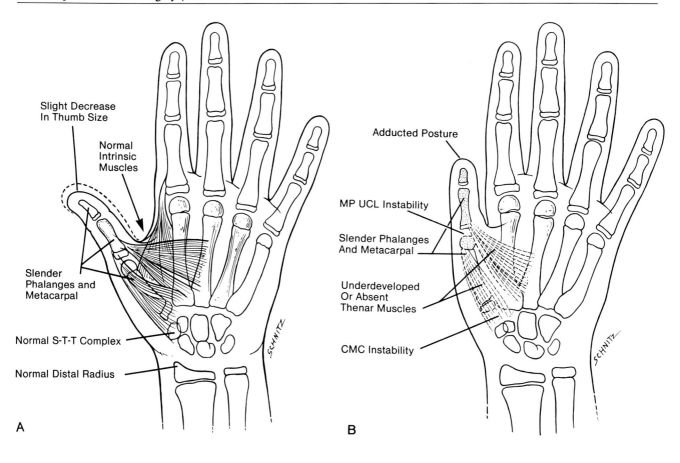

Slight Decrease In Thumb Size
Normal Intrinsic Muscles
Slender Phalanges and Metacarpal
Normal S-T-T Complex
Normal Distal Radius
A

Adducted Posture
MP UCL Instability
Slender Phalanges And Metacarpal
Underdeveloped Or Absent Thenar Muscles
CMC Instability
B

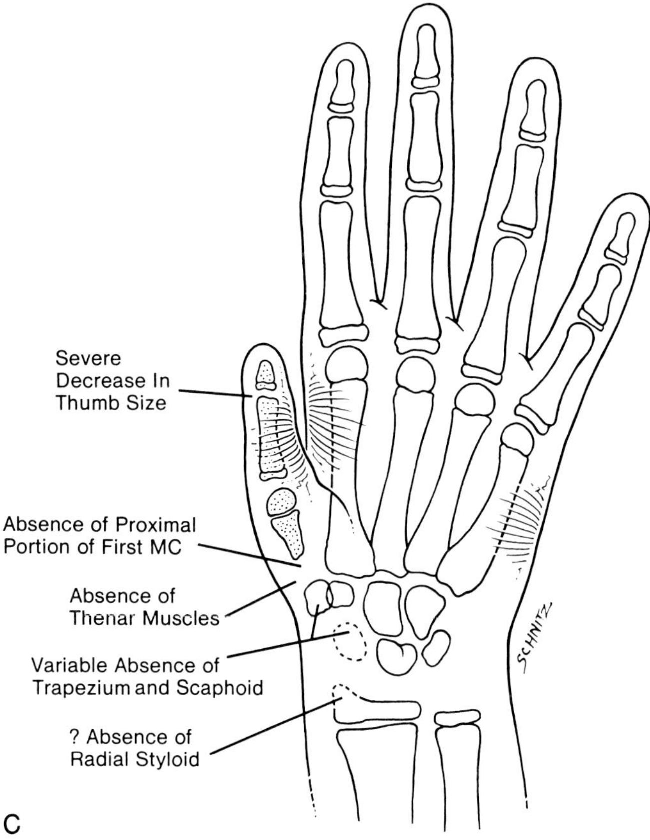

Fig. 57-7. Buck-Gramcko classification of thumb hypoplasia. **(A)** Grade I has an essentially complete complement of bones in the osteoarticular column; thenar and first web space musculature, and joint ranges of motion are normal; only the overall size of the thumb is diminished. **(B)** Grade II is manifest by an even smaller thumb stature than grade I, and either reduction of volume or complete absence of thenar muscles. Because of imbalance between thumb abductors and adductors, first web space contracture is common. The bones of the osteoarticular column are narrow, and instability of the ulnar collateral ligament of the metacarpophalangeal joint is common. Basilar thumb instability may also be found, although the radial carpus (scaphoid, trapezium, and trapezoid) is usually present. **(C)** Grade III is associated with severe first web space contracture secondary to a usually complete absence of thenar muscles. The thumb is short, and global instability of the metacarpophalangeal joint is common. Osseous and articular relationships at the thumb base are variable in their formation. *(Figure continues.)*

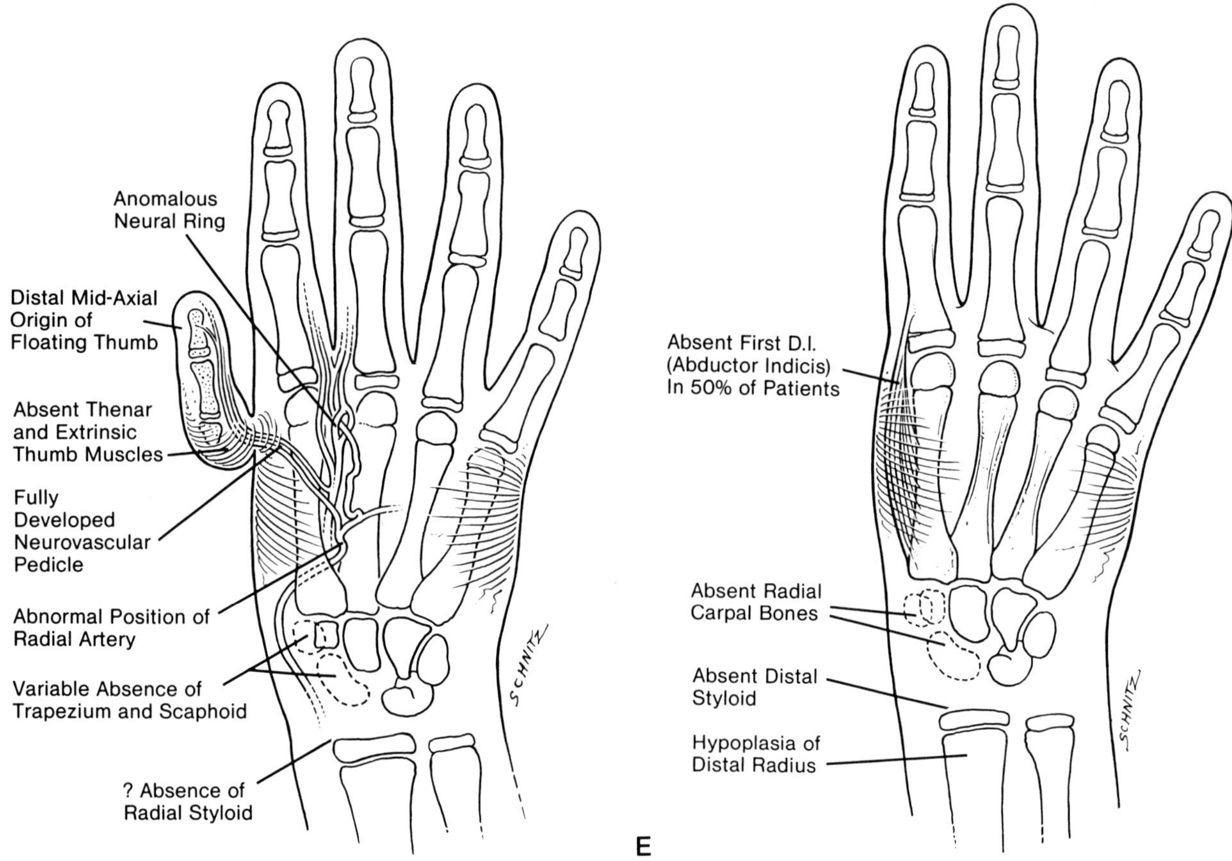

Fig. 57-7 *(Continued).* **(D)** Grade IV is the classic *pouce flottant* (floating thumb). At least one well-formed neurovascular pedicle can be found coursing through the pedicle; the origin of the pedicle is quite distal, along the radial midaxial line. All thenar and adductor thumb musculature is absent, except for the second metacarpal origin of the first dorsal interosseous (abductor indicis). The trapezium and scaphoid are usually absent; the trapezoid is often normal. **(E)** Grade V is complete congenital absence of the thumb (aplasia); even the abductor indicis is absent or deficient in more than 50 percent of cases. The index finger usually undergoes pulp broadening, digital pronation, and index-long finger web space widening, with progressive curvature of the index ray (see Fig. 57-2). These cases are ideal candidates for index finger pollicization.

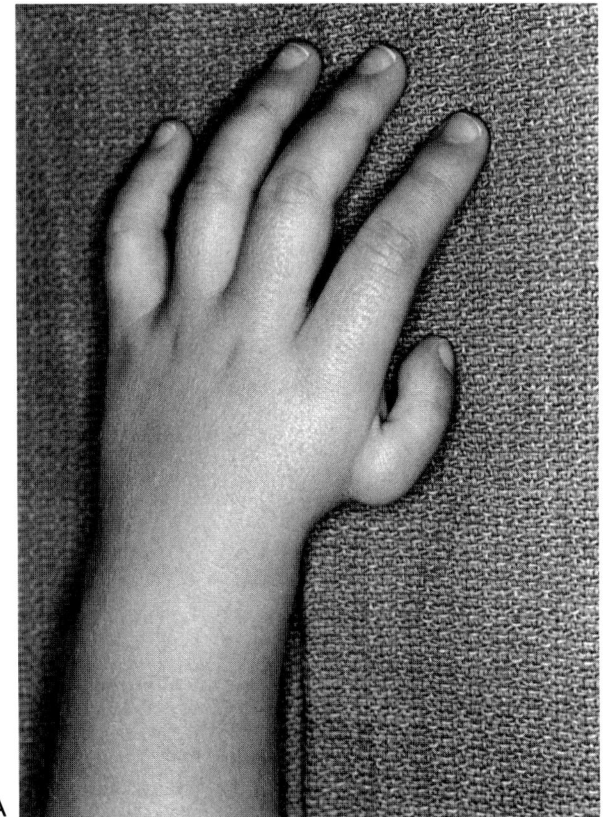

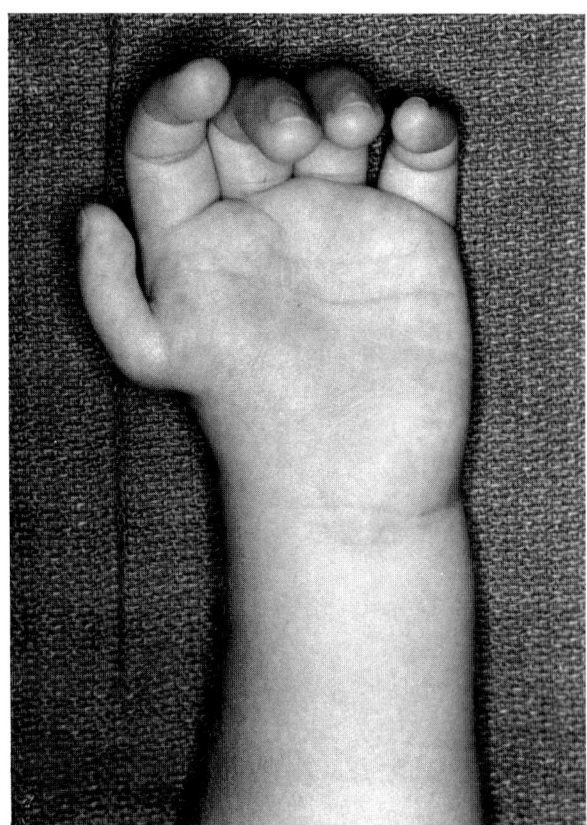

Fig. 57-8. **(A&B)** Absence of an osteoarticular foundation, and a distal/dorsal origin make functional reconstitution of the congenital *pouce flottant* difficult. To achieve prehension, the origin of the thumb unit must be surgically moved more palmar and proximal, and bone grafts used to create a stable base.

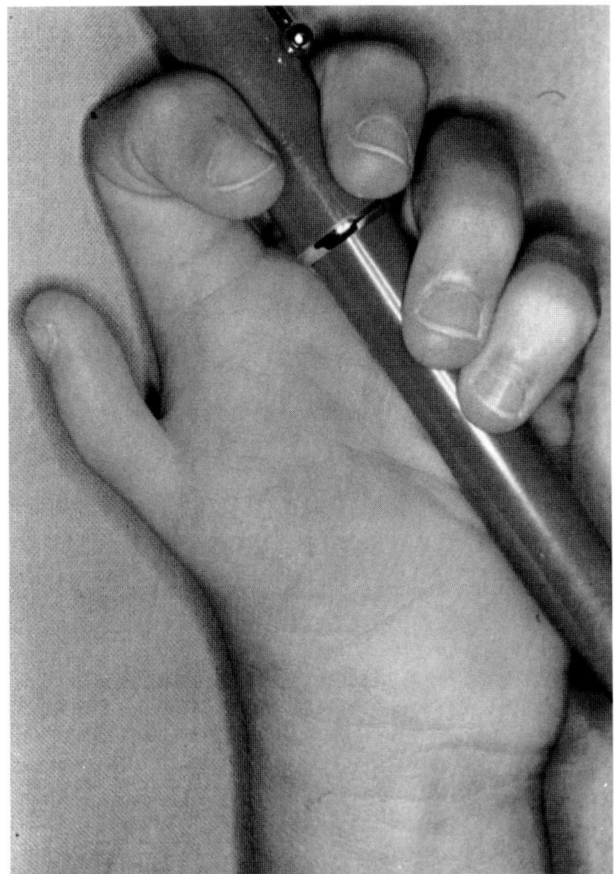

Fig. 57-9. Patients with severe thumb hypoplasia prefer the scissoring action of index-long abduction/adduction for pinch and minor grasp. Left untreated, even the "rich" hypoplastic thumb will frequently be bypassed because of its subnormal stability and mobility, and its reduced cerebrocortical representation.

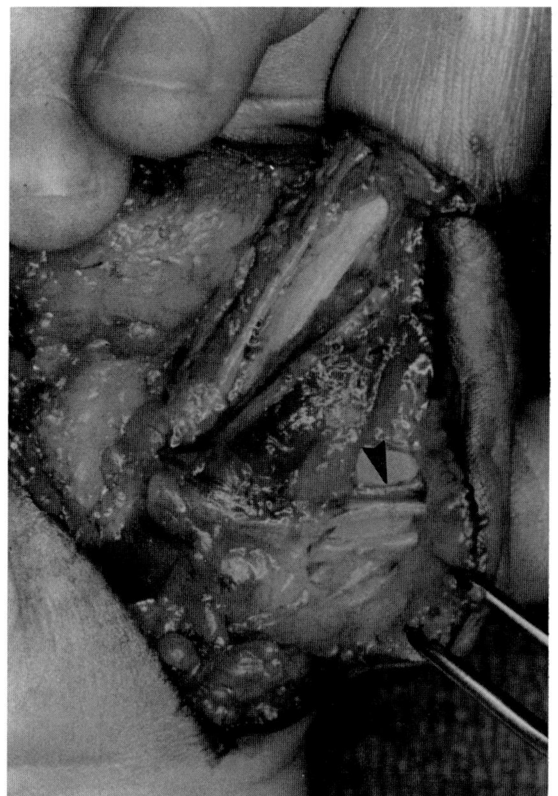

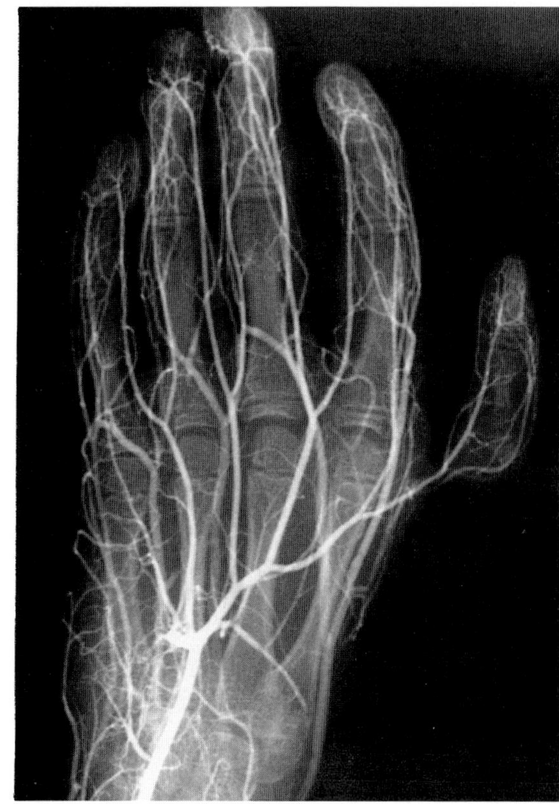

Fig. 57-10. **(A)** In spite of severe underdevelopment and gross instability, the narrow constricting pedicle of the *pouce flottant* has normal digital nerves and vessels; **(B)** arteriogram of a patient with grade IV hypoplasia demonstrates a single large uncompromised digital artery passing through its narrow base.

and proximal locus, ensuring stability by either autogenous corticocancellous iliac crest bone graft or longitudinal fibular strut. Each can be inserted between the base of the index metacarpal and the rudimentary proximal phalanx of the thumb. Concomitant reconstruction of a wide first webspace is obviously necessary. Tajima[125] has advocated the use of a large dorsal skin flap designed over the index metacarpal and proximal phalanx, which can be rotated with the floating thumb to create an acceptable first web; split-thickness skin graft is applied to the flap donor site.

Match[75] reported filleting open the floating unit at the time of pollicization and incorporating the skin of the deficient thumb into the new first web space (Fig. 57-11). Osseous stability in these grade IV hypoplastic thumbs can also be achieved using a free nonvascularized transfer of the MP joint of the fourth toe, potentially providing a degree of thumb mobility. Because of the importance of the five-fingered hand in Japanese culture, techniques oriented towards salvage and reconstruction of the congenital floating thumb have emanated principally from that country. Reconstruction is obviously a major surgical effort, involving efforts to stabilize the digit by bone graft or whole joint transfer, complex skin flaps and grafts, and three subsequent individual tendon transfers as potential balancing motors. Thumb extension can be achieved by transfer of the extensor indicis proprius (EIP); abduction and/or opposition by the Huber transfer[44] of the abductor digiti quinti (modified by Littler[59-61,64]); and flexion/adduction by direct transfer of the ring flexor digitorum superficialis (FDS IV).

The surgeon must realize that results of these reconstructions are disappointing at best. Poor joint development should be an absolute contraindication for tendon transfer. By definition, tendon excursion will be severely limited by poor joint mechanics, and the natural pattern of functional index-long finger scissoring will continue. The potential for index pollicization may also be lost by irreparable surgical damage to skin incurred during primary efforts to make the grade IV hypoplastic thumb functionally useful. None of White's[140] priorities for thumb reconstruction can be met; despite excellent sensibility, opposition cannot be effectively generated from a rigidly fixed thumb base. Pollicization of the index finger becomes a very attractive alternative.

While we are indebted to a great number of contributors over the past 50 years, our current method of pollicization in cases of Blauth[8] types IV and V thumb hypoplasia (*pouce flottant* and complete absence) are based on simple modifications of Buck-Gramcko's technique, suggested more than 20 years ago. Nevertheless, the profound and revolutionary contribu-

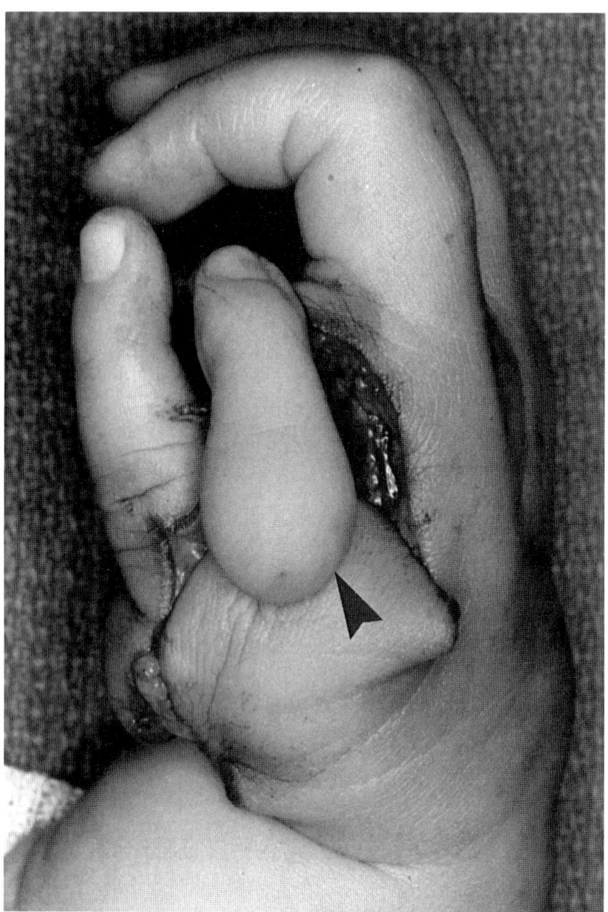

Fig. 57-11. A major contemporary principle of pollicization is construction of a scar-free, contracture-free first web space. If well-planned, the *pouce flottant* can be filleted and its skin effectively used in the process.[75]

tions to pollicization by Gossett, Littler, Zancolli, and Carroll, are worthy of the reader's understanding and appreciation.

Technique of Gosset (1949)

Originally described as a method for utilizing the index ray as a new thumb, Gosset based many of his pollicization principles on experience accumulated during and after World War II. The distal phalanx and nail of the index were first amputated to decrease the overall length of the new thumb. The index was then mobilized by circumscribing its base. A recipient oval skin ellipse, designed over the amputated thumb stump, was proportioned to receive the transferred index ray. The two oval skin incisions were then connected by a single dorsal curvilinear incision, elevated off the first web space, creating a palmar-pedicled commissural flap (Fig. 57-12A). The index finger was carried radially on its neurovascular pedicles (with venae comitantes). A segment of index metacarpal was removed, and the metacarpal head prepared as a slot. It could then be derotated and securely introduced into a reciprocal groove fashioned at the proximal base of the thumb metacarpal; rotation into an appropriate level of thumb pronation was thus assured (Fig. 57-12B & C). Since Gosset's pollicization technique was performed only for cases of traumatic thumb loss, the extensor pollicis longus and brevis could consistently be sutured to the index lateral band and central slip, respectively (Fig. 57-12D).

The principle of a palmar-based transposition flap, dorsally advanced over the path of the ray transfer, is a useful one. Unfortunately, primary closure of the large oval-shaped donor defect was difficult using Gosset's incisions. In spite of attractive drawings made to demonstrate the technique, postoperative web space contracture remained a significant problem (Fig. 57-12E).

Technique of Littler (1953)

Subsequent to his experience in World War II, Littler pointed out the functional inadequacies and cumbersome nature of many digital transposition techniques used to restore thumb function after partial or complete thumb amputation. In detailing the application of the neurovascular island pedicle principles for hand surgery, he emphasized the adequacy of a *single* digital artery and its venae comitantes in preserving circulation to and from the part being mobilized, and went on to suggest that the "probability of digital congestion is reduced if a dorsal vein can be preserved to aid the venous return." He also clearly recognized that although ligating one of the digital arteries to a normal index finger would reduce inflow volume by half (reducing the propensity for venous congestion), the chance of thrombosis of the single remaining artery represented too much risk to the system; he therefore encouraged the employment of *both* neurovascular pedicles during the procedure (Fig. 57-13).

Littler's utilization of the surgical principles of neurovascular island pedicles paved the way to more aggressive skin incisions for pollicizations, which allowed the first web space to remain essentially scar-free (Fig. 57-14A & B and Fig. 57-15A–D). Abduction of the new thumb osteoarticular column was by first dorsal interosseous transfer to the radial border of the index proximal phalanx; the oblique and transverse heads of the adductor pollicis (proximal to the level of injury) would continue to adduct the new thumb. The first palmar interosseous was excised, and the extensor pollicis longus (EPL) sutured under appropriate tension to the distal stump of the extensor digitorum communis (EDC) of the index (Fig. 57-15E). The proximal extensor indicis proprius was woven into the ulnar lateral band, as suggested earlier in France by Gosset (see Fig. 57-12D).

Littler recommended that the power and independence of thumb flexion be enhanced at a later stage by resecting a portion of the flexor digitorum superficialis in the distal forearm, and transferring the flexor pollicis longus at its musculotendinous junction to the index flexor digitorum profundus through the same incision (Fig. 57-15F).

While innovative, and employing a great number of surgical principles still used regularly today, the technique was more appropriate for reconstruction of the thumb following traumatic loss than for congenital absence.

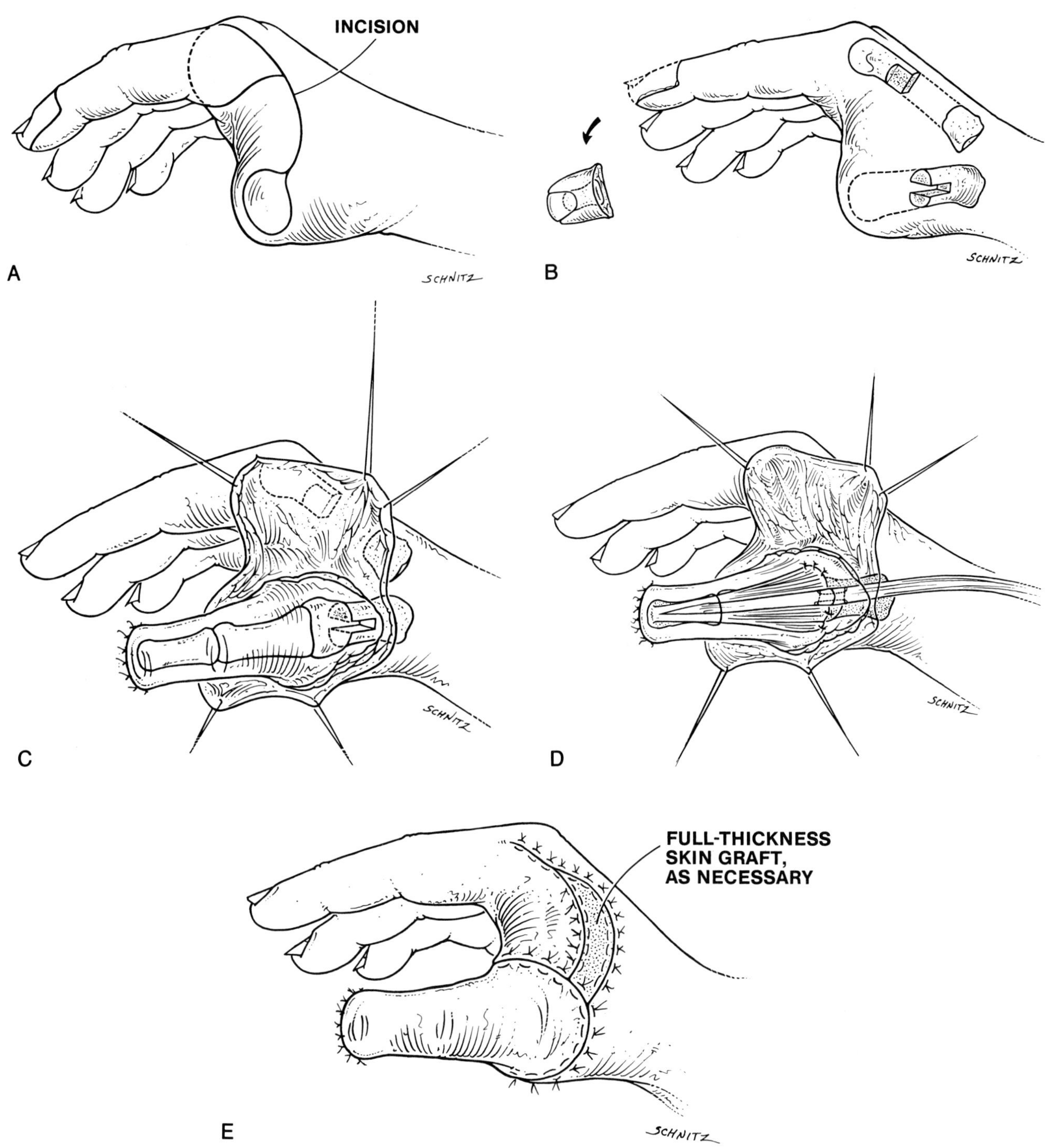

Fig. 57-12. Gosset's technique of pollicization of the index finger: **(A)** The incision created a recipient site for the shortened index finger donor, and established a palmar-pedicle flap for the first web space. **(B)** The nail, nail bed, and distal phalanx were amputated, and resection of the proximal index metacarpal allowed shortening and derotation. **(C)** The base of the retained distal index metacarpal was "slotted" into the base of the thumb metacarpal. **(D)** The pollicized index was motored by EPL transfer to the ulnar lateral band, and EPB into the central slip, because of their consistent availability (see text); **(E)** final closure of the defect with a full-thickness skin graft. Unfortunately, first web space contracture remained a problem using Gosset's technique.

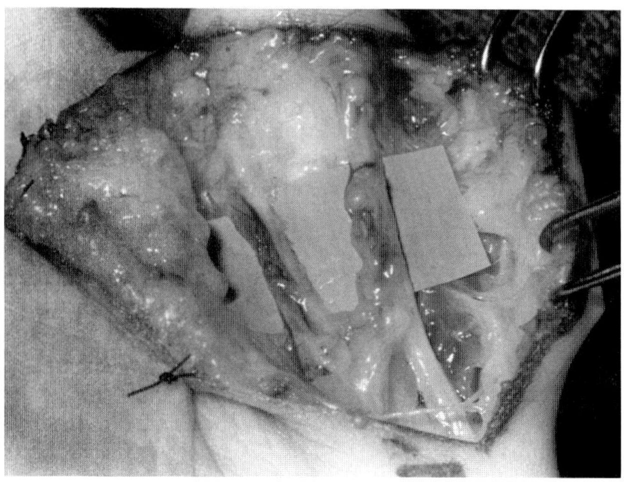

Fig. 57-13. The "standard" use of both neurovascular pedicles of the digit to be pollicized was strongly advocated by Littler[59-61,64] as a means of reducing the risk of thrombosis of a single artery.

Technique of Zancolli (1960)

The first clear separation of problems inherent in thumb reconstruction following trauma and those of congenital failure of formation was made by Zancolli in a short paper in which a single case was presented with a 2-year follow-up. At the time of its publication the technique was considered quite innovative; it is still successfully used in parts of South America and elsewhere 30 years later.

The technique places the first webspace at the level of the PIP joint of the index finger, avoiding an over-lengthened appearance (Fig. 57-16A & B). The head of the index finger metacarpal (separated from its parent bone at the appropriate length), was internally fixed to the trapezoid area of the carpus by percutaneous K-wires (Fig. 57-16C). The appropriate tension and vector of the first dorsal interosseous (once transposition and shortening of the index finger on its neurovascular pedicles had been performed) was established by recessing its entire proximal origin, and transferring it across the proximal palm to the hypothenar fascia on the ulnar border of the hand. This maneuver was performed through a subcutaneous palmar tunnel, leaving the nerve and vascular supply to the muscle intact (Fig. 57-16D).

Zancolli recognized early postoperative redundancy of the relatively lengthened flexors digitorum profundus and superficialis, but recommended that these tendons *not* be shortened; he claimed that the claw deformity "disappeared as these muscles adapted to their new position"[141] (Fig. 57-16E).

Technique of Carroll (1988)

During his 40 years of practice, Carroll treated a large number of congenital anomalies of the upper extremity, and he performed many pollicizations for congenital thumb absence. Skin flaps using his technique were designed to allow mobilization of the donor digit (usually the index finger) on whatever neurovascular pedicle was available. Carroll advocated preoperative arteriography under general anesthesia for evaluation of any potential deficiency of the arterial blood supply, often

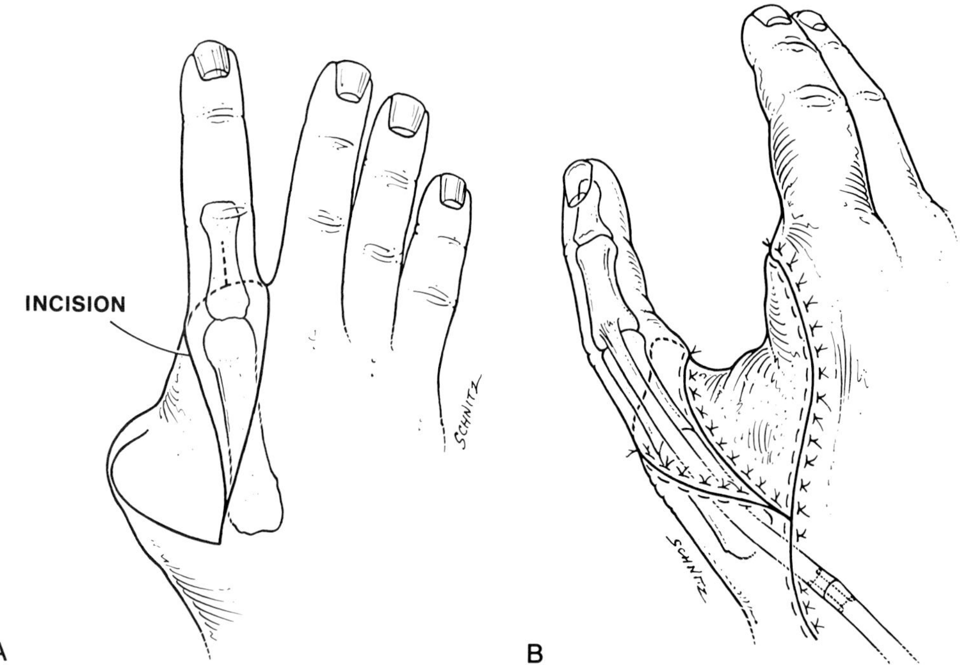

Fig. 57-14. **(A&B)** Transfering the pollicized index finger on long neurovascular pedicles allowed more aggressive skin flaps to be designed; these flaps were specifically fashioned to reduce the propensity for first web scarring, seen prior to this early flap design by Littler (Type I).

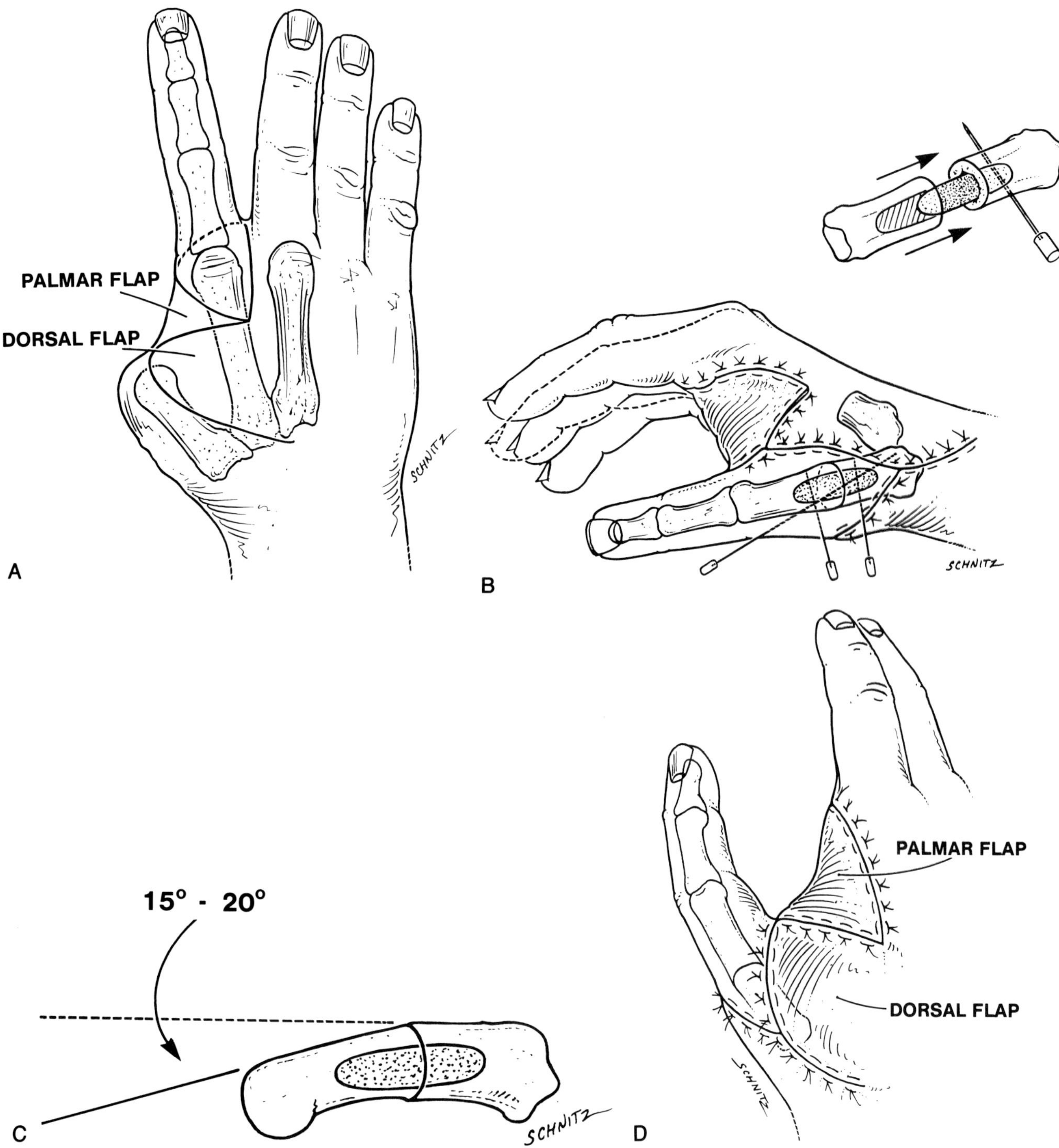

Fig. 57-15. **(A–F)** Littler's pollicization technique. **(A)** The traditional Littler index finger pollicization for traumatic thumb amputation separates Gosset's palmar-based flap into two smaller, but safer flaps: one palmar and one dorsal-based. **(B)** Shortening is achieved by resection of the entire index metacarpal and distal half of the thumb metacarpal, and spares the nail and terminal phalanx (removed in Gosset's original technique). **(C)** A corticocancellous dowel graft can be used to unite the base of the index proximal phalanx and the base of the thumb metacarpal, allowing rotation of the index into a position of 120 degrees pronation and 10 to 15 degrees flexion. Percutaneous K-wires can be used to temporarily secure the graft until union takes place. **(D)** Advancement of the palmar and dorsal flaps into their final position minimizes scarring and contracture in the new first web space between the index and long fingers. *(Figure continues.)*

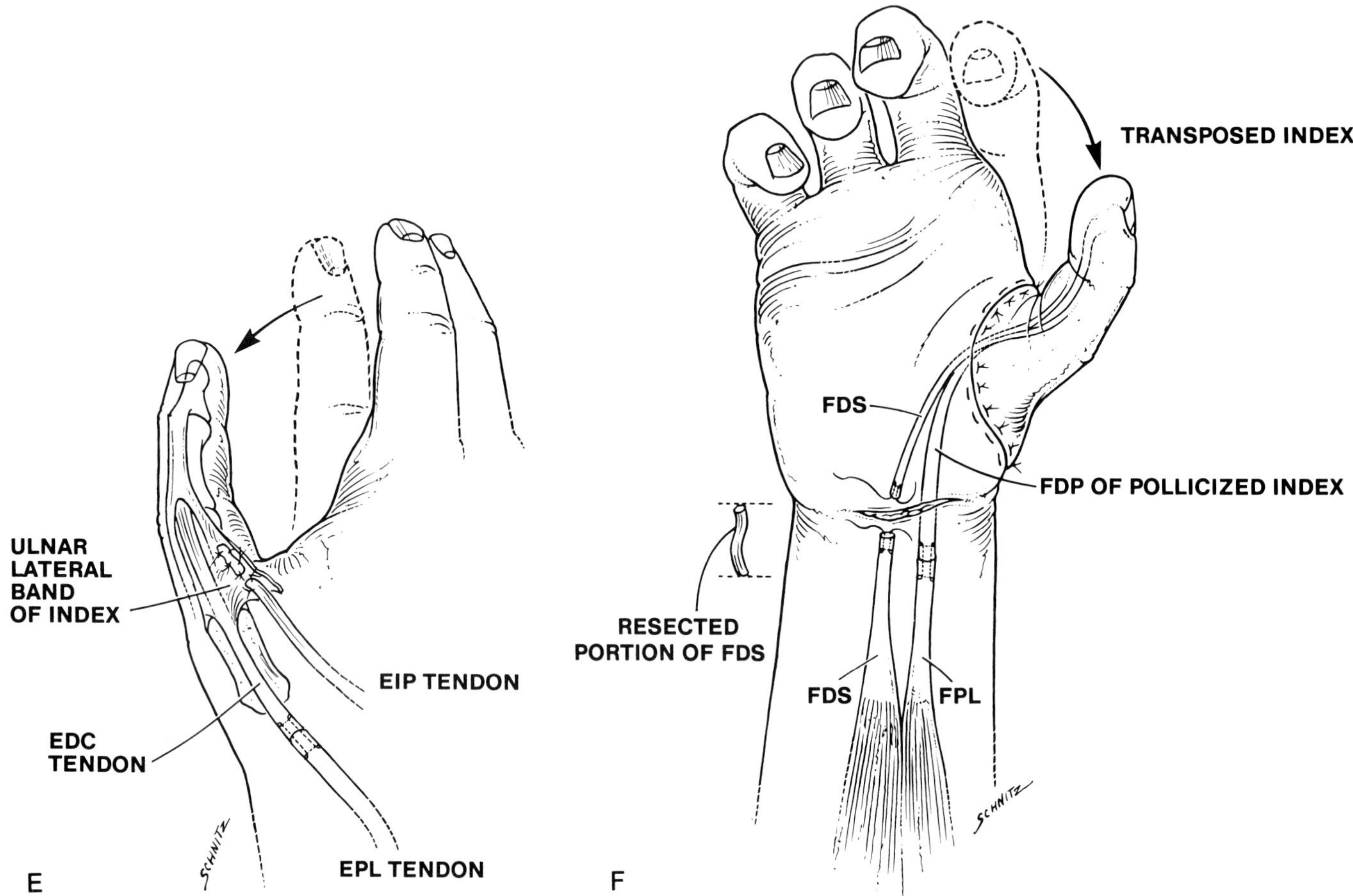

Fig. 57-15 *(Continued).* **(E)** Motoring is achieved by transfer of EIP to the ulnar lateral band (as suggested by Gosset), the EPL to the EDC of the index, and the first dorsal interosseous to the radial border of the index proximal phalanx. The intact oblique and transverse heads of the adductor pollicis continue to adduct the new thumb. **(F)** Flexor power can according to Littler be enhanced at a later stage by shortening FDS of index, and transferring FPL to the index FDP. This entire procedure can be performed through a single small incision at the wrist.

seen in cases of congenital limb deficiency. Once the index pedicle was mobilized, palmar-radial flaps were designed to be transposed distal and dorsal along the radial border of the long finger, covering the donor defect and (theoretically) creating a new first web space (Fig. 57-17A & E). While sound in principle, the first web space was infrequently "scar-free," and contractures sometimes resulted.

Shortening and repositioning of the index osteoarticular column was performed by resecting the majority of its metacarpal diaphysis, and introducing the head directly into the metacarpal base, securely holding it 120 to 140 degrees pronated with percutaneous K-wires (Fig. 57-17B & C). The technique involved shortening the digital extensors a length equal to the amount of the resected metacarpal; shortening of the digital flexors was unnecessary, and "no attempt [was] made to save the action of the lumbrical." [20]

The tendons of insertion of the first palmar and (when present) first dorsal interossei were detached from the base of the index proximal phalanx, and reattached to the index middle phalanx, serving as adductor and abductor of the new thumb, respectively. Carroll suggested that all bone and muscle work be performed first, through the dorsal incision, prior to identification and dissection of the neurovascular pedicles (Fig. 57-17B & D). Transferring the interossei to the index lateral bands was found to be unnecessary; Carroll claimed that extension of the new thumb had "not been a problem." [20]

Authors' Preferred Technique of Pollicization for Congenital Absence of the Thumb (Modified from Buck-Gramcko, 1971)[54]

Many authors have contributed their ideas to the development of sound surgical principles for the creation of a grasping, pinching thumb from a medial digit of less importance. Some contributions have been more applicable to pollicization for traumatic thumb loss, while others have been more appropriately directed towards congenital thumb absence.

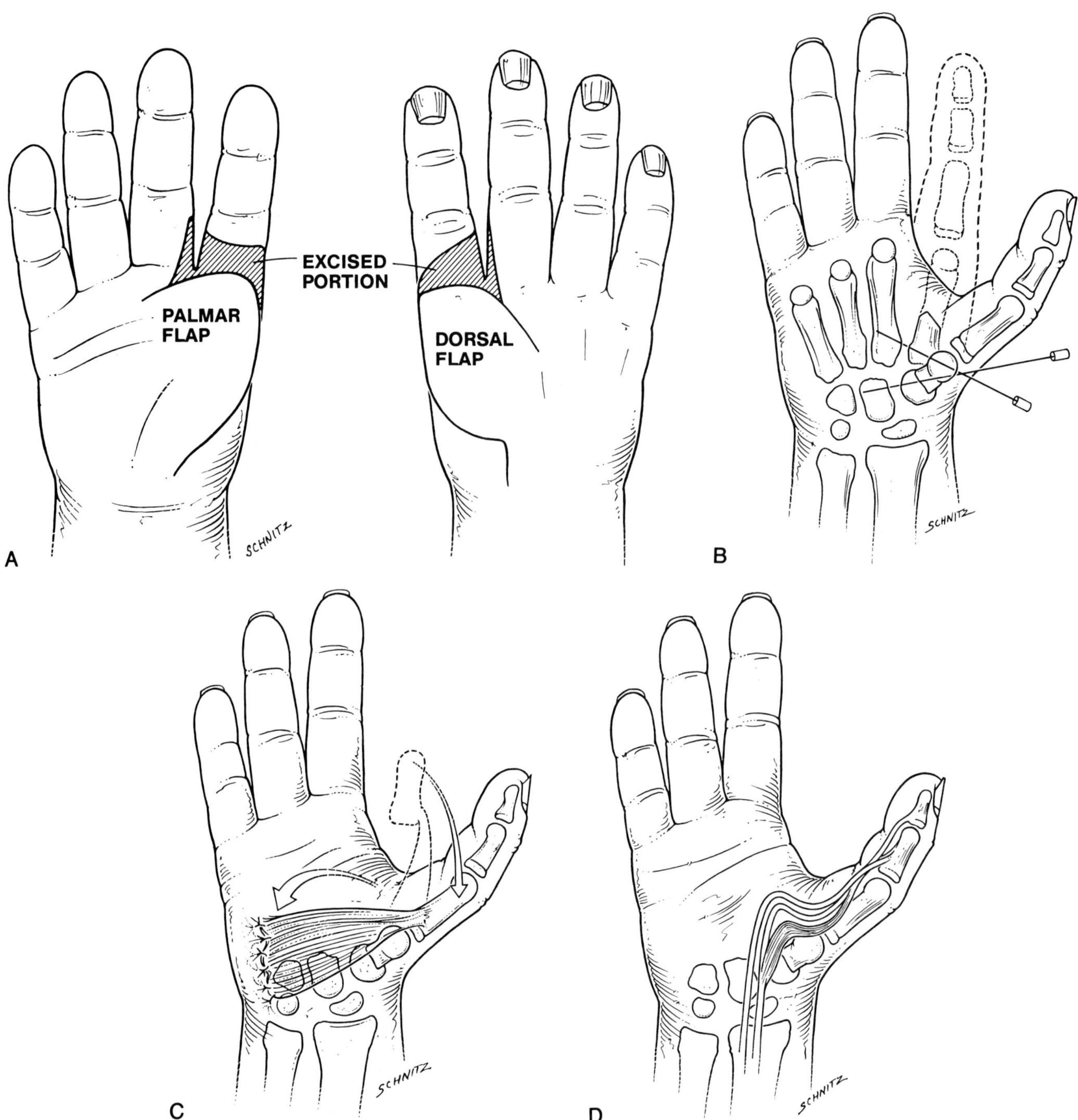

Fig. 57-16. **(A–D)** Zancolli's pollicization technique. Zancolli was the first to publish a technique of pollicization for the *congenitally* absent thumb. **(A)** Incisions involved excision of the area of skin diagrammed, and the creation of broad-based palmar and dorsal flaps; **(B)** The transposed, shortened index finger was anchored to the recipient base of the index osteoarticular column (trapezoid) by percutaneous K-wires; **(C)** The *origin* of the first dorsal interosseous was then transposed across the palm to the hypothenar fascia. **(D)** Redundancy of the extrinsic flexor tendons of the pollicized index finger and the "claw deformity" were left by Zancolli to "disappear as these muscles adapted to their new position."[141]

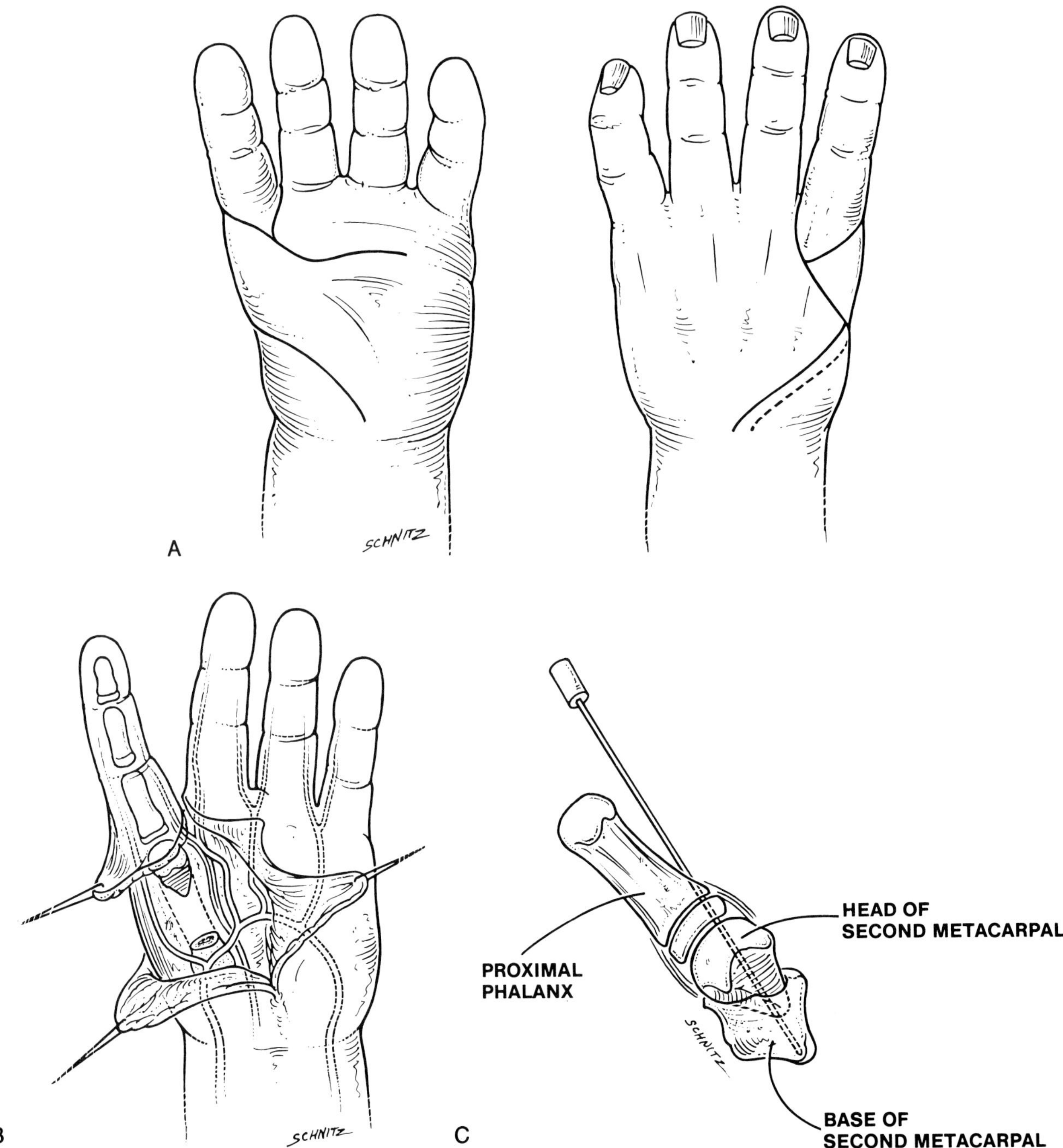

Fig. 57-17. **(A–E)** Carroll's pollicization technique.[20] **(A)** Incisions designed by Carroll for congenital pollicization were intended to result in a relatively contracture-free first web space. **(B)** Carroll recommended that all bone and muscle dissection be performed dorsally first, including resection of the diaphysis of the index finger metacarpal. **(C)** Percutaneous fixation of the contoured metacarpal head to its base was by a single K-wire, often through the entire length of the transposed ray. *(Figure continues.)*

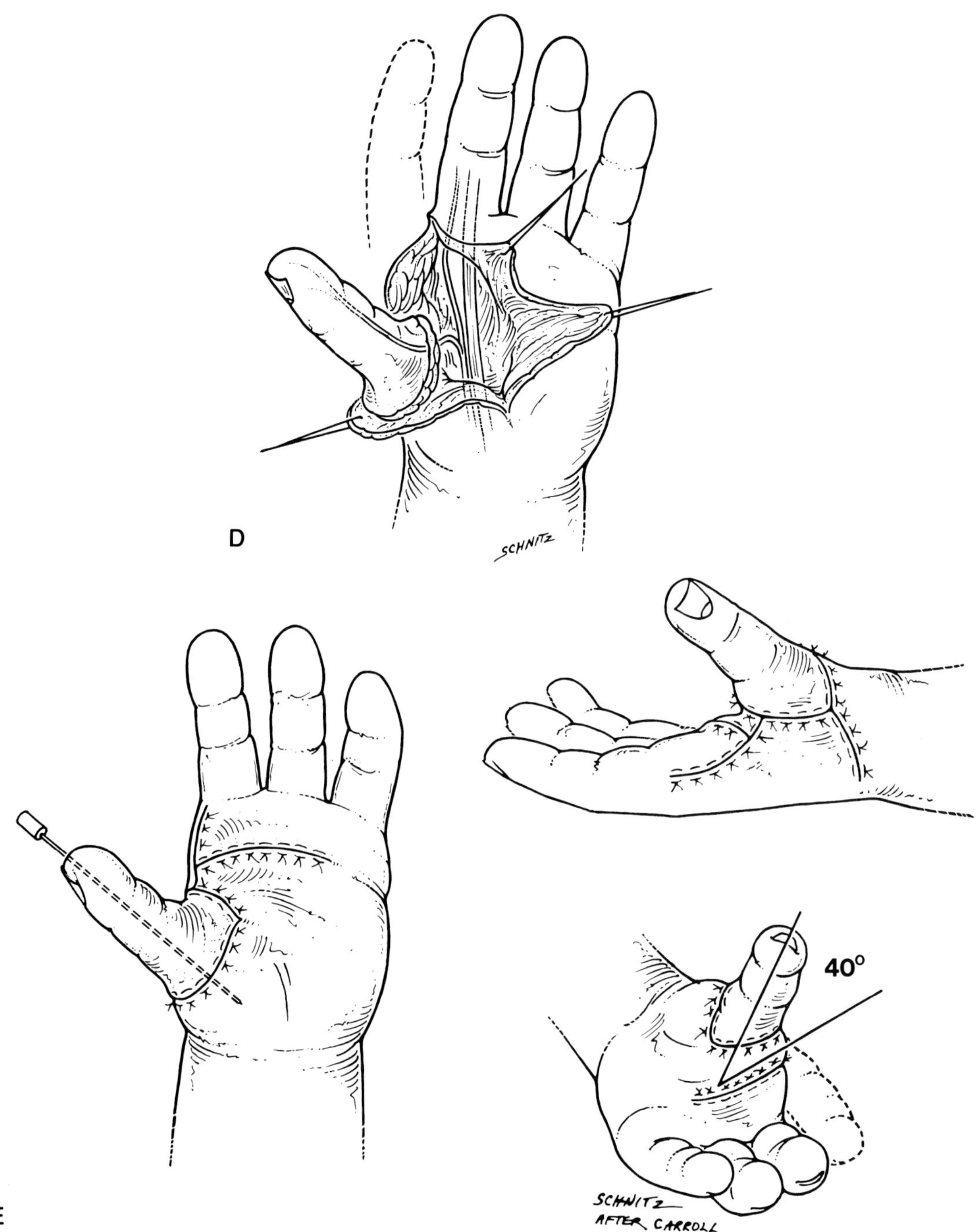

Fig. 57-17 *(Continued).* **(D)** The final position of the pollicized distal index finger ray, stabilized by internal fixation. Carroll believed that transfer of the interossei to the lateral bands was unnecessary and extension of the new thumb was "not a problem."[20] **(E)** Closure of the skin flaps using the Carroll technique of pollicization was felt to provide a contracture-free first web space, although scarring remained problematic in some cases.

Buck-Gramcko's unparalleled experience in congenital reconstruction following the European thalidomide tragedy (see p. 2053) gave him the opportunity to combine the most advantageous principles of previous surgeons' work. Adding his own unique ideas, he was able to create and test what we consider to be the most appropriate technique for index finger pollicization. While fundamentally straightforward and logical, the approach is highly demanding technically. It is wrought with potential complications ranging from weakness and instability of the osteoarticular column, to necrosis of the entire pollicized digit.

Skin Incisions

Of the many technical challenges associated with pollicization, reconstruction of a scar-free first web space remains one of the most demanding. The skin incisions we prefer are basically those of Buck-Gramcko, but are more detailed to ensure greater reliability. If followed precisely, the new thumb will—in essence—have a scar-free first web space, and not require any supplementary skin graft (Fig. 57-18A & B).

The incision begins at the proximal digital crease of the index finger, extending from the radial border of the index-long commissural base to the radial mid-lateral border of the digit. From these two points the incision sweeps dorsal and proximal, converging at a 70-degree angle to a point at the middorsal level of the metacarpal head. Great care must be taken to incise just the skin, avoiding injury to underlying palmar neurovascular structures and dorsal veins. Beginning at a point one-third from the dorsal apex to the radial midlateral line, an antegrade longitudinal incision is made, extending to the index proximal IP joint. This incision allows development of flaps that will create a scar-free first webspace. The two dorsal digital flaps (Fig. 57-19, points A & B) will be elevated, creating a wide separation into which redundant dorsoradial recipient skin can be inset after appropriate contouring at the end of the procedure.

The palmar incision is curvilinear and made in retrograde fashion, extending from the midpoint of the digital crease incision to the distal wrist crease (Fig. 57-19, point A′). The proximal portion is concave radially, establishing the medial border of the recipient site into which the new thumb will be inset (Fig. 57-19, point C to C′).

Neurovascular Dissection

Unlike Carroll's approach to congenital pollicization,[20] we prefer to perform the palmar dissection first (Fig. 57-20A–C), immediately after precise skin incisions have been made. The historic principles of neurovascular island flap-preparation, discussed earlier in this chapter, are employed: in *most* cases of congenital thumb absence, *"pouce flottant,"* or radial club hand with severe thumb involvement, both the radial and ulnar index neurovascular bundles to the index finger will be

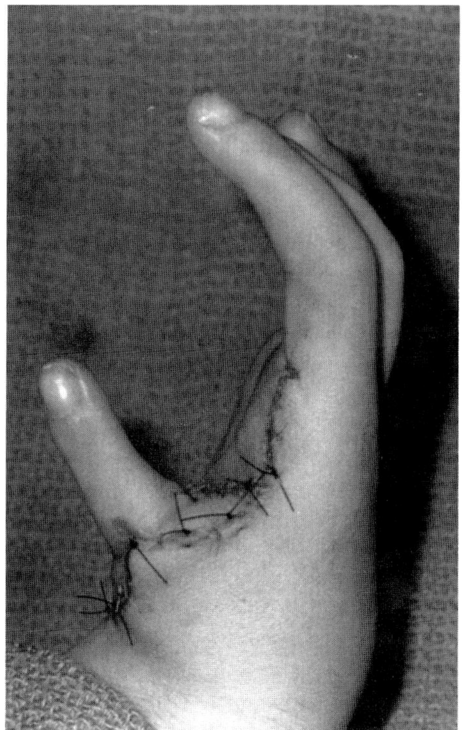
A

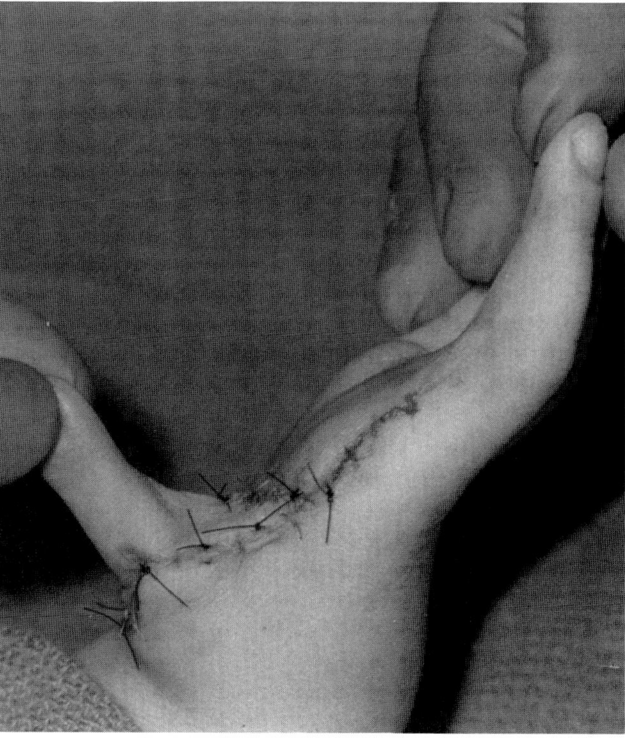
B

Fig. 57-18. **(A&B)** Many surgical designs for skin flaps have been proposed for pollicization over the past half-century. The technique of Buck-Gramcko[13] provides the least propensity for contracture of the first web space, and the fewest incisions transgressing this critical area. These photographs clearly demonstrate both thumb stability and passive extensibility of the Buck-Gramcko-design first web space reconstruction immediately after the operation.

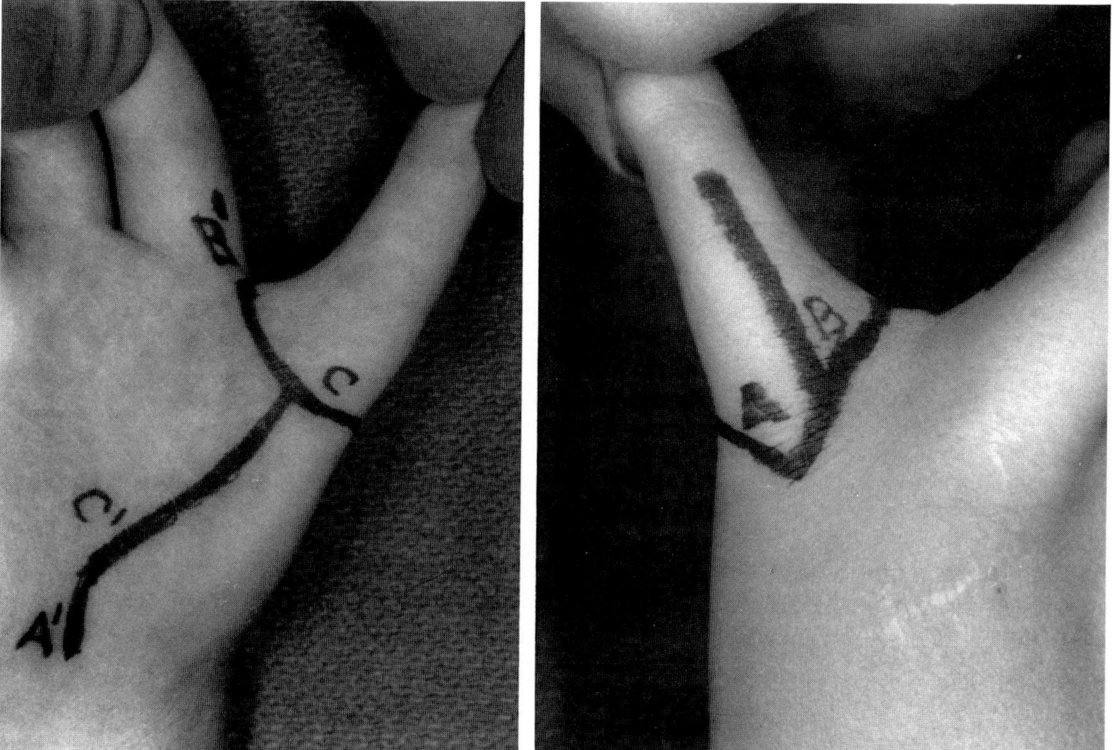

A B

Fig. 57-19. **(A&B)** Buck-Gramcko's incisions. Accurate placement of skin incisions insures the quality of the first web space after the Buck-Gramcko pollicization. The proximal limb of the palmar incision is concave radially (between *A′* and *C′*) to allow the transposed digit to rotate directly into the recipient defect. The index finger circumferential incision is along the proximal digital crease palmarly, and chevron-shaped dorsally (the chevron apex is over the index metacarpal *A*). The antegrade longitudinal incision at *B* starts equidistant between point A and the commissure, and continues distally to the index PIP joint.

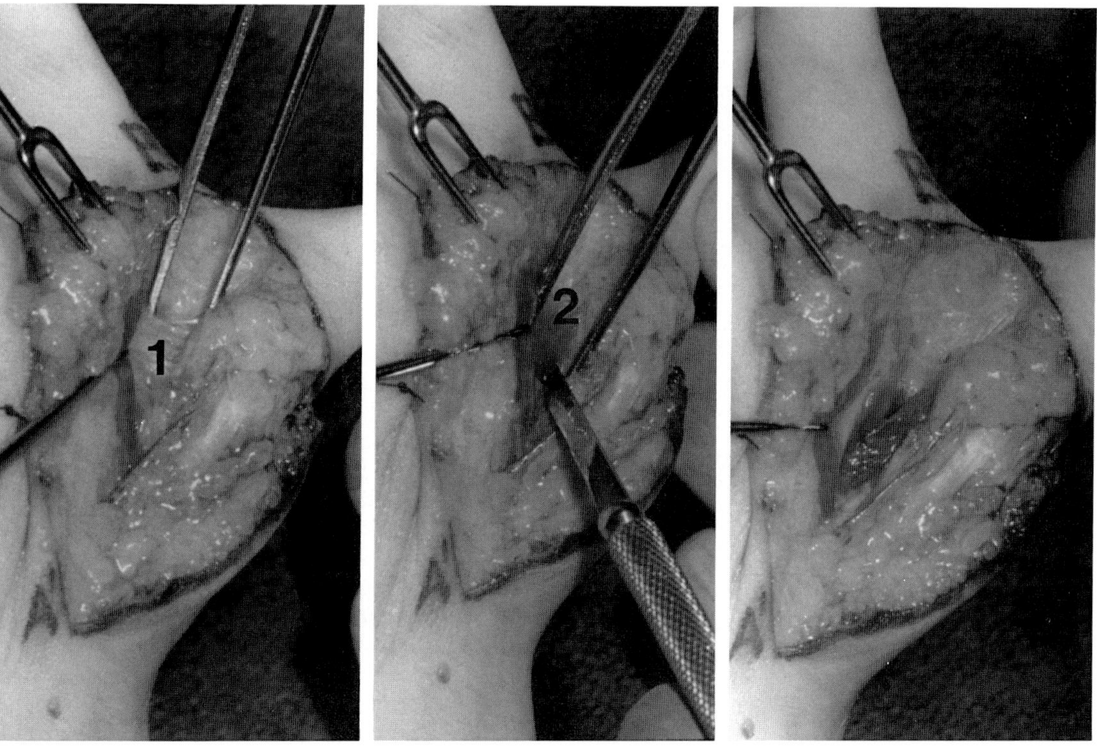

Fig. 57-20. Our preferred approach to congenital pollicization is to perform the palmar dissection first. Once skin incisions have been made and the neurovascular bundles isolated, the lumbrical to the long finger is retracted ulnarward, and the deep transverse metacarpal ligament between index and long fingers *(1)* is transected. *(2)* This maneuver exposes the first palmar and second dorsal interosseous muscles; the former will be used as the adductor of the new thumb.

available for dissection and incorporation into the new thumb circulation. The bifurcation of the common digital artery to the radial border of the long finger is cross-clamped and ligated, enabling the entire common digital vessel to the index-middle web to remain with the index finger (Fig. 57-21). The common digital nerve accompanying this vessel must then be dissected proximally into the two components supplying adjacent borders of the index-long web. This technique enables the index ray to be necessarily shortened without tension on the digital nerves. As Edgerton, et al[25] have pointed out, presence of an anomalous neural ring around the common digital vessel requires even more careful proximal and distal nerve dissection to avoid vessel-kinking with digital shortening.

Both neurovascular bundles are carefully mobilized from the proximal digital crease to the proximal palm, incorporating venae comitantes and as much perivascular fat as possible (see Fig. 57-13). Loupe magnification of 4.0 to 4.5X is critical for precise dissection. While we believe that it *is technically possible* to perform a pollicization relying solely on venous outflow through the venae comitantes, this practice should be discouraged. We concur with Littler, Buck-Gramcko, Carroll, and others, that at least one major dorsal vein should be preserved throughout the case (Fig. 57-22A & B), assuring adequate venous drainage from a new thumb supplied by two arteries. Fortunately, at least one major vein is available during dissection of the index finger.

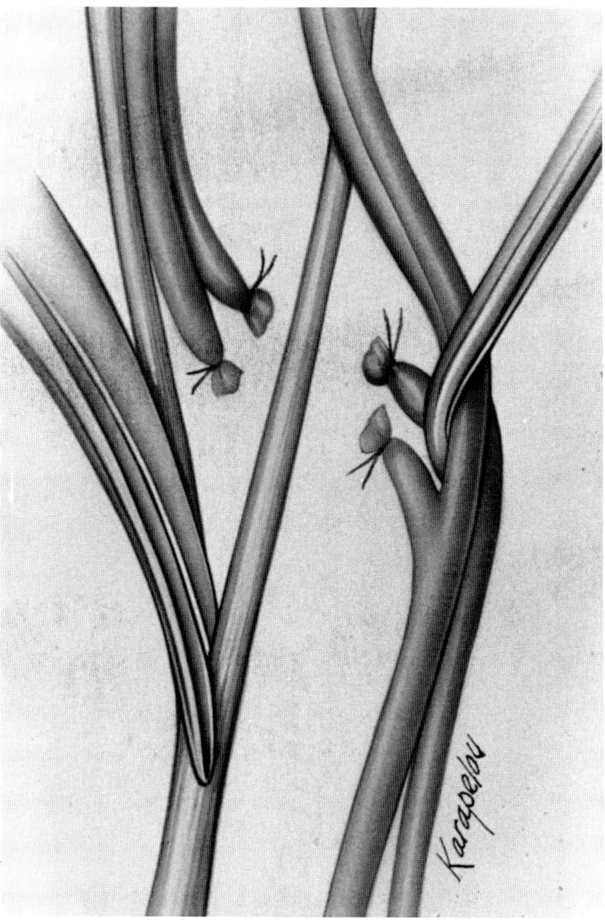

Fig. 57-21. Cross-clamping and ligating the long finger branch of the index-long common digital artery allows the entire common digital vessel to the index-long web space to be carried with the pollicized digit. Recommended strongly by Littler,[60] the technique of pollicizing the index finger on *two* arteries and their venae comitantes reduces the risks of vascular compromise. Note also *longitudinal* division of the common digital nerve done very carefully either with scissors as shown here or with a fine scapel blade.

Metacarpal Shortening, Rotation and Fixation

Good surgical judgment and experience are required to decide on an appropriate length of the new thumb: how much index metacarpal should be resected? We prefer a shorter pollicization to a longer one; the ideal length should bring the distal end of the pollicized index to the middle digital crease of the long finger when the new thumb is adducted. If the index finger to be pollicized is of normal length, we recommend a subcapital resection of the entire metacarpal through the epiphyseal plate (Fig. 57-23A–C). In this manner the MP joint can be preserved, the proximal phalanx hyperextended on the metacarpal head, and the head secured to the cartilaginous mass at the base of the resected index metacarpal. This technique was designed by Buck-Gramcko to eliminate the propensity towards unstable hyperextension of the pollicized digit,[13] often observed if the head is keyed into the metacarpal base directly (see Gosset's technique on page 2054). Hyperextending the proximal phalanx on the metacarpal head before seating the entire ray is a critical part of the procedure, and must be carefully performed (Fig. 57-24A & B). Two sutures of 3–0 braided nylon are placed through the hyperextended metacarpal head along the radial and ulnar collateral ligament borders. These sutures are then passed through the distal carpus to loosely align the new thumb in a pronated posture approximately 160 degrees relative to the plane of the palm. It is not necessary to anchor this relationship securely. The sutures establish only the proper height and position of the new thumb (Fig. 57-25); stability and final resting posture are controlled by carefully setting the tension on all tendon transfers to the new thumb, resulting in 40 degrees abduction, 15 degrees extension, and 120 degrees pronation of the metacarpal (see below). Fibrous ankylosis of the metacarpal head to its new surroundings will occur spontaneously during the early postoperative period (see Postoperative Management).

In spite of Carroll's and others' experience to the contrary, we believe that the metacarpal head of the index finger should be hyperextended prior to its attachment to the radial aspect of the carpus, as described by Buck-Gramcko. Techniques of pollicization that simply shorten the metacarpal by diaphyseal resection, pronating the distal end prior to K-wire fixation (see descriptions above), leave the index MP joint with a physiologic propensity towards hyperextension. While not functionally compromising per se, we find this posture to be aesthetically displeasing, and recommend taking the technical pains to eliminate hyperextensibility inherent in the index MP joint by extending the metacarpal head before suturing it in place against the carpus. This technique simply shifts the index

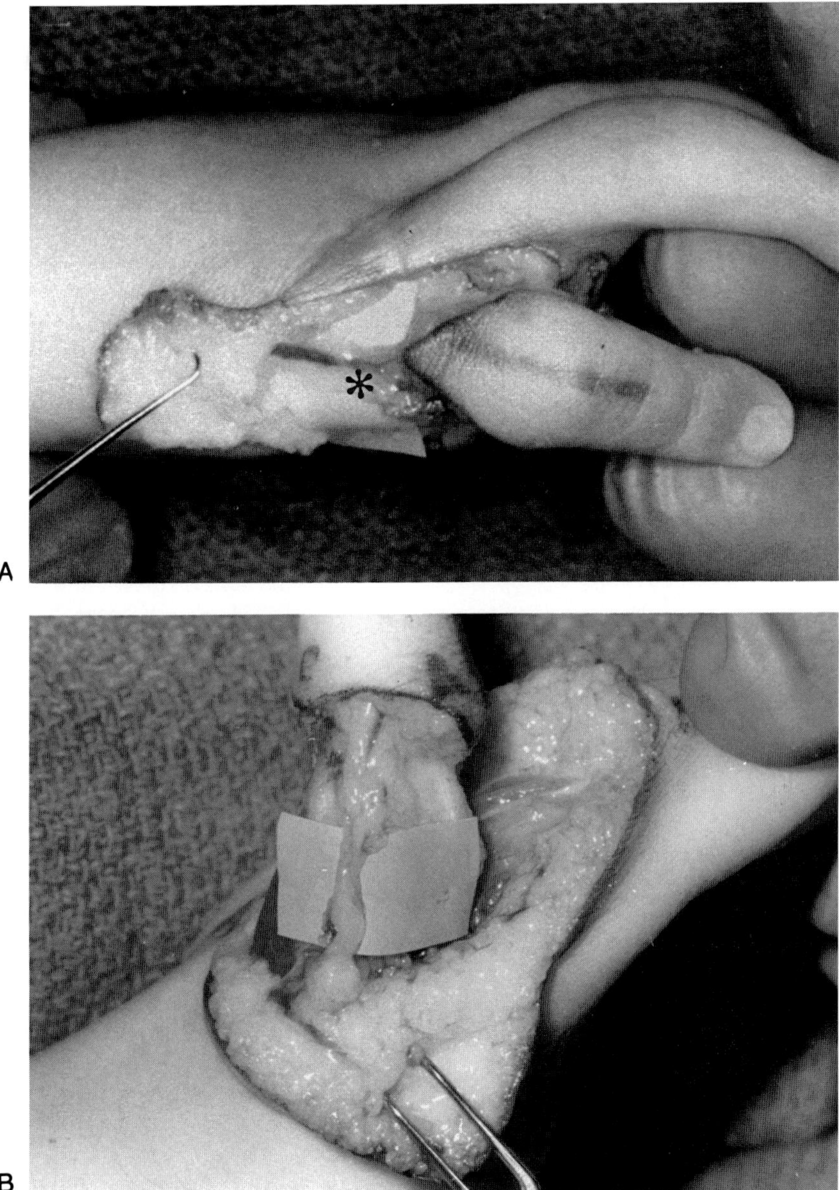

Fig. 57-22. (A&B) Two different cases of index finger pollicization for congenital thumb absence clearly demonstrate the technique and stress the importance of preserving at least one major dorsal vein to facilitate vascular outflow. We discourage sole reliance on the venae comitantes of the digital arteries for outflow. *, main dorsal vein.

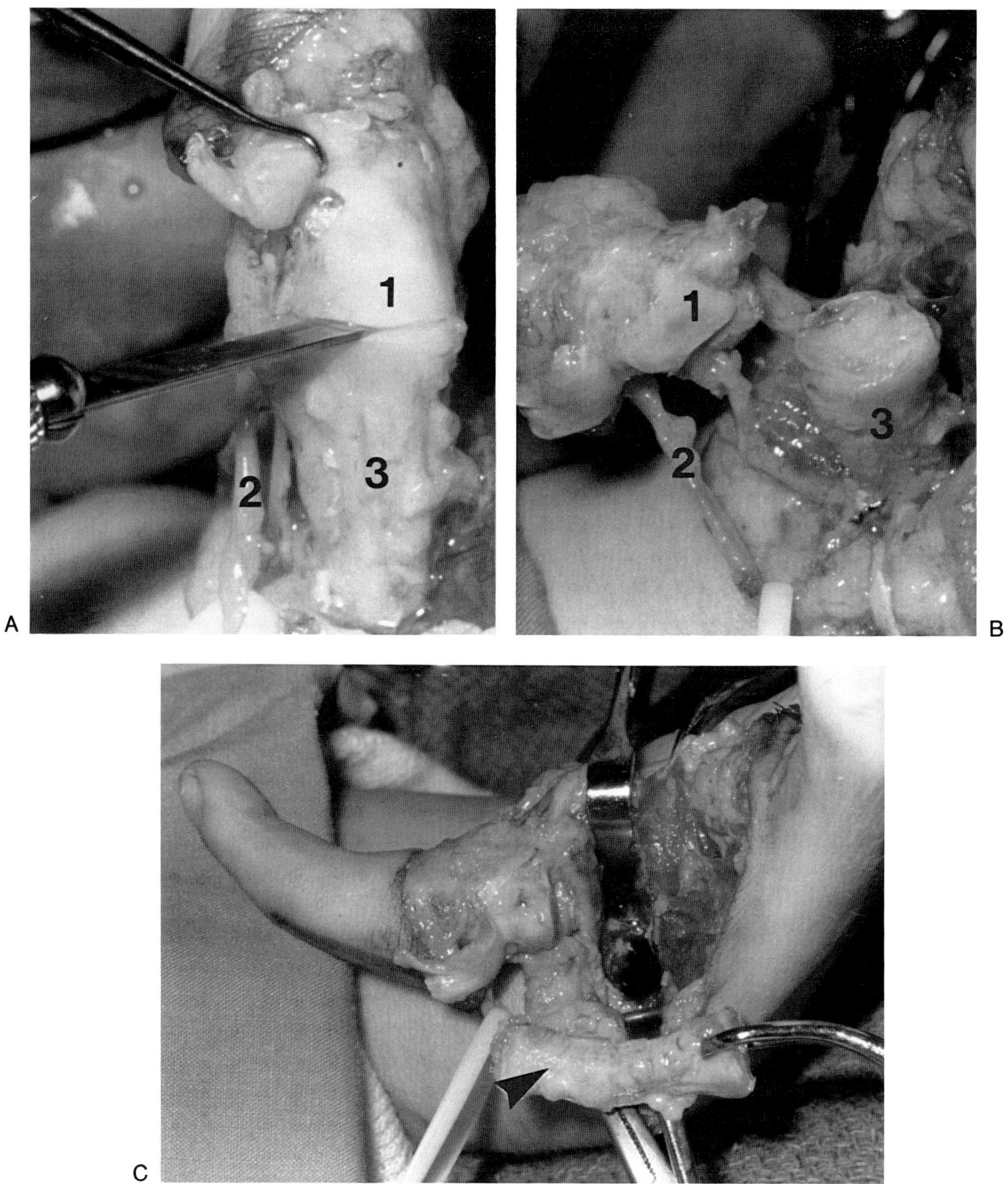

Fig. 57-23. **(A&B)** The index metacarpal *(3)* being separated from its head *(1)* by subcapital resection through the epiphyseal plate [for reference, the radial neurovascular bundle is indicated by *(2)*]. The arrow in **(C)** points to the segment of metacarpal removed when the index finger is of normal length preoperatively.

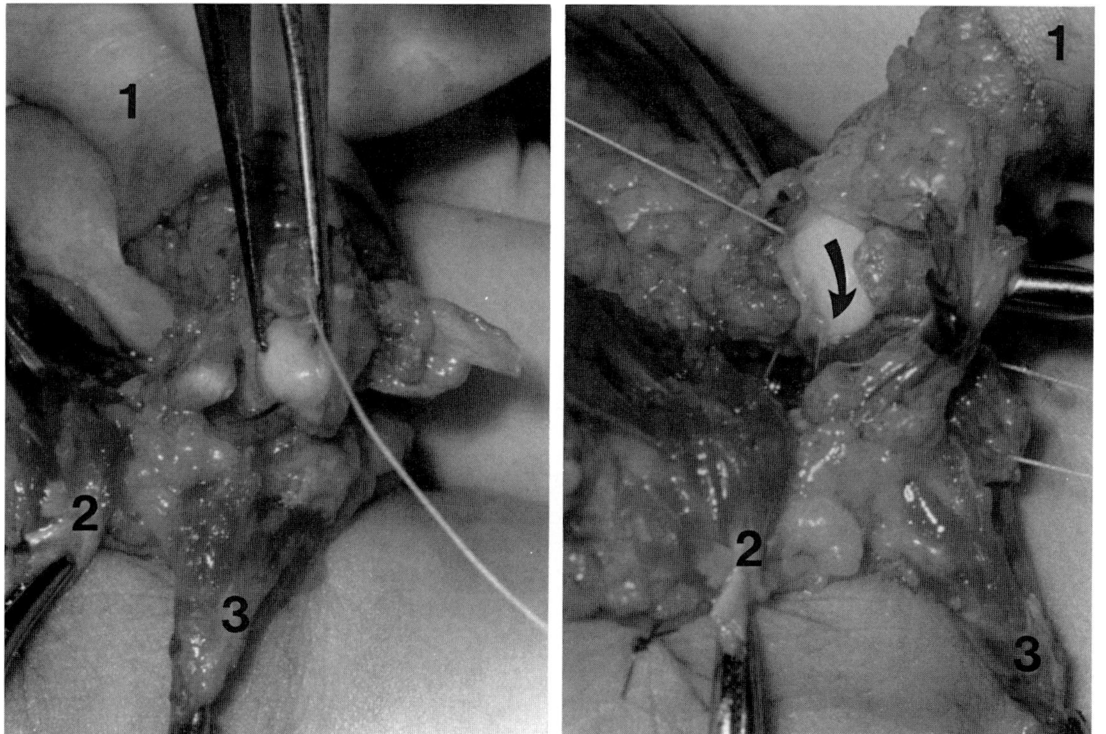

Fig. 57-24. **(A&B)** Only two well-positioned controlling sutures (3–0 braided nylon) are necessary to "anchor" the hyperextended MP joint to the radial base of the distal carpus, after resection of the *entire* proximal index finger metacarpal. While these sutures provide proper initial pronation (160 degrees) and abduction (40 degrees) of the digit to be pollicized *(1)*, final stabilization and position is achieved by the appropriate tension of tendon transfers after the metacarpal head is well seated. The first palmar interosseous *(2)* will be appropriately tensioned for thumb adduction, and the first dorsal interosseous (abductor indicis) *(3)* tensioned for abduction.

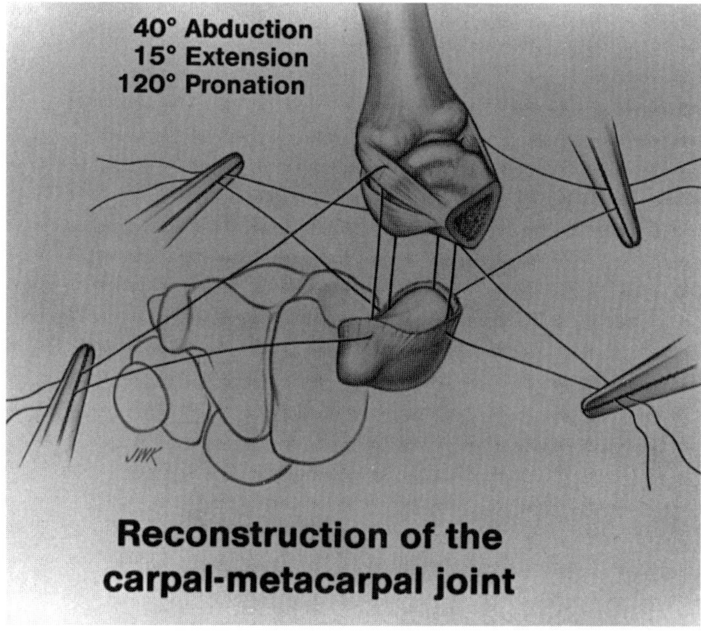

Fig. 57-25. The ideal final resting posture of the pollicized digit is 120 degrees pronation, 40 degrees abduction, and 15 degrees extension. This figure demonstrates the placement of *four* sutures to stabilize the base of the new thumb. This is unnecessary; we now prefer—and advise—the use of only *two* 3–0 braided nylon sutures, placed 180 degrees to each other.

flexion-extension arc of motion into more flexion and less hyperextension; we encourage its use.

In those cases in which the finger to be pollicized is relatively short, we recommend leaving a portion of the base of the resected index metacarpal to add some length, suturing the rotated metacarpal head to the soft tissue sleeve surrounding the metacarpal base. Temporary percutaneous K-wire fixation may be necessary in these cases.

Motoring The Pollicized Digit

Neurovascular pedicle transfer, first recommended in this country by Littler[60] in 1953, is a time-tested principle of digital transposition and pollicization; however, new techniques for motoring the transposed digit are regularly being introduced into the literature. The currently popular intrinsic transfers of first dorsal and first palmar interossei for thumb abduction and adduction, respectively, stem from the accumulated experiences of Riordan and Buck-Gramcko. Under ideal circumstances, when the index finger is essentially normal, we shorten the extensor indicis proprius a length equal to the amount of resected metacarpal, and use this motor as the primary thumb extensor. The EDC is redirected palmarly, acting as an abductor of the new thumb metacarpal. The vector of this motor tends to de-rotate the thumb base from its initially pronated posture of 160 degrees, to a final position of 120 degrees pronation. Abduction and adduction are achieved by transferring the first dorsal interosseous (abductor indicis) and first palmar interosseous, respectively, into the lateral bands of the index finger (Fig. 57-26A & B).

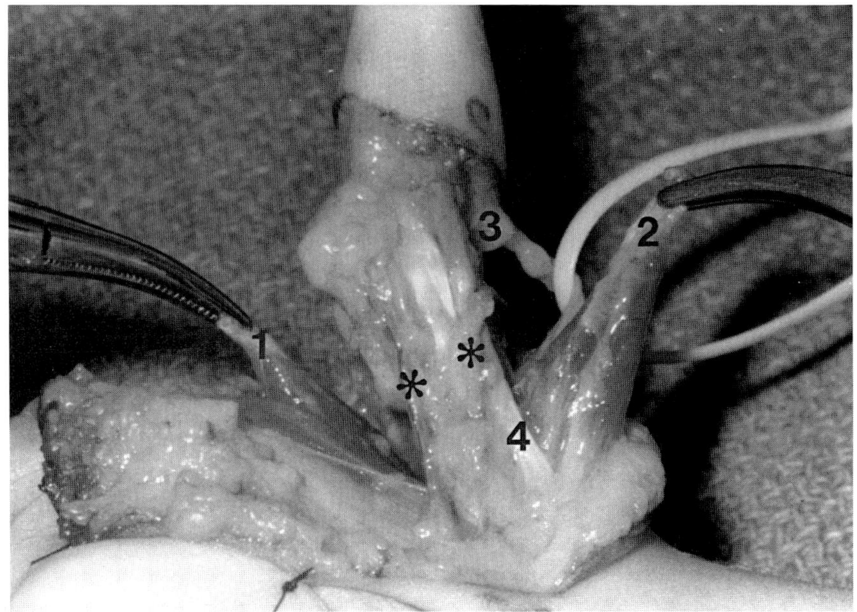

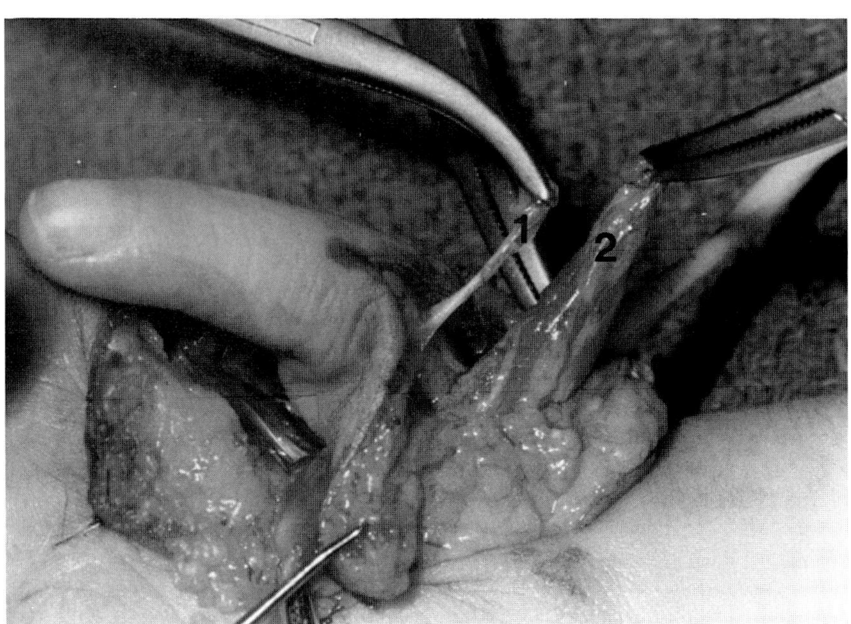

Fig. 57-26. (A&B) Motoring the pollicization. **(A)** The interossei of the index finger are prepared to motor the new thumb: the first palmar interosseous *(1)* will provide adduction, and the first dorsal interosseous (abductor indicis) *(2)* will abduct the pollicized digit (*asterisks* indicate the two preserved neurovascular bundles); *(3)* is the retained dorsal vein; and *(4)* is the intact flexor system of the original index finger. **(B)** The first dorsal interosseous *(2)* is ready for transfer into the radial lateral band *(1)* for future abduction of the pollicization.

The initial longitudinal dorsal incision, extended distally to the PIP joint of the index finger, allows adequate exposure of the dorsal apparatus for complete dissection of the lateral bands. Buck-Gramcko has reported that it is neither necessary to shorten the extrinsic flexor system of the pollicization nor to remove the lumbrical from the index profundus tendon (despite osteoarticular shortening by resection of the entire proximal portion of the index metacarpal). Our own experience with more than 50 pollicizations for congenital deficiency parallels Buck-Gramcko's data, and leaves us with similar impressions: within a few postoperative months, flexor tone returns spontaneously, allowing functional active flexion of the pollicized digit. Buck-Gramcko continues, however, to advise shortening the extrinsic *extensor* tendons (EIP and EDC) by a length equal to the segment of metacarpal removed. Manske and McCarroll[74] disagree with this recommendation and report that in their experience the EIP muscle-tendon unit will also spontaneously absorb the slack of skeletal shortening. They believe that the extensors as well as the flexors should be left surgically unshortened. We have no personal experience with their approach, and continue to use Buck-Gramcko's extensor-shortening recommendations, with predictable functional thumb extension.

The Buck-Gramcko pollicization technique employs distal detachment of the insertions of the abductor indicis (first dorsal interosseous) and first palmar interosseous from the base of the index proximal phalanx. The two motors can then be advanced distally into the radial and ulnar lateral bands (see Fig. 57-26A & B), providing an active abduction-adduction arc. The initial design of skin flaps serves well in accommodating an increased volume of muscle at the metacarpal level, while minimizing scar contracture in the new first webspace. Final tension is adjusted to provide the new thumb metacarpal with a stable resting posture of 40 degrees palmar abduction, 15 degrees extension, and 120 degrees pronation (Fig. 57-27). Internal fixation is not necessary.

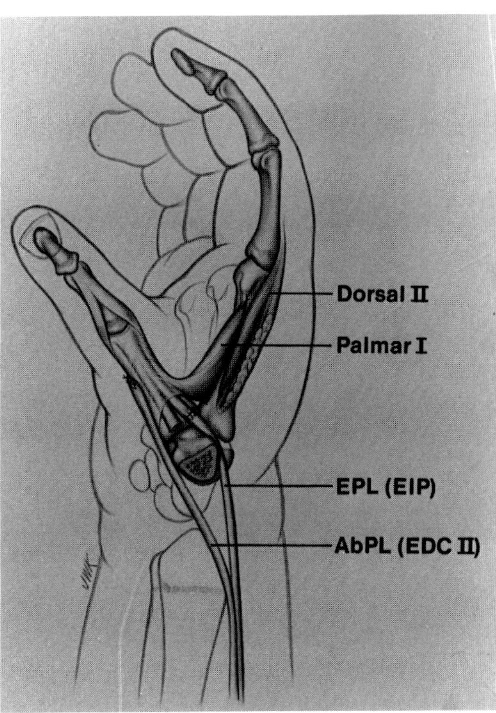

Fig. 57-28. An alternative used by the authors in some cases of complete congenital absence of the abductor indicis muscle involves more distal and palmar advancement of the index finger EDC for abduction; the muscular origin of the first palmar interosseous is detached and advanced distally onto the long finger metacarpal for adduction. No tendon transfer into the lateral bands is necessary using this alternative technique.[54]

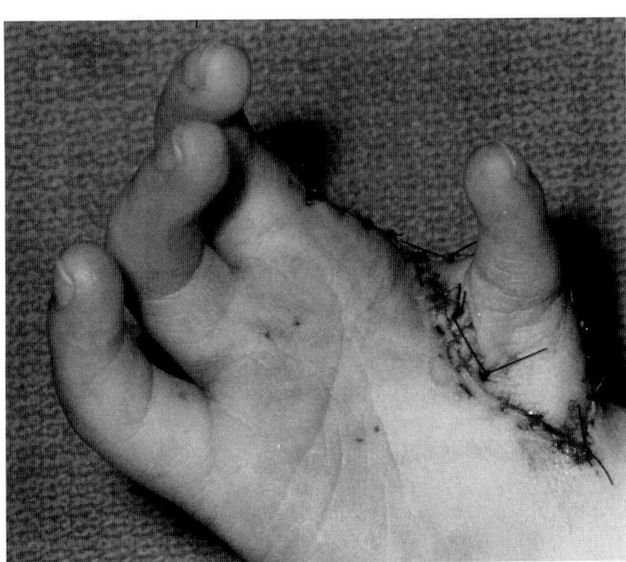

Fig. 57-27. End-stage of the Buck-Gramcko reconstruction: 120 degrees pronation, 40 degrees palmar abduction, 15 degrees extension. *Internal fixation is not necessary.*

The importance of the initial longitudinal dorsal incision on the index finger is readily appreciated (see Fig. 57-19B); it determines how far the lateral bands can be mobilized from the central tendon of the dorsal apparatus, and how far the first dorsal and palmar interossei can be advanced distally.

In personal experience with more than 50 pollicizations performed for congenital thumb deficiency, we have found either hypoplasia or complete absence of the abductor indicis in more than 50 percent. While many of these cases were associated with radial club hands, all could be described by the Blauth[8] thumb hypoplasia classification as stage III, IV, or V (see page 2046). In those cases with absence of the abductor indicis, some active abduction of the pollicization could be achieved by transferring the index EDC more distally onto the palmar border of the proximal phalangeal diaphysis (Fig. 57-28). Later, if necessary, a supplementary opponensplasty could be performed using either the ring flexor digitorum superficialis (FDS IV) or the hypothenar abductor digiti quinti (ABDQ).[44,74] The surgeon must be aware of the potential for major anatomic variations in any type of congenital hand reconstruction, particularly with respect to the availability of useful motors for the pollicized digit. Figure 57-29 points out anatomic variations in a patient in which all structures were

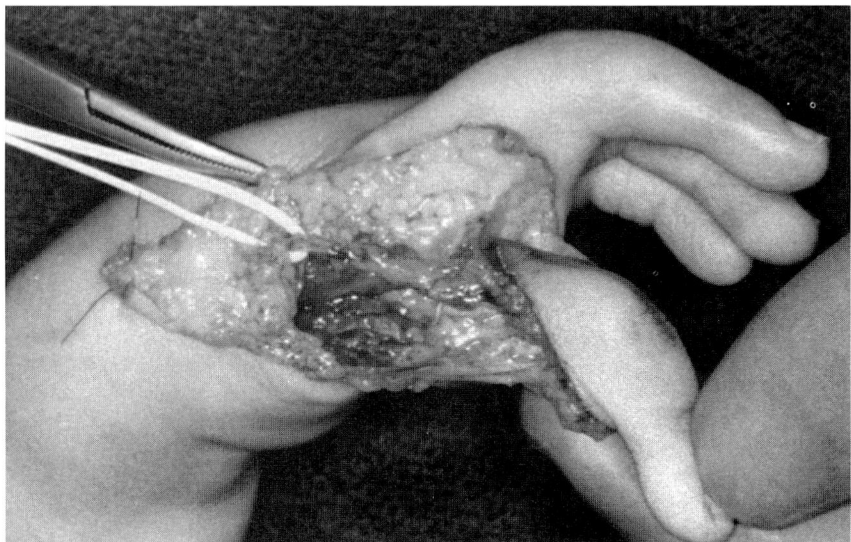

Fig. 57-29. A case of congenital thumb failure of formation. All index finger structures were present at the time of pollicization, except the extrinsic flexor tendons (FDS II, FDP II, lumbrical); the interossei were all normal.

present *except* the extrinsic extensor tendons. Figure 57-30 shows complete absence of extrinsic index flexors in a digit otherwise "rich" in available anatomy. Tendon transfers can always be planned at a later stage for these deficiencies.

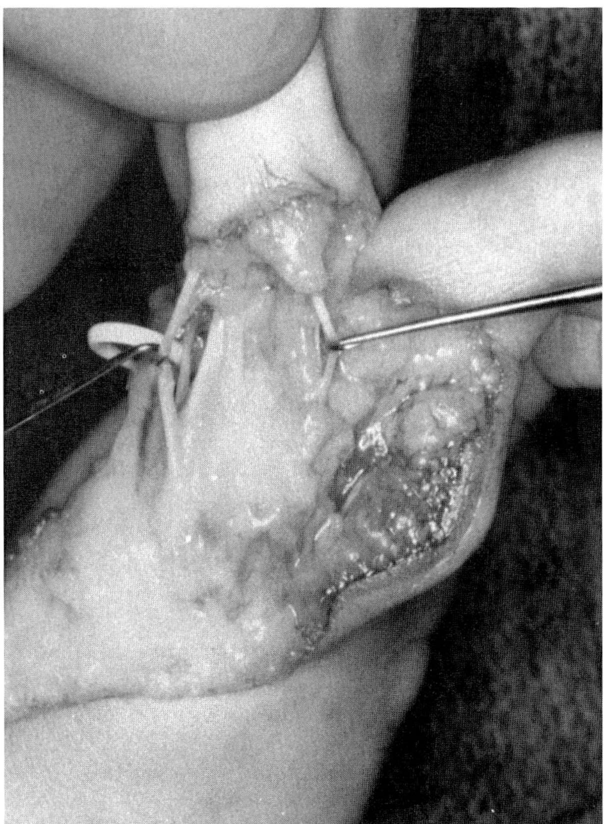

Fig. 57-30. The surgeon must anticipate an entire spectrum of congenital anomalies when performing a pollicization for congenital thumb absence. In this case, extrinsic extensors of the index finger were absent, in spite of *all* other structures being normal.

If present (and if substantial), the abductor indicis should be used for palmar abduction, as Buck-Gramcko and others have detailed; however, distal and palmar advancement of the index EDC should always be considered as an option when a poorly developed abductor indicis is found. Other well-tested techniques we use include FDS IV or ABDQ (Huber) transfers, the EDQP for thumb extension in the absence of extrinsic extensors, or FDS IV in the absence of extrinsic flexors. The surgeon's own ingenuity and skill in selecting the most appropriate transfer will yield the best functional thumb unit.

Skin Closure

One of the most frustrating steps in the pollicization procedure—particularly for the inexperienced hand surgeon—is rearrangement of the designed skin flaps to allow closure without adjunctive skin grafting. Even experienced surgeons worry throughout a case whether or not the flaps will come together "perfectly."

The beauty of Buck-Gramcko's flap design is to maximize the potential for a scar-free first web space, and when his design is used, the web space reconstruction should have a minimal propensity for contracture (see Fig. 57-18A & B). Once the initial flap angles have been rotated into their final transposed positions (see Fig. 57-19A & B), *redundancy* of the proximal flap on the dorsoradial aspect of the webspace can be contoured and debrided. Excess skin and subcutaneous fat is discarded as the flap is rotated into proper alignment. Using the technique of advancement and debridement, the surgeon will find enough tissue available for a "perfect" fit.

Vascularity of the New Thumb

Obviously, the most critical factor involved in pollicization is the circulation of the digit. Even with high technical expertise, compromise to inflow can occur secondary to arterial spasm, a direct consequence of the trauma of dissection. Poor flap design can also result in a suture line that is too tight, compromising inflow to the pollicization. If arterial spasm is present, it is readily seen if the surgeon releases the tourniquet upon completion of the dissection, prior to performing the CMC reconstruction and tendon transfers. We advocate strongly that the inexperienced surgeon release the tourniquet at the completion of the neurovascular pedicle dissection to assure that arterial circulation has not been compromised. In the hands of a more experienced surgeon the procedure may take less than 2 hours to complete; in these cases the tourniquet is usually not released until after the dressing has been applied. Since pollicization as a technique is rather difficult to master, and because recalcitrant situations are frequently encountered, the procedure for congenital reconstruction should be scheduled for at least 4 hours early in one's career, and the tourniquet released once to allow (1) washout of the products of anaerobic catabolism, and (2) check on the viability of the pedicled digit.

Compromise to venous outflow is a much more common problem following the procedure, but one of no less serious consequence. While it may be technically possible to transfer a pedicled digit on a single neurovascular pedicle with its venae comitantes alone, the surgeon should search for, and incorporate in the dissection, at least one dorsal vein to establish a cross-sectional vessel outflow diameter double that of the inflow. This simple relationship between outflow and inflow is similar to the philosophy used in revascularization and replantation surgery.

Postoperative Management

In the operating room, a long arm thumb spica compression dressing is applied, incorporating a dorsal slab of plaster-of-Paris, from the axilla to the midpalm. Vaseline-impregnated fine-mesh gauze is used to cover the wounds, preventing adherence of the dressing. The new thumb can then be held in the anatomic resting position, palmarly abducted 40 degrees, extended 15 degrees, and pronated 120 degrees relative to the plane of the palm. Flexing the elbow 90 degrees within the dressing reduces the child's ability to wiggle out of the immobilization.

The patient is taken to the recovery room after extubation, where careful, regular inspection of the color and turgor of the exposed distal thumb tip should be made. Rapid capillary filling or obvious bluish discoloration indicates venous congestion. This state of compromised vascular outflow should resolve itself quickly when the limb is elevated above heart level. If venous congestion is not relieved with elevation, the dressing must be split open widely to relieve external pressure on the draining digital veins (Fig. 57-31A & B). If necessary, selected sutures should also be removed to relieve skin tension, particularly across the critical dorsal vein. Occasionally, a child will have to be taken back to the operating room, reanesthetized, and the entire wound reopened. An accumulating hematoma or mechanical kinking in the venous system are each factors

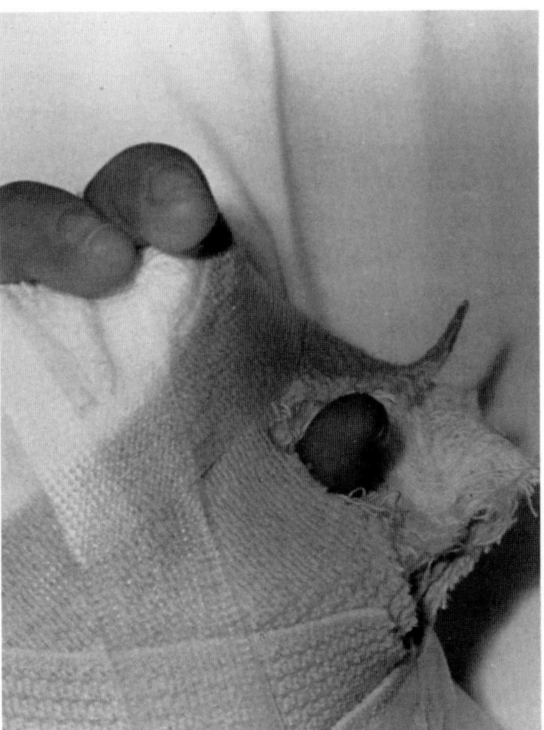
A

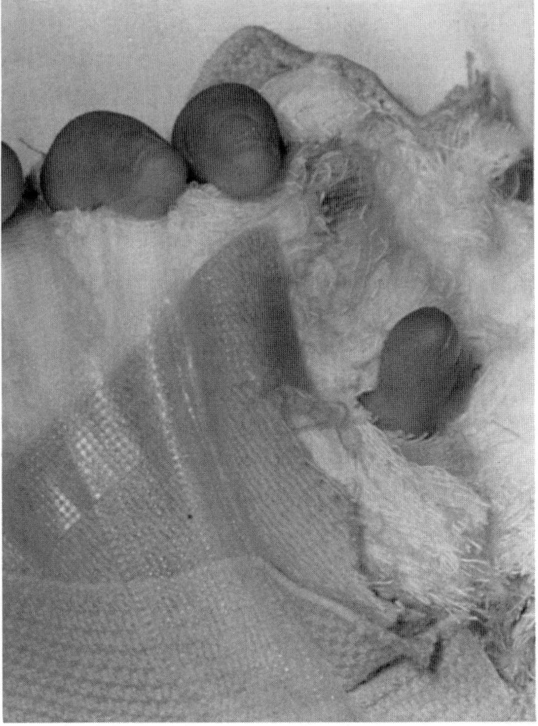
B

Fig. 57-31. (A&B) Marked venous congestion of the thumb in a bulky compression dressing following index finger pollicization. **(A)** With simple splitting of the dressing down to the skin **(B)** drainage is promoted, the congestion quickly resolves, and the vascular status of the new thumb returns to normal. If simple dressing decompression is ineffective, selected sutures should be removed, and consideration given to returning the child to the operating room for vessel exploration.

that might be causing the problem of congestion. The child should remain NPO until the surgeon can be sure that postoperative circulation to and from the thumb is within the limits of normalcy. Only in extreme circumstances should medical-grade leeches be used to help drain a compromised outflow system; these would be cases in which surgical reexploration under anesthesia failed to relieve the morbid vascular status of the digit.

The well-applied long arm (plaster-reinforced) dressing should preclude any need for temporary percutaneous K-wire fixation at the base of the pollicization. After 3 weeks, the dressing and sutures are removed in the office; it is unnecessary to subject the child to the risk of general anesthesia for simple suture removal. We recommend the use of 5-0 absorbable catgut for the skin closure, except at the corners and angles of the flaps, where 5-0 monofilament nylon should be used. The nylon sutures will prevent complete wound dehiscence in the event of an unexpected hematoma.

Between 3 and 6 weeks, a long arm removable splint should be worn. The patient should be encouraged during this time to circumduct the new thumb with active-assisted and gentle passive range of motion exercises. By the end of the third postoperative week tissues between the index metacarpal head and radial aspect of the carpus have fibrosed sufficiently to allow this exercise program to be diligently performed without fear of destabilizing the new thumb. After 6 weeks, a short opponens splint can be substituted for night use only; this should be the only orthotic device needed for the next 6 months.

The differences between postoperative rehabilitation following pollicization for traumatic thumb loss in a child, and the same procedure performed for congenital thumb failure of formation are profound. The former requires little hand therapy to "reeducate" the patient's functional thumb capacity. The thumb is normally represented in the child's cerebral cortex; prehensile tasks rapidly return following the reconstruction.

Congenital reconstruction is quite different: there is little or no thumb cerebrocortical representation; pinch and grasp activities using the new thumb must be learned for the first time. Both surgeon and parents must have patience while rehabilitation slowly progresses. Formal hand therapy may be of great value in training the patient and the patient's parents in the use of the new thumb for pinch and grasp. With rehabilitative consistency, patience, and input from a trained therapist, the patient's frustration can be minimized, and the new thumb progressively incorporated into the complex function of the hand (Fig. 57-32).

Age Considerations

Selection of the most appropriate age for each of the techniques of thumb reconstruction in the congenitally deficient hand remains one of the more controversial facets of hand surgery. While Littler[64,65,67] recommended waiting until the congenitally thumb-deprived child is 2 to 4 years of age before

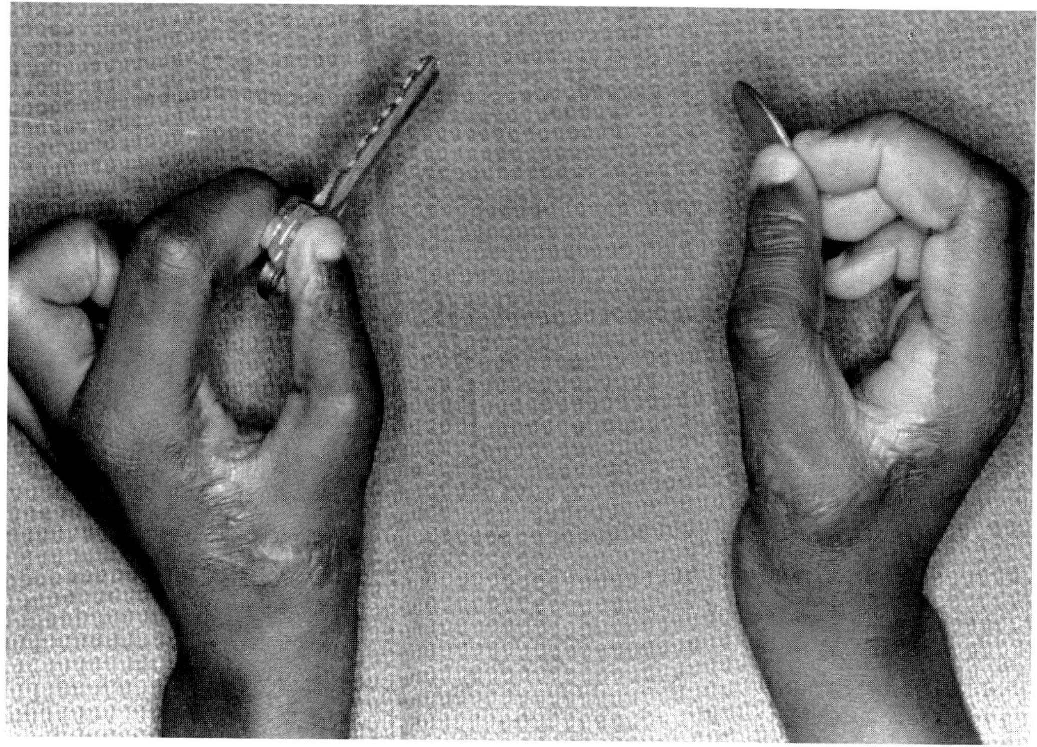

Fig. 57-32. Eight-year follow-up demonstrating excellent reconstitution of pinch function following bilateral index finger pollicizations using the Buck-Gramcko technique. This child had both pollicizations performed prior to age 2, for bilateral congenital failure of thumb formation (grade V hypoplasia).

considering pollicization, Riordan[80,81,115] and Flatt[27] have suggested that the procedure can be performed safely at 6 to 12 months of age. Buck-Gramcko has achieved good results at an even earlier age (D. Buck-Gramcko, M.D: personal communication, 1985). Because the cardiopulmonary system is not well developed until 12 months postpartum, we prefer to wait until the child reaches this age. In addition, since bimanual grasp does not normally develop until 9 to 12 months of age, eagerness to perform the operation should be reserved for a time after this normal developmental landmark has been reached.

Although size itself is not a contraindication to early pollicization, the normal involution of embryonic endosteal circulation during the first year of life makes intraoperative tourniquet control much more effective if the surgeon delays until 1 year of age. By this age an infant's friable arteries and veins have also developed into vessels of substantial thickness. Dissection of the vascular pedicles with low-power magnification (4.0 to 4.5× loupes) is relatively risk-free if careful surgical technique is applied.

What is the appropriate age for pollicization? The surgeon should take into account these four points: development of the cardiopulmonary system, involution of the embryonic endosteal circulation, size of structures and vessel friability, and normal development of bimanual grasp as a functional landmark. Because of these factors, we believe that the optimum time for pollicization, with the least propensity for complications and/or intraoperative difficulty, is when the child is a least 1 year old.[54]

Pollicization remains today one of the premier reconstructive procedures in the hand surgeon's armamentarium. It combines the well-established principles of skeletal stabilization, joint reconstruction, and tendon transfer, with the sophisticated techniques of neurovascular island pedicle design. The procedure becomes an exercise of enormous potential functional benefit for the thumb-deprived patient, whether afflicted by congenital deformity or traumatic loss.

The hand without a thumb is capable of hook function, but pinch and grasp remain primitive unless reconstructive steps are taken. By shortening the index ray and providing a proper degree of abduction and motor balance, the general functional capacity and cosmetic appearance of the hand can be profoundly improved.

PART II: THUMB RECONSTRUCTION FOLLOWING PARTIAL OR COMPLETE TRAUMATIC LOSS

The level of thumb loss is probably the single most important factor in determining the appropriate procedure for thumb reconstruction.[151,270,307,308,328,367,376,378,390,436,442,443,445,446,474–476,491,504,513] For practical purposes the reconstructive needs of the thumb can be best assessed by consideration of the first ray divided into proximal, middle, and distal thirds (Fig. 57-33). In this chapter, we will attempt to define the differing reconstructive needs at each of these levels and de-

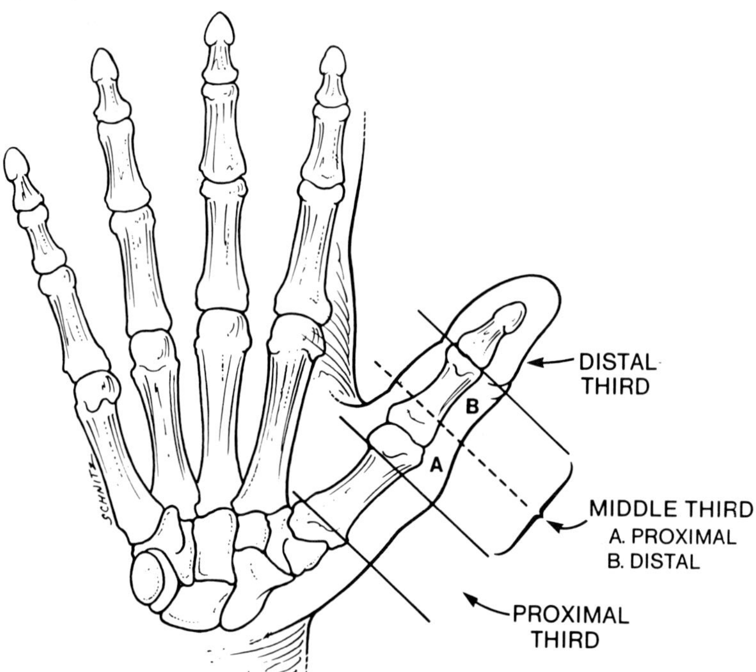

Fig. 57-33. Areas of thumb loss considered in this chapter: distal third, middle third, and proximal third. The middle third is subdivided into *(A)* proximal and *(B)* distal.

scribe in detail the surgical options available. A final section devoted to the metacarpal hand will also be presented.

AMPUTATION THROUGH THE DISTAL ONE-THIRD OF THE FIRST RAY

This level has been described as the "compensated amputation zone."[352] Functional impairment following partial or complete thumb loss in this area is not great, and every effort should be made to restore skeletal stability with painless, well-padded skin and satisfactory sensory perception. Procedures employed to accomplish these goals will vary depending upon the amount and depth of tissue loss, and an attempt should be made to salvage all viable tissues consistent with these objectives. Although injuries to the palmar pad of the distal phalanx of the thumb may be managed by the same coverage techniques that are applicable to fingertip injuries, the approach may be somewhat different as one strives to preserve length.[150,187,199,204,342,375,399,462,473,474,478,482,512]

Small transverse losses of skin and subcutaneous tissue from the terminal aspect of the distal phalanx may be managed by allowing spontaneous healing by secondary intention, free skin grafts,[193,199,471] lateral triangular advancement flaps,[203,249,318,445,506] V-Y advancement flaps,[148,224,231,232,249,307,318,445] or other ingenious techniques.[231,232,249,284,291,296,298,303,352,373,413,419,506,510] The advantage of spontaneous healing or split-thickness skin grafting resides in the ultimate wound contracture, which will result in a minimal defect with near normal sensation preserved.[193,473,474] Advancement of the digital nerves to restore sensation to the distal thumb has also been described,[410] and the free transfer of nerve containing tissues has gained recent popularity.[163,303,339]

When the amount of distal thumb tissue loss has been substantial, when procedures are needed to preserve length, or when there has been significant damage to the digital nerves of the thumb, more extensive coverage procedures may be indicated, including the use of palmar advancement flaps, cross-finger flaps, and, occasionally, neurovascular island pedicle flaps or radial sensory-innervated cross-finger flaps.

Palmar Advancement Flap

Larger avulsions of the thumb pad involving approximately 50 percent of the palmar portion of the distal phalanx are uniquely suitable for the advancement of a palmar flap containing the neurovascular structures with or without proximal skin release and interpositiodal grafting.[249,304,373,374,382,426,442,445,506] First suggested by Moberg,[382] this procedure has the advantage of bringing well-innervated palmar thumb skin distally to resurface the pad lesion, thereby restoring near normal sensory perception with durable skin and subcutaneous tissue. It has been stated that the area that can be resurfaced by this technique is "quarter-sized"[304] or as much as 2 cm,[426] and that flexion of the thumb interphalangeal joint as much as 45 degrees in order to provide sufficient advancement of the flap will not result in a long-term flexion deformity.[304,426] A proximal transverse releasing incision has also been recommended[145,249,442] in order to decrease the need for acute interphalangeal flexion and increase the amount of tissue that can be mobilized.[249,442] The resulting proximal defect may be covered by a full-thickness interpositional graft or allowed to heal secondarily without significant sequelae.[249] Both palmar advancement techniques will be described here in the following sections.

Palmar Advancement Flap without Proximal Releasing Incision (Modified from Keim and Grantham[304] and Posner and Smith[426])

This technique is best for terminal distal phalangeal pad defects of 2 cm or less in length. Under tourniquet hemostasis, necrotic and ragged bone is trimmed from the distal phalanx and thorough soft tissue debridement is carried out (Fig. 57-34A). Midaxial incisions are then made over the radial and ulnar sides of the thumb extending proximally from the lesion to the proximal thumb crease. The palmar flap is then elevated by careful dissection and includes subcutaneous tissue and both neurovascular bundles (Fig. 57-34B). Great care is taken not to disturb the underlying flexor tendon or its sheath. The mobility of the flap is tested by distal traction to determine if any additional soft tissue undermining or releases are necessary. The MP and interphalangeal joints of the thumb are placed in approximately 30 to 45 degrees flexion. The distal edge of the flap is sutured to the remaining nail, nail bed, or terminal skin remnant, and radial and ulnar sutures are used to complete skin closure (Fig. 57-34C).

Palmar Advancement Flap with Proximal Releasing Incision (Modified from Vilain and Michon[506])

This procedure may be used for defects no greater than 2.5 cm in length. Under tourniquet hemostasis, bony fragments are removed and an appropriate debridement of the tip lesion is carried out (Fig. 57-35A). The size of the defect to be covered is measured and will represent the length of the tissue advancement that will be required. Radial and ulnar midaxial incisions are brought proximally from the edges of the lesion to the proximal third of the phalanx. A transverse incision is made between the proximal ends of the lateral incisions and, by carefully elevating the proximal edge of the flap, it is possible to identify and mobilize the neurovascular bundles (Fig. 57-35B). The flap is then raised from distal to proximal bringing with it skin, subcutaneous tissues, and both neurovascular bundles. Care is taken not to violate the sheath of the flexor pollicis longus, and the flap is advanced and sutured in place distally (Fig. 57-35C). A full-thickness skin graft taken from the groin is used to cover the proximal donor area (Fig. 57-35D). It may be necessary for the IP and MP joints of the thumb to be positioned in moderate flexion for several weeks in order to relieve the tension on the neurovascular bundles.

Following either technique, an appropriate compressive dressing is applied and the flap and grafts are inspected at 7 to 10 days. Mobilization of the thumb is begun after 3 weeks, and some splinting may be necessary to recover full joint extension.

The advantage of these procedures is that they bring nor-

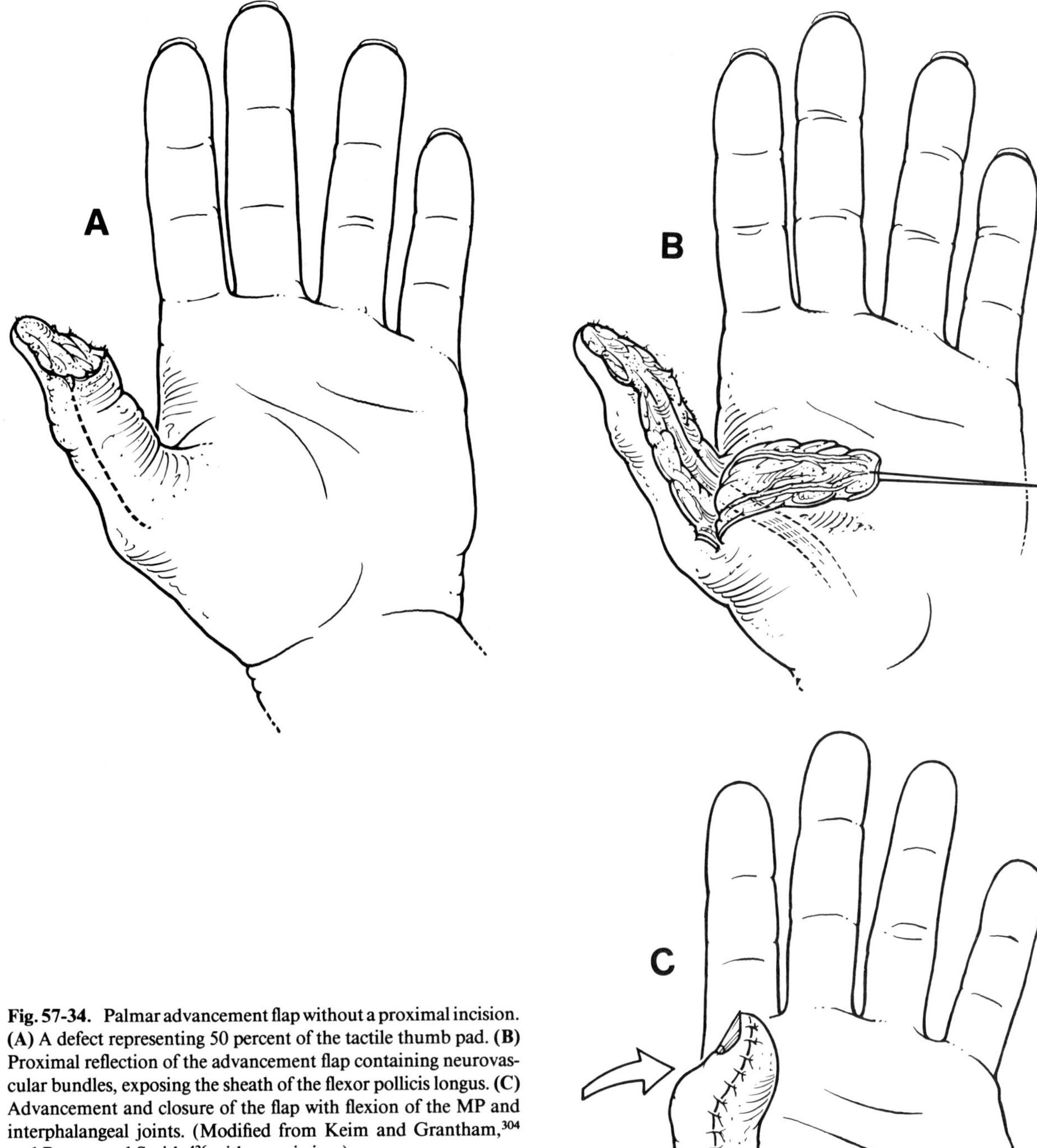

Fig. 57-34. Palmar advancement flap without a proximal incision. **(A)** A defect representing 50 percent of the tactile thumb pad. **(B)** Proximal reflection of the advancement flap containing neurovascular bundles, exposing the sheath of the flexor pollicis longus. **(C)** Advancement and closure of the flap with flexion of the MP and interphalangeal joints. (Modified from Keim and Grantham,[304] and Posner and Smith,[426] with permission.)

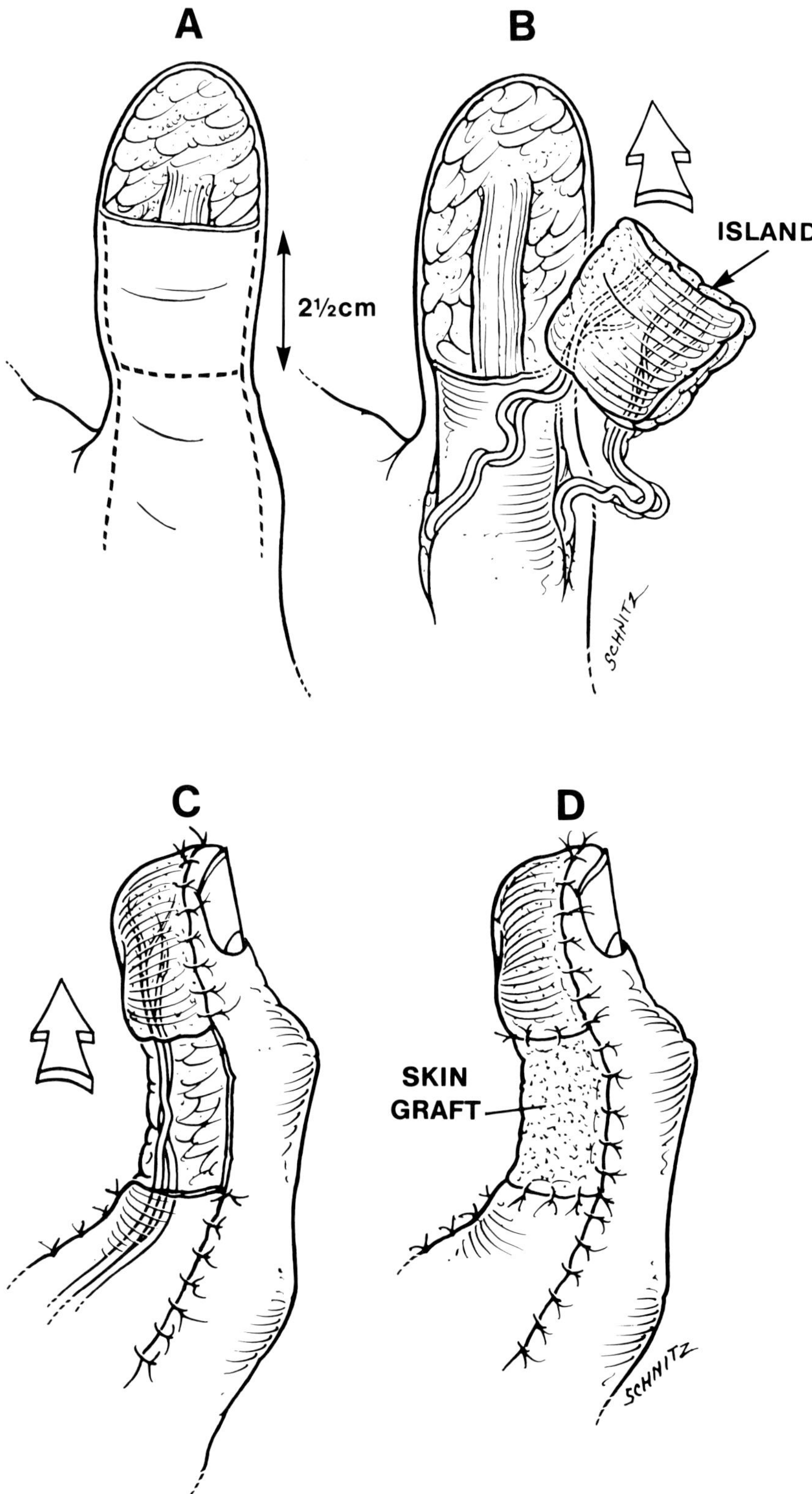

Fig. 57-35. Palmar advancement flap with a proximal releasing incision. **(A)** A 2.5-cm defect of the distal phalangeal thumb pulp, and outlines of incisions for the advancement flap. **(B)** Elevation of the flap and mobilization of neurovascular bundles through the proximal incision. **(C)** Advancement of the flap to close the defect. **(D)** Free skin graft coverage of the proximal donor area. (Modified from Vilain and Michon,[506] with permission.)

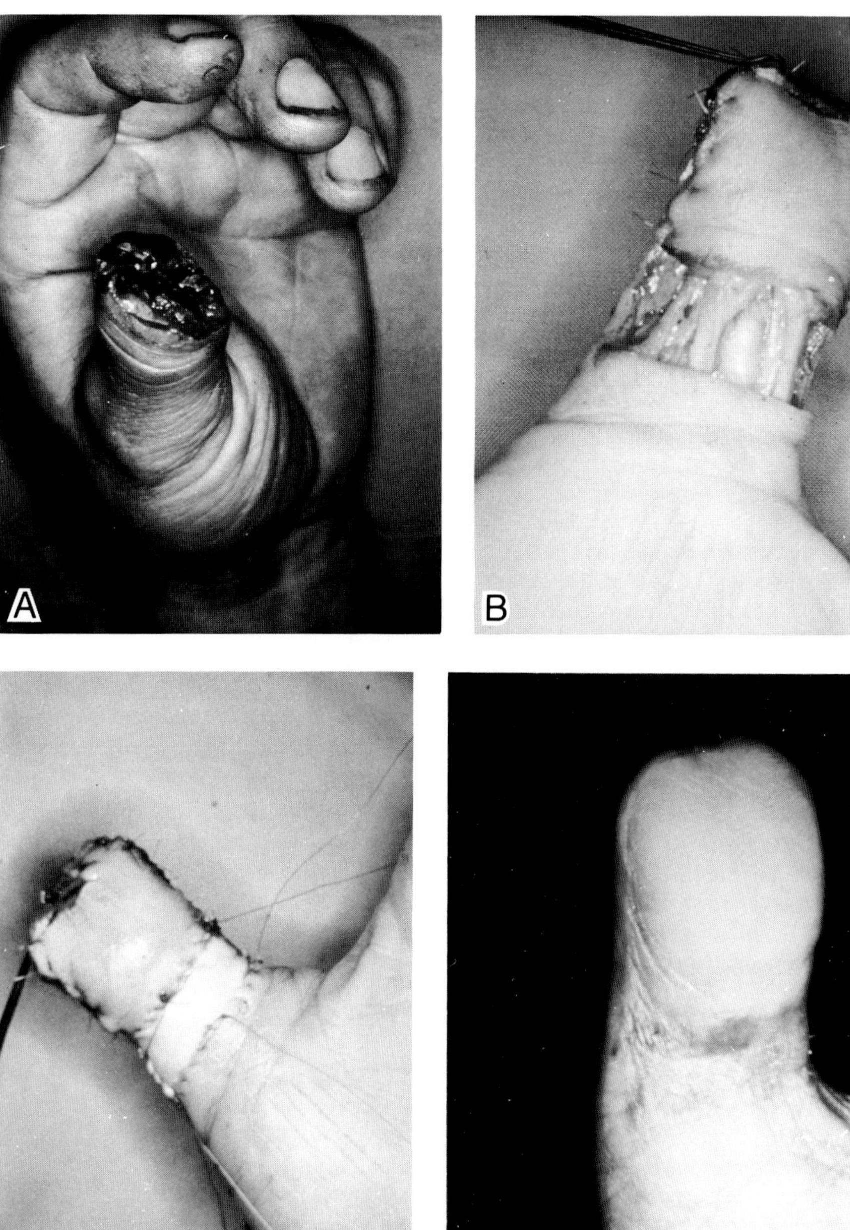

Fig. 57-36. A palmar advancement flap with proximal releasing incision. **(A)** A large oblique avulsion of the palmar thumb pad, including the nail. **(B)** Advancement of the palmar flap following mobilization of the neurovascular bundles. **(C)** Interpositional skin graft over the donor defect. **(D)** Appearance of the flap at 3 months.

mally innervated, well-padded palmar thumb skin for distal coverage of substantial thumb lesions (Fig. 57-36). In addition to their usefulness in the acute situation, they are excellent procedures for thumb resurfacing at a later period when inadequate coverage exists.[374,382,416,442] Disadvantages and complications include the fact that the flaps probably cannot be safely mobilized for more than 2.5 cm or approximately 50 percent of the digital pad of the thumb. There is also a danger of compromising the vascularization of the ungual area, and it is advisable not to dissect the pedicle too far.[506] Sloughing of bits of bone or nail during the immediate postoperative phase has been described,[304] and the possibility of flexion contractures of the IP joints is a concern.[304]

Cross-Finger Flap

When the entire palmar surface of the distal phalanx of the thumb has been avulsed, free grafting will provide inadequate long-term coverage, and palmar advancement becomes technically impossible. A cross-finger flap designed from the proximal phalanx of the index finger will often provide excellent coverage of these lesions with satisfactory skin and subcutaneous tissue, and an adequate sensory recovery is usually achieved.[150,193,206,218,279,280,289,360,361,399,425,427,428,435,441,445,473–475,478,506] Eaton et al[218] suggested that reversed dorsal cross-finger flaps permit more geometric options than can be achieved with conventional methods.

The primary use of a neurovascular island pedicle flap may occasionally be indicated,[479] and other more elaborate procedures, including the use of the tip of the fifth finger,[473] free toe pulp transfers,[332,433,469] a one-stage advancement rotational flap combination,[249,284,298,445] the use of "kite or flag flaps" from the index finger[237,291,384,463,522] a dorsal flap based on the first web space,[360,361] or a flap hinged on the ulnar side of the thumb and rotated distally,[242] are clever procedures that seem to increase the degree of technical difficulty with little if any improvement on the reliable performance of a cross-finger pedicle flap.

Cross-Finger Flap to the Thumb

Under tourniquet hemostasis, small, loose bone fragments are removed and thorough debridement of the distal thumb pad is accomplished. Wound margins are excised and an attempt should be made to convert the lesion into a square or rectangular defect. Using a paper towel, a small pattern is made corresponding in size to the defect and, after bringing the thumb into position against the side of the index finger in order to determine the appropriate level, a donor flap is outlined on the dorsal radial aspect of the proximal phalanx of the index finger (Fig. 57-37A). Because of the unique rotational motion of the thumb, the base of the flap will originate palmar to the midaxial line of the index finger and extend across the dorsum of the proximal phalanx as far as the defect size requires. A slightly oblique configuration to the donor flap will aid in positioning it against the pad lesion.

Incisions are then made along the three borders of the flap, and it is carefully raised across the dorsum of the index finger from the ulnar to the radial side. Subcutaneous tissue is included in the flap, but the filmy peritenon overlying the extensor tendon is preserved. An effort is made to identify and protect small veins in the radial corner of the flap to ensure its viability (Fig. 57-37B).

A near full-thickness skin graft is patterned to fit the donor defect and dissected out of the groin. Some graft excess is retained to provide coverage of the free edge of the pedicle. The graft is then tagged in position and the flap is sutured into the recipient defect on the thumb pad. The graft is then sutured in place, including the ulnar margin of the thumb, to create a completely closed wound (Fig. 57-37C & D). Long tie-over sutures are secured over a moist cotton bolus to create a stent on top of the graft, and a plaster-reinforced, compressive dressing immobilizing the thumb and index, as well as the hand and wrist, is used.

Motion is permitted in the ulnar three fingers to prevent stiffness, and a dressing change at 7 to 10 days is used to assess the viability of the flap and the "take" of the graft. The flap is detached at 3 weeks, and closure of the adjacent margins of the thumb and index finger are carried out at that time.

Satisfactory sensory return has been found in several long-term studies of cross-finger flap performance,[279,419,478] and the technique is reliable, well tolerated by the patient, and provides sufficient padding for long-term heavy thumb use (Fig. 57-38). Disadvantages and complications include the sometimes unsightly defect over the dorsum of the index finger, which may be particularly annoying in children and women, and some occasional problems with digital joint stiffness or thumb web contracture.

Neurovascular Island Pedicle Flap

Permanent sensory loss in the palmar tactile pad of the thumb following irreparable damage of the digital nerves will result in substantial impairment of pinch and grasp function. When local nerve continuity cannot be restored and disability is substantial, it may be appropriate to use a neurovascular island pedicle transfer as first suggested by Moberg[382] and Littler[332] and extended by others.[261,269,271,272,283,316,332-334,373,394,420,439,441,445,470,474,479,495,507] The technique, however, is a very demanding one, and the quality of sensory return has been challenged.[153,394]

Preoperative considerations for this procedure include the selection of a donor digit and the determination of the amount of digital skin and subcutaneous tissue to be brought with the pedicle. If the loss of thumb sensibility has resulted from local injury to the digital nerves of the thumb and there is no concomitant median nerve deficit, then the ulnar aspect of the long finger, by virtue of its freedom from participation in pinch and its long neurovascular pedicle, is an excellent donor choice.

When the procedure is being carried out to restore sensory perception following irreparable median nerve damage, one must use an ulnar nerve-innervated area, such as the ulnar side of the ring finger, as a donor. The amount of tissue taken should correspond with the size of the thumb defect created by removing scarred and insensate tissue, and it is sometimes best to use the "extended" neurovascular island transfer that consists of almost the entire ulnar-palmar half of the donor digit to provide the widest possible areas of sensory restoration.[288,394,439,470,474,495] Several authors[143,211,234,271] have advocated suture of the divided proper digital nerve of the neurovascular island pedicle flap to a previously severed thumb digital nerve to improve sensation. Thompson[490] emphasized that it is not necessary to apply the flap to the absolute tip of the thumb unless it is required for soft tissue coverage and that the position should favor the ulnar side of the thumb. Chen et al[195] reported one case where the entire distal phalanx of the thumb was resurfaced with twin neurovascular island flaps taken from the ulnar and radial sides of the middle and ring fingers.

Neurovascular Island Pedicle Flap (Modified from Reid[437,442,445])

Before beginning, it is necessary to determine the size of the thumb defect to be resurfaced; this measurement will mandate the size of the flap to be used. Because most clinical conditions warrant the use of an extended flap using the entire length of a donor digit, this technique will be described here (Fig. 57-39A).

Under tourniquet hemostasis, the flap is outlined on the ulnar aspect of the donor digit extending from well out on the pad of the distal phalanx along the midline of the palmar aspect of the digit to terminate just short of the proximal digital crease. Small darts are created at the interphalangeal creases, and the flap extends posteriorly beyond the midlateral line to

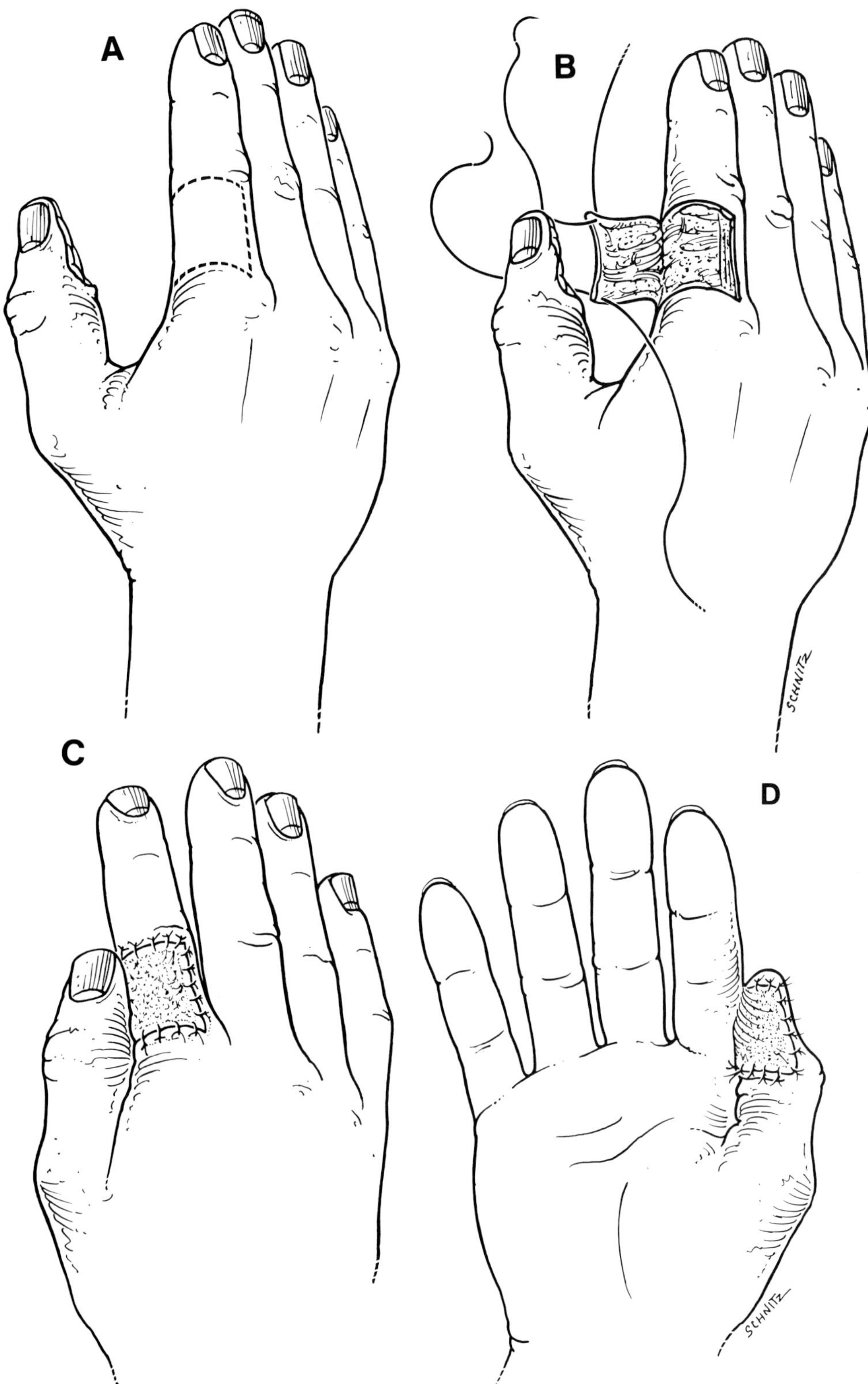

Fig. 57-37. Cross-finger flap from the index finger to the thumb. **(A)** A large defect involving most of the distal pulp of the thumb. Outline of the cross-finger flap on the proximal phalanx of the index finger. **(B)** Placement of the flap on the thumb defect. **(C&D)** Position of the thumb and cross-finger flap with a free graft covering the donor defect.

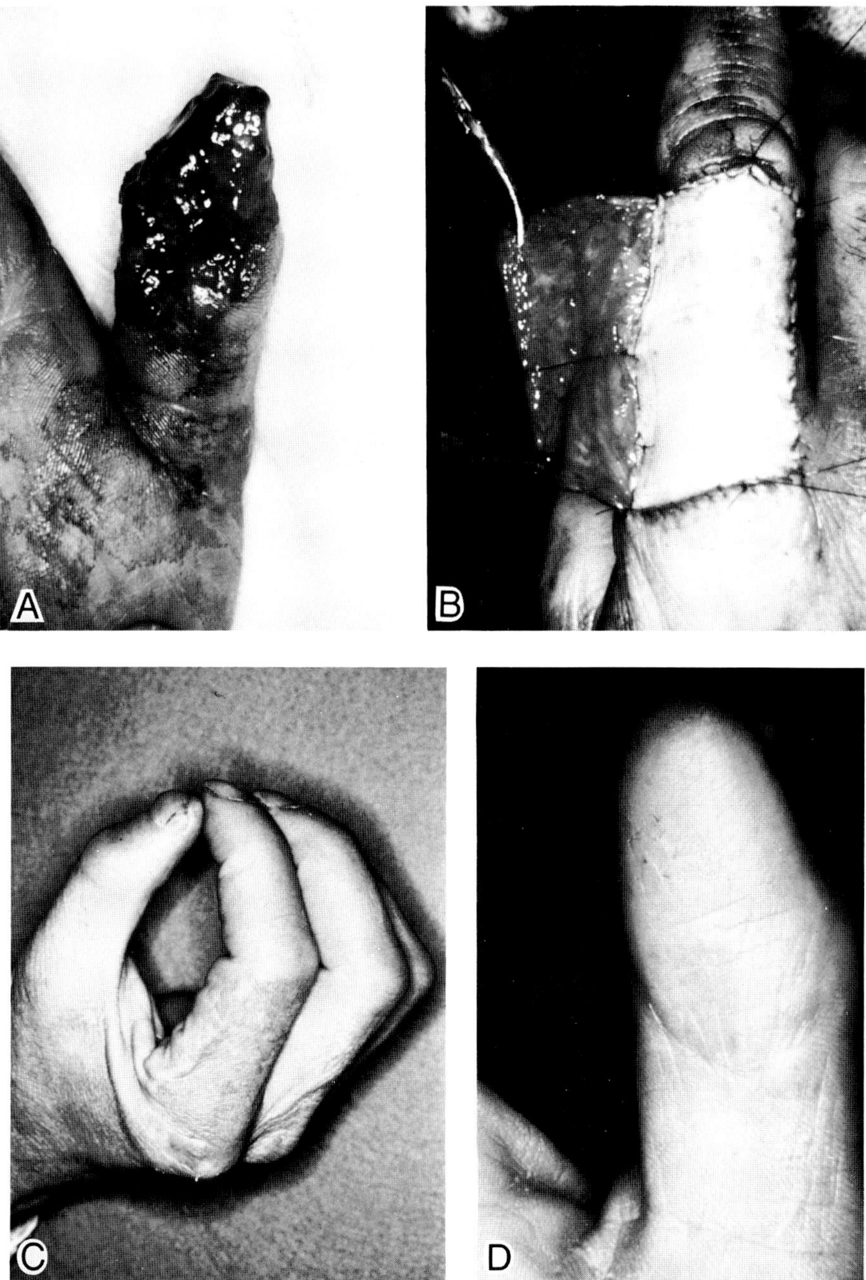

Fig. 57-38. Cross-finger flap coverage of a large thumb defect. **(A)** A large avulsion defect involving the entire palmar aspect of the distal phalanx of the thumb. **(B)** A large cross-finger flap designed from the dorsum of the proximal phalanx of the index finger. The donor site has already been covered with a skin graft. **(C)** Appearance of the thumb and donor defect at 3 months. **(D)** Cosmetic appearance of the thumb pad at 3 months with satisfactory sensation and durable coverage. (From Strickland,[473] with permission.)

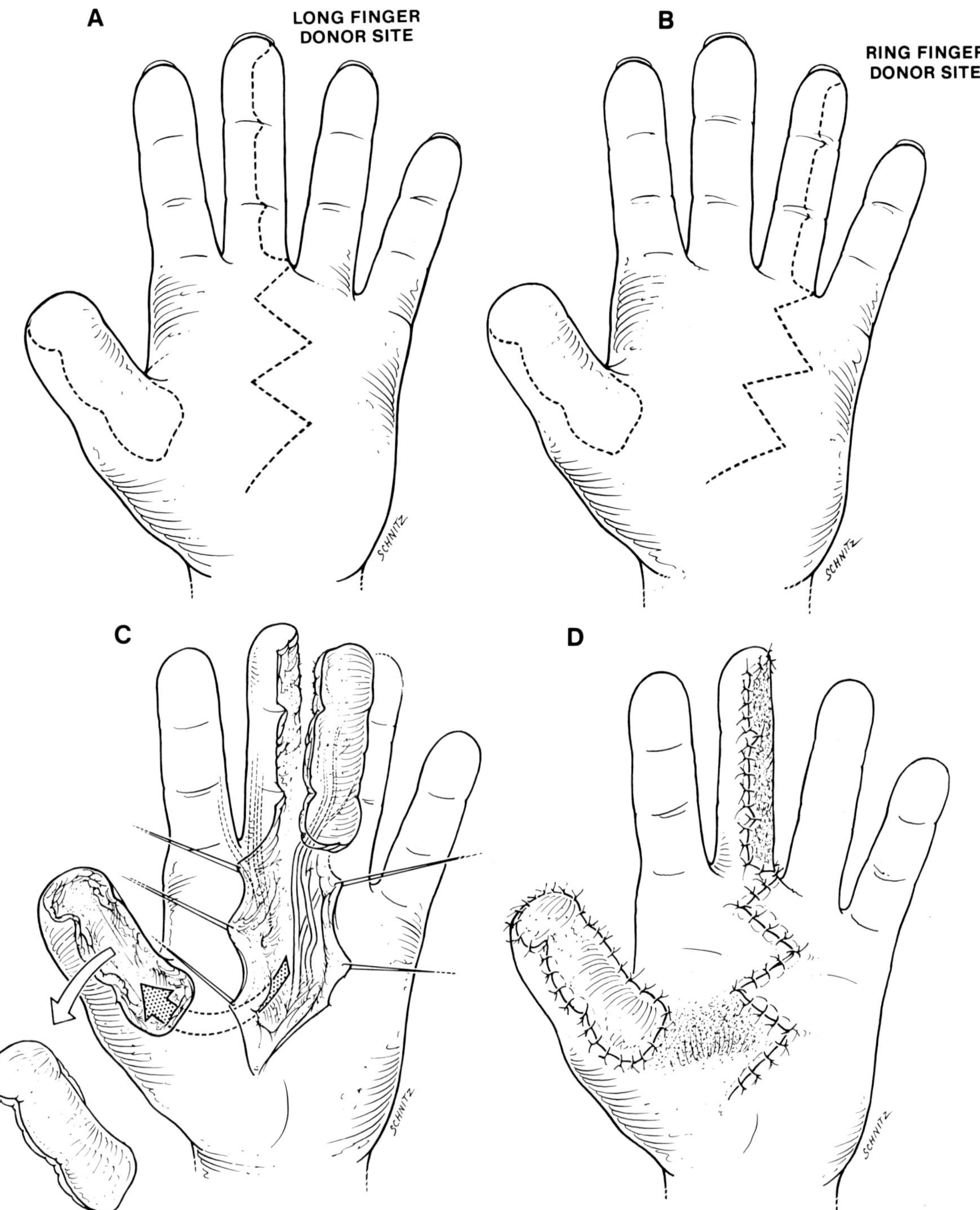

Fig. 57-39. Neurovascular island transfer from either the long or ring finger to provide sensate coverage of the thumb. **(A)** The neurovascular island flap utilizing the ulnar side of the long finger. An extended island flap is designed with an identical defect patterned over the palmar aspect of the thumb. **(B)** The use of the ulnar aspect of the ring finger, which is designed and transferred in an similar manner, is depicted. **(C)** Mobilization of the island flap on its neurovascular pedicle and preparation of the recipient bed on the thumb. Note the areas of undermining required between the palmar and thumb incisions *(dotted arrow)* **(D)** Completed transfer of the neurovascular island flap with a free graft on the donor area of the long finger. Care must be taken to avoid a longitudinal scar along the palmar aspect of the donor finger. (Modified from Reid,[442] with permission.)

the dorsal aspect of the digit. A midlateral proximal continuation is then used to connect the digital incision with a series of palmar zigzag incisions. A paper pattern template with the exact size and configuration of the flap is then used to outline the recipient area on the palmar aspect of the thumb. A proximal connection into the palm is also provided in this area to facilitate passage of the flap. Under magnification, the dissection begins in the palm, and the neurovascular bundle to the web space is identified. The digital artery to the radial side of the adjacent finger is identified and ligated well away from the arterial bifurcation. The digital nerves to the adjacent sides of the long and ring fingers are carefully teased apart well into the midpalm. The artery and nerve to the ulnar side of the donor finger have now been isolated as far as the base of the finger and are then dissected distally into the island flap. Incisions are then made about the entire periphery of the flap, and dissection is dissected distally and carefully continued in a proximal direction, bringing skin, subcutaneous tissue, and the neurovascular bundle, which should be protected by the surrounding soft tissue. The flap is freed on its neurovascular pedicle to the level of the midpalm. Small vascular branches are cauterized and transected during this dissection.

Skin and scar within the previously outlined recipient site on the thumb are excised, and a bridge between the proximal thumb incision and the proximal end of the palmar incision is carefully undermined in an area just below the palmar aponeurosis (Fig. 57-39B). A suture placed in the distal end of the island pedicle flap is used to gently pull the flap from the palmar wound into the thumb wound, with great care taken not to damage or twist the pedicle (Fig. 57-39C). It is important to create some redundancy of the pedicle in order to prevent tension and ensure the viability and sensibility of the flap.

The transferred flap is loosely tagged in place in the recipient defect and the tourniquet is released. Troublesome bleeders are ligated, and the vascularity of the flap can be assessed. Completion of flap suture and the repair of the palmar and proximal digital wounds is carried out at this time. A full-thickness skin graft taken from the groin is then sutured into the donor defect with long tie-overs secured over moist cotton to complete a stent (Fig. 57-39D).

A compressive dressing is applied and shortly thereafter the distal tip of the flap is exposed so that viability can be monitored. Full dressing change at 7 to 10 days is carried out; motion is permitted at 3 to 4 weeks.

This procedure requires careful planning and meticulous dissection. Failure will result in a substantially increased disability for the involved hand. With improvements in digital nerve reconstruction the procedure is used much less today than it was in the past. Complications include partial or complete flap necrosis, failure of the graft, or stiffness of the donor finger. Obviously, the loss of sensate skin in the donor finger is considerable; however, when the indications are appropriate, the restoration of good palmar sensory skin to the critical tactile pad of the thumb is functionally justified. It should be noted, however, that few adults will convert sensory recognition of the transferred flap to that of the thumb.[279,394]

Additional details and illustrations of the neurovascular island flap are presented in Chapter 49.

Radial Sensory-Innervated Cross-Finger Flap

When thumb reconstruction requires substantial resurfacing with innervated skin, a large cross-finger pedicle flap that carries a sensory branch of the radial nerve is an effective alternative to neurovascular island transfer.[142,162,241,277,278,378,431,445,451,508] Transposition of a dorsal sensory branch of the radial nerve was first carried out by Holevich,[278] who recently described a revised procedure designed to provide sensibility to the thumb using a bipedicled neurovascular island flap derived from the dorsoradial surface of the index finger.[414] Techniques for nerve transference together with a cross-finger flap were reported by Adamson,[142] Brallier and Horner,[162] and Gaul.[241] Walker et al[508] have determined that the ultimate sensibility of these flaps is a mixture of the median and radial nerves. Hastings[268] has described a "dual innervated cross finger" or island flap in which the dorsal sensory branch of the index radial digital nerve is repaired to the ulnar digital nerve of the thumb in an effort to improve cortical recognition of the flap as a thumb. Other variations have also been described[201,277,278,378,431,451] and although rarely required, the procedure has a definite place among the reconstructive options for restoration of thumb sensibility.

Radial-Innervated Cross-Finger Flap (Modified from Gaul[241])

Under tourniquet hemostasis the size of the acute defect or the defect to be created in order to provide sensory restoration to the denervated thumb is measured and a pattern created. A suitable flap is then designed over the dorsum of the proximal phalanx of the index finger with its base just palmar to the midlateral line. If necessary, the flap can be extended over the MP joint for resurfacing of larger defects. An oblique incision is designed from the midportion of the transverse base of the flap along the dorsal radial border of the thumb web to a level several centimeters proximal to the midportion of the thumb web (Fig. 57-40A). Dissection is then carried out to delineate a large dorsal sensory branch of the radial nerve which can be followed into the flap. The nerve is carefully mobilized to the proximal aspect of the index incision, and several small branches may require division.

Incisions are made around the edges of the flap and careful dissection is carried out to elevate the flap off the peritendinous tissue over the extensor tendons. When the flap has been mobilized to its base, the thumb is brought along the side of the index finger to check the positioning of the flap into the recipient defect (Fig. 57-40B).

A connecting incision is made along the ulnar border of the thumb and carried proximally to the previous oblique incision extending from the flap. At the time of flap attachment, the nerve is carefully transposed from the dorsum of the index ray to the ulnar thumb incision after undermining has provided a satisfactory trough in which it can lie without tension. Suturing of the ulnar thumb incision and the connecting dorsal radial index incision will secure the position of the nerve, and the defect over the dorsum of the proximal phalanx is covered with

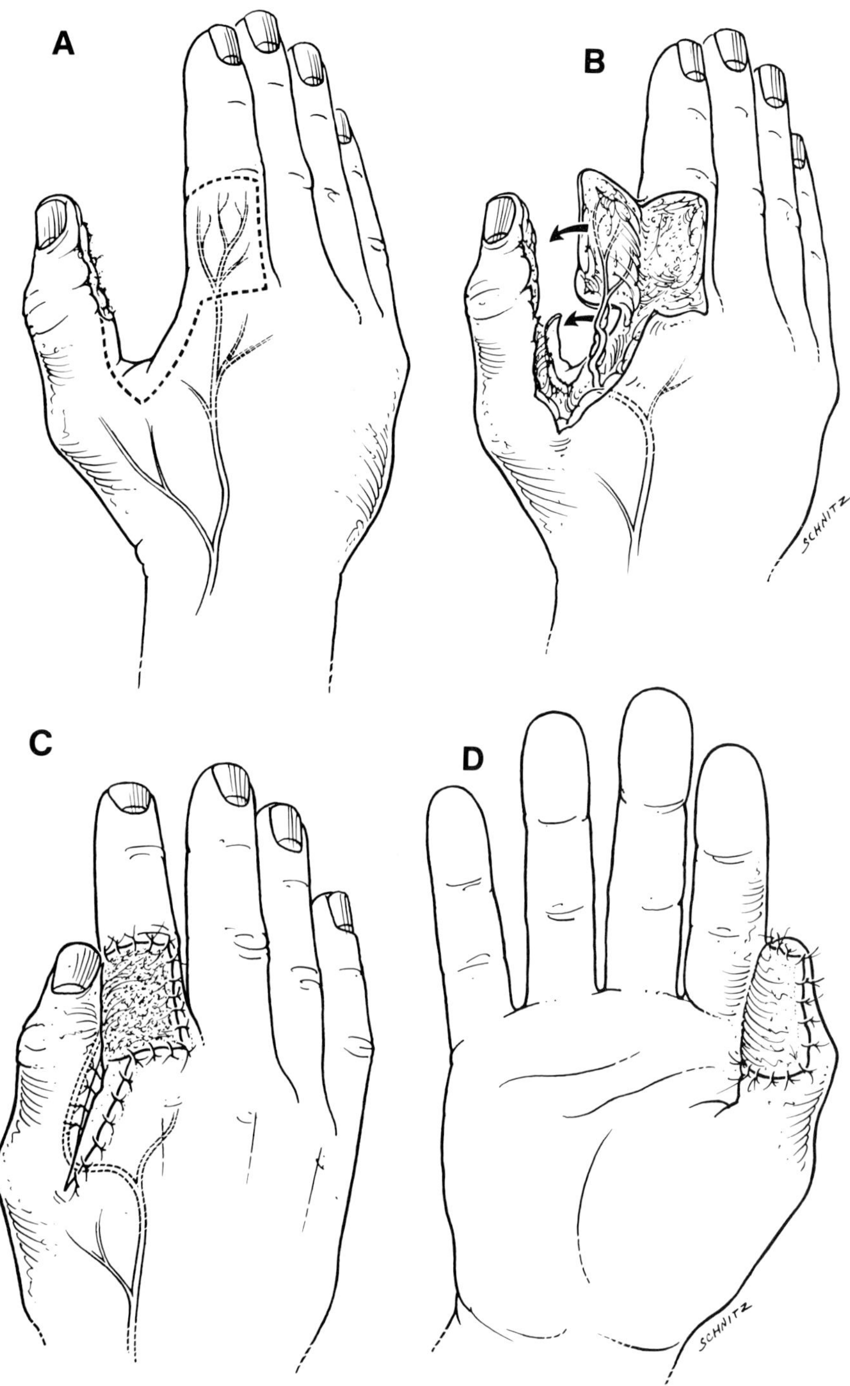

Fig. 57-40. Radial sensory nerve-innervated cross-finger flap. **(A)** Outline of the cross-finger flap with dorsal web incisions connecting to the thumb defect. The incision is made dorsal and proximal to the thumb web to prevent a subsequent scar contracture. The position of the dorsal sensory radial nerve is depicted. **(B)** Reflection of the flap following dissection of the nerve branch. **(C&D)** Position of the thumb and transferred flap with closure of incisions and free graft coverage of the donor defect. (Modified from Gaul,[241] with permission.)

a full-thickness skin graft dissected from the groin area. Sufficient graft is used to provide coverage of the exposed pedicle by suturing into the free ulnar edge of the thumb defect (Fig. 57-40C & D).

A compressive dressing immobilizing the thumb and index fingers as well as the palm and wrist is used for 3 weeks, following which the pedicle is divided and the free opposing edges of the thumb and index finger are closed. Mobilization exercises are initiated, and progressive increments of pressure are permitted against the flap. Complications following this procedure may be those related to damage to the mobilized branch of the radial sensory nerve secondary to undue tension or manipulation. Sensory return may only be protective, and the patient may continue to interpret his thumb sensation as being that of his dorsal index finger. Nonetheless, the radial sensory-innervated cross-finger flap is a useful procedure when faced with irreparable sensory damage to the thumb with no other available source for reconstruction (Fig. 57-41).

Dual Innervated Cross-Finger Flap

In an effort to improve cortical recognition of the flap as a thumb, Hastings[268] designed a "dual innervated cross finger" or island flap in which the dorsal sensory branch of the index radial digital nerve is sutured to the ulnar digital nerve of the thumb.

Dual Innervated Cross-Finger Flap (Hastings[268])

After debridement of the thumb defect, a template is made that is oversized by 20 percent. The thumb is positioned comfortably adjacent to the index, and the pattern is flipped over onto the dorsum of the index. The index cross-finger flap is based at the midaxial line. An incision is made from the proximal aspect of the flap along the radial aspect of the index metacarpal to the recess between the base of the index metacarpal and extensor pollicis longus. A limb is then extended distally along the ulnar aspect of the thumb metacarpal to the MP joint and more distal thumb defect just palmar to the mid axial line (Fig. 57-42).

Flap elevation is initiated distally and dorsoulnarly on the index. This requires incision and electrocauterization or ligation of veins crossing from the flap to the more distal index. The flap is elevated from dorsal to palmar, preserving peritenon of the extensor mechanism and including all neurovascular structures within the flap. Through the connecting incision from the index proximally, flaps are elevated superficial to the neurovascular structures. No attempt is made to separately dissect out the two to four terminal branches of the dorsal sensory radial nerve to the dorsal index. These are included with surrounding fatty tissue, which includes veins and, in most instances, the first dorsal intermetacarpal artery. If the flap is to be transferred as an island pedicle, the intermetacar-

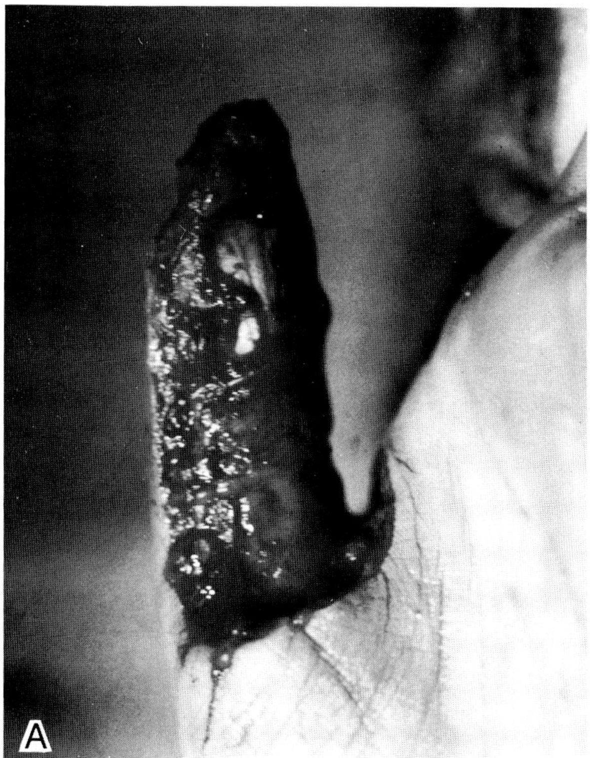

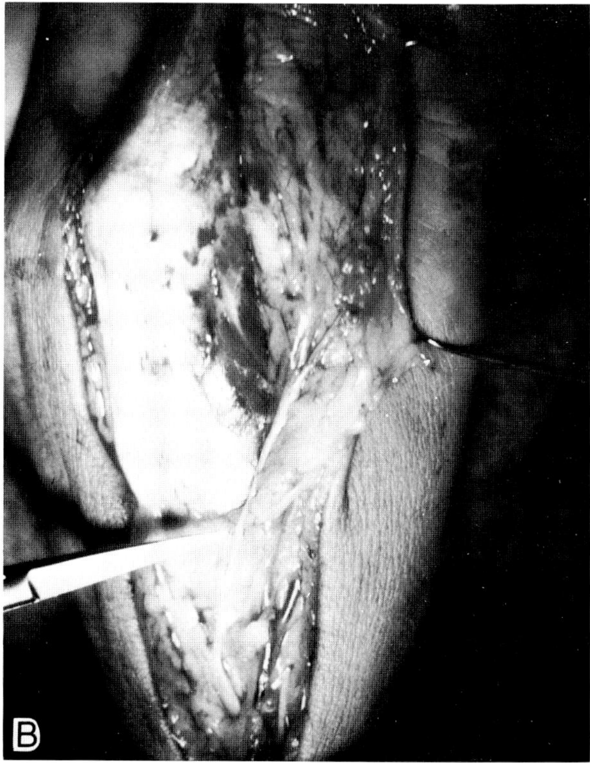

Fig. 57-41. A large radial sensory nerve-innervated cross-finger flap. **(A)** Avulsion of the entire palmar thumb following forceful removal of a circumferential pipe. **(B)** Use of a large sensory-innervated cross-finger flap from the index finger and second metacarpal. Scissors indicate the nerve branch within the flap. *(Figure continues.)*

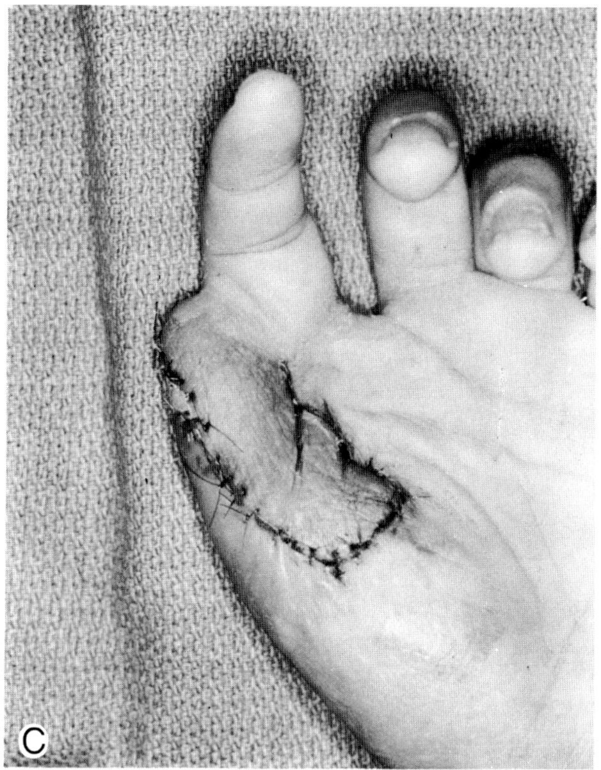

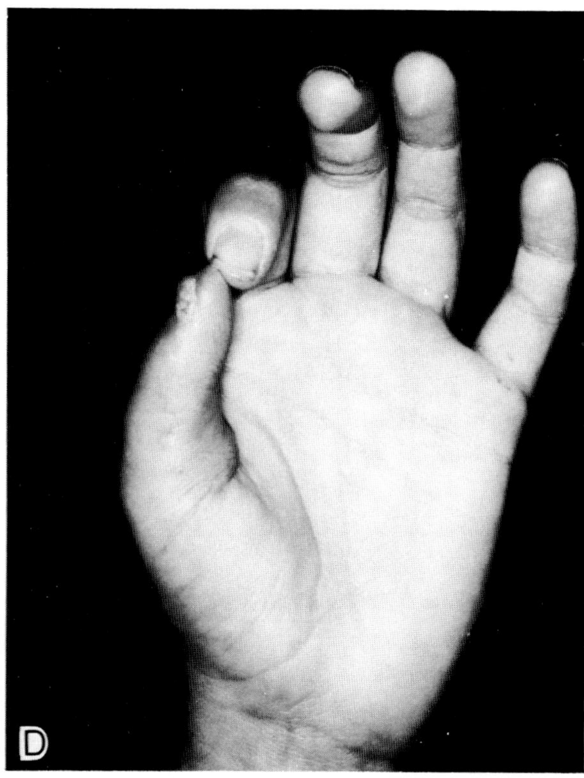

Fig. 57-41 *(Continued).* **(C)** Appearance of the flap on the palmar aspect of the thumb at the time of detachment (3 weeks). **(D)** Appearance of the thumb with satisfactory motion and sensation at 9 months. (From Strickland,[473] with permission.)

pal artery should be identified proximally. As stated by Foucher, the artery most often runs superficial to the fascia,[237] but it may run deep to fascia in 15 percent or consist of two vessels, one superficial and one deep, in 10 percent.[268] At the level of the MP joint, the dorsal branch from the index radial digital nerve is identified and dissected back to its origin. The connecting incision to the thumb is completed, identifying the ulnar digital nerve amputation stump proximal to the thumb defect.

The flap is transposed with the dorsal sensory radial nerve branches and inset radially. By microneurorrhaphy the palmar ulnar digital nerve of the thumb is then sutured to the more distal dorsal sensory nerve branch of the transposed flap (Fig. 57-43). The connecting incisions are closed and donor area skin grafted.

The postoperative care and flap deviation and insetting are identical to the radial innervated cross-finger flap previously described.

Amputation

It may be seen that the reconstructive requirements of the distal one-third of the thumb are those of skeletal stability, durable painless skin and subcutaneous tissues, and satisfactory sensory perception. When sufficient damage has occurred in this area to prejudice any possibility of satisfactory recovery of these requisites, then strong consideration should be given to amputation.[199,225,281,367,462] It is important that closure be carried out using sound amputation principles, including the careful identification and proximal resection of the digital nerves.[199,225,281,367,474] If these techniques are properly carried out, a good stump in the distal third of the thumb can function well with almost no functional disability.[226,352,427,431,441-443,504]

Summary: Reconstruction of the Distal One-Third of First Ray

A number of ingenious procedures may be used to return or improve thumb function following partial or complete loss in the distal one-third of the first ray. The primary goal of most of these procedures is to provide or improve skin coverage using methods that will ensure the return of satisfactory sensation without pain. It is our belief that additional thumb length is not a major consideration at this level, although several of the procedures described here may be used to preserve length without the need to further shorten the bony skeleton. Small lesions may be effectively treated with free skin grafts or by V-Y advancement techniques that have been popularized for other fingertip injuries. The palmar advancement flap is a procedure uniquely suited for the thumb that allows terminal pad defects up to 2.5 cm in size to be covered with well-padded and sensory-innervated skin. For larger lesions, cross-finger flaps have consistently been demonstrated to be reliable methods of

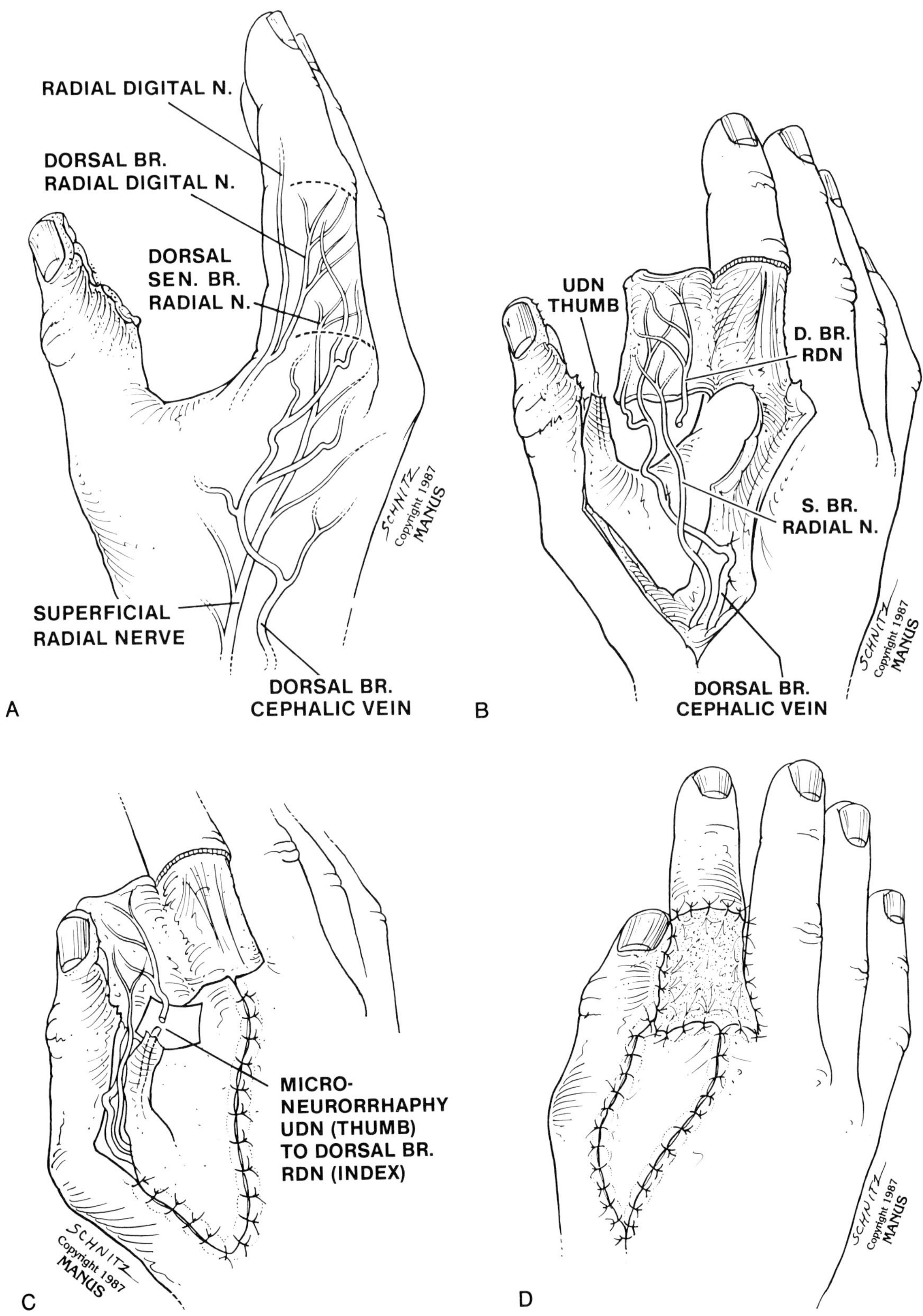

Fig. 57-42. Dual innervated cross finger flap. **(A)** The dorsal sensory branch of the index radial digital nerve predictably innervates the distal dorsal aspect of the index proximal phalanx. **(B)** Elevation of index-to-thumb cross finger flap with joining incisions for transposition of the dorsal sensory branch of radial nerve. **(C)** Microneurorrhaphy of the thumb ulnar digital nerve *(UDN)* to the dorsal branch of index radial digital nerve *(RDN)*. **(D)** Appearance of the flap at closure. (From Hastings.[268])

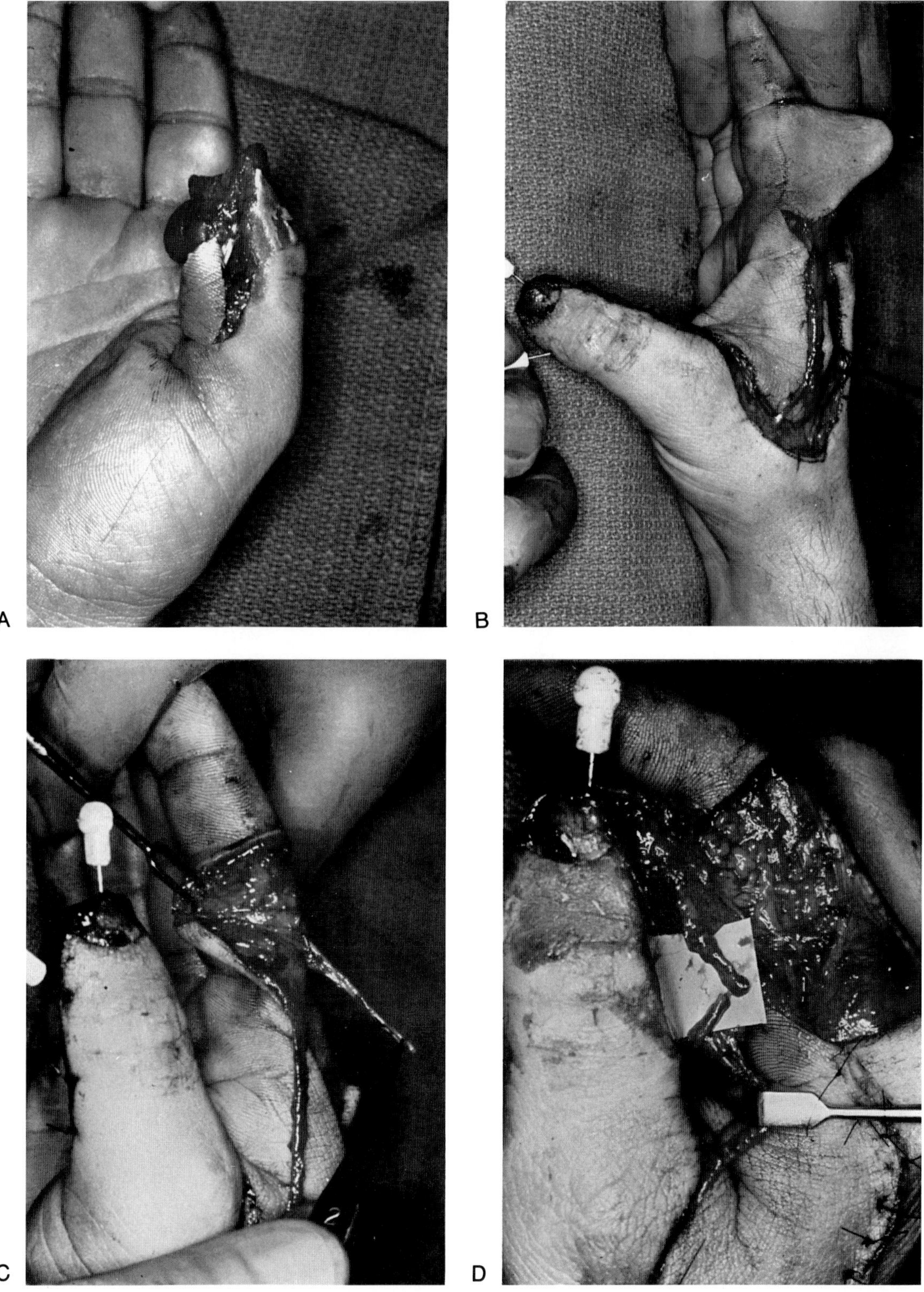

Fig. 57-43. Use of the dual innervated cross-finger flap. **(A)** A crush amputation to the pulp and nailbed of the thumb distal phalanx with proximal phalangeal fracture. **(B)** Dissection of the dorsal sensory radial nerve branches along with surrounding soft tissues to be transposed to the thumb. **(C)** The dorsal branch of index radial digital nerve provides ample pedicle for microneurorrhaphy to the thumb ulnar digital nerve after transposition of the cross-finger flap. **(D)** Microneurorrhaphy of the index dorsal branch of radial digital nerve to the ulnar digital nerve of the thumb. With short regeneration distance, sensory return is rapid, predictable, and cortically perceived as the thumb. *(Figure continues.)*

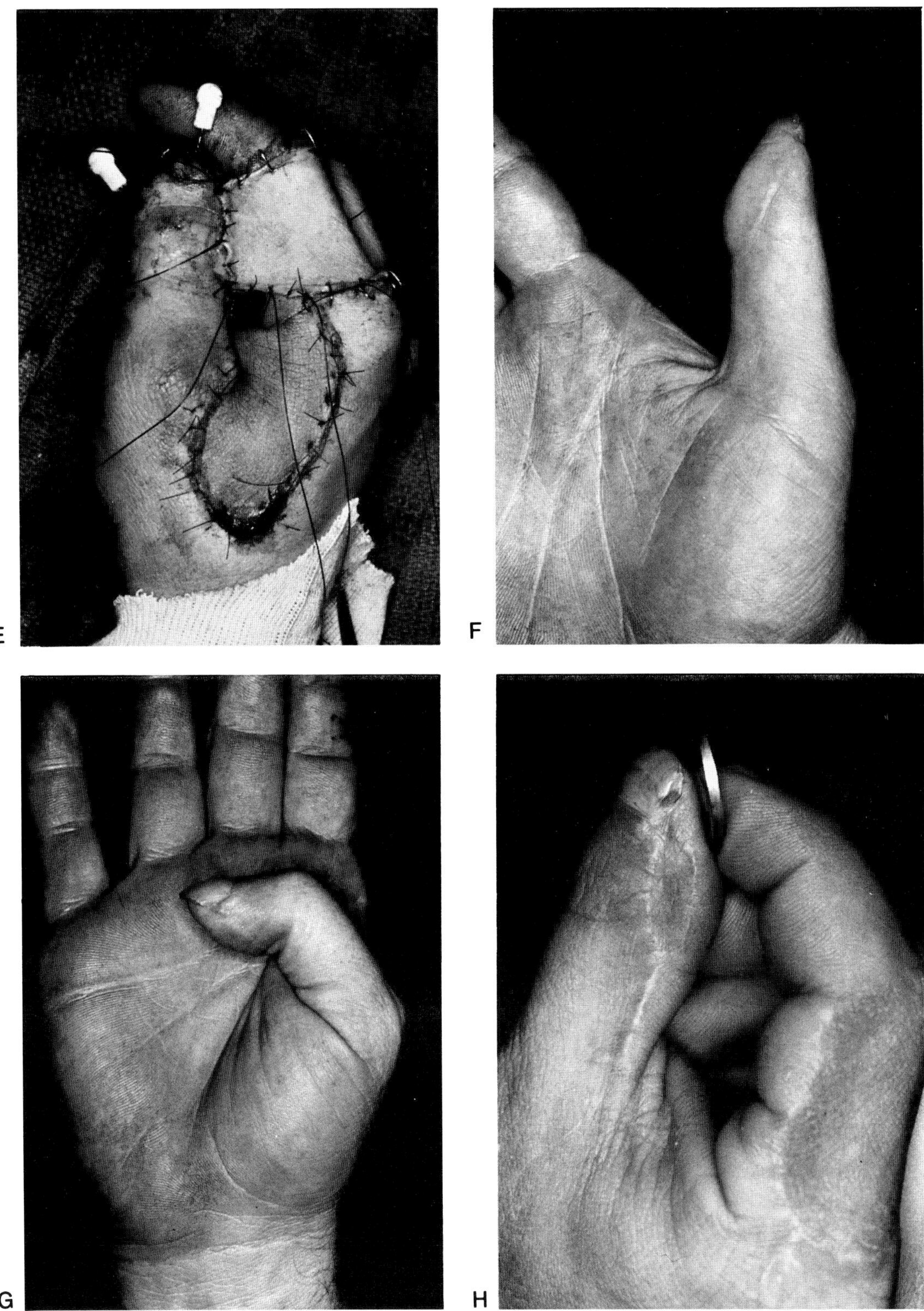

Fig. 57-43 *(Continued).* **(E)** A thick split-thickness skin graft is applied to both the donor area and the intervening pedicle between the index finger and thumb. **(F–H)** Final appearance and function of the resurfaced thumb.

providing durable skin coverage with a reasonable return of sensation. Neurovascular island pedicle flaps and radial sensory-innervated cross-finger flaps are procedures that may be occasionally employed for acute thumb injuries with loss of skin, subcutaneous tissue, and one or both digital nerves. Although these procedures result in varying degrees of impairment to their respective donor areas and often involve some difficulties with patient cortical interpretation, they are time-honored methods of improving function in certain instances of devastating palmar thumb loss, and are best used as secondary restorative methods. The surgeon dealing with lesions in the distal one-third of the thumb ray will have to weigh a number of factors, including the size of the lesion and the nature of neurovascular injury, as well as factors unique to the particular patient, before deciding which method to select.

AMPUTATION THROUGH THE MIDDLE ONE-THIRD OF THE FIRST RAY

Loss of length proximal to the midportion of the proximal phalanx creates problems with dexterous pinch and strong grasping of large objects. Following amputation at this level, most thumbs retain acceptable carpometacarpal rotation and an adequate thumb-index cleft. Functional requirements at this level, therefore, include added length with preservation of sensibility, mobility, stability, and a pain-free status of the thumb. To achieve these goals, a number of procedures have been established that either create relative ray lengthening by deepening the first web space or actually add bony length by a variety of methods.

It must be conceded at this point that the outstanding results achieved by free toe transplant techniques have made those microvascular procedures a strong consideration for reconstruction at this level. In particular, second toe transfer would appear to be an excellent restorative option that can satisfy all the functional requirements of middle-third thumb loss. Sufficient length, adequate sensation, and interdigital joint motion can be predictably reconstructed by this method and, in those patients who are agreeable, it may well be the best procedure. For many patients, however, the use of alternative methods such as those described in the following section may be more desirable. Because of somewhat differing requirements and approaches, the procedures for reconstruction following distal or proximal amputation in the middle one-third of the first ray will be considered separately.

Distal

When unsalvageable amputations occur near the midportion of the proximal phalanx (level B in Fig. 57-33), satisfactory thumb function can usually be achieved by procedures designed to deepen the first web space and create a widened thumb-index interval. These procedures have been called phalangization, and use methods that deepen the interdigital cleft so that the first metacarpal and remaining proximal phalanx are relatively lengthened.[146,165,166,193,218,229,230,258,280,281,286,292,330,331,333,341,367–369,373,376,397,406,407,445,459] This may be accom-

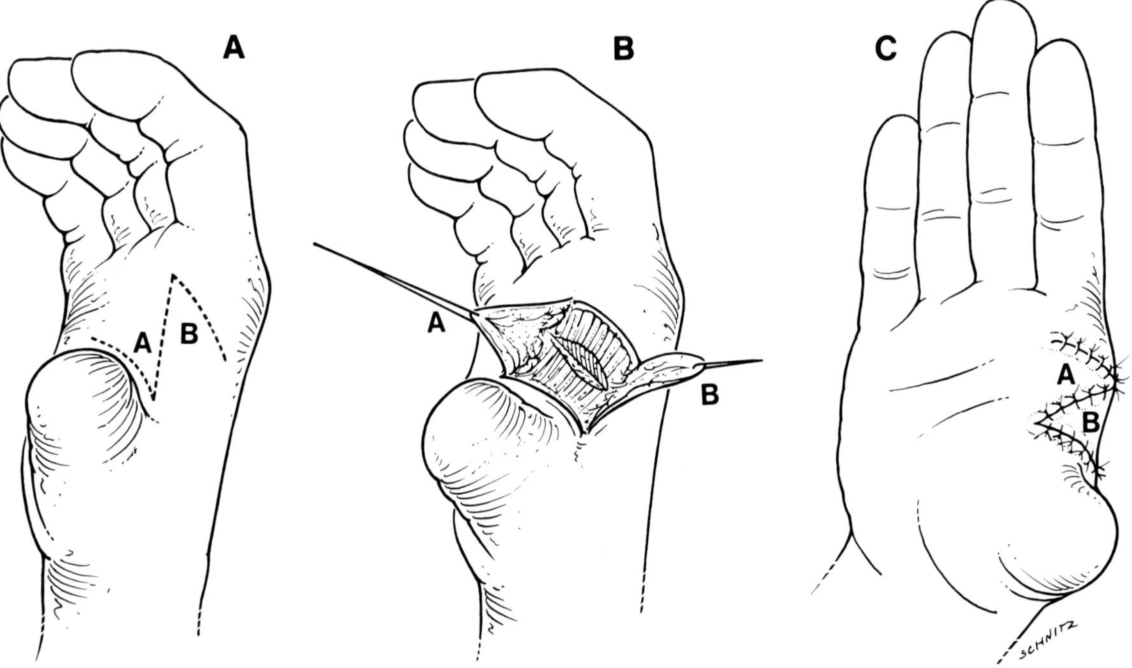

Fig. 57-44. Simple Z-plasty of the thumb web. **(A)** Design of the Z-plasty. The preferred angles are approximately 60 degrees. **(B)** The flaps reflected with partial recession of the web space musculature. **(C)** Appearance of flaps following reversal and suture. Corner sutures are preferred in the tips of the flaps.

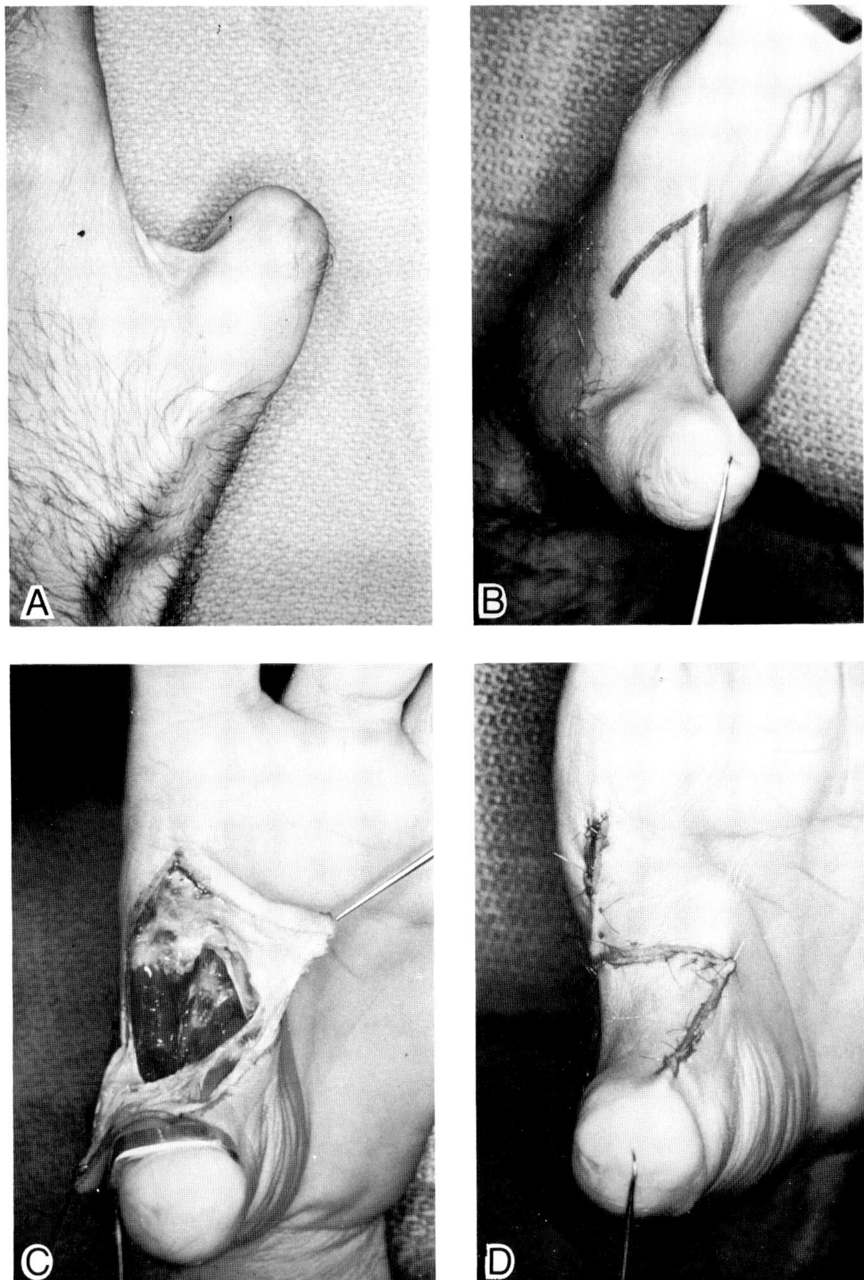

Fig. 57-45. Simple Z-plasty of the thumb web. **(A)** Limited thumb-index cleft following amputation through the midproximal phalanx. **(B)** Design of the Z-plasty. **(C)** Reflection of flaps with partial recession of the first web musculature. **(D)** Appearance of the Z-plasty following reversal and suture of flaps. *(Figure continues.)*

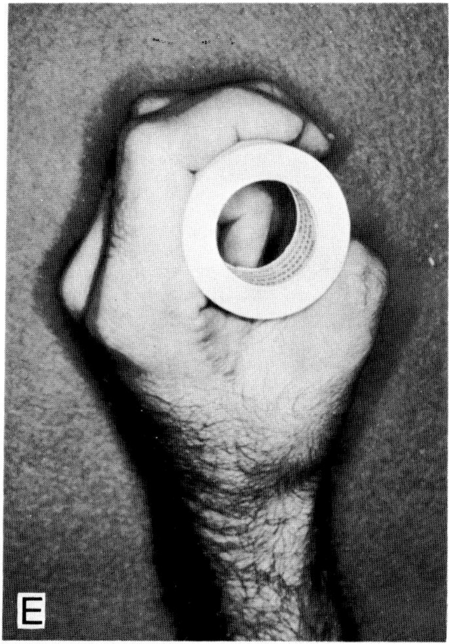

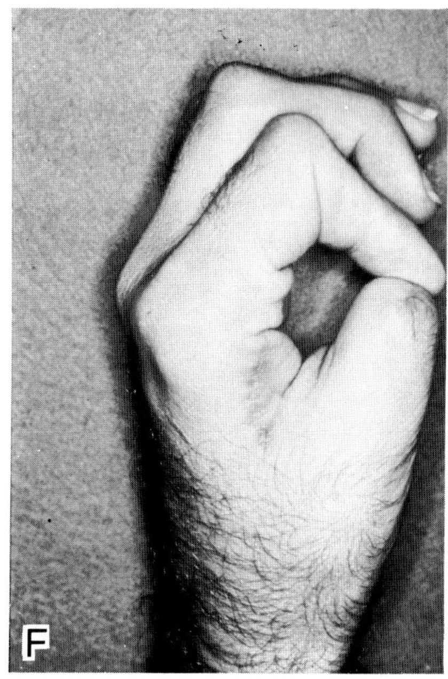

Fig. 57-45 *(Continued).* **(E&F)** Effective deepening of thumb web 3 months postoperatively. (From Strickland,[473] with permission.)

plished by simple web space Z-plasty,[183,229,280,281,373,445,474] a four-flap Z-plasty,[445,474,521] five-flap Z-plasty,[218,317] square flaps,[218] dorsal rotational flap techniques,[166,193,227,333,373,416,445,459,466,471,474,506] remote pedicle flaps,[193,280,281,380,505] radial arm flaps,[218] posterior interosseous flaps,[529] or free flaps such as the lateral arm flap.[456] The indications for these techniques vary according to the residual thumb length, amount of first web contracture, mobility of the first metacarpal, and the condition of the web space skin and muscle.[144,165,166,229,286,330,333,341,376,397,459,471,505]

Z-Plasty Procedures

Simple or four-flap Z-plasty techniques are adequate to achieve web space deepening when (1) at least half of the proximal phalanx remains, (2) the skin is minimally scarred, (3) the first metacarpal is mobile, and (4) there is no muscle contracture.[183,280,281,445,474,521] Although these procedures are relatively simple, it is important that the surgeon understand the concepts of Z-plasty, including proper flap design, mobilization, and repositioning. A thorough discussion of the principles of flap design is found in Chapter 49, but the application of Z-plasties to the thumb web space is presented here.

Simple Z-Plasty of the Thumb Web

Under tourniquet hemostasis, a flap is designed with its longitudinal axis on the distal ridge of the first web space extending from the proximal thumb crease to approximately 1 cm proximal to the proximal digital crease of the index finger at a point that corresponds with the radial confluence of the proximal and middle palmar creases. Oblique proximal palmar and distal dorsal limbs at approximately 60-degree angles are then designed with their length corresponding to the longitudinal incision. Local scar, previous incisions, or possible approaches for other reconstructive procedures may result in the need to reverse the direction of the two oblique limbs (proximal dorsal and distal palmar). Either combination seems to work satisfactorily (Fig. 57-44A).

The flaps are dissected back with careful undermining to avoid vascular compromise. Some additional depth can usually be achieved by a partial recession of the distal edge of the web space musculature (Fig. 57-44B). The flaps are then reversed and sutured in place using corner sutures to prevent tip necrosis (Figs. 57-44C and 57-45).

Four-Flap Z-Plasty of the Thumb Web (Modified from Broadbent and Woolf[163])

Under tourniquet hemostasis, the longitudinal axis of the "Z"-plasty is drawn on the distal edge of the thumb web ridge extending from the ulnar margin of the proximal thumb crease to an area approximately 1 cm proximal to the proximal digital crease of the index finger, corresponding with the confluence of the proximal and middle palmar creases (Fig. 57-46A). Proximal palmar and distal dorsal incisions varying from 90 to 120 degrees are then made with their lengths equaling that of the longitudinal incision. The angles formed by these three lines are then equally divided by an oblique line extending from their apices. These incisions also correspond in length with the other incisions (Fig. 57-46B & C). The flaps are reflected on their bases, elevating skin and a small amount of

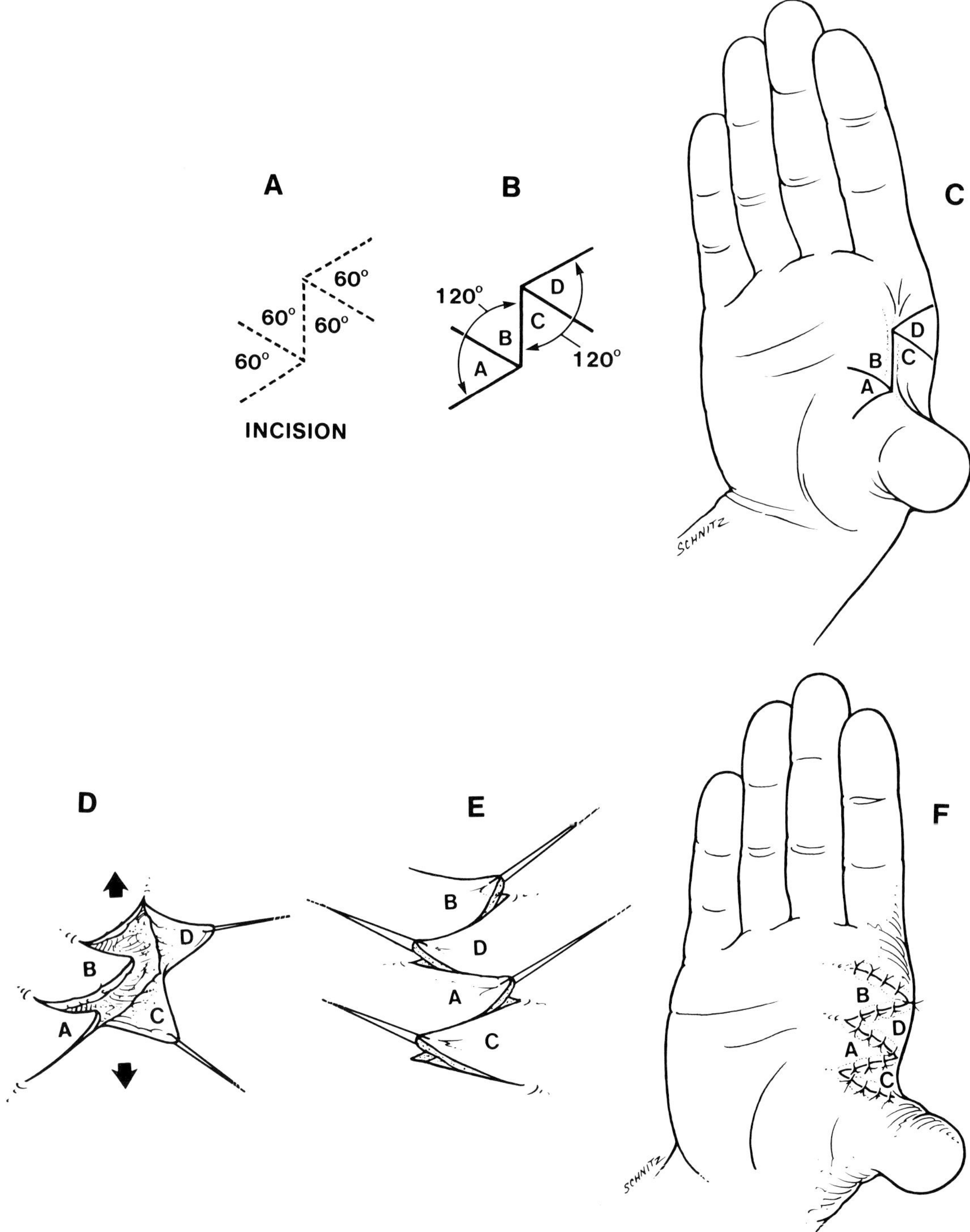

Fig. 57-46. Four-flap Z-plasty of the thumb web. **(A&B)** Two 120-degree angle opposing incisions are bisected to form four 60-degree flaps. **(C)** Design of the flaps in the first web space. **(D)** Incision, elevation, and undermining of the flaps. **(E)** Flap position after interposition. **(F)** Appearance of the thumb web following interposition of the flaps. (Modified from Broadbent and Woolf,[163] with permission.)

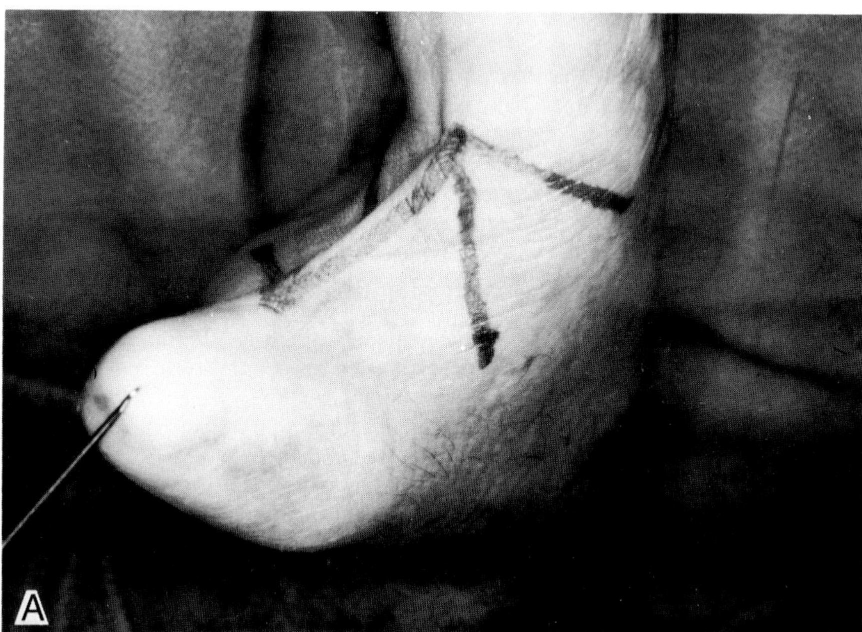

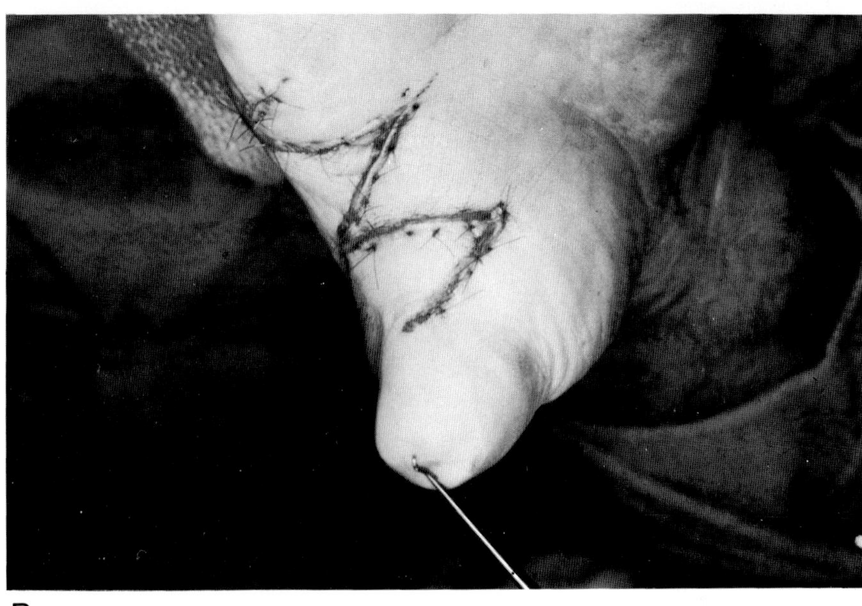

Fig. 57-47. Four-flap Z-plasty of the thumb web. **(A)** Design of flaps (see text and Fig. 57-46). **(B)** Appearance of the thumb web immediately following transposition and suture of the flaps.

subcutaneous tissue. Gentle undermining and a small recession of the thumb web musculature may be carried out to provide further depth.

The flaps are then mobilized and interdigitated so that the common border of the two middle flaps previously formed by the longitudinal line now comes to lie against the proximal and distal incision sites (Fig. 57-46D & E). The proximal palmar and distal dorsal flaps are rotated to the midline and their medial edges, previously formed by the oblique bisecting incisions, are joined. The flaps are then sutured in place without tension. A substantial increase in web depth should be achieved (Fig. 57-46F).

After either Z-plasty technique, a compressive dressing maintaining the expanded web is worn for 7 to 14 days. A small web spacer splint is then utilized for several additional weeks.

These simple skin mobilization techniques, occasionally combined with short distal muscle recession, can provide a reliable deepening of the thumb web and relative lengthening of the shortened thumb. When measured, the gain in depth varies from 1.5 to 2 cm, which should result in improved ability to grasp larger objects (Fig. 57-47). Complications from these techniques should be minimal as long as the surgeon is familiar with this type of skin and soft tissue rearrangement and carries out the procedure in a careful manner.

Dorsal Rotational Flap

On occasion, the injury that has resulted in thumb loss through the proximal phalanx will also result in considerable adjacent tissue injury with involvement of the first web space musculature and an adduction contracture of the first metacarpal. In these instances a more extensive procedure will be necessary to mobilize the first metacarpal and restore the web space. Several dorsal rotational flap techniques have proven effective in deepenitig the first web space, and mobilizing and resurfacing the metacarpal-phalanx unit[166,193,227,333,369,373,416,445,459,466,471,474,506] Sandzen described a pedicle rotated from the dorsum of the thumb ray to cover the defect created by web release.[454,455] Remote sites such as the abdomen,[281,382] arm,[281,506] or chest,[193] have also been sources of thumb web coverage. The advantages of phalangization of the adducted first metacarpal with immediate coverage by a dorsal rotational flap are considerable because of the excellent quality skin with sensory perception that it brings into the web. This technique employs sequential division of all restraining skin, muscle, scar, and capsular adhesions, and can result in a very satisfactory restoration of function.

Phalangization of the First Metacarpal with Dorsal Rotational Flap Coverage (Modified from Brown[166])

Under tourniquet anesthesia, a continuous linear dorsal and palmar incision is carried through the first web, beginning dorsally at the level of the trapeziometacarpal joint and extending along the ulnar border of the first metacarpal to the first MP joint, where it passes through the thumb web and continues palmarward into the palm at the base of the thenar eminence (Fig. 57-48A).

Sharp dissection is continued just ulnar to the extensor pollicis longus and, while protecting sensory branches of the radial nerve, the origin of the first dorsal interosseous muscle is stripped from the metacarpal, or if the muscle has become scarred or fibrotic, it is divided. The radial artery must be identified as it dips between the two heads of the first dorsal interosseous muscle just beyond the trapeziometacarpal joint. By following the artery distally, the princeps pollicis artery can be identified and protected as the border of the adductor pollicis is defined. Both the oblique and transverse heads of the adductor are divided and, by gentle abduction traction on the

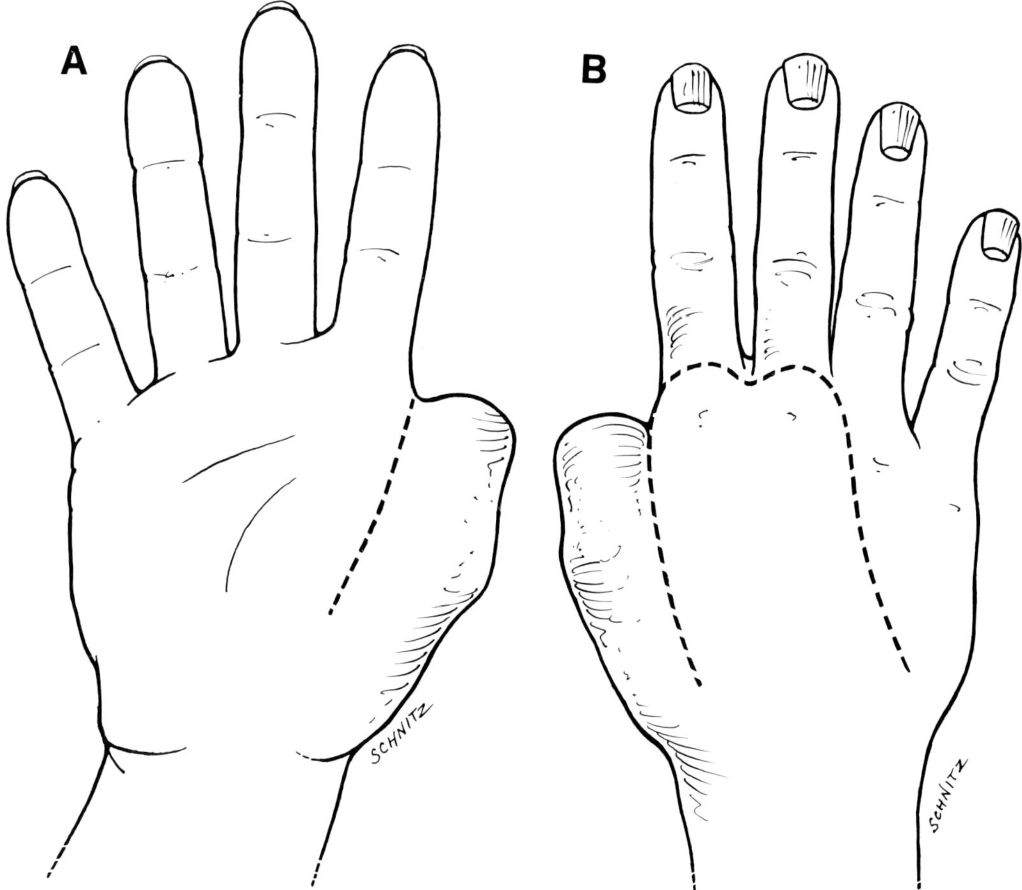

Fig. 57-48. Release of adduction contracture of first web space with dorsal rotational flap coverage. **(A)** The palmar web-dividing incision is a continuous linear incision from the first web space to the thenar crease parallelling the medial margin of the thenar musculature. **(B)** The linear incision over the dorsum of the first web with approximate outline of the dorsal rotational flap. *(Figure continues.)*

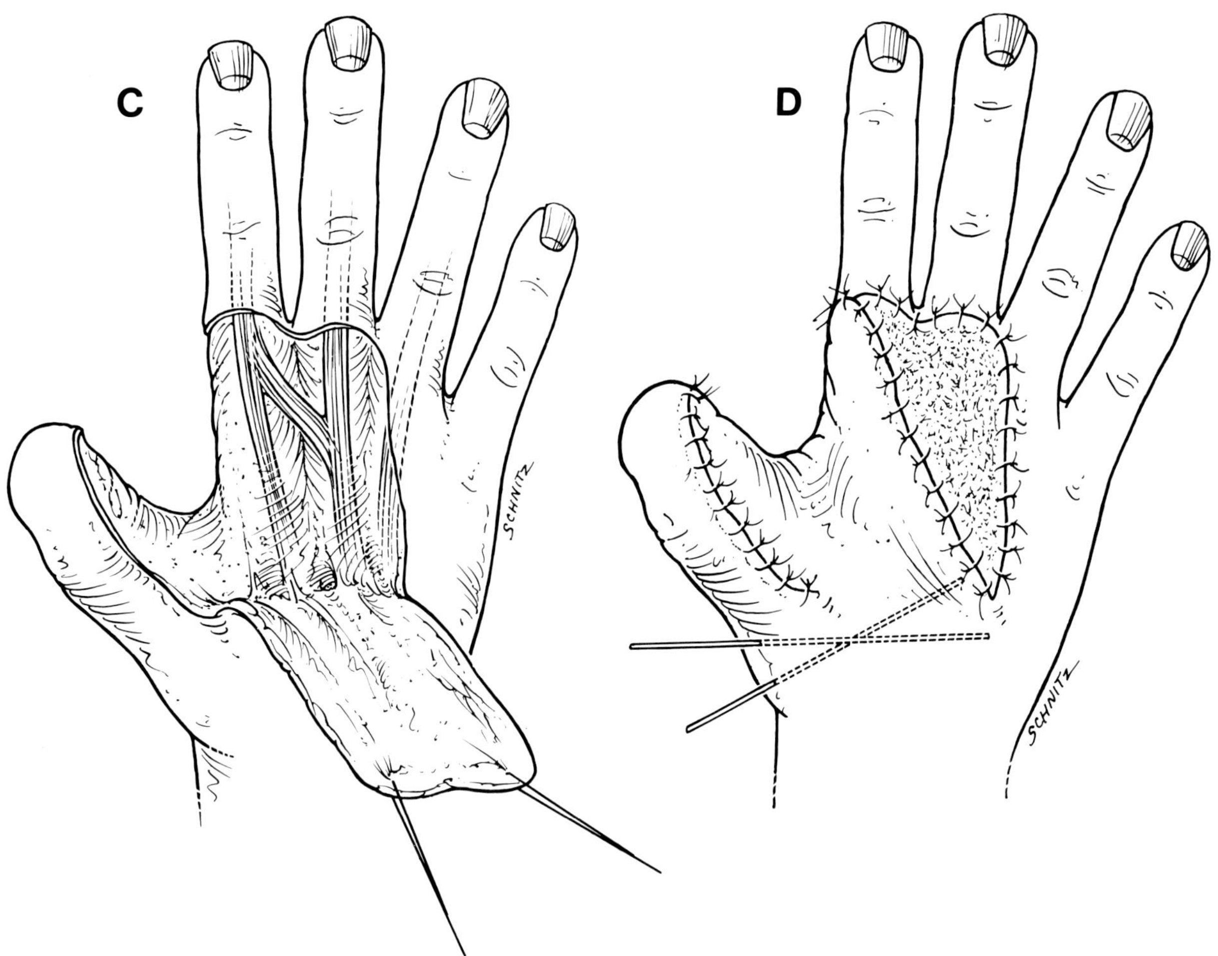

Fig. 57-48 *(Continued).* **(C)** The first web defect following division of restraining skin, soft tissue, and muscle with abduction of the first metacarpal. Elevation of the dorsal rotational flap down to the adventitia overlying the extensor tendons is complete. **(D)** Appearance of the first web following coverage with dorsal rotational flap. K-wires hold the thumb in abduction during healing, and a free skin graft is used to cover the donor defect. (Modified from Brown,[166] with permission.)

first metacarpal, a determination can be made as to the adequacy of first ray mobilization. Stripping of the opponens pollicis muscle may be required in order to mobilize a severely contracted first metacarpal.

In some instances muscle release will not result in complete mobilization of the first metacarpal, and release of the carpometacarpal joint capsule or occasionally trapezial excision may be necessary. The capsule of the trapeziometacarpal joint is opened transversely through a palmar incision, and a similar capsulectomy on the dorsal ulnar side of the joint is sometimes used. The mobilized thumb is stabilized in the corrected position by transfixing the first and second metacarpals through their proximal segments with two nonparallel K-wires (Fig. 57-48D) or with an external fixator (Fig. 57-49A & B).

Tourniquet release is carried out at this point, all brisk bleeders are controlled, and the vascularity of the thumb confirmed prior to reinflation. Trial rotation of a paper pattern placed over the dorsum of the hand will help determine the proper size and configuration of the flap. The incision is continued from the ulnar web and wound dorsally across the radial aspect of the MP joint of the index finger and across the dorsum of the proximal phalanx of that digit. It is then brought proximally over the dorsum of the hand to approximately the base of the fourth metacarpal, although the exact configuration can best be determined by the paper pattern technique just described (Fig. 57-48B). The dorsal flap is dissected free from the peritenon overlying the extensors of the fingers, and although there is minimal interference with the dorsal veins of the hand, a few sizable veins should be ligated distally and brought with the flap (Fig. 57-48C).

Gentle undermining is carried out, and an occasional additional dorsoulnar skin release may be necessary in order to bring the flap into proper position to cover the defect. The flap is then sutured in place and the resulting triangular defect over the dorsoradial hand is covered with either a dissected near full-thickness graft from the groin or a split-thickness graft taken with a dermatome (Fig. 57-48D).

A stent dressing is used over the graft and a small suction

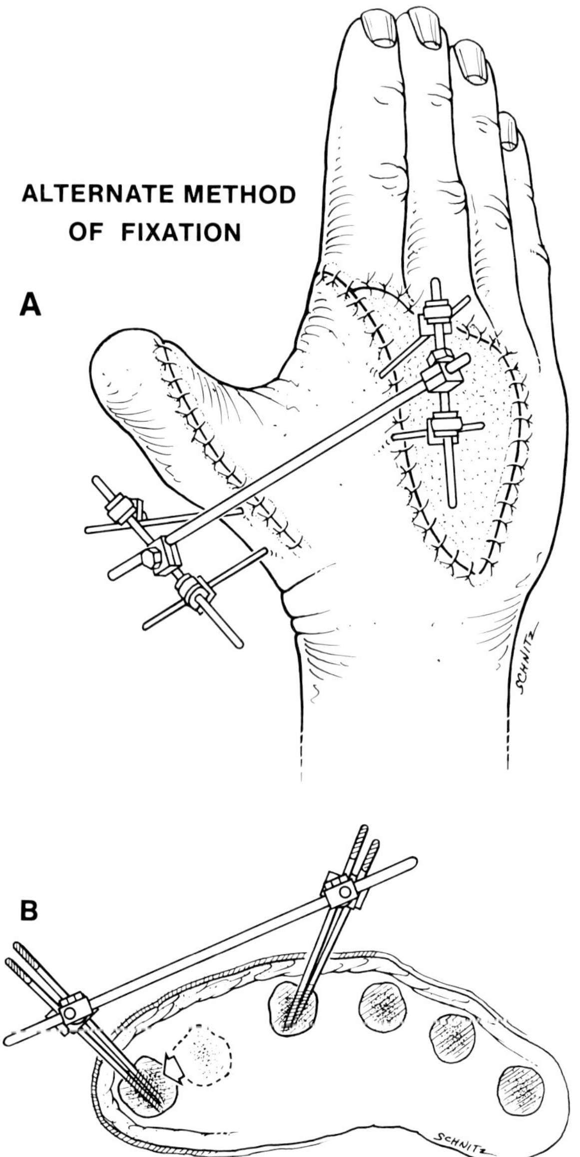

Fig. 57-49. An alternative method of fixation of the first and second metacarpals following first web space deepening. The use of a mini-external fixator is depicted. **(A)** The purchase pins in the lateral aspect of the first metacarpal and dorsum of the second metacarpal with a transfixing bar used to stabilize and maintain the web. **(B)** Transverse section to depict the position of the fixator pins in the metacarpals.

drain is placed beneath the flap for 24 to 48 hours. A voluminous compressive dressing is applied to the hand, wrist, and forearm. The flap and grafts are first checked at 7 to 10 days and the sutures removed at 2 weeks. Although digital mobilization is begun at 2 to 3 weeks, a conforming splint is intermittently used in the first web for 3 months. The pins are removed at 4 to 6 weeks. Continuous monitoring of the web space status will be necessary for 1 year, and night splinting utilizing a web spacer may be necessary throughout that time period.

Long-standing severe adduction contracture of the first metacarpal is a crippling deformity, particularly when a portion of the distal thumb has been lost. Surgical release of the deformity is accomplished by meticulous sequential division of all contracting elements and will result in a substantial skin and soft tissue deficit, which may be well covered by the use of a rotation flap from the dorsum of the hand (Fig. 57-50). Complications include hematoma formation, flap loss, graft failure, or recurrent adduction contracture. If the surgical procedure is carefully carried out with attention to technical detail and proper postoperative care is used, the incidence of these problems should be minimal. Additional reconstructive procedures, such as tendon transfers, may be necessary in order to further enhance thumb function; however, the restoration of the web space and improvement in thumb posture alone should have a profoundly favorable influence on hand performance (Fig. 57-51).

Cross-Arm Flap

When a severe first web space contracture exists with deep muscle and joint contracture and with concomitant compromise of the adjacent dorsal skin, a remote pedicle source must be sought to provide quality coverage following releasing procedures. The cross-arm technique can be used occasionally in these circumstances to provide excellent resurfacing of the first web space.[281,397,445,476] This procedure is excellent both functionally and cosmetically. It provides thin, supple skin, and the contour of the arm is excellent for maintaining the web space while the pedicle is being vascularized.[397] The skin is thin and the subcutaneous layer is also usually thin, and the flap is best taken from the medial aspect of the arm.

First Web Space Deepening with Cross-Arm Flap Coverage

Release of the first web space is carried out in a manner identical to that described for the dorsal rotational flap (Fig. 57-52A). The abducted position of the thumb is maintained by the use of K-wires crossed between the bases of the first and second metacarpals or by the use of an external fixator. The hand is then brought into place against the opposite arm in such a manner that the ulnar border of the hand can rest against the anterior medial surface of the forearm with the thumb comfortably placed around the inner aspect of the upper arm. Patterns are used to design a proximally based triangular flap that can be used to resurface the dorsal half of the divided web space (Fig. 57-52B). The flap is meticulously elevated, including skin and subcutaneous tissue, and temporary split-thickness skin coverage is placed on the arm and palmar hand defects. Moist cotton stent dressings over the graft are important, and the position of the arm is maintained by the use of a plaster Velpeau dressing. At 3 weeks, the patient is returned to surgery and a corresponding triangular flap is designed proximally, which is then dissected out and turned into

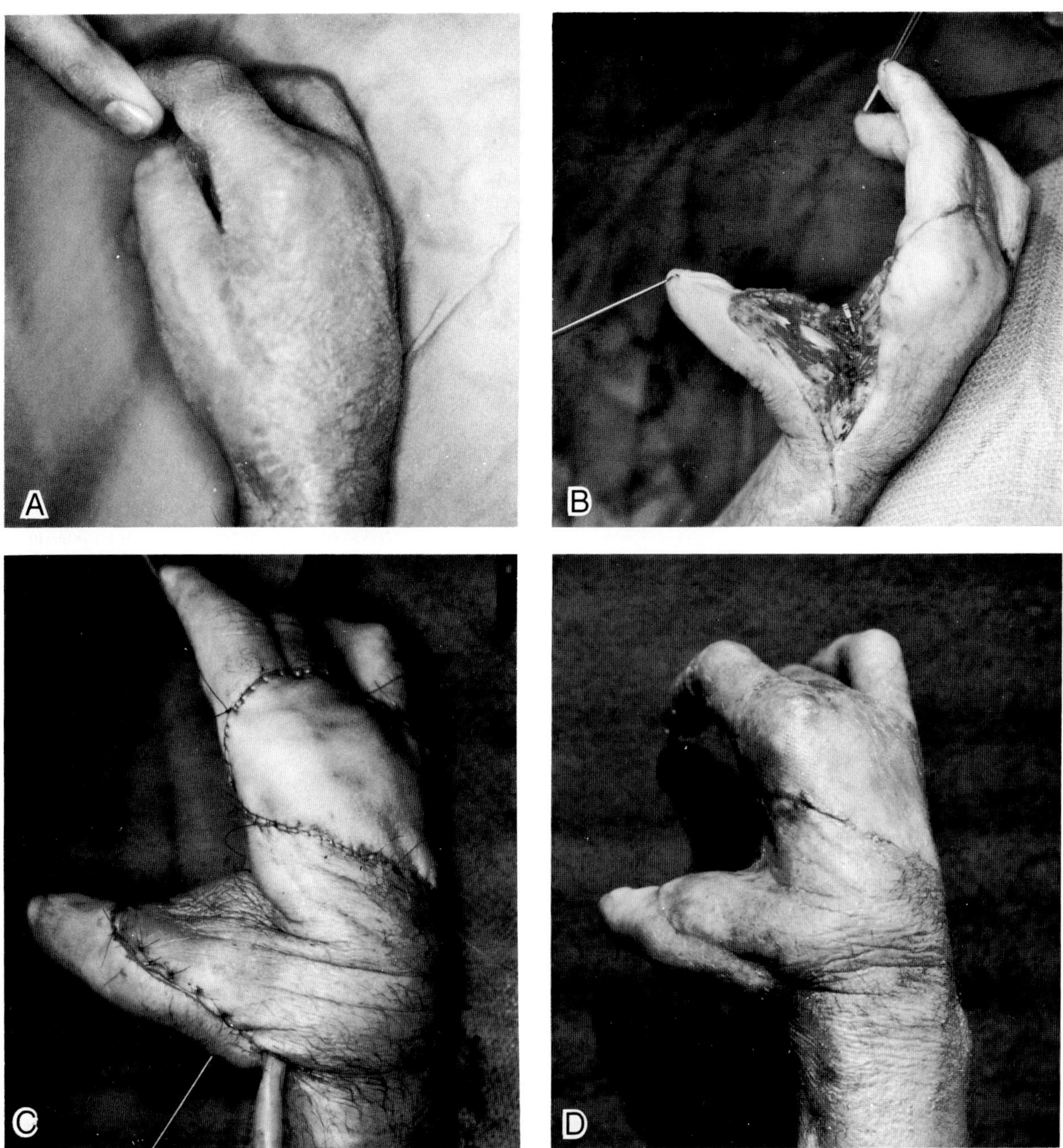

Fig. 57-50. Phalangization of a severely contracted first metacarpal with a dorsal rotational flap. **(A)** Severe, long-standing adduction contracture of the thumb following amputation through the proximal phalanx. **(B)** Appearance of the thumb web following release of skin, soft tissue, web space musculature, and basilar thumb joint. **(C)** Coverage of the thumb web with a large dorsal rotational flap. **(D)** Appearance of the thumb web at 3 months.

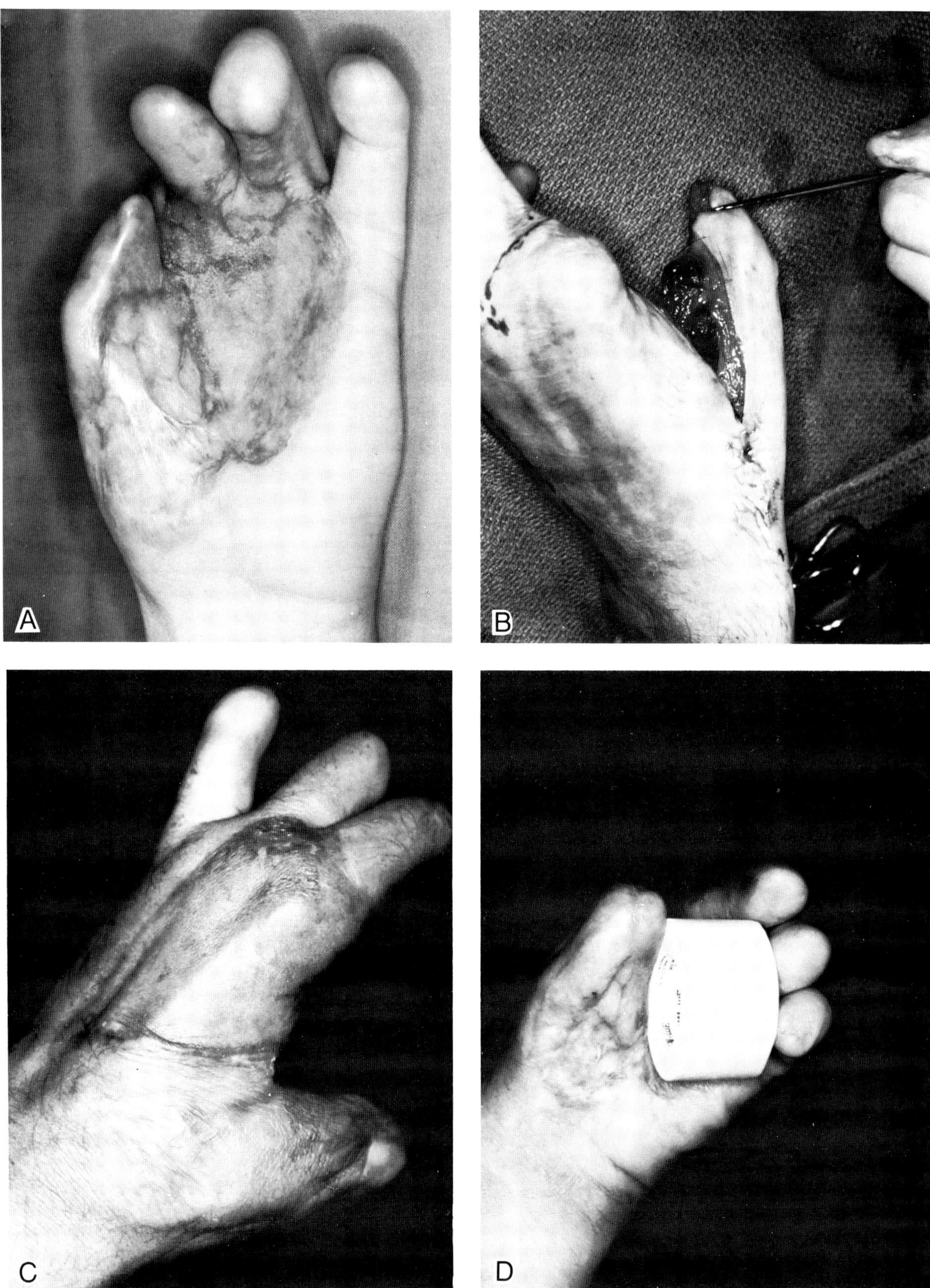

Fig. 57-51. Phalangization of a damaged metacarpal-phalanx unit. **(A)** A tightly contracted thumb metacarpal and proximal phalanx with poor skin coverage following a combination crush-burn injury. **(B)** Mobilization of the metacarpal and division of the contracted web with excision of skin and division of the first dorsal interosseous and adductor pollicis muscles. **(C)** Improved abduction of the phalangized thumb at 4 months. **(D)** Improved grasp and pinch at 4 months. (From Strickland,[473] with permission.)

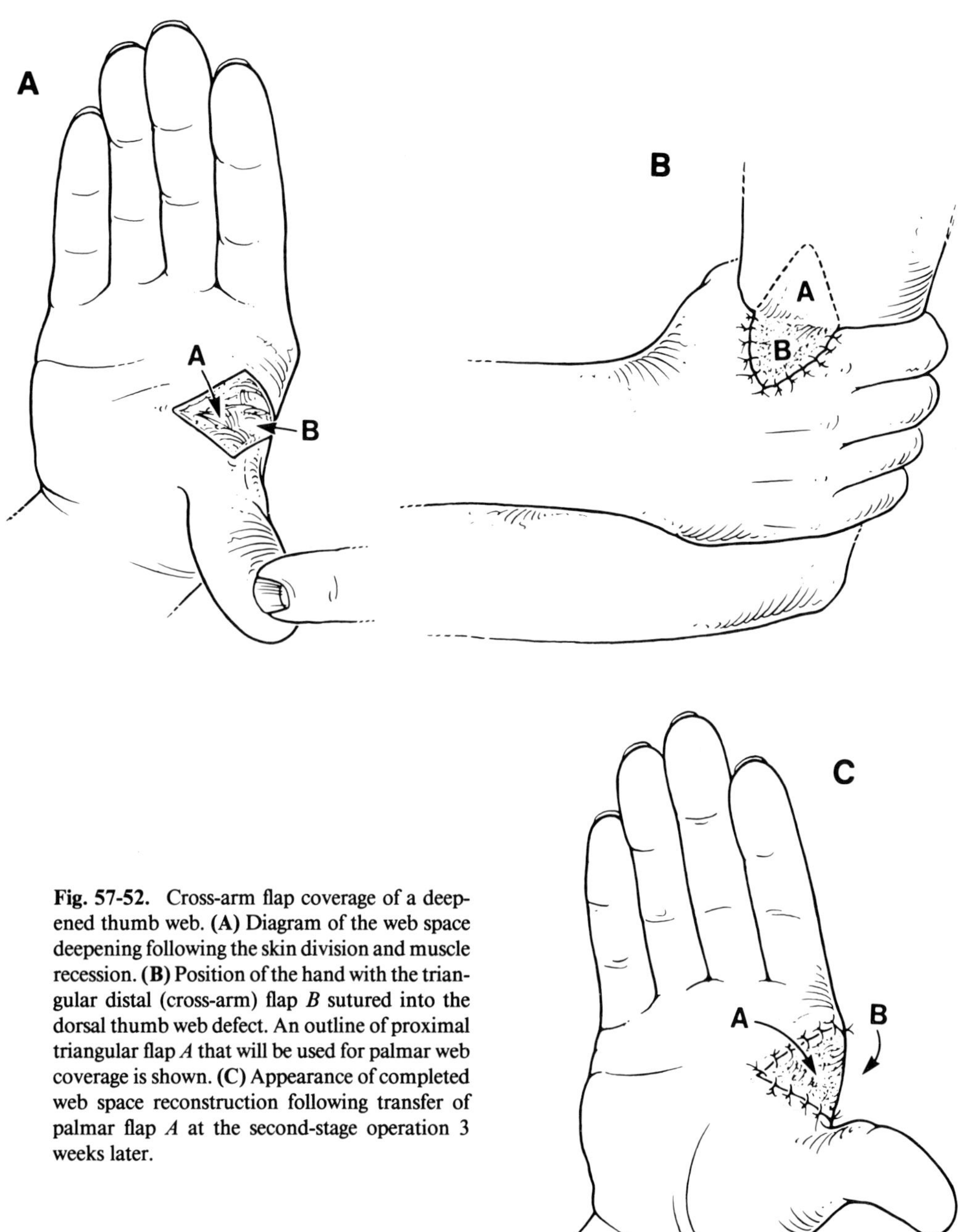

Fig. 57-52. Cross-arm flap coverage of a deepened thumb web. **(A)** Diagram of the web space deepening following the skin division and muscle recession. **(B)** Position of the hand with the triangular distal (cross-arm) flap *B* sutured into the dorsal thumb web defect. An outline of proximal triangular flap *A* that will be used for palmar web coverage is shown. **(C)** Appearance of completed web space reconstruction following transfer of palmar flap *A* at the second-stage operation 3 weeks later.

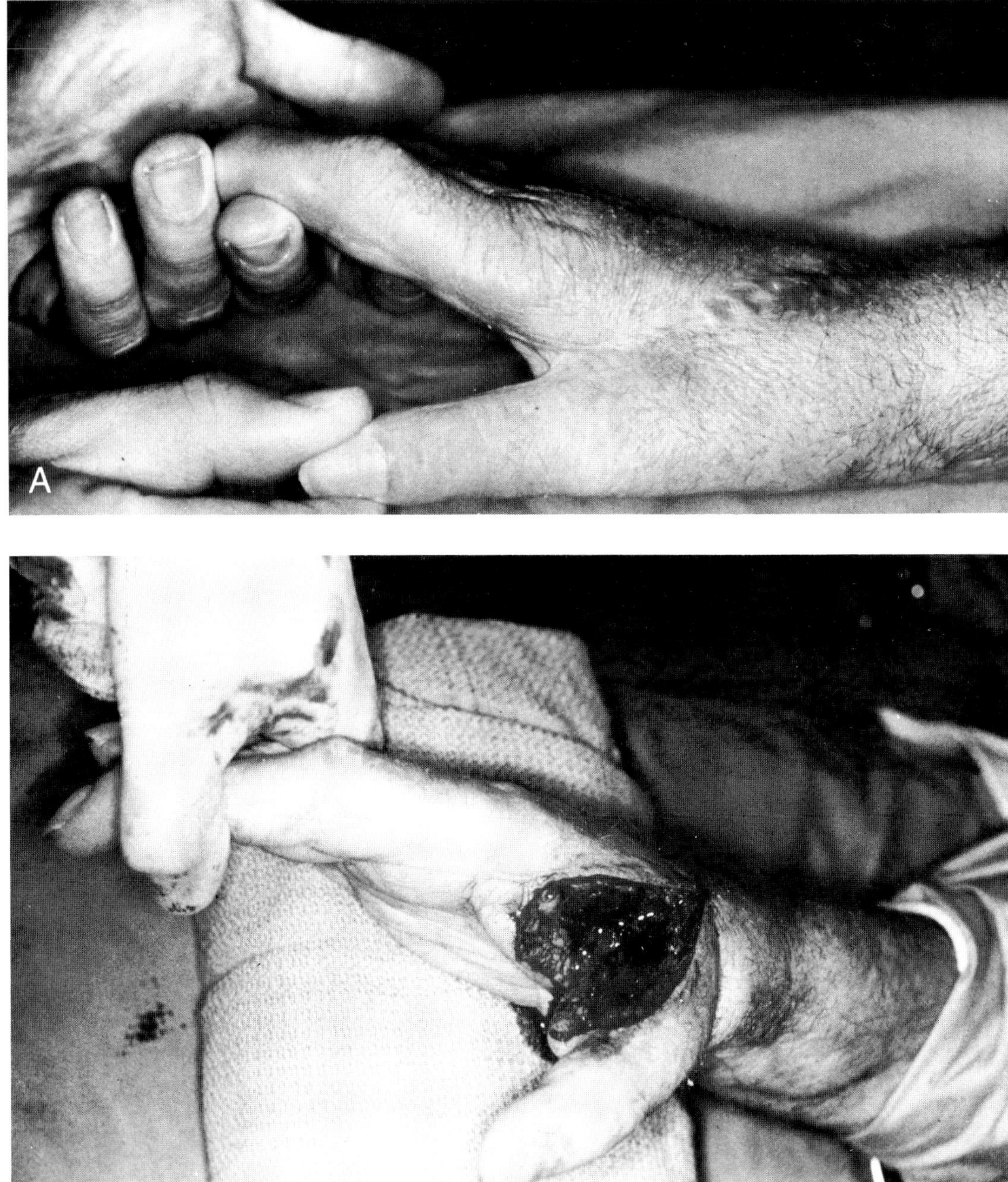

Fig. 57-53. A clinical application of the cross-arm flap technique. **(A)** Tightly contracted first web space with severe injury to dorsal skin. **(B)** Appearance of the thumb web defect following skin, muscle, and scar division. *(Figure continues.)*

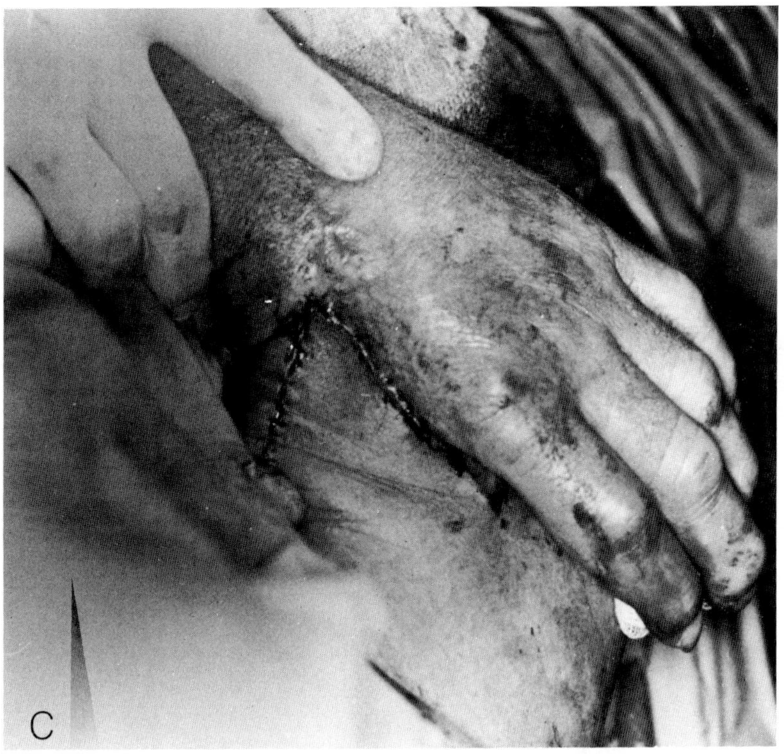

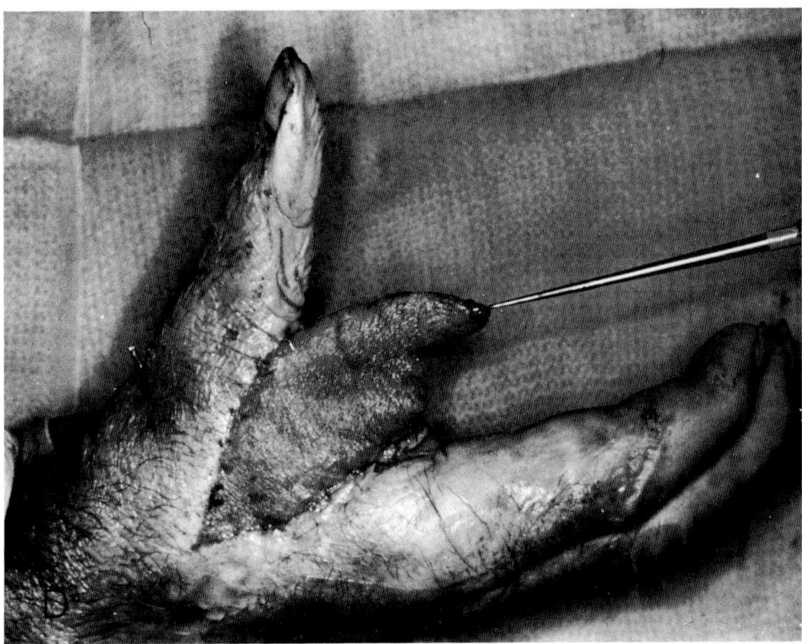

Fig. 57-53 *(Continued).* **(C)** Appearance of the dorsal first web space coverage with the distal triangular upper arm flap. **(D)** At 3 weeks, following satisfactory healing of the dorsal flap, the proximal triangular flap is transposed into the palmar web defect. *(Figure continues.)*

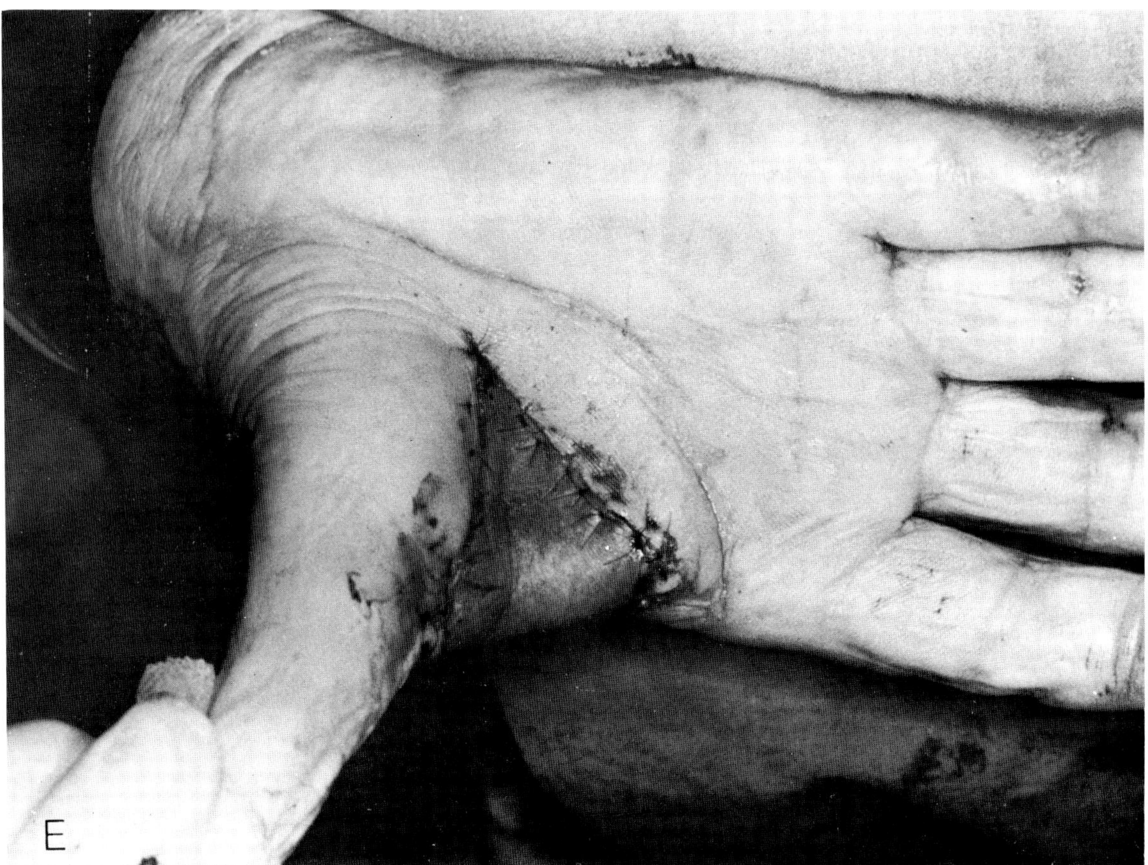

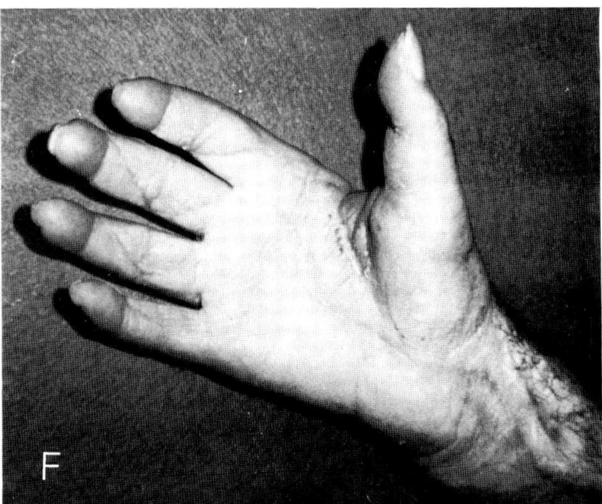

Fig. 57-53 *(Continued).* **(E)** Appearance of palmar web coverage at time of insetting. **(F)** Appearance of the reconstructed first web space using this technique.

the palmar defect after the free graft is excised. Defatting is usually not necessary, and an excellent restoration of the web space can be achieved in this manner (Fig. 57-52C). Maintenance web space splinting using an orthoplast spacer is used for 2 to 3 months after removal of the fixation pins at 6 weeks. This will, hopefully, prevent the recurrence of the adduction deformity secondary to contracture of deep web space scarring.

The cross-arm flap may provide excellent coverage following release of the first web space in patients with amputations of the thumb through the middle one-third of the first ray. The procedure restores excellent skin and subcutaneous tissue both palmarly and distally without the need to use the often compromised dorsal hand skin. It has the disadvantage of a resulting defect on the opposite arm and although it can, in general, maintain the hand in a position of function, it does cause the obvious limitation of upper limb function during the period of obligatory immobilization. The procedure is probably not a good one for women as a scar defect is created in an exposed area. Nonetheless, it has proven to be an effective technique for web space widening and deepening and relative thumb lengthening in certain instances (Fig. 57-53).

Proximal

Thumb loss near the MP joint (level A in Fig. 57-33) may result in a stump that is inadequate to perform many of the important functions of the thumb.[436,438,443,452,474] Approximately 2 cm of added length may substantially improve function, provided there is concomitant restoration of satisfactory sensory perception.[475] In the acute injury in which replantation is not a possibility, autograft techniques have been advocated by some.[245,251,275,398,429,436,439,441,450,519] Skin and subcutaneous tissue are removed from the amputated part, and the remaining thumb consisting of bone and tendon is either replaced primarily or preserved in an abdominal pocket and reattached after several weeks or months. Reconstruction is then carried out with coverage provided by a remote tubed flap, and sensation added later by means of a neurovascular island pedicle flap. Although this procedure is not widely used, it apparently can provide a satisfactory return of thumb function.

The occasional degloving injury of the thumb with loss of all skin and subcutaneous tissue represents a major reconstructive challenge. Unlike the ring finger, the importance of thumb function precludes primary amputation in this type of injury, and because revascularization of the denuded skin is only occasionally successful, even with microvascular techniques, it is necessary to resurface all or part of the thumb and, in most instances, to provide sensory input.[296] The use of a radial island forearm flap[236] or a tubed abdominal pedicle flap followed by the addition of a neurovascular island pedicle flap appears to be the best method of resurfacing following this injury.[436,441] It is usually necessary to remove the distal phalanx to achieve the correct length, and it should be emphasized that the ability to provide sensory perception to the resurfaced thumb is the critical factor in achieving a satisfactory functional state.

When faced with existing deformity created by the loss of the thumb at or near the MP joint, reconstruction may be accomplished by neurovascular free tissue transfers such as the "wraparound great toe flap" originally described by Morrison[389,390] and modified by others.[340,468,493] Alternative methods include pollicization of an injured or partially amputated digit, the use of the "cocked-hat" flap, metacarpal lengthening techniques, or the use of osteoplastic reconstruction involving a bone graft covered by a tubed pedicle flap and the addition of an island pedicle flap. Loda (personal communication, 1992) described a "vascular rein" technique in which the whole or one-half of the distal phalanx (with its nail) of the middle finger is transposed to thumb position on a double vascular loop together with the ulnar digital nerve. The transferred tissue may be added to existing phalangeal bone or added to an interposed bone graft with supplementary skin coverage provided by a dorsal rotational flap. Perhaps the best of all of these methods is the radial forearm island flap or "Chinese flap" recently described by Biemer[155] and Foucher.[236]

Transfer of a Damaged Digit to the Thumb

Not infrequently, injuries that result in the loss of the thumb also cause partial destruction or amputation of adjacent digits, leaving the possibility of transfer of an injured digit or distal metacarpal to the base of the proximal phalanx of the thumb or to the first metacarpal in order to restore length and sensory perception.[181,192–194,196,197,207,208,246,255,256,263,272,293,294,302,331,332,358,365,366,377,385,412,415,416,436,438,439,442,443,445,453,473,475,477,509] The most common associated digital injuries associated with thumb loss are partial or complete amputation of the index or index and long fingers. This creates an ideal situation for pollicization of the index or long finger stump to the thumb remnant. This procedure not only adds length to the thumb but also serves to widen and deepen the first web space by providing a ray resection of the second metacarpal.

When both the thumb and index finger have been lost and there has been damage or partial amputation of the long finger, transposition of the stump of the long finger may be carried out by techniques almost identical to those described for pollicization of the index stump. Occasionally, satisfactory index function will be preserved with damage or amputation to the long finger, making it the best candidate for transposition.

Careful planning is essential before making this composite tissue transfer so that sensation can be preserved and the vascular status of the transferred digit is ensured. Although a transfer of an injured ring or small finger[377] may occasionally be indicated, concomitant damage to the index or long fingers makes them much more frequent candidates for transfer, and the techniques described here will be limited to those two digits.

Pollicization of an Index Finger Stump (Technique of Reid[436,445])

Under tourniquet hemostasis, an incision is designed circumferentially about the base of the index finger, at about the level of the MP joint, that joins as a "V" over the dorsal hand proximal to the midportion of the second metacarpal. An incision originating from the tip of the "V" curves transversely to the ulnar aspect of the first metacarpal. This creates a flap that will be used to cover the new first web (Fig. 57-54A).

Skin flaps are carefully raised with initial dissection carried out palmarly. Under magnification, the digital nerve to the radial side of the index finger is identified together with the radial digital artery. The flexor tendons are identified, and the neurovascular bundle to the index and long fingers is then delineated. Careful dissection will isolate the digital artery to the radial side of the long finger, which is then clamped and ligated well beyond the bifurcation of the common palmar digital artery. Under magnification the digital nerves to the adjacent sides of the index and long finger are carefully teased apart well back into the palm (Fig. 57-54B–D).

By alternating dissection from the palm to the dorsum, the second intermetacarpal space is developed beginning in the web and proceeding proximally. The transverse intermetacar-

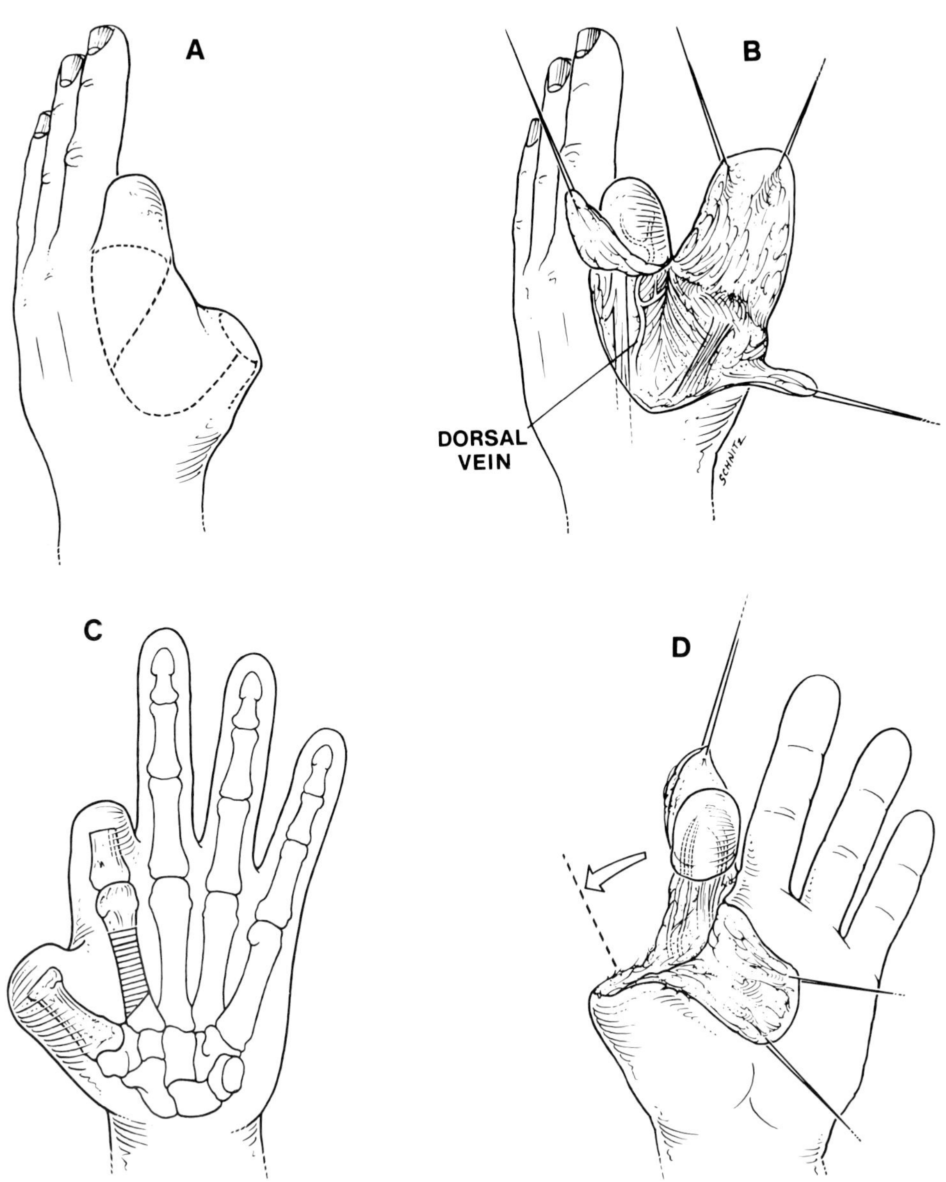

Fig. 57-54. Pollicization of an index finger stump. **(A)** Incisions used for index stump transposition. **(B)** Elevation of flaps and mobilization of the second ray. Identification of a dorsal vein is shown. **(C)** Diagram depicting the areas of the second metacarpal to be divided and excised *(striped)* prior to transfer of the distal metacarpal and proximal phalangeal stump. **(D)** The palmar flap with intact neurovascular bundles and flexor tendons, following division of the radial digital artery to the long finger. *(Figure continues.)*

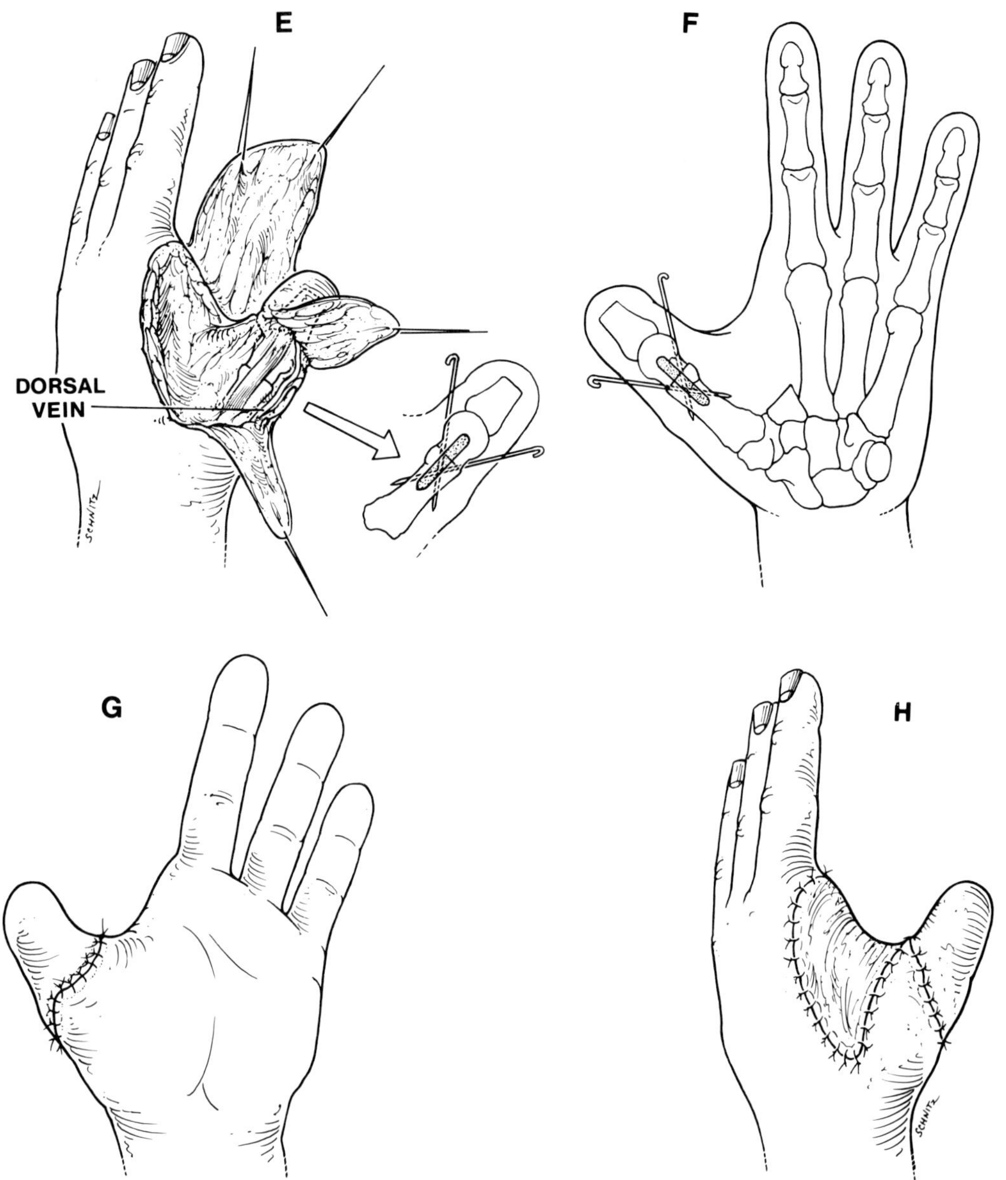

Fig. 57-54 *(Continued).* **(E)** Transfer of the index stump to the first metacarpal, again with preservation of a dorsal vein. Fixation by means of a bone peg and crossed K-wires is shown. **(F)** First and second metacarpal fixation with proximal deletion of the second metacarpal. **(G)** Wound closure on the palmar surface of the transposed index stump. **(H)** The use of the palmar flap to create a thumb-long finger cleft. (Adapted from Reid,[442] with permission.)

pal ligament is divided, and the interossei in the cleft are separated down to the proximal part of the intermetacarpal interval by blunt dissection. Flexor and extensor tendons are left undisturbed.

The index metacarpal is now completely exposed subperiosteally and an osteotome or reciprocating saw is used to divide it obliquely at its base. The amount of additional metacarpal to be removed will depend on the exact level of thumb loss, but is usually just proximal to the metacarpal neck for amputations at the MP joint level. The stump to be pollicized should now be quite mobile, attached only by its two neurovascular pedicles and the flexor and extensor tendons.

At this point the thumb stump is prepared by the removal of all scarred bone and cartilage. At the time of transposition, a small bone peg may be fashioned from the removed section of the second metacarpal and used to traverse the bony juncture (Fig. 57-54E). The limiting factor in the transfer is the length of the neurovascular pedicles, and great care must be taken not to put these structures under tension. Obliquely placed K-wires or a small compression plate are used to secure fixation of the

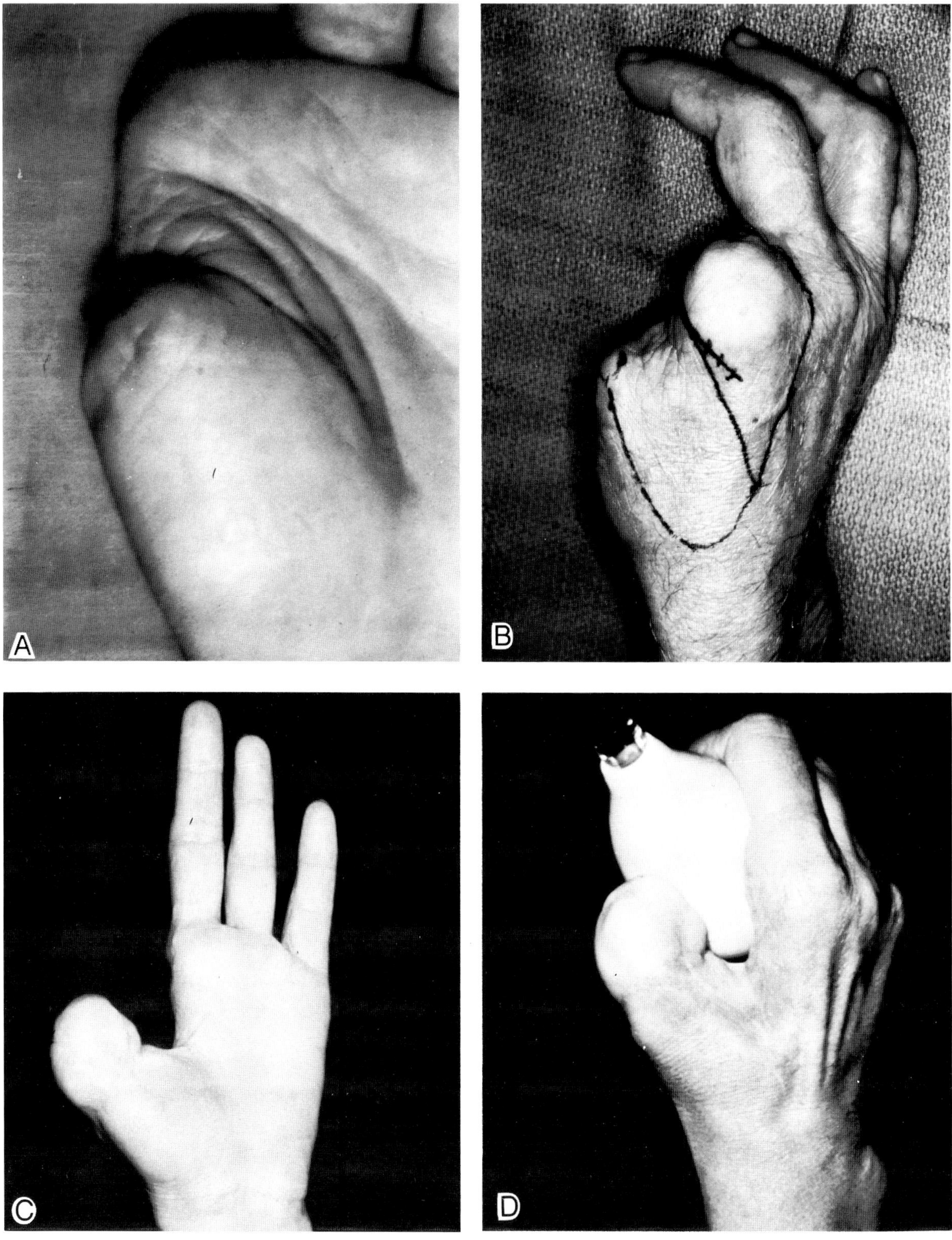

Fig. 57-55. Pollicization of a second metacarpal stump. **(A)** Old amputations of the thumb and index finger through the MP joints. **(B)** Incisions outlined for pollicization of the index stump to the first metacarpal. **(C)** Appearance of the transferred index metacarpal at 6 months. **(D)** Restoration of pinch and grasp following transfer. (From Strickland,[473] with permission.)

transferred digit (Fig. 57-54E). The tourniquet is released to ensure hemostasis and the vascularity of the transferred digital stump. Skin defects are then closed by transposing the lateral flap into the cleft created by transposition (Figs. 57-54G & H and 57-55).

Postoperatively, the hand is kept in a large plaster-reinforced compressive dressing for 2 weeks and a plaster cast is continued until bony union occurs. A light web space maintaining splint should then be worn at least intermittently for several additional months (Fig. 57-56).

Pollicization of the Stump of the Long Finger (Technique of Reid[438,442,445])

Under tourniquet hemostasis, the base of the long finger stump is circumscribed with incisions carried through the second and third webs dorsally to join as a "V" over the midportion of the third metacarpal. A large web flap is designed with its base on the radial aspect of the hand by means of a distal-dorsal incision that continues along the third metacarpal to its base and then slopes radially to the lateral margin of the hand (Fig. 57-57A). The palm is approached through a zigzag incision, and flaps are then carefully raised (Fig. 57-57B). Palmar dissection allows exposure of the neurovascular bundles to the clefts between the index and long and the long and ring fingers, respectively. Under magnification, the digital arterial bifurcations are identified, exposing the proper digital arteries to the ulnar side of the index finger and the radial side of the ring finger, which are carefully ligated and divided well away from the bifurcations (Fig. 57-57C). The common digital nerves are carefully separated from each other well back into the palm.

Alternate dissection on both the palmar and dorsal aspects of the hand is then carried out, and the intermetacarpal ligaments are divided, as are the interossei between the second and third

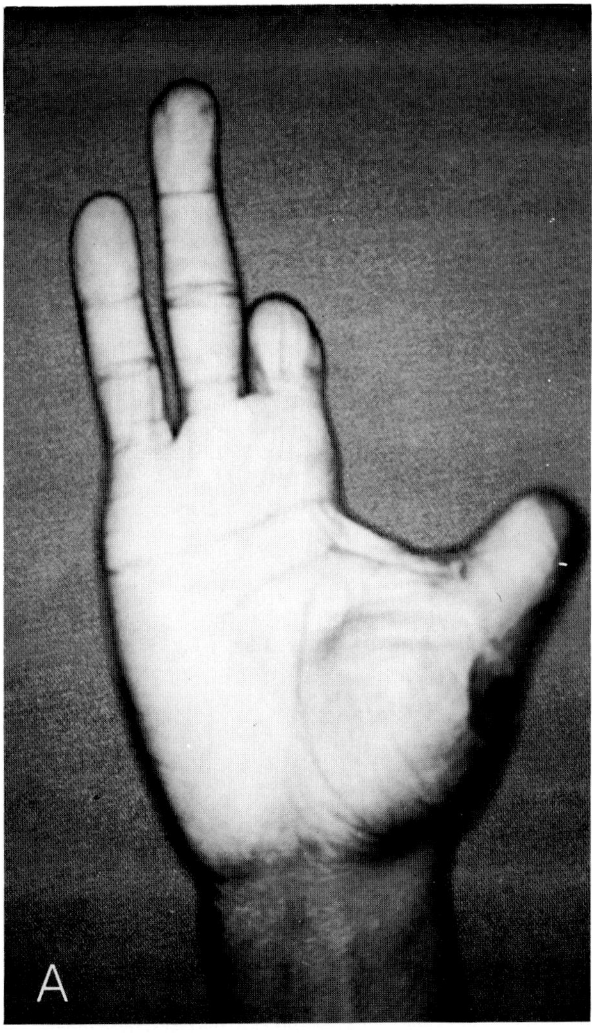

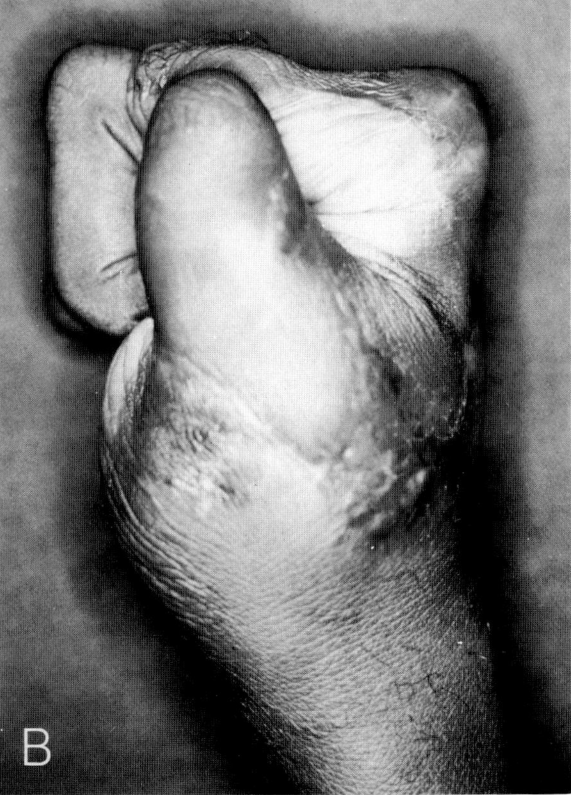

Fig. 57-56. **(A)** Palmar and **(B)** dorsal views of a hand 6 months after pollicization of the stump of the proximal phalanx and MP joint of the index finger.

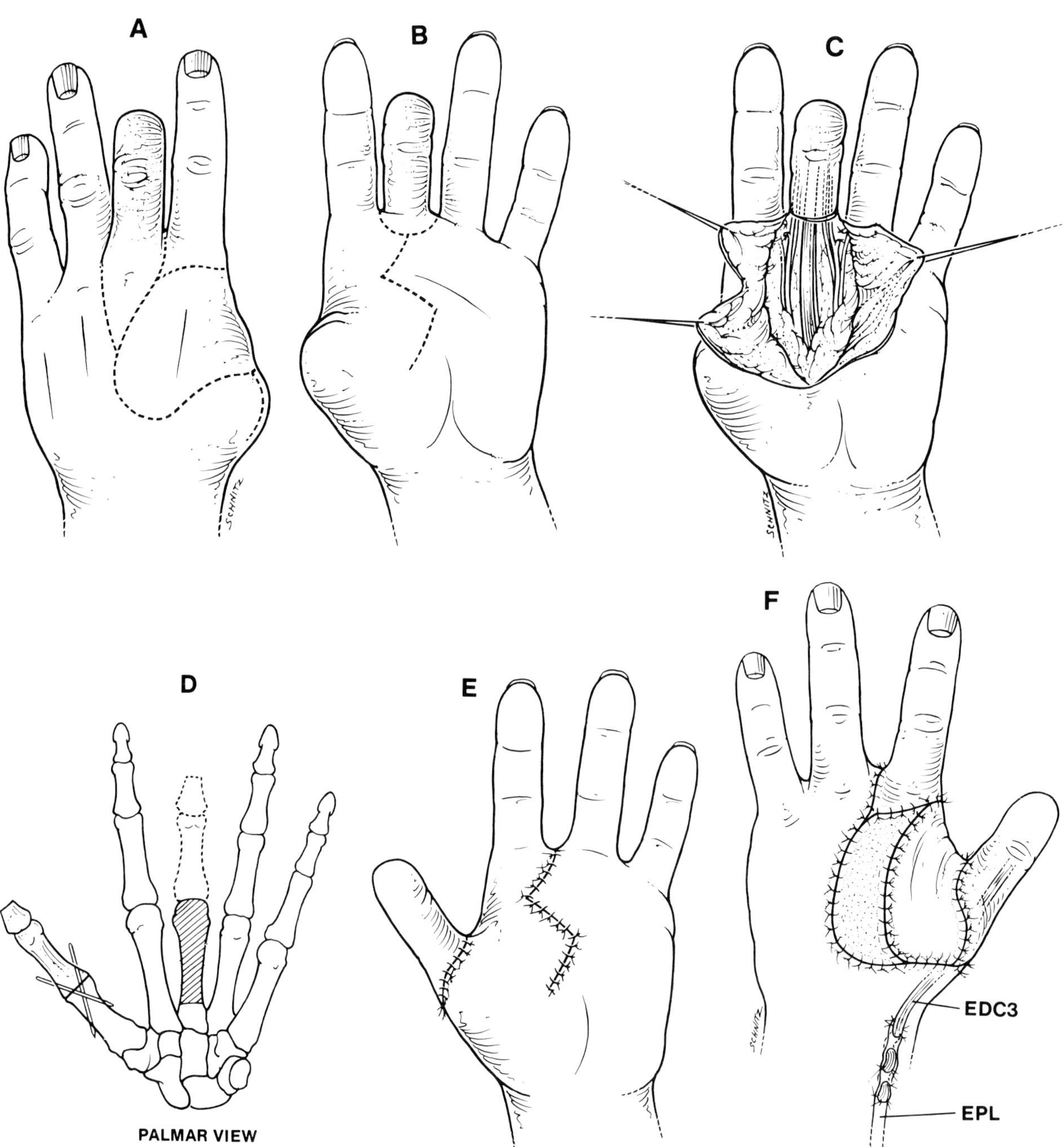

Fig. 57-57. Pollicization of the stump of the long finger. **(A)** Dorsal incision creating a dorsal lateral flap for thumb web coverage. **(B)** Palmar incisions. **(C)** Palmar dissection showing isolation and ligation of the ulnar digital artery to the index finger and the radial digital artery to the ring finger. **(D)** Diagram of bony transfer utilizing phalangeal bone from the long finger stump, with ray excision of the third metacarpal *(stripes)*. **(E)** Closure of the palmar wound following completion of the pollicization. **(F)** Dorsal wounds following completion of web space reconstruction using the dorsal flap with free skin graft coverage of the donor defect proximal to the index finger. Suture of the extensor pollicis longus *(EPL)* to the extensor digitorum communis of the long finger *(EDC3)* is shown. (Modified from Reid,[442] with permission.)

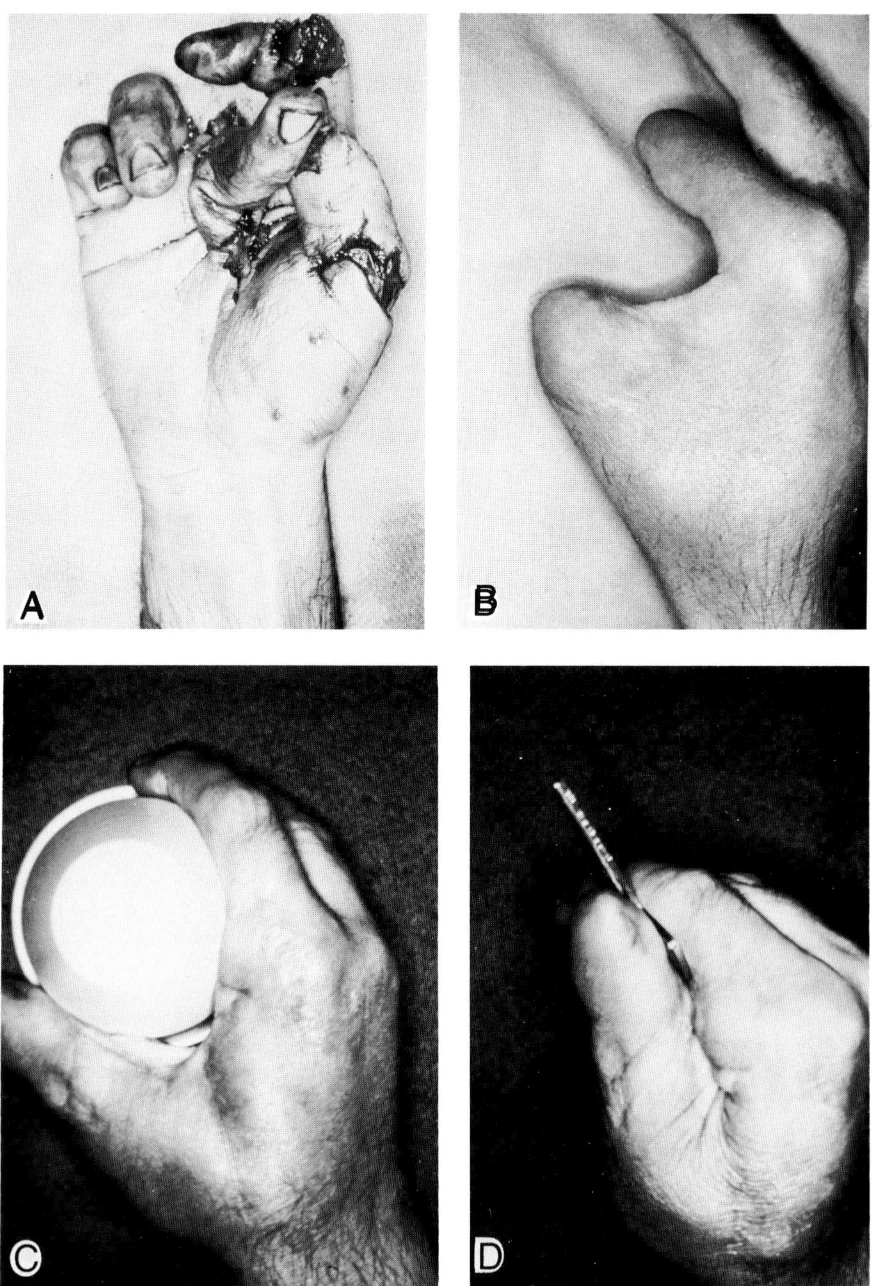

Fig. 57-58. Pollicization of the middle finger stump. **(A)** Mutilating injury of the right hand resulting in amputation of the distal thumb, index ray, and distal two-thirds of the long finger. **(B)** Appearance of the hand prior to pollicization of the long finger stump. **(C&D)** Nine months following transfer of the proximal phalanx of the long finger with satisfactory grasp and pinch. (From Strickland,[473] with permission.)

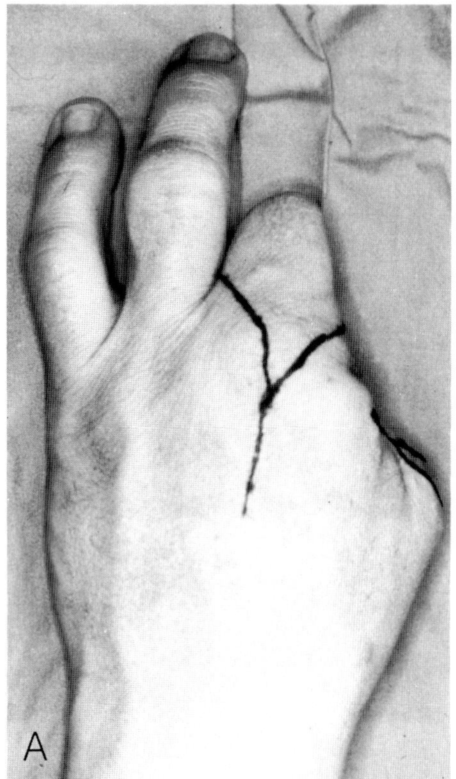

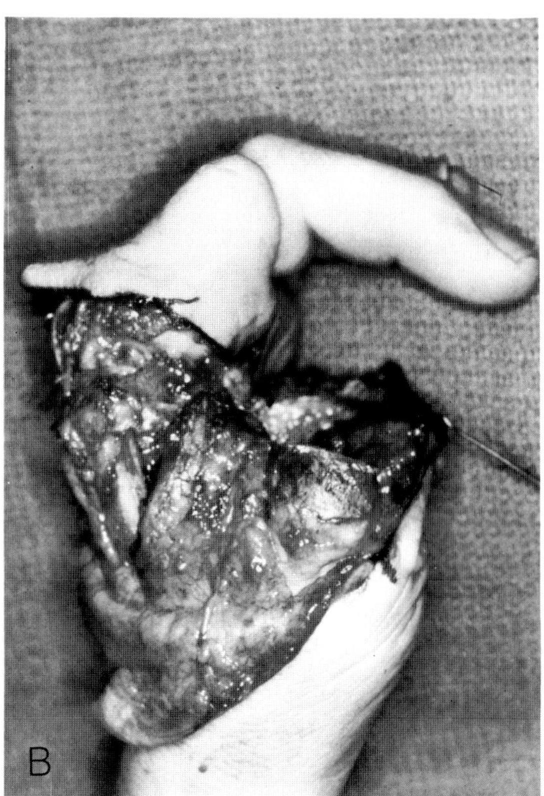

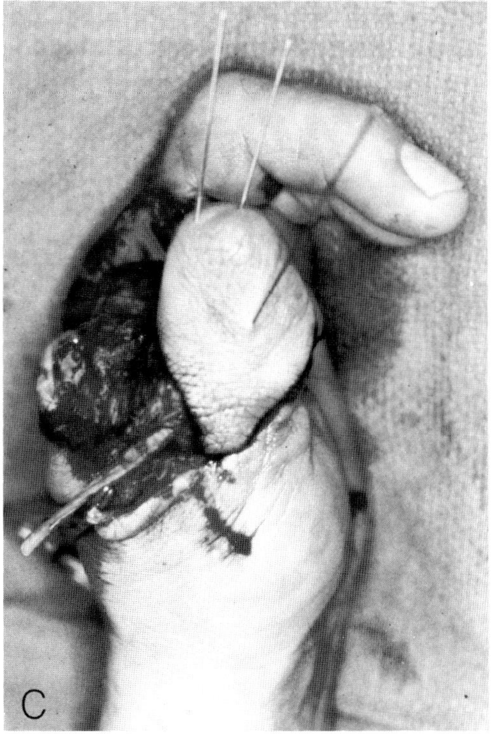

Fig. 57-59. Transposition of a stump of the long finger following traumatic amputation of the thumb through the MP joint and the index finger through the distal second metacarpal. **(A)** Appearance of the dorsal hand with proposed skin incisions. **(B)** Reflection of the dorsal flap, mobilization of the third metacarpal and long finger stump, and preparation of the first metacarpal recipient site. **(C)** Appearance of the long finger stump immediately after transference to thumb position. *(Figure continues.)*

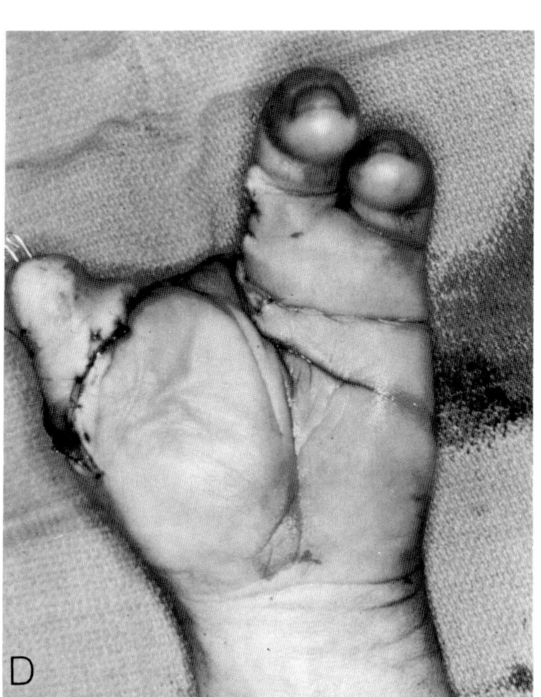

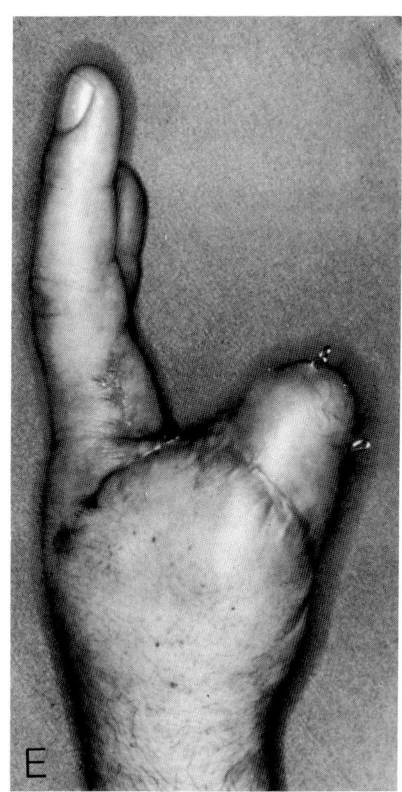

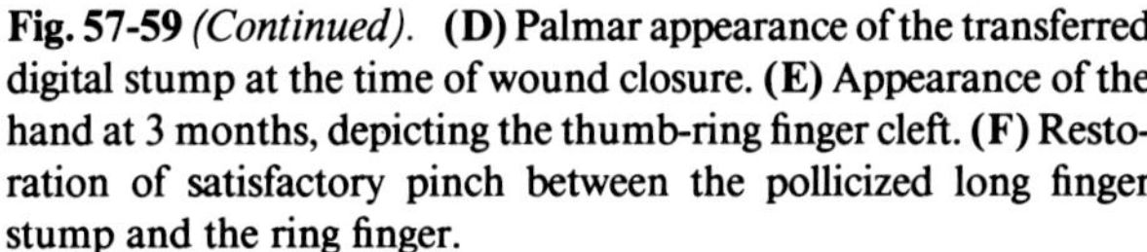

Fig. 57-59 *(Continued).* **(D)** Palmar appearance of the transferred digital stump at the time of wound closure. **(E)** Appearance of the hand at 3 months, depicting the thumb-ring finger cleft. **(F)** Restoration of satisfactory pinch between the pollicized long finger stump and the ring finger.

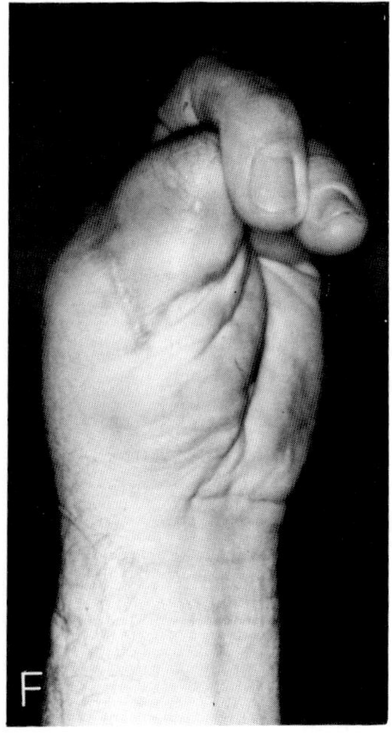

and third and fourth metacarpals. The third metacarpal is exposed dorsally by subperiosteal dissection and divided close to its base or disarticulated at the CMC joint (Fig. 57-57D). The flexor tendons are left intact and will be transferred with the digit. The extensor tendon is divided with sufficient length for subsequent juncture with the stump of the extensor pollicis longus. An appropriate amount of the third metacarpal is then excised, depending upon the bony requirements of the reconstructed thumb.

After ensuring that the neurovascular bundles have been mobilized well into the palm, a subcutaneous tunnel is made to the distal aspect of the first metacarpal, which has been cleared of scar tissue and trimmed to strong, well-vascularized bone. The isolated middle finger stump is then passed through the tunnel, and additional tailoring of the bone ends will be necessary to ensure proper positioning of the pollicized stump.

A small bone peg taken from the resected segment of the third metacarpal shaft is utilized across the site of bone juncture, and K-wires or a small plate are used to secure fixation (Fig. 57-57D). At this point, it may be possible to identify the stump of the extensor pollicis longus and to free it from its scar tissue and trim it to a good tendon. Tendon repair to the extensor tendon of the transferred long finger stump may then be completed under appropriate tension.

The tourniquet should be released to allow for hemostasis and to confirm the vascularity of the transferred digital stump. The lateral flap is now rotated into position to create a web between the reconstructed thumb and index finger. The index and ring fingers are approximated by suturing their opposing deep transverse metacarpal (intervolar plate) ligaments, and closure of the palmar wound and web space are carried out (Fig. 57-57E). The remaining dorsal hand defect is then covered with either a full-thickness skin graft taken from the groin area or a split-thickness skin graft (Figs. 57-57F and 57-58).

A plaster-reinforced compressive dressing is worn for 10 days to 2 weeks, at which time all wounds and the graft are inspected. Casting is continued for approximately 6 more weeks or until good bony union has occurred. A small web-spacer splint may also be used intermittently for several months if necessary.

These techniques utilizing the transference of stumps of injured index or long fingers to create additional thumb length are perhaps the most practical and efficient of all the thumb reconstructive techniques because they utilize functionless and sometimes obstructing parts that, by virtue of their excellent sensibility, can substantially improve function in their new position (Fig. 57-59). The complications of these procedures should not be frequent and would include partial or complete necrosis of the transferred part, nonunion of the bony juncture, and flap or graft necrosis. These complications can usually be avoided by careful attention to technique, particularly the mobilization of the vascular pedicles so that they can be transferred without tension. Preoperative arteriograms are invaluable, particularly when previous palmar injury may have damaged the normal arterial anatomy of the index or long finger stump. With careful planning, precise surgical technique, and appropriate postoperative care, these procedures should have a high degree of predictability and patient acceptance despite the fact that the cosmetic appearance of the reconstructed thumb may be somewhat bulbous.[474]

"Cocked-Hat" Flap

The use of the "cocked-hat" flap as originally suggested by Gillies[247,248] and carried out by Hughes and Moore[285] is an additional reconstructive possibility when thumb amputation is at the MP joint level and an adjacent injured digit is not available for reconstruction. The procedure involves the mobilization of local skin and subcutaneous tissue from the dorsum and lateral aspects of the first metacarpal to cover up to 2.5 cm of iliac bone graft. It may provide a useful increase in thumb length with at least protective sensibility.[228,270,285,288,300,301,348,373,410,436,441-446,466,474,507] Modifications of the procedure have been described.[350] Some surgeons have found the operation disappointing,[307] and it has largely fallen into disuse at this time. Nonetheless, it may occasionally prove valuable when other methods are precluded.

The Gillies "Cocked-Hat" Flap (Modified from Reid[442,445])

Under tourniquet hemostasis, a long curved incision is designed that begins dorsally at the level of the neck of the second metacarpal and curves proximally around the base of the thumb at the level of the carpometacarpal joint to terminate palmarly just distal to the distal edge of the thenar musculature in line with the index finger (Fig. 57-60A).

The flap is dissected distally at the level of the deep fascia exposing the musculature about the first metacarpal. Dissection is continued until the flap is completely mobilized, and great care must be taken in reflecting the flap off the end of the first metacarpal bone where the skin may be quite thin. The flap may now be displaced over the end of the bony stump, and branches of the median nerve supplying the palmar aspect of the thumb should be carefully preserved.

A corticocancellous bone segment, approximately 5 cm long is now taken from the iliac crest (Fig. 57-60B). Using fine power driven burrs, a cortical stem is fashioned out of the proximal portion of the graft, leaving 2 to 2.5 cm to augment metacarpal length. The end of the first metacarpal is prepared by removing scar, cartilage, and dead bone. The cartilage and dead bone in the medullary canal is reamed to receive the graft stem. The graft peg is then inserted and secured in the metacarpal and the distal graft should be trimmed and smoothed. Although pin fixation is not always necessary, longitudinally or obliquely placed K-wires can be used to provide additional graft stability (Fig. 57-60C).

The previously raised flap is now brought back across the graft. It may be necessary to use a short linear incision to facilitate flap placement without damaging the graft. It is important that the skin flap completely cover the bone graft, and flap tension around the graft should not be great to prevent impairment of flap vascularity. The linear incision should be closed and the defect created over the proximal two-thirds of

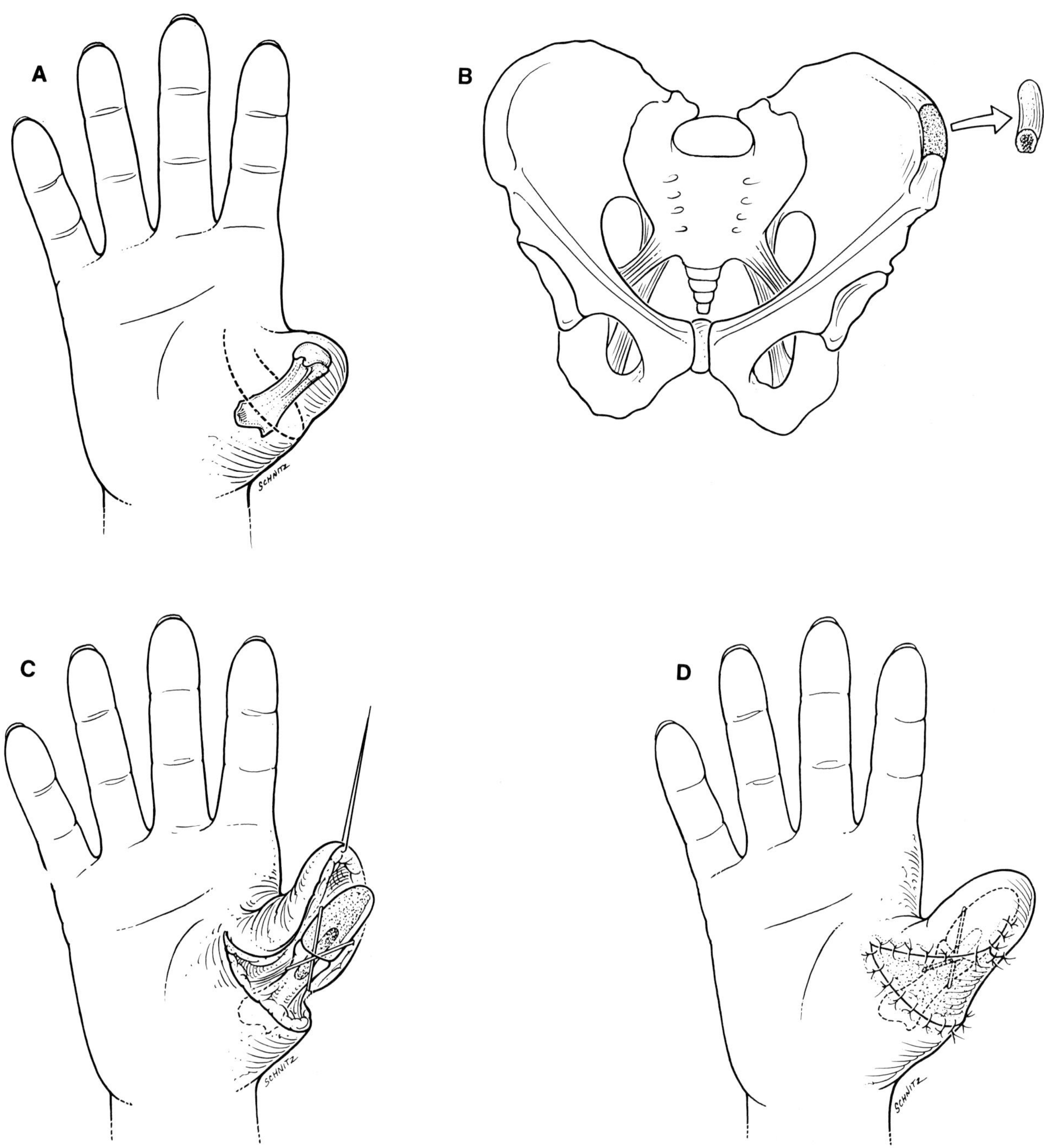

Fig. 57-60. Gillies' "cocked-hat" flap. **(A)** Outline of the incisions around the base of the thenar eminence. **(B)** Tricorticocancellous iliac crest bone graft to elongate first metacarpal. **(C)** The flap is reflected and the graft is in place with crossed K-wire fixation. The graft may be stemmed for insertion into the metacarpal, or a cortical peg may be used to bridge the graft-metacarpal interval, as shown here. **(D)** The flap brought back to cover the bone graft. A free skin graft covers the thumb defect. (Modified from Reid,[442] with permission.)

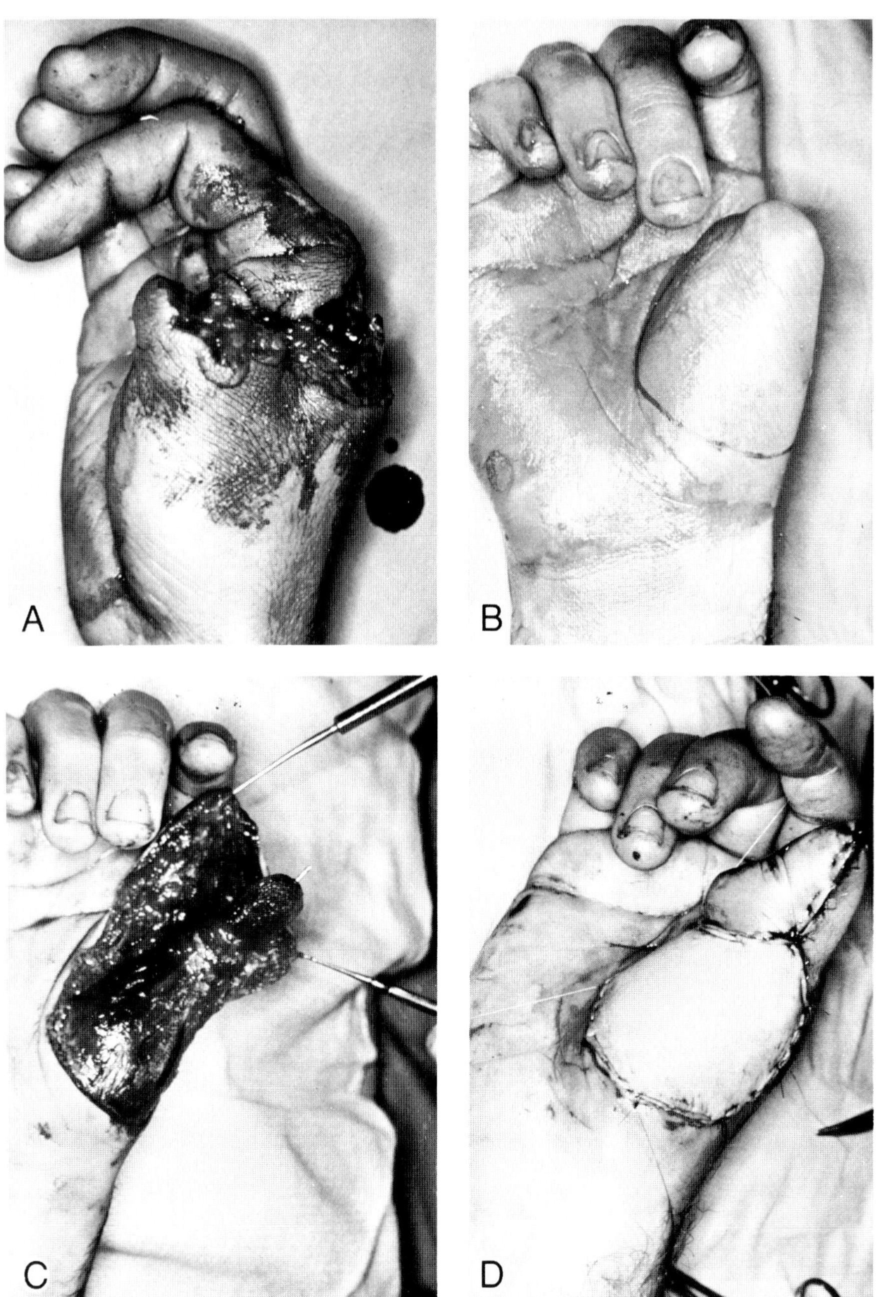

Fig. 57-61. A "cocked-hat" flap. **(A)** Power saw amputation of the thumb at the MP joint with concomitant injury to the index finger. **(B)** Incision to be used for the "cocked-hat" flap. **(C)** The reflected flap with a 2-cm iliac bone graft held in position with K-wires. **(D)** Coverage of the graft with the flap, using a linear releasing incision. Full-thickness skin graft coverage of the donor defect. *(Figure continues.)*

the thumb metacarpal covered either with full-thickness skin dissected from the groin or a split-thickness graft (Fig. 57-60C).

A plaster-reinforced compressive dressing is worn for 7 to 10 days, at which time the flap and graft are inspected. Plaster protection is maintained for approximately 6 weeks or until bony union can be established.

This technique, which involves the use of clever skin mobilization to elongate a metacarpal following thumb loss, has several pitfalls and drawbacks. Sensory perception in the lengthened thumb unit is often marginal because the transference of dorsal metacarpal skin into a palmar position necessitates the division of its proximal skin and dorsal cutaneous nerve contributions. In addition, a convoluted web space is often created by redundant skin and subcutaneous tissue, which are rotated at the time of flap transfer; although this will improve with the passage of time, it creates a somewhat unsatisfactory cosmetic appearance and diminishes the depth of the web. Nonetheless, when other alternatives for thumb lengthening are not available the "cocked-hat" flap may still be a useful technique (Fig. 57-61).

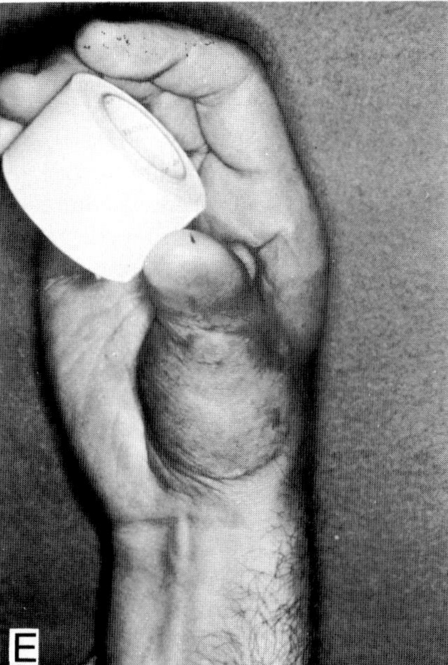

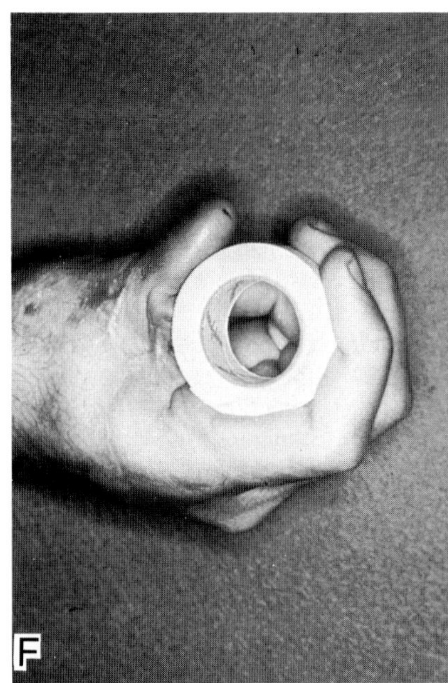

Fig. 57-61 *(Continued).* **(E&F)** Satisfactory function of the lengthened thumb at 6 months. (From Strickland,[473] with permission.)

First Metacarpal Lengthening

The technique of first metacarpal lengthening described and refined by Matev[346–352] and reported with various modifications by others,[160,205,287,289,308,309,392,393,399,434,445,507] has become an excellent method for restoring thumb function following loss at the MP joint level. Usually combined with phalangization techniques, this procedure is often simpler, more reliable, and more esthetically pleasing than other methods of thumb reconstruction at this level. Although the technique usually involves gradual metacarpal distraction over several weeks, some surgeons prefer to accept the bony distraction achieved at osteotomy and insert a bone graft at that time.[172] Technical improvements in the external fixation-distraction apparatus have added to the predictability of this technique. Moy et al[392] stated that while neoosteogenesis frequently occurs in pediatric patients, bone grafting is recommended in individuals 25 years and older with gaps of 3 cm and greater. Although the rate of complications such as tissue necrosis and nonunion are still high, it would appear that with continuing experience this procedure may prove to be the primary reconstructive consideration in this area.

Prerequisites for metacarpal lengthening are the presence of at least two-thirds of the first metacarpal and good skin cover over the stump.[351] The patients must be well versed in the technique and agreeable to participation in the lengthy process of metacarpal elongation.

First Metacarpal Bone Lengthening (Procedure of Matev[351])

Under tourniquet control, a linear incision is made over the dorsum of the first metacarpal, and the bone is exposed by retracting the extensor tendons (Fig. 57-62A). An osteotomy site is selected in the midportion of the first metacarpal, and two K-wires are driven transversely across the bone both proximal and distal to this site. A transverse osteotomy is then carried out with an oscillating saw. Following wound closure, the distraction apparatus is applied to the K-wires but no effort is made to initiate distraction (Fig. 57-62B).

Several days after the osteotomy, gradual lengthening is begun, and the screw of the distraction device is turned sufficiently to provide 1 to 1.5 mm of metacarpal elongation. Gradual lengthening commensurate with patient tolerance is continued for 20 to 35 days, and sites of pin protrusion through the skin are painted with Merthiolate or iodine to minimize superficial infection (Fig. 57-62C).

After the desired lengthening of 1.5 to 4 cm has been achieved, the gap between the fragment ends is filled with a generous corticocancellous iliac bone graft. At the time of bone grafting, the distraction pins may be continued or removed. The graft is secured by means of K-wires or a compression plate (Fig. 57-62D).

In younger patients, spontaneous bone consolidation may occur without bone grafting. However grafting is almost always required in adults. Thumb web deepening by means of Z-plasty techniques is usually effective in providing additional relative thumb length and may be carried out at the time of bone grafting (Fig. 57-62E & F).

Complications of metacarpal lengthening have included pin migration through bone, pin loosening and infection, distal skin slough, and nonunion. Restraint from overzealous initial distraction at the time of surgery or too rapid distraction in the early postoperative period will usually prevent skin problems, and careful doctor-patient monitoring of the gradual distraction process and the status of the apparatus should lessen other problems. When carried out correctly, this procedure provides an excellent elongated and phalangized first metacarpal unit with satisfactory sensation and minimal sacrifice of other tissues (Fig. 57-63).

Osteoplastic Thumb Reconstruction

Thumb reconstruction by means of a bone graft covered by a tubed pedicle flap has long been a technique for thumb reconstruction and has enjoyed varying degrees of popularity among surgeons. Osteoplastic reconstruction historically was first attempted (but apparently abandoned) by Nicoladoni[400] in 1897. Although there were many reports of successful thumb reconstruction prior to 1955 using bone graft and tubed pedicle techniques,[144,151,153,157,215,255,257,342,400,401,418,421,424,442,453,481,511] the results of these techniques were generally considered to be unsatisfactory because they failed to provide adequate sensory perception to the reconstructed thumb and because there was usually a significant resorption of the bone graft insided the pedicle. After the suggestions by Moberg[381,383] and Littler[333,334] that neurovascular island pedicle transfer be used as part of osteoplastic reconstruction of the thumb, many surgeons have developed techniques that have proven to be considerably more successful and predictable.[183,193,196,208,209,223,279,283,326,332,333,337,362,363,373,381,385,386,413,416,439,442,443,445,450,460,467,470,474,475,495,496,503,504] Although occasional reports of this method without the use of neurovascular island transfer still emerge,[163,307] and several have questioned the merit of this multiple staged procedure[373,383,416,457] it has nonetheless retained popularity as a method of thumb reconstruction at the distal metacarpal level when there is good basilar joint motion, the fingers are normal or too badly damaged for transfer, and toe transfers or lengthening techniques are not appropriate.[328]

As osteoplastic reconstruction has been modified over the years, the number of stages and the time interval required to complete thumb reconstruction have been reduced, with most techniques now requiring two stages.[209,283,328,363,386,439,442,443,460,474] Although the tibia[153,342] and clavicle[144,213,363] have been used as the source of bone grafts, iliac bone is thought to be the best for this reconstruction.[283,442,443,460] The use of a large extraperiosteal tricortical graft appears to have diminished the likelihood of bone resorption.[328,386]

The tubed pedicle flap has, in most instances, been raised from the abdomen[306,442] or groin,[364,443,461] although some surgeons have preferred upper chest,[193] deltopectoral,[386] or inframammary[153,213] sources. The use of thinned flaps[193,306,489] has effectively decreased the bulk of the reconstructed thumb unit. Flaps taken concomitantly with the removal of underlying iliac crest[163,186,193,222] or clavicle bone[364] have been suggested to speed union and decrease reabsorption by means of retained vascular connections. The use of a sensory-innervated cross-finger flap in this type of reconstruction[142,326] has also been advocated rather than the use of a neurovascular island flap,[159,261,281,334,366,379,442,444,460,470] and various other ingenious procedures, often using local flaps, have been described.[389,413,422,450,501] Techniques employing free flaps have

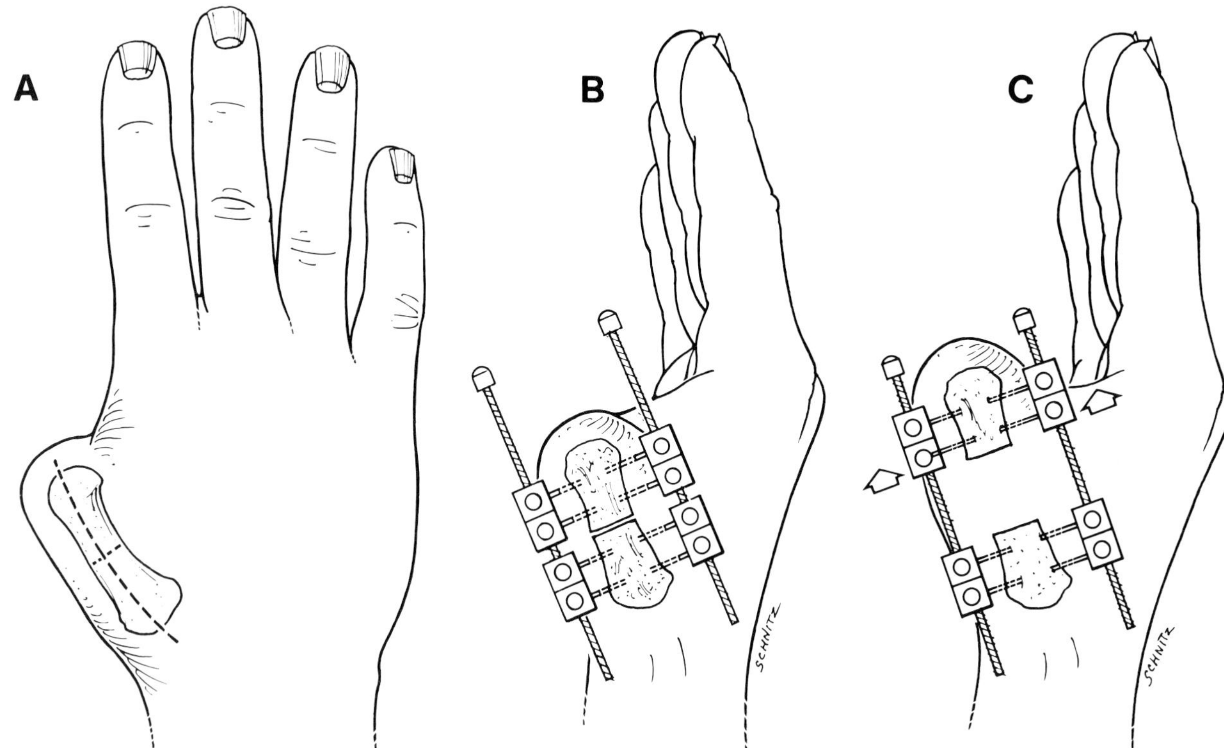

Fig. 57-62. First metacarpal bone lengthening. **(A)** The incision for osteotomy. **(B)** Transverse osteotomy of the midshaft of the first metacarpal with the distraction apparatus in place. **(C)** Gradual widening of the midmetacarpal gap by distraction of the external fixation device. *(Figure continues.)*

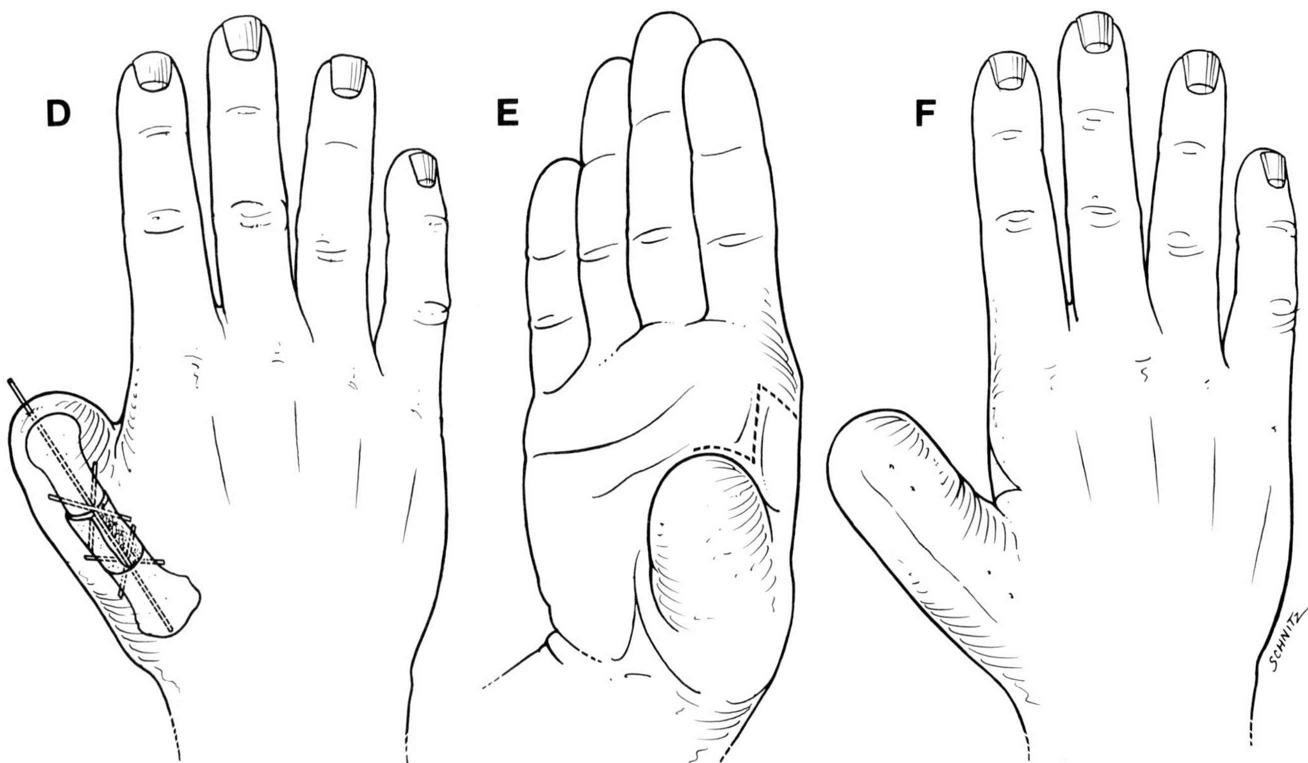

Fig. 57-62 *(Continued).* **(D)** Iliac bone grafting of the defect with K-wire fixation is performed at a second-stage operation after the desired length has been achieved. **(E)** A Z-plasty to deepen the web done at the same time as the bone graft further enhances the functional length of the thumb. **(F)** Appearance of the lengthened first metacarpal. (From the technique of Ivan B. Matev, M.D.)

also been reported[244,262,355,383,390,406,489,520] and have demonstrated their effectiveness in this type of repair.

Two methods of single-stage thumb reconstruction using a composite radial forearm island flap have been described by Biemer[155] and by Foucher et al.[231] Creative extensions and revisions of the radial forearm flap have been reported,[164,189,218,354] and Wendt recently described the successful use of the flap to provide wrap around coverage of an "osteoarthrotendinous" allograft for total thumb reconstruction.[515] Biemer[155] described a one-stage total thumb reconstruction using an osteocutaneous forearm flap, a method first seen in China, where it had been used as a free flap for postburn neck contractures. A composite pedicle containing skin and subcutaneous tissue, a segment of radial bone, a length of the lateral cutaneous nerve of the forearm, and two veins is turned 180 degrees and the radial bone is fixed to the first metacarpal. The digital nerves of the thumb are sutured to the nerves in the flap and vein anastomosis is optional. Foucher's technique[236] is similar and also uses a radial forearm osteocutaneous flap. His method, however, restores sensation by means of a neurovascular island pedicle flap. Matti[354] has also employed a proximal skin-paddle radial-artery island flap in combination with metacarpal transfer or bone grafts to partially reconstruct the thumb.

Osteoplastic Reconstruction of the Thumb (Modified from Simonetta[461])

Stage I (Fig. 57-64A–D). A groin flap as described by McGregor,[363] including the superficial circumflex iliac artery is patterned and raised on the same side as the hand whose thumb is to be reconstructed (see Chapter 49). The flap should have a width of 7.5 cm and a minimum length of 12 cm with its free end positioned over the lateral prominence of the underlying iliac crest. A large extraperiosteal tricortical bone graft is then taken from the iliac crest; the graft should be 7 to 8 mm thick, 5 to 6 cm long, and 1.5 cm wide (Fig. 57-64B).

Preparation of the first metacarpal is carried out under tourniquet hemostasis, beginning with removal of the skin overlying the distal metacarpal and trimming away of scar, cartilage, and dead bone. Generous skin reflection and excision over the first metacarpal is accomplished to increase the vascular contact area of the flap. A small curette is used to fashion a hole in the medullary canal of the metacarpal, and the bone graft is shaped with a motorized burr to produce a stout cortical stem 2 cm in length. The graft is inserted and secured in the metacarpal so that its flattened raw edge is facing the index finger in opposition with the first metacarpal (Fig. 57-64C). Fixation is secured by longitudinally- or obliquely-placed pins. Distal

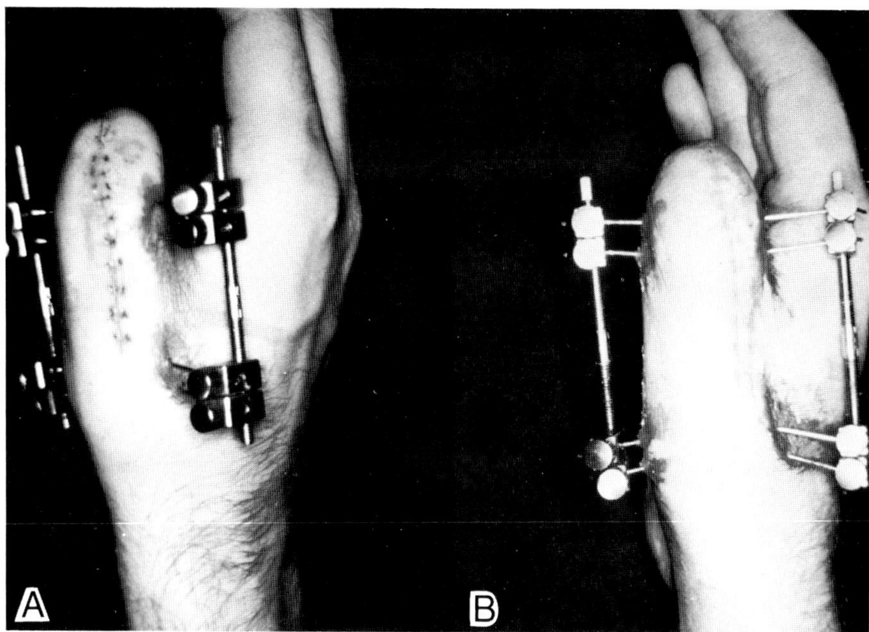

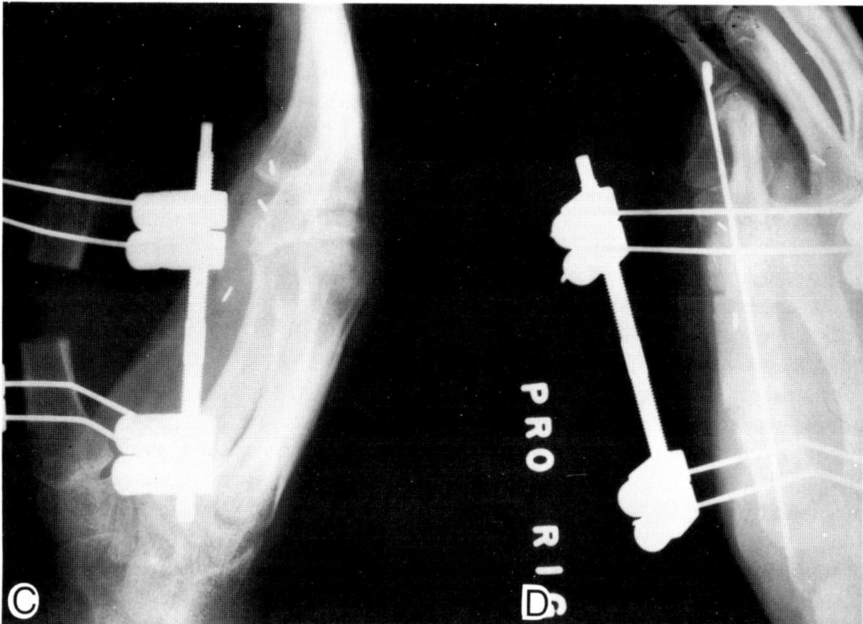

Fig. 57-63. First metacarpal lengthening. **(A)** Amputation through the base of the proximal phalanx. The distraction apparatus in place following osteotomy of the midshaft of the first metacarpal. **(B)** Appearance of the thumb and distraction device at 3 weeks, following gradual lengthening. **(C)** Radiographic appearance of the first metacarpal with approximately 1 cm of distraction lengthening. **(D)** A 1.5-cm iliac bone graft in position at 5 weeks with longitudinal K-wire fixation. *(Figure continues.)*

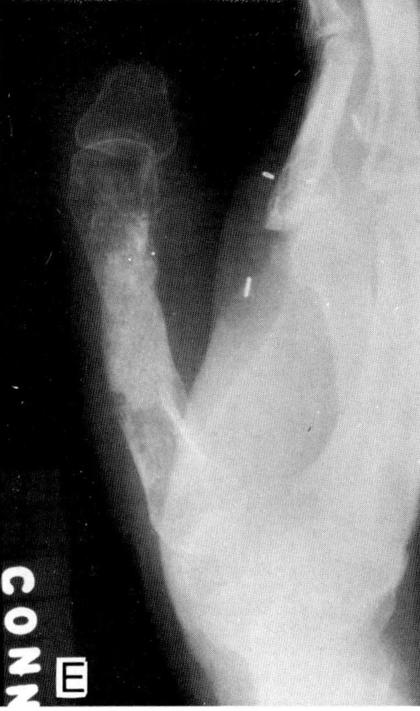

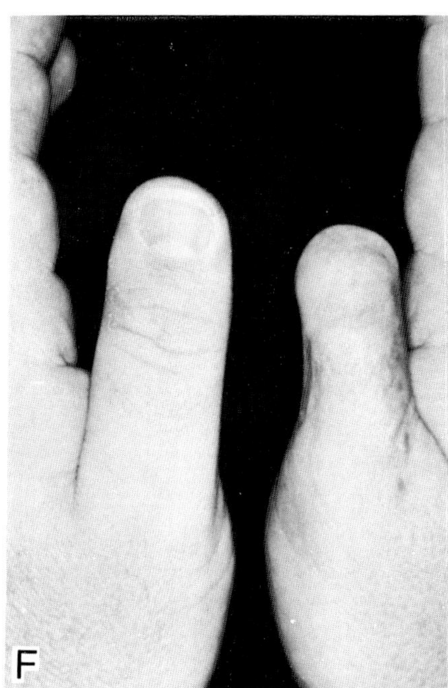

Fig. 57-63 *(Continued).* **(E)** Consolidation of bone graft in the lengthened metacarpal. **(F)** Appearance of the elongated thumb compared with the opposite normal thumb. (Courtesy of J.B. Steichen, M.D.)

shaping and trimming of the graft produces a smooth configuration, and the length should approximate the interphalangeal joint of the normal thumb.

The groin flap is tubed along most of its length and partially defatted distally depending on the amount of subcutaneous fat present. The donor defect is undermined and closed without excessive tension, and the bone graft is inserted into the tube with the suture line coming to lie palmarly in preparation for the insertion of the island flap during the second stage. The free end of the pedicle is then sutured to the expanded metacarpal skin defect (Fig. 57-64D). Care is taken to avoid tension, twisting, or kinking of the pedicle, and a low suction drain is placed in the groin wound for 24 to 48 hours. A soft Velpeau type restraining dressing will comfortably immobilize the arm, and the patient may be ambulatory within several days.

Stage II (Fig. 57-64E–H). Because the excellent blood supply of the groin flap may not satisfactorily stimulate circulation from the hand and because of the limited contact area of the flap to its new blood supply, a partial division of the flap and ligation of the superficial circumflex iliac artery is recommended at 4 weeks.[460] This procedure is carried out under local anesthesia by means of a transverse incision that is made close to the groin connection of the flap at the future site of its division. Following identification and ligation of the artery, a small dressing is applied and, at 6 weeks, division of the tube is completed.

At the time of tube release, an extended neurovascular island flap (see page 2078) is raised from the ulnar aspect of the long finger and dissected well into the palm. A pattern representing the exact configuration of the flap is used to prepare an identical defect on the palmar and distal aspects of the tube with the center of this defect corresponding to the tube suture line (Fig. 57-64E). It should be possible to extend the defect over the distal aspect of the bone graft, and dissection should be carried down to the raw bone on the palmar side of the graft (Fig. 57-64F & G). After appropriate undermining, the island pedicle is passed from the palm into the reconstructed thumb unit and sutured in place, together with the closure of the open end of the tube. A full-thickness skin graft is dissected from the opposite groin and used to cover the donor defect on the ulnar side of the long finger (Fig. 57-64H).

A plaster-reinforced compressive dressing is used postoperatively for 7 to 10 days, and cast immobilization is continued until bony union is complete at 6 to 8 weeks. Gradually increasing use of the reconstructed thumb is then permitted.

Although rarely necessary, this type of thumb reconstruction is fairly rapid and does not require the use of other digits or toes (Fig. 57-65). Its disadvantages lie in the obligatory insult to the long finger and the tendency to continue to perceive the reconstructed thumb unit as the long finger, although this may be a less bothersome phenomenon with the passage of time. The potential complications are numerous and include partial necrosis of the groin flap, loss of blood supply or diminished sensory perception in the neurovascular island flap, failure of the free graft to the long finger, and nonunion of the bone graft. The problem of long-term resorption of the bone graft may also be seen (Fig. 57-66), although the use of an extraperiosteal tricortical graft with direct application of a neurovascular island pedicle seems to have substantially diminished this problem. In the hands of experienced surgeons, this method still rates consideration for thumb reconstruction when the indications are appropriate.

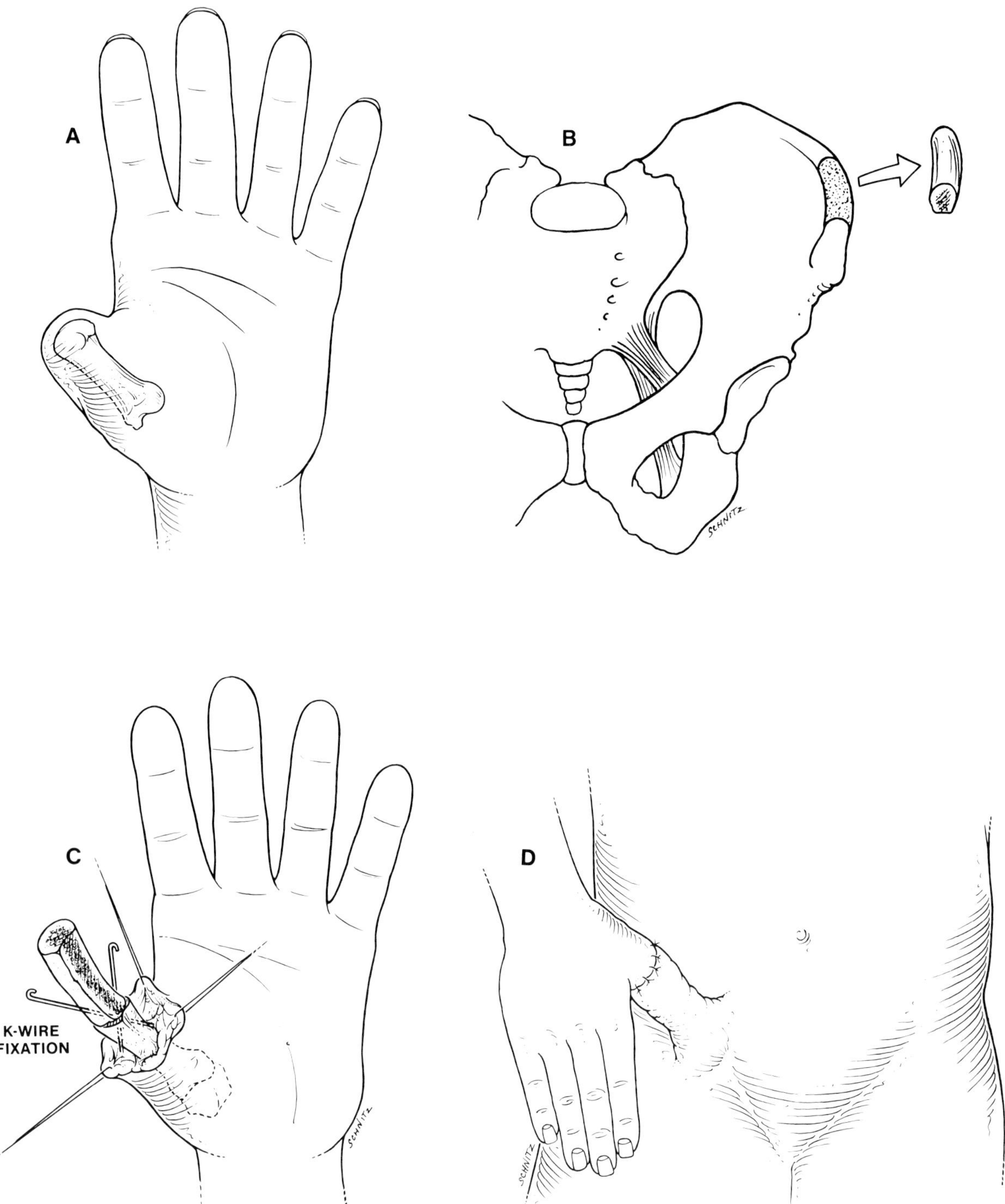

Fig. 57-64. Osteoplastic reconstruction of the thumb. **(A)** Thumb amputation through the metacarpophalangeal joint. **(B)** Site of removal of extraperiosteal tricorticocancellous iliac crest bone graft. **(C)** Preparation of the recipient site with the insertion of the iliac crest graft into the first metacarpal shown here with K-wire fixation. **(D)** Bone graft coverage with a tubed groin flap. *(Figure continues.)*

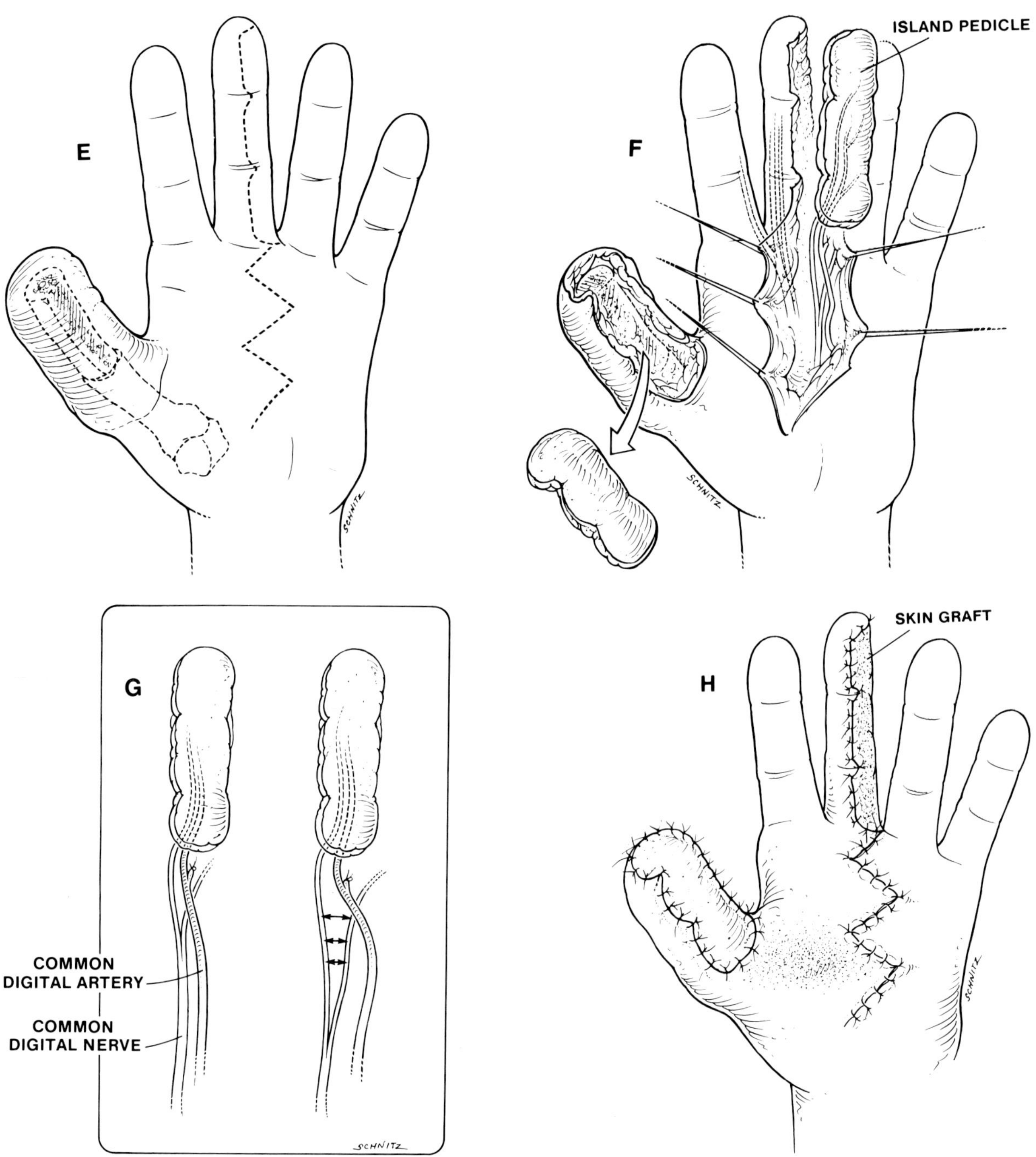

Fig. 57-64 *(Continued).* **(E)** Incisions for the use of an extended neurovascular island pedicle flap to provide vascularized and innervated skin on the palmar aspect of the reconstructed thumb. **(F)** Transference of the neurovascular island flap to the palmar thumb defect at the time of flap detachment. **(G)** Severance of the digital artery to the opposite web and careful intraneural separation of the common digital nerve in preparation for a tension-free transfer of the neurovascular island flap. **(H)** Completion of neurovascular island transfer with a free skin graft to the donor defect in the long finger. (Modified from Simonneta,[461] with permission.)

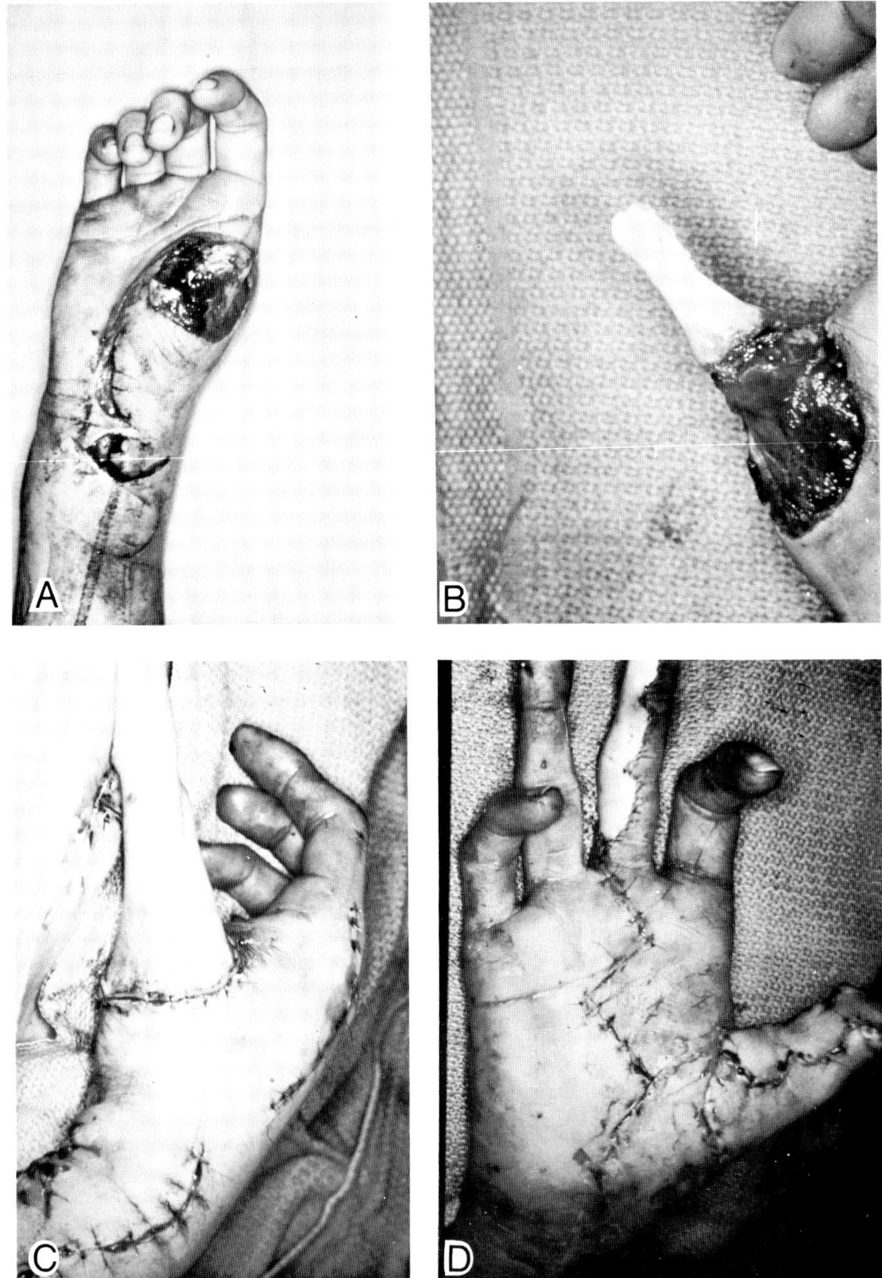

Fig. 57-65. Osteoplastic reconstruction of an amputated thumb. **(A)** Traumatic amputation of the thumb through the first metacarpal. **(B)** Bone graft utilizing the preserved proximal phalanx of the amputated thumb. **(C)** Application of a thin, tubed upper abdominal pedicle flap. **(D)** Transfer of an extended neurovascular island pedicle flap from the ulnar aspect of the long finger at the time of pedicle flap detachment. *(Figure continues.)*

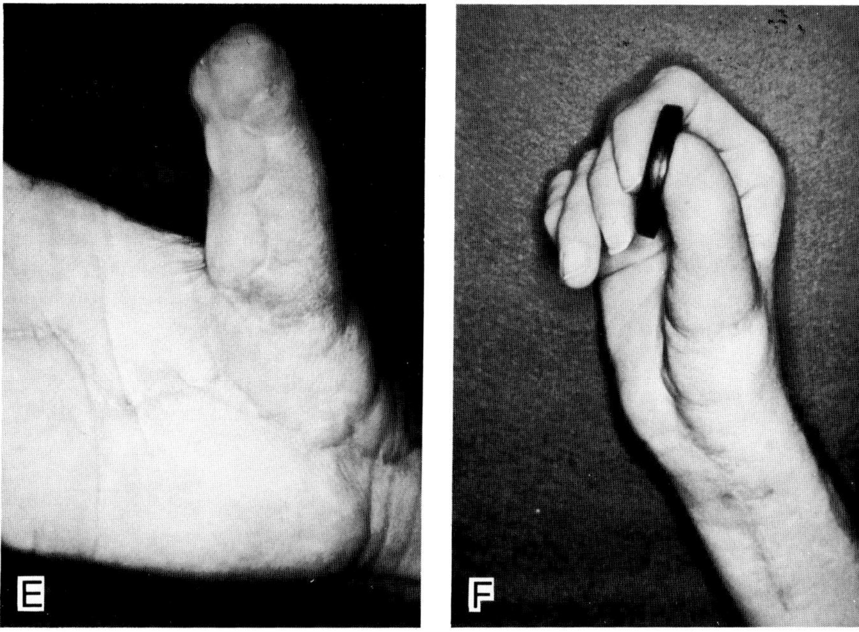

Fig. 57-65 *(Continued).* **(E&F)** Appearance of the thumb unit at 9 months with satisfactory pinch and grasp functions. (From Strickland,[473] with permission.)

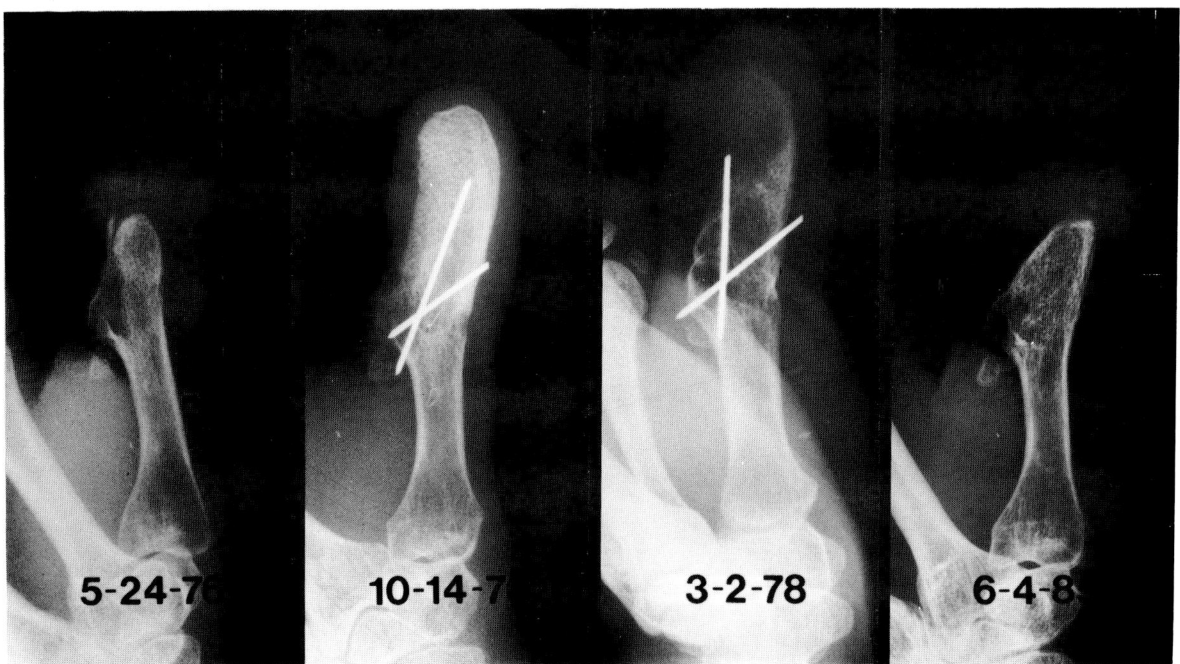

Fig. 57-66. Bone resorption following osteoplastic reconstruction. Shown here are radiographs of the same patient who underwent the osteoplastic reconstruction shown in Figure 57-65. Resorption of the proximal phalangeal bone graft is seen on May 24, 1976, 3 years after osteoplastic reconstruction. A subsequent iliac bone graft is shown shortly after its insertion, on October 14, 1976. Follow-up radiographs on March 2, 1978 and June 4, 1985 again show gradual resorption of the bone graft inside the groin flap.

Composite Radial Forearm Island Flap (Modified from Foucher et al[236])

This procedure has the advantage of providing a well-vascularized skin and bone graft and, with the addition of an extended neurovascular island pedicle flap, avoids the staging necessitated by conventional osteoplastic methods. A prerequisite to the procedure is an arteriogram that demonstrates the competency of the ulnar artery and a superficial palmar arch that provides a strong contribution to the vascularity of all of the digits of the involved hand. The finding of a predominantly radial blood supply or the absence of an ulnar artery would preclude the use of this procedure.

The flap is designed from the palmar and radiodorsal aspect of the forearm, beginning several centimeters proximal to the radial styloid. It should be 7 to 8 cm in length and 6 to 7 cm in width (Fig. 57-67A). After preparation of the distal thumb stump, the flap that includes the radial artery and its venae comitantes is carefully raised. Great care is taken not to damage the cutaneous branches of the radial nerve or the blood supply to the radius just proximal to the styloid process. A small branch from the radial artery is identified as it enters the pronator quadratus muscle and extends down to the periosteum of the radius. This vessel is carefully mobilized and protected, following which a bone graft is osteotomized and elevated from the radius with bone instruments. The length of the graft will vary from 2 to 4 cm depending upon the amount of thumb lengthening desired. The graft should be at least 1.5 cm in width and should be removed in a manner that preserves its vascularity and includes corticocancellous bone from the lat-

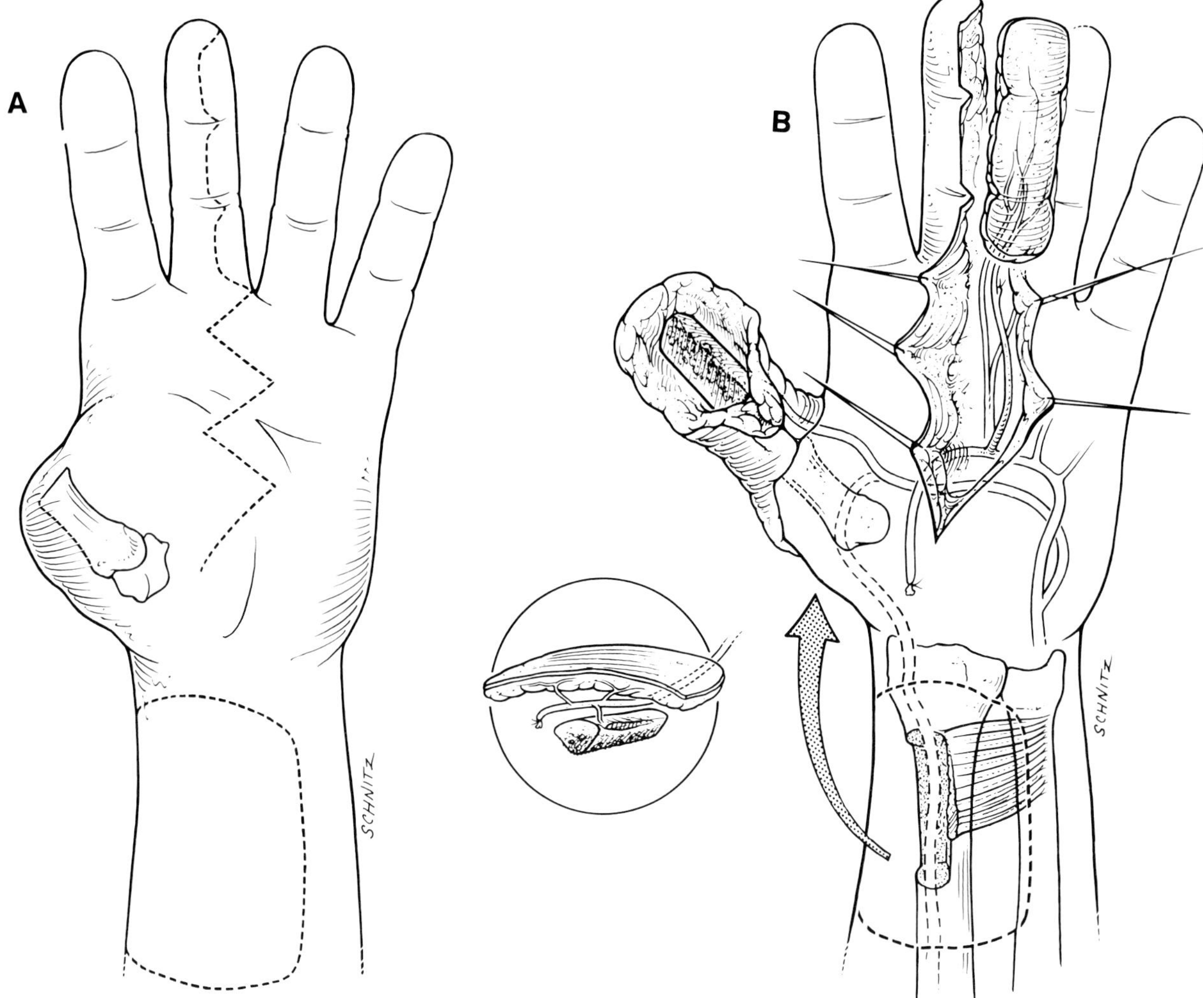

Fig. 57-67. Composite radial forearm flap. **(A)** Incisions to be used for thumb reconstruction using a composite radial forearm island flap and neurovascular island flap taken from the ulnar side of the long finger. The radial flap is approximately 7 × 7 cm and is raised from the distal palmar lateral forearm. **(B)** Elevation of the flap together with a segment of the distal radius with careful preservation of radial artery communications between the skin and bone graft *(inset)*. The artery is ligated proximally, and the flap is tunneled under the first dorsal compartment. The position of the bone graft and the flap are shown. The neurovascular island pedicle flap is raised in preparation for the palmar resurfacing of the reconstructed thumb. *(Figure continues.)*

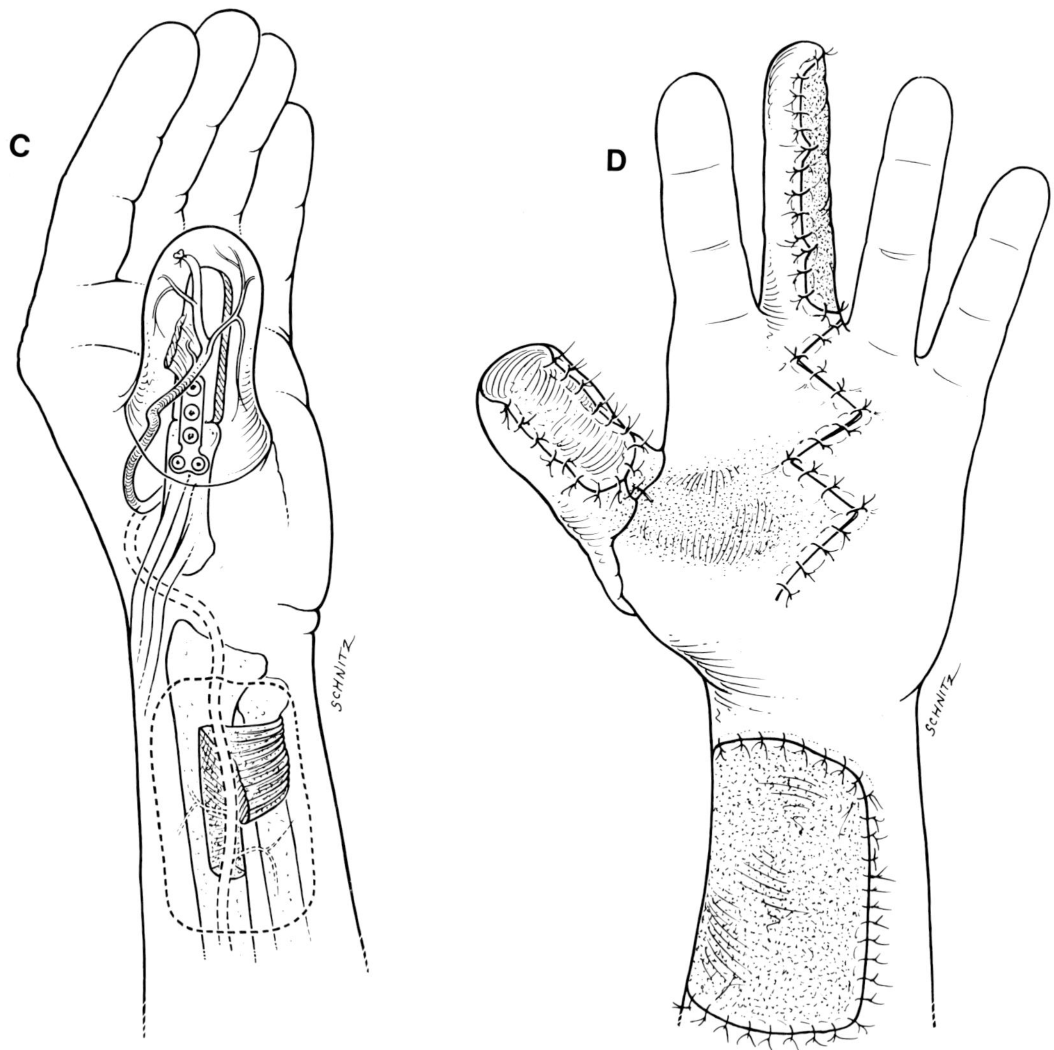

Fig. 57-67 *(Continued).* **(C)** Dorsal appearance of the composite radial forearm flap and bone graft in position, showing a small T plate used for fixation. Note the position of the radial artery. **(D)** Completion of the thumb reconstruction, with skin grafts used to cover the radial side of the long finger and the palmar forearm. (Modified from Foucher et al,[236] with permission.)

eral side of the radius. The radial vessels are ligated proximally, and the entire flap is mobilized as a composite unit to the level of the anatomic snuffbox. The abductor pollicis longus and extensor pollicis brevis tendons are freed proximally by releasing the distal portion of the first dorsal compartment. The composite bone-skin preparation is then passed from palmar to dorsal beneath the abductor pollicis longus, extensor pollicis brevis, and extensor pollicis longus. The flap is then passed under the skin bridge of the first web space to the level of the distal thumb wound. Connecting incisions may be used if scar tissue makes this passage difficult. The bone graft is secured to the metacarpal with its cancellous raw edge facing the index finger with the first metacarpal in opposition. Fixation is secured by longitudinal or obliquely placed pins, or by the use of a small plate. Distal shaping and trimming of the graft assures a smooth configuration. The forearm skin now provides coverage in a near circumferential fashion around the graft and the distal aspect of the remaining metacarpal or proximal phalangeal bone (Fig. 57-67B).

At this point, an extended neurovascular island pedicle flap (described on page 2078) taken from the ulnar side of either the long finger or ring finger is placed on the palmar aspect of the bone graft to provide sensory perception and complete the reconstruction. The radial arm flap is carefully tailored to accept the neurovascular pedicle, and a full-thickness skin graft is used to cover the defect of the donor finger (Fig. 57-67C). Split-thickness skin grafting taken from the opposite anterior thigh is used to close the forearm donor area after adjacent muscle has been mobilized over the defect created by the removal of radial bone (Fig. 57-67D). The tourniquet must be released prior to dressing application to ensure the competency of the blood supply to both flaps, and exploration of the vascular pedicle must be carried out if any problems exist.

A plaster-reinforced compressive dressing is applied and sufficient portions of both flaps are left exposed to allow for continuous monitoring of their vascularity. A dressing change is carried out at 1 week, and a plaster short arm thumb spica cast is applied at 2 weeks and continued for 6 weeks. Additional immobilization may be necessary depending on the appearance of bone healing.

The advantages of the composite radial forearm island flap are considerable. The procedure eliminates the necessity of staging, and the excellent vascularity brought with both flaps minimizes the possibility of flap failure. The technique should prevent bone graft resorption, which is probably the most significant disadvantage of osteoplastic thumb reconstruction (Fig. 57-68).

The disadvantages of the procedure include the fact that there is a considerable cosmetic defect created in the area of forearm flap removal and the possibility of distal radius fracture. Although no microvascular anastomoses are required, the dissection must be carried out under microscopic magnification to ensure that no damage occurs to the radial artery or its venae comitantes and to maintain the vascular supply to the bone graft. When carried out correctly, this procedure would seem to be the most effective means of osteoplastic thumb restoration (Fig. 57-69).

Summary: Reconstruction of the Middle One-Third of the First Ray

It can be seen that the reconstructive options available to the hand surgeon following thumb loss through the middle one-third of the first ray are considerable. Great toe or second-toe transfer may now be reliably carried out by experienced sur-

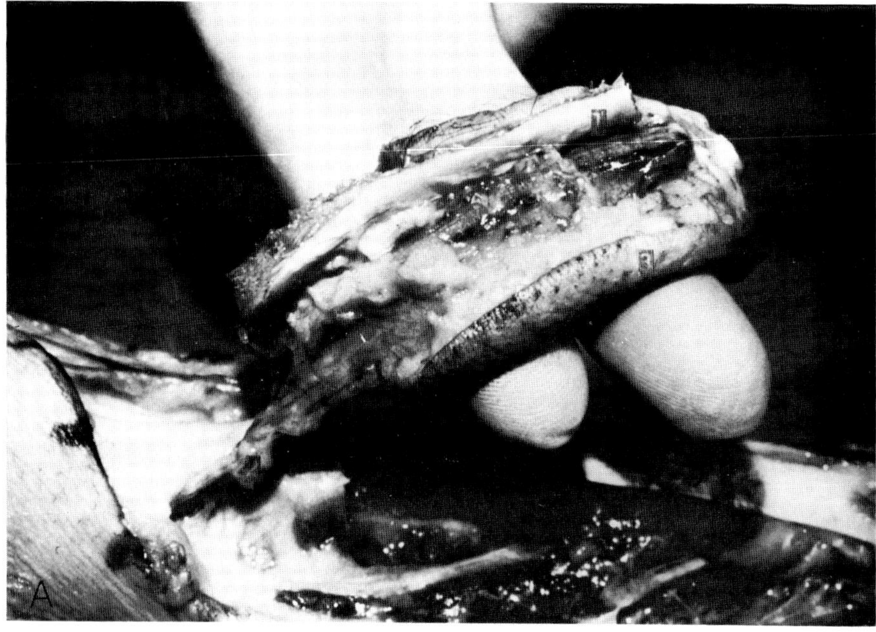

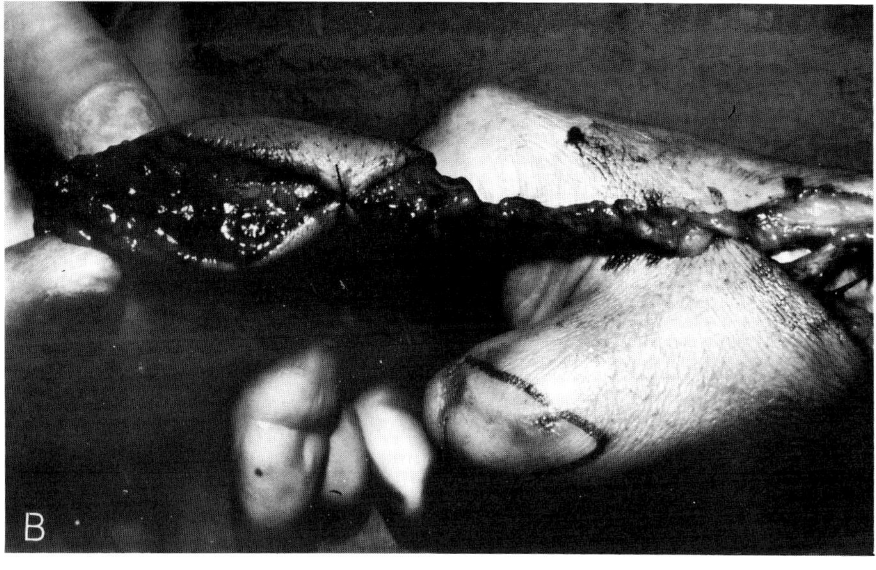

Fig. 57-68. **(A)** Appearance of the composite radial forearm island bone flap on its radial neurovascular pedicle. **(B)** The flap after passage onto the back of the hand in preparation of the distal passage into the thumb. *(Figure continues.)*

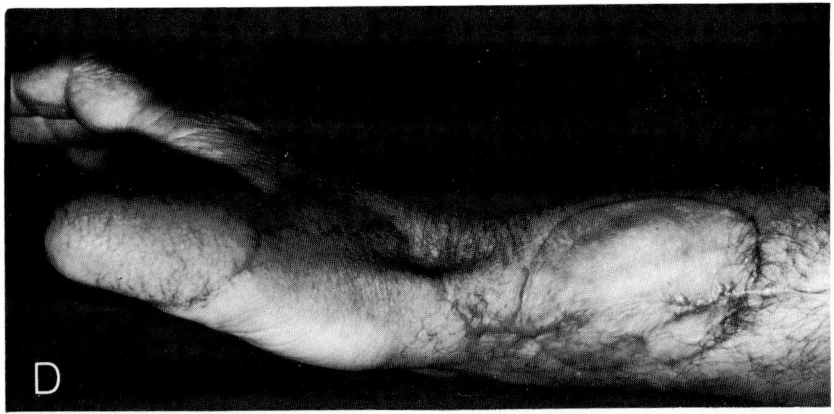

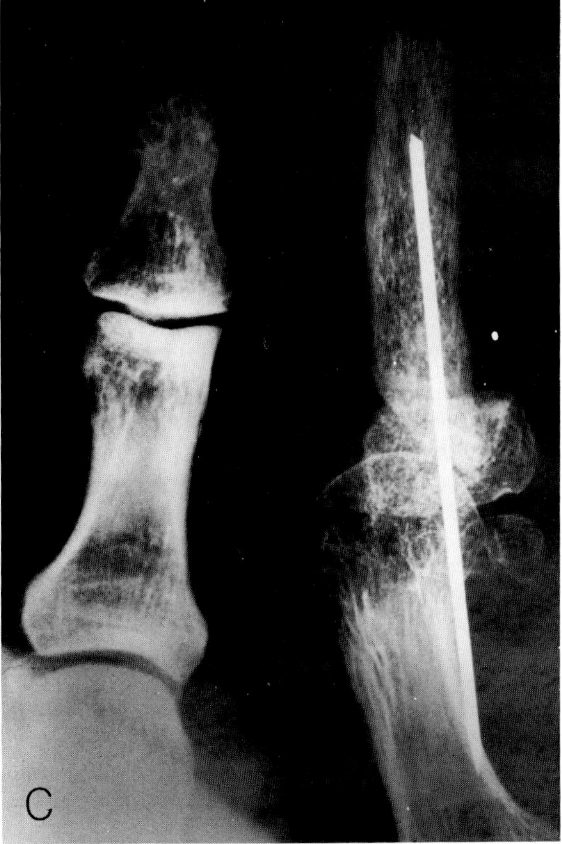

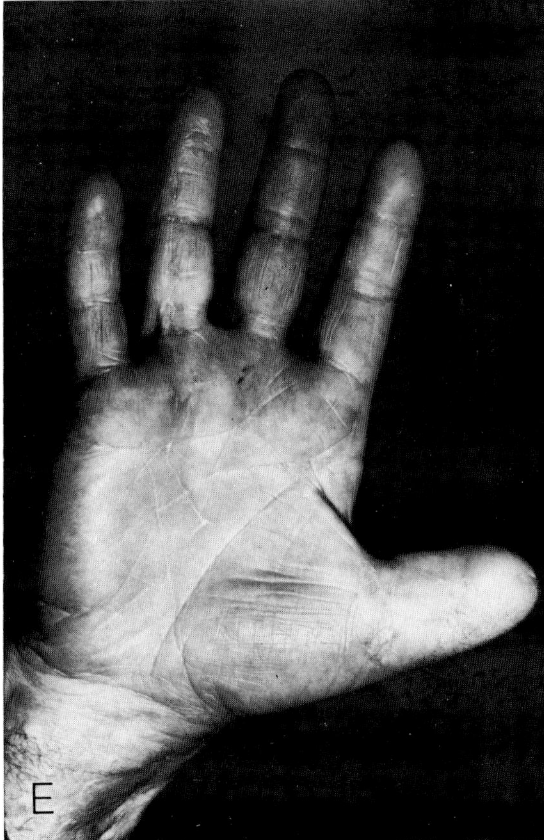

Fig. 57-68 *(Continued).* **(C)** Radiographic appearance of the bone graft after it has been added to the base of the proximal phalanx and fixed with a single longitudinal K-wire. **(D&E)** The appearance of the thumb reconstruction 3 months after the use of a composite radial forearm island bone flap. (Courtesy of Guy Foucher, M.D.)

geons and can effectively restore excellent thumb performance. For middle-third thumb loss, however, other methods may be simpler with fewer risks and a less significant donor deficit.

In addition to the procedures described here, a number of fascinating techniques utilizing microvascular free tissue transfer have already been developed and successfully carried out at microvascular centers.[233,235,239,243,244,250,263,270,271,353,359,364,387,389,394,428,445,499] A particularly impressive technique using a free neurovascular "wraparound flap" from the big toe, which has been described by Morrison and modified by Urbaniak[202,214,389,403,445,449,500] provides the restoration of a nearly normal appearing thumb unit complete with a nail (see Chapter 33). This procedure uses an iliac crest bone graft and a free neurovascular flap from the big toe, vascularized by the first dorsal metatarsal artery. In addition to its cosmetic advantages, the flap returns satisfactory sensation by virtue of suture of the plantar nerves to the digital nerves of the thumb, and

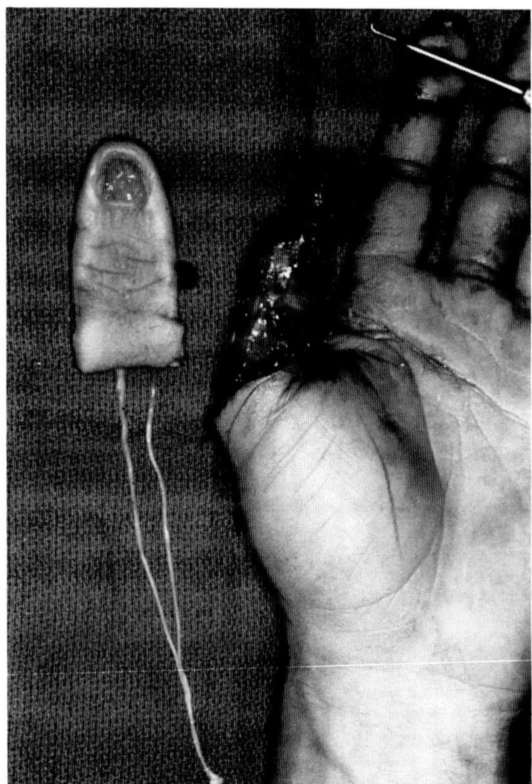

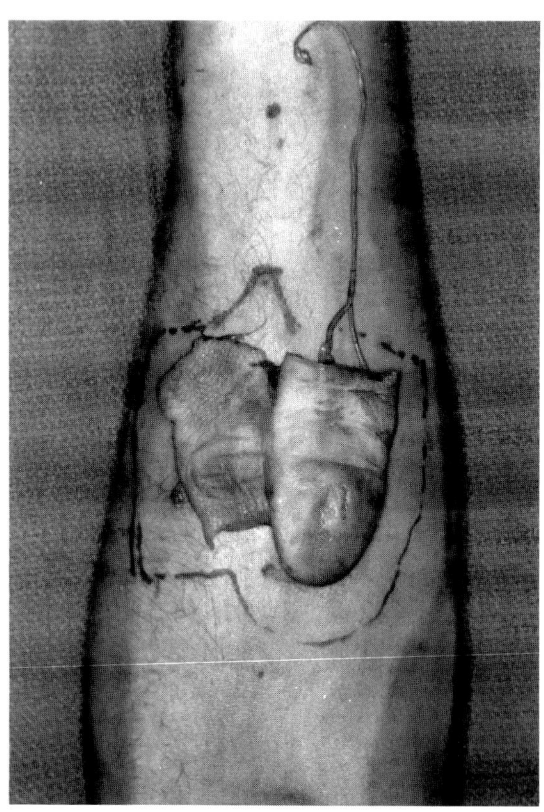

Fig. 57-69. Coverage of a degloved thumb with a patterned radial artery forearm flap. **(A)** This thumb was totally degloved from the MP joint distally, including skin and digital nerves. **(B)** The avulsed skin was used as a pattern for the radial artery forearm flap. Note oversizing of the skin pattern to assure adequate coverage. *(Figure continues.)*

does not involve the complete ablation of the great toe as is necessitated by toe transplantation. Similar thumb reconstructions utilizing free skin flaps from the great toe have also been described by Yu,[524-527] and Huang et al[282] have further modified the method by means of a free pedal neurovascular flap and composite phalanx-joint-tendon homograft. Yu and He[526] have carried the procedure a step further by reconstructing a thumb by transplanting a free skin-nail flap from the big toe and the bones, joints, and tendons of the second toe. The great toe is then resurfaced with the skin-nail flap from the second toe. Second-toe transfer for thumb reconstruction as popularized by Leung[323-325] would seem to be an excellent method for thumb loss through the middle third of the thumb ray. These procedures have reached a degree of reliability that makes them applicable for use by hand surgeons with a higher level of microvascular expertise. They are of extremely long duration and technically demanding, and failure is so catastrophic that they are not justifiable in certain circumstances. With additional technical refinement it is beyond question that the reliability of these and similar procedures will improve to a point where they are a major part of the reconstructive armamentarium of microvascular surgery teams in many areas.

For most amputations in the middle third of the thumb ray, one should try to select the simplest and most reliable procedure compatible with the goals of the patient and the skills of the surgeon. Thumb loss through the proximal half of the proximal phalanx may be best managed by web-deepening techniques such as simple or four-flap Z-plasty. Adduction contractures with extensive involvement of the thumb musculature may require more extensive phalangization using dorsal rotational flaps to achieve first metacarpal positioning and mobility. Thumb loss at the level of the MP joint is probably best managed by metacarpal lengthening or pollicization of the stump of the injured index or long finger. If those options are not available, osteoplastic reconstruction remains as a viable option for thumb reconstruction with the radial island forearm flap offering an excellent method of restoration. If the vascular status of a particular hand precludes the use of the composite radial forearm island flap and it is still deemed appropriate to proceed with osteoplastic reconstruction, the one-stage osteoplastic reconstruction using a free neurovascular dorsalis pedis flap and iliac bone graft combination as described by Doi[213] is probably the best alternative. The "cocked-hat" flap should probably be ranked last among the reconstructive options because of a less than adequate sensory return and marginal appearance.

It should be emphasized that a careful review of these reconstructive possibilities with the patient is the obligation of the surgeon prior to making the final decision. The successful selection and completion of thumb reconstruction using one of

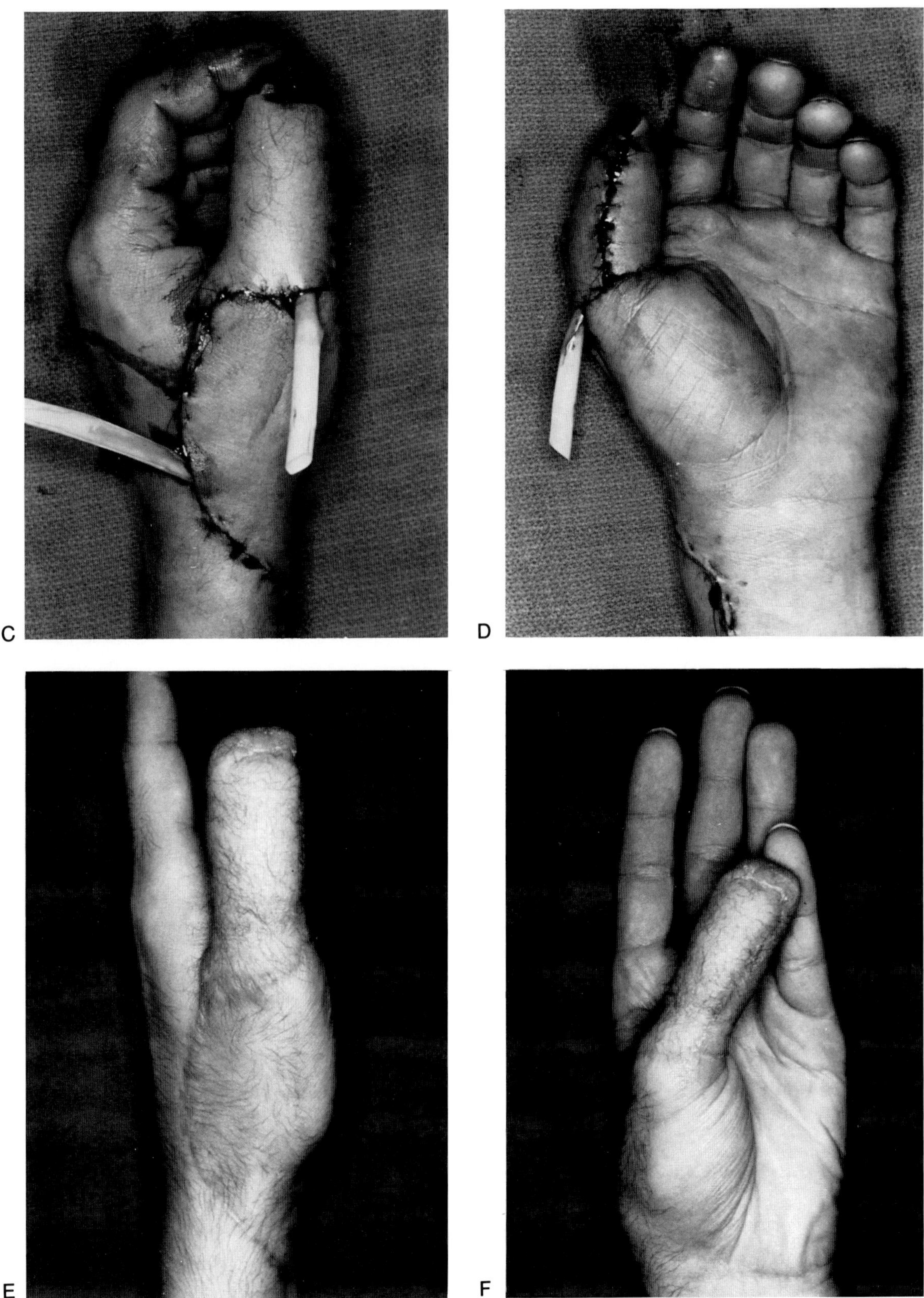

Fig. 57-69 *(Continued).* **(C&D)** The thumb immediately following completion of the radial forearm flap coverage. **(E)** The appearance of the thumb at 3 months. **(F)** The reconstructed thumb demonstrating pinch to the small finger. Sensation could be enhanced with a dual innervated cross finger flap or by an extended neurovascular island pedicle flap. (From Hastings,[268] with permission.)

these procedures should substantially improve the functional capability of the hand with thumb loss in this critical area.

AMPUTATION THROUGH THE PROXIMAL ONE-THIRD OF THE FIRST RAY

When there has been loss of the entire thumb and at least the distal third of the first metacarpal, a procedure designed to provide total thumb reconstruction is necessary. Because the required length of the reconstructed thumb will usually be in excess of 5 cm and because the mobility achieved in a short first metacarpal stump may be limited, the procedures described for middle-third loss are usually not applicable. The use of an adjacent injured digit for thumb reconstruction is possible in the presence of a short first metacarpal stump providing length will be adequate to restore satisfactory thumb function. Pollicization of an injured index finger is the most likely option because it is frequently injured at the time of thumb loss. Severe injury to the second metacarpal or MP joint and to the index intrinsic or extrinsic tendons will render the index finger relatively functionless despite the best management efforts. As long as the neurovascular status of the digit is adequate, transposition of the index finger to the thumb position is an excellent reconstructive procedure. When there has been loss of basilar joint motion, it is desirable for the transferred digit to have at least some motion, preferably at the MP joint, so that power flexion is provided in the transferred position. Even if little or no motion is present in the injured digit, careful attention to positioning can allow it to function as a satisfactory resisting post for the remaining digits.

When the thumb has sustained proximal loss through the first metacarpal and there is no concomitant digital injury, the restoration options are limited to free great toe transfer or pollicization of a normal digit. Great toe transfer is discussed in Chapter 33; although the procedure has been shown to provide an excellent return of thumb function with minimal functional impact on the donor foot, there are often mitigating factors, including patient resistance, that preclude its use. Pollicization of a normal finger on the stump of the metacarpal has the advantages of being a safe, one-stage procedure that maintains satisfactory joint motion and near normal sensation.

Pollicization of a Damaged or Normal Digit

Pollicization of a damaged or normal finger before the advent of neurovascular transfer techniques was an extremely difficult and hazardous operation that required the mobilization of large tissue segments, and the ultimate performance of the transferred digit was often marginal by present standards.[151,207,216,228,229,293,297,385,461,505] In some instances, abdominal flaps were used to fill the cleft left by digital transfer,[216] while in other techniques tendons and nerves were not joined.[505] The first report of true pollicization of an index finger using neurovascular dissection and transfer techniques was in 1949 by Gosset,[252] with similar pollicization of the long finger being carried out shortly thereafter by Hilgenfeldt.[275] Since that time, the procedure has been modified with technical considerations emphasized by Littler,[273,330–332,335–338] and numerous reports concerned with indications, techniques, results, and complications have been published.[147,161,168,174,176,182,185,188,193,203,217,230,231,240,253,258,262,265–267,285,294,295,305,313,320,322,330–332,334–338,362,367,370,373,374,395,396,410,423,438–440,442,443,445,448,457,464,475,496,503,517,518] Although most authors have tended to favor the index finger as the digit to be transferred,[147,188,192,203,210,263,295,313,330,335,337,338,347,362,373,376,445,489,484] the use of the long finger,[275,297,442,443] ring finger,[185,240,253,310,320,322,457,496] and even the small finger,[285,301,305,377] have been advocated. In recent years, careful emphasis on the fundamental priorities of pollicization have been advocated and technical considerations for the restoration of muscle balance, length, and correct rotation have been emphasized.[265,267,335–338,364,445] Contributions by surgeons carrying out pollicization for congenital absence of the thumb have added further technical modifications that are applicable for use following acquired thumb loss.[158,171,173,219,264,319,345,373,441,448,464,478,528]

Pollicization has the advantage of being a one-stage procedure that maintains at least some functional joint motion and has near normal sensation and vascularization.[179] The most frequently injured digit available for transfer is the index finger that has often suffered extensor tendon and second metacarpal damage at the time of amputation of the thumb through the proximal first metacarpal. Predictably, imaginative microvascular surgeons have utilized previously injured digits from the opposite hand for free transfer onto the thumb position.[152,395]

Pollicizations of normal index or ring fingers have emerged as the most popular techniques and each has its advocates. Littler[330–332,335–338] has championed index pollicization on the grounds that it is technically simpler, provides the restoration of excellent thumb function and sensation, and is cosmetically pleasing. Letac and others[185,240,253,320,322,457,507] have suggested that the index finger is too long, and that its deletion deprives the hand of the most important prehensile digit.[322] They prefer ring finger transfer to thumb position, contending that there is a minimal sacrifice of normal hand function and that excellent cosmetic and functional recovery can be achieved. In this section we will describe the techniques for pollicization of an injured or normal index finger and a normal ring finger as perhaps the best alternatives for thumb restoration following proximal loss.

Pollicization of an Injured or Normal Index Finger (Modified from Reid[442,443,445])

Under tourniquet anesthesia, flaps are designed around the base of the index finger and over the second metacarpal, taking into consideration areas of poor skin and scarring secondary to previous trauma. If possible, a racquet-type incision around the base of the index finger commencing palmarly at the proximal digital crease and continuing around the digit to join as a "V" over the midportion of the second metacarpal is used, with a curved connection extending to the base of the metacarpal, where it is sloped laterally to the metacarpal stump area (Fig. 57-70A & B). If previous injury precludes this incision, alternative incisions will be necessary depending on the specific situation.

The flaps are carefully raised and elevated and areas of scar and bone, if present, are removed from the second metacarpal. By dissecting palmarward under the lateral flap, it is possible to identify and protect the radial neurovascular structures to the index finger. The flexor tendon is also freed in the palmar wound and the ulnar neurovascular structures are identified and carefully dissected out under magnification. The digital artery to the radial side of the long finger is identified and divided beyond the bifurcation of the common digital artery. Careful splitting of the common digital nerve to the index and long finger is also carried out well into the palm.

Alternating dissection is carried out both dorsally and palmarly beginning distally at the second web and proceeding proximally. If possible, several dorsal veins to the index finger are mobilized with the ligation of tributaries that would restrict their transfer. The transverse intermetacarpal ligament is divided, and the interossei are separated. As much as possible of the extensor tendon over the dorsum of the second metacarpal is salvaged, and the articular base of the proximal phalanx is transversely removed. The index finger is now free on its neurovascular bundles and the flexor tendon, and is ready for transfer.

The first metacarpal is then prepared and, if it is small or absent, the distal surface of the trapezium is removed to cancellous bone. The medullary cavity of the first metacarpal stump or trapezium is reamed and a small bone peg taken from the excised second metacarpal is interposed into the base of the proximal phalanx of the index finger as it is brought across and secured in position (Fig. 57-70C). Great care should be taken to prevent damage or tension on the index neurovascular structures. It is important that the position of the pollicized digit is in proper abduction, opposition, and pronation. K-wire fixation is used and, if possible, the extensor tendons from the index are joined to the mobilized stump of the extensor pollicis longus.

Because the index finger has been appreciably shortened, it may occasionally be necessary to carry out secondary shortening of the flexor tendons to the index finger. At this stage the tourniquet is released to allow for control of bleeding and to assess the viability of the transferred thumb. Skin closure is completed by transposing the lateral web flap into the new cleft created between the pollicized index and the long finger (Fig. 57-70D).

A plaster-reinforced compressive dressing is worn for 2 weeks, and plaster immobilization of the first metacarpal is maintained until bony union is complete at approximately 6 to 8 weeks. Secondary reconstructive possibilities include shortening of the flexor tendons, tenolysis of the extensor tendon,

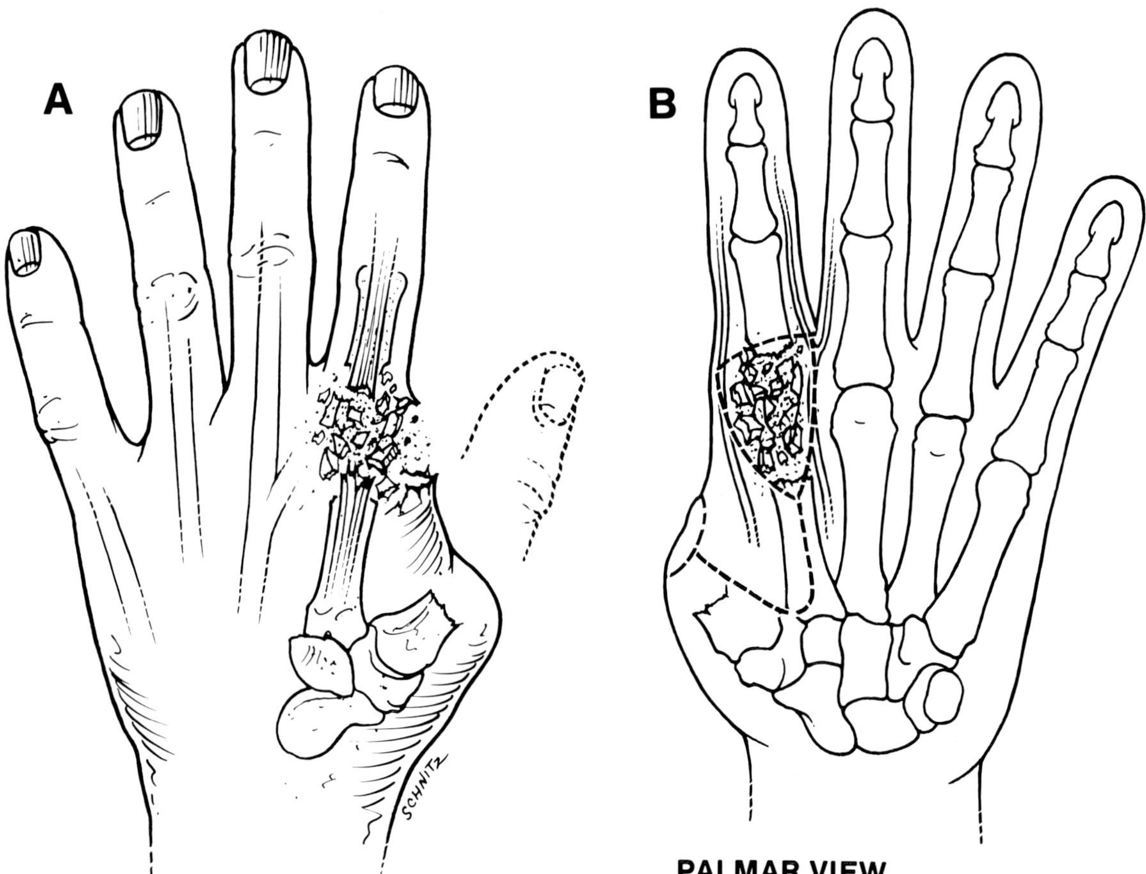

Fig. 57-70. Pollicization of an injured index finger. **(A&B)** Incisions for transfer of the index finger following thumb loss through the proximal part of the metacarpal with damage to the second metacarpal and extensor tendon. Incisions may vary depending on skin conditions. *(Figure continues.)*

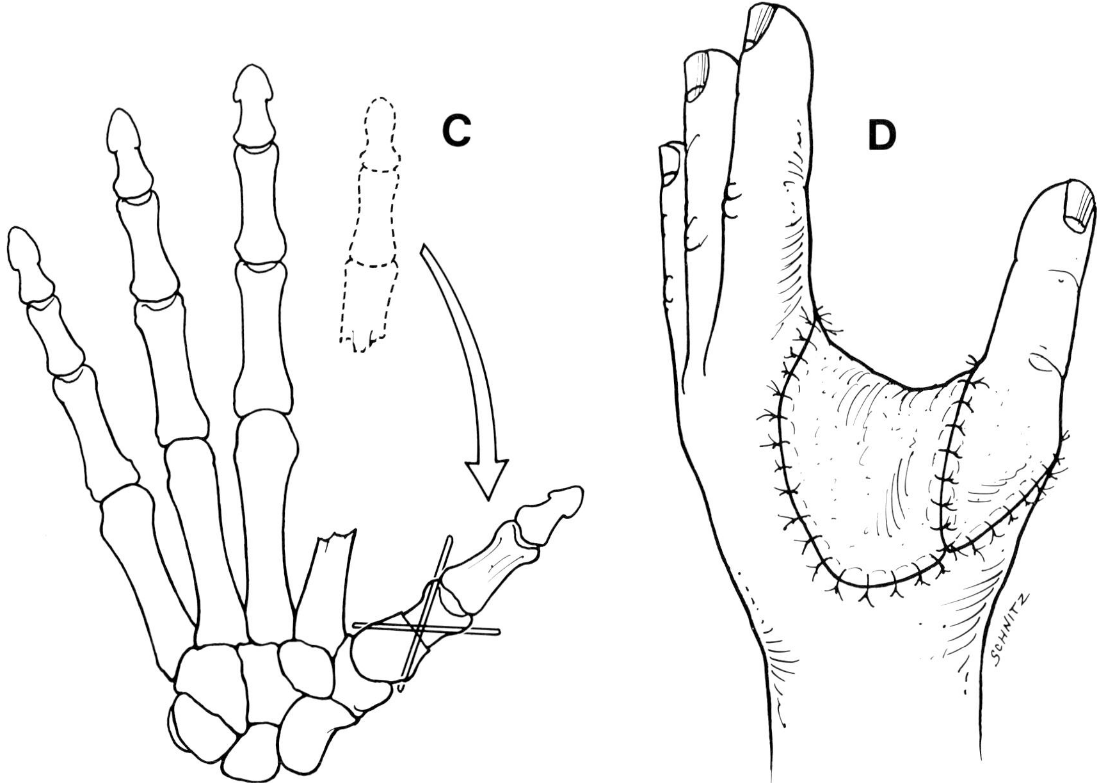

Fig. 57-70 *(Continued).* **(C)** Diagram of bone transfer including proximal, middle, and distal phalanges of the index to first metacarpal base or scaphoid, depending on the level of thumb loss. **(D)** Appearance of the reconstructed thumb following pollicization with the lateral flap used to restore the first web. (Modified from Reid,[442] with permission.)

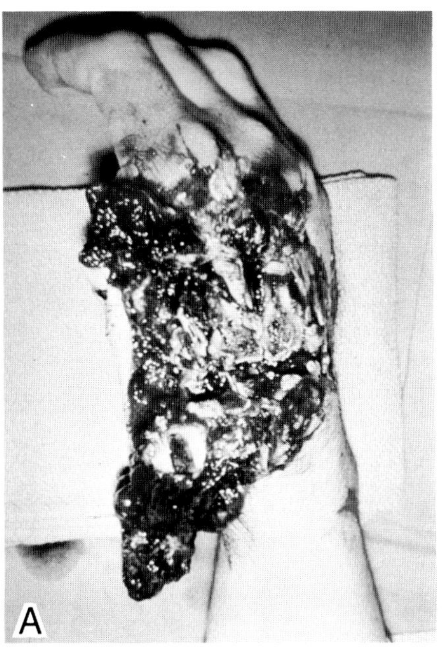

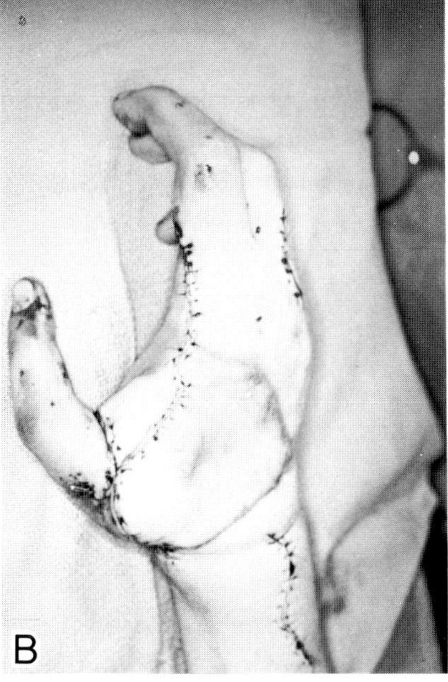

Fig. 57-71. Pollicization of an injured index finger. **(A)** A mutilating injury resulting in thumb amputation and destruction of the second metacarpal and extensor tendons. **(B)** Appearance of the hand at 2 months, immediately following abdominal pedicle resurfacing and pollicization of the damaged index finger ray. *(Figure continues.)*

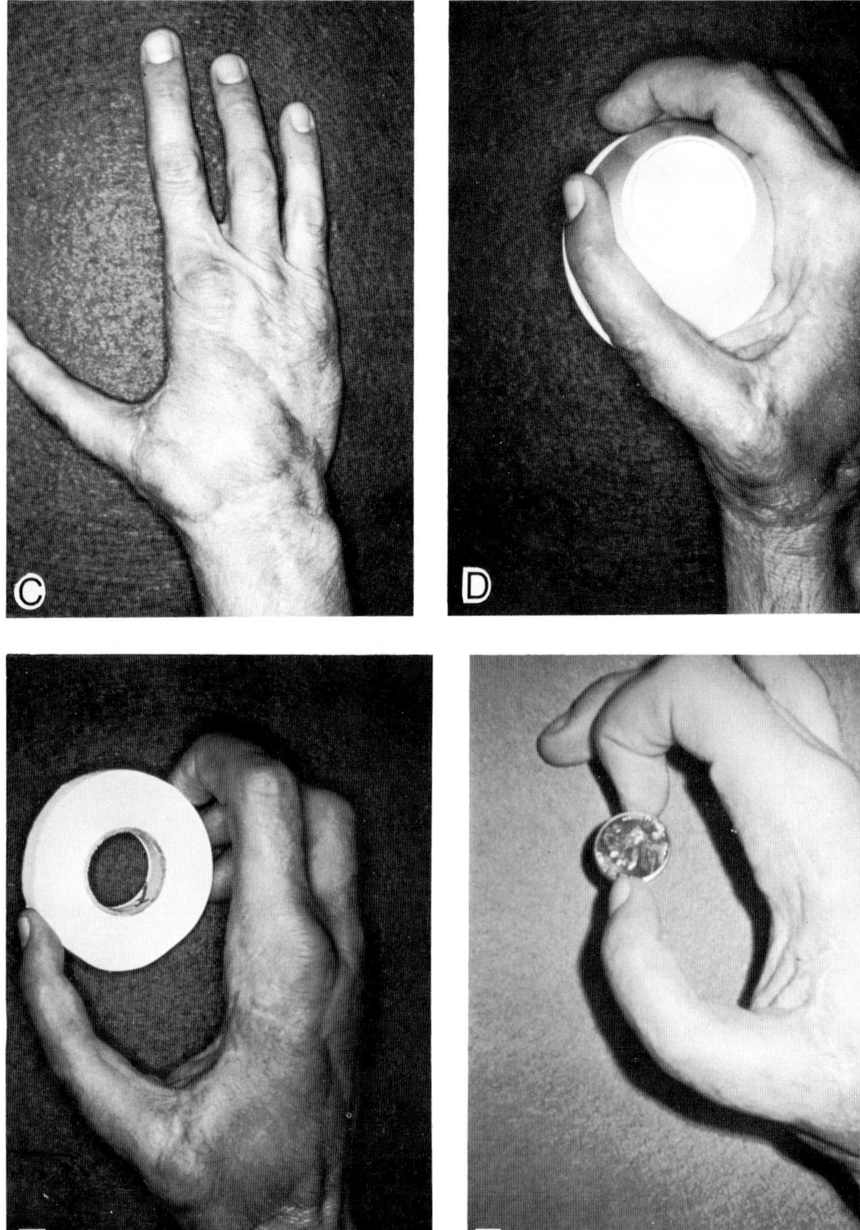

Fig. 57-71 *(Continued).* **(C–F)** Appearance of the hand at 3 years with ability to carry out grasping and pinching activities. (From Strickland,[473] with permission.)

and opponensplasty if all thenar muscle function has been lost and satisfactory basilar joint rotation is retained (Fig. 57-71).

Pollicization of the Ring Finger (Modified from Letac[322])

Under tourniquet anesthesia, palmar incisions are begun at the level of the distal palmar crease and extended on each side of the ring finger through the web to join dorsally over the fourth metacarpal at approximately its midpoint. The dorsal "V" is then continued as a single proximally longitudinal incision to the base of the fourth metacarpal (Fig. 57-72A & B). Flaps are carefully raised and elevated, and palmar dissection is used to carefully identify, mobilize, and preserve the neurovascular bundles. Ligation of the ulnar digital arterial branch to the long finger and the radial digital arterial branch to the small finger is carried out just distal to the bifurcation of the common digital arteries to the third and fourth web spaces respectively (Fig. 57-72C). Careful microscopic splitting of the common digital nerves to the long and ring fingers and to the ring and small fingers is also required in order to assure transfer of the digit across the palm without undue tension on the digital nerves or injury to the remaining nerves to the long and small fingers.

Alternating dissection is carried out both dorsally and palmarly in both the third and fourth web spaces. The transverse

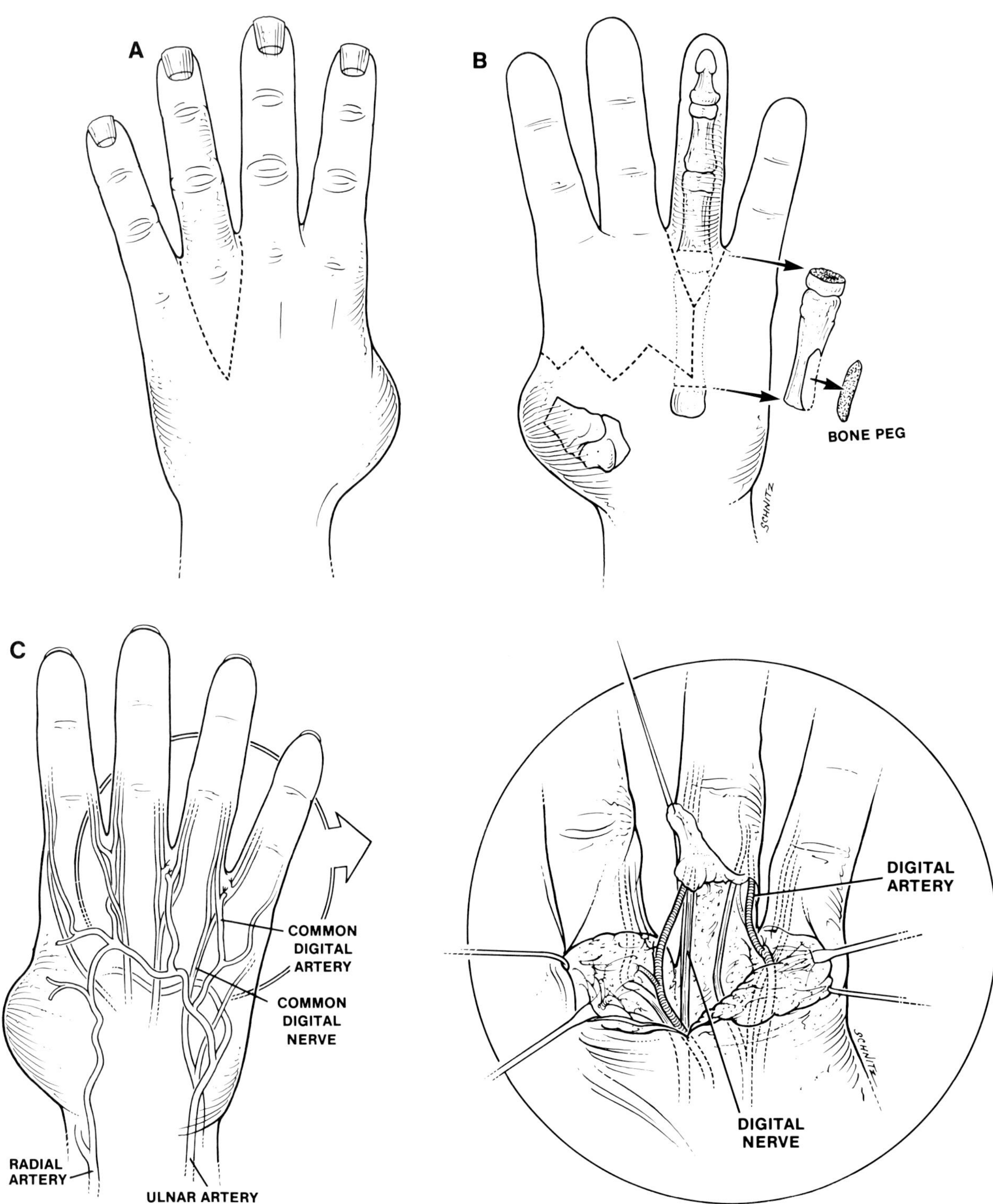

Fig. 57-72. Pollicization of the ring finger. **(A)** Proposed dorsal incision. **(B)** Palmar incision with proposed connecting incision to the thumb. The amount of bone to be resected from the fourth metacarpal and base of the proximal phalanx is shown. A bone peg may be fashioned from the metacarpal to be used at the bone juncture site. **(C)** The division of the proper digital arteries to the ulnar side of the long finger and the radial side of the small finger during the mobilization of the ring finger for transfer is shown. Some proximal separation of the common digital nerves is also necessary to lessen tension on the nerves to the transferred digit *(inset)*. *(Figure continues.)*

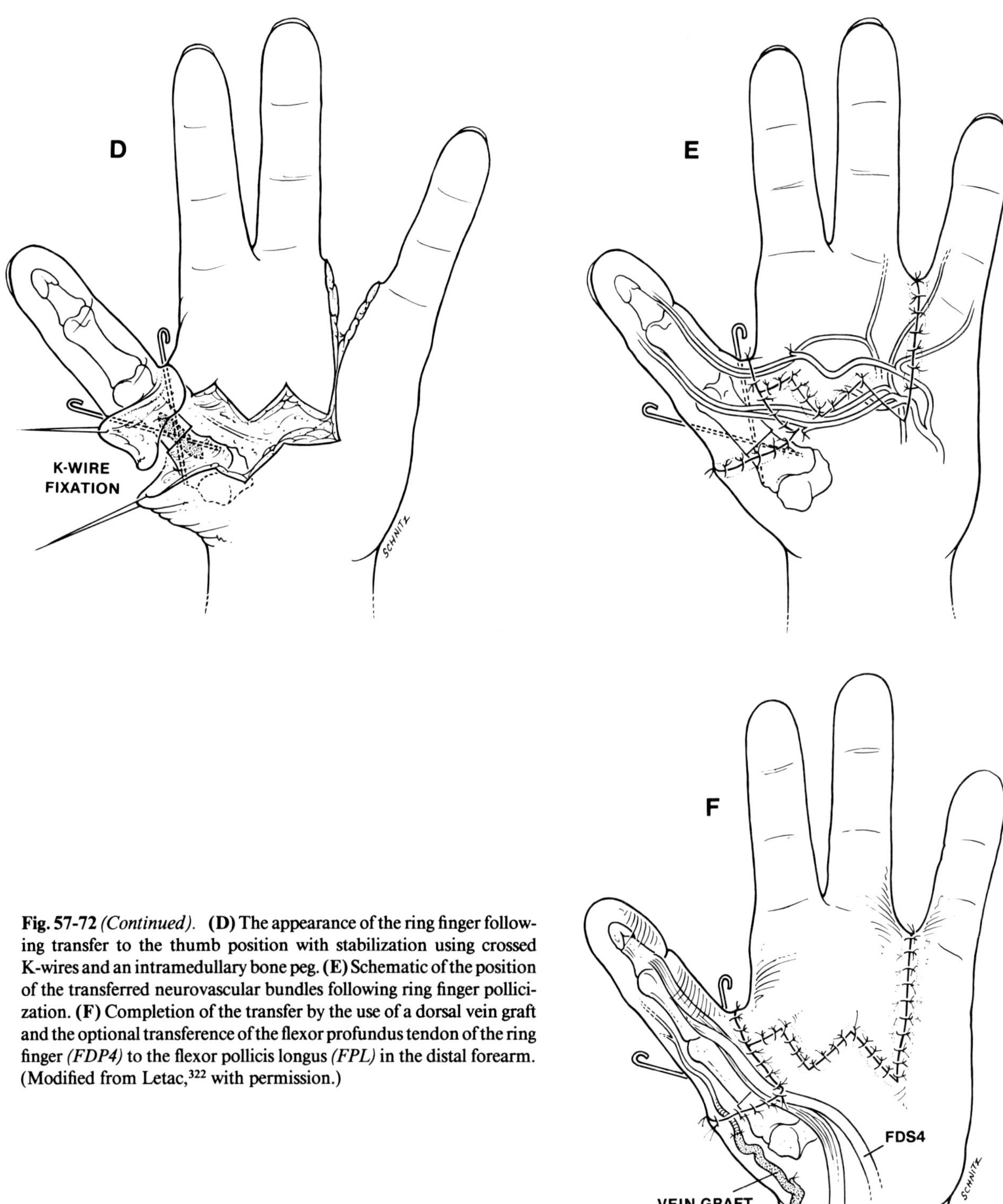

Fig. 57-72 *(Continued).* **(D)** The appearance of the ring finger following transfer to the thumb position with stabilization using crossed K-wires and an intramedullary bone peg. **(E)** Schematic of the position of the transferred neurovascular bundles following ring finger pollicization. **(F)** Completion of the transfer by the use of a dorsal vein graft and the optional transference of the flexor profundus tendon of the ring finger *(FDP4)* to the flexor pollicis longus *(FPL)* in the distal forearm. (Modified from Letac,[322] with permission.)

intermetacarpal ligaments in each space are divided, leaving sufficient length to allow for the joining of the two ligaments following ring finger transfer. The extensor tendon to the ring finger is divided at the base of the fourth metacarpal and mobilized distally to the base of the proximal phalanx. The fourth metacarpal is then stripped of its interosseous attachments and the intrinsic tendons to the ring finger are divided distally. The fourth metacarpal is then osteotomized at its base and removed. The flexor tendons are mobilized to the midpalm and all remaining soft tissue attachments to the ring finger are carefully divided in preparation for its passage across the palm.

The first metacarpal is carefully prepared to receive the transferred ring finger and if it is small or absent the distal surface of the trapezium is removed to cancellous bone. It is possible to ream a small hole in the first metacarpal or in the distal trapezium and to use a bone peg for attachment of the ring finger after its passage. A proximal dorsal extension of the first metacarpal incision is used to identify and mobilize the stump of the extensor pollicis longus, and all scar is removed from the site of thumb amputation, preserving good supple skin for suture to the transferred digit.

Letac[322] described the preparation of a tunnel under the palmar fascia proceeding obliquely from the upper part of the palm to the thumb wound by passing just distal to the thenar eminence. Once established, the tunnel is widened by the use of progressively larger Hager dilators. A strong suture is secured to the end of the mobilized ring finger, passed through the palmar tunnel, and then used to carefully deliver the digit through the tunnel and into thumb position. In its new position the finger will have rotated 100 degrees on its longitudinal axis in order to achieve a satisfactory position with the least tension on the neurovascular pedicles. The articular surface of the proximal phalanx of the ring finger is removed, and appropriate bone removal, contour, and shaping are carried out to assure the proper length and position of the transferred digit. Stabilization of the bony juncture is achieved by K-wires or a small compression plate; the use of an intramedullary peg across the site of bony contact is optional (Fig. 57-72D & E).

The procedure is completed by suture of the extensor tendon of the ring finger to the distal stump of the extensor pollicis longus of the thumb. The tendon juncture is carried out underneath normal skin, with sufficient tension to maintain the ring finger in full extension at PIP and DIP joints. If possible, the remnant of the abductor pollicis brevis tendon may be attached to the intrinsic tendon remnants on the radial side of the transferred ring finger, and on occasion, it may even be possible to suture the remnant of the adductor tendon to the stumps of the intrinsic tendons to the ulnar side of the transferred digit. The tourniquet is then released to confirm the vascularity of the transferred digit and to achieve hemostasis.

Repair of the donor wound is completed after careful repair of the transverse intermetacarpal ligaments to the long and small fingers. This repair as well as the tailoring and closure of the skin between the two digits is carried out in such a manner as to minimize the breadth of the new cleft resulting from the removal of the ring finger and to provide the best possible cosmetic appearance. Finally, closure of the skin at the base of the transferred ring finger is completed, and it is often wise to use several small Z-plasties to avoid a constricting circumferential repair, which might be prejudicial to the vascularity of the transposed digit.

A number of modifications to this technique may be made, depending on the exact level of thumb loss and the nature of the scarring about the first metacarpal stump. Additional skin can be brought with the ring finger transfer if the amount of scarring about the thumb ray is excessive, although this may require some skin grafting in the donor area at the time of closure. Butler[185] has modified the procedure in several ways. His procedure includes a connecting incision between the palmar incision at the base of the ring finger and the stump of the first metacarpal in order to directly visualize and protect the neurovascular bundles at the time of transfer. He also recommended transfer of the MP joint of the transferred digit to replace the lost thumb MP joint and shortening of the transferred digit with a shift of the nail bed and matrix on a palmar pedicle. He emphasized that the profundus tendon to the ring finger must be separated from its close relationship to the profundi of the long and small fingers in order to prevent a checkrein effect that would prevent complete flexion of the small finger. To further obviate this problem, Garcia Velesco[240] recommended severing the flexor tendons in the palm and sacrificing the superficialis, with the profundus tendon being joined to the mobilized stump of the flexor pollicls lollgus at a later operation. I would concur that it may be appropriate to divide the profundus tendon and suture it to the flexor pollicis longus stump but prefer to carry out this transfer at the time of ring finger pollicization (Fig. 57-72F).

A plaster-reinforced compressive dressing is worn for 2 weeks; plaster immobilization of the first metacarpal is maintained until bony union is complete at approximately 6 to 8 weeks following ring finger pollicization. Ring finger motion is commenced at 3 to 4 weeks, although firm compression plate fixation of the bony juncture may permit earlier mobilization.

Utilization of a damaged or poorly functional digit or of a normal index or ring finger may provide an excellent restoration of thumb function when loss has occurred through the proximal portion of the first metacarpal (Fig. 57-73). It is important that arteriographic documentation of at least one good digital artery be obtained prior to the transfer of a previously injured index digit, or the unfortunate loss of the digit might result. The obvious disadvantage of the use of a normal index or ring finger is that there is some inevitable functional consequence to the involved hand and there is controversy as to which digit results in the least loss of hand performance. Both procedures must be done with great technical care to insure that there is no damage to the neurovascular structures in the transferred digit. Although failure to bring dorsal veins with the transferred digit has apparently not resulted in significant outflow problems, recent microsurgical techniques make venous anastomoses, with or without interpositional grafts, a meaningful addition to these procedures.

On occasion, compromised vascular performance may require immediate reexploration of the transferred digit, and if the ring finger has been transferred through a palmar tunnel, it may be necessary to connect the thumb and ring finger wounds in order to decompress a kinked or twisted neurovascular pedicle. Nonunion or delayed union of the bony junction of the thumb and transferred digit may occasionally result in the

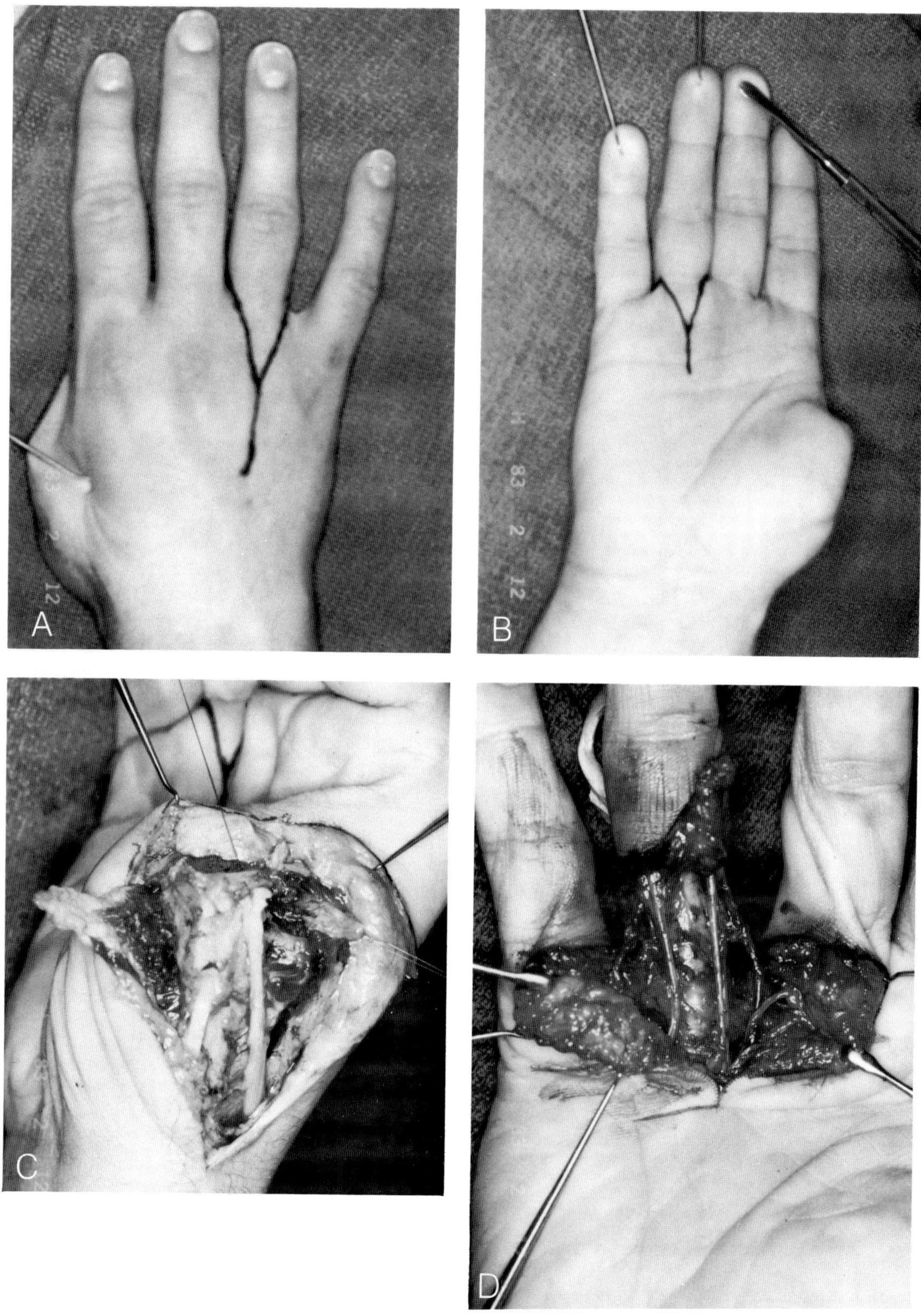

Fig. 57-73. Ring finger pollicization. **(A&B)** Dorsal and palmar incisions. **(C)** Preparation of the recipient area, including trimming of bone and identification of flexor and extensor tendons. **(D)** Palmar dissection with isolation of the neurovascular bundles to the ring finger. *(Figure continues.)*

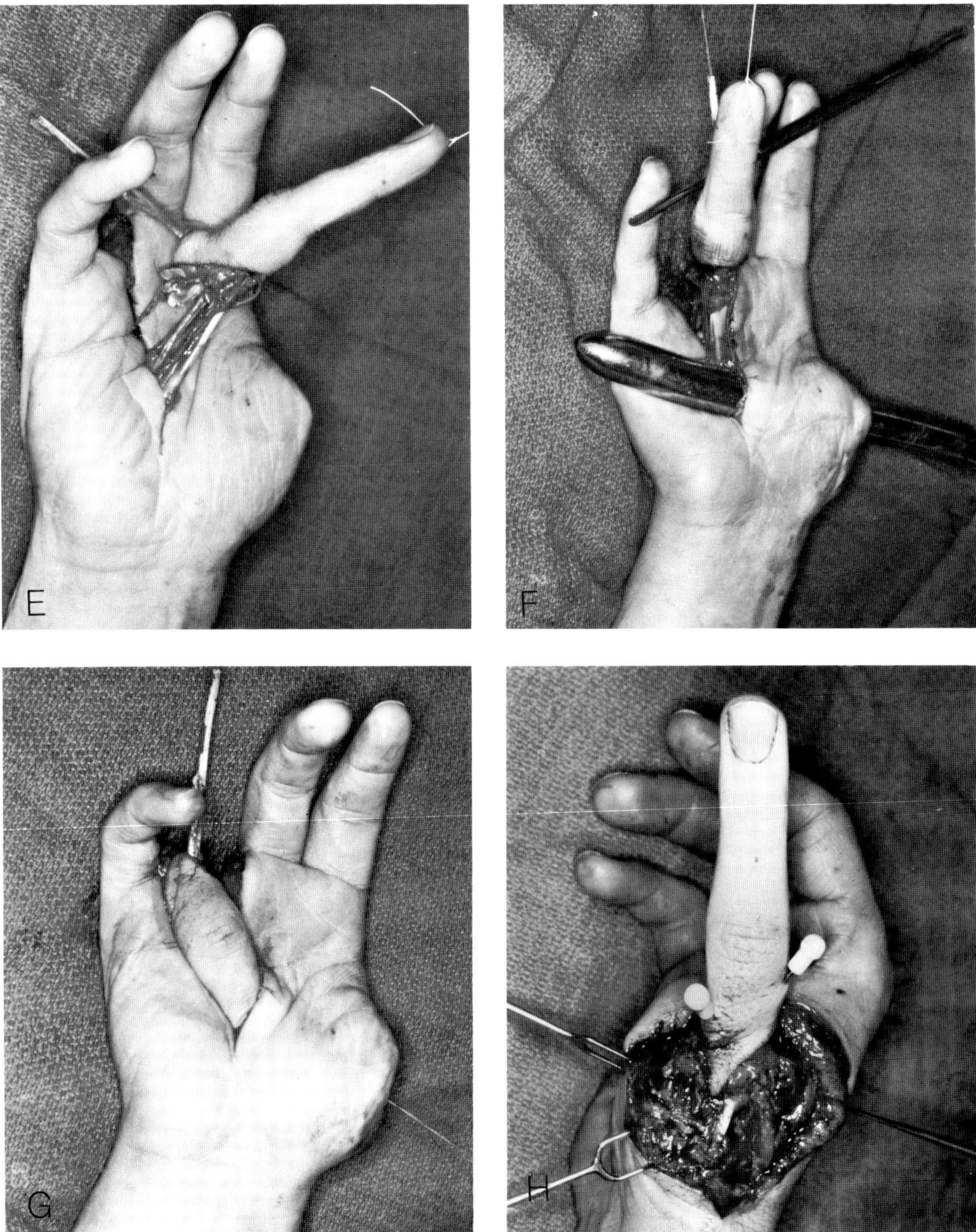

Fig. 57-73 *(Continued).* **(E)** The ring finger mobilized on its flexor tendons and neurovascular bundles. **(F)** Preparation for transpalmar passage of the ring finger using dialators after the method of Letac. Optional connecting incisions may be preferable. **(G)** Careful passage of the ring finger across the palmar tunnel, with care taken to avoid torsion of the neurovascular bundles. **(H)** Positioning of the ring finger on the metacarpal stump with K-wire fixation. *(Figure continues.)*

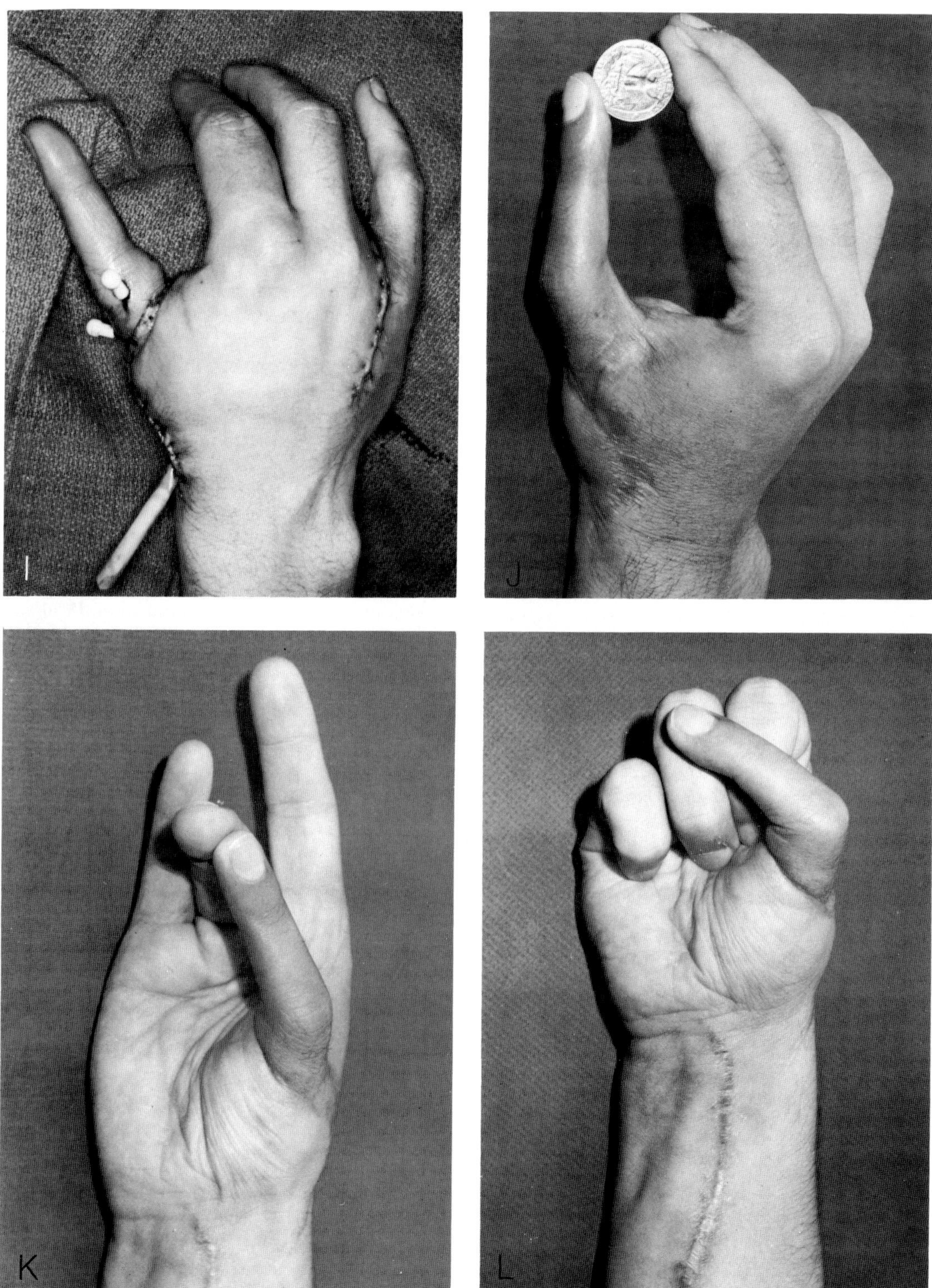

Fig. 57-73 *(Continued).* **(I)** Appearance of the pollicized ring finger with wound closure and tourniquet release. **(J–L)** Appearance and function of the ring finger pollicization at 6 months, with excellent grasp and pinch function.

need for secondary procedures, and tenolysis or opponensplasty may in some instances be required. Nonetheless, digital transfer to the thumb position remains as a very viable alternative to thumb reconstruction following loss at the proximal metacarpal, particularly when factors mitigate against great toe transfer. Although the index and ring fingers have been preferred by most for pollicization, the long or even the small finger may occasionally be utilized.

Free Toe-to-Thumb Transfer

Surgical efforts to transfer a finger from the opposite hand (refs. 167,299,406, Steichen and Strickland: unpublished observations) or toes to replace a thumb have been occasionally carried out since Nicoladoni's first toe-to-hand transfer in 1900.[401] Prior to the advent of predictably successful microvascular anastomoses, the staged transfer of a toe (usually the big toe) to the hand was extremely difficult and fraught with complications. Although hand function may have been improved by this transfer, the technical difficulty, cosmetic appearance, poor sensation, and marginal performance of the transferred part served to prevent this method of reconstruction from becoming popular.[156,191,196,198,238,247,402,523] Following the experimental work of Buncke and Schultz,[178] Cobbett,[200] Buncke,[176-179] O'Brien,[404-409] Tamai,[486] and others[179,190,215,223,233,235,250,274,321,323-325,327,353,356,357,373,375,389,390,411,430,449,472,474,520] have successfully described and refined procedures for the free transfer of toes to the thumb position with vessel, nerve, and tendon repairs. When carried out by skilled microvascular teams, toe-to-thumb transfer has reached the stage of predictability and functional performance where it must be considered as the best reconstructive option for the young patient with thumb loss through the proximal first metacarpal.[171] The technique of O'Brien[406] simplifies the procedure by allowing for transfer of the great toe on the dorsalis pedis artery and dorsal veins, obviating the necessity for the difficult plantar dissection of vascular structures. Candidates for this procedure must be of the proper mental and physical status for the prolonged operation and subsequent rehabilitation and should be aware of the possibility of failure that would compound thumb amputation by the loss of the great toe. As more microvascular centers are established and the repugnance for this procedure on the part of reconstructive hand surgeons diminishes, toe-to-thumb transfer will assume an increasingly important place among the restorative options following thumb loss at a proximal level. Toe-to-thumb transfer is described in detail in Chapter 33.

Summary: Reconstruction of the Proximal One-Third of First Ray

The return of satisfactory thumb function following amputation of the entire thumb and the distal portion of the first metacarpal can be quite challenging. From 4 to 8 cm of additional length must be provided together with satisfactory sensation and strong skeletal stability. The functional result of such reconstruction is greatly enhanced by the retention of good basilar joint motion. Great toe transfer has been demonstrated to be an excellent method of thumb reconstruction in this area, and in appropriate patients it is probably the procedure of choice. Pollicization of an injured digit, however, may often be utilized as an effective means of restoring thumb length and sensibility without the need to sacrifice the great toe. Pollicization of normal digits into thumb position has also been a time honored and effective method of restoring thumb function following proximal loss, and the index and ring finger have probably become the most popular methods of pollicization. In an excellent statistical study attempting to evaluate and compare the results of toe-to-hand transfers and pollicization, Michon et al[372] concluded that:

1. For thumb amputation without injuries to the other fingers either procedure is applicable. Pollicization returns better discriminative sensation and fine motor control, while toe transfer establishes better strength.
2. When other digits are amputated or mutilated, toe transfers are preferable in an effort to maximize strength.
3. For the metacarpal hand, the transfer of one or more toes is the only technique capable of restoring function.

The patient should be allowed to participate in the decision-making process. When duly informed of the alternatives and with a thorough understanding of the anticipated functional gain and problems resulting from toe or digit transfer, a rational decision can be made, and the final results should be quite satisfactory with a high level of patient acceptance.

LOSS OF THUMB AND ALL DIGITS

The occasional amputation of the thumb and all digits result in a catastrophic functional loss to the hand. The reconstructive surgeon faced with this deformity must assess the possibility of restoring two opposable rays with strong motion in at least one. Transfer of one or more toes to the digitless hand has been described, and the evolution of microvascular techniques will undoubtedly add tremendously to the reconstructive options in these unfortunate situations.[520,527] Other methods that provide length by the addition of bone grafts and insensitive abdominal flaps usually provide little long-term functional improvement and should be generally condemned. When there are digital remnants present it may be possible to phalangize mobile metacarpal segments with satisfactory strength achieved to accomplish crude pinch and grasp functions.[359]

Metacarpal Clefting by Phalangization

Procedures described for this situation have been quite varied and have included attempts to further digitalize small phalangeal remnants,[259] first metacarpal phalangization combined with excision of the second metacarpal,[165,193] and excision of the second and the majority of the third metacarpal.[497] Phalangization and osteotomy of the first and fifth metacarpals com-

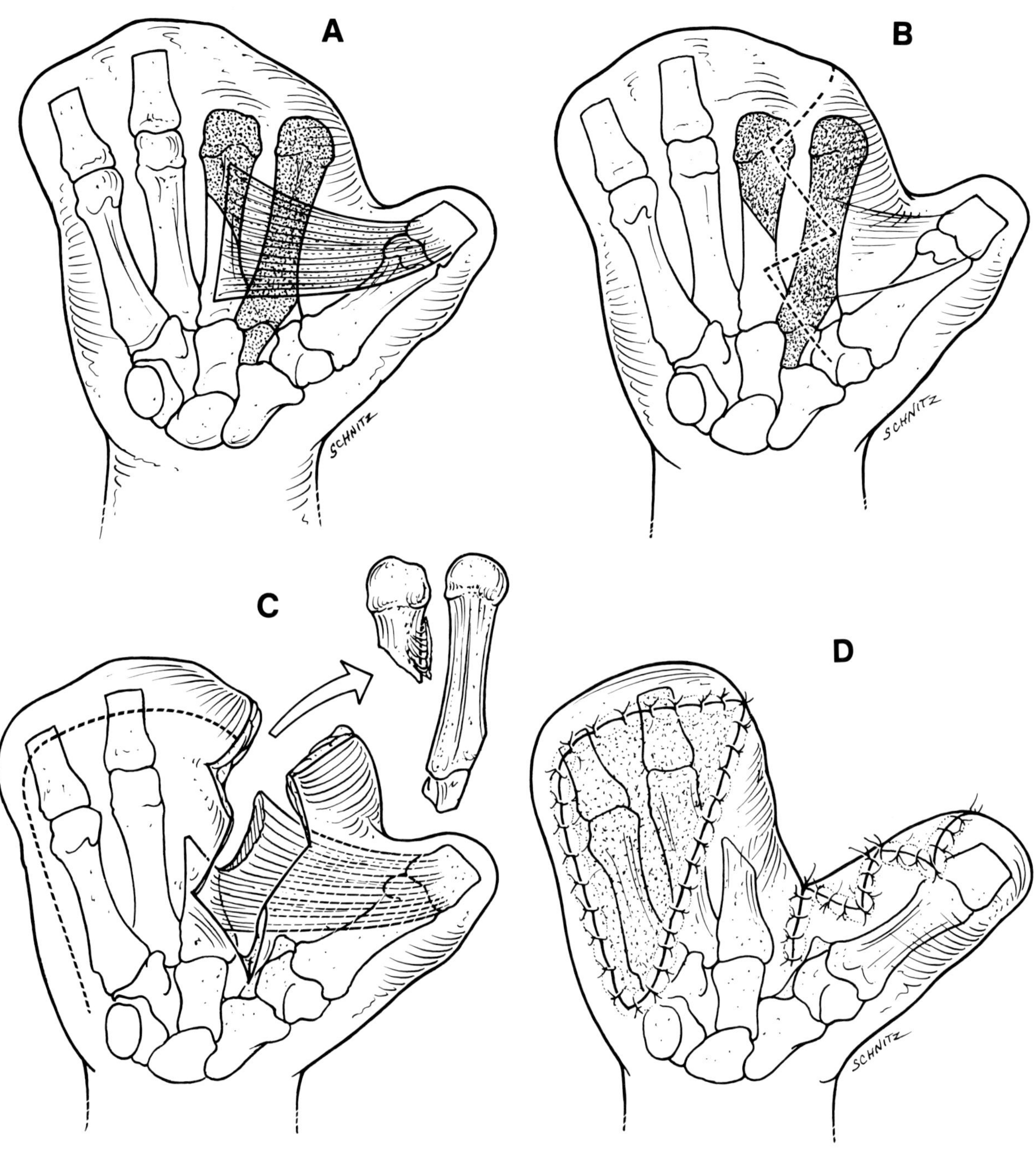

Fig. 57-74. Phalangization of the metacarpal hand. **(A)** Appearance of the metacarpal hand with small proximal phalangeal remnants in the thumb, ring, and small fingers. The shaded areas of the second and third metacarpals are to be excised. **(B)** Zigzag skin incisions over the proposed cleft between the thumb and ring finger remnants. **(C)** Phalangization of the first metacarpal with excision of the second metacarpal, trapezoid, and distal half of the third metacarpal. The origin of adductor pollicis brevis from the proximal half of the third metacarpal is carefully preserved. **(D)** Closure of the ulnar side of the first ray and dorsal rotational flap coverage of the first web. Free skin graft coverage of the donor defect. (Modified from Brown et al,[165] with permission.)

bined with excision of the second and fourth metacarpals have also been advocated[183,497] and more elaborate procedures consisting of a pedicle transfer of the second metacarpal to lengthen the first metacarpal at the time of phalangization have also been carried out.[220,368,369] Further bone-skin gymnastics to provide additional length of the first and third metacarpals have been described,[369] and when a full first metacarpal exists with minimal adjacent metacarpal length, the creation of an ulnar post by osteoplastic means has been devised.[183,368,369] By utilizing these or similar techniques,[183,416] one can hopefully achieve a wide enough cleft for an opening and closing pincher function.

Technical considerations for phalangization procedures following loss of all digits and the thumb include removing enough metacarpal and portions of the distal carpal row to provide a satisfactory cleft, while attempting to preserve as much adductor and abductor pollicis function as possible to ensure the mobility of the first metacarpal ray. In those patients with no phalangeal remnants or short metacarpal segments, the procedure may often prove unsatisfactory, although small

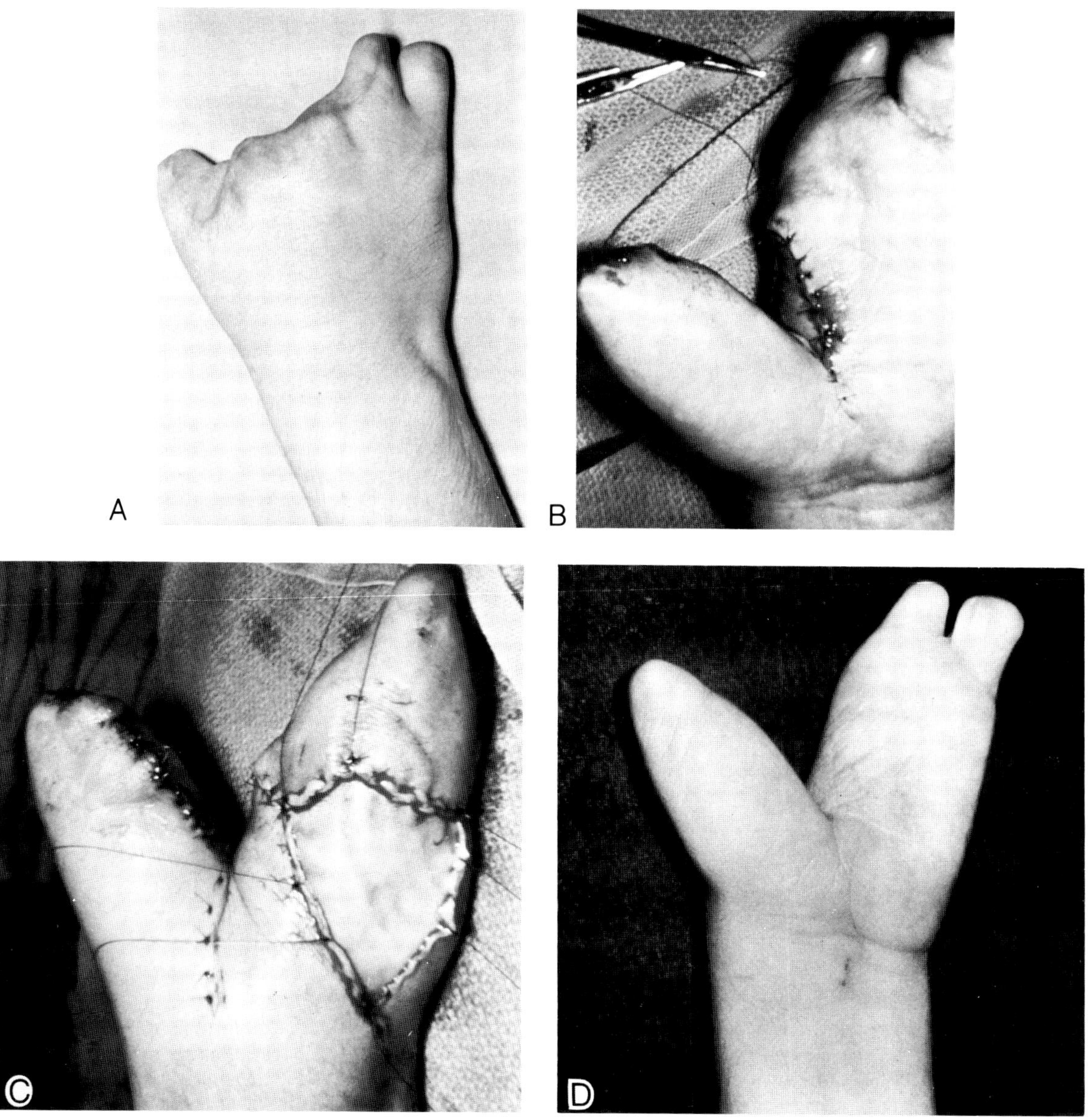

Fig. 57-75. Phalangization of the metacarpal hand. **(A)** Appearance of a hand following amputation of all digits and thumb with short phalangeal remnants present over the first, fourth, and fifth metacarpals. **(B)** Immediately following phalangization of the first metacarpal with midhand clefting permitted by excision of the second metacarpal, the trapezoid, and the distal half of the third metacarpal. **(C)** The dorsal aspect of the hand following first metacarpal closure and rotational flap coverage of the web. Full-thickness skin graft coverage of the donor defect. **(D)** Appearance of the palmar hand at 6 months. *(Figure continues.)*

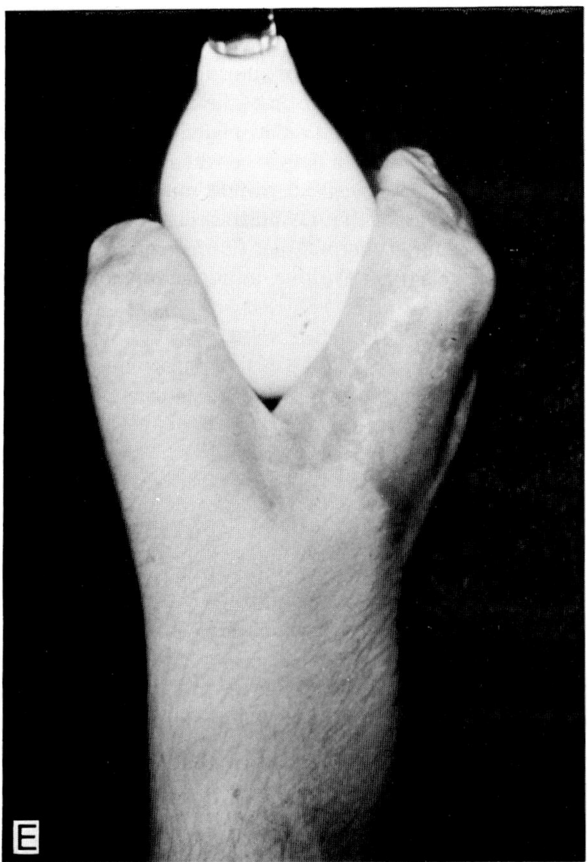

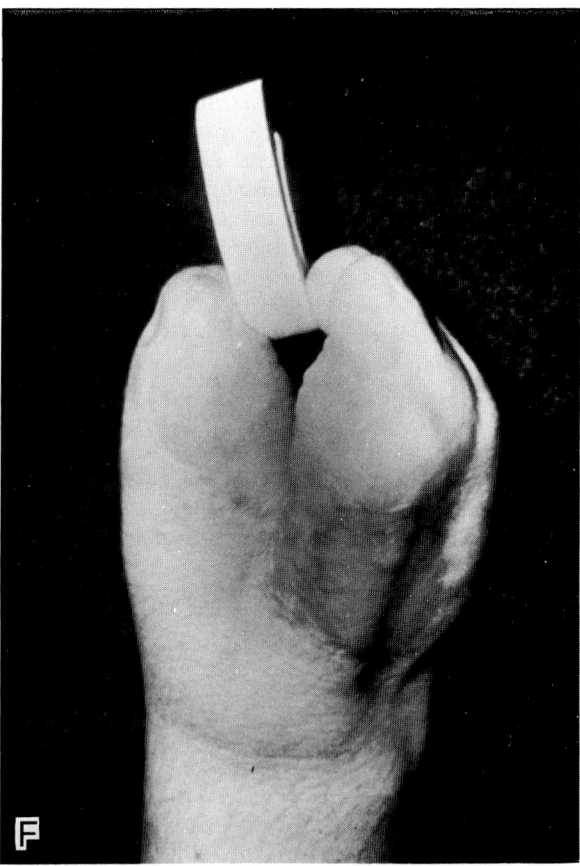

Fig. 57-75 *(Continued).* **(E&F)** Restoration of grasp and pinch functions. (From Strickland,[473] with permission.)

increments of length may occasionally be gained by interpositional or add-on grafting utilizing portions of the metacarpals excised to create a cleft.[317,368,369] It would also appear that metacarpal lengthening techniques previously described on page 2115 may be applicable in these cases in an attempt to substantially elongate the first or first and fifth metacarpals to provide better function. The results of these procedures may prove disappointing if one cannot ensure a satisfactory midray space, opposable strength and motion of at least one ray, and satisfactory sensory perception on opposing sides of the pincer.

Phalangization of the Metacarpal Hand (Modified from Brown[165])

Under tourniquet hemostasis, a linear or zigzag incision designed over the second metacarpal is begun dorsally at the wrist and continued over the metacarpal stump palmarly to the base of the thenar eminence. Flaps are planned to interdigitate with the ulnar side of the mobilized first metacarpal (Fig. 57-74A & B).

The flexor and extensor tendons are carefully dissected off the second and third metacarpals, and the radial digital nerve to the index stump, together with the common digital nerve to the index and long fingers, are transsected proximally near their origins from the median nerve.

If present, the index and long finger flexors are excised proximally and allowed to retract, and the extensor tendons are divided over the distal wrist as well. The second metacarpal and the trapezoid are then excised sharply, and as much as 50 percent of the third metacarpal is removed with an oblique osteotomy. As much adductor origin as possible is preserved, commensurate with the bony excision (Fig. 57-74C).

Following closure of the ulnar side of the mobilized first ray, it is often necessary to create a dorsal rotational flap for coverage of the radial margin of the cleft. A small paper pattern is rotated from the dorsal hand into the defect to determine the appropriate flap size, and the flap is then dissected off the dorsal hand in a manner previously described. A full-thickness skin graft is used to provide coverage for the donor area, and a large compressive dressing is then applied for 7 to 10 days (Fig. 57-74D).

Dressing change at 7 to 10 days is used to determine the condition of the wounds and the dorsal skin graft, and a small web-spreading splint is employed intermittently for several months. The need for additional osteotomy of the fifth metacarpal is determined by observing function following this procedure.

Although producing a crude "lobster claw" type hand, phalangization procedures following loss of the thumb and all digits can be quite rewarding (Fig. 57-75). It should be emphasized that the patient must have maintained mobility of at least the first metacarpal and preferably the first and fourth and fifth metacarpal rays to allow these techniques to return significant function. The need for osteotomy of the fifth metacarpal may have been somewhat overstated in the past, and it should be remembered that with good hypothenar function and basilar joint mobility, these metacarpals normally rotate toward the thumb during normal activity. Preservation of the adductor origin would seem important, although if the thumb amputation is proximal to the MP joint, the adductor insertion has already been lost (Fig. 57-76). The presence of phalangeal remnants on the first and fourth and fifth metacarpals adds considerably to the final function following this type of procedure, and it would, therefore, appear that elongating techniques that add on portions of the second and/or fourth metacarpals to the first and fifth may be of considerable value. The development of metacarpal lengthening techniques and free tissue transfers will undoubtedly have a role in the production of better hand function in these severely handicapped hands in the future.

CONCLUSION

It may be seen from this chapter that there are many esoteric and technically difficult procedures available for the restoration of thumb function following partial or total loss. Emphasis has been placed on careful evaluation of the functional requirements necessitated at each level of thumb amputation, and procedures that best meet those requirements are suggested. A genuine consideration of the specific desires of each patient is mandatory, and it is the obligation of the reconstructive surgeon to explain in detail the realistic goals of each restorative procedure as well as possible complications. A sufficient time interval following thumb amputation should elapse before any secondary reconstructive procedure is undertaken in order for the patient to adjust to the hand function necessitated by thumb loss. This knowledge will help the patient participate in decisions relating to reconstruction. Finally, it should be emphasized that these procedures require not only a cooperative patient but a highly skilled hand surgeon, familiar with intricate reconstructive procedures of this nature, and the availability of a hand rehabilitation unit to aid in the establishment of thumb function following restorative surgery. Any compromise in these basic considerations will almost inevitably lead to disappointing results.

Much of what is written in this chapter is gradually becoming outdated. The explosive improvements in reconstructive procedures brought about by the development of microneurovascular techniques have set the stage for free tissue transfer procedures that have already added dramatically to the ability to return function to this important part of the hand and will continue to do so.

A 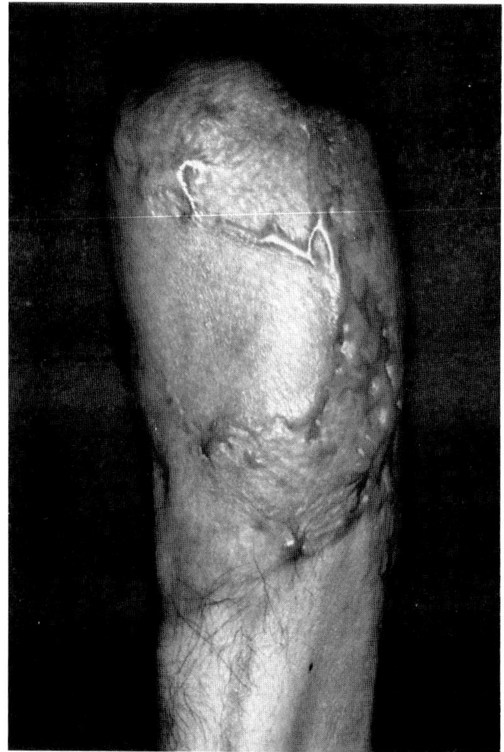

B 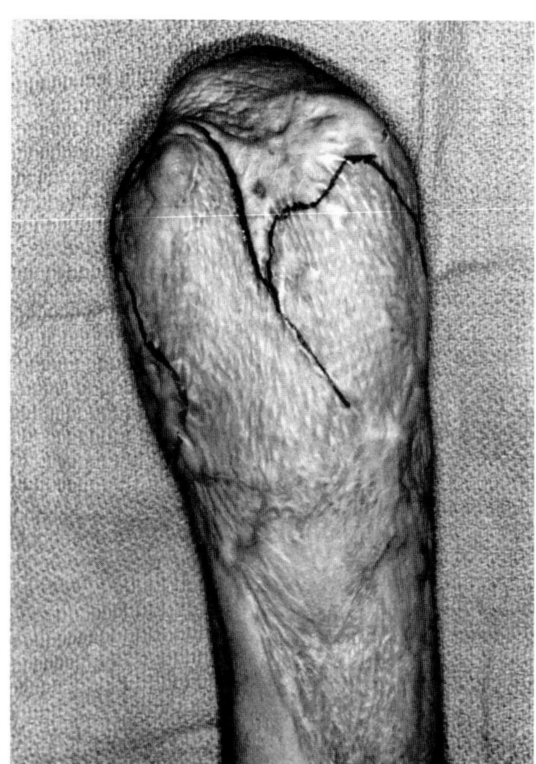

Fig. 57-76. This 31-year-old man suffered a severe degloving injury of his left hand, which was treated with a free fascial scapular flap. Healing was complicated by a partial necrosis, and resurfacing was completed with split-thickness skin grafts. There was amputation of the thumb and all digits through the bases of the proximal phalanges. **(A)** Mitten configuration of the dorsal surface of the remaining hand with no visible phalangeal remnants. **(B)** Palmar surface of the mitten hand with incisions planned for the phalangization procedure. *(Figure continues.)*

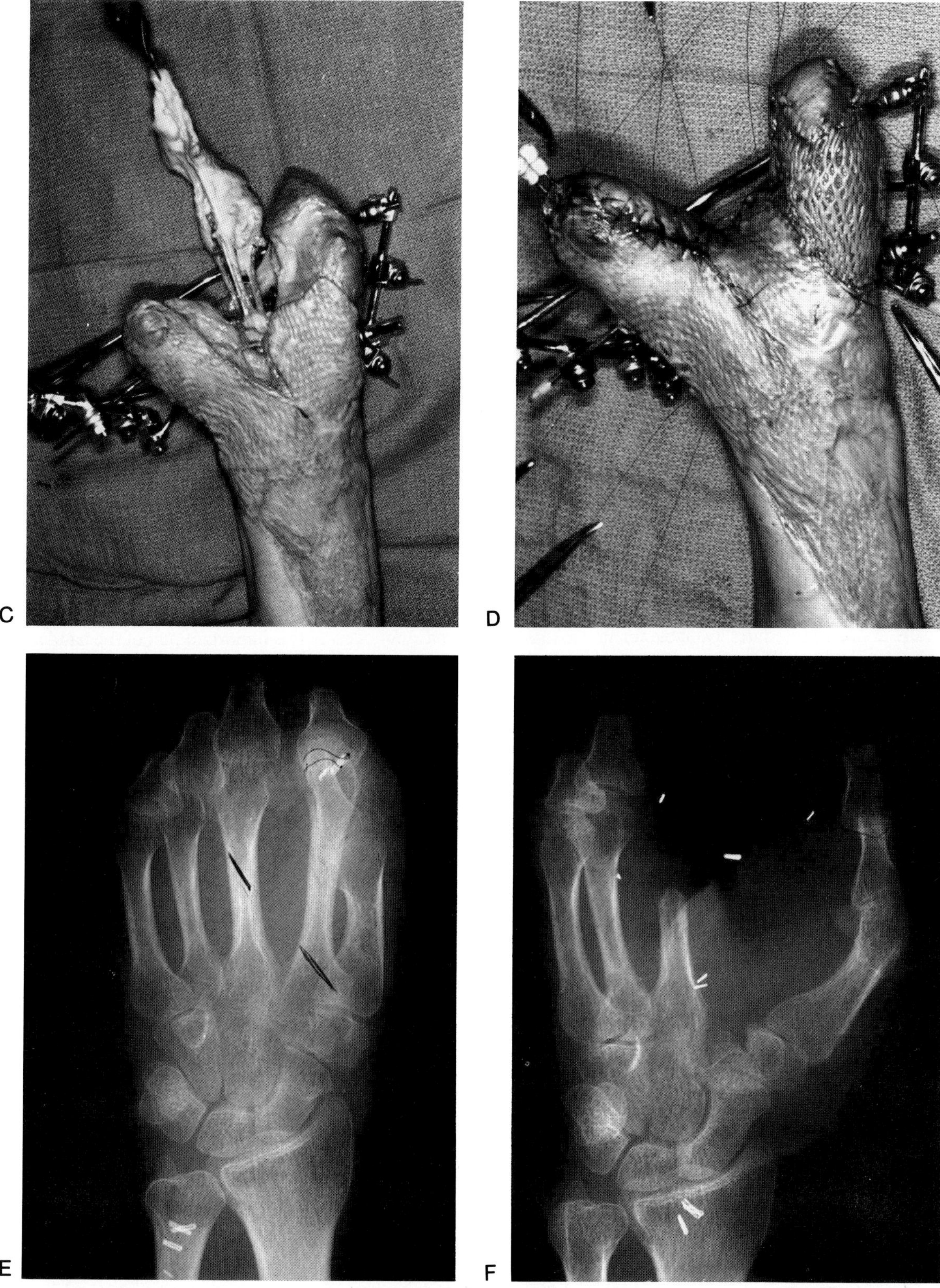

Fig. 57-76 *(Continued).* **(C)** Appearance of the hand during phalangization with excision of a central cleft of skin, scarred subcutaneous tissue, the entire second metacarpal, and 50 percent of the third metacarpal. The proximal phalanx of the index finger was transferred to the proximal remnant of the thumb. **(D)** The appearance of the phalangized hand at the conclusion of the procedure. Note the deepened cleft covered by a dorsal pedicle with meshed graft used to resurface the ulnar post. An external fixator was used to maintain the position of the radial and ulnar posts. **(E)** The preoperative x-rays with planned areas of bone division. **(F)** Postoperative x-rays following removal of fixation pins. Note the lengthened position of the thumb following successful incorporation of the transferred index proximal phalanx. The second metacarpal has been entirely removed, but enough third metacarpal was retained to insure preservation of the adductor origin. *(Figure continues.)*

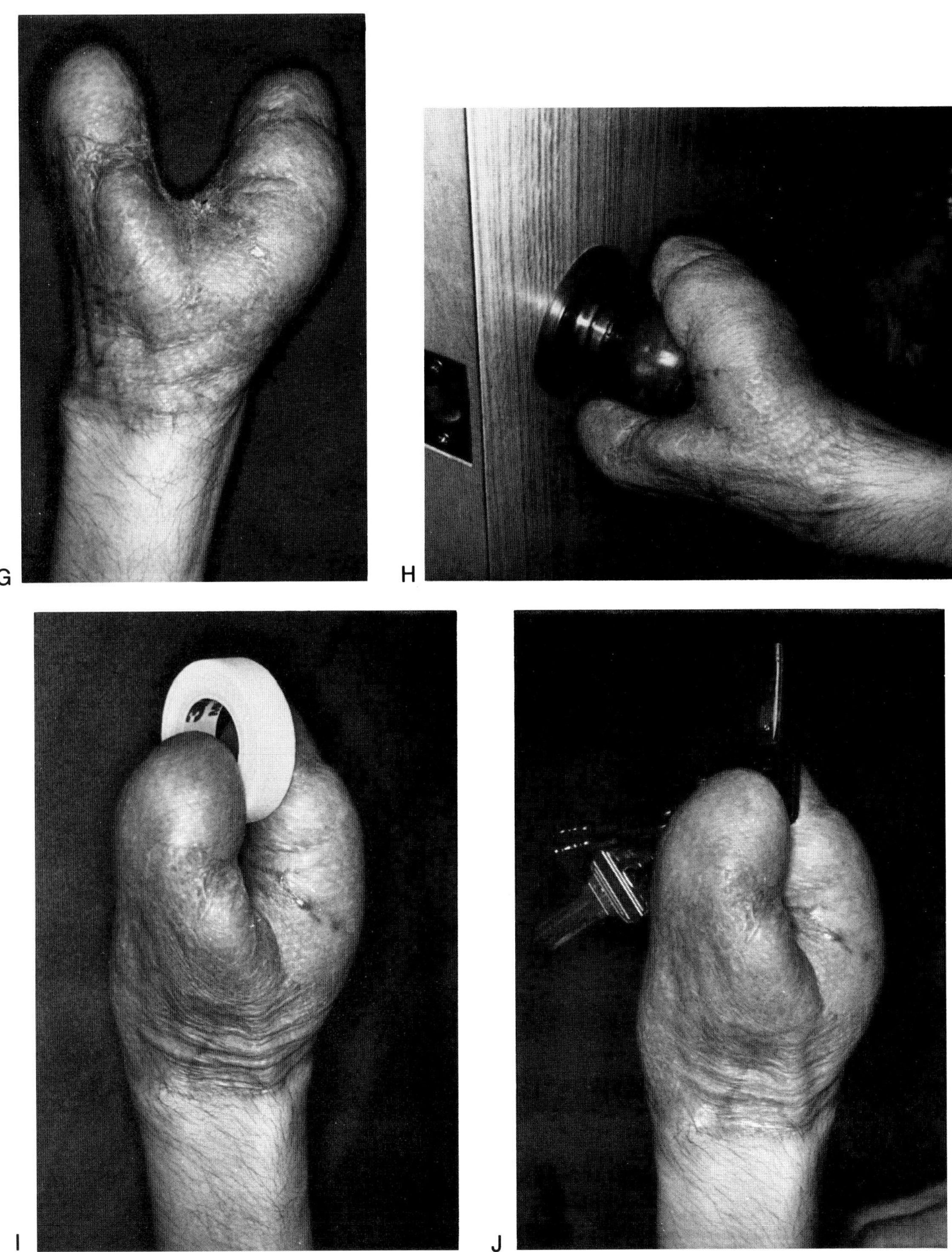

Fig. 57-76 *(Continued).* **(G)** The appearance of the phalangized hand several months later. **(H)** The hand could be effectively used to grasp and turn a door knob. **(I&J)** Pinch capabilities of the reconstructed hand.

REFERENCES

Congenital (Pollicization)

1. Ahstrom JP Jr: Pollicization in congenital absence of the thumb. Curr Pract Orthop Surg 5:1, 1973
2. Albee FH: Synthetic transplantation of tissues to form new finger with restored function of hand. Ann Surg 69:379–383, 1919
3. Banzet P, Le Quang C, Beres J, Mitz V, Lorenceau P, Duforumental C, Vilain R: Analyse des resultats a un an d'une serie de replantation digital. (Analysis of the results at one year of a series of digital reimplantations.) Ann Chir 31:1041–1046, 1977
4. Barsky AJ: Restoration of the thumb by transplantation, plastic repair and prosthesis. Surgery 23:227–247, 1948
5. Barsky AJ: Congenital anomalies of the hand and their surgical treatment. p. 104. Charles C Thomas, Springfield, IL, 1958
6. Barsky AJ: Reconstructive surgery in congenital anomalies of the hand. Surg Clin North Am 39(2):449–467, 1959
7. Biemer E: Vein grafts in microvascular surgery. Br J Plast Surg 30:197–199, 1977
8. Blauth W: Der hypoplastiche daumen. Arch Orthop Unfallchir 62:225, 1967
9. Boca M, Fongo A, Rinaldi F: Pollicizzazione del quatro dito. Bollettino Societa Pediatria Medica y Chirurgica 29:499, 1959
10. Boron R, Fabre A: Technique de reconstruction du pouce. Presse Med 60:1597–1598, 1952
11. Bruner JM: Salvage of the "all-but-amputated" thumb. Plast Reconstr Surg 14:244–248, 1954
12. Büchler U, Phelps DB, Boswick JA: Digital replantation: Guidelines for selection and management. Rocky Mt Med J 74:17–22, 1977
13. Buck-Gramcko D: Pollicization of the index finger: Method and results in aplasia and hypoplasia of the thumb. J Bone Joint Surg 53A:1605–1617, 1971
14. Bunnell S: Reconstructive surgery of the hand. Surg Gynecol Obstet 39:259–270, 1924
15. Bunnell S: Physiological reconstruction of a thumb after total loss. Surg Gynecol Obstet 52:245, 1931
16. Bunnell S: The management of the nonfunctional hand—Reconstruction vs prosthesis. Artif Limbs 4:76–101, 1957
17. Bunnell S: Reconstruction of the thumb. Am J Surg 95:168–172, 1958
18. Butler B Jr: Ring-finger pollicization with transplantation of nail bed and matrix on a volar flap. J Bone Joint Surg 46A:1069–1076, 1964
19. Candiollo I, Rinaldi F: Indagini anatomiche sulla vascolarizzazione arteriosa del IV dito della mano translato sul primo metacarpo (IV dito "pollicization"). G Acad Med Torino 123:82, 1960
20. Carroll RE: Pollicization. pp. 2263–2280. In Green DP (ed): Operative Hand Surgery. 2nd Ed. Churchill Livingstone, New York, 1988
21. Chase RA: An alternate to pollicization in subtotal thumb reconstruction. Plast Reconstr Surg 44:421–430, 1969
22. Chase RA, Milford LW, Goldner JL, Flatt AE, Smith RJ: In thumb repair, is length most crucial? Mod Med 75–79, August 20, 1973
23. Clarkson P: Reconstruction of hand digits by toe transfers. J Bone Joint Surg 37A:270–276, 1955
24. Dunham T: A method for obtaining a skin-flap from the scalp and a permanent buried vascular pedicle for covering defects of the face. Ann Surg 17:677–679, 1893
25. Edgerton MT, Snyder GB, Webb WL: Surgical treatment of congenital thumb deformities (including psychological impact of correction). J Bone Joint Surg 47A:1453–1474, 1965
26. Elsahy NI: Replantation of a completely amputated distal segment of a thumb. Case Report. Plast Reconstr Surg 59:579–581, 1977
27. Flatt AE: The Care of Congenital Hand Anomalies. p. 79. CV Mosby, St Louis, 1977
28. Flynn JE, Burden CN: Reconstruction of the thumb. Arch Surg 85:56–60, 1962
29. Gebauer T, Ihl W: Reparacion del pulgar pro transplante de un dedo de la misma mano. Revista de Orthopedia y Traumatologia, Edicion Latino Americana 1:28, 1955
30. Gersuny R: Kleiner mittheilungen: Plasticher ersatzder Wangen-Shleimbaut. Zentralblatt fur Chirurgie 14:706, 1887
31. Gosset J: La pollicisation de l'index (technique chirurgicale). J Chir (Paris) 65:403, 1949
32. Graham JK: Microsurgery II; Replantation of amputation injuries. J La State Med Soc 130:145–147, 1978
33. Guermonprez F: Sur le prognostic des mutilations de la main. Bulletin de la Societe de Chirurgie Paris 10:363, 1884
34. Guermonprez F: Notes Sure Quelques Resections et Restaurations du Pouce. p. 1. Paris, P. Asselin, 1887
35. Guermonprez F, Derode: Notes Sur Les Indications de la Restauration du Ponce. Toulouse, Imprimerie Pinel, 1889
36. Hamiliton RB, O'Brien BMcC, Morrison A, MacLeod AM: Survival factors in replantation and revascularization of the amputated thumb—10 years experience. Scand J Plast Reconstr Surg 18:163–173, 1984
37. Harrison SH: Restoration of muscle balance in pollicization. Plast Reconstr Surg 34:236–240, 1964
38. Harrison SH: Pollicisation in cases of radial club hand. Br J Plast Surg 23:192–200, 1970
39. Harrison SH: Pollicisation in children. Hand 3:204–210, 1971
40. Hentz VR: Conventional techniques for thumb reconstruction. Clin Orthop 195:129–143, 1985
41. Herausgegeben V, Nigst H, Buck-Gramcko D, Milles H: Handchirurugie in Zwei banden, band II, frische verletzungen und rekonstrauktionen sekindare eingriffe begutachtung. Georg Theime Verlag, Heidelberg, 1983
42. Hilgenfeldt O: Operative Daumenersatz und Seittigung von Griefsverungen bei Fingerverlusten. p. 1. Stuttgart, Enke V, 1950
43. Hirasawa Y, Katsumi Y, Tokioka T: Evaluation of sensibility after sensory reconstruction of the thumb. J Bone Joint Surg 67B:814–819, 1985
44. Huber E: Hilfsoperation bei medianuslahmung. Deutsche Zeitscrift fur Chirurgie 162:271, 1921
45. Huguier PC: Replacement du pouce par son metacarpien, par l'angradissement du premier espace interosseoux. Arch Gen Med (Paris) 1:78, 1874
46. Ikuta Y, Watari S, Kubo T, Oyama K, Hiramatsu K, Nakasaki T, Mouri T, Yoshimura O, Hiramatsu H, Tsuge K: The reattachment of severed fingers. Hiroshima J Med Sci 22:131–154, 1973
47. Isaacs IJ: The vascular complications of digital replantation. Aust NZ J Surg 47:292–299, 1977
48. Jepson PN: Transformation of the middle finger into a thumb. Minn Med 8:552, 1925
49. Joyce JL: A new operation for the substitution of a thumb. Br J Surg 5:499–504, 1917–1918
50. Kelikian H: Congenital Deformities of the Hand and Forearm. p. 825. WB Saunders, Philadelphia, 1974
51. Kelleher JC, Sullivan JG: Thumb reconstruction by fifth digit transposition. Plast Reconstr Surg 21:470, 1958
52. Kleinert HE, Juhala CA, Tsai T-M, Van Beek A: Digital replantation—selection, technique, and results. Orthop Clin North Am 8:309–318, 1977
53. Kleinert HE, Kasdan ML, Romero JL: Small blood-vessel anastomosis for salvage of severely injured upper extremity. J Bone Joint Surg 45A:788–796, 1963

54. Kleinman WB: Management of thumb hypoplasia. Hand Clin 6(4):617-641, 1990
55. Komatsu S, Tamai S: Successful replantation of a completely cut-off thumb. Plast Reconstr Surg 42:374-377, 1968
56. LeTac R: Reconstitution du pouce detruit par pollicization de l'annulaire ou du 5e doigt. Mem Acad Chir (Paris) 78:262, 1952
57. Lichtman DM, Ahbel DE, Brown DE: Thumb reconstruction in the era of microsurgery: Case reports. Military Med 149:246-250, 1984
58. Lister G: The choice of procedure following thumb amputation. Clin Orthop 195:45-51, 1985
59. Littler JW: Subtotal reconstruction of the thumb. Plast Reconstr Surg 10:215-226, 1952
60. Littler JW: The neurovascular pedicle method of digital transposition for reconstruction of the thumb. Plast Reconstr Surg 12:303-319, 1953
61. Littler JW: Neurovascular pedicle transfer of tissue in reconstructive surgery of the hand (abstract). J Bone Joint Surg 38A:917, 1956
62. Littler JW: The prevention and the correction of adduction contracture of the thumb. Clin Orthop 13:182-192, 1959
63. Littler JW: Neurovascular skin island transfers in reconstructive hand surgery. International Society of Plastic Surgery, Transactions. E & S Livingstone, Edinburgh, 1960
64. Littler JW: Digital transposition. In Adams JP (ed.): Current Practice in Orthopaedic Surgery. Vol. 3. CV Mosby, St. Louis, 1960
65. Littler JW: Panel II, Reconstruction of the thumb. Trans Int Soc Plast Surg (Third Congress, Washington, D.C.), 1963
66. Littler JW: Digital transposition. Curr Pract Orthop Surg 3:157, 1966
67. Littler JW: On making a thumb: One hundred years of surgical effort. J Hand Surg 1:35-51, 1976
68. Littler JW: Reconstruction of the thumb in traumatic loss. pp. 3350-3367. In Converse JM (ed): Reconstructive Plastic Surgery. 2nd Ed. WB Saunders, Philadelphia, 1977
69. Littler JW: Discussion of Aston JW Jr, Lankford LL: Use of thin, mobile skin flaps in pollicization of the index finger. Plast Reconstr Surg 63:119, 1979
70. Luksch I: Uber eine nene methode zum ersatz des verlorenen daumens, Verhandelingen der Deutsche Gesellschaft Chirurgie 32:221, 1903
71. Machal H: Beitrag zur daumenplastick. Beitr Klin Chir 114:181, 1919
72. Manketelow RT: What are the indications for digital replantation? Ann Plast Surg 1:336-337, 1978
73. Manktelow RT, McKee NH: Digital replantation: A functional assessment. Can J Surg 22:47-53, 1979
74. Manske PR, McCarroll HR Jr: Abductor digiti minimi opponensplasty in congenital radial dysplasia. J Hand Surg 3:552-559, 1978
75. Match RM: The use of a skin flap from a floating thumb in pollicization of the index. Case report. Plast Reconstr Surg 61:790-792, 1978
76. Matev IB: Thumb reconstruction through metacarpal bone lengthening. J Hand Surg 5:482-487, 1980
77. Matev IB: Reconstructive Surgery of the Thumb. The Pilgrims Press, Brentwood, Essex, England, 1983
78. May JW Jr, Smith RJ, Piemer CA: Toe-to-hand free tissue transfer for thumb construction with multiple digit aplasia. Plast Reconstr Surg 67:205-213, 1981
79. Michon J, Merle M, Bouchon Y, Foucher G: Functional comparison between pollicization and toe-to-hand transfer for thumb reconstruction. J Reconstr Microsurg 1:103-110, 1984
80. Milford L: Congenital anomalies. p. 419. In Crenshaw AH (ed): Campbell's Operative Orthopaedics. 7th Ed. CV Mosby, St. Louis, 1987
81. Milford L: The Hand. 3rd Ed. p. 309. CV Mosby, St. Louis, 1987, p 309
82. Miura T: Use of paired abdominal flaps for release of adduction contractures of the thumb. Plast Reconstr Surg 63:242-244, 1979
83. Moberg E: Discussion of Brooks D: The place of nerve-grafting in orthopaedic surgery. J Bone Joint Surg 37A:305, 1955
84. Moberg E: Aspects of sensation in reconstructive surgery of the upper limb. J Bone Joint Surg 46A:817-825, 1964
85. Moberg E: Discussion following Reid DAC. Pollicization: an appraisal. Hand 1:31, 1969
86. Moore FT: The technique of pollicisation of the index finger. Br J Plast Surg 1:60-68, 1948-1949
87. Morrison WA, O'Brien BM, MacLeod AM: A long-term review of digital replantation. Aust NZ J Surg 47:767-773, 1977
88. Morrison WA, O'Brien BMcC, McLeod AM: Experience with thumb reconstruction. J Hand Surg 9B:223-233, 1984
89. Muller W: Die Angeborenen Fehlbildungen Der Menschlichen, Hand. Thieme, Leipzig, 1937
90. Murray RA: The injured or abnormal thumb: recommendations for treatment. South Med J 52:845-850, 1959
91. Nicoladoni C: Daumenplastik. Wein Klin Wochenschr 10:663, 1897
92. Noesske K: Uber den plastischen ersatz von ganz oder teilweise verlorene fingern, insbesondere des daumens, und uber handtellerplastik. Munch Med Wochenschr 56:1403, 1909
93. O'Brien BM, Black MJM, Morrison WA, MacLeod AM: Microvascular great toe transfer for congenital absence of the thumb. Hand 10:113-124, 1978
94. O'Brien BMcC, MacLeod AM, Sykes PJ, Donahoe S: Hallux-to-hand transfer. Hand 7:128-133, 1975
95. Oudard JS: Greffe de doigts par transplantation. Rev d'Orthop (3rd series) 9:413, 1922
96. Pho RWH, Chacha PB, Yeo KQ: Rerouting vessels and nerves from other digits in replanting an avulsed and degloved thumb. Plast Reconstr Surg 64:330-335, 1979
97. Poznanski AK, Holt JF: The carpals in congenital malformation syndromes. Am J Roentgenol Radium Ther Nucl Med 112:443-459, 1971
98. Pringle RG: Amputations of the thumb. A study of techniques of repair and residual disability. Injury 3:211-217, 1972
99. Pringle RG: Loss of distal thumb need not be severe disability. Mod Med 69, 1972
100. Prpić I: Reconstruction of the thumb immediately after injury. Br J Plast Surg 17:49-52, 1964
101. Ratliff AHC: Amputations of the distal part of the thumb. Hand 4:190-193, 1972
102. Reid DAC: Experience of a hand surgery service. Br J Plast Surg 9:11-24, 1956-1957
103. Reid DAC: Reconstruction of the thumb. J Bone Joint Surg 42B:444-465, 1960
104. Reid DAC: The neurovascular island flap in thumb reconstruction. Br J Plast Surg 19:234-244, 1966
105. Reid DAC: Reconstruction of the thumb. In Pulvertaft RG (ed): Clinical Surgery—The Hand. Butterworths, Washington, 1966
106. Reid DAC: Pollicisation—An Appraisal. Hand 1:27-31, 1969
107. Reid DAC: Thumb injuries. Hand 2:126-129, 1970
108. Reid DAC: Aplasia and hypoplasia of the thumb. pp. 395-397. In Stack HG, Bolton H (eds): The Second Hand Club. British Society for Surgery of the Hand, London, 1975
109. Reid DAC: Reconstruction of the mutilated hand. pp. 184-198. In Rob C, Smith R, Pulvertaft RG (eds): Operative Surgery: The Hand. 3rd Ed. Butterworths, London, 1977

110. Reid DAC: Thumb reconstruction in the mutilated hand with special reference to pollicisation. pp. 81–94. In Campbell Reid DA, Gosset J (eds): Mutilating Injuries of the Hand. Churchill Livingstone, Edinburgh, 1979
111. Reid DAC: The Gillies thumb lengthening operation. Hand 12:123–129, 1980
112. Reid DAC: Surgery of the Thumb. Butterworths, Boston, 1985
113. Rijnders W, Dijkstra R: Survival of the thumb by a vein graft in a case of a severe hand lesion. Hand 8:261–264, 1976
114. Rijnders W, Dijkstra R: Microvasculaire chirurgie bij de primaire dehandeline van ernstige letels man de hand, in het bijonder van de duim. (Microvascular surgery in the primary treatment of severe injuries of the hand, with special emphasis on the thumb.) Ned Tijdschr Geneeskd 121:221–225, 1977
115. Riordan DC: Congenital absence of the radius. J Bone Joint Surg 37A:1129–1140, 1955
116. Schmiedt W: Beitrag zur daumenplastik. Deutsche Z Chir 145:420, 1918
117. Serafin D, Kutz JE, Kleinert HE: Replantation of a completely amputated distal thumb without venous anastomosis. Case report. Plast Reconstr Surg 52:579–582, 1973
118. Shepelmann: Plasticher ersatz bei totaldefekt des rechten daumens. Z Orthop Chir 34:1914, 35:1916, 39:1919
119. Snyder CC, Stevenson RM, Browne EZ Jr: Successful replantation of a totally severed thumb. Plast Reconstr Surg 50:553–559, 1972
120. Stefani AE, Kelly AP: Reconstruction of the thumb: A one-stage procedure. Br J Plast Surg 15:289–292, 1962
121. Strickland JW: Thumb reconstruction. pp. 1563–1618. In Green DP (ed): Operative Hand Surgery. Churchill Livingstone, New York, 1982
122. Strickland JW: Reconstruction of the contracted first web space. pp. 28–32. In Strickland JW, Steichen JB (eds): Difficult Problems in Hand Surgery. CV Mosby, St. Louis, 1982
123. Strickland JW, Dingman DL: Avulsions of the tactile finger pad: An evaluation of treatment. Am Surg 35:756–761, 1969
124. Swanson AB: Levels of amputations of fingers and hand. Consideration for treatment. Surg Clin North Am 44:1115–1126, 1964
125. Tajima T: Classification of thumb hypoplasia. Hand Clin 1(3):577–594, 1985
126. Tamai S: Digit replantation. Analysis of 163 replantations in an 11 year period. Clin Plast Surg 5:195–209, 1978
127. Tanzer RC, Littler JW: Reconstruction of the thumb by transposition of an adjacent digit. Plast Reconstr Surg 3:533–547, 1948
128. Tegtmeier RE, Omer GE, Orgel MG, Moneim MS, Kilpatrick WC: Upper extremity replantation. J Fam Pract 5:539–541, 1977
129. Tsai T: Experimental and clinical application of microvascular surgery. Ann Surg 181:169–177, 1975
130. Tsai T: A complex reimplantation of digits: A case report. J Hand Surg 4:145–149, 1979
131. Tsuge K: The reattachment of severed fingers. Hiroshima J Med Sci 22:131, 1973
132. Tsuyuguchi Y, Masada K, Kawabata H, Kawai H, Ono K: Congenital clasped thumb: A review of forty-three cases. J Hand Surg 10A:613–618, 1985
133. Tubiana R, Duparc J: Restoration of sensibility in the hand by neurovascular skin island transfer. J Bone Joint Surg 43B:474–480, 1961
134. Tubiana R, Stack HG, Hakstian RW: Restoration of prehension after severe mutilations of the hand. J Bone Joint Surg 48B:455–473, 1966
135. Van Beek AL, Wavak PW, Zook EG: Microvascular surgery in young children. Plast Reconstr Surg 63:457–462, 1979
136. Verdan C: The reconstruction of the thumb. Surg Clin North Am 48:1033–1061, 1968
137. Verdan C, Tubiana R, Harrison SH, Littler JW: Panel on reconstruction of the thumb. Transactions of the Third International Congress of Plastic Surgery. Washington, DC 1963
138. Weiland AJ, Villarreal-Rios A, Kleinert HE, Kutz J, Atasoy E, Lister G: Replantation of digits and hands: Analysis of surgical techniques and functional results in 71 patients with 86 replantations. J Hand Surg 2:1–12, 1977
139. Wexler M, Rousso M, Weinberg H, Neuman Z: Experience in reimplantation of amputated digits. Isr J Med Sci 14:1056–1062, 1978
140. White WF: Fundamental priorities in pollicisation. J Bone Joint Surg 52B:438–443, 1970
141. Zancolli E: Transplantation of the index finger in congenital absence of the thumb. J Bone Joint Surg 42A:658–660, 1960

Post-Traumatic

142. Adamson JE, Horton CE, Crawford HN: Sensory rehabilitation of the injured thumb. Plast Reconstr Surg 40:53–57, 1967
143. Adani R, Pancaldi G, Castagnetti C, Zanasi S, Squarzina PB: Neurovascular island flap by the disconnecting-reconnecting technique. J Hand Surg 15B:62–65, 1990
144. Albee FH: Synthetic transplantation of tissues to form new finger with restored function of hand. Ann Surg 69:379–383, 1919
145. Alnot JY, Monod A: Bi-pedicle rectangular palmar advancement flap in distal defects of the fingers. Ann Chir Main 7(2):151–157, 1988
146. Arana GB: Phalangization of the first metacarpal. Surg Gynecol Obstet 40:859–862, 1925
147. Aston JW, Lankford LL: Use of thin, mobile skin flaps in pollicization of the index finger. Plast Reconstr Surg 62:870–872, 1978
148. Atasoy E, Ioakimidis E, Kasdan ML, Kutz JE, Kleinert HE: Reconstruction of the amputated finger tip with a triangular volar flap. J Bone Joint Surg 52A:921–962, 1970
149. Banzet P, Le Quang C, Beres J, Mitz V, Lorenceau P, Duforumental C, Vilain R: Analyse des resultats a un an d'une serie de replantation digital. (Analysis of the results at one year of a series of digital reimplantations.) Ann Chir 31:1041–1046, 1977
150. Barclay TL: The late results of fingertip injuries. Br J Plast Surg 8:38–43, 1955
151. Barsky AJ: Restoration of the thumb by transplantation, plastic repair and prosthesis. Surgery 23:227–247, 1948
152. Bartlett SP, Moses MH, May JW: Thumb reconstruction by free microvascular transfer of an injured index finger. Plast Reconstr Surg 77:660, 1986
153. Beardsley JM, Zecchino U: Reconstruction of the thumb. Am J Surg 71:825–827, 1946
154. Biemer E: Vein grafts in microvascular surgery. Br J Plast Surg 30:197–199, 1977
155. Biemer E, Stock W: Total thumb reconstruction: a one-stage reconstruction using an osteo-cutaneous forearm flap. Br J Plast Surg 36:52–55, 1983
156. Blair VP, Byars LT: Toe to finger transplant. Ann Surg 112:287–290, 1940
157. Blake HE: Notes on the reconstruction of the thumb. Illustrated by a case of group 2. Br J Plast Surg 1:119–122, 1948–1949
158. Blauth W: Prinzipien der pollizisation unter besonderer Beruecksichtigung einerneuen Schnitt fuhrung. (Principles of pollicization with special emphasis on new incision methods.) Handchirurgie 2:117–121, 1970
159. Boe S: The neurovascular island pedicle flap. Acta Orthop Scand 50:67–71, 1979

160. Bolton H: Elongation of the partially amputated thumb. In Stack HG, Bolton H (eds): The Second Hand Club. British Society for Surgery of the Hand, London, 1975
161. Bowe JJ: Thumb construction by index transposition. Plast Reconstr Surg 32:414-424, 1963
162. Bralliar F, Horner RL: Sensory cross-finger pedicle graft. J Bone Joint Surg 51A:1264-1268, 1969
163. Broadbent TR, Woolf RM: Thumb reconstruction with contiguous skin-bone pedicle graft. Plast Reconstr Surg 26:494-499, 1960
164. Brotherston TM, Banerjee A, Lamberty BGH: Digital reconstruction using the distally based osteofasciocutaneous radial forearm flap. J Hand Surg 12B:93-95, 1987
165. Brown H, Welling R, Sigman R, Flynn W, Flynn JE: Phalangizing the first metacarpal. Plast Reconstr Surg 45:294-297, 1970
166. Brown PW: Adduction-flexion contracture of the thumb. Correction with dorsal rotation flap and release of contracture. Clin Orthop 88:161-168, 1972
167. Brownstein ML: Thumb reconstruction by free transplantation of a damaged index ray from the other hand. Case report. Plast Reconstr Surg 60:280-283, 1977
168. Brunelli GA, Grunelli GR: Reconstruction of traumatic abscence of the thumb in the adult by pollicization. Hand Clin 8(1):41-55, 1992
169. Bruner JM: Salvage of the "all-but-amputated" thumb. Plast Reconstr Surg 14:244-248, 1954
170. Büchler U, Phelps DB, Boswick JA: Digital replantation: Guidelines for selection and management. Rocky Mt Med J 74:17-22, 1977
171. Buck-Gramcko D: Pollicization of the index finger: Methods and results in aplasia and hypoplasia of thumb. J Bone Joint Surg 53A:1605-1617, 1971
172. Buck-Gramcko D: Lengthening of first metacarpal in case of loss of thumb and several fingers. Transactions Fifth International Congress Plastic and Reconstructive Surgery. p. 553. Butterworths, London, 1971
173. Buck-Gramcko D: Difficulties in technique of pollicization of the index finger in aplasia of the thumb. In Stack HG, Bolton H (eds): The Second Hand Club. British Society for Surgery of the Hand, London, 1975
174. Buck-Gramcko D: Thumb reconstruction of digital transposition. Orthop Clin North Am 8:329-342, 1977
175. Buckley PD, Smith P III, Dell PC: Thumb Amputation: A review of reconstructive alternatives. Microsurgery 8:140-145, 1987
176. Buncke HJ: Toe digital transfer. Clin Plast Surg 3:49-57, 1976
177. Buncke HJ: Free toe-to-hand transfers. In Daniller AI, Strauch B (eds): Symposium on Microsurgery. CV Mosby, St Louis, 1976
178. Buncke HJ, Buncke CM, Schulz WP: Immediate Nicolandoni procedure in the rhesus monkey or hallus-to-hand transplantation, utilizing microminiature vascular anastomoses. Br J Plast Surg 19:332-337, 1966
179. Buncke HJ, McLean DH, George PT, Creech BJ, Chater NL, Commons GW: Thumb replacement: great toe transplantation by microvascular anastomosis. Br J Plast Surg 26:194-201, 1973
180. Bunnell S: Reconstructive surgery of the hand. Surg Gynecol Obstet 39:259-270, 1924
181. Bunnell S: Physiological reconstruction of a thumb after total loss. Surg Gynecol Obstet 52:245-248, 1931
182. Bunnell S: Digit transfer by neurovascular pedicle. J Bone Joint Surg 34A:772, 1952
183. Bunnell S: The management of the nonfunctional hand—Reconstruction vs prosthesis. Artif Limbs 4:76-101, 1957
184. Bunnell S: Reconstruction of the thumb. Am J Surg 95:168-172, 1958
185. Butler B: Ring-finger pollicization (with transplantation of nail bed and matrix on a volar flap). J Bone Joint Surg 46A:1069-1076, 1964
186. Button M, Stone EJ: Segmental bony reconstruction of the thumb by composite groin flap: a case report. J Hand Surg 5:488-491, 1980
187. Byrne H, Clarkson P: Traumatic amputations of the fingertips. In Flynn JE (ed): Hand Surgery. Williams & Wilkins, Baltimore, 1966
188. Carroll RE: Pollicization. pp. 1619-1634. In Green DP (ed): Operative Hand Surgery. Churchill Livingstone, New York, 1982
189. Chacha B, Soin K, Tan KC: One stage reconstruction of intercalated defect of the thumb using the osteocutaneous radial forearm flap. J Hand Surg 12B:86-92, 1987
190. Chait LA, Fleming J, Becker H: Hallux-to-thumb transfer by microvascular anastomoses. S Afr Med J 52:429-432, 1977
191. Chandler R, Clarkson P: A toe-to-thumb transplant with nerve graft. Am J Surg 95:315-317, 1958
192. Chase RA: An alternate to pollicization in subtotal thumb reconstruction. Plast Reconstr Surg 44:421-430, 1969
193. Chase RA: Atlas of Hand Surgery. Vol. 2. WB Saunders, Philadelphia, 1984
194. Chase RA, Milford LW, Goldner JL, Flatt AE, Smith RJ: In thumb repair, is length most crucial? Mod Med 75-79, 1973
195. Chen H, Noordhoff S: Coverage of the degloved thumb with twin neurovascular island flaps: a case report. Br J Plas Surg 39:255-256, 1986
196. Clarkson P: Reconstruction of hand digits by toe transfers. J Bone Joint Surg 37A:270-276, 1955
197. Clarkson P: On making thumbs. Plast Reconstr Surg 29:325-331, 1962 (Erratum: Plast Reconstr Surg 30:491, 1962)
198. Clarkson P, Furlong R: Thumb reconstruction by transfer of big toe. Br Med J 2:1332-1334, 1949
199. Clifford RH: Evaluation of three methods of finger tip injuries. Arch Surg 65:464-466, 1956
200. Cobbett JR: Free digital transfer. Report of a case of transfer of a great toe to replace an amputated thumb. J Bone Joint Surg 51B:677-679, 1969
201. Cohen BE, Cronin ED: An innervated cross-finger flap for fingertip reconstruction. Plast Reconstr Surg 72:688-697, 1983
202. Coleman DA, Urbaniak JR: Osteocutaneous flaps for thumb and digit reconstruction in unique situations. Hand Clin 1(4):717-728, 1985
203. Colson P, Gangolphe M, Janvier H: Deep burns of both thumbs. Pollicization of the index fingers. Lyon Chir 60:382, 1964
204. Costa H, Smith R, McGrouther DA: Thumb reconstruction by the posterior interosseous osteocutaneous flap. Br J Plast Surg 41:228-233, 1988
205. Cowen N, Loftus J: Distraction-augmentation manoplasty, Orthop Rev 7:45, 1978
206. Curtis RM: Cross finger pedicle flap in hand surgery. Ann Surg 145:650-665, 1957
207. Cuthbert JB: Pollicization of the index finger. Br J Plast Surg 1:56-59, 1948
208. De La Caffiniere JY, Langlais F: Reconstruction du pouce pour mutilation traumatique ancienne. Bilan de 45 pollicisations et 16 lambeau tubules armes. (Reconstructive surgery of the thumb after traumatic amputation). Rev Chir Orthop 64:409-422, 1978
209. De Oliveira JC: Some aspects of thumb reconstruction. Br J Surg 57:85-89, 1970
210. de Saxe BM: Pollicization of the index finger. S Afr Med J 52:710, 1977
211. DeConinck A: Transplantation hetero-digitale avec reinnervation locale. Acta Orthop Belg 41(2):170-176, 1975

212. Dial DE: Reconstruction of thumb after traumatic amputation. J Bone Joint Surg 21:98–100, 1939
213. Doi K, Hattori S, Kawai S, Nakamura S, Kotani H, Matsuoka A, Sunago K: New procedure on making a thumb-one-stage reconstruction with free neurovascular flap and iliac bone graft. J Hand Surg 6:346–350, 1981
214. Doi K, Kuwata N, Kawai S: Reconstruction of the thumb with a free wrap-around flap from the big toe and an iliac-bone graft. J Bone Joint Surg 67A:439–445, 1985
215. Dongyue Y, Yudong G: Thumb reconstruction utilizing second toe transplantation by microvascular anastomosis: Report of 78 cases. Clin Med J 92:295–309, 1979
216. Dunlop J: The use of the index finger for the thumb: Some interesting points in hand surgery. J Bone Joint Surg 5:99–103, 1923
217. Dykes ER: Reconstruction of the thumb. Hawaii Med J 27:33–35, 1967
218. Eaton CJ, Lister GD: Treatment of skin and soft-tissue loss of the thumb. Hand Clin 8(1):71–97, 1992
219. Edgerton MT, Snyder GB, Webb WL: Surgical treatment of congenital thumb deformities (including psychological impact of correction). J Bone Joint Surg 47A:1453–1474, 1965
220. Elsahy NI: Reverse pollicisation for thumb reconstruction. Hand 6:233–235, 1974
221. Elsahy NI: Replantation of a completely amputated distal segment of a thumb. Case Report. Plast Reconstr Surg 59:579–581, 1977
222. Finseth F, May JW, Smith RJ: Composite groin flap with iliac-bone flap for primary thumb reconstruction. Case Report. J Bone Joint Surg 58A:130–132, 1976
223. Finseth F, Buncke HJ: Thumb and digit reconstruction: toe-to-hand microvascular composite tissue transplantation. Int Surg 66:13, 1981
224. Fisher RH: The kutler method of repair of finger tip amputations. J Bone Joint Surg 49A:317–321, 1967
225. Flatt AE: The Care of Minor Hand Injuries. CV Mosby, St Louis, 1963
226. Flatt AE: An indication for shortening of the thumb (description of technique and brief reports of five cases). J Bone Joint Surg 46A:1534–1539, 1964
227. Flatt AE, Wood VE: Multiple dorsal rotation flaps from the hand for thumb web contractures. Plast Reconstr Surg 45:258–262, 1970
228. Floyd WE: Reconstruction of the thumb. J Med Assoc Ga 57:425–429, 1968
229. Flynn JE: Adduction contracture of the thumb. N Engl J Med 254:677–686, 1956
230. Flynn JE, Burden CN: Reconstruction of the thumb. Arch Surg 85:56–60, 1962
231. Foucher G, Braun JB: A new island flap transfer from the dorsum of the index to the thumb. Plast Reconstr Surg 63:344–349, 1979
232. Foucher G, Braun JB, Merle M: Le lambeau 'cerfvolant' (The "skin-kite flap"). Ann Chir 32:593–596, 1978
233. Foucher G, Merle M, Maneaud M, Michon J: Microsurgical free partial toe transfer in hand reconstruction. A report of 12 cases. Plast Reconstr Surg 65:616–627, 1980
234. Foucher G, Braun FM, Merle M, Michon J: La technique du "debranchment-rebranchment" due lambeau en ilot pedicule. Ann Chir 35(4):301–303, 1981
235. Foucher G, Van Genechten F, Merle M, Denuit P, Braun FM, Debry R, Sur H: Toe-to-hand transfers in reconstructive surgery of the hand. Experience with seventy-one cases. Ann Chir Main 3:124–138, 1984
236. Foucher G, Van Genechten M, Merle M, Michon J: Single stage thumb reconstruction by a composite forearm island flap. J Hand Surg 9B:245–248, 1984
237. Foucher G: The kite flap. pp. 355–360. In Tubiana R (ed): The Hand. Vol. II. WB Saunders, Philadelphia, 1985
238. Freeman BS: Reconstruction of thumb by toe transfer. Plast Reconstr Surg 17:393–398, 1956
239. Freiberg A, Manktelow R: The Kutler repair for fingertip amputations. Plast Reconstr Surg 50:371–375, 1972
240. Garcia-Velasco J: Thumb reconstruction using the ring finger. Br J Plast Surg 26:406–407, 1973
241. Gaul JS: Radial-innervated cross-finger flaps from index to provide sensory pulp to injured thumb. J Bone Joint Surg 51A:1257–1263, 1969
242. Gaul JS Jr: A palmar-hinged flap for reconstruction of traumatic thumb defects. Hand Surg 12A:415–421, 1987
243. Gilbert A: Composite tissue transfers from the foot: Anatomic basis and surgical technique. In Daniller AJ, Strauch B (eds): Symposium on Microsurgery. CV Mosby, St Louis, 1976
244. Gilbert A, Tubiana R: Reconstruction of the mutilated hand using microsurgery. pp. 99–103. In Campbell Reid DA, Gosset J (eds): Mutilating Injuries of the Hand. Churchill Livingstone, New York, 1979
245. Gillies H: Autograft of an amputated digit, a suggested operation. Lancet 1:1002–1003, 1940
246. Gillies H, Cuthbert JB: Operation for pollicization of an index finger. Medical Annual, 202. John Wright and Sons, Bristol, 1943
247. Gillies H, Millard DR: The Principles and Art of Plastic Surgery. Little, Brown, Boston, 1957
248. Gillies H, Reid DAC: Autograft of the amputated digit. Br J Plast Surg 7:338–342, 1955
249. Glicenstein J: Finger-tip amputation. pp. 30–35. In Campbell Reid DA, Gosset J (eds): Mutilating Injuries of the Hand. Churchill Livingstone, New York, 1979
250. Gordon L, Rosen J, Alpert BS, Buncke HJ: Free microvascular transfer of second toe ray and serratus anterior muscle for management of thumb loss at the carpometacarpal joint level. J Hand Surg 9A:642–644, 1984
251. Gordon S: Autograft of amputated thumb. Lancet 2:823, 1944
252. Gosset J: La pollicisation de l'index (technique chirurgicale). J Chir 65:403, 1949
253. Gosset J: Reconstruction of the amputated thumb. pp. 70–77. In Campbell Reid DA, Gosset J (eds): Mutilating Injuries of the Hand. Churchill Livingstone, New York, 1979
254. Graham JK: Microsurgery II; Replantation of amputation injuries. J La State Med Soc 130:145–147, 1978
255. Graham WC, Brown JB, Cannon B, Riordan DC: Transposition of fingers in severe injuries of the hand. J Bone Joint Surg 29:998–1004, 1947
256. Graham WC, Riordan DC: Reconstruction of the thumb. NY State J Med 49:49–50, 1949
257. Greeley PW: Reconstruction of the thumb. Ann Surg 124:60–70, 1946
258. Guermonprez F: Notes sur quelques resection et restaurations de ponce. Passelin, Paris, 1887
259. Haas SL: Plastic operation for the loss of all fingers of both hands. Am J Surg 36:720–723, 1937
260. Hamilton RB, O'Brien BMcC, Morrison A, MacLeod AM: Survival factors in replantation and revascularization of the amputated thumb—10 years experience. Scand J Plast Reconstr Surg 18:163–173, 1984
261. Hansen DA: The island-flap in thumb reconstruction. S Afr Med J 47:1936–1938, 1973
262. Harii K, Ohmori K, Torri S, Sekiguchi J: Microvascular free skin flap transfer. Clin Plast Surg 5:239–263, 1978

263. Harkins PD, Raffety JE: Digital transposition in the injured hand. J Bone Joint Surg 54A:1064-1069, 1972
264. Harrison SH: Restoration of muscle balance in pollicization. Plast Reconstr Surg 34:236-240, 1964
265. Harrison SH: Pollicisation in cases of radial club hand. Br J Plast Surg 23:192-200, 1970
266. Harrison SH: Reconstruction of the thumb. In Stack HG, Bolton H (eds): The Second Hand Club. British Society for Surgery of the Hand, London, 1975
267. Harrison SH: Pollicization. In Stack HG, Bolton H (eds): The Second Hand Club. British Society for Surgery of the Hand, London, 1975
268. Hastings H II: Dual innervated index to thumb cross finger or island flap reconstruction. Microsurgery 8:168-172, 1987
269. Henderson HP, Campbell Reid DA: Long-term follow-up of neurovascular island flaps. Hand 12:113-122, 1980
270. Hentz VR: Conventional techniques for thumb reconstruction. Clin Orthop 195:129-143, 1985
271. Hentz VR: Reconstruction of individual digits. Hand Clin 1(2):335-349, 1985
272. Herausgegeben V, Nigst H, Buck-Gramcko D, Milles H: Handchirurugie in zwei banden, band II, frische verletzungen und rekonstrauktionen sekindare eingriffe begutachtung. Georg Theime Verlag, Heidelberg, 1983
273. Herndon JH, Littler JW, Watson FM, Eaton RG: Traumatic amputation of the thumb and three fingers: Treatment by digital pollicization. A case report. J Bone Joint Surg 57A:708-709, 1975
274. Hibi N, Sadahiro T, Iwasaki K, Yagi S, Ikata T, Ogawa Y: Toe-to-hand transfer. Our method and indication. Tokushima J Exp Med 27:69, 1980
275. Hilgenfeldt O: Operative Daumenersatz und Beseitigung von Griefstorungen bei Fingerverlusten. Ferdinand Enke Verlag, Stuttgart, 1950
276. Hirasawa Y, Katsumi Y, Tokioka T: Evaluation of sensibility after sensory reconstruction of the thumb. J Bone Joint Surg 67B:814-819, 1985
277. Hoffman HL: Der sensible gekreuzte Fingerlapen zur Deckung von Spitzendefekten am Daumen (Sensitive cross-finger flap for the covering of fingertip defects on the thumb.) Handchirurgie 1:82, 1969
278. Holevich J: A new method of restoring sensibility to the thumb. J Bone Joint Surg 45B:496-502, 1963
279. Hoskins HD, Curtis RM: The versatile cross-finger pedicle flap (abstract). J Bone Joint Surg 41A:778, 1959
280. Howard LD: Contracture of the thumb web. J Bone Joint Surg 32A:267-273, 1950
281. Howard LD: Plastic Procedures in Hand Surgery. Handout given with AAOS Instructional Course Lectures, 1963
282. Huang SH, Hou MZ, Yan CL: Reconstruction of the thumb by a free pedal neurovascular flap and composite phalanx-joint-tendon homograft: A preliminary report. J Reconstr Microsurg 1:299-303, 1985
283. Hueston J: The extended neurovascular island flap. Br J Plast Surg 18:304-305, 1965
284. Hueston J: Local flap repair of fingertip injuries. Plast Reconstr Surg 37:349-350, 1966
285. Hughes NC, Moore FT: A preliminary report on the use of a local flap and peg bone graft for lengthening a short thumb. Br J Plast Surg 3:34-39, 1950-1951
286. Huguier PC: Replacement of du ponce par son metacarpien, par l'angrandissement du premier espace interosseux. Arch Gen Med 1:78, 1874
287. Hydroop GL: Transfer of a metacarpal with or without its digit, for improving the function of the crippled hand. Plast Reconstr Surg 4:45-58, 1949
288. Ikuta Y, Watari S, Kubo T, Oyama K, Hiramatsu K, Nakasaki T, Mouri T, Yoshimura O, Hiramatsu H, Tsuge K: The reattachment of severed fingers. Hiroshima J Med Sci 22:131-154, 1973
289. Ilizarov GA: Clinical application of the tension-stress effect for limb lengthening. Clin Orthop 250:8-26, 1990
290. Isaacs IJ: The vascular complications of digital replantation. Aust NZ J Surg 47:292-299, 1977
291. Iselin F: The flag flap. Plast Reconstr Surg 52:374-377, 1973
292. Iselin M, Muret F: Restauration du ponce par pollicization du deuxieme metarpien. Presse Med 2:1099, 1937
293. Iselin M: Reconstruction of the thumb. Surgery 2:619-622, 1937
294. Iselin M: Atlas of Hand Surgery. McGraw-Hill, New York, 1964
295. Jeffery CC: A case of pollicisation of the index finger. J Bone Joint Surg 39B:120-123, 1957
296. Jeffs JV, Kemble H: The cone flap for surfacing reconstructing partial digits. Br J Plast Surg 26:163-166, 1973
297. Jepson PN: Transformation of the middle finger into a thumb. Minn Med 8:522, 1925
298. Joshi BB: One-stage repair for distal amputation of the thumb. Plast Reconstr Surg 45:613-615, 1970
299. Joyce JL: A new operation for the substitution of a thumb. Br J Surg 5:499-504, 1917-1918
300. Joyce JL: The results of a new operation for the substitution of a thumb. Br J Surg 16:362-369, 1928-1929
301. Kaplan I: Primary pollicization of injured index finger following crush injury. Plast Reconstr Surg 37:531-535, 1966
302. Kaplan I, Plaschkes J: One stage pollicisation of little finger. Br J Plast Surg 13:272-276, 1960
303. Kartchinov KD: Reconstruction and sensitization of the amputated thumb. J Hand Surg 9A:478-484, 1984
304. Keim HA, Grantham SA: Volar-flap advancement for thumb and finger-tip injuries. Clin Orthop 66:109-112, 1969
305. Kelleher JC, Sullivan JG: Thumb reconstruction by fifth digit transposition. Plast Reconstr Surg 21:470-478, 1958
306. Kelleher JC, Sullivan JG, Baibak GJ, Dean RK: Use of a tailored abdominal pedicle flap for surgical reconstruction of the hand. J Bone Joint Surg 52A:1552-1556, 1970
307. Kelly AP: Subtotal reconstruction of the thumb. Arch Surg 78:582-585, 1959
308. Kessler I: War injuries of the hand with special emphasis to reconstruction of the thumb. Prog Surg 16:89-110, 1979
309. Kessler I, Hecht O, Baruch A: Distraction lengthening of digital rays in the management of the injured hand. J Bone Joint Surg 61A:83-87, 1979
310. Kessler I: Cross transposition of short amputation stumps for reconstruction of the thumb. J Hand Surg 10B:76-78, 1985
311. Kleinert HE, Juhala CA, Tsai T-M, Van Beek A: Digital replantation-selection, technique, and results. Orthop Clin North Am 8:309-318, 1977
312. Kleinert HE, Kasdan ML, Romero JL: Small blood-vessel anastomosis for salvage of severely injured upper extremity. J Bone Joint Surg 45A:788-796, 1963
313. Kojima T, Harase M, Hosoda H: Pollicization. Jpn J Plast Reconstr Surg 13:263-270, 1970
314. Koman LA, Poehling GG, Price JL: Thumb reconstruction—An Algorithm. Orthopaedics 9:873-878, 1986
315. Komatsu S, Tamai S: Successful replantation of a completely cut-off thumb. Plast Reconstr Surg 42:374-377, 1968
316. Krag C, Rasmussen KB: The neurovascular inland flap for protective sensibility of the thumb. J Bone Joint Surg 57B:495-499, 1975
317. Kurtzman LC, Stern PJ, Yakuboff KP: Reconstruction of the burned thumb. Hand Clin 8(1):107-119, 1992
318. Kutler W: A new method for finger-tip amputation. JAMA 133:29-30, 1947

319. Laico J: Total reconstruction of a thumb in a thumbless hand. J Philipp Med Assoc 30:381-387, 1954
320. Langlais F, Gosset J: Results of thumb reconstruction. pp 78-80. In Campbell Reid DA, Gosset J (ed): Mutilating Injuries of the Hand. Churchill Livingstone, New York, 1979
321. Lejeune G, Yoshimura D, Alexandre G: Neo-pouce par transplantation microchirurgicale du second orteil. A propos de deux observations. (Thumb replacement using microsurgical transplantation of the second toe. Apropos of 2 cases.) Bull Mem Acad R Med Belg 133:583-593, 1978
322. Letac R: Pollicization of the ring finger. J Int Coll Surg 22:649-655, 1954
323. Leung PC: Transplantation of the second toe to the hand. A preliminary report of sixteen cases. J Bone Joint Surg 62A:990-996, 1980
324. Leung PC: Thumb reconstruction using second toe transfer. Hand 15:15-21, 1983
325. Leung PC: Thumb reconstruction using second toe transfer. Hand Clin 1:285-295, 1985
326. Lewin ME: Sensory island flap in osteoplastic reconstruction of the thumb. Am J Surg 109:226-229, 1965
327. Lichtman DM, Ahbel DE, Brown DE: Thumb reconstruction in the era of microsurgery: Case reports. Military Med 149:246-250, 1984
328. Lister G: The choice of procedure following thumb amputation. Clin Orthop 195:45-51, 1985
329. Lister G: Reconstruction of the hypoplastic thumb. Clin Orthop 195:52-65, 1985
330. Littler JW: Subtotal reconstruction of the thumb. Plast Reconstr Surg 10:215-226, 1952
331. Littler JW: The neurovascular pedicle method of digital transposition for reconstruction of the thumb. Plast Reconstr Surg 12:303-319, 1953
332. Littler JW: Neurovascular pedicle transfer of tissue in reconstructive surgery of the hand (abstract). J Bone Joint Surg 38A:917, 1956
333. Littler JW: The prevention and the correction of adduction contracture of the thumb. Clin Orthop 13:182-192, 1959
334. Littler JW: Neurovascular skin island transfers in reconstructive hand surgery. International Society of Plastic Surgery, Transactions. E & S Livingstone, Edinburgh, 1960
335. Littler JW: Digital transposition. In Adams JP (ed): Current Practice in Orthopaedic Surgery. Vol. 3. CV Mosby, St Louis, 1960
336. Littler JW: On making a thumb: One hundred years of surgical effort. J Hand Surg 1:35-51, 1976
337. Littler JW: Reconstruction of the thumb in traumatic loss. pp. 3350-3367. In Converse JM (ed): Reconstructive Plastic Surgery. 2nd Ed. WB Saunders, Philadelphia, 1977
338. Littler JW: Discussion of Aston JW Jr, Lankford LL: Use of thin, mobile skin flaps in pollicization of the index finger. Plast Reconstr Surg 63:119, 1979
339. Logan A, Elliot D, Foucher G: Free toe pulp transfer to restore traumatic digital pulp loss. Br J Plast Surg 38:497-500, 1985
340. Lowden IMR, Nunley JA, Goldner RD, Urbaniak JR: The wraparound procedure for thumb and finger reconstruction. Microsurgery 8:154-157, 1987
341. Lyle HHM: The formation of a thumb from the first metacarpus. Ann Surg 76:121-123, 1922
342. Maltz M: Reconstruction of thumb. A new technique. Am J Surg 58:429-433, 1942
343. Manktelow RT: What are the indications for digital replantation? Ann Plast Surg 1:336-337, 1978
344. Manktelow RT, McKee NH: Digital replantation: A functional assessment. Can J Surg 22:47-53, 1979
345. Match RM: The use of a skin flap from a floating thumb in pollicization of the index. Case report. Plast Reconstr Surg 61:790-792, 1978
346. Matev IB: First metacarpal lengthening for thumb reconstruction. Orthop Travmatol Protez 6:11-14, 1969
347. Matev IB: Thumb reconstruction after amputation at the metacarpophalangeal joint by bone lengthening. A preliminary report of three cases. J Bone Joint Surg 52A:957-965, 1970
348. Matev IB: Distraktsionnyi method vosstanovleniia bol'shogo pal'tsa. (Distraction method in the restoration of the thumb.) Orthop Travmatol Protez 34:43-46, 1973
349. Matev I: Gradual elongation of the first metacarpal as a method of thumb reconstruction. pp. 495-496. In Stack HG, Bolton H (eds): The Second Hand Club. British Society for Surgery of the Hand, London, 1975
350. Matev IB: Reconstructive surgery of the thumb. Sofia. Medicina i Fizkultura, 1978
351. Matev IB: Thumb reconstruction through metacarpal bone lengthening. J Hand Surg 5:482-487, 1980
352. Matev IB: Reconstructive Surgery of the Thumb. The Pilgrims Press, Brentwood, Essex, England, 1983
353. Mathes SJ, Vasconez LO: Free flaps (including toe transplantation). pp. 829-859. In Green DP (ed): Operative Hand Surgery. Churchill Livingstone, New York, 1982
354. Matti BA, Quaba A, and Page RE: Partial thumb reconstruction using the proximal skin paddle radial artery island flap. J Hand Surg 11B:35-39, 1986
355. May JW, Chait LA, Cohen BE, O'Brien BM: Free neurovascular flap from the first web of the foot in hand reconstruction. J Hand Surg 2:387-396, 1977
356. May JW, Daniel RK: Great toe to hand free tissue transfer. Clin Orthop 133:140-153, 1978
357. May JW Jr: Aesthetic and functional thumb reconstruction: Great toe to hand transfer. Clin Plast Surg 8:357-362, 1981
358. May JW, Donelan MB, Toth BA, Wall J: Thumb reconstruction in the burned hand by advancement pollicization of the second ray remnant. J Hand Surg 9A:484-489, 1984
359. May JW, Bartlett SP: Great toe-to-hand free tissue transfer for thumb reconstruction. Hand Clin 1:271-284, 1985
360. McFarlane RM: The treatment of major skin loss in the thumb. p. 209. In Stack HG, Bolton H (eds): The Second Hand Club. British Society for Surgery of the Hand, London, 1975
361. McFarlane RM, Stromberg WB: Resurfacing of the thumb following major skin loss. J Bone Joint Surg 44A:1365-1375, 1962
362. McGregor IA: Reconstruction of the thumb. In Gibson T (ed): Modern Trends in Plastic Surgery. Butterworths, London, 1966
363. McGregor IA, Jackson IT: The groin flap. Br J Plast Surg 25:3-16, 1972
364. McGregor IA, Simonetta C: Reconstruction of the thumb by composite bone-skin flap. Br J Plast Surg 17:37-48, 1964
365. Mehrotra ON: Hand reconstruction using a damaged index finger. NZ Med J 86:137-140, 1977
366. Mehrotra ON: Restoration of grasp and pinch in a burnt hand by pollicization of an island flap taken from the same finger. Aust NZ J Surg 47:806-810, 1977
367. Metcalf W, Whalen WP: Salvage of the injured distal phalanx-plan of care and analysis of 369 cases. Clin Orthop 13:114-123, 1959
368. Michon J: Secondary tenolysis after pollicisation. pp. 109-110. In Campbell Reid DA, Gosset J (eds): Mutilating Injuries of the Hand. Churchill Livingstone, New York, 1979
369. Michon J: The metacarpal hand. pp. 60-63. In Campbell Reid DA, Gosset J (eds): Mutilating Injuries of the Hand. Churchill Livingstone, New York, 1979
370. Michon J, Dolich BH: The metacarpal hand. Hand 6:285-290, 1974
371. Michon J, Merle M, Bouchon Y, Foucher G: Functional com-

parison between pollicization and toe to-hand transfer for thumb reconstruction. J Reconstr Microsurg 1:103-110, 1984
372. Michon J, Merle M, Bouchon Y, Foucher G: Thumb reconstruction pollicisation or toe-to-hand transfers. A comparative study of functional results. Ann Chir Main 4(2):98-110, 1985
373. Milford L: The hand. In Edmonson AS, Crenshaw AH (eds): Campbell's Operative Orthopaedics. 6th Ed. CV Mosby, St Louis, 1980
374. Millender LH, Albin RE, Nalebuff EA: Delayed volar advancement flap for thumb tip injuries. Plast Reconstr Surg 52:635-639, 1973
375. Minami A, Usui M, Katoh H, Ishii S: Thumb reconstruction by free sensory flaps from the foot using microsurgical techniques. J Hand Surg 9B:239-244, 1984
376. Minkow FV, Stein F: Phalangization of the thumb. J Trauma 13:648-655, 1973
377. Mischokowsky T: Daumenbildung durch transposition eines beschagigten kleinfingers und interpositions-span nach explosions-verletzung der hand. (Thumb reconstruction by means of transposition of a damaged little finger and interposition splint after an explosion injury to the hand.) Handchirurgie 8:85-88, 1976
378. Miura T: Thumb reconstruction using radial innervated cross-finger pedicle graft. J Bone Joint Surg 55A:563-569, 1973
379. Miura T: Use of paired abdominal flaps for release of adduction contractures of the thumb. Plast Reconstr Surg 63:242-244, 1979
380. Miura T, Kino Y, Nakamura R: Reconstruction of the mutilated hand. Hand 8:78-85, 1976
381. Moberg E: Discussion of paper by Brooks D: The place of nerve grafting in orthopaedic surgery. J Bone Joint Surg 37A:305, 1955
382. Moberg E: Aspects of sensation in reconstructive surgery of the upper limb. J Bone Joint Surg 46A:817-825, 1964
383. Moberg E: Discussion following Reid DAC. Pollicization: an appraisal. Hand 1:31, 1969
384. Molski M, Pisarek W: Functional reconstruction of the palmar surface of the thumb using the neurovascular flap from the index. Acta Chir Plast 31, 3, 1989
385. Moore FT: The technique of pollicisation of the index finger. Br J Plast Surg 1:60-68, 1948-1949
386. Morgan LR, Stein F: Method for a rapid and good thumb reconstruction. Plast Reconstr Surg 50:131-133, 1972
387. Morrison WA, O'Brien BM, Hamilton RB: Neurovascular free foot flaps in reconstruction of the mutilated hand. Clin Plast Surg 5:265-272, 1978
388. Morrison WA, O'Brien BM, MacLeod AM: A long-term review of digital replantation. Aust NZ J Surg 47:767-773, 1977
389. Morrison WA, O'Brien BM, MacLeod AM: Thumb reconstruction with a free neurovascular wrap-around flap from the big toe. J Hand Surg 5:575-583, 1980
390. Morrison WA, O'Brien BM, MacLeod AM: Experience with thumb reconstruction. J Hand Surg 9B:223-233, 1984
391. Moss ALH, Waterhouse N: One stage thumb reconstruction using a previously injured little finger from the contralateral hand. J Hand Surg 10B:73-75, 1985
392. Moy OJ, Peimer CA, Sherwin FS: Reconstruction of traumatic or congenital amputation of the thumb by distraction-lengthening. Hand Clin 8(1):57-62, 1992
393. Mulliken JB, Curtis RM: Thumb lengthening by metacarpal distraction. J Trauma 20:250, 1980
394. Murray JF, Ord JVR, Gavelin GE: The neurovascular island pedicle flap. An assessment of late results in sixteen cases. J Bone Joint Surg 49A:1285-1297, 1967
395. Murray RA: Reconstructive surgery of the hand with special reference to digital transplantation. Br J Plast Surg 34:131, 1946
396. Murray RA: The injured or abnormal thumb: recommendations for treatment. South Med J 52:845-850, 1959
397. Mutz SB: Thumb web contracture. Hand 4:236-246, 1972
398. Nemethi CE: Reconstruction of the distal part of the thumb after traumatic amputation. Restoration of the function and sensation using nerve, tendon, and bone from the amputated portion. J Bone Joint Surg 42A:375-391, 1960
399. Nichols HM: Manual of Hand Injuries. 2nd Ed. Year Book Medical Publishers, Chicago, 1960
400. Nicoladoni C: Daumenplastik. Wein Klin Wochenschr 10:663-670, 1897
401. Nicoladoni C: Daumenplastik fund organischer Ersatz der Fingerspitze (Anticheiroplastik und Daktyloplastik). Arch Klin Chir 61:606-614, 1900
402. Nicoladoni C: Weitere Erfahrungen uber Daumenplastik. Arch Klin Chir 69:695-703, 1903
403. Nunley JA, Goldner RD, Urbaniak JR: Thumb reconstruction by the wrap-around method. Clin Orthop 195:97-103, 1985
404. O'Brien BMcC: One stage toe-to-hand transfer. pp. 182-204. In Microvascular Reconstructive Surgery. Churchill Livingstone, Edinburgh, 1977
405. O'Brien BM: Microvascular surgery—Its present place in reconstructive surgery. Handchirurgie 10:75-76, 1978
406. O'Brien BM, Black MJM, Morrison WA, MacLeod AM: Microvascular great toe transfer for congenital absence of the thumb. Hand 10:113-124, 1978
407. O'Brien BM, Brennen MB, MacLeod AM: Microvascular free toe transfer. Clin Plast Surg 5:223-237, 1978
408. O'Brien BM, MacLeod AM, Morrison WA: Digital replantation. In Campbell Reid DA, Gosset J (eds.): Mutilating Injuries of the Hand. Churchill Livingstone, New York, 1979
409. O'Brien BMcC, MacLeod AM, Sykes PJ, Donahoe S: Hallux-to-hand transfer. Hand 7:128-133, 1975
410. Ogunro O: Restoration of sensibility to a thumb by the technique of digital nerve advancement: a new surgical procedure. J Hand Surg 9A:440-444, 1984
411. Ohmori K, Harii K: Transplantation of a toe to an amputated finger. Hand 7:134-138, 1975
412. Operative technique of pollicization utilizing finger stumps. Chin Med J 92:253-259, 1979
413. Orticochea M: Reconstruction of the thumb using two flaps from the same hand. Br J Plast Surg 24:345-350, 1971
414. Paneva-Holevich E, Holevich Y: Further experience with the bipedicled neurovascular island flap in thumb reconstruction. J Hand Surg 16A:594-597, 1991
415. Parin BV: Reconstruction of Hand Digits (in Russian). Medciz, Moscow, 1944
416. Peacock EE: Reconstruction of the thumb. In Flynn JE (ed): Hand Surgery. Williams & Wilkins, Baltimore, 1966
417. Penteado CV, Masquelet AC, Chevrel JP: The anatomic basis of the fasciocutaneous flap of the posterior interosseous artery. Surg Radiol Anat 8:209, 1986
418. Petersen N: Plastic reconstruction of the thumb. S Afr Med J 17:137-138, 1943
419. Pho RWH: Local composite neurovascular island for skin cover in pulp loss of the thumb. J Hand Surg 4:11-15, 1979
420. Pho RWH, Chacha PB, Yeo KQ: Rerouting vessels and nerves from other digits in replanting an avulsed and degloved thumb. Plast Reconstr Surg 64:330-335, 1979
421. Pierce GW: Reconstruction of thumb after total loss. Surg Gynecol Obstet 45:825-826, 1927
422. Pitzler K: Daumenersatz aus dem zweiten mettelhandknochen. (Thumb replacement with the second metacarpal bone. Split hand formation with extension of the thumb metacarpal bone by Hilgenfeldt.) Bruns Beitr Klin Chir 217:321-329, 1969

423. Pohl AL, Larson DL, Lewis SP: Thumb reconstruction in the severely burned hand. Plast Reconstr Surg 57:320–328, 1976
424. Polonsky B: Reconstruction of a missing thumb. S Afr Med J 23:812–814, 1949
425. Porter RW: Functional assessment of transplanted skin in volar defects of the digits. A comparison between free grafts and flaps. J Bone Joint Surg 50A:955–963, 1968
426. Posner MA, Smith RJ: The advancement pedicle flap for thumb injuries. J Bone Joint Surg 53A:1618–1621, 1971
427. Pringle RG: Amputations of the thumb. A study of techniques of repair and residual disability. Injury 3:211–217, 1972
428. Pringle RG: Loss of distal thumb need not be severe disability. Mod Med 69, 1972
429. Prpić I: Reconstruction of the thumb immediately after injury. Br J Plast Surg 17:49–52, 1964
430. Quang C, Banzet P, Dufourmentel C: Digital reconstruction by microvascular transfer of the second toe. In Campbell Reid DA, Gosset J (eds): Mutilating Injuries of the Hand. Churchill Livingstone, Edinburgh, 1979
431. Rank BK, Wakefield AR: Reconstruction of opposition digits for mutilated hands. Aust NZ J Surg 17:172–188, 1947–1948
432. Ratliff AHC: Amputations of the distal part of the thumb. Hand 4:190–193, 1972
433. Ratcliffe RJ, McGrouther DA: Free toe pulp transfer in thumb reconstruction. Experience in the West of Scotland Regional Plastic Surgery Unit. J Hand Surg 16B:165–168, 1991
434. Reconstruction of missing thumbs with improved "cocked hat" operation. Chin Med J 10:626–627, 1974
435. Reid DAC: Experience of a hand surgery service. Br J Plast Surg 9:11–24, 1956–1957
436. Reid DAC: Reconstruction of the thumb. J Bone Joint Surg 42B:444–465, 1960
437. Reid DAC: The neurovascular island flap in thumb reconstruction. Br J Plast Surg 19:234–244, 1966
438. Reid DAC: Reconstruction of the thumb. In Pulvertaft RG (ed): Clinical Surgery—The Hand. Butterworths, Washington, 1966
439. Reid DAC: Pollicization—An appraisal. Hand 1:27–31, 1969
440. Reid DAC: Thumb injuries. Hand 2:126–129, 1970
441. Reid DAC: Aplasia and hypoplasia of the thumb. pp. 395–397. In Stack HG, Bolton H (eds): The Second Hand Club. British Society for Surgery of the Hand, London, 1975
442. Reid DAC: Reconstruction of the mutilated hand. In Rob C, Smith R, Pulvertaft RG (eds): Operative Surgery: The Hand. 3rd Ed. Butterworths, London, 1977
443. Reid DAC: Thumb reconstruction in the mutilated hand with special reference to pollicisation. pp. 81–94. In Campbell Reid DA, Gosset J (eds): Mutilating Injuries of the Hand. Churchill Livingstone, Edinburgh, 1979
444. Reid DAC: The Gillies thumb lengthening operation. Hand 12:123–129, 1980
445. Reid DAC: Surgery of the Thumb. Butterworths, Boston, 1985
446. Rijnders W, Dijkstra R: Survival of the thumb by a vein graft in a case of a severe hand lesion. Hand 8:261–264, 1976
447. Rijnders W, Dijkstra R: Microvasculaire chirurgie bij de primaire dehandeline van ernstige letels man de hand, in het bijonder van de duim. (Microvascular surgery in the primary treatment of severe injuries of the hand, with special emphasis on the thumb.) Ned Tijdschr Geneeskd 121:221–225, 1977
448. Riordan DC: Cited by Milford L. The Hand. CV Mosby, St Louis, 1971
449. Robbins F, Reece T: Hand rehabilitation after great toe transfer for thumb reconstruction. Arch Phys Med Rehabil 66:109–111, 1985
450. Robinson OG: Primary reconstruction of the thumb using amputated part and tube pedicle flap. South Med J 66:1025–1029, 1973
451. Rybka FJ, Pratt FE: Thumb reconstruction with a sensory flap from the dorsum of the index finger. Plast Reconstr Surg 64:141–144, 1979
452. Sallis JG: Primary pollicisation of an injured middle finger. J Bone Joint Surg 45B:503, 1963
453. Sanders GB: Reconstruction of the thumb. Am J Surg 83:347–351, 1952
454. Sandzen SC: Dorsal pedicle flap for resurfacing a moderate thumb-index web contracture release. J Hand Surg 7:21–24, 1982
455. Sandzen SC: Thumb web reconstruction. Clin Orthop 195:66–81, 1985
456. Scheker LR, Lister DG, Wolff TW: The lateral arm free flap in releasing severe contracture of the first web space. J Hand Surg 13B:146–150, 1988
457. Sels M: Present methods of reconstruction of the amputated thumb. Plast Reconstr Surg 32:672, 1963
458. Serafin D, Kutz JE, Kleinert HE: Replantation of a completely amputated distal thumb without venous anastomosis. Case report. Plast Reconstr Surg 52:579–582, 1973
459. Sharpe C: Tissue cover for the thumb web. Arch Surg 104:21–25, 1972
460. Shaw MH, Wilson ISP: An early pollicization. Br J Plast Surg 3:214–215, 1950–1951
461. Simonetta C: Reconstruction of the thumb by tube pedicle, bone graft and island flap. In Campbell Reid DA, Gosset J (eds): Mutilating Injuries of the Hand. Churchill Livingstone, Edinburgh, 1979
462. Slocum DB: Amputations of the fingers and the hand. Clin Orthop 15:35–59, 1959
463. Small JO, Brennen MD: The first dorsal metacarpal artery neurovascular island flap. J Hand Surg 13B:136–145, 1988
464. Smith RJ, Lipke RW: Treatment of congenital deformities of the hand and forearm. N Engl J Med 300:344–349, 1979
465. Snyder CC, Stevenson RM, Browne EZ Jr: Successful replantation of a totally severed thumb. Plast Reconstr Surg 50:533–559, 1972
466. Spinner M: Fashioned transpositional flap for soft tissue adduction contracture of the thumb. Plast Reconstr Surg 44:345–348, 1969
467. Stefani AE, Kelly AP: Reconstruction of the thumb: A one-stage procedure. Br J Plast Surg 15:289–292, 1962
468. Steichen JB, Weiss A-PC: Reconstruction of traumatic absence of the thumb by microvascular free tissue transfer from the foot. Hand Clin 8(1):17–32, 1992
469. Stern PJ: Free neurovascular cutaneous toe pulp transfer for thumb reconstruction. Microsurgery 8:158–161, 1987
470. Storvik HM: The extended neurovascular island flap in thumb reconstruction. Scand J Plast Reconstr Surg 7:147–149, 1973
471. Strauch B: Dorsal thumb flap for release of adduction contracture of the first web space. Bull Hosp Joint Dis 36:34–39, 1975
472. Strauch B: Microsurgical approach to thumb reconstruction. Orthop Clin North Am 8(2):319–327, 1977
473. Strickland JW: Restoration of thumb function following partial or total amputation. In Hunter JM, Schneider LH, Mackin EJ, Bell JA (eds): Rehabilitation of the Hand. CV Mosby, St Louis, 1978
474. Strickland JW, Dingman DL: Avulsions of the tactile finger pad: An evaluation of treatment. Am Surg 35:756–761, 1969
475. Strickland JW: Thumb reconstruction. pp. 2175–2261. In Green DP (ed): Operative Hand Surgery. 2nd Ed. Churchill Livingstone, New York, 1988
476. Strickland JW: Reconstruction of the contracted first web space.

pp. 28-32. In Strickland JW, Steichen JB (eds): Difficult Problems in Hand Surgery. CV Mosby, St Louis, 1982
477. Strickland JW: Restoration of thumb function following partial or total amputation. In Hunter JM, Schneider LH, Mackin E, Callahan AD (eds): Rehabilitation of the Hand. 2nd Ed. CV Mosby, St. Louis, 1984
478. Sturman MJ, Duran RJ: Late results of finger tip injuries. J Bone Joint Surg 45A:289-298, 1963
479. Sullivan JG, Kelleher JC, Baibak GJ, Dean R, Pinker LD: The primary application of an island pedicle-flap in thumb and index finger injuries. Plast Reconstr Surg 39:488-492, 1967
480. Swanson AB: Levels of amputations of fingers and hand. Considerations for treatment. Surg Clin North Am 44:1115-1126, 1964
481. Szlazak J: Total reconstruction of the thumb. Plast Reconstr Surg 8:67-70, 1951
482. Tajima T: Treatment of open crushing type of industrial injuries of the hand and forearm: Degloving, open circumferential, heat-press, and nail-bed injuries. J Trauma 14:995-1011, 1974
483. Takami H, Takahashi S, Ando M: Subtotal reconstruction of the thumb by transposition of index finger. J Hand Surg 10B:176-178, 1985
484. Takami H, Takahashi S, Ando M: Total thumb reconstruction by an index finger transposition. J Hand Surg 11B:31-34, 1986
485. Tamai S: Digit replantation. Analysis of 163 replantations in an 11 year period. Clin Plast Surg 5:195-209, 1978
486. Tamai S, Hori Y, Tatsumi Y, Okuda H: Hallux-to-thumb transfer with microsurgical technique: A case report in a 45 year old woman. J Hand Surg 2:152-155, 1977
487. Tanzer RC, Littler JW: Reconstruction of the thumb by transposition of an adjacent digit. Plast Reconstr Surg 3:533-547, 1948
488. Tegtmeier RE, Omer GE, Orgel MG, Moneim MS, Kilpatrick WC: Upper extremity replantation. J Fam Pract 5:539-541, 1977
489. Thomas CV: Thin flaps. Plast Reconstr Surg 65:747-752, 1980
490. Thompson James S: Reconstruction of the insensate thumb by neurovascular island transfer. Hand Clin 8(1):99-105, 1992
491. Tsai T: Experimental and clinical application of microvascular surgery. Ann Surg 181:169-177, 1975
492. Tsai T: A complex reimplantation of digits: A case report. J Hand Surg 4:145-149, 1979
493. Tsai T-M, Aziz W: Toe-to thumb transfer: A new technique. Plast Reconstr Surg 88:149-153, 1991
494. Tsuge K: The reattachment of severed fingers. Hiroshima J Med Sci 22:131, 1973
495. Tubiana R: Phalangization of the metacarpals. In Campbell Reid DA, Gosset J (eds): Mutilating Injuries of the Hand. Churchill Livingstone, Edinburgh, 1979
496. Tubiana R, Duparc J: Restoration of sensibility in the hand by neurovascular skin island transfer. J Bone Joint Surg 43B:474-480, 1961
497. Tubiana R, Stack HG, Hakstian RW: Restoration of prehension after severe mutilations of the hand. J Bone Joint Surg 48B:455-473, 1966
498. Ulitskyi G, Malygn G: Roentgenological dynamics of reparative regeneration in lengthening of metacarpals by the distraction method. Acta Chir Plast 15:82, 1973
499. Urbaniak JR: Replantation. In Green DP (ed): Operative Hand Surgery. pp. 811-827. Churchill Livingstone, New York, 1982
500. Urbaniak JR: Wrap-around procedure for thumb reconstruction. Hand Clin 1:259-269, 1985
501. Uzelac O: Reconstruction of the thumb: Another possibility. Br J Plast Surg 23:85-89, 1970
502. Van Beek AL, Wavak PW, Zook EG: Microvascular surgery in young children. Plast Reconstr Surg 63:457-462, 1979
503. Verdan C: The reconstruction of the thumb. Surg Clin North Am 48:1033-1061, 1968
504. Verdan C, Tubiana R, Harrison SH, Littler JW: Panel on reconstruction of the thumb. Transactions of the Third International Congress of Plastic Surgery. Washington, DC, 1963
505. Verrall PJ: Three cases of reconstruction of the thumb. Br Med J 2:775, 1919
506. Vilain R, Michon J: Plastic Surgery of the Hand and Pulp. Masson, New York, 1979
507. Vossmann H, Zellner PR: Verlangerung des ersten Mittelhandknochens bei Verlust des Daumens nach Matev. (Lengthening of the 1st metacarpal according to Matev after loss of the thumb.) Z Plast Chir 3:49-54, 1979
508. Walker MA, Hurley CB, May JW Jr: Radial nerve cross-finger flap differential nerve contribution in thumb reconstruction. J Hand Surg 11A:881-887, 1986
509. Ward JW, Pensler JM, Parry SW: Pollicization for thumb reconstruction in severe pediatric hand burns. Plast Reconstr Surg 76:927-932, 1985
510. Watman RN, Denkewalter FR: A repair for loss of the tactile pad of the thumb. Am J Surg 97:238-240, 1959
511. Weckesser EC: Reconstruction of the distal portion of the thumb. Ohio State Med J 44:602-603, 1948
512. Weckesser EC: Reconstruction of a grasping mechanism following extensive loss of digits. Clin Orthop 15:60-73, 1959
513. Wei J-N, Wang S-H, and Li Y-N: Reconstruction of the thumb. Clin Orthop 215:24-31, 1987
514. Weiland AJ, Villarreal-Rios A, Kleinert HE, Kutz J, Atasoy E, Lister G: Replantation of digits and hands: Analysis of surgical techniques and results in 71 patients with 86 replantations. J Hand Surg 2:1-12, 1977
515. Wendt JR: Transplantation of an osteoarthrotendinous allograft with autogenous soft-tissue coverage for thumb reconstruction. Plast Reconstr Surg 88:713-717, 1991
516. Wexler M, Rousso M, Weinberg H, Neuman Z: Experience in reimplantation of amputated digits. Isr J Med Sci 14:1056-1062, 1978
517. White WF: Pollicisation for the missing thumb, traumatic or congenital. Hand 1:23-26, 1969
518. White WF: Fundamental priorities in pollicisation. J Bone Joint Surg 52B:438-443, 1970
519. Wilson JSP, Braithwaite F: The autografting of an amputated thumb. In Transactions of the Third International Congress of Plastic Surgery. Washington, DC, 1963
520. Wilson CS, Buncke HJ, Alpert BS, Gordon L: Composite metacarpophalangeal joint reconstruction in great toe-to-hand free tissue transfers. J Hand Surg 9A:645-649, 1984
521. Woolf RM, Broadbent TR: The four-flap Z-plasty. Plast Reconstr Surg 49:48-50, 1972
522. Yanai A, Nagata S, Mochizuki M, Tanaka H: Reconstructed thumb tip with a narrow pedicled cross-finger flap. Ann Plast Surg 16(3):261-267, 1986
523. Young F: Transplantation of toes for fingers. Surgery 20:117-123, 1946
524. Yu ZJ, Ho HG, Tang CH: Reconstruction of the thumb by free skin flap of the big toe. J Reconstr Microsurg 1:155-159, 1984
525. Yu ZJ, Ho HG, Tang CH: Microsurgical reconstruction of the amputated hand. J Reconstr Microsurg 1:161-165, 1984
526. Yu ZJ, He HG: Thumb reconstruction with free big toe skin-nail flap and bones, joints, and tendons of the second toe. Report of the cases. Chin Med J 98:863-872, 1985
527. Yu ZJ, He HG: Method of reconstructing thumb, index and/or middle finger for digitless hands. Chin Med J 98:868, 1985
528. Zancolli E: Transplantation of the index finger in congenital absence of the thumb. J Bone Joint Surg 42A:658-660, 1960
529. Zancolli EA, Angrigiani C: Posterior interosseous island forearm flap. J Hand Surg 13B:130-135, 1988

58

Ganglions of the Hand and Wrist

Alexander C. Angelides

GENERAL CONSIDERATIONS

Clinical Characteristics

Ganglions represent 50 to 70 percent of all soft tissue tumors of the hand, and in some series, the percentage is even higher. The soft mucin-filled cyst is usually attached to the adjacent underlying joint capsule, tendon, or tendon sheath. Ganglions are most prevalent in women (3 : 1) and generally occur (70 percent) between the second and fourth decades of life, but they are not rare in children[78,80,100] and have been reported from the first to the eighth decades. Ganglions usually occur singly and in very specific locations, but they have been reported arising from almost every joint of the hand and wrist (Table 58-1). The less common ganglions are often associated with other conditions of the hand (e.g., bossing of the second and third carpometacarpal joints, de Quervain's disease, and Heberden's nodes of the DIP joint), and have been reported to cause clinically significant external pressure on the median and ulnar nerves of the hand.[11,45,76,83,109] Their prevalence make ganglions well recognized by even the inexperienced hand surgeon, and rarely should they be misdiagnosed. The diffuse swelling seen with extensor tenosynovitis, lipomas and other hand tumors, when present over the dorsal aspect of the wrist, can be easily mistaken for a dorsal ganglion.

Their cosmetic presence, pain, and the complaint of weakness are the usual presenting symptoms. A specific antecedent traumatic event is present in at least 10 percent of cases, and repeated minor trauma appears to be an etiologic factor in their development. Malignancy has never been reported. They may appear quite suddenly or develop over several months. There is no correlation with the patient's occupation. Ganglions respond poorly to conservative measures, but do subside with rest, enlarge with activity, and may rupture or disappear spontaneously. While recurrences are rare with proper excision,[3,18,38,59] over 50 percent will recur if improperly and incompletely excised.

Radiographs are usually normal, but intraosseous cysts may be identified and osteoarthritic changes noted in the DIP or carpometacarpal joints. A communication between the joint and cyst is demonstrated with arthrograms[2,8,116] but not with cystograms. A one-way valvular mechanism[60] has, therefore, been postulated, connecting the wrist joint to the cyst.

Microscopic Anatomy

The microscopic description of ganglions is well known, although there is no unanimity of opinion on the interpretation of these findings. Microscopically the main cyst, which may be single or multiloculated, appears smooth, white, and translucent. The wall is made up of compressed collagen fibers and is sparsely lined with flattened cells, without evidence of an epithelial or synovial lining. Recent electromicroscopic studies further confirm these findings.[74,94]

The capsular attachment of the main cyst reveals mucin-filled "clefts," which have been shown by serial sections to intercommunicate,[3] thereby forming a tortuous continuous duct connecting the main cyst with the adjacent underlying joint. The stroma surrounding the intracapsular ducts may show tightly packed collagen fibers or sparsely cellular areas with broken collagen fibers and mucin-filled inter- and extracellular lakes. No inflammatory reaction or mitotic activity is noted.

The contents of the cyst are characterized by a highly viscous, clear, sticky, jellylike mucin made up of glucosamine,

Table 58-1. Ganglions of the Hand and Wrist

Dorsal wrist ganglion
Volar wrist ganglion
Volar retinacular ganglion
  (Flexor tendon sheath ganglion)
Mucous cyst (ganglion of DIP joint)
Other ganglions
  Carpometacarpal boss
  PIP joint
  Extensor tendon
  Miscellaneous locations
    First extensor compartment
      (dorsal retinacular ganglion)
    Carpal tunnel
    Ulnar canal
    Intraosseous ganglion

albumin, globulin, and high concentrations of hyaluronic acid. In some cases the mucin may be blood-tinged. The contents of the cyst are decidedly more viscous than normal joint fluid, but the significance of this is disputed.

Pathogenesis

The etiology and pathogenesis of ganglions remain obscure, and a review of the literature indicates the confusion that exists.[17,35,113] Since Hippocrates offered the first recorded description of "knots of" tissue containing "mucoid flesh," numerous speculative theories with little scientific basis have abounded. This became especially true when the eighteenth and nineteenth century anatomists offered the following hypotheses: (1) synovial herniation (Eller, 1746) or rupture through tendon sheath; (2) synovial dermoid or rest due to "arthrogenesis blastoma cell nests" or embryonic periarticular tissue (Hoeftman, 1876); (3) new growths from synovial membranes (Henle, 1847); and (4) modifications of bursae or degenerative cysts (Vogt, 1881).

Until recently, the most widely accepted theory, initially postulated by Ledderhose (1893) and popularized by Carp and Stout,[15] was that of mucoid degeneration. The fibrillation of collagen fibers, accumulation of inter- and extracellular mucin, and decreased collagen fibers and stroma cells supported this theory. Mucoid degeneration does not explain, however, why the degenerative process is self-limiting and solitary and usually occurs among adolescents and young adults, and why the fluid recurs following aspiration or incomplete excision.

I believe that the stimulating factor for the production of hyaluronic acid (a tissue lubricant) is tissue trauma or irritation, such as stretching of the capsular and ligamentous supporting joint structures. The process is initiated at the synovial-capsular interface. The mucin producing cells may be modified synovial cells, mesenchymal cells, or fibroblasts, which in tissue culture have been found to synthesize hyaluronic acid.[86] The mucin thus formed is visualized as dissecting through the attached joint ligament and capsule to form the capsular ducts seen on histologic sections. The ducts and lakes of mucin eventually coalesce to form the main subcutaneous cyst. The capsular stromal findings are interpreted as secondary to the mucin production and are atrophic in nature. The possibility of an osmotic gradient across the synovial-capsular interface has yet to be investigated.

Although the pathogenesis of ganglions has never been satisfactorily explained, surgical treatment can be undertaken with confidence.

Treatment

Nonoperative Treatment

The high recurrence rate and other complications of surgery have been the main stimuli to seek nonsurgical methods of treatment. Nonsurgical treatment has included digital pressure, rupture with a mallet or Bible, injections of hyaluronidase or sclerosing solutions,[79] subcutaneous tenotome dissection, and cross fixation with a heavy suture. These methods have been discarded and need not be considered except for their historical interest. More recently, the treatment of piercing the ganglion with crossing threads has been resurrected, but again offers little promise of success.[42]

While all nonsurgical methods have limited success, aspiration of the ganglion, puncture of the cyst wall and instillation of lidocaine (Xylocaine) and betamethasone (Celestone) into the capsule or tendon sheath attachments reduces the mass and alleviates symptoms for varying periods of time.[34,98,124] This is especially true with volar retinacular ganglions as well as early occult painful dorsal ganglions of the wrist. Injection and aspiration of volar wrist ganglions must be approached with a great deal of respect because of the adjacent radial artery, and is therefore less commonly performed. I do not use triamcinolone (Kenalog), having seen marked subcutaneous atrophy and skin depigmentation following its use.

The most effective nonsurgical treatment is patient reassurance. An explanation of the condition and assurance of its nonmalignant nature is often the only treatment sought or required. Surgery is best reserved for those patients with persistently symptomatic ganglions.

Operative Treatment

If surgery becomes the treatment of choice, it must be approached with the same seriousness as any other hand operation.[3,18] Ganglions must be excised in a complete surgical suite, under pneumatic tourniquet control and either general or brachial block anesthesia. Intravenous regional anesthesia (Bier block) does not allow release of the tourniquet for adequate hemostasis and is therefore not recommended. The use of ocular loupes or the microscope is encouraged in the surgical excision of all hand tumors. Prior to wound closure, meticulous hemostasis must be assured and the wound should be irrigated copiously with Ringer's lactate, normal saline, and/or antibiotic solution.

Attempts to close the joint capsule are unnecessary and contraindicated. Large or small capsular defects do not lead to joint infections or recurrences. Capsular closures do, however, result in prolonged immobilization and subsequent joint stiffness.

The wound is simply closed with fine, nonabsorbable mattress sutures (such as 5-0 nylon) or more preferably with a pull-out suture. The wound is then supported with Benzoin, Steri-strips, and a bulky, fluffy bandage. A method to keep the hand elevated during the immediate postoperative period is used (such as an upper extremity sling).

Although this approach to a simple nonmalignant lesion may appear radical, it is preferable, for both the patient and physician, to inadequate excision followed by unwarranted recurrences. A cosmetically acceptable scar, with a full range of motion and no complications, should be the goal in all cases.

DORSAL WRIST GANGLION

Clinical Characteristics

The prototype of all ganglions of the hand is the dorsal wrist ganglion, which accounts for 60 to 70 percent of all hand and wrist ganglions. The main cyst is usually directly over the scapholunate ligament (Fig. 58-1) and is easily seen and diagnosed. The cyst may present anywhere else between the extensor tendons, however, and can be connected to the ligament through a long pedicle (Fig. 58-1). Failure to identify this pedicle and its scapholunate ligament attachment contributes greatly to recurrences. Careful preoperative palpation of the cyst with digital compression often reveals the extent of the cyst and the direction of the pedicle. While ganglions have been reported from other carpal joints, these are rare, and attachments to the scapholunate joint must be ruled out before a dissection is considered complete.

Occult Dorsal Carpal Ganglion

Unlike the protruding dorsal ganglion, the smaller, occult dorsal ganglion is easily overlooked and can often only be palpated with the involved wrist in marked volar flexion.[108] Comparison with the opposite normal wrist is helpful. The occult ganglion may be the cause of unexplained wrist pain and is disproportionately tender. Its intimate relationship to the overlying posterior interosseous nerve has been suggested as the etiology of the exquisite pain and tenderness associated with the occult dorsal ganglion.[27] This seems unlikely, however. The differential diagnosis between the painful occult dorsal ganglion, sprains of the scapholunate ligament, and other intercarpal ligaments with early carpal instability is difficult to make, especially following dorsiflexion injuries of the wrist. Dorsal ganglions do occasionally occur in association with an underlying scapholunate diastasis, and they may be blamed for the carpal instability following their excision.[22,31,50] Dorsal prominence of the proximal pole of the scaphoid secondary to intercarpal instability may be confused with a painful occult ganglion and must be diagnosed with appropriate radiographic studies.[8,72,116] to avoid a delay in proper treatment (see Chapter 22). The presence of a ganglion does not exclude other causes of wrist pain, and when appropriate, I am careful to explain to the patient that the preoperative pain may be the result of both a sprain of the scapholunate ligament and the presence of a dorsal ganglion (especially occult ganglions). Excising the ganglion alone might not alleviate all of the patient's preoperative pain. Excision of the posterior interosseous nerve at the level of the radiocarpal joint may help to alleviate pain and add to the patient's postoperative comfort. If other causes of wrist pain and tenderness, especially directly over the scapholunate ligament, can be excluded, the occult dorsal ganglion is best initially treated conservatively with immobilization and steroid injections directly into the dorsal capsule which may also aid in diagnosis.[104]

In those cases where further diagnostic studies are necessary,

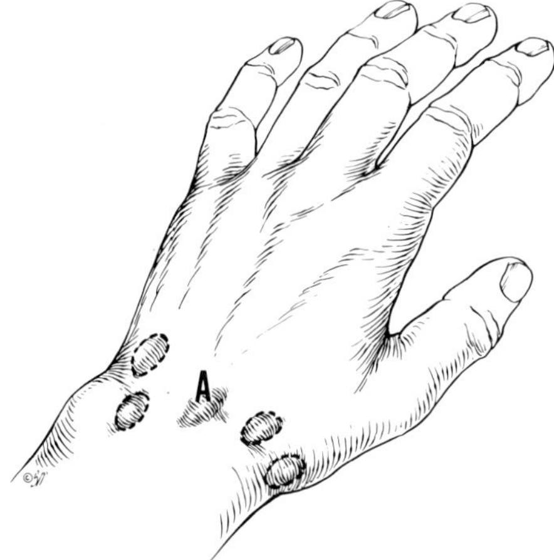

Fig. 58-1. A few of the many possible locations of the dorsal wrist ganglion. **(A)** The most common site, directly over the scapholunate ligament. The others *(dotted circles)* are connected to the scapholunate ligament through an elongaged pedicle.

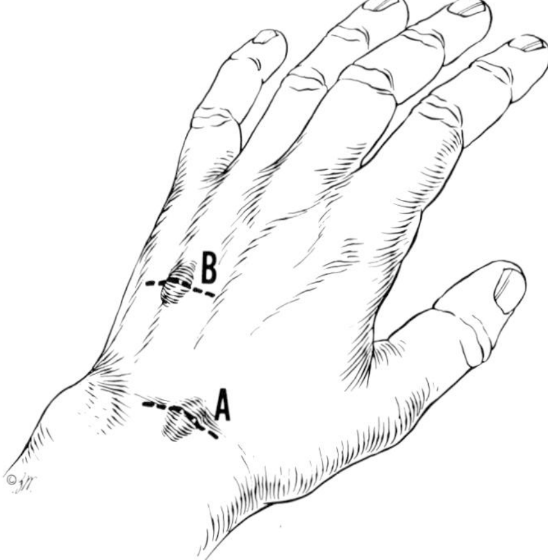

Fig. 58-2. **(A)** A transverse incision over the scapholunate ligament used to expose the typical dorsal ganglion. **(B)** An additional incision to expose a more distant cyst. The main cyst and pedicle are mobilized, passed under the extensor tendons, and delivered through incision *A*.

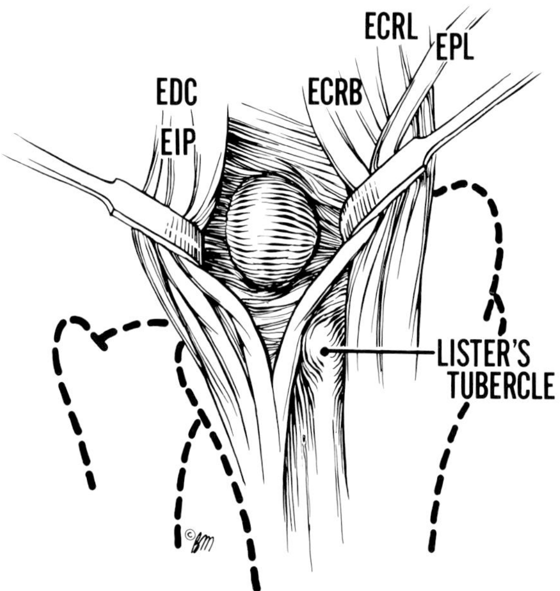

Fig. 58-3. The dorsal ganglion exposed and mobilized between the extensor pollicis longus *(EPL)*, extensor carpi radialis longus *(ECRL)*, and extensor carpi radialis brevis *(ECRB)* radially and the extensor digitorum communis *(EDC)* and extensor indicis proprius *(EIP)* ulnarly.

some authors have found the use of magnetic resonance imaging (MRI), computed tomography (CT) scans, and ultrasonography helpful.[36,46,90,91,96,120] The cost-effectiveness of these studies must be kept in mind.

Chronic tenosynovitis of the extensor tendons may be confused with dorsal wrist ganglion but is easily distinguished by the diffuse nature of the swelling and the puckering seen with digital extension, the so-called tuck sign.

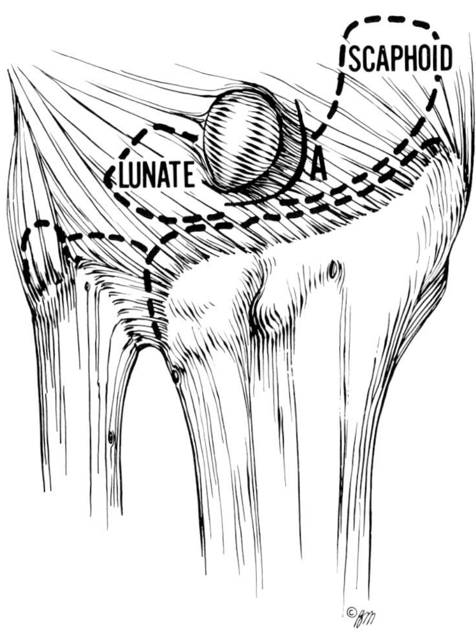

Fig. 58-4. The initial incision through the joint capsule *(A)* to expose the scapholunate ligament attachments and intracapsular cysts.

Operative Technique

Most dorsal ganglions may be approached through a transverse incision over the proximal carpal row, but a modified incision or second transverse incision may be necessary for those ganglions that are not directly over the scapholunate ligament (Fig. 58-2). Typically, the dorsal ganglion appears between the extensor pollicis longus and extensor digitorum communis tendons, which are retracted radially and ulnarly respectively (Fig. 58-3). The main cyst and its pedicle are mobilized down to the underlying joint capsule. With the wrist in volar flexion, the joint capsule is opened along the border of the radius and proximal pole of the scaphoid (Fig. 58-4). The capsule is elevated and retracted distally, exposing the capsular attachments to the scapholunate ligament. Smaller intraarticular cysts are often identified attached to the scapholunate ligament (Fig. 58-5). The capsular incision is then continued around the ganglion, leaving all capsular attachments to the ligament intact (Fig. 58-6). The capsular incision is extended more laterally if any capsular ducts are encountered during this dissection and identified by small amounts of mucin drainage. The ganglion and its capsular attachments are then tangentially excised off the scapholunate ligament (Fig. 58-7). A small mucin-filled duct is invariably seen piercing the transverse fibers of the scapholunate ligament. This duct appears to connect the underlying scapholunate joint with the main cyst. Synovial and capsular attachments along the distal margin of the scapholunate ligament are also excised, giving an unobstructed view of the head and neck of the capitate (Fig. 58-8). If the ganglion ruptures and its anatomic features are lost during the dissection, the dissection should continue until all attachments to the scapholunate ligament have been excised. The excised portion of the joint capsule usually measures approximately 1.0 × 1.5 cm. It is not necessary to cut into the scapholunate ligament nor is it necessary to curette the scapholunate joint.

The tourniquet is released and hemostasis obtained, and then, under tourniquet control, the wound is closed and a dressing applied. Attempts to close the joint capsule either primarily or with fibrous flaps are contraindicated.

Postoperative Care

A bulky dressing extending from the proximal forearm to the MP joints is applied and the hand is elevated. Early finger motion is encouraged. The dressing is reduced by the fifth postoperative day and early wrist motion stressed, especially volar flexion. Sutures are removed 2 weeks postoperatively, and therapy is continued until a full range of motion has been obtained.

Complications

Early recurrences, the most common complication of ganglion surgery, are due to inadequate and incomplete excisions and should rarely occur. Ganglions appearing at the same site years after excision may in fact be new ganglions. Stiffness of the wrist can be avoided by early motion, physical therapy if

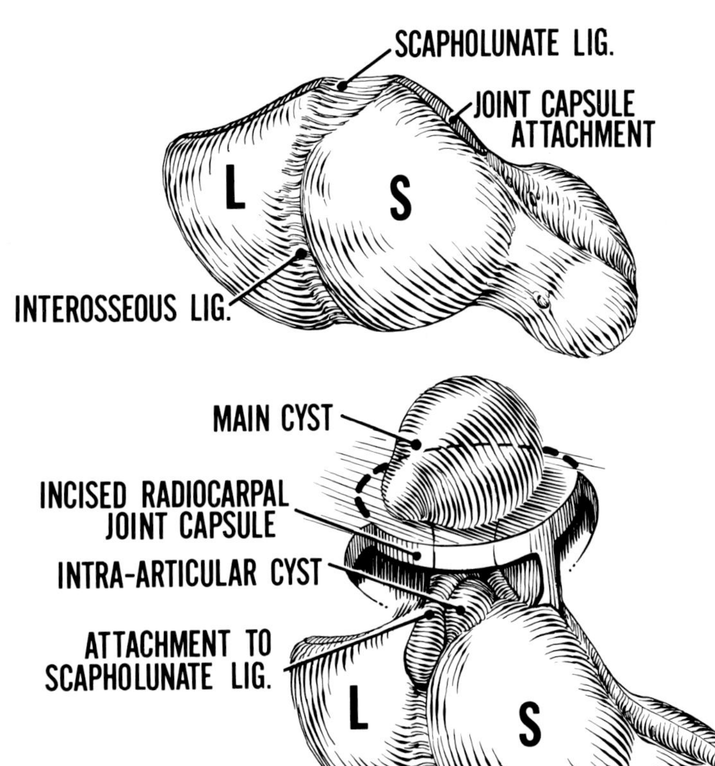

Fig. 58-5. A schematic representation of the cyst in situ. Attachments to the scapholunate ligament are visualized before final excision *(dotted line).*

necessary, and the avoidance of restrictive bandages or casts beyond the first few postoperative days. It is imperative to stress early volar flexion. To avoid keloid or hypertrophic scars, longitudinal incisions across the wrist joint are not made. Awareness and respect for the sensory branches of the radial and ulnar nerves prevent neuroma formation, which often defies effective treatment. I have not seen avascular necrosis of either the lunate or scaphoid or scapholunate dissociation following the above surgical technique.[3,31,119] Ganglions and sprains of the intercarpal ligaments can occur concomitantly following trauma to the wrist and must be distinguished preoperatively.

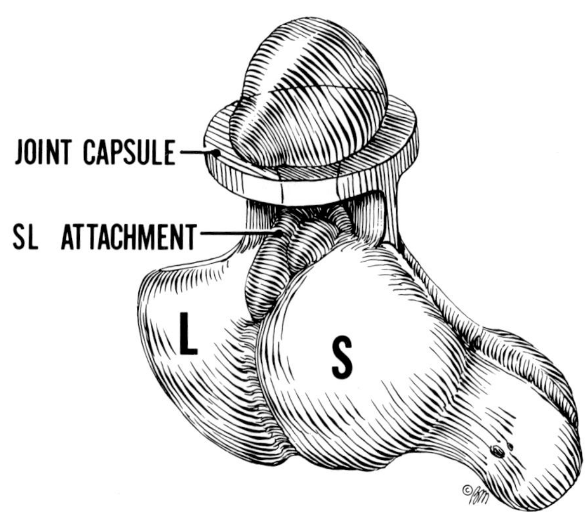

Fig. 58-6. The ganglion and scapholunate *(SL)* attachments are isolated from the remaining, uninvolved joint capsule (not shown).

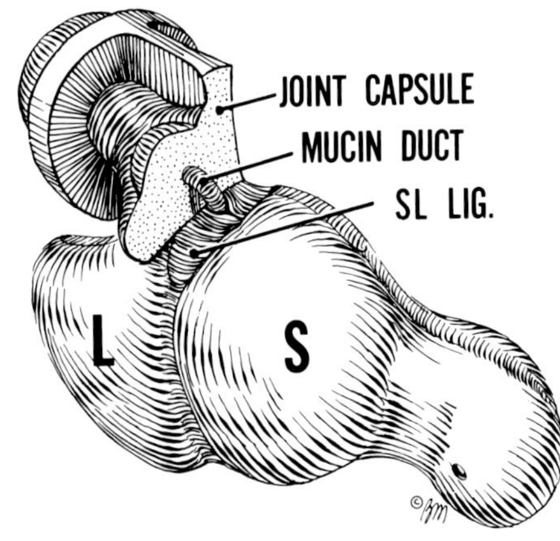

Fig. 58-7. Tangential excision of the ganglion and attachments off the fibers of the scapholunate *(SL)* ligament. A minute mucin duct piercing the fibers of the scapholunate ligament is invariably cut during this dissection.

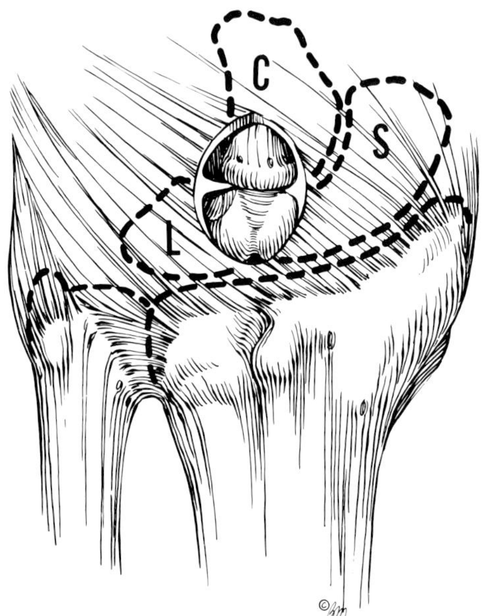

Fig. 58-8. Completed excision of all attachments to the scapholunate *(SL)* ligament and the immediate vicinity. Synovial tissue between the ligament and head of the capitate *(C)* has also been excised. Note that the scapholunate ligaments remain intact.

Recurrent Dorsal Ganglion

The recurrent dorsal ganglion is treated like the primary ganglion, but it can be complicated by more scarring. Old skin incisions are excised and longitudinal scars converted with a Z-plasty. Tendons and nerves are identified and delicately cleaned of scar tissue before dissecting the ganglion itself. Excision can then proceed as described above.

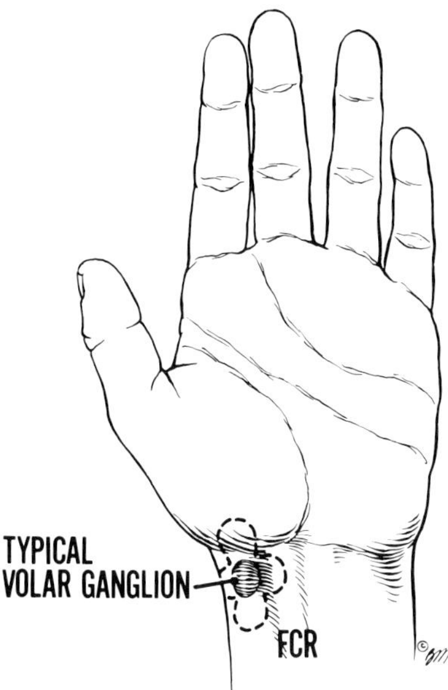

Fig. 58-9. Typical presenting location of the volar wrist ganglion. Possible subcutaneous extensions *(dotted lines)* are often palpable.

VOLAR WRIST GANGLION

Clinical Characteristics

The second most common ganglion of the hand and wrist is the volar wrist ganglion (18 to 20 percent). Most volar ganglions present either directly over the distal edge of the radius, or slightly more distally over the scaphoid tubercle. The former arises from the capsular and ligamentous fibers of the radiocarpal joint and present under the volar wrist crease between the flexor carpi radialis and abductor pollicis longus tendons (Fig. 58-9). The main cyst may be intertwined with the bifurcating branches of the radial artery, making delicate dissection imperative. The other type of volar ganglion arises from the capsule of the scaphotrapezial joint.

While volar ganglions may appear clinically small, they can be surprisingly extensive at surgery. Multiloculated cysts extending under the thenar muscles, along the flexor carpi radialis tendon, into the carpal canal, and under the first extensor compartment adjacent to the dorsal branch of the radial artery as far dorsally as the first web space, may be encountered. These extensions can often be appreciated preoperatively by careful palpation and digital compression of the ganglion.

The importance of the preoperative evaluation of the patency of the radial and ulnar arteries is stressed. Allen's test should be routinely performed and an ulnar artery occlusion excluded. While an occluded ulnar artery is not a contraindication to surgery, the surgeon must be aware of the importance of preserving the radial artery, especially when adherent to the volar ganglion.

Operative Technique

Although the surgical technique of excision of a volar ganglion is similar to that of the dorsal ganglion, the exposure and precise identification of the capsular attachments of the volar ganglion are more difficult. The incision must be planned to allow for extension into the carpal tunnel or base of the thenar muscles (Fig. 58-10). Most difficulties are accentuated by a small transverse incision that does not allow adequate mobilization of adjacent structures.

With the skin flaps retracted, the forearm fascia is incised longitudinally and the dome of the cyst identified and mobilized. Particular care is taken to identify and protect the radial artery, which is often intimately attached to the wall of the ganglion and may even be completely encircled by the ganglion (Fig. 58-11). Magnification is again helpful.

The pedicle is traced to the volar joint capsule (usually the scaphotrapezial or radiocarpal ligament). The joint is opened and explored and the capsular attachments are excised (approximately 3×4 mm). Once the ganglion is excised, the surrounding tissues can be digitally compressed to rule out further mucin-filled pockets. If unidentified extensions are present, they must be excised. Hemostasis, wound lavage, and a simple skin closure (preferably subcuticular) complete the operation. Again, capsular closure is unnecessary and only delays early mobilization.

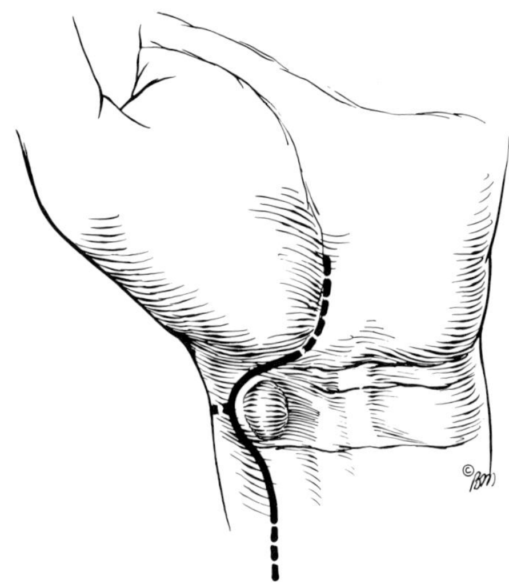

Fig. 58-10. The usual incision to expose the volar ganglion. Extensions proximally, distally, and even radially are possible *(dotted lines)*. Care must be taken to avoid injury to the palmar cutaneous branch of the median nerve if the incision is extended.

Postoperative Care

A bulky bandage and elevation of the hand assure early postoperative comfort. Follow-up care is similar to the dorsal ganglion, and early motion is stressed.

Complications

The complications are similar to those of the dorsal ganglion. Unexpected branches of the radial sensory or lateral antebrachial cutaneous nerves may be injured and lead to troublesome neuromas. Extensions of the routine incision into the carpal canal must avoid injury to the palmar cutaneous branch of the median nerve. Injuries to the radial artery can be microscopically repaired or ligated. While no adverse effects have been reported following ligation of the artery with an intact ulnar artery, I prefer a microvascular repair. Other authors[74] recommend leaving a portion of the cyst wall attached to the artery in order to avoid arterial injury. However, I have never found this to be necessary. Stiffness of the wrist is a much less common occurrence than with the dorsal ganglion, but it can result if early motion is not encouraged. Unpleasant scars are not an uncommon problem on the volar aspect of the wrist, and often they defy "plastic" revisions. Curved incisions appear to provide more consistently attractive scars, especially near the volar wrist creases (see Fig. 58-10).

VOLAR RETINACULAR (FLEXOR TENDON SHEATH) GANGLION

Clinical Characteristics

The third most common ganglion (10 to 12 percent) of the hand is the volar retinacular ganglion arising from the proximal annular ligament (A1 pulley) of the flexor tendon sheath. This ganglion is invariably a small (3 to 8 mm), firm, tender mass palpable under the MP flexion crease (Fig. 58-12). The cyst is attached to the tendon sheath and does not move with the tendon. Needle rupture,[12] followed with a steroid injection and digital massage to disperse the cyst contents, can often delay or obviate the need for surgery. Several attempts at conservative treatment are recommended prior to surgery with the patient's understanding that recurrences may happen. The proximity of the digital nerves must be appreciated.

Operative Technique

The ganglion is approached through a curved or angular incision over the mass (Fig. 58-12). Transverse incisions are more popular but often do not allow adequate exposure without undue skin traction. The incision must also allow identification and mobilization of the radial and ulnar neurovascular bundles. The ganglion can then be traced to the tendon sheath and excised with a small portion of the annular ligament (Fig. 58-13).

The synovial side of the specimen usually reveals a defect in its smooth, white homogeneous surface, suggesting a communication between the tendon space and cyst.

Following skin closure, a simple dressing, allowing early motion, is applied.

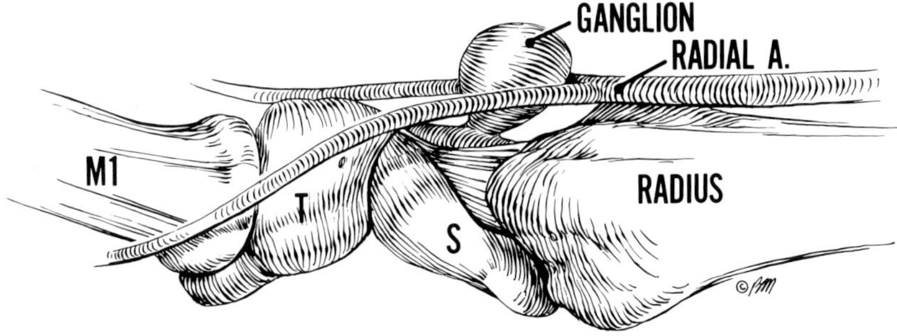

Fig. 58-11. The usual relation of the ganglion to the radial artery and volar joint capsule. (*S*, scaphoid; *T*, trapezium; *M1*, first metacarpal.)

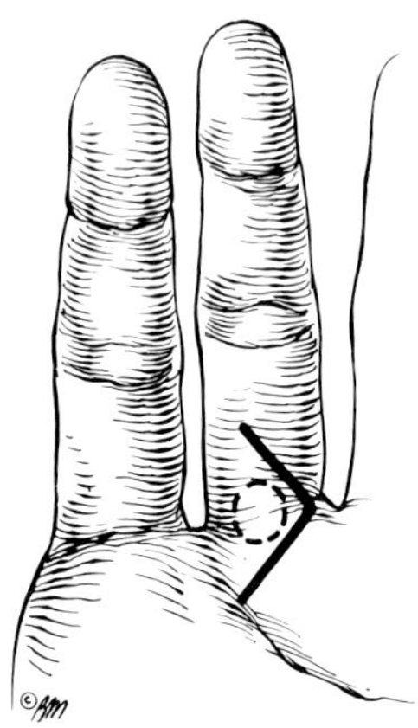

Fig. 58-12. The volar retinacular ganglion palpable over the proximal tendon sheath and an incision for easy exposure.

Complications

Complications and recurrences are rare although injuries of the digital nerves have been reported.

MUCOUS CYST

Clinical Characteristics

The mucous cyst is a ganglion of the DIP joint usually occurring between the fifth and seventh decades. The earliest clinical sign may be longitudinal grooving of the nail, without a visible mass, due to pressure on the nail matrix (Fig. 58-14). Usually, however, the patient is seen after the cyst has enlarged and attenuated the overlying skin. The cyst (3 to 5 mm) usually lies to one side of the extensor tendon and between the dorsal distal joint crease and eponychium. The patient often has Heberden's nodes and radiologic evidence of osteoarthritic changes of the joint. The cyst and osteophytes should both be treated to assure a satisfactory result.[32]

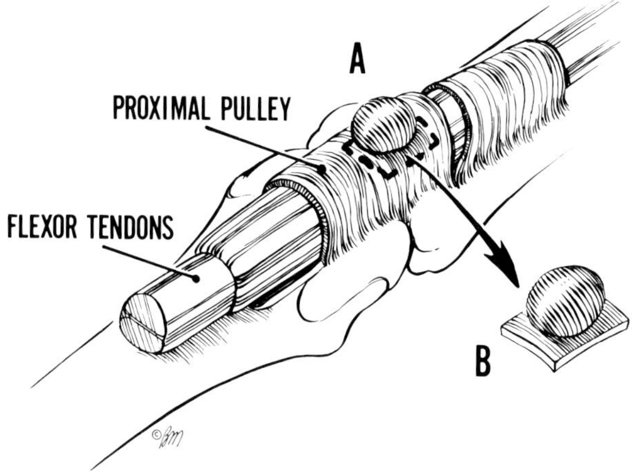

Fig. 58-13. (**A**) The volar retinacular ganglion in situ on the proximal annular ligament (A1 pulley) of the flexor tendon sheath. (**B**) The excised specimen with a surrounding margin of tendon sheath.

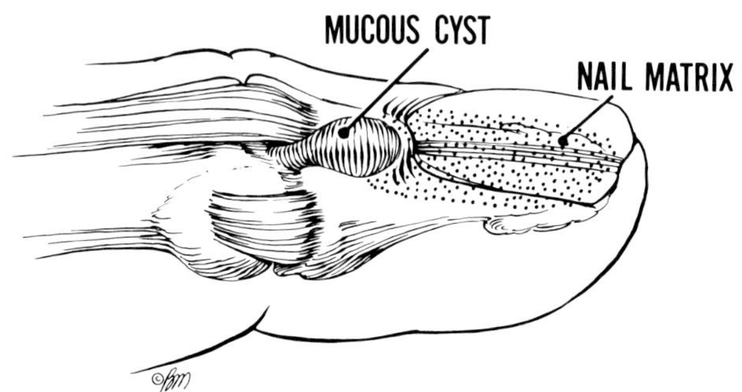

Fig. 58-14. The early mucous cyst resting on the nail matrix may cause longitudinal grooving of the nail in some cases.

Operative Technique

The cyst is approached through an "L"-shaped or curved incision (Fig. 58-15A), and any attentuated or involved skin that cannot be easily separated from the cyst wall is elliptically excised (Fig. 58-15B). The cyst is mobilized, traced to the joint capsule, and excised with the joint capsule (Fig. 58-16A). From a practical point of view, however, all soft tissues between the retracted extensor tendon and adjacent collateral ligament are excised, leaving the DIP joint exposed (Fig. 58-16B). Care is

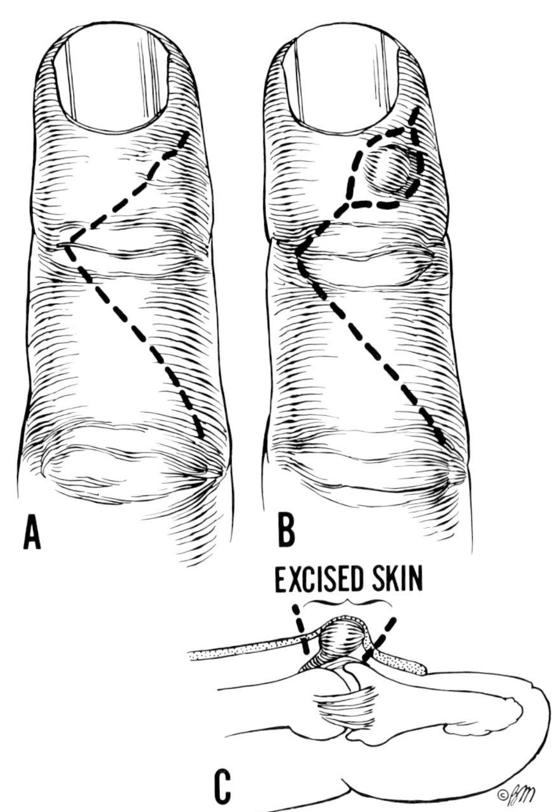

Fig. 58-15. (**A**) The cyst without skin involvement and overlying incision. (**B**) Schematic representation of the extent of the elliptical incision when the skin is attenuated. A skin graft or local rotation flap is usually necessary to close the defect.

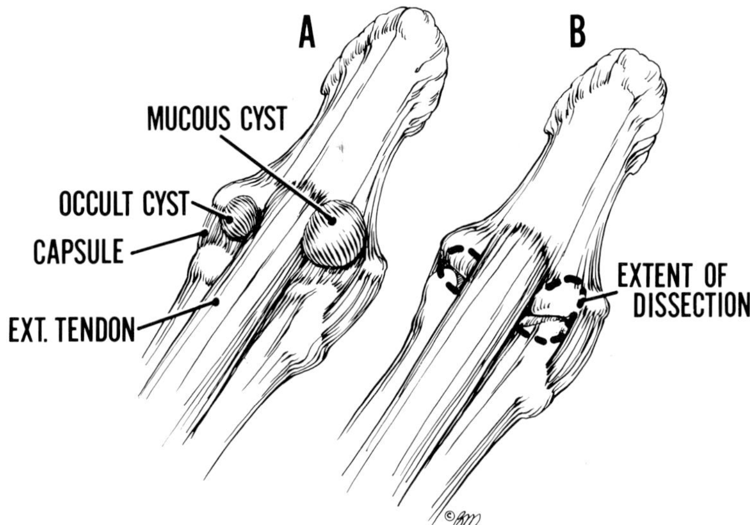

Fig. 58-16. (**A**) The ganglion in situ with its connection to the dorsal joint capsule. A second occult cyst is also illustrated. (**B**) The exposed DIP joint following excision.

taken not to disturb the insertion of the extensor tendon or nail matrix. With the joint extended and tendon dorsally retracted, the opposite side is explored and occult cysts or hypertrophied synovial tissue are excised.

The osteophytes can be excised with a rongeur or a fine power burr (Fig. 58-17). Skin closure may require rotation and advancement of the dorsal skin flap[69] or a full-thickness skin graft. (See Chapter 49 for a discussion of the principles of local rotation flaps.)

Postoperative Care

If a skin graft is used, the distal joint is supported with a cast or splint for 2 weeks. Earlier motion is permitted if a local rotation flap is used. Motion and therapy can then be undertaken until full painless motion has been achieved.

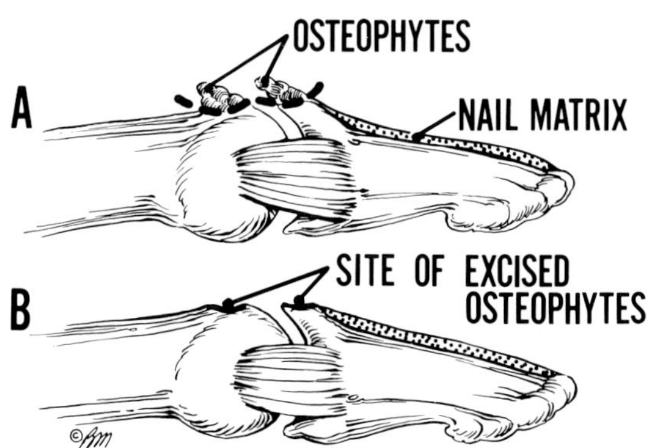

Fig. 58-17. (**A**) The usual osteophytes seen with mucous cysts. (**B**) The extent of dissection, avoiding injury to the nail matrix, insertion of the extensor tendon, and articular surface.

Complications

Recurrences are invariably due to inadequate excision of the involved skin or the capsular attachments of the ganglion and failure to recognize extensions of the ganglion under the extensor tendon to the opposite side. A meticulous dissection and relief of pressure on the nail matrix restore the nail to its normal appearance. Stiffness is rarely a functional problem.

OTHER GANGLIONS OF THE HAND

Dorsal, volar retinacular, and DIP ganglions constitute over 90 percent of the ganglions of the hand. Ganglions do occur at other locations, however, and must be approached with the same care and thoroughness.

CARPOMETACARPAL BOSS

Clinical Characteristics

The dorsal wrist ganglion is most often confused with the carpal boss, so named by the French physician Foille.[25] The carpal boss is an osteoarthritic spur that develops at the base of the second and/or third carpometacarpal joints (Fig. 58-18). A firm, bony, nonmobile, tender mass is visible and palpable at the base of the carpometacarpal joints, especially when the wrist is volar flexed.

Radiologically, the mass is best visualized with the hand in 30 to 40 degrees supination and 20 to 30 degrees ulnar deviation ("carpal boss view").[25]

The boss is more common in women (2 : 1), in the right hand (2 : 1), and between the third and fourth decades. The mass may be asymptomatic, but the patient may complain of considerable pain and aching. A small ganglion is associated with

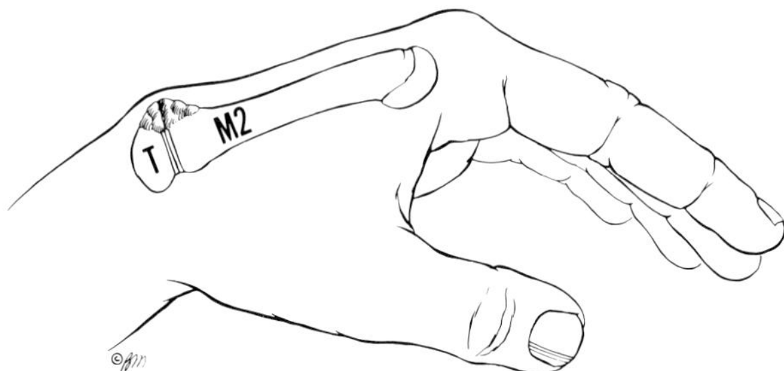

Fig. 58-18. The carpal boss involving the second carpometacarpal joint (*T*, trapezoid).

the carpal boss in 30 percent of cases, adding to its confusion with the more common dorsal wrist ganglion. As with the mucous cyst, successful treatment requires excision of the ganglion as well as the osteoarthritic spurring.

Operative Technique

The mass is approached through a transverse or oblique incision over the bony prominence (Fig. 58-19). The extensor digitorum communis and extensor indicis proprius tendons

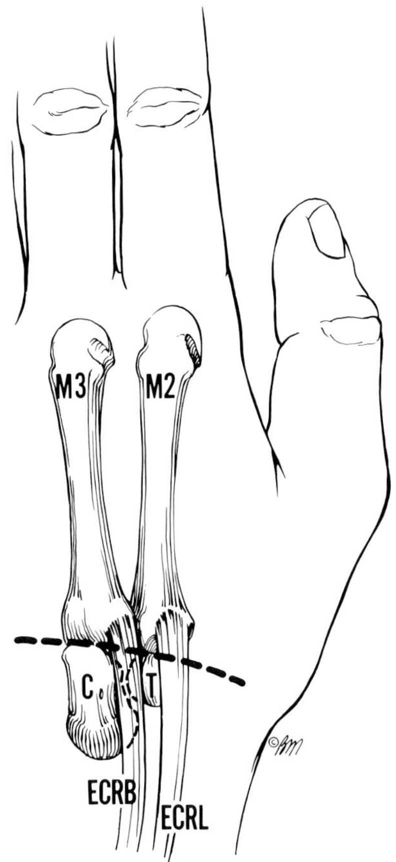

Fig. 58-19. The incision for carpal boss excision, centered over the second and third carpometacarpal joints. (*C*, capitate; *T*, trapezoid; *ECRB*, extensor carpi radialis brevis; *ECRL*, extensor carpi radialis longus.)

are retracted ulnarward. A ganglion, if present, can be mobilized and excised with its capsular attachments. The osteophytes and carpometacarpal joints are approached through a separate longitudinal incision over each involved joint. Subperiosteal dissection exposes the involved joint with the adjacent osteophytes. The osteophytes are then excised with small osteotomes down to normal cartilage. The dissection may involve the second and third carpometacarpal joints individually or all four opposing surfaces together (Fig. 58-20). The surgical area is palpated through the skin to assure the excision of all palpable prominences.

The capsule, periosteum, and any adjacent overlying tendon fibers (extensor carpi radialis longus, extensor carpi radialis brevis) are reapproximated over the joint with a few fine inverting sutures that should not be palpable through the skin.

Postoperative Care

A cast is worn for 4 to 6 weeks to allow for adequate ligamentous healing.

Complications

The most common complication is the persistence of a mass because of excision of the ganglion alone or inadequate excision of the osteophytes. Pain will persist unless all abnormal abutting surfaces have been excised. Dorsal wrist ganglions can present over the carpometacarpal joints and must be distinguished from the carpal boss with its own associated ganglion. Avoidance of injury to branches of the radial and ulnar sensory nerves is again stressed.

PROXIMAL INTERPHALANGEAL JOINT

Clinical Characteristics

Similar to the mucous cyst of the DIP joint, ganglions also occur dorsally over the PIP joint on either side of the extensor tendon. They arise from the joint capsule and usually pierce the oblique fibers between the central slip and lateral band. They are small (3 to 5 mm) and tender and may interfere with joint motion.

Operative Technique

A curved incision over the PIP joint exposes the ganglion (Fig. 58-21). The lateral margin of the lateral band is released from the transverse retaining ligament and retracted dorsally to expose the PIP joint (Fig. 58-22). The pedicle from the main cyst can usually be followed through the extensor system into the joint capsule. A small, elliptical incision through the oblique extensor fibers mobilizes the cyst and pedicle. The entire joint capsule and synovial lining are excised between the

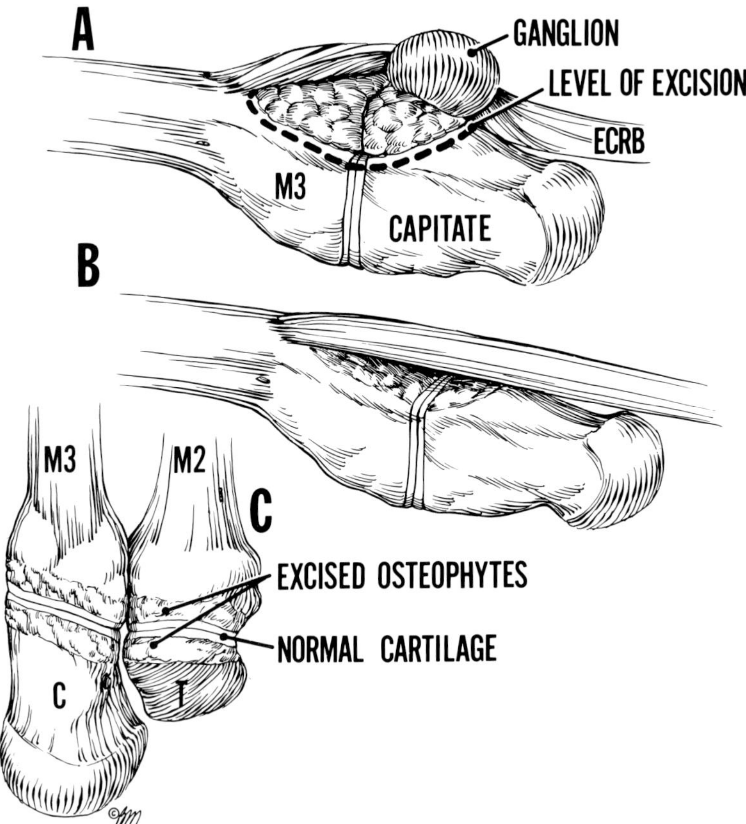

Fig. 58-20. (**A**) The typical carpal boss and associated ganglion. The extent of the bony excision is illustrated. (**B**) Excised osteophytes with periosteum and extensor carpi radialis tendon reapproximated. (**C**) Exposure following excision of osteophytes involving both carpometacarpal joints (attached extensor carpi radialis longus and extensor carpi radialis brevis not illustrated). (*C*, capitate; *T*, trapezoid.)

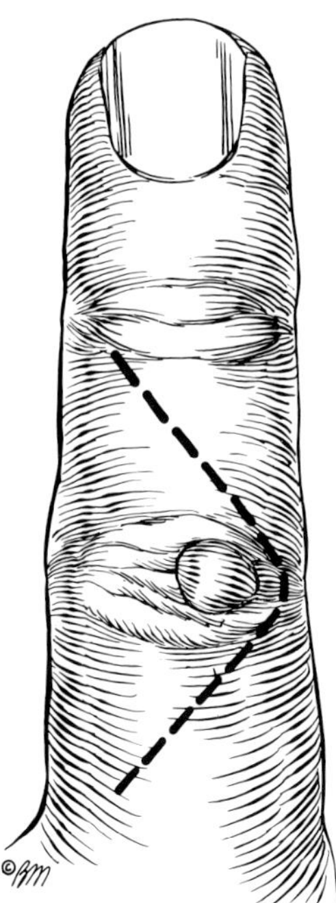

Fig. 58-21. The dorsal PIP ganglion with curved skin incision.

collateral ligament and extensor insertion on the middle phalanx.

Postoperative Care

A simple skin closure and dressing followed by early motion are all that is required.

GANGLIONS OF EXTENSOR TENDONS

Clinical Characteristics

Ganglions do arise on or within extensor tendons.[122] They usually occur over the metacarpals and are distinguished by their proximal motion with the fingers in extension. They can, however, be confused with dorsal wrist ganglions, carpal bossing, or extensor tenosynovitis. The patient may complain of tenderness, aching, or snapping of the tendon with motion.

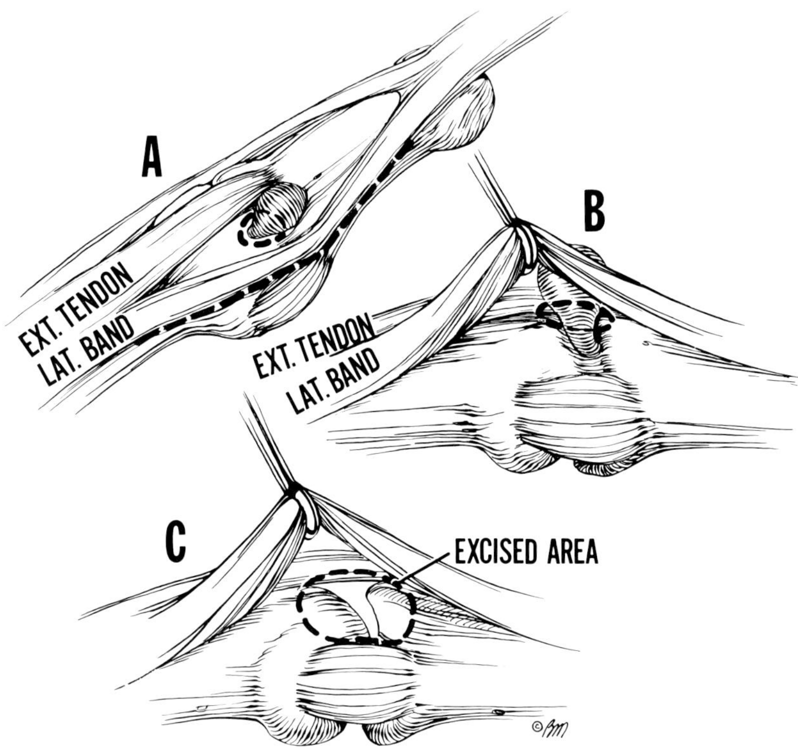

Fig. 58-22. (**A**) A PIP ganglion in situ between the extensor tendon and lateral band. An incision along the lateral border of the lateral band and the base of the pedicle is illustrated with a dotted line. (**B**) The lateral band has been released and elevated to expose the joint capsule and infratendinous portion of the cyst. (**C**) The cyst and joint capsule have been excised, revealing the exposed PIP joint.

Operative Technique

The ganglion is approached through a transverse incision (Fig. 58-23) and the intimate broad attachment to the extensor tendon is readily appreciated. The ganglion is dissected off the extensor tendon with all the synovial tissue surrounding the involved tendon. Rupture of the ganglion is difficult to avoid, but recurrences are rare.

MISCELLANEOUS LOCATIONS

Ganglions have been reported from numerous other locations of the hand and wrist and are often associated with other conditions,[82] including the sites discussed below.

First Extensor Compartment (Dorsal Retinacular) Ganglion

Ganglions attached to the first extensor compartment, similar to the volar retinacular ganglion, are seen in patients with acute stenosing tenosynovitis (De Quervain's disease) (Fig. 58-24). In addition to releasing the tendons (see Chapter 54), therefore, the involved tendon sheath and the ganglion are excised. Injury to the radial sensory nerve and failure to recognize a separate tunnel for the extensor pollicis brevis are the most common complications.

Carpal Tunnel

Symptoms consistent with compression of the median nerve have been reported secondary to ganglions arising from the volar carpus within the carpal canal.[52,65] The volar wrist ganglion can also extend distally and ulnarward to compress the median nerve. All carpal tunnel releases should be accompanied by an exploration of the canal to rule out extrinsic masses, including ganglions.

Ulnar Canal

Ganglions within the ulnar canal (loge de Guyon) can compress the ulnar nerve, leading to motor and/or sensory loss.[11,70,76,109] These ganglions usually arise from joints around the hamate and dissect through the hypothenar muscles or along the motor branch. Ganglions in the palm may lead to an isolated atrophy of the first dorsal interosseous muscle.[83] Early excision is imperative and avoids permanent injury to the ulnar nerve.

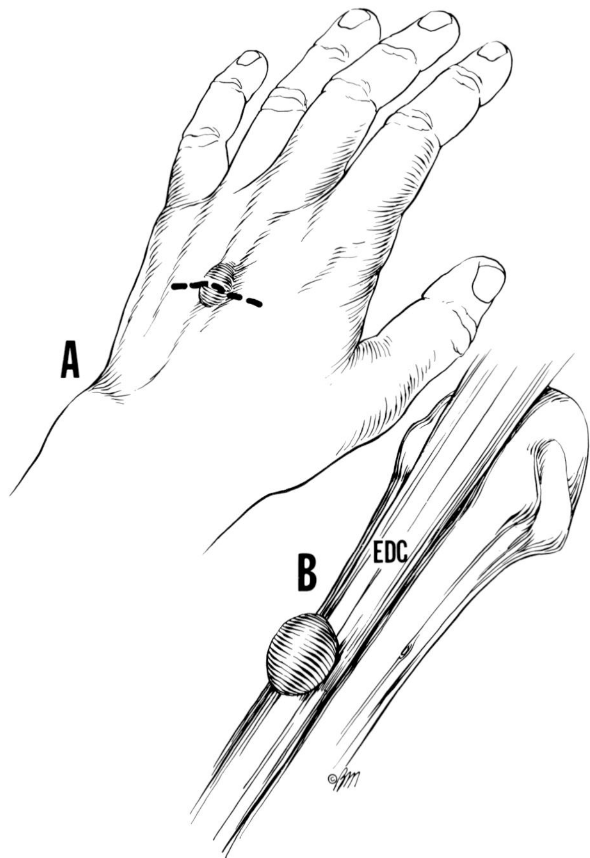

Fig. 58-23. Extensor tendon ganglion. (A) The ganglion, tendon, and overlying skin incision. (B) The ganglion in situ on the extensor tendon (*EDC*, extensor digitorum communis).

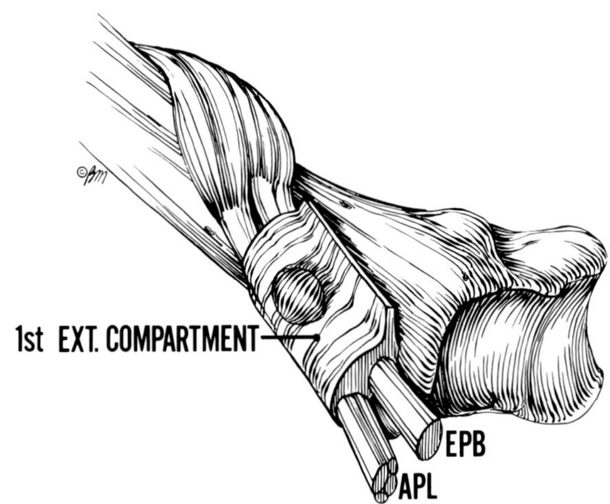

Fig. 58-24. Dorsal retinacular ganglion. The first extensor compartment with attached ganglion. A separate compartment for the extensor pollicis brevis *(EPB)* is illustrated. (*APL*, abductor pollicus longus.)

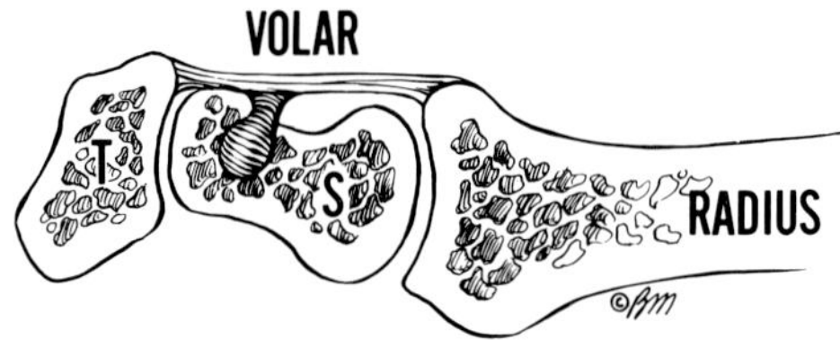

Fig. 58-25. Intraosseous ganglion of the scaphoid with articular communication. This patient complained of localized swelling, erythema, and pain, and was successfully treated with curettage and bone grafting. (*T*, trapezoid; *S*, scaphoid.)

Intraosseous Ganglions

Although they are rare and usually an incidental radiographic finding, intraosseous ganglions are being increasingly recognized as a source of wrist pain.[10,21,35,53,64,92,110] Surgical treatment is best delayed, however, until all other possible etiologic factors for the patient's discomfort have been excluded. When indicated, curettage and bone grafting will adequately treat the condition. A careful exploration of the joint at the time of surgery helps rule out other undiagnosed causes for the patient's symptoms. Communications between the joint cavity and the intraosseous cyst are inconsistently demonstrated (Fig. 58-25). The histologic features of intraosseous ganglions are identical to their soft tissue counterparts.

REFERENCES

1. Anderson CR: Longitudinal grooving of the nails caused by synovial lesions. Arch Dermatol Syphylol 55:828–830, 1947
2. Andren L, Eiken O: Arthrographic studies of wrist ganglions. J Bone Joint Surg 53A:299–302, 1971
3. Angelides AC, Wallace PF: The dorsal ganglion of the wrist: Its pathogenesis, gross and microscopic anatomy, and surgical treatment. J Hand Surg 1:228–235, 1976
4. Arner O, Lindholm A, Romanus R: Mucous cysts of the fingers, report of 26 cases. Acta Chir Scand 111:314–321, 1956
5. Backstrom CG, Linell F, Ostberg G: Cystic myxomatous adventitial degeneration of the radial artery with development of ganglion in connective tissue. Acta Chir Scand 129:447–451, 1965
6. Barnes WE, Larsen RD, Posch JL: Review of ganglia of the hand and wrist, with analysis of surgical treatment. Plast Reconstr Surg 34:570–578, 1964
7. Becker WF: Hydrocortisone therapy in ganglia. Industrial Med Surg 22:555–557, 1953
8. Blair WF, Berger RA, El-Khoury GY: Arthrotomography of the wrist: An experimental and preliminary clinical study. J Hand Surg 10A:350–359, 1985
9. Bourns HK, Sanerkin NG: Mucoid lesions ("Mucoid Cysts") of the fingers and toes. Clinical features and pathogenesis. Br J Surg 50:860–866, 1963
10. Bowers WH, Hurst LC: An intraarticular-intraosseous carpal ganglion. J Hand Surg 4:375–377, 1979
11. Brooks DM: Nerve compression by simple ganglia. J Bone Joint Surg 34B:391–400, 1952
12. Bruner JM: Treatment of "sesamoid" synovial ganglia of the hand by needle rupture. J Bone Joint Surg 45A:1689–1690, 1963

13. Burman M: Semilunar ganglion. Hand 5:256–259, 1973
14. Butler ED, Hamil JP, Seipel RS, De Lorimier AA: Tumors of the hand. Am J Surg 100:293–302, 1960
15. Carp L, Stout AP: A study of ganglion, with special reference to treatment. Surg Gynecol Obstet 47:460–468, 1928
16. Cherry JH, Ghormley RK: Bursa and ganglion. Am J Surg 52:319–330, 1941
17. Clarke WC: The pathogenesis of ganglia, with a description of the structure and development of synovial membrane. Surg Gynecol Obstet 7:56–78, 1908
18. Clay NR, Clement DA: The treatment of dorsal wrist ganglia by radical excision. J Hand Surg 13B:187–191, 1988
19. Constant E, Royer JR, Pollard RJ, Larsen RD, Posch JL: Mucous cysts of the fingers. Plast Reconstr Surg 43:241–246, 1969
20. Constantian MB, Zuelzer WA, Theogaraj SD: The dorsal ganglion with anomalous muscles. J Hand Surg 4:84–85, 1979
21. Crane AR, Scarano JJ: Synovial cysts (ganglia) of bone. J Bone Joint Surg 49A:355–361, 1967
22. Crawford GP, Taleisnik J: Rotatory subluxation of the scaphoid after excision of dorsal carpal ganglion and wrist manipulation-A case report. J Hand Surg 8:921–925, 1983
23. Croft JD, Jacox RF: Rheumatoid "ganglion" as an unusual presenting sign of rheumatoid arthritis. JAMA 203:144–146, 1968
24. Culberg G: Synovial cysts of the wrist and hand. Acta Orthop Belg 43:212–232, 1977
25. Cuono CB, Watson HK: The carpal boss: Surgical treatment and etiological considerations. Plast Reconstr Surg 63:88–93, 1979
26. Dao L: A new method of treatment of ganglions and synovial cysts. J Occup Med 6:217–220, 1964
27. Dellon AL, Seif SS: Anatomic dissections relating the posterior interosseous nerve to the carpus, and the etiology of dorsal wrist ganglion pain. J Hand Surg 3:326–332, 1978
28. DeOrsay RH, MeCray PM, Ferguson LK: Pathology and treatment of ganglion. Am J Surg 36:313–319, 1937
29. Derbyshire RC: Observations on the treatment of ganglia, with a report on hydrocortisone. Am J Surg 112:635–636, 1966
30. Doyle RW: Ganglia and superficial tumors. Practitioner 156:267–277, 1946
31. Duncan KH, Lewis RC Jr: Scapholunate instability following ganglion cyst excision. A case report. Clin Orthop 228:250–253, 1988
32. Eaton RG, Dobranski AI, Littler JW: Marginal osteophyte excision in treatment of mucous cysts. J Bone Joint Surg 55A:570–574, 1973
33. Engle RB: The treatment of myxomatous cutaneous cysts. Radiology 71:93–95, 1958
34. Esteban JM, Oertel YC, Mendoza M, Knoll SM: Fine needle aspiration in the treatment of ganglion cysts. South Med J 79:691–693, 1986
35. Feldman F, Johnson AD: Ganglia of bone: Theories, manifestations and presentations. CRC Crit Rev Clin Radiol Nucl Med 4:303–343, 1973
36. Feldman F, Singson RD, Staron RB: Magnetic resonance imaging of para-articular and ectopic ganglia. Skeletal Radiol 18:353–358, 1989
37. Fisher RH: Conservative treatment of mucous cysts. Clin Orthop 103:88, 1974
38. Flugel M, Kessler K: Follow-up of 425 patients operated for ganglion cysts. Handchir Mikrocher Plast Chir 18:47–52, 1986
39. Fowler AW: Letter. Br Med J 4:558, 1971
40. Fowler AW: Excision of ganglion (letter). Lancet 2:1389, 1973
41. Fowler AW: Ganglia (letter). Br Med J 2:1671–1672, 1977
42. Gama C: New technic for surgical treatment of the wrist ganglion. Int Surg 62:22–23, 1977
43. Gang RK, Makhlouf S: Treatment of ganglia by a thread technique. J Hand Surg 13B:184–186, 1988
44. Ghadially FN, Mehta PN: Multifunctional mesenchymal cells resembling smooth muscle cells in ganglia of the wrist. Ann Rheum Dis 30:31–42, 1971
45. Gillies RM, Burrows C: Nerve sheath ganglion of the superficial radial nerve. J Hand Surg 16B:94–95, 1991
46. Goldman L, Kitzmiller KW: Transillumination for diagnosis of mucinous pseudocysts of the finger (letter). Arch Dermatol 109:576, 1974
47. Gould EP: Treatment of tenosynovitis and ganglion. Br Med J 2:415–416, 1938
48. Grange WJ: Subperiosteal ganglia. J Bone Joint Surg 60B:124–125, 1978
49. Gross RE: Recurring myxomatous cutaneous cysts of the fingers and toes. Surg Gynecol Obstet 65:289–302, 1937
50. Gunther SF: Dorsal wrist pain and the occult scapholunate ganglion. J Hand Surg 10A:697–703, 1985
51. Hand BH, Patey DH: The treatment of ganglion of the wrist. Practitioner 169:195–197, 1952
52. Harvey FJ, Bosanquet JS: Carpal tunnel syndrome caused by a simple ganglion. Hand 13:164–166, 1981
53. Helal B, Vernon-Roberts B: Intra-osseous ganglion of the pisiform bone. Hand 8:150–154, 1976
54. Holm PCA, Pandey SD: Treatment of ganglia of the hand and wrist with aspiration and injection of hydrocortisone. Hand 5:63–68, 1973
55. Hvid-Hansen O: On the treatment of ganglia. Acta Chir Scand 136:471–476, 1970
56. Isaacson NH, McCarty D: Recurring myxomatous cutaneous cyst. Surgery 35:621–623, 1954
57. Iveson JMI, Hill AGS, Wright V: Wrist cysts and fistulae. An arthrographic study of the rheumatoid wrist. Ann Rheum Dis 34:388–394, 1975
58. Jacox HW, Freedman LJ: The roentgen treatment of myxomatous cutaneous cysts. Radiology 36:695–699, 1941
59. Janzon L, Niechajev IA: Wrist ganglia. Incidence and recurrence rate after operation. Scand J Plast Reconstr Surg 15:53–56, 1981
60. Jayson MIV, Dickson AStJ: Valvular mechanism in juxta-articular cysts. Ann Rheum Dis 29:415–420, 1970
61. Jensen DR: Ganglia and synovial cysts, their pathogeneses and treatment. Ann Surg 105:592–601, 1937
62. Johnson WC, Graham JH, Helwig EB: Cutaneous myxoid cyst. A clinicopathological and histochemical study. JAMA 191:15–20, 1965
63. Jordan HM: Ganglion: Twenty-five consecutive cases successfully treated. Lancet 2:242–245, 1893
64. Kenan S, Robin GC, Floman Y: Traumatic intraosseous ganglion. A case report. Bull Hosp Joint Dis Orthop Inst 44:82–85, 1984
65. Kerrigan JJ, Bertoni JM, Jaeger SH: Ganglion cysts and carpal tunnel syndrome. J Hand Surg 13A:763–765, 1988
66. King ESJ: Concerning the pathology of tumors of tendon sheaths. Br J Surg 18:594–617, 1931
67. King ESJ: The pathology of ganglion. Aust NZ J Surg 1:367–381, 1932
68. King ESJ: Mucous cysts of the fingers. Aust NZ J Surg 21:121–129, 1951
69. Kleinert HE, Kutz JE, Fishman JH, McCraw LH: Etiology and treatment of the so-called mucous cyst of the finger. J Bone Joint Surg 54A:1455–1458, 1972

70. Kuschner SH, Gelberman RH, Jennings C: Ulnar nerve compression at the wrist. J Hand Surg 13A:577–580, 1988
71. Lewis OJ, Hamshere RJ, Bucknill TM: The anatomy of the wrist joint. J Anat 106:539–552, 1970
72. Linsheid RL, Dobyns JH, Beabout JW, Bryan RS: Traumatic instability of the wrist. J Bone Joint Surg 54A:1612–1632, 1972
73. Lister GD, Smith RR: Protection of the radial artery in resection of adherent ganglions of the wrist. Plast Reconstr Surg 61:127–129, 1978
74. Loder RT, Robinson JH, Jackson WT, Allen DJ: A surface ultrastructure study of ganglia and digital mucous cysts. J Hand Surg 13A:758–762, 1988
75. Lucas GL: An intratendinous cyst in the extensor digitorum brevis manus tendon. J Hand Surg 4:176–177, 1979
76. Lucas GL: Irritative neuritis of the dorsal sensory branch of the ulnar nerve from underlying ganglion. Clin Orthop 186:216–219, 1984
77. Lyle FM: Radiation treatment of ganglia of the wrist and hand. J Bone Joint Surg 23:162–163, 1941
78. MacCollum MS: Dorsal wrist ganglions in children. J Hand Surg 2:325, 1977
79. Mackie IG, Howard CB, Wilkins P: The dangers of sclerotherapy in the treatment of ganglia. J Hand Surg 9B:181–184, 1984
80. MacKinnon AE, Azmy A: Active treatment of ganglia in children. Postgrad Med J 53:378–381, 1977
81. Matthews P: Ganglia of the flexor tendon sheaths in the hand. J Bone Joint Surg 55B:612–617, 1973
82. McCollam SM, Corley FG, Green DP: Posterior interosseous nerve palsy caused by ganglions of the proximal radioulnar joint. J Hand Surg 13A:725–728, 1988
83. McDowell CL, Henceroth WD: Compression of the ulnar nerve in the hand by a ganglion. J Bone Joint Surg 59A:980, 1977
84. McEvedy BV: The simple ganglion. A review of modes of treatment and an explanation of the frequent failures of surgery. Lancet 266:135–136, 1954
85. McEvedy BV: Simple ganglia. Br J Surg 49:585–594, 1962
86. McEvedy P: Treatment of the simple ganglion by injections. Lancet 2:902–903, 1930
87. Morris CC, Godman GC: Production of acid mucopolysaccharides by fibroblasts in cell cultures. Nature 188:407–409, 1960
88. Nelson CL, Sawmiller S, Phalen GS: Ganglions of the wrist and hand. J Bone Joint Surg 54A:1459–1464, 1972
89. Newmeyer WL, Kilgore ES Jr, Graham WP III: Mucous cysts: The dorsal distal interphalangeal joint ganglion. Plast Reconstr Surg 53:313–315, 1974
90. Ogino T, Minami A, Fukada K, Sakuma T, Kato H: The dorsal occult ganglion of the wrist and ultrasonography. J Hand Surg 13B:181–183, 1988
91. Ogino T, Minami A, Kato H: Diagnosis of radial nerve palsy caused by ganglion with use of different imaging techniques. J Hand Surg 16A:230–235, 1991
92. Pellegrino EA Jr, Olson JR: Bilateral carpal lunate ganglia. Clin Orthop 87:225–227, 1972
93. Posch JL: Tumors of the hand. J Bone Joint Surg 38A:517–540, 1956
94. Psaila JV, Mansel RE: The surface ultra-structure of ganglia. J Bone Joint Surg 60B:228–233, 1978
95. Reef TC, Brestin SG: The extensor digitorum brevis manus and its clinical significance. J Bone Joint Surg 57A:704–706, 1975
96. Reicher MA, Kellerhouse LE: MRI of the Wrist and Hand. Raven Press, New York, 1990
97. Rich RE: Hydrocortisone in the treatment of ganglia. J Med Soc NJ 52:260–261, 1955
98. Richman JA, Gelberman RH, Engber WD, Salamon PB, Bean DJ: Ganglions of the wrist and digits: Results of treatment by aspiration and cyst wall puncture. J Hand Surg 12A:1041–1043, 1987
99. Ronchese F: Treatment of myxoid cyst with flurandrenolone tape. RI Med J 57:154–155, 1974
100. Rosson JW, Walker G: The natural history of ganglia in children. J Bone Joint Surg 71B:707–708, 1989
101. Rudavsky AZ, Moss CM, Strauch B: Scintiangiographic demonstration of bleeding into a wrist ganglion. Hand 9:28–30, 1977
102. Rutherford R: Treatment of ganglion. Br Med J 2:590, 1938
103. Sames CP: The simple ganglion (letter). Lancet 266:317, 1954
104. Sanders WE: The occult dorsal carpal ganglion. J Hand Surg 10B:257–260, 1985
105. Sarma PJ: The injection treatment of ganglions and bursae. Indications and limitations. Surg Clin North Am 20:135–140, 1940
106. Sarpyener MA, Ozurumez O, Seyhan F: Multiple ganglions of the tendon sheaths. J Bone Joint Surg 50A:985–990, 1968
107. Savastano AA: The use of hydrocortisone in office practice. RI Med J 41:80–89, 1958
108. Schajowicz F, Sainz MC, Slullitel JA: Juxta-articular bone cysts (Intra-osseous ganglia). J Bone Joint Surg 61B:107–116, 1979
109. Seddon HJ: Carpal ganglion as a cause of paralysis of the deep branch of the ulnar nerve. J Bone Joint Surg 34B:386–390, 1952
110. Sim FH, Dahlin DC: Ganglion cysts of bone. Mayo Clin Proc 46:484–488, 1971
111. Smith EB, Skipworth GB, VanderPloeg DE: Longitudinal grooving of nails due to synovial cysts. Arch Dermatol 89:364–366, 1964
112. Soren A: Pathogenesis and treatment of ganglion. Clin Orthop 48:173–179, 1966
113. Soren A: Pathogenesis, clinic, and treatment of ganglion. Arch Orthop Traumatic Surg 99:247–252, 1982
114. Stith JS, Browne PA: Extensor digitorum brevis manus. Hand 11:217–223, 1979
115. Subin GD, Mallon WJ, Urbaniak JR: Diagnosis of ganglion in Guyon's canal by magnetic resonance imaging. J Hand Surg 14A:640–643, 1989
116. Tehranzadeh J, Labosky DA, Gabriele OF: Ganglion cysts and tear of triangular fibrocartilages of both wrists in a cheerleader. Am J Sports Med 11:357–359, 1983
117. Thomson A: Case of ganglion with observations upon their method of origin. Rep Edinb Hosp 5:354, 1898
118. Tophøj K, Henriques U: Ganglion of the wrist—A structure developed from the joint. A histological study with serial sections. Acta Orthop Scand 42:244–250, 1971
119. Watson HK, Rogers WD, Ashmead D IV: Reevaluation of the cause of the wrist ganglion. J Hand Surg 14A:812–817, 1989
120. Weiss KL, Beltran J, Lubbers LM: High-field M.R. surface-coil imaging of the hand and wrist. Part II. Pathologic correlations and clinical relevance. Radiology 160:147–152, 1986
121. Woodburne AR: Myxomatous degeneration cysts of skin and subcutaneous tissues. Arch Dermatol Syphylol 56:407–418, 1947
122. Young SC, Freiberg A: A case of an intratendinous ganglion. J Hand Surg 10A:723–724, 1985
123. Zachariae L, Vibe-Hansen H: Ganglia: Recurrence rate elucidated by a follow-up of 347 operative cases. Acta Chir Scand 139:625–628, 1973
124. Zubowicz VN, Ishii CH: Management of ganglion cysts of the hand by simple aspiration. J Hand Surg 12A:618–620, 1987

59

Skin Tumors

Earl J. Fleegler

Tumors involving the skin of the upper extremity are not unusual, but they are frequently neglected by the patient and, on occasion, not appreciated by physicians. Such neoplasms may stop growing before becoming large enough to produce a clinical problem. Others, however, because of size or location, may interfere with gloves, rings, and movement of the fingers. They may produce pain when in confined areas (such as under the fingernail), and/or come to the patient's attention because of deformity. These tumors are often benign, but can be insidious in their development. A variety of neoplasms that produce great difficulty in diagnosis has been encountered under the nail area. However, because these tumors are frequently visible, the alert physician has an opportunity to diagnose and treat them at a relatively early stage. Usually this requires a biopsy in addition to the patient's history and physical examination. Beyond the deforming, annoying, and functionally disturbing nature of some of these tumors, on occasion patients will present with malignant varieties. As in other areas, this last group may produce local destruction, e.g., the basal cell carcinoma, or may be the cutaneous manifestation of other problems, e.g., Kaposi's sarcoma and metastatic tumors. Certain malignancies may tend to recur after what appears to be adequate excision, e.g., the sweat gland tumors,[52] or may even metastasize and threaten limb and life.

In the upper extremity we are fortunate in being able to recognize tumors associated with or predisposing to malignant change, such as the cutaneous horn, possibly the keratoacanthoma, the actinic or solar keratosis, and early in-situ squamous cell carcinomas and melanomas (this is not intended to be a complete list).[21] These factors, coupled with a growing body of knowledge, make it possible for us to diagnose and treat even the more malignant, life-threatening tumors at an earlier stage. It is the opinion of this author that the physician adequately armed with information about these worrisome masses will not fail to adequately biopsy the tumors, even though this produces potential deformity. Those having adequate experience with the disciplines of hand surgery, as well as tumor surgery, will be able to keep such deformity to a minimum. Therefore the introduction to this area will review some pertinent anatomic points.

ANATOMY

Figure 59-1 schematically points out the variety of anatomic architecture that the surgeon encounters in attempting to understand the patient's problem as well as examine and biopsy the lesion. Appreciation of this anatomy may help the surgeon maintain a functioning extremity after appropriate tumor surgery. This information is also necessary in obtaining safe exposure and wound coverage. Emphasis needs to be placed on the complex anatomy of the eponychial fold (Fig. 59-2), where epidermis exists not only on the dorsal exposed skin, but also curves under the fold and proximally. The proximal extent of the major nail growth area—matrix—is quite close to other important anatomic structures (extensor tendon and joint).[53] Figure 59-1 emphasizes the marked difference in the thickness of the epidermis between the thick, protective palmar skin that must resist considerable abrasive and other assaults, and the thinner, more pliable extensor surface skin. The latter contains special structures, such as sebaceous glands and hair follicles, that may be the site of origin from which tumors can grow. Pigment-producing cells—melanocytes—are found in the basal layer of the epidermis, along with the immature keratinocytes that will ultimately mature into the more superficial areas of the epidermis and protective cornified outer layer.

The thick layer subjacent to the epidermis, between it and the subcutaneous fat, is the dermis. This contains skin appendages such as hair follicles and sebaceous glands in the dorsal skin and eccrine sweat glands in the palmar skin. Divided into a superficial, papillary dermis, which projects into the overlying epidermal ridges, and a deeper, reticular dermis that lies over the subcutaneous fat, this area also includes the termina-

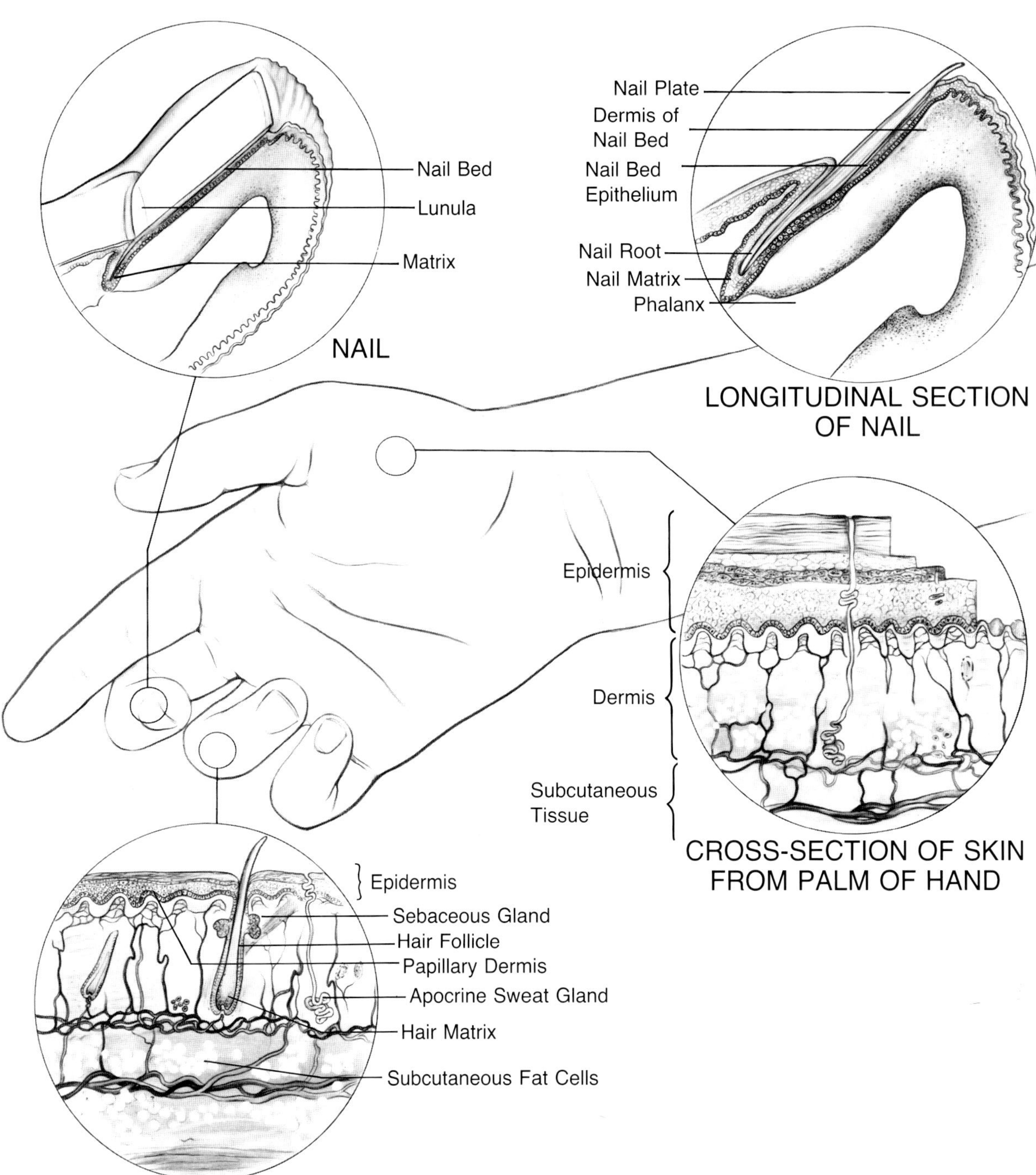

Fig. 59-1. Histologic anatomy of the skin, showing the differences between thick palmar skin and thin skin of the dorsum of the hand.

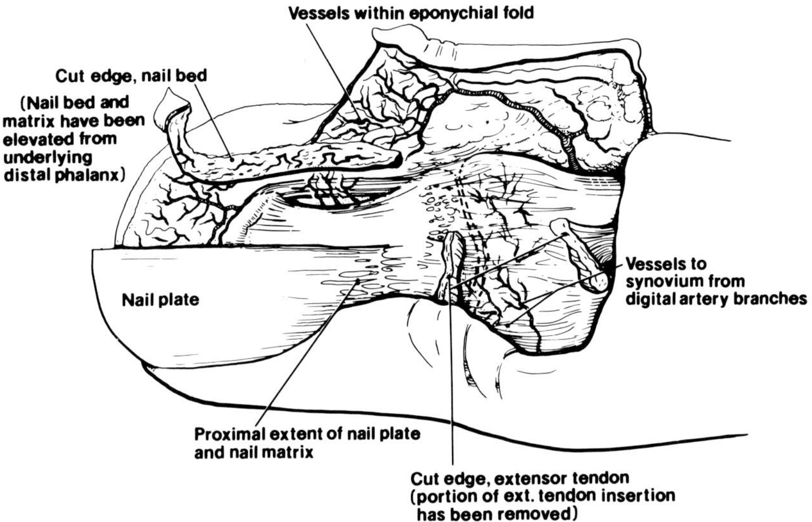

Fig. 59-2. The complex anatomy around the eponychial fold. (Drawing made through operating microscope at 4 × power by Rodney Green, M.D.)

tion of sensory nerve end organs, blood vessels, and lymphatics.[36] Palmar lymphatics not only proceed proximally, deeply with the venous network, but also into the digital web areas and onto the dorsum of the hand. Lymph node drainage areas include the epitrochlear nodes in the vicinity of the medial epicondyle of the humerus, along the cephalic venous drainage in the deltopectoral area, and channels that are associated with major vascular supply to the limb into the axillary area.[28] Squamous cell carcinoma and melanoma are among the more common malignancies that can spread to such regional nodes.

DIFFERENTIAL DIAGNOSIS

Reference to Table 59-1 reminds us of some of the many different types of masses that must be considered in our review of patients' problems.

BENIGN TUMORS OF THE SKIN

Cutaneous Horns

Cutaneous horns (Fig. 59-3) not only bother the patient, are unsightly, and may interfere with hand function, but, on biopsy, may be found to have a variety of skin tumors near their base. While some of these are benign, warty, or keratotic lesions, squamous cell carcinoma may also be found.[4]

Cysts

Some tumors that appear to involve the skin are in fact cysts that originate from underlying anatomic structures. These may produce contour deformities, interfere with hand function because of their physical size or joint involvement, or cause discomfort. Ganglions arising from joints in the hand, ligamentous structures, or the sheaths about tendons can mimic hand tumors. Their smooth, firm, characteristic findings on examination usually produce accurate clinical impressions for the experienced examiner. Those cystic lesions that

Table 59-1. A Partial List of Upper Extremity Tumors Involving the Skin

Benign	Malignant
1. Cysts[a]	1. Basal cell carcinoma
Inclusion cyst	2. Dermatofibrosarcoma
Ganglion	3. Fibrosarcoma
2. Cutaneous horn	4. Kaposi's sarcoma
3. Dermatofibroma	5. Melanoma
4. Dupuytren's fasciitis[a]	6. Metastatic tumors
5. Fibroma	7. Squamous cell carcinoma
6. Giant cell tumor[b]	8. Sweat gland carcinoma
7. Glomus tumor	
8. Gout[a]	
9. Granuloma[a]	
10. Hemangioma	
11. Keratoses	
Actinic	
Seborrheic	
12. Keratoacanthoma[c]	
13. Lipoma	
14. Lymphangioma	
15. Neurofibroma	
16. Nevi	
17. Nodular fasciitis[a]	
18. Sweat gland tumors	

[a] Mass, nontumor
[b] ?Tumor.
[c] Some question exists as to pattern of behavior.

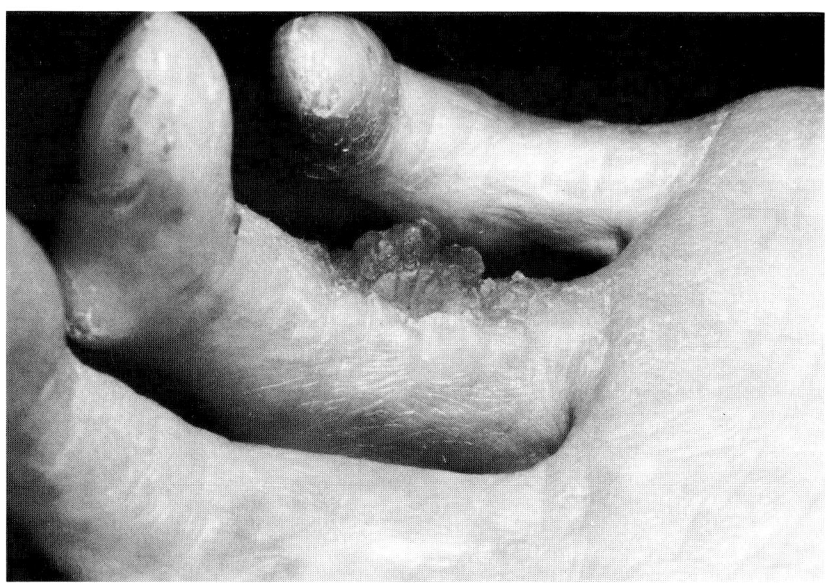

Fig. 59-3. A cutaneous horn arising from an area of irradiated skin.

arise within the skin, e.g., inclusion cysts, can produce similar complaints and physical findings, and are also quite common.[26] Fingertips, especially the tactile surfaces of the hand, and even subungual areas, are locations to keep in mind in the assessment and understanding of these benign masses. Discomfort, deformity, and/or difficulty in diagnosis may lead to the need for a biopsy.

Giant Cell Tumor of Tendon Sheath

Other tumors and tumor-like conditions can also begin deep to the skin, but appear to involve it. The giant cell tumor of tendon sheath, which may arise from a joint, is quite common, as are fibrous neoplasms.[18,26] Although these are benign conditions, their correct differential diagnosis and removal is important because of their tendency to recur and involve more extensive areas of the hand.[6]

Glomus Tumors

Glomus tumors arising from the pericytes in the fingertip or subungual areas that contain arteriovenous communications can produce asymptomatic or painful masses in the distal finger areas. Excisional biopsy usually establishes the diagnosis and is adequate treatment[49] (Fig. 59-4) (see also Chapter 34).

Fibrous Tumors

Fibrous tumors can occur throughout the palm and digits, produce contour deformities that appear to involve the skin, and therefore, enter into the differential diagnosis of tumors of the skin of the upper extremity. These can be especially difficult to evaluate, biopsy, and adequately treat. However, biopsy information is needed to make the correct diagnosis and help one decide whether or not additional patient work-up and surgical treatment are necessary. Figure 59-5 illustrates an enlarging subungual, firm mass of 4 years' duration that was found to be a benign fibroma. Another slow-growing mass (Fig. 59-6), which ultimately came to my attention because of the significant deformity, was found to be a fibrosarcoma. Although fibrosarcomas are considered by some authors to originate more commonly from deep fascial structures, they may also occur in the subcutaneous tissues. As shown in Figure 59-6, they may even develop in the subungual areas. Perhaps their survival rate will be found to be higher when present in one of these more obvious anatomic locations. If primary surgical treatment does not control these tumors, early recurrence will frequently be seen. On occasion, however, recurrence may not come to one's attention until many years later. Fibrosarcomas generally metastasize via the hematogenous route. The lung is the most common site for distant metastatic disease.[33] Although it would be less common to find them metastasizing to regional lymphatics, such areas must be evaluated in the work-up of patients.[18,23] Surgical treatment is still considered the first line of therapy.[22]

Dermatofibroma

Dermatofibroma, usually a small fibrous tissue tumor that involves the skin, is common, and enters into the differential diagnosis between many of the lesions under consideration here, including fibrosarcoma and melanoma.[18,23]

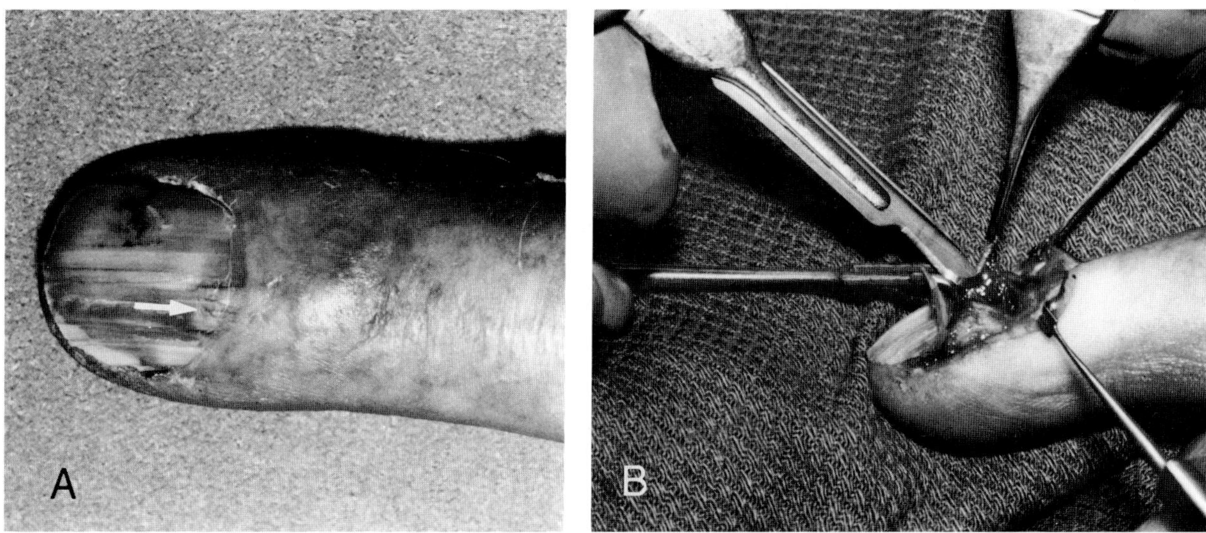

Fig. 59-4. (A) A glomus tumor elevating the subungual area and deforming the eponychial fold and nail plate. The finger also exhibits postradiation skin atrophy. (B) A longitudinal incision "opens" the nail fold skin (held by small retractors), allowing the nail plate to be elevated (and later replaced) to expose the tumor, which is pointed out by the scalpel blade.

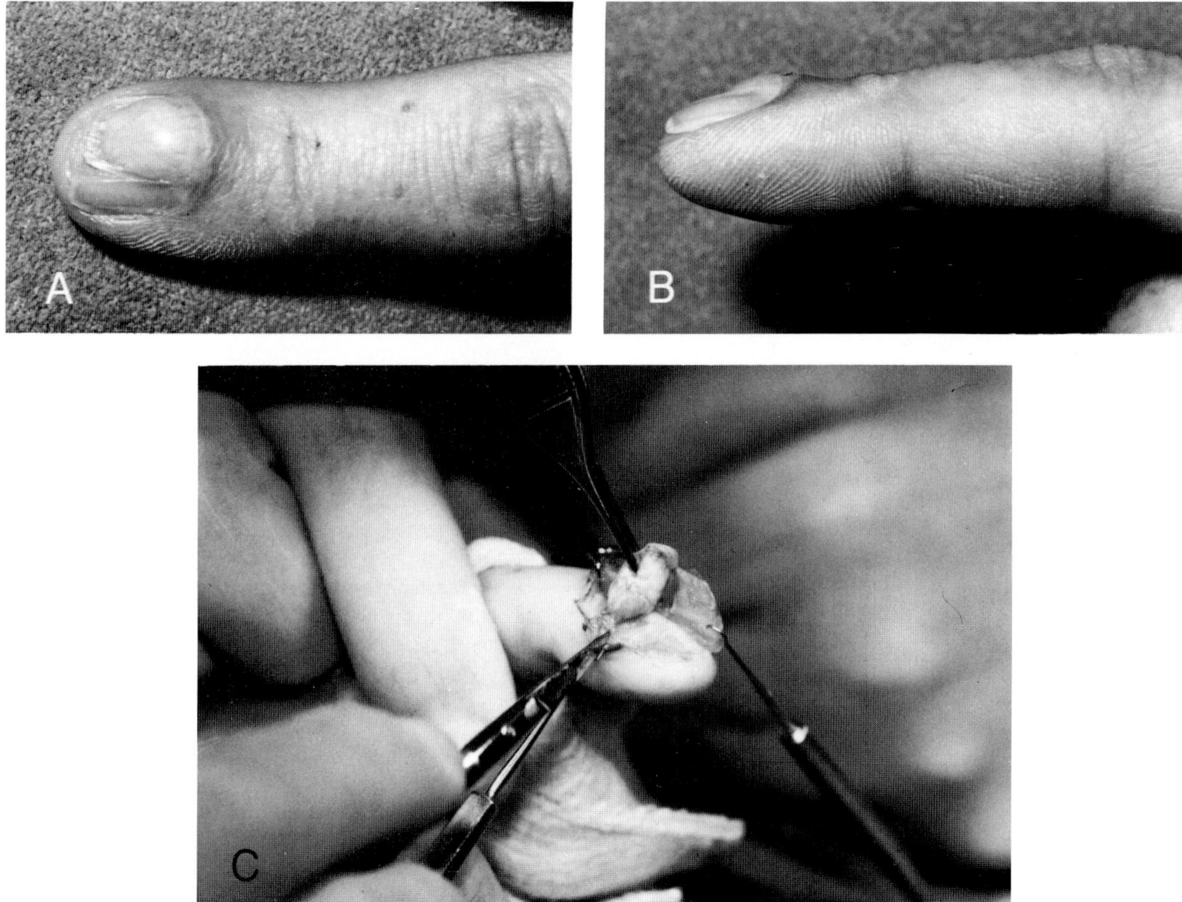

Fig. 59-5. (A) Nail plate deformity in a 28-year-old woman with a slowly enlarging subungual mass. (B) Note secondary elevation of the eponychial fold. (C) An incision was made to elevate the eponychial fold and nail plate to permit biopsy. The nail plate was then used as a "stent" under the eponychial fold to help prevent adhesions between the skin of the fold and the nail bed.

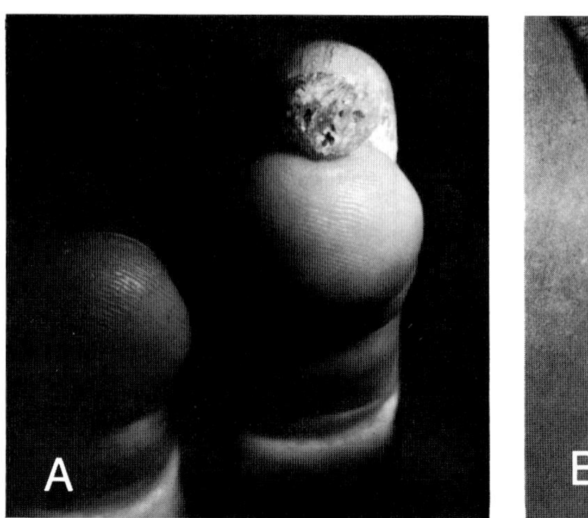

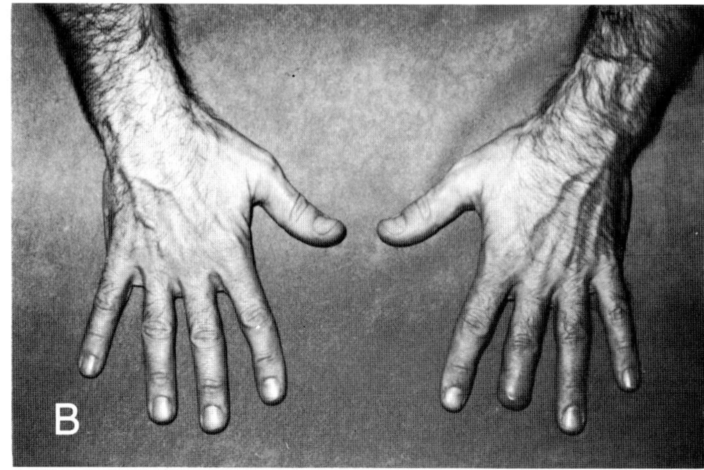

Fig. 59-6. **(A)** A 48-year-old man presented with this unusually large nail deformity. **(B)** Biopsy revealed this to be a fibrosarcoma, and distal phalanx amputation was carried out. There was no evidence of regional or systemic spread of this tumor preoperatively or at follow-up more than 4 years later.

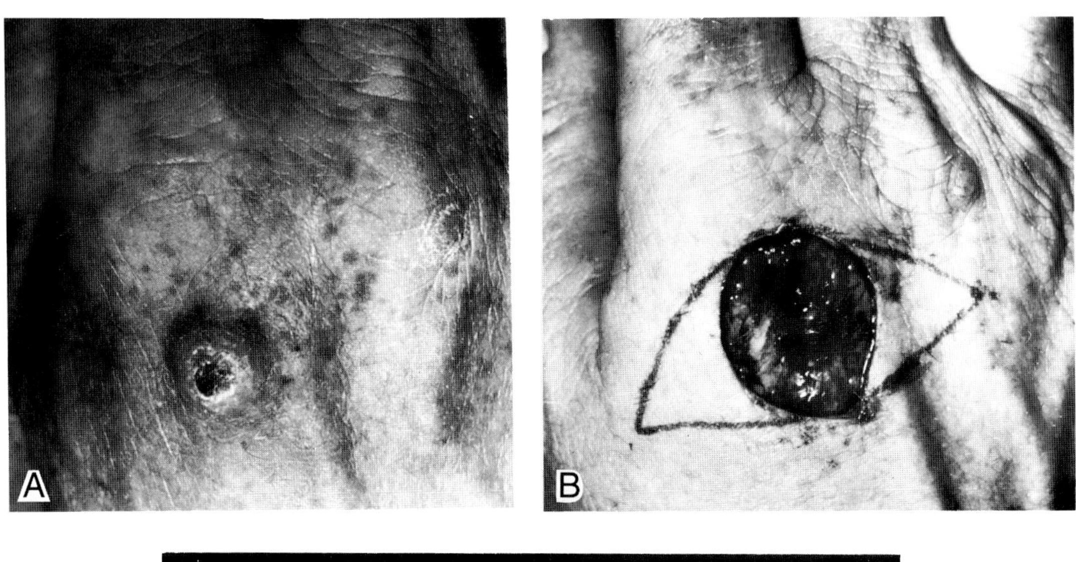

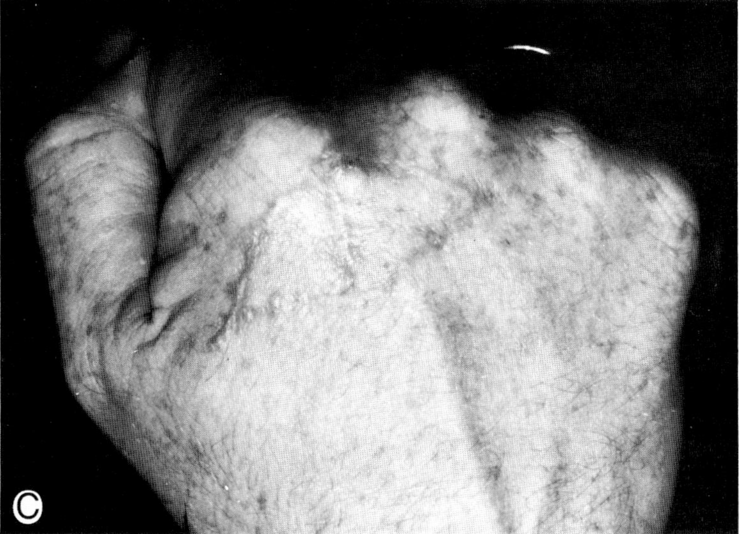

Fig. 59-7. Keratoacanthoma. **(A)** A round, elevated nodular lesion with a central crater. **(B&C)** A biopsy was performed to differentiate this persistent lesion from squamous cell carcinoma (see Fig. 59-9). The V-Y advancement flap may be used for coverage of such defects.

Other Tumors

Clinically, other benign lesions must be understood in order to differentiate them from malignant tumors. Pyogenic granuloma, dermatofibroma, glomus tumor, hemangioma, and a variety of nevi enter into the differential diagnosis of melanoma.[25] Keratoacanthoma (Fig. 59-7) which is still a debated lesion, as well as various keratoses, can resemble or even be a premalignant precursor of squamous cell carcinoma.

Keratoacanthoma

The keratoacanthoma (KA) most commonly presents as an elevated, dimpled, or ulcerated mass that contains a plug of keratin (Fig. 59-7). In my opinion, this is still not a well-understood lesion, but the literature and personal experience lead me to believe that if the clinical and histological appearance are those of the classic KA, then the lesion probably will behave in a benign fashion. However, it may be difficult to distinguish this tumor from a squamous cell carcinoma. The classic description of KA describes its origin as a papular mass that increases in size relatively rapidly (over weeks) and develops a central keratin plug. The tumor is symmetrical and is supposed to spontaneously resolve over months to form a scarred base. However, because of the concerns described above, it has been my practice to carry out excisional biopsy of the mass. When surgical planning and frozen section evaluation reveal that it is a benign tumor and contains an adequate margin of normal tissue around it to feel that it is completely excised, reconstruction can then be done with local flaps or skin graft. In the subungual area, keratoacanthoma again requires biopsy confirmation. It is my recommendation that the area be completely ablated. Evidence is developing in the literature that indicates this may be carried out by either curettage or excision with careful follow-up.[27]

Arsenical Keratoses, Solar Keratoses, and Radiation Injury

Arsenical keratoses (Fig. 59-8), occasionally still seen on the palmar aspects of the hands and plantar surfaces of the feet as well as other areas of the skin, and solar keratoses are premalignant lesions, the eradication of which may prevent a more serious problem. Radiation skin injury (Fig. 59-9) is an insidious, precancerous pathologic alteration that may involve extensive areas of tissue and be difficult to treat. The depth of these lesions is frequently greater than is clinically apparent.

Sweat Gland Tumors

Tumors arising from sweat glands (Fig. 59-10) may be confused with giant cell tumors (Fig. 59-11) that have arisen more deeply and involve the overlying tissues. Both of these lesions may recur locally and involve greater areas of tissue with each recurrence. Surgical treatment must be combined with careful histologic examination in an effort to ascertain whether or not margins of the excised specimen are involved by tumor cells.[52]

MALIGNANT TUMORS OF THE SKIN

The differential diagnosis of skin tumors is frequently a difficult challenge. Since few surgeons have extensive experience with malignant neoplasms of the skin of the hand, it is valuable to be able to recognize serious tumors that can produce metastasis and even death. Recognition of malignant skin neoplasms is the first step, but it is then necessary for adequate resection to be carried out. This in turn creates special challenges in reconstruction in order to minimize deformity and regain as much function as possible.

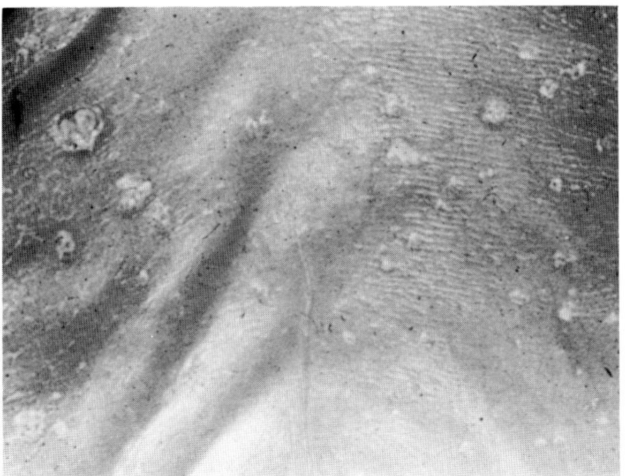

Fig. 59-8. Arsenical keratoses. (Courtesy of Wilma Bergfeld, M.D., Cleveland, Ohio.)

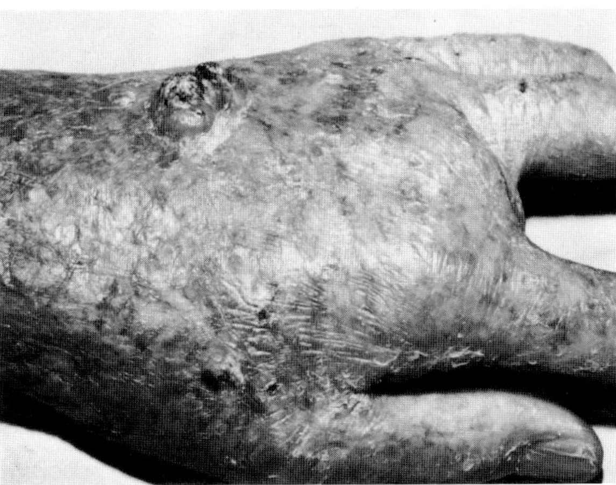

Fig. 59-9. Squamous cell carcinoma arising in an area of radiodermatitis.

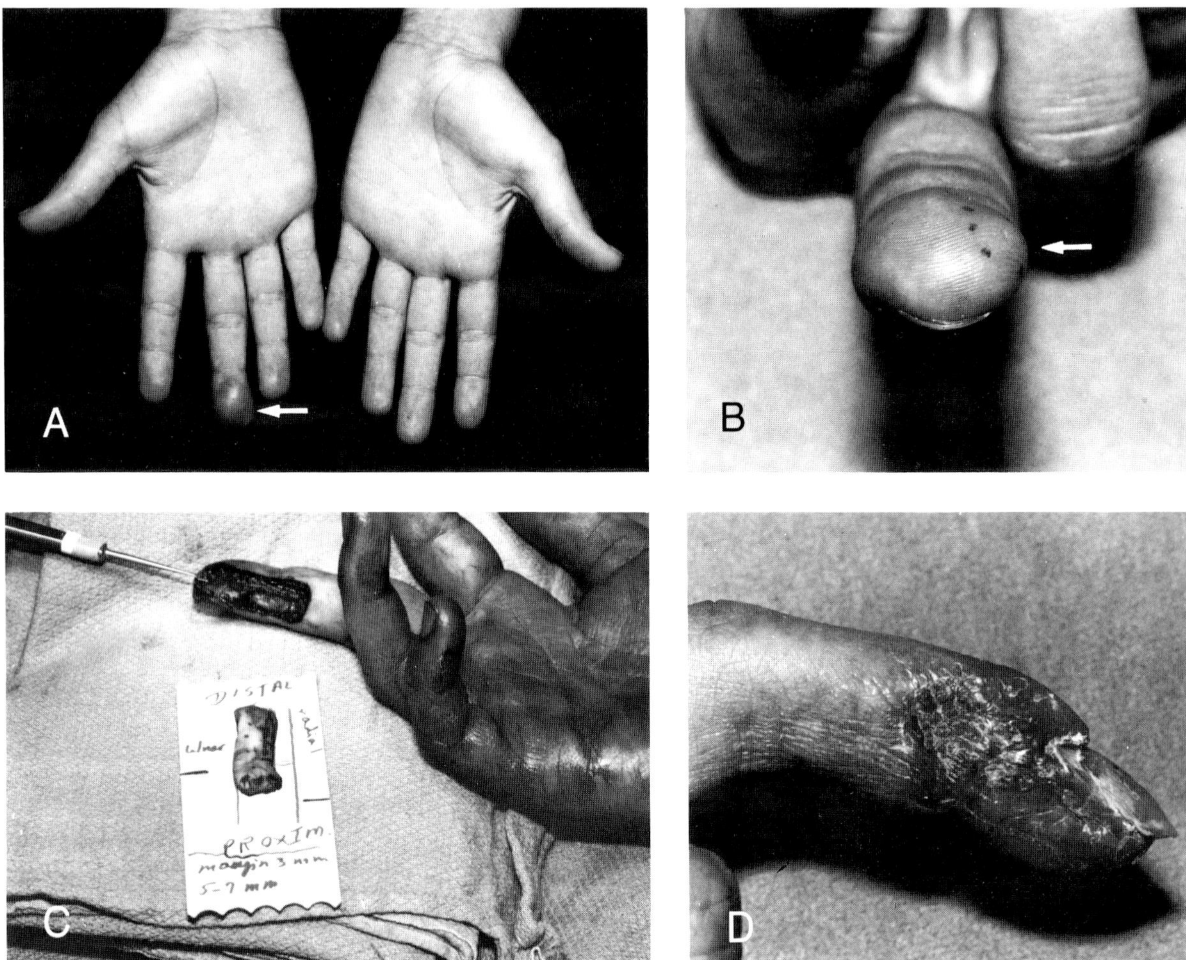

Fig. 59-10. **(A)** A mass arising from the pulp area in the right middle finger *(arrow)* of a 10-year-old girl. **(B)** Recurrence of the tumor was noted approximately 2 years postoperatively. **(C)** After biopsy of presumed recurrent giant cell tumor, the diagnosis of benign sweat gland tumor was made. The biopsy showed involved margins, and reexcision included the surrounding skin and underlying collateral ligament. **(D)** Early postoperative appearance showing split-thickness skin graft.

Malignant tumors arising from the skin of the upper extremity may cause a variety of problems, including local tissue destruction, difficulty in differential diagnosis, metastasis, and even death of the patient. Evaluation of these tumors requires a careful history, physical examination, routine x-ray studies of the involved areas and chest, possible computed tomography or magnetic resonance imaging scans, and evaluation of other possibly related anatomy. Laboratory evaluation should include routine studies, calcium, alkaline phosphatase, and enzymes reflecting possible bone and/or liver involvement. Appropriate isotope studies may also be indicated.

Recognition at an early stage of development with adequate ablation of the tumor and reconstruction of the area offers the clinician an opportunity to achieve an excellent result, frequently with minimal disfigurement. If this early opportunity is lost, the surgeon is faced with increasingly objectionable choices that may result in loss of form and function. Most physicians and patients, even in dealing with later stages of malignancy, accept the necessary disfigurement in order to avoid the less desirable outcome.

Basal Cell Carcinoma

Although basal cell carcinoma is one of the less frequent malignancies of the hand, these potentially destructive, usually nonmetastasizing tumors do occasionally occur in middle-aged and older adults (Fig. 59-12A). These are perhaps seen even more frequently in radiation-damaged skin than in areas without this preexisting alteration. Skin with radiation damage has been associated with other tumors as well, including squamous cell carcinoma and underlying secondary malignancies, including sarcomas of various tissue origins.

Physical characteristics of basal cell carcinoma, although not always specific, include erythematous changes of the skin with

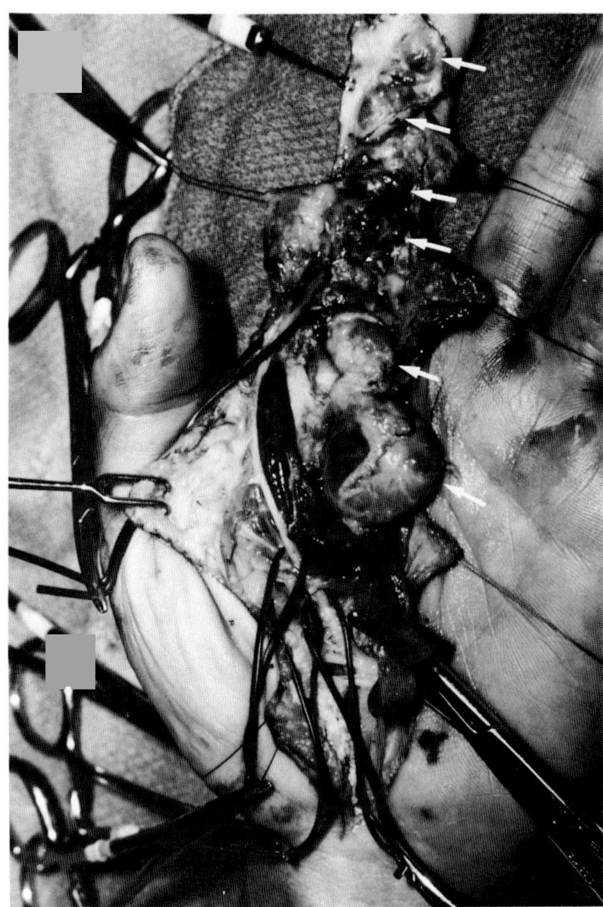

Fig. 59-11. Extensive recurrence of giant cell tumor throughout the index finger is seen in this operative photograph. Arrows point out recurrent tumor.

or without ulceration. On occasion, a raised, pearly edge may also be present.

If treatment is delayed, significant destruction of the skin and its adjacent structures can result. Adequate treatment principles include ascertaining that the margins of resection are free of tumor. Careful preoperative planning of incisions is helpful in ensuring tumor-free margins (Fig. 59-12B). Anatomic orientation of the specimen on a diagram (Fig. 59-12C) helps not only the surgeon, but also the pathologist in ascertaining areas where excision has been inadequate and additional therapy may be needed. Prior to definitive treatment, diagnosis should be established either by incisional or excisional (depending upon size and adjacent structures) biopsy. I recommend following the usual principles of tumor surgery, which include changing of instruments, drapes, gown, and gloves after the ablative phase of the operation. Copious irrigation of wounds is helpful in reducing contamination of the area of excision or remote sites (other concurrent surgical areas) during such surgery. It is emphasized that early treatment of basal cell carcinoma provides the surgeon with an opportunity to achieve a cure and still preserve hand function.

Squamous Cell Carcinoma

Comparison of Figures 59-7 and 59-9 emphasizes the clinical difficulty in diagnosis of squamous cell carcinoma. This tumor, which is one of the most frequent hand malignancies encountered, may range in size from a small, slow-growing lesion (Fig. 59-13) to a huge, ulcerated lesion such as that seen in Figure 59-14. These are malignant tumors with the capacity to metastasize and kill the patient. Therefore, in addition to a history and physical examination it is mandatory to evaluate regional lymphatic drainage. The first avenue of spread from such squamous cell carcinomata, after local extension, is usually to regional lymphatics. Premalignant lesions, e.g., solar keratoses and arsenical keratoses, may be present for a considerable length of time prior to development of malignancy. Indeed, Bowen's disease (carcinoma in situ) (Fig. 59-15), an early form of squamous cell carcinoma that does not yet invade, provides a good opportunity for a cure by excision with margins of normal tissue. The diagnosis of Bowen's disease should alert the clinician to the possibility of underlying malignancies. Magnification is helpful in assessing the advancing edges of this and other tumors at the time of surgical planning.[5]

In a patient with extensive radiodermatitis, such as that shown in Figure 59-9, complete excision of the involved area may be unrealistic. In such patients, reconstruction of the area of ablation of the squamous cell carcinoma can be accomplished with a skin graft. Careful follow-up is mandatory, since new malignant tumors may arise in the remaining areas of radiation damage.

More localized squamous cell carcinomas arising in the subungual areas may be satisfactorily treated with appropriate levels of amputation. For example, the tumor in the fingernail area of a 93-year-old man shown in Figure 59-16 was treated by an amputation at the middle phalanx level. Very small early lesions may occasionally be treated by wide excision, e.g., nail bed and matrix and contiguous areas. However, amputation that provides adequate tumor-free margins (as determined by histopathology) is more frequently required.

The differential diagnosis of nail bed and nail area lesions can be quite challenging. Squamous cell carcinoma of the nail bed may involve contiguous structures, including the underlying bone. Biopsy-proven squamous cell carcinoma of this area frequently requires distal phalangeal amputation.[10] Recent study of our patients with subungual squamous cell carcinomas revealed that some of these are more appropriately reclassified as keratoacanthomas. While some keratoacanthomas will respond to local destructive measures, such as curettage, careful long-term follow-up is mandatory to be certain that one is not dealing with a recurrent benign lesion or even a squamous cell carcinoma. Although metastasis from these fingernail area squamous cell carcinomas is rare, it can occur.

Other areas of the hand involved by squamous cell carcinomas may provide the opportunity for wide excision of the primary tumor, maintaining surgical margins of approximately 2 cm or more of normal tissue with the tumor (see Fig. 59-14). It is difficult to be dogmatic regarding a precise margin of normal tissue to be included around a particular malignancy. This dilemma exists because of the irregular nature of the advancing edge of a malignant tumor. Histopathologic examina-

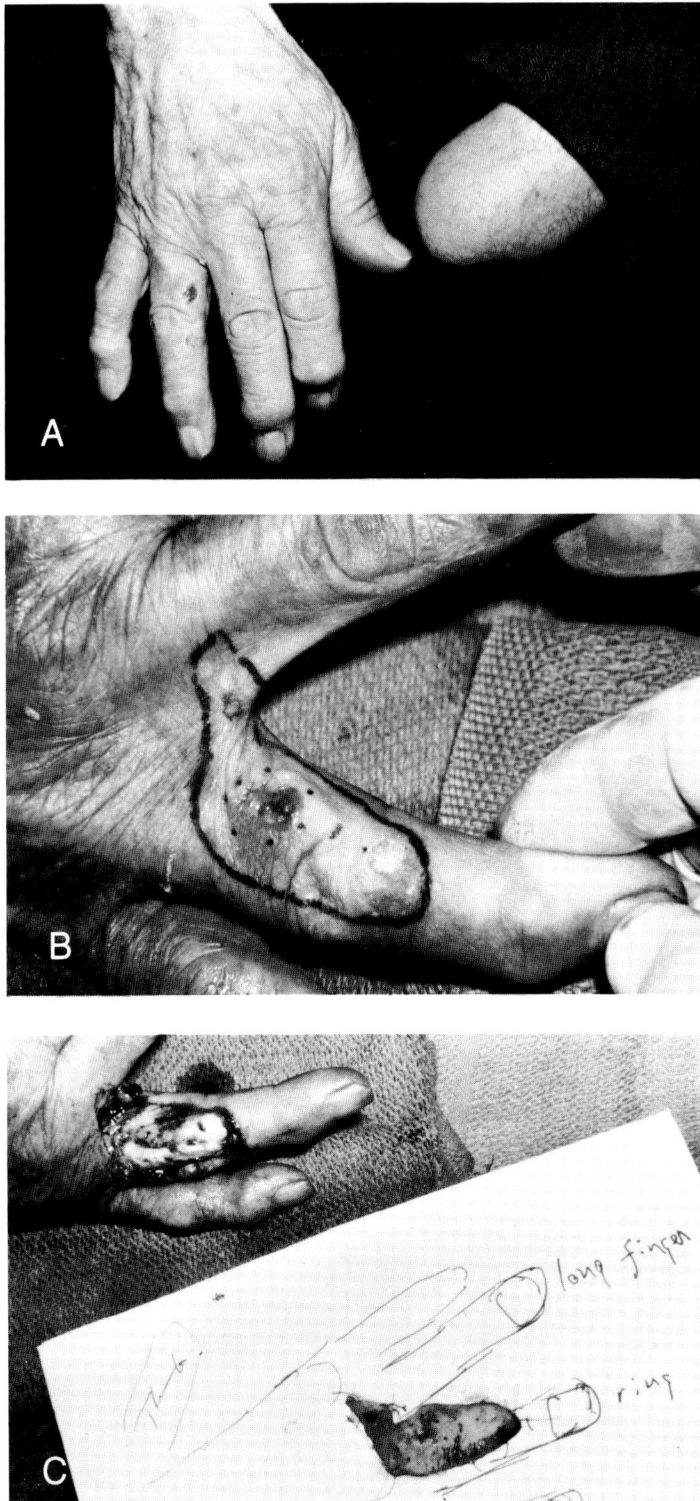

Fig. 59-12. **(A)** An 82-year-old patient with a previous traumatic amputation of the left hand and an elevated, ulcerated lesion of the right ring finger. **(B&C)** Excisional biopsy was done in this patient because adjacent premalignant skin changes, as well as the primary lesion, required treatment. Histologic evaluation of the margins of resection is necessary. Note the important use of the drawing to orientate the specimen for more precise evaluation of the margins. Incisional biopsy, especially when needed to determine type of treatment and to limit tumor seeding, is an appropriate alternative.

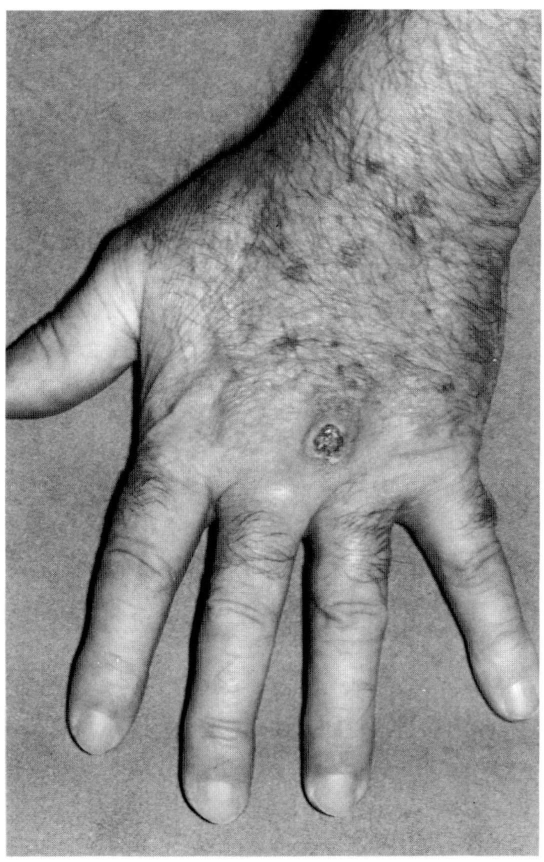

Fig. 59-13. A 76-year-old man with an ulcerated squamous cell carcinoma of 18 months' duration. There were no clinically positive nodes.

tion often requires extensive sampling to ascertain that margins are free of tumor. Regular patient follow-up is important to attempt to detect treatable local recurrence or metastatic disease.

Malignant Melanoma

Malignant melanoma is a treacherous, potentially lethal tumor that has recently shown a marked increase in incidence.[21] Therefore, a brief review of pigmented tumors is presented to introduce this section.

Types of Nevi

Nevi ("moles") are collections of melanocytes that usually appear after birth and may be genetically determined. They include lentigo, junctional, compound, and intradermal moles.[40,45]

Senile lentigo lesions are rather uniformly tan to dark brown and are variable in size. They appear on exposed areas of the body surface and are not unusual on the hands. Such lentigines are flat. They are characterized on histologic examination by an increased number of normal-appearing melanocytes just above the basement membrane. If the physician is secure in diagnosis, he need not treat them.

While some authors have stated that there is a relationship between moles and melanoma, others disagree. Benign moles characteristically have a regular color pattern, and normal skin markings that can usually be observed with the assistance of a magnifying lens. Moles usually are not present at birth but develop early in life and continue to appear as one matures. This can occur at any age, including childhood.[32,35] Congenital melanocytic nevi, especially those larger than 20 cm in diameter, were described by Smith et al as having a 5 percent to 20 percent chance of developing melanoma within the borders of the lesion sometime during the life of that patient.[42,17] Groups of moles may first be noted at puberty or may develop during pregnancy; also, preexisting moles may darken during pregnancy.[12]

Nevi are commonly differentiated by their clinical and histologic pictures as follows: (1) junctional nevi are flat lesions with their nevus cells present in the epidermis above the basement membrane; (2) compound nevi are slightly raised tumors that, on histologic evaluation, have nevus cells present both in the junctional areas and the dermis; (3) intradermal nevi are raised and have their nevus cells within the dermis; and (4) blue nevi are blue or slate blue lesions that have a smooth surface and a uniform color. These last nevi are frequently found on the feet and dorsum of the hands. Their melanocytes are in the deeper dermis. They are benign and only rarely undergo malignant change.[15]

Benign nevi, as well as malignant melanomas, may develop surrounding depigmentation, giving the appearance of a halo nevus.[15]

Types of Melanomas

Lentigo Maligna

Based upon clinical and histologic appearance, a preinvasive, flat pigmented tumor occurring on sun-exposed areas in older individuals is designated as lentigo maligna (melanotic freckle of Hutchinson) (Fig. 59-17A). These lesions are usually small, tan to brown to black, and flat, with very irregular borders. Color changes occur and the lesions slowly grow larger. There are frequently pink areas in such tumors. If the tumor remains untreated, vertical growth and metastasis may occur. It is then called a lentigo maligna melanoma.[16] Excision of a lentigo maligna with a good margin of normal tissue (at least 1 to 2 cm) is the treatment I prefer.

Superficial Spreading Melanoma

Superficial spreading malignant melanoma (Fig. 59-17B) tends to occur in people younger than those who develop lentigo maligna. These melanomas also have a predilection for sun-exposed areas, are somewhat irregular in shape, and frequently have notched borders. A variety of colors may be present, including shades from tan to brown to even gray and black, as well as combinations of red, white, and blue. Areas that become depigmented may present apparent "regression"

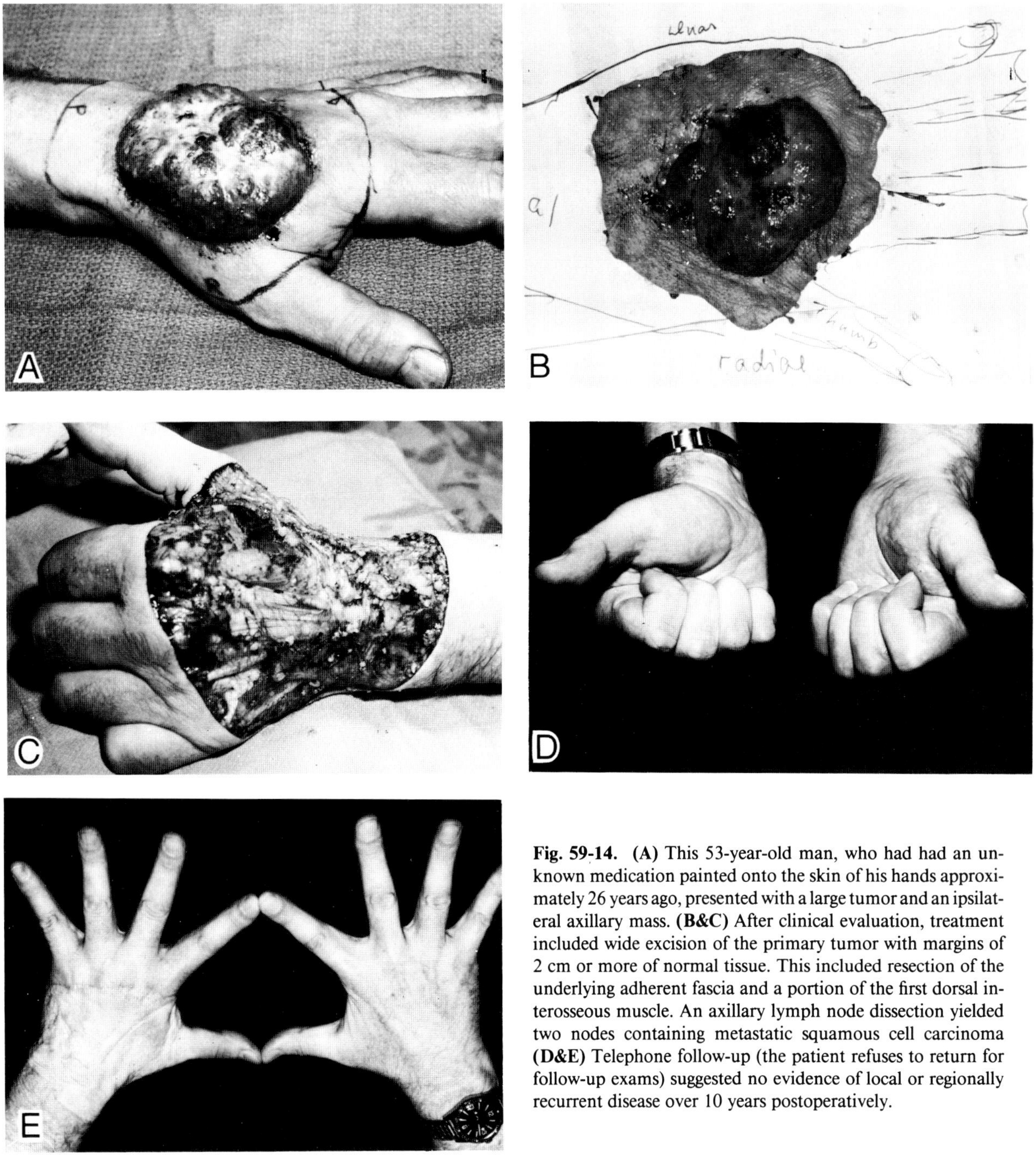

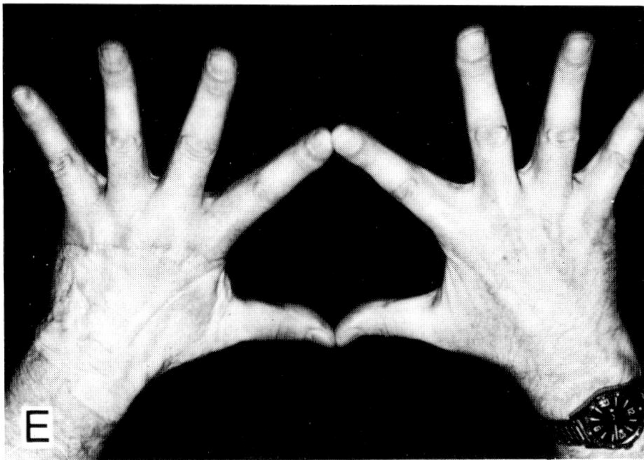

Fig. 59-14. **(A)** This 53-year-old man, who had had an unknown medication painted onto the skin of his hands approximately 26 years ago, presented with a large tumor and an ipsilateral axillary mass. **(B&C)** After clinical evaluation, treatment included wide excision of the primary tumor with margins of 2 cm or more of normal tissue. This included resection of the underlying adherent fascia and a portion of the first dorsal interosseous muscle. An axillary lymph node dissection yielded two nodes containing metastatic squamous cell carcinoma **(D&E)** Telephone follow-up (the patient refuses to return for follow-up exams) suggested no evidence of local or regionally recurrent disease over 10 years postoperatively.

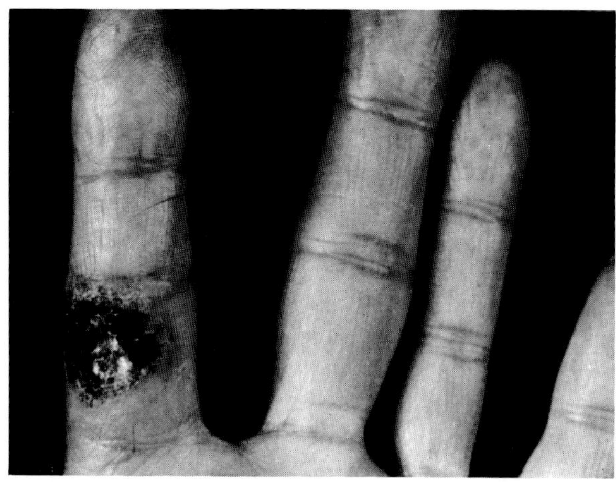

Fig. 59-15. Bowen's disease. (Courtesy of Wilma Bergfeld, M.D., Cleveland, Ohio.)

of the lesion. Even though only scar can be found in areas of "regression," such tumors have been known to metastasize.[37]

Nodular Malignant Melanoma

The development of elevated, or nodular, areas in such lesions (Fig. 59-17C) is evidence that they have evolved into their vertical growth phase. The risk of metastasis is greater once this occurs. Nodular malignant melanomas do not have a recognizable radial growth phase. They are vertically growing lesions and may metastasize at an early stage in their evolution.[42]

Acral Lentiginous Melanoma

Acral lentiginous melanomas (Fig. 59-18) include those that occur on the extremities, as well as the subgroup that are subungual melanomas.[2]

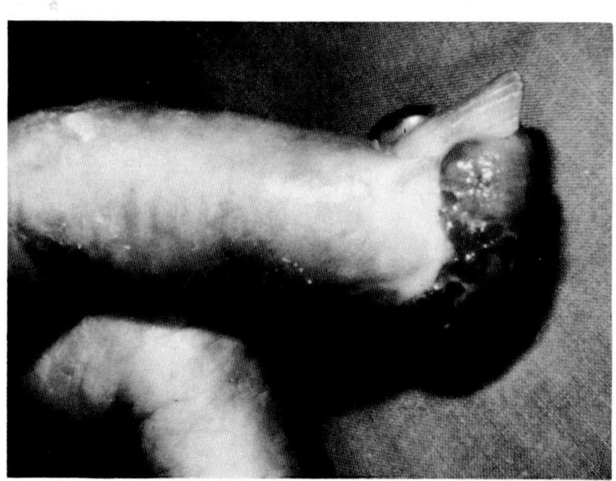

Fig. 59-16. Squamous cell carcinoma of a fingertip that involved the nail area.

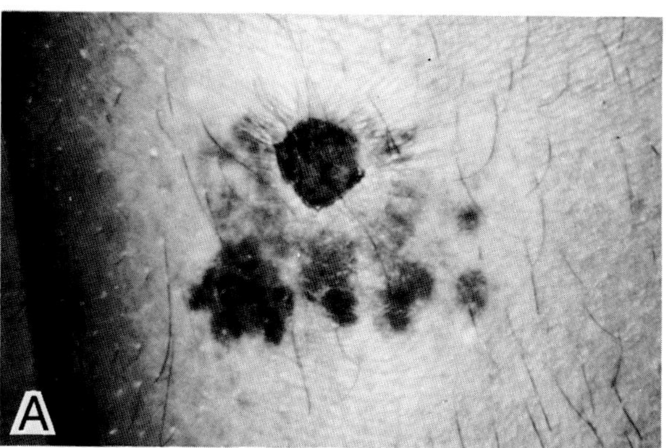

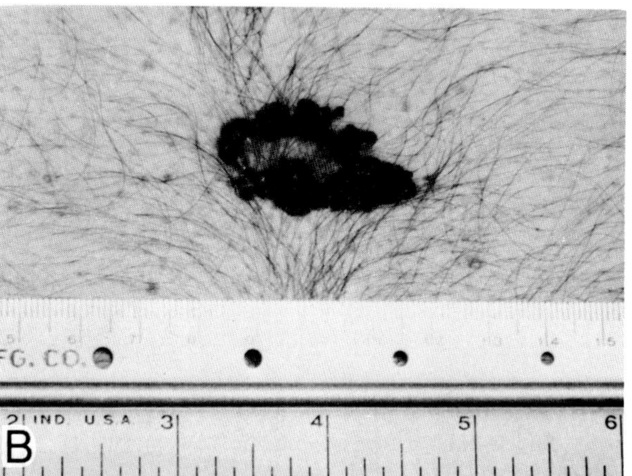

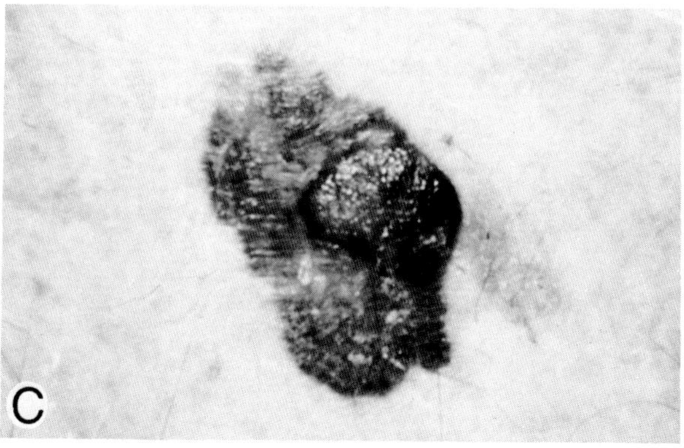

Fig. 59-17. Types of melanomas (see text). **(A)** Lentigo maligna. **(B)** Superficial spreading melanoma. **(C)** Superficial spreading melanoma with nodule.

All subungual melanomas are not as easily recognized as the ones shown in Figure 59-18A and B. This is clearly demonstrated in the case of a 72-year-old woman with only a small area of eponychial staining (Fig. 59-18C). Indeed, many of these are extremely difficult to diagnose. While some physicians advocate ray amputation for biopsy-proven subungual melanomas, the actual level of amputation or resection should be based on a careful evaluation of the tumor (Figs. 59-19 and 59-20). Less essential rays, such as an index finger in an otherwise normal hand, are better completely ablated.

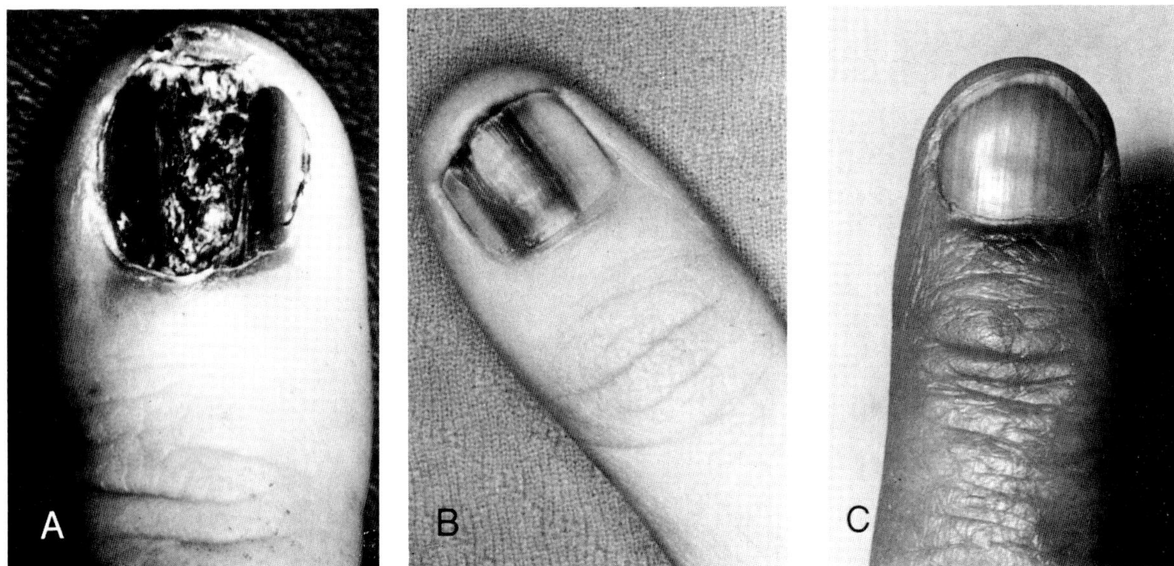

Fig. 59-18. Various presentations of subungual melanomas. Note the eponychial pigmentation in **(C)**. (Fig. A Courtesy of Melvyn Dinner, M.D.)

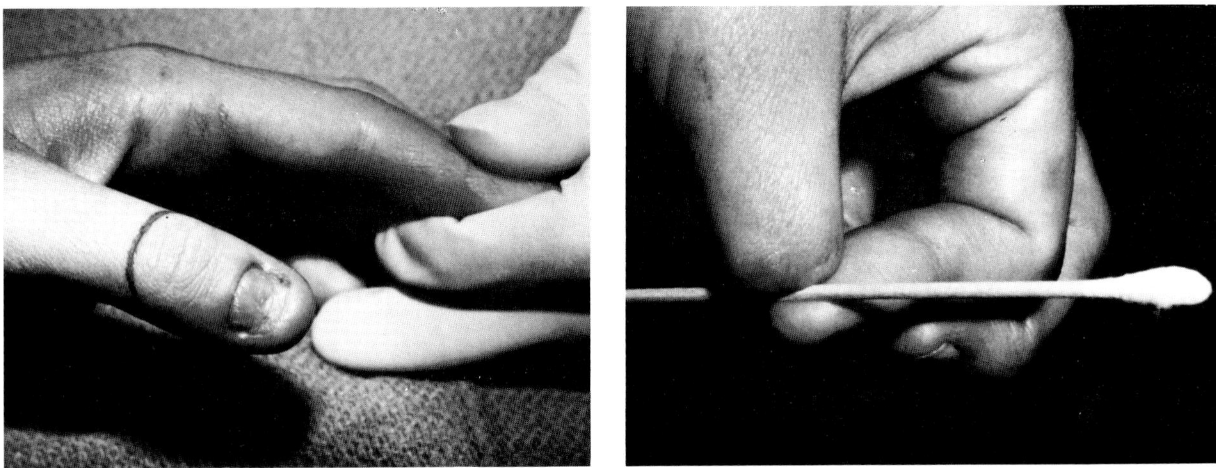

Fig. 59-19. Level of amputation for a patient with subungual melanoma in the thumb.

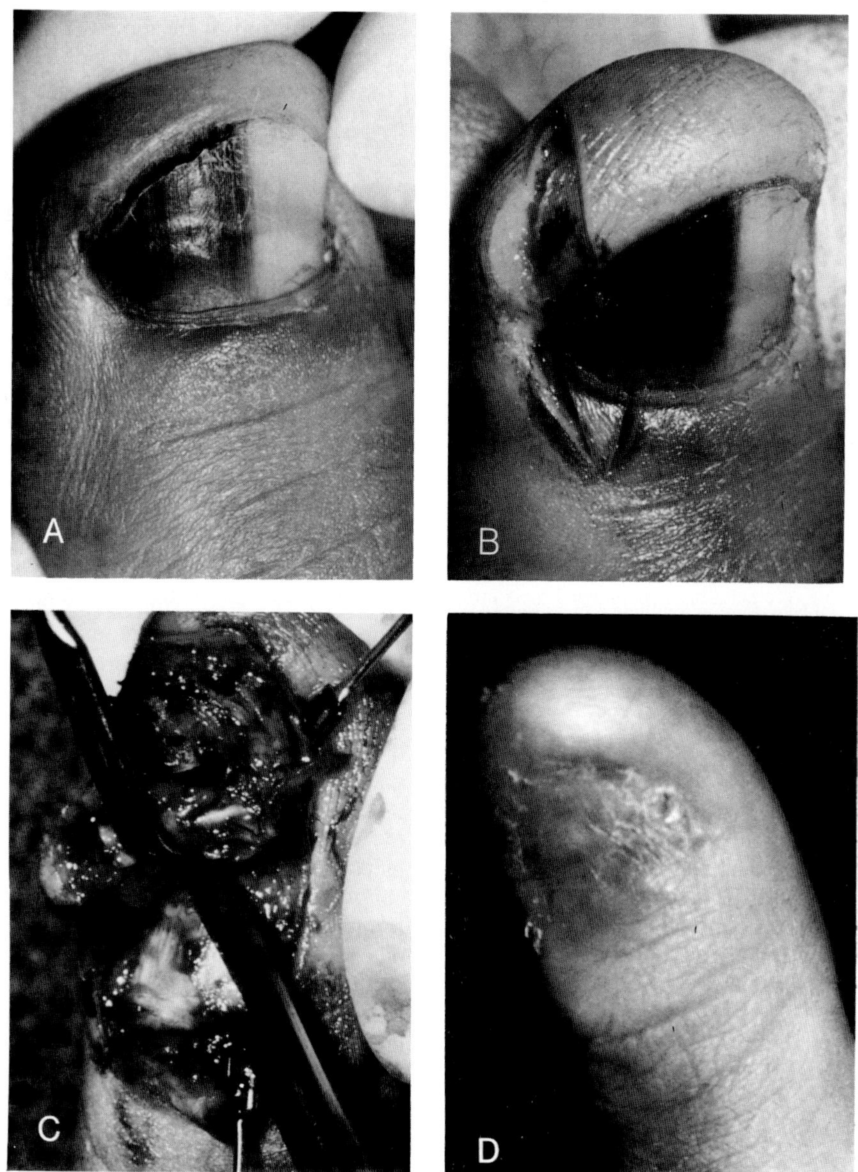

Fig. 59-20. **(A)** This 10-year-old boy presented with an enlarging subungual pigmented tumor of 18 months' duration. **(B)** After clinical evaluation, incisional biopsy, which included the eponychial area, revealed a benign active junctional nevus. **(C)** Treatment included total removal of the lesion and **(D)** skin graft reconstruction.

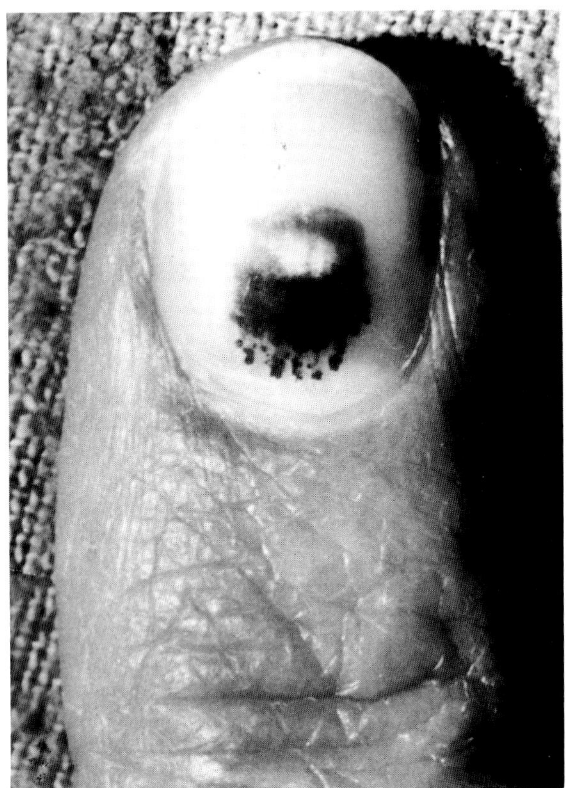

Fig. 59-21. A subungual hematoma resembling a melanoma.

Differential Diagnosis of Melanoma

Figure 59-21 shows a subungual hematoma in a patient who did not have a clear history of trauma. Because the lesion had been persistent, biopsy was necessary to establish its correct diagnosis. A careful history frequently helps clarify the confusion surrounding a post-traumatic pigment change in the subungual area.

The differential diagnosis of a pigmented tumor can be difficult. What looks like a nodular melanoma may be a benign lesion and vice versa.[26]

Melanoma Classification and Staging

Clark's classification (Fig. 59-22), proposed in 1967, divides melanomas according to their level of invasion. This is helpful in understanding their clinical behavior. Level I tumors are those that are confined to the epidermis ("in situ"). Level II refers to penetration into the papillary dermis. Level III lesions fill and expand the papillary dermis. Level IV melanomas invade the reticular dermis. Level V tumors extend into the subcutaneous fat.[7,13]

Breslow contributed significantly to our understanding of the behavior of melanomas when he classified the microscopic invasion by measuring the thickness between the granular layer of the epidermis and the depth of the tumor extension with an ocular micrometer.[8]

Some authors believe that thickness yields better prognostic information than does level. There is some evidence that patients whose primary tumor involves the upper extremity have a better prognosis than those with melanomas arising in other sites.[7]

Clinical staging of melanoma (Table 59-2) is also important in treatment choice and follow-up review.[1]

Preoperative Evaluation

According to some investigators, complete evaluation for metastatic malignant melanoma should include a careful history that also seeks information concerning family history.

A thorough physical examination, chest radiograph, and routine laboratory studies complete the minimal requirements for this evaluation. Examination of these patients must include a complete inspection of their skin. Therefore, they must be undressed and carefully inspected. Appropriate regional lymphatic drainage areas should be examined. Decisions about whether or not various scans or other special studies are done depend upon the circumstances of the individual patient.

Biopsy

Controversy exists concerning the appropriate means of biopsying a suspected melanoma. Small punch, shave, or frozen section biopsies may provide inadequate information. With large lesions, such as that shown in Figure 59-23, it is sometimes preferable to do an incisional biopsy and wait for the definitive pathology before proceeding with surgical treatment. Whether incisional or excisional biopsy techniques are used, adequate specimens should include tissue that will allow the pathologist to evaluate lateral and deep margins. The biopsy should be taken from that part of the tumor that is considered thickest and most characteristic of the pathology. In my opinion, it is helpful, not only in choosing the type of biopsy, but in planning appropriate future surgical treatment, for the treating surgeon to perform the initial biopsy. It may be difficult to know how deep and what tissue was transgressed in a three-dimensional plane when a punch-type biopsy was carried out by other than the treating surgeon. Indeed, even the treating surgeon may have difficulty knowing the depth that a punch achieved. Generally, excisional biopsies encompassing the tumor are preferred. However, large lesions may be evaluated by a carefully planned incisional biopsy.

Operative Treatment

The extent of surgical treatment of a given melanoma must be worked out on an individual basis. At this time it is difficult to present hard and fast rules for this. Use of all the information available, including the history, physical findings, biopsy findings, interpretation in light of Clark's and Breslow's levels and measurements, as well as evaluation of regional nodes and the patient in general, will help the clinician to arrive at a satisfac-

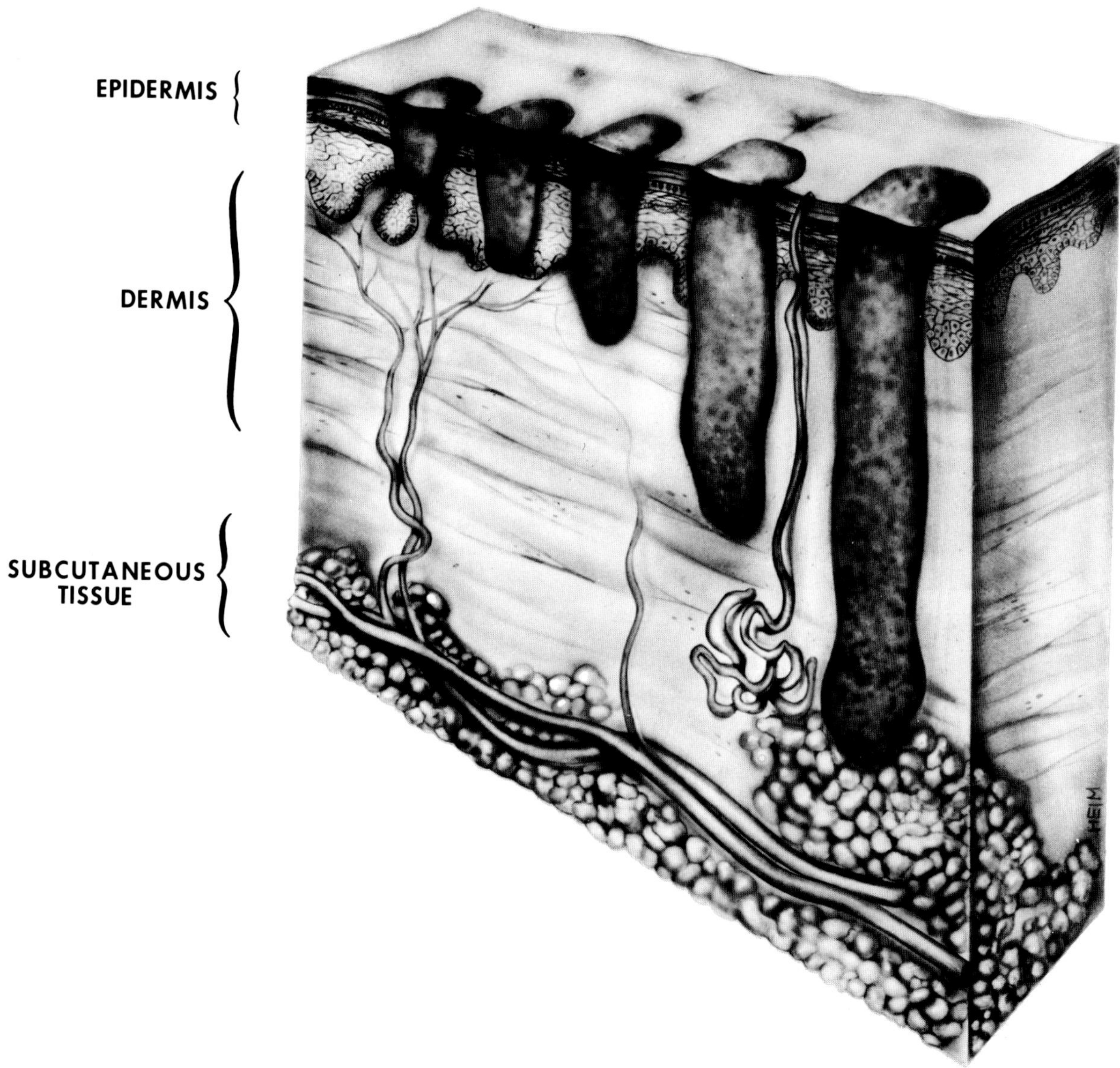

Fig. 59-22. Clark's classification of melanoma according to level of invasion.

Table 59-2. Clinical Staging of Melanoma

Stage I	Primary lesions with or without satellites within 5 cm of the primary lesion
Ia	Designates local recurrence of a primary melanoma[42]
Stage II	Spread to a single draining regional lymph node area or in transit skin metastases beyond 5 cm from the primary lesion
Stage III	Involvement of two or more lymph node groups, disseminated skin involvement, or visceral metastases

(From Clark et al,[12] with permission.)

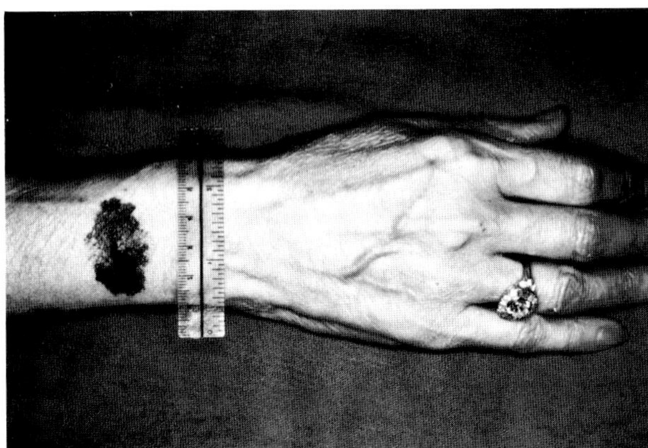

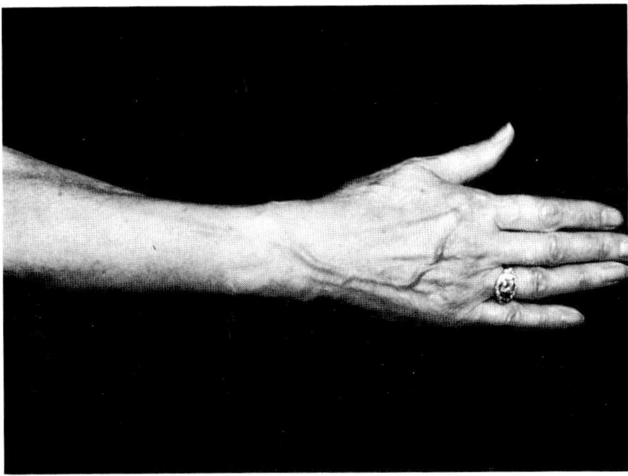

Fig. 59-23. This 66-year-old woman underwent an excisional biopsy of a lesion that clinically appeared to be a melanoma. Frozen section evaluation of the wrist lesion was read as benign. Although the patient had undergone a radical mastectomy on the same side as her wrist lesion excision, a subsequent metastatic tumor to her lung was found to be a melanoma. Review of the hand and metastatic tumor, including that done by the AFIP in Washington D.C., reversed the original impression and read this as a melanoma. After additional treatment with resection for the pulmonary lesion and various forms of immuno- and chemotherapy, including C. parvum and D.T.I.C., she has shown no evidence of melanoma 10 years postoperatively.

tory approach to treatment. Records with regard to measurements or margins, follow-up information, and an open mind to new findings in the literature will help revise future treatment plans for these serious malignancies.[3,46,47] It should be emphasized that the management of patients with melanoma is still controversial (Fig. 59-24). Continued prospective studies and long-term review are still required, because recurrences can occur many years following excision of a melanoma.

Management of Patients with Malignant Melanomas

Total patient-oriented care requires a sympathetic, informed approach by a team of physicians who can provide current diagnostic and treatment modalities for these serious conditions. The increasing incidence of these tumors, particularly melanomas, emphasizes the necessity for us to restudy this subject. Earlier lesion detection might produce cures for otherwise doomed patients. Patient examination frequently requires a total body inspection, even though a specific area is brought to the physician's attention. In certain instances relatives must also be examined. Although chemotherapy, immunotherapy, and radiotherapy are still in their investigative phases, these treatment modalities should be kept in mind.[11] Specialists in these areas involved in the treatment teams may offer patients increased hope.

Preventive care is still the best approach. We must educate ourselves and our patients to recognize the various premalignant conditions.[14,32,45] Undue sun exposure should be discouraged, and environmental protection from further deterioration in natural solar radiation barriers must be a common concern.

Sweat Gland Carcinoma

Although sweat gland tumors appear to be relatively uncommon, they are important because of the difficulty in differentiating them from other lesions. These include the common giant cell tumors and other benign lesions already described, as well as malignancies including basal cell carcinoma, squamous cell carcinoma, melanoma, and metastatic malignant tumors to the skin from sites including the breast, salivary glands, lung, and other areas.[9,48]

Classification

One method of classification groups these tumors based on biologic behavior. Knowledge of the histologic subtype of the tumor is important because it is associated with a different biologic behavior. Those in the low malignant potential category include mucinous carcinoma, aggressive digital papillary adenoma, and adenoid cystic carcinoma. The high malignant potential group includes eccrine poroma, acrospiroma, mixed tumor, spiradenoma, and cylindroma.[19,41] Those that have a higher propensity for metastatic disease to regional lymph nodes include apocrine carcinomas, malignant cylindromas, mixed tumors, and acrospiroma. Therefore, some have sug-

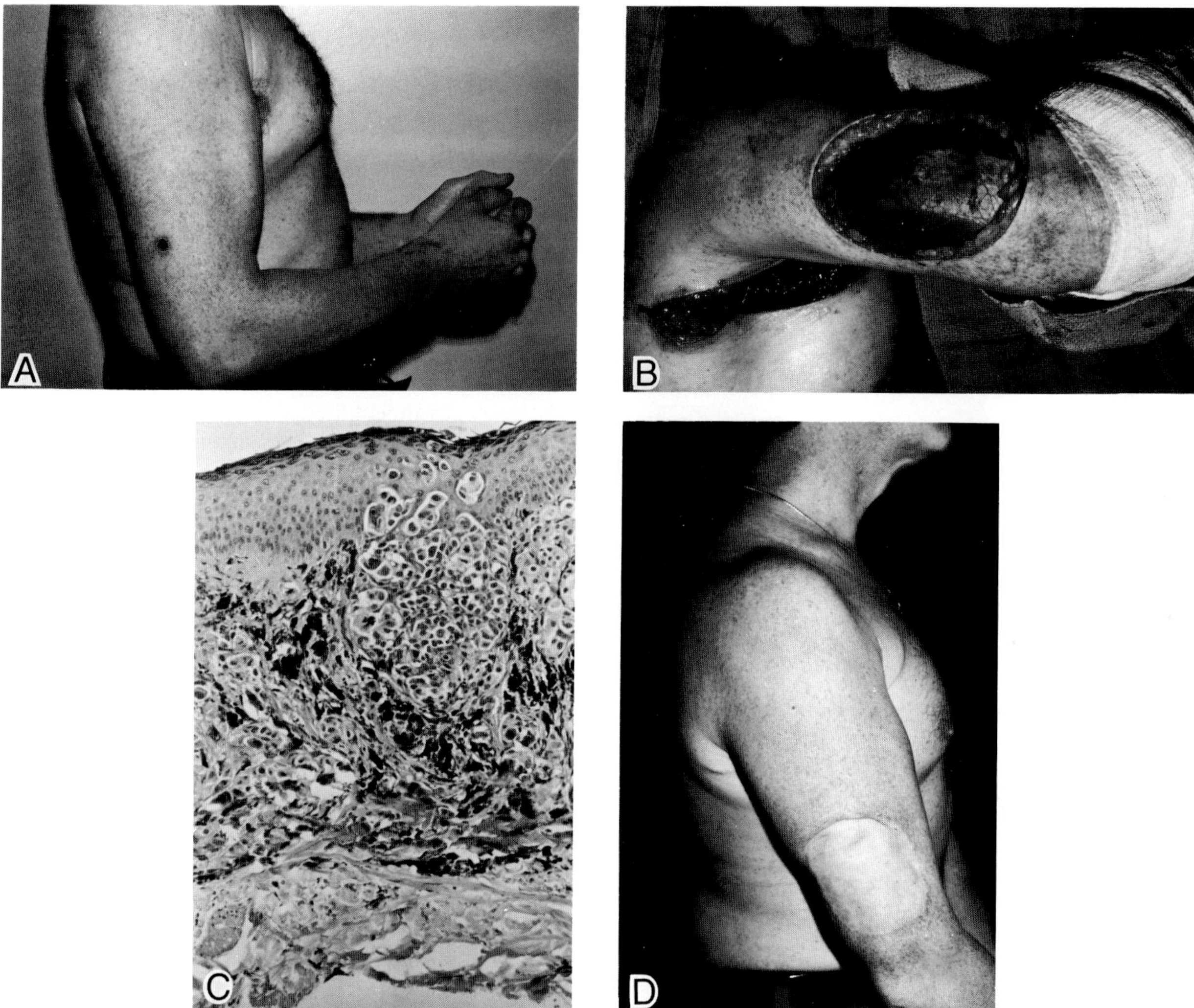

Fig. 59-24. This 43-year-old man had a biopsy-proven Level III to IV (Breslow 1.74 mm) melanoma. **(A)** Because the lesion was thought to be in the high-risk group, which raised the question of metastasis to the regional nodes, the patient, after evaluation, was treated with a wide reexcision of the biopsy site **(B)** and regional lymphadenectomy. **(C)** The histologic appearance of the tumor. **(D)** Three years postoperatively the patient is free of any evidence of melanoma.

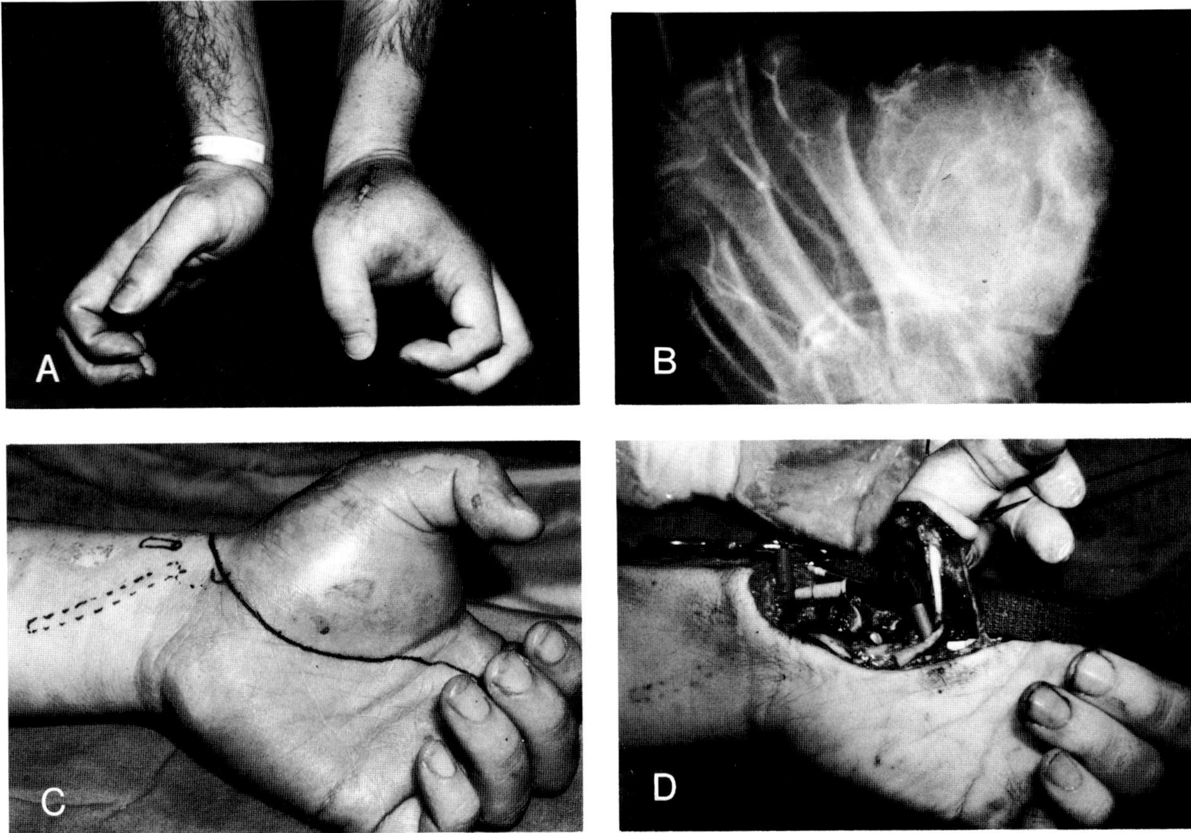

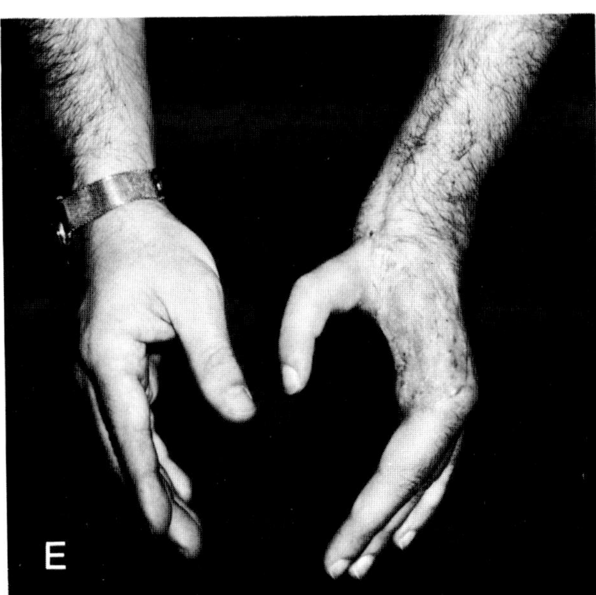

Fig. 59-25. **(A)** The biopsy site of recurrent tumor in the left hand of a 30-year-old right-handed man. This tumor was first noted and excised at age 13, recurred, and was reexcised at age 18. A third excision for recurrence was carried out at age 23, again followed by recurrence, pain, and interference with grip at age 30. **(B)** A preoperative angiogram revealed involvement of vessels to the thumb and index finger by the tumor. **(C)** Tumor also involved the deep palmar arch, requiring interpositional vein grafting, because there was no superficial arch. **(D)** The revascularized index finger, which was outside of the tumor resection site, was utilized for immediate pollicization. **(E)** The tumor was read as a chondrosarcoma on incisional biopsy. However, review of the entire specimen after en-bloc resection lead to a diagnosis of cutaneous mixed tumor (chondroid syringoma), probably malignant. Follow-up information is not available as the patient left town without a forwarding address.

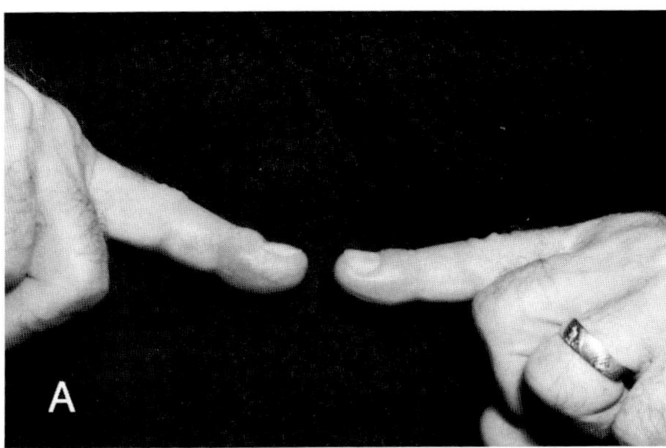

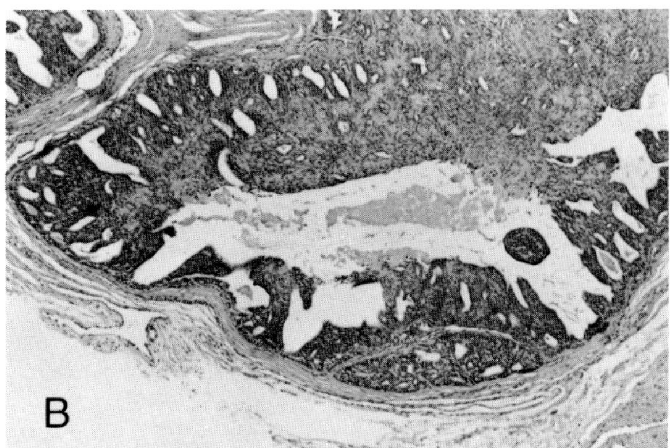

Fig. 59-26. (**A**) This 67-year-old man presented with a 2-year history of slowly growing tumor on the ulnar side of the distal phalanx, especially in the nail fold area. This had blue and erythematous discoloration. (**B**) Low power microscopic examination of the tumor revealed a glandular pattern described by the AFIP as an "aggressive digital papillary adenoma," with the additional comment that "occasional cases of underlying bone involvement and metastasis to the lung have occurred and those lesions are regarded as aggressive digital papillary adenocarcinoma."

gested elective lymph node dissection for patients afflicted with this group. Certain malignant subtypes are noted for their benign precursor lesions; these include apocrine carcinoma, malignant acrospiroma, malignant spiradenoma, and dermal cylindroma.[19,41]

Pattern of Spread

The history of the evolution of these tumors becomes important, in my opinion, in the differential diagnosis. They are frequently very slow-growing, although they may have rapid growth phases and may metastasize. Metastatic disease in those cases reviewed in the literature has been relatively common to the regional lymph nodes, as well as by blood-borne routes to bone, skin, lung, and even the brain and kidneys.[38]

Clinical Picture

Sweat gland tumors of the hand are most often found involving the palms. Examination may reveal a firm nodular or multiple nodular mass, which, at least initially, is usually painless. There may be an erythematous or violaceous color. Ulceration usually is not a common feature, at least early. Recurrence after excision is not unusual.[20] Although frequently of limited size, recurrent lesions may become quite large before evidence of metastasis is found (Fig. 59-25).[44]

Treatment

Evaluation and treatment require careful history and physical examination (which must include evaluation of sites that are potential primary sources for tumors that may be confused with sweat gland tumors, such as the breast). This should then be followed by appropriate biopsy. Surgical treatment requires complete tumor removal with safe, tumor-free margins. Some authors have recommended regional lymph node dissections. There is no good evidence at the present time to my knowledge that radiotherapy or chemotherapy has a major role to play[1,38,48] (Fig. 59-26). These tumors may be extremely aggressive, possibly following a long, indolent course.[44]

Kaposi's Sarcoma and AIDS

This tumor not only enters into the differential diagnosis of lesions of the hand and upper extremity, but also brings in an increasingly important relationship, that of acquired immune deficiency syndrome (AIDS).

Unlike some of the tumors previously mentioned that can frequently be cured by early recognition and treatment, Kaposi's sarcoma may be seen in a setting that presently defies cure. The subtle presentations of this tumor, problems in differential diagnosis, and its association with the as yet incurable disease AIDS make recognition of this lesion important. Although more common in other areas, e.g., the lower extremities, Kaposi's sarcoma has now been recognized in the hand as well.[30,51] Although there is a form of this tumor seen without an AIDS relationship, AIDS must be considered when bluish-red or dark brown plaques or nodules are presented for evaluation (Fig. 59-27). These skin changes may be annular, serpiginous, bluish-red patches. Later there may be lymphadema of the involved extremity (especially lower extremity). Lymph nodes may be enlarged, and viscera, such as the gastrointestinal tract, liver, lungs, and heart, may be involved.[34] In Keith and Wilgis's case[30] the patient presented with what appeared to be a chronic paronychial infection. Examination revealed a nontender purple plaque involving the eponychial area of the little finger. In addition to intraoperative cultures, a biopsy of the area was obtained. Subsequently the diagnosis of AIDS-related Kaposi's sarcoma was confirmed with a positive HTLV-3 test.

A relationship to AIDS, a disease causing a profound defect in cellular immunity, brings up many other implications.[39] These include other malignancies and the spectrum of oppor-

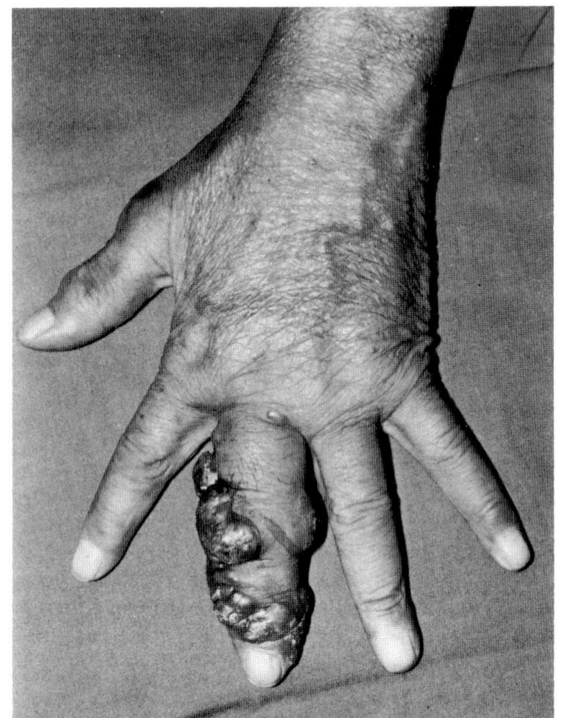

A

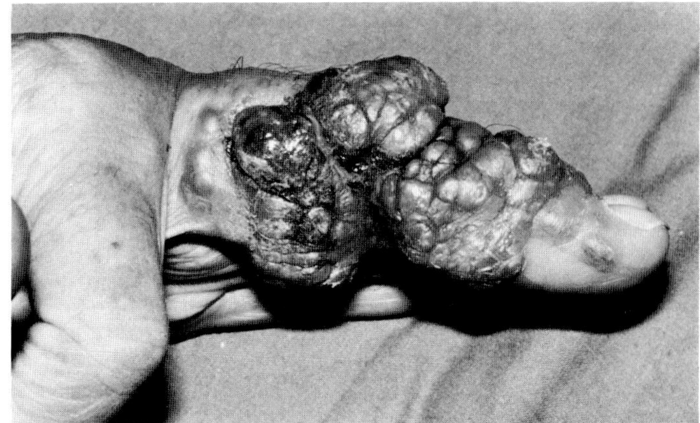

B

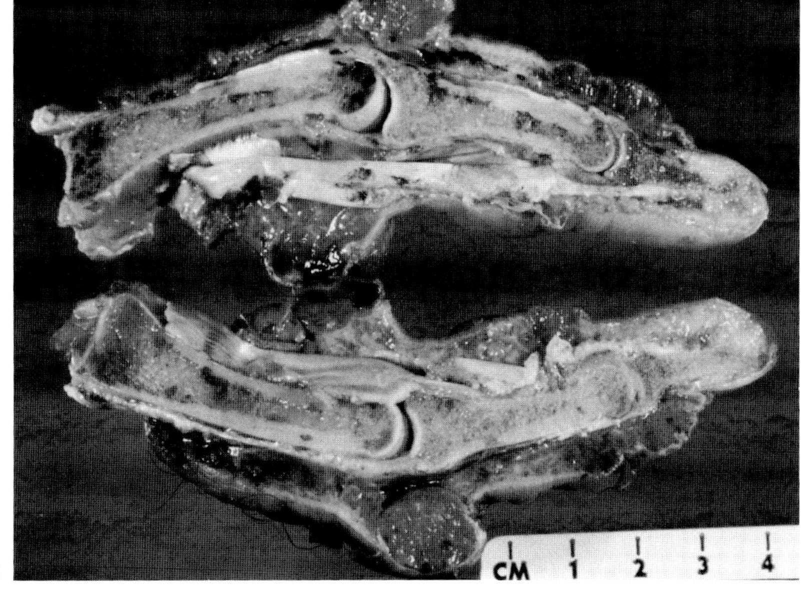

C

Fig. 59-27. **(A&B)** Clinical example of hand involvement in Kaposi's sarcoma in an elderly male. Gross longitudinal section of the tumor **(C)** demonstrates the classic appearance of the nodular formation associated with the later stages of this entity. This figure demonstrates Kaposi's sarcoma in a non-AIDS patient.

tunistic infections that can be involved with the ultimate demise of these unfortunate patients.

SUMMARY

Recognition of this spectrum of problems should help us in our management and advice to patients presenting with "lumps" in the upper extremity. Proper treatment of annoying benign lesions and early recognition and treatment in order to provide a cure where it is yet possible for malignant tumors results from such recognition. Let us hope that continuing efforts in the areas where cure is not yet possible will improve survival and contribute to overall patient welfare.

REFERENCES

1. Adeyemi-Doro HO, Durosimi-Etti FA, Olude O: Primary malignant tumors of the hand. J Hand Surg 10A:815–820, 1985
2. Arrington JH, Reed RJ, Ichinose H, Krementz ET: Plantar lentiginous melanoma: A distinctive variant of human cutaneous malignant melanoma. Am J Surg Pathol 1:131–142, 1977
3. Balch CM: Surgical management of regional lymph nodes in cutaneous melanoma. J Am Acad Dermatol 3:511–524, 1980
4. Bart RS, Andrade R, Kopf AW: Cutaneous horn. Acta Derm Venereol (Stockh) 48:507–515, 1968
5. Beasley RW, Ristow BVW: Malignant tumors of the hand. pp. 1435–1440. In Andrade R, Gumport S, Popkin G, Rees T (eds): Cancer of The Skin. WB Saunders, Philadelphia, 1976
6. Biddulph S: Giant cell tumor of synovium. In Bogumill GB, Fleegler EJ (eds), Tumours of the Hand and Upper Limb. Churchill Livingstone, Edinburgh, 1992
7. Blois MS, Sagebiel RW, Abarbanel RM, Caldwell TM, Tuttle MS: Malignant melanomas of the skin. 1. The association of tumor depth and type, and patient sex, age, and site with survival. Cancer 52:1330–1341, 1983
8. Breslow A: Thickness, cross sectional areas and depth of invasion in the prognosis of cutaneous melanoma. Ann Surg 172:902–915, 1970
9. Brown E, Ariano L: Histologic diagnosis of benign adnexal skin tumors. An algorithmic approach. J Am Acad Dermatol 12:350–358, 1985
10. Carroll RE: Squamous cell carcinomas of the nail bed. J Hand Surg 1:29–97, 1976
11. Chaudhuri PK, Walker MJ, Briele HA, Beattie CW, Das Gupta TK: Incidence of estrogen receptor in benign nevi and human malignant melanoma. JAMA 244:791–793, 1980
12. Clark WH, Ainsworth AM, Bernardino EA, Yang CHY, Mihm MC, Reed RJ: The developmental biology of primary human malignant melanomas. Semin Oncol 2:83–103, 1975
13. Clark WH Jr, From L, Bernardino EA, Mihm MC: The histogenesis and biologic behavior of primary human malignant melanomas of the skin. Cancer Res 29:705–727, 1969
14. Clark WH, Goldman LI, Mastrangelo MJ: Human Malignant Melanoma. Grune & Stratton, New York, 1979
15. Clark WH, Mihm MC Jr: Moles and malignant melanoma. pp. 491–511. In Fitzpatrick TB, Arndt KA, Clark WH Jr, Eisen AZ, VanSchott EJ, Vaugh JH (eds): Dermatology in General Medicine. McGraw-Hill, New York, 1971
16. Clark WH, Mihm MC: Lentigo maligna and lentigo maligna melanoma. Am J Pathol 55:39–54, 1969
17. Consensus conference: Precursors to malignant melanoma. JAMA 251:1864–1866, 1984
18. Cooper PH: Fibroma of tendon sheath. J Am Acad Dermatol 11:625–628, 1984
19. Cooper PH: Carcinoma of sweat glands. Pathol Annu, Part 1, 22:83–124, 1987
20. El-Domeiri AA, Brasfield RD, Huvos AG, Strong EW: Sweat gland carcinoma: A clinicopathologic study of 83 patients. Ann Surg 173:270–274, 1971
21. Elwood JM, Lee JAAH: Recent data on the epidemiology of malignant melanoma. Semin Oncol 2:149–154, 1975
22. Enzinger FM, Weiss SW: Soft Tissue Tumors, pp. 103–124. CV Mosby, St Louis, 1983
23. Enzinger FM, Weiss SW: Benign fibrohistiocytic Tumors. pp. 223–251. In Soft Tissue Tumors. 2nd Ed. CV Mosby, St. Louis, 1988
24. Enzinger FM, Weiss SW: Soft Tissue Tumors. 2nd Ed. pp. 102–135. CV Mosby, St. Louis, 1988
25. Fitzpatrick T, Gilchrest B: Dimple sign to differentiate benign from malignant pigmented cutaneous lesions. N Engl J Med 2962:1518, 1977
26. Fleegler EJ: Tumors involving the skin of the upper extremity. Hand Clin 3:197–212, 1987
27. Fleegler E, Sood R, Zienowicz R, Bergfeld W, Lucas A, Turgeon K: Benign tumors of the skin of the upper extremity. In Bogumill GB, Fleegler EJ (eds): Tumours of the Hand and Upper Limb, Churchill Livingstone, Edinburgh, 1992
28. Haagensen CD: The upper extremity pp. 399–436. In Haagensen CD, Feind CR, Herter FP, Slanetz CA Jr, Weinberg JA: The Lymphatics in Cancer. WB Saunders, Philadelphia, 1972
29. Hamm JC, DeFranzo AJ, Argenta LC, White W: Keratoacanthoma necessitating metacarpal amputation. J Hand Surg 15A:980–986, 1990
30. Keith JE, Wilgis EFS: Kaposi's sarcoma in the hand of an AIDS patient. J Hand Surg 11A:410–413, 1986
31. Kopf AW, Bart RS, Rodriquez-Sains RS, Ackerman AB: Malignant Melanoma. pp. 154–156. Mason, New York, 1979
32. Kopf AW, Hellman LJ, Rogers GS, Gross DF, Rigel DS, Friedman RS, Levenstein M, Brown J, Golomb FM, Roses DF, Gumport SL, Mintzis MM: Familial malignant melanoma. JAMA 256:1915–1919, 1986
33. Laskin, Weiss: Fibrous lesions of the upper extremity. In: Bogumill GB, Fleegler EJ (eds): Tumours of the Hand and Upper Limb. Churchill Livingstone, Edinburgh, 1992
34. Lever WF: Histopathology of the Skin. 6th Ed. pp. 636–647. JB Lippincott, Philadelphia, 1983
35. Lund HZ, Kraus JM: Melanotic Tumors of the Skin. AFIP Fascicle 3, 1962
36. Lever WF, Schaumburg-Lever G: Histology of the skin. Ch. 3. pp. 9–43. In Histopathology of the Skin. 7th Ed. JB Lippincott, Philadelphia, 1990
37. McGovern VJ: Spontaneous regression of malignant melanoma. Pathology 7:91–99, 1975
38. Morris DM, Sanusi ID, Lanehart WH: Carcinoma of eccrine sweat gland: Experience with chemotherapy, autopsy findings in a patient with metastatic eccrine carcinoma, and a review of the literature. J Surg Oncol 31:26–30, 1986
39. Muggia F, Lonberg M: Kaposi's sarcoma and AIDS. Med Clin North Am 70:1, 1986
40. Odland GF, Short JM: Structure of the skin. pp. 39–41. In Fitzpatrick TB, Arndt KA, Clark WH Jr, Eisen AZ, VanScott EJ, Vaughn JH (eds): Dermatology in General Medicine. McGraw-Hill, New York, 1971
41. Santa-Cruz DJ: Sweat gland carcinomas, comprehensive review. Semin Diagn Pathol 4(1):38–74, 1987

42. Smith AA, Smith DJ Jr, Robson MC, Beatty E: Melanoma of the upper extremity. In Bogumill GB, Fleegler EJ (eds): Tumors of the Hand and Upper Limb, Churchill Livingstone, Edinburgh, 1992
43. Smith JW, Guthrie RH: Tumors of the hand. pp. 641-649. In Grabb WC, Smith JW (eds): Plastic Surgery. 3rd Ed. Little, Brown, Boston, 1979
44. Sood R, Fleegler EJ, Tuthill R: Sweat gland tumors of the hand—work in progress
45. Stegmaier OC, Montgomery H: Histopathologic studies of pigmented nevi in children. J Invest Dermatol 20:51-64, 1953
46. Veronesi U, Adamus J, Bandiera DC, Brennhovd IO, Caceres E, Cascinelli N, Claudio F, Ikonopisov RL, Javorski VV, Kirov S, Kulakowski A, Lacour J, Lejeune F, Mechl Z, Morabito A, Rode I, Sergeev S, vanSlooten E, Szczgiel K, Trapeznikov NN, Wagner RI: Inefficacy of immediate node dissection in Stage I melanoma of the limbs. N Engl J Med 297:627-630, 1977
47. Veronesi U, Adamus J, Bandiera DC, Brennhovd IO, Caceres E, Cascinelli N, Claudio F, Ikonopisov RL, Javorski VV, Kirov S, Kulakowski A, Lacour J, Lejeune F, Mechl Z, Morabito A, Rode I, Sergeev S, vanSlooten E, Szczgiel K, Trapeznikov NN, Wagner RI: Delayed regional lymph node dissection in Stage I melanoma of the skin of the lower extremities. Cancer 49:2420-2430, 1982
48. Wick MR, Goellner JR, Wolfe JT, Su DWP: Adnexal carcinomas of the skin. 1. Eccrine carcinomas. Cancer 56:1147-1162, 1986
49. Wilgis EFS: Vascular Injuries and Diseases of the Upper Limb, Little, Brown, Boston, 1983
50. Wilgis EFS: Tumors of the hand and upper limb—malignant lesions of the vessels. In Bogumill GB, Fleegler EJ (eds): Tumours of the Hand and Upper Limb. Churchill Livingstone, Edinburgh, 1992
51. Witt JD, Jupiter JB: Kaposi's sarcoma in the hand seen as an arteriovenous malformation. J Hand Surg 16A:607-609, 1991
52. Yaremchuk MJ, Elias LS, Graham RR, Wilgis EFS: Sweat gland carcinoma of the hand: Two cases of malignant eccrine spiradenoma. J Hand Surg 9A:910-914, 1984
53. Zook EG: Anatomy and physiology of the perionychium. Hand Clin 6:1-7, 1990

60

Aggressive and Malignant Musculoskeletal Tumors: Principles of Diagnosis and Management

Clayton A. Peimer
Harold M. Dick
Owen J. Moy

The problems of tumor management are complex, challenging, and sometimes frustrating. Considerable skill and thought are needed to solve problems, treat the patient as well as the tumor, and still salvage both survival and function. Because anatomy, biology, and surgery must be integrated, we have made the decision to divide our work into two chapters. We begin with principles.

Campanacci organized somatic cell disorders into three major classifications[6]:

1. *Hyperplasia* is an accumulation of cells resulting from accelerated proliferation.
2. *Hamartoma* is a congenital error in which an island of tissue is excluded from regional organization. However, it has a structure similar to the tissue of origin. The lesion is often multicentric and/or hemicorporal in its location. Both hyperplasias and hamartomas stop growing at musculoskeletal maturity.
3. *Neoplasia* is a new cellular growth that proceeds to grow and expand in an atypical, autonomous, and progressive manner.

Neoplasms are usually classified in two categories, benign and malignant; in musculoskeletal tissues, malignancies may also be subdivided into low grade and high grade. (Tables 60-1, 60-2) Cellular growth in benign neoplasms is autonomous, organized, and orderly, and it proceeds at a much slower rate than in malignant tumors. Benign lesions may be expansile and sometimes encapsulated. No distant spread occurs, and local recurrence is relatively more unusual in benign than in malignant lesions.

Malignant neoplasia is characterized by a rapid growth rate, atypical cellularity, and poor cell differentiation. Local growth

Table 60-1. Skeletal Tumors

Differentiation or Histogenesis	Benign	Low-grade Malignancy	High-grade Malignancy
Fibrous and histiocytic	Histiocytic fibroma Benign fibrous histiocytoma Giant cell tumor Desmoid fibroma	Grades 1, 2 fibrosarcoma	Grades 3, 4 fibrosarcoma Malignant fibrous histiocytoma
Cartilaginous	Exostosis Hemimelic epiphyseal dysplasia Chondroma Chondroblastoma Chondromyxoid fibroma	Grades 1, 2 central chondrosarcoma Peripheral chondrosarcoma Periosteal chondrosarcoma Clear cell chondrosarcoma Fibrocartilaginous mesenchymoma	Grade 3 central chondrosarcoma Mesenchymal chondrosarcoma
Osseous	Osteoma Osteoid osteoma Osteoblastoma Fibrous dysplasia Osteofibrous dysplasia	Parosteal osteosarcoma Periosteal osteosarcoma Low-grade central osteosarcoma	Classical osteosarcoma Hemorrhagic osteosarcoma Small cell osteosarcoma Osteosarcomatosis
Emopoietic			Lymphoma Plasmacytoma (Leukemia, Hodgkin)
Vascular	Hemangioma Lymphangioma	Low-grade hemangioendothelioma Hemangiopericytoma	High-grade hemangioendothelioma Hemangiopericytoma
Nervous	Neurinoma Neurofibroma		Ewing's sarcoma (?)
Adipose	Lipoma		Liposarcoma
Mixed		Adamantinoma (?)	Malignant mesenchymoma
Notochordal		Chordoma	

(Modified from Campanacci,[6] with permission.)

is aggressive and infiltrative; there are only "pseudocapsules." Such tumors are likely to spread as blood-borne metastases, and local recurrence is high after excision unless a wide margin of normal tissue is included in the resection. "Low grade" malignancies are midway in a continuum between benign and virulently malignant tumors; they grow more slowly, infiltrate early, but are not as likely to metastasize as to recur locally. It must be remembered that neither all generic categories nor all isolated case illustrations are consistent with these classifications.

Many benign tumors of the hand or forearm require no treatment, can be diagnosed clinically, and are asymptomatic. However, if a lesion increases in size or becomes symptomatic, or if the physical or radiographic appearance suggests an aggressive process, appropriate staging studies, including obtaining tissue for diagnosis, must be done.[4,5,7,9,10,12,14–16,18,31,39,40] Unfortunately, lumps and growths that look innocent may not necessarily be so; every tumor ought to be considered potentially troublesome—to function, if not to survival. Surgeons need to be familiar with the range of possible diagnoses. A physician is not justified in advising a patient that a mass ought to be "left alone" until the proper diagnosis is established by all appropriate means. Any tumor with an unclear diagnosis on the basis of nonsurgical evaluation should be biopsied. If the biopsy proves the tumor to be benign, no further surgery may be necessary. If a malignant or an aggressive nonmalignant lesion is identified, further management is required.

The presence of a mass without apparent cause away from synovium (a significantly reactive tissue), is potentially worrisome. Tumors that are symptomatic or continue to grow need to be diagnosed and classified as to stage. The clinical and family history, physical characteristics of the tumor, and data from laboratory and imaging studies provide at least the basis of a clinical impression. If the *precise* diagnosis is unclear after such a complete work-up, a carefully planned biopsy is required to avoid hazards of misdiagnosis and its complications.

CLASSIFICATION AND STAGING OF TUMORS

Managing tumors of the hand and upper extremity does not differ significantly from managing tumors in other parts of the musculoskeletal system. Correct treatment must always take into consideration the size and location of the growth, the histologic grade and clinical behavior, and the potential for metastases.[10,14–18,31,37,39,40] Although tumor-specific and histo-

Table 60-2. Tumors of Soft Tissue

Differentiation or Histiogenesis	Benign	Low-grade Malignancy	High-grade Malignancy
Fibrous	Fibromatosis (subdermic, digital, aponeurotic, congenital) Desmoid tumor	Grades 1, 2 fibrosarcoma Infantile fibrosarcoma	Grades 3, 4 fibrosarcoma
Fibrohistiocytic	Benign fibrous histiocytoma	Dermatofibrosarcoma protuberans Atypical fibroxanthoma	Malignant fibrous histiocytoma (pleomorphic storiform, myxoid, giant cell, angiomatoid, histiocytic)
Adipose	Lipoma (angiolipoma, spindle-cell, pleomorphic, lipoblastoma, lipoblastomatosis, intranervous, lipomatosis, hibernoma)	Liposarcoma (well-differentiated, myxoid)	Liposarcoma (pleomorphic, round cell, dedifferentiated)
Smooth muscular	Leiomyoma (vascular, deep)	Grades 1, 2 leiomyosarcoma	Grades 3, 4 leiomyosarcoma
Striated muscular	Rhabdomyoma (adult fetal, genital, cardiac)		Rhabdomyosarcoma (embryonal, alveolar, pleomorphic)
Vascular	Angiomas and angiodysplasias Glomus tumor Epithelioid hemangioma Hemangiopericytoma	Low-grade hemangioendothelioma Kaposi's sarcoma Hemangiopericytoma	High-grade hemangioendothelioma Kaposi's sarcoma Hemangiopericytoma
Synovial			Synovial sarcoma
Nervous	Neurinoma Neurofibroma		Malignant neurinoma Peripheral neuroepithelioma
Cartilaginous		Myxoid chondrosarcoma Synovial chondrosarcoma	Mesenchymal chondrosarcoma
Osseous			Osteosarcoma
Uncertain	Intramuscular myxoma Giant cell tumor		Malignant granular cell tumor Ewing's sarcoma Alveolar sarcoma Epithelioid sarcoma Clear cell sarcoma of the tendons and aponeurosis

(Modified from Campanacci,[6] with permission.)

logically identifiable data are presented in the next chapter, an understanding of certain principles and guidelines is essential.

Histologic Grade

The histologic grade (G) of a neoplasm is determined by the malignant characteristics of tissue obtained with a biopsy. Accepted classification is as follows:

Classification	Description
G_0	Benign.
G_1	Low-grade. Few cells, much stroma, little necrosis, mature cells, fewer than five mitoses per high-power field.
G_2	High-grade. Many cells, little stroma, much necrosis, immature cells, more than ten mitoses per high-power field.

Benign tumors can be classified into three stages[16]:

Latent/stage I tumors do not merit treatment; they usually heal spontaneously and/or remain unchanged.

Active/stage II benign neoplasms grow within a limited zone and are contained by natural barriers; if surgery is required, these tumors are most often controlled by intralesional or marginal excision.

Locally aggressive/stage III benign tumors may both grow and spread beyond natural barriers; excision requires a wide surgical margin or en bloc resection for local cure.

To avoid confusion and differences of opinion about malignant bone tumors, it has become important to establish specific grading criteria for tumors. A classification scheme based on a modified staging system for bone sarcomas was estab-

Table 60-3. Surgical Stages

Stage	Grade	Site
IA	Low (G_1)	Intracompartmental (T_1)
IB	Low (G_1)	Extracompartmental (T_2)
IIA	High (G_2)	Intracompartmental (T_1)
IIB	High (G_2)	Extracompartmental (T_2)
III	Any (G) Regional or distant metastasis (M)	Any (T) Regional or distant metastasis (M)

(Adapted from Enneking et al,[18] with permission.)

lished by the American College of Surgeons Joint Committee on Cancer and End Results Reporting in 1977. It was proposed by W.F. Enneking at the University of Florida and agreed upon by the Musculoskeletal Tumor Society (MSTS) in 1979 (Table 60-3).

The pathologist and surgeon must agree upon a surgical grade (G_1 or G_2) of malignancy based primarily on the histologic features of the tumor and also on its gross pathologic appearance, the clinical setting, and the radiologic appearance. The histologic grade is agreed upon only following a representative biopsy and careful scrutiny by an experienced musculoskeletal pathologist. It must be emphasized that the clinical and radiologic status are also very important parameters for determining the final tissue diagnosis and surgical grade.

There are, therefore, two grades of malignant tumors: G_1—low-grade malignancy with rare likelihood of metastasis and frequent local recurrence, and G_2—high-grade malignancy with frequent blood-borne metastases. The so-called "low-grade" malignant tumors can also metastasize but, more typically, are less likely to metastasize early in their course. The assignment of a grade to a particular tumor is neither easy nor exact because grading criteria are not quantifiable. Cellular morphology, anaplasia, necrosis, mitoses, and tissue of origin must all be considered descriptive. The assignment of grade may also be influenced by clinical behavior. Tumors that are known to be exceptionally dangerous (such as synovial and epithelioid sarcomas) will most properly be classified into a higher grade than their histology would indicate. Two other criteria are important: T, which represents the size and site of the tumor; and M, which designates the presence of detectable metastases.

Location (Site)

Enneking has drawn attention to the fact that the size of the lesion is not always a matter of the "bigger the badder." For example, synovial sarcoma can be less than 1 cm at presentation, yet survival rates are among the worst of any soft tissue tumor; low-grade cartilage tumors may double in size, and yet not metastasize. Regardless of size, if the tumor is limited to a single anatomic compartment, it will usually be resectable. At the same time it will be possible to preserve the extremity, as is the case when highly malignant tumors involve the distal phalanges and other acral parts. The basis of defining a "compartment" is the recognition that certain natural anatomic barriers exist that will temporarily contain and delay the spread of a pathologic process, such as infection and neoplasia. For example, an intraosseous tumor contained by the cortices and intramedullary canal of a tubular bone would be (defined as) "intracompartmental." However, if this tumor perforates into the surrounding soft tissues (or the reverse for a soft tissue tumor), it would then be considered "extracompartmental," as it has already crossed a natural barrier. Computed axial tomography (CT) and magnetic resonance imaging (MRI) enable us to estimate the size and location of a tumor, permitting more accurate preoperative planning than was previously possible.

Metastases

The third criterion for malignant tumor classification identifies patients in whom the tumor has already metastasized to other sites. The final system therefore appears as three stages, with stage III including all patients with distant metastases, regardless of the other parameters (Table 60-3). Lymph node involvement is always a very important finding, since primary musculoskeletal neoplasms rarely spread to regional nodes. As fewer than 5 percent of patients with such sarcomas develop lymph node metastases during their course, the differential diagnosis of extremity tumors with possible nodal metastases always must be expanded to include carcinomas and melanomas. Notably, however, metastases to lymph nodes are significantly more prevalent with rhabdomyosarcoma (all types), epithelioid sarcoma, clear cell sarcoma, and synovial sarcoma.

Once the appropriate staging studies are completed, the surgeon will know the anatomic characteristics (the T) of the lesion and whether metastases (the M) are absent or present. A differential diagnosis can then be formulated and the biopsy planned.

EVALUATION PROTOCOL

There are no precise physical characteristics that clearly distinguish aggressive and malignant tumors from benign and reactive lesions. The only definitive test is histologic evaluation of biopsy material. However, because hand tumors may produce such significant dysfunction, and inadequate or unnecessarily aggressive surgery also presents risks, biopsy must be the final step in obtaining a diagnosis. All nonsurgical studies should be completed before surgical biopsy (Fig. 60-1).

Laboratory Studies

Laboratory studies should include serum calcium, phosphorus, blood urea nitrogen, and creatinine to evaluate the possibility of metabolic bone disease. The serum alkaline phosphatase will be elevated in metabolic bone disease and in some malignancies. A serum immunoelectrophoresis will determine if multiple myeloma is present. The hematologic profile and

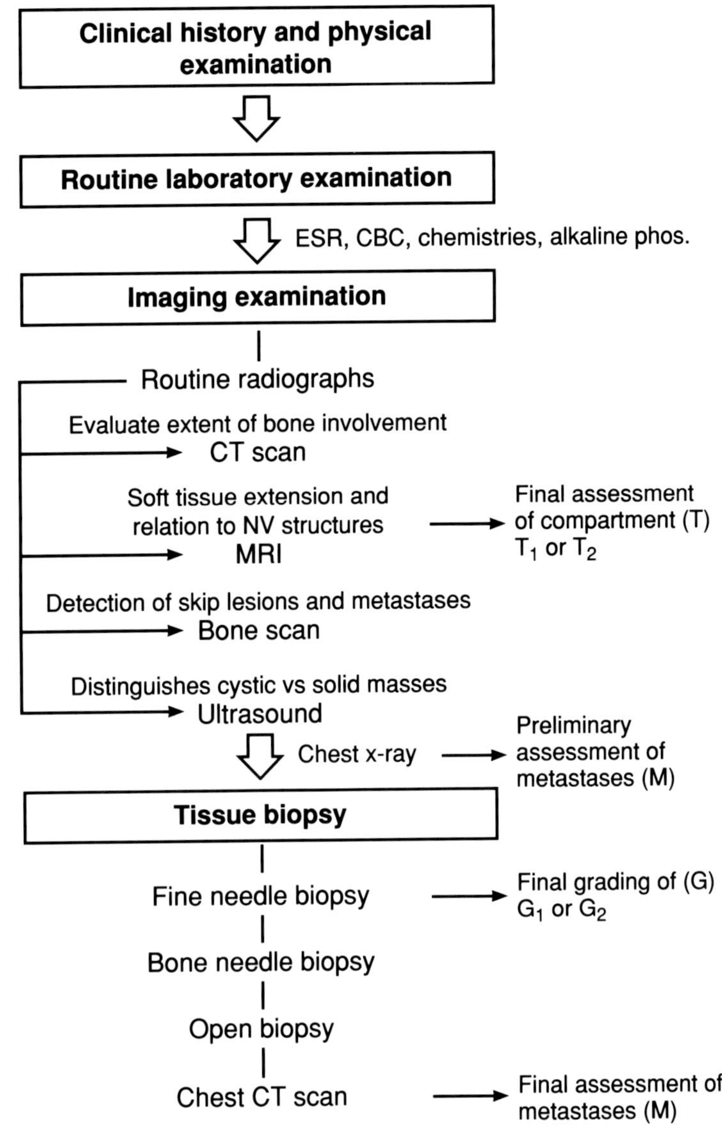

Fig. 60-1. Suggested evaluation protocol for suspected musculoskeletal neoplasms.

the erythrocyte sedimentation rate will be abnormal in the presence of many neoplastic and infectious processes. A urinalysis may detect an occult hypernephroma. Antinuclear antibodies and rheumatoid factor may be positive in patients who have upper extremity swelling secondary to rheumatoid disease.

Diagnostic Imaging

A variety of diagnostic imaging techniques permit us to analyze and localize the size and extent of the lesion and its impingement on normal anatomy. Although imaging does not typically offer a specific diagnosis, it provides important clues in the evaluation, analysis, and work-up of a specific patient.

Plain Radiographs and Tomograms

Plain films afford the best possible resolution and detail of bone and adjacent soft tissues. The anatomic region in question should be fully visualized on all radiographs and tomograms, and this is achieved by taking an adequate number of views. Plain x-rays are the standard for predicting the presence and location of bony involvement. Linear tomography produces images at varying depths and is somewhat useful in studying specific bone tumors.

Computed Tomography

Although conventional radiographs offer significant spacial information, the higher resolution of CT produces images useful specifically in localizing small tumors within a bone and in identifying soft tissue extension or calcifications within such growths. Because of its ability to discriminate varying densities, a CT scan allows visual separation between the medullary canal, cortex, and surrounding soft tissues, often providing critical information concerning anatomic location (T) for tumor staging. Plain chest films should always be done before biopsying a suspected malignancy; chest CT scans are useful for staging histologically defined malignant tumors, but are not used for prebiopsy screening studies.

Arthrography

Arthrography has limited value but may be useful in delineating involvement of synovium by adjacent bone and soft tissue tumors as well as synovial cysts. If combined with CT images, arthrograms can offer excellent detail of joint surfaces and can be of special value, for example, in revealing synovial chondromatosis and differentiating it from chondrosarcoma.

Scintigraphy

Radionuclide "bone scan" imaging can be very helpful in detecting primary and metastatic tumors. However, the phenomenon of increased radiopharmaceutical pooling (increased uptake) in a particular bone or soft tissue area is not at all specific or diagnostic. The technique has two time-variable phases. Within minutes after injection, conditions associated with an increased vascularity show abnormally high uptake (trauma, infection, and neoplasia). Later, the isotopes are actively concentrated; in the skeleton, pooling occurs in woven (new) bone, so that any process that forms immature bone would be associated with increased uptake on films done 2 or 3 hours after injection. Radioisotope scans are probably most helpful to demonstrate lesions that may not have been suspected clinically or in anatomic sites not seen on initial images that focused only on the symptomatic region. These findings may be important in patient management, and they have the potential to alter biopsy or therapeutic plans significantly.

Angiography

Angiography is a technique that has been very important historically for evaluating the vascular supply of tumors and the effect of tumors on surrounding structures. However, for most situations, this same information is available by noninvasive or minimally invasive means, such as the combination of CT, MRI, and scintigraphic studies.

Magnetic Resonance Imaging

MRI is a technique that depends on sophisticated computers to produce excellent delineation of soft tissue contrast as well as images in axial, coronal, and sagittal views. For MRI studies, electromagnets generate strong fields that cause cellular nuclei to "wobble" or "vibrate" at specific frequencies. A number of technical factors affect the MRI signal, including echo time (TE), pulse or repetition time (TR) longitudinal or spin-lattice relaxation (T1) and spin-spin relaxation (T2).

Briefly, one needs to know that short TR and TE times accentuate T1 differences; long TR and TE times accentuate T2 differences. The majority of soft tissue tumors have a low signal intensity (i.e., appear darker) on T1-weighted scans and a high signal intensity (i.e., appear brighter or whiter) on T2-weighted studies. Specific problems such as hematoma, lipoma (or liposarcoma), hemangioma or conditions that involve hemorrhage into an existing tumor zone are known to have a high signal on T1 weighted scans. Obviously, the potential value of MRI is entirely lost in a region recently subjected to prior biopsy, trauma, or other surgery.

Sonography

Sonograms produce images from a differential pattern of transmitted and received echos. Compared to CT and MRI, sonography produces less detail with respect to precise anatomic relationships and tumor margins. Echo patterns of solid masses are nonspecific, but fluid-filled lesions (even deep ones) can be easily differentiated from solid tumors. Sonograms are extremely inexpensive in comparison to the cost of CT and MRI and may be more useful than either for distinguishing reactive and cystic processes.

BIOPSY

The biopsy is the last stage of diagnostic management. Biopsy surgery should be planned as carefully as the definitive operation.[31,39] The exact technique used is influenced by history, location, and size of the mass as well as the experience of the surgeon and the pathologist.

Needle Biopsy

Needle biopsy has an extremely limited role in the diagnosis of lesions in the hand and upper extremity, although it can be helpful in obtaining information on deep or inaccessible tumors in other locations. It is also useful in confirming the histology of a recurrent or metastatic lesion. Needle biopsy produces only a small and often fragmented tissue sample that may be impossible to diagnose or grade accurately. Even if the core biopsy seems clearly diagnosable, the tissue volume may not be representative of the tumor, leading to the possibility of overgrading or undermanagement.

Open Biopsy

Open surgical biopsy is a complex procedure, but one that plays a critical role in determining treatment outcome for aggressive and malignant tumors.[31,39,40] During the biopsy, the patient and surgeon must be prepared for the unexpected. Institutions or clinicians who are not prepared or able to complete all diagnostic studies *and also* provide definitive surgical and medical/adjunctive management are best advised to refer patients *before* the biopsy is performed.

Hand surgery is most safely and efficiently performed in a bloodless field. The use of a pneumatic tourniquet is acceptable both during open biopsy and surgical treatment of tumors and neoplasms. Unless the physician is entirely certain that the lesion is benign, limb exsanguination is contraindicated before tourniquet inflation because of the risk of seeding or dislodging tumor cells (a caveat that applies equally to the seeding of bacteria from infections or infected tumors). An entirely satisfactory field is achievable by elevating the arm for about 3 to 4 minutes before inflating the tourniquet. Likewise, use of intravenous anesthesia (Bier block technique), a method that also requires pretourniquet exsanguination, is not appropriate for tumor biopsy or treatment of aggressive bone or soft tissue neoplasms.

A frozen section is necessary at the time the biopsy is performed to determine whether an adequate specimen has been sampled so that permanent light and special microscopic evaluations can be carried out subsequently. It is rare to find a pathologist who can consistently provide accurate histologic analysis of a frozen specimen dependable enough to begin treatment.[31,39,40] The definitive treatment plan should be decided upon only after results of all permanent sections, electron microscopic studies, and special tissue techniques are complete and reported. *All* biopsies should be cultured (and all cultures should be biopsied). Although plain chest radiographs are taken before biopsy, chest CT is performed to stage a diagnosed lesion. If the tumor is aggressive or malignant, the biopsy tract itself will be contaminated with tumor cells. Preferred biopsy incisions are therefore longitudinal and carefully placed so as to permit their complete excision without having to extend a dissection margin simply to accommodate a badly placed biopsy incision (Fig. 60-2).

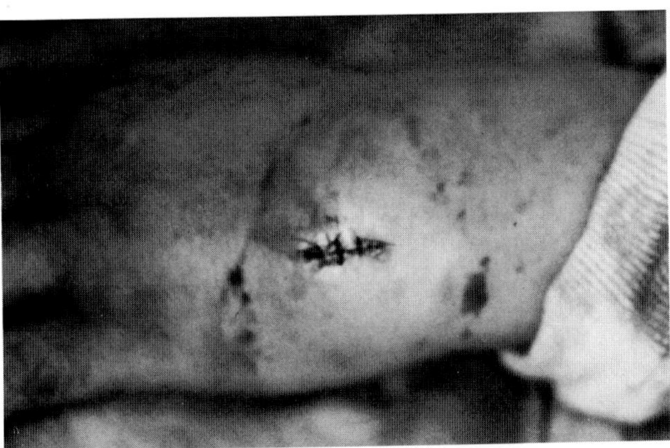

Fig. 60-2. An open incisional biopsy was performed for a rapidly growing hand lesion. The biopsy site is contaminated with tumor cells; the incision is oriented longitudinally and will be excised as part of the definitive procedure performed later. Frozen section at biopsy verified adequacy of the specimen sample.

Incisional Biopsy

Incisional biopsy is frequently the most appropriate technique for diagnosis of bone and soft tissue masses. It requires excision of an adequate tissue sample that is minimally manipulated and suture-tagged for orientation. Frozen sections are important to determine specimen sample adequacy. The biopsy incision is located to afford the *most* direct route to the tumor, thereby assuring that the fewest tissue planes are disturbed or contaminated.

Correct surgical technique for biopsy is different from all typical surgical dissections. Biopsy involves a *direct* approach via longitudinal incision *through* muscle and other tissues that overlie the mass. Biopsy technique does *not* include spreading or extensive and vigorous retraction, which has the potential to contaminate a widened area. However, adequate visualization during biopsy, as is true of any operation, is critical. Because the biopsy tract is cell-contaminated, an approach through a muscle sacrifices only one plane, whereas spreading techniques (i.e., moving muscles aside) contaminates not only the muscle that is retracted but all surrounding structures. Postsurgical hemostasis is essential to avoid hematoma, which potentially can lead to cellular spread beyond the primary site and biopsy tract. Once the wound is dry and hemostasis secure following tourniquet release, the wound is closed, not drained. Postbiopsy surgical care is otherwise routine while the surgeon awaits the definitive histologic findings.

Excisional Biopsy

Excisional biopsy involves complete removal of a lesion without a significant margin of normal tissue. It is a technique that should be reserved for very small lesions (a diameter smaller than 1 to 2 cm) to avoid compromising subsequent surgical procedures. When necessary, excised skin or other superficial lesions (sites) may be either left open or temporarily covered by a synthetic semi-occlusive material until the definitive biopsy results are available.

DEFINITIVE TREATMENT

General Plan of Tumor Excision

Benign Tumors

Nonaggressive, benign neoplasms are usually removed simply by marginal or intralesional operations such as "shelling out" or curettage. If there is a question about the adequacy of resection, or of the tissue margins—and the diagnosis is already confirmed—a frozen section may be of great assistance for intraoperative sampling of the margins.

Malignant Tumors

In the management of malignancies of the upper limb, preservation of function is secondary to eradication of the disease process.[43] The hand surgeon who undertakes management of a neoplasm must have a thorough understanding of the tumor's biological behavior, its patterns of local and metastatic spread, and its response to radiotherapy and chemotherapy. Radiation and chemotherapy may allow the surgeon to use less radical tumor margins so that amputation may be avoided and function may be restored.[10,14,15,28,33,38,41,48,49] However, the risk of unnecessary sacrifice of tissue must be balanced against the need for adequate resection because local recurrence of sarcoma carries such a grave prognosis.[7] One of the major problems in assessing outcome has been the lack of a common procedural language regarding surgical methods; however, uniform use of the Enneking terminology as recommended by the MSTS will provide such a means of communication[16] (Table 60-4).

Treatment should not begin until a neoplasm has been diagnosed definitively and the results of all preoperative studies, including biopsy, are verified. The assumption that a problem can be "handled" by a relatively simple extirpation in the absence of complete diagnostic data is neither justified nor defensible. The risks associated with soft tissue extension from a tumor-contaminated field are too great. Because most tumors are benign, cystic, and nonproblematic, the outcome of those few that are aggressive or truly malignant may be disastrous if we become too casual or complacent. When a malignant tumor or aggressive nonmalignant lesion is identified, carefully planned treatment is required not only to preserve a maximal degree of hand function but also to save the patient's life. Function is secondary to survival[1,10,23,27,31,42,43] (Fig. 60-3A–H).

The hand surgeon who seeks to treat a specific neoplasm must have not only a general understanding of the concepts and principles of tumor management, but also a detailed knowledge of this tumor's biology, histologic and clinical behavior, tendency to spread locally and widely, and potential response to adjunctive measures. All of these considerations may bear significantly on proposed surgical margins and long-term functions.[10,14,15,28,33,38,41,48,49] These issues will be discussed in detail with respect to important and serious growths later in the next chapter. In this section, we will focus on surgical paradigms since the resection that permits a local recurrence may condemn the patient to a far worse prognosis than would otherwise occur.[3,7,12,19–21,29,36,39]

According to MSTS criteria, compartmental resection and radical excision cannot yet be applied to the hand.[12,13] Most hand tumors occur in spaces rather than in compartments, and although metacarpal excisions may remove a compartment for a IA or IIA bone tumor, extirpation of the entire flexor surface or above-elbow amputation would be required to remove the compartment if the neoplasm arises on a digital flexor. Presently there are no data to support a conclusion that the MSTS definitions should be applied uniformly to all parts of an acral compartment. Since the flexor tenosynovium is continuous in the thumb and little finger, but not in the index, middle, and ring fingers, there may be differences in management that can be prudently used with such variations in location. A soft tissue tumor that develops along the dorsum of the wrist requires surgical extirpation of the extensors of several fingers and/or the thumb but not necessarily of the entire muscle compartment proximally or distally. Functional restoration can be achieved via tendon grafts, transfers, or free muscle flaps. True radical excision may be impractical if function of any kind is to be salvaged in lesions of the hand and forearm, and it may be that a 3- to 5-cm margin of normal tissue, especially with tumors that are sensitive to adjuncts, will be safe and allow secondary reconstruction.[11,13,14,26,30,32,34,35,42,47] The extent of surgical resection for aggressive tumors is dependent on the histologic diagnosis, location, and size. Although there are no data to support the hypothesis that smaller tumors may be safely resected with smaller margins, the general principles of tumor biology apply.[11–14,26,32,35,42] Remote tissues, except when provided by microvascular transfer,[24,50,51,52] should be avoided because of the risk of transferring malignant cells via tissue/flap pedicles.

Table 60-4. Surgical Procedures for Extremity Sarcomas

Margin	Surgical Method: Limb-salvage	Surgical Method: Amputation	Plans of Dissection	Microscopic Appearance
Intralesional	Debulking, piecemeal excision/curettage	Translesional amputation	Within tumor (palliative)	Tumor at all margins
Marginal	Marginal en bloc excision	Marginal amputation	Within tumor "reactive zone"	Reactive tissue (± microextensions of tumor)
Wide	Wide en bloc excision	Wide through-bone amputation	Through normal tissue but within compartment	Normal tissue (± "skip lesions")
Radical	En bloc resection of entire compartment	Extraarticular disarticulation	Normal tissue—extracompartmental	Normal tissue

(Adapted from Enneking,[17] with permission.)

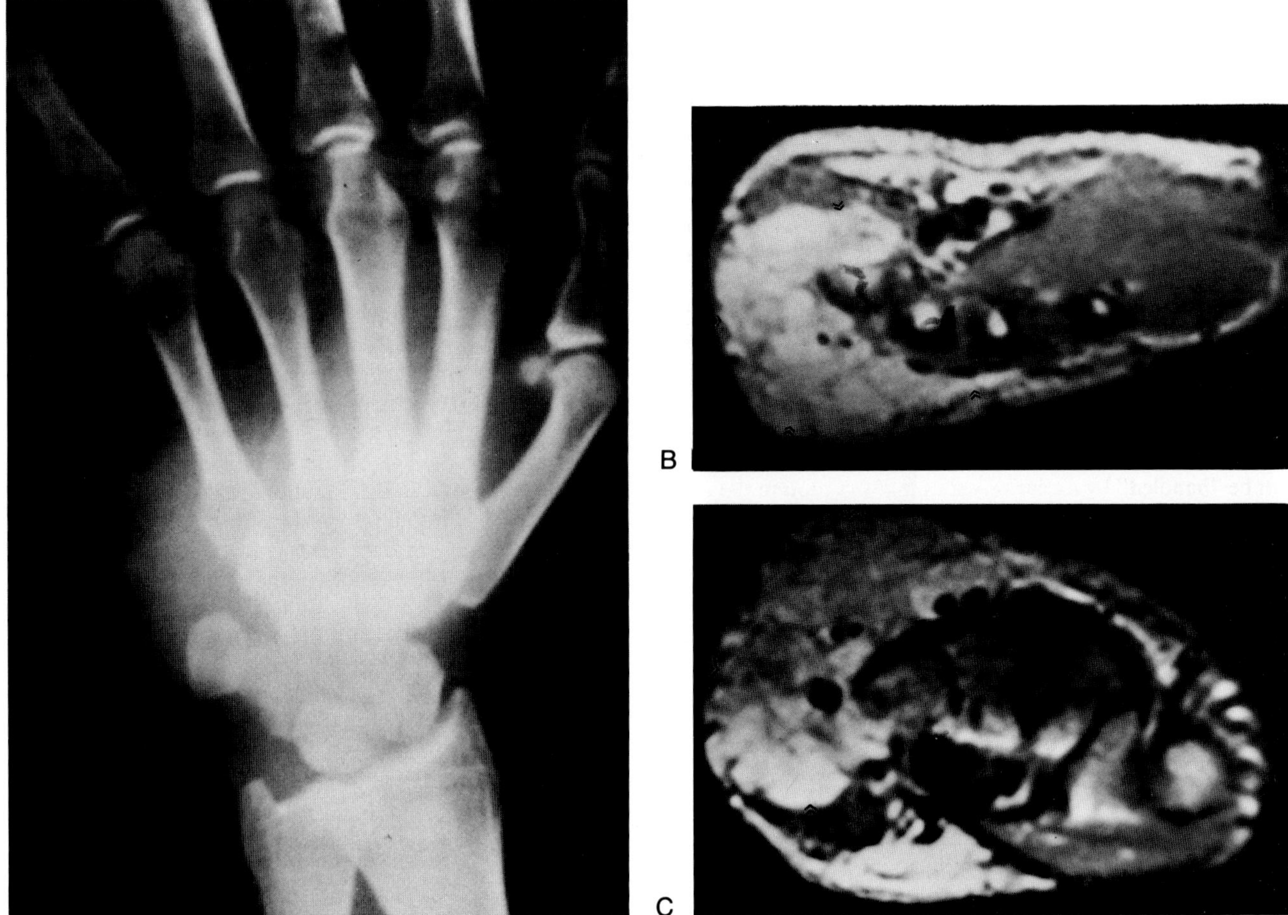

Fig. 60-3. A 39-year-old construction laborer reported an 8-month history of an enlarging mass following an injury at work. Plain radiographs (**A**) demonstrated only a soft tissue shadow, but MRI (**B&C**) revealed a solid tumor extending along the dorsal subaponeurotic space to at least the third metacarpal and with possible invasion of the carpal tunnel *(arrows)*. *(Figure continues.)*

Principles of Excision for Specific Sites

Malignant Bone and Soft Tissue Tumors of the Distal Phalanx

Malignant soft tissue tumors in the distal phalanx typically involve skin and bone[8,21] (Fig. 60-4A–C). Safe removal may require excision at the distal interphalangeal (DIP) joint; occasionally a lesser segment may need to be excised when the lesion, such as a nail bed carcinoma, is more superficial and slow growing. A small portion of dorsal or palmar skin might be used as a local flap in order to cover the middle phalanx after DIP joint disarticulation. In such an instance, the distal phalanx and DIP joint are sacrificed if the lesion involves or threatens enough tissue, while retaining the tissues at a safe distance from the tumor site. Indeed, if the tumor involves both the dorsal and palmar surfaces of soft tissue as well as bone, a more proximal transosseous amputation through the middle phalanx is required. In every case, the proximal end of the excision margin should be biopsied and inspected by frozen section at operation and later by permanent technique histology in order to assure the safety of the level of removal.

Malignant distal phalangeal lesions require removal with an appropriate cuff of contiguous soft tissue. Lower-grade bone tumors may be managed by distal phalangeal amputation including a soft tissue cuff 1 to 2 cm proximal to the intraosseous tumor, a level that requires transosseous resection through the middle phalanx. It is unlikely that such lesions could be safely removed by DIP disarticulation alone. Cases that present with pathologic fractures or extracompartmental extension (coming from or into bone) usually require removal of the finger at or proximal to PIP level, or even ray resection.

Malignant Tumors of the Middle Phalanx

Malignant and aggressive soft tissue tumors in the middle phalanx and those proximal to the region of the DIP joint require amputation at MP joint or metacarpal level (i.e., ray

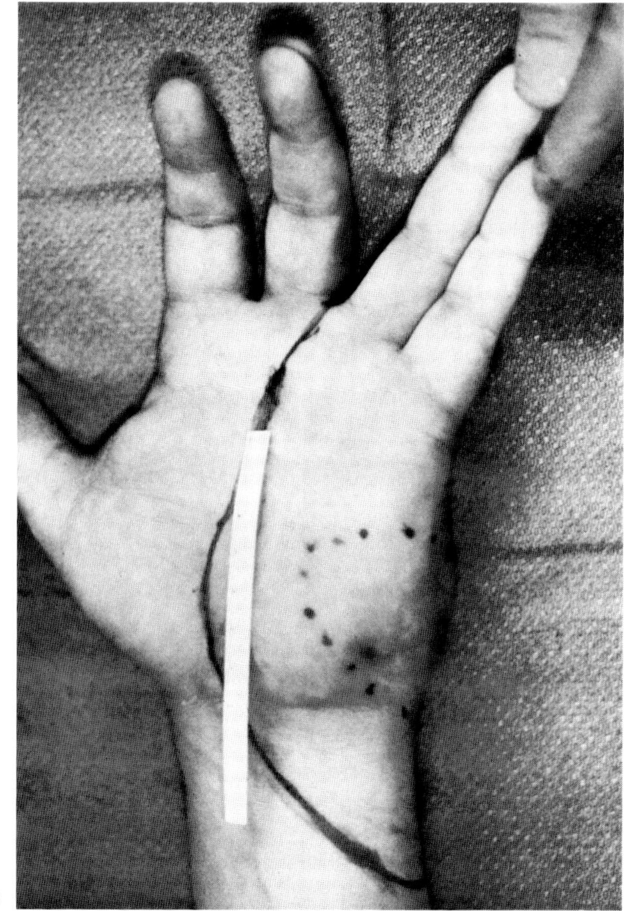

D

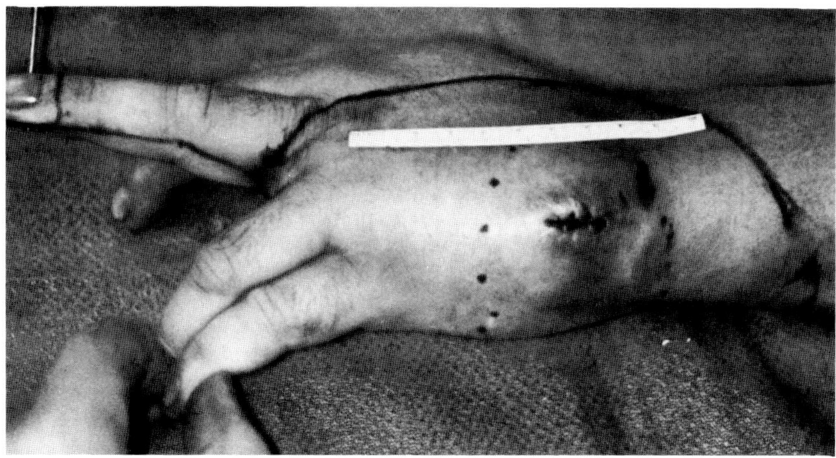

E

Fig. 60-3 *(Continued).* After completion of preoperative studies, incisional biopsy revealed a malignant fibrous histiocytoma. Partial hand amputation was planned **(D&E),** anticipating resection of the second through fifth metacarpals with bone graft to preserve index length, plus coverage of the ulnar palm with an axial filet flap of the middle finger. *(Figure continues.)*

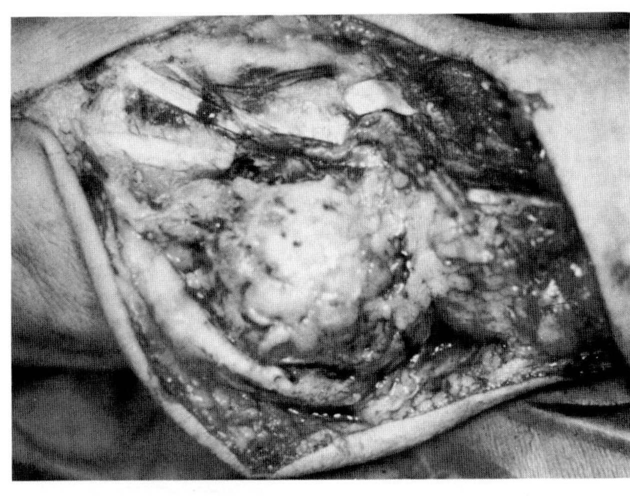
F

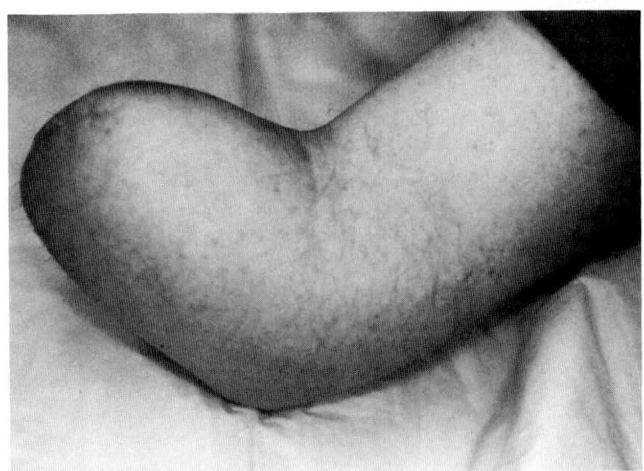
G

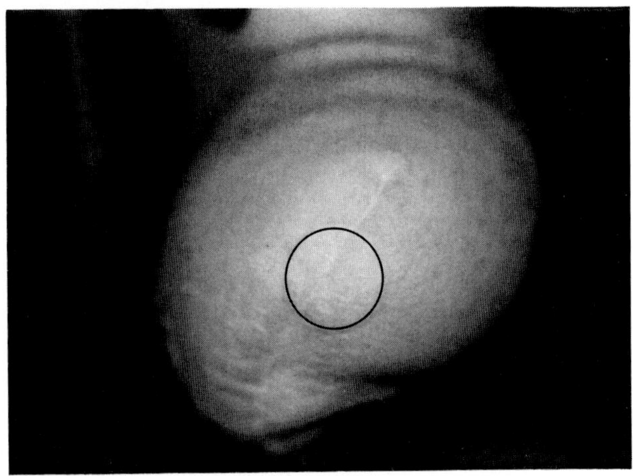
H

Fig. 60-3 *(Continued)*. **(F–H):** At surgery, the tumor was found to have invaded the second dorsal compartment **(F)** as well as the carpal tunnel. In order to control the tumor, the planned procedure was abandoned (this possibility had been explained to the patient preoperatively) and a below elbow amputation performed **(G)**. Multiple biopsies of the forearm and amputated limb, plus later detailed pathologic dissection, revealed no evidence of tumor proximal to the wrist. The patient received chemotherapy and did well. Thirteen months after amputation, however, he noted a firm nodule at the stump suture line **(H**—outlined). When biopsied, this proved to be a regional metastasis from his original tumor. An elbow disarticulation was performed, followed by local radiation and additional chemotherapy. (Courtesy of Edward Diao, M.D.)

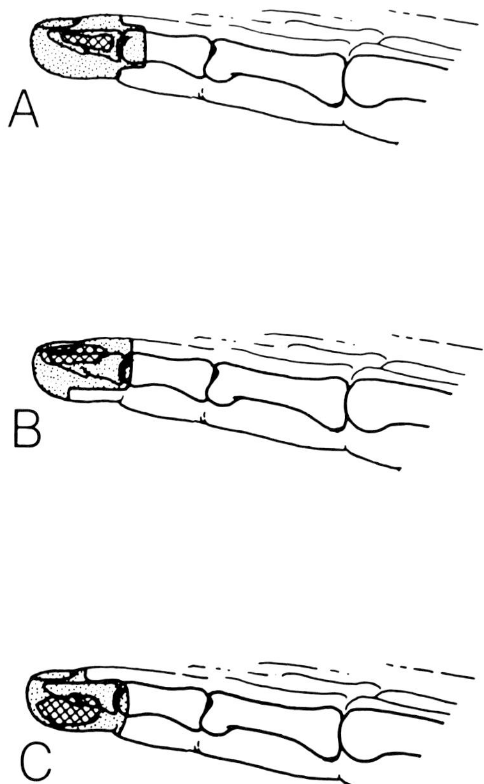

Fig. 60-4. Malignant lesions of the terminal segment of the finger generally require amputation at or proximal to the DIP joint. **(A)** Intraosseous distal phalangeal tumors are amputated at or proximal to the joint, with combined dorsal and volar flap closure. **(B)** Dorsal lesions are treated by appropriate tumor excision and volar flap closure. **(C)** After removal of a palmar tumor, dorsal flap closure may be possible.

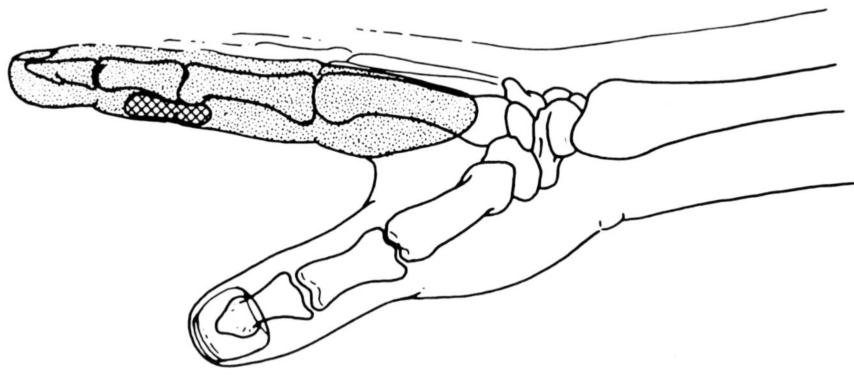

Fig. 60-5. Tumors of the soft tissue at the middle phalangeal and PIP joint level are best treated by ray resection.

resection) (Fig. 60-5). In this instance MP joint disarticulation should allow at least a 2- to 3-cm margin of normal tissue. However, functional and aesthetic considerations strongly recommend ray resection (Fig. 60-6). In theory, bone tumors involving the proximal and middle phalanges may be excised and replaced with bone graft (allograft) if the lesion is not aggressive and if it has not extended into the soft tissues. However, ray resection is a actually a far more practical, functional alternative if both the proximal and middle phalanges are involved. For tumors that have spread beyond bone via fracture or by slow, progressive extension, ray amputation is clearly indicated whereas local excision is not.

Amputations of the central rays (middle and ring fingers) may be reconstructed by primary transposition of the adjacent border digit or by ligamentous reconstruction. (See Chapter 3 on amputation techniques.) MP joint disarticulation is rarely a safe, practical, functional, or aesthetic choice for treating tumors at these levels.

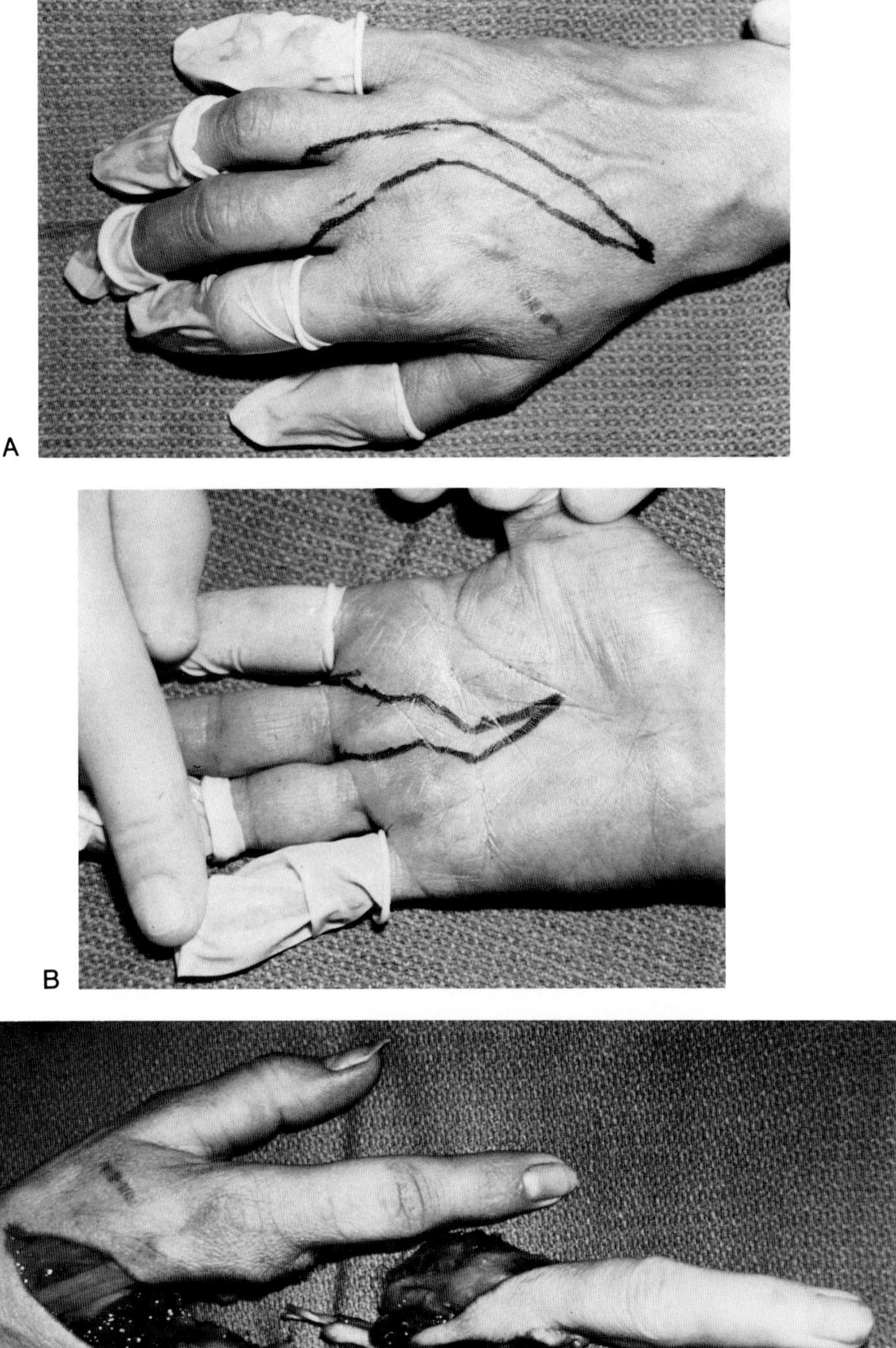

Fig. 60-6. **(A)** Excisional biopsy of a mass on the ulnar surface of the middle finger revealed a fibrosarcoma. **(B)** Ray resection was performed. **(C)** Third ray resection included contiguous intraosseous muscles. *(Figure continues.)*

D

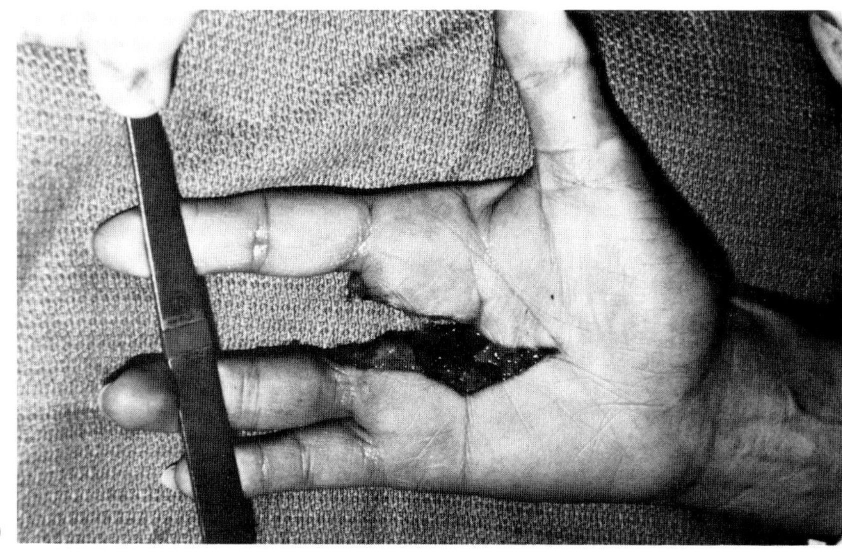

E

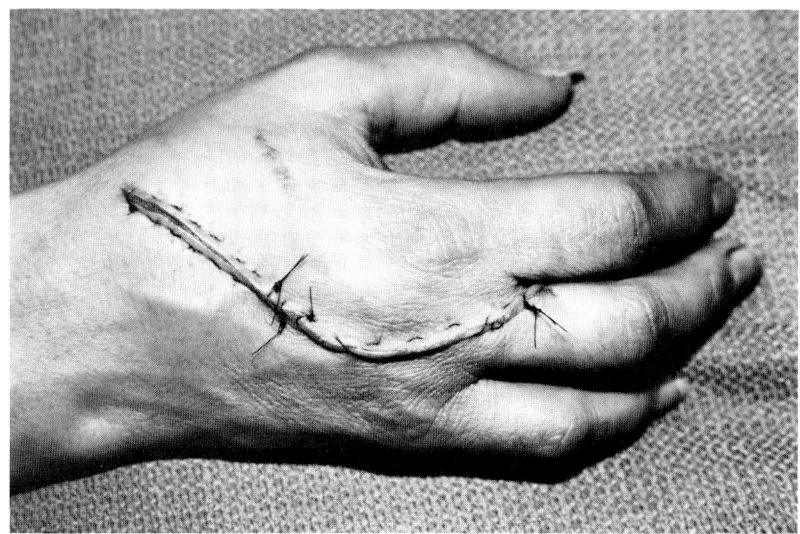

F

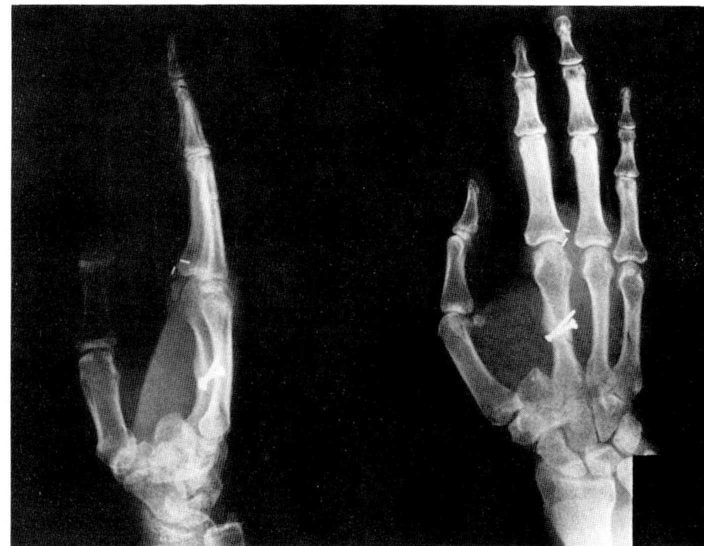

Fig. 60-6 *(Continued).* **(D&E)** The second metacarpal was transposed to the third metacarpal base. **(F)** Postoperative radiograph. *(Figure continues.)*

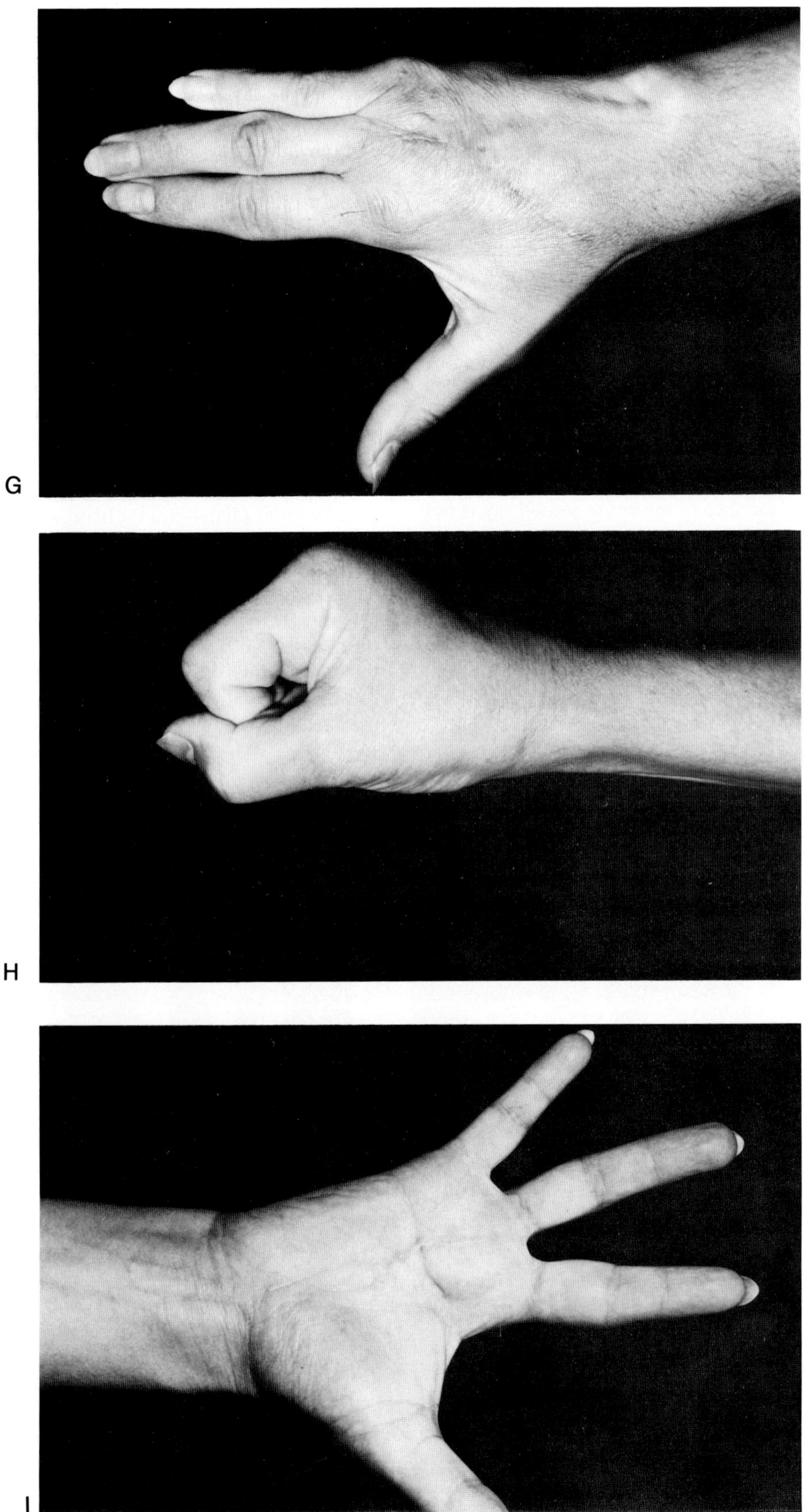

Fig. 60-6 *(Continued).* **(G–I)** Appearance following rehabilitation. Function and aesthetic appearance were retained.

Tumors of the First Metacarpal

Intracompartmental first metacarpal malignancies may be treated by osseous excision and autogenous or allograft replacement (Fig. 60-7). Following removal, biopsies should be taken from the soft tissue bed surrounding the excised bone, and the metacarpal also carefully studied to exclude breakthrough. Replacement by metatarsal or metacarpal allograft, or fibular or iliac autograft, may be considered in appropriate circumstances.[29,44,46] Autografting should be done utilizing a second, separate surgical setup to avoid cross contamination of the bone donor site. Osteoarticular allografts may be unstable, and arthrodesis may be required at the trapeziometacarpal articulation.

If a bone tumor has broken into soft tissue, a more radical resection is required, including the entire first ray, and/or larger portions of the web and second metacarpal in order to gain a safe margin. If part of the second metacarpal is resected, the "floating index" thereby produced can be considered for direct pollicization if sacrifice of the entire second ray is not required.[10,22]

Tumors of the Finger Metacarpals

Aggressive and malignant bone tumors of the second through fifth metacarpals generally require en bloc bone excision. Curettage can be complicated by intermediate or late recurrence[1] (Fig. 60-8). A more important treatment decision may be whether removal of one metacarpal alone is possible or whether removal of an entire ray, or pair of rays, is best. Ray excision is usually best for lesions of the second and fifth metacarpals (Fig. 60-9). With the additional consideration of ray transposition, the principles governing removal of the third and fourth rays are no different from those governing the second and fifth. If allograft metatarsal has been used, carpometacarpal arthrodesis, and MP ligament reconstruction or silicone arthroplasty may be practical. Whatever level is chosen for reconstruction, it is essential that an adequate, safe margin of normal tissue first be excised en bloc with the tumor.

Aggressive tumors of the second through fifth metacarpals, which have invaded soft tissue or sustained pathologic fractures, often require excision not only of the involved ray but also of the contiguous ray(s) radial and ulnar to the involved digit. A malignant tumor of the second metacarpal that extends into the soft tissues may necessitate removal of the second and third rays, or of the first through third rays, while preserving soft tissue of the middle finger as a filet flap to resurface the radial side of the hand. A similar technique can be employed on tumors on the ulnar side of the hand. If the second, third, and fourth rays must be removed, the best strategy is usually to osteotomize and supinate the fifth metacarpal to promote effective oppositional pinch and grasp to the thumb. If a tumor of the fourth metacarpal requires removal of the third through fifth ray, the radial aspect of the middle finger or a filet of that digit on its radial neurovascular pedicle can be used to close the ulnar side of the hand. Tumors of the fifth

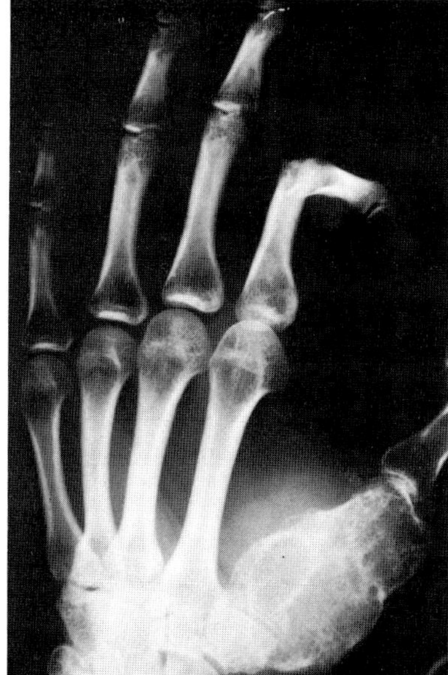

A

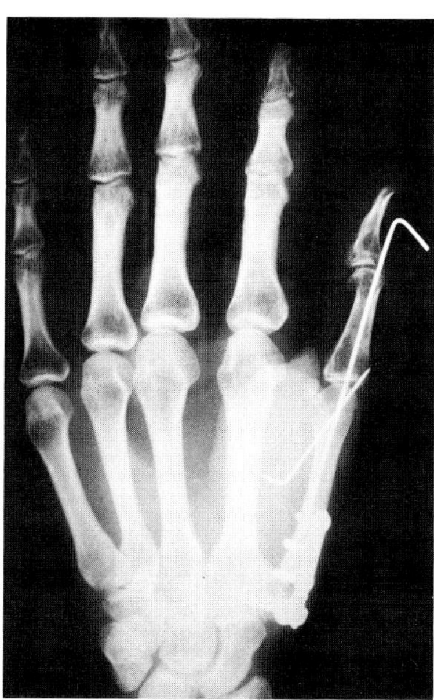

B

Fig. 60-7. **(A)** Recurrent tumor in the first metacarpal following excision of an enchondroma proved to be a low-grade chondrosarcoma. **(B)** The first metacarpal and distal trapezium were removed with contiguous soft tissues and replaced by an allograft, MP reconstruction, and CMC joint arthrodesis.

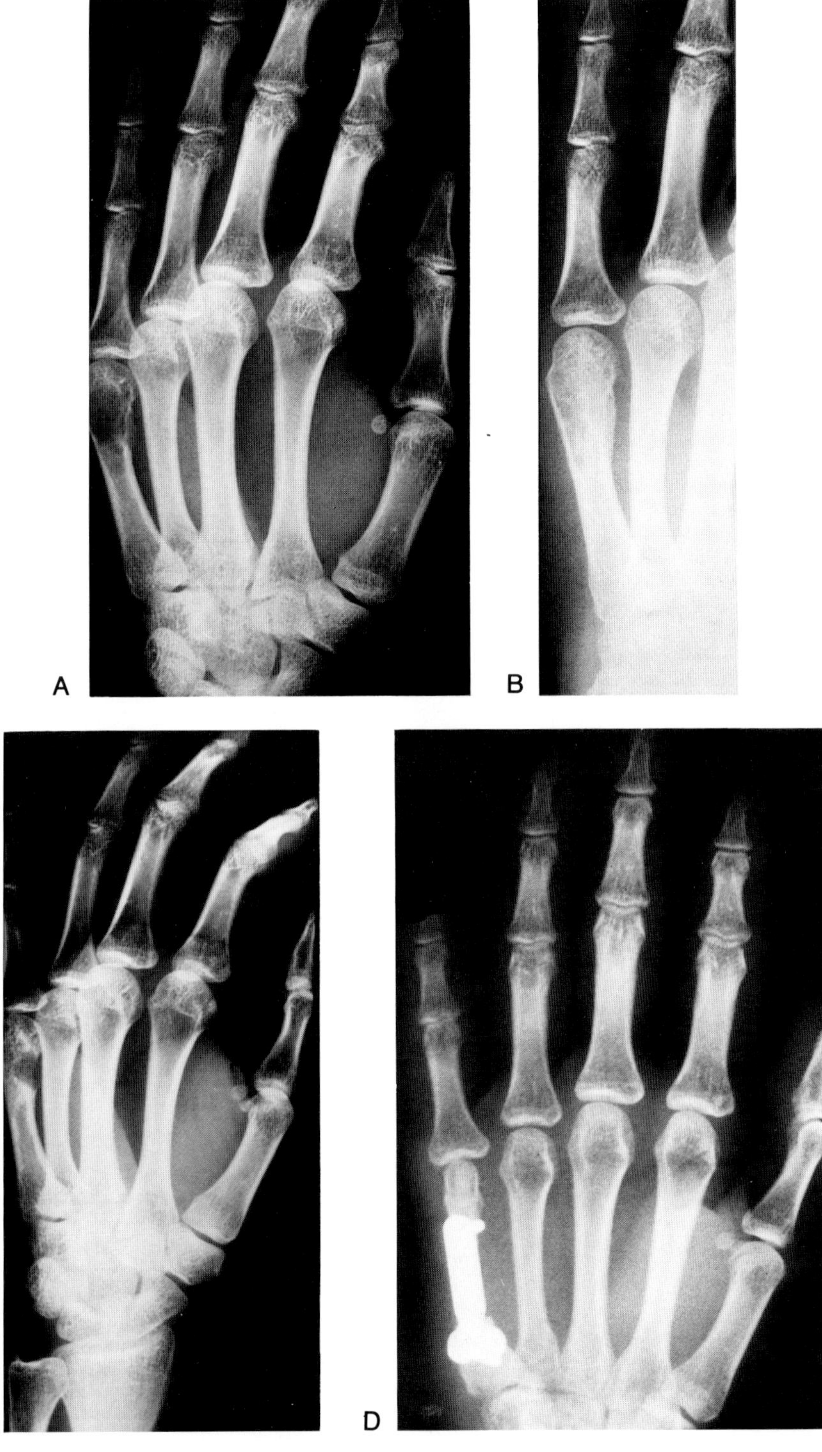

Fig. 60-8. **(A)** Giant cell tumor of the fifth metacarpal in a 17-year-old woman. **(B)** Six months after curettage and bone graft, there was no evidence of recurrent tumor. **(C)** One year later, symptoms and radiographs showed a recurrent lytic lesion. **(D)** The fifth metacarpal was removed and replaced with a metatarsal allograft shown here 1 year after reconstruction.

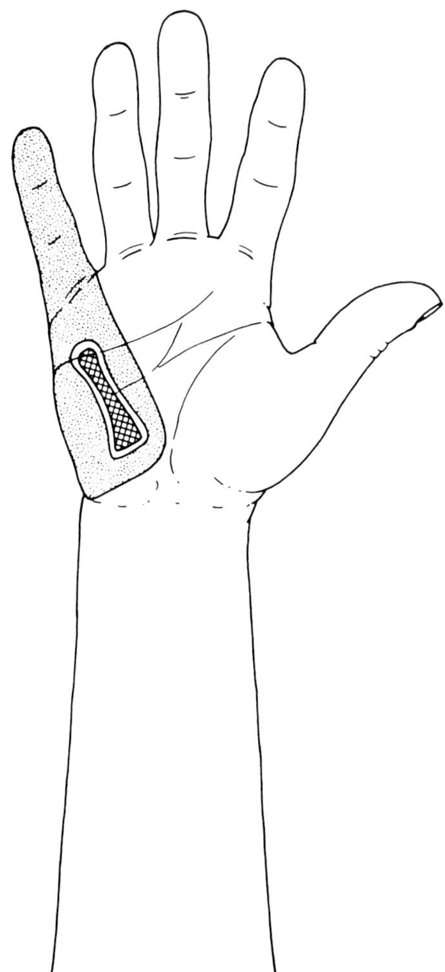

Fig. 60-9. Malignant tumors of the fifth metacarpal can be treated by ray excision.

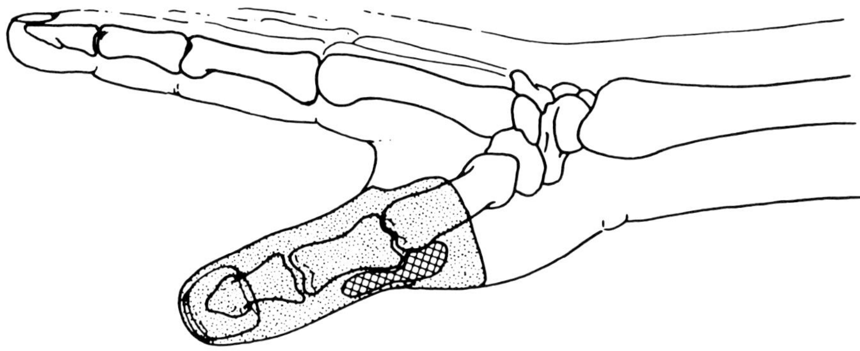

Fig. 60-10. Malignant soft tissue tumors adjacent to the thumb MP joint require amputation through the metacarpal; more aggressive and extensive tumors may require removal of the entire ray, possibly contiguous with the second metacarpal.

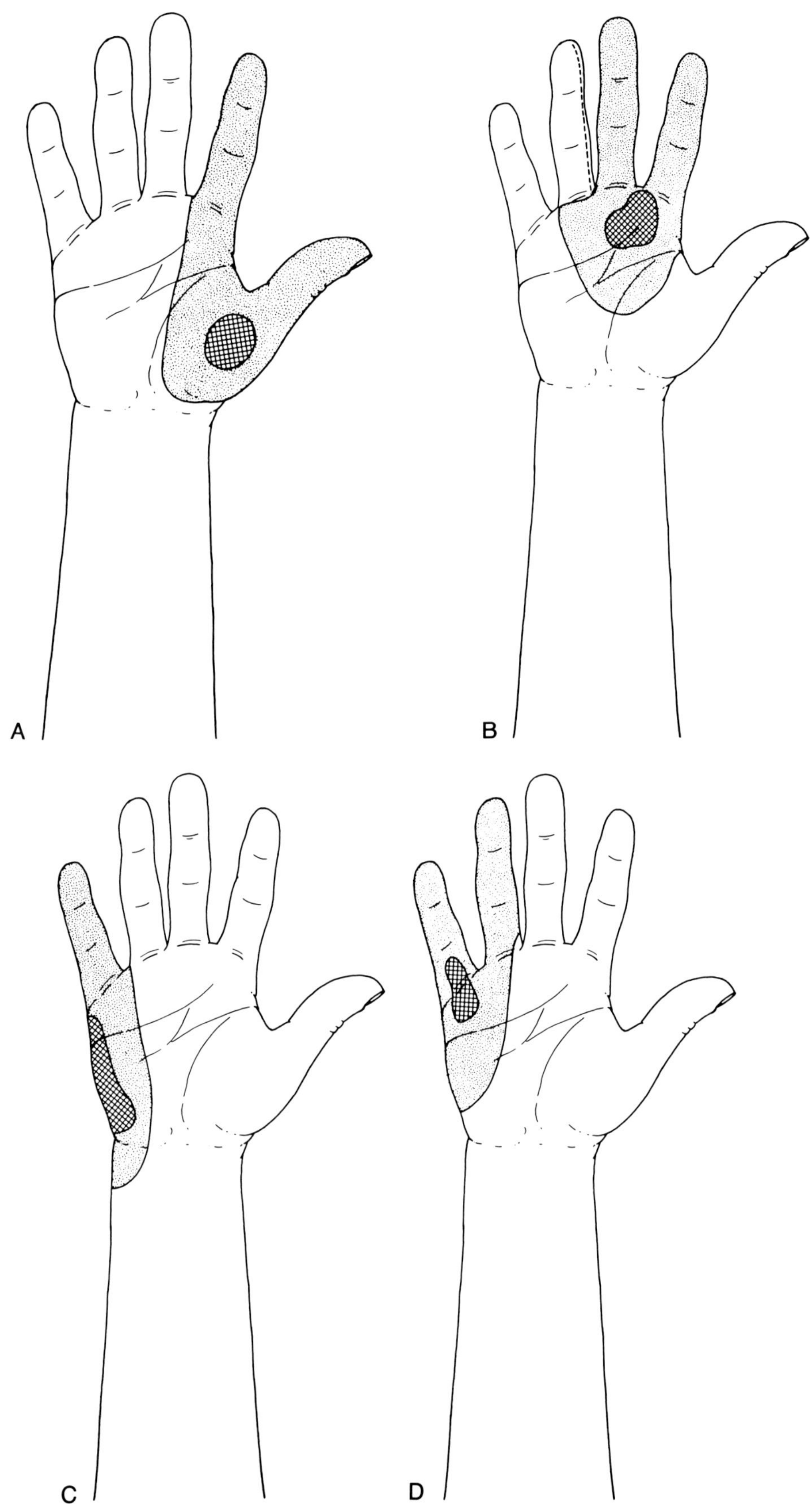

Fig. 60-11. (A) Tumors located between the first and second metacarpals may require amputation of both rays for adequate local control. **(B)** Tumors between the second and third metacarpals require removal of both rays. **(C)** Lesions of the ulnar border of the hand can be treated by fifth ray resection and local flap or skin graft closure. **(D)** Large and more aggressive lesions or those extending more radially may need removal of both the fourth and fifth rays.

metacarpal require excision of at least the fourth and fifth rays and similar skin coverage potentially possible from the ring finger, or as a rotation flap from the dorsum of the hand, or a combination of the two.

If a malignant tumor has broken into the midpalm and extended across the metacarpals, removal of all digital rays may be needed to gain an adequate soft tissue margin. Retention of a sensate and relatively mobile thumb may be considerably more aesthetic and functionally satisfactory than a forearm or wrist level amputation.[45] However, if a tumor extends proximally from the metacarpals, a more proximal level of hand, wrist, or forearm amputation is required for safe tumor management (see Fig. 60-3A–H).

Soft tissue tumors in the palm or on the dorsum of the hand, as well as metacarpal tumors, usually require at least a partial hand amputation. If treated by only local or limited excision, the chance of recurrence and metastasis may be enhanced; below elbow amputation is necessary to treat these larger tumors. It is unusual for an aggressive soft tissue tumor to be adequately removed by a truly local en bloc excision. At a minimum, aggressive soft tissue tumors, like bony tumors, require ray resection or removal of multiple rays (Figs. 60-10 to 60-12). Central palmar lesions usually require sacrifice of three rays; those on the border are more likely than those in the center to be salvageable by removing only two rays. In the presence of proximal, broader, and larger lesions, all four digits or the entire hand may be sacrificed to save the patient.

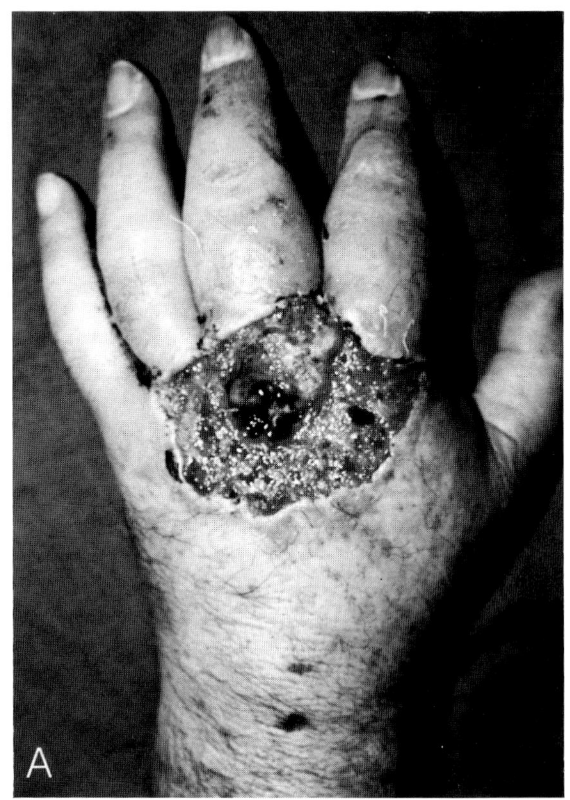

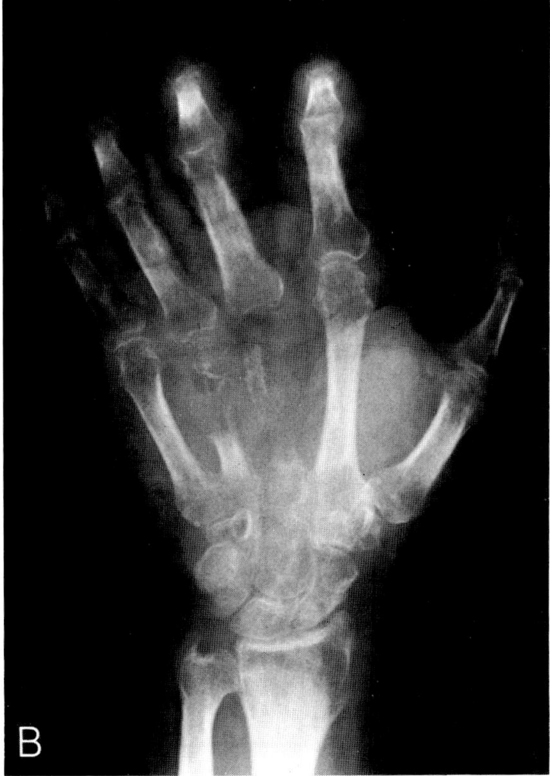

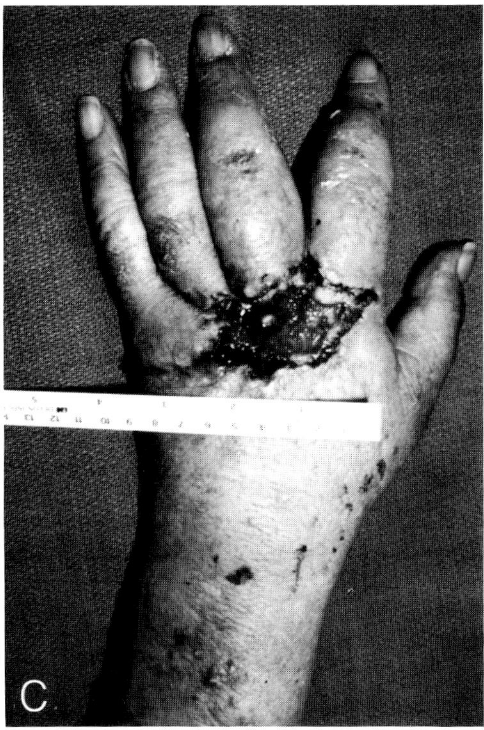

Fig. 60-12. **(A&B)** This neglected squamous cell carcinoma progressed to invade and destroy the third and fourth metacarpals. **(C)** After staging to rule out metastases, the patient received intravenous cyst-platinum, with a resultant decrease in tumor size. *(Figure continues.)*

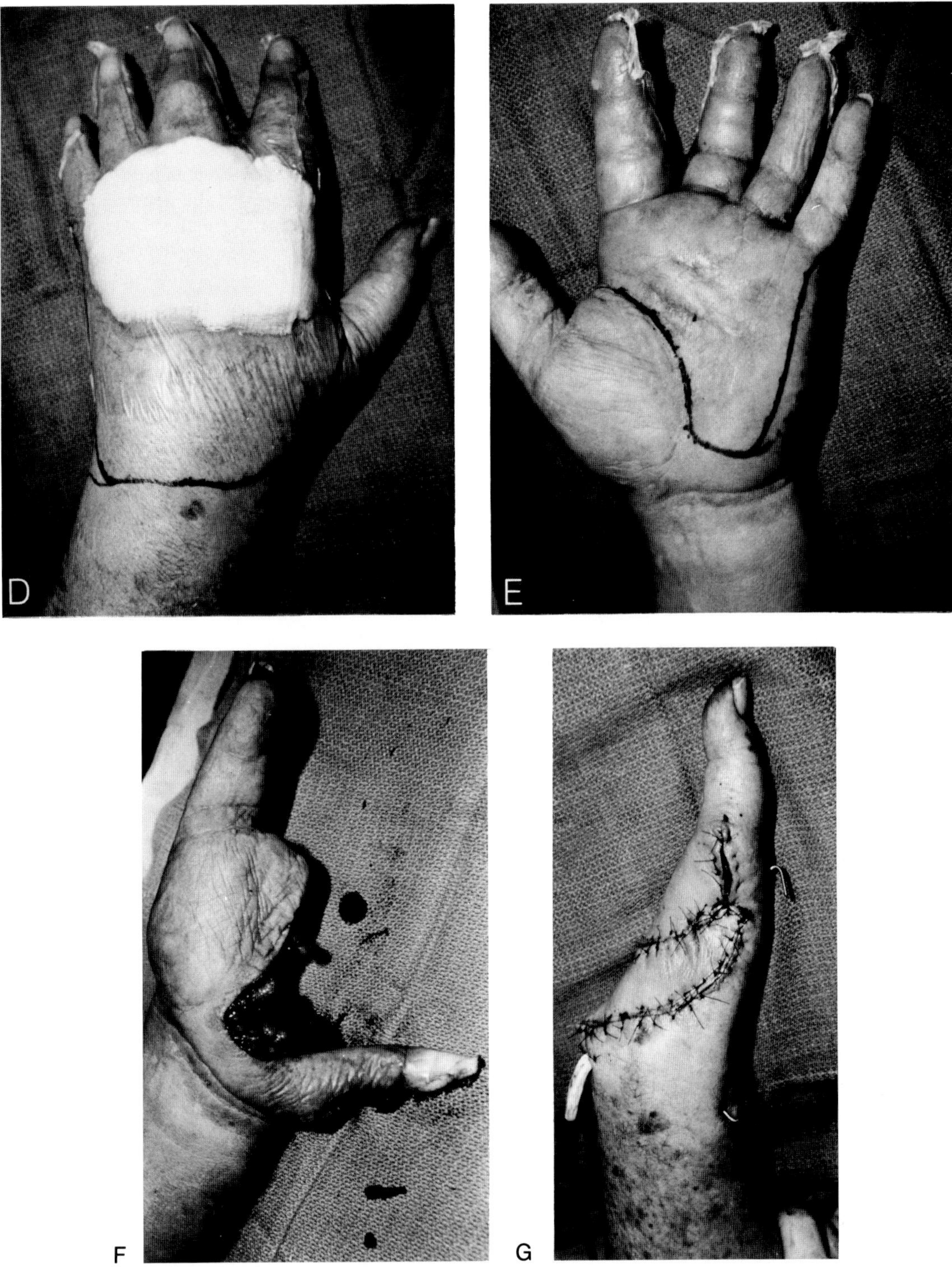

Fig. 60-12 *(Continued).* **(D–G)** The tumor was removed by partial hand resection, retaining the ulnar skin in order to resurface the border of the thumb. Axillary node dissection was negative.

Tumors of the Wrist and Distal Forearm

Malignancies of the proximal palmar hand and volar wrist should not be treated with local excision. A dissection that attempts to "salvage" the median nerve or one or two flexors in the middle of an expanding tumor or reactive zone is likely only to spread the disease. Correct surgical and medical principles of tumor removal and care should be followed (Figs. 60-13 to 60-15).

Tumors that arise on the dorsum may allow preservation of the hand if staging studies show that the lesion has not penetrated into the palm, and the excision margin verifies a safe plane of normal tissue. Isolated intraosseous carpal lesions that have not invaded soft tissue are rare but may be excised locally. The carpals are intraarticular, so the onset of symptoms is usually associated with synovitis and joint invasion; therefore below elbow amputation is likely to be necessary.

Growths on the volar aspect of the distal forearm generally require above or below elbow amputation since it is not easy to excise a tumor adequately and still preserve function in and distal to this region following removal of all flexor muscles and tendons, the median and ulnar nerves, and vessels. If a tumor arises in a location that does not specifically involve the ulnar nerve and artery, it may be possible to save a portion of the hand and wrist along with the neurovascular bundle and to consider later reconstruction after longitudinal hemiamputa-

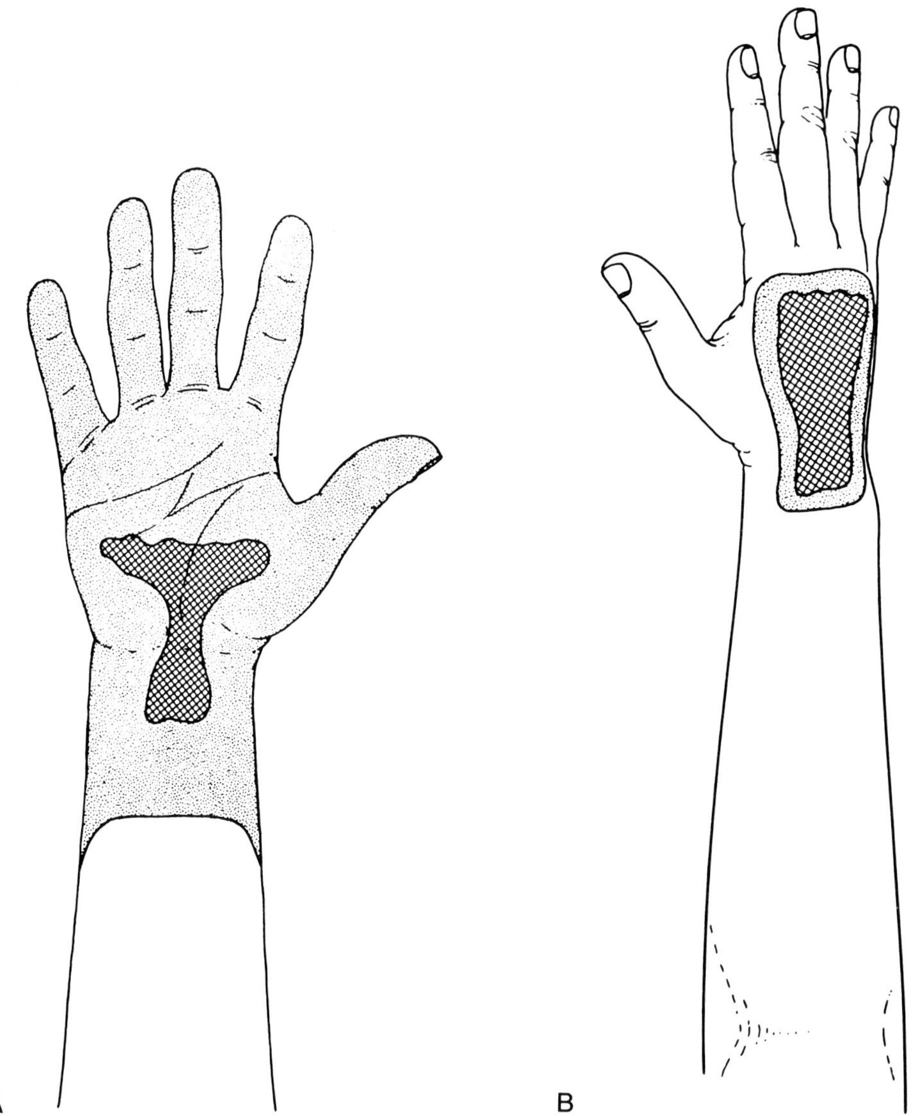

Fig. 60-13. **(A)** Tumors on the proximal volar palm often involve the flexor tendons and median and ulnar nerves; forearm or wrist level amputation is usually required. **(B)** Lesions on the dorsum of the hand may not necessarily invade vital neurovascular structures and can be adequately resected en bloc followed by secondary reconstruction.

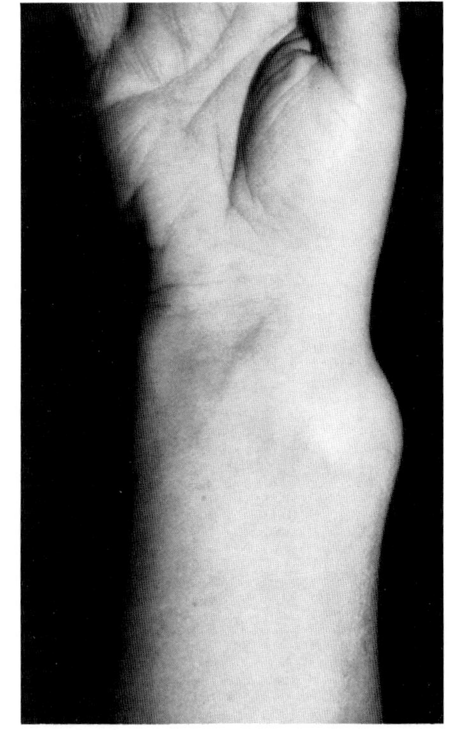

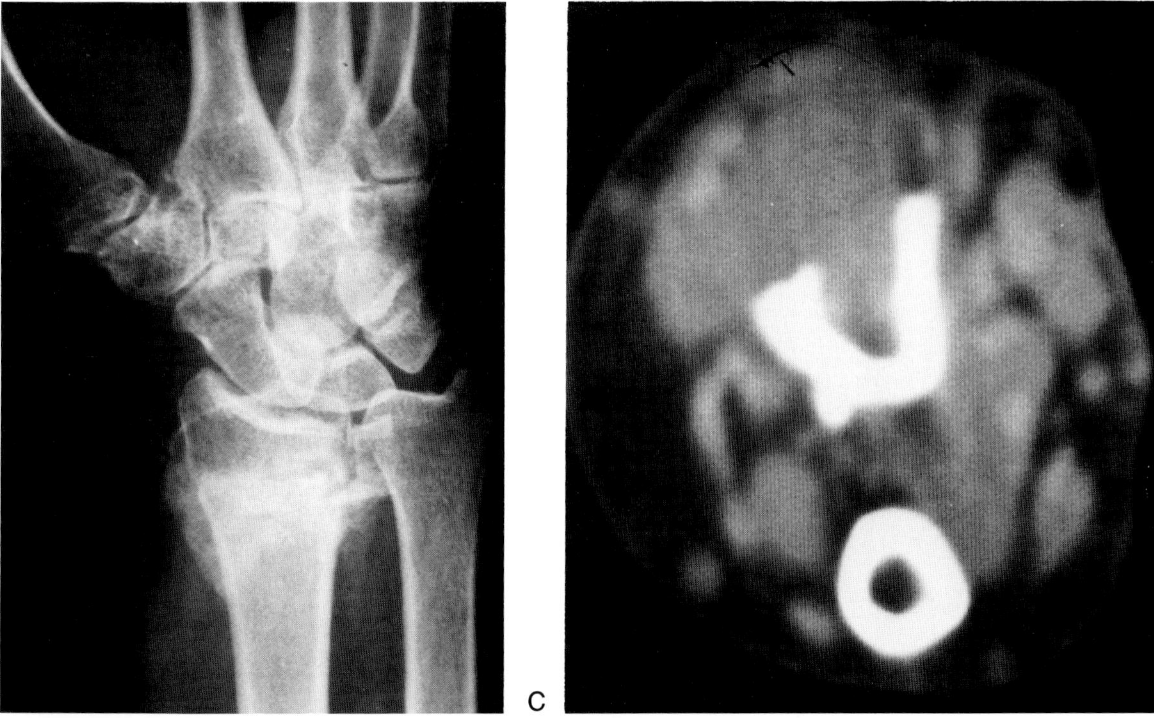

Fig. 60-14. **(A&B)** A soft tissue mass of the volar forearm was discovered following treatment and healing of a now apparently pathologic fracture of the distal radius. **(C)** CT scan demonstrates bony invasion. Biopsy revealed fibrosarcoma now properly considered Stage IIB. *(Figure continues.)*

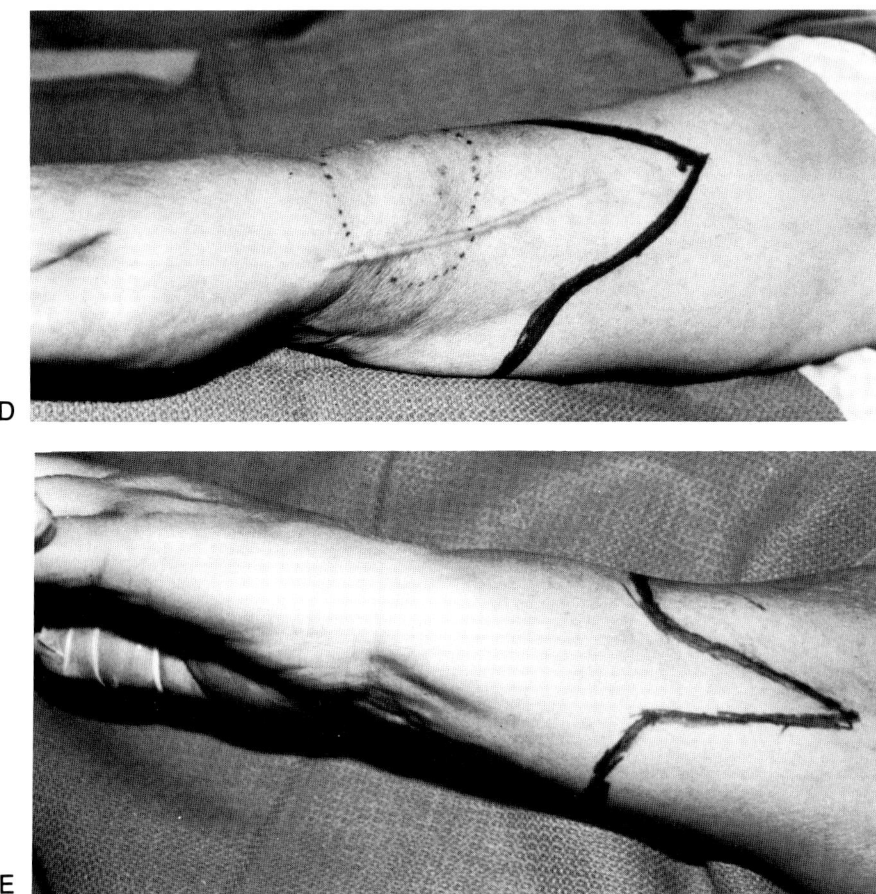

Fig. 60-14 *(Continued).* The tumor was treated by generous below elbow amputation with flaps designed to excise the prior overly generous biopsy incision *(dotted lines).*

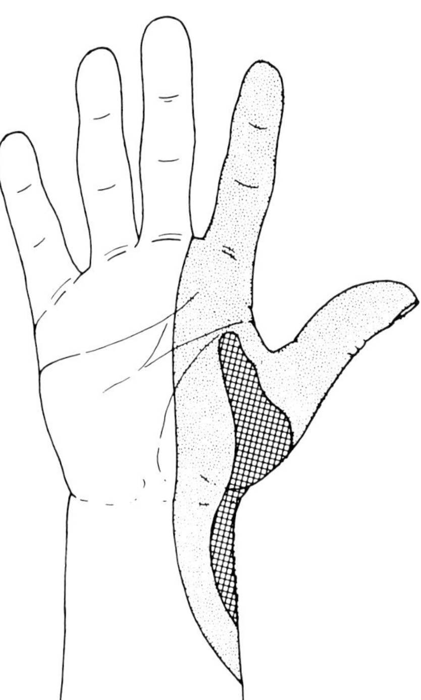

Fig. 60-15. Aggressive tumors of the radial side of the distal forearm may require amputation of the thumb and index rays as well as the contiguous radial wrist, at a minimum.

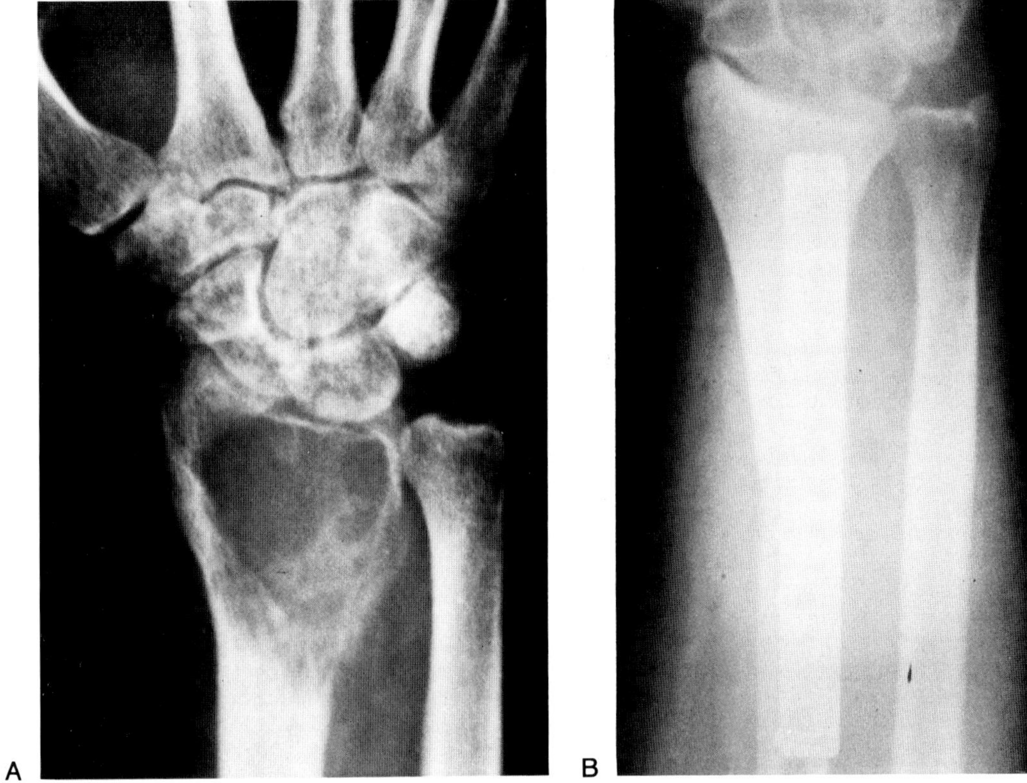

Fig. 60-16. **(A)** Stage I Angiosarcoma of the right distal radius. **(B)** Surgical management by en bloc radial excision and allograft replacement.

tion. Treatment of tumors arising on the radial side of the distal forearm varies according to lesion size and exact location (Figs. 60-16 and 60-17). In many situations, as is true of lesions on the volar side, amputation is probably preferable when all criteria are considered. Tumors on the extreme ulnar side of the wrist may be handled in a way that mirrors those on the radial aspect.

Intracompartmental lesions still within the distal radius or ulna can be treated by intercalary excision of the bone and allograft or autograft replacement.[1,30,34,47] In such a situation, transosseous excision must include biopsy of the medullary canal from the retained segment(s) as well as the resected piece. Tumors that have invaded tissues or crossed compartments extensively require (above or below elbow) amputation.

Wherever a tumor is located, treatment must be individualized to achieve the goal of functional restoration without risking local recurrence and later distant spread. Since we lack control over the site and origin of the neoplasm, the surgeon's responsibility is confined to intelligent management and treatment, adhering to the proper principles of care.

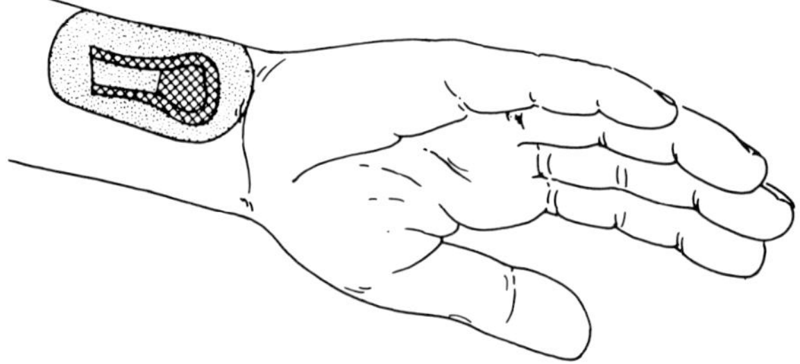

Fig. 60-17. Intraosseous tumors of the distal ulna can be managed by en bloc excision without bone replacement.

ACKNOWLEDGMENTS

The authors are deeply indebted to the seminal work in this area presented in the chapter written for the previous edition by Waldo E. Floyd, III and the late Richard J. Smith. We have preserved and retained, wherever possible, the written text and illustrations from that work, seeking only to update and integrate them into a current plan of diagnostic and surgical management. We also acknowledge the editorial work of Frances Sherwin, M.A., without whom this chapter would not have been effectively completed.

REFERENCES

1. Adeyemi-Doro HO, Durosimi-Etti FA, Olude O: Primary malignant tumors of the hand. J Hand Surg 10A:815-820, 1985
2. Averill RM, Smith RJ, Campbell CJ: Giant cell tumors of the bones of the hand. J Hand Surg 5:39-50, 1980
3. Beasley RW, Ristow BvB: Malignant tumors of the hand. pp. 1434-1440. In Andrade R, Gumport SL, Popkin GL, Rees TD (eds): Cancer of the Skin. WB Saunders, Philadelphia, 1976
4. Bernardino ME, Jing B, Thomas JL, Lindell MM, Zorhozs J: The extremity soft tissue lesion: A comparative study of ultrasound, CT and xeroradiography. Diag Radiol 139:53-59, 1981
5. Bowden L, Booher RJ: The principles and technique of resection of soft parts for sarcoma. Surgery 44:963-977, 1958
6. Campanacci M: Bone and Soft Tissue Tumors. pp. 1-90. Springer-Verlag, New York, 1990
7. Cantin J, McNeer GP, Chu FC, Booher RJ: The problem of local recurrence after treatment of soft tissue sarcoma. Ann Surg 168:47-53, 1968
8. Carroll RE: Squamous cell carcinoma of the nail bed. J Hand Surg 1:92-97, 1976
9. Clifford RH, Kelly AP: Primary malignant tumors of the hand. Plast Reconstr Surg 15:227-232, 1955
10. Consensus Conference: Limb-sparing treatment of adult soft-tissue sarcomas and osteosarcomas. JAMA 254:1791-1796, 1985
11. Cooley SGE: Tumors of the hand and forearm. pp. 3449-3506. In Converse JM (ed): Reconstructive Plastic Surgery. 2nd Ed. Vol. 6. WB Saunders, Philadelphia, 1977
12. Creighton JJ Jr, Peimer CA, Mindell ER, Boone DC, Karakousis CP, Douglass HO: Primary malignant tumors of the upper extremity: Retrospective analysis of one hundred twenty-six cases. J Hand Surg 10A:805-814, 1985
13. Dobyns JH: Hand reconstruction after tumor excision. pp. 11:123-136. In Evarts CM (ed): Surgery of the Musculoskeletal System. Vol. 4. Churchill Livingstone, New York, 1983
14. Eilber FR, Eckhardt J, Morton DL: Advances in the treatment of sarcomas of the extremity—Current status of limb salvage. Cancer 54:2695-2701, 1984
15. Eilber FR, Morton DL, Eckhardt J, Grant T, Weisenburger T: Limb salvage for skeletal and soft tissue sarcomas. Multidisciplinary preoperative therapy. Cancer 53:2579-2584, 1984
16. Enneking WF: Musculoskeletal Tumor Surgery. Churchill Livingstone, New York, 1983
17. Enneking WF: Staging of musculoskeletal neoplasms. In: Current concepts of diagnosis and treatment of bone and soft tissue tumors. Springer-Verlag, Heidelberg, 1984
18. Enneking WF, Spanier SS, Goodman MA: Current concepts review: The surgical staging of musculoskeletal sarcoma. J Bone Joint Surg 62A:1027-1030, 1980
19. Enneking WF, Spanier SS, Goodman MA: A system for the surgical staging of musculoskeletal sarcoma. Clin Orthop 153:106-120, 1980
20. Enzinger FM, Weiss SW: Soft Tissue Tumors. CV Mosby, St. Louis, 1983
21. Fleegler EJ: Soft tissue tumors. Part II: Skin tumors. pp. 1660-1677. In Green DP (ed): Operative Hand Surgery. Churchill Livingstone, New York, 1982
22. Forsythe RL, Bajaj P, Engeron O, Shadid EA: The treatment of squamous cell carcinoma of the hand. Hand 10:104-108, 1978
23. Frassica FJ, Amadio PC, Wold LE, Dobyns JH, Linscheid RL: Primary malignant bone tumors of the hand. J Hand Surg 14A:1022-1028, 1989
24. Hausman M: Microvascular applications in limb sparing tumor surgery. Orthop Clin North Am 20(3):427-437, 1989
25. Hoopes JE, Graham WP, Shack RB: Epithelioid sarcoma of the upper extremity. Plast Reconstr Surg 75:810-813, 1985
26. Kendall TE, Robinson DW, Masters FW: Primary malignant tumors of the hand. Plast Reconstr Surg 44:37-40, 1969
27. Kilgore ES, Graham WP III: The Hand, Surgical and Non-Surgical Management. p. 346. Lea & Febiger, Philadelphia, 1977
28. Lindberg RD, Martin RG, Romsdahl MM, Barkley HT: Conservative and postoperative radiotherapy in 300 adults with soft-tissue sarcomas. Cancer 47:2391-2397, 1981
29. Littler JW: Metacarpal reconstruction. J Bone Joint Surg 29:723-737, 1947
30. Mankin HJ, Fogelson FS, Thrasher AZ, Jaffer F: Massive resection and allograft transplantation in the treatment of malignant bone tumors. N Engl J Med 294:1247-1255, 1976
31. Mankin HJ, Lange TA, Spanier SS: The hazards of biopsy in patients with malignant primary bone and soft-tissue tumors. J Bone Joint Surg 64A:1121-1127, 1982
32. Palmieri TJ: Chondrosarcoma of the hand. J Hand Surg 9A:332-338, 1984
33. Patel MR, Desai SS, Gordon SL: Functional limb salvage with multimodality treatment in epithelioid sarcoma of the hand: A report of two cases. J Hand Surg 11A:265-269, 1986
34. Peimer CA, Schiller AL, Mankin HJ, Smith RJ: Multicentric giant-cell tumor of bone. J Bone Joint Surg 62A:652-656, 1980
35. Peimer CA, Smith RJ, Sirota RL, Cohen BE: Epithelioid sarcoma of the hand and wrist: Patterns of extension. J Hand Surg 2:275-282, 1977
36. Rosenberg SA, Suit HD, Baker LH: Sarcomas of soft tissues. p. 315. In de Vita VT, Hellman S, Rosenberg SA (eds): Cancer: Principles and Practice of Oncology. JB Lippincott, Philadelphia, 1985
37. Russell WO, Cohen J, Enzinger F, Hajdu SI, Heise H, Martin RG, Meissner W, Miller WT, Schmitz RL, Suit HD: A clinical and pathological staging system for soft tissue sarcomas. Cancer 40:1562-1570, 1977
38. Shimm DS, Suit HD: Radiation therapy of epithelioid sarcoma. Cancer 52:1022-1025, 1983
39. Simon MA: Current concepts review—Biopsy of musculoskeletal tumors. J Bone Joint Surg 64A:1253-1257, 1982
40. Simon MA, Enneking WF: The management of soft tissue sarcomas of the extremities. J Bone Joint Surg 58A:317-327, 1976
41. Simon MA, Nachman J: Current concepts review. The clinical utility of preoperative therapy for sarcomas. J Bone Joint Surg 68A:1458-1463, 1986
42. Smith RJ: Complications of surgical treatment of tumors of the hand. pp. 286-293. In Boswick JA (ed): Complications in Hand Surgery. WB Saunders, Philadelphia, 1986
43. Smith RJ: Tumors of the hand: Who is best qualified to treat tumors of the hand? (editorial). J Hand Surg 2:251-252, 1977
44. Smith RJ, Brushart TM: Allograft bone for metacarpal reconstruction. J Hand Surg 10A:325-334, 1985
45. Smith RJ, Dworecka F: Treatment of the one digit hand. J Bone Joint Surg 55A:113-119, 1973
46. Smith RJ, Gumley GJ: Metacarpal distraction lengthening. Hand Clin 1(3):417-429, 1985
47. Smith RJ, Mankin HJ: Allograft replacement of the distal radius for giant cell tumor. J Hand Surg 2:299-309, 1977
48. Suit HD, Mankin HJ, Wood WC, Proppe KH: Preoperative, intraoperative and post operative radiation in the treatment of primary soft tissue sarcoma. Cancer 55:2659-2667, 1985
49. Suit HD, Proppe KH, Mankin HJ, Woods WC: Pre-operative

radiation therapy for sarcoma of soft tissue. Cancer 47:2269–2274, 1981

50. Usui M, Ishii S, Yamamura M, Minami A, Sakuma T: Microsurgical reconstructive surgery following wide resection of bone and soft tissue sarcomas in the upper extremities. J Reconstr Microsurg 2:77–84, 1986
51. Weiland AJ, Kleinert HE, Kutz JE, Daniel RK: Free vascularized bone grafts in surgery of the upper extremity. J Hand Surg 4:129–144, 1979
52. Weingrad DW, Rosenberg SA: Early lymphatic spread of osteogenic and soft tissue sarcomas. Surgery 84:231–240, 1978

61

Tumors of Bone and Soft Tissue

Clayton A. Peimer
Owen J. Moy
Harold M. Dick

The focus of this chapter is on neoplasms common to the hand, specifically those characterized by unusual diagnoses, biologic behaviors, or treatment. Information unique to a particular lesion is presented to enable the reader to relate principles and guidelines outlined in Chapter 60 to a particular clinical case, histologic diagnosis, or lesional problem. Hand tumors include soft- and hard-tissue neoplasms, reactive nodules and cysts, rheumatoid and other systemic connective tissue proliferations and calcifications, bone spurs, and foreign body reactions.[10,19,21,26,32,34,50,53,87,90,107,118,135,198] Surgeons treating hand tumors must be cognizant of the range of possibilities. Therefore, each section of this chapter is organized in a similar fashion, beginning with common, benign lesions, proceeding to more troublesome and locally aggressive tumors, and finally ending the section with aggressive and malignant neoplasms.

Musculoskeletal Tumor Society (MSTS) staging methods will make analysis of present and future treatment more logical and, therefore, more useful. However, data on various large multi-institutional series of cases are not yet available. At this time what exactly constitutes a "safe margin" and how much function must be sacrificed to save the life of the patient have not been established indisputably.[56,67] At the present time there are insufficient data to support application to the hand of the principle of anatomic compartmentalization (based on the presence of tissue barriers that resist tumor cell extension and invasion), which governs tumor management in other sites of the body. The most important principle is that a generous margin must not be compromised if it endangers the primary goal of surgery, which is to cure the tumor. In the interests of prudence, surgery currently is supplemented and enhanced by adjunctive protocols, more frequently now including preoperative ("neoadjuvant") administration.

SOFT TISSUE LESIONS

Reactive Tumors

Ganglion and Mucous Cysts

Ganglion and mucous cysts, among the most common tumors (masses) in the hands, are discussed in detail in Chapter 58.

Epidermal Inclusion Cysts

Although epidermal inclusion cysts are less common than joint and tendon ganglia, they are not rare. The origin of these tumors is an injury that implants epithelial cells into the subcutaneous tissue. These cells survive, grow, produce carotene, and slowly enlarge to a significant size over months or years. If they become large enough, they can interfere with function or aesthetics. Typically, they are painless unless located in an area that sustains an injury, in which case there may be local hemorrhage and pain.

Inclusion cysts present as relatively globular, freely mobile masses that are firm or hard on examination. They usually do not transilluminate, even on the dorsum of the hand. If they arise in a fixed location, for example near the nail, or are limited by digital fascia, they may produce secondary bone erosion (Fig. 61-1). A history of even minor open injury should suggest an inclusion cyst as a possible diagnosis.

Careful surgical excision, which avoids rupture of the tumor sac and spillage of contents, is curative. The surgeon must avoid damaging surrounding anatomy and must thoroughly curette any intraosseous portion of the tumor.[26,34,40,78,90,198,235,247]

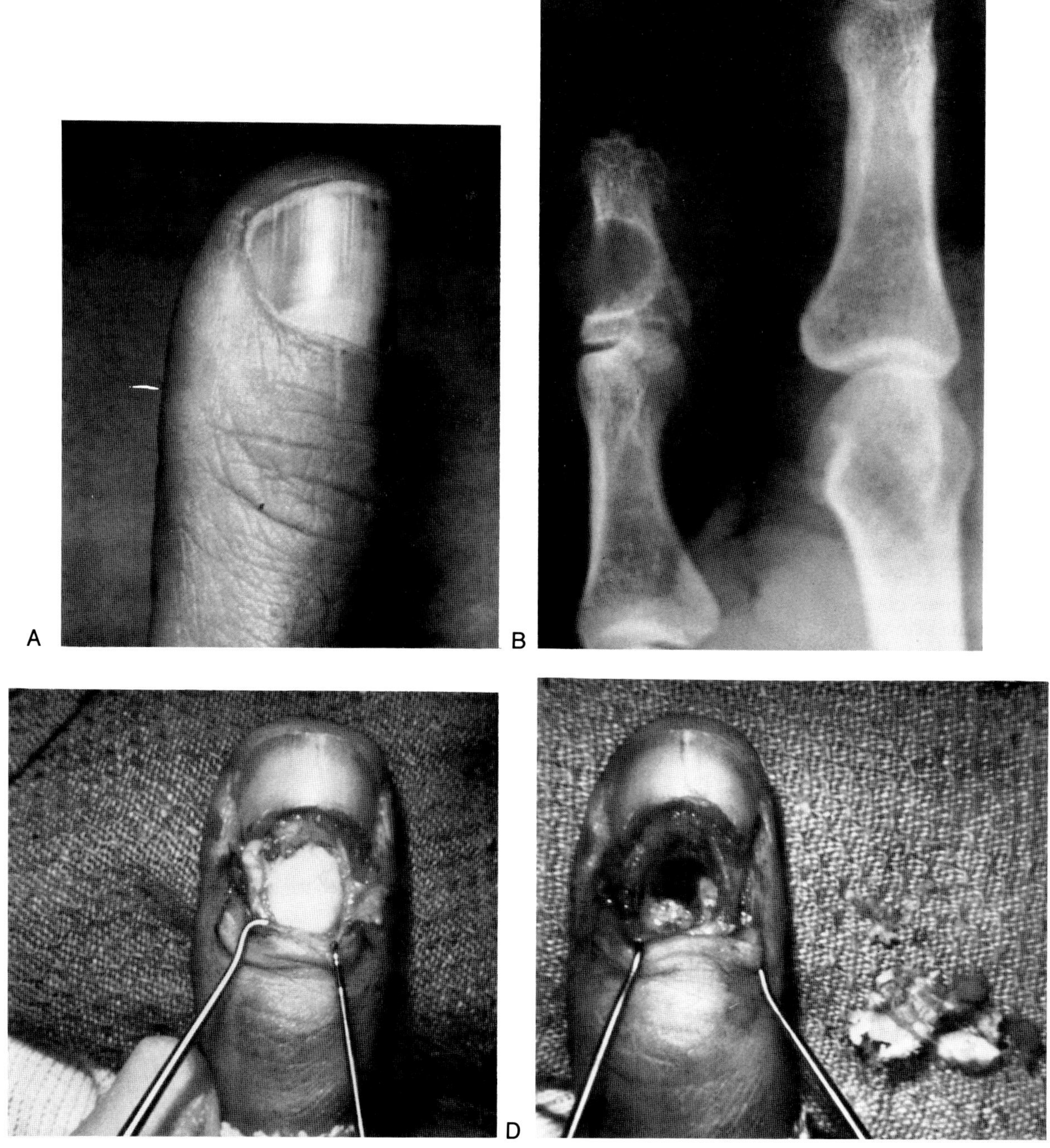

Fig. 61-1. A 53-year-old salesman reported that an enlarging deformity of the thumb **(A)** had progressed slowly for some time following a crush injury that occurred at least 18 months earlier. Radiographs showed a well-circumscribed distal phalangeal lesion with a reactive endosteal cortical rim **(B)** typical of bone reaction to a slowly growing soft tissue tumor. **(C&D)** Excisional biopsy revealed an inclusion cyst that was successfully treated by removal and phalangeal curettage.

Foreign Body Lesions

Other tumors, also traumatic in origin, in reality may be a response to retained foreign body material. Even benign and supposedly noninflammatory particulate matter, such as glass or steel, materials which are not inherently cytotoxic, may incite at least an end-stage fibrous encapsulation. Such a response, which is common to vertebrate and invertebrate species, is the host's method of isolating recognized extraneous tissue. Toxic material produces a prolonged inflammatory response indistinguishable clinically from any other cause of local cellular death, such as infection or burns. These lesions are usually relatively superficial in location. If the size of nontoxic particles is small enough, the result may be a locally mediated cellular inflammatory response.[145,190,191]

It is important to establish the etiology of these lesions. A history of local trauma and identification of the foreign body with radiographs or other imaging studies may provide this information,[212] but it may be impossible to distinguish preoperatively with assurance between an inclusion cyst and a foreign body reaction. In either case, careful, thorough local excision results in cure of the problem.

Fat Tumors

Lipoma/Lipofibroma

Lipoma, and its slightly more reactive or traumatized analog, lipofibroma, are very common, painless soft tissue masses that have a characteristic soft or spongy consistency on palpation, especially recognizable if they arise in superficial tissues. Lipomata located in deeper tissues, and beneath muscle or muscular planes, feel considerably less distinct or firm. Typically, the patient presents with a gradually enlarging, soft, painless mass. Radiographs reveal a fat or water density.

These tumors are composed of normal fat cells, which are thinly encapsulated and sometimes lobulated. They often look much like the surrounding subcutaneous tissues in the upper limb, but because large deposits of fat are unusual in the hand, identification during dissection is usually easy. Excision may be difficult if the tumor has been ignored for years and has become very large, completely surrounding or displacing tendons, vessels, and nerves. Although intrinsically asymptomatic, these tumors may compress nerves, producing secondary symptoms.[127,263] Simple, local excision is all that is required; however, removal may present a technical challenge if neurovascular structures are involved.[28,69,104,111,127,137,149,153,168,196] Lipoma and lipofibroma have no tendency to undergo malignant change.

Liposarcoma

Liposarcoma is an extremely uncommon tumor in the upper extremity, although it is one of the more common soft tissue sarcomas in adults. The histologic picture varies from well-differentiated lipoma-like and myxoid tumors to very cellular pleomorphic malignancies. The clinical behavior closely parallels its variable histology in that the well-differentiated forms are low-grade malignancies that rarely metastasize, whereas anaplastic ones are highly aggressive, tend to recur and metastasize frequently.[49,203,223,234] Wide or radical surgical excision plus local radiotherapy (especially if margins are compromised, and for the myxoid variety) is a valuable primary and adjunctive combination. Data on the efficacy of chemotherapy are insufficient to recommend or reject it.[46,223]

Synovial Tumors

Giant Cell Tumor of Tendon Sheath

Among the most common solid neoplasms in the hand, the giant cell tumor of tendon sheath may be a misnomer, as is its frequent synonym, fibroxanthoma or tendon sheath xanthoma. Although commonly found in association with tendon sheaths and joints, strictly speaking, these tumors may have few giant cells and no tendon sheath. Jaffe believed that this is a localized variant of *pigmented villonodular tenovagosynovitis.*[118]

Giant cell tumor of tendon sheath is generally considered to be a reactive lesion, the biologic behavior of which may vary from entirely quiescent to locally invasive. Typically, following a relatively short history (several months), the patient presents complaining of the presence of a slowly enlarging, painless mass. The tumor is usually found fixed to underlying tissue rather than to skin and subcutaneous plane, most commonly on the palmar surface of the fingers, hand, and wrist (Fig. 61-2). Secondary nerve compression, bone invasion, or joint destruction may have occurred. Such a clinical presentation should suggest the possibility of this tumor.[120,125,170,215,253]

At operation, the lesion is yellowish, orange, or brown, with areas of gray, frequently lobulated and somewhat gritty. Histologic studies are required to make the diagnosis and to distinguish it from xanthoma tuberosum, a metabolic disease of patients with familial hypercholesterolemia, in which the fatty deposits infiltrate throughout tissues rather than remaining regionalized.

Synovial Sarcoma, Epithelioid Sarcoma, and Clear-cell Sarcoma

Epithelioid sarcoma, synovial sarcoma, and clear-cell sarcoma may be among the most frequent primary malignancies of the upper extremity, especially in the soft tissues distal to the elbow.[9,11,23,24,25,28a,31,35,36,54,57,75,77,83,89,94,101,108,150,167,179,185,188,193,199,200,214,223,239,242,250]

These tumors are discussed under a single heading because of their similar aggressive and capricious behavior, local invasion, and the unusual risks of metastases directly to local and regional lymph nodes. These tumors are often confusing in appearance and presentation, and variable in their method of spread. An otherwise benign looking, solid, soft tissue lesion of the hand and wrist should be approached with caution and a significant index of suspicion because it may be one of these tumors. At a minimum, wide en bloc excision is required; more radical excision or amputation may be indicated, de-

A
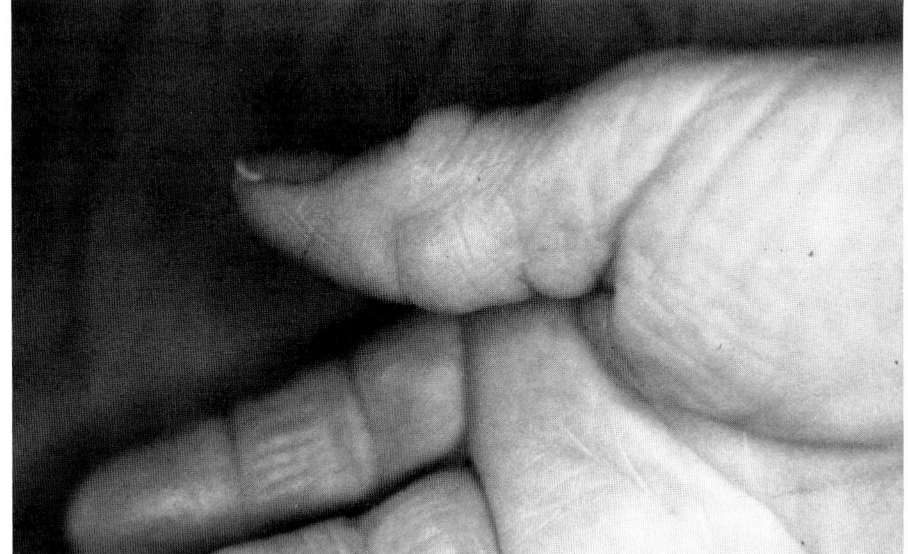

B
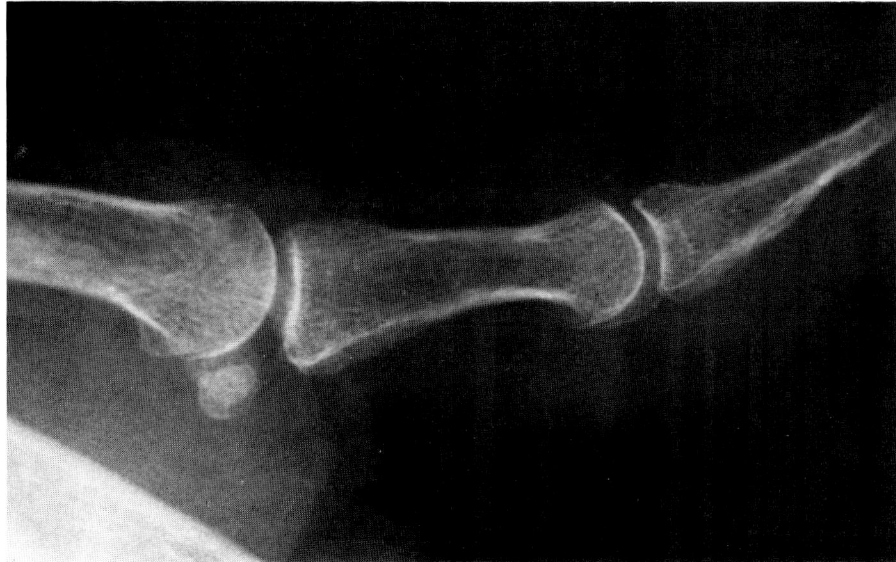

Fig. 61-2. A 61-year-old woman complained of a slowly growing thumb mass **(A)**, which now interfered with function. Radiographs **(B)** and bone scan (not shown) were negative. The patient's insurance company refused MRI evaluation despite the preoperative impression that the lesion involved both dorsal and palmar surfaces, a more worrisome finding. At excision, the specimen was found to involve both the flexor pollicis longus tendon sheath and IP joint, extending into the dorsal subcutaneous tissues. All resected specimens were consistent with giant cell tumor of tendon sheath.

pending on tumor location and stage. Axillary node dissection is strongly advised regardless of clinical and even lymphangiographic findings. Response to radiation therapy has been reported to be positive in some cases. The role of systemic chemotherapy has not yet been clearly defined in a significant series.[47,63,78,101,185]

Whether these tumors begin in the superficial subcutaneous tissues or, more deeply, in association with tendon and/or synovial cells is not known. Early in the history, the epithelioid sarcoma, especially, may present as a skin plaque or nodule that later ulcerates. Misdiagnoses include granulomatous inflammation; chronic ulcers, or infected and degenerated/ulcerating warts; nodular fasciitis; and tenosynovitis; the malignant nature may not be (fully) recognized histologically. These tumors may spread along fascial planes and tendon sheaths, to skin, scalp, and by vascular invasion as well as to lymph nodes.

The prognosis of these lesions may be quite variable because they are often characterized by multiple local recurrences, late distant recurrences, and unusual secondary sites. While Enzinger[78] has reclassified clear-cell sarcoma as a malignant melanoma of soft parts (in an effort to explain its rather bizarre metastatic sites), that same consideration may yet need to be given to the other two lesions as well.

Nerve Tumors

Schwannoma/Neurilemoma

The Schwannoma/neurilemoma is a relatively common, solitary, benign tumor arising from the Schwann cell in nerve trunks or branches. It occurs frequently on the flexor surface.[76,103,112,195,204,225,236] These tumors are generally fewer than 3 to 4 cm in diameter; larger masses should always be viewed with a high index of suspicion, of course. Presenting symptoms are usually from nerve compression with this relatively eccentric, typically well defined, slow growing tumor. Although the lesion can often be shelled out surgically without postsurgical nerve impairment, removal may require microscopic dissection to prevent iatrogenic injury to compressed, secondarily atrophic adjacent fascicles. Tumors involving small nerves may not be technically amenable to excision by dissection, but may require en bloc excision and nerve reconstruction by advancement or grafting if appropriate.

Neurofibroma/von Recklinghausen's Disease/ Neurofibrosarcoma

Neurofibroma is a diffuse growth of Schwann cells, fibrous tissue, and axons, which may occur as solitary or multiple lesions (the latter in von Recklinghausen's disease). When isolated, the solitary tumor tends not to recur following excision. Multiple plexiform neurofibromata cannot be easily enucleated from nerves, and their excision requires segmental nerve resection if dictated by local symptoms or nerve destruction. Because of the difficulty of surgery, even for the isolated tumors, most authors believe that removal is warranted only if a particular tumor begins to grow and produce symptoms, or shows signs of malignant degeneration.[27,141,204]

Malignant schwannoma develops from benign lesions in patients with von Recklinghausen's disease and may more properly be considered neurofibrosarcoma. An isolated neurofibrosarcoma may develop from a neurofibroma, but it is also known to arise without a precursor. Exceedingly wide ablation, radical excision, and amputation are the surgical treatments of choice.[79,207] This tumor is not generally considered responsive to systemic chemotherapy, and neither is it radiosensitive.[27]

Lipofibromatous Hamartoma

Lipofibromatous hamartoma, especially of the median nerve, presents as a slowly growing and painless mass that is often first noted in childhood. It has the same symptoms as carpal tunnel syndrome. Treatment is best limited to carpal tunnel release, occasionally with epineurotomy. Rarely, if ever, is intraneural dissection advisable.[1,154,189,210,211] A consequence of these very uncommon tumors is gradual, progressive, local neurologic deterioration.

Granular Cell Myoblastoma

Granular cell myoblastoma is a very rare tumor generally believed to arise from neural elements.[237] It may occur anywhere and at almost any age. Wide local or en bloc excision generally prevents recurrence. Malignant degeneration is unexpected but considered possible.

Muscle Tumors

Pseudo-hypertrophy

Pseudo-hypertrophy is neither frequently recognized nor commonly reported, although we have identified this lesion in several patients who have had prior direct trauma to the first web. This lesion probably represents a gradation in the continuum of denervation and scarring. These patients present with a localized swelling or sense of fullness, and the problem may be indistinguishable clinically from a deeper neoplasm such as a lipoma. The lesion should be distinguishable from a real neoplasm by MRI evaluation (Fig. 61-3). Biopsy reveals reactive, swollen denervated muscle cells.

Treatment is expectant. Muscle excision is not recommended, and patients eventually respond to rest and antiinflammatory medication. Resumption of activities, especially gripping, pinching, and lifting, tends to aggravate the symptoms early in the course. In the long-term, symptoms subside, and the localized swelling becomes an accepted part of the post-traumatic residua. The most difficult part of dealing with this lesion is getting the patient to accept the diagnosis and the somewhat protracted and annoying, but benign, course.

Rhabdomyosarcoma

Rhabdomyosarcoma is an uncommon, but well known childhood tumor. It arises from striated muscle stem cells and is often aggressively malignant. There are four cell types: alveolar, botryoid, embryonal, and pleomorphic. Rhabdomyosarcoma not only spreads directly and regionally, but also metastasizes to local or regional lymph nodes, and may even involve bone marrow.[12,106,109,121,139,152,157,161,176,230,241]

Significant benefit can be derived from the use of systemic combined chemotherapy protocol in the treatment of rhabdomyosarcoma. The positive role of radiation therapy is evident.[51,109,121,158,161,218] The combination of wide en bloc or radical surgical measures and adjuvants has been helpful for many with this serious childhood sarcoma (Fig. 61-4).

Fibromatoses

The tumors included in this category are, in general, some of the most common neoplastic and reactive lesions in the hand and may be the source both of great concern and confusion for the treating surgeon and pathologist. An experienced pathologist is probably the most important member of the team treating the patient with a growing fibrous tumor. These lesions cover the entire spectrum of histologic and clinical behavior, from those that are quiescent, entirely benign, and localized to those that are locally invasive and frankly malignant. Their histology does not necessarily predict or anticipate the eventual course and outcome.[148,220]

Keloid, Fasciitis, and Fibromatosis

Keloid is a post-traumatic phenomenon, generally occurring in patients aged 10 to 25 years, and frequently in African-Americans, other dark-skinned individuals, and those with a family history of the problem. Keloids may continue to grow for months or years, or they may involute spontaneously. Surgical excision and radiation are rarely more than temporarily successful, although sometimes they are helpful. Intradermal steroid injection plus elastic garments/appliques may be helpful in some cases. Fasciitis is commonly post-traumatic, and occurs in the same age group as keloids.[100,197]

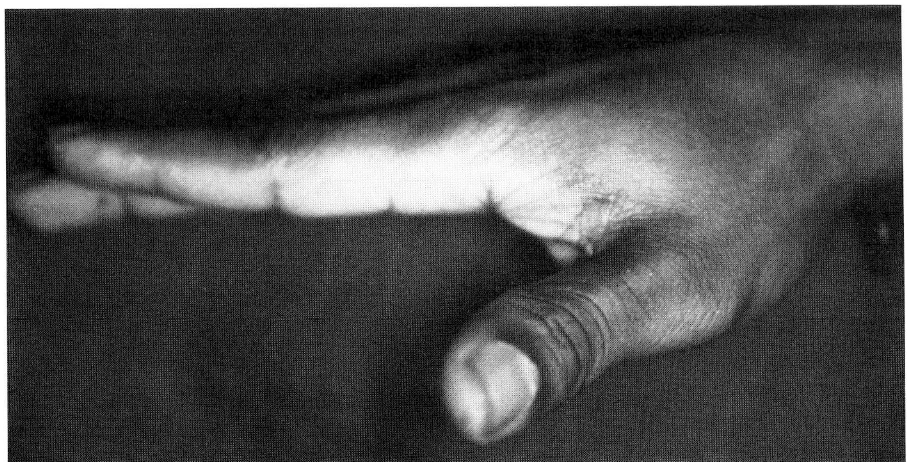
A

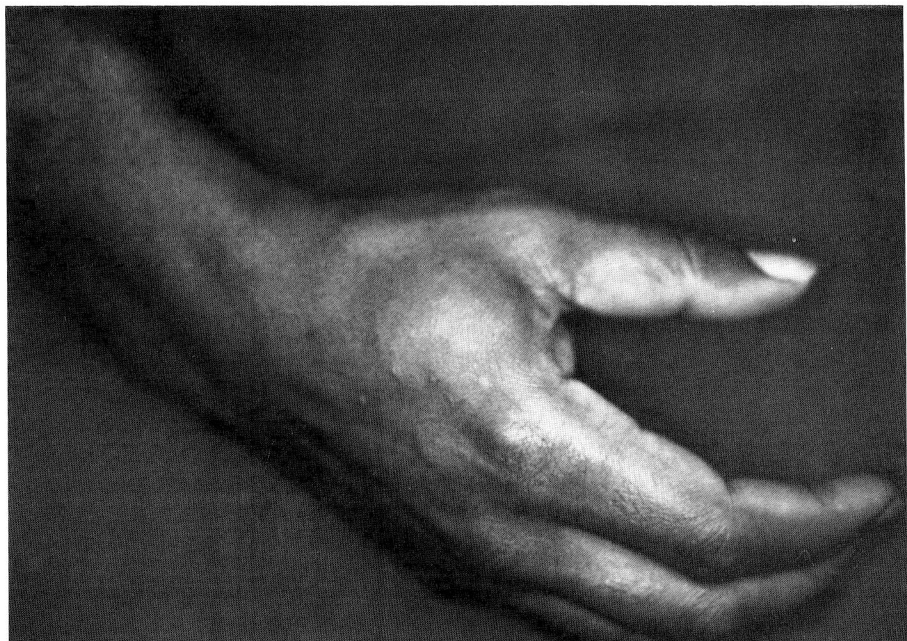
B

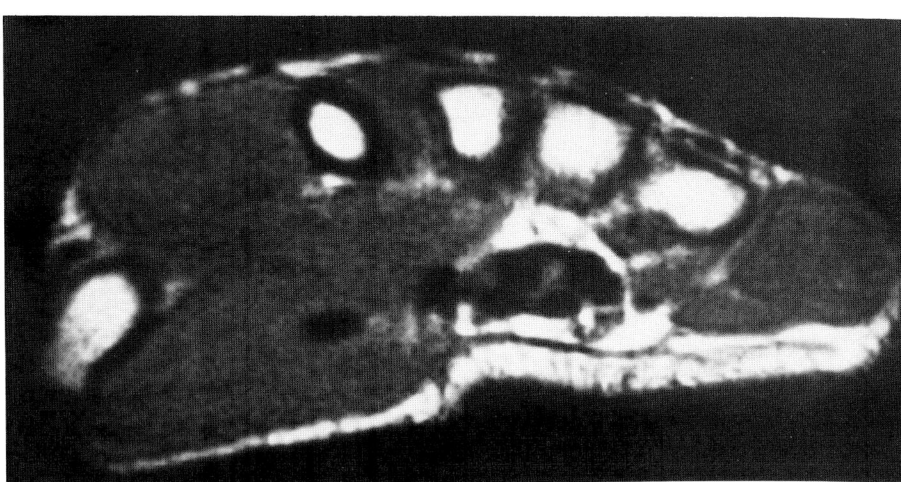
C

Fig. 61-3. This young laborer complained of first web enlargement **(A&B)** and discomfort that progressed for several months following a crush contusion at work. Once fully present, however, the mass did not continue to grow. The enlarged area in the first web was soft but firm and minimally tender. MRI **(C)** did not disclose a discrete mass, but enlargement of the superficial portion of the first dorsal interosseous muscle is clear, consistent with the diagnosis of post-traumatic muscular pseudohypertrophy.

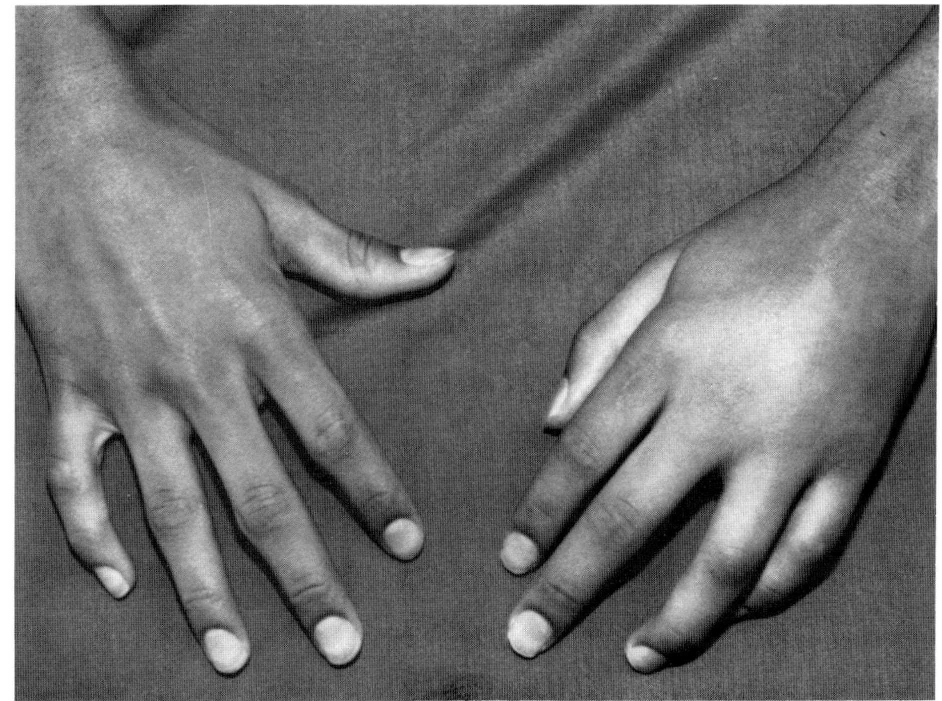

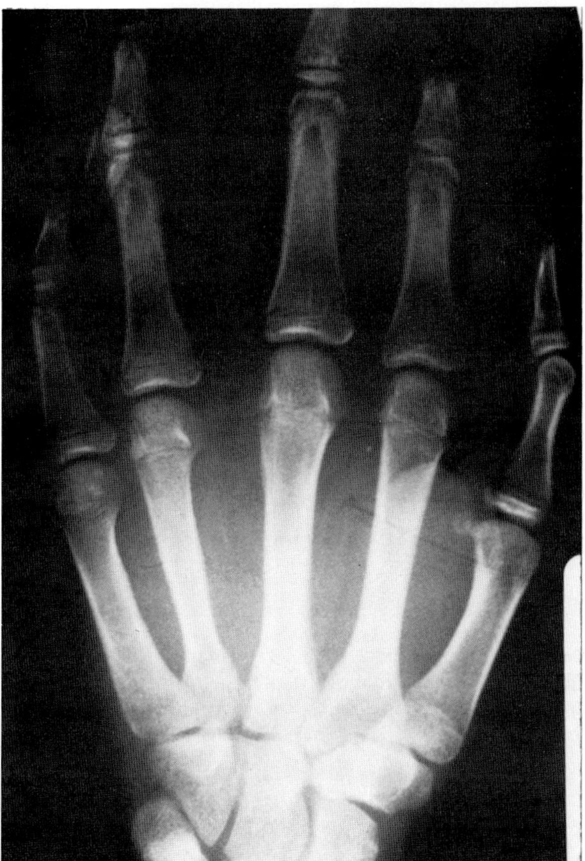

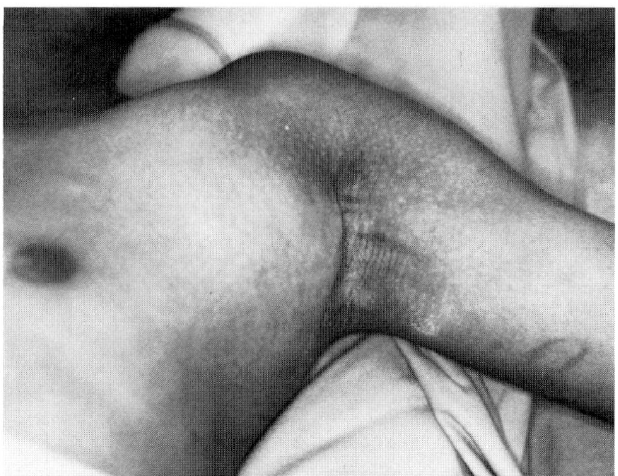

Fig. 61-4. This 14-year-old boy complained of rapid onset of pain and swelling in the left hand **(A)** after a minor injury during a basketball game 2 months earlier. His ER radiographs were interpreted as negative, but at the time of this examination, obvious swelling and firm enlargement of the left hand were present, and plain radiographs revealed widening of the third/fourth intermetacarpal space **(B).** Axillary examination **(C)** revealed a mildly tender, but very firm and definite enlargement. Chest radiographs were negative. *(Figure continues.)*

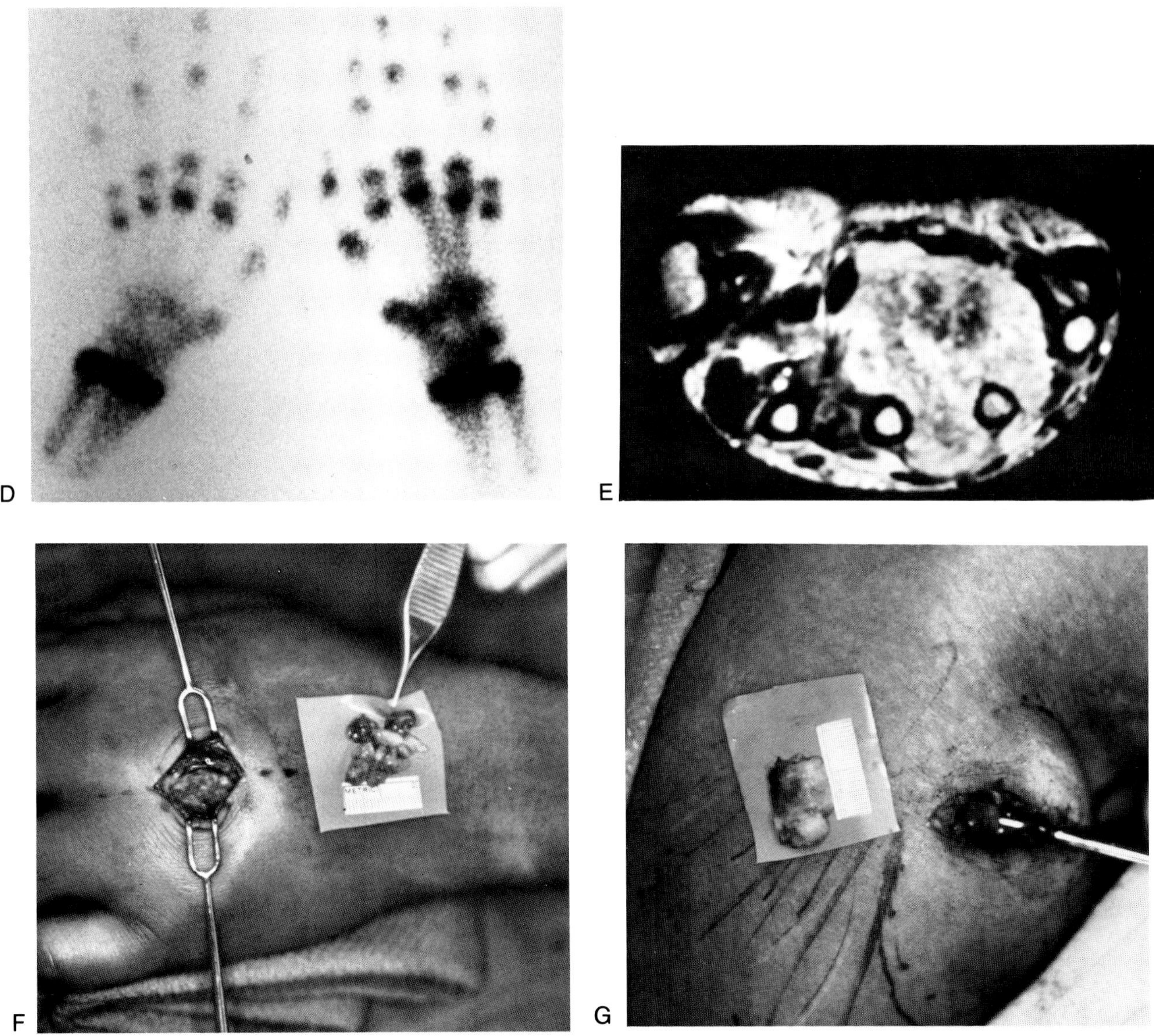

Fig. 61-4 *(Continued).* Tc-99 bone scan **(D)** showed some increased uptake in the involved metacarpals and web. MRI **(E)** showed a solid tumor invading the entire midpalm and hand. Simultaneous incisional biopsies of the left hand **(F)** and axilla **(G)** disclosed a similar whitish, firm tumor thought to be malignant on frozen section, and diagnosed as embryonal type rhabdomyosarcoma on permanent sections. This tumor, like synovial, clear cell and epithelioid sarcomas, is unusual in its tendency to metastasize to regional lymph nodes.

Fibroma

Fibroma is a benign, encapsulated lesion which, if completely excised, has a very low recurrence rate. Tumors arise from tendons/tendon sheaths (tenosynovial), or they occur adjacent to fingernails (periungual)[55] (Fig. 61-5).

Dermatofibroma/Juvenile Aponeurotic Fibroma

Dermatofibromas and juvenile aponeurotic fibromas are locally infiltrative and recurrent fibrotic lesions. Included in this category are subdermal fibromatosis of infancy, infantile dermatofibromatosis, juvenile aponeurotic fibroma, and palmar fibromatosis (i.e., Dupuytren's, Lederhose's, and Peyronie's). Surgery is primarily for diagnosis of dermatofibroma and juvenile aponeurotic fibroma, in which recurrences and local extension can be significantly problematic. Recurrent enlargement and extension may interfere with function (Fig. 61-6). The clinical course may be aggressive; accurate histologic diagnosis depends on tissue examination as well as communication between surgeon and pathologist, since the histologic examination must distinguish these from aggressive fibromatosis, fibrosarcoma, and fibrous histiocytoma. Benign forms tend to recur locally if incompletely excised, and new lesions may appear. The exact course depends on the tumor diagnosis and age. Juvenile lesions may regress spontaneously.[2,43,74,116,117,133,172,231,232] Surgery for Dupuytren's disease is described in Chapter 13.

Extraabdominal Desmoid/ Desmoplastic Fibroma

Extraabdominal desmoid tumors are potentially very aggressive but nonmetastatic. They are likely to recur. Typically, they occur in young patients, especially males. Effective treatment requires wide local en bloc excision or even amputation in progressive and aggressive cases. Careful, repeated postoperative observation and examination of the line of excision at nearby tissues is required because of the tendency of this tumor to recur locally. Recurrences should be treated promptly by repeat local excision, because a slow and progressive course with deep and expanding extension is the rule. The lesions are notable because they are considerably more aggressive clinically than histologically, sometimes behaving exactly like low-grade fibrosarcomas. Indeed, over a prolonged and extended course, transformation is certainly not unknown.[93,180,205,217]

Fibrous Histiocytoma

Fibrous histiocytomas are most common in males in the fourth decade.[100] These lesions have both benign and malignant variations. The benign form, which is not rare in the hand (and is also known to occur about the knee) has about a 10 to 15 percent incidence of recurrence after excision. Marginal or wide en bloc excision is indicated, especially for large lesions.

Malignant fibrous histiocytoma is an uncommon tumor, which has received considerable attention in the literature recently even though it was described clearly three decades

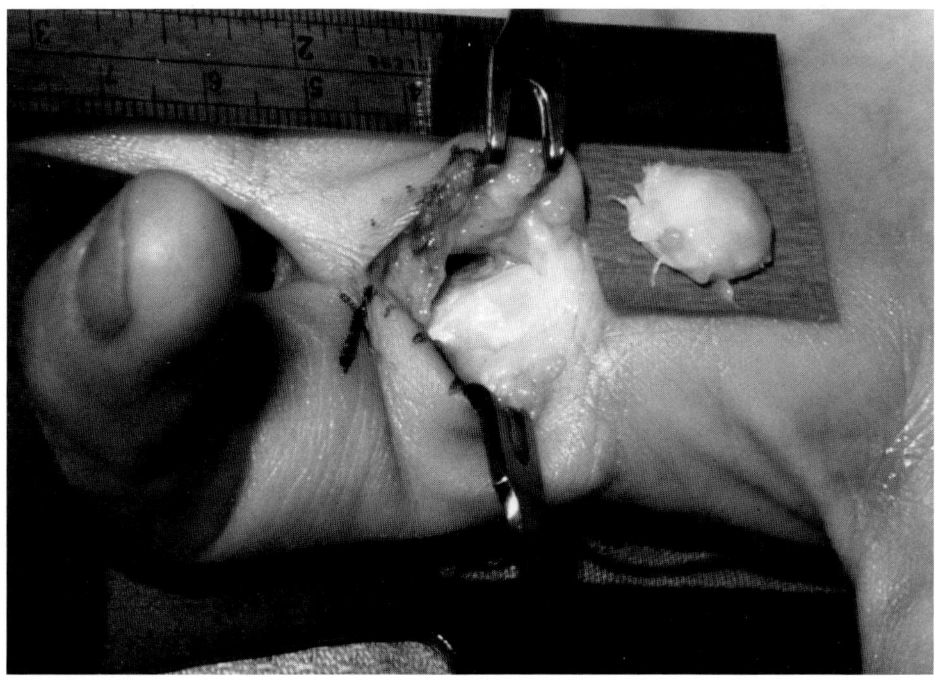

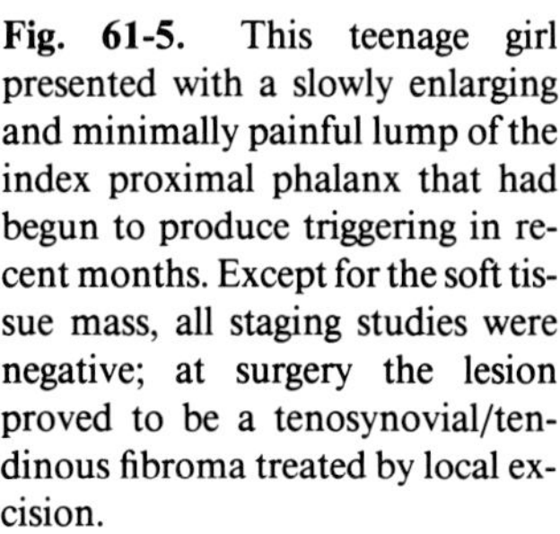

Fig. 61-5. This teenage girl presented with a slowly enlarging and minimally painful lump of the index proximal phalanx that had begun to produce triggering in recent months. Except for the soft tissue mass, all staging studies were negative; at surgery the lesion proved to be a tenosynovial/tendinous fibroma treated by local excision.

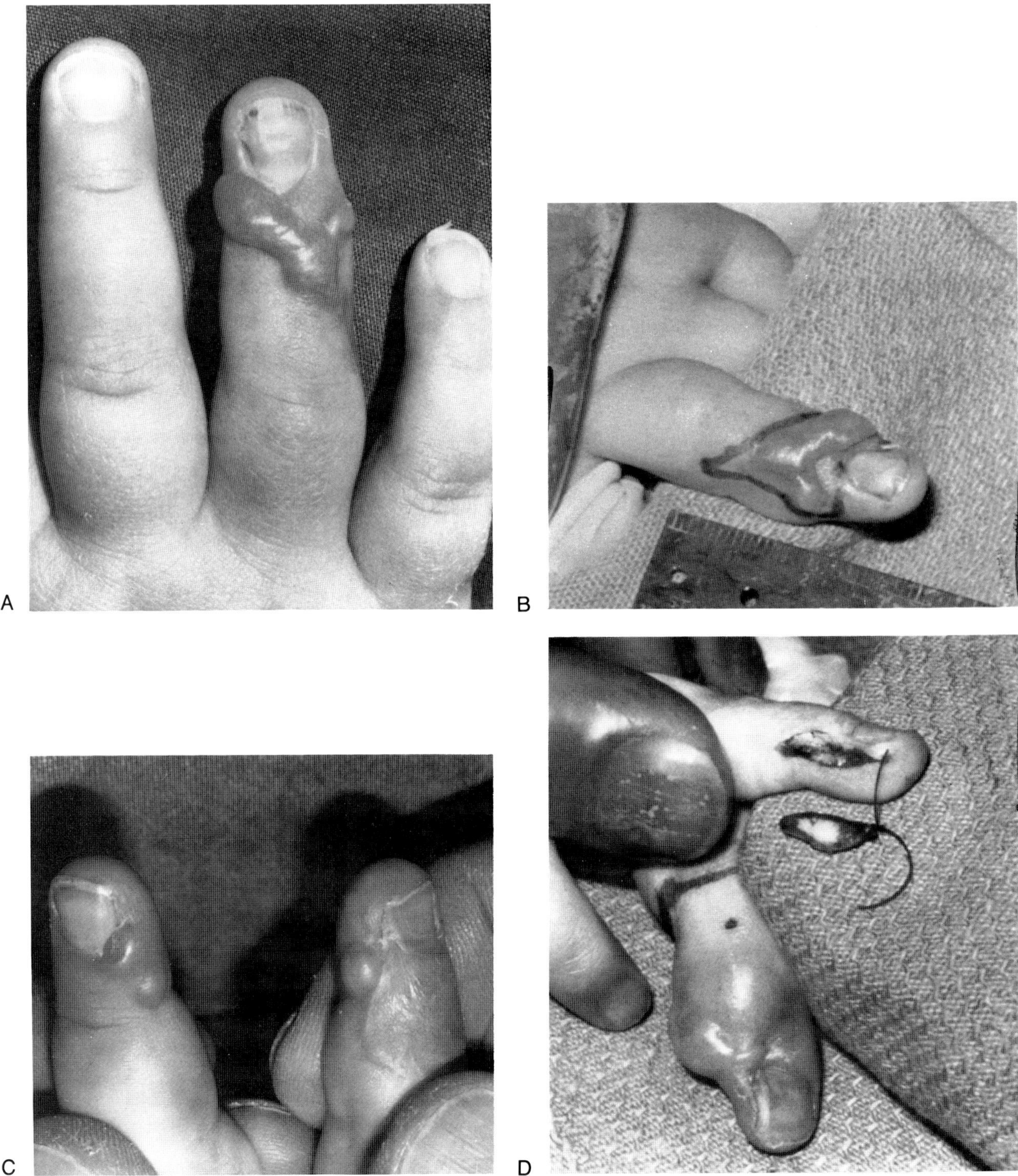

Fig. 61-6. **(A)** This 3-year-old boy was examined for progressively enlarging recurrence of a juvenile aponeurotic fibroma 9 months after local excision and skin grafting. **(B)** Marginal en bloc excision and skin graft were performed; frozen and permanent sections showed the resection lines to be clear of invasion. He did well for 6 months, but 1 year postsurgery, he returned with a recurrent lesion on the ring finger and a similar growth on the middle finger **(C)**. Both tumors were excised en bloc and skin grafted **(D)**. Resection margins were clear on frozen and permanent sections, and initially he did well. He was lost to follow-up for 2 years, but then returned with a small growth on the ring finger, this time on the ulnar side. In addition, there was a large, disfiguring, and extensive tumor of the middle finger, which was found to invade tendon, sheath, and joint, necessitating ablation. The histologic diagnosis remained unchanged and the patient has had no further recurrences.

ago.[121] Whether it is of fibrous or histiocytic origin is still subject to some pathologic debate. However, its clinical course has been correlated to size and location.[33,68,102,114,129,140,164,175,213,245,248,256,259] Appropriate surgical interventions for this lesion include radical local excision, wide en bloc excision, and amputation. There is limited literature on the results of chemotherapy, although significant benefit was obtained in at least one series.[16] In other series, sensitivity to radiation therapy has been positive. The most useful scenario probably includes wide excision at a minimum, followed by postoperative radiation at about 6 to 8 weeks. The combination of surgery, local radiation, and chemotherapy may be the most appropriate approach for this significantly aggressive malignant tumor.[16,20,39,229,251,255]

Fibrosarcoma

Fibrosarcoma is a true malignancy that is at the severe end of the continuum of fibromatous diagnoses. However, even within this category, lesions may be graded; the tumor may be relatively quiescent or truly aggressive and lethal. Fibrosarcomata arise in areas that have been previously or even chronically affected by trauma, burns and scar, or prior surgery. This lesion has a more aggressive propensity for recurrence and spread than fibromatous lesions discussed previously in this section.[45,61,78,80,87,115,147,201,202,258]

Treatment varies by location and grade. At a minimum, en bloc or radical excision, or even amputation, may be necessary.[194] Although the value of chemotherapy has not been clearly established, radiotherapy has a positive role.[257]

Vascular Tumors

These reactive neoplastic lesions, including hemangiomata, false aneurysms, glomus tumors, and angiosarcomas, are covered in Chapter 62. Kaposi's sarcoma is discussed in Chapter 59.

TUMORS OF BONE AND CARTILAGE

Cartilage

Chondroma

Extraosseous and endosteal (i.e., enchondromatous) cartilage tumors are the most common primary neoplasms of the skeleton of the hand. Most frequently, a solitary enchondroma is found in young adults. Virtually unique to the phalanges and metacarpals, it is extremely rare in the carpal bones.[3,118,155,159,160,165,184,198] Almost all of these lesions present as pathologic fractures, although incidental discovery from radiographs taken for other reasons occurs. Very small tumors may need only periodic observation; large lesions and those associated with fractures should be treated. Radiographically, with or without fracture, the neoplasm has a characteristic appearance, which includes metaphyseal and/or diaphyseal radiolucence, most often with thinning and expansion of the

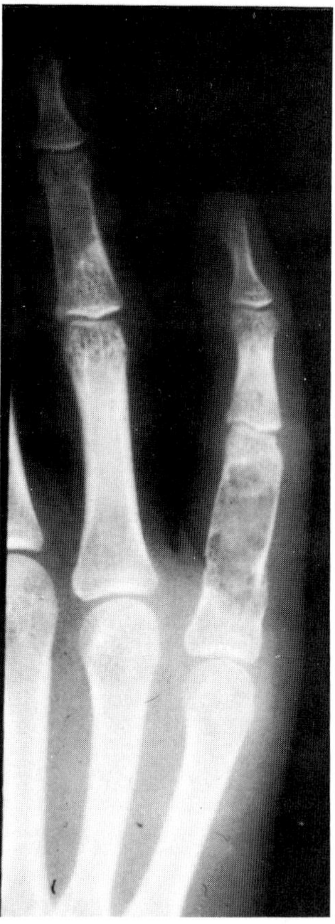

Fig. 61-7. A 25-year-old man with painful swelling of the proximal phalanx of the little finger presented after a minor injury. The pathologic fracture was due to a relatively osteolytic lesion that shows speckled calcification typical of a benign enchondroma. He was treated with curettage and bone grafting.

bony cortex, and speckled calcifications locally or throughout (Fig. 61-7).

The occurrence of a fracture through the tumor is unlikely to result in spontaneous resolution and healing of the lesion as the fracture heals. These slowly growing, locally destructive tumors can be treated by curettage. The addition of autogenous bone graft is appropriate to increase the rate of bone reconstitution if the tumor is relatively large. Recurrence is unusual.

There is some debate as to whether to treat these tumors and the pathologic fracture at the time of presentation, or to allow the fracture to heal and then perform surgery later to treat the lesion. We prefer to treat both the lesion and the fracture simultaneously so that there is only one rather than two periods of disability. The addition of internal fixation (i.e., K-wires) plus a bone graft is needed for some of these cases to stabilize the curetted and fractured bone. In our experience, delaying treatment of these lesions may not only prolong the disability but retard the diagnosis in the unusual circumstance that the tumor proves to be other than an enchondroma.

The surgical approach is generally through a dorsal or dorsallateral incision. Autogenous and allograft bone has been used in addition to plaster and methylmethacrylate to fill the defects

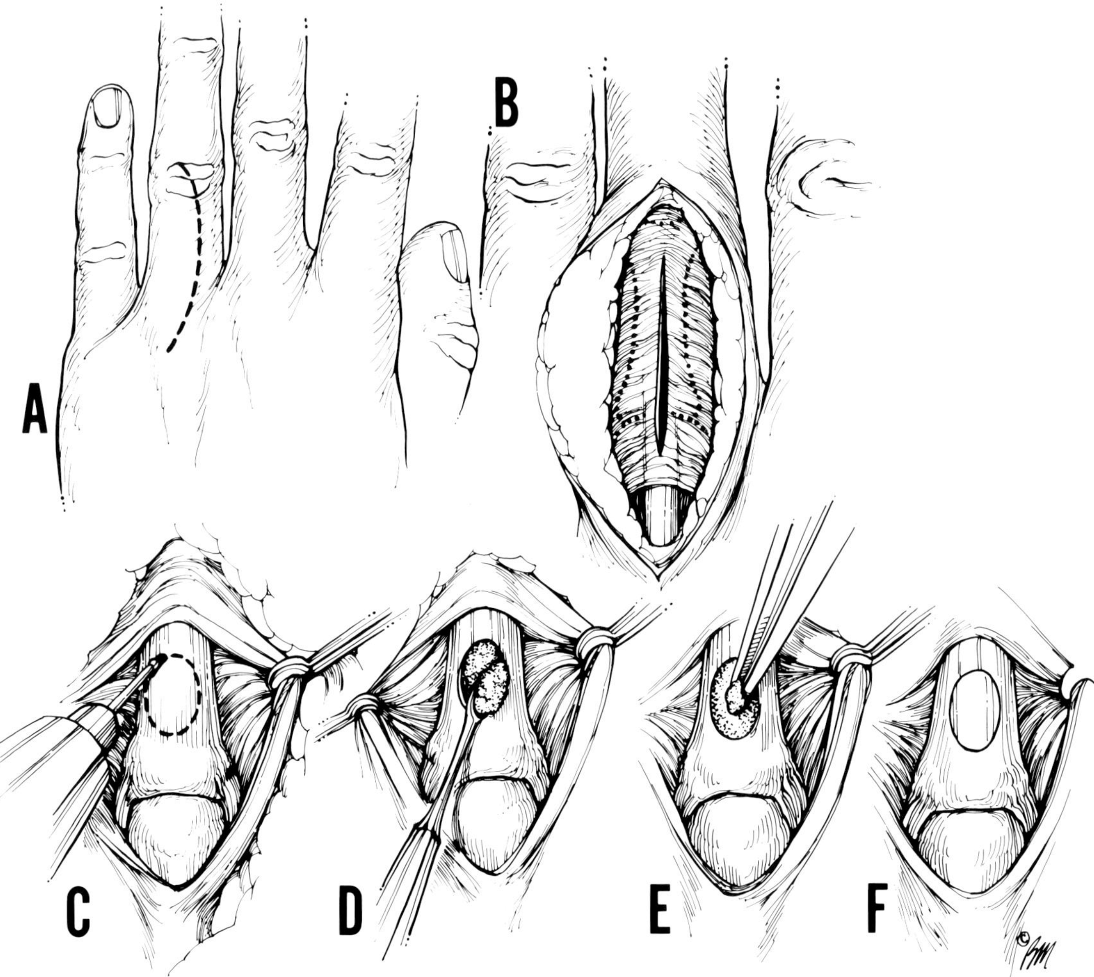

Fig. 61-8. Technique of curettage and bone grafting for benign tumors, such as enchondromata.

(Fig. 61-8). Healed tumors rarely recur, although when they do, some cellular atypia (usually without significant mitoses) is expected.[18,113,142,245,251,262]

Multiple Enchondromatosis (Ollier's Disease)

Multiple enchondromata, although far less common than solitary lesions, tend to be larger and associated with deformities of the axial skeleton.[243] Multiple lesions have a considerably greater risk of degeneration into chondrosarcoma, and therefore this possibility should be considered if known tumors become painful, enlarged, or are associated with a sudden onset of symptoms and/or deformity (Fig. 61-9). If any one of these symptoms is present, incisional biopsy is indicated. Treatment should be deferred until a histologic diagnosis is definitive. Enchondromata of the larger tubular bones should be considered as probable chondrosarcomas. Low-grade chondrosarcomas or (much more often) somewhat atypical enchondroma of the phalanges and metacarpals are likely to be entirely benign.

Osteochondromas

Both solitary and multiple exostoses may arise in the bones of the hand. They are often hereditary and widespread, which may cause generalized and significant skeletal deformities.[85,130,138,155,160,169] These cartilaginous tumors are characterized by the aberration of secondary bone mass production via enchondral ossification. The base stalk is bone, and the cap of cartilage continues to enlarge as the child grows. Although the hand bones are considerably less commonly involved than the radius and ulna, most cases have symptoms caused by the presence of a bony mass (Fig. 61-10).

The aim of treatment is to remove the space-occupying tumor, and at the same time to preserve surrounding soft tissues and uninvolved skeleton. Malignant transformation is extremely uncommon in hand lesions. The real problem presented by these tumors may be the need for reconstructive surgery to restore functional alignment of the bone or joints. Therefore, although benign, these tumors can be very troublesome and should be carefully watched if not excised. Delay of treatment until epiphyseal closure is complete may not be possible if the neoplastic growth produces an angular deformity or if it blocks joint motion.

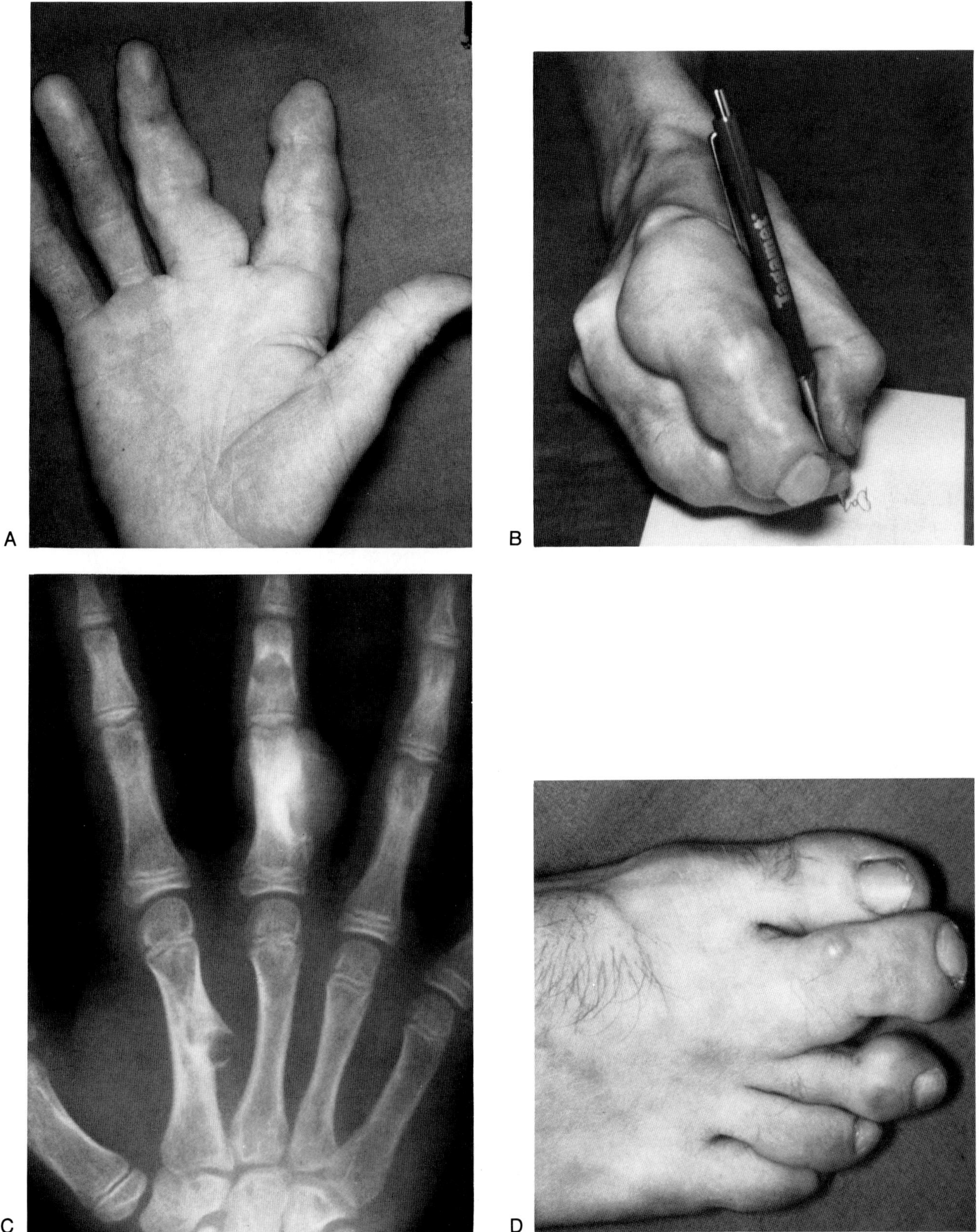

Fig. 61-9. This 24-year-old right-handed Amish farmer had a family history of slowly deforming and enlarging growths of the acral skeleton. He had exosteal and endosteal cartilaginous growths on his right index and middle fingers **(A–C)**, and second and third toes **(D)**. Although he declined treatment on multiple occasions, he remained asymptomatic over prolonged periodic evaluations.

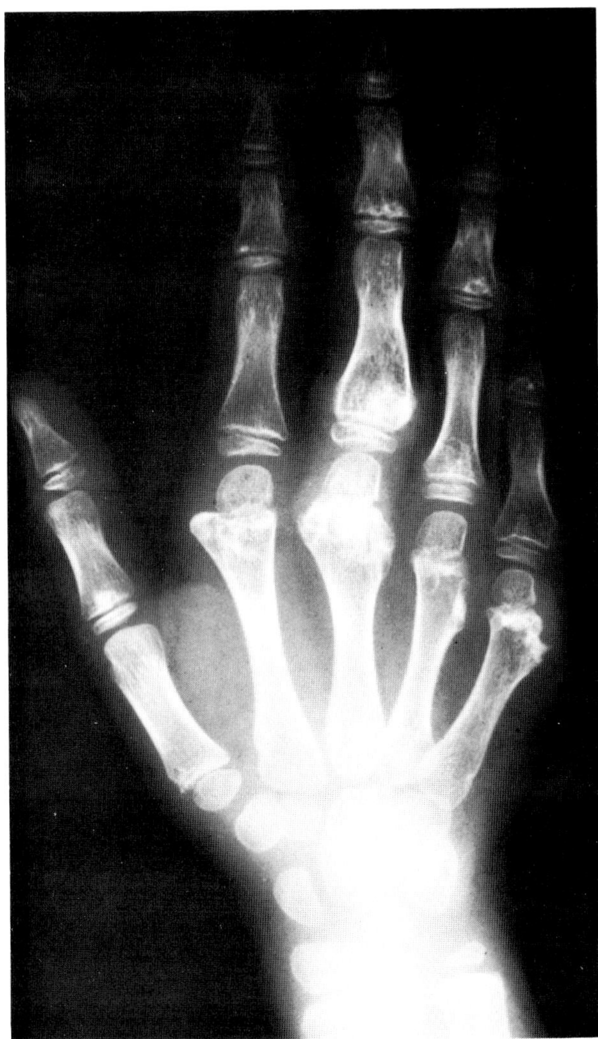

Fig. 61-10. Osteochondroma. A 10-year-old girl with multiple osteochondromas. The hand was asymptomatic without deformity or restricted motion. No treatment is indicated at this time.

Chondromyxoid Fibroma

Chondromyxoid fibroma is an unusual lesion that rarely arises in the hand but may occur in the forearm; it affects a population similar to that with giant cell tumor of bone (see page 2241), for which it may be mistaken radiographically. Unlike giant cell tumors, these lesions generally respond very well to curettage; typically bone graft is needed.[8]

Chondrosarcoma

Chondrosarcoma, a very rare tumor in the hand, when it does occur, is generally seen in patients well over 40, and more typically in the elderly. The most common hand site is in the proximal phalanx, but locations are essentially the same as enchondromata.[37,44,58,59,62,96,124,126,128,132,146,178,181,183,186,219,224,249,253,261] The presentation is similar to enchondroma, but the tumor is generally larger and is longstanding, and it has frequently been ignored (Fig. 61-11).

Mild cellular atypia in chondral lesions is not necessarily a cause for concern. These tumors may be identified histologically more often than is realized, especially if a recurrence following treatment of enchondromas has occurred. Because it is generally a very slow growing tumor, it is best treated by en bloc excision (if it is purely intraosseous) or by ray resection. In appropriate circumstances, allograft replacement of a larger bone may be considered. Because it is not a very aggressive malignancy, the role of radiation and chemotherapy is extremely limited. The prognosis is excellent.

Calcific Lesions

Periosteal and extraosseous (soft tissue and subcutaneous) calcifications are more common in the hand in relation to systemic collagen/connective tissue diseases than following trauma. Although calcinosis circumscripta is not rare in systemic lupus erythematous, dermatomyositis, and other diseases, it is not properly labeled neoplastic.

Bone Tumors

Unicameral (Solitary) Bone Cysts

Unicameral (solitary) bone cysts are entirely benign, cystic lesions, which although rare in the bones of the hands, are more common in the distal radius. These eccentric metaphyseal lesions appear radiolucent, and may first be seen following pathologic fracture through a thinned cortex (Fig. 61-12). These tumors have no known potential for malignant deterioration.[38,155,159,160]

Injection treatment has been suggested for these cysts. The method requires radiographic control and the use of a #15 Craig needle with stylet attached to a 5-cc syringe plus a #18 gauge needle on a 5-cc syringe. Both needles are positioned to enter the cyst; aspirated cyst fluid should be sent for laboratory analysis (cells, culture, and blood chemistry). After evacuation, 40 to 80 mg of methlyprednisilone is injected through the larger Craig needle; injection of up to 200 mg has been reported for large cysts. Some fluid extravasation is expected; a compression dressing is applied. Radiographs are taken about every 6 weeks; healing occurs after about 8 to 12 weeks; the method may be repeated two or three times, if indicated. Treatment by intraosseous injection of methylpredinisilone offers an alternative method to surgical curettage and grafting via a cortical window[216] (Fig. 61-13).

If injection fails, or if a lesion is rather large, thorough curettage to remove the cyst lining is important. Radiation therapy is contraindicated. Spontaneous healing has been reported in some cases.

Osteoid Osteoma

Osteoid osteoma, a benign bone forming tumor, which most typically presents as a painful but radiographically obscure lesion in the young individual, is most common during the first

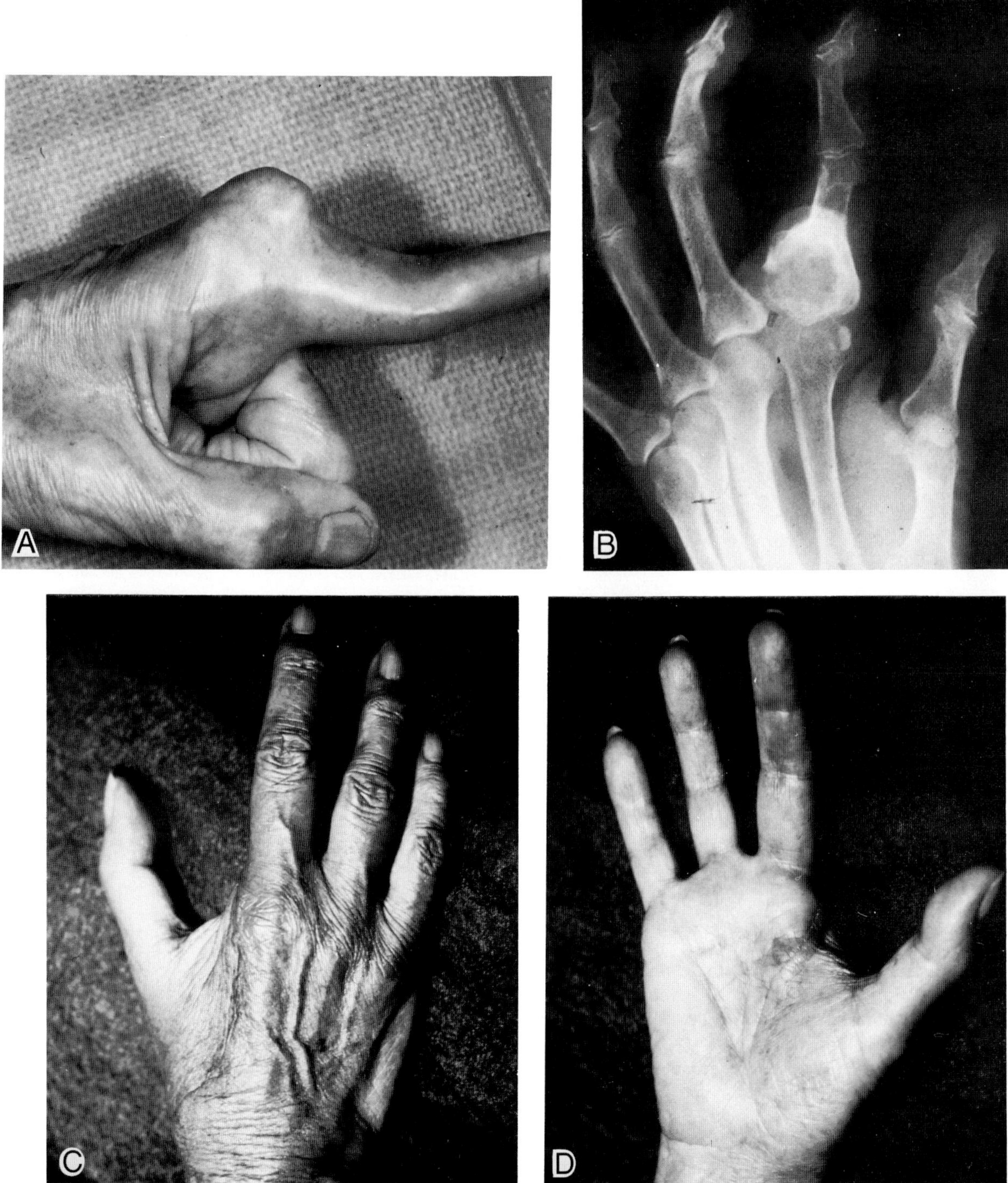

Fig. 61-11. A 69-year-old woman with recently noticed swelling and enlargement of the proximal phalanx of the left index. Preoperative staging studies and biopsy revealed a stage IIB chondrosarcoma, which was successfully treated by ray resection.

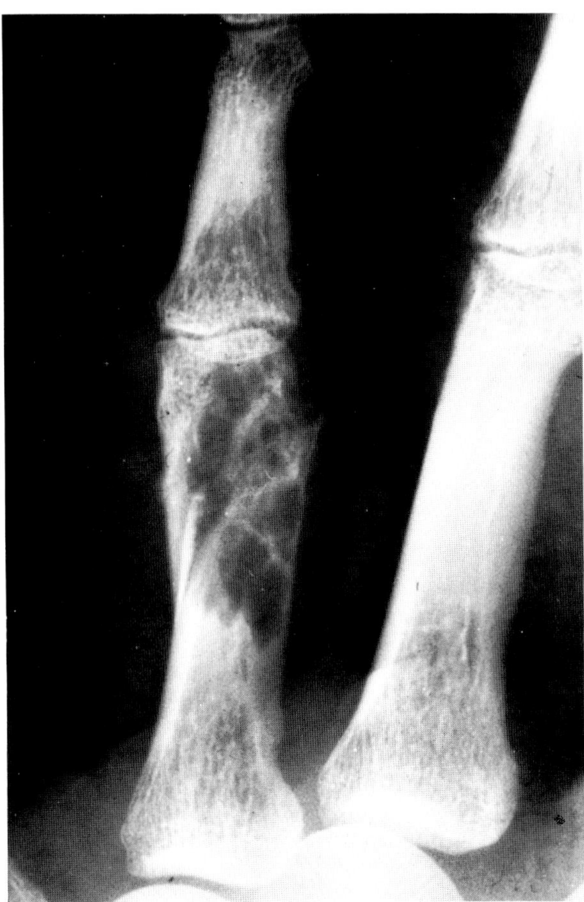

Fig. 61-12. Solitary (unicameral) bone cyst. An 18-year-old man with a pathologic fracture through a bone cyst. Biopsy revealed a cavity with fluid present. Treatment was curettage and bone grafting with an excellent prognosis.

20 years of life. This neoplasm has been reported in metaphyseal and diaphyseal regions of bones of the hand as well as in the carpals and in the larger bones of the axial skeleton. The "classic history" includes pain relief with aspirin, although this is actually rather variable. If seen on radiographs, the characteristic appearance is an eccentric area of cortical sclerosis surrounding a radiolucent zone with a dense nidus. The lesion does not exceed 1 cm in diameter and may require CT scan, bone scintigraphy, and/or tomography for definite visualization[59,71,92,144,166,240] (Fig. 61-14).

Probably the most difficult part of the treatment is making the diagnosis. Cure without recurrence is to be expected after complete excision of the nidus via a cortical window. The entire nidus must be removed; if not, symptoms will not improve or will rapidly recur.[4,6,29,48,71,162,166,174,177,243,260]

Osteoblastoma

Osteoblastoma, a rare benign tumor that is usually larger than 2 cm in diameter, is characterized by osteoid and woven bone production.[173] The tumor is most frequently found in the spine (posterior elements), but other sites include the long bones and phalanges. The histology is similar to that described for osteoid osteoma, but it is important that the tumor be distinguished from osteosarcoma. The differentiation between osteoblastoma and osteoid osteoma is usually based on location and size. The osteoblastoma is more commonly centered in the medullary portion of bones, whereas osteoid osteomas tend to be located in the shaft, juxtacortically, or intracortically. Osteoid osteomas are usually smaller. Standard treatment for this tumor is curettage and bone grafting. In circumstances where the lesion has recurred or has become locally destructive, cure may require bone resection with extensive (corticocancellous) autografts or allografts.

Aneurysmal Bone Cyst

Aneurysmal bone cysts (ABC) are very rare tumors in the hand, although they are not unusual in the spine and more proximal long bones. They are most common in the second to third decades. A benign hemorrhagic and cystic bone lesion, this tumor has a tendency to recur locally.[17,38,88,99,105,123]

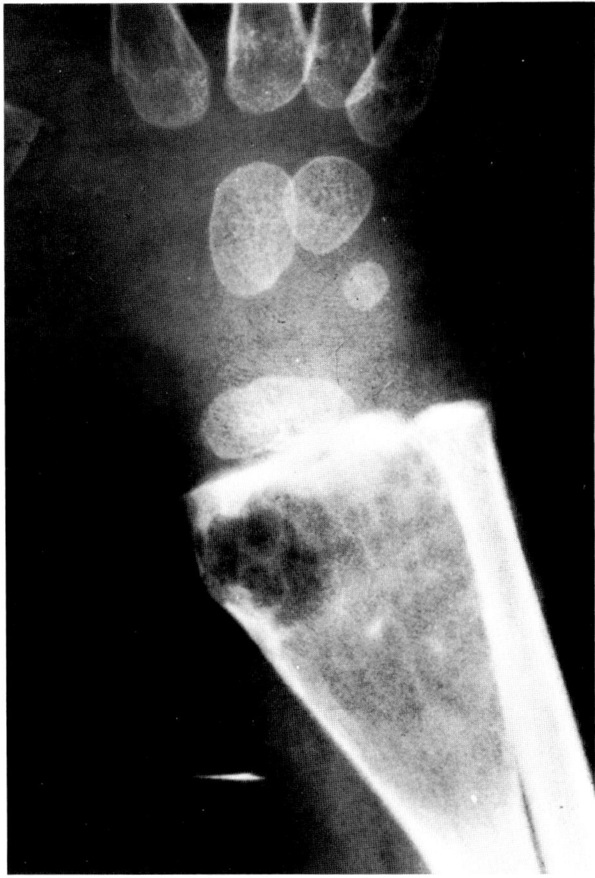

Fig. 61-13. Solitary (unicameral) bone cyst. A 4-year-old boy with a more classic picture of a bone cyst present in the metaphysis of the distal radius. Treatment was curettage and bone grafting.

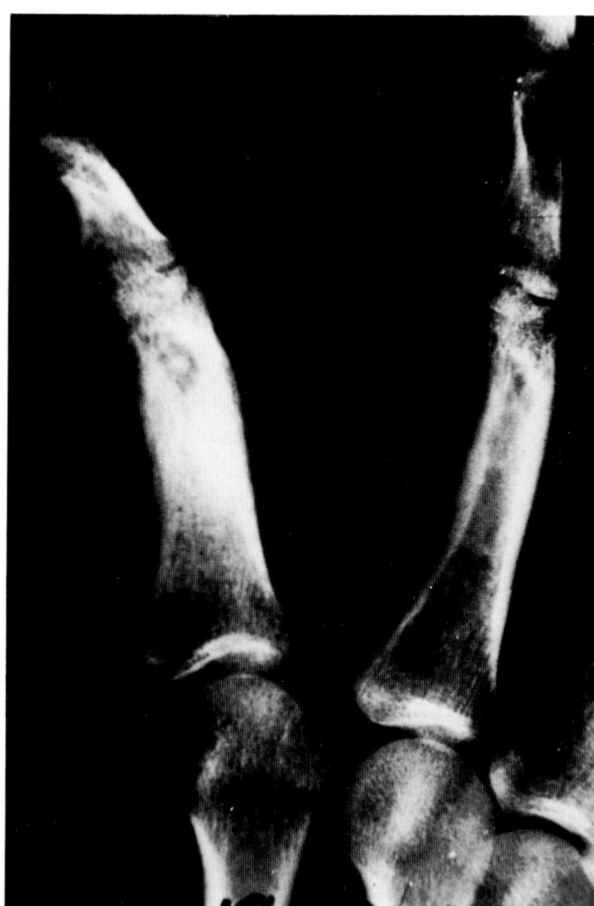

Fig. 61-14. Osteoid osteoma. A 19-year-old woman with a painful proximal phalanx, dramatically relieved with aspirin. Note the classic sclerotic cortical area with a radiolucent nidus. Complete relief of pain followed local resection of the tumor nidus.

Although benign, ABC's may be very aggressive, grow rapidly, and invade locally. Surgical resection requires en bloc bone excision to prevent or minimize recurrence, and with osseous replacement by strut grafts or allograft bone. Ray resection should probably be reserved for only the largest of these lesions, and then perhaps only in recurrent cases[70,86,123] (Fig. 61-15).

Giant Cell Tumor of Bone

Giant cell tumor of bone is infrequent in the hand but is not uncommon in the distal radius. It is more likely to occur in the young adult than in other age groups. The presenting symptoms are pain and swelling that may be accompanied by pathologic fracture. Although it may present as a solitary lesion, it has been reported in the hand more frequently with multifocal giant cell tumors of bone.[13,60,119,163,192,206,221,225,227,233] Therefore, bone scintigraphy is very important in the routine workup of these patients to exclude the possibility of multicentric lesions.

Radiographically, this tumor is typically seen as an eccentric, expansile, radiolucent lesion of the epiphyseal portion of a tubular bone. Although it is unusual for other lytic lesions to involve the subchondral region, the fact that this tumor typically does may be a characteristic radiographic feature of this diagnosis (Fig. 61-16).

These tumors have a very high incidence of local recurrence. Although curettage with or without bone grafting may be appropriate for giant cell tumor of bone in other locations, we recommend that these tumors be treated by excision (ray resection or en bloc removal) and by replacement with autogenous bone graft, vascularized fibular graft, or allograft (as appropriate). On the basis of available literature, it is really not possible to recommend curettage and grafting of the lesions in the hand as a method likely to produce cure. The use of Jaffe's histologic criteria to "grade" these tumors is no longer justified because of a lack of relation to their clinical behavior.[13,122] Although distant metastases from multiply operated lesions in larger bones are rare, they are not unknown.

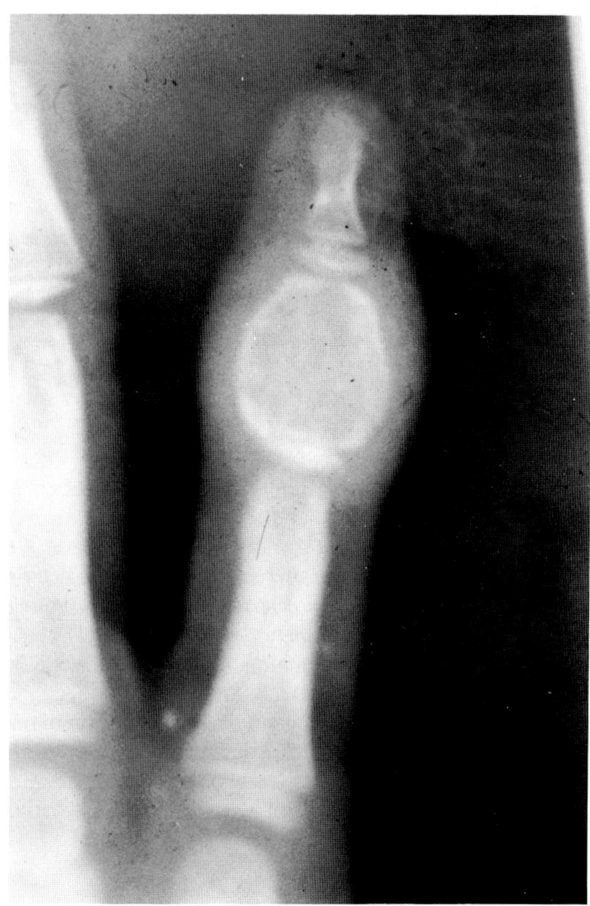

Fig. 61-15. This teenage boy had a rapid course of pain and swelling in the finger accompanied by the radiographs showing expansile "blowout" osteolytic destruction of the middle phalanx. Biopsy revealed an aneurysmal bone cyst, which was treated by excision and grafting.

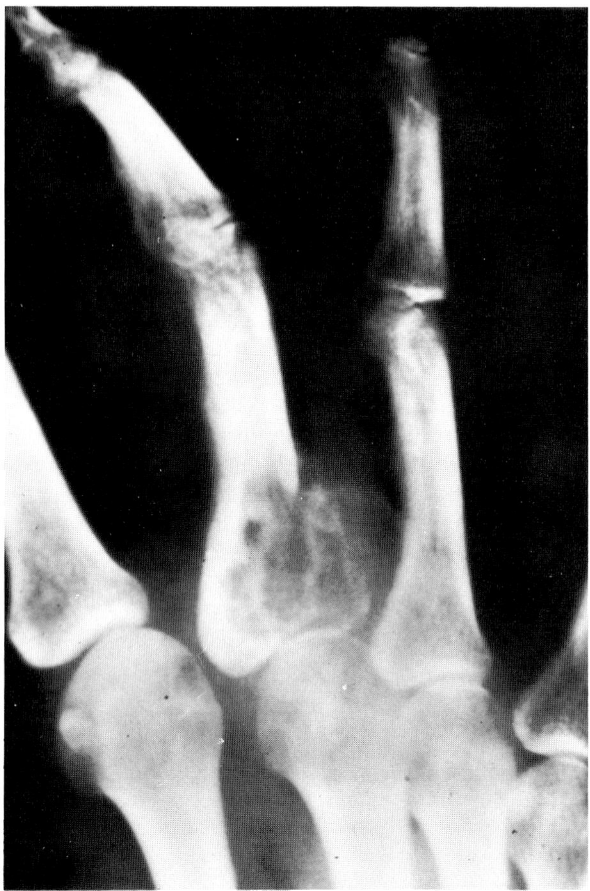

Fig. 61-16. This 25-year-old man presented with a pathologic fracture through an eccentric osteolytic epiphyseal lesion of the proximal phalanx of the middle finger; after staging studies it was diagnosed as giant cell tumor of bone at incisional biopsy.

Osteogenic Sarcoma

Osteogenic sarcoma, an extremely uncommon tumor in the hand, occurs during the first and second decades in metacarpals and proximal phalanges.[7,42,84] It presents as a progressively painful, swollen mass and is characterized by a rapid course. Radiographs reveal a sclerotic, expansile, destructive bone lesion (Fig. 61-17). At biopsy, the histologic differential between this tumor and osteoblastoma may be challenging or frankly difficult. Treatment of osteogenic sarcoma requires aggressive wide en bloc excision, radical removal, or amputation of multiple rays. Adjuvant chemotherapy including consideration of preoperative adjuvants (neo-adjuvants) should be strongly encouraged for all cases. The beneficial role of radiation therapy is not firmly established.[14,15,64,91,151,208]

Ewing's Sarcoma

Ewing's sarcoma is an extremely rare malignant tumor of the hand skeleton that may occur in young patients, usually in the first decade of life. It has been reported in the phalanges and metacarpals, often with a soft tissue component.[66,72,73,80,134] As is true of other neoplastic problems, this tumor may present as an inflammatory process that includes pain, swelling, and erythema. Fever and elevated sedimentation rate are not rare. This tumor has a round cell origin. Radiographs demonstrate a destructive lytic lesion and swelling of the soft tissue (Fig. 61-18).

Incisional biopsy followed by wide en bloc resection or amputation are appropriate. The tumor is radiosensitive, and adjuvant chemotherapy is also recommended.[64,80,143,222,236] Surgical treatment is often more practical than other modalities, especially if radiation would include uninvolved tissues, such as nerves, that may be sensitive to fibrosis, especially in a child. Chances of survival if this lesion occurs in the hand may be better than if it occurs elsewhere, possibly because of earlier recognition when it is small in size.

Metastatic Tumors

Skeletal metastases are rare below the elbow and may occur in patients with other primary malignancies, especially kidney, colon, breast, and lung tumors.[5,30,52,58,110,131,136,187,208,228,262] In-

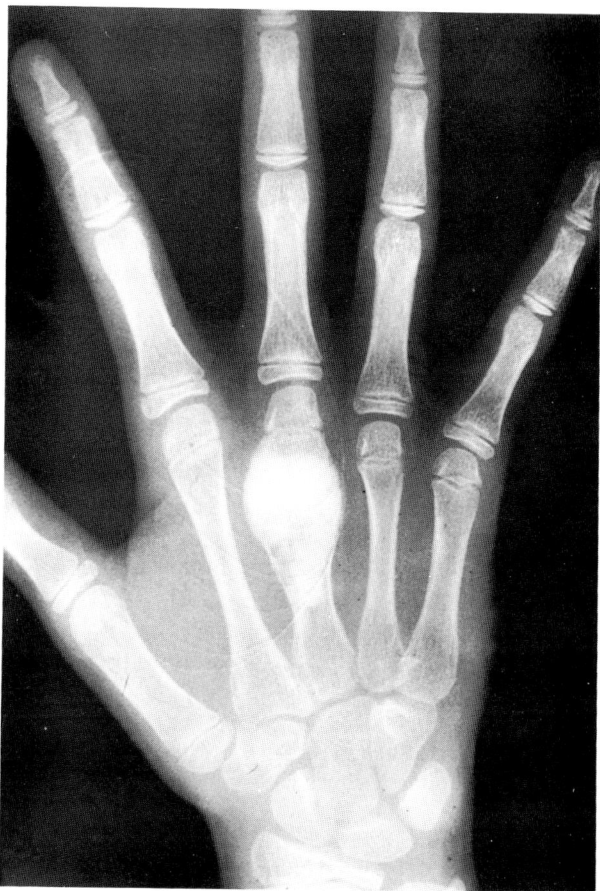

Fig. 61-17. This 7-year-old girl experienced swelling and pain of the right third metacarpal. Biopsy and staging studies disclosed a stage IIB osteosarcoma treated by third ray resection.

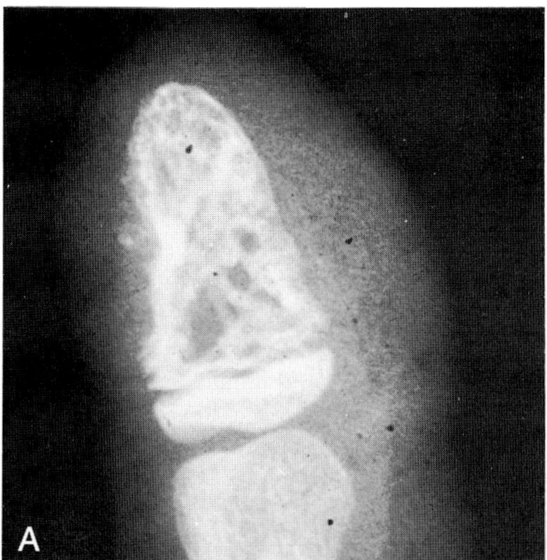

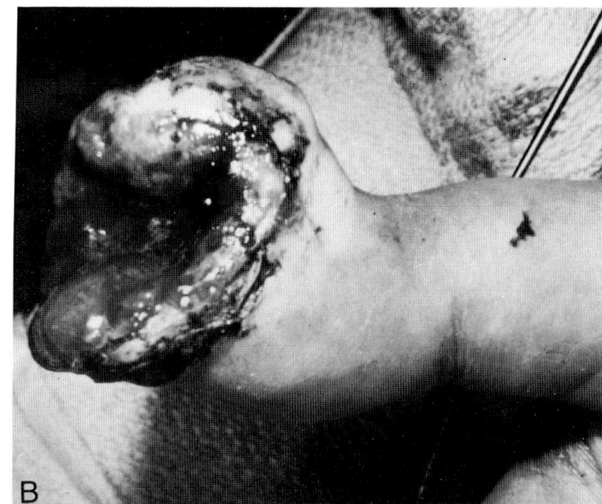

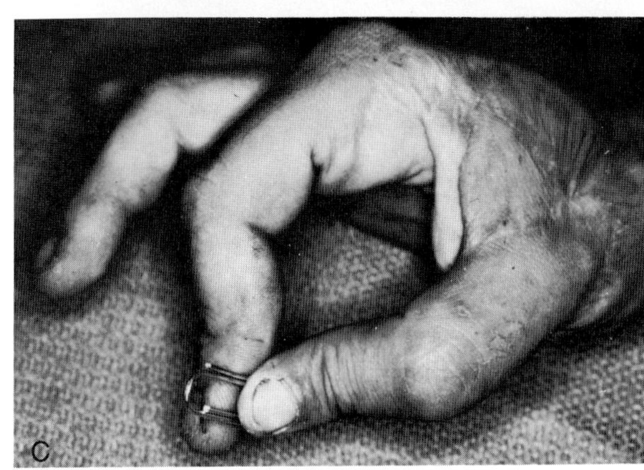

Fig. 61-18. This 10-year-old boy experienced progressive pain and swelling in the distal segment of his thumb with irregular osteolysis (**A**). Incorrectly diagnosed as a felon, the finger was incised and drained without success. Cultures were negative and pathology revealed an Ewing's sarcoma, which was then treated by thumb MP joint disarticulation (**B**). Two years later there was no evidence of recurrence or metastases. Pollicization was therefore performed (**C**) and he remains disease-free long-term.

terestingly, the distal phalanx is the most common location in the hand for metastatic lesions, whereas the carpal bones are the most uncommon sites.

The clinical presentation may be suggestive of an infection, especially if the primary tumor is still silent; symptoms include progressive pain, swelling, and erythema, and radiographs usually disclose a radiolucent, destructive bone process (Fig. 61-19). The diagnosis is confirmed by biopsy, which can be with needle technique after the primary lesion has already been diagnosed. Of course, standard biopsy protocol should be followed if a distant primary site is unknown (see Chapter 60).

Choices of treatment vary depending on the overall status of the patient and the primary tumor. Commonly, local radiotherapy or palliative digit and/or ray amputation are appropriate. In all cases, it should be clear that this presentation is an ominous prognostic sign and that the majority of patients with hand metastases do not survive more than about 6 months.

SUMMARY

Our goal in writing this chapter has been to provide information on diagnosis and treatment (including protocols and methods), providing paradigms for management with respect to the various lesions of the soft tissues, bone, and cartilage of the hand. Although these generalizations and principles are important, each case is different and must be handled in the way most likely to produce a cure and to salvage maximum function if at all possible.

It is essential that surgeons treating tumors of the hand are prepared to examine, biopsy, diagnose, and remove these lesions appropriately. The surgeon who biopsies these tumors should be prepared to treat them. However, hand surgeons treating bone and soft tissue tumors should be part of a team that includes knowledgeable radiologists, pathologists, and oncologists. Although the hand surgeon is often the physician to whom the patient presents, in some centers or cases it may be better for the team leader to be a physician who specializes in the treatment of tumors. The team should jointly plan the combination of resection, reconstruction, and adjuvant therapy, thus assuring as much as possible that errors of omission and mistakes of commission are minimized. Balancing each consideration and priority is not easy. However, the ultimate priority is tumor cure. In some cases, it may be reasonable to perform surgical reconstruction at the time of excision; in others reconstruction may be a separate stage performed later for a patient who is likely to survive and use the hand. Although the landscape is ever changeable, the principles of care and the outcome goals are not.

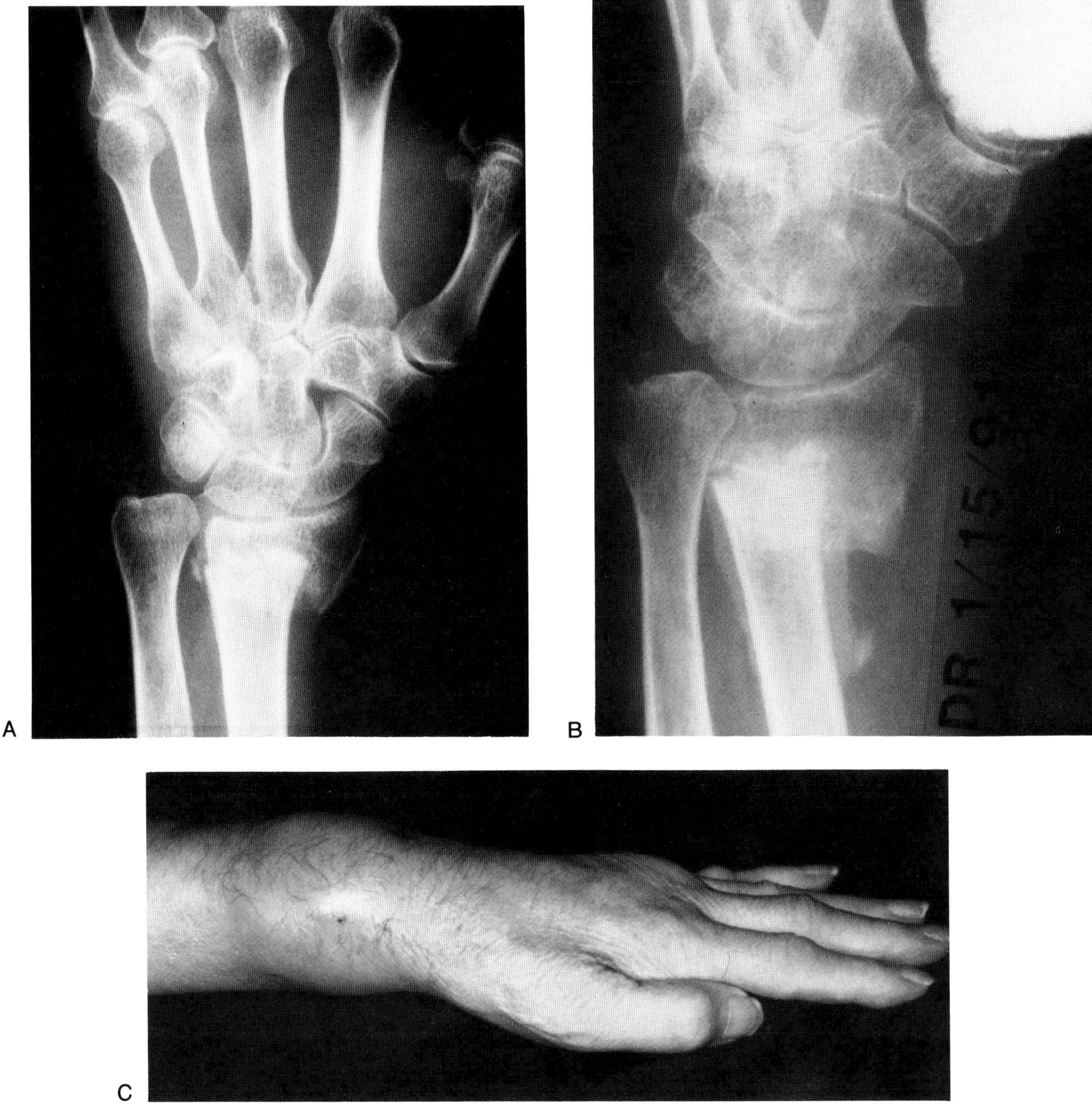

Fig. 61-19. This 54-year-old woman fell and sustained an extra-articular distal radius fracture **(A),** which healed uneventfully **(B).** **(C–E)** However, 3 months later she returned complaining of increasing pain and swelling accompanied by an enlarging mass **(C)** and obvious osteolysis of the radius *(Figure continues.)*

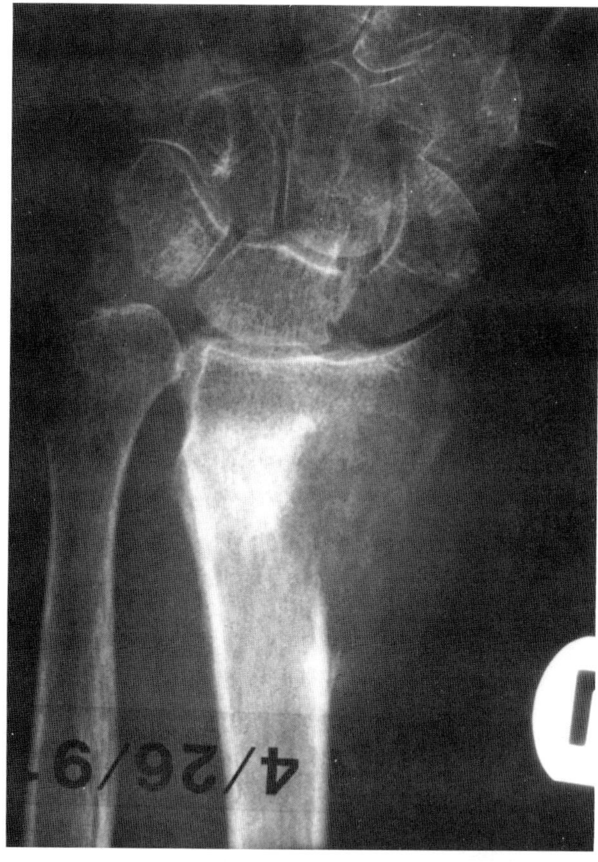

D

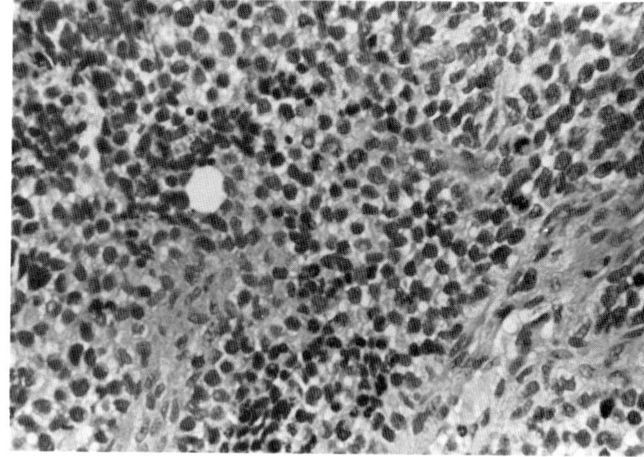

E

Fig. 61-19 *(Continued).* **(D)** Carcinoma of the lung was diagnosed with biopsy **(E)**. She was treated by systemic chemotherapy and local radiation. (Courtesy of Robert Lifeso, M.D.)

ACKNOWLEDGMENTS

The authors acknowledge the editorial work of Frances Sherwin, M.A., without whom this chapter would not have been effectively completed.

REFERENCES

1. Abu Jamra FN, Rebeiz JJ: Lipofibroma of the median nerve. J Hand Surg 4:160, 1979
2. Adeyemi-Doro HO, Olude O: Juvenile aponeurotic fibroma. J Hand Surg 10B:127-128, 1985
3. Alawneh I, Giovanini A, Willmen HR, Peters H, Kuhnelt F, Shubert HJ: Enchondroma of the hand. Int Surg 62:218-219, 1977
4. Allieu Y, Lussiez B, Benichou M, Cenac P: A double nidus osteoid osteoma in a finger. J Hand Surg 14A:538-541, 1989
5. Amadio PC, Lombardi RM: Metastatic tumors of the hand. J Hand Surg 12A:311-316, 1987
6. Ambrosia JM, Wold LE, Amadio PC: Osteoid osteoma of the hand and wrist. J Hand Surg 12A:794-800, 1987
7. American Joint Committee for Cancer Staging and End Results Reporting: Manual for Staging Cancer. pp. 1-2. Whiting Press, Chicago, 1977
8. Anderson WJ, Bowers WH: Chondromyxoid fibroma of the proximal phalanx. A tumour that may be confused with chondrosarcoma. J Hand Surg 11B:144-146, 1986
9. Andrew TA: Clear cell sarcoma of the hand. Hand 14:200-203, 1982
10. Angelides AC, Wallace PF: The dorsal ganglion of the wrist: Its pathogenesis, gross and microscopic anatomy and surgical treatment. J Hand Surg 1:228, 1976
11. Archer IA, Brown RB, Fitton JM: Epithelioid sarcoma in the hand. J Hand Surg 9B:207-209, 1984
12. Ariel IM, Briceno M: Rhabdomyosarcoma of the extremities and trunk: Analysis of 150 patients treated by surgical resection. J Surg Oncol 7:269-287, 1975
13. Averill RM, Smith RJ, Campbell CJ: Giant-cell tumors of the bones of the hand. J Hand Surg 5:39-50, 1980
14. Bacci G, Dallar D, Bertoni F, Fontana M, Campanacci M, Pignatti G, Mercuri M, Bacchini P, Avella M: Primary chemo-delayed surgery for telangiectatic osteogenic sarcoma of the extremities. J Chemother 1(3):190-196, 1989
15. Bacci G, Dallar D, DiScioscio M, Caldora P, Picci P, Ferrari S, Malaguti C, Avella M, Prasad R: Importance of dose intensity in neoadjuvant chemotherapy of osteosarcoma. J Chemother 2(2):127-135, 1990
16. Bacci G, Springfield D, Capanna R, Picci P, Bertoni F, Campanacci M: Adjuvant chemotherapy for malignant fibrous histiocytoma in the femur and tibia. J Bone Joint Surg 67A:620-625, 1985

17. Barbieri CH: Aneurysmal bone cyst of the hand. An unusual situation. J Hand Surg 9B:89-92, 1984
18. Bauer RD, Lewis MM, Posner MA: Treatment of enchondromas of the hand with allograft bone. J Hand Surg 13A:908-916, 1988
19. Beasley RW, Ristow BvB: Malignant tumors of the hand. pp. 1434-1440. In Andrade R, Gumport SL, Popkin GL, Rees TD (eds): Cancer of the Skin. WB Saunders, Philadelphia, 1976
20. Benjamin RS, Chawla SP, Plager C, Papadopoulis NE, Yap BS, Ayala AG, Wallace S, Saunders PP, Murray JA: Primary malignant fibrous histiocytoma of bone—A chemotherapy-responsive tumor. Proc Am Assn Cancer Res 24:144, 1983
21. Besser E, Roessner A, Brug E, Erlemann R, Timm C, Grundmann E: Bone tumors of the hand. A review of 300 cases documented in the Westphalian Bone Tumor Register. Arch Orthop Trauma Surg 106:241, 1987
22. Bickerstaff DR, Harris SC, Kay NRM: Osteosarcoma of the carpus. J Hand Surg 13B:303-305, 1988
23. Black WC: Synovioma of the hand. Report of a case. Am J Cancer 28:481-484, 1936
24. Bliss BO, Reed RJ: Large cell sarcomas of tendon sheath. Malignant giant cell tumors of tendon sheath. Am J Clin Pathol 49:776-781, 1968
25. Bloustein PA, Silverberg SG, Waddell RW: Epithelioid sarcoma. Case report with ultrastructural review, histogenetic discussion, and chemotherapeutic data. Cancer 38:2390-2400, 1976
26. Bogumill GP, Sullivan DJ, Baker GI: Tumors of the hand. Clin Orthop 108:214-222, 1975
27. Bojsen-Moller M, Myhre-Jensen O: A consecutive series of 30 malignant schwannomas. Acta Path Microbiol Immunol Scand 92A:147-155, 1984
28. Booher RJ: Lipoblastic tumors of the hands and feet. A review of the literature and a report of 33 cases. J Bone Joint Surg 47A:727-740, 1965
28a. Bos GD, Pritchard DJ, Reiman HM, Dobyus JH, Ilstrup DM, Landon GC: Epithelioid sarcoma. An analysis of fifty-one cases. J Bone Joint Surg 70:862-870, 1988
29. Bowen CVA, Dzus AK, Hardy DA: Osteoid osteomata of the distal phalanx. J Hand Surg 12B:387-390, 1987
30. Brason FW, Eschner EG, Sanes S, Milkey G: Secondary carcinoma of the phalanges. Radiology 57:864-867, 1951
31. Bryan RS, Soule EH, Dobyns JH, Pritchard DJ, Linscheid RL: Primary epithelioid sarcoma of the hand and forearm. A review of thirteen cases. J Bone Joint Surg 56A:458, 1974
32. Bryan RS, Soule EH, Dobyns JH, Pritchard DJ, Linscheid RL: Metastatic lesions of the hand and forearm. Clin Orthop 101:167-170, 1974
33. Bullon A, Nistal M, Razquin S, Novo A, Fregenal J, Regadera J: Malignant fibrous histiocytoma in a child's hand. J Hand Surg 11A:744-748, 1986
34. Butler ED, Hamill JP, Seipel RS, DeLorimier AA: Tumors of the hand—A ten year survey and report of 437 cases. Am J Surg 100:293-302, 1960
35. Button M: Epithelioid sarcoma. A case report. J Hand Surg 4:368, 1979
36. Cadman NL, Soule EH, Kelly PJ: Synovial sarcoma. An analysis of 134 tumors. Cancer 18:613-627, 1965
37. Calvert PT, MacLellan GE, Sullivan MF: Chondrosarcoma of the thumb. A case report of treatment with preservation of function. J Hand Surg 10B:415-417, 1985
38. Campanacci M, Capanna R, Picci P: Unicameral and aneurysmal bone cysts. Clin Orthop 204:25-36, 1986
39. Campanna R, Bertoni F, Bacchini P, Bacci G, Guerra A, Campanacci M: Malignant fibrous histiocytoma of bone. The experience at the Rizzoli Institute. Report of ninety cases. Cancer [in press]
40. Carroll RE: Epidermal (epithelial) cyst of the handskeleton. Am J Surg 85:327, 1953
41. Carroll RE: Osteoid osteoma in the hand. J Bone Joint Surg 35A:888-893, 1953
42. Carroll RE: Osteogenic sarcoma in the hand. J Bone Joint Surg 39A:325-331, 1957
43. Carroll RE: Juvenile aponeurotic fibroma. Hand Clin 3:219-224, 1987
44. Cash SL, Habermann ET: Chondrosarcoma of the small bones of the hand: Case report and review of the literature. Orthop Review XVII(4):365-369, 1988
45. Castro EB, Hajdu SI, Fortner JG: Surgical therapy of fibrosarcoma of extremities: A reappraisal. Arch Surg 107:284-286, 1973
46. Chang HR, Gaynor J, Tan C, Hajdu S, Brennan MF: Multifactorial analysis of survival in primary extremity liposarcoma. World J Surg 14:610-618, 1990
47. Chase DR, Enzinger FM: Epithelioid sarcoma: Diagnosis, prognostic indicators, and treatment. Am J Surg Pathol 9:241-263, 1985
48. Chen SC, Caplan H: An unusual site of osteoid osteoma in the proximal phalanx of a finger. J Hand Surg 14B:341-344, 1989
49. Chung CK, Stryker JA, Zaino R, Sears HF: Liposarcoma after asbestos exposure. Pa Med 85:47-48, 1982
50. Clifford RH, Kelly AP: Primary malignant tumors of the hand. Plast Reconstr Surg 15:227-232, 1955
51. Cohen M, Ghosh L, Schafer M: Congenital embryonal rhabdomyosarcoma of the hand and Apert's syndrome. J Hand Surg 12A:614-617, 1987
52. Colson GM, Willcox A: Phalangeal metastases in bronchogenic carcinoma. Lancet 1:100-102, 1948
53. Cooley SGE: Tumors of the hand and forearm. pp. 3449-3506. In Converse JM (ed): Reconstructive Plastic Surgery, 2nd Ed. Vol. 6. WB Saunders, Philadelphia, 1977
54. Cooney TP, Hwang WS, Robertson DI, Hoogstraten J: Histopathology 6:163-190, 1982
55. Cooper PH: Fibroma of tendon sheath. J Am Acad Dermatol 11:625-628, 1984
56. Creighton JJ Jr, Peimer CA, Mindell ER, Boone DC, Karakousis CP, Douglass HO: Primary malignant tumors of the upper extremity: Retrospective analysis of one hundred twenty-six cases. J Hand Surg 10A:805-814, 1985
57. Cugola L, Pisa R: Synovial sarcoma: with radial nerve involvement. J Hand Surg 10B:243-244, 1985
58. Culver JE, Sweet DE, McCue FC: Chondrosarcoma of the hand arising from a pre-existent benign solitary enchondroma. Clin Orthop 113:128-131, 1975
59. Dahlin DC: Bone Tumors. Charles C Thomas, Springfield, Illinois, 1957
60. Dahlin DC: Giant-cell-bearing lesions of bone of the hands. Hand Clin 3(2):291-297, 1987
61. Dahlin DC, Ivins JC: Fibrosarcoma of bone. A study of 114 cases. Cancer 23:35-41, 1969
62. Dahlin DC, Salvadore AH: Chondrosarcomas of bones of the hand and feet. A study of 30 cases. Cancer 34:755-760, 1974
63. Dick HM: Synovial sarcoma of the hand. Hand Clin 3(2):241-245, 1987
64. Dick HM, Angelides AC: Malignant bone tumors of the hand. Hand Clin 5(3):373-381, 1989
65. Dick HM, Bigliani LU, Michelsen Y, Stinchfield FE: Adjuvant arterial embolization in the treatment of benign primary bone tumors in children. Orthop Trans 1:249, 1977
66. Dick HM, Francis KC, Johnston AD: Ewing's sarcoma of the hand. J Bone Joint Surg 53A:345-348, 1971
67. Dobyns JH: Hand reconstruction after tumor excision. pp.

11:123–136. In Evarts CM (ed): Surgery of the Musculoskeletal System. Vol 4. Churchill Livingstone, New York, 1983

68. Dock W, Hajek P, Wittich G, Kumpan W, Grabenwoger F: Primary malignant fibrous histiocytoma of a metacarpal bone: A new localization. Br J Radiol 62:940–942, 1989
69. Dooms GC, Hricak H, Sotlitto RA, Higgins CB: Lipomatous tumors with fatty component: MR imaging potential and comparison of MR and CT results. Radiology 157:479–483, 1985
70. Dossing KV: Aneurysmal bone cyst of the hand. Scand J Plast Reconstr Hand Surg 24:173–175, 1990
71. Doyle LK, Ruby LK, Nalebuff EG, Belsky MR: Osteoid osteoma of the hand. J Hand Surg 10A:408–410, 1985
72. Dreyfuss UY, Auslander L, Bialik V, Fishman J: Ewing's sarcoma of the hand following recurrent trauma. A case report. Hand 12:300–303, 1980
73. Dryer RF, Buckwalter JA, Flatt AE, Bonfiglio M: Ewing's sarcoma of the hand. J Hand Surg 4:372–374, 1979
74. Eisenbaum SL, Eversmann WW Jr: Juvenile aponeurotic fibroma of the hand. J Hand Surg 10A:622–625, 1985
75. Enjoji M, Hashimoto H: Diagnosis of soft tissue sarcomas. Path Res Pract 178:215, 1984
76. Enneking WF: Musculoskeletal Tumor Surgery. Churchill Livingstone, New York, 1983
77. Enzinger FM: Epithelioid sarcoma. A sarcoma simulating a granuloma or a carcinoma. Cancer 26:1029–1041, 1970
78. Enzinger FM, Weiss SW: Soft Tissue Tumors. CV Mosby, St. Louis, 1983
79. Epstein MJ: Malignant schwannomas of the hand. A review. Bull Hosp Joint Dis 32:136, 1971
80. Euler E, Wilhelm K, Permanetter W, Kreusser Th: Ewing's sarcoma of the hand: Localization and treatment. J Hand Surg 15A:659–662, 1990
81. Eyre-Brook AL, Price CHG: Fibrosarcoma of bone. Review of fifty consecutive cases from the Bristol bone tumour registry. J Bone Joint Surg 51B:20–37, 1969
82. Finci R, Gültekin N, Günhan Ö, Demiriz M, Somuncu I: Primary osteosarcoma of a phalanx. J Hand Surg 16B:204–207, 1991
83. Fisher ER, Horvat B: The fibrocytic derivation of the so-called epithelioid sarcoma. Cancer 30:1074–1081, 1972
84. Fleegler EJ, Marks KE, Sebek BA, Groppe CW, Belhobek G: Osteosarcoma of the hand. Hand 12:316–322, 1980
85. Fogel GR, McElfresh EC, Peterson HA, Wicklund PT: Management of deformities of the forearm in multiple hereditary osteochondromas. J Bone Joint Surg 66A:670–680, 1984
86. Frassica FJ, Amadio PC, Wold LE, Beabout JW: Aneurysmal bone cyst: Clinicopathologic features and treatment of ten cases involving the hand. J Hand Surg 13A:676–683, 1988
87. Frassica FJ, Amadio PC, Wold LE, Dobyns JH, Linscheid RL: Primary malignant bone tumors of the hand. J Hand Surg 14A:1022–1028, 1989
88. Fuhs SE, Herndon JH: Aneurysmal bone cyst involving the hand. A review and report of two cases. J Hand Surg 4:152–159, 1979
89. Gabbiani G, Fu Y, Kaye GI, Lattes R, Majno G: Epithelioid sarcoma. A light and electron microscopic study suggesting a synovial origin. Cancer 30:486–499, 1972
90. Gaisford JC: Tumors of the hand. Surg Clin North Am 40:549–566, 1960
91. Gebhart MJ, Lane JM: Management of bone sarcomas at Memorial Sloan-Kettering Cancer Center. World J Surg 12:299–306, 1988
92. Ghiam GF, Bora FW: Osteoid osteoma of the carpal bones. J Hand Surg 3:280–283, 1978
93. Goellner JR, Soule EH: Desmoid tumors. An ultra-structural study of eight cases. Hum Pathol 11:43–50, 1980
94. Goodwin DRA, Salama R: Synovial sarcoma of the finger. Hand 14:198–199, 1982
95. Goorin AM, Andersen JW: Experience with multiagent chemotherapy for osteosarcoma. Improved outcome. Clin Orthop 270:22–28, 1991
96. Gottschalk RG, Smith RT: Chondrosarcoma of the hand. Report of a case with radioactive sulphur studies and review of literature. J Bone Joint Surg 45A:141–150, 1963
97. Greene TL, Strickland JW: Fibroma of tendon sheath. J Hand Surg 9A:758–760, 1984
98. Greyson-Fleg RT, Reichmister JP, McCarthy EF, Freedman MT: Post traumatic osteochondroma. Can Assoc Radiol J 38:195–198, 1987
99. Guy R, Langevin R, Raymond O, Martineau G: Phalangeal aneurysmal bone cyst. Union Med Can 86:866, 1957
100. Hajdu SI: Pathology of Soft Tissue Tumors. Lea & Febiger, Philadelphia, 1979
101. Hajdu SI, Shiu MH, Fortner JG: Tendosynovial sarcoma. A clinicopathologic study of 136 cases. Cancer 39:1201–1217, 1977
102. Hankin FM, Hankin RC, Louis DS: Malignant fibrous histiocytoma involving a digit. J Hand Surg 12A:83–86, 1987
103. Harkin JC: Differential diagnosis of peripheral nerve tumors. pp. 657–668. In Omer GE, Spinner M (eds): Management of Peripheral Nerve Problems. WB Saunders, Philadelphia, 1980
104. Harrington AC, Adnot J, Chesser RS: Infiltrating lipomas of the upper extremity. J Dermatol Surg Oncol 16(9):834–837, 1990
105. Harto-Garofalides G, Rigopoulos C, Fragiadakis E: Aneurysmal bone cyst of the proximal phalanx of the thumb. Successful replacement by tibial autograft. Clin Orthop 54:125–129, 1967
106. Hays DM, Sutow WW, Lawrence W Jr, Moon TE, Tefft M: Rhabdomyosarcoma: Surgical therapy in extremity lesions in children. Orthop Clin North Am 8(4):883–902, 1977
107. Healy JH, Turnbull ADM, Miedema B, Lane JM: Acrometastases. A study of twenty-nine patients with osseous involvement of the hands and feet. J Bone Joint Surg 68A:743, 1986
108. Heppenstall RB, Yvars MF, Chung SMK: Epithelioid sarcoma. Two case reports. J Bone Joint Surg 54A:802–806, 1972
109. Heyn RM, Holland R, Newton WA Jr, Tefft M, Breslow N, Hartmann JR: The role of combined chemotherapy in the treatment of rhabdomyosarcoma in children. Cancer 34:2128–2141, 1974
110. Hicks MC, Kalmon EH, Glasser SM: Metastatic malignancy to phalanges. South Med J 57:85–88, 1964
111. Hoehn JG, Farber HF: Massive lipoma of the palm. Ann Plast Surg 11:431–433, 1983
112. Holdsworth BJ: Nerve tumors in the upper limb. A clinical review. J Hand Surg 10B:236–238, 1985
113. Hsueh S, Cruz JS: Cartilaginous lesions of the skin and superficial soft tissue. J Cutaneous Pathol 9:405–416, 1982
114. Hubbard LF, Burton RI: Malignant fibrous histiocytoma of the forearm: Report of a case and review of the literature. J Hand Surg 2:292–296, 1977
115. Ivins JC, Dockerty MB, Ghormley RK: A fibrosarcoma of the soft tissues of the extremities: A review of seventy-eight cases. Surgery 28:495, 1950
116. Iwasaki H, Kikuchi M, Eimoto T: Juvenile aponeurotic fibroma: An ultrastructural study. Ultrastruct Pathol 4:75–83, 1983
117. Iwasaki H, Kikuchi M, Ohtsuki I, Enjoji M, Suenaga N, Mori R: Infantile digital fibromatosis. Cancer 1:1653–1661, 1983
118. Jaffe HL: Tumors and Tumorous Conditions of Bone. Lea & Febiger, Philadelphia, 1958
119. Jaffe HL, Lichtenstein L, Portis R: Giant cell tumor of bone. Arch Pathol 30:993–1031, 1940

120. Jaffe HL: Metabolic, Degenerative and Inflammatory Disease of Bones and Joints. Lea & Febiger, Philadelphia, 1972
121. Jaffe N, Filler RM, Farber S, Traggis DG, Vawter GF, Tefft M, Murray JE: Rhabdomyosarcoma in children. Improved outlook with a multidisciplinary approach. Am J Surg 125:482-487, 1973
122. Jaffe N, Frei E, Trageis D, Bishop Y: Adjuvant methotrextate and citrovorum factor treatment of osteogenic sarcoma. New Engl J Med 291:994-997, 1974
123. Johnston AD: Aneurysmal bone cyst of the hand. Hand Clin 3(2):299-310, 1987
124. Jokl P, Albright JA, Goodman AH: Juxtacortical chondrosarcoma of the hand. J Bone Joint Surg 53A:1370-1377, 1971
125. Jones FE, Soule EH, Coventry MB: Fibrous xanthoma of synovium (giant-cell tumor of tendon sheath, pigmented nodular synovitis). A study of one hundred and eighteen cases. J Bone Joint Surg 51A:76-86, 1969
126. Justis EJ Jr, Dart RC: Chondrosarcoma of the hand with metastasis: A review of the literature and case report. J Hand Surg 8:320-324, 1983
127. Kalisman M, Dolich BH: Infiltrating lipoma of the proper digital nerves. J Hand Surg 7:401-403, 1982
128. Karabela-Bouropoulou V, Patra-Malli F, Agnantis N: Chondrosarcoma of the thumb: An unusual case with lung and cutaneous metastases and death of the patient 6 years following treatment. J Cancer Res Clin Oncol 112:71-74, 1986
129. Karev A: Malignant histiocytoma of the arm in a four year old boy. Hand 11:106-107, 1979
130. Karr MA, Aulicino PL, DuPuy TE, Gwathmey FW: Osteochondromas of the hand in hereditary multiple exostosis. Report of a case presenting as a blocked proximal interphalangeal joint. J Hand Surg 9A(2):264-268, 1984
131. Karten I, Bantfeld H: Bronchogenic carcinoma simulating early rheumatoid arthritis. JAMA 179:162-164, 1962
132. Kasdan ML, Chipman JR, Kasdan AS: Massive chondrosarcoma of the hand. J Ky Med Assoc 85:126-129, 1987
133. Kawabata H, Masada K, Aoki Y, Ono K: Infantile digital fibromatosis after web construction in syndactyly. J Hand Surg 11A:741-743, 1986
134. Kedar A, Bialik V, Fishman J: Ewing sarcoma of the hand. Literature review and a case report of nonsurgical management. J Surg Oncol 25:25-27, 1984
135. Kendall TE, Robinson DW, Masters FW: Primary malignant tumors of the hand. Plast Reconstr Surg 44:37-40, 1969
136. Kerin R: Metastatic tumors of the hand. J Bone Joint Surg 40A:263-278, 1958
137. Kernohan J, Dakin PK, Quain JS, Helal B: An unusual "giant" lipofibroma in the palm. J Hand Surg 9B:347-348, 1984
138. Kettlekamp DB, Mills WJ: Tumors and tumor-like conditions of the hand. N Y State J Med 66:363-372, 1966
139. Keyhani A, Booher RJ: Pleomorphic rhabdomyosarcoma. Cancer 22:956-967, 1968
140. Kim K, Goldblatt PJ: Malignant fibrous histiocytoma cytologic, light microscopic and ultrasound studies. Acta Cytol 26:507-511, 1982
141. Kleinman GM, Sanders FJ, Gagliari JM: Plexiform schwannoma. Clin Neuropath 4:265-266, 1985
142. Kuur E, Hansen SL, Lindequist S: Treatment of solitary enchondromas in fingers. J Hand Surg 14B:109-112, 1989
143. Lacey SH, Danish EH, Thompson GH, Joyce MJ: Ewing sarcoma of the proximal phalanx of a finger. A case report. J Bone Joint Surg 69A:931-934, 1987
144. Lamb DW, DelCastillo F: Phalangeal osteoid osteoma in the hand. Hand 13:291-295, 1981
145. Lammers RL: Soft tissue foreign bodies. Ann Emerg Med 17:1336-1347, 1988
146. Lansche WE, Spjut HJ: Chondrosarcoma of the small bones of the hand. J Bone Joint Surg 40A:1139-1144, 1958
147. Larsson S, Lorentzon R, Boquist L: Fibrosarcoma of bone. A demographic, clinical and histopathological study of all cases recorded in the Swedish cancer registry from 1958 to 1968. J Bone Joint Surg 58B:412-417, 1976
148. Lattes R: Tumors of the Soft Tissue. Atlas of Tumor Pathology. Second series. Fascicle 1/revised. Armed Forces Institute of Pathology, 1983
149. Leffert RD: Lipomas of the upper extremity. J Bone Joint Surg 54A:1262, 1972
150. Lindberg T: Treatment of localized soft tissue sarcomas in adults at M.D. Anderson Hospital and Tumor Institute. Cancer Treat Symptoms 3:59, 1985
151. Link MP, Goorin AM, Horowitz M, Meyer WH, Belasco J, Baker A, Ayala A, Shuster J: Adjuvant chemotherapy of high-grade osteosarcoma of the extremity. Updated results of the multi-institutional osteosarcoma study. Clin Orthop 270:8-14, 1991
152. Linscheid RL, Soule EH, Henderson ED: Pleomorphic rhabdomyosarcomata of the extremities and limb girdles. A clinicopathological study. J Bone Joint Surg 47A:715-726, 1965
153. Louis DS, Hankin FM: Benign nerve tumors of the upper extremity. Bull NY Acad Med 61:611-619, 1985
154. Louis DS, Hankin FM, Greene TL, Dick HM: Lipofibromas of the median nerve: Long-term follow-up of four cases. J Hand Surg 10A:403-408, 1985
155. Lucas GL: Hand tumors. A quick guide to types and treatment. Res Staff Phys 25:76-91, 1979
156. MacLellan DI, Wilson FC Jr: Osteoid osteoma of the spine. A review of the literature and report of six new cases. J Bone Joint Surg 49A:111-121, 1967
157. Mahour GH, Soule EH, Mills SD, Lynn HB: Rhabdomyosarcoma in infants and children: A clinicopathologic study of 75 cases. J Pediatr Surg 2:402-409, 1967
158. Mandell L, Ghavimi F, LaQuaglia M, Exelby P: Prognostic significance of regional lymph node involvement in childhood extremity rhabdomyosarcoma. Med Pediatr Oncol 18:466-471, 1990
159. Mangini U: Tumors of the skeleton of the hand. Bull Hosp Joint Dis 28:61-103, 1967
160. Mason ML: Tumors of the hand. Surg Gynecol Obstet 64:129-148, 1937
161. Maurer HM, Moon T, Donaldson M, Fernandez C, Gehan EA, Hammond D, Hays DM, Lawrence W Jr, Newton W, Regab A, Raney B, Soule EH, Sutow WW, Tefft M: The intergroup rhabdomyosarcoma study. A preliminary report. Cancer 40:2015-2026, 1977
162. McCarten GM, Dixon PL, Marshall DR: Osteoid osteoma of the distal phalanx: A case report. J Hand Surg 12B:391-393, 1987
163. McDonald DJ, Sim FH, McLeod RA, Dahlin DC: Giant-cell tumor of bone. J Bone Joint Surg 68A:235, 1986
164. McDowell CL, Henceroth WD: Malignant fibrous histiocytoma of the hand: A case report. J Hand Surg 2:297-298, 1977
165. McGrath MH, Watson HK: Late results with local bone graft donor sites in hand surgery. J Hand Surg 6:234-237, 1981
166. Meng Q, Watt I: Phalangeal osteoid osteoma. Br J Radiol 62:321-325, 1989
167. Miettinen M, Virtanen I: Synovial sarcoma: A misnomer. Am J Pathol 117:18, 1984
168. Mikhail IK: Median nerve lipoma in the hand. J Bone Joint Surg 46B:726, 1964

169. Moore JR, Curtis RM, Wilgis EFS: Osteocartilaginous lesions of the digits in children: An experience with 10 cases. J Hand Surg 8:309–315, 1983
170. Moore JR, Weiland AJ, Curtis RM: Localized nodular tenosynovitis: Experience with 115 cases. J Hand Surg 9A:412–417, 1984
171. Mortensen NHM, Kuur E: Aneurysmal bone cyst of the proximal phalanx. J Hand Surg 15B:482–483, 1990
172. Mortimer G, Gibson AAM: Recurring digital fibroma. J Clin Pathol 35:849–854, 1982
173. Mosher JF, Peckham AC: Osteoblastoma of the metacarpal. A case report. J Hand Surg 3:358–360, 1978
174. Muren C, Höglund M, Engkvist O, Juhlin L: Osteoid osteomas of the hand. Report of three cases and review of the literature. Acta Radiol 32:62–66, 1991
175. Mutale CB, Patil PS, Patel JB: Malignant fibrous histiocytoma of the second metacarpal. J Hand Surg 11B:149–150, 1986
176. Mutz SB, Curl W: Alveolar cell rhabdomyosarcoma of the hand: Case report with four year survival and no evidence of recurrence. J Hand Surg 2:283, 1977
177. Nakatsuchi Y, Sugimoto Y, Nakano M: Osteoid osteoma of the terminal phalanx. J Hand Surg 9B:201–203, 1984
178. Nelson DL, Abdul-Karim FW, Carter JR, Makley JT: Chondrosarcoma of small bones of the hand arising from enchondroma. J Hand Surg 15A:655–659, 1990
179. Nelson FR, Crawford BE: Epithelioid sarcoma. A case report. J Bone Joint Surg 54A:798–801, 1972
180. Nichols RW: Desmoid tumors: A report of thirty-one cases. Arch Surg 7:227–236, 1923
181. Nigrism M, Ferraro A, DeCristofaro R, Picci P: Condrosarcoma della mano e del piede. Chir Organi Mov LXXV:315–323, 1990
182. Okunieff PG, Suit HD: Extremity preservation by combined modality treatment of sarcomas of the hand and wrist. Int J Radiat Oncol Biol Phys 2:1923–1929, 1986
183. Olszewski W, Woyke S, Musiatowicz B: Fine needle aspiration biopsy cytology of chondrosarcoma. Acta Cytol 27:345–349, 1983
184. Pack GT: Tumors of the hands and feet. Surgery 5:1–26, 1939
185. Pack GT, Ariel IM: Synovial sarcoma (malignant synovioma). A report of 60 cases. Surgery 28:1047–1084, 1950
186. Palmieri TJ: Chondrosarcoma of the hand. J Hand Surg 9A:332–338, 1984
187. Panebianco AC, Kaupp HA: Bilateral thumb metastasis from breast carcinoma. Arch Surg 96:216–218, 1968
188. Patchefsky AS, Soriano R, Kostianovsky M: Epithelioid sarcoma. Ultrastructural similarity to nodular synovitis. Cancer 39:143–152, 1977
189. Patel ME, Silver JW, Lipton DE, Pearlman HS: Lipofibroma of the median nerve in the palm and digits of the hand. J Bone Joint Surg 61A:393–396, 1979
190. Peimer CA: Long-term complications of trapeziometacarpal silicone arthroplasty. Clin Orthop 220:86–98, 1987
191. Peimer CA, Medige J, Eckert BS, Wright JR, Howard CS: Reactive synovitis after silicone arthroplasty. J Hand Surg 11A:624–638, 1986
192. Peimer CA, Schiller AL, Mankin HJ, Smith RJ: Multicentric giant-cell tumor of bone. J Bone Joint Surg 62A:652–656, 1980
193. Peimer CA, Smith RJ, Sirota RL, Cohen BE: Epithelioid sarcoma of the hand and wrist: Patterns of extension. J Hand Surg 2:275–282, 1977
194. Pennington DG, Marsden W, Stephens FO: Fibrosarcoma of metacarpal treated by combined therapy and immediate reconstruction with vascularized bone graft. J Hand Surg 16A:877–881, 1991
195. Phalen GS: Neurilemmomas of the forearm and hand. Clin Orthop 114:219, 1976
196. Phalen GS, Kendrick JI, Rodriguez JM: Lipomas of the upper extremity. A series of 15 tumors of the hand and wrist and 6 tumors causing nerve compression. Am J Surg 121:298–305, 1971
197. Poppen NK, Niebauer JJ: Recurring digital fibrous tumor of childhood. J Hand Surg 2:253, 1977
198. Posch JL: Tumors of the Hand. In Flynn JE (ed): Hand Surgery. 2nd Ed. Williams & Wilkins, Baltimore, 1975
199. Povysil C: Synovial sarcoma with squamous metaplasia. Ultrastruct Pathol 7:207–213, 1984
200. Prat J, Woodruff JM, Marcove RC: Epithelioid sarcoma. An analysis of 22 cases indicating the prognostic significance of vascular invasion and regional lymph node metastasis. Cancer 41:1472–1487, 1978
201. Pritchard DJ, Sim FH, Ivins JC, Soule EH, Dahlin DC: Fibrosarcoma of bone and soft tissues of the trunk and extremities. Orthop Clin North Am 8(4):869–881, 1977
202. Pritchard DJ, Soule EH, Taylor WF, Ivins JC: Fibrosarcoma—A clinicopathologic and statistical study of 199 tumors of the soft tissues of the extremities and trunk. Cancer 33:888–897, 1974
203. Reedick RL, Michelitch H, Triche TJ: Malignant soft tissue tumors (malignant fibrous histiocytoma, pleomorphic liposarcoma, and pleomorphic rhabdomyosarcoma): An electron microscopic study. Hum Pathol 10:327–343, 1979
204. Rinaldi E: Neurilemomas and neurofibromas of the upper limb. J Hand Surg 8:590–593, 1983
205. Ritter MA, Marshall JL, Straub LR: Extra-abdominal desmoid of the hand. A case report. J Bone Joint Surg 51A:1641, 1969
206. Roberts A, Long J, Wickstrom J: A metacarpal giant cell tumor, a sternal osteoblastoma and a public osteogenic sarcoma in the same patient. South Med J 69:660–662, 1976
207. Rogalski RP, Louis DS: Neurofibrosarcomas of the upper extremity. J Hand Surg 16A:873–876, 1991
208. Rosen G, Murphy ML, Huvos AG, Guttierez M, Marcove RC: Chemotherapy, en bloc resection and prosthetic bone replacement in the treatment of osteogenic sarcoma. Cancer 37:1–11, 1976
209. Rosenberg SA, Tepper J, Glatstein E, Costa J, Young R, Baker A, Brennan MF, Demoss EV, Seipp C, Sindelar WF, Sugarbaker P, Wesley R: Prospective randomized evaluation of adjuvant chemotherapy in adults with soft tissue sarcomas of the extremities. Cancer 52:424–434, 1983
210. Rowland SA: Lipofibroma of the median nerve in the palm. J Bone Joint Surg 49A:1309, 1967
211. Rowland SA: Case report: Ten year follow-up of lipofibroma of the median nerve in the palm. J Hand Surg 2:316, 1977
212. Russell RC, Williamson DA, Sullivan JW, Suchy H, Suliman O: Detection of foreign bodies in the hand. J Hand Surg 16A:2–11, 1991
213. Rydholm A, Mandahl N, Heim S, Kreicbergs A, Willen H, Mitelman F: Malignant fibrous histiocytomas with a 19p+ marker chromosome have increased relapse rate. Genes Chromosom Cancer 2:296–299, 1990
214. Santiago H, Feinerman LK, Lattes R: Epithelioid sarcoma. A clinical and pathologic study of nine cases. Hum Pathol 3:133–147, 1972
215. Sapra S, Prokopetz R, Murray AH: Giant cell tumor of tendon sheath. Int J Dermatol 28:587–590, 1989
216. Scaglietti O, Marchetti PG, Bartolozzi P: The effects of methylprednisolone acetate in the treatment of bone cysts. Results of three years follow-up. J Bone Joint Surg 61B:200–204, 1979

217. Schenkar DL, Kleinert HE: Desmoplastic fibroma of the hand. Case report. Plast Reconstr Surg 59:128–133, 1977
218. Schovartsmann G, Spittle MF: Embryonal rhabdomyosarcoma of the hand. Clin Oncol 10:73–78, 1984
219. Scott ADN, Crane P, Staunton MD: Chondrosarcoma—local recurrence and systemic embolization. J R Soc Med 83:48–49, 1990
220. Seel DJ, Booher RJ, Joel R: Fibrous tumors of musculoaponeurotic origin. Surgery 56:497–504, 1964
221. Shaw JA, Mosher JF: A giant-cell tumor in the hand presenting as an expansile diaphyseal lesion. Case report. J Bone Joint Surg 65A:692–695, 1983
222. Shirley SK, Gilula LA, Vietti TJ, Thomas PR, Siegal GP, Reinus WR, Kissane JM, Nesbit ME: Ewing's sarcoma in bones of the hands and feet: A clinicopathologic study and review of the literature. J Clin Oncol 3(5):686–696, 1985
223. Simon MA, Enneking WF: The management of soft tissue sarcomas of the extremities. J Bone Joint Surg 58A:317–327, 1976
224. Sivridis E, Verettas D: Chondrosarcoma in the distal phalanx of the ring finger. Acta Orthop Scand 61:183–184, 1990
225. Smith RJ, Brushart TM: Allograft bone for metacarpal reconstruction. J Hand Surg 10A:325–334, 1985
226. Smith RJ, Lipke RW: Surgical treatment of peripheral nerve tumors of the upper limb. pp. 694–711. In Omer GE Jr, Spinner M (eds): Management of Peripheral Nerve Problems. WB Saunders, Philadelphia, 1980
227. Smith RJ, Mankin HJ: Allograft replacement of the distal radius for giant cell tumor. J Hand Surg 2:299–309, 1977
228. Smithers DW, Woodhouse Price LR: Isolated secondary deposit in a terminal phalanx in a case of squamous-cell carcinoma of the lung. Br J Radiol 18:299–300, 1945
229. Soule EH, Enriguez P: Atypical fibrous histiocytoma, malignant histiocytoma, and epithelioid sarcoma: A comparative study of 65 tumors. Cancer 30:128–143, 1972
230. Soule EH, Geitz M, Henderson ED: Embryonal rhabdomyosarcoma of the limbs and limb-girdles. A clinicopathologic study of 61 cases. Cancer 23:1336–1346, 1969
231. Specht EE, Konkin LA: Juvenile aponeurotic fibroma. The cartilage analogue of fibromatosis. JAMA 234:626–629, 1975
232. Specht EE, Staheli LT: Juvenile aponeurotic fibroma. J Hand Surg 2:256, 1977
233. Srivastava TP, Tuli SM, Varma BP, Gupta S: Giant cell tumor of metacarpals. Indian J Cancer 12:164–169, 1975
234. Stout AP: Liposarcoma—the malignant tumor of lipoblasts. Ann Surg 119:86–107, 1944
235. Stout AP: Tumors of soft tissue. AFIP Atlas of Tumor Pathology, Fascicle 1, First Series, Armed Forces Institute of Pathology, Washington, DC
236. Strege DW, Hanel DP, Vogler C, Schajowicz F: Ewing sarcoma in a phalanx of an infant's finger. J Bone Joint Surg 71A:1262–1265, 1989
237. Strickland JW, Steichen JB: Nerve tumors of the hand and forearm. J Hand Surg 2:285, 1977
238. Strong EW, McDivitt RW, Brasfield RD: Granular cell myoblastoma. Cancer 25:415–422, 1970
239. Sugarbaker PH, Auda S, Webber BL, Triche TJ, Shapiro E, Cook WJ: Early distant metastases from epithelioid sarcoma of the hand. Cancer 48:852–855, 1981
240. Sullivan M: Osteoid osteoma of the fingers. Hand 3:175–180, 1971
241. Sutow WW, Sullivan MP, Ried HL, Taylor HG, Griffith KM: Prognosis in childhood rhabdomyosarcoma. Cancer 25:1384–1390, 1970
242. Swift JE, Blend MJ, Berkerman C, DasGupta TK, Greager JA: Detection of pulmonary metastases in a patient with synovial cell sarcoma using In-111 monoclonal antibody 19-24. Clin Nucl Med 15:227–230, 1990
243. Szabo RM, Smith B: Possible congenital osteoid-osteoma of a phalanx. A case report. J Bone Joint Surg 67A:815–816, 1985
244. Takigawa K: Chondroma of the bones of the hand. A review of 110 cases. J Bone Joint Surg 53A:1591–1600, 1971
245. Taxy JB, Battifora H: Malignant fibrous histiocytoma. An electron microscopic study. Cancer 40:254–267, 1977
246. Tordai P, Hoglund M, Lugnegård H: Is the treatment of enchondroma in the hand by simple curettage a rewarding method? J Hand Surg 15B:331–334, 1990
247. Totty WGc, Murphy WA, Lee JKT: Soft tissue tumors. Radiology 160:135–140, 1986
248. Tracy T Jr, Neifield JP, DeMay RM, Salzberg AM: Malignant fibrous histiocytomas in children. J Pediatr Surg 19:81–83, 1984
249. Trias A, Basora J, Sanchez G, Madarnas P: Chondrosarcoma of the hand. Clin Orthop 134:297–300, 1978
250. Tsujimoto M, Ueda T, Nakashima H, Hamada H, Ishiguro S, Aozasa K: Monophasic and biphasic synovial sarcoma. An immunohistochemical study. Acta Pathol Jpn 37(4):597–604, 1987
251. Urban C, Rosen G, Huvos AG, Caparros B, Cacavia A, Niremberg A: Chemotherapy of malignant fibrous histiocytoma of bone. A report of five cases. Cancer 51:795–802, 1983
252. Urist MR, Kovacs S, Yates KA: Regeneration of an enchondroma defect under the influence of an implant of human bone morphogenetic protein. J Hand Surg 11A:417–419, 1986
253. Vanel D, Coffre C, Zemoura L, Oberlin O: Chondrosarcoma in children subsequent to other malignant tumours in different locations. Skeletal Radiol 11:96–101, 1984
254. Vidyasagar JVS, Sharma S, Krishnakumar S, Veliath AJ: Giant cell tumour of tendon sheath. Indian J Pathol Microbiol 32:50–54, 1988
255. Weiner M, Sedlis M, Johnston AD, Dick HM, Wolff JA: Adjuvant chemotherapy of malignant fibrous histiocytoma of bone. Cancer 51:25–29, 1983
256. Weiss SW, Enzinger FM: Malignant fibrous histiocytoma. An analysis of 200 cases. Cancer 41:2250–2266, 1978
257. Widerow AD: Fibrosarcoma of the hand. S Afr J Surg 26:118–120, 1988
258. Wilkins RM, McLeod RA, Reiman HM, Pritchard DJ: Fibrosarcoma. Orthopedics 8:141–143, 1985
259. Wiss DA: Malignant fibrous histiocytoma. J Surg Oncol 22:228–230, 1983
260. Wiss DA, Reid BS: Painless osteoid osteoma of the fingers. J Hand Surg 8:914–917, 1983
261. Wu KK, Frost HM, Guise EE: A chondrosarcoma of the hand arising from an asymptomatic benign solitary enchondroma of 40 years' duration. J Hand Surg 8:317–319, 1983
262. Wu KK, Guise ER: Metastatic tumors of the hand. A report of six cases. J Hand Surg 3:271–276, 1978
263. Wulle C: On the treatment of enchondroma. J Hand Surg 15B:320–330, 1990
264. Zahrawi F: Acute compression ulnar neuropathy at Guyon's canal resulting from lipoma. J Hand Surg 9A:238–240, 1984

62

Vascular Disorders

William L. Newmeyer

Vascular disorders of the hand are uncommon in comparison with other problems of the hand, and they are less common than vascular problems found elsewhere in the body. Ischemic pain is the most usual presenting complaint, along with the physical manifestations of pallor and gangrene.[1,24] The presence of a mass, with or without pain and tenderness, is the second most common presenting complaint.[20] The mass may be soft or hard, have a bruit or thrill, and coexist with ischemic digits.

Several review studies of upper extremity vascular problems report a variety of causes,[10,15,17,18,23,28] but the fundamental theme in all of them is the problem of ischemia. Vascular disorders of the upper extremity may be conveniently grouped into eight categories: (1) ulnar artery and other local artery thrombosis; (2) aneurysms; (3) iatrogenic, accidental, and deliberate injuries; (4) ischemic digits from emboli; (5) vascular compression in the neck; (6) Raynaud's phenomenon and related disorders; (7) vascular tumors; and (8) congenital and acquired arteriovenous fistulas.

Treatment of these problems requires a detailed knowledge of the arterial anatomy of the hand and a familiarity with vascular diagnostic techniques.

ARTERIAL ANATOMY OF THE HAND

Arterial blood in quantities sufficient to support an actively functioning hand comes via radial and ulnar arteries. In very few hands, a large median artery may carry a significant amount of oxygenated blood. The classical arterial pattern is well described in various articles and texts[2,4,11,22] and is shown in Figure 62-1, adapted from the classic paper by Coleman and Anson.[4] When an accident or an iatrogenic event is imposed on a hand with arterial anatomy that varies from normal, with the assumption that the normal exists, ischemic or even gangrenous digits may be the result.

The ulnar and radial arteries are the terminal branches of the brachial artery in the upper volar forearm. The highest branch of the ulnar artery is the common interosseous, which divides within 1 or 2 cm of its origin to form the volar and dorsal interosseous arteries. The median artery is a branch of the former and may persist as a very large vessel.[19]

At the wrist, the ulnar artery enters the hand through the canal of Guyon[5,11] accompanied only by the ulnar nerve that lies ulnar to it. The bony limits of this canal are the hook of the hamate radially and distally, and the pisiform, ulnar and about 2 cm proximal to the hook of the hamate. The "floor" and radial side of this canal are formed by the pisohamate ligament, which is an extension of the transverse carpal ligament. A fascial extension of the flexor carpi ulnaris running from the pisiform to the hook of the hamate forms the "roof" or volar aspect of the canal. The only other volar coverings are the palmaris brevis muscle, subcutaneous fat, and skin. When the nerve and vessel emerge from beneath the overhanging pisiform, protection is poor and the structures are vulnerable to blunt injury.

The ulnar artery is usually the main source of the superficial palmar arch, which in turn is usually the source of most of the volar digital arteries. However, significant variation from normal may exist (Figs. 62-2 and 62-3). In Figure 62-2 the superficial arch is "complete," in that arteries to all five digits arise from the arch. However, the arch may be dependent on only one artery (Fig 62-2B and E) or any one of two (Fig. 62-2A and C) or any one of three (Fig. 62-2D). A "complete" arch exists in about 80 percent of hands.

Figure 62-3 demonstrates arches that are "incomplete." In these hands, diminished flow in the ulnar, radial, or, rarely, median artery would seriously compromise the arterial supply to some digits, with the possibility of gangrene and loss of one or more digits.

The radial artery at the wrist generally gives off a volar carpal artery, which crosses the pronator quadratus and joins a branch of the ulnar artery (and sometimes a branch of the volar

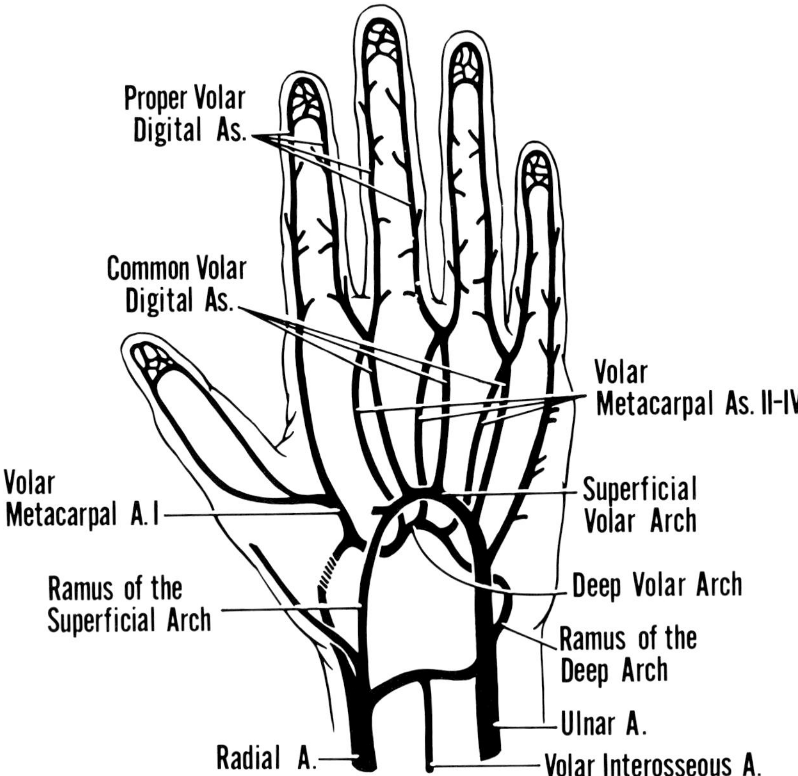

Fig. 62-1. "Typical" or "usual" patterns of the deep and superficial arterial arches of the hand and the arrangement of the digital arteries. (Adapted from Coleman and Anson,[4] with permission.)

interosseous artery) to form a transverse arch.[11] This arch, in conjunction with dorsal arterial branches, is important in the blood supply to the carpal bones.

The most important branches of the radial artery are the superficial and deep ones. The former contributes to the superficial palmar arch from its radial side. The latter pursues a course dorsally, deep to the tendons of the first dorsal compartment, passes through the anatomic snuffbox (where it is usually easily palpated), and terminates into the deep palmar arch, the princeps pollicis artery, and often a large branch to the index finger.[21] The usual pattern of the hand in its most typical form is seen in Figures 62-4 and 62-5.

It is most important for the hand surgeon to be acutely aware of the variability of the arterial anatomy of the hand. Collateral circulation may save a hand,[7] but it should never be blindly relied upon to do so.

In the latter half of the 1980s a number of workers have added considerably to our knowledge of vascular anatomy in the hand. Both radiographic studies and microdissection of injected specimens have been performed, often in conjunction with each other. Ikeda et al[9] studied 220 cadaver hands and found a somewhat lower incidence of incomplete arches than did Coleman and Anson. Work has been done on specific areas of the hand in order to provide a better map for microvascular surgeons for replantations and free tissue transfers.[3,6,12,13,26,27] For the same reason the venous anatomy of the digits is attracting increasing attention. Several recent studies[14,16,26] have nicely demonstrated the predominance of the dorsal venous system of the digits while noting the presence of a palmar system that can provide drainage via a link between the two.

DIAGNOSTIC TECHNIQUES FOR VASCULAR DISORDERS[53]

Vascular problems can be evaluated by one of three techniques: (1) noninvasive, requiring only skillfully applied knowledge—the history and physical examination[61]; (2) noninvasive, involving some type of instrumentation[108]; and (3) invasive, involving injection of some type of dye or radioactive substance with the use of a measuring or recording device.

History and Physical Examination

When obtaining the history from a patient with suspected vascular disease, it is very important to ask about any possible extrinsic causes of vascular insufficiency including a history of smoking, chronic use of vasoconstrictive drugs, systemic diseases, a history of cold exposure, and either chemical or traumatic industrial exposure. One should query the patient about any tendency toward hand pallor with cold exposure or emotional upset. The examiner should note any history of open or closed trauma to the limb or masses in the limb present from childhood.

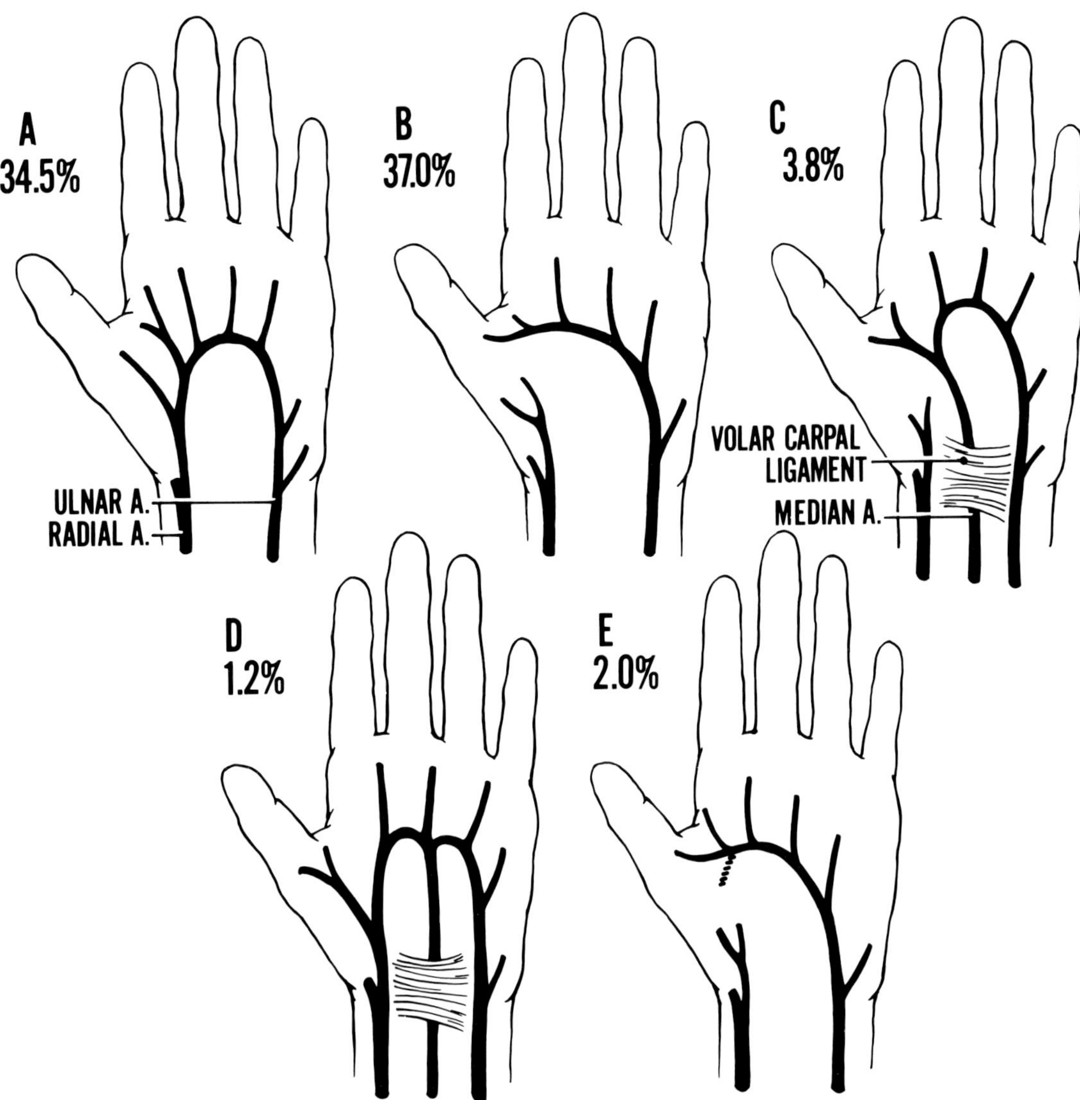

Fig. 62-2. Five variations of a complete superficial arch (i.e., one that gives off arteries to each of the digits) as found in dissections by Coleman and Anson. About 80 percent of hands (78.5 percent in this series) have a complete arch. Note that a complete arch may be discontinuous. (Adapted from Coleman and Anson,[4] with permission.)

A surprising amount of information can be gleaned just by looking at the involved hand. To be noted especially are areas of pallor, cyanosis, hyperemia, trophic ischemic changes (and their exact location), sclerodactyly, location and character of masses (particularly whether or not they pulsate), and presence or absence of scars. By combining a careful history concerning the onset of the problem with the circumstances under which it arose, the observer can usually place the pathologic condition into the category of either congenital or acquired, as well as differentiate local from systemic and tumor from occlusive arterial conditions.

Physical examination will help to elucidate the problem further. Is the mass soft and compressible? (probably a hemangioma); is it pulsatile with systole? (probably an aneurysm); does it have a continuous thrill? (probably an arteriovenous fistula); is it tender? (thrombosed arteries often are). All of the patient's upper extremity pulses should be evaluated. The examiner should start at the neck and palpate subclavian, axillary, brachial, ulnar, radial at the wrist and in the snuffbox, and the digital arteries of involved digits. Comparative blood pressure recordings should be taken in each arm (Fig. 62-6).

By taking blood pressures in the arm and digits, a useful ratio known as the digital brachial index (DBI) may be obtained. This is the digital pressure divided by the brachial pressure. According to Sumner[95] the DBI in normal subjects averages 0.97 (range, 0.78 to 1.27). Patients with obstruction between brachial and digital vessels will have a low DBI but it may be normal in patients with vasospastic disease.

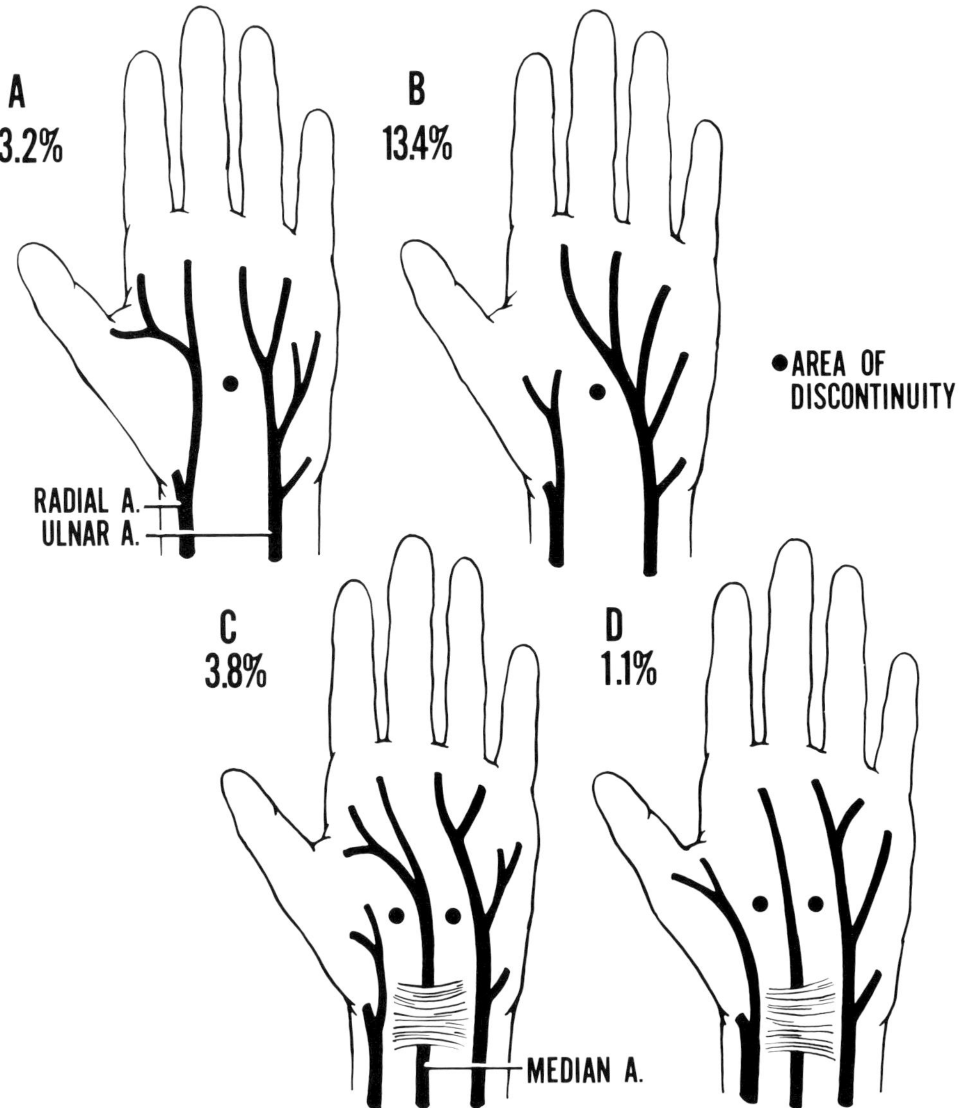

Fig. 62-3. About 20 percent of hands have incomplete superficial arches, with five varieties found by Coleman and Anson. (Adapted from Coleman and Anson,[4] with permission.)

Allen's Test

Allen's test is the most widely known and useful test to evaluate the relative contribution of radial and ulnar arteries to normal and/or pathologic anatomy.[29] The test demonstrates a principle enunciated by McGregor and Morgan[71]; namely that of the dynamically equilibrated watershed between two vascular beds, in this case those of the radial and ulnar arteries. Ordinarily there is little mixing between the two but, if one is shut off or its pressure reduced, the potential for substantial flow from the other exists and in clinical situations usually takes place.

As described by Allen, the radial artery of each wrist is compressed, the subject makes a fist to exsanguinate the hand, and circulation is evaluated and compared after release of the arteries in each hand. This test has been modified somewhat in common use today. Usually, both ulnar and radial arteries of the same hand are compressed by the examiner at the wrist, and the patient makes a fist two or three times to exsanguinate the hand. The patient then opens the hand without extending the fingers forcibly. The hand should be opened about 90 percent. Opening the digits into forcible extension will prevent normal arterial inflow and give a false positive test.[42,45]

One artery is released at a time, and the time of arterial filling, as well as the precise area filled, is noted. The test is then repeated with the other artery.

By convention a positive Allen test is one in which there is no arterial flush in the hand within a short time. Gelberman and Blasingame[45] studied 800 hands and found the average filling time via the radial artery to be 2.4 ± 1.2 seconds and for the

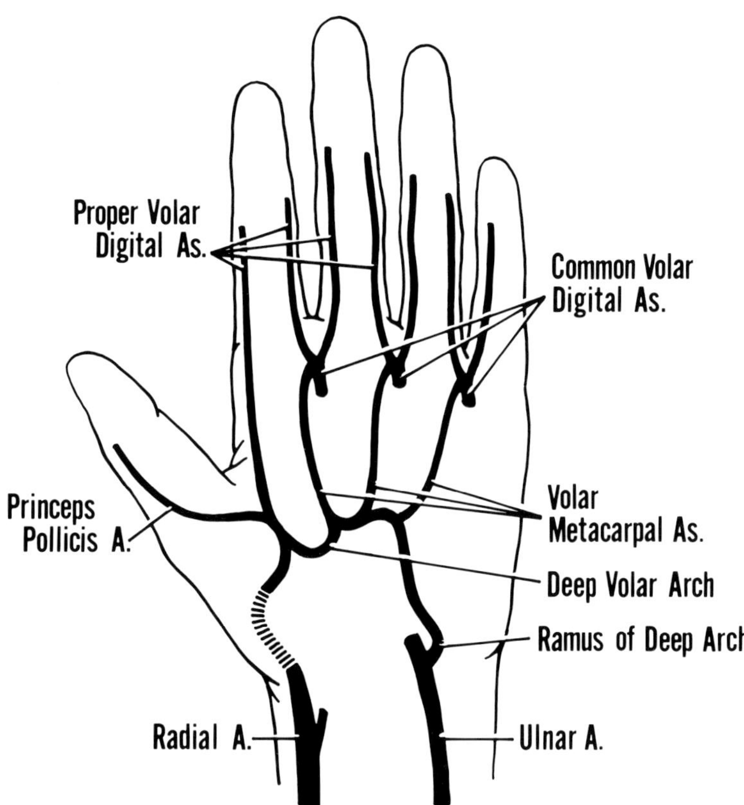

Fig. 62-4. The most common pattern of the deep arch. Note the branches that anastomose with common digital arteries distally. It is the presence of these branches, as well as the often present direct radial branch into the superficial arch, that allows the hand to survive so well, *in most instances,* following division of either radial or ulnar artery without repair. (Adapted from Coleman and Anson,[4] with permission.)

ulnar artery 2.3 ± 1.0 seconds. They noted that 7 percent of ulnar arteries and 2 percent of radial arteries failed to fill the hand completely within 6 seconds. One should be wary of sacrificing either artery unless the fill via the other one is quite rapid.

Since Allen's test may need to be performed on unconscious or otherwise noncooperative patients, some ingenious ways to make it a totally passive test have been devised. Barber, Wright, and Ellis[31] locate and mark the radial artery, put a blood pressure cuff on, and exsanguinate the arm with a rubber bandage. The cuff is then inflated above systolic pressure and the rubber bandage removed. The premarked radial artery is compressed digitally and the cuff deflated. The pattern and time of arterial fill in the hand show the extent to which the ulnar artery supplies the hand.

Ramanathan, Chalon, and Turndorf,[79] noting that the radial artery will continue to pulsate distal to digital occlusion if the superficial arch is complete, performed a modified Allen's test by distally occluding both arteries, releasing the ulnar artery and palpating a radial pulse distal to the site of the still-occluded radial artery. In 20 subjects tested, 19 hands had continued radial pulsation. The Doppler ultrasonic scanner may be used in a passive Allen's test. In addition to uses noted above, the passive variants of Allen's test are useful in heavily pigmented hands in which the arterial flush is not always easily and readily seen. Scavenius et al[82] have described a quantitative Allen's test performed by measuring digital systolic pressure before and during compression of either radial or ulnar arteries. In normal subjects, the pressure drops less than 25 percent.

A number of workers have voiced concern about the accuracy of the Allen test.[32,50,51,52,83] Levinsohn et al[59] studied four methods of performing the Allen test. Using the standard subjective method they found eleven abnormal (false positive) patterns, but by using digital systolic blood pressure found only three abnormals. Use of a laser Doppler flowmeter gave the same results as digital systolic blood pressures and they found this to be the easiest and best technique. Using a pulse oximeter, the instrument indicated normals (i.e., false negatives) in two of the three found by the Doppler and digital pressure recordings to be abnormal. While other authors have relied on the pulse oximeter[68,81] this study would indicate a precautionary note on its use in this particular application.

McGregor[70] did an interesting and somewhat puzzling analysis investigating the accuracy of the Allen test, using fluorescein angiography to study six patients in whom the subjective test indicated nonpatent radial arteries. In each case cannulation of the radial artery and injection of the dye indicated perfusion of only the radial side of the hand and thumb. But with the ulnar artery occluded, the dye spread through the

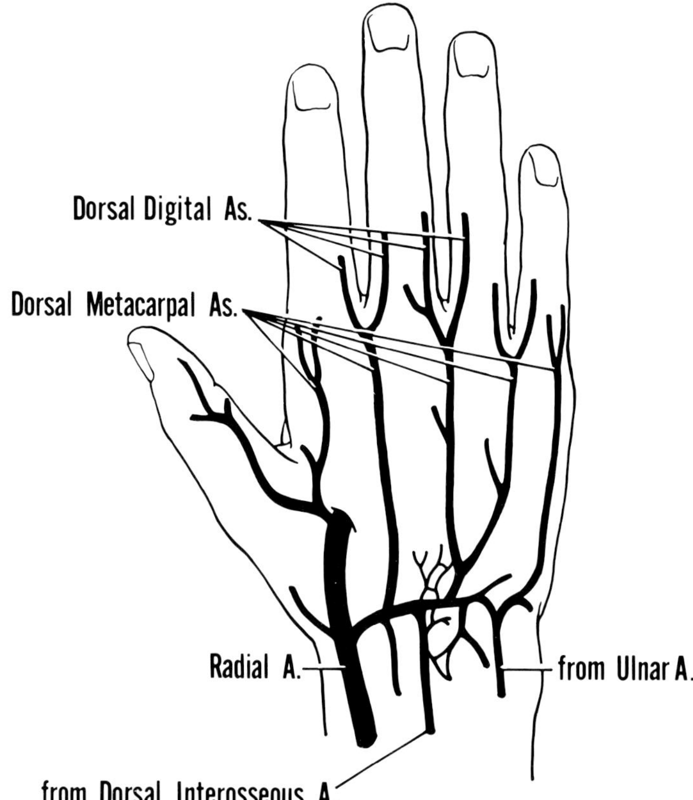

Fig. 62-5. The typical dorsal arterial pattern. These vessels may be critical for hand survival (even through marginal) when both radial and ulnar arteries are divided and neither is repaired. These arteries allow surgical development of dorsal vascular pedicles for various revascularization procedures. (Adapted from Coleman and Anson,[4] with permission.)

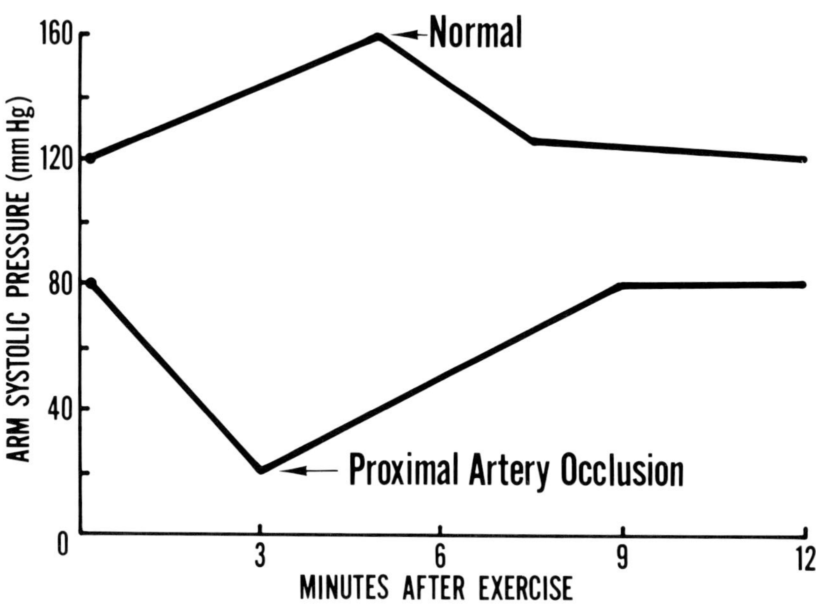

Fig. 62-6. Blood pressure studies after exercise in a normal limb and in one with proximal arterial occlusion. (Adapted from Gross and Louis,[47] with permission.)

entire hand. In these six cases there would appear to be a shift of the dynamic equilibrium between the ulnar and radial beds to answer a physiologic need. The Allen test gave a false positive which forces the surgeon to err on the side of providing more blood supply rather than the dangerous false negative which gives a false sense of security.

Noninvasive Instrument Techniques

The Doppler Scanner

The most useful noninvasive device to evaluate blood flow in the upper extremity is the Doppler ultrasonic scanner. It was developed in the early 1960s[92,103,104] and came into wide use in the 1970s.

The simplest Doppler available today is similar to the one shown in Figure 62-7B and is available for about $335. An instrument that combines a Doppler with a plethysmograph is a good deal more expensive and will cost $2500 or more.

The basic instrument consists of two piezoelectric crystals, one to emit an ultrasound beam and one to receive the altered sound as it is reflected back to the device. The ultrasound waves are of low intensity (1 to 10 MHz). A sound-conducting gel is applied to the hand, and the beam passes through the tissues to an underlying blood vessel, where its frequency is shifted by an amount porportional to the flow velocity of the blood. The receiving crystal gathers in the sound of altered frequency mixed with that of the transmitted frequency to produce an audible signal. The pitch of the signal varies with the velocity of the blood flow.[91,92] In simpler terms, it can be said that the louder the signal, the greater the blood flow. The signal may also be electronically put on an oscilloscope for a visual display of the pulse wave and may be recorded. A recording from a normal subject is seen in Fig. 62-8. Detailed normal and pathologic recording patterns are shown in Figure 62-9. Absence of a signal over a vessel is evidence of no flow or a very low flow.

Most Dopplers emit a continuous wave of sound. The pulsed Doppler is a more sophisticated laboratory device, which may

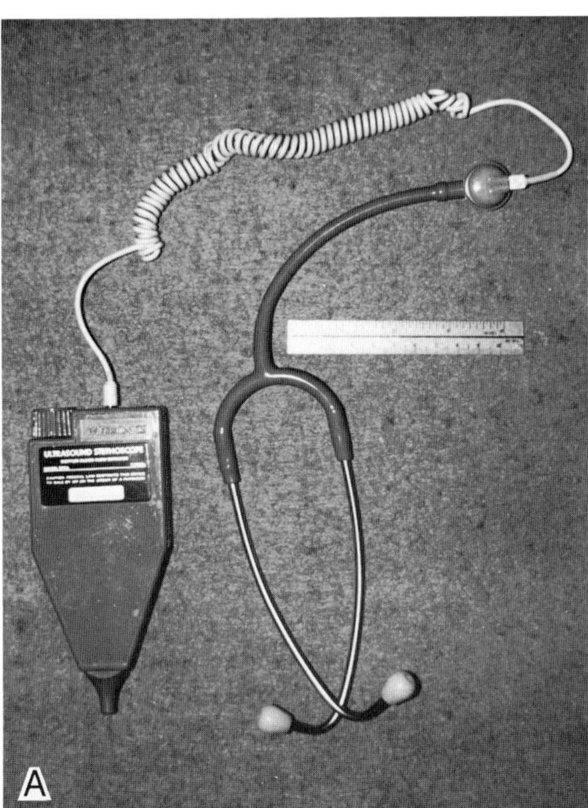

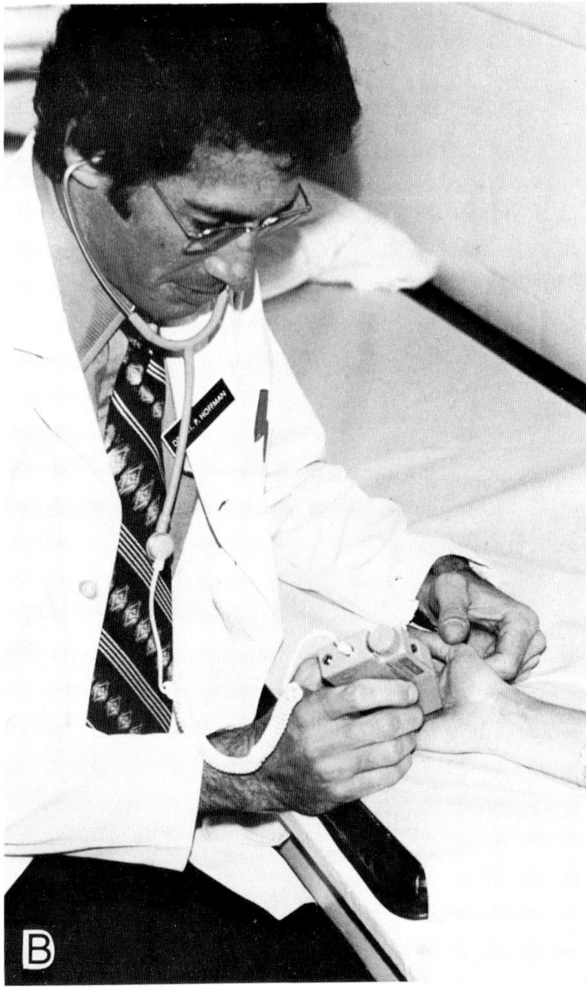

Fig. 62-7. **(A)** A typical portable Doppler ultrasonic scanner with a stethoscope attachment. **(B)** The device is easy to use, the main requirements being some knowledge of surface anatomic landmarks over arteries and a little patience.

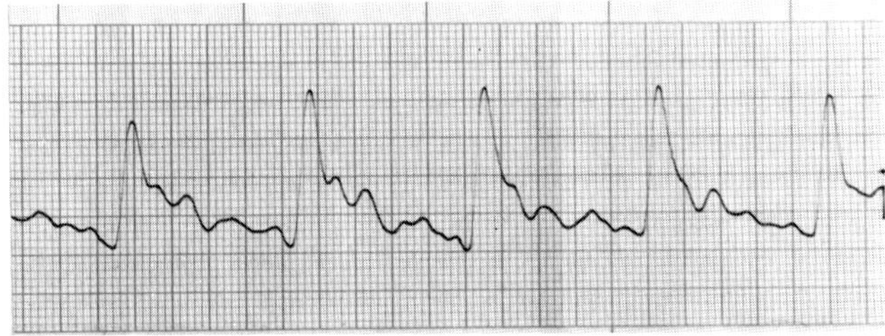

Fig. 62-8. A waveform recorded with a Doppler scanner from the digit of a normal 49-year-old man.

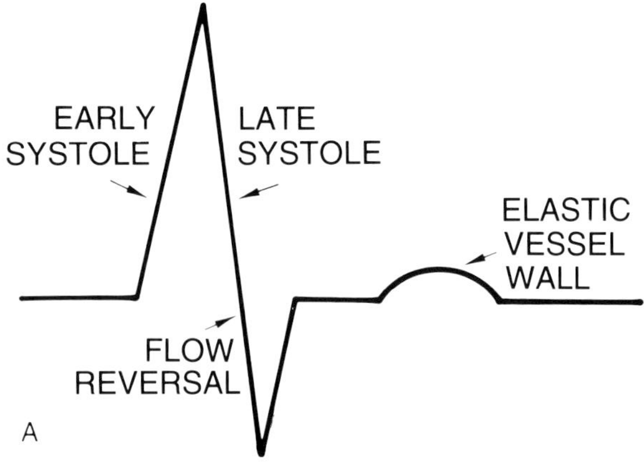

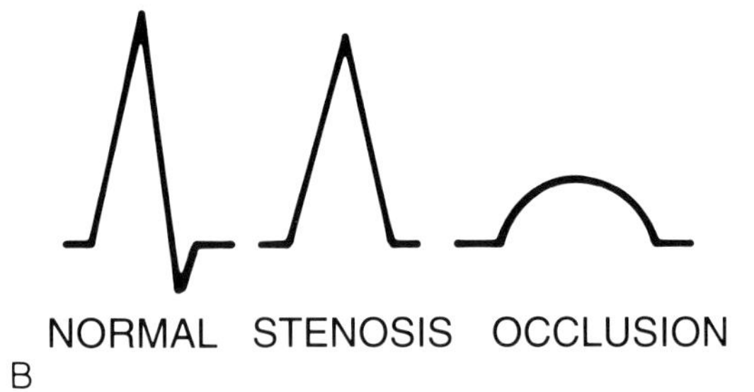

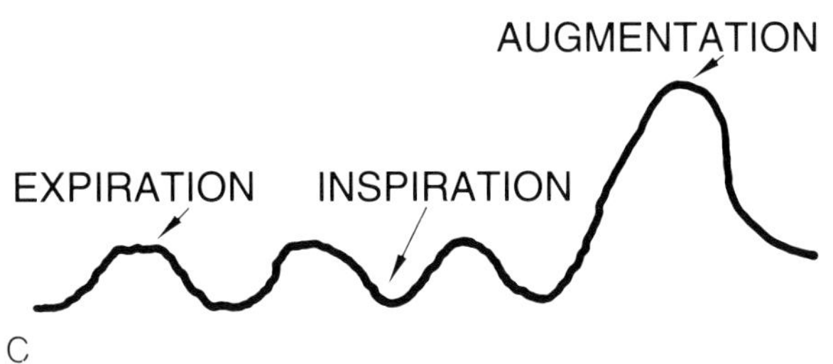

Fig. 62-9. Normal and obstructive arterial patterns **(A&B)** and a normal venous pattern **(C)** recorded on an oscilloscope from a Doppler scanner. Venous augmentation is achieved by squeezing the limb distal to the position of the probe to accelerate venous return. (Adapted from Gross and Louis,[47] with permission.)

be used to give a three-dimensional view of an artery. This is particularly useful determining the degree of obstruction in a partially occluded artery.[72] Blair, Green and Omer[35] have used a pulsed ultrasound Doppler (20 MHz) velocity meter (PUDVM) to obtain information about average blood velocities and vessel lumen diameters in small blood vessels. Using the velocity profiles obtained, blood flow in human digital arteries may be quantitated.[36] Several authors[88,102,105] have compared the Doppler to other noninvasive techniques, including plethysmography, thermography, and radionuclide scans, and have found that Doppler gives the most specific and most useful information.

The Doppler may be sterilized and used intraoperatively to help in localizing small arteriovenous fistulas.[34] Perhaps the most useful application of the Doppler is in evaluating the arterial anatomy in a normal hand in which cannulation or other procedures that could damage an artery are contemplated. Studies by Mozersky and colleagues[72] and by Little and colleagues[62] confirmed what Coleman and Anson demonstrated in their dissections (see Fig. 62-1). This noninvasive technique allows, with a high degree of accuracy, the prediction of the importance of an artery to hand survival.

Gross and Louis[47] did a Doppler assessment of 38 patients with obscure symptoms that were thought to be of vascular origin. Eighteen of the patients had angiography before or after the Doppler study, and in each case the presence or absence of hemodynamically significant vascular occlusion was predicted or confirmed by the study. The other 20 patients had normal Doppler studies and avoided the expense and risks of angiography. They demonstrated the usefulness of the Doppler in the evaluation of venous disease.

DiBenedetto et al[38] have also found the Doppler to be a very accurate alternative to angiography. Dooley et al[39] assessed the accuracy of the duplex scanner in predicting the patency of microvascular anastomoses with a duplex scanner. This instrument utilizes a B-mode ultrasound imager to locate the vessel of interest and a bi-directional Doppler to determine the blood flow. This instrument correctly predicted 27 of 27 patent arteries but only 8 to 11 partially occluded arteries and 28 of 32 totally occluded arteries.

Plethysmography

Plethysmos is a Greek word meaning "an enlargement." Plethysmography is the determination of the varying size of an organ according to the amount of blood it contains. A standard blood pressure device is a simple, analog type of plethysmograph. Instruments available today are considerably more sophisticated than this.

Plethysmographs falls into one of several categories.[93] Water-filled instruments measure volume change directly by fluid displacement. Air-filled plethysmographs measure volume changes indirectly. With a change of volume from blood inflow in the limb being studied, there is a change of pressure in the captive air of an applied cuff, and this can be measured and recorded. Strain gauge plethysmographs are fine rubber tubes filled with mercury (or an indium-gallium alloy), which makes contact with copper electrodes at each end of the

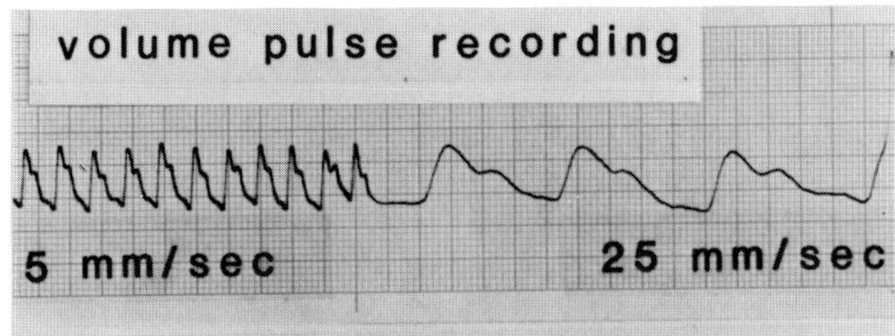

Fig. 62-10. A waveform recorded with a pneumoplethysmograph of the same subject shown in Figure 62-8.

tube.[78,90,94,96,101] The resistance of the gauge varies with its length, so changes in limb circumference will be reflected in a change of voltage, and this change is read out on the recording device in the familiar wave form (Fig. 62-10). Impedance plethysmographs measure changes in electrical resistance from electrodes applied directly to the skin.

The photoplethysmograph (PPG) is a device that emits light outside the visible spectrum (either ultraviolet or infrared). This light emission is reflected off red blood cells and back to a detection photodiode, making it somewhat similar to a Doppler device. It must be placed very close to surface blood vessels (4 to 6 mm) and, therefore, the nail bed or a finger pad is most often used.[86] The amount of light reflected back varies proportionally to the blood flow, and this information can be recorded in the familiar wave form that varies with the strength of the pulse being measured. A typical wave form can be recorded (Fig. 62-11).

Instruments now commercially available are quite compact, with a central unit that can interpret and print information from a pneumoplethysmograph, a photoplethysmograph or a Doppler probe. The received signal is printed on a roll of moving paper in the familiar pulse volume wave (Figs. 62-8, 62-10, and 62-11). The Doppler signal may also be presented as an audible signal.

Ultrasound Imaging

Diagnostic ultrasound units emit very high frequency sound waves that may be aimed to penetrate into living tissues, where they are reflected according to the density of the tissue they encounter. Upon return to a receiving probe, they are subjected to computer analysis for interpretation. In the upper extremity, high frequency waves with better resolution may be used, because less penetration is required than in other parts of the body. Overall contours of different tissues can be identified to evaluate objects of interest, such as aneurysms and vascular anastomoses.[48,54,74]

Cold Stress Testing

Cold exposure of the whole body, of an involved extremity, or of a part of the body remote from that extremity may cause a drop of finger pulp temperature and symptoms of pain. The magnitude of the signs and the severity of the symptoms are related to various pathological entities. This response to stress may be useful for identifying pathological processes in the vascular system and isolating surgically correctable lesions from others.

Koman[32] and co-workers have identified three characteristic temperature response curves (Fig. 62-12). Using a modified refrigerator in which the hands are sealed off through portholes and temperatures recorded via a telethermometer from small surface temperature probes, they found that Type I patients (normal controls, persons who have recovered following arterial injury, or those in an early postsympathectomy stage) had baseline temperature of 30°C or greater, that digital skin temperature dropped only 2° to 5°C during cooling, and that there was a rapid return of temperatures to baseline values in the rewarming period. These patients had little or no pain during the test.

Type II patients (those with isolated nerve injury, those in an intermediate stage following sympathectomy, or those with fair collateral circulation following injury) had a baseline temperature a bit below 30°C, had a significant lowering of digital temperature (8° to 10°C or more) during cooling, and regained normal temperature much more slowly than Type I patients. These patients had moderate pain during the test.

Type III patients had arterial insufficiency, a chronic sympathectomy effect, combined arterial and peripheral nerve injury, or vasospastic disease. They had a baseline temperature of 28.5°C or less. During the cooling phase of the test, digital temperatures dropped to the range of 8° to 13°C, and they regained normal temperatures very slowly in the rewarming phase of the test. They experienced severe pain during the test.

It was found that this dynamic test is a useful diagnostic tool in differentiating vasomotor dysfunction from psychologic or strictly mechanical problems, as well as being helpful in assessing the effect of treatment of vasomotor problems. Exposing a hand to cold results, as one might expect, in a decrease of the volume of the pulse, as shown in Figure 62-13.

Other Noninvasive Techniques

These include standard x-rays and the techniques derived from them, including xerography,[589] computerized tomography,[575] and magnetic resonance imaging[76]. These are all techniques that define a mass with a greater or lesser degree of accuracy. Because of the dynamic nature of many vascular

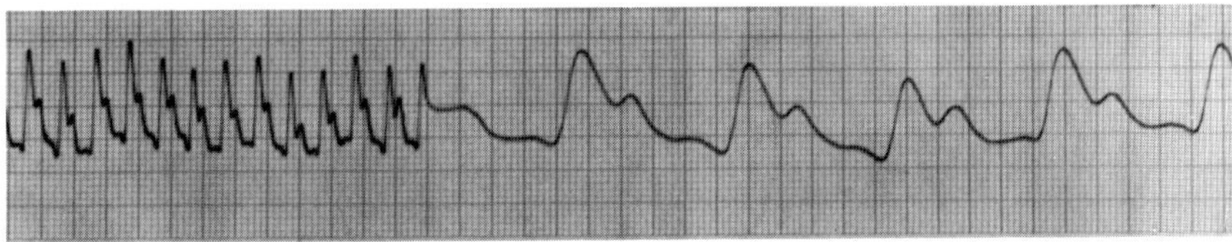

Fig. 62-11. A photoplethysmograph recording of the same subject shown in Figures 62-8 and 62-10.

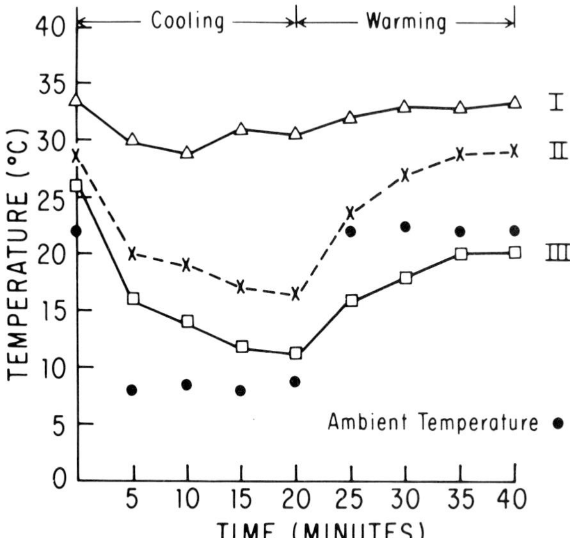

Fig. 62-12. Temperature response curves of three different types of patients upon exposure to a standard cold environment (see text for details). (From Koman et al,[55] with permission.)

lesions, other techniques based on that dynamism would appear to have greater efficacy.

Invasive Techniques

Arteriography

Arteriography is the most dramatic and visually evocative of all techniques for studying the vascularity of the upper extremity.[41,58,87,99] It is not without hazards (see section on iatrogenic injuries). Allen and Camp[30] did the first peripheral arterial studies in living subjects in 1935, using thorium dioxide. They cannulated the brachial artery for injection of the dye. The injection was made with a blood pressure cuff inflated just above systolic pressure. They noted pain with injection, especially if there was extravasation of dye, and a need for very rapid exposure of the x-ray plates after injection. Rapid cassette changers and magnetic tape recording have helped to overcome this latter problem today. Allen and Camp found that this method was most useful in the study of congenital problems, conditions with altered vessel lumen, and for the determination of the degree of collateral circulation.

Seldinger[86] introduced his technique in 1953. This consists of cannulating a vessel with a hollow needle containing a sterile wire, removal of the cannulating needle, and introduction of a plastic catheter over the wire. The method offers some distinct advantages over injection via a cannulating needle: (1) the catheter may be advanced from an easily accessible artery to almost any desired location; (2) the risk of extravasation is nil; (3) the patient may be placed in any desired position; and (4) the cathter may be left in place for repeat studies. In the upper extremity, perhaps the biggest advantage is the ability to visualize the more proximal vessels, starting with the subclavian artery. Vessel obstruction in the neck may affect the hand quite seriously, and this will not be appreciated unless proximal studies are performed.

All dyes used for arteriography contain iodine. Conventional agents (diatrizoic or iothalamic acid) are negatively charged in solution and use sodium or meglumine or a mixture as a balancing agent. This results in a markedly hypertonic solution (up to 2000 mOsm compared to 300 mOsm for blood). New agents (iohexol, iopamidol, and ioxaglate) are nonionic, have about one half of the ismolarity of the older agents, and are much safer than the older agents, but are 15 to 25 times as expensive.[33] The danger with the older agents is systemic reaction. Available evidence indicates that the contrast medium does not damage microvessel endothelium if injection pressures are not excessive.[77,85] However, the contrast agent may extravasate and cause a major skin slough. Loth and Jones[62] treated five patients with a significant extravasation and found that early drainage (within 6 hours) gave excellent results. Approximately 20 to 40 cc are used to visualize the vascularity of an extremity. Priscoline may be used to dilate the vessels and prevent arterial spasm.[87] Premedication is essential[67] and regional or general anesthesia is used on occasion. Performing the arteriogram under brachial or stellate ganglion block has the distinct advantage of dilating the vessels and providing better visualization of the more distal arteries. Alternatively, an intravenous regional sympathetic block may be used in conjunction with general anesthesia to achieve maximal vasodilatation.[98] A rapid cassette changer or, more likely, magnetic tape is used to get serial views of the vascular tree in arterial and venous phases (Fig. 62-14A and B). The technique is most useful in acute trauma with vascular compromise,[63,64,75] acquired[28] and congenital[56] tumors, and condi-

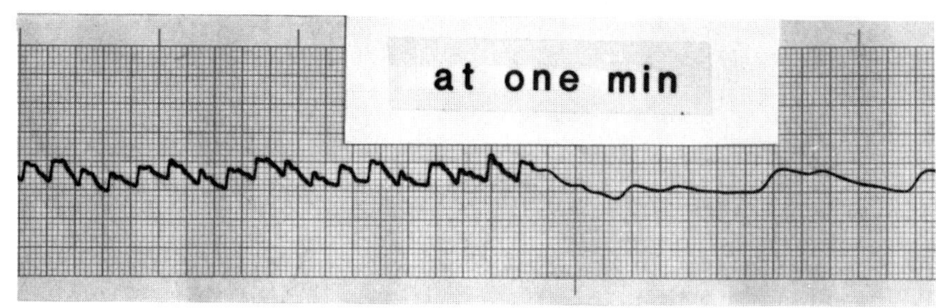

Fig. 62-13. The effect of cold on digital pulse volume recorded with a photoplethysmograph on the subject shown in Figure 62-8. This was recorded 1 minute after a 2-minute long immersion of the subject's entire hand in a water bath at 4°C.

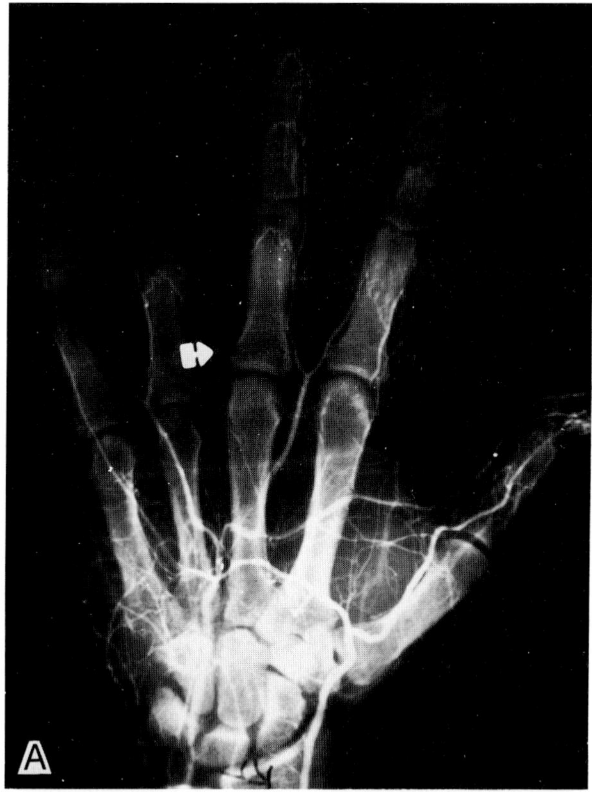

Fig. 62-14. The arterial (A) and venous (B) phases of an arteriogram. A lesion present on the ulnar side of the long finger fails to be demonstrated in A and B *(arrows)*. However, with closed-system venography (C), the lesion is well seen. The radiograph in C has been reversed in the photograph, but the ulnar side is marked for clarification. (Courtesy of WW Eversmann, MD.)

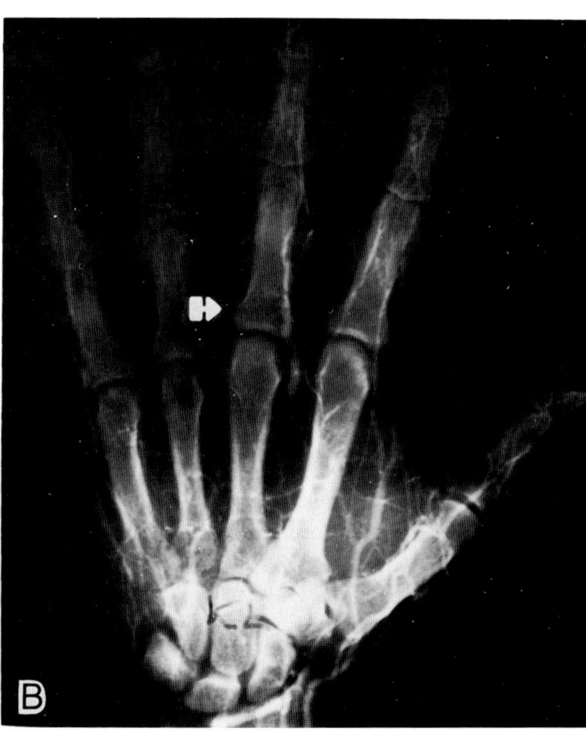

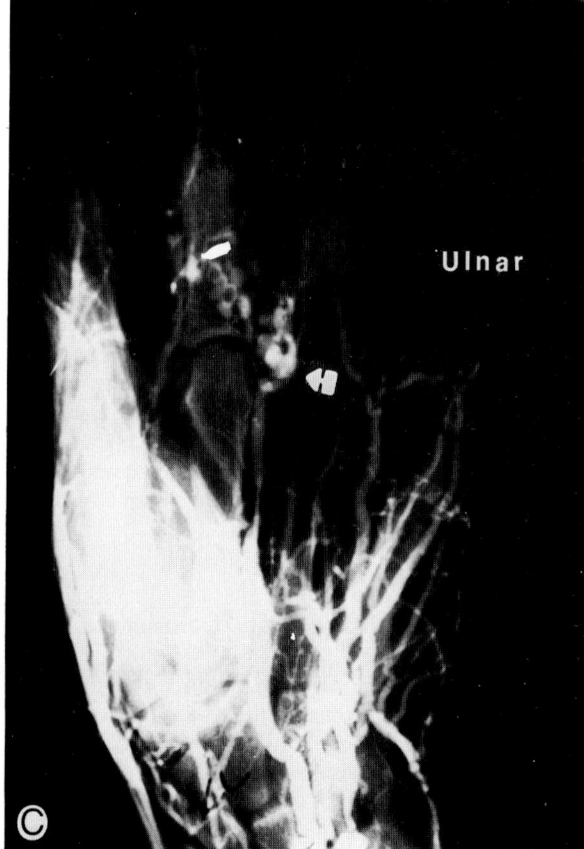

tions caused by vascular compromise in the neck. With vascular tumors that appear normal on the arteriogram, venography with direct venous injection into an exsanguinated arm may clearly delineate the lesion[24] (Fig. 62-14C).

Subtraction arteriography is a technique that is being reborn, thanks to computers. Basically, subtraction techniques record images prior to contrast injection and then following contrast injection, all of the images that are irrelevant for that study, such as bone and soft tissue shadows, are eliminated. The film subtraction technique was cumbersome and, because arterial catheter techniques gave such good pictures, it fell by the wayside. However, with the ability to record and subtract digitally, there is now renewed interest in subtraction arteriography.[37] Although ideally it is done by intravenous injection, many radiologists have found that much better images are obtained if the injection is done via a catheter placed in an artery. Much smaller doses of contrast medium are required than with standard arteriograms.

Radionuclide Imaging

A very accurate and useful picture of hand vasculature can be obtained by this technique.[43,97] The study is done in a three-phase fashion.[69] The first phase is done almost immediately after injection of the dye. Whether one calls it dynamic radionuclide imaging (DRI)[56] or a radionuclide angiogram (RNA),[66] the picture obtained shows the outline of the filling arteries, which is at least a good qualitative angiogram and may eliminate the need for further, more invasive studies. The second phase, the so-called "blood pool" image, is taken immediately at the conclusion of the first and provides information about relative perfusion of the digits. The third phase, obtained at 3 or 4 hours after injection, gives information about bones and joints; i.e., the information one would expect from a standard bone scan.

Technitium-labeled red cells have been used to evaluate hemangiomas.[60]

Other Methods

Careful skin temperature measurements in a temperature-controlled environment may provide useful information regarding hand circulation.[40] Infrared thermography has been used, but it appears to be a test that is only a supplement to other techniques.[57,80] An injection of fluorescein allows assessment of upper extremity vascularity,[65] the technique has limited application because of its complexity.

Summary of Diagnostic Techniques

A careful history and physical examination in a room with a comfortable ambient temperature is the cornerstone of vascular diagnosis. The examination should emphasize careful pulse evaluation of all levels and with the extremity in different positions. This is correlated with blood pressures done at several levels. These steps should be sufficient to identify any obstructive lesion in the neck and in the larger vessels to wrist level. To identify obstructive lesions distal to the wrist the Doppler and possibly pneumoplethysmograph should be utilized. If an obstructive lesion is suspected, arteriography should follow. If no obstructive lesion is found a cold tolerance test, as well as studies for collagen vascular disease, may be utilized to delineate the problem.

ULNAR ARTERY AND OTHER LOCAL ARTERY THROMBOSIS

There is a certain overlap in the next four sections of this chapter (ulnar and other local arterial thrombosis, aneurysms, other vascular trauma, and embolic problems). In each of these trauma may play a significant role. Arterial obstruction, with secondary ischemia of digit or digits, is usually the central problem, and either mechanical or chemical relief of the obstruction is often the first line of invasive treatment. Primary or secondary microemboli often cause or intensify the ischemia in the digits. Arterial resection with vein grafting is often necessary, and the techniques of this are discussed in detail in Chapter 26. The use of streptokinase or urokinase may have a role in the treatment of these problems; this is discussed in the section on embolic problems.

Considering the impatient proclivities of humans and the hard, superficial canal through which the ulnar artery enters the hand, it is not surprising that this artery should be damaged from time to time. Conn, Bergan, and Bell[117] coined the phrase "hypothenar hammer syndrome" to describe the signs and symptoms associated with ischemia of the hand and fingers secondary to repetitive blunt trauma of the distal ulnar artery and superficial volar arch against the hook of the hamate bone. Von Rosen[152] in 1933 described a case of thrombosis of the ulnar artery following a contusion of the overlying hand. The patient was cured by resection of the thrombosed artery and lysis of the ulnar nerve. He postulated that intimal damage to the artery would result in thrombosis, while damage to the media would result in a true aneurysm.

Other authors have emphasized the close etiologic association of ulnar artery thrombosis and true aneurysms of the ulnar artery following either single or multiple episodes of blunt trauma.[118,140,180] Anomalous hypothenar muscles may cause ulnar artery thrombosis and ulnar nerve symptoms.[115,153] Okihiro's syndrome (manifested in the hand by hypothenar hypoplasia) makes the ulnar artery more susceptible to thrombosis due to blunt trauma because of the lack of normal protection.[108]

Afflicted people will seek help because of (1) a tender, painfull mass in the hypothenar area of the hand; (2) ischemic symptoms of pain with pallor or even early gangrene; (3) numbness due to nerve compression in one or more branches of the ulnar nerve; or (4) a combination of the above.[114,124,125,134,137,141] Cold sensitivity and even cold intolerance in the involved digits (Raynaud's phenomenon) may be part of the complaint.[154] Certainly, a patient with unilateral Raynaud's phenomenon should have the status of the ulnar artery evaluated, especially if only the ulnar two or three digits are involved. Generally, nerve involvement is to one or more of the sensory branches of the ulnar nerve, but compression of the motor branch of the median nerve from ulnar artery thrombosis has been reported.[107]

Most of the patients with ulnar artery thrombosis are men of working age who have jobs in which the hands are subjected to blunt trauma.[146] Little and Ferguson[133] studied a large group of men who worked in a vehicle maintenance shop and found that 11 of 79 men (14 percent) who admitted to using their hand as a hammer had evidence of ulnar artery occlusion, and all of them were symptomatic. In some cases, no specific episode of trauma could be recalled by the patient, but, in the absence of any other cause, it may be assumed that a forgotten blow to the hand initiated the problem (Fig. 62-15).

While the problem is unusual in women, it may occur under certain circumstances. Eguro and Goldner[119] reported a case in a 70-year-old woman who compressed and thrombosed first one and then the other ulnar artery over a 2-year period from the pressure of her cane in the palms.

The radial artery seems to be less prone to "spontaneous" thrombosis than the ulnar artery, but it may occur in the snuff box where the extensor pollicis longus crosses the artery.[145] (Fig. 62-16). It also has been reported as a result of compression by a ganglion.[127]

A curious and very unusual cause of local arterial thrombosis is local giant cell inflammatory arterial disease. This is usually seen in the temporal arteries, but may appear elsewhere. Bugg, Coonrad, and Grimm[113] reported three cases of such a problem in the hand. Their patients were all men in the third and fourth decades of life. There was one case each of a thrombosed radial, median, and ulnar artery. Resection was curative in each instance. Histologic examination of the resected arteries revealed an inflammatory reaction mainly in the media, with foreign body giant cells in each case. A condition that may be related or identical is polymyalgia arteritica. Thompson, Simmons, and Smith[149] reported a case with bilateral subclavian artery occlusion and hand ischemia. In their case, giant cells were also seen in the histologic sections.

Paletta reported a curious case of thrombosis of the subclavian and axillary veins with gangrene of the hand.[142] It was associated with an ipsilateral squamous cell carcinoma of the bronchus.

Thrombosis of the median artery may cause digital ischemia[106] or carpal tunnel symptoms.[132] A mass in the area of the ulnar artery is not necessarily thrombosis of that vessel, but may be due to thrombosis of the vena comitantes, in which case resection is the clear operative choice and is curative.[122]

Diagnosis

The correct diagnosis should be strongly suspected from the history. Examination should include a careful Allen's test,[107] both by inspection and with the Doppler. If the ulnar artery is thrombosed, compression of the radial artery will obliterate the superficial arch pulse. Angiography is seldom necessary.[130] Occasionally, thrombosis of the artery is associated with a fracture of the hook of the hamate.[125]

The differential diagnosis includes the gamut of ischemic diseases of the upper extremity, but once the problem has been localized to the area of the distal ulnar artery–superficial arch, the only other possibilities that need to be considered are an aneurysm, a ganglion,[110] band constriction of the artery,[120] and embolization. Preoperative diagnosis of any one of the first three would not change the operative plan in any way. A careful history should enable one to diagnose the latter preoperatively.

Treatment

Although various indirect methods of treatment, including vasodilators,[154] stellate ganglion block,[117,154] cervicodorsal sympathectomy,[117] and chemical clot lysis,[116] have been used in treating the problem, the usual and recommended treatment is direct surgical attack. Leriche, Fontaine, and Dupertuis[131] stated the rationale for resection of the lesion: "We believe that an obliterated artery functionally ceases to be an artery but becomes a diseased plexus of sympathetic nerve fibers, provoking distal vasospasm in the anastomotic network of vessels." It should be noted that resection of the offending segment of thrombosed artery also removes a probable source of showers of microemboli, and this may be as important or more important than the sympathectomy effect.

Numerous reports support the contention that simple resection of the lesion is curative.[123,136,138,154] However, Kleinert and Volianitis[128] in 1965 suggested that thrombectomy and restoration of blood flow is a preferable method of treatment. Given, Puckett, and Kleinert[121] reviewed 46 cases in 1978. Sixteen of these patients had resection of their lesions with an excellent or improved result in ten (63 percent). Six patients had thrombectomy with two excellent, two improved, and two unimproved results. Fourteen patients had lesion resection and anastomosis with eight excellent and six improved results. Eight patients had lesion resection and arterial reconstruction with a vein graft, with three excellent, four improved, and one unimproved results. They concluded that an attempt to reestablish blood flow is worthwhile, even though the patency rate in the 28 patients with arterial reconstruction was only 50 percent. Koman and Urbaniak[129] reported their analysis of 28 patients with proved ulnar artery thrombosis and concluded that there is no single proven treatment regimen. They presented a treatment algorithm based on the needs of the patient. Mehloff and Wood[139] reviewed eight patients in whom they had resected a thrombosed ulnar artery, replacing it with a vein graft. Seven of the grafts stayed patent with four excellent and three good results. They found the best results in nonsmokers, patients with only one episode of trauma, and those with pre-operative symptoms of less than 5 months' duration.

The evidence that vascular reconstruction is helpful in achieving an excellent result is significant if not overwhelming. There is probably little to lose and possibly much to gain by reconstituting the arterial system in either an ulnar or radial artery that has been interrupted by thrombosis. In most cases a vein graft will be necessary because several centimeters of thrombosed artery will have to be resected. Median arteries are very rare, and the need to reconstruct a thrombosed median artery must be based on the anatomy in an individual patient. Even when thrombosis of an arterial repair or graft occurs as

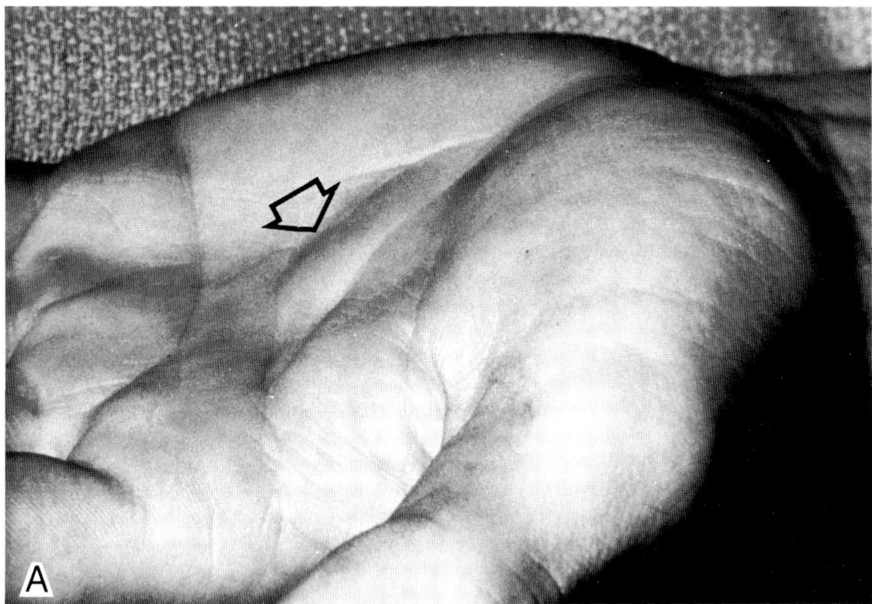

Fig. 62-15. This 22-year-old man was employed as a bicycle messenger and frequently put considerable pressure on his palms. He developed a tender mass in his midpalm *(arrow)* **(A)**. *(Figure continues.)*

manifested by a positive Allen's test, the results are usually good, in that symptoms of ischemia and nerve compression are alleviated.

Operative Technique

The operative approach to the ulnar artery is through a zig-zag incision over Guyon's canal. The ulnar nerve, including the motor branch that arises from the dorsal aspect of the nerve and may be relatively hidden from view, must be carefully protected throughout the procedure. After identification and resection of the thrombosed segment, the proximal and distal arterial stumps are ligated with a 5-10 nonabsorbable material other than silk. If arterial anastomosis is to be done, an 8-0 or 9-0 nonabsorbable vascular suture material is used. Either high magnification loupes (6×) or an operating microscope must be used. (The details of microvascular repair and reconstruction are described in Chapter 26.)

Postoperatively, the usual bulky protective hand dressing is used. I also recommend low molecular weight Dextran (500 cc daily for 3 days)[107] and aspirin (600 mg daily for 10 days).

Early postoperative complications include thrombosis of the arterial repair or graft.[151] If this occurs, no further operative intervention is indicated unless there is ischemia of the digits. Suture line ruptures with or without pseudoaneurysm formation must be handled operatively. Infections are treated in the usual fashion, with care taken to make sure arterial ends are securely ligated. Long-term complications are uncommon, but ulnar nerve entrapment may occur and require a neurolysis.[116]

Impact and Vibratory Arterial Trauma

Lowrey, Chadwick, and Waltman[135] studied young professional baseball catchers, ages 20 to 28, for evidence of arterial injury in the index fingers of each hand, with the noncatching hand being used as a control. They used Allen's test with and without the Doppler and found that only 9 of 22 players had normal circulation to the left index (catching hand) finger. All but one of the right index fingers were found to be normal. Each of these nine men used extra padding in his catcher's mitt.

There are several reports of vibrating pneumatic tools causing vascular problems in the digits of the hand in which the tool is held.[118,144,147,148] The critical speed of the tool to initiate the problem is between 2000 and 3000 motions per minute. The clinical picture is Raynaud's phenomenon, aggravated by exposure to cold, often appearing many months after the use of the tool. There is no apparent cure; the patients must change jobs and avoid cold exposure.

ANEURYSMS IN THE UPPER EXTREMITY

Most aneurysms seen in the upper extremity are caused by trauma.[221] Ho et al[185] reported 30 lesions seen in 28 patients over a 10-year period. All but two were the result of trauma, and the cause of those two was unknown. Twenty were false aneurysms, seven true aneurysms, two listed as mycotic, and one unknown. Mycotic aneurysms in the upper extremity are

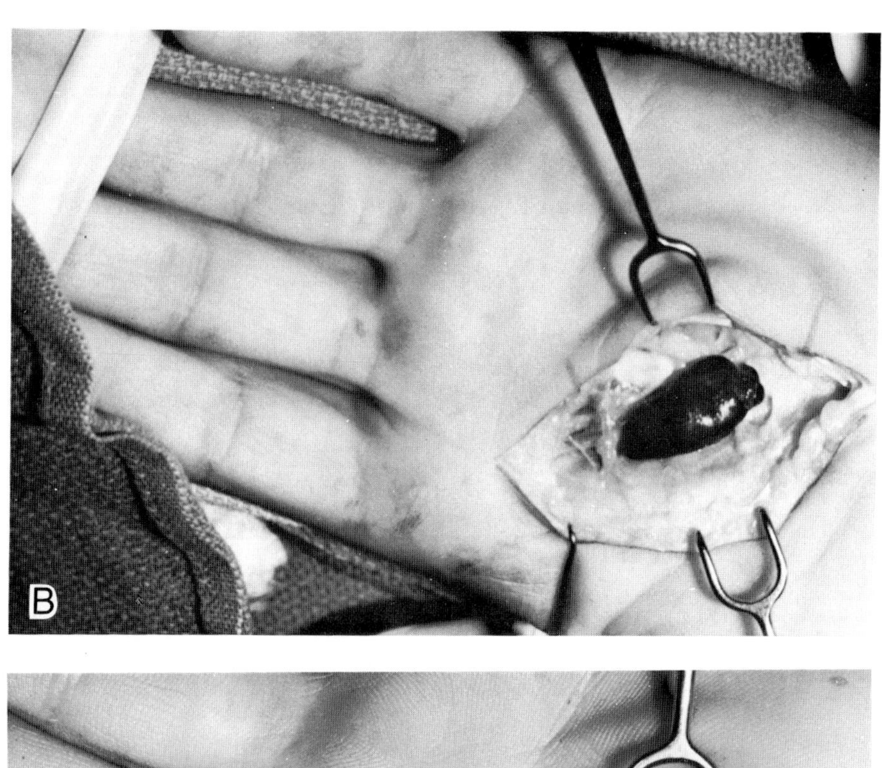

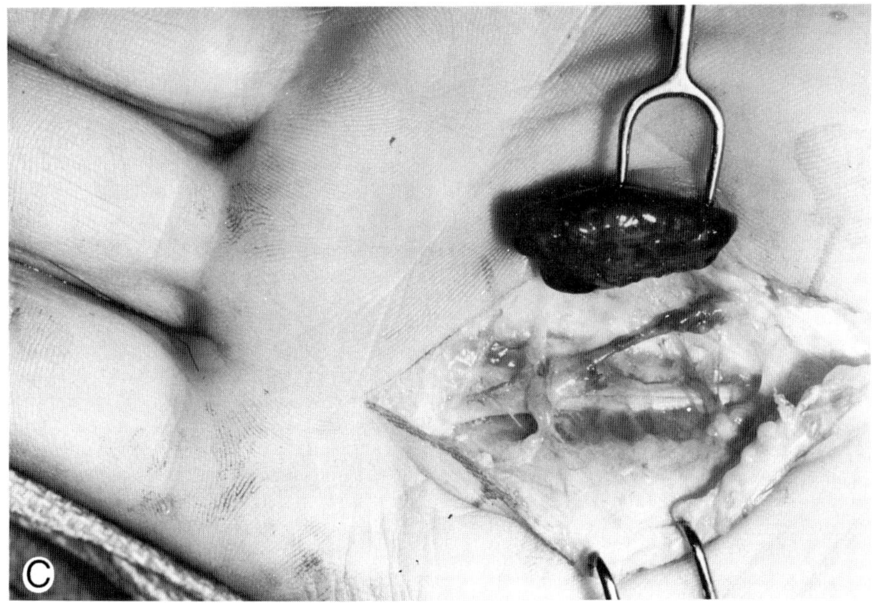

Fig. 62-15 *(Continued).* The mass was found to be a thrombosed dilated common digital artery **(B&C).** The lesion was resected and the arterial ends were ligated. No ischemic signs or symptoms were present pre- or postoperatively. (Courtesy of ES Kilgore, Jr, MD.)

generally due to injection of illicit drugs[184] but may be caused by septic emboli[160] or organisms introduced by penetrating trauma.[215] In a wartime situation, upper and lower extremities have equal risk of arterial injury that will result in an aneurysm or a traumatic arteriovenous fistula,[161,207a,211] while in peacetime the upper extremity arteries are more prone to these lesions. Arteriosclerotic aneurysms are very rare in the upper extremities, but are seen in the lower extremities with regularity.[168] Aneurysms can be either true or false (pseudo)[180,190,231] (Fig. 62-17).

Aneurysms are seen at every level of the upper extremity but are more common at the wrist[185,214] and in the digital arteries.[164,182,227,228] Venous aneurysms (apparently due to penetrating trauma) have been seen in the upper extremity but are very rare.[209,229] Resection without reconstruction is the treatment of choice for venous aneurysms.

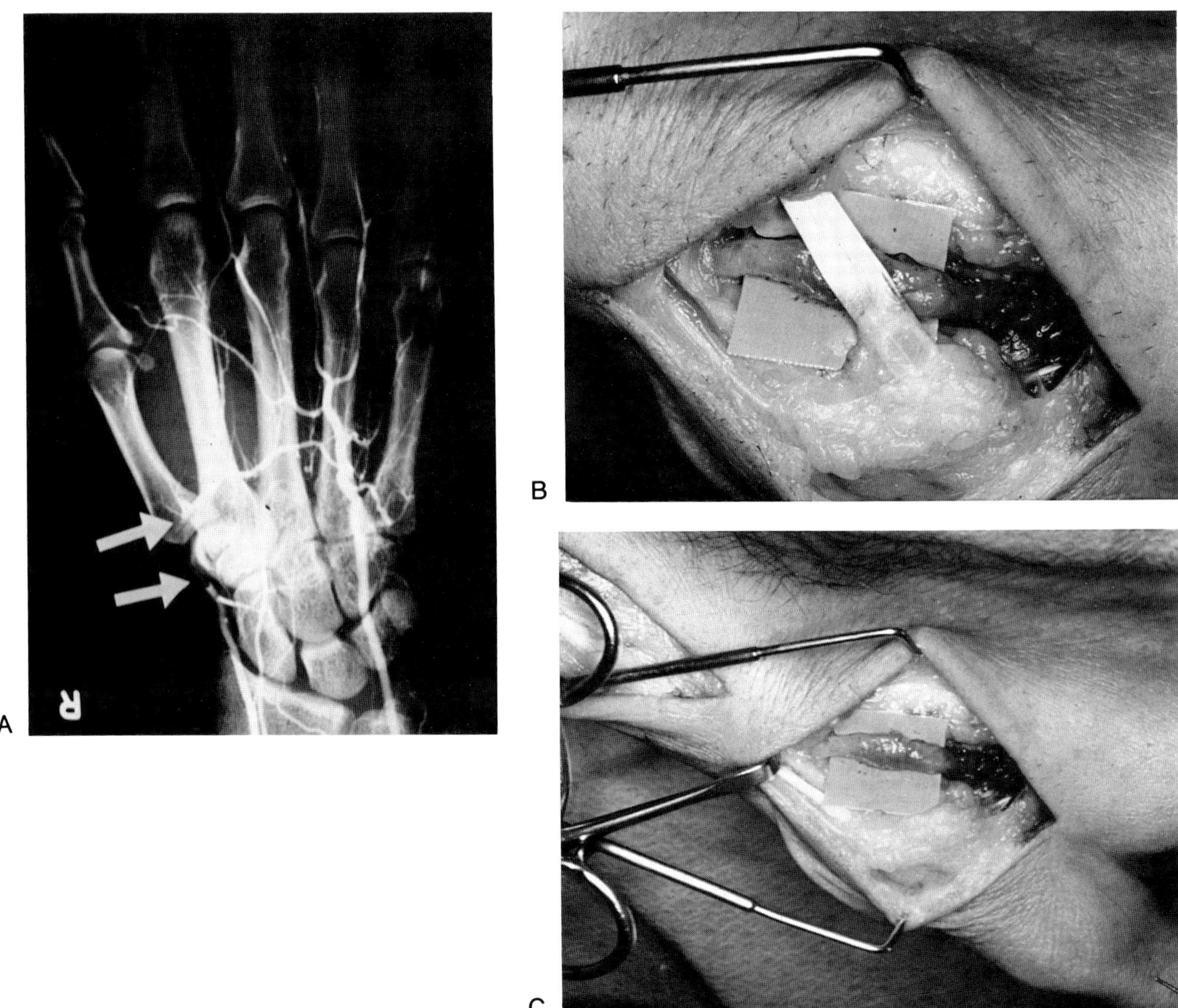

Fig. 62-16. **(A)** Arteriogram of a 58-year-old man with ischemic changes in the tip of his left index finger. Arrows show the extent of the thrombosis in the radial artery. **(B)** The thrombosed section of the artery lies directly beneath the extensor pollicis longus (EPL) tendon. **(C)** The EPL tendon has been retracted and the thrombosed section of the artery is clearly seen. It was resected and replaced with a vein graft. The patient had complete resolution of his ischemic symptoms. (Case and photographs kindly provided by William E. Sanders, MD.)

True Aneurysms

A true aneurysm is one that contains some elements of the three layers of the arterial wall. It is usually a fusiform aneurysm and arises as a consequence of a weakness in the arterial wall, due to either trauma or disease.[156,165,168,187,191,204,220,222] In the upper extremity, trauma is by far the more common cause. There are a few reports of arteriosclerotic aneurysms,[195,226] although trauma may even play a role in some of these.[219] "Spontaneous" aneurysms have been reported, and the case most often cited is that reported by Griffiths[181] in 1897 in a 23-year-old woman. This patient had an ulnar artery aneurysm with no evidence of other vascular disease. He concluded that the lesion "is an instance of sub-acute localised [sic] endarteritis deformans with extension into and almost complete disappearance of the muscle fibers and of the elastic membrane." In reviewing the paper, one cannot help but feel that an episode of unrecognized blunt trauma is the more likely cause.

There are few reports of mycotic aneurysms,[179,188,230] and in one of these, the infection was clearly superimposed on an already existing arteriosclerotic aneurysm.[210] True aneurysms may arise from granulomatous arteritis[192]

A true aneurysm resulting from trauma may follow either single episodes of blunt injury[164,174] or arise from the repeated use of the hand as a hammer.[199,201,218] The latter condition has been termed the "hypothenar hammer syndrome" (see preceding section on local artery thrombosis, page 2262). Traction on an upper extremity may weaken an arterial wall and

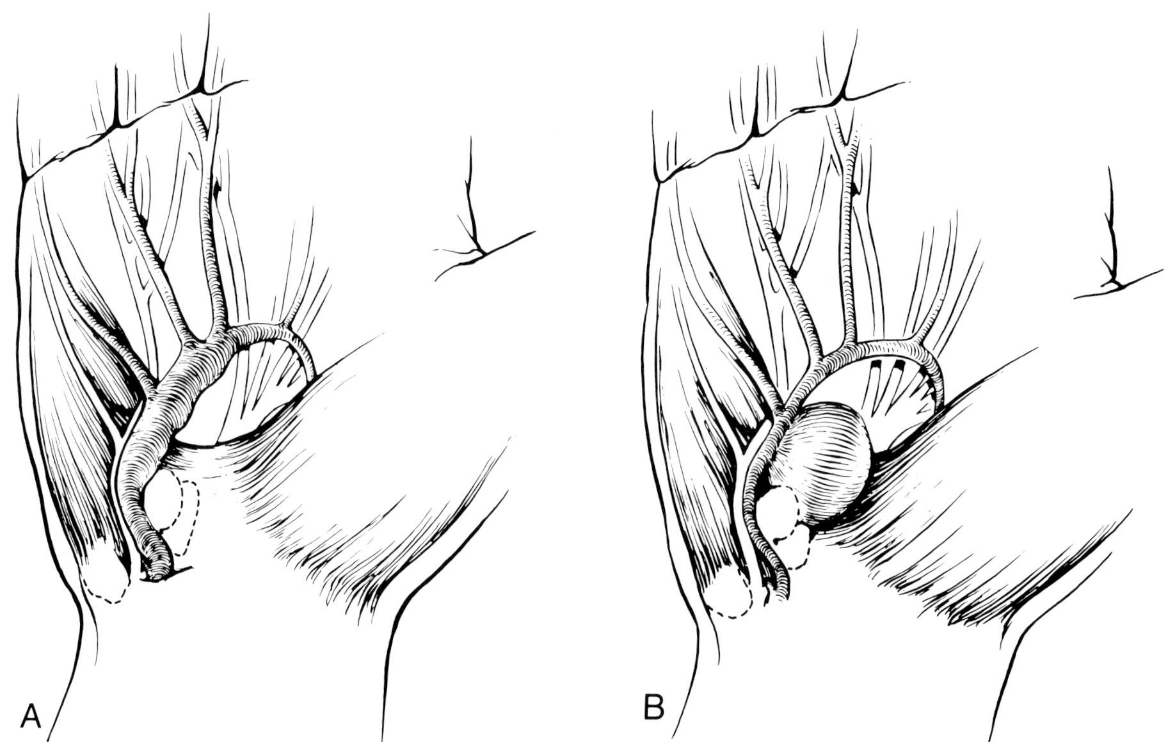

Fig. 62-17. **(A)** A true aneurysm. Note the fusiform shape involving the entire artery. **(B)** A false aneurysm. Note the saccular form involving only one side of the artery. (From Green,[180] with permission.)

allow aneurysm formation.[217] Axillary compression in patients on crutches should not be overlooked as a cause of axillary artery aneurysms.[155,212]

False (Pseudo) Aneurysms

This variety of aneurysm occurs as a result of penetrating trauma with arterial perforation.[157,167,171,173,176,193,194,202,207,213,216,224] Pseudoaneurysms are more common in the hand than are true aneurysms. Following perforation of the artery, a hematoma forms between the wall of the artery and the tissues surrounding the artery.[159] The flowing arterial blood slowly carves a cavity in the hematoma through the arterial hole. Over a period of time (usually weeks, but it may take days or months), this cavity becomes lined with endothelium and the hematoma slowly becomes replaced with fibrous scar tissue[157,175] (Fig. 62-18).

Pseudoaneurysms may follow any type of penetrating trauma, but perhaps the most typical situation is one in which a narrow, long, sharp object, such as a piece of glass or a knife, perforates the skin over an artery to an unknown depth. The profuse bleeding that follows the injury is controlled by pressure, the skin wound is closed, and the patient is sent on his way. Within the next few weeks or months, a pulsatile mass appears beneath the skin wound (Fig. 62-19).

These lesions may also follow operative procedures during which there has been an inadvertent injury to an artery.[172] They may be caused by implanted hardware.[200] This injury may occur even more often in extremity surgery because it is not recognized in the bloodless field with the tourniquet inflated.[183,186] Certainly, this is not a reason to stop using the tourniquet as some have advocated,[225] but it is a strong argument for releasing the tourniquet prior to skin closure when the operative procedure has been near a major artery. Pseudoan-

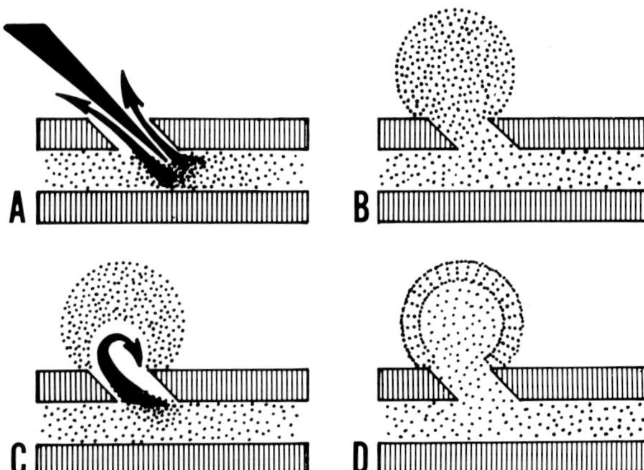

Fig. 62-18. Mechanism of false aneurysm formation. **(A)** The artery is punctured on one side. **(B)** A hematoma forms, stopping the leak. **(C)** The continued flow of arterial blood carves a cavity in the hematoma. **(D)** The cavity becomes lined with endothelium, and the hematoma wall is slowly replaced by collagen to form scar.

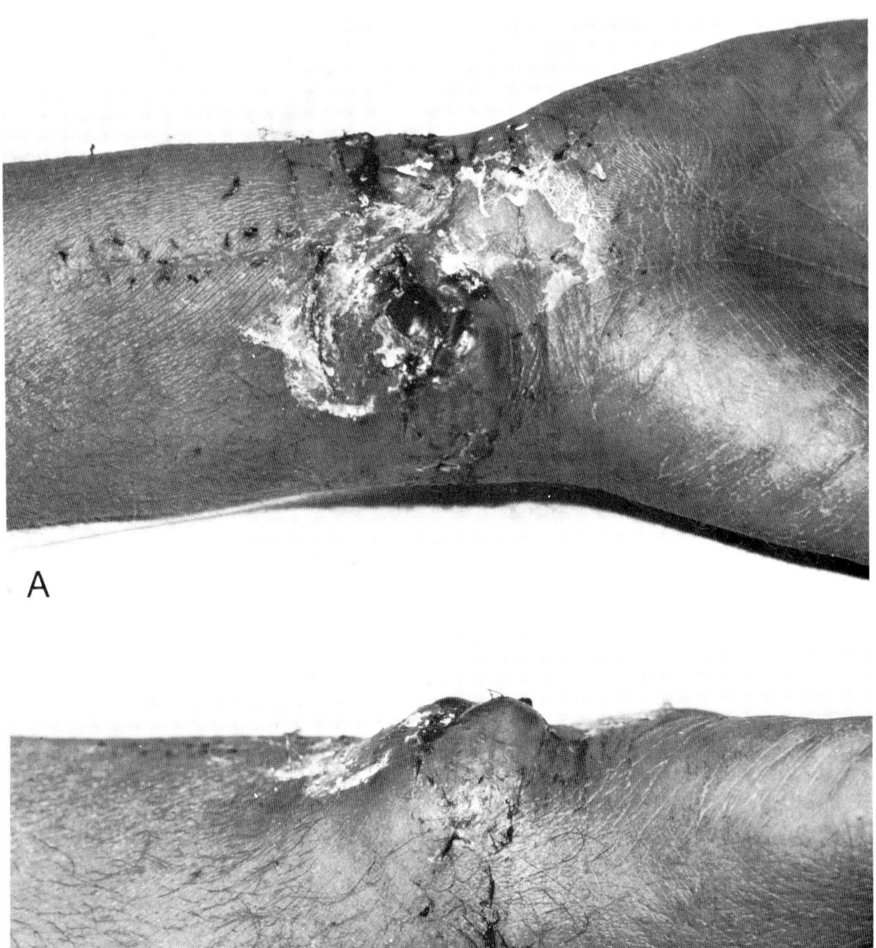

Fig. 62-19. **(A)** One month after a volar wrist laceration involving nerves, tendons, and arteries, this 26-year-old woman presented with the sudden onset of a pulsatile mass at the radial end of her traumatic wound scar. This was erythematous and slightly tender as well as pulsatile. **(B)** It is seen more dramatically on the lateral view. *(Figure continues.)*

eurysms have also developed following fractures, presumably caused either by a bone spike at the time of injury or during manipulative reduction.[170] They have been reported to result from a bone spike of an osteochrondroma.[203] Diagnostic arterial punctures may give rise to this lesion.[197,208] An aneurysm of the radial artery had been caused by a single puncture for de Quervain's disease.[223] Aneurysms may also occur at an arterial anastomosis line.[177] Although usually one of the larger arteries at the wrist or in the palm is affected, digital arteries may form aneurysms following surgery or trauma.[158,186]

Diagnosis of Aneurysms

From the foregoing, it is apparent that an accurate, careful history is often the critical factor in making the correct diagnosis. The patient will most frequently complain of a pulsatile mass that is often painful and tender. However, if the aneurysm is small or deep, the first signs and symptoms may be pallor and pain in the digits due to embolic showers following thrombosis in the aneurysm.[198,217] This can give rise to Raynaud's phenomenon[178] or even to irreversible ischemia and gangrene, requiring amputation[205] (Fig. 62-20). If there is local nerve compression, numbness may be present in one or more digits distal to the lesion.[189,206] There may be a bruit and/or thrill over the aneurysm that is systolic rather than continuous, as it is with an arteriovenous fistula. An aneurysm may be quite erythematous and mimic an abscess, or it may resemble a bone tumor.[162]

Examination should include a careful palpation of all the pulses in the upper extremity, and they should be compared with the opposite upper extremity. Allen's test should be performed, both in the usual manner and using the various modifications described earlier. This can be done both with pal-

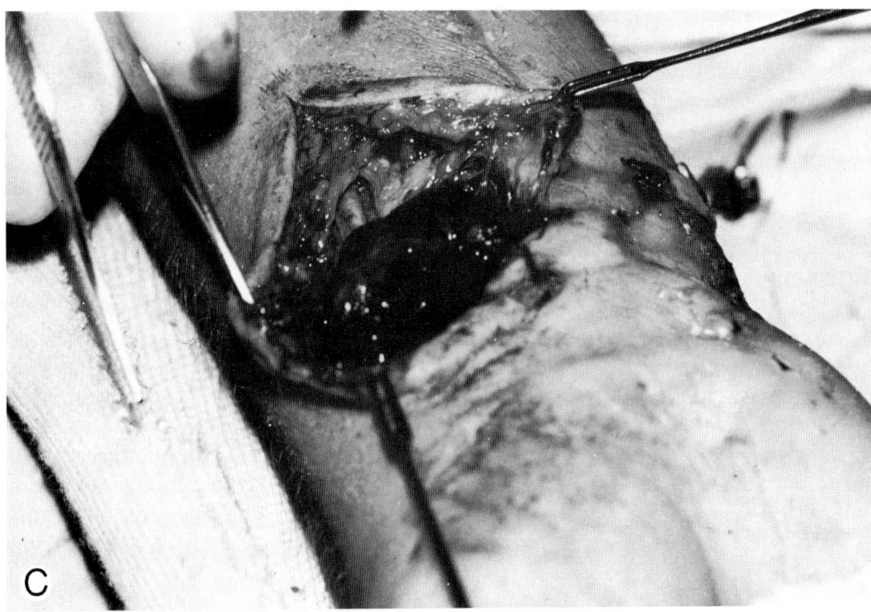

Fig. 62-19 *(Continued).* **(C)** An intraoperative photograph showing the large hematoma of the early pseudoaneurysm. Resection of the ragged arterial ends and end-to-end anastomosis were done with loupe magnification using 8–0 nylon. The deep arch Doppler impulse, absent preoperatively, was restored immediately after surgery. One month later the patient had a warm hand, a palpable pulse in the snuffbox, and evidence of good arterial fill via the radial artery by the digital Allen's test. This patient dramatically illustrates the need to identify the arteries in a major wrist laceration and the efficacy of arterial repair.

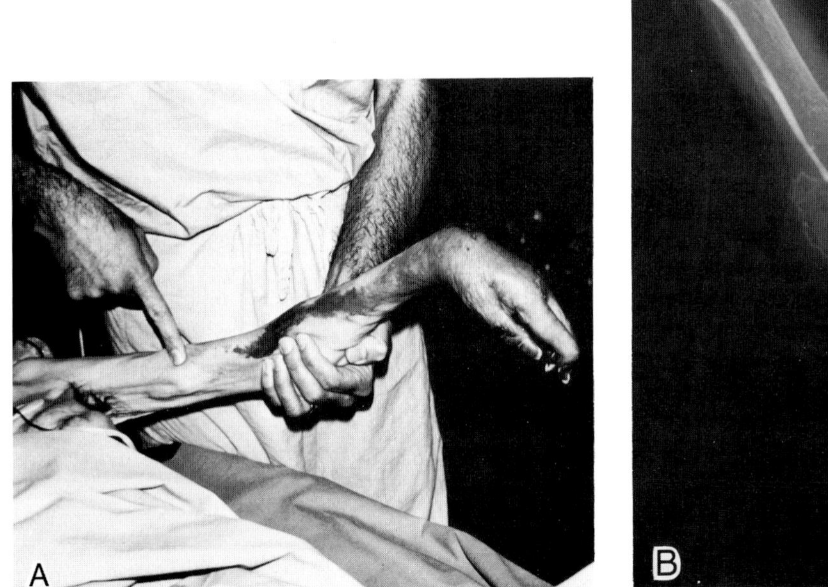

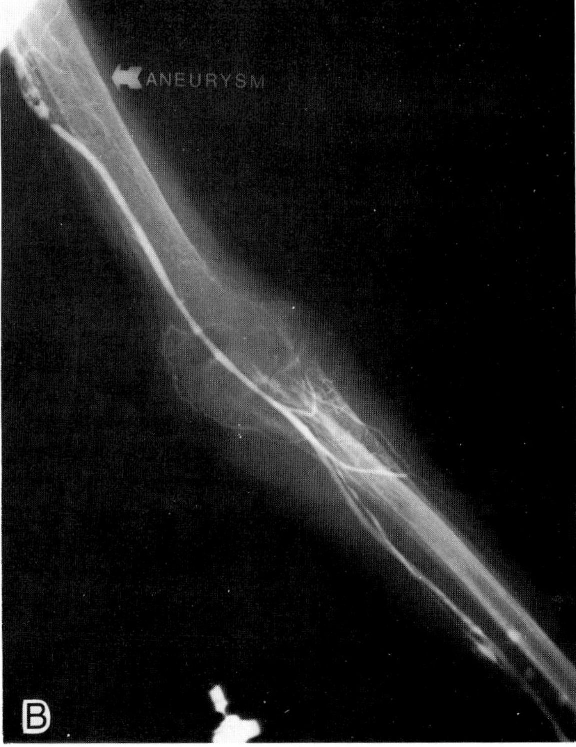

Fig. 62-20. This 58-year-old man had an arteriosclerotic aneurysm of his midbrachial artery (**A,** pointing finger, and **B** on the arteriogram). For a variety of reasons, no treatment was given. The aneurysm thrombosed, presumably threw off emboli, and the distal extremity became gangrenous. Above-elbow amputation was necessary.

pation and with the Doppler. Angiography is usually not necessary, either for the diagnosis or to plan the operative treatment, but it may be useful in some situations. An example of an indication for a preoperative arteriogram is a patient with an ulnar artery aneurysm at the wrist, in whom Allen's test shows diminished or absent filling from the radial artery (Fig. 62-21).

Treatment of Aneurysms

Historically, larger aneurysms of the upper extremity have been treated with either obliterative or restorative endoaneurysmorrhaphy.[161,196] Those aneurysms of the smaller arteries of the wrist and hand have been treated with indirect techniques, such as stellate ganglion block and cervicodorsal sympathectomy (see section on local artery thrombosis). For the most part, however, aneurysms at the wrist and distally have been surgically treated directly.[180,190] The only real argument about

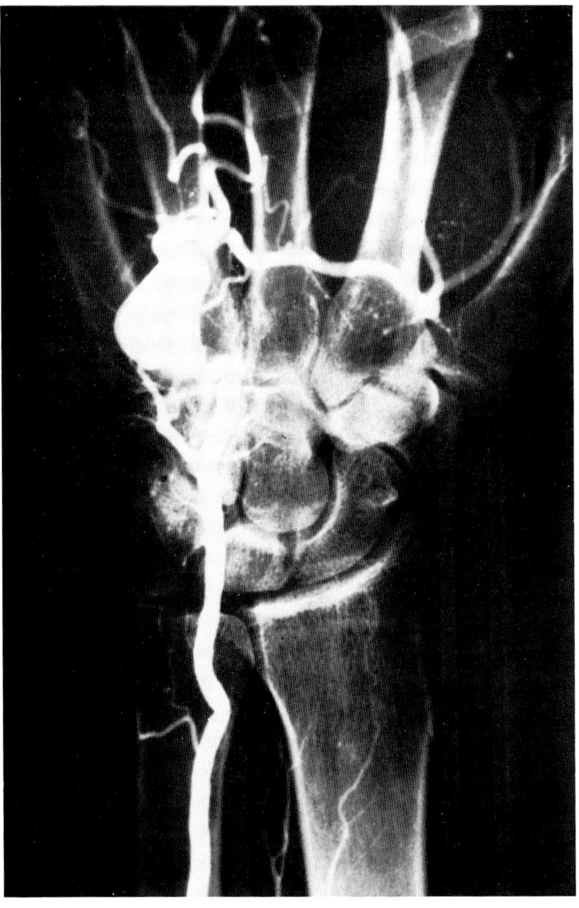

Fig. 62-21. A 56-year-old man presented with a very large aneurysm arising from the ulnar artery. Preoperative Allen's test revealed that he had *no* filling through the radial artery, and therefore this arteriogram was done. The findings here suggest that the operative risk outweighs the potential benefits of the operation. This is an example of an indication for an arteriogram in a patient with an aneurysm. (Courtesy of DP Green, MD.)

their treatment today is whether to simply resect the aneurysm and ligate the arterial ends or to resect the aneurysm and reconstruct the artery. Certainly, if there is evidence that the wrist artery not involved with the aneurysm provides an insufficient blood supply to the hand, every effort should be made to reconstruct the artery after resection of the aneurysm. This would be more important in patients with arteriosclerotic aneurysms, who presumably have arteriosclerosis of other hand vessels. It is true in any patient who has an incomplete vascular arch.

If direct arterial reconstruction is not possible, a vein graft will be used to span the gap, using the techniques described in Chapter 26. If the uninvolved artery appears to provide an adequate blood supply to the hand, resection and ligation are simpler and faster techniques. Certainly, the results from this have been excellent in numerous case reports.[163,166,170] The patient shown in Figure 62-20 provides an excellent example of the advisability of arterial reconstruction. Particularly in longstanding aneurysms where the distal blood supply is adequate, simple resection of the aneurysm and ligation of the arterial stumps is all that is required.[214]

Postoperatively, I prefer a bulky, compressive short arm plaster shell dressing. Following reconstruction, the same regimen as previously outlined is used. The two major complications are infection and, with repair or graft, thrombosis. Infection could, of course, lead to another false aneurysm which would have to be treated with resection and ligation, as well as antibiotics and the usual wound care. If thrombosis occurs, further operations are probably not advisable unless there is frank distal ischemia.

ARTERIAL INJURIES — IATROGENIC, ACCIDENTAL, AND DELIBERATE

This section includes a miscellaneous collection of traumatic arterial problems that merit special mention, more because of their cause than because of the specific condition that results. There is obviously some overlap with the section on local artery thrombosis, aneurysms, and traumatic arteriovenous fistulas. The first to be discussed here and the most important problem in this group is iatrogenic arterial injury from indwelling or single, brief cannulations. The second problem discussed is intraarterial injury from injections of artery-destroying substances. Most of these injuries are self-inflicted, but a few are iatrogenic. Third is a discussion of accidental and iatrogenic arterial injury, to stress again the principles of management of acute injuries. Finally, several miscellaneous problems will be briefly mentioned.

Cannulation Injuries

Radial artery cannulation has become such a common procedure in patients who are critically ill or are undergoing major chest, abdominal or intracranial surgery that sometimes little thought is given to the possible disastrous results of the cannulation procedure[233,242,248,256,272,296] (Fig. 62-22). Fortunately

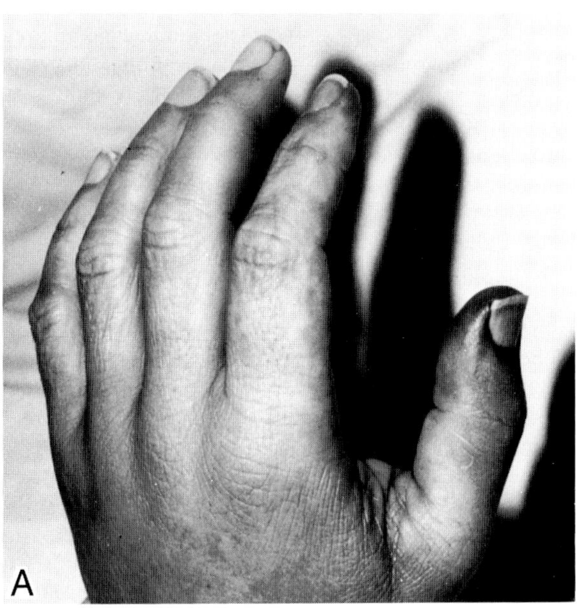

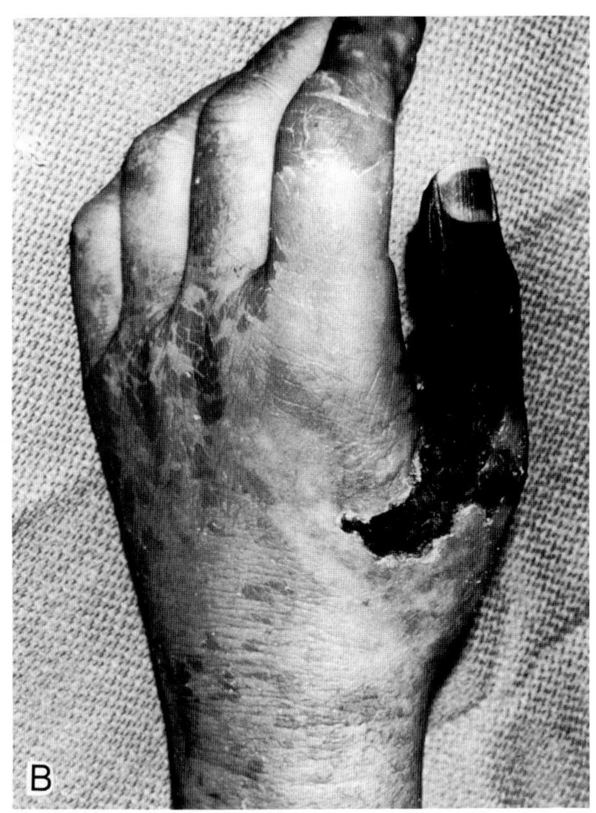

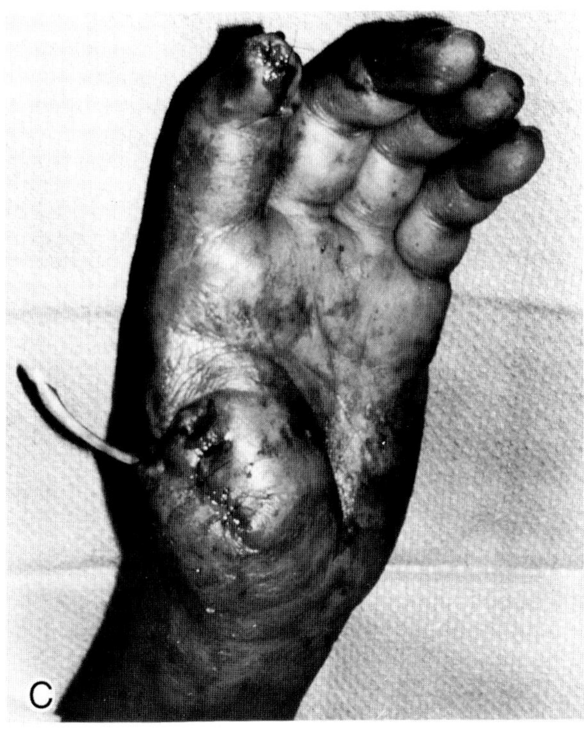

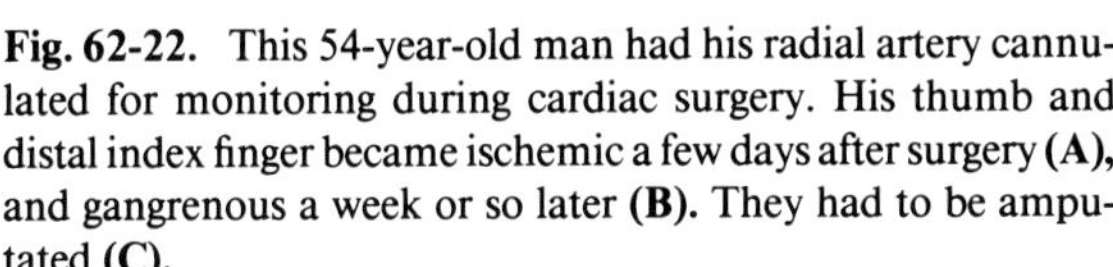

Fig. 62-22. This 54-year-old man had his radial artery cannulated for monitoring during cardiac surgery. His thumb and distal index finger became ischemic a few days after surgery **(A)**, and gangrenous a week or so later **(B)**. They had to be amputated **(C)**.

these disasters are rare,[213,257,269,281,290,301] but that is little comfort to a patient with a gangrenous thumb. Bedford and Ashford[239] found that pretreatment with aspirin will reduce the incidence of postcannulation thrombosis.

A careful assessment of the circulation of the hand with the Doppler scanner prior to cannulation is the most important step in preventing loss of digits. Mandel and Dauchot[275] studied 1000 patients who had a radial artery cannulation. They did very careful Doppler assessment prior to insertion, used 20-gauge catheters, and had only two serious complications. One patient required embolectomy and the other radial artery reconstruction.

Several studies[235,238,259] indicate that smaller catheters (20-gauge rather than 18) result in significantly fewer complications. Downs and co-workers[252] found that 20-gauge Teflon catheters maintained with constant irrigation caused a much lower incidence of radial artery thrombosis than heparin-impregnated polyethylene catheters. One report favored the use of the brachial artery rather than the radial to achieve a lower complication rate.[234] The incidence of postcannulation occlusion is directly related to the duration of cannulation. Bedford and Wollman[240] studied 105 patients and found that 40 (38 percent) had a temporary thrombosis following cannulation. In cannulations of less than 20-hour duration, this incidence was 25 percent, at 20 to 40 hours, 50 percent; and over 40 hours, 93 percent. Most of these thrombi will recanalize and cause no long-term problems, but if the vascular arches are incomplete and part of the hand is rendered totally ischemic, recanalization will be too late to prevent gangrene. Other factors leading to complications are hypotensive episodes, use of vasoconstrictive drugs, the coexistence of vasospastic (Raynaud's) disease, a tendency to thrombosis, diabetes, severe arteriosclerosis, and thoracic outlet syndrome.[257,274,288]

Bedford[237] evaluated two groups of 35 patients each. In one group, the catheter was withdrawn with pressure on the wound for a few minutes. In the second group, the artery was digitally occluded proximally and distally and negative pressure was applied to the catheter by an attached syringe during withdrawal. In many instances, this would draw out the often-present thrombus, and a much lower rate of vessel occlusion was observed.

Hand surgeons are usually asked to see these patients when ischemia and/or impending or even frank gangrene is already present. A patient in this situation obviously has inadequate circulation to the ischemic part of the hand. An attempt at thrombolysis with streptokinase or urokinase should be made via the affected artery. This may be dramatically helpful (see discussion of thrombolysis in the section on Emboli), but if this is not successful a direct approach will have to be used. At this stage an arteriogram via the femoral artery is helpful if the patient is not too ill have this procedure. If it appears that there is still a chance for some salvage of digits or digits I recommend an exploration of the involved artery on an urgent basis. Axillary or supraclavicular block is the anesthetic of choice because of the sympathectomy effect of either. A Bier block is contraindicated. The first effort should be with a Fogarty catheter to try to clean out thrombotic material. The smallest Fogarty is size 2 Fr, which is about 0.67 mm. At this point if there is no relief of the ischemia consideration has to be given to a more radical procedure, i.e., resection and vein graft. This is why a preoperative arteriogram is very useful, because this cannot be done unless the information gleaned from an arteriogram is available.

Injuries following cannulation for arteriography are less common than those done for monitoring, because the duration of cannulation is short and arteriography via an upper extremity artery is done far less frequently than cannulation for monitoring. If there is ischemia of the hand and digits following arterial puncture for arteriography, the chance of a vessel injury that is surgically correctable and will lead to either short-term gangrene or long-term claudication if not corrected is high.[241,245,275,292] In this situation, the artery should be explored, and whether the problem is a thrombus or an arterial tear with an obstructing flap, it should be corrected.[269,270]

Accidental and Deliberate Intraarterial Injections

These injuries may occur iatrogenically when an artery is mistaken for a vein. Hazlett[264] pointed out that this may be easy to do if the ulnar artery is located quite superficially, as it was in almost 3 percent of 730 limbs he studied. Usually, Pentothal is the substance injected and the only immediate clue to the mistaken route of access may be the delay in loss of consciousness. Other medications accidently injected intraarterially include promazine (Sparine), dextroamphetamine (Dexedrine), sodium sulfobromazine,[255] penicillin,[291] depomedrone,[297] propylhexedrine (Benzedrex used in nasal inhalers),[247] and dextropropoxyphene[293] (Darvon).

Engler and colleagues[255] had difficulty reproducing the problem seen clinically in humans in experimental animals unless the artery proximal to the injection was occluded. They postulated that proximal occlusion allowed delivery of an undiluted, highly irritating bolus. The mechanism of injury may be mechanical from precipitated crystals, a chemical endarteritis, or an aggregation of blood elements.[249] Burn[243] found that pretreatment of mice with reserpine could prevent gangrene of tails from injection of the tail artery with thiopentone. Since reserpine is known to cause disappearance of noradrenaline from tissues, he concluded that thiopentone caused damage by stimulating release of noradrenaline. Probably several of these mechanisms operate in concert to produce the clinical picture.

The clinical picture is one of immediate, intense, burning pain, sometimes followed by an arterial flush that is then replaced by blanching and subsequent cyanosis.[263,264] Gangrene follows. Zachary et al[302] noted the role of the potent vasoconstrictor and platelet aggregator, thromboxane, and achieved some good results by using methimazole and topical aloe vera.

Immediate conservative measures include intraarterial vasodilators or thrombolytic agents (see following section), anticoagulation with heparin, stellate ganglion block, and systemic vasodilators.[263,264] Because the arterial changes are both chemical arteritis and mechanical blockade, the advisability of direct surgical approach to the involved vessel is not clear-cut. However, if there is not a very prompt early response to the indirect measures, I favor arteriotomy with insertion of a small Fogarty catheter to try to pull out any thrombotic material. There is little to lose by this maneuver and much to gain.

With drug addicts the injected substance may or may not be known by the injector. There are recent reports of injection of propylhexedrine[247] and dextropropoxyphene.[293] In addition to the uncertain identity of the injected substance, it may be impure and the patient is often not seen for days and weeks, by which time the artery is probably irretrievably occluded. Charney and Stern[246] treated five drug addict patients in whom it was difficult to obtain the mechanism of injury. Two required amputation of portions of digits, one resolved with a stellate ganglion block and two resolved with vein grafts. Often, all that can be done with these pathetic but exasperating people is to wait for the demarcation line of the gangrene and to amputate the nonviable tissue.[249,282,283,288]

Schanzer, Gribetz, and Jacobson[291] struck a pessimistic note on this entire problem: "the end result seems to depend more on the severity of the original damage than on the therapeutic measures applied."

Accidental and Operative Vascular Trauma

Perry, Thal, and Shires[287] analyzed 508 arterial injuries in a civilian practice. Of these, 442 were to the extremities and 236 to the upper extremity (53 percent). Most of these were to the brachial (78), radial (58), and ulnar (39) arteries. Almost 40 percent were accompanied by a major venous or nerve injury. The authors noted that most of the injuries were from "aggressive acts of violence." They listed seven criteria that should alert the surgeon to arterial injury and the need for exploration: (1) decreased or absent distal pulse; (2) history of persistent arterial bleeding; (3) large or expanding hematoma; (4) major hemorrhage with hypotension; (5) bruit at or distal to the artery; (6) injury to an anatomically related nerve; and (7) anatomic proximity of the wound to a major artery.

Arterial injuries resulting in distal ischemia require urgent treatment. Gordon[262] has demonstrated in rats that warm ischemia of the quadriceps femoris of more than 1 hour results in severe histological changes in muscle. As would be expected, this has been borne out by clinical studies.[273,276] Often, the severity of the injury will mandate urgent surgical treatment, even in the absence of distal ischemia.[278,279] If physical signs are inconclusive regarding the need for surgery but the proximity of the wound to a major vessel indicates a high probability of injury, angiography is indicated.[277,294]

Major arterial injury may be caused by a closed injury such as a dislocated shoulder,[268] a fractured clavicle,[299] a fractured proximal humerus,[271a] or a large exostosis of the proximal humerus.[284] Nonpenetrating trauma in the neck and shoulder region may cause injury to the subclavian artery with potentially catastrophic consequences.[303] Iatrogenic vascular injury occurring in extremity surgery is not uncommon.[250,254,295] Holt[266] evaluated a large number of arterial injuries occurring during orthopaedic operations. Not surprisingly, most of the upper extremity iatrogenic injuries were sustained during ganglionectomy. Most of the arteries were ligated after injury and an untoward result was uncommon.

Following injury to the brachial artery, restoration of arterial flow by repair or graft is advised by most authors to avoid possible short-term arm loss, which is unusual, and long-term claudication problems, which are common.[207] At a more distal level the need for arterial repair or reconstruction depends on the local situation and the severity of the injury. In some situations the need is obvious and acute[262a] while in others it is not necessary for survival of the parts, but without repair or reconstruction symptoms of chronic ischemia may ensue.[245]

Gelberman and co-workers[259] reviewed forearm arterial injuries and found that single, unrepaired arterial injuries caused modest consistent alteration of hand vascularity but few clinical signs of ischemia or of cold intolerance. If combined with nerve injury, especially injury to the median nerve, the hands did have a decreased vascularity that could be quite disabling, but the arterial injury had no effect on the rate or completeness of nerve recovery. However Leclercq et al[271b] studied 64 patients with ulnar nerve injuries, in which the ulnar artery was intact in 34 and severed in 45. In those patients with the artery severed it was ligated in eight, repaired with a graft in eight and repaired directly in 29. The authors noted that the clinical results for both sensory and motor recovery were superior when the vascular repair remained intact as compared to those in which repair was not done or the artery thrombosed.

Studies of repair of single artery lacerations in the dog showed a high rate of thrombosis, probably due to high distal stump pressure.[260] This finding has been confirmed in a three-center study on humans with radial and/or ulnar artery lacerations.[201] In this latter study, it was found that operative technique, back pressure in distal arterial stumps, and the extent of hand ischemia relative to its normal blood supply (i.e., the local vascular arch anatomy) are the most important determinants of vessel patency following repair. Recent experimental[298] and clinical[285] studies of single wrist level artery repairs have reported an approximately 50 percent long-term patency rate.

When any hand, wrist, forearm, or arm laceration is explored, I strongly recommend exposure and identification of any significant artery that may be involved. If the superficial palmar arch is divided and there is flow from both sides, only ligation is required. If not, repair should be undertaken. In the wrist and forearm, the status of radial and ulnar arteries (and median, if present) should be ascertained. If the arteries are divided, I favor direct arterial repair or repair by graft of at least one, usually the ulnar, or both if possible. If this course is not chosen, the surgeon should at least identify and ligate both ends of each artery to avoid the early postoperative problem of bleeding and the later problem of aneurysm formation. Even if the artery is totally divided, retracted and clotted, occasionally a rebleed will require another trip to the operating room. It is far better to take a few extra minutes the first time than to subject the patient to a second operation.

Miscellaneous Problems

An excessively tight bandage, neglected tourniquet, or other constrictive device should never be overlooked as a cause of vascular compromise, especially in a digit.[280] Obviously, the treatment for this is prevention.

Extravasation of potent vasoconstrictive drugs may cause vascular embarrassment. Denkler and Cohen[251] treated a premature infant with this problem with topical nitroglycerin ointment with good results. Abu-Nema et al[232] cared for two patients with a jellyfish sting that resulted in severe hand ischemia. Thrombolysin with intraarterial urokinase was curative in each case. Johnson et al[268a] treated an infant whose upper limbs underwent in utero ischemic necrosis from oligohydramnios and compression. Amputation was necessary.

A patient with an unusual mass in the hand should always be questioned about other systemic diseases. A pseudocyst has been reported in the hand of a mechanic with hemophilia.[235] Trauma, even trivial, may compromise an artery in an already tight position and cause impending gangrene without actual thrombosis.[244] Surgical correction of the local problem with appropriate systemic support is the treatment of choice.

EMBOLI TO UPPER EXTREMITY VESSELS

Hand surgeons will rarely see a patient with an acute embolic problem in the upper extremity. The reason is that most of these patients have either severe cardiac disease, generalized arteriosclerosis, or both, and when the problem occurs, it will be obvious to those who are caring for the patient's heart or vascular disease, and referral will be to a vascular surgeon. This may be just as well, because the brain, abdominal viscera, and lower extremities may also be involved.

Champion and Gill[310] reported seven cases of upper limb arterial embolus and reviewed a number of other studies. Approximately 15 percent of all emboli lodge in the upper extremity. The source of these can be either cardiac or a major artery.[318] The heart is at least twice as common a source.[304,331] The usual cardiac problems are atrial fibrillation or a recent myocardial infarction. Arterial thrombi giving off showers of emboli may be caused by thoracic outlet syndrome, arteriosclerotic plaques, mechanical problems in a graft, or trauma.[305,306,325,331,332] An unusual cause is heparin-induced thromboembolism.[308,325] An ulnar artery aneurysm may be the source of emboli.[323] Acute vasospasm in the upper extremity may be mistaken for embolism.[317]

The presenting symptoms are somewhat different from the two sources. An embolus from the heart is a *macroembolus,* and it causes a sudden, acute obstruction at a fairly proximal level manifested by the "five Ps": pain, pallor, pulselessness, paresthesia, and paralysis.[333] Arterial emboli are *atheroemboli* or *thromboemboli* and are more likely to throw off showers of microemboli with much more subtle symptoms. The symptoms from this latter cause may be Raynaud's phenomenon.[306] This is one reason why every patient who presents with the phenomenon needs a careful evaluation for a mechanical causation. The presentation of an embolus may be quite unusual and striking. Bashir[307] reported the case of a 45-year-old man who lost consciousness and woke up with a painful left hand and a gangrenous left thumb and index finger. An extensive investigation was not done, but he was presumed to have a left subclavian artery thrombus with emboli to the brain and hand.

Diagnosis of upper extremity embolus is made with the usual sequence of evaluation and studies. Arteriography is often crucial in the diagnosis, and it should be done from the groin approach so that all upper extremity vessels from the subclavian distally are visualized.

Treatment[329]

Some emboli or thrombi, especially those in veins, do dissolve or at least retract markedly.[314] In the arteries, when there is impending gangrene distally, the leisurely approach of watchful waiting must be abandoned and a more aggressive one pursued. Surgery is the usual treatment of choice, and the approach to be used is proximal arteriotomy with embolectomy.[304,309,310] In 1963, Fogarty and colleagues[315,316] revolutionized this treatment with the introduction of the catheter with an inflatable balloon (the Fogarty catheter). These are now available in sizes small enough to be passed into the superficial and deep vascular arches in the hand. Local anesthesia may be used for this approach.

Cooney, Wilson, and Wood[311] studied fibrinolytic agents in small vessels (internal diameter 0.8 to 1.5 mm) in dogs and found its efficacy to be doubtful. However, Puckett and coworkers[328] found streptokinase to improve the blood flow and tissue survival in ischemic epigastric flaps in rats. Kakkasseril et al[321] found streptokinase to be most effective in occluded native arteries and autogenous vein grafts, and least effective in prosthetic grafts. In the upper extremity, and especially in the hand, the use of thrombolytic agents in the desperate situation where a surgical approach is not possible or feasible is clearly indicated.[320,327] Thrombolysin (streptokinase and plasminogen) is administered into the involved artery directly, with close monitoring of the clotting factors.[319,343] Kartchner and Wilcox[322] used this method in a series of patients with impending digital gangrene and were able to achieve an excellent result in eight hands and a good one in two.

Parkhouse and Smith[326] found streptokinase useful in salvaging a replanted thumb. Both Jelalian et al[320] and Tisnado et al[334] have suggested guidelines for the administration of streptokinase. It is delivered via the affected vessel proximal to the clot. Usually a loading dose of 50,000 to 100,000 IU is injected over the first 30 to 60 minutes followed by a maintenance dose of 5000 IU/hour until the affected part is perfused. Fibrinogen levels (normal 165 to 365 mg/dl) are closely monitored, and if the level drops below 110 to 150, the hourly dose is halved. If it falls below 100, the streptokinase is stopped until fibrinogen values have recovered to a safe level. Both streptokinase, which is a purified bacterial growth elaborated by group C beta-hemolytic streptococci, and urokinase obtained from human kidney tissue cultures are used clinically for thrombolysis. Each of them converts plasminogen to the enzyme plasmin, which degrades fibrin clots and other plasma proteins. These are very potent drugs and there is always the danger of significant bleeding problems developing, although these should be minimal when the drug is perfused directly into a limb artery.

Following treatment by whichever method, the patient should be anti-coagulated with heparin for about 7 to 10 days.[312,319,324] If all else fails, stellate ganglion block may be done to relieve acute symptoms of pain, and cervicodorsal sympathectomy may give long-term relief from symptoms due to small vessel occlusion.[312]

VASCULAR COMPRESSION (THORACIC OUTLET SYNDROME) AND OTHER VASCULAR PROBLEMS IN THE NECK

When searching for an obscure cause of digital ischemia or for the cause of upper extremity venous occlusion, a vascular constriction in the neck should always be considered.[347,356] Thoracic outlet syndrome is usually thought of as a nerve constriction problem, and symptoms of nerve compression are more common than those of vascular constriction. Kelly[348] reviewed a personal series of 304 patients and found 12 (4 percent) with venous obstruction and none with symptoms due to major arterial occlusion. Adson,[336] however, found 52 of 142 patients had vascular compression symptoms. Gross and colleagues[343] analyzed 43 patients with upper extremity arterial insufficiency. In their series, these 43 patients comprised only 0.9 percent of all vascular cases and only 19 of the 43 had a problem in the neck (the other problems were in the arm and due mostly to postangiography injury). Of the 19 patients with vascular problems in the neck, 15 were due to arteriosclerosis and 4 to trauma. This should give the reader some idea of the rarity of the problem.

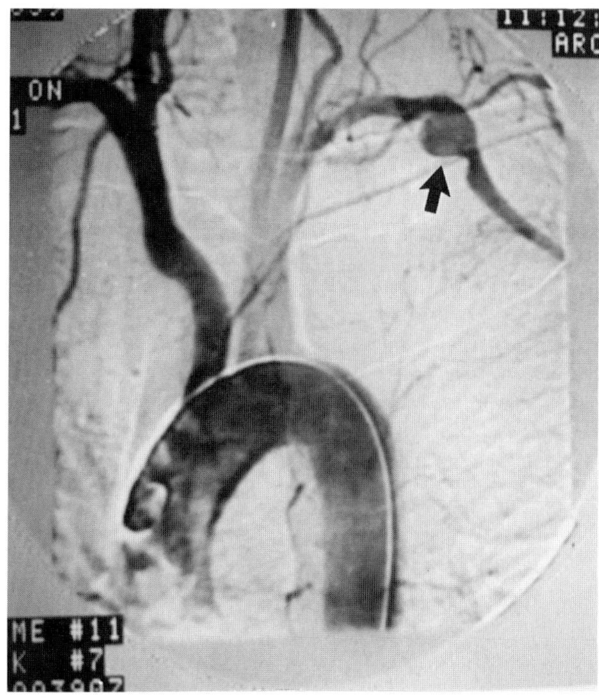

Fig. 62-24. The arteriogram of a 53-year-old woman who had gone from doctor to doctor complaining of hand pain until a careful examination finally revealed a markedly diminished radial pulse. Noninvasive vascular studies confirmed an occlusive lesion in the neck, which was eventually shown to be an aneurysm on arteriogram *(arrow)*. Resection of the lesion and replacement by a graft was curative.

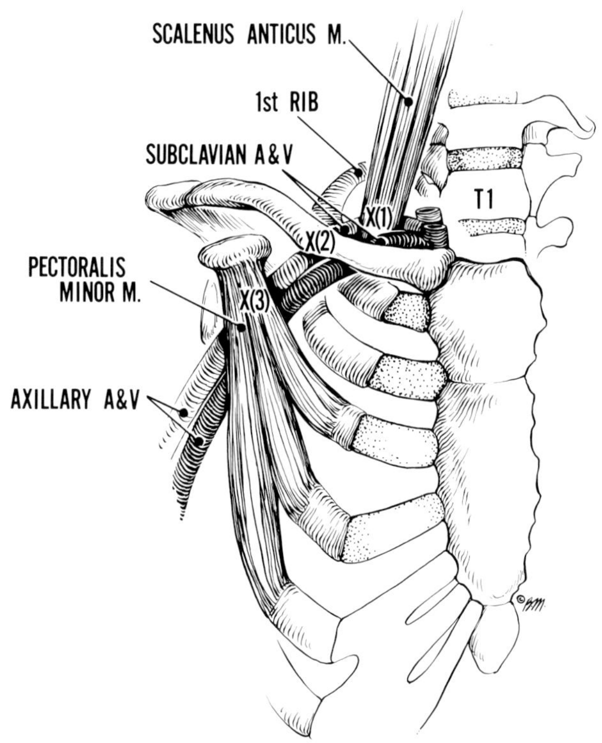

Fig. 62-23. The neck should always be considered in vascular problems of the upper extremity. The three usual sites of vascular compression are at X(1), X(2), and X(3) (see text). Arterial compression is possible at all three sites, but venous compression usually only at the distal two.

Figure 62-23 shows the points at which the artery and vein may become obstructed.[317] The highest or most proximal point, X(1), is where the artery crosses over the first rib in exiting from the thoracic cavity. It lies behind the scalenus anticus muscle, while the vein lies anterior to that structure. At this point, the fibrous band that attaches a cervical rib to the first rib may squeeze the neurovascular structures from behind. The second point of potential constriction, X(2), is between the clavicle and the first rib, and the third, X(3), is posterior to the origin of the pectoralis minor muscle.

Vascular compression, manifested by digital gangrene, may be caused at Point X(1), either with or without a cervical rib present,[340,357,360,363] or the principal manifestation may be only Raynaud's phenomenon.[340,341] The vein is more likely to be occluded at Point X(2) or X(3), but arterial occlusion is possible at all three.[353] For compression to occur at one of these points, either abnormal bony or fibrous structures must be present, the scalenus anticus must be hypertrophied, or some abnormal stress must be placed on the structures.[341,345] A rudimentary first rib may form a plate complex with the second rib that compresses the axillary artery causing upper extremity ischemia.[339] Aneurysms may be caused by compression in the same area[342a] (Fig. 62-24). Actions that precipitate the problem include prolonged abnormal hyperabduction of the arm (as, for example, in painters or mechanics under a car on a rack) or

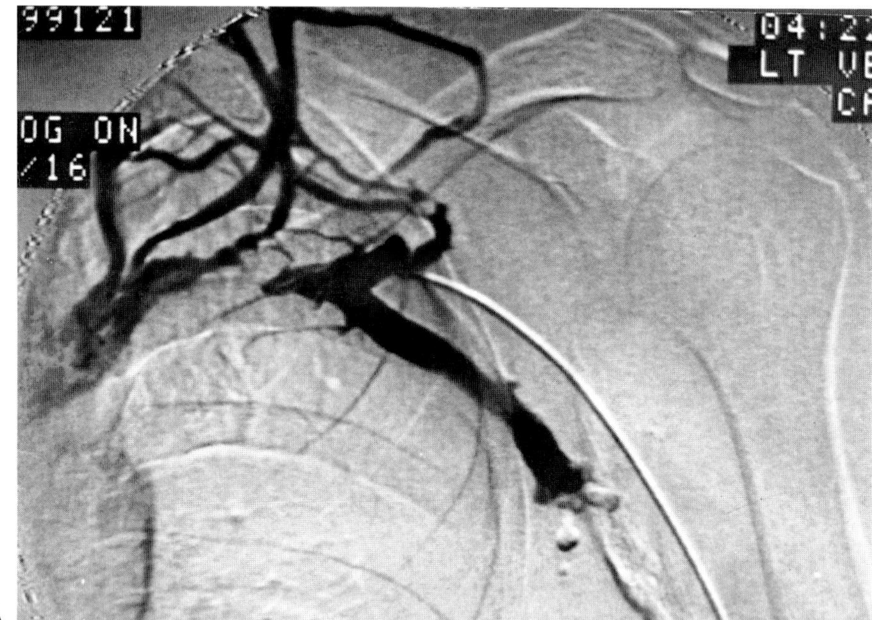

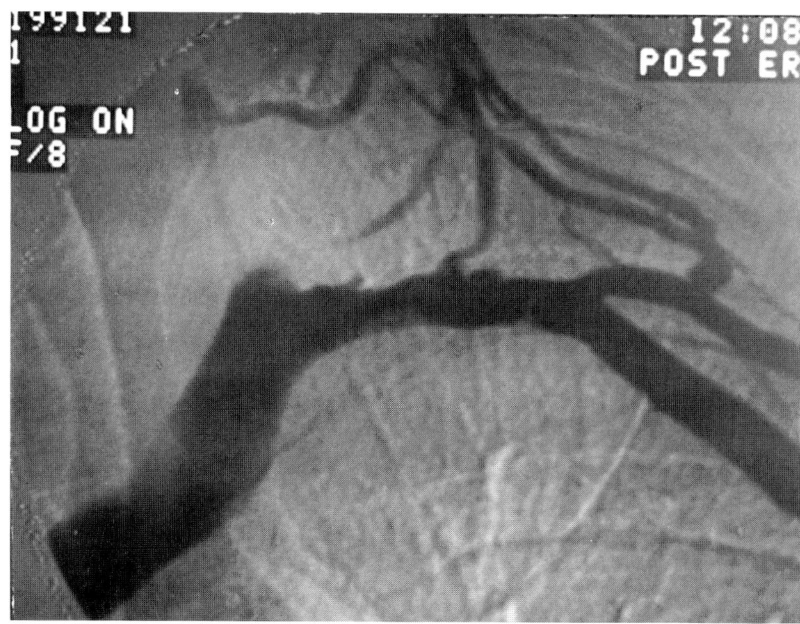

Fig. 62-25. **(A)** This 30-year-old man was putting on a sweater when he noted pain, swelling, and tightness in his left upper extremity. The physical examination suggested venous obstruction, which led to this venogram showing complete occlusion of the axillary-subclavian vein complex. **(B)** Urokinase was delivered through the venogram catheter and the thrombosis was completely cleared.

holding the arm in this position while sleeping.[366] Effort-related or spontaneous compression of the axillary-subclavian vein complex is known as Paget-Schroetter syndrome[350] and may occur with as benign an action as abducting the upper extremities at the shoulders to put on a sweater, as happened to the patient shown in Figure 62-25.

Vascular problems in the neck may arise as a consequence of catheters placed in the subclavian vein. Davis et al[342] reported three cases of subclavian vein stenosis developing 3 to 6 months after prolonged placement (> 15 days) of a catheter for dialysis. This was manifested by massive upper extremity edema. I have seen one similar case.

By contrast, situations can arise in which a primary upper extremity problem may cause a loss of blood flow to the brain. Hunter et al[346] reported a case of subclavian steal following a carotid-subclavian bypass for arm claudication. Argenta and coworkers[338] described a patient with massive hand trauma due to a severe upper extremity traction injury. The patient required a lengthy operation under general anesthesia to reconstruct the hand, and neurologic signs of a right hemiparesis were not apparent until the day after injury. They urged careful preoperative neurologic evaluation in similar cases.

Diagnosis

Diagnostic maneuvers to elicit signs of neurovascular compression in the neck include the following tests.

Adson's Maneuver. The arm of the side affected is placed on the sitting patient's thigh with the forearm supinated. The patient turns his head *to* the affected side and extends the neck while holding his breath. A positive test is obliteration of the radial pulse.[336]

The Hyperabduction (Wright) Maneuver.[366] The patient places the extremity in full abduction and reaches back as far as he can. The test should be done both passively and actively, as the former may be negative and the latter positive. Radial pulse obliteration alone is not particularly meaningful, but loss of the pulse with concomitant reproduction of symptoms is a positive test. Creation of a bruit in the supraclavicular area adds further evidence of vessel constriction.

The "At Attention Test." This is performed by having the patient thrust the shoulders down and back, as when standing stiffly at attention or when carrying a backpack.[359] This test particularly narrows the costoclavicular space [Point X(2) in Fig. 63-23]. Again, a positive test is radial pulse obliteration.

Normal, or at least asymptomatic, persons may have their radial pulse obliterated by these maneuvers. They should probably be wary about occupations involving overhead work, avoid sleeping with their arms "over the head," and be wary of placing unusual stress on the shoulder girdle, as may occur in carrying backpacks.

Work-up in patients suspected of vascular compression in the neck should include the three maneuvers described above, as well as the routine vascular work-up. A plain anteroposterior radiograph of the neck should be taken to look for a cervical rib. Arteriography or venography will often be necessary to make a definite diagnosis.[351] Comparative measurement of venous pressures in each arm may be useful if venous obstruction or occlusion is suspected. One way, noted by Wiseheart,[365] to distinguish obstruction in the neck from distal arterial obstruction is that reactive hyperemia is more pronounced in the latter. One should always rule out hysterical (factitious) edema in evaluation of possible venous obstruction.[364]

Treatment

Once a diagnosis is established, surgical removal of the offending structures (first rib, cervical rib, middle third of the clavicle, scalenus anticus muscle, or fibrous band) should be undertaken.[337,358,360] Stallworth and Horne[362] evaluated 1140 patients with thoracic outlet syndrome and found that 194 required surgery. Soft tissue release resulted in improvement in 173 of 180, and bone resection in 6 of 14. Horowitz[345] made a plea for very specific use of transaxillary rib resection for thoracic outlet syndrome, to avoid severe and permanent damage to the brachial plexus. If arterial obstruction is present, thromboendarterectomy or interposition graft may be done.[349,352] If symptoms persist, cervicodorsal sympathectomy may help alleviate hand pain and ischemia.[349] Occasionally, a bypass arterial graft will be required to restore arterial blood flow.[355]

Chronic venous obstruction should be approached in the same way, that is, by removal of the constricting structures and by thrombectomy.[335] Rowen, Dorsey, and Hepps[359] found that thrombectomy was often not successful and that long-term anticoagulation and the wearing of a compressive upper extremity garment may be necessary.

RAYNAUD'S PHENOMENON AND RELATED OCCLUSIVE AND VASOSPASTIC PROBLEMS[384,432]

To include a section on ischemic disease of the hand not correctable by surgery in a text on operative hand surgery is almost a contradiction at the outset. Not only is this group of disorders not generally amenable to surgery, but one of the most common alleviatory surgical procedures is a cervicodorsal sympathectomy, which is out of the province of most hand surgeons. Yet, this large group of diseases exists, causes great grief and misery to those who suffer from them, and must be considered. The hand surgeon will be asked to see patients with the complications of this group of diseases and treat the end-stage gangrene by amputating digits or a hand. The patients may also be seen on referral from a family or general practitioner or from an internist for evaluation of ulcers, joint stiffness, and pain.

Raynaud's Phenomenon

This phenomenon was named after Maurice Raynaud, who described asphyxia and symmetrical gangrene of the digits in 1862.[390] Raynaud's phenomenon is a pallor of the digits with or without cyanosis upon exposure to cold. The thumbs are usually spared. Paresthesias or hypesthesias are common in involved digits. An attack is followed, upon rewarming, by an intense hyperemia and a gradual return to normal. Characteristically, the hands are normal between attacks.

The phenomenon may occur because of one of three situations: (1) blood pressure decreases and blood flow ceases when a critical closing pressure of the vessel is reached; (2) vessel constriction reaches a point where blood flow ceases; or (3) an increase of blood viscosity causes a sluggish flow, which finally ceases.[433] These three factors may function individually or together to cause an attack. Raynaud's phenomenon caused by proximal vascular obstruction would be an example of the first type. Idiopathic Raynaud's or that due to a collagen disease would be an example of the second mechanism. Raynaud's caused by cryoglobulinemia is an example of the third.

Whether the fault is with vasomotor overactivity or with faulty vessels has been an area of some disagreement. Lewis and Pickering[429] believed that the fault is with the vessels. Mendlowitz and Naftchi[437] studied 20 patients with Raynaud's disease under stabilized conditions by administering *l*-norepinephrine intravenously, and concluded that attacks are produced by either in the setting of vascular obstruction with normal vasomotor factors operating or by heightened vasomotor factors acting upon normal vessels.

People susceptible to attacks of Raynaud's phenomenon have an abnormal response to cold.[411] Bollinger and Schlumpf[379] measured digital blood flow in three groups of normal patients: young men, young women, and postmenopausal women. They compared digital blood flow in these three groups with that in a group of patients with Raynaud's disease and found that flow was significantly higher in the men and postmenopausal women at rest and following 3 minutes of circulatory arrest than it was in either the normal young women or in the Raynaud's group. These latter two groups had similar flow patterns. Wouda found the same thing.[467] McGrath and Penny[433] have summarized current data about the mechanisms responsible for Raynaud's phenomenon, and it is safe to say that a number of factors may operate to cause Raynaud's phenomenon. These may be either local or systemic, and the only common denominator is low or stopped blood flow in the digits provoked by cold exposure, or, in certain instances, by emotional stress. The similarities between the appearance of the digits in an acute Raynaud's attack and those in profound hypovolemic shock are striking. The use of dopamine, a naturally occurring catecholamine that is a very potent vasoconstrictor, may cause irreversible digital ischemia in patients already in shock.[404]

The diagnosis of Raynaud's phenomenon is usually made on clinical grounds. In a doubtful situation, putting the patient's hand in cold water (or, better yet, exposing the patient to a cold environment) should confirm the diagnosis. Arteriography would appear to offer little in the way of specific information, but may serve to confirm that the problem is secondary to a proximal vascular obstruction.[423] Plethysmography serves only to confirm the presence or absence of proximal occlusive disease.[468]

Clinical Patterns of Raynaud's Phenomenon

Raynaud's phenomenon, without a demonstrable or causative disease, is known as primary Raynaud's phenomenon or, more commonly, as Raynaud's disease. When the phenomenon is associated with or caused by a disease, it is known as Raynaud's syndrome or secondary Raynaud's phenomenon. For convenience, the terms Raynaud's disease and Raynaud's syndrome will be used here.

Raynaud's Disease

This condition is seen mainly in young women,[372,376,401,412] often having its onset in the late teens. Attacks are precipitated by cold exposure and, very commonly, by emotional upset. Allen and Brown[369] in 1932 established the criteria that must be met to confirm a diagnosis of the disease: (1) intermittent attacks of discoloration of the acral parts; (2) symmetrical or bilateral involvement; (3) absence of clinical occlusion of peripheral arteries; (4) gangrene or trophic changes, when present, are limited to the distal digital skin; (5) symptoms present for a minimum of 2 years; (6) absence of an organic disease to which the vasomotor changes may be attributed; and (7) strong predilection for females.

In two large series of cases, females predominated by 3 : 1[372] and 4 : 1.[412] Sixty percent of patients had the onset of the disease between ages 11 and 30, 80 percent between 11 and 40. Cold always precipitates an attack; emotional upset will do so 60 percent of the time. While symptoms may have their onset in women at menopause, they will almost always disappear after menopause.[376]

Raynaud's Syndrome

Velayos and colleagues[463] classified Raynaud's syndrome into two categories: that associated with a connective tissue disorder and that associated with some other disease. When the association is with a connective tissue disease, there is once again a preponderance of females, but when associated with another disease, the male-female distribution is about equal.

Numerous authors have emphasized the need for a careful work-up to rule out other diseases associated with the syndrome, because many of them carry a far more serious prognosis than Raynaud's disease and many of them are treatable when diagnosed.[380,389,399,440,450,461]

The list of associated or causative diseases is a long one.[407] A number of them are mentioned elsewhere in this chapter, because they are caused by intrinsic or extrinsic vascular obstruction amenable to surgical correction; these include Raynaud's syndrome caused by neurovascular compression, obstructive arterial disease, and vibrational occupational disease.

Foremost among the diseases causing Raynaud's syndrome are the collagen diseases.[367] The syndrome forms part of the symptom complex of the less virulent or CREST form of scleroderma,[462] i.e., (C) calcinosis; (R) Raynaud's; (E) esophageal motility changes; (S) sclerodactyly; (T) telangiectasia. Carpal tunnel syndrome has been reported as the initial manifestation of scleroderma.[373] An unusual location for calcifications is the digital nerve.[447] The hand of a woman with scleroderma and ischemic fingertip changes is shown in Figure 62-26. Gahhos et al[347] have outlined a treatment program for the difficult problem of sclerodermal finger ulcers, which appears to have general applicability to patients with vasospastic finger ulcers from other causes.

Jones and his co-workers[418–420] have treated a large number of patients with scleroderma who have hand problems and have analyzed the problems very thoroughly. In general, their conclusions are similar to others, i.e., meticulous care of ischemic digits is the most important measure, but they have had success with revascularization procedures in a few patients.

In one series,[377] 50 percent of patients with systemic lupus erythematosus whose hands were affected were disabled because of Raynaud's syndrome. Patients with polyarteritis,[374] mixed connective tissue disease,[428] rheumatoid arthritis, der-

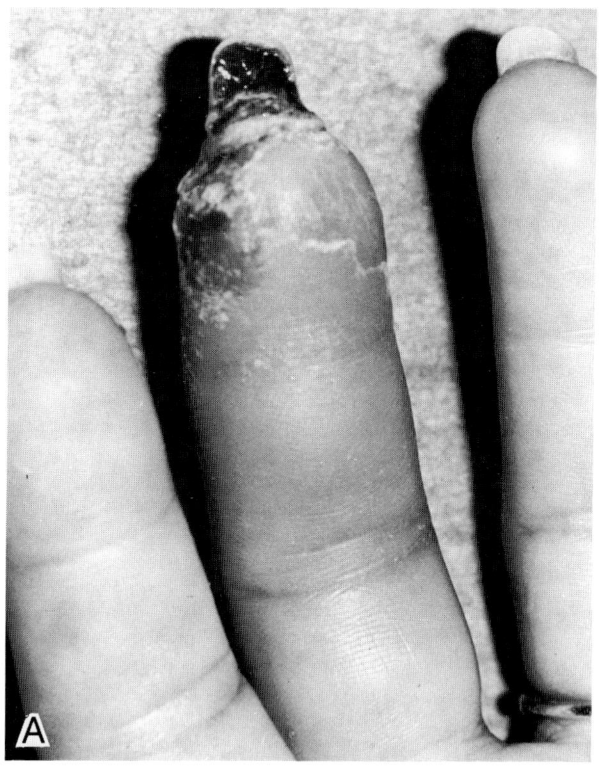

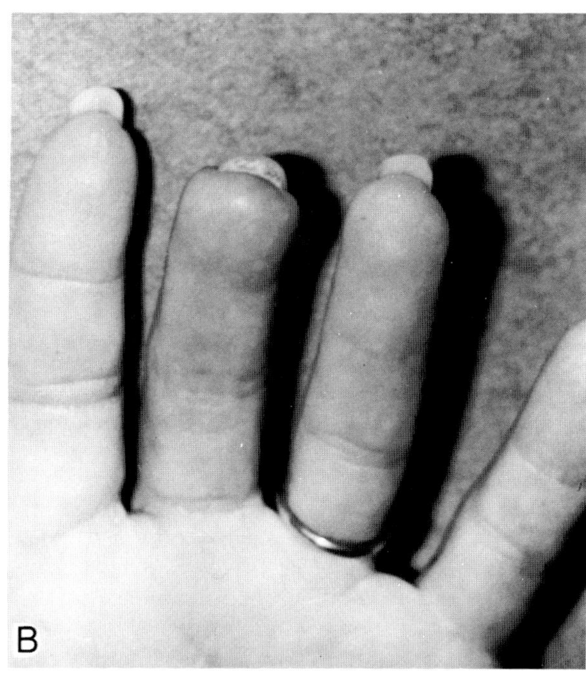

Fig. 62-26. **(A)** This 54-year-old woman developed ischemic changes in her left long fingertip without evidence of central vascular disease. A diagnosis of scleroderma was made. **(B)** Conservative debridement and time resulted in a healed finger. Like most ischemic lesions, this was intensely painful and tender.

matomyositis, and polymyositis[433] may also exhibit Raynaud's phenomenon.

Porter and colleagues[448] studied 100 patients with the phenomenon. Twenty-eight had scleroderma, 10 had systemic lupus erythematosus, and 43 had miscellaneous autoimmune disease. Of the remaining 19 who were diagnosed as having Raynaud's disease, 14 had isolated serologic abnormalities. As the scope of our laboratories broadens and our ability to make more definitive diagnosis improves, the number of patients misdiagnosed as having Raynaud's disease will decrease.

A group of diseases that are sometimes associated with Raynaud's phenomenon are those in which increased blood viscosity is a significant factor. These include polycythemia and cryoglobulinemia. The latter has been reported to cause ischemia severe enough to require digital amputation.[416] A patient in whom increased blood viscosity may have contributed to a severe, limb-threatening vasospasm is shown in Figure 62-27.

Acrocyanosis is an unusual condition in which the hands and feet become cyanotic. It has been reported in young women[400] and in older women.[391] In young patients, it is apparently more of an annoyance than a threat. In older patients, there is occasional partial digital loss from gangrene.

The work-up of a patient with Raynaud's phenomenon should be systematic and complete. It starts with a careful history, paying particular attention to (1) family history of vasospastic problems; (2) occupational history, especially exposure to cold or the use of vibrating tools; and (3) medication and chemical exposure history. A careful physical examination should be done, with close attention to pulses and the condition of the skin. Laboratory studies should include a complete blood count with an erythrocyte sedimentation rate, urinalysis, protein electrophoresis, antinuclear antibody factor, rheumatoid factor, cryoproteins, and cold agglutinins. Appropriate radiographs should be obtained.[434]

Features that suggest Raynaud's syndrome rather than Raynaud's disease include (1) age at onset over 40 and no sex predilection; (2) absence of peripheral pulses; (3) marked nail and nail fold changes; (4) Rapid progression of digital ischemia; (5) asymmetric involvement of digits; (6) systemic symptoms; (7) anemia and elevated sed rate; and (8) other skin changes, such as purpura and telangiectasia.[434]

Treatment

When Raynaud's phenomenon is not caused by a correctable lesion, such as a constricted or thrombosed artery or a neurovascular compression syndrome, a variety of other treatments, none of them perfect, may be used. As in all other vasospastic conditions, tobacco smoking must be stopped.[383,406,439]

Several investigators have noted good results with reserpine. Kontos and Wasserman[426] found that patients with Raynaud's phenomenon who were treated with reserpine had a markedly

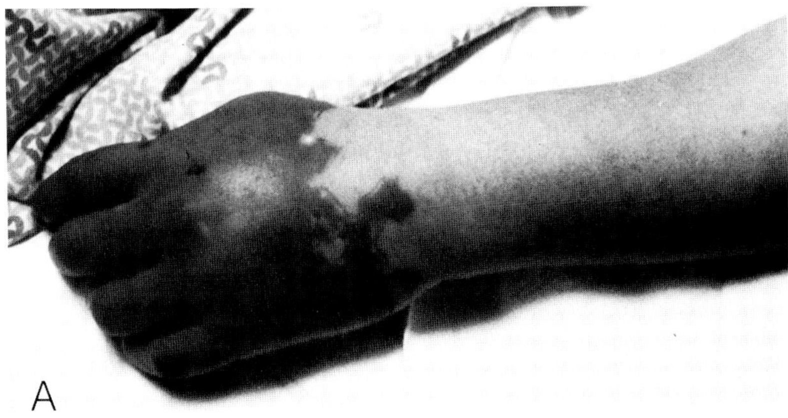

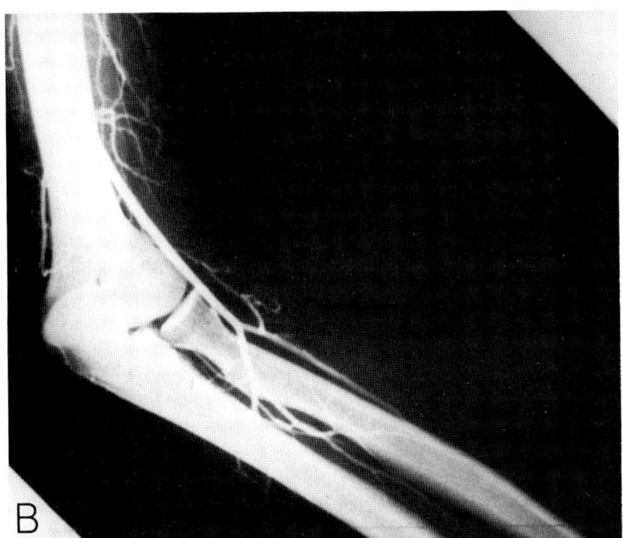

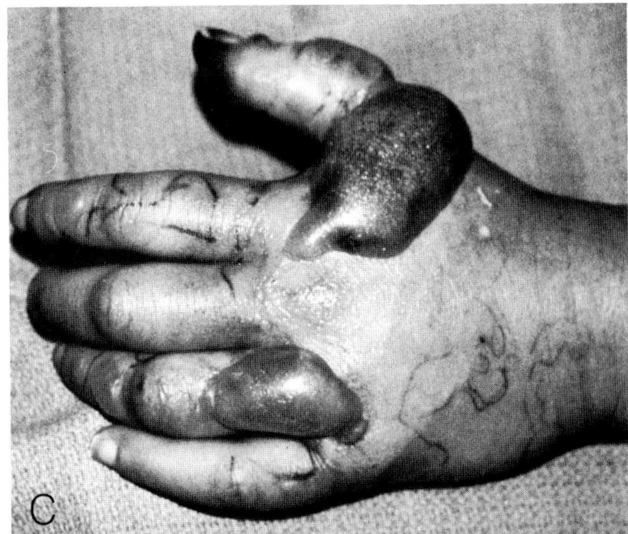

Fig. 62-27. **(A)** The hand of a 20-year-old woman 12 hours after admission to a hospital because of coma due to diabetic acidosis, with blood sugar level of 1700 mg%. **(B)** An arteriogram of the same patient a few hours later. Priscoline was used in an attempt to cause vasodilatation. **(C)** The same patient's hand $3\frac{1}{2}$ days after treatment with intravenous nitroprusside. See text for more details.

reduced response to intraarterial vasoconstrictors. Willerson and colleagues[466] found that only patients with very extensive obstructive disease did not respond to the drug. Romeo and co-workers[453] used intraarterial reserpine in 18 patients with either Raynaud's disease or Raynaud's phenomenon. Two-thirds of them had some positive response with minimal side effects and an average duration of clinical effectiveness of 7 months.

Porter and colleagues[449] noted improvement in Raynaud's symptoms with both guanethidine and phenoxybenzamine. They treated a total of 23 patients (most of them with the syndrome) and had good or excellent clinical results in 19. Most of the patients were treated with the former drug. Sonneveld et al[457] studied the effects of guanethidine regional intravascular sympathetic blocks in 11 patients by measurement of transcutaneous PO_2(TcPO). They found increased PO_2 levels and decreased symptoms in eight, and no change in the other three patients. At this time, this drug is available only for oral use (as Ismelin) in the United States, but the intravenous application may become available in the future. Waldo[464] found striking improvement with the use of prazosin in a patient with advanced changes of Raynaud's phenomenon. All of these drugs find their primary use as antihypertensive agents, and at least some of them are catecholamine inhibitors.

The calcium channel blocker nifedipine has recently become available for the treatment of hypertension and has found some use in vasospastic disorders. Kemerer et al[421] successfully used this drug to treat one patient with ergotism (from Cafergot), which had caused severe ischemia of the left lower extremity. Roseheffer and co-workers[452] treated 15 Raynaud's patients with nifedipine and found a good response in some and no response in others. They could not explain the individual variation, but concluded that it is a useful drug in this problem. Pentoxyfylline is said to improve red cell flexibility and may have a role in problems of increased blood viscosity.

In a situation of acute, severe vasospasm of uncertain cause, sodium nitroprusside[375] given intravenously may be limb-saving (see Fig. 62-27).

Low molecular weight Dextran has been used in a series of patients with scleroderma.[414,441] It was given at 5- to 8-week intervals in the winter and at long intervals in the summer. Decrease of ischemic pain and healing of ulcers was noted in 10 of 12 patients. A study on the use of biofeedback was conducted under the auspices of the National Institutes of Health[395] and 19 of 20 patients reported subjective improvement. Talpos and colleagues[458] reported striking improvement in five patients who had not responded to other forms of treatment by means of plasmapheresis. I have seen one patient with scleroderma whose chronic digital ulcers healed and whose pain vanished after treatment with this modality. However, Klinenberg and Wallace[425] reported no improvement in two patients they treated with this technique.

An indirect surgical approach to Raynaud's is cervicodorsal sympathectomy.[431] This has been done for many years via a variety of surgical approaches. Adson and Brown[368] reported an excellent result in one patient who had a bilateral sympathectomy from the posterior approach. The difficulty of this route has discouraged most others from using it. Palumbo has written extensively about upper dorsal sympathectomy, and states that Horner's syndrome can be avoided in most instances if only the lower one-third of the stellate (first dorsal) ganglion is removed.[442–444] He is very enthusiastic about the operation and favors the transthoracic route. Another approach is the cervical, which gives good exposure to the stellate ganglion but makes removal of the T3 and T4 ganglions difficult. The transaxillary approach, when used in conjunction with first rib resection, is said to give excellent exposure.

De Takats believes that the most important aspect of this operation is the proper selection of patients. He stated that failure is foreordained if a sympathectomy is done on a patient with "incipient, latent, or unrecognized collagen disease." He obtained excellent results in patients with Raynaud's due to obstructive vascular disease (Buerger's disease, embolic, and thrombotic disease) and in patients with Raynaud's who were demonstrated to have a diencephalic discharge.[388] He stated that the T1–T5 segment must be removed to get a reliable upper extremity sympathetic paralysis.[387]

The results of sympathectomy are mixed at best. Gifford, Hines, and Craig[402] found that only 54 percent of women (37 of 68) with Raynaud's disease who had the operation had a good long-term result. Most of those who did not have a good long-term result had a good short-term result, with a relapse in the first 1 to 2 years. Seventy-two percent of patients with Raynaud's syndrome had a poor result. Kirtly and colleagues[424] did 104 sympathectomies in 76 patients and noted most of the poor results in patients with a collagen disease. Baddeley,[371] in a series of 64 patients with Raynaud's disease, found about 50 percent good results after 6 years. Johnston, Summerly, and Birnstingl[417] reported results that are in general agreement with the others cited. McLaughlin[436] proposed an interesting procedure for patients too ill to undergo a surgical sympathectomy, namely, infusion of lidocaine via a catheter placed adjacent to the stellate ganglion. He stated that he had used this for as long as 5 days.

Flatt presented an intriguing new approach to sympathectomy at the digital level.[396] A 3- to 4-mm length of the proper digital artery is stripped of as much adventitia as possible without compromising the vessel.[446] He reported on eight patients that were followed for 1 to 12 years. All had relief of symptoms and an increase in skin temperature, except one woman with Raynaud's disease who had a relapse. Egloff, Mifsud, and Verdan[392] have treated 13 patients with digital artery sympathectomies and reported good to excellent results. Morgan and Wilgis[438] evaluated this technique experimentally in a rabbit ear model and noted good results, i.e., the sympathectomized ears remained warm. Wilgis[465] has emphasized the need for careful preoperative evaluation in patients being considered for digital artery sympathectomy. He notes that they must experience improvement in response to cold stress following digital blockade to be considered candidates for this type of operative treatment.

Other diagnoses include post-cold injury, post-traumatic vasospasm, and scleroderma. The magnitude of this procedure is considerably less than that of a cervicodorsal sympathectomy, and this approach offers a much more discrete attack when only one or two digits are affected with vascular compromise or trophic changes.

It is difficult to predict with precision whether or not a patient with Raynaud's phenomenon will eventually develop a collagen disease, although they certainly must be considered a high-risk group. Physical findings are not always as helpful as one might expect. Farmer, Gifford, and Hines[394] studied 71 patients with Raynaud's disease and sclerodactyly and found that only three of them developed scleroderma.

Other Vasospastic Diseases

Buerger's disease,[381] or thromboangiitis obliterans, is not often seen in the upper extremities. It is an inflammatory thrombosis seen mostly in young men[410] who are very heavy smokers,[456] and is characterized by a relentless progression of ischemic changes that are arrested if smoking is stopped.

Constam[385] reported the disease in the upper extremities of 24 of 94 patients studied at the Mayo Clinic. The diagnosis was made on the basis of pulseless vessels, signs of vascular insufficiency, and vasomotor phenomena. McKuseck and colleagues[435] in 1962 studied 12 patients with arteriography. All were men (ages 15 to 43), all were smokers, and, of the four biopsied, all had histologically proven inflammatory disease of the arteries. The only practical treatment is to stop smoking. Ischemic lesions are treated as local conditions dictate.

There are scattered reports[415] in the literature of serious medical illnesses that are preceded or accompanied by a fairly fulminant Raynaud's syndrome with ischemic or even gangrenous changes in digits. Hawley, Johnston, and Rankin[409] reported six such cases, all of them in women who subsequently developed a malignancy. Only three of their patients were smokers. Andrasch and colleagues[370] noted a similar problem in a patient who subsequently developed a renal neoplasm. Raynaud's syndrome has been the harbinger of hepatitis[386] and an accompanist of chronic renal failure.[403] Elderly patients with acute medical illness of no more specific diagnosis than multiple organ failure may develop the problem in one

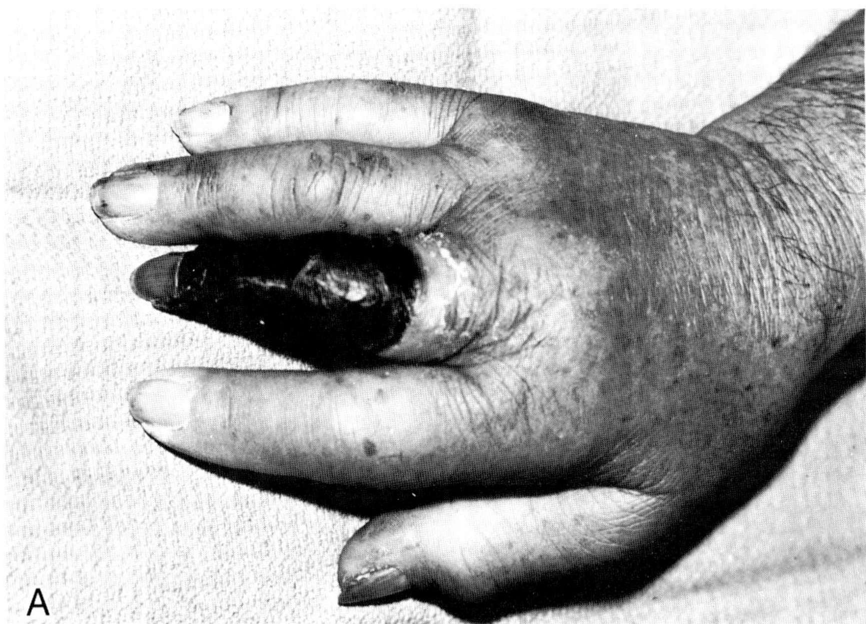

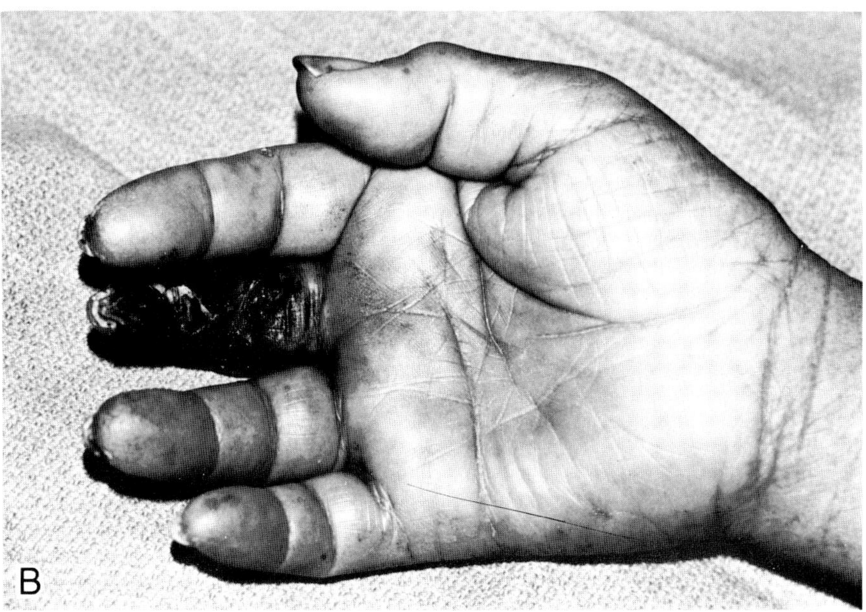

Fig. 62-28. This 75-year-old woman was admitted to a hospital because of general debility and an ischemic long fingertip. **(A&B)** No cause for the ischemia could be found and it progressed relentlessly. *(Figure continues.)*

or more extremities.[405] The hand of an elderly woman with such a problem is seen in Figure 62-28. The problem may also be encountered at the other end of the age spectrum with gangrene in the hand of a newborn.[413,455] Giant cell arteritis may be the cause of symptomatic occlusive disease at the level of the subclavian and axillary arteries,[451] as well as causing occlusive vascular symptoms in the hand.[113] A variety of other rather rare diseases, including Wegner's granulomatosis, polyarteritis nodosa, and Takayasu's arteritis may manifest themselves in the upper extremity vascular system.[445] Patients with hyperparathyroidism[378] and patients on dialysis with possible iron overload from transfusions may develop ischemic changes in the extremities.[454a] Workers exposed to vinyl chloride may also develop ischemic problems in the digits.[393]

Several drugs taken systemically have been implicated in causing gangrenous changes in the hand. Ergotamine, taken for migraines, is the most common.[395,422,459] Neoarsphenamine, when used for the treatment of syphilis, is reported to have caused gangrene in a hand.[430]

Unfortunately, there is little reconstructive surgery available for the hand surgeon to perform in this group of diseases. The operations to be done are usually amputations (see Chapter 3).

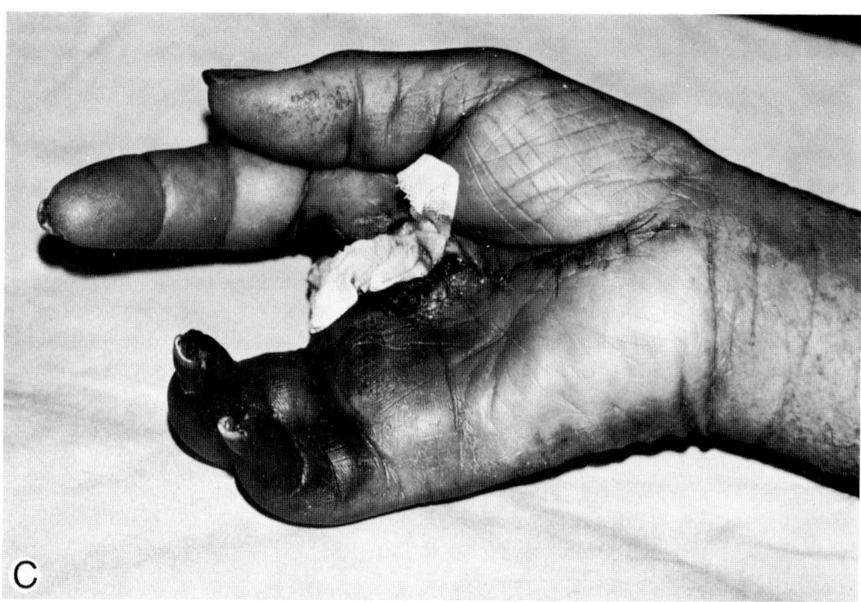

Fig. 62-28 *(Continued).* **(C)** Shortly after long finger amputation, the ring and little fingers became gangrenous. Eventually midforearm amputation was necessary, at which time the radial and ulnar arteries were found to be thrombosed. She died a few months later, but no explanation for this phenomenon could be found.

Any amputation performed should be at a level of assured vascularity with absolutely no tension on the flaps. A very loose closure or leaving the wound open is preferable to attempting to achieve a finely tailored stump in these ischemic digits. Most of the other procedures for these disorders are outside the purview of most hand surgeons. As a group, however, hand surgeons should be able to offer some diagnostic insight about any problem that manifests itself in the hand, and perhaps be able to suggest diagnostic and therapeutic steps to help the patient.

Atherosclerosis is very uncommon in the upper extremities. It may be found in the large vessels at the base of the neck and in the axilla.[408,427] Clinical manifestation of the disease in the hand itself is very rare, particularly when contrasted with the frequency of its presence in the lower extremity. Taylor et al[460] found evidence of this disease in digital arteries in 5 of 37 patients with small artery occlusive disease, seen in a 7-year period in a center renowned for a study of vascular problems. Caffee and Master[382] treated three patients with severe atherosclerotic disease in the upper extremity by bypass vein grafts from the forearm to the superficial palmar arch.

VASCULAR TUMORS

The final two sections of this chapter discuss vascular tumors and arteriovenous fistulas. Vascular tumors include hemangiomas, glomus tumors, malignant vascular tumors, lymphangiomas, and miscellaneous vascular lesions. Hemangiomas and congenital arteriovenous fistulas have much in common etiologically, and the reader may wish to skip ahead and briefly review the section on etiology of congenital arteriovenous fistulas at this time (see page 2289).

Butler and colleagues[483] reported on 437 hand tumors and noted only 36 vascular tumors of any description (8 percent). Twenty-six of these were angiomas, four glomus tumors, four pyogenic granulomas, and two traumatic aneurysms. Stack,[562] in reporting on 300 hand tumors, found only 15 (5 percent) vascular tumors, including six hemangiomas, six pyogenic granulomas, one traumatic aneurysm, one organized hematoma, and one thrombophlebitis migrans. Palmieri[541] reported a very large series of subcutaneous hemangiomas seen over a 10-year period. He noted that these 160 patients accounted for 8 percent of all hand tumors seen during this period. Johnson et al[511] by contrast, found that only 3.3 percent of 543 hand tumors were vascular.

Hemangiomas

Classification and Origin

Skin and Subcutaneous Hemangiomas

Basically, there are cavernous hemangiomas, capillary hemangiomas, and a mixture of these.[492,498,510,535,539,568,572,577] Elkin and Cooper[492] noted that hemangiomas are tumors of independently growing blood channels that probably have their origin as embryonic rudiments of mesodermal tissue. In a study of 93 hemangiomas of the extremities, Johnson, Ghormley, and Dockerty[510] found that 33 percent were manifest at birth and 57 percent by age 30. Watson and McCarthy[577] studied 1056 patients at Memorial Hospital in New York who were seen between 1931 and 1939. These patients had 1363 lesions, 1243 of them being cavernous (952) or capillary (291) hemangiomas. There were 55 lymphatic tumors. Of the remaining 65 lesions, most can be placed into either capillary or cavernous classifications. These authors also noted a striking association between young age and the time when the lesion was first noted. Seventy-three percent were seen at birth and 85 percent by age one.

Morris[573] made an extensive study of hemangiomas and offered the very useful functional classification of involuting and noninvoluting tumors. All involuting lesions are present at birth or noted soon thereafter, grow rapidly for 4 to 6 months, at which time they begin to involute, and generally disappear by age seven. He noted, as did Watson and McCarthy, that the head and neck are the most common locations, but that a significant number is seen in the extremities. Lister,[523] in a literature search and in personal experience with 77 children having 93 strawberry nevi (capillary hemangiomas), noted in 1938 that "no exception has been found to the rule that nevi which grow rapidly during the early months of life subsequently retrogress and disappear of their own accord, on the average by the fifth year of life." Others share this view.[520]

Morris[573] and Blackfield and colleagues[478-480] found that the ratio of involuting to noninvoluting tumors in all patients is 4:1 or more. The involuting type may be either capillary (Fig. 62-29), cavernous, or mixed. Cavernous hemangiomas will not involute, but subcutaneous capillary hemangiomas, which look cavernous, usually will. The noninvoluting type may also be either capillary or cavernous. However, there are some useful guidelines to distinguish between involuting and noninvoluting. Noninvoluting capillary hemangiomas invariably are the so-called port wine stain, or nevus flammeus.[522] This is a broad, flat lesion, usually on the face but sometimes on the extremities, that looks like a red, splotchy stain. It is almost impossible to eradicate and is best left alone and hidden with cosmetics. The noninvoluting cavernous type will almost always have a significant element of an arteriovenous fistula.

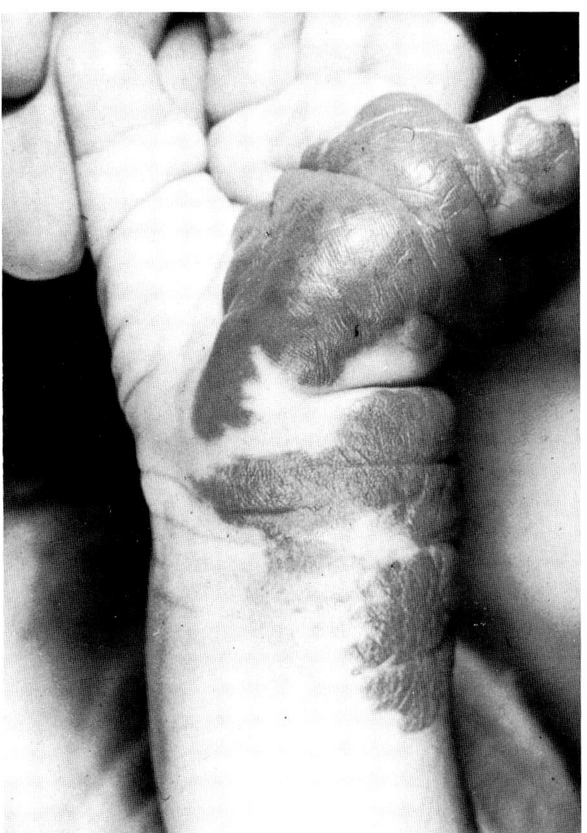

Fig. 62-29. This 5-month-old child had a strawberry hemangioma (involuting capillary hemangioma) that was entirely gone by the age of five. (Courtesy of WJ Morris, MD.)

These lesions, which account for most of the hemangiomas seen in the upper extremity, are all either in the skin or subcutaneous tissue. There are several other hemangiomas of the upper extremity that merit mention, not because they are of another type, but because of their association with various tissues or unusual syndromes.

Skeletal Muscle Hemangiomas

Watson and McCarthy[577] found only 10 skeletal muscle hemangiomas in 1363 vascular lesions. Allen and Enzinger[471] analyzed 89 cases in the files of the Armed Forces Institute of Pathology and identified three types: small vessel, large vessel, and mixed. The small vessel tumors were usually diagnosed as vascular, only by their histologic appearance, while the other two could be grossly identified as vascular tumors. The different types do not carry any marked prognostic differences.

These lesions are probably congenital in origin.[512,521,557] They are seen in a variety of locations,[405,457] with no special predilection for the upper extremity. When found in the upper extremity, they may be in either intrinsic[487] or extrinsic musculature.[495] Wood[578] reported three patients with hemangiomas associated with bone lesions. He observed that patients with bone lesions combined with hemangiomas merit close observation, because malignant transformation and/or fractures of bones weakened by the hemangiomas may occur.

Hemangiomas may infiltrate not only the muscle but also other adjacent tissues and be extremely difficult to extirpate without sacrificing normal structures.[532,556]

Other Hemangiomas

Hemangiomas may be physically associated with the median nerve, causing a carpal tunnel syndrome[518,542,543] (Fig. 62-30), or seen with cranial or other peripheral nerves.[519,524,537] Maffucci's syndrome, an unusual condition, is the association of skeletal chondromas and soft tissue angiomas.[488,508] In an entity known as phantom disease of bone, in which the bone is dissolved, the lesion is histologically a hemangioma and has been described in the hand.[571,578] Thrombocytopenic purpura associated with a large hemangioma was first described by Kasabach and Merritt in 1940.[515] It is thought that platelets become sequestered in the sluggish blood in the hemangioma.[530] Straub et al[569] studied a patient with a giant hemangioma, and their results "suggest that a localized rather than a generalized process of fibrin formation is responsible for the coagulation abnormalities and the hemorrhagic diathesis." Resolution of the hemangioma resolves the problem of the thrombocytopenia.

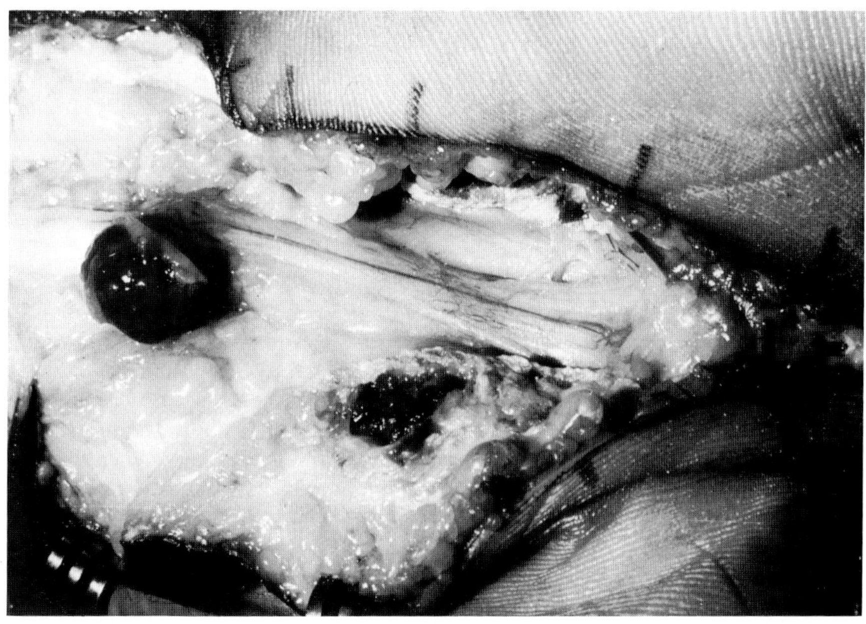

Fig. 62-30. This well-localized hemangioma in the carpal tunnel caused pressure on the median nerve and a clinical carpal tunnel syndrome. (Courtesy of ES Kilgore, Jr, MD.)

An hemangioma has been found in a middle phalanx[570] and in a metacarpophalangeal joint,[494] where it caused locking.

Diagnosis of Hemangiomas

Knowledge of the time of appearance of the lesion is most important in its diagnosis and prognosis. Sometimes hemangiomas are associated with trauma, [476,510] but trauma is probably the uncovering event rather than the inciting event.

By far, the most common symptoms are pain and discomfort or fullness in the affected area.[512] A mass is almost always present and may be cutaneous, subcutaneous, or deep. It may be spongy and compressible or quite firm.[521] The mass may increase in size with warm weather or with menstruation.[481]

Cutaneous lesions will have some red hue. Subcutaneous lesions will often be a splotchy blue color (Fig. 62-31). If the hemangioma is in a muscle whose action can be easily isolated, there will be loss of discrete function.[529] Such a case has been described involving the common profundus muscle belly.[507] Not only was there loss of terminal phalangeal flexion, but a flexion deformity developed.

If a thrill or bruit is felt or heard, the lesion is better classified with arteriovenous fistulas. The relationship between hemangiomas and arteriovenous fistulas is a very close one, and the lesions are probably different manifestations of the same embryonic development gone awry.

Radiographs of the lesions will often show a soft tissue mass, and calcifications are commonly noted in the mass.[487,554] Arteriography may help to visualize the lesion (see page 2260), but this test is not often done because the diagnosis of hemangioma may not be entertained preoperatively. Certainly, with any large tumor that is apparently vascular in origin, an effect to visualize it angiographically should be made.[528]

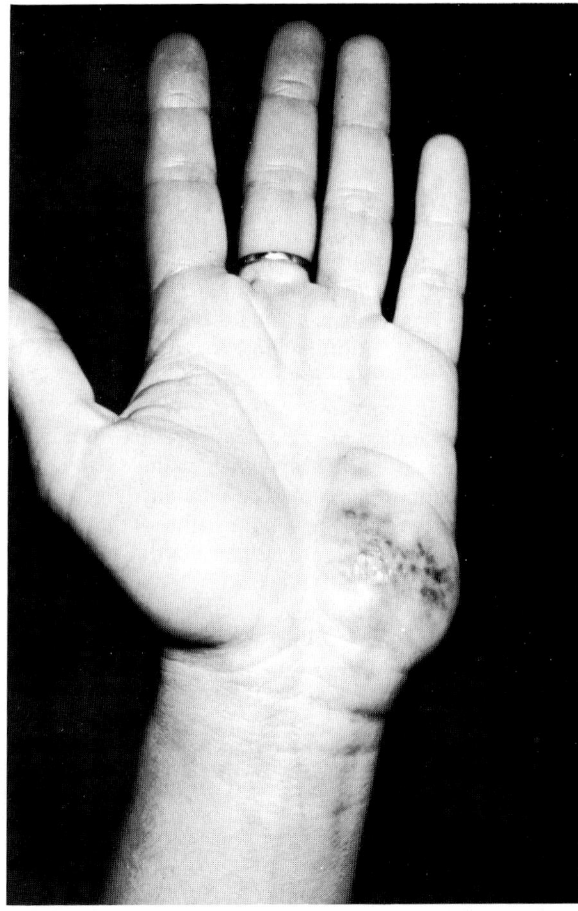

Fig. 62-31. This 40-year-old man has a static cavernous hemangioma of the hand. He is not eager to have surgery done.

Treatment of Hemangiomas

It is obvious from the preceding discussion that hemangiomas that make their appearance at birth or soon thereafter should be left alone, since most of them will involute. Occasionally, large involuting tumors will cause problems of ulceration and bleeding, and these complications must be dealt with in a conservative fashion, realizing that they are only stopgap maneuvers. Before Lister's[523] observations became known, there was a tendency to be surgically aggressive with these lesions,[485] but on the basis of current knowledge, early operative treatment should not be done.

The fortuitous disappearance of a hemangioma in an adult following visualization with radiopaque dye has been reported.[545] However, this does not appear to be a method that can be relied upon. Radiation therapy has been used, but as Watson and McCarthy[577] note, its success is inversely related to the age of the patient. The disappearance of lesions in young children given radiation therapy is probably due to the natural course of the lesion, as much as to the radiation administered. Because of the well-known adverse effects of radiation, especially in the young, this treatment is to be discouraged. Owens and Stephenson[538] reported on the use of sodium morrhuate injections with good results, but their patients were mostly young and the lesions would probably have regressed spontaneously.

Cryosurgery has been used for intraoral hemangiomas that were not amenable to surgical treatment, with good results and minimal complications noted.[509] Apfelberg and co-workers have used the argon laser for treatment of capillary hemangiomas in infants[473] and the YAG laser for treatment of these lesions in one child and seven adults.[474] In the latter cases only one excision was noted to be total. Zarem and Edgerton[491,579] found that systemic cortisone induces resolution of cavernous hemangiomas. Miller, Smith, and Schochat[531] found long-term compression therapy a useful adjunct in controlling large hemangiomas. They postulated that this method may induce earlier resolution in involuting tumors and reduce the size of noninvoluting tumors, at least temporarily. They stressed that custom-fitted garments must be worn.

Surgical extirpation is the treatment of choice for noninvoluting lesions, except for the capillary hemangioma known as the port wine stain, which should be left alone. The success of surgical excision is related more to the nature of the lesion than to anything else. If the lesion is well localized, the surgery will almost always be successful (Fig. 62-32). If the lesion is ill-defined and infiltrative, recurrence is common, and additional surgical procedures are often necessary. Johnson, Ghormley, and Dockerty,[510] in treating 70 circumscribed and 20 diffuse lesions, had to perform 46 operations on the 20 patients with diffuse lesions, including three amputations. Allen and Enzinger,[471] in their review, noted a minimum recurrence rate of 9 percent with the large vessel group, 20 percent in the small vessel group, and 28 percent in the mixed vessel group.

When the initial surgery is done, feeding and drainage vessels should be carefully isolated and ligated.[499] The lesion should be excised in toto, sparing crucial structures. Occasionally, a two-stage procedure is indicated — the first to ligate vessels and the second to remove the lesion — but this is much more likely to be necessary with an arteriovenous fistula.

If there is a small recurrent tumor, it should be excised when it appears, as this is often curative.[487,505] If the lesion is very extensive, amputation may be required as the primary operation.[501,551]

Glomus Tumors

Of all the vascular tumors of the upper extremity, this is the one that excites the most interest. The reasons for this are manifold: it is rare, it presents with a striking clinical picture, and when correctly treated, the cure rate is close to 100 percent.

Masson[526] described a tumor of the neuromyoarterial apparatus, which he called the glomus (hence, glomus tumor) in 1924. It is a normal structure whose function is to regulate temperature.[567] Popoff[546] described the apparatus and its function in 1934. He found that it consisted of five parts: (1) an afferent artery; (2) Sucquet-Hoyer canal (the arteriovenous channel); (3) neuroreticular and vascular structures around these canals; (4) an outer layer of lamellated collagenous tissue; and (5) primary collecting veins. He noted that the glomus exists in large numbers beneath nails and in finger pads, and in lesser but still substantial numbers elsewhere in the hands and feet.

Murray and Stout[536] in 1942 identified the characteristic epithelioid cell of the glomus tumor as being derived from the pericyte of Zimmerman. These cells have a wide distribution in the body. This fact explains the wide distribution of glomus tumors. This cell is also the one from which the very rare hemangiopericytoma tumor arises.[552,565,574] Glomus tumors have a highly organized architecture, are encapsulated, and have a large number of nerves associated with them, while hemangiopericytomas are less defined.[566] There is a striking increase in the number of nerves either in[482] or adjacent to[558] the lesion, which explains the great sensitivity of glomus tumors.

Clinical Patterns of Glomus Tumors

Patients with these tumors present with the triad of pain, tenderness, and cold sensitivity.[484] Pain is the first symptom to appear. The tenderness is very striking and specific. If a patient complains persistently of a consistently painful, tender area around the distal finger, a very careful examination using the head of a pin to palpate may uncover one very tender spot. The patient will complain of a lancinating, burning pain and will pull the finger away. Even if no mass is visible, the evidence for a glomus tumor is very good.[559] Cold may also set off the attacks of severe paroxysmal pain.

In appearance, a glomus tumor may suggest a small hemangioma.[470] The tumor may cause ridging of the nail. A radiograph may show indentation of the distal phalanx from the pressure of the tumor.[497] The tumor may be seen in children,[517] although it is more common in adults. Multiple tumors may be seen in one fingertip. Plewes[544] reported four separate ones in the finger pulp of a 16-year-old boy. In the hand, these tumors have been found in the body of the distal phalanx[486] and in the head of a metacarpal,[553] as well as associated with pacinian hyperplasia.[503] Joseph and Posner[513] reported three patients

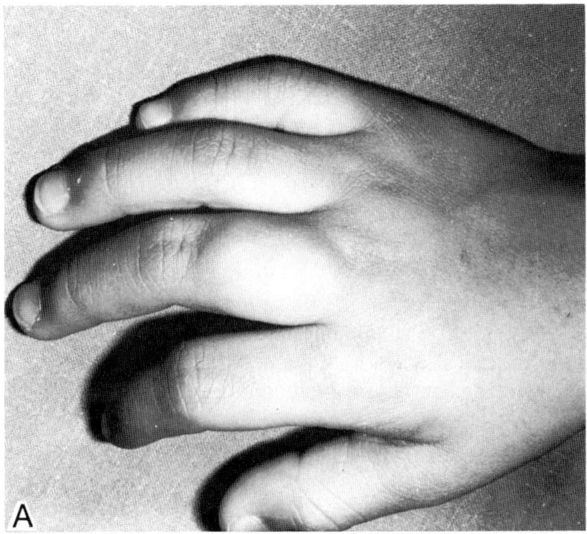

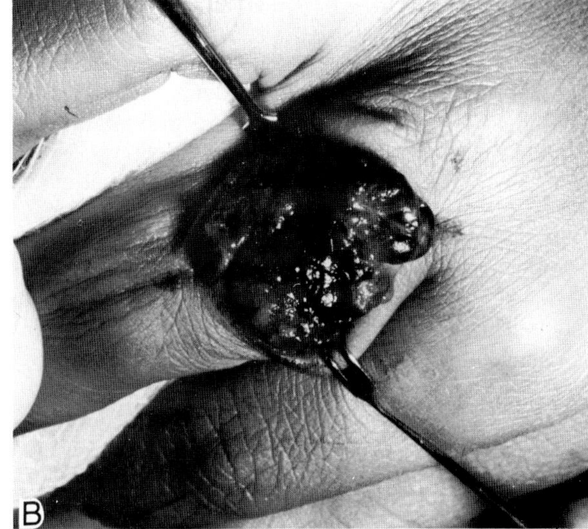

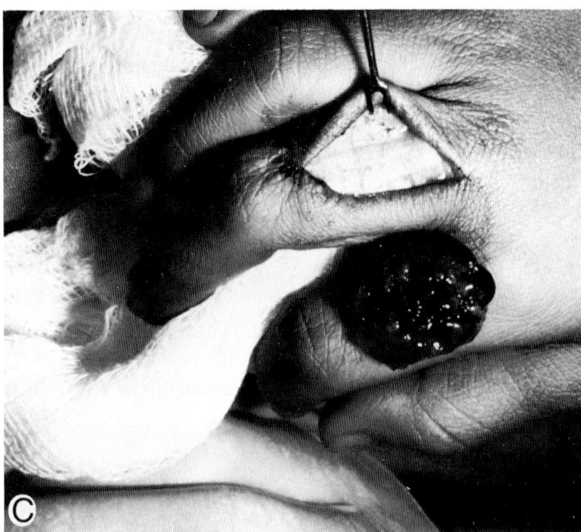

Fig. 62-32. **(A)** This 5-year-old presented with a soft mass on the dorsum of the long finger. **(B&C)** Operative exposure showed it to be a small, well-circumscribed hemangioma that was easily removed. It might well have involuted if it had been left alone.

with glomus tumors of the wrist. The tumor is seen in whites, orientals, and blacks.[560] Shugart, Soule, and Johnson[558] reviewed 74 glomus tumors in 74 patients and found a male-to-female ratio of 1.7 : 1. They found only 19 (26 percent) of these tumors to be subungual, but 54 (74 percent) were in the upper extremity. Other locations include the neck, thigh, knee, leg, foot, and toes. Mason and Weil[525] reported a patient with the tumor at the knee, and Grauer and Burt[502] saw two patients with glomus tumors in the penis.

Treatment of Glomus Tumors

The treatment of glomus tumors is surgical extirpation. The lesion should be identified with magnification (surgical loupes) and totally excised. Even though the lesion is usually distal and small, I recommend a regional anesthetic rather than local infiltration so that the lesion may be carefully dissected out of the surrounding tissues. If the location of the lesion is subungual, the nail should be removed and the nail bed incised and meticulously repaired after tumor removal with fine (5-0 and 6-0) absorbable sutures. If this treatment is carried out, the problem will be solved. However, as Carroll and Berman[484] have observed, it is easy for the unwary surgeon to operate right on top of the lesion and overlook it, leaving the patient unrelieved of his misery.

Malignant Hemangiomas

It is very rare for hemangiomas to become malignant.[498] There are two basic types of malignant hemangiomas: angiosarcoma and Kaposi's sarcoma.[437] Both are more common in adult white males and are seen in the extremities.

Angiosarcomas are red vascular tumors that metastasize.[575]

The biologic behavior of these tumors is variable,[564] and if they are treated early with wide excision, a cure is often achieved.[568]

According to Baxt, Mori, and Hoffman,[475] Kaposi's sarcoma is "an indolent growth of vascular tissues found in the skin of middle-aged men, starting typically in the extremities and spreading to other cutaneous sites and to the viscera." The lesions are small, bluish-red to dark brown plaques and nodules.[522] The clinical course is variable, and the disease may pursue a long indolent course or it may be fatal in a fairly short time.[568] With the advent of AIDS in the last 10 years this tumor has become much more common and has been reported in the hand literature.[516] Baxt, Mori, and Hoffman described a case in a young man with an aneurysm of the ulnar artery caused by the disease. Resection of the aneurysm resulted in total remission of the disease.[475]

Lymphangiomas

These tumors are a rare subgroup of the uncommon hemangiomas.[568] Wegner (cited by Watson and McCarthy[577]) classified lymphangiomas into three types: simple lymphangiomas, cavernous lymphangiomas, and cystic lymphangiomas (cystic hygromas). There seems to be general agreement on this classification, although Watson and McCarthy[577] described two additional categories that are subdivisions of the cavernous lymphangioma: cellular or hypertrophic lymphangioma and diffuse systemic lymphangioma.

Simple lymphangiomas border on being just simple lymphangiectasia. The lesions are small and well circumscribed with a wartlike appearance and have little tendency to grow. They may be treated by local excision.

Cavernous lymphangioma is the commonest variety. The lesion appears at birth or shortly thereafter, and consists of dilated lymphatic sinuses. They may become quite massive and involve an entire upper extremity. Elements of hemangiomas may be present. This can be a very difficult lesion to remove, and occasionally an extensive amputation is needed.[481,496,504,548] Radiation may be helpful in controlling recurrences, which are common.[550,577]

Cystic hygromas occur in the neck or, rarely, the axilla.[550] They arise from the primitive jugular sacs, are present at birth, and grow rapidly. Treatment is by surgical excision.[577]

Lymphangiosarcoma is seen in upper extremities that have had massive lymphedema for many years. This is typically in the woman with postmastectomy lymphedema. Cure is by radical surgery (i.e., forequarter amputation).[489,555,563] The lesion has been reported in a patient who had a congenital lymphangioma and never had irradiation.[534]

Other Benign Vascular Tumors

Hemangioendothelioma is a very rare, probably benign, vascular tumor that may be seen in the hand.[469,534] It may be confused with angiosarcoma, and the precise line between benign and malignant is difficult to draw with these tumors.[495]

Vascularized hamartomas also are lesions that may be symptomatic in the upper extremity when there is hemorrhage in them.[477,514] Eosinophilic granuloma is a bone destructive lesion that has been reported in the hand.[540] Tumors that may be mistaken for hemangiomas are infiltrating angiolipomas[576] and angiolymphoid hyperplasia.[506] They must be completely excised. The latter lesion may be mistaken for AIDS-related Kaposi's sarcoma, but a negative HIV test will aid in the correct diagnosis.[549]

Other Vascular Lesions

Telangiectasia is a dilatation of small vessels in or near the skin. Spittell[561] listed four types: (1) simple telangiectasia, (2) senile telangiectasia, (3) cutaneous arterial spiders, and (4) hereditary hemorrhagic telangiectasia.

The first two types are of little clinical significance and occur in adults, often with some obvious inciting cause. The third type is of interest mainly because of its association with hepatic disease. The fourth type is important because of lesions in mucous membranes, which may bleed massively. Lesions of the hands are troublesome rather than dangerous.

The pyogenic granuloma is an accretion of inflammatory granulation tissue that has been found intravenously in the hand[472,490], but is more commonly seen in a chronic wound at the end of a digit (Fig. 62-33). Excision with cauterization of the vascular bed is generally curative.

ARTERIOVENOUS FISTULAS

When one looks at a river safely and peacefully confined to its normal bed, it is hard to imagine the wild ferocity it may attain at flood time. Similarly, when one looks at a normal

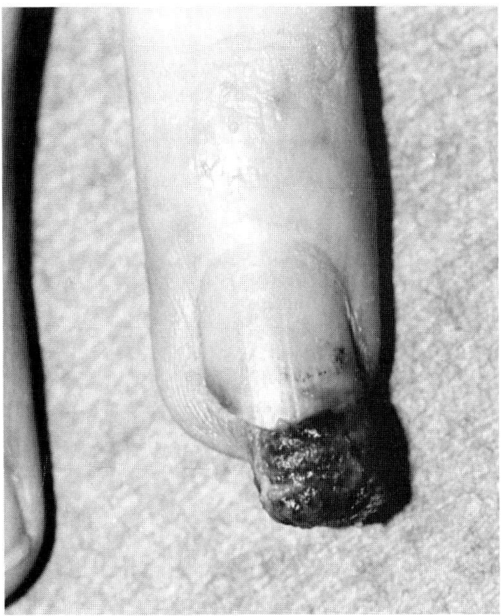

Fig. 62-33. A 25-year-old man had a minor laceration on his fingertip which led to this ugly lesion some weeks later. Although it looks rather alarming, it is a simple pyogenic granuloma.

upper extremity, it is hard to imagine the increased girth it may attain with the swollen, pulsatile vessels that may exist with an arteriovenous fistula. The normal in each case is hardly noticed; the abnormal prints itself indelibly on the observer's mind.

An arteriovenous fistula[601,659,660,666] is a communication between artery and vein that short-circuits the normal capillary circulation. It is usually an abnormal finding, but in fetal life the ductus arteriosus and in postnatal life the glomus are examples of normal arteriovenous fistulas. Abnormal congenital arteriovenous fistulas characteristically have multiple small connections between arterial and venous circulation.[468,546,595,609,649] An acquired fistula usually has a single connection that is easily identified surgically. Acquired fistulas are invariably traumatic and are caused by a penetrating injury that pierces a vein and an artery where they lie in close juxtaposition. This same type of injury may result in a false aneurysm if the artery alone is injured. Today, a third category (a subcategory of the acquired type) exists—the surgical arteriovenous fistula created for chronic renal dialysis.

William Hunter is given credit for first accurately describing a traumatic arteriovenous fistula in 1757.[625] He noted the bruit and thrill over the fistula, the dilating pulsating veins, and the proximal arterial enlargement.

Congenital Arteriovenous Fistulas

Etiology

We owe our present concept of the etiology of congenital arteriovenous fistulas to Florence Sabin[647] and HH Woollard.[668] In the late nineteenth and early twentieth centuries, there was a lively controversy in embryology regarding the development of the vascular system in limbs. On the one hand was the idea that blood vessels originate as definite formed tubes, and on the other was the idea that a primitive vascular network formed and from this, the venous and arterial systems differentiated. Woollard, acknowledging his debt to Sabin and especially to HM Evans, formulated his ideas and expressed them in a paper in 1922. He identified three separate stages in the development of individual arterial tubes: (1) the stage of the capillary net; (2) the retiform stage, characterized by enlarged tubes showing island formation, coalescence, and a tendency to fuse; and (3) the formation of definite vascular stems.

Reinhoff[646] studied chick embryos and observed a capillary network that was first entirely arterial undergo transformation and assume a venous character brought about by the formation of new connections between the original capillary network and venous trunks. He wrote, "the capillary network which previously served as an arterial channel now serves as a venous channel." He commented on a letter sent to him by Sabin, in which she described her observation of the development of an arteriovenous fistula in a chick embryo injected with a bacterial broth. He concluded that (1) congenital vascular anomalies may be predominantly venous or arterial, or have significant components of each; (2) congenital arteriovenous fistulas may be continuous or discontinuous with the main vessel; and (3) all congenital vascular tumors are due to embryonic persistence, and that this includes congenital hemangiomas.

If we accept these findings, situations observed clinically become clear or at least comprehensible. The findings show the definite common etiology of congenital arteriovenous fistulas and congenital hemangiomas.[665] The reason for the multiple small connections of congenital arteriovenous fistulas becomes obvious.

The most frustrating and confusing aspect that the student of congenital vascular problems confronts is the bewildering number of categories into which the problems are classified.[622] Reid[645] in 1925 stated, "From a study of the reported cases of cirsoid aneurysm [sic, cirsoid aneurysm—pulsating angioma, racemose aneurysm, aneurysm by anastomosis] and of my own cases [sic, arteriovenous fistulas], I cannot escape the conclusion that there is no difference between this condition and arterio-venous aneurysm, except that cirsoid aneurysm has been applied to that condition which results where abnormal arterio-venous communications occur in the more peripheral and smaller vessels." Commenting further on the etiology of angiomas, he noted that, "I cannot escape the conclusion that they are dilations of the small arteries and veins caused by a traumatic or congenital abnormal communication between the smallest arteries and veins." His obvious conclusion was that cirsoid aneurysm and angiomas are not neoplastic growths.

De Takats[598] reported on five patients with vascular anomalies of the extremities and stated, "most angiomas are only angiectasias" (i.e., dilatation of blood vessels). However, he went on to list five types with physically descriptive but etiologically unenlightening terminology. He concluded that "none of these vascular tumors are true growths but all are due to faulty development, and the variations encountered are due to the stage of vascular development in which the aberration from normal occurred." Thus, capillary angiomas (vascular nevi) are localized remnants of arrest at Woollard's stage one and are harmless unless traumatized. Congenital arteriovenous fistulas and diffuse phlebectasia come from arrest in the retiform or second stage. Malan and Puglionisi,[626,627] in a massive, two-part study published in 1964 and 1965, evaluated congenital angiodysplasias of the extremities. They stated that the problems are either genetic or caused in utero. They acknowledged the importance of the work of Sabin, Woollard, and Reinhoff as the factor in primary morphogenesis. They found that the vascular malformations may be either dysplasias (normal formations with structural deviations) or hamartias (anomalous formations of normally present tissues). The dysplasias are the ectatic (dilated) vessels seen in many arteriovenous fistulas. Angiomas are hamartias. Secondary factors that influence the development of vascular malformations include local hemodynamic factors, local trauma, and local infections.

Malan and Puglionisi grouped the abnormalities into the following four categories:

I. Venous dysplasias
II. Arterial dysplasias (very rare)
III. Arteriovenous dysplasias
IV. Mixed angiodysplasias

Each of these groups has one or more subcategories. Of particular interest, because it is the group that affects the upper extremity, is Group III. It consists of two main subgroups, congenital arteriovenous troncular fistulas (CAVF) and arteriovenous angiomas (AVAN). These lesions may be either active or hypoactive. Twenty-four CAVF and four AVAN were active, the remainder hypoactive.

Szilagyi and colleagues[657] in 1965 reported 33 cases of peripheral arteriovenous fistulas and proposed the following classification:

Designation	Embryonic Arrest Stage
Hemangioma	Stage I
Microfistulous avf	Stage II
Macrofistulous avf	Stage III

avf = arteriovenous fistula.

The reason for dwelling on the problem of etiology and classification is that it is an area of endless confusion. The terms encountered (racemose aneurysm, cirsoid aneurysm, troncular fistula, arterialized cavernous hemangioma, etc.) imply a vast number of different kinds of lesions, when the difference is really one of degree. It is a continuous spectrum with a unitary source.

When any single problem is encountered, a very useful approach is to evaluate the lesion as in the following manner.

1. Depth—Skin or subcutaneous?
2. Color—Red (capillary), blue (venous), or blue-red (arterial)?
3. Containment—Circumscribed or massive and infiltrating?
4. Arteriovenous shunt (bruit or thrill) by examination, Doppler, or arteriogram?

On the basis of the answers to the above questions, it should be possible to classify the lesion as primarily capillary, venous, arterial, or a combination of these. The old terms will persist and they are certainly useful for their descriptive qualities, but for the surgeon seeing an occasional congenital vascular problem, this approach should make it easier to classify the lesion.

Hemodynamic and Physical Changes of Arteriovenous Fistulas

The extent of the hemodynamic changes that occur depends on the size of the fistula. The changes include an increase in the heart rate, a decrease in the blood pressure, a decrease in the peripheral vascular resistance, and an increase in the circulating blood volume. These changes come about as the body adjusts to supply two vascular circuits—the normal and the fistulous.[611,612,634] With a large arteriovenous fistula, proximal compression of the feeding artery will cause a decrease in the heart rate that is sometimes quite dramatic with a large shunt. This is known as Branham's bradycardic sign.[586,612] When a shunt is closed, the heart rate drops and the blood pressure increases transiently.

In association with a long-standing arteriovenous shunt, there will be marked dilatation of the artery proximal to the fistula, even extending to the heart.[608] The walls of veins involved in the fistula become thickened with more elastic tissue (become "arterialized"), and the arteries undergo "venization,"[640,643] Many observers have commented on the increased length of affected limbs, although this is not a universal finding with congenital fistulas.[614,639,663] This would occur in an acquired fistula only if it were in a child and of long duration.

Increased skin temperature in the limb around the fistula is commonly found.[610,662] Distally, however, the temperature may be cooler, and trophic changes of ischemia are often seen. This is due to both the paucity of oxygenated blood going distally (a steal syndrome[626]) and to the impedance of venous return due to increased pressure on the venous side.[639,583] Bertelsen and Dohn[583] proposed that the massive shunt of blood that causes the distal ischemia may stimulate the formation of collateral circulation, which only complicates the situation by drawing even more blood into the fistulous extremity. Lewis[624] supported this contention.

Cardiac hypertrophy and heart failure may occur with upper extremity[628] arteriovenous fistulas, but this probably does not happen with those fistulas distal to the elbow. Creech, Gantt, and Wren[594] noted that the hemodynamic effect of a fistula is limited by its size, which can be no greater than the diameter of the feeding artery. They found that only 15 percent of arteriovenous fistulas produced systemic effects, and stated, "those peripheral to the brachial and popliteal arteries never produce systemic effects."

Diagnosis of Congenital Arteriovenous Fistulas

Congenital arteriovenous fistulas are not common, and most reports about them come either from large referral centers or include only a few cases. The limbs, head, and neck are involved more often than the major body cavities—the upper extremity in 30 to 60 percent of cases.[591,604,614,618,621–623,644,657]

Diagnosis should not be too difficult when the patient seeks help because of symptoms from an arteriovenous fistula. The history is extremely important. Most patients will acknowledge that they "knew something was wrong" or "knew something was there" at a fairly early age. Around 50 percent of the lesions become manifest before the age of two, and 60 percent by the age of 10.[614,626] Trauma may either cause the lesions to become more serious or cause the patients to notice them.[546,596] In patients who first notice the lesion after the age of 10, a typical story is an episode of blunt trauma to a digit or the hand in the teen-age years, with a small mass becoming noticeable. Pain and swelling become more persistent in the twenties, and the patient eventually seeks medical help.[586,605,669]

Varices, a common complaint in the lower extremity, are not so common in the upper extremity, and their presence should make one consider an arteriovenous fistula at once. A typical situation is seen in Figure 62-34. Patients will complain of enlargement of the hand or forearm (about 50 percent), pain (about 40 percent), or a mass (about 30 percent).[593] Other

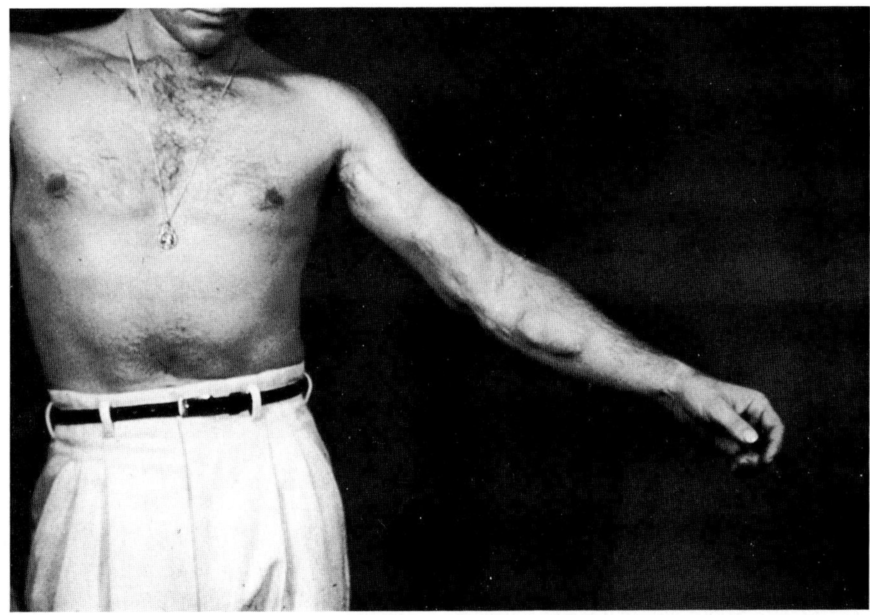

Fig. 62-34. This young man had an arteriovenous fistula of his left upper extremity. The venous ectasia was more pronounced than the arteriovenous shunt. At the time the photograph was taken the patient was relatively asymptomatic. (Courtesy of WJ Morris, MD.)

presenting complaints include ischemic ulcers,[596] limb warmth,[614] paresthesias, and hyperhidrosis.[593]

The physical signs are much as one would expect. The limb is enlarged and there is a mass, or at least enlarged blood vessels, discernible in most cases. It is common for the patients to have, or to have had, a cutaneous vascular malformation.[593,626,663] Skin stasis and trophic changes may be present, especially distal to the lesion. Bruits and thrills are not always present with congenital arteriovenous fistulas. They are present with the large or active ones, and a careful search with a Doppler may reveal microfistulas that are not otherwise obvious. Other physical findings occasionally present include edema, a positive Branham's sign, secondary joint stiffness, and a decrease or loss of pulses distal to the lesion. Bleeding from an arteriovenous malformation (AVM) has been reported to have caused an acute posterior interosseous nerve palsy.

As in many other vascular lesions, the Doppler scanner and arteriography are the two most helpful techniques. Certain lesions, such as the microfistulas of the Klippel-Trenaunay syndrome[641] (a triad of cutaneous hemangioma, atypical varicose veins, and limb hypertrophy), can be found in no other way. The Doppler may also be taken into the operating room to make sure lesions are not overlooked.[653]

A plain radiograph should always be taken. It will show a soft tissue mass in about 65 percent of cases and calcifications in the mass (from phleboliths) in about 50 percent of cases. Other findings that may be seen include new bone formation and bone erosion.[89,584] Cabbabe[590] has found xeroradiography to be useful in providing information about bony involvement in cases of congenital AVMs.

Arteriography should always be done in patients with these lesions.[613,633] The striking finding on arteriography is the filling of the deep venous system almost simultaneously with that of the arterial system, with puddling of the dye in the malformation[619] (Fig. 62-35). The distal vascular tree fills slowly and poorly. Bliznak and Staple[584] identified four different radiologic patterns of congenital arteriovenous fistulas:

	Feeding Artery	Shunt	Veins
Localized arteriovenous malformation	Large	Rapid	Dilated
Diffuse arteriovenous malformation	Large	Rapid	Dilated
Small vessel malformation	Normal	Slight	Normal
Venous malformation	Normal	None	Huge

From the 18 cases on which they reported, these various categories do not seem to carry a marked prognostic significance. Venograms are required to visualize a venous deformity, and the technique of closed-system venography may be useful (see the section on diagnostic techniques).

Blood on the venous side of an arteriovenous fistula has a higher than normal oxygen content, and several workers have used this fact in diagnosis.[589,590,661,663] It appears mostly to confirm what can be determined more easily by other methods. Yao and co-workers[670] have used plethysmography in patients with arteriovenous fistulas and have demonstrated increased blood flow to the skin in all of the patients studied. This also appears to be a confirmatory rather than primary diagnostic tool.

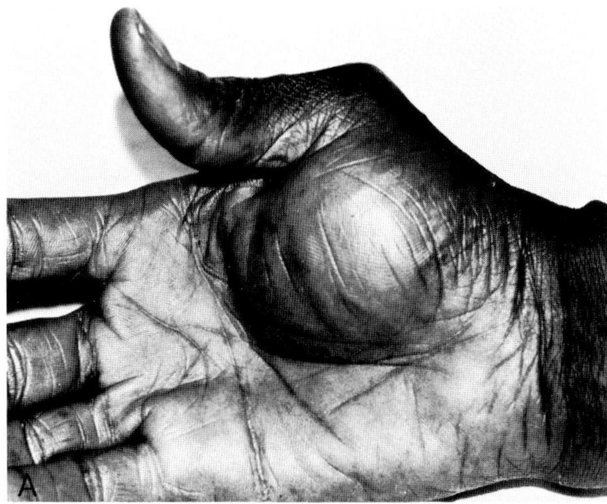

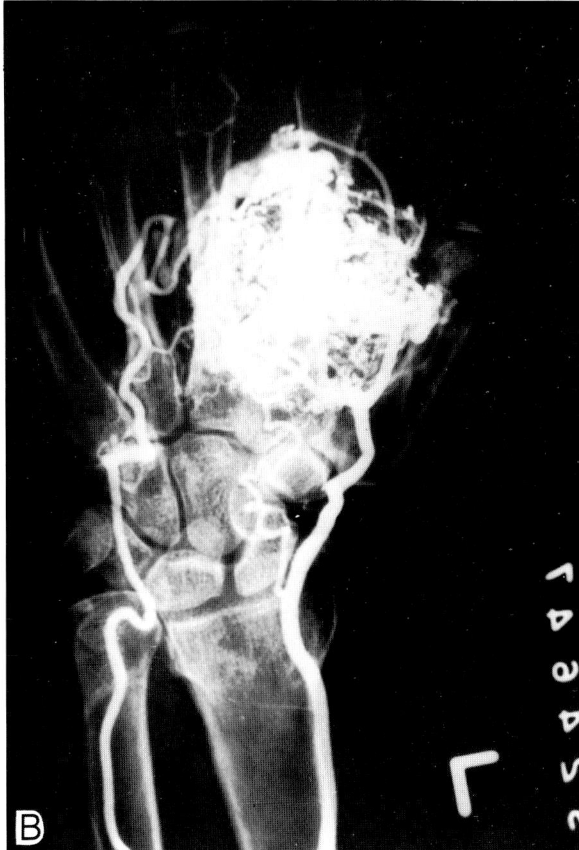

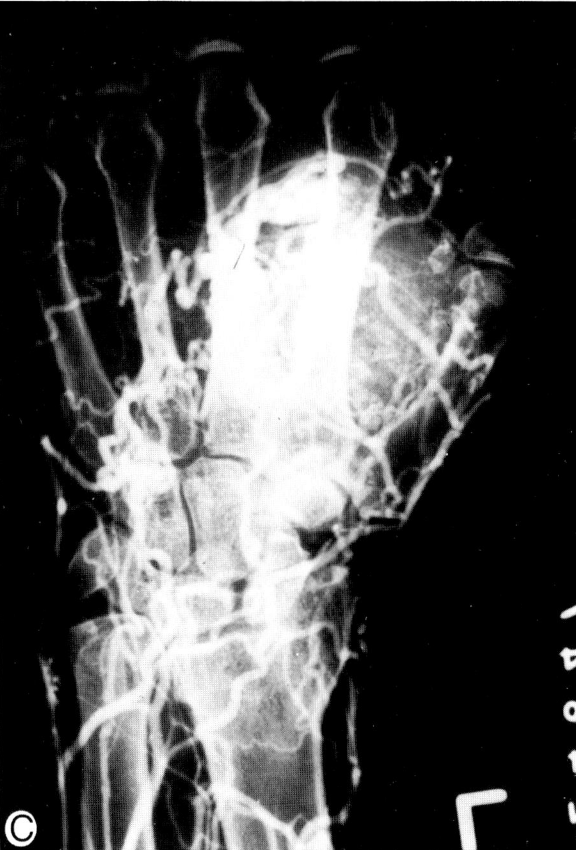

Fig. 62-35. **(A)** This 44-year-old man has a relatively small, asymptomatic, and static arteriovenous fistula of his left hand. Arteriograms in the arterial **(B)** and venous phases **(C)** show the rapid shunt, pooling in the fistula and paucity of distal circulation.

Operations for Congenital Arteriovenous Fistulas

These are difficult lesions to cure surgically or in any other manner. A quote from Szilagyi and colleagues[656] summarizes the almost universal opinion of surgeons who have dealt with this problem: "The most impressive lesson taught by this study was the realization of the futility of any attempt to cure by surgical means any but the simplest and most sharply localized of these lesions."

Pemberton and Saint[639] outlined four possible operative approaches to congenital arteriovenous fistulas:

1. Excision of the fistulous tract with the feeding artery and draining vein;
2. Ligation of the fistulous tract;
3. Restorative angiorrhaphy by
   (a) division of the fistula and repair of both vessels,
   (b) transverse closure of the fistula, and
   (c) Endoaneurysmorrhaphy; and
4. Quadruple ligation—ligation of each vessel, proximal and distal to the fistula.

Unfortunately, all of these methods are dependent on the presence of a single, easily isolated fistula, which is almost never the case with a congenital problem. Pemberton and Saint condemn proximal ligation of the feeding artery, because this procedure invariably causes the collaterals present to feed into the fistulous tract, decreasing the amount of blood going to the distal limb and causing gangrene of all or part of it.

Gelberman and Goldner[602] listed three surgical options: (1) excision of the fistula in one, two, or more stages; (2) ligation of feeding arteries and communicators; and (3) amputation of the part. Their first option is the one used by most surgeons,[595,596,598,661] with the amputation of a digit (digits), hand, or arm always being a very real possibility[582,667,669] (Fig. 62-36). The second option would obviously be part of any excision, but ligation by itself is often of limited value. Amputation may have to be very extensive to cure a lesion (or save a life), and may include the entire shoulder girdle on occasion.[615] For a vivid description of the problems encountered with a larger arteriovenous fistula, the reader is referred to the account by Bernheim.[582]

Nisbet[635] offered the insight that one of the problems with eradication of a congenital arteriovenous fistula is the extension of the lesion into bone. He proposed a staged procedure, in which the surgeon first removes all of the soft tissue portion of the lesion and ligates all feeders going into the bone; then excises the lesion in the bone, packing the resultant defect with cancellous chips; and finally restores the limb by a bone graft. This is a variation of the staged procedure and may have to be terminated by amputation if the lesion gets out of hand.

Although these lesions are not malignant in the usual sense of the word, they are locally infiltrative and aggressive.[602,623,628,630]

Operative intervention often seems to enhance their extension or to activate more proximal, previously quiescent portions of the lesion.

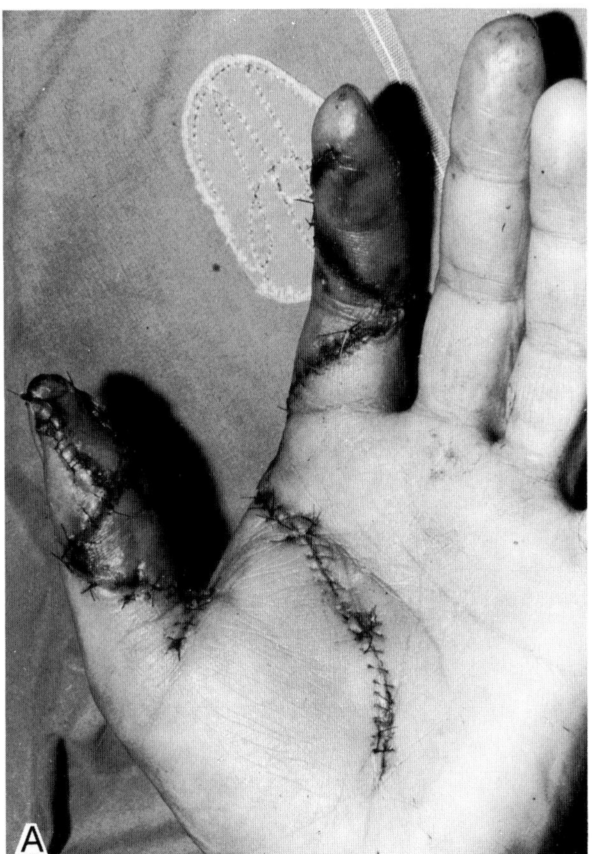

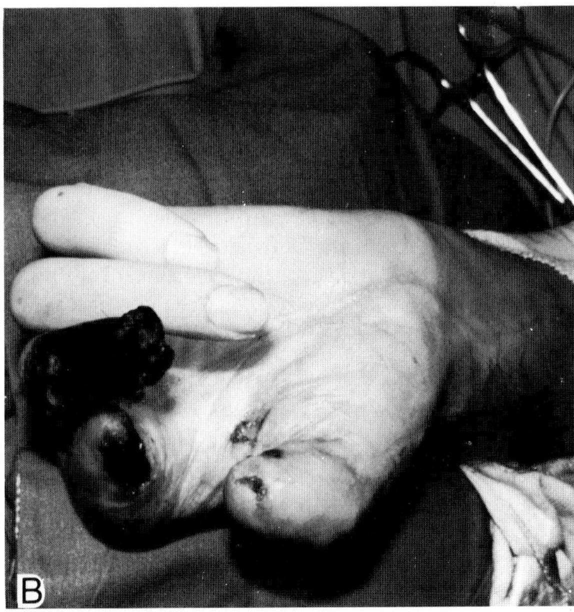

Fig. 62-36. This young man had an enlarging arteriovenous fistula on the radial side of his left hand. An extensive resection was done **(A)**, but distal ischemia occurred requiring piecemeal amputations **(B)**. Eventually amputation at the midforearm level was necessary to control pain. (Courtesy of LO Vasconez, MD.)

Nonoperative Approaches

Mikkelsen[631] reported an apparent cure of a multiply recurring lesion in a 21-year-old woman, 4 years after irradiation with 4500 rads. She had had seven or eight prior operative procedures in an attempt to remove a large congenital arteriovenous fistula of the upper extremity. At the time Mikkelsen made his report, the patient had no symptoms, but the lesion was still present. Recurrence of symptoms seemed likely, but the procedure at least delayed very radical surgery for more than 4 years.

A procedure that has been used for treatment of arteriovenous malformations mostly in the head, neck, and major body cavities is intraarterial embolization.[581,599,603,606,609,617,632,637,651] A catheter is placed by the Seldinger technique into a main feeding artery of the lesion, and emboli of autogenous muscle or some other substance to promote local intravascular clotting is injected. An effort is made to save the feeding artery in case a second or third treatment is necessary. The patient typically has ischemic pain after the procedure and this may be quite severe. Often the lesion can be brought under control or reduced to a size where it is amenable to surgery.

Table 62-1. Differential Features in Congenital Versus Acquired Ateriovenous Fistula

	Congenital	Acquired
History		
Noted early in life	Often	
Noted after vague injury	Often	
Seen after penetrating injury	No	Only
Symptoms		
Mass, fullness, discomfort	Often	Often
Signs		
Mass	Yes	Yes
Warm limb	Yes	Yes
Limb longer	Often	No
Distal ischemia	Sometimes	Sometimes
Bruit and thrill	Sometimes	Usually
Scar of trauma	No	Yes
Arteriogram		
Large, single feeder	Sometimes	Yes
Rapid shunting	Sometimes	Yes
Treatment		
Conservative often best	Yes	No
May need multiple stages	Yes	No
May require amputation	Yes	No
Single stage, straightforward	Rarely	Usually

Acquired Arteriovenous Fistulas

Acquired arteriovenous fistulas are either traumatic or surgical. One traumatic cause, bloodletting, is fortunately no longer with us.[636] The patient with this lesion invariably has a history of a penetrating injury,[580,588,597,600,650,654] although May et al[630] reported a case of an acquired lesion from closed blunt trauma at the base of a thumb that apparently was an arteriovenous fistula. The lesion, at least in the early stages, is well-localized and amenable to surgical correction fairly easily. The hemodynamic changes and consequent physical findings are similar to those of congenital arteriovenous fistulas (Table 62-1).

The diagnostic maneuvers and operative approaches are the same as those used in congenital lesions, but in these the direct approach to the fistulas has some practical reality. It is wise to operate on these lesions at an early date after injury, because in long-standing acquired fistulas, irreversible degenerative changes in the arterial wall may make surgery technically more difficult and predispose to a postoperative aneurysm or thrombosis. Replacement of the artery may even become necessary.[625]

Surgical Arteriovenous Fistulas

Brescia and co-workers[587] in 1966 developed an internal shunt to overcome some of the problems of external shunts.[638] Both shunts are, of course, used for chronic renal dialysis. Since 1966, many modifications of the shunt have been described.[658] All of the problems seen with congenital or traumatic arteriovenous fistulas are seen with surgical shunts.[592] These include "arterialization" of veins with development of atherosclerosis,[652] the various manifestations of distal ischemia,[607,620,629,655] and hand swelling from increased venous pressure.[648] The possibility of congestive heart failure has been considered, but no evidence has been found.[616]

Hand surgeons may be called upon to see these patients from complications of the shunt or for an unrelated hand problem in the hand of the shunted arm. The shunt here is obviously not the problem, but rather the solution to another problem, and taking it down is not usually a therapeutic possibility. If surgery is required in one of these hands, it is best to do it without a tourniquet inflated. The tourniquet may be put in place and used if absolutely necessary, but if it is inflated, the surgeon must be prepared to unclot the shunt at the conclusion of the procedure.

ACKNOWLEDGMENT

William E. Sanders, MD, is a surgeon with a great interest in vascular problems of the upper extremity and he went to extraordinary lengths to give me data and his clear thinking on some important aspects of this fascinating topic. I am most grateful to him for his input.

Summary of Recommended Treatment of Arteriovenous Fistula

I. Careful history and physical examination
  A. Congenital versus acquired
  B. Assess extent of the lesion

II. Studies
  A. Careful assessment with the Doppler
  B. Plain radiographs
  C. Arteriogram

III. Treatment—congenital
  A. Consider conservative treatment with a limb compression garment
  B. If well localized, excise the lesion in one or two stages. Be prepared to reconstitute an artery to prevent ischemia
  C. If the lesion is infiltrative but advanced in size, or symptoms force surgery, have the patient prepared for multistage surgery and for a possible amputation (see Fig. 62-34)
  D. If the lesion involves one or two digits extensively, strongly consider one or two ray amputations to ablate the lesion entirely
  E. In an extensive lesion, especially if the patient is adamantly opposed to amputation, consider intraarterial embolization

IV. Treatment—acquired
  A. Direct surgical approach with sacrifice of the artery if vascularity is very good without it. For example, one digital, radial, or ulnar artery might be sacrificed
  B. Direct surgical approach with arterial reconstitution if there is any question about the importance of the artery for distal blood supply. Direct repair or a graft may be used as indicated

V. Postoperative treatment is the same as that after any other hand procedure with or without arterial repair

REFERENCES

Introduction and Anatomy

1. Bergan JJ, Conn J, Trippel OH: Severe ischemia of the hand. Ann Surg 173:301–307, 1971
2. Calenoff L: Angiography of the hand: Guidelines for interpretation. Radiology 102:331–335, 1972
3. Chaudakshetrin P, Kumar VP, Satku K, Pho RWH: The arteriovenous pattern of the distal digital segment. J Hand Surg 13B:164–166, 1988
4. Coleman SS, Anson BJ: Arterial patterns in the hand based upon a study of 650 specimens. Surg Gynecol Obstet 113:409–424, 1961
5. Denman EE: The anatomy of the space of Guyon. Hand 10:69–76, 1978
6. Earley MJ: The arterial supply of the thumb, first web and index finger and its surgical application. J Hand Surg 11B:163–174, 1986
7. Edwards EA: The anatomy of collateral circulation. Surg Gynecol Obstet 107:183–194, 1958
8. Edwards EA: Organization of the small arteries of the hand and digits. Am J Surg 99:837–846, 1960
9. Ikeda A, Ugawa A, Kazihara Y, Hamada N: Arterial patterns in the hand based on a three-dimensional analysis of 220 cadaver hands. J Hand Surg 13A:501–509, 1988
10. Jarrett F, Hirsch SA: Current diagnosis and management of upper extremity ischemia. Surg Annu 15:207–228, 1983
11. Kaplan EB: Functional and Surgical Anatomy of the Hand. 2nd Ed. pp. 143, 187. JB Lippincott, Philadelphia, 1965
12. Kleinert JM, Fleming SG, Abel CS, Firrell J: Radial and ulnar artery dominance in normal digits. J Hand Surg 14A:504–508, 1989
13. Leslie BM, Ruby LK, Madell SJ, Wittenstein F: Digital artery diameters: An anatomic and clinical study. J Hand Surg 12A:740–743, 1987
14. Lucas GL: The pattern of venous drainage of the digits. J Hand Surg 9A:448–450, 1984
15. McCarthy WJ, Flinn WR, Yao JST, Williams LR, Bergan JJ: Result of bypass grafting for upper limb ischemia. J Vasc Surg 3:741–746, 1986
16. McCormack LJ, Cauldwell EW, Anson BJ: Brachial and antebrachial arterial patterns: A study of 750 extremities. Surg Gynecol Obstet 96:43–54, 1953
17. McNamara MF, Takaki HS, Yao JST, Bergan JJ: A systematic approach to severe hand ischemia. Surgery 83:1–11, 1978
18. Mills JL, Friedman EI, Taylor LM Jr, Porter JM: Upper extremity ischemia caused by small artery disease. Ann Surg 206:521–528, 1987
19. Moss SH, Schwartz KS, von Drasek-Ascher G, Ogden LL II, Wheeler CS, Lister GD: Digital venous anatomy. J Hand Surg 10A:473–482, 1985
20. Neviaser RJ, Adams JP: Vascular lesions in the hand. Curr Manage Clin Orthop 100:111–119, 1974
21. Parks BJ, Arbelaez J, Horner RL: Medical and surgical importance of the arterial blood supply of the thumb. J Hand Surg 3:383–385, 1978
22. Patten BM: Morris' Human Anatomy. 11th Ed. pp. 679–690. Blakiston, New York, 1953
23. Pin PG, Sicard GA, Weeks PM: Digital ischemia of the upper extremity: A systematic approach for evaluation and treatment. Plast Reconstr Surg 82:653–657, 1988
24. Short DW: Occlusive vascular lesions. Hand 4:100–106, 1972
25. Smith DO, Oura C, Kimura C, Toshimori K: Artery anatomy and tortuosity in the distal finger. J Hand Surg 16A:297–302, 1991
26. Smith DO, Oura C, Kimura C, Toshimori K: The distal venous anatomy of the finger. J Hand Surg 16A:303–307, 1991
27. Strauch B, deMoura W: Arterial system of the fingers. J Hand Surg 15A:148–154, 1990
28. Wilgis EFS: Evaluation and treatment of chronic digital ischemia. Ann Surg 193:693–698, 1981

Diagnostic Studies

29. Allen EV: Thromboangitis obliterans: Methods of diagnosis of chronic occlusive arterial lesions distal to the wrist with illustrative cases. Am J Med Sci 178:237–244, 1929
30. Allen EV, Camp JD: Arteriography. A Roentgenographic study of the peripheral arteries in the living subject following their injection with a radio-opaque substance. JAMA 104:618–624, 1935

31. Barber JD, Wright DJ, Ellis RH: Radial artery puncture. A simple screening test of the ulnar anastomotic circulation. Anesthesia 28:291-292, 1973
32. Bauman DP: The specificity of the Allen test in obliterative vascular disease. Angiology 5:36-38, 1954
33. Bettmann MA: Radiographic contrast agents—A perspective. N Engl J Med 317:891-893, 1987
34. Bingham HG, Lichti E: Use of the ultra sound transducer (Doppler) to localize peripheral and arteriovenous fistulae. Plast Reconstr Surg 46:151-154, 1970
35. Blair WF, Greene ER, Omer GE Jr: A method for the calculation of blood flow in human digital arteries. J Hand Surg 6:90-96, 1981
36. Blair WF, Morecraft RJ, Brown TD, Gabel RH: Transcutaneous blood flow measurements in arteries of the human hand. J Hand Surg 16A:169-175, 1991
37. Brody WR, Enzmann DR, Miller DC, Guthaner DF, Pelc NJ, Keyes GS, Riederer SJ: Intravenous arteriography using digital subtraction techniques. JAMA 248:671-674, 1982
38. DiBenedetto MR, Nappi JF, Ruff ME, Lubbers LM: Doppler mapping in hypothenar syndrome: An alternative to angiography. J Hand Surg 14A:244-246, 1989
39. Dooley TW, Welsh CF, Puckett CL: Noninvasive assessment of microvessels with the duplex scanner. J Hand Surg 14A:670-673, 1989
40. Ebel A, Rose OA, Raab K: The use of an environmental temperature vasomotor test in the evaluation of peripheral arterial disease. Angiology 12:310-315, 1961
41. Edwards EA: The status of vasography. N Engl J Med 209:1337-1343, 1933
42. Ejrup B, Fischer B, Wright IS: Clinical evaluation of blood flow to the hand: The false-positive Allen test. Circulation 33:778-780, 1966
43. Ernst D, Hurlow RA, Strachan CJL, Chandler ST: The assessment of digital vessel disease by dynamic hand scanning. Hand 10:217-225, 1978
44. Geiser JH, Eversmann WW Jr: Closed system venography in the evaluation of upper extremity hemangiomas. J Hand Surg 3:173-178, 1978
45. Gelberman RH, Blasingame JP: The timed Allen test. J Trauma 21:477-479, 1981
46. Greenhow DE: Incorrect performance of Allen's test: Ulnar artery flow presumed inadequate. Anesthesiology 37:356-357, 1972
47. Gross WS, Louis DS: Doppler hemodynamic assessment of obscure symptomatology in the upper extremity. J Hand Surg 3:467-473, 1978
48. Hashway T, Raines J: Real-time ultrasonic imaging of the peripheral arteries: Technique, normal anatomy and pathology. Texas Heart Institute Bull 7:257-265, 1980
49. Herzberg DL, Schreiber MH: Angiography in mass lesions of the extremities. Am J Roentgenol 111:541-546, 1968
50. Hirai M: Digital blood pressure and arteriographic findings under selective compression of the radial and ulnar arteries. Angiology 31:21-31, 1980
51. Hirai M, Kawai S: False positive and negative results in Allen test. J Cardiovas Surg 21:353-360, 1980
52. Husum B, Berthelsen P: Allen's test and systolic arterial pressure in the thumb. Br J Anaesth 53:635-637, 1981
53. Koman LA: Diagnostic study of vascular lesions. Hand Clin 1:217-231, 1985
54. Koman LA, Bond MG, Carter RE, Poehling GG: Evaluation of upper extremity vasculature with high-resolution ultrasound. J Hand Surg 10A:249-255, 1985
55. Koman LA, Nunley JA, Goldner JL, Seaber AV, Urbaniak JR: Isolated cold stress testing in the assessment of symptoms in the upper extremity: Preliminary communication. J Hand Surg 9A:305-313, 1984
56. Koman LA, Nunley JA, Wilkinson RH Jr, Urbaniak JR, Coleman RE: Dynamic radionuclide imaging as a means of evaluating vascular perfusion of the upper extremity: A preliminary report. J Hand Surg 8:424-434, 1983
57. Koob E: Infra-red thermography in hand surgery. Hand 4:65-67, 1972
58. Laws JW, El Sallab RA, Scott JT: An arteriographic and histological study of digital arteries. Br J Radiol 40:740-747, 1967
59. Levinsohn DG, Gordon L, Sessler DI: The Allen's test: Analysis of four methods. J Hand Surg 16A:279-282, 1991
60. Levy I, Danziger Y, Mechlis-Frish S, Lubin E, Mimouni M: Technetium-labeled red blood cell imaging to evaluate soft tissue hemangioma of the hand. Pediatric Dermatol 5:47-49, 1988
61. Little JM, Zylstra PL, West J, May J: Circulatory patterns in the normal hand. Br J Surg 60:652-655, 1973
62. Loth TS, Jones DEC: Extravasations of radiographic contrast material in the upper extremity. J Hand Surg 13A:395-398, 1988
63. Love L, Braun T: Arteriography of peripheral vascular trauma. Am J Roentgenol 102:431-440, 1968
64. Lumpkin MB, Logan WD, Couves CM, Howard JM: Arteriography as an aid in the diagnosis and localization of acute arterial injuries. Ann Surg 147:353-358, 1958
65. Lund F: Fluorescein angiography especially of the upper extremities. Acta Chir Scand (suppl) 465:60-70, 1976
66. Mackinnon SE, Holder LE: The use of three-phase radionuclide bone scanning in the diagnosis of reflex sympathetic dystrophy. J Hand Surg 9A:556-563, 1984
67. Marshall TR, Neustadt D, Chumley WF, Kasdan ML: Hand arteriography. Radiology 86:299-302, 1966
68. Matsuki A: A modified Allen's test using a pulse oxymeter (letter). Anaesth Intensive Care 16:126-127, 1988
69. Maurer AH, Holder LE, Espinola DA, Rupani HD, Wilgis EFS: Three-phase radionuclide scintigraphy of the hand. Radiology 146:761-775, 1983
70. McGregor AD: The Allen test—An investigation of its accuracy by fluorescein angiography. J Hand Surg 12B:82-85, 1987
71. McGregor IA, Morgan G: Axial and random pattern flaps. Br J Plast Surg 26:202-213, 1973
72. Mozersky DJ, Buckley CJ, Hagood CO, Capps WF Jr, Dannemiller FJ Jr: Ultrasonic evaluation of the palmar circulation. A useful adjunct to radial artery cannulation. Am J Surg 126:810-812, 1973
73. Mozersky DJ, Hokanson DE, Baker DW, Sumner DS, Strandness DE Jr: Ultrasonic arteriography. Arch Surg 103:663-667, 1971
74. Myhre HO, Kroes AJ: Ultrasound in the study of peripheral blood circulation. Acta Chir Scand (suppl) 488:1-98, 1979
75. O'Gorman RB, Feliciano DV, Bitondo CG, Mattox KL, Burch JM, Jordan GL Jr: Emergency center arteriography in the evaluation of suspected peripheral vascular injuries. Arch Surg 119:568-573, 1984
76. Pearce WH, Rutherford RB, Whitehill TA, Davis K: Nuclear magnetic resonance imaging: Its diagnostic value in patients with congenital vascular malformations of the limbs. J Vasc Surg 8:64-70, 1988
77. Peimer CA, Eckert BS: Microvascular response to angiography. J Hand Surg 7:4-10, 1982
78. Phelps DB, Rutherford RB, Boswick JA Jr: Control of vasospasm following trauma and microvascular surgery. J Hand Surg 4:109-117, 1979
79. Ramanathan S, Chalon J, Turndorf H: Determining patency of

palmar arches by retrograde radial pulsation. Anesthesiology 42:756–758, 1975
80. Robins B, Bernstein A: Comparative studies of digital plethysmography and infra-red thermography in peripheral vascular diseases. Angiology 21:349–354, 1970
81. Rozenberg B, Rosenberg M, Birkhan J: Allens's test performed by pulse oximeter. Anaesthesia 43:515–516, 1988
82. Scavenius M, Fauner M, Walther-Larsen S, Buchwald C, Nielsen SL: A quantitative Allen's test. Hand 13:318–320, 1981
83. Schwartz R, Cooper WM: The Allen test in polycythemia: The presence and interpretation of positive and negative reactions. Angiology 3:317–322, 1952
84. Seldinger SI: Catheter replacement of the needle in percutaneous arteriography. Acta Radiol 39:368–376, 1953
85. Sheppard JE, Dell PC: The effect of preoperative arteriography on vascular endothelium and replant survival in rabbit ears. J Hand Surg 8:145–153, 1983
86. Smith DJ Jr, Bendick PJ, Madison SA: Evaluation of vascular compromise in the injured extremity: A photoplethysmographic technique. J Hand Surg 9A:314–319, 1984
87. Soila P, Wegelius U, Sirkka-Maija V: Notes on the technique of angiography of the upper extremity. Angiology 14:297–305, 1963
88. Soulen RL, Lapayowker MS, Tyson RR, Korangy AA: Angiography, ultrasound and thermography in the study of peripheral vascular disease. Radiology 105:115–119, 1972
89. Staple TM: Vascular radiological procedures in orthopedic surgery. Clin Orthop 107:48–61, 1975
90. Strandness DE Jr, Bell JW: Peripheral vascular disease. Diagnosis and objective evaluation using a mercury strain gauge. Ann Surg (suppl) 161:1–35, 1965
91. Strandness DE Jr, McCutcheon EP, Rushmer RF: Application of transcutaneous Doppler flowmeter in evaluation of occlusive arterial disease. Surg Gynecol Obstet 122:1039–1045, 1966
92. Strandness DE Jr, Schultz RD, Sumner DS, Rushmer RF: Ultrasonic flow detection. A useful technic in the evaluation of peripheral vascular disease. Am J Surg 113:311–320, 1967
93. Sumner DS: Volume plethysmography in vascular disease: An overview. pp. 97–118. In Bernstein EF (ed): Noninvasive Diagnostic Techniques in Vascular Disease. 3rd Ed. CV Mosby, St. Louis, 1985
94. Sumner DS: Mercury strain-gauge plethysmography. pp. 133–150. In Bernstein EF (ed): Noninvasive Diagnostic Techniques in Vascular Disease. 3rd Ed. CV Mosby, St Louis, 1985
95. Sumner DS: Noninvasive assessment of upper extremity and hand ischemia. J Vasc Surg 3:560–564, 1986
96. Sumner DS, Strandness DE Jr: An abnormal finger pulse associated with cold sensitivity. Ann Surg 175:294–298, 1972
97. Sy WM, Bay R, Camera A: Hand images: Normal and abnormal. J Nucl Med 18:419–424, 1977
98. Vaughan RS, Lawrie BW, Sykes PJ: Use of intravenous regional sympathetic block in upper limb angiography. Ann R Coll Surg Engl 67:309–312, 1985
99. Wegelius U: Angiography of the hand. Acta Radiol (suppl) 315, 1972
100. Wilgis EFS, Jezic D, Stonesifer GL Jr, Classen JN, Sekercan K: The evaluation of small vessel flow: A study of dynamic noninvasive techniques. J Bone Joint Surg 56A:1199–1206, 1974
101. Wilkins RW, Doupe J, Newman HW: The rate of blood flow in normal fingers. Clin Sci 3:403–411, 1938
102. Yao JST: New techniques in arterial evaluation. Arch Surg 106:600–604, 1973
103. Yao JST, Bergan JJ: Application of ultrasound to arterial and venous diagnosis. Surg Clin North Am 54:23–38, 1974
104. Yao JST, Gourmos C, Papathanasiou K, Irvine WT: A method for assessing ischemia of the hand and fingers. Surg Gynecol Obstet 135:373–378, 1972
105. Yao JST, Needham TN, Gourmous C, Irvine WT: A comparative study of strain gauge plethysmography and Doppler ultrasound in the assessment of occlusive arterial disease in the lower extremity. Surgery 71:4–9, 1972

Ulnar and Other Artery Thrombosis

106. Aulicino PL, Klavans SM, DuPuy TE: Digital ischemia secondary to thrombosis of a persistent median artery. J Hand Surg 9A:820–823, 1984
107. Barker NW, Hines FH Jr: Arterial occlusion in the hands and fingers associated with repeated occupational trauma. Mayo Clin Proc 19:345–349, 1944
108. Barre PS, Keith MW, Sobel M, Rashad FA, Shields RW Jr: Vascular insufficiency in Okihiro's syndrome secondary to hypothenar hammer syndrome. J Hand Surg 12A:401–405, 1987
109. Bell GE, Goldner JL: Neuropathy of the median nerve. South Med J 49:966–972, 1956
110. Benedict KT Jr, Chang W, McCready FJ: The hypothenar hammer syndrome. Radiology 111:57–60, 1974
111. Bergan JJ, Trippel OH, Kaupp HA, Kukal JC, Nowlin WF: Low molecular weight Dextran in treatment of severe ischemia. Arch Surg 91:338–341, 1965
112. Boyle JC, Smith NJ, Burke FD: Vibration white finger. J Hand Surg 13B:171–176, 1988
113. Bugg EI, Coonrad RW, Grimm KB: Giant cell arteritis—an acute hand syndrome. J Bone Joint Surg 45A:1269–1272, 1963
114. Butsch JL, Janes JM: Injuries of the superficial palmar arch. J Trauma 3:505–516, 1963
115. Carneirio RS, Mann RJ: Occlusion of the ulnar artery associated with an anomalous muscle: A case report. J Hand Surg 4:412–414, 1979
116. Cho KO: Entrapment occlusion of the ulnar artery in the hand. J Bone Joint Surg 60A:841–843, 1978
117. Conn J Jr, Bergan JJ, Bell JL: Hypothenar hammer syndrome: Post traumatic digital ischemia. Surgery 68:1122–1128, 1970
118. Costigan DG, Riley JM Jr, Coy FE Jr: Thrombofibrosis of the ulnar artery in the palm. J Bone Joint Surg 41A:702–704, 1959
119. Eguro H, Goldner JL: Bilateral thrombosis of the ulnar arteries in the hands. Case report. Plast Reconstr Surg 52:573–578, 1973
120. Foster EJ, Palmer AK, Levinsohn EM: Hamate erosion: An unusual result of ulnar artery constriction. J Hand Surg 4:536–540, 1979
121. Given KS, Puckett CL, Kleinert HE: Ulnar artery thrombosis. Plast Reconstr Surg 61:405–411, 1978
122. Gonzalez MH, Hall RF Jr: Thrombosis of the vena comitantes of the ulnar artery. J Hand Surg 15A:773–776, 1990
123. Goren ML: Palmar intramural thrombosis in the ulnar artery. Calif Med 89:424–425, 1958
124. Herndon WA, Hershey SL, Lambdin CS: Thrombosis of the ulnar artery in the hand. J Bone Joint Surg 57A:994–995, 1975
125. Jackson JP: Traumatic thrombosis of the ulnar artery in the palm. J Bone Joint Surg 36B:438–439, 1954
126. Jelalian C, Mehrhof A, Cohen IK, Richardson J, Merritt WH: Streptokinase in the treatment of acute arterial occlusion of the hand. J Hand Surg 10A:534–538, 1985
127. Kelly GL: Radial artery occlusion by a carpal ganglion. Plast Reconstr Surg 52:191–193, 1973
128. Kleinert HE, Volianitis GJ: Thrombosis of the palmar arterial arch and its tributaries: Etiology and newer concepts in treatment. J Trauma 5:447–457, 1965
129. Koman LA, Urbaniak JR: Ulnar artery insufficiency: A guide to treatment. J Hand Surg 6:16–24, 1981

130. Lawrence RR, Wilson JN: Ulnar artery thrombosis in the palm. Case report. Plast Reconstr Surg 36:604–608, 1965
131. Leriche R, Fontaine R, Dupertuis SM: Arterectomy with follow-up studies on 78 operations. Surg Gynecol Obstet 64:149–155, 1937
132. Levy M, Pauker M: Carpal tunnel syndrome due to a thrombosed persisting median artery. A case report. Hand 10:65–68, 1978
133. Little JM, Ferguson DA: The incidence of the hypothenar hammer syndrome. Arch Surg 105:684–685, 1972
134. Little JM, Grant AF: Hypothenar hammer syndrome. Med J Aust 1:49–53, 1972
135. Lowery CW, Chadwick RO, Waltman EN: Digital vessel trauma from repetitive impact in baseball catchers. J Hand Surg 1:236–238, 1976
136. Malloch JD: Palmar arch thrombosis. Br Med J 2:28, 1962
137. Mansfield JP: Traumatic thrombosis of the ulnar artery in the palm. J Bone Joint Surg 36B:438–439, 1954
138. Martin AF: Ulnar artery thrombosis in the palm. A case report. Clin Orthop 17:373–376, 1960
139. Mehlhoff TL, Wood MB: Ulnar artery thrombosis and the role of interposition vein grafting: Patency with microsurgical technique. J Hand Surg 16A:274–278, 1991
140. Millender LH, Nalebuff EA, Kasdon E: Aneurysms and thromboses of the ulnar artery in the hand. Arch Surg 105:686–690, 1972
141. Paaby H, Stadil F: Thrombosis of the ulnar artery. Acta Orthop Scand 39:336–345, 1968
142. Paletta FX Jr: Venous gangrene of the hand. Plast Reconstr Surg 67:67–69, 1981
143. Parkhouse N, Smith PJ: The use of streptokinase in replant salvage. J Hand Surg 16B:53–55, 1991
144. Peters FM: A disease resulting from the use of pneumatic tools. Occup Med 2:55–56, 1946
145. Richards RR, Urbaniak JR: Spontaneous retrocarpal radial artery thrombosis: A report of two cases. J Hand Surg 9A:823–827, 1984
146. Teece LG: Thrombosis of the ulnar artery. Aust NZ J Surg 19:156–157, 1949
147. Teisinger J: Vascular disease disorders resulting from vibrating tools. J Occup Med 14:129–133, 1972
148. Telford ED, McCann MB, MacCorma DH: "Dead hand" in users of vibrating tools. Lancet 2:359–360, 1945
149. Thompson JR, Simmons CR, Smith LL: Polymyalgia arteritica with bilateral subclavian artery occlusive disease: A case report. Radiology 101:595–596, 1971
150. Tisnado J, Bartol DT, Cho S-R, Vines FS, Beachley MC, Fields WR: Low-dose fibrinolytic therapy in hand ischemia. Radiology 150:375–382, 1984
151. Trevaskis AE, Marcks KM, Pennisi AM, Berg EM: Thrombosis of the ulnar artery in the hand. A case report. Plast Reconstr Surg 33:73–76, 1964
152. Von Rosen S: Ein fall von Thrombose in der Arteria Ulnaris nach Einwirkung von stumpfen Gewalt. Acta Chir Scand 73:500–506, 1933
153. Weeks PM, Young VL: Ulnar artery thrombosis and ulnar nerve compression associated with an anomalous hypothenar muscle. Plast Reconstr Surg 69:130–131, 1982
154. Zweig J, Lie KK, Posch JL, Larsen RD: Thrombosis of the ulnar artery following blunt trauma to the hand. J Bone Joint Surg 51A:1191–1198, 1969

Aneurysms

155. Abbott WM, Darling RC: Axillary artery aneurysms secondary to crutch trauma. Am J Surg 125:515–520, 1973
156. Aulicino PL, Hutton PMJ, DuPuy TE: True palmar aneurysms—A case report and literature review. J Hand Surg 7:613–616, 1982
157. Baird RJ, Doran ML: The false aneurysm. Can Med Assoc J 91:281–284, 1964
158. Baruch A: False aneurysm of the digital artery. Hand 9:195–197, 1977
159. Beck WC: Experiences with pulsating hematoma. Am J Surg 73:580–587, 1947
160. Berrettoni BA, Seitz WH Jr: Mycotic aneurysm in a digital artery: Case report and literature review. J Hand Surg 15A:305–308, 1990
161. Bigger IA: Treatment of traumatic aneurysms and arteriovenous fistulas. Arch Surg 49:170–179, 1949
162. Bowie DC, Kay AW: Traumatic false aneurysm simulating bone sarcoma. Br J Surg 36:310–311, 1949
163. Bradley RM: Aneurysms of the palmar arteries. Milit Surg 97:486–489, 1945
164. Brunelli G, Vigasio A, Battiston B, Guizzi P, Brunelli F: Traumatic aneurysms of two proper digital arteries in the same patient: A case report. J Hand Surg 13B:345–347, 1988
165. Carmichael R: Gross defects in the muscular and elastic coats of the larger cerebral arteries. J Pathol Bacteriol 57:345–351, 1945
166. Carneiro RDS: Aneurysm of the wrist. Plast Reconstr Surg 54:483–489, 1974
167. Cawley JJ: Acute traumatic aneurysm of the palm. Am J Surg 74:98–99, 1947
168. Crawford ES, DeBakey ME, Cooley DA: Surgical considerations of peripheral arterial aneurysms—Analysis of 107 cases. Arch Surg 78:226–237, 1959
169. Dangles CJ: True aneurysm of a thumb digital artery. J Hand Surg 9A:444–445, 1984
170. Davis CB, Fell EH: Traumatic aneurysm as a complication of supracondylar fracture of the humerus. Arch Surg 62:358–364, 1951
171. Duchateau J, Moermans J-P: False aneurysm of the radial artery. J Hand Surg 10A:140–141, 1985
172. Elkin DC: Aneurysm following surgical procedures. Report of five cases. Ann Surg 127:769–779, 1948
173. Engelman RM, Clements JM, Hermann JB: Stab wounds and traumatic false aneurysms in the extremities. J Trauma 9:77–87, 1969
174. Fowler IC, Workman CE: Aneurysm of the ulnar artery due to blunt trauma of the hand. Mo Med 61:927–929, 1964
175. Fraser GA: Traumatic aneurysms and arteriovenous fistulae. Vasc Surg 4:258–268, 1970
176. Gage M: Traumatic arterial aneurysm of the peripheral arteries. Am J Surg 59:210–231, 1943
177. Gardener TJ, Brawley RK, Gott VL: Anastomotic false aneurysms. Surgery 72:474–478, 1972
178. Gaylis H, Kushlick AR: Ulnar artery aneurysms of the hand. Surgery 73:478–480, 1973
179. Goadby HK, McSwiney RR, Rob CG: Mycotic aneurysm. St Thomas Hosp Reports 5:44–52, 1949
180. Green DP: True and false traumatic aneurysms in the hand: Report of two cases and review of the literature. J Bone Joint Surg 55A:120–128, 1973
181. Griffiths JA: A case of spontaneous aneurysm of the ulnar artery in the palm. Excision of the aneurysm. Recovery. Br Med J 2:646–647, 1897
182. Hall RF Jr, Watt DH: Osseous changes due to a false aneurysm of the proper digital artery: A case report. J Hand Surg 11A:440–442, 1986
183. Hentz V, Jackson I, Fogarty D: Case report: False aneurysm of the hand secondary to digital amputation. J Hand Surg 3:199–200, 1978

184. Ho PK, Yaremchuk MJ, Dellon AL: Mycotic aneurysms of the upper extremity, report of two cases. J Hand Surg 11B:271–273, 1986
185. Ho PK, Weiland AJ, McClinton MA, Wilgis EFS: Aneurysms of the upper extremity. J Hand Surg 12A:39–46, 1987
186. Hueston JT: Traumatic aneurysm of the digital artery: A complication of fasciectomy. Hand 5:232–234, 1973
187. Imahori S, Bannerman RM, Grat CJ, Brennan JC: Ehlers-Danlos syndrome with multiple arterial lesions. Am J Med 47:967–977, 1969
188. Johnson JR, Ledgerwood AM, Lucas CE: Mycotic aneurysm—New concepts in therapy. Arch Surg 118:577–582, 1983
189. Kalisman M, Laborde K, Wolff TW: Ulnar nerve compression secondary to ulnar artery false aneurysm at the Guyon's canal. J Hand Surg 7:137–139, 1982
190. Kleinert HE, Burget GC, Morgan JA, Kutz JE, Atasoy E: Aneurysms of the hand. Arch Surg 106:554–557, 1973
191. Layman CD, Ogden LL, Lister GD: True aneurysm of digital artery. J Hand Surg 7:617–618, 1982
192. Leitner DW, Ross JS, Neary JR: Granulomatous radial arteritis with bilateral nontraumatic, true arterial aneurysms within the anatomic snuffbox. J Hand Surg 10A:131–135, 1985
193. Louis DS, Simon MA: Traumatic false aneurysms of the upper extremity. J Bone Joint Surg 56A: 176–179, 1974
194. Lyle HHM: Aneurism of the palmar arches with a report of an aneurism of the deep arch cured by excision. Ann Surg 80:347–362, 1924
195. Malt S: An arteriosclerotic aneurysm of the hand. Arch Surg 113:762–763, 1978
196. Matas R: An operation for the radical cure of aneurysms based upon arterrioraphy. Ann Surg 37:161–196, 1903
197. Mathieu A, Dalton B, Fishcer JE: Expanding aneurysm of the radial artery after frequent puncture. Anesthesiology 38:401–403, 1973
198. May JW, Grossman JAI, Costas B: Cyanotic painful index and long fingers associated with an asymptomatic ulnar artery aneurysm: Case report. J Hand Surg 7:622–625, 1982
199. Mays ET: Traumatic aneurysm of the hand. Am Surg 36:552–557, 1970
200. Meyer TL, Slager RF: False aneurysm following subtrochanteric osteotomy. J Bone Joint Surg 46A:581–582, 1964
201. Middleton DS: Occupational aneurysm of the palmar arteries. Br J Surg 21:215–218, 1933
202. Milling MAP, Kinmonth MH: False aneurysm of the ulnar artery. Hand 9:57–59, 1977
203. Mukerjea SK: Traumatic aneurysm of the popliteal artery due to osteochondroma. Br J Surg 54:810–811, 1967
204. Mukerjea SK: Occupational true aneurysm of the ulnar artery in the palm. Br J Surg 58:934, 1971.
205. Narsete EM: Traumatic aneurysm of the radial artery: A report of three cases. Am J Surg 108:424–427, 1964
206. O'Connor RL: Digital nerve compression secondary to palmar aneurysm. Clin Orthop 83:149–150, 1972
207. Orhewere FA: Post-traumatic aneurysm of the radial artery at the wrist. Br Med J 2:1501–1502, 1966
207a. Pemberton JdeJ, Black BM: Surgical treatment of acquired aneurysm and arteriovenous fistula of peripheral vessels. Surg Gynecol Obstet 77:462–470, 1943
208. Perdue GD, Smith RB III: Postangiographic false aneurysms of the femoral artery. JAMA 223:1511, 1973
209. Perler BA: Venous aneurysm: An unusual upper-extremity mass. Arch Surg 125:124, 1990
210. Poirier RA, Stansel HC Jr: Arterial aneurysms of the hand. Am J Surg 124:72–74, 1972
211. Pratt GH: Surgical treatment of peripheral aneurysms. Surg Gynecol Obstet 75:103–109, 1942
212. Reid MR: Aneurysms in the Johns Hopkins Hospital. All cases treated in the surgical service from the opening of the hospital to January 1922. Arch Surg 12:1–74, 1926
213. Robb D, McKechnie WR, Guthrie DW: Peripheral aneurysms of traumatic origin: Cases occurring in brachial, radial and ulnar arteries. Aust NZ J Surg 12:147–148, 1942
214. Rothkopf DM, Bryan DJ, Cuadros CL, May JW Jr: Surgical management of ulnar artery aneurysms. J Hand Surg 15A:891–897, 1990
215. Sadove RC: Traumatic infected pseudoaneurysm of the hand. J Hand Surg 15A:906–909, 1990
216. Sanchez A, Archer S, Levine NS, Buchanan RT: Traumatic aneurysm of a common digital artery—A case report. J Hand Surg 7:619–621, 1982
217. Sharp WV, Hansel JR: Aneurysm of the brachial artery: Case report of an unusual pathogenesis. Ohio State Med J 63:1177–1178, 1967
218. Short DW: Occupational aneurysm of the palmar arch: Report of a case. Lancet 2:217–218, 1948
219. Shucksmith HS, Fitton JM, Glanville JN: Ununited fracture of the scaphoid complicated by aneurysms of the radial artery. Br J Surg 56:937–938, 1969
220. Smith JW: True aneurysms of traumatic origin in the palm. Am J Surg 104:7–13, 1962
221. Spittel JA Jr: Aneurysms of the hand and wrist. Med Clin North Am 42:1007–1010, 1958
222. Spittel JA Jr, Janes JM: Aneurysm of the ulnar artery: Report of a case. Mayo Clin Proc 32:295–298, 1957
223. Sterling AP, Haberman ET: Traumatic aneurysms of the radial artery. Hand 7:294–296, 1975
224. Suzuki K, Takahashi S, Nakagawa T: False aneurysm in a digital artery. J Hand Surg 5:402–403, 1980
225. Thio RT: False aneurysm of the ulnar artery after surgery employing a tourniquet. Am J Surg 123:604–605, 1972
226. Thorrens S, Trippel OH, Bergan JJ: Arteriosclerotic aneurysms of the hand. Excision, restoration of continuity. Arch Surg 92:937–939, 1966
227. Turner S, Howard CB, Dallimore NS: A case report of a true aneurysm of a digital artery. J Hand Surg 9B:205–206, 1984
228. Tyler G, Stein A: Aneurysm of a common digital artery: Resection and vein graft. J Hand Surg 13B:348–349, 1988
229. Watson MD, Kaye JJ: Traumatic venous aneurysm presenting as a ganglion cyst. A case report. J Bone Joint Surg 70A:1248–1250, 1988
230. Weintraub RA, Abrams HL: Mycotic aneurysms. AJR 102:354–362, 1968
231. Zuckerman IC, Proctor SE: Traumatic palmar aneurysms. Am J Surg 72:52–56, 1946

Other Vascular Trauma

232. Abu-Nema T, Ayyash K, Wafaii IK, Al-Hassan J, Thulesius O: Jellyfish sting resulting in severe hand ischaemia successfully treated with intra-arterial urokinase. Injury 19:294–296, 1988
233. Baker RJ, Chunprapaph B, Nyhus LM: Severe ischemia of the hand following radial artery catheterization. Surgery 80:449–457, 1976
234. Barnes RW, Foster EJ, Janssen GA, Boutros AR: Safety of brachial artery catheters as monitors in the intensive care unit—Prospective evaluation with the Doppler ultrasonic velocity detector. Anesthesiology 44:260–264, 1976
235. Bayer WL, Shea WD, Szeto ILF, Curiel DC, Lewis JH: Excision of a pseudo cyst of the hand in a hemophiliac (PTC deficiency). J Bone Joint Surg 51A:1423–1427, 1969
236. Bedford RF: Radial arterial function following percutaneous

cannulation with 18 and 20 gauge catheters. Anesthesiology 47:37–39, 1977

237. Bedford RF: Removal of radial artery thrombi following percutaneous cannulation for monitoring. Anesthesiology 46:430–432, 1977
238. Bedford RF: Wrist circumference predicts the risk of radial artery occlusion after cannulation. Anesthesiology 48:377–378, 1978
239. Bedford RF, Ashford TP: Aspirin pretreatment prevents post-cannulation radial-artery thrombosis. Anesthesiology 51:176–178, 1979
240. Bedford RF, Wollman H: Complications of percutaneous radial artery cannulation: An objective study in man. Anesthesiology 38:228–236, 1973
241. Bell JW: Treatment of post catheterization injuries. Ann Surg 155:591–598, 1962
242. Brown AE, Sweeney DB, Lumley J: Percutaneous radial cannulation. Anesthesia 24:532–536, 1969
243. Burn JH: Why thiopentone injected into an artery may cause gangrene. Br Med J 2:414–416, 1960
244. Cameron BM: Occlusion of the ulnar artery with impending gangrene of the fingers. Relieved by section of the volar carpal ligament. J Bone Joint Surg 36A:406–408, 1954
245. Cameron JD, Stein F, Kinmonth MH, Parkes A, Stack G, McGregor I, Corbett JR: Cases of severe vascular injury to the hand. Hand 2:74–78, 1970
246. Charney MA, Stern PJ: Digital ischemia in clandestine intravenous drug users. J Hand Surg 16A:308–310, 1991
247. Covey DC, Nossaman BD, Albright JA: Ischemic injury of the hand from intra-arterial propylhexedrine injection. J Hand Surg 13A:58–61, 1988
248. Crossland SG, Neviaser RJ: Complications of radial artery catheterization. Hand 9:287–290, 1977
249. Daniel DD: The acutely swollen hand in the drug user. Arch Surg 107:548–551, 1973
250. Dehne E, Kriz FK: Slow arterial leak consequent to unrecognized arterial laceration. J Bone Joint Surg 49A:372–377, 1967
251. Denkler KA, Cohen BE: Reversal of dopamine extravasation injury with topical nitroglycerine ointment. Plast Reconstr Surg 84:811–813, 1989
252. Downs JB, Chapman RL, Hawkins IF: Prolonged radial-artery catheterization: An evaluation of heparinized catheters and continuous irrigation. Arch Surg 108:671–673, 1974
253. Downs JB, Rackstein AD, Klein EF Jr, Hawkins IF Jr: Hazards of radial artery catheterization. Anesthesiology 38:283–286, 1973
254. Dumanian AV, Kelikian H: Vascular complications of orthopedic surgery. J Bone Joint Surg 51A:103–108, 1969
255. Engler HS, Freeman RA, Kanavage CB, Ogden LL, Moretz WH: Production of gangrenous extremities by intra-arterial injection. Am Surg 30:602–607, 1964
256. Evans D, Ozer S: A simple method of arterial cannulation. Can Anaesth Soc J 17:181–182, 1970
257. Falor WH, Hansel JR, Williams GB: Gangrene of the hand: A complication of radial artery cannulation. J Trauma 16:713–716, 1976
258. Gardner RM, Schwartz R, Wong HC, Burke JP: Percutaneous indwelling radial artery catheters for monitoring cardiovascular function. N Engl J Med 290:1227–1231, 1974
259. Gelberman RH, Blasingame JP, Fronek A, Dimick MP: Forearm arterial injuries. J Hand Surg 4:401–408, 1979
260. Gelberman RH, Gould RN, Hargens AR, Vande Berg JS: Lacerations of the ulnar artery: Hemodynamic, ultrastructural, and compliance changes in the dog. J Hand Surg 8:306–309, 1983
261. Gelberman RH, Nunley JA, Koman LA, Gould JS, Hergenroeder PT, MacClean CR, Urbaniak JR: The results of radial and ulnar arterial repair in the forearm—Experience in three medical centers. J Bone Joint Surg 64A:383–387, 1982
262. Gordon L, Buncke HJ, Townsend JJ: Histological changes in skeletal muscle after temporary independent occlusion of arterial and venous blood supply. Plast Reconstr Surg 61:576–580, 1978
262a. Greenberg BM, Cuadros CL, Jupiter JB: Interpositional vein grafts to restore the superficial palmar arch in severe devascularizing injuries of the hand. J Hand Surg 13A:753–757, 1988
263. Hager DL, Wilson JN: Gangrene of the hand following intraarterial injection. Arch Surg 94:86–89, 1967
264. Hazlett JW: The superficial ulnar artery with reference to accidental intra-arterial injection. Can Med Assoc J 61:289–293, 1949
265. Herman BE: Salvage of an arm with brachial to radial artery graft. Arch Surg 91:342–343, 1965
266. Hoht RP: Arterial injuries occurring during orthopedic operations. Clin Orthop 28:21–37, 1963
267. Inahara T: Arterial injuries of the upper extremities. Surgery 51:605–610, 1962
268. Jardon OM, Hood LT, Lynch RD: Complete avulsion of the axillary artery as a complication of shoulder dislocation. J Bone Joint Surg 55A:189–192, 1973
268a. Johnson D, Rosen JM, Khoury M, Stevenson D: Infarction of the upper limbs associated with oligohydramnios and intrauterine compression. J Hand Surg 13A:408–410, 1988
269. Katz AM, Birnbaum M, Moylan J: Gangrene of the hand and forearm; a complication of radial artery cannulation. Crit Care Med 2:370–372, 1974
270. Kitzmiller JW, Hertzer NR, Beven EG: Routine surgical management of brachial artery occlusion after cardiac catheterization. Arch Surg 117:1066–1071, 1982
271a. Laverick MD, D'Sa AAB, Kirk SJ, Mollan RAB: Management of blunt injuries of the axillary artery and the neck of the humerus: Case report. J Trauma 30:360–361, 1990
271b. Leclercq DC, Carlier AJ, Khuc T, Depierreux L, Lejeune GN: Improvement in the results in sixty-four ulnar nerve sections associated with arterial repair. J Hand Surg 10A:997–999, 1985
272. Llamas R, Gupta SK, Baum GL: A simple technique for prolonged arterial cannulation. Anesthesiology 31:289–291, 1969
273. MacGowan W: Acute ischemia complicating limb trauma. J Bone Joint Surg 50B:472–481, 1968
274. Machleder HI, Sweeney JP, Barker WF: Pulseless arm after brachial artery catheterization. Lancet 1:407–409, 1972
275. Mandel MA, Dauchot PJ: Radial artery cannulation in 1,000 patients: Precautions and complications. J Hand Surg 2:482–485, 1977
276. McQuillan WM, Nolan B: Ischaemia complicating injury. A report of thirty-seven cases. J Bone Joint Surg 50B:482–492, 1968
277. Menzoian JO, Doyle JE, LoGerfo FW, Cantelmo N, Weitzman F, Sequiera JC: Evaluation and management of vascular injuries of the extremities. Arch Surg 118:93–95, 1983
278. Menzoian JO, Doyle JE, Cantelmo NL, LoGerfo FW, Hirsch E: A comprehensive approach to extremity vascular trauma. Arch Surg 120:801–805, 1985
279. Meyer JP, Lim LT, Schuler JJ, Castronuovo JJ, Buchbinder D, Woelfel GF, Flanigan DP: Peripheral vascular trauma from close range shotgun injuries. Arch Surg 120:1126–1131, 1985
280. Miller TA, Haftel AJ: Iatrogenic digital ischemia. West J Med 122:183–184, 1975
281. Miyasaka K, Edmonds JF, Conn AW: Complications of radial artery lines in the paediatric patient. Can Anaesth Soc J 23:9–14, 1976
282. Nach RL, Lohman H: Gangrene of the hand following traumatic occlusion of the radial and ulnar arteries. NY State J Med 48:2173–2175, 1948

283. Nathan P: Intra-arterial injection of barbiturate. Hand 7:175–178, 1975
284. Nevelsteen A, Pype P, Broos P, Suy R: Brachial artery rupture due to an exostosis: Brief report. J Bone Joint Surg 70B:672, 1988
285. Nunley JA, Goldner RD, Koman LA, Gelberman R, Urbaniak JR: Arterial stump pressure: A determinant of arterial patency? J Hand Surg 12A:245–249, 1987
286. Page CP, Hagood CO Jr, Kemmerer WT: Management of post catheterization brachial artery thrombosis. Surgery 72:619–623, 1972
287. Perry MO, Thal ER, Shires GT: Management of arterial injuries. Ann Surg 173:403–408, 1971
288. Petrie PWR, Lamb DW: Severe hand problems in drug addicts following self administered injections. Hand 5:130–134, 1973
289. Rich NM, Baugh JH, Hughes CW: Acute arterial injuries in Vietnam: 1000 cases. J Trauma 10:359–369, 1970
290. Samaan HA: The hazards of radial artery pressure monitor. J Cardiovasc Surg 12:342–347, 1971
291. Schanzer H, Gribetz I, Jacobson JH II: Accidental intra-arterial injection of penicillin G. JAMA 242:1289–1290, 1979
292. Scharzer LA, Baker WH: Non-thrombotic arterial occlusion. Arch Surg 106:349, 1973
293. Siana JE, Stovring JO: Intra-arterial injection of dextropropoxyphene into hand arteries. J Hand Surg 14B:43–44, 1989
294. Smith RF, Elliott JP, Hageman JH, Szilagyi DE, Xavier AO: Acute penetrating arterial injuries of the neck and limbs. Arch Surg 109:198–205, 1974
295. Stein AH Jr: Arterial injury in orthopedic surgery. J Bone Joint Surg 38A:669–676, 1956
296. Swanson E, Freiberg A, Salter DR: Radial artery infections and aneurysms after catheterization. J Hand Surg 15A:166–171, 1990
297. Taweepoke P, Frame JD: Acute ischaemia of the hand following accidental radial artery infusion of Depo-Medrone. J Hand Surg 15B:118–120, 1990
298. Trumble T, Seaber AV, Urbaniak JR: Patency after repair of forearm arterial injuries in animal models. J Hand Surg 12A:47–53, 1987
299. Tse DH, Slabaugh PB, Carlson PA: Injury to the axillary artery by a closed fracture of the clavicle. J Bone Joint Surg 62A:1372–1374, 1980
300. Winegarner FC, Baker AG Jr, Bascom JF, Jackson GF: Delayed vascular complications in Vietnam casualties. J Trauma 10:867–873, 1970
301. Yee J, Westdahl PR, Wilson JL: Gangrene of the forearm and hand following use of radial artery for intra-arterial transfusion. Ann Surg 136:1019–1023, 1952
302. Zachary LS, Smith DJ Jr, Heggers JP, Robson MC, Boertman JA, Niu X-T, Schileru RE, Sacks RJ: The role of thromboxane in experimental inadvertent intra-arterial drug injections. J Hand Surg 12A:240–245, 1987
303. Zelenock GB, Kazmers A, Graham LM, Erlandson EE, Cronenwett JL, Whitehouse WM Jr, Wakefield TW, Lendenauer M, Stanley JC: Nonpenetrating subclavian artery injuries. Arch Surg 120:685–692, 1985

Embolic Problems

304. Baird RJ, Lajos TZ: Embolism to the arm. Ann Surg 160:905–909, 1964
305. Bandyk DF, Thiele BL, Radke HM: Upper extremity emboli secondary to axillofemoral graft thrombosis. Arch Surg 116:393–395, 1981
306. Banis JC Jr, Rich N, Whelan TJ: Ischemia of the upper extremity due to non cardiac emboli. Am J Surg 134:131–139, 1977
307. Bashir AH: Spontaneous radial hemi-amputation of the left hand. Case report. Hand 9:65–66, 1977
308. Bell WR, Tomasulo PA, Aving BM, Duffy TP: Thrombocytopenia occurring during the administration of heparin. A prospective study in 52 patients. Ann Intern Med 85:155–160, 1976
309. Billig DM, Hallman GL, Cooley DA: Arterial embolism: Surgical treatment and results. Arch Surg 95:1–6, 1967
310. Champion HR, Gill W: Arterial emboli to the upper limb. Br J Surg 60:505–508, 1973
311. Cooney WP III, Wilson MR, Wood MB: Intravascular fibrinolysis of small vessel thrombosis. J Hand Surg 8:131–138, 1983
312. Dale WA, Lewis MR: Management of ischemia of the hand and fingers. Surgery 67:62–79, 1970
313. Dellon AL, Curtis RM, Chen C: Prevention of femoral vein occlusion by local injection of thrombolysin in the rat. J Hand Surg 4:121–128, 1979
314. Editorial: The behavior of thrombi. Arch Surg 105:681–682, 1972
315. Fogarty TJ, Cranley JJ, Krause RJ, Strasser ES, Hafner DD: A method for extraction of arterial emboli and thrombi. Surg Gynecol Obstet 116:241–244, 1963
316. Fogarty TJ, Daily PO, Shumway NE, Krippaehne W: Experience with balloon catheter technic for arterial embolectomy. Am J Surg 122:231–237, 1971
317. Gardner C: Traumatic vasospasm and its complications. Am J Surg 83:468–470, 1952
318. Haimovici H: Peripheral arterial embolism; a study of 330 unselected cases of embolism of the extremities. Angiology 1:20–45, 1950
319. Holm J, Schersten T: Anticoagulant treatment during and after embolectomy. Acta Chir Scan 138:683–693, 1950
320. Jelalian C, Mehrhof A, Cohen IK, Richardson J, Merritt WH: Streptokinase in the treatment of acute arterial occlusion of the hand. J Hand Surg 10A:534–538, 1985
321. Kakkasseril JS, Cranley JJ, Arbaugh JH, Roedersheimer LR, Welling RE: Efficacy of low dose streptokinase in acute arterial occlusion and graft thrombosis. Arch Surg 120:427–429, 1985
322. Kartchner MM, Wilcox WC: Thrombolysis of palmar and digital arterial thrombosis by intra-arterial thrombolysin. J Hand Surg 1:67–74, 1976
323. Lawhorne TW, Sanders RA: Ulnar artery aneurysm complicated by distal embolization: Management with regional thrombolysis and resection. J Vasc Surg 4:663–665, 1986
324. Maxwell TM, Blaisdell FW, Olcutt C: Vascular complications of drug abuse. JAMA 221:343–344, 1972
325. Moore JR, Weiland AJ: Heparin-induced thromboembolism: A case report. J Hand Surg 4:382–385, 1979
326. Parkhouse N, Smith PJ: The use of streptokinase in replant salvage. J Hand Surg 16B:53–55, 1991
327. Persson AV, Thompson JE, Patman RD: Streptokinase as an adjunct to arterial surgery. Arch Surg 107:779–784, 1973
328. Puckett CL, Misholy H, Reinisch JF: The effects of streptokinase on ischemic flaps. J Hand Surg 8:101–104, 1983
329. Ricotta JJ, Scudder PA, McAndrew JA, DeWeese JA, May AG: Management of acute ischemia of the upper extremity. Am J Surg 145:661–666, 1983
330. Sachatello CR: Technique for subclavian, axillary and brachial embolectomy. Arch Surg 97:836–838, 1968
331. Sachatello CR, Ernst CB, Griffen WO Jr: The acutely ischemic upper extremity. Selective management. Surgery 76:1002–1009, 1974
332. Schmidt FE, Hewitt RL: Severe upper limb ischemia. Arch Surg 115:1188–1191, 1980
333. Thompson JE: Acute peripheral arterial occlusion. N Engl J Med 290:950–952, 1974

334. Tisnado J, Bartol DT, Cho S-R, Vines FS, Beachley MC, Fields WR: Low-dose fibrinolytic therapy in hand ischemia. Radiology 150:375–382, 1984

Occlusive Disease Outside the Hand

335. Adams JT, DeWeese JA, Mahoney EB, Rob CG: Intermittent subclavian vein obstruction without trauma. Surgery 63:147–165, 1968
336. Adson AW: Surgical treatment for symptoms produced by cervical ribs and the scalenus anticus muscle. Surg Gynecol Obstet 85:687–700, 1947
337. Adson AW, Coffey JR: Cervical rib; a method of anterior approach for relief of symptoms by division of the scalenus anticus muscle. Ann Surg 85:839–857, 1927
338. Argenta LC, Duus EC, Lane GA: Carotid injury and cerebral infarction in a revascularization hand injury case. J Hand Surg 8:935–937, 1983
339. Baumgartner F, Nelson RJ, Robertson JM: The rudimentary first rib: A cause of thoracic outlet syndrome with arterial compromise. Arch Surg 124:1090–1092, 1989
340. Beyer JA, Wright IS: The hyperabduction syndrome with special reference to its relationship to Raynaud's syndrome. Circulation 4:161–172, 1951
341. Craig WMcK, Knepper PA: Cervical rib and the scalenus anticus muscle. Ann Surg 105:556–563, 1937
342. Davis D, Petersen J, Feldman R, Cho C, Stevick CA: Subclavian venous stenosis: A complication of subclavian dialysis. JAMA 252:3404–3406, 1984
342a. Fidler MW, Helal B, Barwegen MGMH, Van Dongen RJAM: Subclavian artery aneurysm due to costoclavicular compression. J Hand Surg 9B:282–284, 1984
343. Gross WS, Flanigan DP, Kraft RO, Stanley JC: Chronic upper extremity arterial insufficiency: Etiology, manifestations and operative management. Arch Surg 113:419–423, 1978
344. Hewitt RL: Acute axillary vein obstruction by the pectoralis minor muscle. N Engl J Med 279:595, 1968
345. Horowitz SH: Brachian plexus injuries with causalgia resulting from transaxillary rib resection. Arch Surg 120:1189–1191, 1985
346. Hunter G, Palmaz JC, Carson SN, Lantz BMT: Surgically induced carotid subclavian steal syndrome: Diagnosis by video dilution technique. Arch Surg 118:1325–1329, 1983
347. Judy KL, Heymann RL: Vascular complications of thoracic outlet syndrome. Am J Surg 123:521–531, 1972
348. Kelly TR: Thoracic outlet syndrome: Current concepts of treatment. Ann Surg 190:657–662, 1979
349. Kleinert HE, Cook FW, Kutz JE: Neurovascular disorders of the upper extremity. Treated by trans-axillary sympathectomy. Arch Surg 90:612–616, 1965
350. Kunkel JM, Machleder HI: Treatment of Paget-Schroetter syndrome: A staged, multidisciplinary approach. Arch Surg 124:1153–1157, 1989
351. Lang EK: Arteriography and venography in the assessment of thoracic outlet syndrome. South Med J 65:129–137, 1972
352. Laroche GP, Bernatz PE, Joyce JW, MacCarty CS: Chronic arterial insufficiency of the upper extremity. Mayo Clin Proc 51:180–186, 1976
353. McGowan JM: Cervical rib: The role of the clavicle in occlusion of the subclavian artery. Ann Surg 124:71–89, 1946
354. McGowan JM, Velinsky M: Costo clavicular compression. Arch Surg 59:62–73, 1949
355. Moseley HS, Porter JM: Femoral-axillary artery bypass for arm ischemia. Arch Surg 106:347–348, 1973
356. Rapp JH, Reilly LM, Goldstone J, Krupski WC, Ehrenfeld WK, Stoney RJ: Ischemia of the upper extremity: Significance of proximal arterial disease. Am J Surg 152:122–126, 1986
357. Rob CG, Standeven A: Arterial occlusion complicating thoracic outlet compression syndrome. Br Med J 2:709–712, 1958
358. Roos DB: Trans-axillary approach for first rib resection to relieve thoracic outlet syndrome. Ann Surg 163:354–358, 1966
359. Rowen M, Dorsey TJ, Hepps SA: Primary venous obstruction of the upper extremity. West J Med 118:18–23, 1973
360. Schein CJ, Haimovici H, Young H: Arterial thrombosis associated with cervical ribs: Surgical considerations. Surgery 40:428–443, 1956
361. Swinton NW Jr, Hall RJ, Baugh JH, Blake HA: Unilateral Raynaud's phenomenon caused by cervical-first rib anomalies. Am J Med 48:404–407, 1970
362. Stallworth JM, Horne JB: Diagnosis and management of thoracic outlet syndrome. Arch Surg 119:1149–1151, 1984
363. Telford ED, Stopford JSB: The vascular complications of cervical rib. Br J Surg 18:557–564, 1930–31
364. Williams C: Hysterical edema of hand and forearm. Ann Surg 111:1056–1064, 1940
365. Wisehart JD: Patterns of reactive hyperemia in the hand. Am Heart J 60:116–120, 1960
366. Wright IS: The neurovascular syndrome produced by hyperabduction of the arms: The immediate changes produced in 150 normal controls and the effects on some persons of prolonged hyprabduction of the arms as in sleeping and certain occupations. Am Heart J 29:1–19, 1945

Systemic Diseases

367. Abramson DI: Connective tissue disorders. In Circulatory Diseases of the Limbs: A Primer. 1st Ed. Grune & Stratton, Orlando, 1978
368. Adson AW, Brown GE: Raynaud's disease of upper extremities: Successful treatment by resection of sympathetic cervicothoracic and second thoracic ganglions and intervening trunk. JAMA 92:444–449, 1929
369. Allen EV, Brown GE: Raynaud's disease: A clinical study of 147 cases. JAMA 99:1472–1478, 1932
370. Andrasch RH, Bardana EJ, Porter JM, Pirofsky B: Digital ischemia and gangrene preceding renal neoplasm. Arch Int Med 136:486–488, 1976
371. Baddeley RM: The place of upper dorsal sympathectomy in the treatment of primary Raynaud's disease. Br J Surg 52:426–429, 1965
372. Balas P, Tripolitis AJ, Kaklamanis P, Mandalaki T, Paracharalampous N: Raynaud's phenomenon: Primary and secondary causes. Arch Surg 114:1174–1177, 1979
373. Barr WG, Blair SJ: Carpal tunnel syndrome as the initial manifestation of scleroderma. J Hand Surg 13A:366–368, 1988
374. Belsole RJ, Lister GD, Kleinert HE: Polyarteritis: A cause of nerve palsy in the extremity. J Hand Surg 3:320–325, 1978
375. Berenbom L, Geltman EM: Congestive heart failure. pp. 90–91. In Campbell JW, Frisse M (eds): Manual of Medical Therapeutics. 24th Ed. Little, Brown, Boston, 1983
376. Blain A III, Coller FA, Carver GB: Raynaud's disease: A study of criteria for prognosis. Surgery 29:387–397, 1951
377. Bleifeld CJ, Inglis AE: The hand in systemic lupus erythematosus. J Bone Joint Surg 56A:1207–1216, 1974
378. Blumberg A, Weidmann P: Successful treatment of ischaemic ulceration of the skin in azotaemic hyperparathyroidism with parathyroidectomy. Br Med J 1:552–553, 1977
379. Bollinger A, Schlumpf M: Finger blood flow in healthy subjects of different ages and sex and in patients with primary Raynaud's disease. Acta Chir Scand 465:42–47, 1976

380. Bouhoutsos J, Morris T, Martin P: Unilateral Raynaud's phenomomenon in the hand and its significance. Surgery 82:547–551, 1977
381. Buerger L: Thrombo-angitis obliterans: A study of the vascular lesions leading to presenile spontaneous gangrene. Am J Med Sci 136:567–580, 1908
382. Caffee HH, Master NT: Atherosclerosis of the forearm and hand. J Hand Surg 9A:193–196, 1984
383. Clyne CAC, Arch PJ, Carpenter D, Webster JHH, Chant DB: Smoking, ignorance and peripheral vascular disease. Arch Surg 117:1062–1065, 1982
384. Coffman JD, Davies WT: Vasospastic diseases: A review. pp. 123–146. Progress in Cardiovascular Diseases. Vol. 18. Grune & Stratton, Orlando, 1975
385. Constram GR: Primary involvement of the upper extremities in thromboangitis obliterans (Buerger's disease). Am J Med Sci 174:530–536, 1927
386. Cosgriff TM, Arnold WJ: Digital vasospasm and infarction associated with hepatitis B antigenemia. JAMA 235:1362–1363, 1976
387. de Takats G: Discussion of Management of ischemia of the hand and fingers. Surgery 67:77–79, 1970
388. de Takats G, Fowler EF: Raynaud's phenomenon. JAMA 179:1–8, 1962
389. Eastcott HHG: Dead fingers. Practitioner 218:662–668, 1977
390. Editorial: Episodic digital vasospasm: The legacy of Maurice Raynaud. Lancet 1:1039–1040, 1977
391. Edwards EA: Remittent necrotizing acrocyanosis. JAMA 161:1530–1534, 1956
392. Egloff DV, Mifsud RP, Verdan Cl: Superselective digital sympathectomy in Raynaud's phenomenon. Hand 15:110–114, 1983
393. Falappa P, Magnavita N, Bergamaschi A, Colavita N: Angiographic study of digital arteries in workers exposed to vinyl chloride. Br J Ind Med 39:169–172, 1982
394. Farmer RG, Gifford RW Jr, Hines EA Jr: Raynaud's disease with sclerodactylia: A followup study of 71 patients. Circulation 23:13–15, 1961
395. Fitzgerald B: Saint Anthony's fire or carpal tunnel syndrome? (A case of iatrogenic ergotism). Hand 10:82–86, 1978
396. Flatt AE: Digital artery sympathectomy. J Hand Surg 5:550–556, 1980
397. Gahhos F, Ariyan S, Frazier WH, Cuono CB: Management of sclerodermal finger ulcers. J Hand Surg 9A:320–327, 1984
398. Gerber L: Biofeedback for patients with Raynaud's phenomenon. JAMA 242:509–510, 1979
399. Gifford RW Jr: The clinical significance of Raynaud's disease. Med Clin North Am 42:963–970, 1958
400. Gifford RW Jr: Arteriospastic disorders of the extremities. Circulation 27:970–975, 1963
401. Gifford RW Jr, Hines EA Jr: Raynaud's disease among women and girls. Circulation 16:1012–1021, 1957
402. Gifford RW Jr, Hines EA Jr, Craig WMcK: Sympathectomy for Raynaud's phenomenon: Follow up study of 70 women with Raynaud's disease and 54 women with secondary Raynaud's phenomenon. Circulation 17:5–13, 1958
403. Gipstein RM, Coburn JW, Adams DA, Lee DBN, Parsa KP, Sellers A, Suki WN, Massry SG: Calciphylaxis in man: A syndrome of tissue necrosis and vascular calcification in 11 patients with chronic renal failure. Arch Int Med 136:1273–1280, 1976
404. Golbrandson FL, Lurie L, Vance RM, Vandell RF: Multiple extremity amputations in hypotensive patients treated with dopamine. JAMA 243:1145–1146, 1980
405. Goodwin JN, Berne TV: Symmetrical peripheral gangrene. Arch Surg 108:780–784, 1974
406. Hansteen V: Medical treatment in Raynaud's disease. Acta Chir Scand (suppl) 465:87–91, 1976
407. Hardy JD, Conn JH, Fain WR: Nonatherosclerotic occlusive lesions of the small arteries. Surgery 57:1–13, 1965
408. Harris RW, Andros G, Dulawa LB, Oblath RW, Salles-Cunha SX, Apyan R: Large vessel arterial occlusive disease in symptomatic upper extremity. Arch Surg 119:1277–1282, 1984
409. Hawley PR, Johnston AW, Rankin JT: Association between digital ischemia and malignant disease. Br Med J 3:208–212, 1967
410. Hershey FB, Pareira MD, Ahlvin RC: Quadrilateral peripheral vascular disease in the young adult. Circulation 26:1261–1269, 1962
411. Hillestad L: Blood flow in vascular disorders. A plethysmographic study. Acta Med Scan 188:185–189, 1970
412. Hines EA Jr, Christensen NA: Raynaud's disease among men. JAMA 129:1–4, 1945
413. Hoffman S, Valderrma E, Gribetz I, Strauss L: Gangrene of the hand in a newborn child. Hand 6:70–73, 1974
414. Holti G: The effect of intermittent low molecular weight Dextran infusions upon digital circulation in systemic sclerosis. Br J Dermatol 77:560–568, 1965
415. Hussey HH: Digital gangrene (Editorial). JAMA 236:2656, 1976
416. Hutchinson JH, Howell RA: Cryoglobulinemia: Report of a case associated with gangrene of the digits. Ann Int Med 39:350–357, 1953
417. Johnston EMN, Summerly R, Birnstingl M: Prognosis in Raynaud's phenomenon after sympathectomy. Br Med J 1:962–964, 1965
418. Jones NF, Imbriglia JE, Steen VD, Medsger TA: Surgery for scleroderma of the hand. J Hand Surg 12A:391–400, 1987
419. Jones NF, Raynor SC, Medsger TA: Microsurgical revascularization of the hand in scleroderma. Br J Plast Surg 40:264–269, 1987
420. Jones NF: Ischemia of the hand in systemic disease: The potential role of microsurgical revascularization and digital sympathectomy. Clin Plast Surg 16:547–556, 1989
421. Kemerer VF Jr, Dagher FJ, Pais SO: Successful treatment of ergotism with nifedipine. AJR 143:333–334, 1984
422. Kenney FR: Gangrene of the hand following treatment for pruritis of hepatotoxic origin. N Engl J Med 235:35–39, 1946
423. Kent SJS, Thomas ML, Browse NL: The value of arteriography of the hand in the Raynaud's syndrome. J Cardiovasc Surg 17:72–80, 1976
424. Kirtley JA, Riddell DH, Stoney WS, Wright JK: Cervicothoracic sympathectomy in neurovascular abnormalities of the upper extremities. Ann Surg 165:869–879, 1967
425. Klinenberg JR, Wallace D: Plasmapheresis in Raynaud's disease. Lancet 1:1310–1311, 1978
426. Kontos HA, Wasserman AJ: Effect of reserpine on Raynaud's phenomenon. Circulation 39:259–266, 1969
427. Laroche GP, Bernatz PE, Joyce JW, MacCarty CS: Chronic arterial insufficiency of the upper extremity. Mayo Clin Proc 51:180–186, 1976
428. Lewis RA, Adams JP, Gerber NL, Decker JL, Parsons DB: The hand in mixed connective tissue disease. J Hand Surg 3:217–222, 1978
429. Lewis T, Pickering GW: Observations upon maladies in which the blood supply to digits ceases intermittently or permanently and upon bilateral gangrene of digits; observations relevant to so called "Raynaud's disease." Clin Sci 1:327–366, 1934
430. Lindstrom LI: A case report of fulminant occlusive arterial disease with gangrene of the extremities due to neoarsphenamine intoxication. Acta Chir Scand 100:509–514, 1950
431. Lord JW: Post traumatic vascular disorders and upper extremity sympathectomy. Orthop Clin North Am 1:393–398, 1970

432. Machleder H: Vaso-occlusive disorders of the upper extremity. Curr Probl Surg 25:7-67, 1988
433. McGrath MA, Penny R: The mechanisms of Raynaud's phenomenon: Part I. Med J Aust 2:328-333, 1974
434. McGrath MA, Penny R: The mechanisms of Raynaud's phenomenon: Part II. Med J Aust 2:367-375, 1974
435. McKuseck VA, Harris WS, Ottesen OE, Goodman RM: The Buerger syndrome in the United States: Arteriographic observations with special reference to involvement of the upper extremities and the differentiation from atherosclerosis and embolism. John Hopkins Hosp Bull 110:145-176, 1962
436. McLaughlin J: Discussion of Cervicothoracic sympathectomy in neurovascular abnormalities of the upper extremities. Ann Surg 165:878-879, 1967
437. Mendlowitz M, Naftchi N: The digital circulation in Raynaud's disease. Am J Cardiol 4:580-584, 1959
438. Morgan RF, Wilgis EFS: Thermal changes in a rabbit ear model after sympathectomy. J Hand Surg 11A:120-124, 1986
439. Mosely LH, Finseth F: Cigarette smoking: Impairment of digital blood flow and wound healing in the hand. Hand 9:97-101, 1977
440. Nielsen SL: Raynaud's phenomenon in obliterative arterial disease of the upper extremity. Acta Chir Scand 465:33-36, 1976
441. Nordlind K, Berglund B, Swanbeck G, Hedin H: Low molecular weight dextran therapy for digital ischaemia due to collagen vascular disease. Dermatologica 163:353-357, 1981
442. Palumbo LT: Upper dorsal sympathectomy without Horner's syndrome. Arch Surg 71:743-751, 1955
443. Palumbo LT: A new concept of the sympathetic pathways to the eye. Surgery 42:740-748, 1957
444. Palumbo LT, Lulu DJ: Transthoracic upper dorsal sympathectomy. Surgery 53:563-566, 1963
445. Paulus H, Kono D: Upper extremity manifestations of systemic vascular disorders. In Machleder HI (ed): Vascular Disorders of the Upper Extremity. Futura Publishing, Mt Kisco, NY, 1983
446. Pick J: The Autonomic Nervous System: Morphological, Comparative, Clinical, and Surgical Aspects. JB Lippincott, Philadelphia, 1970
447. Polio JL, Stern PJ: Digital nerve calcification in CREST syndrome. J Hand Surg 14A:201-203, 1989
448. Porter JM, Bardan EJ Jr, Baur GM, Wesche DH, Andrasch RH, Rosch H: The clinical significance of Raynaud's syndrome. Surgery 80:756-764, 1976
449. Porter JM, Snider RL, Bardana EJ, Rosch J, Eidemiller LR: The diagnosis and treatment of Raynaud's phenomenon. Surgery 77:11-23, 1975
450. Richards RL: Raynaud's syndrome. Hand 4:95-99, 1972
451. Rivers SP, Baur GM, Inahara T, Porter JM: Arm ischemia secondary to giant cell arteritis. Am J Surg 143:554-558, 1982
452. Rodeheffer RJ, Rommer JA, Wigley F, Smith CR: Controlled double-blind study of nifedipine in the treatment of Raynaud's phenomenon. N Engl J Med 308:880-883, 1983
453. Romeo SG, Whalen RE, Tindall JP: Intra-arterial administration of reserpine: Its use in patients with Raynaud's disease or Raynaud's phenomenon. Arch Int Med 125:825-829, 1970
454. Rubinger D, Friedlaender MM, Silver J, Kopolovic Y, Czaczkes WJ, Popovtzer MM: Progressive vascular calcification with necrosis of extremities in hemodialysis patients: A possible role of iron overload. Am J Kidney Diseases 7:125-129, 1986
455. Shaffer WO, Aulicino PL, DuPuy TE: Upper extremity gangrene of the newborn infant. J Hand Surg 9A:88-90, 1984
456. Silbert S: Etiology of thromboangiitis obliterans. JAMA 1295-1299, 1945
457. Sonneveld GJ, van der Meulen JC, Smith AR: Quantitative oxygen measurements before and after intravascular guanethidine blocks. J Hand Surg 8:435-442, 1983
458. Talpos G, White JM, Horrocks M, Cotton LT: Plasmapheresis in Raynaud's disease. Lancet 1:416-417, 1978
459. Tator CH, Heimbecker RO: Unilateral arm ischemia due to ergotamine tartrate. Can Med Assoc J 95:1319-1321, 1966
460. Taylor LM, Baur GM, Porter JM: Finger gangrene caused by small artery occlusive disease. Ann Surg 193:453-461, 1981
461. Thulesius O: Primary and secondary Raynaud's phenomenon. Acta Chir Scand 465:5-6, 1976
462. Tuffanelli DL, Winkelmann RK: Diffuse systemic scleroderma; A comparison with acrosclerosis. Ann Int Med 57:198-203, 1962
463. Velayos EE, Robinson H, Porciuncula FU, Masi AT: Clinical correlation analysis of 137 patients with Raynaud's phenomenon. Am J Med Sci 262:347-356, 1971
464. Waldo R: Prazosin relieves Raynaud's vasospasm. JAMA 241:1037, 1979
465. Wilgis EFS: Digital sympathectomy for vascular insufficiency. Hand Clin 1(2):361-367, 1985
466. Willerson JT, Thompson RH, Hookman P, Herdt J, Decker JL: Reserpine in Raynaud's disease and phenomenon. Ann Int Med 72:17-27, 1970
467. Wouda AA: Raynaud's phenomenon: Photoelectric plethysmography of the fingers of persons with and without Raynaud's phenomenon during cooling and warming up. Acta Med Scand 201:519-523, 1977
468. Zweifler AJ: Detection of occlusive arterial disease in the hand in patients with Raynaud's phenomenon. Acta Chir Scand 465:48-52, 1976

Vascular Tumors

469. Acharya G, Merritt WH, Theogaraj SD: Hemangioendotheliomas of the hand: Case reports. J Hand Surg 5:181-182, 1980
470. Adair FE: Glomus tumor: A clinical study with a report of ten cases. Am J Surg 25:1-6, 1934
471. Allen PW, Enzinger FM: Hemangioma of skeletal muscle: An analysis of 89 cases. Cancer 29:8-22, 1972
472. Anderson WJ: Intravenous pyogenic granuloma of the hand. J Hand Surg 10A:728-729, 1985
473. Apfelberg DB, Greene RA, Maser MR, Lash H, Rivers JL, Laub DR: Results of argon laser exposure of capillary hemangiomas of infancy—Preliminary report. Plast Reconstr Surg 67:188-193, 1981
474. Apfelberg DB, Maser MR, Lash H, White DN: YAG laser resection of complicated hemangiomas of the hand and upper extremity. J Hand Surg 15A:765-773, 1990
475. Baxt S, Mori K, Hoffman S: Aneurysm of the hand secondary to Kaposi's sarcoma. J Bone Joint Surg 57A:995-997, 1975
476. Ben-Menachen Y, Epstein MJ: Post traumatic capillary haemangioma of the hand: A case report. J Bone Joint Surg 56A:1741-1743, 1974
477. Binns M, Noble J, Marcuson R: Arterio-venous hamartoma of the hand. J Hand Surg 9B:349-350, 1984
478. Blackfield HM, Morris WJ, Torrey FA: Visible hemangiomas: A preliminary statistical report of a 10 year study. Plast Reconstr Surg 26:326-329, 1960
479. Blackfield HM, Torrey FA, Morris WJ, Low-Beer BVA: The management of visible hemangiomas. Am J Surg 94:313-320, 1957
480. Blackfield HM, Torrey FA, Morris WJ, Low-Beer BVA: The conservative treatment of hemangiomas in infants and children. J Int Coll Surg 30:255-260, 1958
481. Blair WF, Buckwalter JA, Mickelson MR, Omer GE: Lymphangiomas of the forearm and hand. J Hand Surg 8:399-405, 1983
482. Blanchard AJ: The pathology of glomus tumors. Can Med Assoc J 44:357-360, 1941

483. Butler ED, Hamill JP, Seipel RS, DeLorimer AA: Tumors of the hand: A ten year survey and report of 437 cases. Am J Surg 100:293–302, 1960
484. Carroll RE, Berman AT: Glomus tumors of the hand. Review of the literature and report on 28 cases. J Bone Joint Surg 54A:691–703, 1972
485. Chamberlain RH, Pendergrass EP: Some considerations regarding the treatment of hemangiomas. Pa Med J 51:867–869, 1948
486. Chan C-W: Intraosseous glomus tumor—Case report. J Hand Surg 6:368–369, 1981
487. Chen VT: Haemangioma of adductor pollicis. Hand 9:187–194, 1977
488. Chen VT, Harrison DA: Maffucci's syndrome. Hand 10:292–298, 1978
489. Dembrow VD, Adair FE: Lymphangiosarcoma in the post mastectomy lymphedematous arm: Case report of a ten year survivor treated by interscapulo thoracic amputation and excision of local recurrence. Cancer 14:210–212, 1961
490. DiFazio F, Mogan J: Intravenous pyogenic granuloma of the hand. J Hand Surg 14A:310–312, 1989
491. Edgerton MT: The treatment of hemangiomas with special reference to the role of steroid therapy. Ann Surg 183:517–530, 1976
492. Elkin DC, Cooper FW Jr: Extensive hemangioma: report of cases. Surg Gynecol Obstet 84:897–902, 1947
493. Fergusson ILC: Haemangiomata of skeletal muscle. Br J Surg 59:634–637, 1972
494. Fernandez GN: Locking of a metacarpo-phalangeal joint caused by a haemangioma of the volar plate. J Hand Surg 13B:323–324, 1988
495. Finsterbush A, Husseini N, Rousso M: Multifocal hemangioendothelioma of bones in the hand—A case report. J Hand Surg 6:353–356, 1981
496. Fonkalsrud EW, Coulson WF: Management of congenital lymphedema in infants and children. Ann Surg 177:280–285, 1973
497. Fragiadakis EG, Giannikas A: Glomus tumors in the fingers. Hand 3:172–174, 1971
498. Geschickter CF, Keasby LE: Tumors of blood vessels. Am J Cancer 23:568–591, 1935
499. Glanz S: The surgical treatment of cavernous hemangiomas of the hand. Br J Plast Surg 22:293–301, 1969
500. Goetsch E: Hygroma colli cysticum and hygroma axillare. Arch Surg 36:394–477, 1938
501. Goidanich IF, Campanacci M: Vascular hamartoma and infantile angioectatic osteohyperplasia of the extremities. J Bone Joint Surg 44A:815–842, 1962
502. Grauer RC, Burt JC: Unusual location of glomus tumor: report of two cases. JAMA 112:1806–1810, 1939
503. Greider JL, Flatt AE: Glomus tumor associated with pacinian hyperplasia—A case report. J Hand Surg 7:113–117, 1982
504. Harkins GA, Sabiston DC Jr: Lymphangioma in infancy and childhood. Surgery 47:811–822, 1960
505. Harkins HN: Hemangioma of a tendon or tendon sheath. Report of a case with a study of 24 cases from the literature. Arch Surg 34:12–22, 1937
506. Hendricks MW, Moore MM, Dell PC: Angiolymphoid hyperplasia with eosinophilia: A case report. J Hand Surg 10A:286–288, 1985
507. Holden CEA: Haemangioma of flexor digitorum profundus. Hand 4:42–44, 1972
508. Howard FM, Lee RE Jr: The hand in Maffuci syndrome. Arch Surg 103:752–758, 1971
509. Jarzab G: Clinical experience in the cryo-surgery of hemangioma. J Maxillofac Surg 3:146–149, 1975
510. Johnson EW Jr, Ghormley RK, Dockerty MB: Hemangiomas of the extremities. Surg Gynecol Obstet 102:531–538, 1956
511. Johnson J, Kilgore E, Newmeyer W: Tumorous lesions of the hand. J Hand Surg 10A:284–286, 1985
512. Jones KG: Cavernous hemangioma of striated muscle—a review of the literature and a report of 4 cases. J Bone Joint Surg 35A:717–728, 1953
513. Joseph FR, Posner MA: Glomus tumors of the wrist. J Hand Surg 8:918–920, 1983
514. Joseph FR, Posner MA, Terzakis JA: Compartment syndrome caused by a traumatized vascular hamartoma. J Hand Surg 9A:904–907, 1984
515. Kasabach HH, Merritt KK: Capillary hemangioma with extensive purpura. Am J Dis Child 58:1063–1070, 1940
516. Keith JE Jr, Wilgis EFS: Kaposi's sarcoma in the hand of an AIDS patient. J Hand Surg 11A:410–413, 1986
517. Kohout E, Stout AP: The glomus tumor in children. Cancer 14:555–566, 1961
518. Kojima T, Ide Y, Marumo E, Ishikawa E, Yamashita H: Hemangioma of median nerve causing carpal tunnel syndrome. Hand 8:62–65, 1976
519. Kon M, Vuursteen PJ: An intraneural hemangioma of a digital nerve—A case report. J Hand Surg 6:357–358, 1981
520. Lampe I, Latourette HB: Management of hemangiomas in infants. Ped Clin North Am 6:511–528, 1959
521. LaSorte AF: Cavernous hemangioma of striated muscle; review of the literature and report of a case. Am J Surg 100:593–596, 1960
522. Lever WF, Schaumburg-Lever G: Tumors of vascular tissue. pp. 591–617. In Histopathology of the Skin. 5th Ed. JB Lippincott, Philadelphia, 1975
523. Lister WA: Natural history of strawberry nevi. Lancet 1:1429–1434, 1938
524. Losli EJ: Intrinsic hemangiomas of the peripheral nerves. A report of two cases and a review of the literature. Arch Pathol 53:226–232, 1952
525. Mason ML, Weil A: Tumor of a subcutaneous glomus: Tumor glomique; tumeur du glomus neuromyo-arteriel; subcutaneous painful tubercle; angiomyo-neurome; subcutaneous glomal tumor. Surg Gynecol Obstet 58:807–816, 1934
526. Masson P: Le glomus neuromyo-arteriel des regions tactiles et ses tumeurs. Lyon Chirurgical 21:257–280, 1924
527. McCarthy WD, Pack GT: Malignant blood vessel tumors. A report of 56 cases of angiosarcoma and Kaposi's sarcoma. Surg Gynecol Obstet 91:465–482, 1950
528. McNeill TW, Chan GE, Capek V, Ray RD: The value of angiography in the surgical management of deep hemangiomas. Clin Orthop 101:176–181, 1974
529. McNeill TW, Ray RD: Hemangioma of the extremities: Review of 35 cases. Clin Orthop 101:154–166, 1974
530. Milikow E, Asche T: Hemangiomatosis, localized growth disturbance and intra-vascular coagulation disorder presenting with an unusual arthritis resembling hemophilia. Radiology 97:387–388, 1970
531. Miller SH, Smith RL, Shochat SJ: Compression treatment of hemangiomas. Plast Reconstr Surg 58:573–579, 1976
532. Milner RH, Sykes PJ: Diffuse cavernous haemangiomas of the upper limb. J Hand Surg 12B:199–202, 1987
533. Moss ALH, Ibrahim NBN: Lymphangiosarcoma of the hand arising in a pre-existing non-irradiated lymphangioma. J Hand Surg 10B:239–242, 1985
534. Moss LA, Stueber K, Hafiz MA: Congenital hemangioendothelioma of the hand—A case report. J Hand Surg 7:53–56, 1982
535. Mulliken JB, Glowacki J: Hemangiomas and vascular malformations in infants and children: A classification based on endothelial characteristics. Plast Reconstr Surg 69:412–420, 1982
536. Murray MR, Stout AP: Glomus tumor; investigation of its distri-

bution and behavior; and identity of its "epithelioid" cell. Am J Pathol 18:183–203, 1942

537. Nagay L, McCabe SJ, Wolff TW: Haemangioma of the digital nerve: A case report. J Hand Surg 15B:487–488, 1990
538. Owens N, Stephenson KL: Hemangioma: An evaluation of treatment by injection and surgery. Plast Reconstr Surg 3:109–123, 1948
539. Pack GT, Miller TR: Hemangioma classification, diagnosis and treatment. Angiology 1:405–426, 1950
540. Palmer RE: Eosinophilic granuloma of the hand: Case report. J Hand Surg 9A:283–285, 1985
541. Palmieri TJ: Subcutaneous hemangiomas of the hand. J Hand Surg 8:201–204, 1983
542. Patel CB, Tsai T-M, Kleinert HE: Hemangioma of the median nerve: A report of two cases. J Hand Surg 11A:76–79, 1986
543. Peled I, Iosipovich Z, Rousso M, Wexler MR: Hemangioma of the median nerve. J Hand Surg 5:363–365, 1980
544. Plewes B: Multiple glomus tumors; four in one finger tip. Can Med Assoc J 44:364–365, 1941
545. Pomeranz MM, Tunick IS: Visualization and obliteration of angiomata by radioopaque solutions. Ann Surg 114:1050–1059, 1941
546. Popoff NW: The digital vascular system: With reference to the state of the glomus in inflammation, arteriosclerotic gangrene, diabetic gangrene, thromboangitis obliterans and super numeray digits in man. Arch Pathol 18:295–330, 1934
547. Prosser AJ, Burke FD: Haemangioma of the median nerve associated with Raynaud's phenomenon. J Hand Surg 12B:227–228, 1987
548. Ravitch MM: Radical treatment of massive mixed angiomas (hemolymphangiomas) in infants and children. Ann Surg 134:228–243, 1951
549. Risitano G, Gupta A, Burke F: Angiolymphoid hyperplasia with eosinophilia in the hand: A case report. J Hand Surg 15B:376–377, 1990
550. Russo PE, Dewar JP: Congenital lymphangioma. Am J Roentgenol 85:726–728, 1961
551. Schatten WE, Kramer WM, Thomas LB: Multiple cavernous hemangiomas involving veins of an upper extremity. Report of a case treated by extensive local resection. Ann Surg 148:104–110, 1958
552. Schiffman KL, Harris DCM, Hooper G: Hemangiopericytoma of the median nerve. J Hand Surg 13A:75–78, 1988
553. Serra JM, Muirragui A, Tadjalli H: Glomus tumor of the metacarpophalangeal joint: A case report. J Hand Surg 10A:142–143, 1985
554. Scott JES: Hemangiomata in skeletal muscles. Br J Surg 44:496–501, 1957
555. Scott RB, Nydick I, Conway H: Lymphangiosarcoma arising in lymphedema. Am J Med 28:1008–1012, 1960
556. Shajrawi I, Dreyfuss UY, Stahl S, Boss JH: Intramuscular haemangioma of the forearm. J Hand Surg 15B:362–365, 1990
557. Shallow TA, Eger SA, Wagner FB Jr: Primary hemangiomatous tumors of skeletal muscle. Ann Surg 119:700–740, 1944
558. Shugart RR, Soule EH, Johnson EW Jr: Glomus tumors. Surg Gynecol Obstet 117:334–340, 1963
559. Sibulkin D, Healy WV: Invisible glomus tumor. Arch Surg 109:111–112, 1974
560. Silva JF, Saw HS: Solitary glomus tumors of the fingers. Hand 6:204–207, 1974
561. Spittell JA Jr: Tumors of blood and lymph vessels. In Fairbairn JF, Juergens JL, Spittell JA Jr (eds): Allen-Barker-Hines, Peripheral Vascular Disease. 4th Ed. WB Saunders, Philadelphia, 1972
562. Stack HG: Tumors of the hand. Br Med J 1:919–922, 1960
563. Stewart FW, Treves N: Lymphangiosarcoma in post mastectomy lymphedema; a report of six cases in elephantiasis chirurgica. Cancer 1:64–81, 1948
564. Stout AP: Hemangioendothelioma: A tumor of blood vessels featuring vascular endothelial cells. Ann Surg 118:445–462, 1943
565. Stout AP: Hemangiopericytoma: A study of 25 new cases. Cancer 2:1027–1035, 1949
566. Stout AP: Tumors featuring pericytes. Glomus tumors and hemangiopericytomas. Lab Invest 5:217–223, 1956
567. Stout AP: Tumors of the neuromyo-arterial glomus. Am J Cancer 24:255–272, 1935
568. Stout AP, Lattes R: Tumors of the Soft Tissues. pp. 67–81; 145–156. Second Series, fas.one. Armed Forces Institute of Pathology, Washington DC, 1967
569. Straub PW, Kessler S, Schreiber A, Frick PG: Chronic intravascular coagulation in Kasabach-Merritt syndrome. Arch Int Med 129:475–478, 1972
570. Thomas AMC, Mulligan PJ, Jones EL: Benign haemangioma of bone in a middle phalanx. J Hand Surg 15B:484–486, 1990
571. Tunon JB, Gonzalez FP: Angiomatosis of the metacarpal skeleton. Hand 9:88–91, 1977
572. Upton J, Mulliken JB, Murray JE: Classification and rationale for management of vascular anomalies in the upper extremity. J Hand Surg 10A:970–974, 1985
573. Vasconez L, Morris WJ, Owsley JQ Jr: Skin tumors. pp. 997–1000. In Dunphy JE, Way LW (eds): Current Surgical Diagnosis. 4th Ed. Lange Medical Publications, Los Altos, 1979
574. Vathana P: Primary hemangiopericytoma of bone in the hand: A case report. J Hand Surg 9A:761–764, 1984
575. Ward GE, Jonas AF Jr: Metastasizing hemangioma simulating an aneurysm. Arch Surg 36:330–335, 1938
576. Walling AK, Companioni GR, Belsole RJ: Infiltrating angiolipoma of the hand and wrist. J Hand Surg 10A:288–291, 1985
577. Watson WL, McCarthy WD: Blood and lymph vessel tumors. A report of 1056 cases. Surg Gynecol Obstet 71:569–588, 1940
578. Wood VE: Hemangioma with bone lesions. J Hand Surg 7:287–290, 1982
579. Zarem HA, Edgerton MT: Induced resolution of cavernous hemangiomas following prednisone therapy. Plast Reconstr Surg 39:76–83, 1967

Arteriovenous Malformations

580. Beall AC Jr, Harrington OB, Crawford ES, DeBakey ME: Surgical management of traumatic arteriovenous aneurysms. Am J Surg 106:610–618, 1963
581. Bennett JE, Zook EG: Treatment of arteriovenous fistulas in cavernous hemangiomas of the face by muscle emolization. Plast Reconstr Surg 50:84–87, 1972
582. Bernheim BM: Congenital arteriovenous fistula in left brachial artery and vein with secondary arterial blood supply to arm. Ann Surg 81:465–469, 1925
583. Bertelsen A, Dohn K: Congenital arteriovenous communications of the extremities: Clinical and patho-physiological investigations. Acta Chir Scand 105:448–459, 1953
584. Bliznak J, Staple TW: Radiology of angiodysplasias of the limb. Radiology 110:35–44, 1974
585. Bogumill GP: Clinico-pathological correlation in a case of congenital arterio-venous fistula. Hand 9:60–64, 1977
586. Branham HH: Aneurismal varix of the femoral artery and vein following a gunshot wound. Int J Surg 3:250–251, 1890
587. Brescia MJ, Cimino JE, Appel K, Hurwich BJ: Chronic hemodialysis using veni puncture and a surgically created arteriovenous fistula. N Engl J Med 275:1089–1092, 1966

588. Broder HM, Caughran JH: Traumatic arteriovenous aneurysm of the foot. J Bone Joint Surg 39A:427–430, 1957
589. Brown GE: Abnormal arteriovenous communication diagnosed from the oxygen content of the blood of regional veins. Arch Surg 18:807–810, 1929
590. Cabbabe EB: Xeroradiography as an aid in planning resection of arteriovenous malformations of the upper extremities. J Hand Surg 10A:670–674, 1985
591. Callander CL: Study of arteriovenous fistula with an analysis of four hundred and forty seven cases. Johns Hopkins Hosp Rep 19:259–358, 1920
592. Connolly JE, Brownell DA, Levine EF, McCart PM: Complications of renal dialysis access procedures. Arch Surg 119:1325–1328, 1984
593. Coursley G, Ivins JC, Barker NW: Congenital arteriovenous fistulas in extremities: Analysis of 69 cases. Angiology 7:201–217, 1956
594. Creech O Jr, Gantt J, Wren H: Traumatic arteriovenous fistula at unusual sites. Ann Surg 161:908–920, 1965
595. Cross FS, Glover DM, Simeone FA, Oldenbury FA: Congenital arteriovenous aneurysms. Ann Surg 148:649–665, 1958
596. Curtis RM: Congenital arteriovenous fistulae of the hand. J Bone Joint Surg 35A:917–928, 1953
597. David VC: Aneurysm of the hand. Arch Surg 33:267–275, 1936
598. deTakats G: Vascular anomalies of the extremities. Surg Gynecol Obstet 55:227–237, 1932
599. Dotter CT, Goldman ML, Rosch J: Instant selective arterial occlusion with isobutyl 2-cyanoacrylate. Radiology 114:227–230, 1975
600. Freeman NE: Arterial repair in the treatment of aneurysms and arteriovenous fistulae. A report of eighteen successful restorations. Ann Surg 124:888–919, 1946
601. Fry WJ: Surgical considerations in congenital arteriovenous fistula. Surg Clin North Am 54:451–454, 1978
602. Gelberman RH, Goldner JL: Congenital arteriovenous fistulas of the hand. J Hand Surg 3:451–454, 1978
603. Gomes AS, Busuttil RW, Baker JD, Oppenheim W, Machleder HI, Moore WS: Congenital arteriovenous malformations: The role of transcatheter arterial embolization. Arch Surg 118:817–825, 1983
604. Gomes MR, Bernatz PE: Arteriovenous fistulas: A review and ten year experience at the Mayo Clinic. Mayo Clin Proc 45:81–103, 1970
605. Greenhalgh RM, Rosengarten DS, Calnan JS: A single congenital arteriovenous of the hand. Br J Surg 59:76–78, 1972
606. Griffin JM, Vasconez LO, Schatten WE: Congenital arteriovenous malformations of the upper extremity. Plast Reconstr Surg 62:49–58, 1978
607. Haimov M, Baez A, Neff M, Slifkin R: Complications of arteriovenous fistulas for hemodialysis. Arch Surg 110:708–712, 1975
608. Halsted WS: Congenital arteriovenous and lymphatico-venous fistulae. Unique clinical and experimental observations. Am Surg Assoc Trans 37:262–272, 1919
609. Hamby WB, Gardner WJ: Treatment of pulsating exopthalmos. Arch Surg 27:676–685, 1933
610. Harris KE, Wright GP: A case of hemangiectatic hypertrophy of a limb and observations upon rate of growth in the presence of increased blood supply. Heart 15:141–149, 1930
611. Holman E: Abnormal arteriovenous communications. Great variability of effects with particular reference to delayed development of cardiac failure. Circulation 32:1001–1009, 1965
612. Homan E: Abnormal Arteriovenous Communications. 2nd Ed. Charles C Thomas, Springfield, IL, 1968
613. Horton BT, Ghormley RK: Congenital arteriovenous fistulae of the extremities visualized by arteriography. Surg Gynecol Obstet 60:978–983, 1935
614. Horton BT: Hemihypertrophy of extremities associated with congenital arteriovenous fistulas. JAMA 98:373–377, 1932
615. Hurwitt ES, Johnston A: Interscapulothoracic amputation for diffuse angiomatous malformation. Ann Surg 142:115–120, 1955
616. Johnson G Jr, Blythe WB: Hemodynamic effects of arteriovenous shunts used by hemodialysis. Ann Surg 171:715–721, 1970
617. Joyce PF, Sundaram M, Riaz MA, Wolverson MK, Barner HB, Hoffman RJ: Embolization of extensive peripheral angiodysplasias. Arch Surg 115:665–668, 1980
618. Kaplan EN: Vascular malformation of the extremities. pp. 144–161. In Williams HB (ed): Symposium of Vascular Malformations and Melanotic Lesions. CV Mosby, St Louis, 1983
619. Kittredge RD, Kanick V, Finby N: Arteriovenous fistulas. Am J Roentgenol 100:431–435, 1967
620. Leb DE, Sharma JK: Clubbing secondary to an arteriovenous fistula used for hemodialysis. JAMA 240:142–143, 1978
621. Leonard FC, Vassos GA Jr: Congenital arteriovenous fistulation of the lower limb. N Engl J Med 245:885–888, 1951
622. Lewis DDW: Congenital arteriovenous fistulae. Lancet 2:621–628, 1930
623. Lewis DDW: Congenital arteriovenous fistulae. Lancet 2:680–685, 1930
624. Lewis T: The adjustment of blood flow to the affected limb in arteriovenous fistula. Clin Sci 4:277–285, 1940
625. Lindenauer SM, Thompson NW, Kraft RO, Fry WJ: Late complications of traumatic arteriovenous fistulas. Surg Gynecol Obstet 129:525–532, 1969
626. Malan E, Puglionisi A: Congenital angiodysplasias of the extremities (Note I: Generalities and classification; venous dysplasias). J Cardiovasc Surg 5:87–130, 1964
627. Malan E, Puglionisi A: Congenital angiodysplasias of the extremities (Note II: Arterial and venous haemolymphatic dysplasias). J Cardiovasc Surg 6:255–345, 1965
628. Matas R: Congenital arteriovenous angioma of the arm: Metastases eleven years after amputation. Ann Surg 111:1021–1045, 1940
629. Matolo N, Kastagir B, Stevens L, Chrysanthakopoulos S, Weaver DH, Klinkman H: Neurovascular complications of brachial arteriovenous fistula. Am J Surg 121:716–719, 1971
630. May JW, Atkinson R, Rosen H: Traumatic arteriovenous fistula of the thumb after blunt trauma: A case report. J Hand Surg 9A:253–255, 1984
631. Mikkelsen W: Discussion of Congenital arteriovenous anomalies of the limbs. Arch Surg 111:430, 1976
632. Moore JR, Weiland AJ: Embolotherapy in the treatment of congenital arteriovenous malformations of the hand: A case report. J Hand Surg 10A:135–139, 1985
633. Murphy TO, Margulis AR: Roentgenographic manifestations of congenital peripheral arteriovenous communications. Radiology 67:26–33, 1956
634. Nakano J, DeSchryver C: Effects of arteriovenous fistula on systemic and pulmonary circulation. Am J Physiol 207:1319–1324, 1964
635. Nisbet NW: Congenital arteriovenous fistula in the extremities. Br J Surg 41:658–661, 1954
636. Norris G: Varicose aneurism at the bend of the arm: Ligature of the artery above and below the sac; secondary hemorrhages with a return of the aneurismal thrill on the tenth day; cure. Am J Med Sci 5:27–30, 1843
637. Olcott C IV, Newton TH, Stoney RJ, Ehrenfeld WK: Intra-arterial embolization in the management of arteriovenous malformations. Surgery 79:3–12, 1976

638. Ozeran RS, Gral T, Gordon HE: Long term experience with arteriovenous shunt for hemodialysis. Am Surg 38:259-267, 1972
639. Pemberton JdeJ, Saint JH: Congenital arteriovenous communications. Surg Gynecol Obstet 46:470-483, 1928
640. Petrovsky BV, Milonov OB: "Arterialization" and "venization" of vessels involved in traumatic arteriovenous fistulae. Aetiology and pathogenesis (an experimental study). J Cardiovasc Surg 8:396-407, 1967
641. Pisko-Dubienski ZA, Baird RJ, Wilson DR, Bayliss CE, Gardiner JH, Sepp H: Identification and successful treatment of congenital microfistulas with the aid of directional Doppler. Surgery 78:564-572, 1975
642. Regan PJ, Roberts JO, Bailey BN: Acute posterior interosseous nerve palsy caused by bleeding from an arteriovenous malformation. J Hand Surg 16A:272-273, 1991
643. Reid MR: The effect of arteriovenous fistula upon the heart and blood vessels: An experimental and clinical study. Bull Johns Hopkins Hosp 31:43-50, 1920
644. Reid MR: Studies on abnormal arteriovenous communications acquired and congenital. I. Report of a series of cases. Arch Surg 10:601-638, 1925
645. Reid MR: Abnormal arteriovenous communications, acquired and congenital. II. The origin and nature of arteriovenous aneurysms, cirsoid aneurysms and simple angiomas. Arch Surg 10:996-1009, 1925
646. Reinhoff WF Jr: Congenital arteriovenous fistula: An embryological study with the report of a case. Bull Johns Hopkins Hosp 35:271-284, 1924
647. Sabin FR: Origin and development of the primitive vessels of the chick and of the pig. Contrib Embryol 6:61-124, 1917
648. Santiago Delpin EA: Swelling of the hand after arteriovenous fistula for hemodialysis. Am J Surg 132:373-376, 1976
649. Seeger SJ: Congenital arteriovenous anastomoses. Surgery 3:264-305, 1938
650. Seeley SF, Hughes CW, Cook FN, Elkin DC: Traumatic arteriovenous fistulas and aneurysms in war wounded. Am J Surg 83:471-479, 1952
651. Stanley RJ, Cubillo E: Non-surgical treatment of arteriovenous malformations of the trunk and limb by transcatheter arterial embolization. Radiology 115:609-612, 1975
652. Stehbens WE, Karmody AM: Venous atherosclerosis associated with arteriovenous fistulas for hemodialysis. Arch Surg 110:176-180, 1975
653. Stephenson HE Jr, Lichti EL: Application of the Doppler ultrasonic flowmeter in the surgical treatment of arteriovenous fistula. Am Surg 37:537-538, 1971
654. Stewart FT: Arteriovenous aneurism treated by angeiorrhaphy. Ann Surg 57:574-580, 1913
655. Storey BG, George CRP, Stewart JH, Tiller DJ, May J, Sheil AGR: Embolic and ischemic complications after anastomosis of radial artery to cephalic vein. Surgery 66:325-327, 1969
656. Szilagyi DE, Elliott JP, DeRusso FJ, Smith RF: Peripheral congenital arteriovenous fistulas. Surgery 57:61-81, 1965
657. Szilagyi DE, Smith RF, Elliott JP, Hageman JH: Congenital arteriovenous anomalies of the limbs. Arch Surg 111:423-429, 1976
658. Tellis VA, Kohlberg WI, Bhat DJ, Driscoll B, Veith FJ: Expanded polytetrafluroethylene graft fistula for chronic dialysis. Ann Surg 189:101-105, 1979
659. Upton J, Mulliken JB, Murray JE: Classification and rationale for management of vascular anomalies in the upper extremity. J Hand Surg 10A:970-975, 1985
660. Upton J: Vascular malformations of the upper limb. pp. 381-399. In Mulliken JB, Young AE (eds): Vascular Birthmarks: Hemangiomas and Malformations. WB Saunders, Philadelphia, 1988
661. Veal JR, McCord WM: Congenital abnormal arteriovenous anastomoses of the extremities with special reference to diagnosis by arteriography and by the oxygen saturation test. Arch Surg 33:848-866, 1936
662. Wakim KG, Janes JM: Influence of arteriovenous fistula on the distal circulation in the involved extremity. Arch Phys Med Rehab 39:431-434, 1958
663. Ward CE, Horton BT: Congenital arteriovenous fistulas in children. J Pediatr 16:746-766, 1940
664. Weber FP: Hemangiectatic hypertrophy of limbs—Congenital phlebarteriectasisa and so called congenital varicose veins. Br J Child Dis 15:13-17, 1918
665. Webster GV: Discussion of Congenital arteriovenous fistulae of the hand. J Bone Joint Surg 35A:926-927, 1953
666. Weinberg M Jr, Steiger Z, Fell EH: Unusual congenital anomalies of the arteriovenous system. Surg Clin North Am 40:67-74, 1960
667. Wilbur DL: Multiple aneurysms of the arteries of the right arm associated with fistula and arterial embolism: Report of a case. Am J Med Sci 180:221-232, 1930
668. Wollard HH: The development of the principal arterial stems in the forelimb of the pig. Contrib Embryol 14:139-154, 1922
669. Wright LT, Logan AC: Congenital arteriovenous aneurysm of right upper extremity. Am J Surg 48:658-663, 1940
670. Yao ST, Needham TN, Lewis JB, Hobbs JT: Limb blood flow in congenital arteriovenous fistula. Surgery 73:80-84, 1973

Index

Page numbers followed by f *indicate figures; those followed by* t *indicate tables*

E

G

H

J

K

L

N

S

T

U

V